EMBRYOLOGY FOR SURGEONS

The Embryological Basis for the Treatment of Congenital Anomalies

2ND EDITION

EDITORS-IN-CHIEF

JOHN ELIAS SKANDALAKIS, M.D., Ph.D., F.A.C.S.

CHRIS CARLOS DISTINGUISHED PROFESSOR AND DIRECTOR
THE ALFRED A. DAVIS RESEARCH CENTER FOR SURGICAL ANATOMY AND TECHNIQUE AND
THE THALIA AND MICHAEL CARLOS CENTER FOR SURGICAL ANATOMY AND TECHNIQUE
EMORY UNIVERSITY SCHOOL OF MEDICINE
SENIOR ATTENDING SURGEON
PIEDMONT HOSPITAL
ATLANTA, GEORGIA;
CLINICAL PROFESSOR OF SURGERY
THE MEDICAL COLLEGE OF GEORGIA
AUGUSTA, GEORGIA

STEPHEN WOOD GRAY, A.B., M.A., Ph.D.

PROFESSOR AND ASSOCIATE DIRECTOR (EMERITUS)
THE ALFRED A. DAVIS RESEARCH CENTER FOR SURGICAL ANATOMY AND TECHNIQUE AND
THE THALIA AND MICHAEL CARLOS CENTER FOR SURGICAL ANATOMY AND TECHNIQUE
EMORY UNIVERSITY SCHOOL OF MEDICINE
ATLANTA, GEORGIA;
CONSULTANT TO PIEDMONT HOSPITAL
MEDICAL STAFF FOR CONGENITAL ANOMALIES
ATLANTA, GEORGIA

ASSOCIATE EDITORS

RICHARD R. RICKETTS, M.D.; J. ALEXANDER HALLER, JR., M.D.
THOMAS S. PARROTT, M.D., F.A.A.P., F.A.C.S.
CONSTANTINE MAVROUDIS, M.D.
LEE JOHN SKANDALAKIS, M.D., F.A.C.S.
CHARLES N. PAIDAS, M.D.

CONSULTANTS

GENE L. COLBORN, Ph.D.; THOMAS R. GEST, Ph.D.;
MARGARET L. KIRBY, Ph.D.; THOMAS A. WEIDMAN, Ph.D.

EMBRYOLOGY FOR SURGEONS

The Embryological Basis for the Treatment of Congenital Anomalies

2ND EDITION

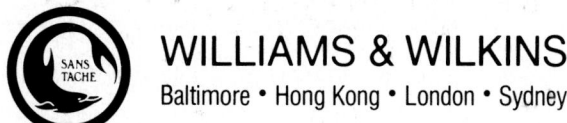

WILLIAMS & WILKINS

Baltimore • Hong Kong • London • Sydney

Editor: Charles W. Mitchell
Project Manager: Victoria M. Vaughn
Copy Editor: Kathleen Marks
Designer: Dan Pfisterer
Illustration Planner: Ray Lowman

Copyright © 1994
Williams & Wilkins
428 East Preston Street
Baltimore, Maryland 21202, USA

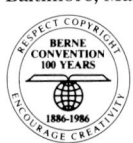

Accurate indications, adverse reactions, and dosage schedules for drugs are provided in this book, but it is possible that they may change. The reader is urged to review the package information data of the manufacturers of the medications mentioned.

Printed in the United States of America

First Edition 1972

Library of Congress Cataloging-in-Publication Data
Embryology for surgeons / edited by John E. Skandalakis, Stephen W. Gray.—2nd ed.
    p. cm.
    Rev. ed of: Embryology for surgeons / Stephen Wood Gray, John Elias Skandalakis. 1972.
    Includes bibliographical references and index.
    ISBN 0-683-07756-2
    1. Abnormalities, Human.   2. Embryology, Human.   3. Anatomy, Surgical and topographical.   I. Skandalakis, John Elias, 1920-   .
II. Gray, Stephen Wood, 1915-   .   III. Gray, Stephen Wood, 1915- Embryology for surgeons.
    [DNLM: 1. Abnormalities—surgery. 2. Abnormalities—embryology.
QS 675 E53 1993]
QM691.E93 1993
616'.043'0246171—dc20
DNLM/DLC
for Library of Congress   93-34518
                                                                      CIP
                                                          93 94 95 96 97
                                                          1 2 3 4 5 6 7 8 9 10

In Appreciation and Gratitude

to Alfred A. Davis

whose support made this

publication possible

PREFACE TO THE SECOND EDITION

Several years ago, my son, Lee, and I (J.E.S.) visited Dr. Robert E. Gross, one of the
fathers of pediatric surgery, on his farm in Brattleboro, Vermont. We spent most of
the day with this giant. To borrow from Churchill, this is the man who burned with
the flame of pediatric surgery. We discussed many things. Toward the end of our
conversation he penetrated me with his eyes and said, "You have an obligation to
the children with congenital anomalies, to the medical profession of today and
tomorrow, and an obligation to yourself that you must have a second edition of your
Embryology for Surgeons very soon. It is a must."

For a second time, we attempt to reveal the drama of the child with congenital
malformations. The anarchy of tissues resulting in congenital deformities of varying
magnitude is the focus of our work. Our goal is to enable the student, the resident,
and the pediatric surgeon to analyze the etiological morphology of congenital anomalies, a difficult and complex task since most human malformations are of unknown
etiology, tales of unfathomable and unsolved problems. The teaching of the anatomy
of the normal and the anatomy of the abnormal has become the stepchild of basic
science, a phenomenon still present in our medical schools. Both these queens,
Anatomy and Embryology, are in disgrace but still in splendor. We hope our small
contributions will shift the pendulum to the right direction.

Since the first edition, pediatric surgery has changed dramatically. The failures of
yesterday have yielded to the triumphs of today. We have seen advances in every
branch of the pediatric sciences from fetal surgery to transplantation. T.K. Whipple
was quite right when he stated, "What they dreamed, we live, and what they lived,
we dream." We can only imagine that in the third edition of this book, we will perhaps present the realizations of today's dreams.

Despite the fact that the authorship of this book belongs, for all practical purposes, to the Editors-In-Chief, a tremendous amount of work was done by our Associate Editors and Contributors. With the Associate Editors, we decided to retain the
format of the first edition, in most cases, and for historical reasons, to keep the original writing, adding any new work, treatment, philosophy, and ideas about the
embryological and anatomical basis of congenital anomalies. We report some modern embryological advances, noting that experiments and observations in given animals demonstrate embryological changes as well as physiological developments.
However, we do not know if this learning may be applied to humans during intrauterine or early neonatal life. At the same time, we want to emphasize that there still
is not a final answer in many problems. We hope this will not confuse the reader. We
do consider this book a reference book for the old as well as for the new.

Neither Dr. Gray nor I could rewrite this book as well as we originally wrote it—
20 years ago! In a previous publication, we used the phrase "springtime of our senil-
ity." Dr. Gray and I are at this point, but our co-workers are not. They added their

salt and pepper to make a more tasty digestion of reading. Therefore, we believe our decision to include additional contributors to be the right one, since we want to pair and link the past with the present in a most acceptable way. We are deeply grateful to all who contributed, advised, consulted and edited. To all of them belong the Aristotelian:

> *Pleasure is the actions of the present*
> *the hope of the future*
> *and the remembrance of things past*

There are some changes of note in the Second Edition. We have expanded our coverage of congenital anomalies by including several new chapters. Additions include chapters on teratomas, conjoined twins, the peritoneum. The chapters on spleen and body asymmetry were separated.

Variation is defined as deviation from typical, and *anomaly* is marked deviation from normal standards. Therefore, with this confusing definition, we decided to include some anatomical variations in some chapters, such as chapters on the liver and pancreas.

Like the First Edition, this is not a book of pediatric surgery, and the short clinical presentations are included with each topic only to complete the picture but not to give details. To give a lot of details is impossible. The summary of the few we did was done with a hope that the reader would approve our selections.

A weekday edition of the *New York Times* contains more information than the average person was likely to have in a lifetime in 17th century England. The information available today about our subject is immense. Thus, we hope that our selections are the right and the best ones, and their inclusion in this volume is successful.

In the preface of our First Edition, we wrote: "We believe that within a few more years surgery will be devoted almost entirely to the correction of congenital malformations and to the repair of traumatic injuries." If such an evolutionary process will take place, the authors and contributors of this book can repeat happily the poem of Melisanthi:

> *I close my eyelids: deep in me the light*
> *I open them, light everywhere around me*
> *I say then: Sun, what splendid death now might*
> *in such a divine flood of light, find me.*

When paraphrased, the poem reminds of what we hope to accomplish with this revised edition—to give splendid *life* in newborns with congenital anomalies.

> *I close my eyelids: deep in me the light*
> *I open them, light everywhere around me*
> *I say then: Sun, what splendid* life *now might*
> *in such a divine flood of light, find me.*

The following letter by Dr. Gross, and the repeated requests by several pediatric surgeons, also stimulated us enough to start the Second Edition—which we hope will fulfill the expectations of the reader.

JOHN E. SKANDALAKIS, M.D., Ph.D.
STEPHEN W. GRAY, Ph.D.
Editors-In-Chief

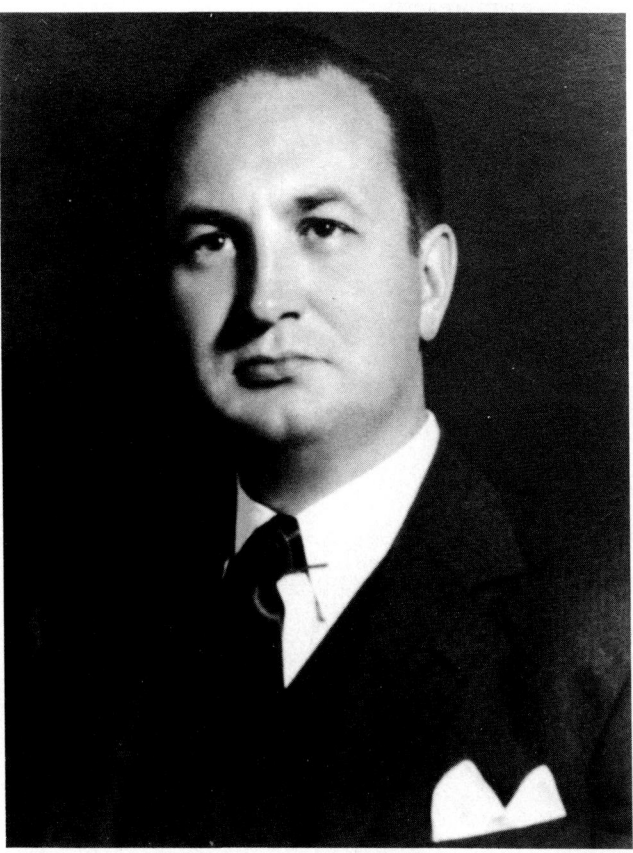

Robert E. Gross (1904–1988)

Box 493, Brattleboro, Vermont 05301

May 10, 1979

Dear Dr. Skandalakis—

Dr. Houpis delivered the book to me, and I must say that I was really overwhelmed! You are most kind and generous to give me the book. And my admiration for the volume is very great and very real. You could not have given it to anyone who would appreciate it more!

Human embryology—and the aberrations of it which can occur—have long been of tremendous interest and importance to me. This you can surely understand because all of my professional life has been devoted to surgery of infancy and childhood—and a considerable portion of this meant the handling of a wide variety of anomalies. In my first year of medical school at Harvard, there was an excellent course in embryology, richly augmented by demonstrations at the Children's Hospital clearly showing the many ways that nature could go wrong in developing the human body. The combustion of an interest in embryology and the challenge of surgery for youngsters made it clear to me what my life's work would be.

While I had long been in the habit of referring to individual published articles on various anomalies I was about to attack, I have never seen anything like the book you have brought forth, encompassing such wide territory. It is obviously a masterpiece and a classic contribution. It is an astounding compilation. So wonderfully complete, handsomely illustrated, and superbly published. I cannot tell you how very much I admire and value it.

You have been most cordial in sending the *Embryology for Surgeons* to me—and I really feel overcome each time I think about it.

With kindest regards

Robert E. Gross

PREFACE TO THE FIRST EDITION

Most of us are born normal. We conform to the morphologic pattern of our species and sex and begin life with the proper equipment to perform the necessary and expected functions. Minor variations in structure are frequent, but unless they are a threat to life, to adequate functioning or to acceptable appearance and behavior, they are usually of little concern to the individual.

It is the infant who is abnormal at birth or who fails to develop normally that is a source of concern to his parents, to the surgeon who must try to correct his defect and to the anatomist who wishes to understand how his abnormality occurred.

The purpose of this book is to provide the anatomist and the surgeon with an organized account of many of the malformations that can arise during the gestation of a human being. Against a background of normal embryology, we have described the specific pathological conditions and critically reviewed the embryogenesis of a large number of congenital defects. We have tried to place them in their proper perspective, supplying estimates of their frequency, their distribution within the population and their prognosis. Finally, we have discussed their diagnosis and the principles underlying their surgical correction. In nonbiological terms, this book may be considered a "failure analysis" of human development.

Embryology for Surgeons was selected for the title because we hope that the broad view of human development defects presented here may open up new surgical vistas and provide new insights into the mechanisms of human malformation.

We do not intend this to be a book on pediatric surgery; excellent texts in that field already exist. The sections on treatment are only indications of the ends to be achieved, not specific directions for surgery.

With Dr. Warren H. Cole[a] we wish to emphasize the surgeons of today that the surgeons of tomorrow will increasingly perform the operations mentioned here. They will certainly refine these procedures, and they will design new ones. We believe that within a few more years surgery will be devoted almost entirely to the correction of congenital malformations and to the repair of traumatic injuries. It is for the surgeons of tomorrow that this book is written.

STEPHEN W. GRAY
JOHN E. SKANDALAKIS

---

[a]Cole WH. Foreword. In Thorek P. Anatomy in Surgery, 2nd ed. Philadelphia: JB Lippincott, 1962.

ACKNOWLEDGMENTS

We are indebted to the readers of the First Edition of *Embryology for Surgeons*. The popularity of the book has been due to the acceptance of it by readers around the world. It is a herculean task to prepare a book of such a wide spectrum. Rapid advancement in many areas results in the inevitable omission of the very latest references in some chapters. We thank all the readers for their understanding in this matter. Further, we remind them that the aim of this work is to offer the nonspecialist a synthesis that will not go out of date too quickly.

We would like to pay special tribute to all those professionals who collaborated with us to produce this revision. A book of this scope would have been impossible without their cooperation. The delays encountered in the preparation of this book have proven a great nuisance to many, including those contributors who maintained our original schedule and who have had to revise their chapters. We are grateful for their willing cooperation.

We wish to acknowledge the contributions of the large number of individuals who gave permission to reproduce illustrations from their published works.

Special recognition and gratitude is given to Mr. Richard Parker and Ms. Carol Froman who, although joining us at the midpoint of the production process, performed the endless editorial tasks required to complete this edition. They made many worthwhile suggestions that improved the book. We wish to also recognize Ms. Cynthia Painter, Ms. Martha Hagan, and Mr. Mark Barbaree for their assistance in performing noneditorial tasks.

We would like to express our gratitude to Ms. Victoria Vaughn, Project Manager of Williams & Wilkins, for her assistance throughout the publishing process.

CONTRIBUTORS

Bruce H. Broecker, M.D.
Clinical Associate Professor of Surgery (Urology)
Emory University School of Medicine
Atlanta, Georgia

Gene L. Colborn, Ph.D.
Professor of Anatomy
Director of Center for Clinical Anatomy
The Medical College of Georgia
Augusta, Georgia

Thomas F. Dodson, M.D.
Assistant Professor of Surgery
Emory University School of Medicine
Atlanta, Georgia

Thomas R. Gest, B.S., M.S., Ph.D.
Assistant Professor of Anatomy
The Medical College of Georgia
Augusta, Georgia

Stephen Wood Gray, A.B., M.A., Ph.D.
Professor and Associate Director (Emeritus)
The Alfred A. Davis Research Center for Surgical Anatomy and Technique and
The Thalia and Michael Carlos Center for Surgical Anatomy and Technique
Emory University School of Medicine
Consultant to Piedmont Hospital Medical Staff for Congenital Anomalies
Atlanta, Georgia

J. Alexander Haller, Jr., M.D.
Professor of Pediatric Surgery
Pediatrics & Emergency Medicine
The Johns Hopkins University School of Medicine
Baltimore, Maryland

Margaret L. Kirby, A.B., Ph.D.
Regents Professor
The Medical College of Georgia
Augusta, Georgia

Constantine Mavroudis, M.D.
Professor of Surgery
Northwestern University Medical School
Division Head and A.C. Buehler Professor of Cardiovascular-Thoracic Surgery
Children's Memorial Hospital
Chicago, Illinois

Charles N. Paidas, M.D.
Assistant Professor
Surgery, Pediatrics and Oncology
The Johns Hopkins University School of Medicine
Baltimore, Maryland

Thomas S. Parrott, M.D., F.A.A.P., F.A.C.S.
Clinical Associate Professor of Surgery (Urology)
Emory University School of Medicine
Atlanta, Georgia

Daniel Dale Richardson, B.A., M.D.
Surgical Resident
Emory University School of Medicine
Atlanta, Georgia

Richard R. Ricketts, M.D.
Associate Professor of Surgery
Emory University School of Medicine
Chief of Surgery
Egleston Hospital for Children
Atlanta, Georgia

William M. Scaljon, B.S., M.S., M.D.
Attending Urologist
Piedmont Hospital
Atlanta, Georgia

Mark E. Silverman, M.D.
Professor of Medicine (Cardiology)
Emory University School of Medicine
Chief of Cardiology
Piedmont Hospital
Atlanta, Georgia

John Elias Skandalakis, M.D., Ph.D., F.A.C.S.
Chris Carlos Distinguished Professor and Director
The Alfred A. Davis Research Center for Surgical Anatomy and Technique and
The Thalia and Michael Carlos Center for Surgical Anatomy and Technique
Emory University School of Medicine
Senior Attending Surgeon
Piedmont Hospital
Atlanta, Georgia
Clinical Professor of Surgery
The Medical College of Georgia
Augusta, Georgia

Lee John Skandalakis, M.D., F.A.C.S.
Clinical Assistant Professor
The Alfred A. Davis Research Center for Surgical Anatomy and Technique and
The Thalia and Michael Carlos Center for Surgical Anatomy and Technique
Emory University School of Medicine
Attending Surgeon
Piedmont Hospital
Atlanta, Georgia

Panagiotis N. Symbas, M.D.
Professor of Surgery (Cardiothoracic)
Emory University School of Medicine
Atlanta, Georgia

Jane L. Todd, M.D.
Assistant Professor
Department of Pediatrics
Emory University School of Medicine
Atlanta, Georgia

N. Wendell Todd, M.D., F.A.C.S.
Associate Professor of Surgery (Otolaryngology) and Pediatrics
Emory University School of Medicine
Atlanta, Georgia

Thomas A. Weidman, B.S., M.S., Ph.D.
Associate Professor of Anatomy
The Medical College of Georgia
Augusta, Georgia

Willis H. Williams, M.D.
Professor of Surgery (Cardiothoracic)
Emory University School of Medicine;
Chief, Cardiothoracic Surgery
Egleston Hospital
Atlanta, Georgia

CONTENTS

Preface to the Second Edition . . . . *vii*
Preface to the First Edition . . . . *xi*
Acknowledgments . . . . *xiii*
Contributors . . . . *xv*

chapter 1
THE SURGEON AND THE PROBLEM 1
John E. Skandalakis / Stephen W. Gray
Editorial Comments: *J. Alexander Haller, Jr. / Charles N. Paidas*

chapter 2
PHARYNX AND ITS DERIVATIVES 17
John E. Skandalakis / Stephen W. Gray / N. Wendell Todd

chapter 3
ESOPHAGUS 65
John E. Skandalakis / Stephen W. Gray / Richard R. Ricketts
Editorial Comments: *J. Alexander Haller, Jr. / Charles N. Paidas*

chapter 4
PERITONEUM 113
John E. Skandalakis / Stephen W. Gray / Richard R. Ricketts. / Daniel D. Richardson

chapter 5
STOMACH 150
John E. Skandalakis / Stephen W. Gray / Richard R. Ricketts
Editorial Comments: *J. Alexander Haller, Jr. / Charles N. Paidas*

chapter 6
SMALL INTESTINES 184
John E. Skandalakis / Stephen W. Gray / Richard R. Ricketts / Daniel D. Richardson
Editorial Comments: *J. Alexander Haller, Jr. / Charles N. Paidas*

chapter 7
COLON AND RECTUM 242
John E. Skandalakis / Stephen W. Gray / Richard R. Ricketts
Editorial Comments: *J. Alexander Haller, Jr. / Charles N. Paidas*

chapter 8
LIVER 282
John E. Skandalakis / Stephen W. Gray / Richard R. Ricketts / Lee J. Skandalakis
Editorial Comments: *J. Alexander Haller, Jr. / Charles N. Paidas*

chapter 9
EXTRAHEPATIC AND BILIARY DUCTS 296
John E. Skandalakis / Stephen W. Gray / Richard R. Ricketts / Lee J. Skandalakis / Thomas F. Dodson
Editorial Comments: *J. Alexander Haller, Jr. / Charles N. Paidas*

chapter 10
SPLEEN 334
Lee J. Skandalakis / Stephen W. Gray / Richard R. Ricketts / John E. Skandalakis

chapter 11
PANCREAS 366
John E. Skandalakis / Stephen W. Gray / Richard R. Ricketts / Lee J. Skandalakis
Editorial Comments: *J. Alexander Haller, Jr. / Charles N. Paidas*

chapter 12
LARYNX 405
N. Wendell Todd / John E. Skandalakis / Stephen W. Gray
Editorial Comments: *J. Alexander Haller, Jr. / Charles N. Paidas*

chapter 13
TRACHEA AND LUNGS 414
John E. Skandalakis / Stephen W. Gray / Panagiotis N. Symbas
Editorial Comments: *J. Alexander Haller, Jr. / Charles N. Paidas*

chapter 14
PULMONARY CIRCULATION 451
John E. Skandalakis / Stephen W. Gray / Panagiotis N. Symbas

chapter 15
DIAPHRAGM 491
John E. Skandalakis / Stephen W. Gray / Richard R. Ricketts
Editorial Comments: *J. Alexander Haller, Jr. / Charles N. Paidas*

chapter 16
ANTERIOR BODY WALL 540
John E. Skandalakis / Stephen W. Gray / Richard R. Ricketts / Lee J. Skandalakis

chapter 17
KIDNEY AND URETER 594
Thomas S. Parrott / John E. Skandalakis / Stephen W. Gray
Editorial Comments: *Thomas S. Parrott*

chapter 18
BLADDER AND URETHRA 671
Thomas S. Parrott / Stephen W. Gray / John E. Skandalakis
Editorial Comments: *Thomas S. Parrott*

chapter 19
SUPRARENAL GLAND 718
*John E. Skandalakis / Stephen W. Gray / William M. Scaljon /
Thomas S. Parrott / Richard R. Ricketts*
Editorial Comments: *Thomas S. Parrott*

chapter 20
OVARY AND TESTIS 736
*John E. Skandalakis / Stephen W. Gray / Thomas S. Parrott /
Richard R. Ricketts*
Editorial Comments: *Thomas S. Parrott*

chapter 21
MALE REPRODUCTIVE SYSTEM 773
John E. Skandalakis / Stephen W. Gray / Bruce H. Broecker
Editorial Comments: *Thomas S. Parrott*

chapter 22
FEMALE REPRODUCTIVE SYSTEM 816
Stephen W. Gray / John E. Skandalakis / Bruce H. Broecker
Editorial Comments: *Thomas S. Parrott*

chapter 23
SEX DETERMINATION 848
John E. Skandalakis / Stephen W. Gray / Thomas S. Parrott
Editorial Comments: *Thomas S. Parrott*

chapter 24
LYMPHATIC SYSTEM 877
John E. Skandalakis / Stephen W. Gray / Richard R. Ricketts
Editorial Comments: *J. Alexander Haller, Jr. / Charles N. Paidas*

chapter 25
PERICARDIUM 898
Willis H. Williams / Stephen W. Gray / and John E. Skandalakis
Editorial Comments: *Constantine Mavroudis*

chapter 26
HEART 912
*Jane L. Todd / Mark E. Silverman / Margaret L. Kirby / Stephen W.
Gray / John E. Skandalakis*
Editorial Comments: *Constantine Mavroudis*

chapter 27
CORONARY VESSELS 958
John E. Skandalakis / Stephen W. Gray / Mark E. Silverman
Editorial Comments: *Constantine Mavroudis*

chapter 28
THORACIC AND ABDOMINAL AORTA 976
John E. Skandalakis / Stephen W. Gray / Panagiotis N. Symbas
Editorial Comments: *Constantine Mavroudis*

chapter 29
SUPERIOR AND INFERIOR VENA CAVAE . . .1032
John E. Skandalakis / Stephen W. Gray / Panagiotis N. Symbas
Editorial Comments: *Constantine Mavroudis*

chapter 30
ANOMALIES OF SITUS AND SYMMETRY 1052
Stephen W. Gray / John E. Skandalakis / Richard R. Ricketts

chapter 31
TERATOMA 1060
Richard R. Ricketts / Stephen W. Gray / John E. Skandalakis
Editorial Comments: *J. Alexander Haller, Jr. / Charles N. Paidas*

chapter 32
CONJOINED TWINS 1066
Richard R. Ricketts / Stephen W. Gray / John E. Skandalakis
Editorial Comments: *J. Alexander Haller, Jr. / Charles N. Paidas*

chapter 33
**INTRAUTERINE SURGERY FOR THE
CREATION AND STUDY OF CONGENITAL
ANOMALIES** 1079
J. Alexander Haller, Jr. / Charles N. Paidas
Editorial Comments: *John E. Skandalakis*

Index 1085

CHAPTER 1

THE SURGEON AND THE PROBLEM

John Elias Skandalakis / Stephen Wood Gray

Where there is love for humanity, there is also love for the art of medicine.
—*HIPPOCRATES*

The surgeon is both a human being and a scientist with a desire to help and to understand the unknown. Both spring from a deep responsibility to the patient, to his or her family, and to society, as well as to the progress of medical science. This last desire has produced the triumphal march of pediatric surgery, led by such gifted people as Ladd, Gross, Potts, Swenson, and many others, named in subsequent chapters, who used the scalpel to conquer anomalies that previous generations had considered inoperable. Thus satisfying the desire for progress has enabled the surgeon to satisfy the desire to help.

We are living in a new era. We agree with Lister and Irving that the neonatologist plays a profound role in the survival of the child with multiple anomalies (1). Today neonatology and pediatric surgery work together to produce better results. Of course, we also agree with Rickham that the ethical development of the medical profession parallels scientific development (2).

While most anatomic congenital anomalies in liveborn babies can be surgically corrected with no visible traces, there still exists a small percentage of babies with severe and multiple anomalies who, after palliation or even functional correction, are still distressingly and obviously malformed. With this small percentage the drama and the agony begins—a drama of great magnitude and an agony coupled with constant anxiety. The cast in the drama includes the physician, the family, the surgeon, and the infant.

In most cases the first witnesses to the tragedy of the infant with Down's syndrome or the infant born without extremities or with meningocele are the obstetrician and his or her team. When the pediatrician arrives, the discussion begins of what to say to the family and how to say it. Carefully selecting their words, one or both physicians explain the situation to the family. The first response—shock—is soon replaced by questions for advice. If surgical solutions are recommended, the surgeon who is called in will be the senior member of the medical team, with the responsibility of outlining possibilities to the family. Whatever these are, when the prognosis has been made, the various solutions outlined, and the family members are ready to make their decision, what questions must the surgeon ask? If the parents of a severely deformed baby ask the surgeon's advice about whether an attempt should be made for a possible life-saving operation that has a poor prognosis, what shall he or she say? If the parents decide on no operation and the child dies, will the surgeon condemn them?

Keeping in mind the social, economic, and psychologic problems arising when normal children live under the same roof with a malformed child, should the surgeon advise the family to isolate the deformed baby in a special institution?

In this poignant drama, the surgeon's response to the parents' cry, "What do you advise, doctor?," is perhaps best expressed by Potts, who tells one unfortunate family: "I cannot answer your question. You talk it over and let us know your decision. Whatever you decide . . . will be right" (3). The medicophilosopher Potts states that it is impossible not to add that, if the parents are young, their chances of having a number of healthy children is excellent.

What can the rest of the cast in this drama say?

Parents:	Our poor baby! How can we keep him? How can we let him go? How can we live with our decision?
Infant:	Please leave me alone to die in peace. I don't want to be a burden to my parents and to society. You know that because of my deformities I'll bring unhappiness to my parents, embarrassment to my brothers and sisters, and misery to myself. Society will isolate me. The joy of playing, the joy of creativity, and finally the joy of love will be denied me. Please leave me alone.
Doctor (human being):	You are right. I do understand you. Let me talk to your family and I am sure they will decide the best for all of you.
Doctor (scientist):	I have to proceed, and I promise to do my best. My duty and responsibility is to preserve life. I have to try— to try with deep respect for the dig-

1

nity of human life. Who knows, perhaps the experience with you could be a life-saving experience for another unfortunate baby? I have to create and refine surgical judgment and technique. I am not using you as an experimental animal, but as a means to scientific prosperity.

This double personality of the surgeon is responsible for the brilliant and successful drama of pediatric surgery. New technical devices, plastic surgery, improvement in surgical aids and skills, and transplantation allow us to save the lives of mutilated and deformed babies.

McCormick talks, among other things, about meaningful lives and quality of life and generally supports care and love for the deformed (4). (The ancient Spartan ancestors of one of the editors [JES] believed that the deformed child should not live; by order of the state, they threw all the deformed infants into the Keas outside of the city. Both Aristotle and Plato supported this practice.)

Singer supports the idea that each human being has the right to the highest quality of life he or she can achieve (5). The medicolegal problems of today are very complex, occasionally enigmatic, and many times incomprehensible for the responsible general physician, neonatologist, and pediatric surgeon. The surgeon's dilemma is augmented by several classifications of the selection of cases for surgery. Rickham supports an old classification, which reads as follows (2):

Class 1: Infants who are likely to be completely cured by surgery
Class 2: Infants who, after treatment, will be handicapped to some extent but may still be able to lead a relatively normal life
Class 3: Infants who, after treatment, will have severe physical handicaps and will have to lead a more or less sheltered life
Class 4: Infants in classes 1 to 3 who, in addition, are of subnormal intelligence but can be trained up to a point
Class 5: Infants in classes 1 to 3 who, in addition are severely mentally defective and leading a "vegetable" existence

Still we, the editors, support what we stated 20 years ago—that a healthy, honest dialogue between physicians and family is necessary and that, finally, the decision—any decision—should be up to the family and not to the courts.

EDITORIAL COMMENT

Perhaps the ancient and fundamental guideline for all physicians is still "first do no harm," and in the management of newborn infants with congenital abnormalities incompatible with meaningful life, the decision, although anguishing, must include doing no harm to sib-

lings and total family as well as to society. This is a tremendous burden but one that pediatric surgeons must bear in greatest humility (JAH/CNP).

Knowledge of the embryogenesis of each defect or malformation will help the surgeon in this great obligation. The remainder of this book gives the picture of the "known" so that the surgeon may proceed to the "unknown." As Claude Bernard said, "Man may learn nothing unless he proceeds from the known to the unknown."

INCIDENCE OF CONGENITAL ANOMALIES

Defective embryonic development is not limited by geography, race, or social class. In every pregnancy it lurks as a small but sinister possibility. The first question a mother asks, whether aloud or to herself, is, "Is my baby normal?"

To determine the risk of having a malformed baby (or of losing one late in pregnancy), we need to know how many abnormal infants are conceived and how many of these are born alive.

For the first question we have only a little data. Based on estimates of fetal loss and infant death (6), Stickle has constructed a curve of the outcome of pregnancies for 92 weeks after conception (Fig. 1.1) (7). Up to the 42nd week of gestation, there are 295 deaths per 1000 conceptions. This means that from 800,000 to 1 million pregnancies end in death before birth each year in the United States. Stickle suggests that from 50 to 75% of these deaths are caused by fetal maldevelopment (7). This is, of course, only an educated guess. A breakdown of the leading causes of infant mortality is provided in Figure 1.2. Hertig and his colleagues have observed that some loss of fertilized ova occurs so early that clinical pregnancy has not been established (8). Among 36 developing ova between 36 hr and 17 days of age, they found 13 to be abnormal. Witschi has estimated that about 58% of eggs that have been in contact with sperm fail to implant or are lost before the next menstrual period (Fig. 1.3) (9).

The proportion of abnormal live births seems to be easier to demonstrate. Indeed, the incidence of some common anomalies readily diagnosed at birth can be determined with precision. However, the overall frequency of malformations is still unknown because of a variety of complicating factors. Owens stated that the Office of Health Economics in London in 1920 reported that approximately 1:30 infant deaths were due to a malformation, whereas in 1990 about 1:4 were (10).

The earliest serious efforts to attack the problem were those of Murphy (11), who in 1936 tabulated the anomalies among more than 130,000 births in Philadelphia, and of Malpas (12), who in 1937 examined the records of nearly 14,000 births in Liverpool. Many subsequent stud-

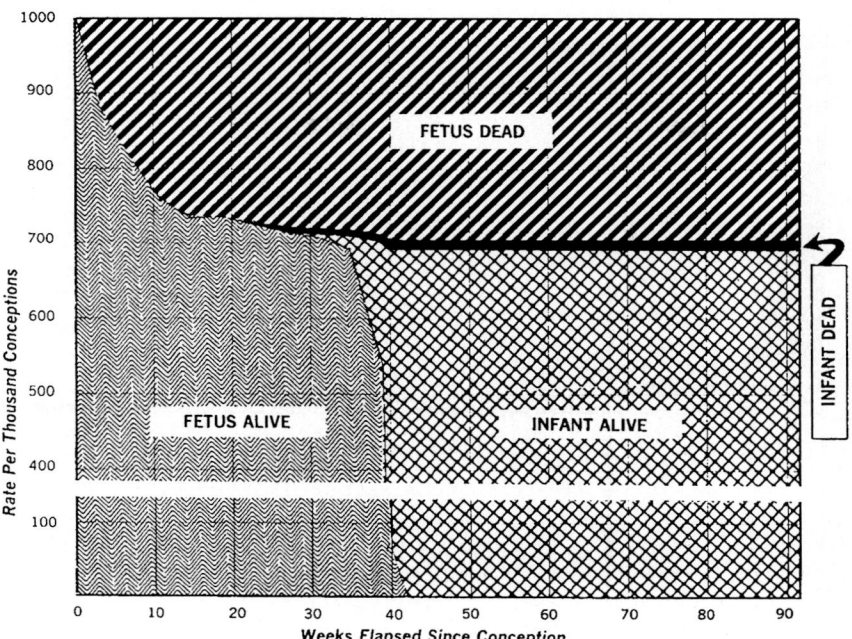

Figure 1.1. Cumulative outcome of 1000 pregnancies by weeks after conception. By week 44 there will have been 705 live births of which 13 infants have died after having been born alive. The remaining 295 will have died before birth.

(From Stickle G. Defective development and reproductive wastage in the United States. Am J Obstet Gynecol 1968;100:442–447.)

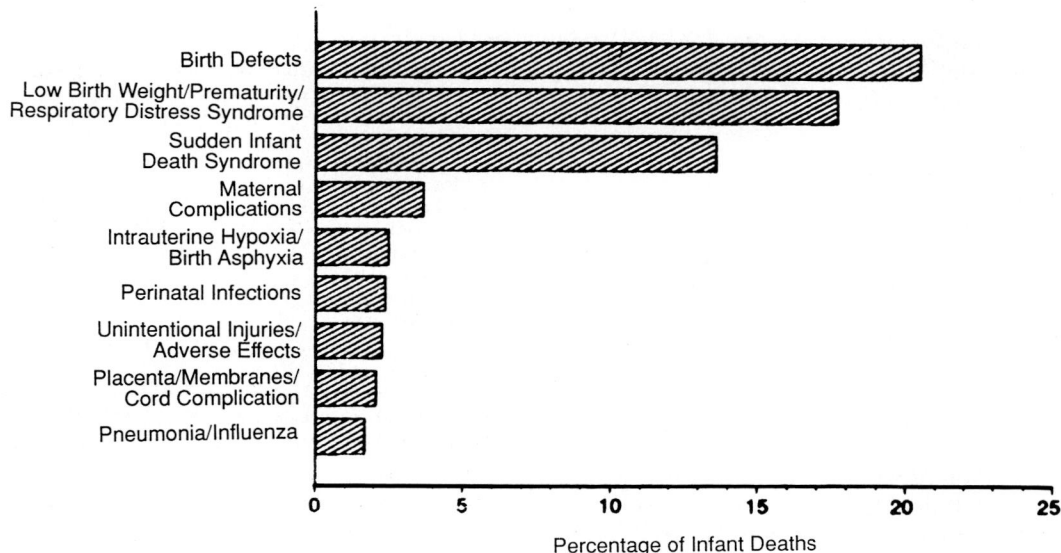

Figure 1.2. Leading causes of infant mortality. (From CDC. Contribution of birth defects to infant mortality—United States, 1986. MMWR 1989;38(37):633.)

ies, both large hospital series and whole country series, have since been published.

Under the auspices of the World Health Organization (WHO), a series of over 400,000 births from around the world was reported in standardized terms; the report was published by Stevenson et al. in 1966 (13). In this series, the overall incidence of anomalies was 1.27% of live births.

In 1967 Kennedy tabulated the results of 238 statistic studies of malformations, including the WHO data, arranging them by country and by the methods by which the data were recorded (14). Values ranged from 0.83%

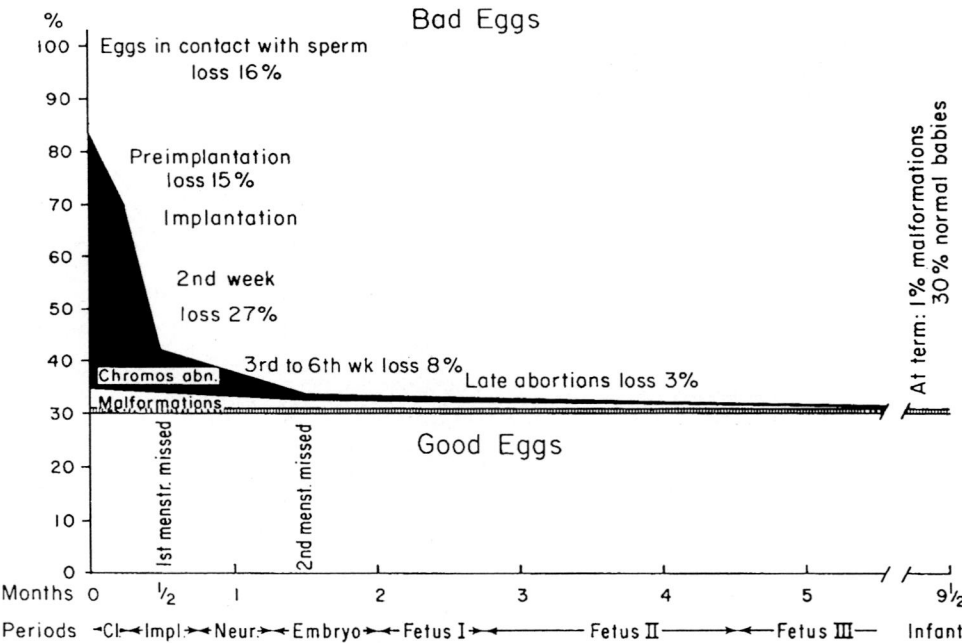

Figure 1.3. Graph of postovulatory survival and development in humans. Baselines give age and developmental periods (*Cl*, cleavage; *Impl.*, implantation; *Neur.*, neurula). Under assumed favorable conditions, 30% of eggs develop to normal babies ("good eggs"); 1% become liveborn infants with cognitive defects (hatched), or in which about 1:25 have chromosome anomalies; 69% perish, being resorbed or aborted: This class, summarily designated as "malformations," may be chromosomally normal *(white)* or anomalous *(black)*. (From Witschi E. Teratogenic effects from overripeness of the egg. In: Fraser FC, McKusick VA, eds. Congenital malformations. Proceedings of the Third International Conference. Amsterdam: Excerpta Medica, 1970.)

(based on birth certificate information) to 4.5% (based on intensive examination). Over 20 million births in 46 countries were involved. The reader should consult Kennedy's paper for references to individual studies in particular areas.

Despite the magnitude of this survey, the reported results vary so widely among countries and even among hospitals in the same country that no clear picture of the geographical distribution of congenital malformations emerges.

An example of a thorough, modern study of the occurrence of malformations is the Metropolitan Atlanta Congenital Malformation Program that began in 1967. The incidence of malformations has been 28:1000 total births. However, since only diagnoses made during the first week of life are tabulated, the data is heavily weighted in favor of gross external deformities and internal anomalies incompatible with extrauterine life.

In 1990 Lynberg and Khoury compiled a listing of birth defects as the cause of death in 7678 infants (Table 1.1) (15). Owens refers to incidence and prevalence, and he clearly defines incidence as "the number of new cases per unit time per unit population (usually annual cases per 1000)" and prevalence as "the number of cases of a disease at any one time per unit population (usually per 1000)" (10). He continues to explain that "prevalence will be influenced by the mortality of the particular disease studied" (Tables 1.2 and 1.3.)

Table 1.1.
Birth Defects as Underlying Cause of Infant Deaths, by Organ System (n = 7678)[a]

Defect	Percentage
Cardiovascular system	41.7
Central nervous system	16.6
Chromosomal anomalies	9.4
Musculoskeletal system	8.4
Respiratory system	6.5
Genitourinary system	6.0
Digestive system	1.9
Other	9.7
TOTAL	100.0

[a]Data compiled from Lynberg MC, Khoury MJ. CDC surveillance summaries. 1990;39(SS-3):1–12.

Table 1.2.
Most Common Congenital Malformations[a]

Neural tube defect
Facial clefts
Down's syndrome
Clubfoot
Congenital dislocation of the hip
Ventricular septal defects
Hypospadias
Polydactyly/syndactyly

[a]From Owen JR. Incidence and causation of congenital defects. In: Lister J, Irving IM, eds. Neonatal surgery. 3rd ed. Boston: Butterworths, 1990.

Table 1.3.
Birth Prevalence of Some Surgical Malformations, Liverpool and Environs, 1979–1983 (Per 1000 Live and Stillbirths)[a,b]

Oesophageal atresia	0.27
Duodenal stenosis	0.11
Jejunal atresia	0.03
Ileal atresia	0.01
Hirschsprung's disease	0.06
Anorectal atresia	0.36
Diaphragmatic hernia	0.22
Exomphalos	0.26
Gastroschisis	0.10
Hydronephrosis	0.12
Ectopia vesicae	0.05
Urethral valves	0.01

[a]From Owen JR. Incidence and causation of congenital defects. In: Lister J, Irving IM, eds. Neonatal surgery. 3rd ed. Boston: Butterworths, 1990.
[b]There were 101,816 total births over this time in the geographical area under surveillance.

Some Factors Affecting Epidemiologic Data

In addition to the usual problems of reporting diseases, such as the standardization of terms, allowance for non-hospitalized cases and national idiosyncrasies, the epidemiology of congenital malformations presents its own special difficulties.

Degree of Severity

Abnormal development expresses itself in a spectrum from trivial to lethal. The thoroughness with which one should record the trivial becomes a problem. In some series only "significant" anomalies have been recorded (16–17), but there is no obvious division between "significant" and "insignificant" anomalies. Tracheoesophageal fistula is surely significant, but what can be said of a septate uterus? We do not criticize the choice of these work-

ers; we use their data only to show the difficulties of the problem.

Lethality Estimates

Birth defects were the leading cause of infant deaths in the United States in 1986, amounting to one-fourth of all such deaths (Fig. 1.4) (18). This percentage has been increasing for at least 50 years, a phenomenon not due to an increase in birth defects but rather to a decrease in deaths of premature infants and other critically ill newborns. This decrease has slowed down in recent decades (19).

In 1990 Lynberg and Khoury estimated that about 80,000 infants are born each year with a major birth defect (15). Of these about 6000 will die in the first 28 days of life and another 2000 will be dead by the end of the first year of life. The remaining 72,000 live with greater or lesser handicaps that will affect them throughout the rest of their lives.

Age at Examination

The time at which the patient is examined greatly affects the number of anomalies detected. Lethal anomalies expressed early in fetal life result in spontaneous abortions. These are rarely counted in any series. Less severe but equally lethal anomalies may allow the fetus to survive in utero, but it may be unable to cope with the requirements of extrauterine life. In this group are stillborn infants, which are included in only a few series. Two series totaling 10,633 stillbirths showed 13.3% to be malformed (19–20).

Inspection of a newborn infant will reveal any gross deformations and anomalies such as imperforate anus. Within a few hours, intestinal atresias, tracheoesophageal

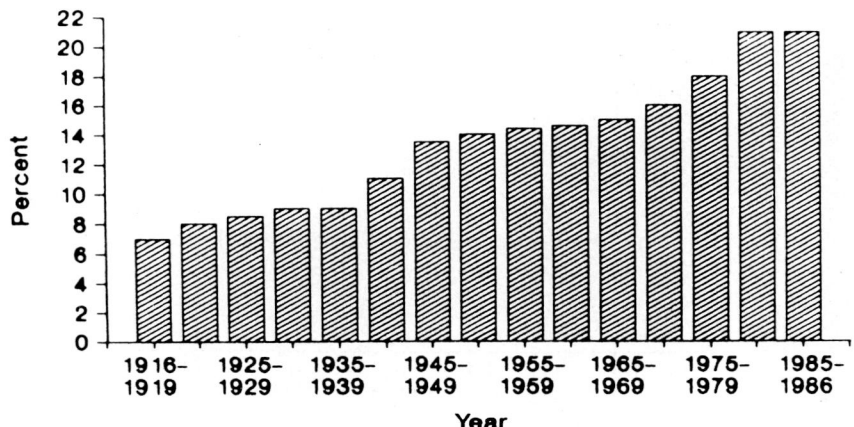

Figure 1.4. Infant deaths in the United States (1918–1986) ascribed to birth defects. (From CDC. Contributions of birth defects to infant mortality–United States, 1986. MMWR 1989;33(37):633.)

fistulae, and some heart defects will be apparent, if present. These early presenting anomalies will probably be entered in the records, but late-presenting defects will not be entered on birth records. Many heart defects will not appear at once. Ectopic ureters will be discovered only after toilet training starts. Undescended testes will not be of concern for a few months; and renal anomalies often will be undetected until puberty or even later. This situation has been documented by Lock and his associates (21). Among 176 infants of rubella-exposed mothers, there were 32 definite and 27 suspected anomalies found on examination at 4 to 12 months of age. Reexamination of the infants at 16 to 25 months of age showed that 7 of 27 suspected anomalies were definitely present and that there were 12 more definite anomalies, most of them serious, that had not been found nor suspected at the earlier examination.

The delay in diagnosis is well illustrated by the experience with congenital heart disease in California reported by Yerushalmy (22). The incidence of heart defects reported at birth was less than 4:1000, but the cumulative rate rose to 11:1000 by the time the same group of children reached the age of 3 years (Fig. 1.5).

Undiscovered Anomalies

In addition to malformations that manifest themselves too early or too late in development to be recorded at birth, there is a large group of anomalies that give their possessors no trouble in the normal course of events, but that may surprise the surgeon at the operating table. An azygos lobe of the lung, an unusual configuration of the biliary tract, an absent kidney, or an accessory spleen produce no functional disorders, yet they represent deviations from normal development as real as those that produce disabling anomalies.

Multiple Anomalies

Lastly, there is the problem of multiple anomalies in the same individual. Two examples from our own experience illustrate the problem:

Among 43 cases of intestinal stenosis or atresia, 18 had no other defect (42%), 16 had one other defect, 6 had two other defects, 2 had three other defects, and 1 had four other defects. Among 264 infants with Down's syndrome, 136 had no other defect (51.5%), 111 had one other defect, 14 had two other defects, 1 had three other defects, and 2 had four other defects.

Deciding how these cases should be counted is not easy. A good series must distinguish between the number of malformed infants and the number of malformations.

We have tried to present in this book some ideas of the relative incidence of the malformations discussed. In the synoptic table, we have listed the specific malformations as "common," "uncommon," "rare," or "very rare." These terms are relative to the total number of malformations that occur, not to the total number of live births.

CLASSIFICATION OF CONGENITAL ANOMALIES

Numerous attempts have been made to classify the great variety of human malformations on a morphologic basis. None has been successful. Groups of defects in one area

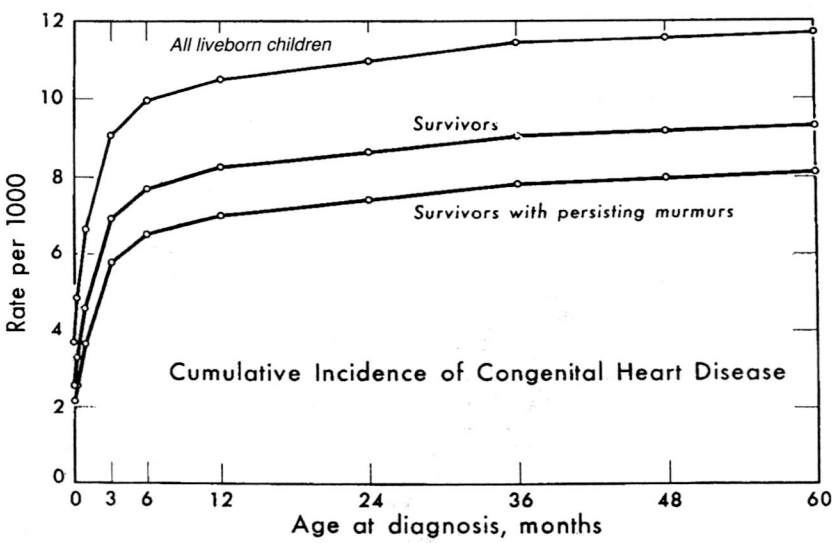

Figure 1.5. Cumulative incidence of congenital heart disease by age at diagnosis in 19,000 California children. (From Yerushalmy J. The California child health and development studies: study design and some illustrative findings on congenital heart disease. In: Fraser FC, McKusick VA, eds. Congenital malformations. Proceedings of the Third International Conference. Amsterdam: Excerpta Medica, 1970.)

can sometimes be organized, especially when they represent a range of mild to severe manifestations of the same basic developmental error. In other areas, no such groups can be established. Multiple anomalies and the frequent association of morphologically and functionally unrelated defects seem to defy logical analysis.

We have chosen to discuss anomalies by anatomical organs and systems without overlooking syndromes that transcend these divisions. We have attempted to identify specific entities and to show their relationships wherever possible.

ETIOLOGY OF CONGENITAL ANOMALIES

The human embryologist usually has to be content with describing the steps by which a malformation develops. Rarely can he or she say how the error occurred. The embryologist is not even able to describe the development in some cases and must then rely on speculation to "reconstruct the crime."

Our best estimate suggests that the etiology of human malformations may be distributed as follows: 15% are of demonstrable genetic origin (i.e., gene makeup); 10% result from chromosomal aberrations; 10% are of viral or teratogenic origin; and 65% are of unknown origin. Most of the latter group probably "result from complicated interactions between genetic predispositions and subtle factors in the intrauterine environment" (23). Some remain attributable to simple mechanical accidents in utero.

Many congenital anomalies can be reproduced in experimental animals, and much has been learned by this method. Unfortunately, to produce an anomaly by experimental means is no evidence that a similar anomaly is produced by the same mechanism spontaneously.

A number of human anomalies are not duplicated in animals either spontaneously or by teratogens. This fact, together with the rarity of most anomalies, leaves the embryologist with little to do but observe and apply general principles to the specific cases.

EDITORIAL COMMENT

While many human congenital abnormalities do not occur in animals, pediatric surgical investigators have been able to create models of major human life-threatening congenital abnormalities in experimental animals. Diaphragmatic hernia, gastroschisis, and intestinal atresia, among others, have been established as animal models for the study of the pathophysiology of these major anomalies, and this has led to a better understanding of the management of human babies born with these conditions (JAH/CNP).

That experimentally induced abnormal development depends less on the nature of the insult than on the time at which it is applied has been known for many years. For this reason efforts have been made to determine at which time during development specific malformations occur.

Ingalls has tabulated the defects that he believes arise in specific weeks of gestation (24). His principle is good but is subject to false interpretation. The "critical time" must be considered as the latest possible time at which the teratogen could have acted. Almost certainly it has acted much earlier. We know that, in many cases, cellular determination takes place some time before there is morphologic evidence of an organ (25). Of course, if the error lies in the genes or in anomalous chromosomes, the time at which the malformation becomes manifest bears no relationship to the primary cause.

GESTATIONAL AGE AT WHICH MALFORMATIONS OCCUR

Stevenson and his colleagues, examining 483 malformed infants, concluded that 67.7% of the malformations had occurred in the first month of gestation, 23.2% in the second month, and only 9.1% after the second month (13). Of these infants, 68.7% survived, 24.8% were stillborn, and 6.5% died in the neonatal period.

We have already seen (p. 4) that reliable estimates of malformation cannot be made by observations on newborn infants alone. To approach the problem in another way, we tabulated the 203 anomalous conditions embraced in the first edition of this book by the gestational week or month (fertilization age) in which they probably occurred. Thus we are considering disease entities rather than patients. Each of these entities permits at least some of its victims to be born alive. None are uniformly fatal in utero. Figure 1.6 shows that, by far, the greatest number of these defects have their morphologic beginning in the third to tenth weeks of development.

Lumping all these lesions together is unreasonable, of course. Thirty-nine must be classed as very rare; 69 are rare; 44 are uncommon; and 51 may be considered common. To correct for the relative incidence, we have arbitrarily weighted the data, assigning a value of 1 to the very rare defects, multiplying the rare anomalies by 10, the uncommon by 100, and the common by 1000. The results are shown in Figure 1.7. That we have not appreciably changed the picture by weighing the data is apparent. The common anomalies have much the same distribution as do the rarer ones.

A picture of defects that are lethal in utero certainly would show a much higher incidence in the first few weeks of gestation. Furthermore, some anomalies—but not all—certainly have their true genesis a week or so earlier than their anatomic manifestation. Finally, congenital defects other than those considered in this book may possibly have a different distribution. Their analysis must await further study.

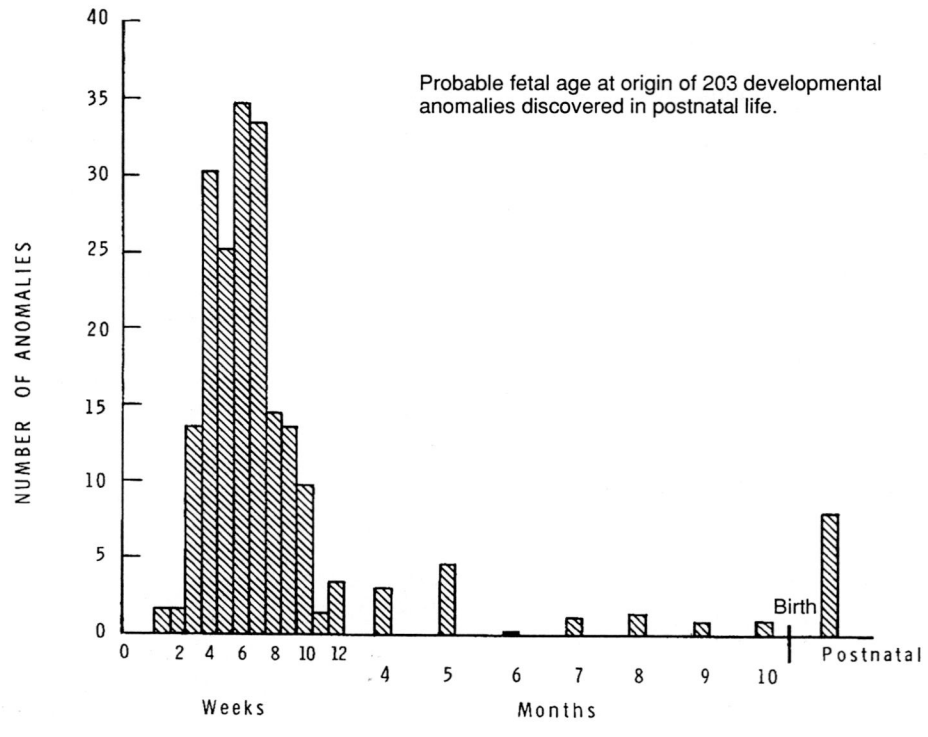

Figure 1.6. The probable age at which developmental errors arise to produce 203 of the different congenital anomalies discussed in this book. Only anomalies that may be present in postnatal life are included.

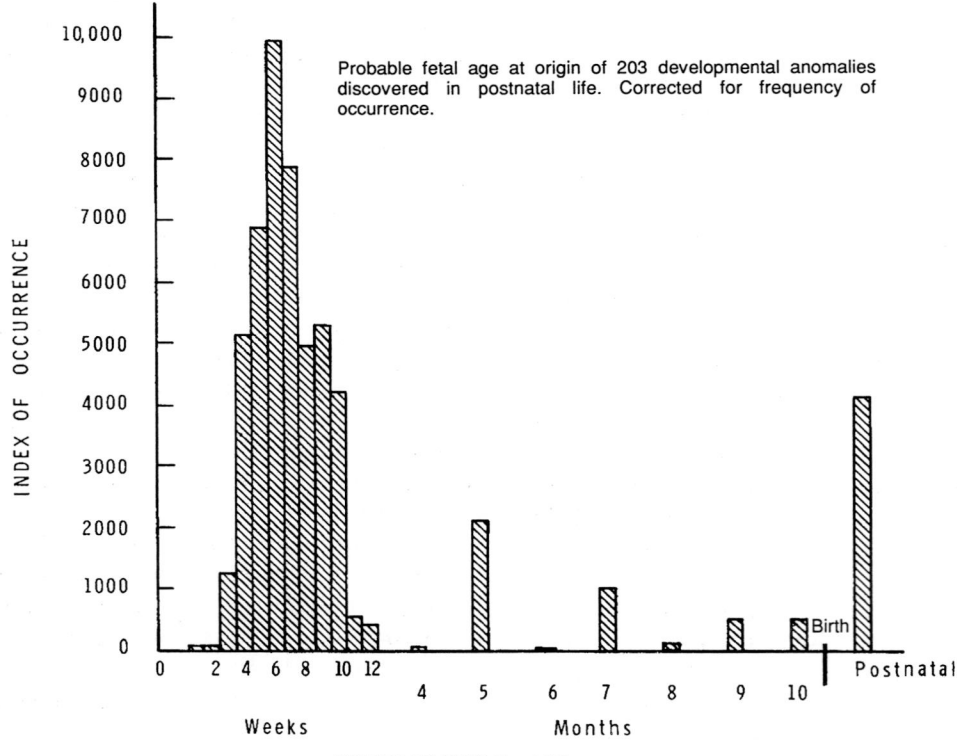

Figure 1.7. The same data as in Figure 1.6, corrected for relative frequency of occurrence of the anomalies. The index of occurrence was obtained by assigning a value of 1 to very rare anomalies, multiplying the rare by 10, the uncommon by 100, and the common by 1000.

NORMAL EMBRYONIC DEVELOPMENT

There is an orderliness to organogenesis, without the strict programming of an assembly line. Development resembles a group of friends walking toward a common destination (birth), where they will perform coordinated duties (postnatal life). Some individuals may be at the head of the group, whereas others may fall behind. Some may lead at one time and drop back in the group later; their relative positions are variable within limits. Occasionally, one may fail to start (agenesis); others may drop out on the way, never to catch up (developmental arrest). An unfortunate one may be struck down along the route (fetal accident). Some may arrive at their destination lame and weary and unable to contribute their share to the activities (defective development).

In many such journeys the weather may be good and the path smooth; the entire group may arrive intact. In a few cases the weather may be unfavorable, and some individuals may fail to reach the destination (teratogenic influences). Even more often the group may include infirm individuals unable to complete the journey even in the best weather (genetic defects).

In our presentation of the malformations of each organ or system we shall briefly describe the normal developmental sequence in terms of the age or size of the embryo.

Age and Size of the Embryo

The complete histories of embryos, especially young ones, rarely are known. A negligible number can be dated absolutely from conception and only a few more from menstrual history. In general, the most available index of age is the size of the embryo.

However, even size is not an absolute measure. Not all embryos of the same size are identically developed: Embryonic development does not proceed in a rigorous, mechanical pattern.

At certain ages development proceeds faster than at others. During the fourth and fifth weeks the embryo grows only about 3 mm in length from 2 to 5 mm, but many fundamental events take place. During this period the number of mesodermal somites formed is a more accurate measure of development than is length. Again, the curvature of the embryo makes an accurate determination of its length difficult. An embryo is relatively straight for a short while after the beginning of development; then it begins to curve ventrally to fit the chorionic vesicle. The best measurement yet found is the crown-rump length, which is measured from the vertex of the head to the rump (Fig. 1.8). The gravest drawback is that this dimension is the chord of a semicircle and therefore is extremely sensitive to alteration in curvature. The advantage of this measurement is the ease with which it can be obtained. Other measurements have been pro-

posed but are rarely used. (Mall describes these in Chapter 8 of Keibel and Mall's *Manual of Human Embryology* [26].)

Another source of error is fixation. Measurements are assumed to be made on fresh specimens. These are not always possible to obtain, and the fixed (or even already sectioned) embryo may be all that is available. Calculations from such material are unreliable. In most instances, however, one must accept the measurement given by the particular investigator describing the embryo; it may be wrong, but there can be no appeal after years have elapsed.

The earliest effort of any significance to correlate length and developmental level of embryos with gestational age was that of His in 1880 (27), but very few young embryos were available at that time. In 1918 Mall constructed a table of size and estimated age from about 1000 embryos and fetuses (28). Among these were 26 with a known menstrual age and 7 with a reasonably certain fertilization age. When the age of the former is corrected to fertilization age by subtracting 14 days, the agreement with modern data is reasonably good. The 7 with known fertilization age are very close to the expected size.

Beginning in 1942 Streeter, Mall's successor at the Carnegie Institution, approached the problem by describing in some detail human embryos at 23 arbitrarily chosen stages of development. The first nine stages, starting with the one-cell stage, were never completely described because of a scarcity of material. The stages from early somite formation to about 30 mm in length are described as "horizons" X through XXIII (29–33). The term *horizon* proposed by Streeter in 1942 was soon replaced by *stage*. Table 1.4 lists the Carnegie Stages, the appearance of somites, crown-rump length, Streeter's estimated age in days, and pertinent gross landmarks.

Streeter's own age estimates, supplemented in the earlier stages by those of Davies (34), are listed, as are estimates by Arey (35), Patten (36), and Witschi (37). Many standard texts and atlases, such as that of Blechschmidt (38), follow Streeter's age estimates. One advantage of Streeter's system is that it fixes attention on size and developmental levels, whereas actual age remains flexible and responsive to new data.

Streeter's approach takes into consideration the inherent variations among embryos. In most of the stages there is a reasonable size range given and the emphasis is on the mean development of all systems rather than on specific developmental events.

Subsequent authors have considered Streeter's ages for horizons XIV to XXII to be too low. The most thoroughly documented series is that of Witschi, who thought that earlier estimates relied too heavily on correlations between human embryos and those of the Rhesus monkey (37). Witschi's stages, while more detailed than those of

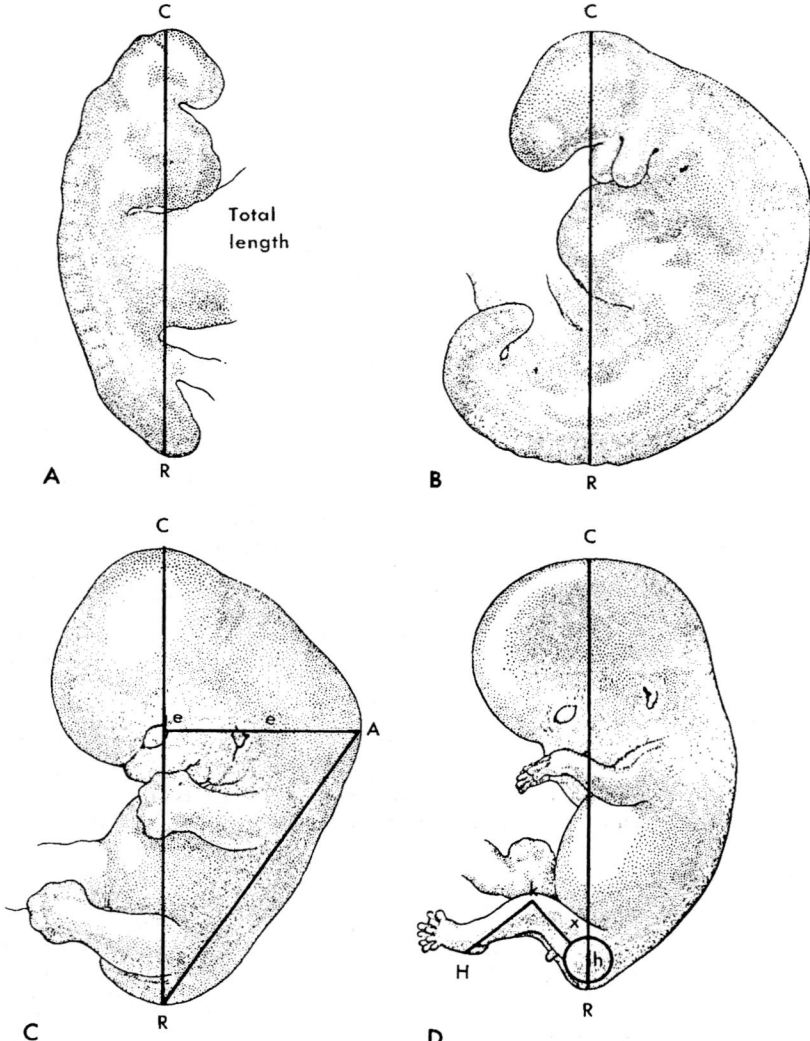

Figure 1.8. Four ways in which embryos may be measured. **A,** Total length of very young, relatively straight embryos. At this stage, the number of somites is a better index of age than is size. **B,** Crown-rump length (C-R), the most widely used dimension of embryos. **C,** Spinal length, measured from base of skull (A) to rump (R); A is established by line e-e through the eye and ear. **D,** Standing height, useful for comparison of older fetuses with postnatal size. The arc of the circle centered on the hip joint (h) and coinciding with the curve of the rump establishes the point x. The distance x-k-H is added to the crown-rump length to give the standing height. (From Davies J. Human developmental anatomy. New York: Ronald Press, 1963.)

Arey (35) and Patten (36), are in essential agreement with them. Until there is a larger collection of dated human embryos from the first 9 weeks of gestation available for study, Witschi's estimates of age appear to be the more soundly based. These estimates may be found in the handbooks of the Federation of American Societies for Experimental Biology (39, 40), as well as in Witschi's own text (37).

The size of the fetus after the 10th week becomes even more difficult to determine. Because babies are born in different sizes, there is an increasing variance in size with fetal age. Again, once the fetus is outside the mother's uterus, the curvature is altered, and the crown-rump measurement can no longer be measured precisely. A third source of error lies in the fact that spontaneously aborted fetuses may have suffered retardation of growth from the very abnormalities that caused them to abort. Table 1.5 shows estimates from several sources.

Weight is a better measure of the fetus than is length, although great variations are encountered in different published series, such as is illustrated by Gruenwald (41). His own data, based on over 12,500 consecutive births at Sinai Hospital, are shown in abbreviated form in Table 1.6. Note that age is counted from the last menstrual period and is not the fertilization age.

Thus the problem of using age and size of embryos is acknowledged. We sympathize with the casual reader of human embryology texts, who often feels frustrated by the terminology of the embryologist. In a discussion of a particular developmental event the reader expects to be

Table 1.4.
Developmental Stages in Human Embryos

Carnegie Stage	Pair of Somites	Size (mm)	Age (Days)	Features
1		0.1–0.15	1	Fertilization
2		0.1–0.2	1½–3	From 2 to about 16 cells
3		0.1–0.2	4	Free blastocyst
4		0.1–0.2	5–6	Attaching blastocyst
5		0.1–0.2	7–12	Implanted, although previllous
5a		0.1	7–8	Solid trophoblast
5b		0.1	9	Trophoblastic lacunae
5c		0.15–0.2	11–12	Lacunar vascular circle
6		0.2	13	Chorionic villi: primitive streak may appear
6a				Chorionic villi
6b				Primitive streak
7		0.4	16	Notochordal process
8		1.0–1.5	18	Primitive pit; notochord and neurenteric canals; neural folds may appear
9	1–3	1.5–2.5	20	Somites first appear
10	4–12	2–3.5	22	Neural folds begin to fuse; 2 pharyngeal bars; optic sulcus.
11	13–20	2.5–4.5	24	Rostral neuropore closes; optic vesicle.
12	21–29	3–5	26	Caudal neuropore closes; two to four pharyngeal bars; upper limb buds appearing
13	30 (?)	4–6	28	Four limb buds; lens disc; otic vesicle
14		5–7	32	Lens pit and optic cup; endolymphatic appendage distinct
15		7–9	33	Lens vesicle; nasal pit; antitragus beginning; hand plate; trunk relatively wider; future cerebral hemispheres distinct
16		8–11	37	Nasal pit faces ventrally; retinal pigment visible in intact embryo; auricular hillocks beginning; foot plate
17		11–14	41	Head relatively larger; trunk straighter; nasofrontal groove distinct; auricular hillocks distinct; finger rays
18		13–17	44	Body more cuboidal; elbow region and toe rays appearing; eyelid folds may begin; tip of nose distinct; nipples appear; ossification may begin
19		16–18	47½	Trunk elongating and straightening
20		18–22	50½	Upper limbs longer and bent at elbows
21		22–24	52	Fingers longer; hands approach each other, feet likewise
22		23–28	54	Eyelids and external ear more developed
23		27–31	56½	Head more rounded; limbs longer and more developed

[a]From O'Rahilly R, Muller F. Developmental stages in human embryos. Washington: Carnegie Institution of Washington, 1987.

Table 1.5.
Comparison of Fetal Measurements from the Eighth to the Fortieth Week of Gestation

Fertilization Age — Lunar Months	Weeks	Crown-Rump Length (mm) Streeter (1920)[a]	Patten (1968)[b]	Arey (1965)[c]	Witschi (1962)[d]	Crown-Heel (Body Extended) Length (mm) Arey (1965)[c]	Boyd (1941)[e]	Rule of Haase (1875)[f]
2	8	23	28–30	23	22–26	30	26	40
	9		39–41					
	10		51–53		40–50			
	11		64–66					
3	12	74	77–79	56		73	90	90
	13		91–93					
	14		105–107					
	15		119–121					
4	16	116	132–134	112		157	167	160
	17		147					
	18		160					
	19		173					
5	20	164	185	160	160–200	239	243	250
	22		208					
6	24	208	230	203		296	311	300
7	28	247	270	242		355	371	350
8	32	283	310	277		409	424	400
9	36	321	346	313		458	470	450
	38		362					
10	40	362		350	320–400	500	510	500

[a]Streeter GL. Weight, sitting height, etc., and menstrual age of the human embryo. Contrib Embryol Carnegie Inst Wash 11:143–170, 1920.
[b]Patten BM. Human embryology. 3rd ed. New York: McGraw-Hill, 1968.
[c]Arey LB. Developmental anatomy: a textbook and laboratory manual of embryology. 7th ed. Philadelphia: WB Saunders, 1965.
[d]Witschi E. Characterization of developmental stages: man. In: Altman PL, Dittmer DS, eds. Growth, including reproduction and morphological development. Washington, DC: Federal American Society Experimental Biology, 1962.
[e]Boyd E. Outline of physical growth and development. Minneapolis: Burgess, 1941.
[f]Arey LB: Developmental anatomy: a textbook and laboratory manual of embryology. 7th ed. Philadelphia: WB Saunders, 1965.

Table 1.6.
Single Birth Weight in Relation to Gestational Age[a]

Weeks from Last Menstrual Period	Standard Deviation from Mean (g)			Percentiles		
	−1	Mean	+1	25	50	75
28	750	1050	1400	850	1080	
30	1000	1380	1750	1150	1350	
32	1340	1750	2150	1500	1750	
34	1720	2170	2610	1920	2240	
36	2150	2610	3080	2380	2650	
38	2560	3050	3480	2780	3030	3330
40	2830	3280	3720	3000	3260	3570
42	2930	3400	3860	3100	3370	3700
44+	2930	3420	3740	3100	3420	3750

[a]Adapted from Gruenwald P. Growth of the human fetus. I. Normal growth and its variations. Am J Obstet Gynecol 1966;94:1112–1119.

told *when* the event occurs. Instead of this, he or she often gets a linear measurement such as 6.3 mm, a value such as 10 somites, or occasionally a reference such as horizon XII. In this book, embryo size is given as *crown-rump length* unless otherwise specified. Age is given as *fertilization age*, arbitrarily set at 14 days after the onset of the last menstrual period.

EDITORIAL COMMENT

Another important confounding variable in the measurement of the size of the developing human fetus is that the mother's health greatly influences the size of the developing baby. Various toxic substances, including drugs, have a profound influence on the size of the fetus and the clinical term "small for gestational age" is a very significant one to neonatologists. It may have a profound impact on the viability of the otherwise normally formed fetus, much less than on the newborn infant who has major congenital abnormalities. The evolving field of prenatal diagnostic studies has contributed greatly to our understanding of fetal development because consecutive sonographic studies reveal the growth pattern of an individual fetus (and thus may pinpoint evidence of failure to thrive in utero) and have significant impact on obstetrical management of the mother and baby (JAH/CNP).

General

Jaubert and Danel made a prophetic statement about the regulation of embryonal development starting to surface by better knowledge of the growth factors:

> The regulation of embryonal development is beginning to surface. Growth factors are involved in a multistep process [43]. The blastocyst of the mouse elaborates three growth factors: two transforming growth factors (TGF-α and TGF-β) and the platelet derived growth factor A (PDGF-A) [44]. On one hand, these factors act on the blastula itself as mitotic and differentiating agents, and on the other hand, they

induce early angiogenesis and deciduation of the uterus for nesting. At the blastulation stage, in Xenopus, fibroblast growth factor (FGF) and TGF-β induce mesoderm differentiation [45]. Later on, after implantation in the endometrium, there is an intermingling of embryonal and maternal derived growth factors acting on the embryo. For example, stimulation by PDGF-A induces the expression of *c-myc* oncogene in the receptive cells [46]. An enhanced *c-myc* expression is found in the intestine (30 per 100 cells) and lung (20 per 100 cells) of the human embryo [47]. Other growth factors may stimulate various oncogenes. The action of growth factors and of the surrounding connective tissue on cell differentiation is called *paracrine action,* in contrast to the endocrine action of hormones [43]. For insects, it is demonstrated that specialized organizers (Homeo box) with a segmental (metameric) specificity are switched on for a while during differentiation (42).

It is not within the scope of this book, which is written for clinicians, to present deep embryologic problems or to elaborate on phenomena in which clinicians are uninterested. However, the editors are happy to mention theories and pragmata for future embryology, the possibility of explanation of the pathogenesis of congenital anomalies, and perhaps the postulation of their prevention.

THE TRIUMPH OF SURGERY WITH CONGENITAL ANOMALIES

Sen Gupta submitted a unique case he encountered in his practice in Calcutta. We present this case to emphasize that there are triumphs in surgery over congenital anomalies. At the same time, we express our appreciation and gratitude to Gupta and his staff for permitting us to present this case.

Clinical Features

A 22-year-old married female with atypical idiopathic female intersex (23), used to defecate, micturate, menstruate, and copulate through the anal orifice (Fig. 1.9).

Investigations confirmed a female with 46XX and normal secondary sex characteristics. There was a normally developed labia majora, absence of the perineal body, and fusion of the pudendal cleft. There was displacement of the labia minora into the anorectal wall with the urethral and vaginal orifices ectopically shifted inside the rectum 5 cm cephalic to the anal canal. The patient also had marked clitoromegaly with megalourethra, bicornuate uterus, bilateral tubal blockage, and septate vagina, without somatic anomalies.

A surgical correction was performed by replacing the vagina and urethra from the anorectal wall to near normal anatomical position by an abdominoperineal approach. This was followed by excision of the phallus and ablation of the phallic urethra. Hysteroplasty and tuboplasty were performed 3 months later (Figs. 1.10 to 1.15). The patient conceived 15 months after the last operation and was delivered by caesarean section of a healthy 2.5-kg female baby.

Embryogenesis

There is a diversity of opinion about the embryological etiology of multiple malformations involving only the genitourinary organs. Howard and Hinman suggested that the incomplete union between the müllerian ducts and the urogenital sinus induces uninhibited development of an accessory phallic urethra (48). The degree of female masculinization is the result of complex biochemical and tissue interaction. The presence of testosterone and its conversion to dihydrotestosterone by 5-α reductase in these tissues are responsible for the development of the male phenotype; this is correlated with androgen dosages, length of administration, and stage of pregnancy when administered (49).

Bellinger and Duckett (50), Belis and Hrabovsky (49), Howard and Hinman (48), and Jones and Scott (51) stress poorly delineated local factors and suggest that the abnormal descent of the müllerian ducts in the urorectal septum causes posterior displacement of the vagina and urethra, allowing the development of the accessory phallic urethra with unusually prominent clitoris. Turnock and Rickwood suggested that it is the presence of both phallic and vulval urethral orifices that distinguished masculinization in adrenogenital syndrome from the urethralization of the female phallus (52). They postulated that failure of differentiation of pericloacal mesoderm, owing to a late arrival and incomplete fusion of the müllerian

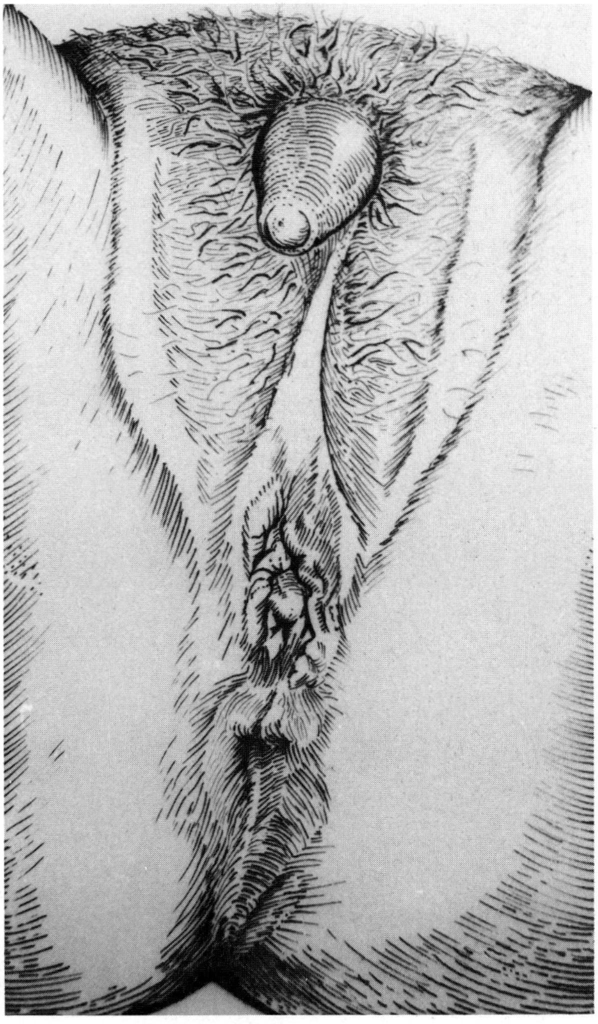

Figure 1.9. External genitalia showing well-developed labia majora, obliterated pudendal cleft, part of the labia minora projecting into anorectal wall; a large phallus situated at the upper part of the labia majora with a small urethral opening at the tip.

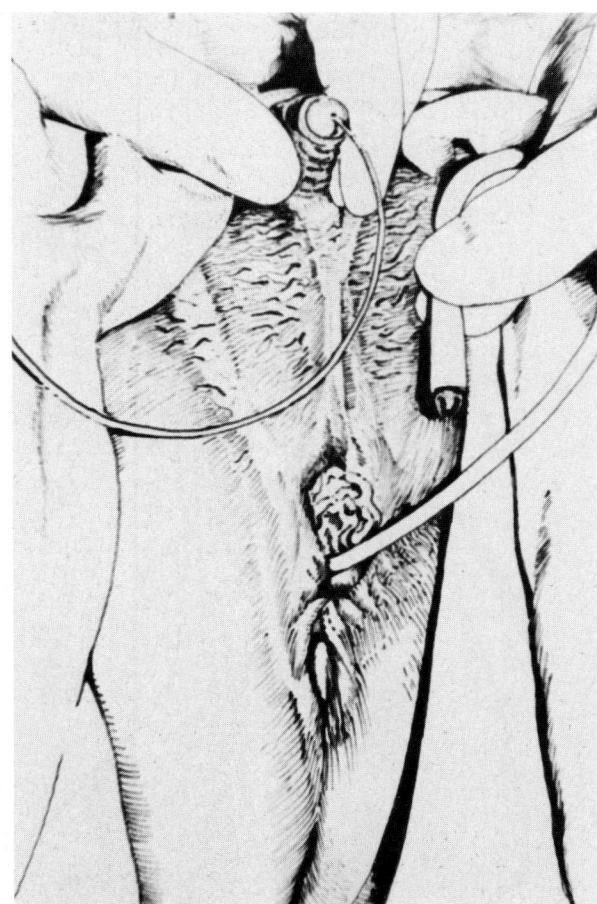

Figure 1.10. Polythene tube through the phallic urethra in situ; rubber catheter through anus into ectopic urethral opening in rectum; drop of urine coming out through the rubber catheter.

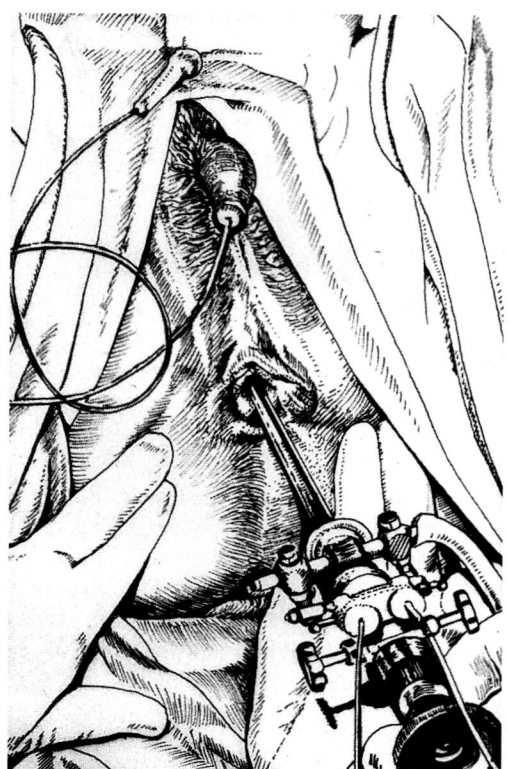

Figure 1.11. Cystocope through ectopic urethra in rectum; ureteric catheter negotiated for retrograde pyelogram; polythene tube through phallic urethra in situ.

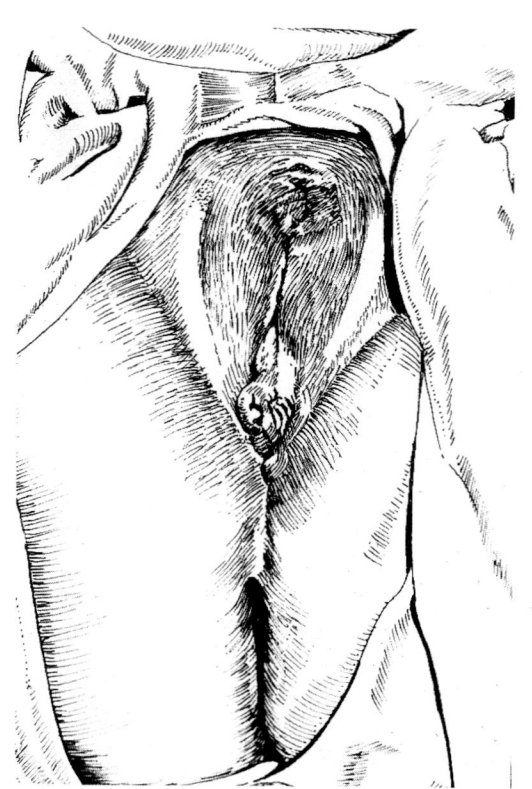

Figure 1.12. Scar at the cephalic end of the labia majora shows site of excision of phallus; labia minora is near anatomical position; newly built perineum demonstrated.

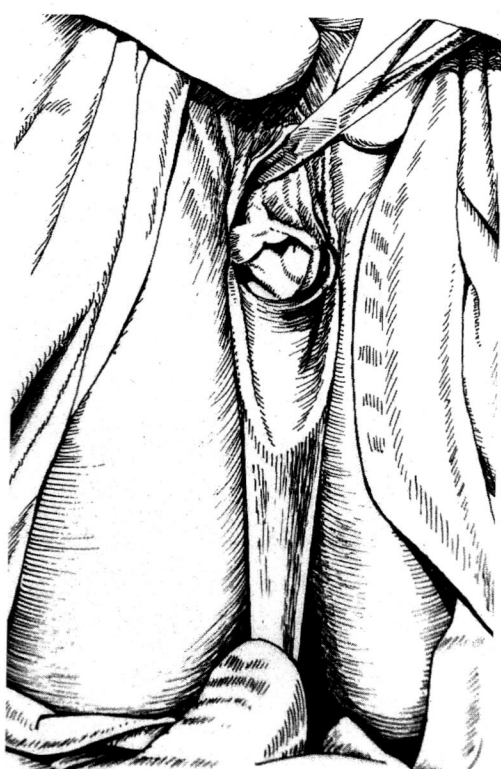

Figure 1.13. Speculum in vagina; normal anatomical criteria, except a sagittal septum.

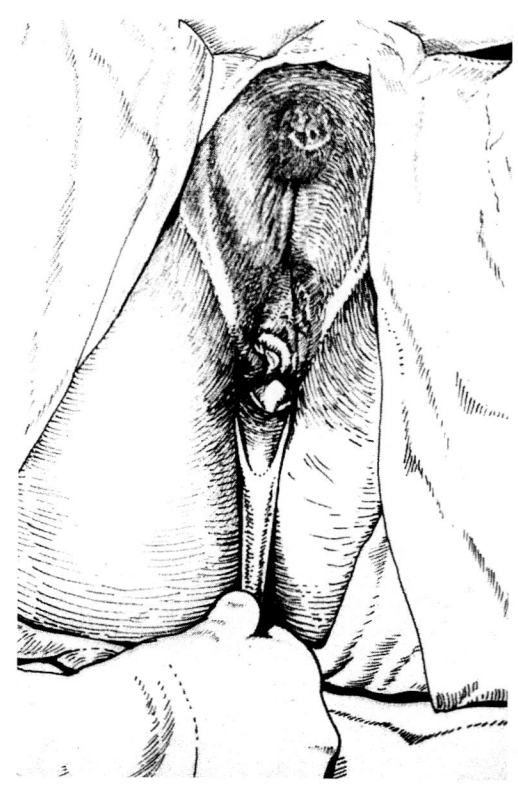

Figure 1.14. Sagittal septum high up, shown with speculum in vagina.

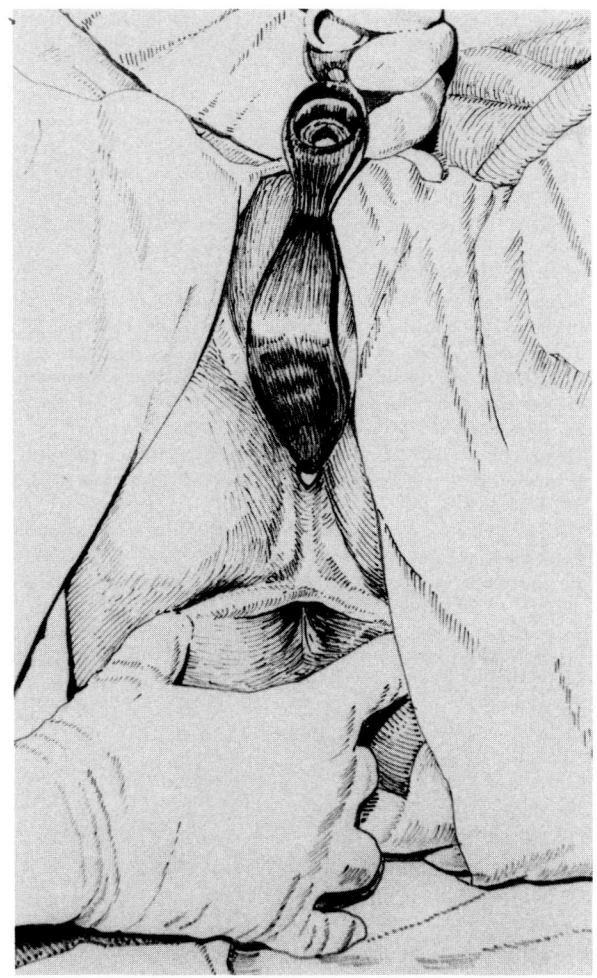

Figure 1.15. Newly built perineum and anus with retractor in vagina.

ducts, might be the cause of such defects. They also confirmed the suggestion of Bellinger and Duckett that the clitoris is prominent because urethralization prevents the development of a normal female ventral chordee (50).

Surgical correction of multiple urogenital anomalies in atypical idiopathic female intersex, followed by successful outcome of pregnancy, is not recorded in the literature.

REFERENCES

1. Lister J, Irving IM. Preface to the third edition. In: Lister J, Irving IM, eds. Neonatal surgery. 3rd ed. Boston: Butterworths, 1990.
2. Rickham PP. The ethics of surgery in newborn infants. In: Lister J, Irving IM, eds. Neonatal surgery. Boston: Butterworths, 1990.
3. Potts WJ. The surgeon and the child. Philadelphia: WB Saunders, 1959.
4. McCormick RA. To save or let die: the dilemma of modern medicine. JAMA 1974;229:172–176.
5. Singer P. Sanctity of life or quality of life? Pediatrics 1983;72:128–129.
6. Erhardt CL. Pregnancy losses in New York City. Am J Public Health 1963;53:1337–1352.
7. Stickle G. Defective development and reproductive wastage in the United States. Am J Obstet Gynecol 1968;100:442–447.
8. Hertig AT. Traumatic abortion and prenatal death of the embryo. In: Hertig AT. Prematurity, congenital malformation and birth injury. New York: Association for the Aid of Crippled Children, 1953:174–176.
9. Witschi E. Teratogenic effects from overripeness of the egg. In: Fraser FC, McKusick VA, eds. Congenital malformations. Proceedings of the Third International Conference. Amsterdam: Excerpta Medica, 1970.
10. Owens JR. Incidence and causation of congenital defects. In: Lister J, Irving IM, eds. Neonatal surgery, 3rd ed. Boston: Butterworths, 1990.
11. Murphy DP. Congenital defects: incidence among the siblings of the first congenitally malformed children in 275 families. JAMA 1936;106:457.
12. Malpas P. The incidence of human malformation and the significance of changes in the maternal environment in their causation. J Obstet Gynaecol Br Commw 1937;44:434–454.
13. Stevenson AC, Johnston HA, Stewart MIP, Golding DR. Congenital malformations: a report of a series of consecutive births in 24 centres. Bull WHO 1966;34(suppl):1–127.
14. Kennedy WP. Epidemiologic aspects of the problem of congenital malformations. Birth Defects 1967;3:1–18.
15. Lynberg MC, Khoury MJ. CDC Surv Summ 1990;39(SS-3):1–12.
16. Wallace HM, Hoenig L, Rich H. Newborn infants with congenital malformations or birth injuries. Am J Dis Child 1956;529–541.
17. Shapiro S, Ross LJ, Levine HS. Relationship of selected prenatal factors to pregnancy outcome and congenital anomalies. Am J Public Health 1965;55:268–282.
18. Centers for Disease Control. Contribution of birth defects to infant mortality, United States, 1986. MMWR 1989;38(37):633.
19. Simpson Maternity Hospital. Annual reports, 1938–1948, 1955–1963. Edinburgh: Simpson Medical Hospital.
20. Saxen L, Haro S. Congenital malformations of newborn infants in Finland, 1957–1962. Duodecim (Helsinki) 1964;80:257–263.
21. Lock FR, Gatling HB, Wells HB. Difficulties in the diagnosis of congenital abnormalities: experience in a study of the effect of rubella on pregnancy. JAMA 1961;178:711–714.
22. Yerushalmy J. The California child health and development studies: study design and some illustrative findings on congenital heart disease. In: Fraser FC, McKusick VA, eds. Congenital malformations. Proceedings of the Third International Conference. Amsterdam: Excerpta Medica, 1970.
23. Fraser FC. Causes of congenital malformations in human beings. J Chronic Dis 1959;10:97–110.
24. Ingalls T. Epidemiology of congenital malformations. In: Mechanisms of congenital malformations. Proceedings of the Second Scientific Conference of the Association for the Aid of Crippled Children, New York, 1954:10–20.
25. De Haan RL. Morphogenesis of the vertebrate heart. In: De Haan RL, Ursprung H, eds. Organogenesis. New York: Holt, Rinehart, & Winston, 1965.
26. Keibel F, Mall EP, eds. Manual of human embryology. Vol 1. Philadelphia: JB Lippincott, 1910.
27. His W. Anatomie menschlicher Embryonen. Leipzig: FCW Vogel, 1880–1885.
28. Mall FP. One the age of human embryos. Am J Anat 1918;23:397–422.
29. Streeter GL. Developmental horizons in human embryos: description of age group XI, 13 to 20 somites and age group XII, 21 to 29 somites. Contrib Embryol Carnegie Inst Wash 1945;30:211–251.
30. Streeter GL. Developmental horizons in human embryos: age

group XIII and XIV. Contrib Embryol Carnegie Inst Wash 1945;31:27–63.

31. Streeter GL. Developmental horizons in human embryos: Description of age groups XV, XVI, XVII, and XVIII. Contrib Embryol Carnegie Inst Wash 1948;32:133–204.

32. Streeter GL. Developmental horizons in human embryos: Description of age groups XIX, XX, XXI, XXII, and XXIII, being the fifth issue of a survey of the Carnegie collection prepared for publication by Herser CH, Corner GW. Contrib Embryol Carnegie Inst Wash 1951;34:165–196.

33. Heuser CH, Corner CW. Developmental horizons in human embryos: description of age group X, 4 to 12 somites. Contrib Embryol Carnegie Inst Wash 1957;36:31.

34. Davies J. Human developmental anatomy. New York: Ronald Press, 1963.

35. Arey LB. Developmental anatomy: a textbook and laboratory manual of embryology. 7th ed. Philadelphia: WB Saunders, 1965.

36. Patten BM. Human embryology. 3rd ed. New York: McGraw-Hill, 1968.

37. Witschi E. Development of vertebrates. Philadelphia: WB Saunders, 1956.

38. Blechschmidt E. The stages of human development before birth. Philadelphia: WB Saunders, 1961.

39. Witschi E. Characterization of developmental stages: man. In: Altman PL, Dittmer DS, eds. Growth, including reproduction and morphological development. Washington, DC: Federal American Society Experimental Biology, 1962.

40. Witschi E. Characterization of developmental stages. In: Altman PL, Dittmer DS, eds. Biology data book. Washington, DC: Federal American Society for Experimental Biology, 1962.

41. Gruenwald P. Growth of the human fetus. I. Normal growth and its variations. Am J Obstet Gynecol 1966;94:1112–1119.

42. Jaubert F, Danel C. Discussion: intrathoracic malformations of foregut derivatives. In: Fallis JC, Filler RM, Lemoine G, ed. Pediatric thoracic surgery. New York: Elsevier, 1991:72–74.

43. Milner RDG, Hill DJ. Fetal growth signals. Arch Dis Child 1989;65:53–57.

44. Rappolee DA et al. Developmental expression of PDGF, TGF-α, and TGF-β genes in preimplantation mouse embryos. Science 1988;241:1823–1825.

45. Mercola M, Melton DA, Stiles CD. Platelet-derived growth factor A chain is maternally encoded in xenopus embryos. Science 1988;241:1223–1225.

46. Schmid P, Schulz WA, Hameister H. Dynamic expression pattern of the *myc* protooncogene in midgestation mouse embryos. Science 1989;243:226–229.

47. Pfeifer-Ohlsson S et al. Cell–type-specific pattern of *myc* protooncogene expression in developing human embryos. Proc Natl Acad Sci USA 1985;82:5050–5054.

48. Howard FS, Hinman F Jr. Female pseudohermaphroditism with supplementary phallic urethra: report of two cases. J Urol 1951;65:439–452.

49. Belis JA, Hrabovsky EE. Idiopathic female intersex with clitoromegaly and urethral duplication. J Urol 1979;122:805–808.

50. Bellinger MF, Duckett JW. Accessory phallic urethra in the female patient. J Urol 1982;127:1159–1164.

51. Jones HW Jr, Scott WW. Hermaphroditism, genital anomalies and related endocrine disorders. 2nd ed. Baltimore: Williams & Wilkins, 1971:275.

52. Turnock RR, Rickwood AMK. Urethralisation of the female phallus: a rare form of intersex. Br J Urol 1987;59:481–482.

CHAPTER 2

THE PHARYNX AND ITS DERIVATIVES

John Elias Skandalakis / Stephen Wood Gray / Norman Wendell Todd

With malleus
Aforethought
Mammals
Got an earful
Of their ancestors'
Jaw.
—*JOHN M. BURNS. EVOLUTION OF AUDITORY OSSICLES.*
BIOGRAFFATI: A NATURAL SELECTION. 1975.
WW NORTON, NEW YORK

DEVELOPMENT

The embryonic foregut, that portion of the primitive gut cranial to the open midgut, differentiates into pharynx, esophagus, stomach, and the cranial half of the duodenum. The development of the pharynx precedes that of the more caudal organs. The pharynx occupies most of the foregut during the first few weeks of development (Fig. 2.1, *A* and *B*).

Between the fourth and sixth weeks, the cranial portion of the foregut changes from a flattened tube into a complicated series of structures, some of which are reminiscent of the primordia of the respiratory apparatus of aquatic vertebrates (Fig. 2.1, *C* and *D*). These structures indicate the fundamental plan of the vertebrate body, but in mammals either the structures become rearranged and adapted to new functions or they disappear, leaving only occasional vestiges. In the human pharynx, this transitory branchial pattern is almost wholly obliterated by the seventh week of embryonic life. (Note that the term *branchial* is used throughout this text in referring to structures reminiscent of the gills of adult nonmammalian aquatic vertebrates. We have chosen the term *branchial* rather than *pharyngeal* because we consider branchial to often be more descriptive and appropriate. Ontogeny does not recapitulate phylogeny. However, the perspectives of comparative anatomy and comparative embryology are interesting and illuminating. Our goal is to provide a clinically applicable account of the ontogenetic origin of humans.)

The structures formed from the pharynx may be divided into the lateral branchial apparatus, consisting of paired endodermal pharyngeal pouches and corresponding ectodermal branchial clefts with mesodermal branchial arches between consecutive pairs, and the unpaired ventral endodermal floor, which produces the following derivatives: the tongue, thyroid gland, larynx, and trachea.

The pharyngeal region, because of its complexity and its phylogenetic significance, has received more attention from embryologists than have most other regions of the body. In the 1820s Rathke described the pharynx of the pig (1), and von Baer described the clefts of the human embryo (2). In 1832 Von Ascherson related cervical cysts to anomalous closure of the clefts (3).

With the development of evolutionary phylogeny by Haeckel under the influence of Darwin, there was great interest in pharyngeal embryology. The wax reconstruction method was applied to human and animal embryos by His (4), Born (5), Piersol (6), and others during the 1880s and in more detail by Wenglowski in 1912 and 1913 (7, 8). The work of Wenglowski and of Grosser, cited in the *Manual of Human Embryology*, edited by Keibel and Mall (9), remains authoritative today. Many of the references to 19th century work on pharyngeal embryology may be found in the review by Lyall and Stahl (10).

When interest in phylogeny began to decline during the 20th century, the rise of endocrinology brought renewed attention to the pharyngeal derivatives. The work of Weller (11), Kingsbury (12–14) and Norris (15, 16) was largely devoted to elucidating the embryogenesis of the thyroid, parathyroid, and thymus glands. In addition, interest in the formation of cystic anomalies has been maintained by Frazer (17), Garrett (18), Hendrick (19), and Albers (20).

First Four Branchial Arches, Clefts, and Pouches

The branchial apparatus is marked externally by four ectodermal branchial clefts on each side of the human embryo in the region of the pharynx (Fig. 2.2, *A*). Inter-

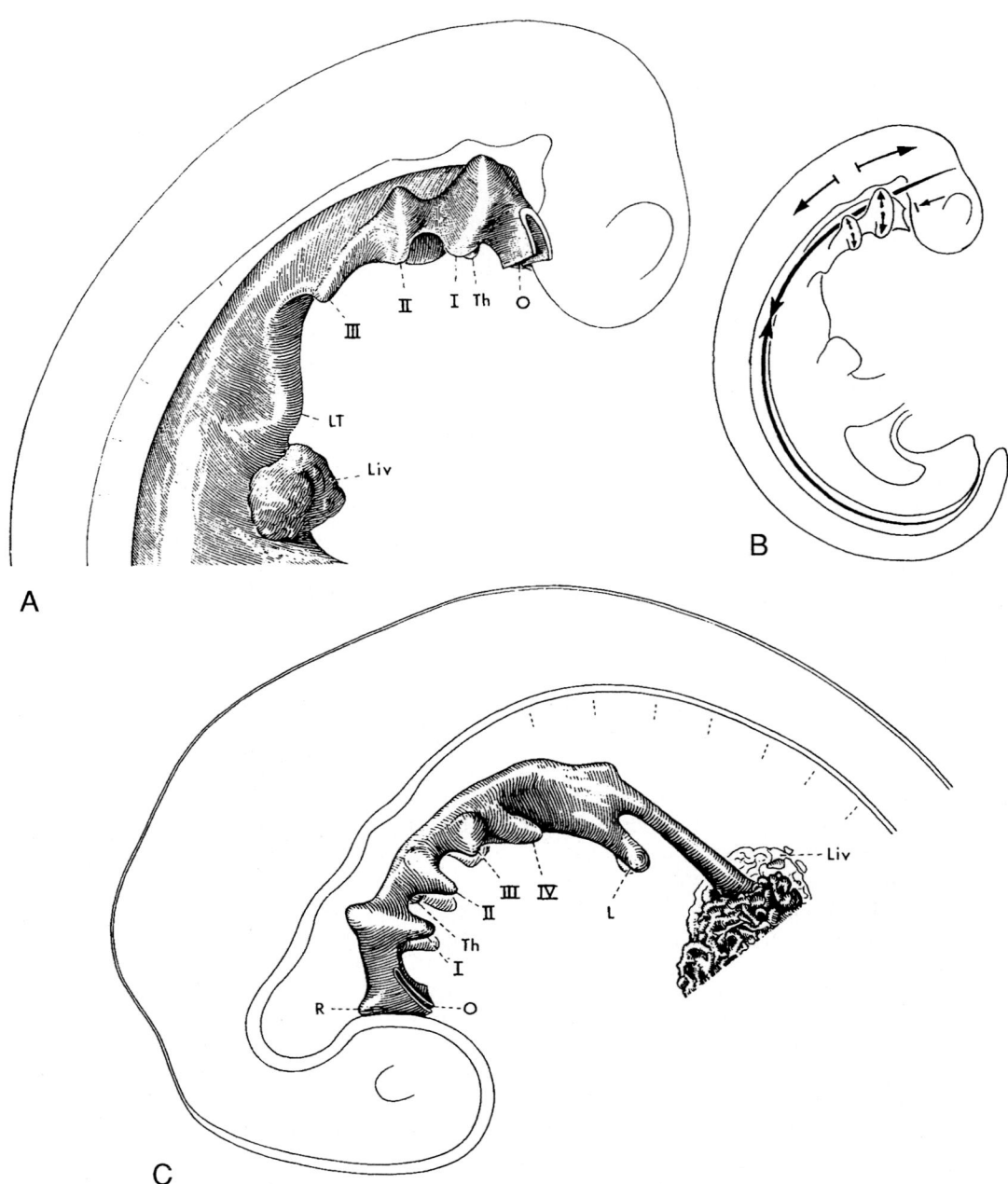

Figure 2.1. Development of the pharynx. **A**, The foregut of a 2.5-mm human embryo. The first three branchial pouches are present, and the laryngotracheal diverticulum is indicated. **B**, Chief directions of growth in the embryo at 2.5 mm. **C**, The foregut of a 4.2-mm human embryo. Four pouches are present, and the lung buds have formed. **D**, Lateral and ventral views of the pharyngeal endoderm of a 4-mm human embryo. The areas of contact between pouch endoderm and cleft ectoderm (closing plates) are shown as flattened surfaces. (**A**, **B**, and **C**, From Blechschmidt E. The stages of human development before birth. Philadelphia: WB Saunders, 1961; **D**, from Hamilton WJ, Boyd JD, Mossman HW. Human embryology, 3rd ed. Baltimore: Williams & Wilkins, 1962 after Weller GL. Development of the thyroid, parathyroid, and thymus glands in man. Contrib Embryol Carnegie Inst Wash 1933;24:141)

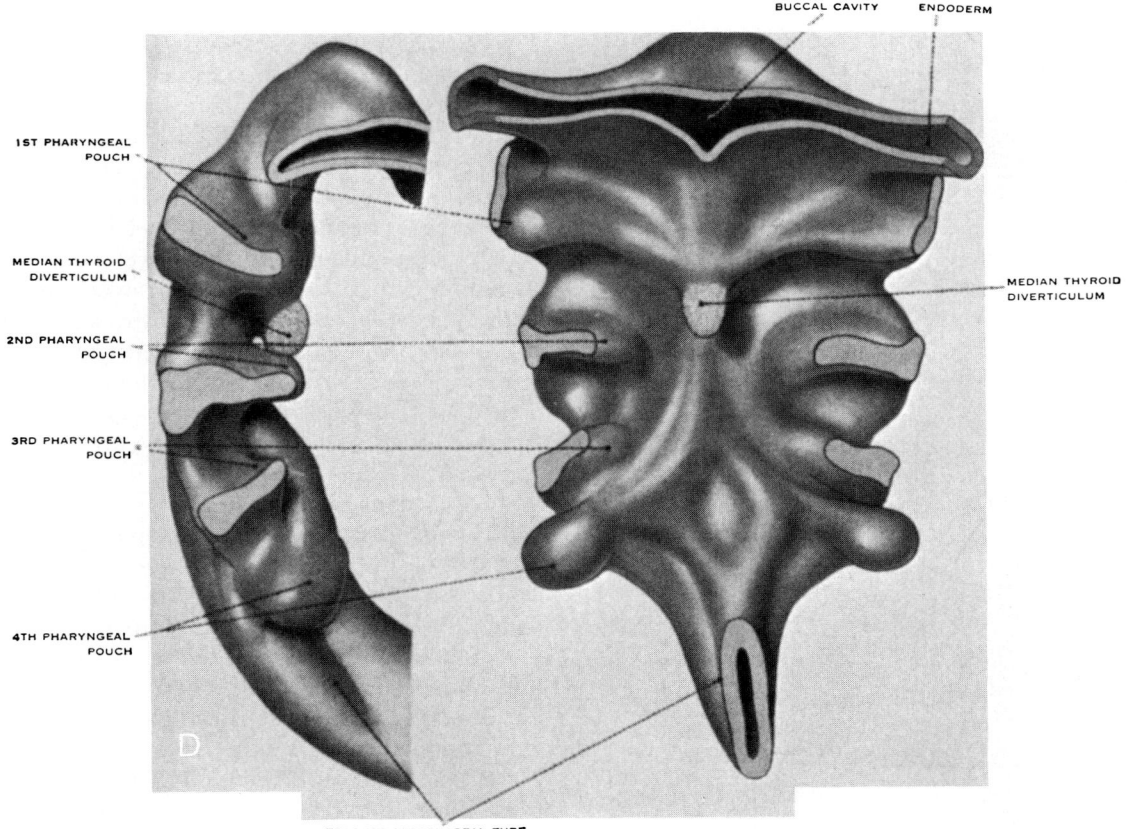

BUCCAL CAVITY   ENDODERM

1ST PHARYNGEAL
POUCH

MEDIAN THYROID
DIVERTICULUM

2ND PHARYNGEAL
POUCH

3RD PHARYNGEAL
POUCH

4TH PHARYNGEAL
POUCH

MEDIAN THYROID
DIVERTICULUM

D

TRACHEO-OESOPHAGEAL TUBE

Figure 2.1 —*continued*

nally, the embryonic pharynx, which begins at the sto-modeal plate, is evaginated into five lateral pharyngeal pouches, of which the first four correspond to the external branchial clefts (Fig. 2.2, *B*). Between consecutive cleft-pouch sets is a mesodermal branchial arch. In each arch there is typically a skeletal element, an aortic arch connecting the ventral and dorsal aortae, and the primordia of nerves and muscles.

In fishes, the thin plate of tissue separating each cleft from its corresponding pharyngeal pouch (Fig. 2.2, *C*) is resorbed to create a true gill slit. Such openings are transitory in terrestrial vertebrates, and in the human embryo they are only occasionally formed during the short period in which the branchial apparatus is at its maximum development.

Of the four branchial clefts visible in the fifth week, only the most dorsal portion of the first cleft persists: the external auditory canal. The corresponding portion of the first pharyngeal pouch becomes the eustachian tube and the cavity of the middle ear, whereas the closing plate between pouch and cleft is represented by the tympanic membrane (Fig. 2.3).

The obliteration of the remaining branchial clefts takes place during the sixth and seventh weeks. The sec-

ond cleft is obliterated by fusion of the second and third arches, and the third and fourth clefts are obliterated by the fusion of the third and fifth arches. The fourth arch is covered and does not reach the surface (17, 18, 21).

The cervical sinus of His, formed by the second arch growing caudally to fuse with the fifth arch, usually has only a transitory existence between the 10-mm and 12-mm stages (i.e., conceptual ages 6 to 7 weeks) (Fig. 2.4, *A* to *E*). The cervical sinus, which amounts to an ectodermal pit, is bordered caudally and dorsally by the V-shaped epipericardial ridge. The epipericardial ridge is formed by proliferating mesoderm, which differentiates into the sternomastoid-trapezius complex of muscles, the infrahyoid muscles, and the muscles of the floor of the mouth and tongue. The nerves of the epipericardial ridge are properly spinal, rather than cranial, nerves: the spinal accessory and the hypoglossal. The caudal growth of the second branchial arch, which is innervated by the facial nerve, is reminiscent of the teleosts' operculum, which overhangs the underlying gill slits. Thus the embryo at the conceptual ages of 6 to 7 weeks resembles the elasmobranchs. With caudal overgrowth of the second arch, the human embryo is reminiscent of the bony fishes (22).

Because the changes in the neck region are so exten-

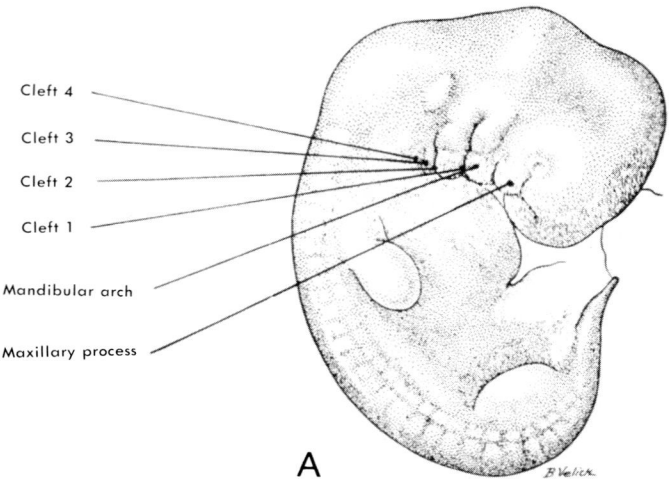

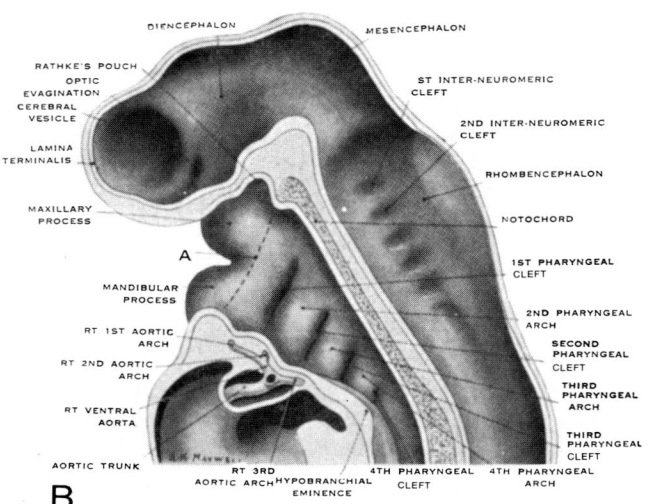

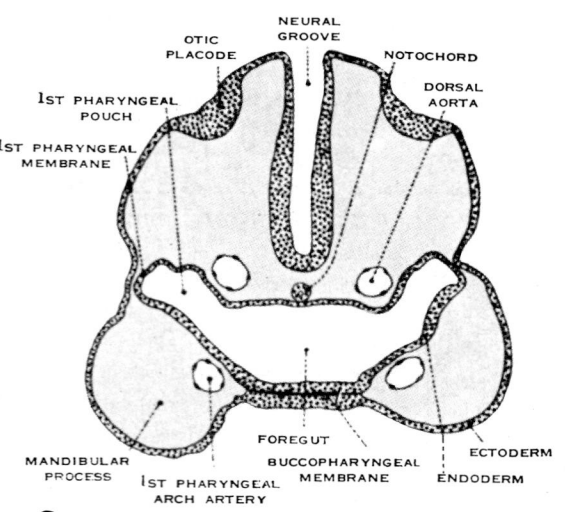

sive, it is not easy to determine the location of the obliterated embryonic clefts and arches in the adult. The site of the first cleft follows the caudal and posterior borders of the mandible and terminates dorsally at the external auditory meatus. The site of the ventral end of the second cleft is under the jaw, and the cleft extends dorsally toward the mastoid process. The anterior portion of the neck, bound laterally by the sternocleidomastoid muscles, thus corresponds to the third arch. On the mistaken assumption that the second arch overgrows the caudal arches like the operculum of fish, some writers have attributed this region to the second arch (23). Ventrally, the site of the third and fourth clefts (cervical sinus, in sensu) (17), may be as low as the suprasternal notch; its dorsal course passes beneath the sternocleidomastoid muscle (Fig. 2.5).

In the adult pharynx, the site of the first branchial pouch is indicated by the eustachian tube, and the second by the tonsillar fossa. The site of the third pouch is apparently near the entry (i.e., cephal end) of the pyriform sinus. The supposed site of the fourth pouch is near the apex (i.e., caudal extent) of the pyriform sinus. The fifth and sixth pouches may be related to the laryngeal ventricle, but there is no consensus (Fig. 2.6, A to D).

A number of adult structures are derived from the embryonic clefts, pouches, and arches of the pharyngeal region (Fig. 2.7, A to C). They are shown in Table 2.1. Of these, we discuss here the pouches and clefts, the parathyroid glands, the thymus glands, the ultimobranchial bodies, and the thyroid gland. In Chapter 28, "The Thoracic and Abdominal Aorta," we discuss the aortic arches and the development of the vessels.

Parathyroids

The parathyroids arise from the dorsal endoderm of pharyngeal pouches III and IV. As a result of their subsequent positions in the adult, parathyroid III develops into the inferior parathyroids and parathyroid IV into the superior parathyroids.

Figure 2.2. Development of the pharynx. **A**, embryo at 5 mm (fifth week), showing maximum external development of the branchial region. **B**, Human embryo at 4.2 mm sectioned sagitally to show the four arches and four clefts from the inside of the pharynx. The dashed line (A) represents the boundary between ectoderm and endoderm. **C**, Semischematic transverse section through the first pouch and cleft, showing the closing plate of endoderm and ectoderm. Such closing plates rupture to form gill slits in fishes and amphibians. They rarely rupture in human embryos. The buccopharyngeal membrane (stomodeum) is also shown. (**A**, From Davies J. Human developmental anatomy. New York: Ronald Press, 1963; **B** and **C**, from Hamilton WJ, Boyd JD, Mossman HW. Human embryology, 3rd ed. Baltimore: Williams & Wilkins, 1962.)

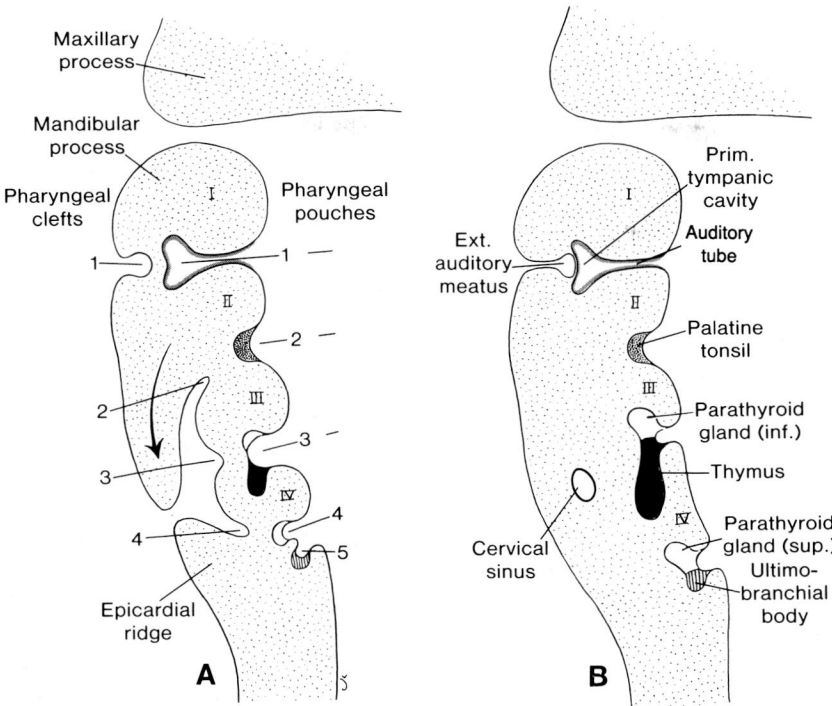

Figure 2.3. **A**, Schematic representation of the development of the pharyngeal clefts and pouches. Note that the second arch grows over the third and fourth arches, thereby burying the second, third, and fourth pharyngeal clefts. **B**, The remnants of the second, third, and fourth pharyngeal clefts form the cervical sinus. Note the structures formed by the various pharyngeal pouches. (From Sadler TW. Langmen's Medical embryology. 6th ed. Baltimore: Williams & Wilkins, 1990:306.)

Parathyroid III differentiates as a solid, spherical, epithelial thickening on the anterior face of the dorsal part of the third pouch just as the pouch becomes constricted off from the pharynx at the end of the sixth week (9 to 12 mm) (24). This detached portion of the pouch contains the parathyroid primordium dorsally and the as yet undifferentiated primordium of the thymus ventrally. It is bound laterally by a portion of cleft IV, which is itself detached from the skin.

The association of parathyroid III with the developing thymus persists until the eighth week (20 mm) or later (Fig. 2.8 *A* to *F*). Usually, parathyroid III descends only as far as the lower border of the thyroid gland and becomes adherent to the thyroid capsule by the end of the seventh week (24). The third pouch parathyroids sometimes descend with the thymus into the mediastinum.

Parathyroid IV, which develops from the dorsal portion of the fourth pouch at about the same time, remains at a higher level because it is not associated with the migrating thymus gland (Fig. 2.9, *A* to *C*).

In both parathyroid primordia—that is, III and IV—the proliferating cells resemble the chief cells of the mature parathyroid. The oxyphil cells appear only several years after birth.

DEFINITION OF NORMAL PATHWAYS OF PARATHYROID TRAVEL

Superior: Descent from the fourth pouch to the posterior surface of the thyroid gland at the vicinity of the cricothyroid junction. Because of the embryonic relation of parathyroid IV to the lateral thyroid anlage, their anatomic closeness in later life is expected.

Inferior: Descent from the third pouch to the posterolateral surface of the inferior thyroid pole. Because of the embryonic relation of parathyroid III to the thymus, it is not surprising that the inferior parathyroid occasionally follows the thymic pathway into the chest.

A picturesque mnemonic based on the embryology of the parathyroids and thymus may assist in remembering the various locations of the parathyroid and thymus glands. Granberg et al. (25) suggest the analogy of traveling from one's home. The gland may not travel far from its origin in the branchial pouch ("the garage") (Fig. 2.10); it may travel along its usual route ("the highway") during ontogenesis; or it may travel a seldom-taken path ("the country road"). The superior parathyroid glands, which arise from pouch IV, almost always take a short highway. They usually are found laterally in the upper portion of the lobe of the thyroid gland. The inferior

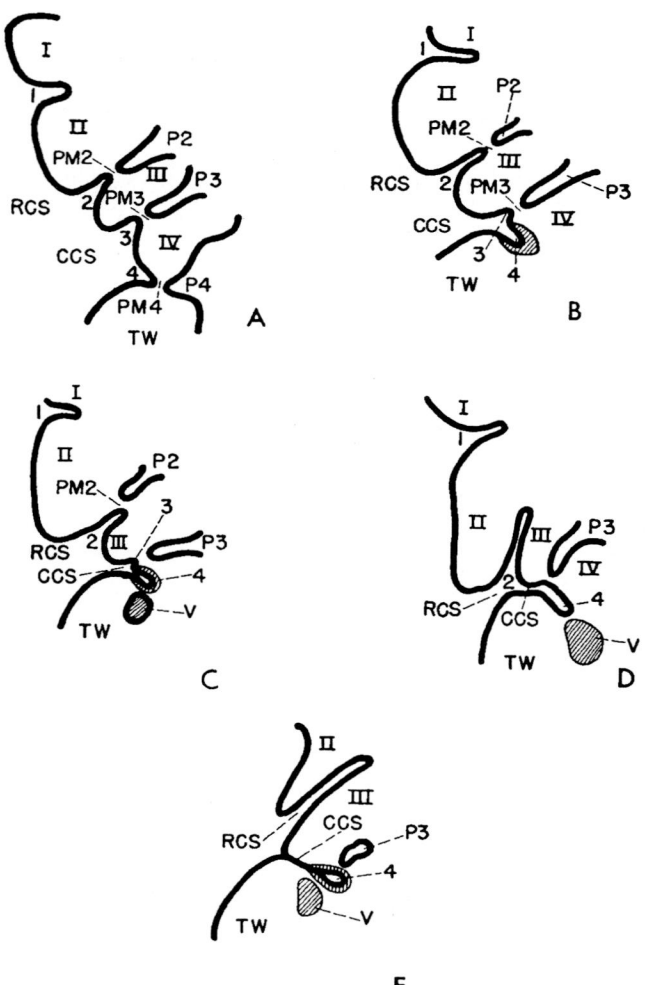

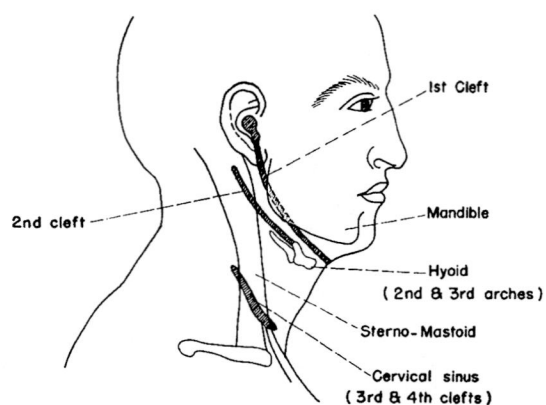

Figure 2.5. Presumptive sites in the adult of the embryonic branchial clefts. (From Proctor B. Lateral vestigial cysts and fistulas of the neck. Laryngoscope 1955;65:355–401; after Keith A. Human embryology and morphology, 6th ed. London: Edward Arnold, 1948.)

Figure 2.4. Fate of the branchial clefts and the cervical sinus in the human embryo. Frontal sections through the left pharyngeal wall: **A**, at 6 mm; **B**, at 8 mm; **C**, at 9 mm; **D**, at 10.5 mm; **E**, at 12 mm. Note that the third arch is never fully covered by the second arch, so that the "cervical sinus" consists of a rostral portion (the second cleft) and a caudal portion (the third and fourth clefts). *I-IV*, Branchial arches; *1-4*, branchial clefts; *P2-P4*, tips of corresponding pharyngeal pouches; *PM2-PM4*, closing plates between clefts and pouches; *TW*, thoracic wall; *RCS*, rostral cervical sinus; *CCS*, caudal cervical sinus; *V*, vagus nerve. (From Proctor B. Lateral vestigial cysts and fistulas of the neck. Laryngoscope 1955;65(6):363; after Garrett FD. Development of the cervical vesicles in man. Anat Rec 1948;100:111.)

caudal pharyngeal pouch complex (9). The amalgam forming the human lateral thyroid anlage has two important anatomic features: (*a*) parathyroid glands IV, which do not descend and are called the "superior" parathyroids, and (*b*) the parafollicular C cells, which produce calcitonin.

Thymus

The thymus arises as a pair of primordia from the ventral portion of the third pharyngeal pouch. At about the 10-mm stage, the third pouch has separated from the pharynx and lies in contact with cleft IV, which has itself lost its connection with the skin. The dorsal portion of the pouch has begun to differentiate into parathyroid III. During the seventh and eighth weeks, the thymus elongates caudally and ventromedially until, by the end of the eighth week, the advancing ends of the primordia meet and fuse at the level of the upper margin of the arch of the aorta (11). The midline fusion involves only the connective tissue of the organ; the parenchyma of the two sides do not fuse (28). The shape and dimension of the adult thymus gland are variable (Fig. 2.11).

Unlike the parathyroids, which are solid from their first appearance, the thymus primordia retain a lumen—the thymopharyngeal duct, which is pinched off from the third pouch—until after medial fusion of its two halves (Fig. 2.9, *A* to *C*).

Norris (29) concluded from his studies that the ectodermal cervical sinus disappeared by uniting with the endodermal primordium, thereby forming the cortical layer of the thymus. He believed that Hassall's corpuscles originated from this ectodermal component. However, neither earlier students of the human thymus (11, 30) nor later ones have agreed with Norris. The cervical sinus, which is essentially the lumina of clefts III and IV, seems to vanish completely.

parathyroid glands, which arise from pouch III, take a longer highway and are most commonly located at the lower border of the thyroid or in the thyrothymic ligament. The inferior glands often travel beyond their usual highway, and their "country road" may lead into the chest. The "highway" for the thymus is into the anterosuperior mediastinum.

The human lateral thyroid anlage is an amalgam from the fourth and fifth branchial pouches (26). The amalgam, which includes the ultimobranchial body (also known as the telopharyngeal body), has been termed the

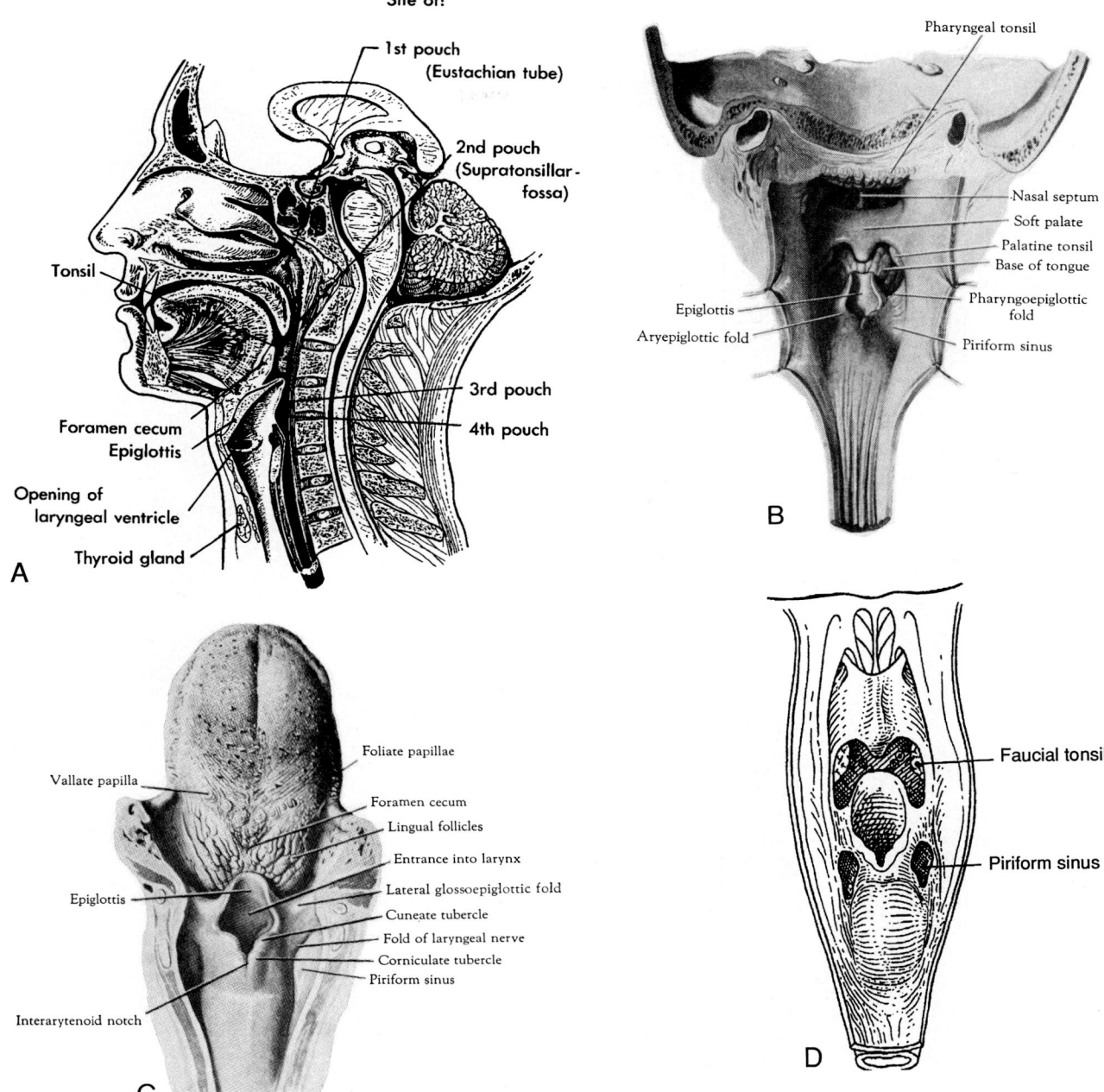

Figure 2.6. **A**, Presumptive sites in the adult of the embryonic pharyngeal pouches. **B**, A child's pharynx, exposed and opened from behind. (The pharyngoepiglottic fold is correctly termed the *lateral glossoepiglottic fold*.) **C**, Tongue and entrance into the larynx. **D**, An adult's pharynx, exposed and opened from behind. (**A**, From Gardiner ED, Gray DJ, O'Rahilly R. Anatomy, 3rd ed. Philadelphia: WB Saunders, 1969; **B** and **C**, from Sicher H, and Tandler J. Anatomie für zahnärtze. Vienna and Berlin: Julius Springer, 1928.)

Present views of the origin and nature of Hassall's corpuscles suggest a quite different explanation. By the ninth week (25 mm), the endodermal epithelial cells are seen to form vesicular outgrowths from the original primordium. These outgrowths, primarily tubular but secondarily compressed and distorted, appear as "corpuscles" in two-dimensional histologic sections (31). This concept of the nature of Hassall's corpuscles was originally proposed in 1903 by Schambacher (32), but it was forgotten until revived by recent interest in the thymus, arising from new concepts of its function (33).

By the end of the ninth week, lymphocytes appear in increasing numbers in the mesenchyme surrounding the endodermal thymus. The thymus primordium acquires a

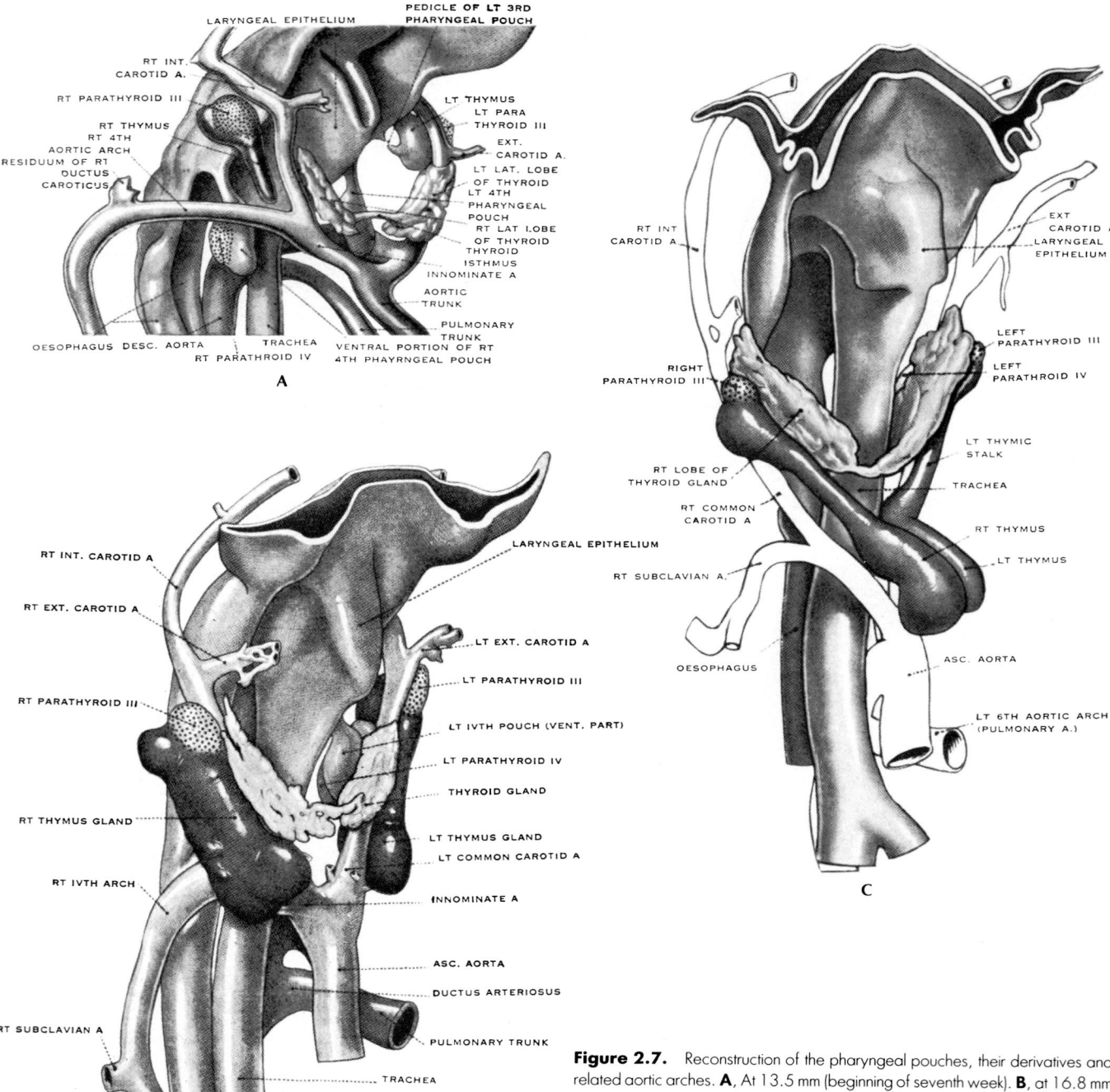

Figure 2.7. Reconstruction of the pharyngeal pouches, their derivatives and related aortic arches. **A**, At 13.5 mm (beginning of seventh week). **B**, at 16.8 mm (beginning of eighth week). **C**, at 23 mm (end of eighth week). (From Hamilton WJ, Boyd JD, Mossman HW. Human embryology, 3rd ed. Baltimore: Williams & Wilkins, 1962; after Weller GL. Development of the thyroid, parathyroid, and thymus glands in man. Contrib Embryol Carnegie Inst Wash 1933;24:141.)

Table 2.1.
Derivatives of Branchial Arches, Clefts, and Pouches

		Dorsal	Ventral	Midline Floor of Pharynx
I	Arch	Incus body	Meckel's cartilage	Body of tongue
	External maxillary artery	Malleus head	Malleus	
	Nerve V	Pinna		
	Cleft	External auditory canal	—	—
	Pouch	Eustachian tube	—	—
		Middle ear cavity		
		Mastoid air cells		
II	Arch	Stapes	Styloid process	Root of tongue
	Stapedial artery		Hyoid (lesser horn and part of body)	Foramen cecum
	Nerves VII and VIII			Thyroid gland's median anlage
	Pouch	Palatine tonsil	—	—
		Supratonsilar fossa		
III	Arch	—	Hyoid (greater horn and part of body)	—
	Internal carotid artery		Part of epiglottis	
	Nerve IX			
	Pouch	Inferior parathyroid	Thymus	—
		Pyriform fossa		
IV	Arch	—	Thyroid cartilage	—
	Arch of aorta (L)		Cuneiform cartilage	
	Part of subclavian artery (R)		Part of epiglottis	—
	Nerve X			
	Pouch	Superior parathyroid (lateral anlage of thyroid gland)	Thymus (inconstant)	—
V	Arch		—	—
	Pouch	Ultimobranchial body (lateral anlage of thyroid gland)	—	—
VI	Arch		Cricoid	—
	Pulmonary artery		Arytenoid	
	Ductus arteriosus (L)		Corniculate cartilage	
	Nerve X (recurrent laryngeal)			

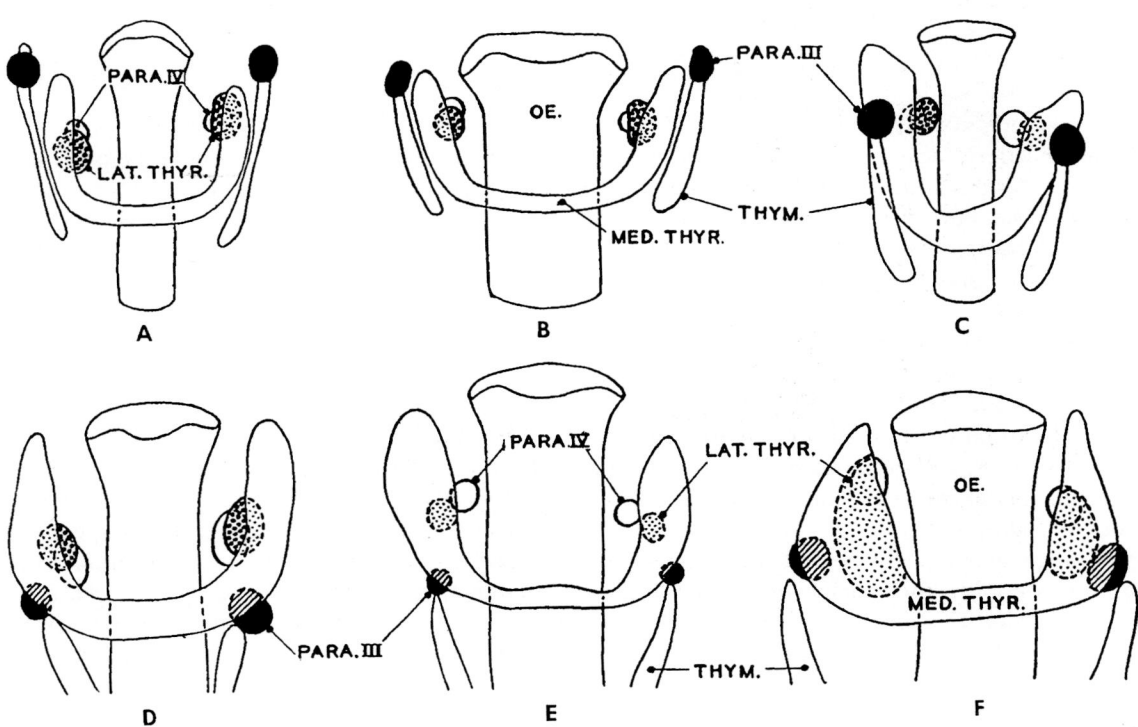

Figure 2.8. The descent of the thymus and parathyroid III in relation to the thyroid gland and parathyroid IV in six human embryos. Parathyroid III thus becomes the "inferior parathyroid." Note that the ultimobranchial body is labeled "lateral thyroid" in these drawings. **A,** Human embryo at 15 mm; **B,** at 16 mm; **C,** at 17 mm; **D,** at 16 mm; **E,** at 20 mm, **F,** at 24 mm. In **D, E,** and **F** parathyroid III has reached its definitive position. (From Norris EH. Parathyroid glands and lateral thyroid in man: their morphogenesis, histogenesis, topographic anatomy and prenatal growth. Contrib Embryol Carnegie Inst Wash 1937;26:247–294.)

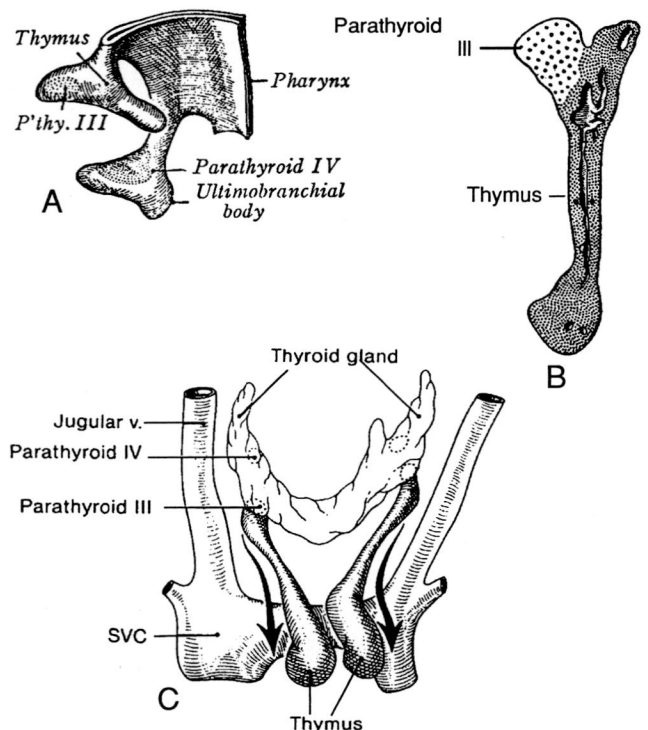

Figure 2.9. **A**, The third and fourth pharyngeal pouches at 10 mm. **B**, The derivatives of the third pouch, showing the lumen of the thymopharyngeal duct. **C**, The descent of the thymus at the end of the second month. The cranial ends of the thymus will disappear; the descending caudal ends will form the definitive thymus. Note that parathyroid III, attached to the thymus, has descended to a site below that of parathyroid IV. *SCV*, superior vena cava. (**A** and **B**, From Arey LB. Developmental anatomy, 7th ed. Philadelphia: WB Saunders, 1965:239; **C**, modified from Arey LB. Developmental anatomy, 6th ed. Philadelphia: WB Saunders, 1954:235.)

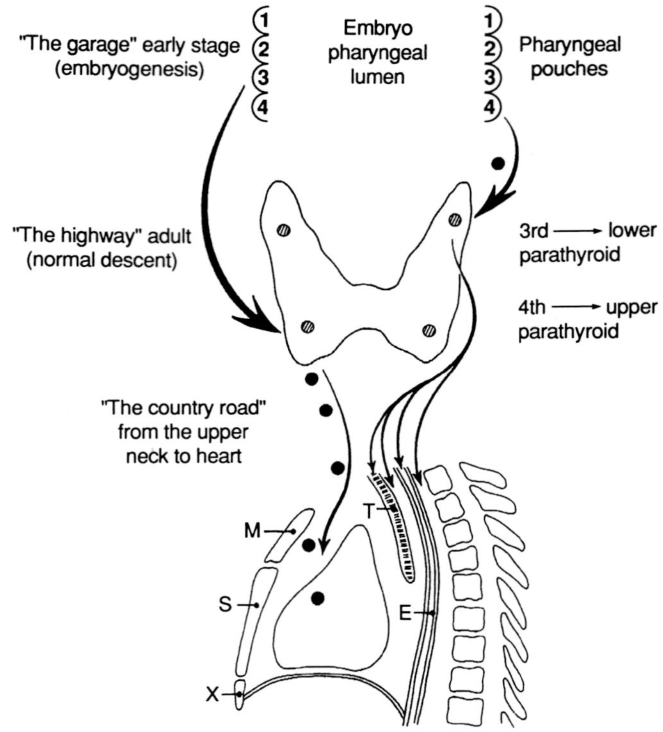

Figure 2.10. Embryogenesis, descent, and localization of the parathyroid glands. The gland may be found close to its origin in the pharyngeal pouch (*"the garage"*) along the line of descent (*"the highway"*), or far down in the thymus. The most common location is at the lower border of the thyroid or in the thyrothymic ligament. The thymus is like an index finger pointing to the gland. (Adapted from Granberg PL, Cedermark B, Farnebo LO, Hamberger B, Werner S: Parathyroid tumors. In: Hickey RC, ed. Current problems in cancer. Chicago, Yearbook Medical, 1985:IX(11):18.)

scalloped border where mesenchyme with blood vessels grows inward, whereas the endodermal component grows outward. The endodermal tissue, in the form of compressed tubules, thus becomes surrounded by accumulations of lymphocytes, which form the thymic lobules.

The lymphocytes are of mesenchymal origin. Precursor stem cells are attracted from the circulation into the microenvironment of the thymus, and the thymus is filled with an increasing number of T-cell precursors and their offspring. The number of T lymphocytes increases during gestation. Neonates delivered prematurely have subnormal numbers of T lymphocytes.

On morphologic grounds it is possible to see a similarity between the adenoids, the faucial tonsils, the lingual tonsils, and the thymus. In a sense, the thymus can be considered part of Waldeyer's ring of lymphoid tissue and called the "mediastinal tonsil." The embryologist notes, of course, that the origin of each of these structures involves the branchial endoderm.

Papiernik (34) and Haynes (35) believe that the mature thymus is in situ by the 15th or 20th gestational week, therefore being the first of the lymphoid organs to develop. Bockman and Kirby (36) give evidence that the neural crest may act as an organizer of an interaction between the primordium of the epithelium and the invading mesenchyme.

Caudal Pharyngeal Pouch Complex

Because seven gill slits are present in primitive vertebrates (elasmobranchs, of which sharks are examples), the earlier embryologists, under the influence of Müller and Haeckel's views of phylogenetic recapitulation, searched mammalian embryos for vestiges of clefts and pouches behind the four that are clearly demarcated. These caudal pharyngeal structures are small, transient, inconstant, and variable from one mammalian species to another; hence, our knowledge of the epithelial derivatives of pouches IV and V remains almost as limited as it was a

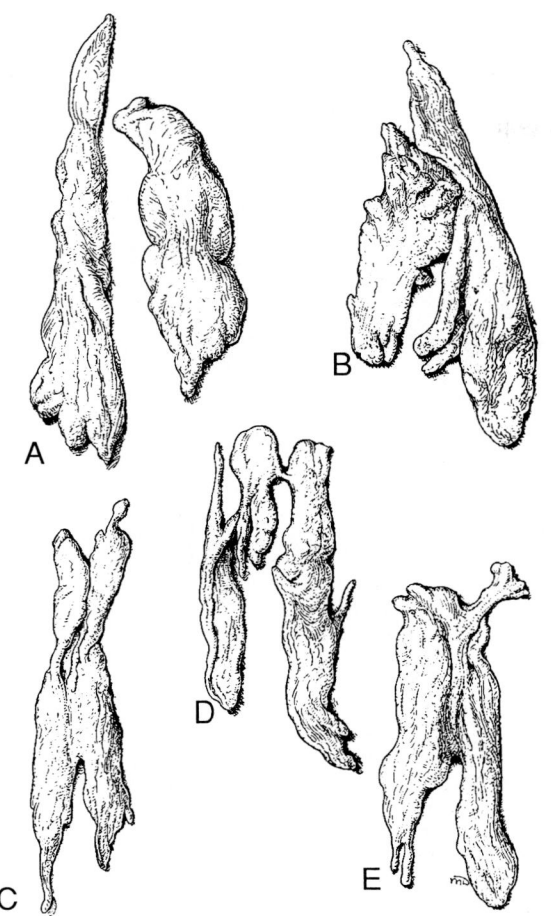

Figure 2.11. Variations in form and dimension of the adult thymus. The two lobes may be separate or united only by connective tissues. (From Anson BJ. An atlas of human anatomy, 2nd ed. Philadelphia: WB Saunders, 1963:258.)

plex'' (9), a move for which many subsequent writers have been grateful.

The ventral portion of pouch IV, like that of pouch III, can produce thymus tissue. Studying infants, Ellis and Knight (37) found that some superior parathyroid glands include thymus histologically: 4:55 left superior parathyroids; 8:55 right superior parathyroids. Such accessory thymus tissue probably does not persist into maturity.

The epithelial body formed by the most caudal pouches is the so-called ultimobranchial or telopharyngeal gland. In humans, this gland forms from derivatives of the ventral portion of pouches IV and V (Fig. 2.12). In nonmammalian vertebrates, the ultimobranchial glands remain separate and discrete from the thyroid gland.

In humans, the ultimobranchial body (caudal pharyngeal pouch complex), in addition to joining parathyroid IV, fuses and eventually becomes lost in the developing thyroid gland. (Fig. 2.12). Because of this union, in 1883,

Born introduced the term *lateral thyroid primordia* for these products of pouches IV and V (5).

The implications of the term *lateral thyroid primordia* have produced much debate. The great embryologist His once believed in lateral thyroid primordia (4), but later altered his view (38). Weller (11) thought as much as 33% of the thyroid originated from the ultimobranchial bodies (Fig. 2.12). Norris (24) considered their contribution to be about 16%. Kingsbury (13, 14) believed that the ultimobranchial bodies joined the thyroid, degenerated, and contributed nothing. Rogers (39) suggested that the lateral contributions from pouches IV and V develop into thyroid follicles by induction of the median thyroid, if they are closely associated with it, and into thymus tissue (thymus IV), if they are not so associated. Ramsay (125) showed by in vitro studies of mouse embryos that the ultimobranchial bodies do not become thyroid tissue in the absence of the median thyroid.

The ultimobranchial bodies have been shown to be responsible for the production of the calcium-regulating hormone, calcitonin (41, 42). In the mammal, the parafollicular C cells of the thyroid have been shown to produce calcitonin (43, 44).

There is evidence in both humans and other vertebrates that the ectodermal neural crest contributes to the development of the ultimobranchial gland (36, 45).

Thyroid Gland

The thyroid gland develops from two anlages: the larger median anlage, and the paired smaller lateral anlages. The median anlage, recognizable by the end of the third week, forms the bulk of the thyroid gland (Fig. 2.13). It presents histologically as an epithelial thickening in the ventral pharyngeal wall, in an area known as the tuberculum impar, at the level of the second branchial arch. Its first appearance is (variably) as a shallow depression with thickened epithelium, as a single diverticulum, or as a paired diverticulum.

Immediately after its appearance, the developing thyroid comes into contact with the aortic sac of the developing heart, which lies just beneath the pharynx (Fig. 2.14). Division into lateral lobes, if not present from the beginning, occurs so early that it is impossible to say whether the human thyroid arises singly or as a paired organ (11) (Fig. 2.15). Although the median stalk usually has a lumen, the thyroglossal duct, it does not extend into the lateral lobes.

Elongation of the embryo, together with the rostral growth of the tongue and pharynx, leaves the thyroid gland caudal to its point of origin. In the adult tongue, the origin of the median thyroid anlage is marked by the foramen cecum. Early in the fifth week, the attenuated

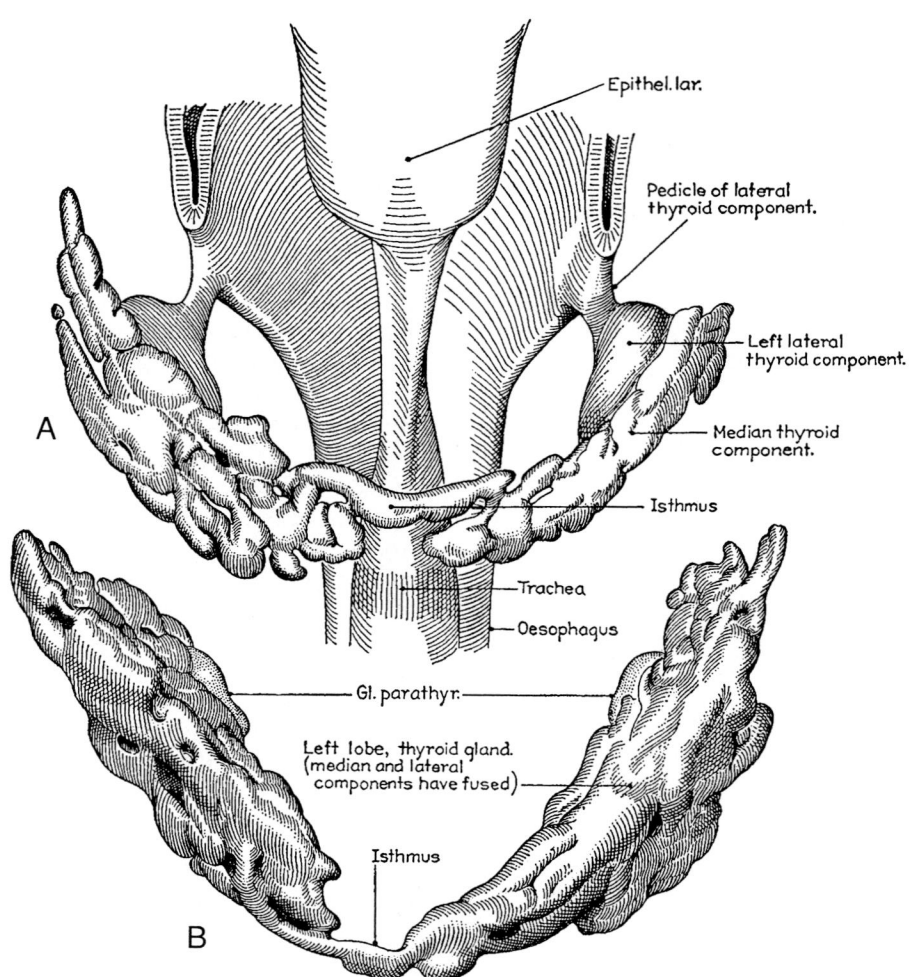

Figure 2.12. **A**, The relationship of the ultimobranchial bodies to the developing thyroid gland at 16 mm. **B**, At 23 mm. The ultimobranchial bodies are labeled "lateral thyroid component" in keeping with Weller's views. (From Weller GL. Development of the thyroid, parathyroid, and thymus glands in man. Contrib Embryol Carnegie Inst Wash 1933;24:105.)

duct loses its lumen and shortly afterwards breaks into fragments (16, 46).

The anlage of the hyoid bone appears adjacent to the thyroglossal duct or its remnants. Usually the thyroglossal duct is just anteroventral to the hyoid, but sometimes the duct (or its remnants) passes through or just dorsal to the hyoid. The rostral and caudal ends of the degenerating thyroglossal duct may completely regress or may persist as a cord. Most often, the rostral portion forms a short diverticulum at the foramen cecum, and the caudal remnant becomes a thickened cord that develops into thyroid tissue, manifesting as the pyramidal lobe of the thyroid gland (Fig. 2.16). Two pyramidal lobes may be present, suggesting that the primordium was paired. The foramen cecum is present in about two-thirds of individuals and is a 2- to 3-mm deep diverticulum in about one-sixth of individuals. A pyramidal lobe is present in about half of individuals.

The developing thyroid gland soon becomes an irregular, plate-like mass ventral to the trachea. Through lateral growth, two wings of tissue come to lie parallel and ventromedial to the elongating thymus glands. The wings are attached to each other across the midline by the isthmus, to which the remains of the thyroglossal duct may attach as the pyramidal lobe. By the seventh week, the tips of the lateral lobes extend to the parathyroid primordia of the third pouch (Fig. 2.12).

Until the eighth week, the thyroid tissue consists of plates of epithelial cells. The plates are of varying thickness and irregularly arranged, with occasional thin spots and fenestrae. The first follicles form from the epithelial plates at the beginning of the second month (24 mm) (16), and by the third month the plates have been converted entirely into follicles. Subsequent follicle formation takes place by budding or division of these primary follicles.

Follicle formation is preceded by the appearance of an

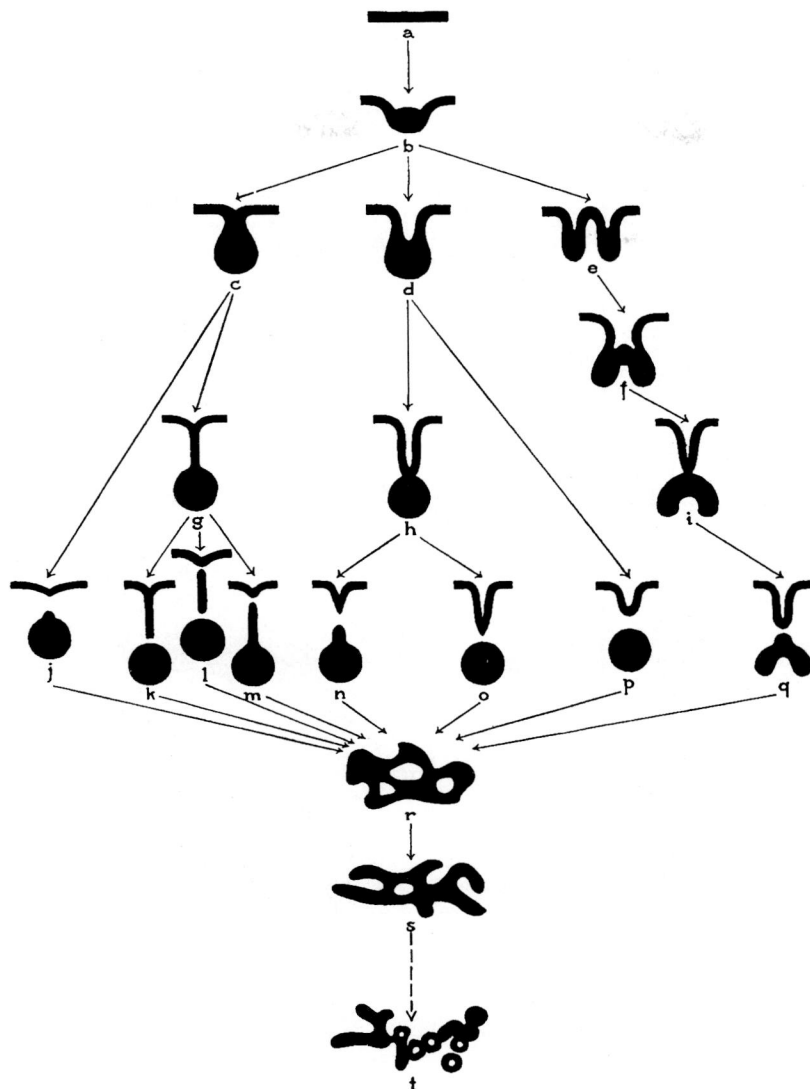

Figure 2.13. Variations in the early development stages of the thyroid gland. All seem to produce a normal adult gland. (From Norris EH. The early morphogenesis of the human thyroid gland. Am J Anat 1918;24:4.)

intracellular PAS-positive material (47). Bierring and Shepard (48) have described intracellular canaliculi with microvilli, which open at the apex and which are in contact with similar structures in adjacent cells. These spaces become confluent and form the lumen of the developing follicles. Desmosomes connect the cells to keep the follicular contents from escaping. During the 11th and 12th weeks, all the stages of follicle formation may be observed at the same time.

The greatest increase in follicle number takes place in the fourth month; the later gain in size of the thyroid is by an increase in the size of existing follicles. Colloid appears in the follicles during the 11th week. Evidence of thyroxine comes with the appearance of colloid.

Studies on fetal rodents (49, 50) indicate that iodine

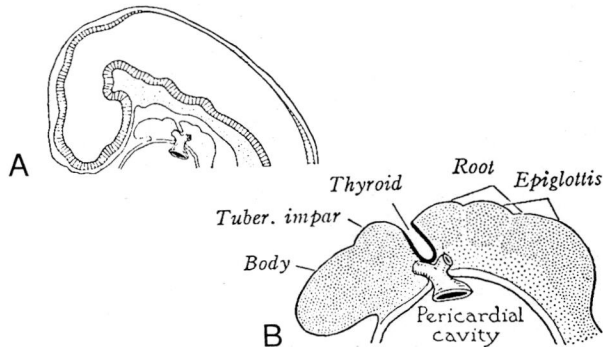

Figure 2.14. The origin of the thyroid primordium from the floor of the pharynx, showing its relationship to the tongue, aorta and pericardium (fourth week). (From Arey LB. Developmental anatomy, 7th ed. Philadelphia: WB Saunders, 1965:233.)

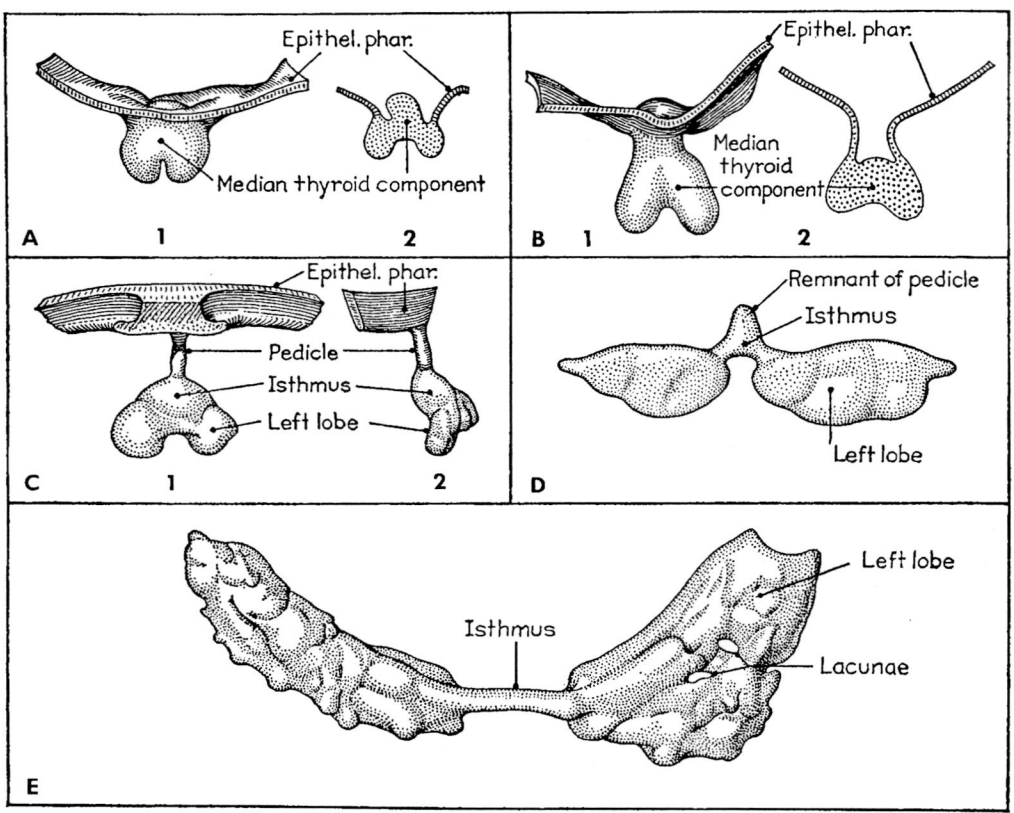

Figure 2.15. Stages in the development of the thyroid gland. **A.1**, Thyroid primordium and pharyngeal epithelium of a 4.5-mm human embryo. **A.2**, section through the same structure, showing raised central portion. **B.1**, Thyroid primordium of a 6.5-mm embryo. **B.2**, section through same structure. **C.1**, Thyroid primordium of an 8.2-mm embryo, beginning to descend. **C.2**, Lateral view of same structure. **D**, Thyroid primordium of an 11-mm embryo. The connection with the pharynx is broken, and the lobes are beginning to grow laterad. **E**, Thyroid gland of a 13.5-mm embryo. The lobes are thin sheets curving around the carotid arteries. Several lacunae are present in the sheets, which are not to be confused with follicles. (From Weller GL. Development of the thyroid, parathyroid, and thymus glands in man. Contrib Embryol Carnegie Inst Wash 1933;24:101.)

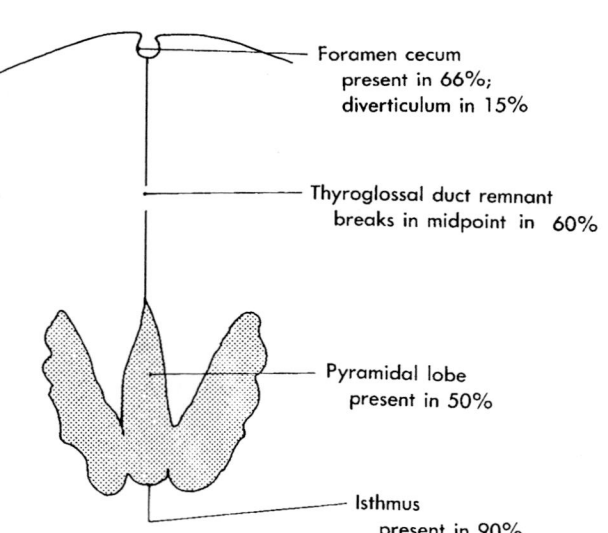

Figure 2.16. Normal vestiges of thyroid development. Presence or absence of these is not of clinical significance.

accumulation in the form of monoiodotyrosine and diiodotyrosine begins before follicle formation. In the chick, iodine concentration also is demonstrable at the very beginning of colloid accumulation (i.e., before follicle formation) (51).

LiVolsi (52) divides the histologic differentiation of the human fetal thyroid into three stages:

1. Precolloid (7 to 13 weeks)
2. Colloid (13 to 14 weeks)
3. Follicular (after 14 weeks)

The final form of the thyroid gland is not constant (Fig. 2.17). Variations of the pyramidal lobe have already been mentioned. The isthmus is absent in about 10% of individuals examined, and the left or right lobe may be small or completely absent. Thyroidal hemiagenesis, in which one of the lobes fails to develop, is rare.

The lateral thyroid anlage, which originates from the ventral portion of the fourth pharyngeal pouch, becomes attached to the posterior surface of the thyroid during the fifth week (11) (Fig. 2.12). Weller (11), Kingsbury

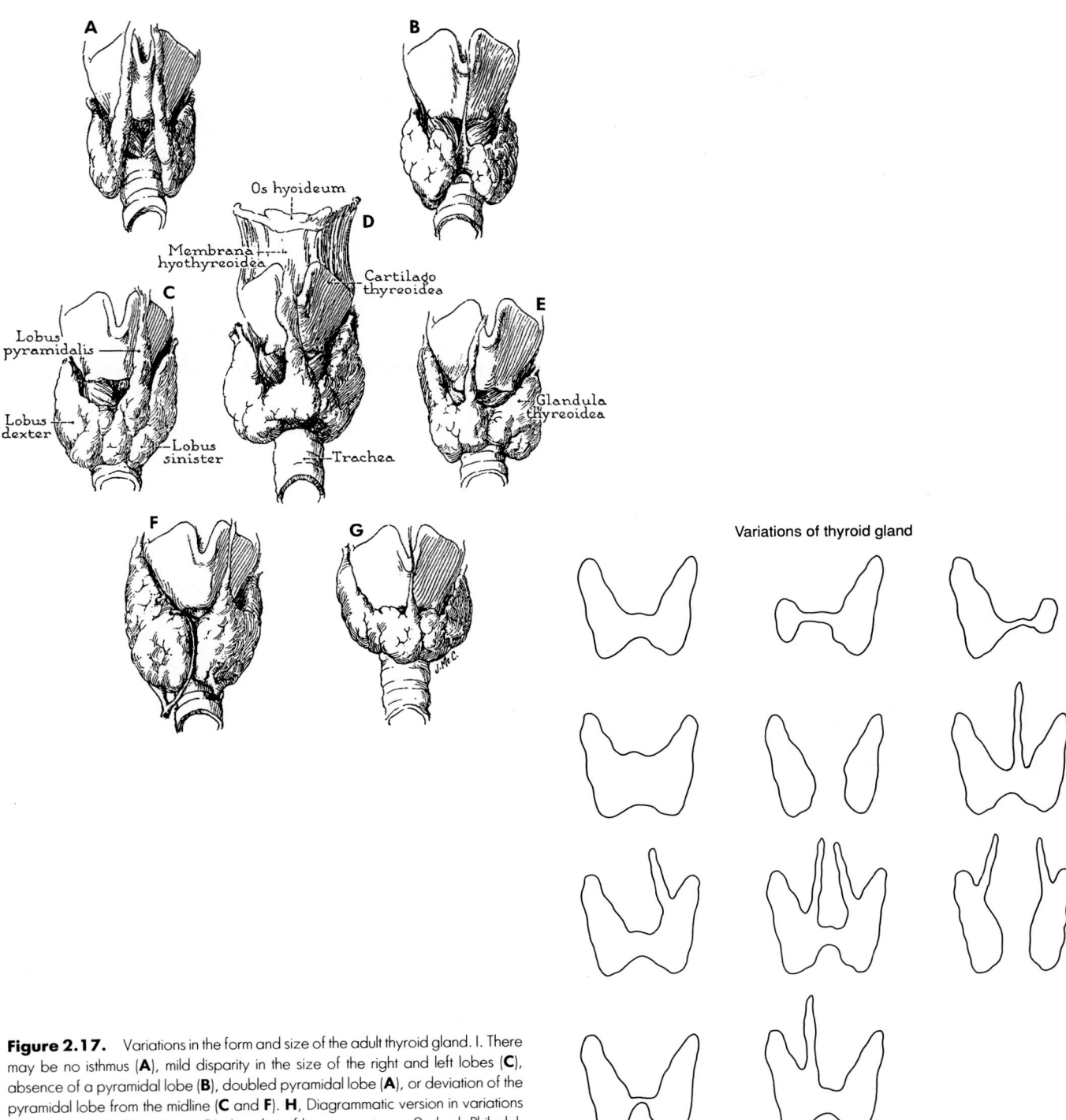

Figure 2.17. Variations in the form and size of the adult thyroid gland. I. There may be no isthmus (**A**), mild disparity in the size of the right and left lobes (**C**), absence of a pyramidal lobe (**B**), doubled pyramidal lobe (**A**), or deviation of the pyramidal lobe from the midline (**C** and **F**). **H**, Diagrammatic version in variations of form. **A** to **G**, (From Anson RJ. An atlas of human anatomy, 2nd ed. Philadelphia: WB Saunders, 1963.)

(13), and Norris (24), as well as Toran-Allerand (53), estimate that the lateral thyroid anlage contributes perhaps 1 to 30% to the thyroid weight. The causes of the fusion of the median and lateral anlages are unknown (13, 54).

Sugiyama (26) speculates that the migration of the ultimobranchial body controls the growth of the median anlage, or that growth of the median anlage laterally and caudally inhibits future expansion of the ultimobranchial body. The lateral thyroid anlage provides the parafollicular C cells that produce calcitonin (see "Lateral Aberrant Thyroid Tissue" later in this chapter).

In summary, remember:

1. The inferior parathyroids develop from the epithelium of the dorsal wing of the third pharyngeal pouch.
2. The superior parathyroids develop from the epithelium of the dorsal wing of the fourth pharyngeal pouch.
3. The thymus develops from the epithelium of the ventral wing of the third pharyngeal pouch.
4. A small part of the thymus perhaps also develops from the epithelium of the ventral wing of the fourth pharyngeal pouch.
5. The ultimobranchial body is the product of the ventral portion of the fourth pharyngeal pouch as well as, perhaps, the product of the fifth pharyngeal pouch. In humans, the fifth pouch and the dorsal portion of the fourth pouch are best termed the "caudal pharyngeal pouch complex."
6. The thyroid gland is formed by the median thyroid anlage and from the lateral thyroid anlage (the fourth and fifth branchial pouch complex) right and left, which together form the ultimobranchial body that produces the C (parafollicular) cells.

Critical Events in Development

Deviations from normal critical events in development (Table 2.2) during these times may result in an unde-

Table 2.2.
Critical Events in Human Pharyngeal Development

Event in Human Pharyngeal Development	Gestational Age (Weeks)
Descent of the median thyroid anlage	4
Obliteration/fragmentation of thyroglossal duct	5
Obliteration of branchial clefts and pouches	6–7
Fusion of median and lateral thyroid anlages	7
Fusion of right/left thymus primordia	8

scended or partially descended thyroid, branchial sinuses or cysts, or fistulae, and nontypical locations for the parathyroid and thymus glands.

ANOMALIES OF THE LATERAL BRANCHIAL APPARATUS

Cystic and Fistular Remnants of the Branchial Apparatus

ANATOMY

In addition to the normal derivatives left behind by the transitory branchial apparatus of the embryo, occasionally epithelium-lined cysts, sinuses, and fistulae result (Fig. 2.18) (Table 2.3). The specific origin of these structures has received great attention, yet much is unknown and much more is still speculative. In this discussion of branchial remnants, we try to distinguish among those items that seem to be well understood, unknown, and speculative.

First Cleft and Pouch Defects.

Congenital Auricular Pits. There is no consensus that these minute pits, sinuses, and cysts in the skin, near the anterior border of the ascending limb of the helix, represent branchial defects. Since the mid–1800s they have

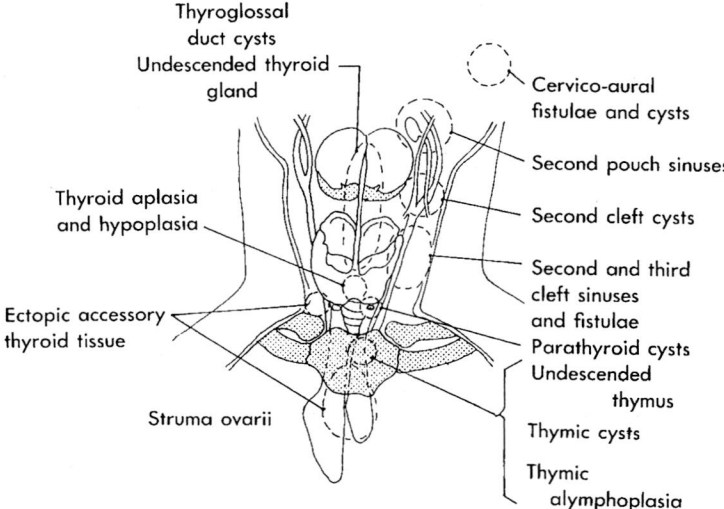

Figure 2.18. Sites of developmental anomalies of the pharynx and its derivatives.

Table 2.3.
Anomalies of the Pharynx and Its Derivatives

Anomaly	Origin of Defect	First Appearance	Sex Chiefly Affected	Relative Frequency	Remarks
Congenital auricular pits	3rd month	Any age	Equal	Very common	Said to show a familial tendency
Cervicoaural fistulae, sinuses and cysts (1st cleft defects)	7th or 8th week	Childhood	Equal	Rare	Anatomically related to the facial nerve
2nd cleft and pouch defects	6th or 7th week	Childhood	Equal	Uncommon	Said to show a familial tendency
Cysts of the parathyroid glands	Possibly 7th week	Adulthood	Female	Very rare	May not be of embryonic origin
Thymic aplasia	Unknown	Shortly after birth	Equal	Very rare	Lobdell-DiGeorge anomaly
Cysts of the thymus	Possibly 7th week	Childhood or later	Unknown	Very rare	May not be of embryonic origin
Undescended thymus	8th to 9th week	Infancy or childhood	Female	Very rare	
Agenesis, aplasia and hypoplasia of the thyroid	Unknown	Infancy	Female	Rare	
Undescended (lingual) and partially descended thyroid	3rd to 4th week	After puberty	Female	Rare to very rare	
Thyroglossal duct cysts	5th week	Childhood or later	Male	Common	Not congenital
Lateral accessory thyroid	Before 7th week	Adulthood	Female	Rare	Many prove to be metastatic
Inferior accessory thyroid	3rd week	Late adulthood	Female	Uncommon	Acquired form more common
Intratracheal thyroid	3rd week	Adulthood	Female	Rare	
Struma ovarii	Unknown	Adulthood	Female only	Rare	Unrelated to development of normal thyroid

been considered to be related to the first branchial cleft, representing ectodermal folds sequestered during fusion of the six hillocks that form the pinna (Fig. 2.19). Although His, the great German embryologist of the nineteenth century, considered the first and second arches to contribute equally to the hillocks, the present consensus is that the tragus comes from the first arch and the remainder of the pinna from the second arch. All of the muscles of the pinna—both those that connect it to the skull and the scalp and those that extend from one part of the pinna to another part—are innervated by the facial nerve, which is the nerve of the second branchial arch. It should be noted that the hillocks may be transitory and incidental, rather than fundamental to the formation of the pinna. Reptiles, avians, and amphibians, none of which develop distinct pinnae, have the six embryonic hillocks (55).

Once considered rare, preauricular pits were found in 0.84% of 53,257 newborns in a multiinstitutional multiracial study in the United States. If syndrome cases are excluded, preauricular pits are about 40 times more common than branchial cleft sinus. A slight familial tendency was noted: 6.26% of the newborns with a preauricular sinus had an affected first- or second-degree relative. The preauricular pits were bilateral in 46% of familial cases, but only 29% of isolated cases. Of unilateral preauricular pits in newborns, 55% were on the right side and 45%

were on the left side. The unilateral distribution (left versus right) was independent of case type (isolated or familial). The male/female ratio was 111:100. The occurrence in blacks was more than four times that of whites (56).

Preauricular pits are lined with skin and may extend deeply, making a tortuous and branching course. Occasionally these lesions communicate, either primarily or after infection, with the external auditory canal. Preauricular pits are typically asymptomatic and require no treatment, unless they become infected. In such cases, extirpation of the entire sinus or cyst may be necessary. Infection should be cleared before operation.

Cervicoaural, Fistulae, Sinuses, and Cysts. The dorsal end of the first branchial cleft has been thought to remain open, becoming the external auditory canal. This statement is correct as regards the cartilaginous portion of the external auditory canal. The early embryonic intimate relation of the first branchial cleft with the first branchial pouch (Fig. 2.3, *B*) is transient. About the eighth week, mesenchymal proliferation closes the medial portion of the first branchial cleft. At about the 28th week of development, a lumen forms in this epithelial strand. Thus the canal that persists after about the seventh week is the anlage of the cartilaginous canal, and the recanalized epithelial strand becomes the bony ear canal (55).

There seem to be two types of defects involving the first branchial cleft (57). Each type is rare. Such defects

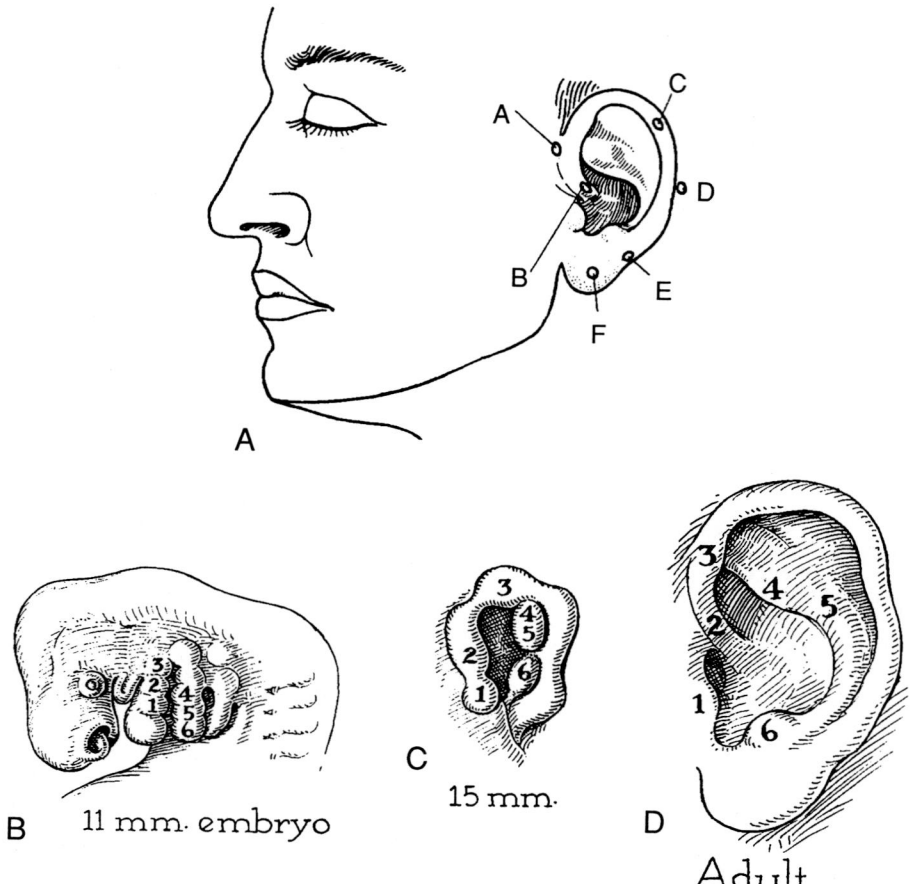

Figure 2.19. **A**, Sites of congenital auricular pits. Sites *B–F* are rare. **B** to **D**, Development of the external ear from the first (mandibular) and second (hyoid) branchial arches surrounding the first branchial cleft. Failure of complete fusion of any adjacent tubercles may result in an epithelium-lined sinus. (**A**, From Aird I. Ear-pit (congenital aural and preauricular fistula). Edinb Med J 1946;53(9):499; after

Congdon ED et al. Human congenital auricular and juxta-auricular fossae, sinuses and scars (including so-called aural and auricular fistulae) and bearing of their anatomy upon the ones of their genesis. Am J Anat 1932;51:439–463; **B** to **D**, from Anson BJ. An atlas of human anatomy, 2nd ed. Philadelphia: WB Saunders, 1963:66.)

are lined by skin and are usually diagnosed after infection. The first type, which may be considered a defect of the dorsal end of the cleft, manifests as a cyst, sinus, or fistulous tract medial to the conchal cartilage, extending into the retroaural crease and routing parallel to the cartilaginous ear canal (Fig. 2.20, *A*).

The other type, which may be considered a defect of the ventral end of the first branchial cleft, manifests as a cyst, sinus, or fistula inferior to the cartilaginous external ear canal and intimately located within the substance of the parotid gland. The lesion variably routes medial or lateral to the facial nerve and may split the trunk of the facial nerve (57) (Fig. 2.20, *B*). Remember that the newborn baby has no mastoid process, and the stylomastoid foramen is subcutaneous. Therefore the facial nerve is very superficial.

Treatment consists of complete excision of the epithelial walls of the fistula, cyst, or sinus. It is important to

note that, for each type of cervicoaural defect, the relationship to the facial nerve cannot be predicted preoperatively. Especially in cases of infection, identification of the facial nerve outside the stylomastoid foramen may be difficult. In some of these cases, the facial nerve is best found within the mastoid, then followed out the stylomastoid foramen, and then followed as it relates to the lesion.

First Pouch Defects. The ventral portion of the first branchial pouch, which blends with the dorsal portion of the second pouch, very rarely manifests anomaly. Wilson (58) reported a case of apparent persistence of the pouch: "The opening of the sinus was found to be a slit of about ½ inch in length just below and behind the eustachian cushion." At least 24 cases of branchiogenic nasopharyngeal cyst have been reported (59, 60).

The dorsal portion of the first branchial pouch, which persists as the eustachian tube, commonly manifests a

FIRST CLEFT
TYPE I SCHEMATIC

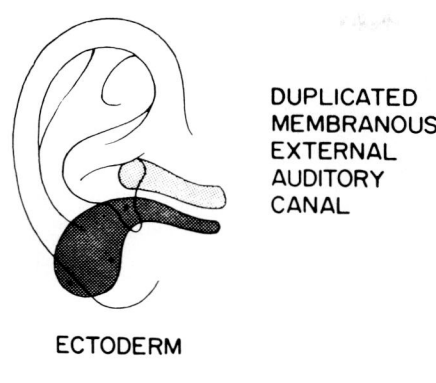

DUPLICATED
MEMBRANOUS
EXTERNAL
AUDITORY
CANAL

ECTODERM

A

FIRST CLEFT
TYPE II SCHEMATIC

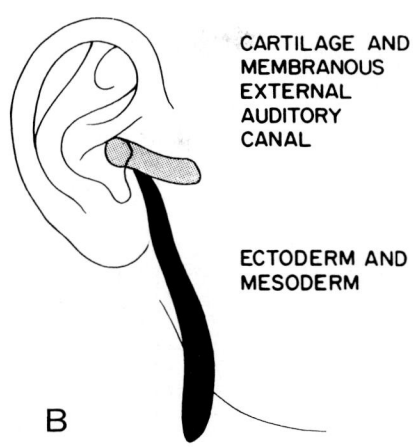

CARTILAGE AND
MEMBRANOUS
EXTERNAL
AUDITORY
CANAL

ECTODERM AND
MESODERM

B

Figure 2.20. **A**, This schematic illustration denotes a type I duplication of the membranous external auditory canal. There may be a slight cartilage tag deformity of the conchal or tragal cartilages. This lesion is principally a duplication anomaly of the membranous external auditory canal. The main cystic mass of the anomaly may be placed anterior and inferior to the ear lobe associated with the parotid gland. Note the three dots indicating possible sinus drainage areas. The external auditory canal and middle ear are normal. **B**, Type II duplication anomalies are depicted schematically. There may be a sinus stoma in the external membranous auditory canal and the upper neck as well. This may be a rather massive lesion. The middle ear is normal. It may be located medially or lateral to the facial nerve or split its main trunk. (From Work WP: Newer concepts of first branchial cleft defects. Laryngoscope 1972;82(9):1583.)

bilateral anomaly. Eustachian tubes that are short in length and have large caliber (at bougie measurement) are associated with otitis media (61).

Second Cleft and Pouch Defects.

Complete Fistulae. Essentially all complete branchial fistulae derive from the ventral portion of the second branchial cleft and pouch. They are rare. Typically, the external opening is in the lower third of the neck on the line of the anterior border of the sternocleidomastoid muscle (Fig. 2.5). The cutaneous orifice may be pigmented. If infection of a bulbous portion of the tract requires incision and drainage, there may be an additional cutaneous opening higher in the neck.

The fistula passes through the subcutaneous tissue and routes caudal to the caudal extent of the platysma muscle and through the deep fascia to reach the carotid sheath. Above the hyoid, the tract turns medially, beneath the stylohyoid and the posterior belly of the digastric muscle. It passes in front of (i.e., over) the hypoglossal nerve and between the bifurcation of the external and internal carotid arteries. It enters the pharynx as a slit on the anterior face of the cephalad half of the posterior pillar of the faucial tonsil (Fig. 2.21, *A* and *B*). Occasionally, the pharyngeal opening is into the tonsil itself.

Sinuses Opening into the Pharynx. These are quite rarely identified. Just as described for a complete fistula of the second branchial pouch-cleft, these open onto the anterior face of the upper half of the posterior tonsil pillar or into the tonsil itself. The sinuses are lined by ciliated epithelium, and the wall typically contains lymphoid tissue.

Sinuses Opening through the Skin of the Neck. External sinus tracts are rare and cannot be assigned to a specific branchial cleft unless traced relative to the structures within the neck. They usually occur along the anterior border of the sternocleidomastoid muscle in the caudal third of the neck and terminate in a cystic dilation. Both stratified squamous and ciliated epithelium may be present.

Many external sinuses are not congenital but result from previous incision of an infected branchial cyst.

Cysts. The second pouch cyst may present clinically in the pharynx as bulging in the posterior pillar of the faucial tonsil.

Most of the cysts encountered along the second pouch-cleft occur in the neck. They are lined by stratified squamous epithelium and are remnants of the second cleft. The cyst may extend between the external and internal carotid arteries (62) (Fig. 2.22).

Because the dorsal portion of pouch II blends with the ventral portion of pouch I, there is controversy about which pouch contributes to branchiogenic nasopharyngeal cysts (see the discussion of first pouch defects).

Third Cleft and Pouch Defects.

A complete fistula of the third pouch and cleft has yet to be reported. Such a fistula would pass below the glossopharyngeal nerve, over the superior laryngeal nerve, and

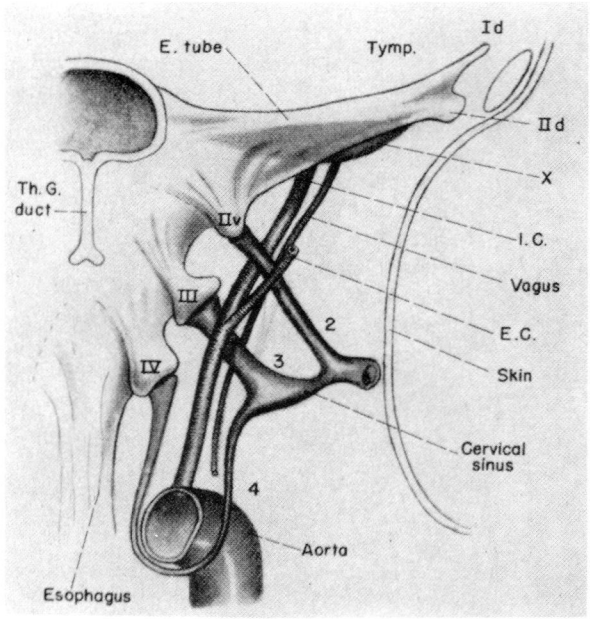

A

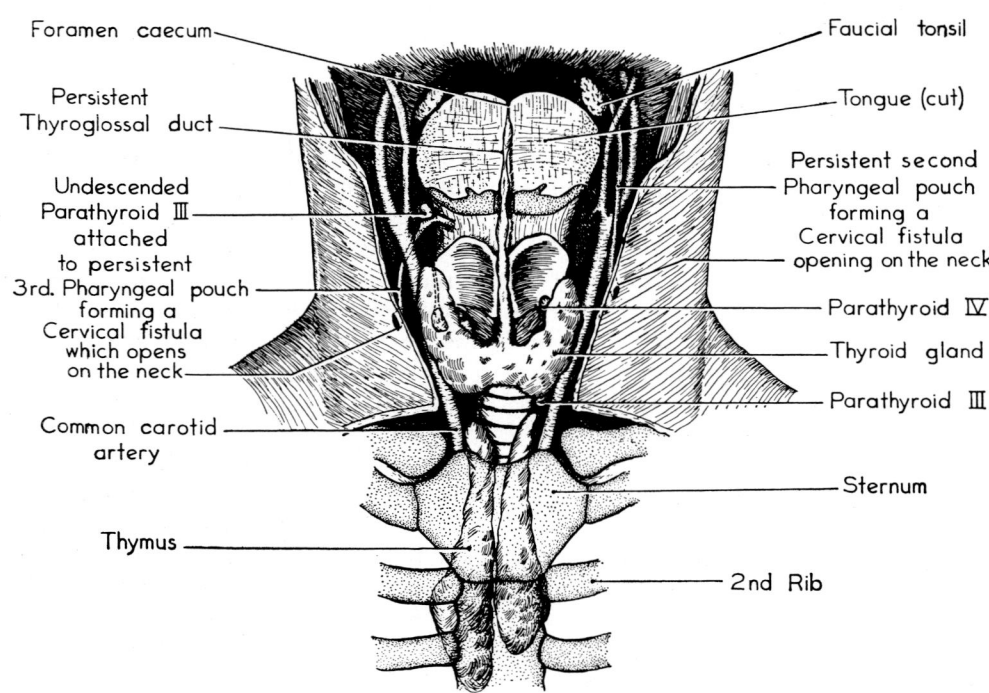

B

Figure 2.21. **A**, Schematic diagram of vestigial remains of branchical pouches and clefts and their relationships to main arteries and nerves. **B**, Sites of fistulous tracts of the second and third branchial clefts in the adult neck. In this figure, the jaw has been removed and the root of the tongue transected at the level of the foramen cecum. An undescended parathyroid III and a persistent thyroglossal duct are also shown. *Id, IId,* dorsal angles of first and second pouches; *IIv, III, IV,* derivatives of ventral angles of second, third and fourth pouches; *2–4,* ductlike remnants of second, third and fourth branchial clefts; *X,* endodermal cells cut off from the lower part of the eustachian tube (E. tube); *E. C.,* external carotid artery; *I. C.,* internal carotid artery; *Th. G.,* thyroglossal duct. **C**, Anatomical relationships of probable course of fourth branchial fistula. (**A**, From Davies J. Human developmental anatomy. New York: Ronald Press, 1963; **B**, from Patten BM. Human embryology, 3rd ed. New York: McGraw-Hill, 1968; **C**, from Liston SL. Fourth branchial fistula. Otolaryngol Head Neck Surg 1981;89(4):521.)

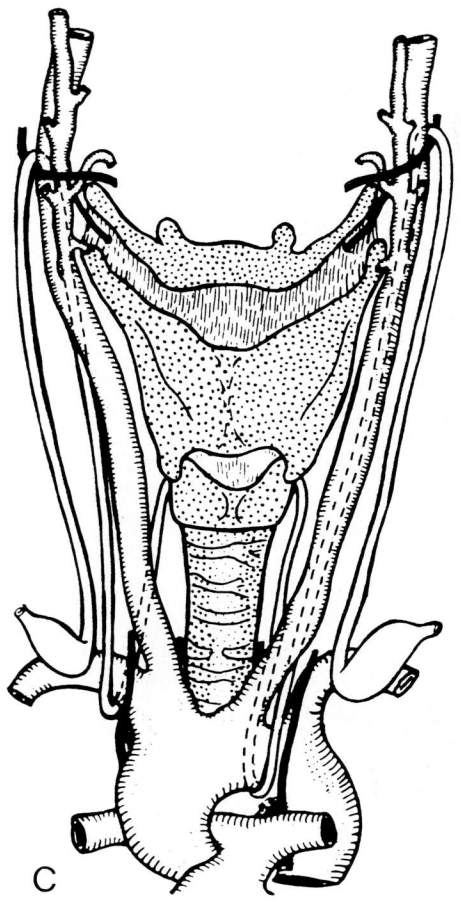

C

Figure 2.21—*continued*

posteromedial to the internal carotid artery to pierce the thyroid membrane laterally just cephalad to the superior laryngeal nerve, opening into the pharynx in the upper part of the piriform recess (Fig. 2.21, *A* and *B*).

Internal sinus tracts from the third pouch have been reported (63). There is debate whether these are, in fact, attributable to the fourth pouch. Miyauchi et al. (63) found the "internal fistula originating from the apex of the left piriform sinus in all cases" and the fistula to route inferior to the superior laryngeal nerve. Nevertheless, they (63) suggest that two findings, one anatomic and one histologic, support their contention of third pouch origin. The anatomic finding is that the superior parathyroid gland, which is of pouch IV origin, was located normally in their five patients. The histologic finding is that thymic tissue was found along the fistula in two patients. Neither concern of Miyauchi et al. seems rigorous: The superior parathyroid derives from the dorsal portion of pouch IV; thymic tissue develops from pouch IV, too, in about 10% of infants (37).

Parke and Settles (64) report bilateral third pharyngeal (branchial) pouch sinuses in a 71-year-old male cadaver. They summarize reported cases of third pouch pharyngeal sinuses (Table 2.4).

Cysts lying deep to the internal carotid artery and intimately associated with the vagus nerve are probably remnants of the third cleft or pouch.

The thymopharyngeal duct, which is the lumen of the primitive thymus, arises from the third pouch. A persistence of the thymopharyngeal duct was thought by Wenglowski in 1913 to be related to most branchial cysts (8). However, subsequent interpretations (e.g., Wilson [58], Zarbo et al. [65]) consider that only a very few cysts deep to the infrahyoid muscles can be attributed to the thymopharyngeal duct.

For a discussion of the agenesis of third pouch derivatives, see the section on Lobdell-DiGeorge syndrome.

Fourth Cleft and Pouch Defects.

A complete fistula of the fourth pouch and cleft has yet to be reported. The route of such a fistula is, of course, speculative. Presumably, from the apex of the pyriform sinus, the fistula would route through the cricothyroid membrane caudal to the cricothyroid muscle (innervated by the superior laryngeal nerve, which is the nerve of the fourth arch), then descend in the tracheoesophageal groove to loop around (i.e., from dorsal to ventral) the artery of the fourth arch (on the right side, the subclavian; on the left side, the ligamentum arteriosum). From there it would travel cephalodorsally to the carotid, to loop over (from medial to lateral) the hypoglossal nerve (a nerve of a postbranchial somite), then to descend in the neck between the strap musculature and the platysma, to a cutaneous fistula low in the neck anterior to the sternocleidomastoid muscle (66) (Fig. 2.21, *C*).

Very few sinuses or cysts can plainly be attributed to the fourth branchial pouch-cleft apparatus. What some have considered pouch IV internal sinuses are considered by others to be of pouch III origin (see the discussion in "Third Cleft and Pouch Defects"). Interestingly, of the 62 cases reported in the English literature by 1990, all but two were on the left side (63, 67). The lesion usually becomes symptomatic before the age of ten years, often presenting as suppurative thyroiditis.

CLINICAL CLASSIFICATION

The terminology of branchial pouch-cleft remnants is straightforward.

A **fistula** is a patent, duct-like structure having both an external (cutaneous) and internal (pharyngeal) orifice. The internal orifice is often difficult to identify and must be diligently sought.

An **external sinus** is a blindly ending space extending

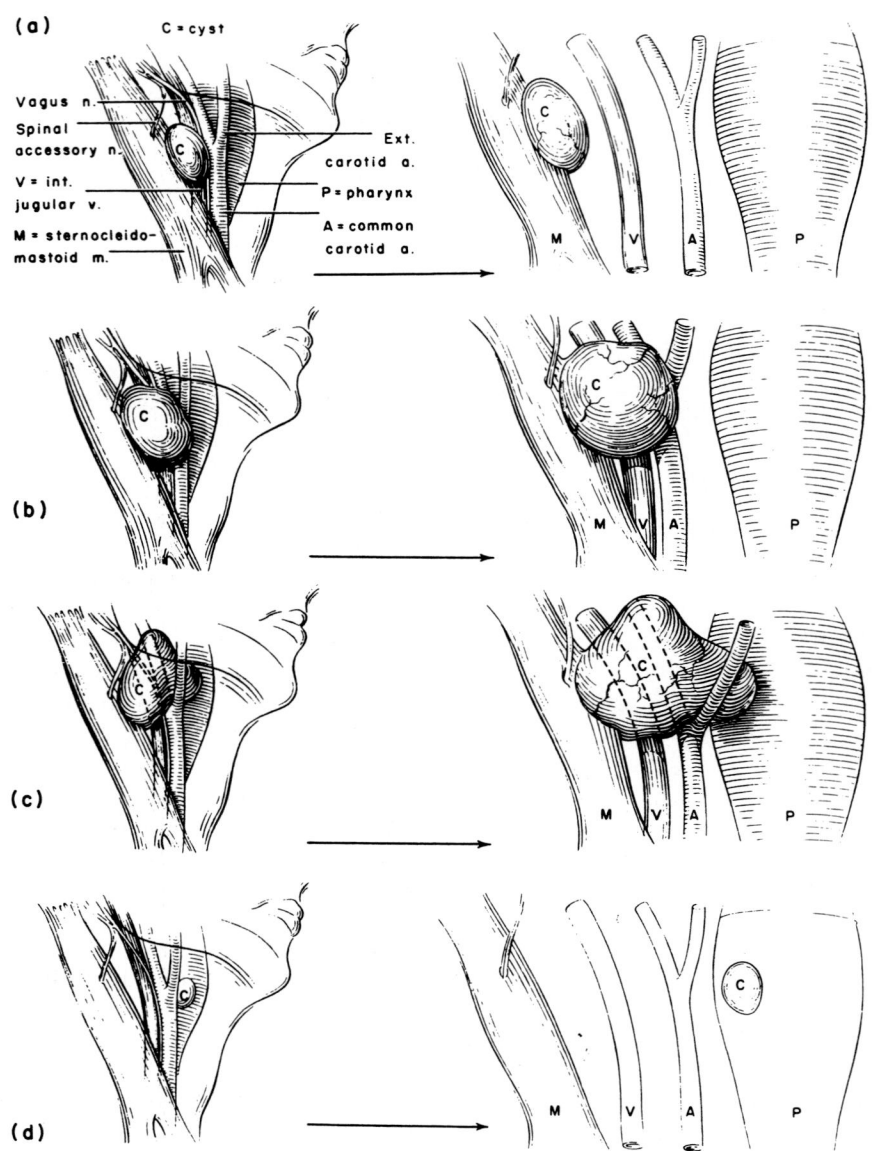

Figure 2.22. (**a**), Type I is found superficially on the anterior border of the sternocleidomastoid muscle beneath the cervical fascia. It probably has its origin from a remnant of the external tract connecting the cervical sinus to the external surface. (**b**), Type II, the most common type, lies deep to the investing fascia, is in contact with the great vessels, and may be adherent to the internal jugular vein. It probably originates from a persistent cervical sinus. (**c**), Type III is similar to type II except that it passes between the internal and external carotid arteries and extends to the pharyngeal wall. It probably originates from a dilated second external pharyngeal duct. (**d**), Type IV is found adjacent to the pharyngeal wall medial to the great vessels. It probably has its origin from a remnant of the internal pharyngeal duct. (From Montgomery WW. Surgery of the upper respiratory system, Vol 2. Philadelphia: Lea & Febiger, 1973:151.)

inward from an opening in the skin; it is thought to represent a nonobliterated branchial cleft.

An **internal sinus** is a blindly ending space extending outward from an opening in the pharynx; it is thought to represent a nonobliterated branchial pouch.

Cysts are ovoid or spherical spaces lying along the track of a branchial fistula, but having no communication with the pharynx or skin. Almost all cystic remnants of the branchial apparatus are derived from the second pouch-cleft. They may be found anywhere along the pathway of a second pouch-cleft fistula (Fig. 2.21, *B*).

In summary, clinical fistulous passages of branchial origin are of two types:

1. Cervicoaural fistulae extend from the medial extent of the cartilaginous ear canal to the skin near the angle of the

Table 2.4.
Previously Reported Cases of Third Pouch Pharyngeal Sinuses[a]

Author	Year	Case (age in years)	Description
Godley & Bucknall	1901	Male, 31	Clinical and surgical observation of large unilateral sinus
Douglas	1918	Male, 45	Clinical observation; large unilateral sinus discharged into pharynx when compressed
Thompson & Aberd	1927	Male, 35	Surgical exposure of sinus extending from hyoid bone to thyroid cartilage
Raven	1933	Infant (sex not given)	Autopsy showed left sinus from pyriform recess chronically inflamed epithelium
Buckstein & Reich	1950	Male, 54	Radiological demonstration of bilateral sinuses causing dysphagia
Buckstein & Reich	1950	Male, 45	Radiological demonstration of bilateral sinuses causing dysphagia
Kaufman	1956	Male, 75	Radiological demonstration of 4-cm unilateral pouch opening into vallecula
McMyn	1957	Female, 33	Pouch opened from vallecula and entrapped food
Fowler	1962	Male, 19	Radiological and surgical observation of 2×4-cm sinus opening into vallecula

[a]From Parke WW, Settles HE. Third pharyngeal pouch sinuses: report of a bilateral case with a review of the embryology and literature. Clin Anat 1991;4:285–297.

jaw, or medial to the conchal cartilage to the retroaural skin. Originating from the first branchial cleft, these cervicoaural fistulae are rare. They are often contiguous to the facial nerve (Fig. 2.20).

2. Lateral cervical fistulae extend from the skin overlying the anterior border of the sternocleidomastoid muscle, to open into the pharynx on the anterior aspect of the posterior faucial pillar. These originate from the second branchial pouch and cleft (Fig. 2.21, B). The minute cutaneous opening is typically in the lower third of the neck; openings more cephalad are usually the result of incision and drainage of an abscess involving the fistulous tract. There is, as yet, no reported case of a complete third or fourth branchial fistula.

EXTERNAL SINUSES

External sinuses, if congenital, have the same openings on the skin as do fistulae. In many cases a cyst has been converted to a sinus by surgical incision. Congenital external sinuses are nearly always of first or second cleft origin. Although a few may be of third or fourth cleft origin, this is usually impossible to prove.

INTERNAL SINUSES

The most common internal sinuses open into the region of the tonsillar fossa; they are of second pouch origin. Very rarely, there is a sinus opening into the pyriform sinus: a third pouch sinus opens into the cephal portion of the pyriform sinus; a fourth pouch sinus opens into the apex (i.e., caudal end) of the pyriform sinus.

EMBRYOGENESIS

In general, the origin of branchial fistulae, sinuses, and cysts from remnants of the transitory branchial apparatus is quite clear. However, two concepts put forward in the past should be modified.

Prior to the studies of Frazer in the 1920s (17), all clinical branchial sinuses were thought to form by the oper-

culum-like growth of the second arch entrapping the ectoderm of the second, third, and fourth clefts (Fig. 2.3). Frazer emphasized the anatomic relationships of branchial sinuses to the external and internal carotid arteries (68). Since the 1920s, almost all branchial cysts and external sinuses are attributed to the second cleft. Very few branchial cysts and external sinuses are attributable to clefts III and IV being overgrown by the third arch (68).

Another source of confusion came from the emphasis of Wenglowski in 1913 (8) that a persistent thymic duct accounts for congenital neck cysts, fistulae, and sinuses. The fact that no fistulae and few internal sinuses open into the pharynx at the pyriform fossa indicates that few branchial remnants can be attributed to persistent thymic duct. The consensus for the past half century is that only a very few cysts can be attributed to the thymopharyngeal duct (58, 65).

HISTORY

Lahey and Nelson (69) credit Hunczowski with having first described a cervical fistula in 1789. In 1832 Von Ascherson (3) related such anomalies to the branchial apparatus. The subsequent history of studies in this area involves the names of great embryologists of the 19th and early 20th centuries. Reviews of the subject by Proctor, Wilson, and Lyall and Stahl (10, 58, 70) have widened our knowledge of the embryology, diagnosis, and treatment of this condition.

INCIDENCE

Branchial cysts occur much more often (perhaps five times more) than do sinuses. Of the branchial sinuses, external are much more frequent than internal sinuses. Complete fistulae are rare. Branchiogenic anomalies are less than half as common as thyroglossal duct cysts. A review of surgical admissions to one charity and two private hospitals in Atlanta for the years 1954 to 1972 revealed that only about 10% of the non-thyroid neck masses could be considered congenital: 63% thyroglossal duct cyst, 25% branchiogenic anomaly, and 12% cystic hygroma (71).

SYMPTOMS

External sinuses or fistulae are present at birth. The rate is reported as 2.25:10,000 births (56). Cysts may be found at any age. A familial tendency has been suggested.

Internal sinuses may be asymptomatic and discovered only incidentally (58, 64) (Fig. 2.21, B). If the internal orifice does not drain readily, the sinus may distend, with resultant encroachment on the pharyngeal lumen, dysphagia, or hoarseness. If the orifice is large, debris (including food particles) may accumulate, and the patient may complain of a foul taste or halitosis.

Cysts manifest as swellings in the neck along the anterior border of the sternocleidomastoid muscle. They may fluctuate in size. If the change in size is dramatic, an open communication into the pharynx should be suspected. Cysts are mobile and usually painless. Discovery may follow trauma to the neck or an upper respiratory tract infection.

BRANCHIOGENIC CARCINOMA

The question of whether or not malignancy occurs in branchial remnants continues to be controversial. In 1950 Martin et al. (72) specified the criteria for branchial cleft carcinoma: (a) the tumor must occur along the anterior border of the sternocleidomastoid muscle; (b) histologically, the tumor must be consistent with an origin from tissue known to be present in branchial vestigia; (c) 5-year follow-up does not reveal a primary tumor; and (d) "the best criterion of all would be the histologic demonstration of a cancer developing in the wall of an epithelial-lined cyst in the lateral aspect of the neck." According to Michaeau et al. (73), "few if any of the purported examples of this entity fulfill the four criteria."

DIFFERENTIAL DIAGNOSIS OF NECK MASSES

With only a history and physical examination, neck masses are challenging to diagnose. Fiberoptic and Hopkins rod endoscopy (available since the 1970s) are helpful. Radionucleotide imaging (i.e., technetium sulfur colloid [Tc 99m]; iodohippurate sodium I 131 and 123) is excellent in identifying functional thyroid tissue. Computed tomography (CT) and magnetic resonance imaging (MRI) are increasingly useful.

Among cystic swellings, thyroglossal duct cysts are more medial (although not always exactly midline) than are branchiogenic cysts. Thyroglossal duct cysts typically move with the hyoid, as noted during swallowing or tongue protrusion. Cysts of the second cleft usually do not move during swallowing or tongue protrusion. With transillumination, cystic hygroma is translucent, but branchial and thyroglossal duct cysts are opaque. Fine-needle aspiration to acquire specimens for cytologic study is often helpful.

Infection may make the initial diagnosis of a branchial cyst, sinus, or fistula difficult. There is limited usefulness of radiopaque contrast-medium injection into a sinus or fistula. Complete filling may be difficult to achieve; thus portions of the lesion may not be visualized. Also, there is the potential for creating and visualizing an iatrogenic "false space."

Neck Mass "Rule of 7"
The usual inflammatory mass has been present for 7 days.
The usual neoplastic mass has been present for 7 months.
The usual congenital mass has been present for 7 years.
Of congenital masses, 70% are thyroglossal duct cysts.

TREATMENT

The only effective treatment of branchial remnants is complete excision of the walls of the cyst, sinus, or fistula. The remnants should be removed early in life to minimize infection. However, if infection occurs, it should be allowed to subside before operation. Scarring from prior infection usually makes the surgery more difficult and risky. The aspiration of accumulated secretions provides only temporary relief. Surgical drainage increases the risk of chronic infection. Sclerosing solutions are considered unsafe for use in the neck.

A number of methods have been advocated for clearly delineating the tract to be excised. When gently used, a probe (e.g., lacrimal) or catheter (e.g., Fogarty) is helpful. Some surgeons prefer methylene blue injection.

A longitudinal neck incision should be avoided because of subsequent scar contracture. If the external orifice is low in the neck, it may be excised by an elliptical incision and the tract dissected cephalad. A second, more cephalad, transverse neck incision may be necessary.

A dissection of a fistula of the second cleft and pouch from the lower neck to the upper portion of the faucial tonsil requires skill, patience, and a thorough knowledge of the anatomy of the neck. The internal jugular vein, the internal and external carotid arteries, and the vagus, hypoglossal, and superior laryngeal nerves must be identified and avoided.

PARATHYROID GLANDS

History

The parathyroid story is fascinating. The parathyroid glands were discovered by anatomists, and the implications of their function were made by surgeons. After clinical measurements of serum calcium levels became widely available, hyperparathyroidism was increasingly diagnosed. Surgeons, frustrated by the difficulties of locating the culprit hyperfunctioning glands, have restudied the anatomy and embryology. Milestones in the history of the parathyroids are shown in Table 2.5 (74, 75).

Variations in Location of Parathyroid Glands

The location and number of parathyroid glands are highly variable. There are usually two pairs, one caudal to the other, on the posterior surface of the thyroid gland. The superior pair tends to lie at the level of the lower border of the cricoid cartilage, whereas the lower pair tends to lie at the caudal margin of the thyroid gland. In about 10% of persons, the lower pair lies caudal to the thyroid.

The ontogenic locations of the parathyroid glands have been beautifully presented by Granberg et al. (25), who continued the work of Sandstrom (76). The parathyroid glands are considered to migrate from their "garages" (i.e., the third and fourth branchial pouches) along "highways" in the neck (Fig. 2.10). The highway for parathyroids IV is short and well defined, ending at the thyroid gland's upper third. In contrast, for parathyroids III, the highway is longer, typically terminating at the thyroid gland's lower third. We enhance the mnemonic of the "country road," which takes a parathyroid gland to an uncommon location. Any parathyroid that travels off the highway onto a country road reaches an ectopic location (Fig. 2.23). The superior glands (i.e., parathyroids IV) descend to the posterior surface of the thyroid gland in the vicinity of the caudal edge of the cricoid cartilage. The lateral thyroid anlage, which arises from the ventral portion of pouch IV, blocks the caudally pointed highway. The inferior parathyroids descend from pouch III along a relatively long highway. Because of the embryonic relationship of parathyroids III to the thymus, parathyroids III occasionally follow the thymus into the anterior mediastinum. The thymus, or a fibrous remnant of the thymus, "is like an index finger pointing to the (inferior, i.e., parathyroid III) gland" (25) (Fig. 2.10).

Variations in parathyroid gland location have been detailed in several large studies, both cadaver (77–80) and surgical (81, 82). Based on these reports of more than 1300 dissections, the consensus is that the superior parathyroids are located at the junction of the cricoid and thyroid cartilages close to the thyroid gland in about 80% of cases; in 15 to 20% of cases they lie more cranially behind the upper pole of the thyroid gland. Fewer than 1% of superior parathyroids are within the substance of the thyroid gland, or posteriorly in the retropharyngeal or retroesophageal space (80) (Fig. 2.23, A).

For ontogenic reasons, the inferior parathyroid glands have a wider distribution than do the superior glands.

Table 2.5.
Milestones in the History of Knowledge of the Parathyroid Glands[a]

Year	Researcher	Discovery
1880	Sandstrom (Uppsala)	Discovered parathyroid glands
1891	Von Recklinhausen (Strassburg)	Described the osteitis fibrosa cystica of hyperparathyroidism
1901	Loeb (New York)	
1903	Askanazy (Konigsberg)	Suggested a relation between parathyroid tumor and osteitis fibrosa cystica
1906	Erdheim (Vienna)	Confirmed relation between parathyroid gland and calcium metabolism; observed compensatory hypertrophy of parathyroid gland and osteomalacia
1908	MacCallum & Voegtlin (Baltimore)	Observed low serum calcium in hypoparathyroidism; tetany relieved by calcium injection
1915	Schlagenhaufer (Vienna)	Showed that tumor rather than compensatory hypertrophy is present in osteitis fibrosa cystica
1924	Hanson (U.S. Army)	Extracted parathyroid hormone
1925	Collip (Edmonton)	Extracted parathyroid hormone
1925	Mandl (Vienna)	First removal of parathyroid adenoma
1926	Collip (Edmonton)	Showed elevated serum calcium in hyperparathyroidism
1926	DuBois (New York)	Diagnosed hyperparathyroidism in patient with osteitis fibrosa cystica; surgically removed mediastinal parathyroid adenoma
1938	Gilmour (London)	Classic anatomy studies; gross and histical
1959	Lobdell (New York)	Reported newborn with agenesis of parathyroid and thymus glands
1965	DiGeorge (Philadelphia)	Clinically associated congenital hypocalcemia, aplasia of the thymus, and defective cellular immunity
1968	Alveryd (Stockholm)	Surgical anatomy
1976	Wang (Boston)	Surgical anatomy
1984	Akerström (Uppsala)	Surgical anatomy
1987	Gaz (Boston)	Unusual gland location in surgical patients

[a]Modified from Gray SW et al. Parathyroid glands. Am Surg 1976;42:653–656 and from Albright F: A page out of the history of hyperparathyroidism. J Clin Endocrinol 1948;8:637–657.

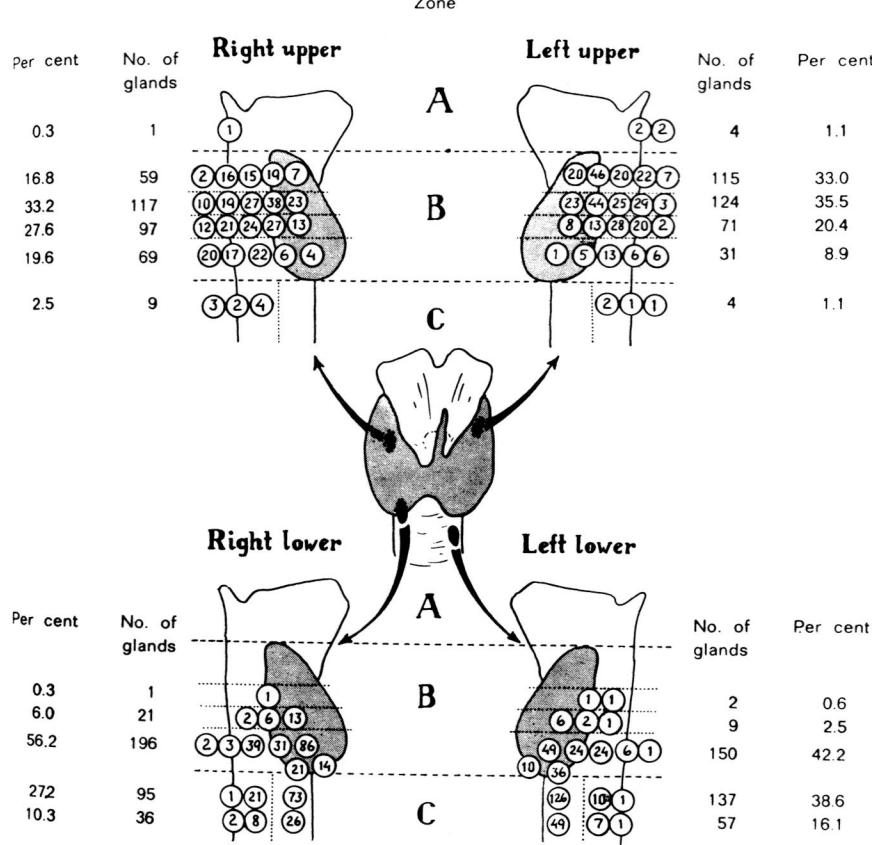

Figure 2.23. The positions of 1405 parathyroid glands identified at 354 autopsies. The locations of the upper and lower glands on the right and left sides are indicated in separate schematic drawings, which show a lateral view of the larynx and trachea with the thyroid gland mobilized and dislocated ventrally and medially. Three zones (A, B, and C) are indicated *(dashed lines)* in relation to the thyroid gland. In zone B, which represents the level of the thyroid, the *dotted hor-* *izontal lines* indicate the midline of the zone and the boundaries of its upper, middle and lower thirds. The ventral and dorsal extents of the trachea below the thyroid (C) are separated *(dotted vertical line)*. The number of glands in various areas of the zones is noted in *circles*. Parathyroids situated >2 cm below the lower pole of the thyroid are included in the most *caudal circles.* (From Alveryd A. Parathyroid gland in thyroid surgery. Acta Chir Scand 1958;389(suppl):21.)

The most common location (40 to 61%) is adjacent (i.e., caudal, dorsal, or lateral) to the lower pole of the thyroid gland. In a high proportion of cases (26 to 39%), the inferior gland is in or close to the thyrothymic ligament or in the cervical extension of the thymus. The frequency of mediastinal parathyroids is probably less than 3%. (The 11% rate of mediastinal parathyroid in the Emory University clinical series, as reported by Conn et al. (82), is probably attributable to referral bias.) Of mediastinal parathyroid glands, a large majority are in the thymus.

In addition to the common ectopic sites involving the thymic and lateral thyroid anlage tracts, parathyroid glands have been found at other sites: posterior to the pharynx and esophagus, anterior to the thymus, with the great vessels, on the pleural surface of the pulmonary hilum, or rarely in the posterior mediastinum. Rarer ectopic sites for parathyroid glands include the isthmus of the thyroid, the anterior capsule of the thyroid (83), the submucosa of the pharynx (85), the lateral triangle of the neck (84, 86), and the areolar tissue of the pericardium (84). Their presence in the posterior mediastinum usually results from postnatal mechanical displacement (87). Guided by the work of Norris in 1937 (24), Udekwu et al. (84) suspected that their two cases of parathyroid gland lateral to the carotid might have been attributable to the division of the primordial gland into two sections by the passage of the carotid artery trunk.

The embryologic origin of a parathyroid gland found within the thyroid gland, with the thyroid issue truly surrounding the parathyroid gland, is uncertain. Gaz et al. (81) suggested that parathyroid IV sometimes migrates into the thyroid, as does parathyroid III into the thymus. Although Gilmour, in his study of parathyroids in 428 autopsies (77), found two cases in which a parathyroid gland was within the thyroid and completely covered by the thyroid tissue, the frequency of these occult glands is not known. Feliciano found parathyroid pathology in an intrathyroid position in 5 of his 100 patients undergoing cervical exploration for hypoparathyroidism (88). Farr and his colleagues found 10 examples among 100 patients with parathyroid tumors (89). To the embryologist, it seems probable that intrathyroid parathyroid glands are merely deep within a sulcus of the thyroid, as suggested by Black and Haynes (90). The surgeon, of course, cares only that such glands are invisible. We think that clinically few intrathyroid parathyroid glands are discovered in the absence of disease.

The locations of parathyroid glands are apparently not related to the number of glands. For supernumerary glands, about two-thirds occur with the thyrothymic ligament or in the cervical extension of the thymus gland (Fig. 2.23).

Akerström et al. (80) found symmetry in the position of the superior parathyroid glands on the left and right sides in about 80% of cases and, for the inferior glands, in about 70%.

The anatomic distribution of adenomatous parathyroid glands, demonstrated in Fig. 2.24, is similar to that of nonadenomatous glands (77, 91).

In our own research regarding the thyroid gland in 50 cadavers, most of the superior parathyroids were located at the middle third and most of the inferior at the lower third of the thyroid gland (74) (Table 2.6).

Variations in Number of Parathyroid Glands

Based on cadaver studies (77–80) the consensus is that about 91% of persons have four parathyroid glands. Of

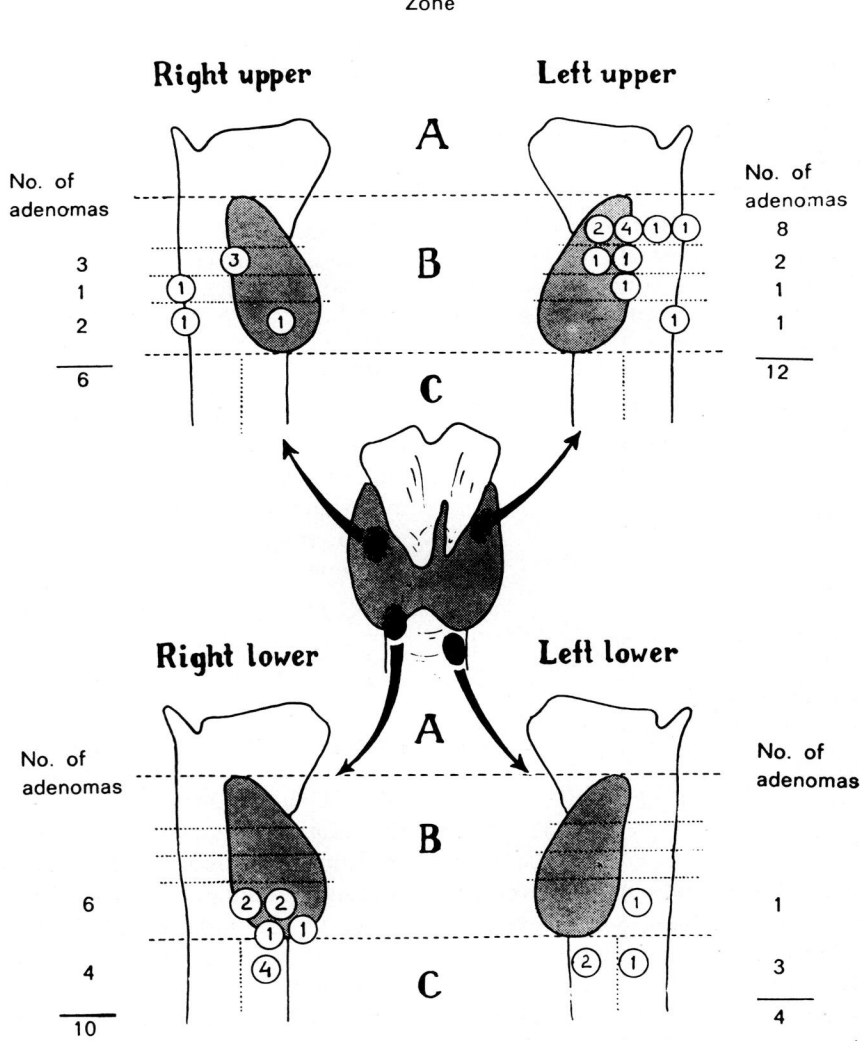

Figure 2.24. The positions of 32 parathyroid glands with adenoma identified in 27 cases at 354 autopsies. The positions of the upper and lower glands on the right and left sides are indicated in separate schematic drawings. (From Alveryd A. Parathyroid gland in thyroid surgery. Acta Chir Scand 1968;389(suppl):25.)

Table 2.6.
Location of Parathyroids in 50 Cadavers[a,b]

Location on Thyroid Gland	Superior Parathyroids	Inferior Parathyroids
Upper third	8	2
Middle third	80	12
Lower third (or below inferior pole)	12	86
TOTAL	100	100

[a]From Gray SW et al. Parathyroid glands. Am Surg 1976;42:653–656.
[b]Note that only four parathyroids glands were sought. As soon as we located the four glands, we did no further exploration for supernumerary glands. No pathological conditions were found in these 200 glands.

the approximately 9% with a nonstandard number, about 0.1% have two, 4% have three, 4.4% have five, 0.3% have six, and 0.2% have seven or more.

Akerström et al. (80) recognized three types of supernumerary glands: (a) the true supernumerary gland, weighing more than 5 mg; (b) the rudimentary, less than 5 mg in weight and closely located to a normal gland; and (c) the divided or split gland. The frequency of each type of supernumerary gland is 5%, 2%, and 6%, respectively.

Because patients without hyperparathyroidism do not undergo surgical exploration of their parathyroid glands, there is limited clinical information on patients with two or fewer parathyroid glands. Congenital absence or hypoplasia of the parathyroid glands does occur and is attributed to failure of differentiation of the endoderm of branchial pouches III and IV. The result is congenital hypoparathyroidism, manifesting as hypocalcemia in the newborn. This congenital anomaly, which typically also involves thymic hypoplasia and conotruncal cardiac defects, is known by the eponym DiGeorge, the describing pediatrician (92).

Geometric Shapes and Sizes of the Parathyroid Glands

Akerström et al. (80) report in their study of 503 cadavers that five-sixths of parathyroid glands are oval, spheric, or bean-shaped; a minority are elongated or bi- or multilobated (Fig. 2.25). The normal parathyroid gland, stripped of fat, measures $5 \times 3 \times 1$ mm.

Weight of the Parathyroid Glands

Gilmour (93) reported the weights of the parathyroids of 145 male cadavers as 26.4 mg for the upper glands and 34 mg for the lower glands. He found slightly higher weights for parathyroid glands of the 100 females: 32 mg for the upper glands and 39.2 mg for the lower glands. Alveryd (78) reported normal values for 50 cadavers, who had neither skeletal nor kidney changes. The mean weight

of the superior glands was 19.3 ± 0.9 mg and, for the inferior glands, was 25.5 ± 1.3 mg. Wang (79) found that "without exception, a piece of parathyroid tissue sank in normal saline solution, whereas a fatty globule was found to float. This observation serves to differentiate a globule of fat from a parathyroid gland."

Vascular Supply of the Parathyroid Glands

The largest series (354 postmortem subjects) analyzing the parathyroid vascular supply is that of Alveryd (78). Both the superior and inferior parathyroids are usually supplied by the inferior thyroid artery: 86.1% on the right side, 76.8% on the left. "In the majority of cases in which the inferior thyroid artery [is absent], both the upper and the lower parathyroid [are] supplied by the superior thyroid artery" (78) (Fig. 2.26, A and B; Table 2.7). Wang (79), who studied 160 postmortem subjects, suggested that "the vascular pedicle may serve as a guide in the identification of a low-lying . . . parathyroid IV" (Fig. 2.27, A and B). DeLattre et al. (94) found that the blood supply seemed to originate as follows:

Superior parathyroids:
77.1%—Inferior thyroid artery
15.3%—Anastomosis of both inferior and superior thyroid arteries
Inferior parathyroids:
90.3%—Inferior thyroid artery

Color

The color of the parathyroid glands has been variously reported as yellow, red, and tan. Perceived color depends, among other things, on the spectrum of the illumination source. (The red-emphasizing tungsten operating room lights have mostly been replaced by noble gas illumination.) Nevertheless, our experience is that the color of the parathyroids varies with age. In the newborn, they are gray and semitransparent. In children, they are pink. In adults, as fat content increases, they are yellow.

Cysts of the Parathyroid Glands

ANATOMY OF PARATHYROID CYSTS

The adult parathyroid glands usually, if not always, contain microscopic (about 10 μm in diameter) cystic vesicles or clear columnar epithelial cells. Some vesicles are larger (30 to 40 μm) and contain colloid reminiscent histologically of thyroid follicles (95). Even larger cysts, visible to the naked eye, are occasionally observed. Very rarely, they become several centimeters in diameter. Most of the large cysts are associated with the inferior pair of parathyroid glands.

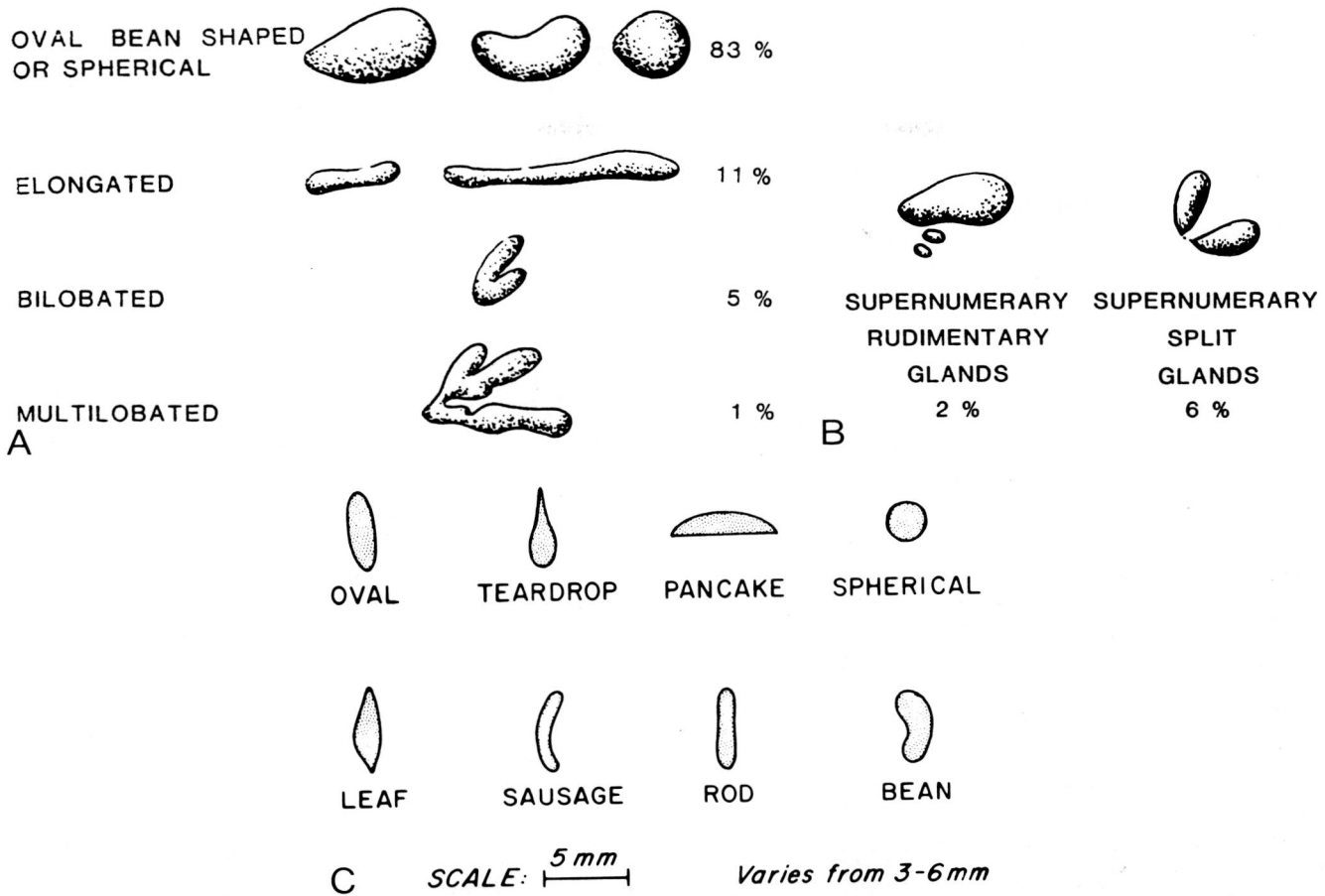

Figure 2.25. **A**, Different shapes of parathyroid glands and their frequencies. **B**, Two different types of supernumerary glands and their frequencies. Proper supernumerary glands—that is, weighing more than 5 mg, located well away from the other four glands—were seen in 5% (not illustrated). **C**, Variations in shape of normal parathyroid glands. (**A** and **B**, From Akerström G, Malmaeus J, Bergstrom R. Surgical anatomy of human parathyroid glands. Surgery 1984;95:15; **C**, from Wang CA. The anatomic basis of parathyroid surgery. Ann Surg 1976;183:273.)

Table 2.7.
Variations in Vascular Supply of 1405 Parathyroids Identified at 354 Autopsies.[a,b]

	Right Side			Left Side		
	1 Parathyroid	2–3 Parathyroids	TOTAL	1 Parathyroid	2–3 Parathyroids	TOTAL
Inferior thyroid artery	12.4[c]	86.4	98.8	20.1[c]	76.8	96.9
Superior thyroid artery	8.7	0.6	9.3	15.0	2.8	17.8
Thyroid ima artery	0.6		0.6	0.6		0.6
Artery from larynx, trachea, esophagus, or mediastinum	1.7		1.7	2.0		2.0

[a]From Alveryd A. Parathyroid gland in thyroid surgery. Acta Chir Scand 1968;389 (suppl):1-120.
[b]The figures indicate the frequency in percent of total number of cases.
[c]Includes 10 cases (right side) and 13 cases (left side) in which only one gland was identified.

EMBRYOGENESIS OF PARATHYROID CYSTS

At least four theories have been offered to explain parathyroid cysts. The embryologic theory is that the cysts represent persistent remnants of the lumen of the branchial pouch from which the parathyroid gland was derived. Another theory is that they are cystic enlargements of the Kursteiner canals of the parathyroid capsule; however, Kursteiner canals normally disappear at birth, and no cysts have been reported in children. A third theory is that a cyst may form by progressive enlargement of a microcyst or by coalescence of microcysts. The fourth and probably the most attractive theory is that parathyroid

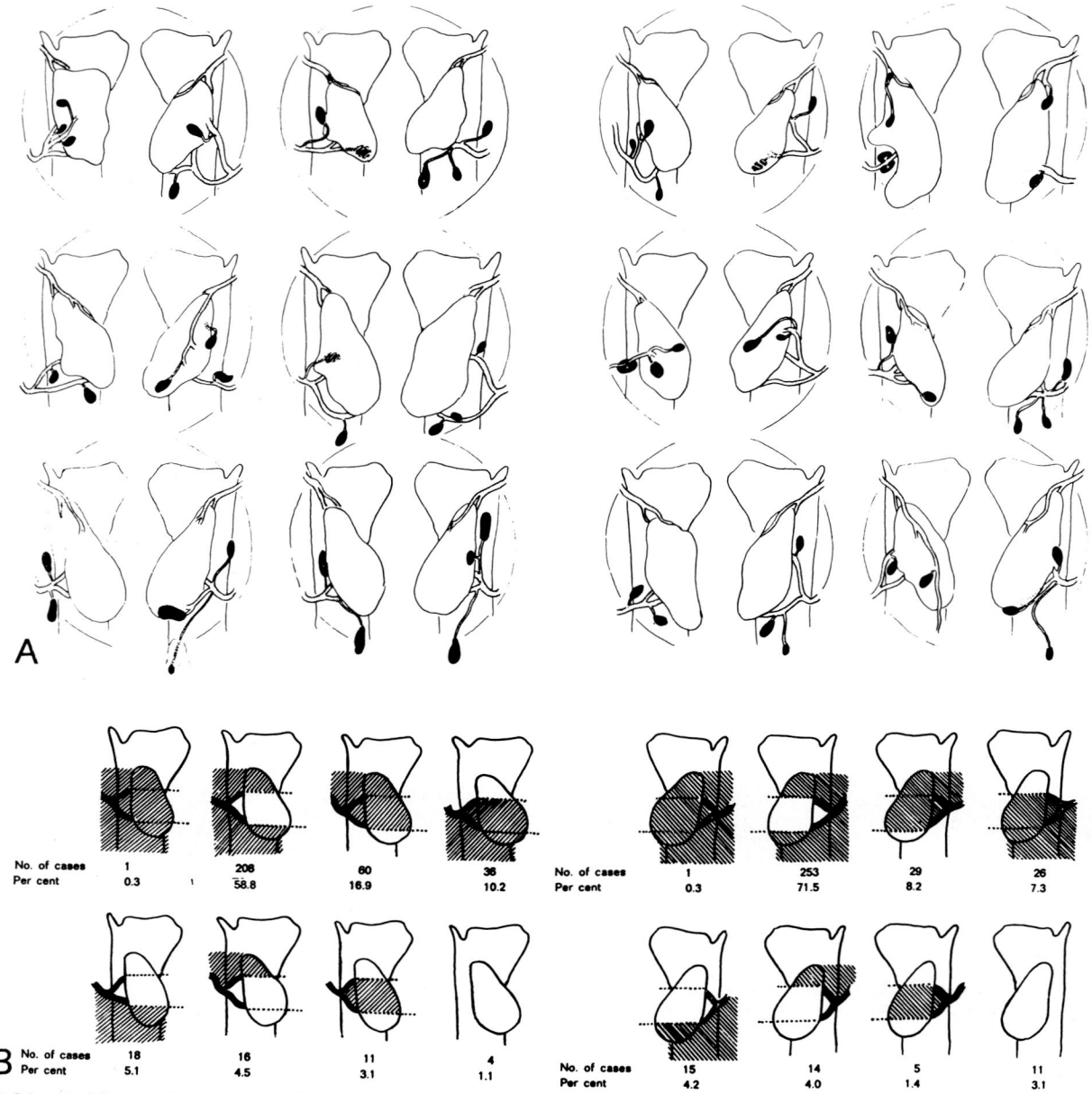

Figure 2.26. **A,** Schematic drawings showing the positions of the parathyroid glands and their vascular supply in 12 cases with 5 parathyroids without adenoma. The right and left parathyroids are indicated separately in each case. **B,** Variations in the location of the parathyroid glands in relation to the inferior artery on both sides in 354 cases with 2–5 glands. The schematic drawings show a lateral view of the larynx and trachea with the thyroid mobilized and dislocated ventrally and medially. *Dotted horizontal lines* indicate the levels of the entrance of the uppermost and lowermost branches of the inferior artery in the thyroid parenchyma. The *hatched areas* indicate the location of the parathyroids. For the sake of completeness, the cases without an inferior thyroid artery are also registered in separate drawings, but in these the location of the parathyroid is not shown. (From Alveryd A. Parathyroid gland in thyroid surgery. Acta Chir Scand 1968;389(suppl):1–120.)

cysts develop by acute cystic degeneration of parathyroid adenomas (96).

HISTORY AND INCIDENCE OF PARATHYROID CYSTS

The first parathyroid cyst was described in 1880 by the Swedish anatomist Sandstrom (76); in 1905 it was again described by Goris (97). Perdue and Martin tabulated the reported cases up to 1959, finding 24 in living patients, in addition to a case of their own (98). In 1985 Ferrara et al. (99) reported 149 cases from the world literature, three of them being their own. In 1988 Lange et al. reported two additional cases (100). The ages of affected patients range from 16 to 79 years, with the greatest number of patients being in their thirties. More females than

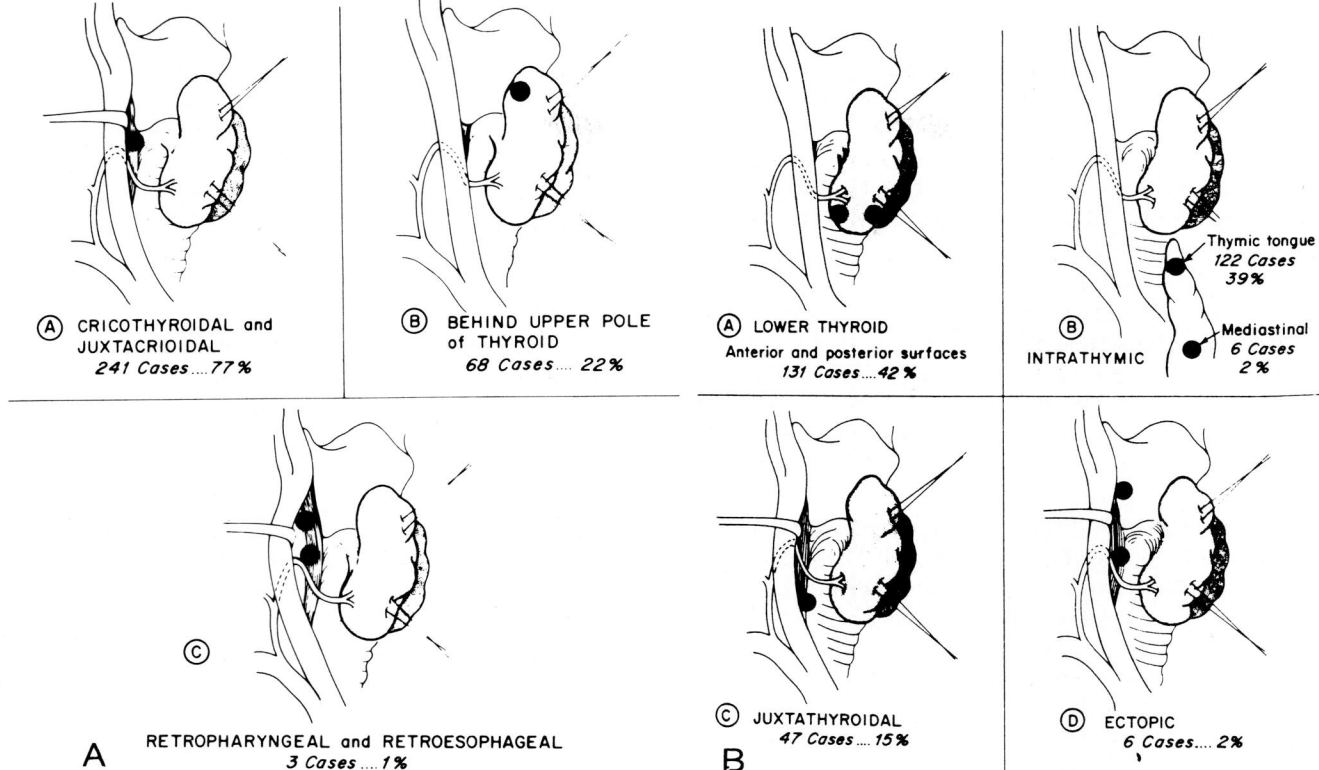

Figure 2.27. **A**, *A to C*, Anatomic distribution of 312 upper parathyroid glands (parathyroid IV). **B**, *1 to 4*, Anatomic distribution of 312 lower parathyroid glands (parathyroid III). (From Wang CA. The anatomic basis of parathyroid surgery. Ann Surg 1976;183:271–275.)

males are affected. More cysts are on the left than the right (101, 102).

SYMPTOMS AND DIAGNOSIS OF PARATHYROID CYSTS

A painless swelling of the neck may simulate a branchial cyst or nodular goiter. Dyspnea, voice changes, and dysphagia have also been reported. Hyperparathyroid activity has been increasingly associated with parathyroid cysts. Calandra et al. (96) reported that 10 of their 11 parathyroid cyst patients had hyperparathyroidism. Although the diagnosis of parathyroid cyst may be suggested from the symptoms, physical findings, and imaging studies, the diagnosis can be confirmed only by histologic identification of parathyroid tissue in the wall of the cyst (103).

TREATMENT

Treatment is excision of the cyst.

THYMUS

Thymus Aplasia

Congenital deficiency of the thymus is rare. The thymus, if indeed present, is small and often ectopic with thick connective tissue septa. Reticular cells and large thymocytes are present, but neither lymphocytes nor Hassall's corpuscles can be found. Congenital thymic deficiency is almost always associated with congenital parathyroid deficiency. Newborns with congenitally deficient thymus and parathyroid glands frequently have anomalies involving contiguous branchial arches and pouches. This constellation of anomalies may be termed the Lobdell-DiGeorge anomaly.

In 1959 Lobdell reported on a newborn with tetany, hypocalcemia, hypoparathyroidism, copious mucopurulent nasal discharge, and pneumonia (104). The autopsy findings included agenesis of the parathyroid and thymus glands and double aortic arch. In 1965 DiGeorge mentioned the thymic-dependent immune deficit of four similar infants (92). Since kudos belong to both men, we like the eponym Lobdell-DiGeorge for this anomaly.

The Lobdell-DiGeorge anomaly is a polytropic developmental field defect focused on the third branchial pouch, with variable cephalad and caudad extension. With the constraints that the field defect be contiguous (involvement of more than one branchial arch or pouch requires involvement of all intervening arches or pouches) and complete (all derivatives of an affected pouch or arch are deficient), in 1987 Thomas et al. (105)

recognized 38 different combinations of the anomaly. The patient typically presents as a neonate with hypocalcemia and repeated infections with microorganisms uncommonly found in the baby with immunocompetent T lymphocytes.

The anomalies found with involvement of caudad branchial arches are those of the conotruncus, usually truncus arteriosus or interrupted aortic arch. The anomalies found with involvement of the cephalad arches include ear anomalies, cleft palate, and characteristic facies (malar hypoplasia, prominent nose with broad nasal root, and hypertelorism).

Stevens et al. (106) reported a case of DiGeorge anomaly with velocardiofacial syndrome. They do not consider the DiGeorge anomaly to be a "distinct syndrome of a single origin but rather a heterogeneous developmental field defect."

Freedom et al. (107) reported DiGeorge infants have a deficiency of C cells of the thyroid gland. These data support the notion that abnormal ultimobranchial body becomes part of the lateral thyroid anlage.

The Lobdell-DiGeorge anomaly can be caused by a number of different mendelian, toxic, metabolic, and chromosomal factors. A problem at chromosome 22 has been suggested (108, 109). The anomaly may be considered to be one of the migrational abnormalities of neural crest cells (110).

Thymus Hyperplasia

There are two types of thymus hyperplasia: true hyperplasia and lymphofollicular hyperplasia. Characteristically, true thymic hyperplasia has an increase in the size and weight of the thymus gland but a normal (for patient's age) microscopic appearance. True thymus hyperplasia has been attributed to a number of items (e.g., decrease of greatly elevated endogenous or exogenous corticosteroid level; viral infection; thyrotoxicosis; sarcoidosis; Beckwith-Wiedemann syndrome; and treatment of a child for hypothyroidism), none of which are considered to be related to an ontogenetic thymus anomaly. Thymus lymphofollicular hyperplasia, which is defined only histologically, has been associated with an even larger number of etiologic factors, none of which can be attributed to an embryological anomaly (111).

Cysts of the Thymus

ANATOMY OF THYMIC CYSTS

Thymic cysts may be considered to be congenital, acquired, or related to thymic neoplasms. Congenital thymic cysts may be small and embedded in the thymus, or they may be large with thymus tissue in the wall. Cysts have been found in the neck, in the mediastinum, and along the ontogenetic migration pathway of the thymus

gland. Practically, the thymic line is similar to the parathyroid line from the upper neck to the superior anterior mediastinum, very rarely in the posterior mediastinum (112), and down to the diaphragm. The size of the cyst may be 15 cm. The cysts are usually solitary.

Most inflammatory thymic cysts have been attributed to symphilitic infection—the so-called Dubois' abscess (113). Radiation and chemotherapy have been implicated as etiologic factors for acquired thymic cysts (114).

EMBRYOGENESIS OF THYMIC CYSTS

It is easy to assign an embryonic origin to thymic cysts. They may represent persistence of the thymopharyngeal duct, which normally obliterates. Zarbo et al. (65) report "a cystic thymopharyngeal duct (probe patent to the pharynx) in association with an undescended solid thymus-parathyroid complex." A related theory is that congenital thymic cysts arise from degenerated Hassall's corpuscles. Shier (33) contends that Hassall's corpuscles derive from epithelium of the thymopharyngeal duct. Additional support for the congenital nature of thymic cysts is offered by the fairly common association of parathyroid tissue with thymic cysts: Guba et al. (115) report such an association in 5 of their 16 cases.

Multilocular thymic cysts in the anterior mediastinum, in addition to being diagnostically and therapeutically problematic, have features of both congenital and acquired origin. These cysts may appear invasive on gross inspection, have variegated microscopic features, and may be found with thymic tumors. Suster and Rosai (116) suggest that these cysts are pathogenetically analogous to a variety of cystic lesions of the head and neck: (a) branchial cleft cysts that often present clinically after an upper respiratory tract infection; (b) the branchial cleft-like cysts in thyroid glands affected by Hashimoto's or other types of thyroiditis; and (c) the so-called benign lymphoepithelial cysts of the parotid gland. Suster and Rosai (116) propose that the common denominator is the induction of cystic transformation in branchial pouch-derived epithelium by an acquired inflammatory process.

INCIDENCE OF THYMIC CYSTS

Cysts of the thymus that are large enough to attract the attention of the patient are extremely rare. Most thymic cysts are in the mediastinum (117). Thymic cysts are known to occur in the neck. Through 1978, Guba et al. (115) collected 72 histologically confirmed cases of cervical thymic cyst. About three-fourths of patients with histologically proven cervical thymic cyst are less than 20 years of age at presentation (115). Most mediastinal thymic cysts occur in adults (114).

SYMPTOMS AND DIAGNOSIS OF THYMIC CYSTS

Cervical thymic cysts are typically firm, nonmoveable, nontender masses that have been present for a few months. They may simulate goiter. Probably half of cervical thymic cysts extend by direct extension or by connection to a solid cord or vestigial remnant of thymus into the mediastinum (115). Mediastinal thymic cysts are usually asymptomatic and are found incidentally on radiographic examination.

TREATMENT OF THYMIC CYSTS

Excision of the cyst is the treatment of choice.

Variations in Location: Undescended, Accessory

The most common example of undescended thymus is the attenuated finger of thymic tissue that points and sometimes connects by fibrous tissue to the inferior parathyroid gland (Figs. 2.7 and 2.9, C).

The descent of the thymus into the mediastinum rarely fails to take place. Rare cases are reported in infancy and childhood (118–120). The finding of the thymus along the line of normal descent may be explained by two mechanisms. The first is failure of the unilateral gland to descend. Another, and seemingly more common mechanism, is sequestration of thymic tissue along the normal pathway of descent; this mechanism explains the so-called accessory thymus. If ectopic thymus is identified as a neonate's only thymus, then excision would comprise the child's immunologic development.

Accessory thymus may also originate from branchial pouch IV (37). Such origin may explain the rare reports of thymus attached to the superior parathyroid glands or embedded in the thyroid gland (121).

Thymus tissue in the neck may manifest as a noncystic tumor. Chan and Rosa (122) suggest four clinicopathologic entities ranging from the benign "ectopic hamartomatous thymoma" to the ectopic cervical thymoma to the malignant "spindle epithelial tumor with thymus-like differentiation" and "carcinoma showing thymus-like differentiation."

Thymus tissue is quite rarely found beyond recognized migration routes from branchial pouches III and IV. Thymus involving the lung and pericardium almost always has a pedicle connecting to recognizable thymus in the anterior mediastinum (123). Nevertheless, Bar-Ziv et al. (124) report a 3 × 5 × 2-cm accessory thymus that was posterior to the superior vena cava and separate from the normal thymus.

History

The history of the thymus, as reviewed by Jean-Claude Givel (40), is summarized in Table 2.8. The etymology of "thymus" is interesting. There are two theories, each colorful and each deriving from the identically spelled (but differently accented) ancient Greek word *qumos*. One theory suggests that the term arose from the gland's resemblance to the leaves of an herb of the genus *Thymus,* which is used as a flavoring in cooking. The other theory is that the term comes from a word meaning emotion or courage, since the gland is closely located to the heart (126), which the ancient Greeks considered to be the center of emotions.

Table 2.8.
Milestones in the History of Surgical Knowledge of Thymus[a]

Year	Researcher	Knowledge
1470–1550	Berengario da Carpi (Italy)	First anatomical description
1614	Felix Platter (Switzerland)	Thymus death in infants
1832	Sir Astley Paston Cooper (London)	First account of tumor in thymus
1845	A. Restelli	Experimental thymectomy
1849	Arthur Hill Hassall (Britain)	Thymic histology
1858	Friedleben	Experimental thymectomy
1899	Herman Oppenheim (Germany)	Thymic tumor and myasthenia gravis
1910	Victor Veau	Partial thymectomy
1911	Ernst F. Sauerbruch (Switzerland)	Thymectomy for myasthenia gravis
1917	E.T. Bell	Collected 28 cases of myasthenia gravis
1918	Crotti (Ohio)	Radiation for treatment of thymic hyperplasia
1939	Alfred Blalock (Nashville)	First successful case of thymectomy (benign cystic tumor) associated with myasthenia gravis
1944	Hyde et al (Texas)	Total removal of cervical thymic cyst
1946	Sir Geoffrey Keynes (Britain)	Surgical removal of thymus gland by sternal division, with emphasis on blood supply of thymus

[a]Data from Givel JC. Surgery of the thymus. Berlin: Springer-Verlag, 1990.

THYROID

Classification of Anomalies

With present knowledge, the classification of thyroid congenital anatomical anomalies is difficult and, in some regards, impossible. This is because of the dual embryogenesis of the gland: the medial and lateral anlages become intermingled. We present a classification that is imperfect but acceptable for clinical and mnemonic activities. Our classification is based on the thyroid anlage(s), if any, involving the anomaly. Thus we consider four categories: Both median and lateral anlages are involved; just the median anlage is involved; just the lateral anlage is involved; and neither anlage is involved (Table 2.9).

BOTH MEDIAN AND LATERAL ANLAGES INVOLVED

The weight of a normal thyroid gland is 14.5 g in women, 18 g in men. Evidence of cyclic alterations of thyroid size

Table 2.9.
A Classification of Congenital Anomalies of the Thyroid Gland[a]

Both Median and Lateral Anlages	Median Anlage	Lateral Anlage	Neither Anlage

A. Variable shape and weight
B. Symmetry
C. Total thyroid agenesis
D. One lobe absent
E. Pyramidal lobe
   1. Absent
   2. From the right lobe
   3. From the left lobe
   4. From the isthmus
	A. Agenesis
	   1. Isthmus: thick, thin, absent
	   2. Bilobed partial
	   3. Unilateral
	   4. Pyramidal lobe
	   5. Short
	   6. Long
	   7. Right or Left
	   8. Thyroglossal duct
	B. Anomalies of descent along the thyroid line
	   1. Lingual
	   2. Sublingual
	   3. Prelaryngeal
	C. Accessory ectopic
	   (i.e., outside the pathway of descent)
	    1. Mediastinal
	    2. Intratracheal
	    3. Lateral to jugular
	    4. Ovarian
	    5. Sella turcica
	    6. Retrotracheal
	    7. Preaortic
	    8. Pericardial
	    9. Cardiac
	   10. Portal hepatis
	   11. Gallbladder
	   12. Groin
	   13. Intralaryngeal
	   14. Intraesophageal
	   15. Intralymph node
		A. Nonfusion with median anlage
		B. Cysts with squamous epithelial lining
		C. Solid cell rests: C cells
		D. Agenesis: Lobdell-DiGeorge syndrome
		E. Pharyngeal pouches remnants
		   1. Thymic
		   2. Parathyroid
		   3. Ultimobranchial body
		F. Ectopic thyroid tissue in fat, muscles
		G. Fat, muscle cartilage within the thyroid gland
		H. Lateral aberrant thyroid not within the capsule of medially located lymph nodes
			A. Vessels
			   1. Artery
			   2. Vein
			   3. Lymph
			B. Muscles
			C. Nerves

[a]This classification is based on the thyroid anlage(s), if any, involving the anomaly.

during the menstrual cycle has been reported in healthy women (127). Symmetry, shape, and weight depend not only on sex but also on endocrinological activity.

Occasionally, one lobe is absent, which means that part of the median anlage (total right or left) and total lateral anlage (right or left) are not developed (74, 128–133). Again, it depends on which anlage or which part of the anlage is absent or if both anlages are absent. Therefore total or partial thyroid agenesis may take place in such areas as the isthmus, the lobes, or the pyramidal lobe.

The two lobes of the thyroid gland are not always symmetrical, something observed in the laboratory and operating room. The asymmetry does not mean disease; however, investigation is indicated. In a study in the last century of thyroid morphology in children, Marshall found 7% of the cadavers to have one lobe larger than the other, and in 7% the isthmus was entirely absent (134) (Fig. 2.17).

MEDIAN ANLAGE ANOMALIES

Agenesis. Total agenesis of products of the median thyroid anlage is an extremely rare phenomenon. Partial absence is common, especially of the isthmus (in 10% of persons). The variable thickness and thinness of the isth-

mus should be remembered, especially at thyroid surgery, laryngotracheoplasty, and tracheotomy. The pyramidal lobe, present in about 50% of cases, may be short or long and springing from the isthmus or from the right or left lobe. The foramen cecum is absent in about 34% of cases, and the foramen diverticulum is absent in about 85% of cases (135) (Fig. 2.16).

Most embryologic catastrophes of the median anlage that come to the surgeon's attention probably happen between 7 to 13 weeks of gestation—that is, in the pre-colloid stage, rather than in the colloid or follicular stage.

Anomalies of Descent along the Thyroid Line. The anomalies of descent of the median anlage may be divided into two parts: the proximal group, which occur above the normal location of the gland, and the distal anomalies below the normal location. We accept without question the proximal anomalies such as (a) thyroglossal duct, (b) lingual thyroid gland, and (c) sublingual thyroid gland (Fig. 2.28). However, we have some doubts about the distal anomalies (Figs. 2.29 and 2.30).

Distal thyroid gland, with co-existent low hyoid bone and larynx (intrathoracic cricoid cartilage) was reported by Soliman (136). Are the distal anomalies an extension of the thyroid line with the heart, since the heart is so

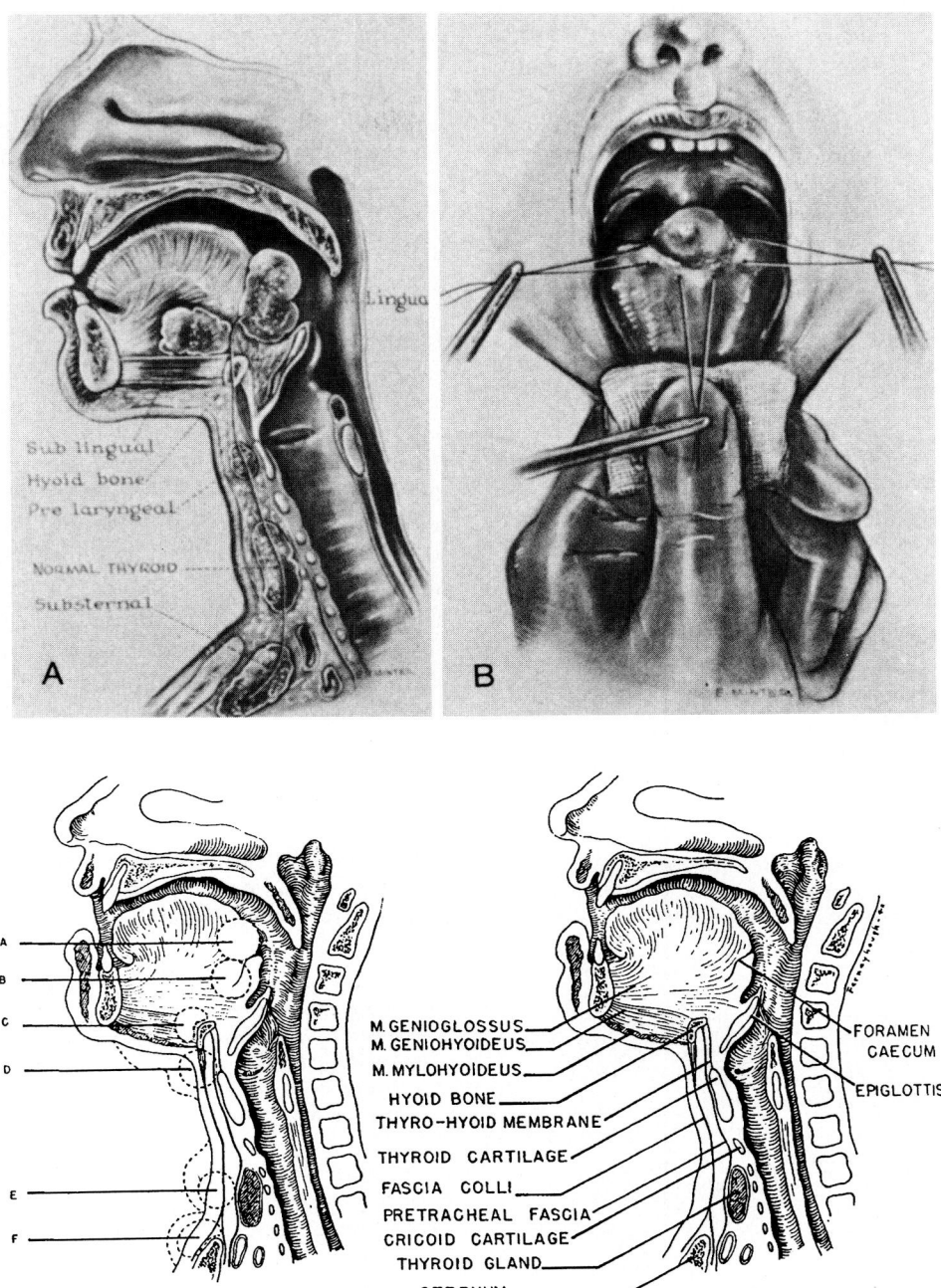

Figure 2.28. Ectopic thyroid gland. **A**, Sites along the path of descent of the thyroid from the foramen cecum (lingual thyroid) to the normal location. Hyperdescent to a site beneath the sternum is also indicated. **B**, The method of exposure of a lingual thyroid gland and the scheme for control of hemorrhage. **C**, Various locations of thyroglossal duct cysts. *A*, In front of the foramen cecum; *B*, at the foramen cecum; *C*, above the hyoid bone; *D*, below the hyoid bone; *E*, in the region of the thyroid gland; *F* at the suprasternal notch. About 50% of the cysts are located at *D*, below the hyoid bone. (**A** and **B**, From Lemmon WT, Paschal GW Jr. Lingual thyroid. Am J Surg 1941;52:1; **C**, from Ward GE, Hendrick JW, Chambers RG. Thyroglossal tract abnormalities: cysts and fistulas. Surg Gynecol Obstet 1949;89:728.)

close to the pharyngeal apparatus? Or, are the distal anomalies just as McGregor and DuPlessis (137) reported—a weakness of the false capsule of the thyroid at its posterior part, permitting thyroid tissue to overdescend? If the latter is true, then retrosternal or mediastinal thyroid should be connected with the mother gland. If not, then perhaps the distal thyroid is ectopic.

LATERAL THYROID ANLAGE ANOMALIES

The lateral thyroid anlage derives from the caudal pharyngeal pouch complex, which includes the ultimobranchial body. Unfortunately and confusingly, Weller in 1933 used the term "lateral thyroid" (11). We prefer

more descriptive wording: caudal pharyngeal pouch complex that migrates into the developing thyroid.

The lateral thyroid anlage apparently does not produce thyroid follicles in *Homo sapiens,* but does so in the dog (138). In humans, the lateral anlage contributes C cells and solid cell nests. The lateral anlage probably contributes minimally to total thyroid weight; estimates range from less than 1% to as much as 30% (52). Godwin (139) demonstrated that isolated ultimobranchial cells do not form thyroid follicles.

The solid cell nests of the lateral anlage initially appear as the so-called central epithelial cysts; the cysts normally disappear. In the normally fused thyroid gland, solid cell nests can be found in the posterior aspect (both lateral and medial) of each thyroid lobe (26). With nonfusion of the median and lateral anlages, there is not a physiologic deficit: The C cells are present, and the solid cell nests are present. If the median and lateral thyroid anlages do not fuse, the ultimobranchial portion may manifest as a cystic mass (26, 53, 140) or as masses of nonfunctioning cells with the potential to become neoplastic (53).

If the lateral thyroid anlage is absent, the contributions of the ultimobranchial body are lacking—that is, the parafollicular C cells and the solid cell nests are absent (see the discussion of the Lobdell-DiGeorge anomaly).

THYROID ANOMALIES ATTRIBUTABLE TO NEITHER ANLAGE

These anomalies are the various anatomies of the vessels (arteries, veins, lymphatics), nerves, and muscles that relate to the thyroid gland.

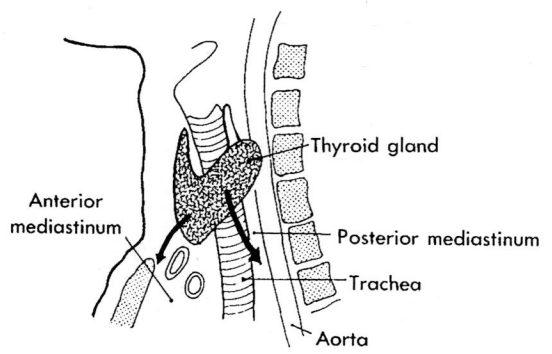

Figure 2.29. Intrathoracic thyroid tissue. Thyroid tissue originating from the isthmus or lower pole of the gland may enter the anterior mediastinum, whereas tissue arising more laterally may enter the posterior mediastinum.

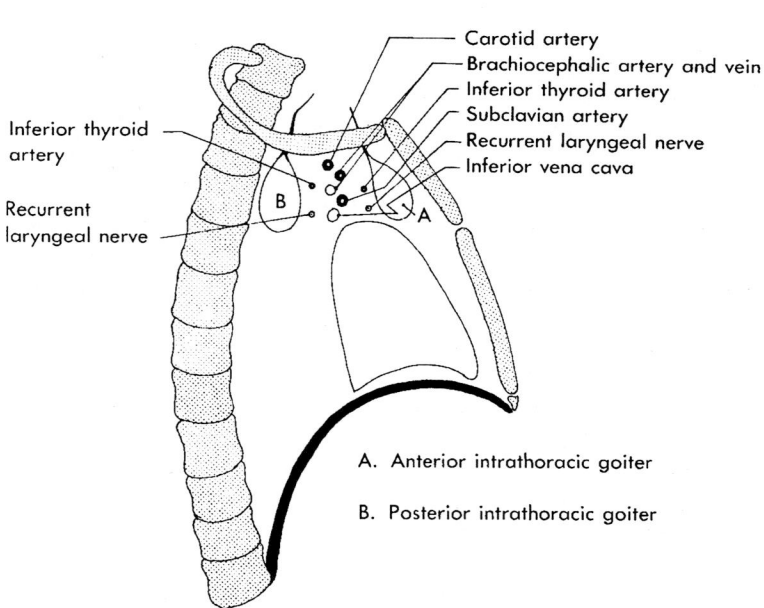

Figure 2.30. Diagram of the thorax viewed laterally, showing the vessels and nerves in the superior mediastinum which must be considered in a surgical approach to intrathoracic thyroid tissue. The relations of the structures are only approximate. Thyroid tissue originating from the isthmus or lower pole of the gland may enter the anterior mediastinum (A), whereas tissue arising more laterally may enter the posterior mediastinum (B).

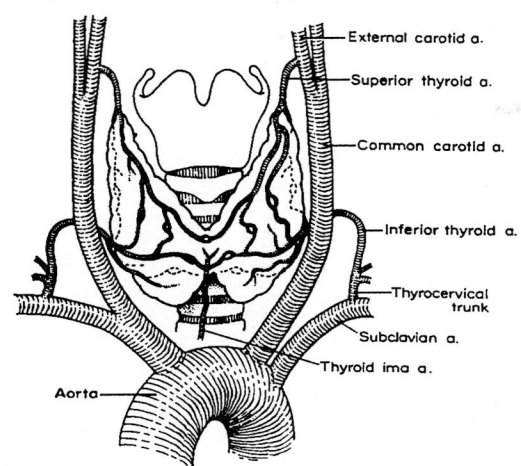

Figure 2.31. The arterial supply of the thyroid gland. A thyroid ima artery is only occasionally present. (From Tzinas S et al. Vascular patterns of the thyroid gland. Am Surg 1976;42:640.)

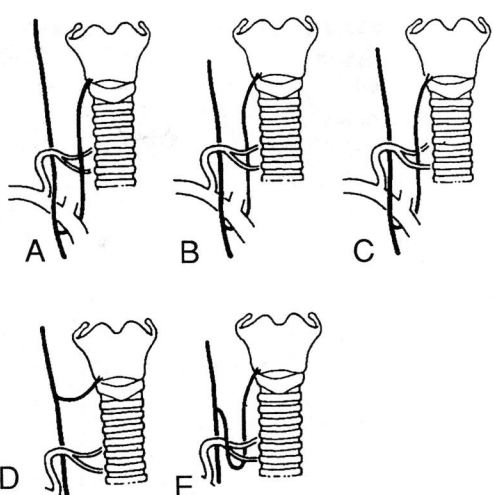

Figure 2.32. Possible relationship of the inferior thyroid artery to the recurrent laryngeal nerve. **A** to **C**, Common variations. **D** and **E**, Represent "non-recurrent" laryngeal nerves. (From Tzinas S et al. Vascular patterns of the thyroid gland. Am Surg 1976;42:640.)

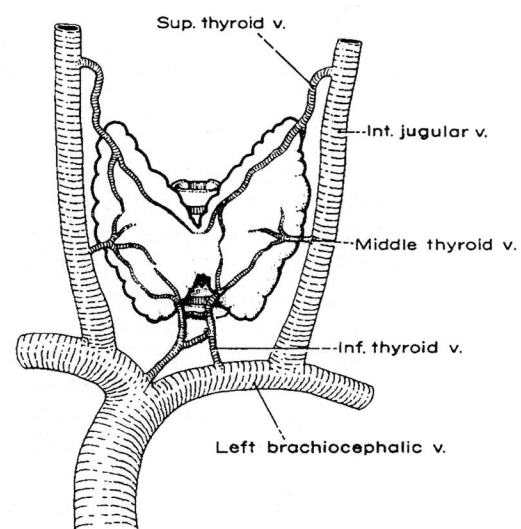

Figure 2.33. The venous drainage of the thyroid gland. The inferior thyroid veins are quite variable. (From Tzinas S et al. Vascular patterns of the thyroid gland. Am Surg 1975;42:641.)

Arteries of the Thyroid.
The thyroid gland, one of the most vascularized tissues in the body, is supplied by two paired arteries and some accessory arteries (141) (Fig. 2.31). With the ligation of all major thyroid arteries in "total" thyroidectomy, the parathyroid glands—as well as remaining thyroid tissue— seemingly receive adequate blood from tracheal anastomoses of the thyroid vessels with the bronchial, inferior laryngeal, or tracheoesophageal arteries.

Superior Thyroid Artery. The superior thyroid artery is usually the second branch of the external carotid artery but may arise from the bifurcation or from the common carotid artery just below the bifurcation (Fig. 2.31).

Inferior Thyroid Artery. The inferior thyroid artery usually arises from the thyrocervical trunk. In about 17% of cases it arises directly from the subclavian artery. In fewer than 1% of cases, the inferior thyroid artery arises from the vertebral artery, in common with the vertebral artery from the subclavian artery, or directly from the aortic arch (142).

The inferior thyroid artery divides into two or more branches as it crosses the ascending recurrent laryngeal nerve. The nerve may lie anterior or posterior to the artery or may pass between its branches (Fig. 2.32).

The inferior thyroid artery may be doubled or absent. If the artery is absent, branches from the ipsilateral superior thyroid artery or the contralateral inferior thyroid artery take its place. Enlargement of one inferior thyroid artery should suggest the presence of parathyroid adenoma on that side.

Thyroid Ima Artery. The thyroid ima artery (Fig. 2.31) is an accessory artery to the thyroid gland that may arise from the brachiocephalic artery, the right common carotid artery, the aortic arch, or rarely the internal thoracic artery or a mediastinal artery. Various authors have reported the frequency of the thyroid ima artery as from 1.5 to 12.2%. The vessel may be as large as an inferior thyroid artery. The thyroid ima artery has been reported to vascularize a parathyroid adenoma (143).

Veins of the Thyroid.
The veins of the thyroid gland form a plexus (thyroid plexus) lying in the substance and on the surface of the gland. This plexus is drained by three pairs of veins (Fig. 2.33).

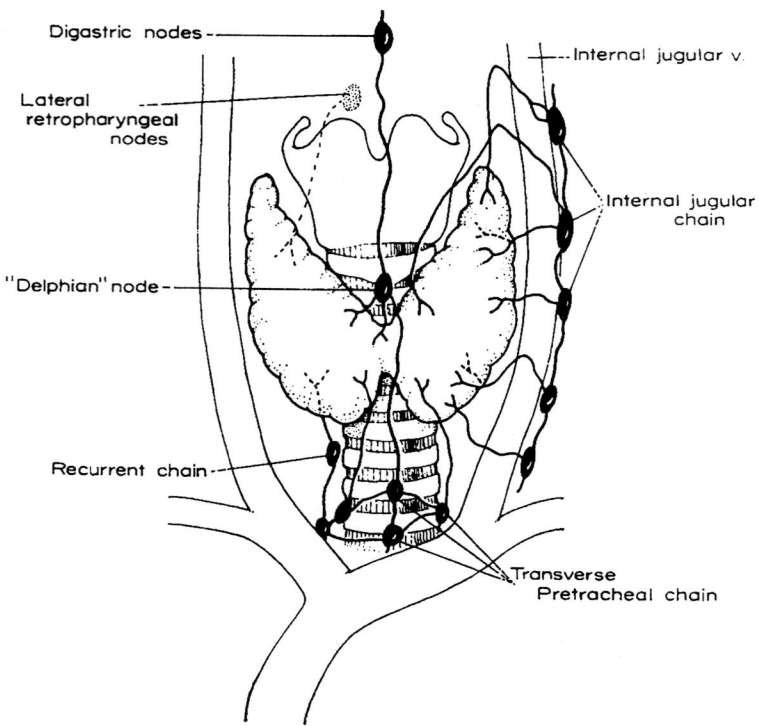

Figure 2.34. The lymphatic drainage of the thyroid gland after the description of Rouvière. (From Tzinas S et al. Vascular patterns of the thyroid gland. Am Surg 1976;42:643.)

Superior Thyroid Vein. The superior thyroid vein accompanies the superior thyroid artery. The superior thyroid vein is the most constant of the thyroid veins and is the only one accompanied by an artery.

Middle Thyroid Vein. The middle thyroid vein arises on the lateral surface near the junction of the middle and lower one third of the thyroid gland. This vein is frequently absent and occasionally doubled. In the latter case, the extra vein lies inferior to the normal site, the "fourth" thyroid vein of McGregor and DuPlessis (137).

Inferior Thyroid Vein. This is the largest and most variable of the thyroid veins; the right and left sides are usually asymmetrical. When a common trunk is formed, it is called the thyroid ima vein.

Lymphatics of the Thyroid.
They travel upward, downward into the mediastinum, and laterally to the posterior triangle. The recipient lymph nodes are the deep cervical nodes, the paraesophageal nodes, and nodes of the posterior triangle (144). The thyroid, from a lymphatic standpoint, is the "gypsy" of the neck (Fig. 2.34).

Nerves Adjacent to the Thyroid Gland.
Although these nerves do not supply the thyroid gland per se, they are certainly important surgically. Injury to one or more of these nerves may induce airway obstruction, vocal fold paralysis, hoarseness, and choking.

The recurrent laryngeal nerves are asymmetrical (Fig.

2.35). On the right, the nerve branches from the vagus as it crosses anterior to the right subclavian artery; the nerve then loops around the artery posteriorly and ascends in the tracheoesophageal groove, passing posterior to the right lobe of the thyroid gland to enter the larynx behind the cricothyroid articulation and the inferior cornu of the thyroid cartilage.

On the left, the recurrent laryngeal nerve arises where the vagus crosses the arch of the aorta. It loops under the aorta and ascends in the tracheoesophageal groove, posterior to the left lobe of the thyroid gland, to enter the larynx on the left side. Both nerves cross the inferior thyroid artery or its branches near the lower border of the middle one-third of the thyroid gland.

The recurrent laryngeal nerve may divide before entering the larynx. Probably only one of the branches carries motor fibers; the others are sensory. The surgeon must preserve all branches.

There are at least four variations in the course of the recurrent nerve. One is major and the others are minor, but each increases the liability of injury to the nerve during thyroid surgery (Fig. 2.23 and Table 2.10).

Nonrecurrent Inferior Laryngeal Nerve. In a few patients, perhaps as many as 1:100, the right inferior laryngeal nerve arises from the vagus at the level of the cricoid cartilage and passes almost directly to the larynx close to the inferior thyroid vessels (Fig. 2.32, *D*). In such cases the

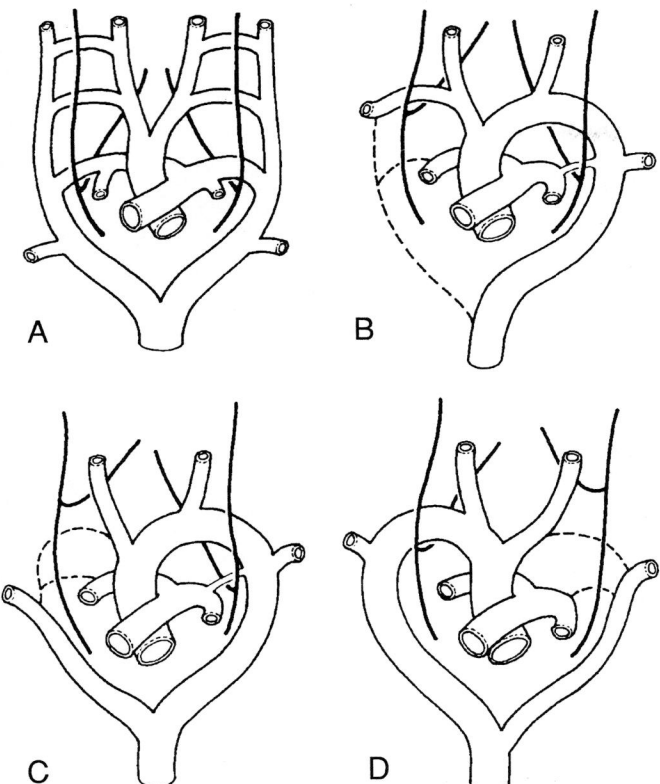

Figure 2.35. **A**, Embryonic stage. The recurrent nerves loop under the distal sixth (pulmonary) aortic arches. **B**, Normal adult. On the right the nerve loops under the subclavian artery; on the left it loops under the ductus arteriosus. **C**, With a retroesophageal subclavian artery arising from the descending aorta, the right nerve is nonrecurrent. **D**, With a right aortic arch the left nerve is nonrecurrent. (From Skandalakis JE et al. The recurrent laryngeal nerve. Am Surg 1976;42:630–631.)

Table 2.10.
Recurrent Laryngeal Nerve in the Presence of Aortic Arch Anomalies[a]

Vascular Anomaly	Recurrent Nerves
Normal aortic arch Normal right subclavian artery	Both nerves recurrent
Normal aortic arch Retroesophageal right subclavian artery	Left nerve recurrent Right nerve direct
Right aortic arch Other vessels normal, but reversed	Both nerves recurrent

Right aortic arch
Retroesophageal left
  subclavian artery
	Left nerve direct
	Right nerve recurrent around
	  aorta

Right aortic arch
Retroesophageal left
  subclavian artery
Left ligamentum arteriosum
	Left nerve recurrent around
	  ligamentum arteriosum
	Right nerve recurrent around
	  aorta

Double aortic arch	Left nerve recurrent around
	  left aorta[b]
	Right nerve recurrent around
	  right aorta[b]

[a]From Gray SW et al. Embryological considerations of thyroid surgery. Am Surg 1976;42(9):625.
[b]One "aorta" may be reduced to a fibrous remnant, the ductus arteriosus.

right subclavian artery arises from the descending aorta and turns to the right posterior to the esophagus. As this vascular anomaly (known as aberrant right subclavian) is rarely symptomatic, the thyroid surgeon will rarely be aware preoperatively of the nonrecurrence of an inferior laryngeal nerve.

Quite less common than 1:100 is a nonrecurrent left inferior laryngeal nerve. The arterial anatomy in this circumstance involves a right-sided aortic arch and a retroesophageal aberrant left subclavian artery (Fig. 2.35, *D*). Stedman (145) described the first such case in a cadaver, and Pemberton and Stalker (146) presented the first surgical case. Henry et al. (147) presented 19 cases of nonrecurrent inferior laryngeal nerve identified in 3791 cases in 7 years of thyroid and parathyroid surgery: 0.54% of right inferior laryngeal nerves and 0.07% of left inferior laryngeal nerves. On 6961 neck explorations for thyroid and parathyroid disease, Proye et al. found 0.8% of persons to have nonrecurrent right inferior laryngeal nerve, but none on the left side (148).

Ascending Course of the Recurrent Laryngeal Nerve. In its ascending course, the recurrent laryngeal nerve is surrounded by loose connective tissue, usually thicker on the right than on the left. This layer of fascia also encloses the trachea and inferior thyroid veins. In the middle third of its ascending course, the nerve may lie in the tracheo-esophageal groove, medial to the suspensory ligament of the thyroid (ligament of Berry), within the ligament (peritracheal), or within the substance of the thyroid gland. In the upper third of its ascent, the nerve becomes parallel and closely applied to the trachea.

We have examined the course of the recurrent laryngeal nerves in 62 male and 40 female cadavers. In approximately one half, the nerves lay in the groove between the trachea and esophagus. In the other half, the nerves lay anterior or posterior to the groove, either lateral to the esophagus, lateral to the trachea in the suspensory ligament of Berry, or anterolateral to the trachea in the substance of the thyroid gland (Fig. 2.36, *A* and *B*). Our findings in 204 nerves of 102 cadavers are summarized in Table 2.11 (149). In general, the left recurrent nerve is more closely applied to the trachea than is the right nerve in the lower part of its ascending course. At the level of the lower pole of the thyroid, the right nerve is separated from the trachea and slightly more anterior than is the left recurrent laryngeal nerve.

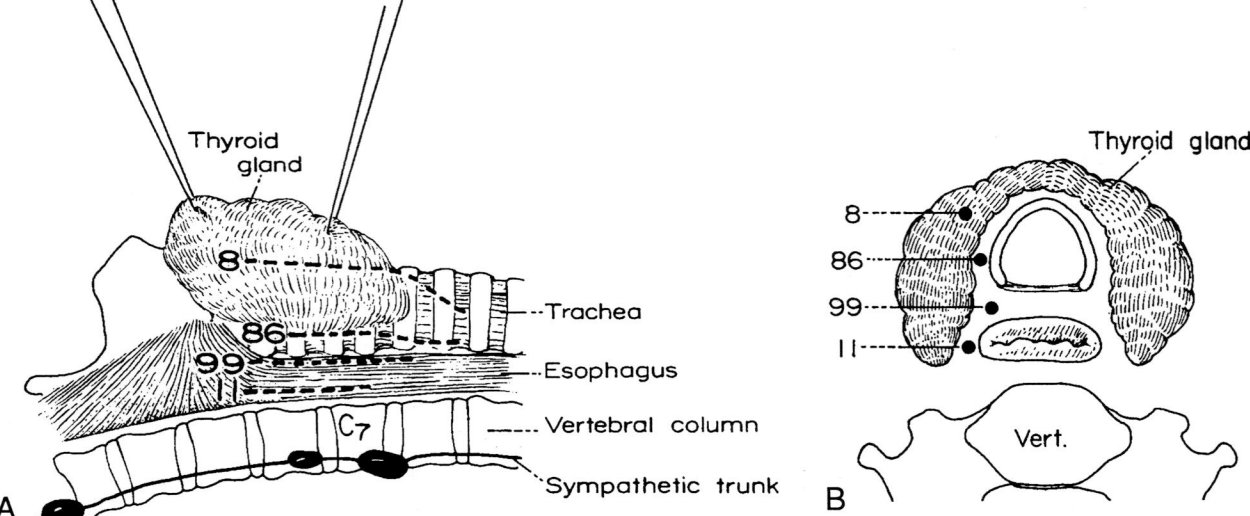

Figure 2.36. The course of the recurrent layngeal nerve at the level of the thyroid gland in 102 cadavers. In about one half of the cases the nerve lay in the groove between trachea and esophagus. **A**, Lateral view. **B**, Cross-sectional view. (From Skandalakis JE et al. The recurrent laryngeal nerve. Am Surg 1976;42:629–634.)

Table 2.11.
Relationship of Recurrent Laryngeal Nerve to Tracheoesophageal Groove[a]

Position	Number		Percent Total
	Right	Left	
In the tracheoesophageal groove	42	57	48.5
Posterior to the groove (periesophageal)	5	6	5.4
Anterior to the groove			
In the suspensory ligament anterior to the groove (peritracheal)	50	36	42.2
In the thyroid parenchyma	5	3	3.9
TOTAL	102	102	100.0

[a]From Skandalakis JE et al. The recurrent laryngeal nerve. Am Surg 1976;42:629–634.

Relationship of the Recurrent Laryngeal Nerve to the Inferior Thyroid Artery. As the recurrent laryngeal nerve ascends toward the middle one-third of the thyroid gland, it crosses the inferior thyroid artery. The nerve may lie in front of, behind, or between the branches of the artery. In a study of 253 cadavers, Reed found 28 variations of the artery-nerve relationship (150). For the clinical surgeon, three of the variations are important (Fig. 2.32). Among the 102 cadavers we examined, the nerve passed behind the artery in a simple majority of cases. The relative incidence of types agreed roughly with that found in 1236 bodies described by other writers (Table 2.12). On the right, the nerve most frequently lay between arterial branches (48%); on the left, it was usually behind the artery (64%).

The So-Called Multiple Recurrent Laryngeal Nerves. The authors feel that the expression "I found two or three recurrent laryngeal nerves" is embryologically and ana-

Table 2.12.
Relationship of Recurrent Laryngeal Nerve and Inferior Thyroid Artery[a]

Relation	Per Cent Frequency			
	102 Cadavers			1246 Cases from Literature[b]
	Right	Left	Both Sides	Both Sides
Nerve anterior to artery	31.4	9.8	20.6	21.1
Nerve posterior to artery	19.6	63.7	41.6	50.4
Nerve between branches of artery	48.0	26.5	37.3	24.8
Nonrecurrent nerve and other	1.0	—	0.5	3.6
	100.0	100.0	100.0	99.9

[a]From Skandalakis JE et al. The recurrent laryngeal nerve. Am Surg 1976;42:629–634.
[b]From Berlin DD. The recurrent laryngeal nerves in total ablation of the normal thyroid gland. Surg Gynecol Obstet 1935;60:19; Fowler CH, Hanson WH. Surgical anatomy of the thyroid gland with special reference to the relations of the recurrent laryngeal nerve. Surg Gynecol Obstet 1929;49:59; Reed AF. The relations of the inferior laryngeal nerve to the inferior thyroid artery. Anat Rec 1943;85:17; Wade JSH. Vulnerability of the recurrent laryngeal nerves at thyroidectomy. Br J Surg 1955;43:164.

tomically incorrect; rather, it is just a myth. Normally the recurrent nerve bifurcates to an anterior and posterior branch prior to or after its entry to the larynx. Sometimes, however, the recurrent laryngeal nerve divides into two, three, or more branches low in the neck.

Superior Laryngeal Nerve. The superior laryngeal nerve

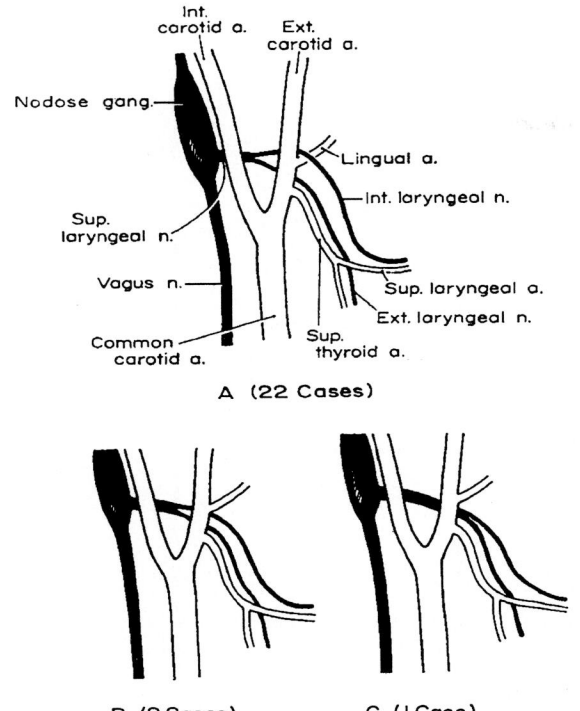

Figure 2.37. Branching of the superior laryngeal nerve into internal and external branches and their relation to the branching of the carotid artery. **A,** The most usual type. The external branch of the nerve crosses the external carotid artery above the origin of the lingual nerve. **B,** The external branch of the nerve crosses the external carotid artery below the origin of the lingual nerve. **C,** The superior laryngeal nerve divides after passing medial to the external carotid artery. (From Droulias C et al. The superior laryngeal nerve. Am Surg 1976;42:636.)

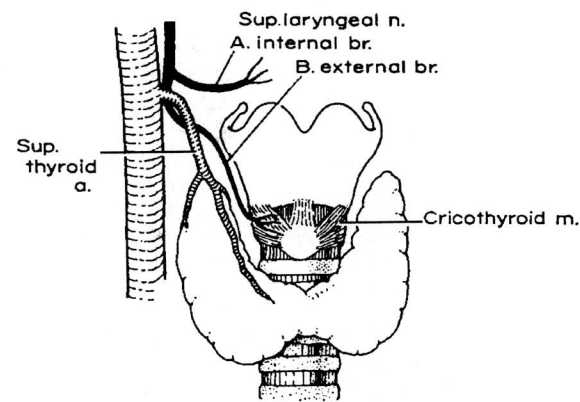

Figure 2.38. Relationship of the internal and external branches of the superior laryngeal nerve to the superior thyroid artery and the superior pole of the thyroid gland. (From Droulias C et al. The superior laryngeal nerve. Am Surg 1976;42:636.)

arises from the inferior (nodose) ganglion of the vagus nerve just outside the jugular foramen of the skull. The nerve passes medial to the carotid arteries. It divides, at the level of the superior cornu of the hyoid bone, into a large, sensory, internal laryngeal nerve and a smaller motor, external laryngeal nerve to the cricothyroid muscle (Figs. 2.37 and 2.38). In our study (151), in 23 out of 24 cadavers examined, the bifurcation of the nerve lay within the bifurcation of the internal and external carotid arteries. In one case it bifurcated medial to the external carotid artery (Fig. 2.36). In two cadavers the internal branch of the nerve crossed the external carotid between the origin of the lingual artery and that of the superior thyroid artery. In 22 cadavers the nerve crossed the artery above the origin of the lingual artery (151).

The internal branch (1 to 2 mm in diameter [152]) of the superior laryngeal nerve passes beneath the thyrohyoid muscle and pierces the thyrohyoid membrane above the inferior pharyngeal constrictor muscle (Fig. 2.38). The nerve is accompanied by the superior laryngeal artery. After entering the larynx, this sensory nerve divides into a number of branches to the mucosa of the larynx down to the level of the true vocal folds.

The external branch of the superior laryngeal nerve,

together with the superior thyroid vein and artery, passes beneath the sternothyroid muscle into the sternothyroid-laryngeal triangle of Moosman and DeWeese (152) (Fig. 2.39). The triangle is formed by the sternohyoid muscle anterosuperiorly, the inferior pharyngeal constrictor and the cricothyroid muscles posteromedially, and the superior pole of the thyroid gland. In this triangle the nerve is usually medial; the superior thyroid vein is lateral; and the artery is between them. The nerve then passes anteriorly beneath the vessels into the lower part of the thyropharyngeal muscle and then inferior to enter and innervate the cricothyroid muscle (Fig. 2.38). In some cases the nerve enters the cricothyroid muscle directly without passing between fibers of the thyropharyngeal muscle. Occasionally, the nerve descends on the anterosuperior surface of the thyroid, crossing anterior to anterior branches of the superior thyroid artery before entering the thyropharyngeal muscle.

The external laryngeal nerve usually lies in close association with the inferior pharyngeal constrictor muscle. In most cases the surgeon can develop a plane of dissection between the thyroid sheath and the true thyroid capsule, thus separating the vessels from the nerve (Fig. 2.39). Moosman and DeWeese found 79% of 200 cadavers to have the nerve surgically separate from, and posteromedial to, the superior thyroid vessels (152).

Levator Glandulae Thyroideae Muscle.
The authors have never noted any case of this peculiar muscle which, according to Hollinshead (153), is an occasional muscular slip or paired slips from the hyoid bone to one or both lobes of the thyroid.

Anomalies of Descent of the Median Anlage

LINGUAL THYROID

The term "lingual thyroid" refers to an entire thyroid gland that has failed to descend to its normal cervical

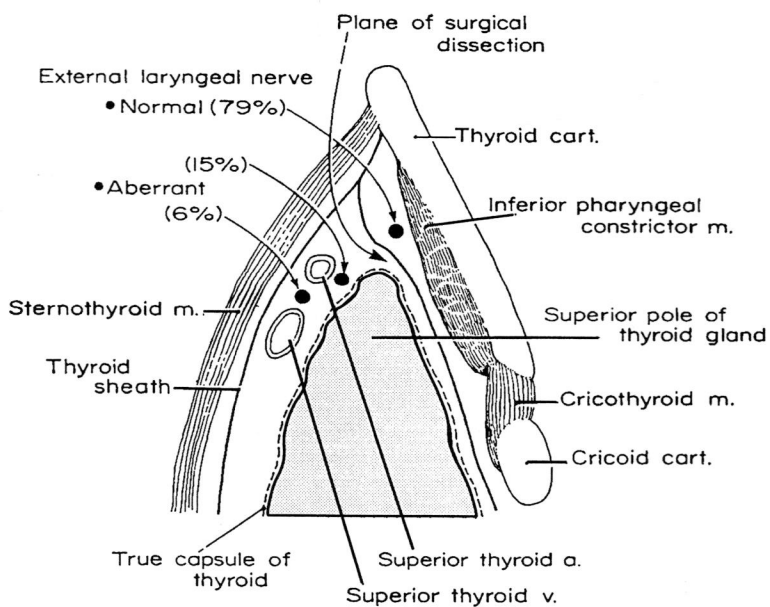

Figure 2.39. Schematic frontal section through the triangle of Moosman and DeWeese. The triangle is formed by the sternothryoid muscle anterosuperiorly and the inferior constrictor and cricothyroid muscles posteriorly, and the base is occupied by the superior pole of the thyroid gland. The external branch of the superior laryngeal nerve is usually (79%) posteromedial to the plane of surgical dissection. (From Droulias C et al. The superior laryngeal nerve. Am Surg 1976;42:637; modified from Mossman DA, DeWeese MS. The external laryngeal nerve as related to thyroidectomy. Surg Gynecol Obstet 1968;127:1013.)

location; thyroglossal duct remnants at the foramen cecum of the tongue are not included in the term. Lingual thyroids lie within the tongue subjacent to the mucosa, at the normal location of the foramen cecum (Fig. 2.28). The lingual thyroid is typically that patient's only thyroid tissue.

Embryogenesis. The lingual thyroid represents successful development of the median primordium, but subsequent failure of duct formation later in the third week of gestation. The lingual thyroid has failed to descend in the sense that it remains close to its site of origin, the foramen cecum. The normally descended thyroid gland lies caudal to its level of origin in the pharynx, but quite cephalad with respect to the ventral aorta. In a sense the foramen cecum ascends, and the lingual thyroid represents an unusually ascended thyroid, rather than an undescended thyroid gland.

Incidence. By 1984 there were about 400 cases of lingual thyroid reported in the North American and European literature (154). The female/male predominance is about 3:1, similar to the ratio for the occurrence of agenesis of a thyroid lobe.

Symptoms. Hypothyroidism often occurs in patients with lingual thyroid (155). Other symptoms may include dyspnea, dysphonia, a sensation of tongue fullness, and choking. Nevertheless, most cases are incidently discovered, with the lingual thyroid being asymptomatic (156). Lingual thyroid with associated epiglottis has been reported (154).

Diagnosis. Radioactive iodine scintigraphy is useful and will determine the presence of other thyroid tissue in the patient's neck. Pertechnetate uptake in the major and minor (e.g., lingual) salivary glands prompts confusion; therefore, ^{123}I scanning is indicated when the question is lingual thyroid. CT and MRI are useful, but not definitive for thyroid malignancy.

Treatment. Hormonal therapy (levothyroxine) shrinks the lesion. Surgery is reserved for cases with airway or swallowing obstruction or if there is a question of malignancy.

PARTIALLY DESCENDED THRYOID GLAND ("SUBLINGUAL THYROID GLAND")

Very rarely, the developing thyroid gland begins to descend but fails to reach its normal location. Such arrested descent leaves the gland at or just below the hyoid bone, where it forms a median protuberance of the neck. It is much less common than lingual thyroid.

The partially descended thyroid gland is of importance because it resembles the much more common thyroglossal cyst, and the gland may inadvertently be removed surgically before it is recognized as the patient's only thyroid tissue. Ectopic thyroid misdiagnosed preoperatively as thyroglossal cyst has an incidence of 1 to 2% in most series (157). The preoperative diagnosis of partially descended thyroid gland can be certain only when radioactive iodine (^{123}I, preferably) is positive. To alleviate the need to scan all patients, Radkowski et al. (157) suggest that a high-risk

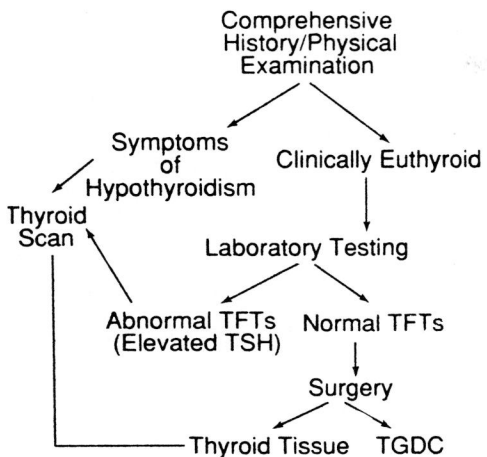

Anterior Midline Neck Swelling

Figure 2.40. Anterior midline neck swelling. *TFTs* thyroid function testings; *TSH,* thyroid stimulating hormone; and *TGDC,* thyroglossal duct remnant/cyst. (From Radkowski et al. Thyroglossal duct remnants: preoperative evaluation and management. Arch Otolaryngol Head Neck Surg 1991;117:1381.)

Table 2.13.
Reported Cases of Thyroglossal Duct Associated Carcinoma[a]

Histology:	Papillary carcinoma	99
	Adenocarcinoma	2
	Malignant struma	1
	Squamous cell carcinoma	7
	TOTAL (reported cases)	109
Female/Male	66:42 (1 unknown)	
Age	6 to 81 years	
History of neck radiation		3

[a]Adapted from LiVolsi VA. Surgical pathology of the thyroid. Philadelphia: WB Saunders, 1990.

group may be identified (Fig. 2.40). The schema of Radkowski et al. is predicated on the high incidence of laboratory-identifiable hypothyroidism in patients with ectopic thyroid (157).

Analogous to patients with lingual thyroid, the primary treatment of partially descended thyroid is hormonal (levothyroxine).

THYROGLOSSAL DUCT CYST

The normal remnants of the thyroglossal duct are the foramen cecum of the tongue and the pyramidal lobe of the thyroid gland (Fig. 2.16). Cysts ranging from a few millimeters to several centimeters in diameter may form anywhere along the pathway of persisting duct from the tongue to the usual location of the thyroid gland. The cysts are usually located near the hyoid bone (Fig. 2.28). They typically occur in the midline, but may be paramedian. Thyroid tissue is found in about one-fifth of the thyroglossal duct cyst specimens (158–160).

In some patients with thyroglossal duct cysts, there is an opening through the skin as a result of operative drainage or spontaneous perforation following infection. Such a thyroglossal duct sinus tract is subject to infection.

The tract or tracts of the thyroglossal duct cyst almost always distort the architecture of the hyoid bone (159). Multiple tracts, or "lateral branches," above the hyoid bone have been recognized for years (161).

Embryogenesis. The undifferentiated epithelium of the thyroglossal duct is subject to different induction fields at its two ends. Proximally at the foramen cecum, it differentiates into tongue mucosa; distally into thyroid tissue, the pyramidal lobe. Normally, the midportion of the duct

remains as a discontinuous microscopic tube of undifferentiated epithelium passing through or near the hyoid bone (162).

Cysts do not arise from a primary failure of the thyroglossal duct to close, as Kostanecki and Mielecki (163) originally supposed. Cysts form when the epithelial cells cease to remain inactive. The cause of the induction of cystic changes in the ductular structures, usually toward the type of cells normally found in the pharynx, is unknown. Once acquired, secretory activity of the duct cells does not disappear; therefore drainage of the cyst will not result in obliteration. Secretory activity of thyroglossal duct cells may begin at any time, even late in life (164).

History. The thyroglossal duct was first described in 1723 by Vater (165), who used the term "lingual duct." Following the studies of His in 1885 and 1891 (4, 38), it was often called the canal of His.

Incidence. Thyroglossal duct cysts are three times more common than branchial cysts (166). The male/female preponderance is slight, about 60:40 (157, 167), but unexplained. A familial occurrence has been reported (168). A few cysts are present at birth; most develop during childhood; the remainder may appear in adults of any age (164).

Symptoms, Signs, and Differential Diagnosis. The patient with thyroglossal duct cyst usually seeks medical attention because of a disfiguring lump in the anterior of the neck near the hyoid bone. The tumor moves with swallowing and is nontender (unless infected). The lesion may be paramedian. The differential diagnosis must include partially descended thyroid gland, accessory thyroid nodule, dermoid cyst, midline thyroid adenoma, inflammatory lymph node, and lipoma. (The importance of preoperatively recognizing the partially descended thyroid gland is discussed in the section on "Lingual Thyroid.") Carcinoma arising in association with thyroglossal cyst is rare; just over 100 cases have been reported in the English literature (52) (Table 2.13).

Treatment. Treatment requires surgical removal of the entire tract. The operation of choice was popularized in 1920 by Sistrunk (161). Although Sistrunk removed about one-fourth of an inch of hyoid bone, currently more hyoid is often removed: "at least 1.5 cm of the bone and related periosteum" (158) or "the body of the hyoid" (167). The suprahyoid duct should be removed in a core of tissue "without any attempt to isolate the duct" (161); this item of technique has been repeatedly emphasized (158, 167). Sistrunk opened into the mouth to remove the foramen cecum. However, Solomon and Rangecroft, in reporting 300 cases over nearly 30 years, state "entry into the mouth is usually unnecessary" (158).

Recurrence rates of 5 to 7% in primary cases are reported, notwithstanding all the attention to meticulous and thorough dissection (158, 159, 167). In addition to incomplete dissection, recurrence may be related "to young age [of patient], skin involvement by the cyst, lobulation of the cyst, and rupture of the cyst" (167). After reexcision, the recurrence rates are 25 to 30% (158, 167). Certainly, the first operation offers the best chance for successful removal of a thyroglossal duct cyst.

Perhaps one fourth of patients with a preoperative diagnosis of thyroglossal duct cyst are found pathologically to have something else (e.g., dermoid cyst or lymphadenitis). In their review of 75 cases, deMello et al. found six cysts with features of both dermoid and thyroglossal duct cyst (160). We agree with deMello that cysts clinically simulating thyroglossal duct cysts "should be treated with the Sistrunk procedure to avoid incomplete excision" (160).

Malignancy. Malignancy in thyroglossal duct cyst is quite rare—about 100 reported cases (52, 169) (Table 2.13). Medullary carcinoma is not reported in thyroglossal duct. Here, embryology and pathology are in full agreement: The origin cells of medullary carcinoma, that is, the parafollicular C cells, arise from the lateral thyroid anlage.

Accessory Ectopic Thyroid Tissue

Unusually placed thyroid tissue is considered to be "accessory ectopic" when it is found in locations outside the normal pathway of embryonic development (Fig. 2.41). To which anlage can we attribute these rare occurrences? The median anlage is excluded because, by definition, accessory ectopic thyroid tissue is outside the path of thyroid ontogeny. Although in 1937 Norris concluded that the lateral thyroid anlage persists in humans (24) and that it differentiates into follicular elements, LiVolsi (52) considers its follicle contributions to be unclear. In dogs, however, the lateral anlage does produce follicles (138).

Accessory ectopic thyroid tissue may be functional. A scintigram following administration of radioactive iodine

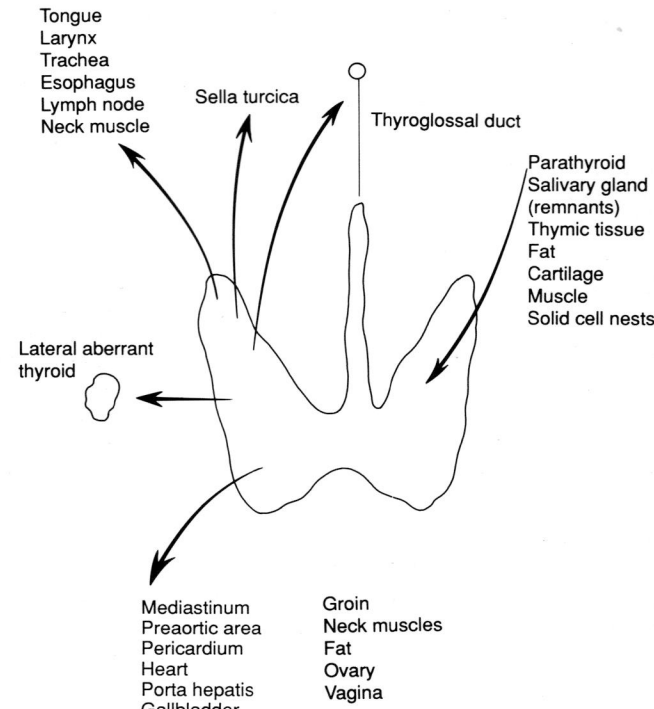

Figure 2.41. Possible sites of accessory ectopic thyroid tissue.

may verify the thyroid nature of suspected tissue and determine the presence of a normally situated thyroid gland.

Accessory ectopic thyroid tissue has been found in at least 13 locations (Table 2.9).

Intrathoracic thyroid tissue for which the blood supply comes from the thoracic vessels is very rare. The explanation for the occurrence of such tissue is that it remained attached to the pericardium or to the great vessels during the period of cervical elongation. In humans, intrathoracic thyroid tissue is usually considered to be a distal (or caudal) extension along the thyroid line: The thyroid tissue is in the anterior mediastinum, connects to cervical thyroid tissue, and gets its blood supply from the inferior thyroid artery. Alosco et al. report a retrotracheal goiter (8 cm in diameter) for which the blood supply came from the inferior thyroid artery (171). Intrapericardial thyroid tissue is quite rare in humans, but not infrequent in dogs.

Intratracheal thyroid tissue occurs in two separate fashions. The more common is that of contiguous growth into the tracheal lumen, from a normally located thyroid gland (172, 174). True ectopic intratracheal thyroid tissue is quite rare, but may account for 6 to 7% of all primary endotracheal tumors (175). However, Grillo had none in his series of 110 primary tracheal tumors (174). The endoscopic appearance is reminiscent of hemangioma, but the mass is not as compressible with the endoscope.

Lateral aberrant thyroid tissue is defined as thyroid tissue located lateral to the jugular vein (52). Such tissue continues to be a problem for the surgeon, the pathologist, and (of course) the patient. Lateral aberrant thyroid tissue manifests morphologically in three ways. First, such tissue may be a nodule attached to the main gland by connective tissue. Such islands of thyroid tissue, pulled away from the main body of the gland during development, are normal. Second, lateral thyroid tissue may be found within lymph nodes or within remnants of nodes. Clinically, a cervical lymph node containing thyroid follicles should be regarded as metastatic thyroid carcinoma. Notwithstanding this practical imperative, heterotopic thyroid tissue in cervical lymph nodes is recognized: Sawicki et al. (173) identified six cases in which the thyroid gland was normal at 5-μm sections. The third morphological group of laterally aberrant thyroid tissue is inexplicable except as congenital. Rubenfeld et al. apparently describe the first patient whose lateral aberrant thyroid tissue was the only thyroid tissue that the person possessed (170).

The ovarian thyroid (struma ovarii) is the most astonishing of the thyroid ectopias. It is not a true congenital anomaly and is not related to the anatomic thyroid gland. Thyroid tissue in the ovary is associated with dermoid cysts and teratomata. Woodruff et al. (176) estimate struma ovarii to exist in 0.2 to 1.3% of all ovarian tumors; in these cases 5 to 6% are bilateral and about 5% have functioning thyroid tissue. Hyperthyroidism in struma ovarii has been reported (178). Malignancy may occur in as many as 5% of cases of ovarian struma (179). Papillary carcinoma of struma ovarii can metastasize (52, 177).

Ectopic thyroid tissue in the sellar region has been documented; the thyroid gland itself was of normal size and weight, and serial sectioning did not reveal a tumor (180). Thyroid and gastric fundal epithelium has been reported in the gallbladder (181). Ectopic thyroid and parathyroid tissue has been found in the vagina (182). A congenital anomaly of thyroid follicles intermingled with skeletal muscle was described by Gardiner (183).

REFERENCES

1. Rathke H. Nova Acta Phys Med Bonn, 1828.
2. Von Baer CE. De ovi mammalium et hominis genesi. Epistolamad academian imperialem scientiarum petropolitanam. Leipzig (Lipsiae): Vossi L, 1827.
3. Von Ascherson FM. De fistulis colli congenitis adjecta fissurarum branchialium in mammalibus avibus historia succincta. Berlin: (Berolini): Jonas CH, 1832.
4. His W. Anatomie menschlicher embryonem. III. Zur Geschichte. Leipzig: FCW Vogel, 1885.
5. Born G. Über die derivate der embyonalen schlundbogen und schlundspalten bei säugetieren. Arch Mikr Anat 1883;22:271–318.
6. Piersol GA. Ueber die entwicklung der embryonalen schlundspalten und ihre derivate bei säugethieren. Zeit Wiss Zool 1888; 47.
7. Wenglowski R. Ueber die halsfisteln und cysten. Arch Klin Chir 1912;98:151–208.
8. Wenglowski R. Ueber die halsfisteln und cysten. Arch Klin Chir 1913;100:789–892.
9. Grosser O. The development of the pharynx and of the organs of respiration. In: Keibel F, Mall FP, eds. Manual of human embryology. Vol 1. Philadelphia: JB Lippincott, 1912;446–473.
10. Lyall D, Stahl WM. Lateral cervical cysts, sinuses and fistulas of congenital origin. Int Abstr Surg 1956;102:417–434.
11. Weller GL Jr. Development of the thyroid, parathyroid and thymus glands in man. Contrib Embryol Carnegie Inst Wash 1933;24:93–142.
12. Kingsbury BF. The development of the human pharynx. Am J Anat 1915;18:329–386.
13. Kingsbury BF. On the fate of the ultimobranchial body within the human thyroid. Anat Rec 1935;61:155–173.
14. Kingsbury BF. The question of a lateral thyroid in mammals with special reference to man. Am J Anat 1939;65:333–359.
15. Norris EH. The morphogenesis of the follicles in the human thyroid gland. Am J Anat 1916;20:411–448.
16. Norris EH. The early morphogenesis of the human thyroid gland. Am J Anat 1918;24:443–466.
17. Frazer JE. The disappearance of the precervical sinus. J Anat 1926;61:132–143.
18. Garrett FD. Development of the cervical vesicles in man. Anat Rec 1948;100:101–113.
19. Hendrick JW. Differential diagnosis of neck tumors. South Med J 1952;45:1019–1027.
20. Albers GD. Branchial anomalies. JAMA 1963;183:399–409.
21. Misugi K. The process of closure of the precervical sinus in the chick embryo. Yokohama Med Bull 1960;11:33–47.
22. Davies J. Embryology and anatomy of the head, neck, face, palate, nose and paranasal sinuses. In: Paparella MM, Shumrick DA, eds. Otolaryngology. Philadelphia: WB Saunders, 1980;63–123.
23. Bill AH Jr. Cysts and sinuses of the neck of thyroglossal and branchial origin. Surg Clin North Am 1956;36:1599–1611.
24. Norris EH. The parathyroid glands and lateral thyroid in man: their morphogenesis, histogenesis, topographic anatomy and prenatal growth. Contrib Embryol Carnegie Inst Wash 1937;26(159):247–294.
25. Granberg PL et al. Parathyroid tumors. Curr Probl Cancer 1985;9(11):1–52.
26. Sugiyama S. The embryology of the human thyroid gland including ultimobranchial body and others related. Ergebn Anat Entwickl Gesch 1971;44(H2):6–11.
27. Sadler TW. Langman's medical embryology. 6th ed. Baltimore: Williams & Wilkins, 1990.
28. Siegler R. The thymus and the unicorn: two great myths of gross anatomy. Anat Rec 1969;163:264.
29. Norris EH. The morphogenesis and histogenesis of the thymus gland in man: in which the origin of the Hassall's corpuscle of the human thymus is discovered. Contrib Embryol Carnegie Inst Wash 1938;27:191–207.
30. Hammar JA. Zur gröberen morphologie und morphogenie der menschenthymus. Anat Hefte 1911;43:201–242.
31. Shier KJ. The morphology of the epithelial thymus: observations on lymphocyte-depleted and fetal thymus. Lab Invest 1963;12:316–326.
32. Schambacher A. Über die persistenz von drüsenkanälen in der thymus und ihre beziehung zur entstehung der hassallschen körperchen. Virchow Arch Pathol Anat 1903;172:368.
33. Shier KJ. The thymus according to Schambacher: medullary ducts

and reticular epithelium of thymus and thymomas. Cancer 1981;48:1183–1199.

34. Papiernik M. Ontogeny of the human lymphoid system: study of the cytological maturation and the incorporation of tritiated thymidine and uridine in the foetal thymus and lymph node and in the infantile thymus. J Cell Physiol 1972;80:235–242.

35. Haynes BF. Phenotypic characterization and ontogeny of components of the human thymic microenvironment. Clin Res 1984;32(5):500–507.

36. Bockman DE, Kirby ML. Dependence of thymus development on derivatives of the neural crest. Science 1984;223:498–500.

37. Ellis HA, Knight B. Parathyroid and cervical thymus in sudden unexpected death in infancy. Pediatrics 1969;44:225–233.

38. His W. Der tractus thyreoglossus und seine beziehungen zum zungenbein. Arch Anat Physiol 1891;8:74.

39. Rogers WM. The fate of the ultimobranchial body in the white rat (mus norvegicus albinus). Am J Anat 1927;38:349–377.

40. Givel JC. Surgery of the thymus. Berlin: Springer-Verlag, 1990.

41. Copp DH, Cockcroft DW, Kueh Y. Calcitonin from ultimobranchial glands of dogfish and chickens. Science 1967;158:924–925.

42. Robertson DR. The effect of extirpation and transplantation of the ultimobranchial glands on calcitonin secretion. Anat Rec 1968;160:416.

43. Pearse AGE, Carvalheira AF. Cytochemical evidence for ultimobranchial origin of rodent thyroid C cells. Nature 1967;214:929–930.

44. Bussolati G, Pearse AGE. Immunofluorescent localization of calcitonin in the "C" cells of pig and dog thyroid. J Endocrinol 1967;37:205–209.

45. Merida-Velasco JA, Garcia-Garcia JD, Espin-Ferra J, Linares J. Origin of the ultimobranchial body and its colonizing cells in human embryos. Acta Anat 1989;135:325–330.

46. Sgalitzer KE. Contribution to the study of the morphogenesis of the thyroid gland. J Anat 1941;75:389–405.

47. Shepard TH, Andersen H, Andersen HJ. Histochemical studies of the human fetal thyroid during the first half of fetal life. Anat Rec 1964;149:363–380.

48. Bierring F, Shepard TH. The thyroid. In: DeHaan RL, Ursprung H, eds. Organogenesis. New York: Holt Rinehart & Winston, 1965.

49. Carpenter E. Development of fetal rat thyroid with special reference to uptake of radioactive iodine. J Exp Zool 1959;142:247–257.

50. Birnie JH, Mapp FE. Thyroid function in fetal rats. Fed Proc 1961;20:201.

51. Wollman SH, Swilling E. Radioiodine metabolism in the chick embryo. Endocrinology 1953;52:526–535.

52. LiVolsi VA. Surgical pathology of the thyroid. Philadelphia: WB Saunders, 1990.

53. Toran-Allerand CD. Normal development of the hypothalamic pituitary-thyroid axis. In: Ingbar SH, Braverman LE, eds. Werner's the thyroid. 5th ed. Philadelphia: JB Lippincott, 1986:7–23.

54. Arey LB. Developmental anatomy. Philadelphia: WB Saunders, 1965:241–243.

55. Van De Water TR, Noden DM, Maderson PFA. Embryology of the ear: outer, middle and inner. Otologic Med Surg 1988;I:3–27.

56. Melnick M, Myrianthopoulos NC. External ear malformations: epidemiology, genetics and natural history. Birth Defects 1979:15 (9).

57. Work WP. Newer concepts of first branchial cleft defects. Laryngoscope 1972;82:1581–1593.

58. Wilson CO. Lateral cysts and fistulas of the neck of developmental origin. Ann R Coll Surg Engl 1955;17:1–26.

59. Taylor JNS, Burwell RG. Branchiogenic nasopharyngeal cysts. J Laryngol 1954;68:667–679.

60. Nicolai P et al. Nasopharyngeal cysts: report of seven cases with review of the literature. Arch Otolaryngol Head Neck Surg 1989;115:860–864.

61. Todd NW, Martin WS. Relationship of eustachian tube bony landmarks and temporal bone pneumatization. Ann Otol Rhinol Laryngol 1988;97:277–280.

62. Montgomery WW. Surgery of the upper respiratory tract. Vol 2. Philadelphia: Lea & Febiger, 1973.

63. Miyauchi A et al. Piriform sinus fistula: a route of infection in acute suppurative thyroiditis. Arch Surg 1981;116:66–69.

64. Parke WW, Settles HE. Third pharyngeal pouch sinuses: report of a bilateral case with review of the embryology and literature. Clin Anat 1991;4:285–297.

65. Zarbo RJ, McClatchey KD, Areen RG, Baker SB. Thymopharyngeal duct cyst: a form of cervical thymus. Ann Otol Rhinol Laryngol 1983;92:284–289.

66. Liston SL. Fourth branchial fistula. Otolaryngol Head Neck Surg 1981;89:520–522.

67. Godin MS et al. Fourth branchial pouch sinus: principles of diagnosis and management. Laryngoscope 1990;100:174–178.

68. Frazer JE. The nomenclature of diseased states caused by certain vestigial structures in the neck. Br J Surg 1923;11:131–136.

69. Lahey FH, Nelson HF. Branchial cysts and sinuses. Ann Surg 1941;113:508–512.

70. Proctor B. Lateral vestigial cysts and fistulas of the neck. Laryngoscope 1955;65:355–401.

71. Gray SW, Skandalakis JE, Androulakis JA. Nonthyroid tumors of the neck. Contemp Surg 1985;26:13–24.

72. Martin H, Morfit HM, Ehrlich H. The case for branchiogenic cancer (malignant branchioma). Ann Surg 1950;132:867–887.

73. Micheau C, Klijanienko J, Luboinski B, Richard J. So-called branchiogenic carcinoma is actually cystic metastases in the neck from a tonsillar primary. Laryngoscope 1990;100:878–883.

74. Gray SW et al. Parathyroid glands. Am Surg 1976;42:653–656.

75. Albright F. A page out of the history of hyperparathyroidism. J Clin Endocrinol 1948;8:637–657.

76. Sandstrom J. On a new gland in man and several mammals (glandulae parathyroeoideae). Upsala Lk-Fren Frh 1879–80;15:441.

77. Gilmour JR. The gross anatomy of the parathyroid glands. J Pathol Bact 1938;46:133–149.

78. Alveryd A. Parathyroid gland in thyroid surgery. Acta Chir Scand (supp) 1968;389:1–120.

79. Wang CA. The anatomic basis of parathyroid surgery. Ann Surg 1976;183:271–275.

80. Akerström G, Malmaeus J, Bergstrom R. Surgical anatomy of human parathyroid glands. Surgery 1984;95:14–21.

81. Gaz RD, Doubler PB, Wang CA. The management of 50 unusual hyperfunctioning parathyroid glands. Surgery 1987;102:949–957.

82. Conn JM, Goncalves MA, Mansour KA, McGarity WC. The mediastinal parathyroid. Am Surg 1991;57:62–66.

83. Heinbach WF. A study of the number and location of the parathyroid glands in man. Anat Rec 1933;57:251–257.

84. Udekwu AO, Kaplan EL, Wu TC, Arganini M. Ectopic parathyroid adenoma of the lateral triangle of the neck: report of two cases. Surgery 1987;101:114–118.

85. Herrold KM, Rabson AS, Ketcham AS. Aberrant parathyroid gland in pharyngeal submucosa. Arch Pathol 1961;71:60–62.

86. Carty SE, Norton JA. Management of patients with persistent or recurrent primary hyperthyroidism. World J Surg 1991;15:716–723.

87. Janelli DE. The parathyroid glands, with special emphasis on surgical aspects. Int Abstr Surg 1956;102:105–126.

88. Feliciano DV. Parathyroid pathology in an intrathyroidal position. Am J Surg 1992;164:496–500.

89. Farr HW. Hyperparathyroidism and cancer. Cancer 1976;26:66–109.

90. Black BM, Haynes AL. Intrathyroid hyperfunctioning parathyroid adenomas: report of two cases. Proc Staff Meet Mayo Clin 1949;24:408.

91. Lunghi F, DiFranco R, Lunghi M, Perin B. Ectopic parathyroid adenoma of the lateral triangle of the neck. Acta Otorhinolaryngol Ital 1988;8:533–538.

92. DiGeorge AM. Discussion: cellular basis of immunity. J Pediatr 1965;67:907–908.

93. Gilmour JR. The weight of the parathyroid glands. J Pathol Bact 1937;44:431–462.

94. DeLattre JF, Flament JB, Palot JP, Pluot M. J Dhir (Paris) 1982;119(11):633–641.

95. Gilmour JR. The normal histology of the parathyroid glands. J Pathol Bact 1939;48:187–222.

96. Calandra DB et al. Parathyroid cysts: a report of eleven cases including two with hyperparathyroid crisis. Surgery 1983;94:887–892.

97. Goris C. Extirpation de trois lobules parathyroidiens kystiques. J Clin Ann Soc Belge Chir 1905;5:394.

98. Perdue GD, Martin JD. Parathyroid cysts: report of a case. Am Surg 1959;25:698–701.

99. Ferrara BE, Haze ll S, Parker TH. Parathyroid cyst. South Med J 1985;78:528–532.

100. Lange CK, Palepu S, Fontana FL. Parathyroid cysts. Contemp Surg 1988;33:69–71.

101. Shields TW, Staley CJ. Functioning parathyroid cyst. Arch Surg 1961;82:937–942.

102. McGinty CP, Lischer CE. The surgical significance of parathyroid cysts. Surg Gynecol Obstet 1963;117:703–708.

103. Petri N, Holten I. Parathyroid cyst: report of a case in the mediastinum. J Laryngol Otol 1990;104:56–57.

104. Lobdell DH. Congenital absence of parathyroid glands. Arch Pathol 1959;67:412–414.

105. Thomas RA, Landing BH, Wells TR. Embryologic and other developmental considerations of thirty-eight possible variants of the DiGeorge anomaly. Am J Med Genet 1987;3(supp):43–66.

106. Stevens CA, Carey JC, Shigeoka AO. DiGeorge anomaly and velocardiofacial syndrome. Pediatrics 1990;85:526–305.

107. Freedom RM, Rosen FS, Nadas AS. Congenital cardiovascular disease and anomalies of the third and fourth pharyngeal pouch. Circulation 1972;46.

108. Dallapiccola B, Marino B, Giannotti A, Valorani G. DiGeorge anomaly associated with partial deletion of chromosome 22: report of a case with x/22 translocation and review of the literature. Ann Genet 1989;32:92–96.

109. de la Chapelle A, Herva R, Koivisto M, Aula P. A deletion in chromosome 22 can cause DiGeorge syndrome. Hum Genet 1981;57:253–256.

110. Jones MC. The neurocristophathies: reinterpretation based upon the mechanism of abnormal morphogenesis. Cleft Palate 1990;27:136–140.

111. Hofmann WJ, Moller P, Otto HF. Hyperplasia. In: Givel J-C, ed. Surgery of the thymus. Berlin: Springer-Verlag, 1990:63ff.

112. Terribile V. Su di un caso di pancreatite fetale associata ad anomalia timica. Boll Soc Ital Pat 1967;10:46–48.

113. Leong ASY. Thymic cysts. In: Givel JC, ed. Surgery of the thymus. Berlin: Springer-Verlag, 1990:71–77.

114. Scully RE, Mark EJ, McNeely BU. Case records of the Massachusetts General Hospital (case #47). N Engl J Med 1982;307:1391–1397.

115. Guba AM Jr, Adam AE, Jaques DA, Chambers RG. Cervical presentation of thymic cysts. Am J Surg 1978;136:430–436.

116. Suster S, Rosai J. Multilocular thymic cyst: an acquired reactive process: study of 18 cases. Am J Surg Pathol 1991;15:388–398.

117. Indeglia RA, Shea MA, Grage TB. Congenital cysts of the thymus gland. Arch Surg 1967;94:149–152.

118. Spigland N, Bensoussan AL, Blanchard H, Russo P. Aberrant cervical thymus in children: three case reports and review of the literature. J Pediatr Surg 1990;25:1196–1199.

119. Civi I, Kurtay M, Civi S. Bilateral thymus found in association with unilateral cleft lip and palate. Plast Reconstr Surg 1989;83:143–47.

120. Dado DV, Gonzalez-Crussi F. Bilateral ectopic thymus gland tissue associated with the cleft lip and palate. Plast Reconstr Surg 1989;84:376.

121. Gilmour JR. Some developmental abnormalities of the thymus and parathyroids. J Pathol Bact 1941;52:213–218.

122. Chan JKC, Rosai J. Tumors of the neck showing thymic or related branchial pouch differentiation: a unifying concept. Hum Pathol 1991;22:349–367.

123. Ceuppens H. Thymic cyst in an unusual site. Neth J Surg 1984;36:17–19.

124. Bar-Ziv J, Barki Y, Itzchak Y, Mares AJ. Posterior mediastinal accessory thymus. Pediatr Radiol 1984;14:165–167.

125. Ramsay AJ. Experimental studies on the developmental potentialities of the third pharyngeal pouch in the mammalian embryo (mouse). Anat Rec 1950;106:234.

126. Crotti A. Thyroid and thymus. Philadelphia: Lea & Febiger, 1918:536.

127. Hegedus L, Hansen JM, Veiergang D, Karstrup S. Does prophylactic thyroxine treatment after operation for non-toxic goiter influence thyroid size? Br Med J [Clin Res] 1987;294:801–803.

128. Gaby M. The role of thyroid dygenesis and maldescent in the etiology of sporadic cretinism. J Pediatr 1962;60:830–835.

129. Harada T et al. Fatal thyroid carcinoma: anaplastic transformation of adenocarcinoma. Cancer 1977;39:2588–2596.

130. Burman KD, Adler RA, Wartofsky L. Hemiagenesis of the thyroid gland. Am J Med 1975;58:143–146.

131. Melnick JC, Stemkowski PE. Thyroid hemiagenesis (hockey stick sign): a review of the world literature and report of four cases. J Clin Endocrinol Metab 1981;52:247–252.

132. Piera J, Garriga J, Calabuig R, Bargallo D. Thyroidal hemiagenesis. Am J Surg 1986;151(3):419–421.

133. Greening WP, Sarker SK, Osborne MP. Hemiagenesis of the thyroid gland. Br J Surg 1980;67:446–448.

134. Marshall CF. Variations in the form of the thyroid gland in man. J Anat Physiol 1895;29:234.

135. Gray SW, Skandalakis JE. Embryology for surgeons: the embryological basis for the treatment of congenital defects. 1st ed. Philadelphia: WB Saunders, 1972.

136. Soliman SM. Thyroid cartilage at the suprasternal notch with low situated thyroid gland. J Laryngol Otol 1988;102:476–478.

137. McGregor AL, Duplessis DJ. A synopsis of surgical anatomy. 10th ed. Baltimore: Williams & Wilkins, 1969.

138. Kameda Y, Shigemoto H, Ikeda A. Development and cytodifferentiation of C cell complexes in dog fetal thyroids: an immunohistochemical study using anti-calcitonin, anti-C-thyroglobulin and anti-19S thyroglobulin antisera. Cell Tissue Res 1980;206:403–415.

139. Godwin MC. The mammalian thymus IV: the development in the dog. Am J Anat 1939;64:165–201.

140. Janzer RC, Weber E, Hedinger C. The relation between solid cell nests and C-cells of the thyroid gland. Cell Tissue Res 1979;197:295–312.

141. Tzinas S et al. Vascular patterns of the thyroid gland. Am Surg 1976;42:639–644.

142. Sartor K, Freckmann N, Boker DK. Related anomalies of origin of left vertebral and left inferior thyroid arteries: report of three cases. Neuroradiol 1980;19:27–30.

143. Krudy AG, Doppman JL, Brennan MV. The significance of the thyroid ima artery in arteriographic localization of parathyroid adenomas. Radiology 1980;45–51.

144. Rouviere H. Anatomy of the human lymphatic system. Ann Arbor, MI: Edwards Bros, 1938.

145. Stedman GW. Singular distribution of some of the nerves and arteries in the neck and the top of the thorax. Edin Med Surg J 1823;19:564.

146. Pemberton J de J, Stalker LK. Cysts, sinuses, and fistulae of the thyroglossal duct. Ann Surg 1940;111:950–957.

147. Henry JF, Audiffret J, Plan M. The nonrecurrent inferior laryngeal nerve: apropos of 19 cases including 2 on the left side. J Chir (Paris) 1985;122(6–7):391–397.

148. Proye CAG, Carnaille BM, Goropoulos A. Nonrecurrent and recurrent inferior laryngeal nerve: a surgical pitfall in cervical exploration. Am J Surg 1991;162(11):495.

149. Skandalakis JE et al. The recurrent laryngeal nerve. Am Surg 1976;42:629–634.

150. Reed AF. The relations of the inferior laryngeal nerve to the inferior thyroid artery. Anat Rec 1943;85:17–23.

151. Droulias C et al. The superior laryngeal nerve. Am Surg 1976;42:635–638.

152. Moosman DA, DeWeese MS. The external laryngeal nerve as related to thyroidectomy. Surg Gynecol Obstet 1968;127:1011–1116.

153. Hollinshead WN. Anatomy for surgeons: the head and neck. 2nd ed. New York: Harper & Row, 1968.

154. Baldwin RL, Copeland SK. Lingual thyroid and associated epiglottitis. South Med J 1988;81:1538–1541.

155. Charkes ND. Thyroid and whole-body imaging. In: Ingbar SH, Braverman LE, eds: Werner's the thyroid. 5th ed. Philadelphia: JB Lippincott, 1986.

156. Haddad A, Frenkiel S, Costom B, Shapiro R, Tewfik T. Management of the undescended thyroid. J Otolaryngol 1986;15:373–376.

157. Radkowski D et al. Thyroglossal duct remnants: preoperative evaluation and management. Arch Otolaryngol Head Neck Surg 1991:117:1378–1381.

158. Solomon J, Rangecroft L. Thyroglossal duct lesions in children. J Pediatr Surg 1984;19:555.

159. Hoffman MA, Schuster SR. Thyroglossal duct remnants in infants and children: reevaluation of histopathology and methods for resection. Ann Otol Rhinol Laryngol 1988;97:483–486.

160. deMello DE, Lima JA, Liapis H. Midline cervical cysts in children: thyroglossal anomalies. Arch Otolaryngol Head Neck Surg 1987;113:418–420.

161. Sistrunk WE. The surgical treatment of cysts of the thyroglossal tract. Ann Surg 1920;71:121–122.

162. Stahl WM Jr, Lyall D. Cervical cysts and fistulae of thyroglossal tract origin. Ann Surg 1954;139:123–128.

163. Kostanecki K, Mielecki A. Die angebornen Kiemenfisteln des merschen. Virchow Arch Path Anat 1890;120:385–436 and 1890;121:55–87.

164. Katz AD, Hachigian M. Thyroglossal duct cysts: a thirty year experience with emphasis on occurrence in older patients. Am J Surg 1983;155:741–743.

165. Vater A. Regiae Magnae Britanniae Societati dicata, qua ductus salivalis in lingua, noviter antehac detectus, nunc elucidatus, confirmatus, novisque, experimentis adstructus, in publicum prodit, ac simul varia observata et experimenta circa ductus excretorios tonsillarum ac glandulae thyroideae exponuntur [Dissertation]. Accessit catalogus Societatis regiae Wittenberg [Wittenbergae], Gerdesiae, 1723.

166. Skandalakis JE, Godwin JT, Androulakis JA, Gray SW. The differential diagnosis of tumors of the neck. In: Ariel IM, ed. Progress in clinical cancer. New York: Grune & Stratton, 1970:141–159.

167. Hawkins DB, Jacobsen BE, Klatt EC. Cysts of the thyroglossal duct. Laryngoscope 1982;92:1254–1258.

168. Ashworth JT Jr. Three generations of thyroglossal duct remnant in one family. J Family Pract 1979;8:624–625.

169. Fernandez JF et al. Thyroglossal duct carcinoma. Surgery 1991;110(6):928–934.

170. Rubenfeld S et al. Ectopic thyroid in the right carotid triangle. Arch Otolaryngol Head Neck Surg 1988;114:913–915.

171. Alosco T, Eisenberg B, Keller SM. Retrotracheal goiter. South Med J 1990;83:239–240.

172. Donnegan JO, Wood MD. Intratracheal thyroid: familial occurrence. Laryngoscope 1985;95:6–8.

173. Sawicki MP, Howard TJ, Passaro E Jr. Heterotopic tissue in lymph nodes: an unrecognized problem. Arch Surg 1990;125(10):1394–1398.

174. Grillo HC. Tracheal surgery. Scand J Thorac Cardiovasc Surg 1983;17:67–77.

175. Fish J, Moore RM. Ectopic thyroid tissue and ectopic thyroid carcinoma. Ann Surg 1963;157:212–222.

176. Woodruff JD, Rauh JT, Markley RL. Ovarian struma. Obstet Gynecol 1966;27:194–201.

177. Rosenblum NG et al. Malignant struma ovarii. Gynecol Oncol 1989;32:224–227.

178. Kempers RD et al. Struma ovarii: ascitic, hyperthyroid and asymptomatic syndromes. Ann Intern Med 1970;72:883–892.

179. Yannopoulos D, Yannopoulos K, Ossowski R. Malignant struma ovarii. Pathol Ann 1976;11:403–413.

180. Ruchti C, Balli-Antunes M, Gerber HA. Follicular tumor in the sellar region without primary cancer of the thyroid: heterotopic carcinoma? Am J Clin Pathol 1987;87:776–780.

181. Curtis LE, Sheahan DG. Heterotopic tissues in the gallbladder. Arch Pathol 1969;88:677–683.

182. Kurman RJ, Prabha AC. Thyroid and parathyroid glands in the vaginal wall. Am J Clin Pathol 1973;59:503–507.

183. Gardiner WR. Unusual relationships between thyroid gland and skeletal muscle in infants. Cancer 1956;9:681–691.

CHAPTER 3

THE ESOPHAGUS

John Elias Skandalakis / Stephen Wood Gray / Richard Ricketts

Hitherto the esophagus has had no patron. It has been used, and sometimes ill-used and ignorantly used, by physicians, otolaryngologists, thoracic surgeons, general surgeons and ontologic surgeons even today.
—*R.G. ELMSLIE IN* SURGERY OF THE ESOPHAGUS,
G.G. JAMIESON, ED. *(1988)*

DEVELOPMENT

The cranial end of both the esophagus and trachea becomes demarcated with the appearance of a median ventral diverticulum of the foregut about 22 or 23 days after fertilization. The embryo at this stage is about 3 mm long and approximately 10 somites are visible (stage 10). Shortly after the formation of this diverticulum, the spindle-shaped enlargement of the stomach appears immediately posterior to it. The esophagus will develop from the small area of endoderm between the tracheal diverticulum and the stomach dilation. The endoderm in this area has two to three layers of low columnar cells, whereas that of the rest of the foregut has but one layer.

The tracheal diverticulum rapidly becomes a groove in the floor of the esophagus, and elongation of both structures begins. Ridges of cells appear on the lateral walls, and beginning at the posterior end of the tracheal groove, the union of these ridges divides the foregut into tracheal (ventral part) and esophageal channels (dorsal part) (1) (Fig. 3.1). At the distal end of the tracheal primordium, the lung buds are visible. Although separation proceeds toward the head, simultaneous elongation of both trachea and esophagus prevents the completion of the process before 34 to 36 days of age (stage 17) (Fig. 3.2). By this stage, the beginning of the submucosal and muscular layers of both esophagus and trachea are visible. The elongation involves first the lower portion of the esophagus and later the upper portion (2). At the level of the tracheal bifurcation, the diameter is reduced so that it actually is smaller than it was at an earlier stage. It is here that most esophageal atresias occur.

Elongation of the esophagus appears to carry the stomach primordium down 16 segments to a position below the forming diaphragm. This apparent descent is actually accomplished by growth of the body craniad, away from the transverse septum and pericardium. Elongation results from "ascent" of the pharynx, rather than "descent" of the stomach (Fig. 3.3 and Fig. 5.1).

The final length of the esophagus is not attained until the seventh week, at which time the abdominal portion of the esophagus is relatively longer than in the adult.

In the newborn infant, the esophagus is slightly more than one-fourth the combined length of the head and trunk. According to Hillemeier (3), at birth the esophagus measures approximately 8 to 10 cm, from the cricoid cartilage to the diaphragm, and it doubles in length during the first few years of life. Lymph capillaries first appear in the submucosa of the esophagus at 3 and 4 months of life (4).

The walls of the esophagus receive both sympathetic and parasympathetic innervation from both myenteric and submucosal plexuses. Parasympathetic innervation of the esophagus is by the vagus nerve with the upper portion being supplied by the recurrent pharyngeal nerves and the vagus below. Sympathetic innervation is from the mediastinal branches of the thoracic sympathetic trunk and from the celiac plexus (3).

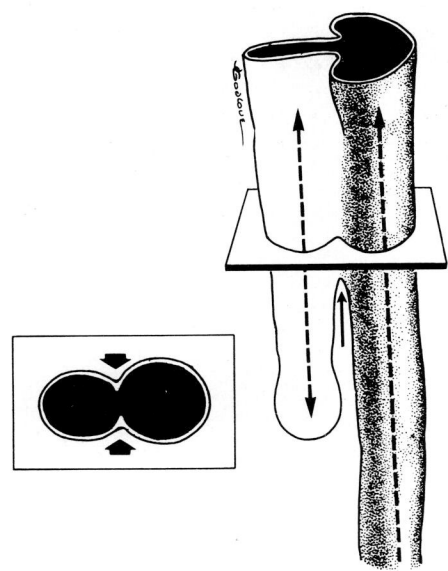

Figure 3.1. Division of the primitive foregut, with stippled area showing the future esophageal portion. *Arrows* indicate the local morphogenetic movements.

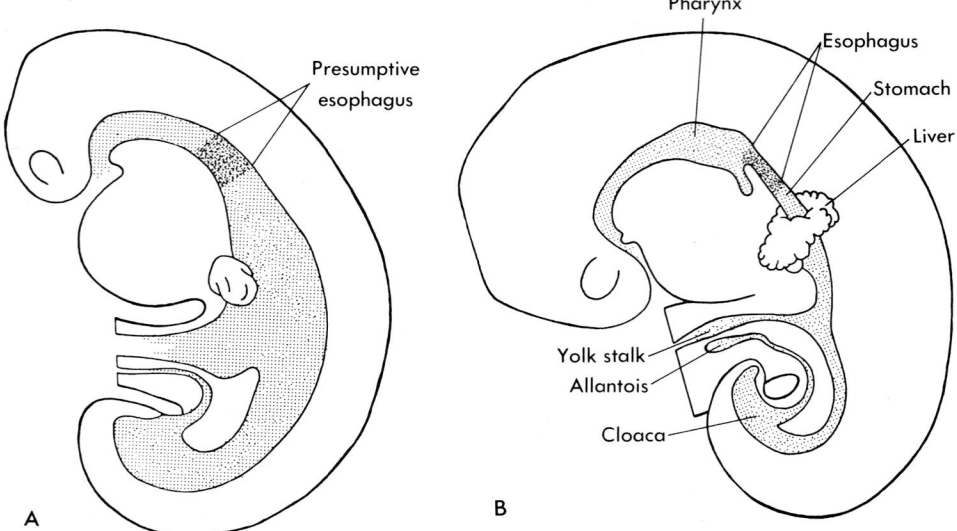

Figure 3.2.   Elongation of the esophagus by cranial growth of the embryonic body. **A**, At 2.5 mm (fourth week). **B**, At 4.2 mm (fifth week). (After Blechschmidt E. The stages of human development before birth. Philadelphia; WB Saunders 1961.)

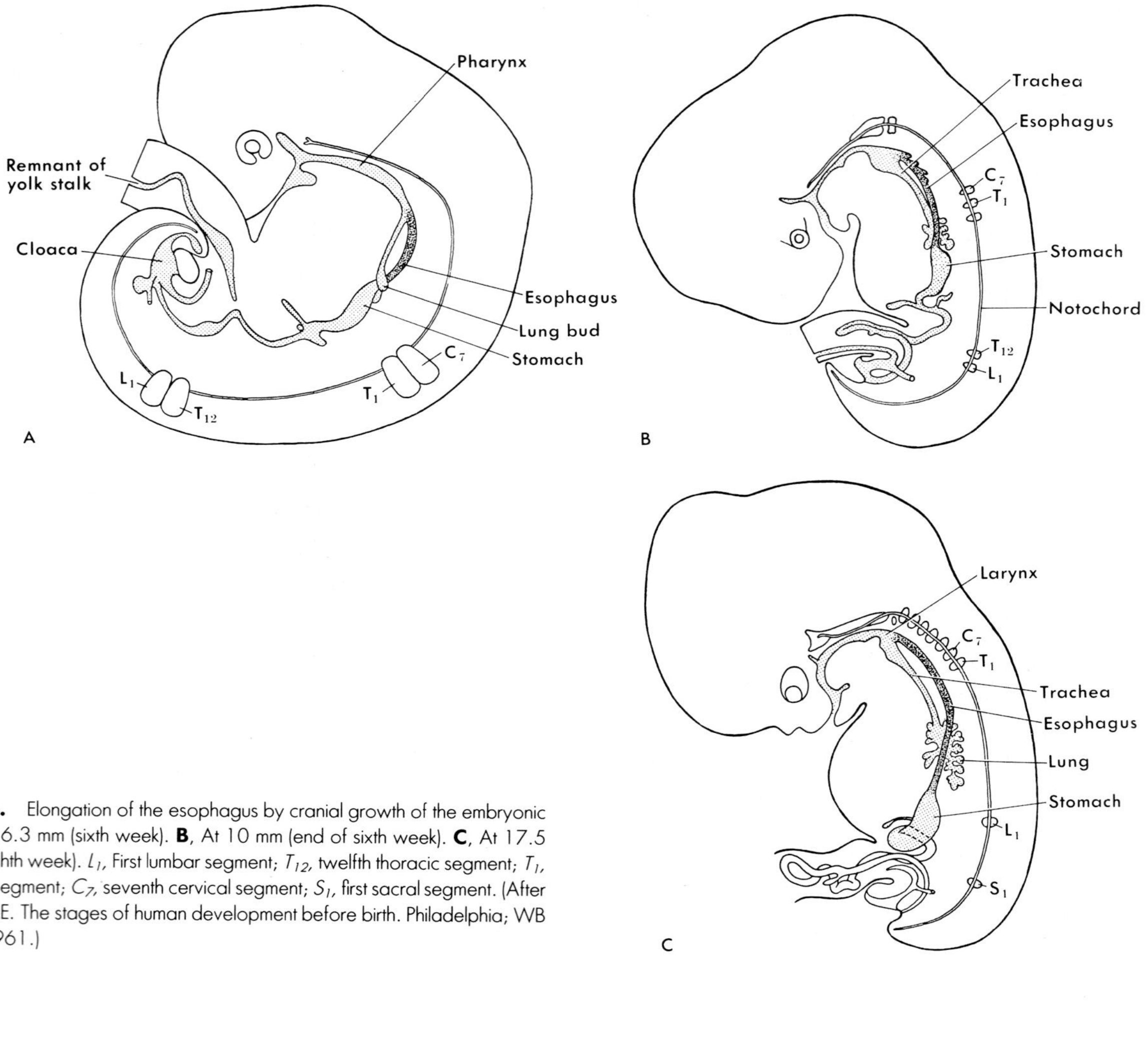

Figure 3.3.   Elongation of the esophagus by cranial growth of the embryonic body. **A**, At 6.3 mm (sixth week). **B**, At 10 mm (end of sixth week). **C**, At 17.5 mm (early eighth week). L_1, First lumbar segment; T_{12}, twelfth thoracic segment; T_1, first thoracic segment; C_7, seventh cervical segment; S_1, first sacral segment. (After Blechschmidt E. The stages of human development before birth. Philadelphia; WB Saunders, 1961.)

The circular muscle coat of mesoderm (mesenchyme) appears early in the sixth week (9 mm), and before the end of the week, branches of the vagus nerves having terminal groups of cells are found just outside the circular musculature. These are the ganglion cells of the myenteric plexus. Blood vessels enter the submucosa from the aorta during the seventh week. The longitudinal musculature is indicated by the ninth week (30 mm), but it is not a definite layer until the 12th week (55 mm). The muscularis mucosae is first differentiated at the lower end in the fourth month and becomes complete a few weeks later.

The esophageal lumen, round at first, becomes flattened dorsoventrally above and laterally below during the fifth week. Longitudinal folds, which are often taken to be random foldings of the wall of a collapsed organ, appear in a definite pattern. Four primary folds are present by the 10th week. The dorsal and ventral folds develop caudad from the upper end and the lateral folds develop cephalad from the lower end. By about the 12th week, the lumen of the esophagus in transverse section has assumed the form of a Greek cross. In the lower third, the ridges rotate 90 degrees clockwise (looking caudad). This is a continuation of the rotation of the stomach, which begins before the esophageal folds are formed. During the fifth month, secondary folds appear by similar processes (Fig. 3.4).

During the seventh and eighth weeks, the esophageal epithelium proliferates until the lumen is nearly filled with cells. Irregular spaces within the cellular mass form communication channels; complete occlusion of the lumen does not normally occur in humans. A solid stage in the development of the esophagus was described by Kreuter in 1905 (5), but its existence was disproved shortly thereafter by Forssner (6) and Schridde (7). However, the rare occurrence of a mucosal diaphragm across the lumen of the esophagus suggests that occlusion may occasionally take place.

By the 10th week, the vacuoles have disappeared, and a single lumen is restored. The superficial layer of epithelial cells has become ciliated chiefly on the infolded ridges. Ciliated cells increase up to the fifth prenatal month.

During the fourth month of gestation, the ciliated epithelium begins to be replaced, starting in midesophagus, by islands of stratified squamous epithelium. Patches of ciliated epithelium may be present at birth although usually these are seen only in premature infants (8). At birth, only a few papillary ridges attach the epithelium to the lamina propria mucosae. These increase during the first postnatal year.

Small areas of columnar cells near the two ends of the esophagus are not replaced by stratified squamous epi-

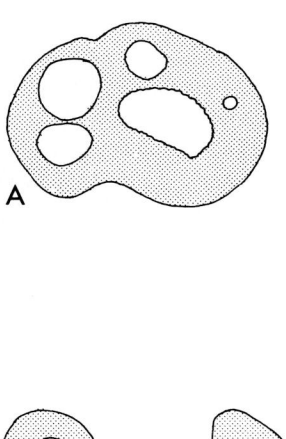

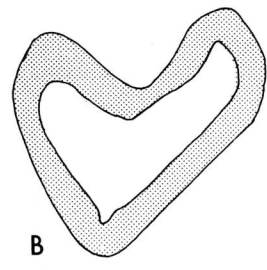

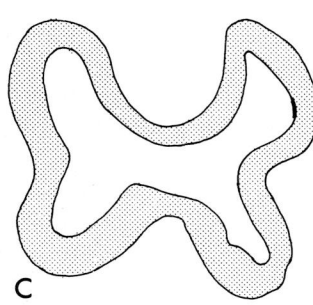

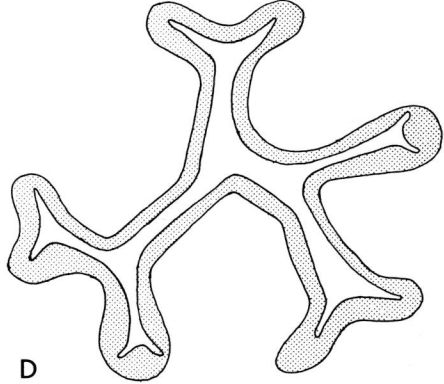

Figure 3.4. Changes in the shape of the esophageal lumen. **A**, At 19 mm (eighth week). **B**, At 37 mm (ninth week). **C**, At 42 mm (late ninth week). **D**, At 120 mm (about the 15th week). (Adapted from Lewis FT. The development of the diges- tive tract and of the organs of respiration: the development of the oesophagus. In Keibel F, Mall FP, eds. Human Embryology, Vol II, Philadelphia: JB Lippincott, 1912.)

thelium; from these come the superficial esophageal glands. Near term the deep esophageal glands appear from similar areas between primary folds.

Piekarsky and Stephens (9) believe that the co-existence of other defects is due to damage of the mesenchymal tissue of the fourth week of gestation.

Reduction in birth weight is associated with intrauterine esophageal obstruction as reported by the experimental work in rabbits by Wesson et al. (10).

Further details concerning the development of the esophagus may be found in the work of Johnson (11), Johns (12), and Botha (13).

Remember:

1. Genesis of esophageal stenosis, atresia, and tracheoesophageal fistula is most likely caused by (*a*) incomplete recanalization of the esophageal lumen or (*b*) deviation of the retroesophageal septum posteriorly, resulting in a faulty partition of the foregut (laryngotracheal tube).

2. Hydramnios or polyhydraminos (excess of amniotic fluid between 1500 to 2000 ml, according to Sadler [14]) is present with atresia due to the inability of the fetus to swallow amniotic fluid into the gastrointestinal tract and secondary collection of the fluid in the amniotic sac (big uterus), moving to the placenta and finally to the maternal circulation.

Critical Events in Development

Two events in the development of the esophagus are of special interest because of the frequency with which they may result in malformations. One is the partitioning of

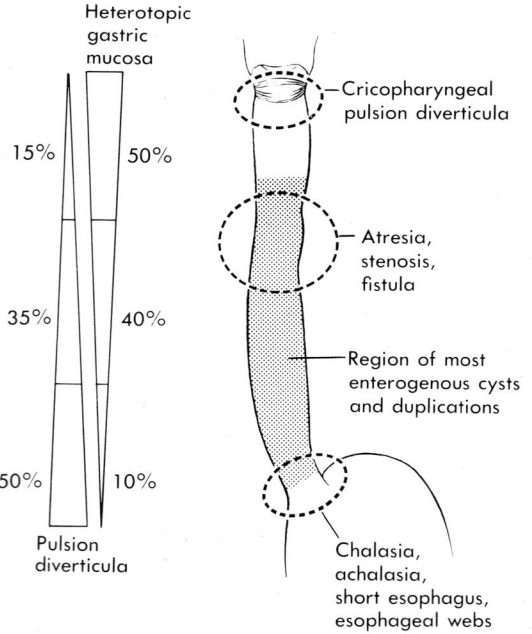

Figure 3.5. Usual location of malformations of the esophagus.

the foregut into esophagus and trachea during the fourth week, which may result in a wide variety of defects if the process fails to proceed normally. The second, a much less dramatic event, is the formation of the cardiac junction. Although not mechanically complicated, this involves coordination between the development of the esophagus, stomach, and diaphragm and the autonomic innervation of these structures. In this area, apparently insignificant developmental variations from the sixth week until birth can result in physiologic problems that may harass their victim throughout life (Fig. 3.5).

ANOMALIES OF THE ESOPHAGUS

Common esophageal anomalies and their characteristics are summarized in Table 3.1. Anomalies and related lesions of the lower esophageal segment and cardiac orifice are given later in this chapter (see Table 3.5).

Esophageal Stenosis, Atresia, and Tracheoesophageal Fistula

ANATOMY

The embryonic separation of the trachea from the esophagus, a major developmental maneuver, provides considerable opportunity for malformation to occur. A number of defects of common embryonic origin, but with different clinical manifestations, are known. They may be divided roughly into the following groups (Fig. 3.6): (*a*) partial or complete failure of trachea and esophagus to separate; (*b*) partial or complete absence of the trachea; (*c*) partial or complete absence of the esophagus; (*d*) atresia of the esophagus without tracheal fistula; (*e*) atresia of the esophagus with tracheal fistula; (*f*) tracheoesophageal fistula without esophageal atresia; and (*g*) stenosis of the esophagus.

Failure of Separation of Trachea and Esophagus (Persistent Foregut). Very rarely, the trachea may fail to separate from the esophagus along its entire length (15, 16) or only the cephalic portions of the two organs remain joined. Failure of separation does not affect differentiation; hence, the "esophagotrachea" has ciliated epithelium and cartilaginous rings anteriorly and stratified squamous epithelium and muscle posteriorly (Fig. 3.7, *A*). This anomaly is discussed in more detail in the section on laryngotracheoesophageal cleft later in this chapter.

Failure of separation at only the cephalic end results in cleft larynx and is discussed in Chapter 12, "The Larynx."

A curious case is known in which three tracheoesophageal fistulae were present without esophageal atresia. This represents a stage between complete failure of septation and the usual type of tracheoesophageal fistula (17).

Table 3.1.
Anomalies of the Esophagus

Anomaly	Origin of Defect	First Appearance	Sex Chiefly Affected	Relative Frequency	Comments
Esophageal atresia, stenosis, and tracheoesophageal fistula	21 to 34 days	At birth	Equal	Common	—
Laryngotracheoesophageal cleft	3rd to 5th week	At birth	Equal	Rare	Type I to IV (larynx to bronchi)
VACTERL associations	Variable; 3 to 5 wk	At birth	Equal	10 to 23% of esophageal atresia/ TEE[a]	—
Esophageal webs and rings	7th wk(?) (if congenital)	Any age	Male	Rare	May never produce symptoms
True duplication	7th wk	Any age	?	Very rare	May never produce symptoms
Enterogenous cysts	End of 3rd wk	Birth to any age	Female(?)	Rare	
Diverticula (excluding traction diverticula)	5th mo to birth(?)	Any age	Male	Uncommon	Muscular weakness may exist indefinitely without herniation occurring
Heterotopic mucosa	5th mo to birth	Any age (if at all)	Equal(?)	Common	May never produce symptoms
Congenital short esophagus	7th wk	Birth to any age	Male	Rare	May never produce symptoms
Achalasia	Late 6th wk(?)	Infancy	Equal	Uncommon	Cases appearing in later life are not of embryonic origin
Chalasia	Late 6th wk(?)	Shortly after birth	Equal	Very common	Resolves spontaneously in most cases as LES matures

[a]From Chittmittrapap S, Spitz L, Kiely EM, Brereton RJ. Oesophageal atresia and associated anomalies. Arch Dis Child 1989;64:364–368.

Absence of the Trachea. (See also Chapter 13, "The Trachea and Lungs," for a discussion of tracheal atresia.) Even more rare is the differentiation of the entire foregut into esophagus with only vestigial tracheal structure developing. In some cases bronchi may arise directly from the esophagus (18) (Fig. 3.7, *B*); in others, the trachea, if formed, failed to develop and the bronchi are blind (19) (Fig. 3.7, *C*).

EDITORIAL COMMENT

Very few cases of absence of the trachea have been reported, probably because these infants all die at birth or are stillborn. There are examples of severe tracheal stenosis which can result in severe respiratory distress with a very high mortality. Successful cases of tracheal reconstruction have been reported recently. We corrected a very tight tracheal stenosis at carina (the opening was less than 2 mm. in diameter) by placing the child on ECMO and repairing the tracheal stenosis with resection and primary anastomosis. The baby was kept on ECMO for a few days to allow for healing of the tracheal anastomosis and then was successfully decannulated. While the baby had continuing problems with bronchomalacia, she eventually recovered from this serious complication. The technique of cardiopulmonary bypass has also been reported for the use of tracheal reconstruction, either on a congenital or traumatic basis, but this carries with it the significant problem of prolonged cardiopulmonary bypass or immediate cessation with positive pressure ventilation through the fresh tracheal anastomosis. We believe the use of ECMO may be a better alternative because it avoids positive pressure ventilation and its stresses on the new tracheal suture line (JAH/CNP).

Absence of the Esophagus. If the entire foregut differentiates into trachea, there may be complete absence of the esophagus. A strip of stratified squamous epithelium on the posterior tracheal wall may represent the suppressed esophagus (1), or there may be a fibrous cord indicating failure of the esophageal primordium to develop (Fig. 3.8, *A*).

More commonly, either the upper end or both upper and lower ends of the esophagus are present, with a fibrous band representing the remainder of the organ. In less extreme forms, the condition grades into segmental atresia (Fig. 3.8, *B* and *C*).

Atresia of the Esophagus. Atresia may be of two types. The usual type is segmental, with the atretic portion of the esophagus absent or represented by a fibrous cord (Fig. 3.8, *B* and *C*). A second, much rarer type is produced by a membranous diaphragm at any level of the esopha-

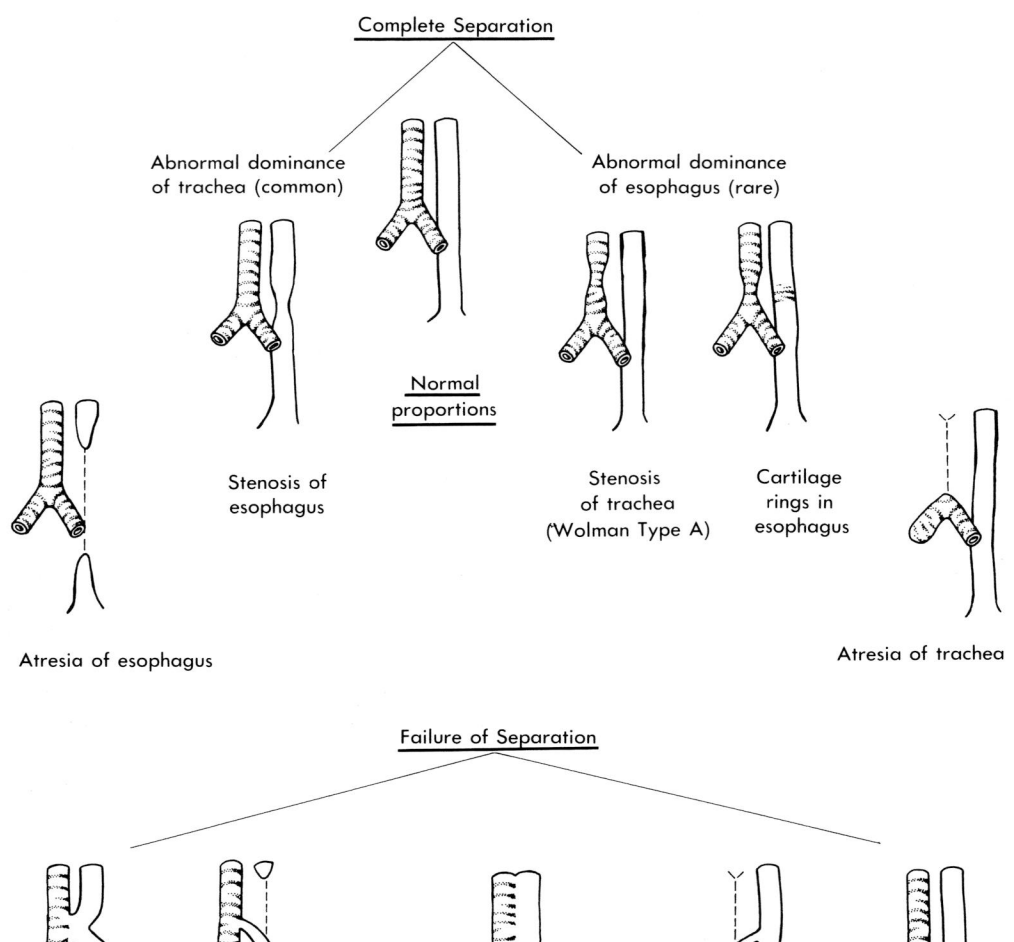

Figure 3.6. Patterns of developmental errors in the division of the primitive foregut.

gus (Fig. 3.8, *D* and *E*) (20). Although the diaphragmatic type produces the same symptoms as the segmental type, it may not have the same origin as other defects of the tracheoesophageal complex. (See section on esophageal webs.)

EDITORIAL COMMENT

Tracheal atresia is rarely diagnosed prenatally because it does not interfere with normal differentiation and development of the fetus. However, esophageal atresia is very commonly diagnosed prenatally because it obstructs the swallowing mechanism and therefore amniotic fluid cannot be swallowed into the gastrointestinal tract for normal physiologic absorption. As a result, in a high percentage of pregnancies in which the fetus has esophageal atresia, significant polyhydramnios will be present and is an indication for prenatal sonography and/or amniocentesis. The diagnosis of esophageal atresia prenatally alerts the neonatal surgical team and the neonatology team to be present at the time of birth of the baby, so that early definitive diagnosis and operative correction can be carried out (JAH/CNP).

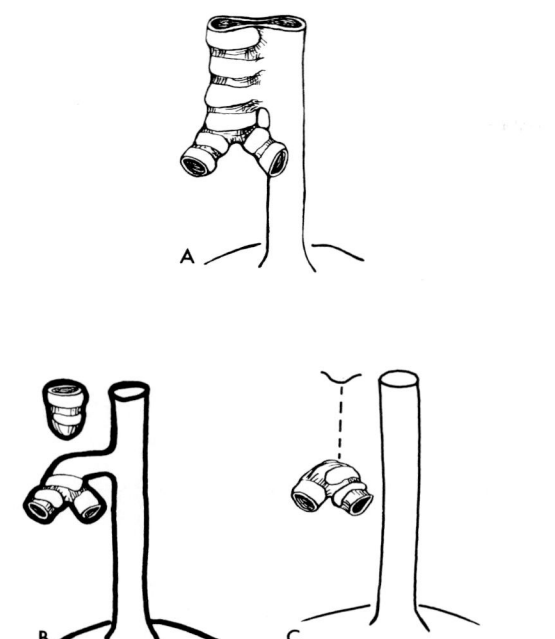

Figure 3.7. Defects of separation of the trachea and esophagus. **A,** Failure of the lateral ridges to fuse. **B,** Partial failure of the trachea to form, as well as failure of complete separation. **C,** Partial failure of the trachea to form, with normal esophagus. In this and in Figures 3.8 to 3.10, the more frequent anomalies are drawn in heavier lines.

Atresia of the Esophagus with Tracheoesophageal Fistula. In this form of defect, the upper or lower portion of the esophagus opens into the trachea (Fig. 3.9, *A* and *B*) or occasionally into a bronchus (Fig. 3.9, *C*), whereas the other portion ends blindly. In some cases both segments of the esophagus open into the trachea (Fig. 3.9, *D* and *E*). Most frequently, however, the upper esophageal segment is blind, and the lower segment opens off the trachea near the carina (Fig. 3.9, *B*).

A few cases have been reported in which the esophagus, although atretic, is also redundant, with the blind end of the cranial segment extending past the fistulous end of the caudal segment almost to the diaphragm (21–25). These cases have sometimes mistakenly been considered duplications of the esophagus (Fig. 3.9, *F*).

In most of these cases there is a muscular continuity of the esophagus and the cephalic segment is usually dilated. The junction of the fistula with the esophagus appears to be higher than usual (25). Almost certainly, these are examples of diaphragmatic atresia above a tracheoesophageal fistula (Fig. 3.9, *G*) in which the blind cranial segment has continued to elongate after atresia occurred. The defect has been found in identical twins (26).

Tracheoesophageal Fistula without Esophageal Atresia. Both the esophagus and trachea may be normally developed, with a large or small fistula connecting them at midesophagus (Fig. 3.10, *A*). More commonly, the fistula is in the cervical portion of the esophagus (Fig. 3.10, *A*). Multiple fistulae are known (17). The fistulous connection may be

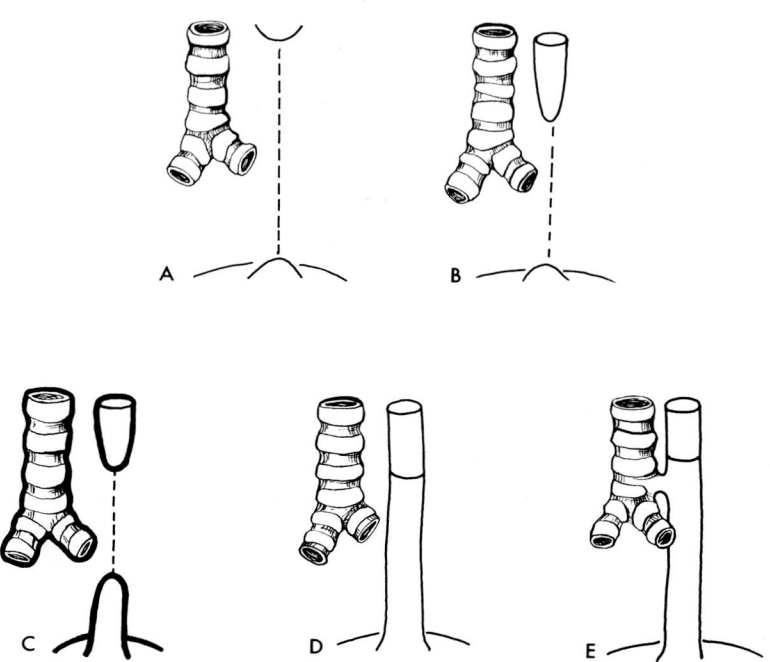

Figure 3.8. Atresia of the esophagus. **A,** Complete absence. **B,** Absence of the distal esophagus. **C,** Absence of the middle third of the esophagus. **D,** Mem- branous atresia of the esophagus without tracheosophageal fistula. **E,** Membra- nous atresia with fistula.

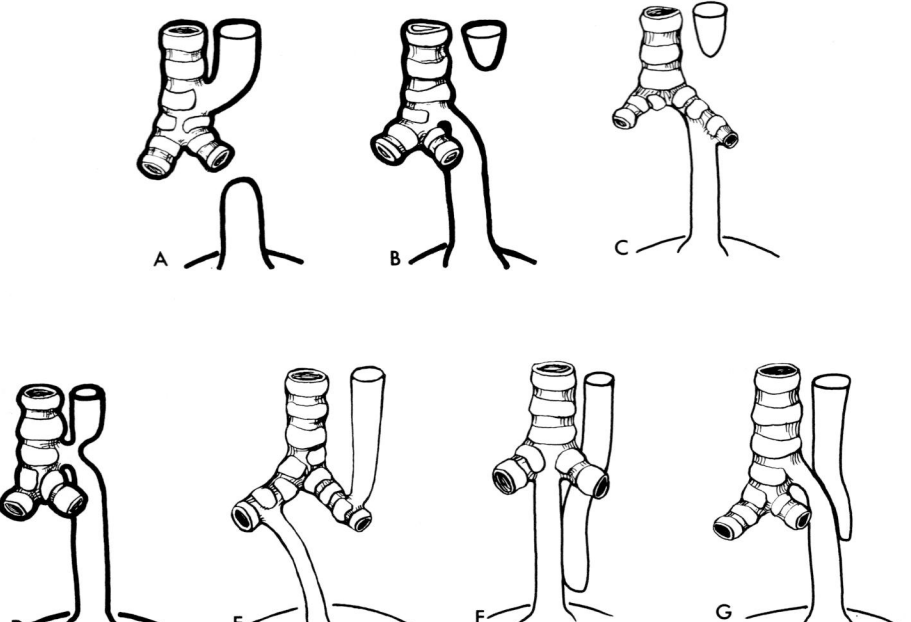

Figure 3.9. Atresia of the esophagus with fistula. **A**, Fistula from the upper esophageal segment. **B**, Fistula from the lower esophageal segment. **C**, Fistula from the lower segment to a bronchus. **D** and **E**, Fistula from both upper and lower segments. **F** and **G**, Fistulae from lower segment with elongated upper segment. In **G**, the wall between the two segments is a mucosal diaphragm. The muscularis is not interrupted. **C**, **E**, **F**, and **G** are rare.

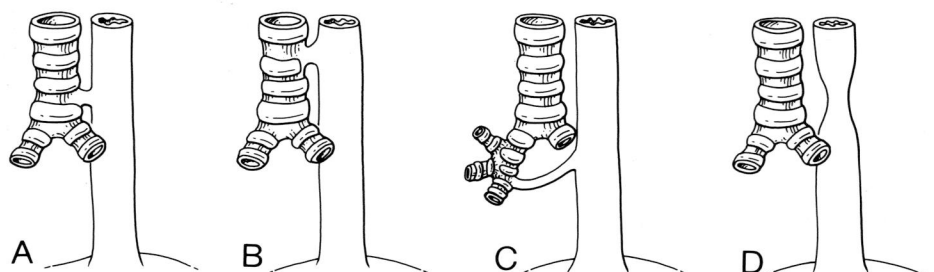

Figure 3.10. **A** to **C**, Fistulae without esophageal atresia. **D**, Esophageal stenosis without fistula.

with a main bronchus or even with a lobar bronchus rather than with the trachea (Fig. 3.10, *C*). In 1964 Frater and Dowdle (27) noted 16 cases of bronchoesophageal fistula in the literature, some of which escaped diagnosis in infancy.

EDITORIAL COMMENT

Tracheoesophageal fistulae without esophageal atresia has been referred to as **H**-type fistula with the cross-arm of the **H** being the fistula between the esophagus and the trachea. Other authors have noted that this fistula is not horizontal, but usually runs from the cephalad end of the trachea to the caudad end on the esophagus. These fistulae are more properly referred to as **N**-type fistulae since there is no obstruction present in the esophagus and no airway problem intrinsically. These infants are not diagnosed at birth, but only after they have had recurring episodes of aspiration

and dysphagia. The diagnosis is best made radiologically by passing a small catheter to the level of the esophageal fistula and injecting water-soluble contrast medium, which usually refluxes up the fistula and delineates the communication. At the time of operative correction, it may be helpful to use the fiberoptic bronchoscope before intubation, and identify the tracheal side of the fistula and insert a small filiform catheter or a small ureteral catheter which helps in the identification of the fistula at the time of the cervical expiration to divide the fistula. All tracheoesophageal fistulae of H-type can be successfully approached with a cervical expiration and do not require a thoracotomy. Rarer bronchoesophageal H-type fistulae will of course require a formal thoracotomy (JAH/CNP).

Stenosis of the Esophagus. The mildest form of the esophageal lesion in this complex of anomalies is stenosis of the middle third of the esophagus (Fig. 3.10, *D*). It

Table 3.2.
Classification of Types of Tracheoesophageal Fistula, Esophageal Atresia, and Stenosis[a]

	Figure	Vogt (1929)	Ladd and Swenson (1949)	Gross (1953)	Stephens et al. (1956)	Approximate Frequency
Failure of separation of trachea and esophagus	3.7, A					Very rare
Absence or atresia of trachea	3.7, B and C					Very rare
Anomalous origin of bronchus	3.10, B					Very rare
Absence of esophagus	3.8, A	I				Rare
Esophageal atresia without fistula	3.8, B to D	II	1	A	B	7.7%
Esophageal atresia with fistula	3.9, A	IIIa	2	B	E	0.8%
	3.9, E		4			Rare
	3.9, B, C, F, and G	IIIb	3	C	A	86.5%
	3.8, E	IIIe	5	D	D	0.7%
	3.9, D					
Fistula without esophageal atresia	3.10, A to C			E	C	4.2%
Esophageal stenosis	3.10, D			F		13%

[a]Revised from first edition with data from Holder TM, Cloud DT, Lewis JE, Jr, Pilling GP, IV. Esophageal atresia and tracheoesophageal fistula: a survey of its members by the surgical section of the American Academy of Pediatrics. Pediatrics 1964;34:542–549.

comprises about 13% of lesions in this region. Congenital stenoses at other levels of the esophagus are of different origin. It should be kept in mind that most esophageal stenoses in children and adults are acquired rather than congenital.

SYSTEMS OF CLASSIFICATION AND RELATIVE FREQUENCY OF THE TYPES OF DEFECTS

Several systems have been developed to classify these lesions. Table 3.2 compares the designations most widely used in the literature. The relative frequencies of the types are based on five of the larger series (28–31).

Holder et al. (30) reported the following statistics in 1000 infants: esophageal atresia with distal tracheoesophageal fistula, 86.5%; esophageal atresia without tracheoesophageal fistula, 7.7%; tracheoesophageal fistula without esophageal atresia (H-type), 4.2%; esophageal atresia with fistula between the upper esophageal pouch and trachea, 0.8%; and esophageal atresia with fistula to both pouches, 0.7%.

Using a large number of case descriptions from 1673 to 1973, in 1976 Kluth (32) classified tracheoesophageal defects into 10 types and 88 subtypes. Many of the latter are unique. Kluth's classification suggests that any imaginable configuration has happened or may happen. Figure 3.11 illustrates Kluth's findings, which may be summarized as follows: Among lesions of the middle esophagus, atresia is more common than stenosis; tracheal fistula accompanies most atresias; and the fistula is usually from the lower esophageal segment in the presence of an atresia but from the cervical esophagus when no atresia is present.

In spite of the above statements, the surgeon must keep in mind that variations, even among the most com-

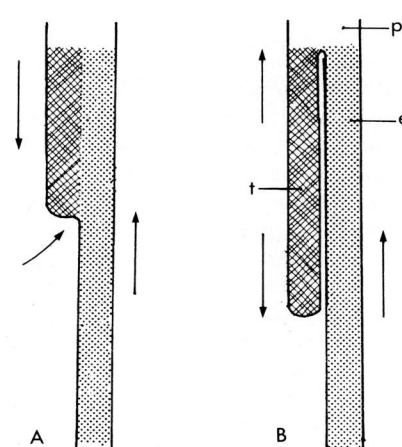

Figure 3.11. Division of the foregut. **A** and **B**, Normal formation of the esophagus and trachea. *p*, Pharynx, *e*, esophagus; *t*, trachea. *Arrows* indicate direction of growth. (After Gruenwald P. A case of atresia of the esophagus combined with tracheoesophageal fistula in a 9 mm human embryo, and embryological explanation. Anat Rec 1940;*78*:293–302.)

mon type, may require that changes in procedure be adopted for each particular patient.

EMBRYOGENESIS

Division of the foregut into the trachea and esophagus involves three simultaneous but independent processes:

1. Appearance of separate organ-forming fields, probably from the mesoderm, on opposite sides of the foregut: These will control the differentiation of the endoderm, anteriorly (ventrad) into the tracheal mucosa and posteriorly (dorsad) into the esophageal mucosa
2. Appearance of the lateral ridges, which project into the lumen to physically separate the tracheal and esophageal tubes

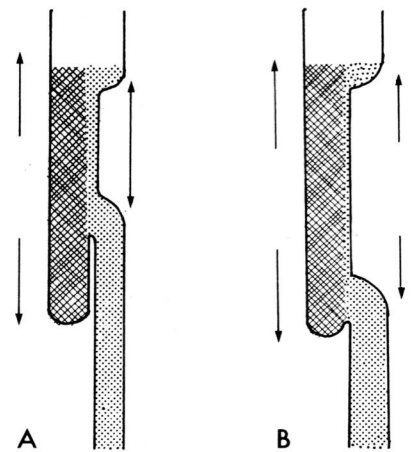

Figure 3.12. Division of the foregut. **A** and **B**, Abnormal formation producing atresia of the esophagus and tracheoesophageal fistula. *Arrows* indicate direction of growth. Compare with Figure 3.11. (After Gruenwald P. A case of atresia of the esophagus combined with tracheoesophageal fistula in a 9 mm human embryo, and embryological explanation. Anat Rec 1940;*78*:293–302.

3. Elongation of both tracheal and esophageal primordia: Should the balance between the organ-forming fields be upset, the division of endoderm will become inequitable. In such cases it is usually the tracheal field that dominates the esophageal field. Esophageal atresia—either complete (Fig. 3.8, *A*) or segmental (Fig. 3.8, *B* and *C*)—results when a disproportionate amount of endoderm becomes organized into the trachea, leaving too little from which to form an esophagus (Fig. 3.12). In a few rare cases (33–37) mesenchyme, under the influence of presumptive tracheal epithelium that remained with the esophagus, has formed cartilage in the esophageal wall (Fig. 3.6). Apparently, it is more difficult to preserve an esophagus than to form a trachea.

Even though the balance between organ-forming fields remains normal, the lateral ridges may fail to form or to fuse completely. The extreme case is seen in Figure 3.7, *A*, in which no separation has occured.

The minimal defects are of two varieties:

1. Arrest of Cranial Growth of the Septum: The septum between the trachea and esophagus grows craniad and may stop before it reaches its normal point of termination. Fusion has failed to keep up with the elongation process. Such a developmental arrest produces a laryngeal cleft. If the septum stops at a more caudal level, the cleft may extend down the trachea, forming a laryngotracheoesophageal fistula, or cleft. Defects of this type are very rare and are discussed later in this chapter.

2. Local Failure of Fusion of the Lateral Ridges: If fusion fails to occur with no other changes taking place, a simple tracheoesophageal fistula without esophageal atresia results (Fig. 3.10, *A*). More often, the unclosed portion falls under the influence of the tracheal mesoderm, and a short section of the foregut becomes entirely trachea with

a corresponding segment of esophagus absent. A fistula to the upper portion, lower portion, or both is present as well. It is these more common lesions with which the surgeon is chiefly concerned (Fig. 3.9, *A–C*).

A number of suggestions have been put forward to account for this constellation of defects. Atresia has been explained as the persistence of a hypothetic stage in which epithelial proliferation reduced the esophagus to a solid cord of cells, which later became recanalized. Although it has been disproved many times, this theory still is mentioned.

Mechanical pressure from the developing heart (38) or from fluid in the transitory pneumoenteric recess (39) has also been held responsible for inducing these defects. Anomalous blood vessels were reported at the site of atresia by Fluss and Poppen (40), who suggested that pressure from these vessels causes the defect. Actually, this theory was proposed as long ago as 1906 by Keith (41), who attributed some atresias to the presence of an aberrant right subclavian artery; however, this vessel is not in the proper location at the time of the formation of the trachea to account for the atresia. When aberrant arteries are found in postnatal life, they may cause esophageal or tracheal compression, but they have not produced atresia.

A more reasonable explanation on a mechanical level is that cell proliferation in the foregut fails to keep up with the elongation produced by growth of more dorsal structures, and the resulting attenuation of the tubular foregut permits the dorsal as well as the ventral cells to differentiate into tracheal tissue (Fig. 3.12).

Separation of the trachea and esophagus normally takes place in the fourth week after fertilization. The larger the communication between the two tubes, the earlier the defect is presumed to have occurred. Tracheoesophageal fistulae are not known to occur spontaneously in other mammals. Kalter (42) produced esophageal atresias ranging to complete absence of the esophagus in mice that had extreme riboflavin deficiency, but the trachea and bronchi were normal and no fistula developed. In 1948 Warkany et al. (43) mentioned one example of tracheoesophageal fistula among 50 rats born to mothers reared on a vitamin–A-deficient diet. (See also Chapter 13, "The Trachea and Lungs," Fistula of the Trachea.)

ASSOCIATED ANOMALIES

About 50% of infants with esophageal atresia or tracheoesophageal fistula have other anomalies (44). Holder et al. (30) reviewed 1058 cases of esophageal atresia with and without fistula and found 48% with additional congenital anomalies. Infants having a fistula of both segments of the esophagus or having a fistula without atresia had a much lower incidence of associated anomalies than those with other lesions (44).

Table 3.3.
Associated Anomalies of Esophageal Atresia and
Tracheoesophageal Fistula[a,b]

	Holder (%)	Chittmittrapap (%)
Gastrointestinal	28	27
Heart	24	29
Genitourinary	13	14
Musculoskeletal	11	10
Central nervous system	7	
Facial	6	
Others	12	

[a]From Holder TM, Cloud PT, Lewis JE, Jr, Pilling GP, IV. Eosphageal atresia and tracheoesophageal fistula: a survey of its members by the surgical section of the American Academy of Pediatrics. Pediatrics 1964;34:542–549.
[b]From Chittmittrapap S, Spitz L, Kiely EM, Brereton RJ. Oesophageal atresia and associated anomalies. Arch Dis Child 1989;64:364–368.

Chittmittrapap and colleagues at Great Ormond Street (45) found a similar incidence of associated anomalies in 253 infants treated between January 1980 and December 1987. The distribution of associated anomalies in these series are presented in Table 3.3.

Of 233 gastrointestinal anomalies in Holder's series (30), 99 were imperforate anus with or without fistula. This is the most common single defect associated with esophageal lesions. Down syndrome also is not unusual, and an association with trisomy of chromosome 18 has been suggested (46).

Hydramnios is frequently encountered in infants with esophageal atresia; the inability to swallow and excrete or absorb the fluid permits its accumulation. Scott and Wilson (47) suggest that hydramnios is the cause of the high percentage of prematurity in such infants. One out of twelve to fifteen infants with polyhydramnios is found to have esophageal atresia (47, 48).

EDITORIAL COMMENT

Polyhydramnios is more frequently absent clinically in patients with esophageal atresia and tracheoesophageal fistula, apparently because the fetus can swallow amniotic fluid through the trachea down through the fistula and into the gastrointestinal tract where it can be absorbed. On the other hand, if the fistula is quite small, then the baby effectively has pure esophageal fistula with no access to the gastrointestinal tract for amniotic fluid absorption. Such babies would be expected to have polyhydramnios as a complication, since amniotic fluid constitutes a minor but significant component of nutrition for the developing fetus. When esophageal atresia is present and polyhydramnios results, the fetus is unable to receive amniotic fluid nutrition, and therefore there can be failure to thrive in utero as one cause of small for gestational age babies (JAH/CNP).

In 1937 de Snoo (49) made an antenatal diagnosis of atresia by injecting saccharine into the amniotic sac and failing to recover it in the maternal urine. Esophageal atresia is now frequently diagnosed antenatally because of the widespread use of fetal ultrasound, particularly in the presence of maternal polyhydramnios.

Greenwood and Rosenthal (50) stated that 30% of babies with esophageal atresia have some cardiac malformations. Andrassy and Mahour (51) reported that 12% of cases with esophageal atresia have also some anal anomalies. Bond-Taylor, Starer, and Atwell (52) discussed the associated vertebral anomalies, and Schiffman et al. (53) present a case of tracheal agenesis associated with esophageal atresia and distal tracheoesophageal fistula.

VACTERL Anomalies of the Foregut. In 1973 Quan and Smith (54) suggested a broad spectrum of associated malformations that might or might not appear together, and they arranged the most important of these defects into the acronym *VATER:*

> *V*ertebral defects
> *A*nal atresias
> *T*racheoesophageal fistula
> *E*sophageal atresia
> *R*enal defects

Quan and Smith (54, 55) introduced the concept of association to include a nonrandom occurrence of a number of malformations. There was no family history of malformations, no recognizable teratogen involved, and no chromosomal abnormality observed. Two patients in Quan and Smith's series had four or more VATER defects, and seven had three or more.

Other anomalies tacked onto the original five (56) include single umbilical artery and ventricular septal defect. Fernbach (57) reported that eight of twenty newborns with VATER association had urethral abnormalities such as megalourethra, duplication, valve, stricture, and hypospadias. The currently used acronym is the VACTERL syndrome (*v*ertebral, *a*norectal, *c*ardiac, *tra*cheoesophageal, *r*enal, *ra*dial, *l*imb) (44, 45). Physicians working with patients with these syndromes emphasize that VACTERL is not a regular syndrome but rather a nonrandom association with an unknown etimology (58–60).

The appearance of any of the characteristic VACTERL defects should stimulate a search for other such defects. The likelihood of one anomaly occurring in the presence of any other is depicted in Figure 3.13.

HISTORY

The history of esophageal fistulae and atresias was covered in detail by Ashcraft and Holder in 1969 (61) and Myers in 1986 (62). A case of esophageal atresia is said to have been seen by Durston in 1670 (63), and the earliest tracheoesophageal fistula was described by Thomas Gibson in 1696 (64). His excellent description is quoted at

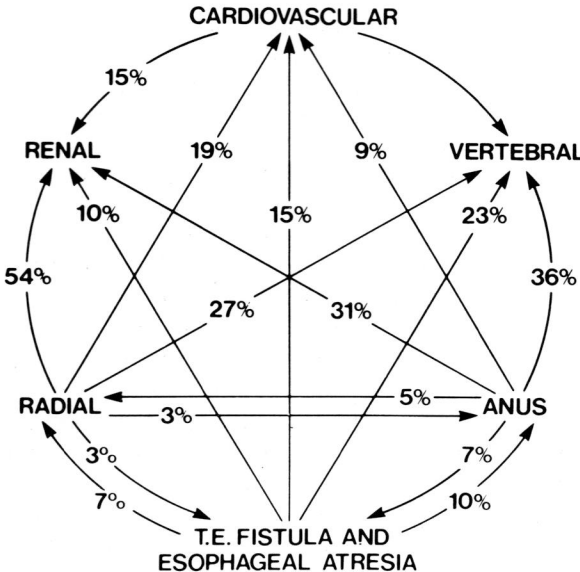

Figure 3.13. VACTERL association "circle." (From de Lorimier AA, Harrison MR. Esophageal atresia: embryogenesis and management. Surgery 1985; 9:250–257.)

Table 3.4.
Reports of Tracheoesophageal Fistula

Report	Incidence	Author
	Live births	
Brooklyn, 1952–1955	1:2000	Shapiro et al., 1958[a]
England, 1935–1942	1:2630	Turner, 1946[b]
Netherlands	1:4000	Pinxter and Rutten, 1963[c]
Boston	1:5083	Ingalls and Prindle, 1949[d]
Washtenaw County, Michigan	1:4425	Haight, 1957[e]
Finland	1:3000	Sulamaa et al., 1951, and Louhimo and Lindahl, 1983[f]
Australia	1:4500	Myers, 1979[g]

[a]Shapiro RN, Eddy W, Fitzgibbon J, O'Brien G. The incidence of congenital anomalies discovered in the neonatal period. Am J Surg 1958;96:396–400.
[b]Turner GG. Injuries and diseases of the esophagus. London: Cassell & Co, 1946.
[c]Pinxter PRJ, Rutten APM. Ervaringen met de behandeling van aangeboren slokdarmetresie. Nederl T Geneeck 1963;107:1790–1795.
[d]Ingalls TH, Prindle RA. Eosophageal atresia with tracheoesphageal fistula: epidemiologic and teratologic implications. N Engl J Med 1949;240:987–995.
[e]Haight C. Some observations of esophageal atresia and tracheoesophageal fistula of congenital origin. J Thorac Surg 1957;34:141–172.
[f]Sulamaa M, Gribenberg L, Alvenainen EK. Prognosis and treatment of congenital atresia of the esophagus. Acta Chir Scand 1951;102:141–157; and Louhimo I, Lindahl H. Esophageal atresia: primary results of 500 consecutive treated patients. J Pediatr Surg 1983;18:217.
[g]Myers NA. Oesophageal atresia with distal tracheoesophageal fistula—a longterm follow-up. Prog Pediatr Surg 1977;10:15.

length almost three centuries later by Ingalls and Prindle (39). By 1880 Mackenzie (65) had found 42 cases in the literature since 1670. Rosenthal (1) reviewed 255 cases, and Lanman (66) estimated that there were at least 500 cases in the literature. In contrast, the first example of fistula without atresia was not found until 1873 (67).

Tracheoesophageal fistula was treated unsuccessfully by gastrectomy by Steele in 1888 (68), and failure accompanied all subsequent efforts until 1939, although Lanman in 1940 (66) had two patients who lived 15 and 32 days, respectively. In 1919 Plass (69) reported a mean survival of 4.8 days and a maximum of 14 days in untreated cases.

In 1939 Leven (70) in St. Paul and Ladd (71) in Boston each independently achieved success with multiple-stage operations involving closure of fistula, gastrostomy, marsupialization of the upper blind pouch, and subsequent construction of an antesternal esophagus. In 1941 Haight and Towsley (72) performed a single-stage, end-to-end anastomosis of the esophagus within the mediastinum.

INCIDENCE

There is considerable variation in the frequency with which tracheoesophageal anomalies have been reported (Table 3.4).

Brown and Brown (73) suggested that there is some evidence of localization in space and time. A statistic analysis of 98 cases in England between 1950 and 1958 indicated a clustering in time more marked than could be accounted for by random distribution. No seasonal pattern is visible, but there may be a relationship to an epidemic maternal infection (74).

Sex Ratio. In most series of tracheoesophageal anomalies, there is a slight preponderance of males. Among a total of 392 cases, 59% were male. The male to female ratio in cases of stenosis is nearly equal.

Maternal Age. The age of the mother is a factor in this anomaly. In 1949 Ingalls and Prindle (39) found that mothers over 30 years of age gave birth to 35.2% of all babies, but that they have 45.3% of the babies with tracheoesophageal fistula. The risk is low for the first pregnancy but increases sharply with each succeeding pregnancy. The investigators found no increase in spontaneous abortions among mothers of affected infants, but hydramnios and abnormal placentation were significantly more frequent. Interestingly, no animal species is known to carry this defect.

Familial Incidence. Reports of two affected siblings in the same family have been published (66, 75, 76), and in 1880 Mackenzie (65) reported a father who had two children with atresia by different wives. Children with successful repair of this defect have now reached reproductive age.

Hansmann et al. (77) reported the occurrence of tracheoesophageal fistula in three consecutive siblings. Haight (78) presented his observations on familial esophageal atresia and tracheoesophageal fistula believing in developmental rather than genetic origin. Engel et al. (79) reported esophageal atresia with tracheoesophageal fistula in mother and child. German et al. (80) reported

102 patients with esophageal atresia with a 9% incidence of twinning. David and O'Callaghan (81) reported twinning and esophageal atresia. King et al. (82) reported a case in twins in which only one had the VACTERL syndrome. The correlation of genetics and esophageal anomalies is still unclear.

After studying cases of families with these defects, Chen et al. (83) postulated that these are not a genetic phenomenon but rather a developmental environmental phenomenon because identical twins originate within 2 weeks of fertilization, and trachea and esophagus develop two weeks later.

Kiesewetter (84) supports a possible genetic factor; Ozimek (85), an environmental one (infectious hepatitis); and Dennis et al. (86), a genetic factor. Randolph (87) believes that external agents have a greater impact on the development of the esophagus.

Tracheoesophageal Fistula in Adults. Occasionally, a fistula without esophageal atresia escapes detection in infancy. Several such fistulae have been reported in children (88, 89). Even more striking are fistulae that remain undiscovered until adulthood: Le Roux and Williams (90) reported three such cases and tabulated 23 others from the literature. The oldest patient was 63 years of age.

Most of these fistulae gave evidence of their existence only through frequent respiratory infection and chronic cough; in a few cases they were revealed only at autopsy. In one patient the diagnosis was made by bronchoscopy although, as retrospective study of previous x-ray films suggested, the correct diagnosis could have been made earlier.

SIGNS AND SYMPTOMS

From the clinical standpoint, infants with tracheoesophageal defects may be divided into five groups, each with well-differentiated symptoms (Fig. 3.14 and Table 3.5).

Group I. When simple atresia is present, the diagnosis can be made immediately after birth by routinely attempting to pass a suction catheter through each nostril into the stomach. The baby's nostrils and mouth are filled with unswallowed saliva. If the baby is fed, the first sips of formula are regurgitated. The milk is uncoagulated, having never reached the stomach. Esophageal atresia should be suspected at once; failure to pass a catheter confirms the diagnosis. In addition, fetal lanugo hair, normally swallowed with amniotic fluid before birth, is not present in the meconium stool when atresia without fistula exists. Coughing and choking may result from aspiration of fluid when feeding is attempted; however, it is less constant than in group III, in which a direct communication exists from esophagus to trachea, and cyanosis is less marked. If

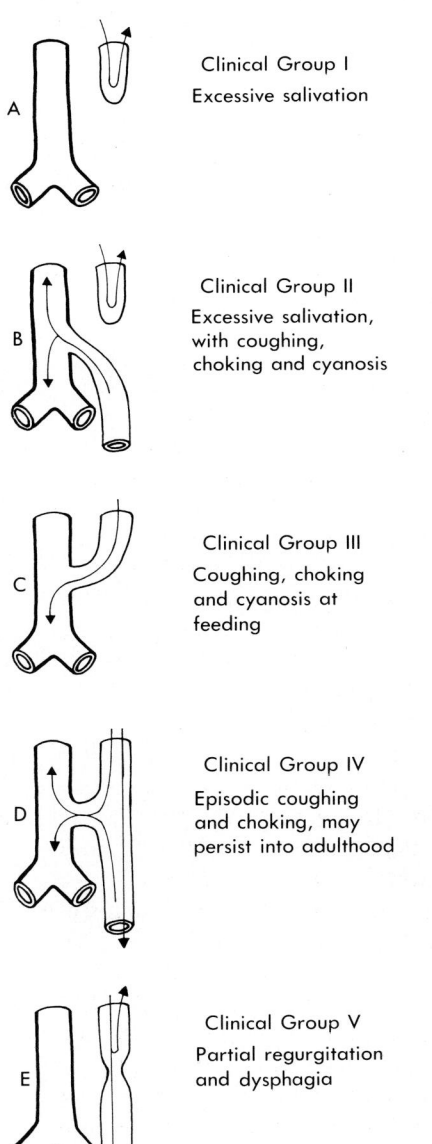

Clinical Group I
Excessive salivation

Clinical Group II
Excessive salivation, with coughing, choking and cyanosis

Clinical Group III
Coughing, choking and cyanosis at feeding

Clinical Group IV
Episodic coughing and choking, may persist into adulthood

Clinical Group V
Partial regurgitation and dysphagia

Figure 3.14. Differential diagnosis among the five clinical groups of esophageal defects.

Table 3.5.
Tracheoesophageal Defects: Signs and Symptoms

Clinical Group	Symptoms	Probable Pathologic Conditions
I	Excessive salivation	Atresia only (Figs. 3.8, A to D and 3.14, A)
II	Excessive salivation with coughing, choking, and cyanosis	Atresia with distal fistula (Figs. 3.9, B, C, F, and G, and 3.14 B)
III	Coughing, choking, and cyanosis	Atresia with proximal fistula (Figs. 3.9, A, and 3.14 C)
IV	Some episodic coughing, choking, and cyanosis	Fistula only (Figs. 3.10, A and B, and 3.14 D)
V	Partial regurgitation and dysphagia	Stenosis (Figs. 3.10, C, and 3.14, E)

the diagnosis is not made early (within 3 days), the prognosis is grave and death may ensue from dehydration, starvation, and pneumonitis.

Group II. Into this group—those with atresia of the upper esophageal segment and fistula of the lower segment—fall about 75% of all cases of tracheoesophageal anomalies and about 90% of tracheoesophageal fistulae. The atretic upper segment produces the same picture of salivation and immediate regurgitation as that found in patients in group I. In addition, gastric fluid entering through the distal fistulous portion produces respiratory distress with cyanosis even when no vomitus has been inhaled. As some air may enter the intestinal tract during expiration, abdominal distension often occurs and air may be present on x-ray. Death from pneumonitis is the outcome of this condition if it is left untreated.

Group III. Among this group, respiratory distress is the first symptom. The infant's sipping of formula results not in regurgitation but in coughing and choking. The baby's color changes from pink to light blue as he becomes cyanotic for a few seconds because of laryngeal spasm. Again the outcome is fatal pneumonitis. In the cases in which both segments of the esophagus communicate with the trachea, the symptoms usually spring from the fistula of the upper segment.

Group IV. In this group—those with fistula only—the size of the fistula governs the onset and severity of symptoms. Large patency may cause enough of the esophageal contents to pass into the trachea and produce symptoms similar to those found in group II. A smaller fistula may produce repeated episodes of pneumonitis in infancy, along with a persistent cough. The pediatrician must keep this anomaly in mind when examining older children as well. A few such cases have given little trouble even into adulthood because mucosal folds may block the entrance to the fistula. The chest surgeon should also keep the possibility of an occult fistula in mind when treating an adult for bronchiectasis of unknown etiology.

Group V. Stenosis without tracheal communication is the second most common condition among esophageal defects although it is not often clinically significant. Symptoms depend somewhat on the diameter of the stenotic segment. Regurgitation of part of each feeding, with failure to gain weight, is the most constant picture in affected infants. Symptoms become more marked when the diet begins to include solid food. Dysphagia may be the complaint in older children. Occasionally, the dilation above the stenosis may become large enough to produce pressure on the trachea. Pulmonary symptoms, which are common in the other types, are much rarer although aspiration pneumonitis is always a danger when frequent vomiting takes place.

Holinger et al. (91) describe cases in which the epithelium of the stenotic segment appears denuded. They suggest the etiologic factor is a failure of epithelialization; however, because an epithelial tube is the earliest manifestation of the esophagus, the absence of epithelium can only have been acquired secondarily.

DIAGNOSIS

Clinical diagnosis may be confirmed by esophageal catheterization, x-ray examination with or without contrast media, and esophagoscopy or bronchoscopy.

Esophageal catheterization is easily accomplished by means of a soft French No. 10 catheter. An inability to pass the catheter confirms the diagnosis of defects of groups I or II. The operator must, however, be alert to the possibility that the catheter has reached the stomach by passing down the trachea and across the fistula into the distal esophagus. Such an occurrence can be dangerously misleading.

Chest x-ray films confirm the existence of pneumonitis and show the location of the tip of the catheter. The abdominal x-ray film demonstrates the presence (Fig. 3.15) or absence (Fig. 3.16) of air in the gastrointestinal tract and, hence, the possible existence of a fistula below the atresia (group II).

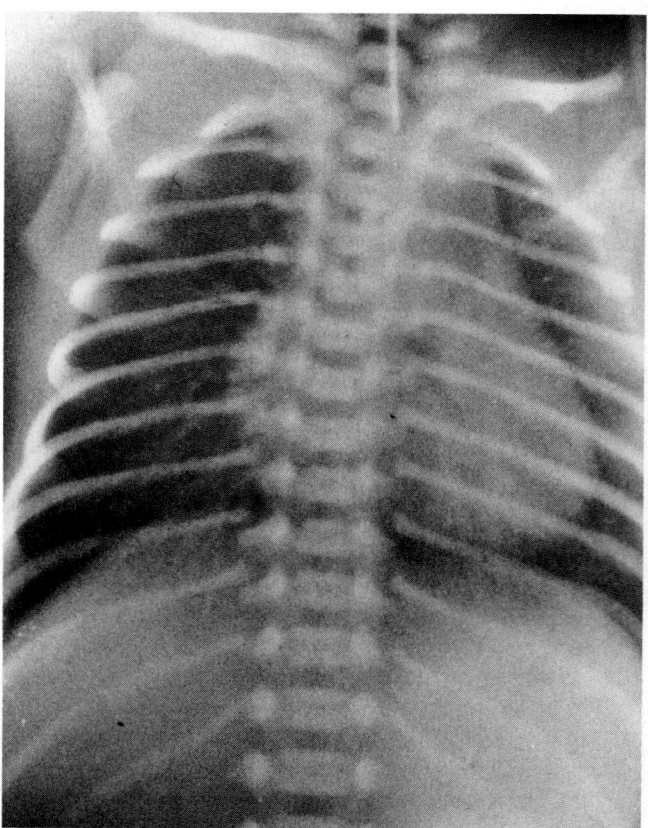

Figure 3.15. Esophageal atresia with distal tracheoesophageal fistula. Note gas in gastrointestinal tract.

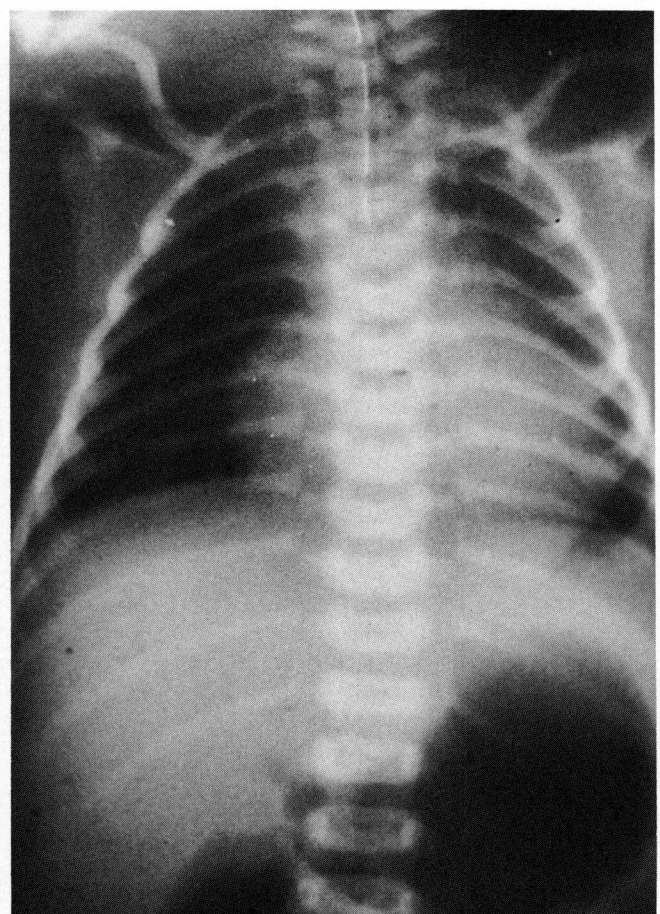

Figure 3.16. Esophageal atresia without tracheoesophageal fistula. Note ''gasless'' abdomen.

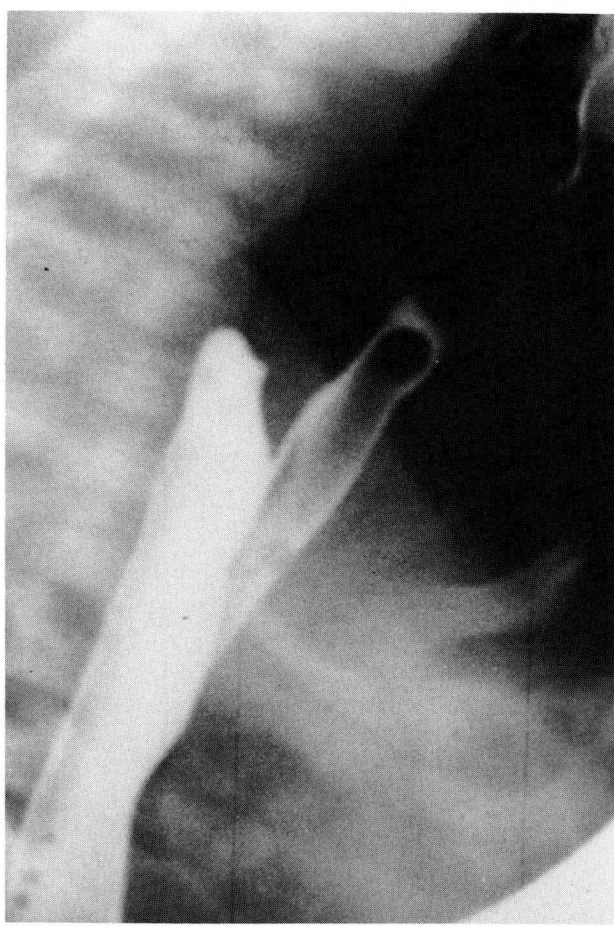

Figure 3.17. Tracheoesophageal fistula without atreasia (H type).

Using a contrast medium enables one to visualize either a blind sac (group I or II), the bronchial tree (group III or IV) (Fig. 3.17), a stenotic segment (group V), or an apparently normal esophagus. In the latter case the possibility of a small fistula cannot be ruled out. The picture also distinguishes between a true stenotic segment and achalasia with cardiac stricture as the cause of the regurgitation.

In general, contrast agents should be avoided. If desired, 1 to 2 cc of dilute barium given under fluoroscopic control is sufficient to demonstrate a proximal fistula. The barium should be aspirated after the study. Water-soluble contrast agents are contraindicated because their high osmolarity causes a severe chemical pneumonitis if they are aspirated into the tracheobronchial tree.

An air study alone may be adequate for demonstrating the pathologic situation. It avoids possible respiratory embarrassment resulting from the use of viscid contrast media.

TREATMENT

Atresia and Fistula. Scarcely 50 years have passed since the only treatment possible for a simple atresia was permanent gastrostomy and esophagostomy and since the only prospect in cases of esophageal fistula was, inevitably, death from pneumonitis. Present principles of treatment for each type of lesion are outlined in Table 3.6.

Anastomosis.
The multiple-stage operations of Ladd (66) and Leven (65), the first to be successful, quickly gave way to the intrathoracic, one-stage, two-layer telescoping, end-to-end anastomosis developed by Haight (89). Currently, a single-layer end-to-end anastomosis is most often used. The operation consists of division and ligation of the fistula and repair of the tracheal defect, followed by end-to-end anastomosis of the upper and lower esophageal segments. Dilation of the lower segment is usually necessary for satisfactory union. Some surgeons perform gastrostomy at the same time to avoid the injurious effects of vomiting (92), whereas others believe that gastrostomy

Table 3.6.
Synopsis of Esophageal Atresias and Tracheoesophageal Fistulas

Symptom Group and Frequency	Pathology	Onset of Symptoms	Symptoms	
			Early	Late
I 4 to 6%	Atresia: Total, segmental, membranous	1st day of life	Excessive salivation and regurgitation[a]	Dehydration, starvation
II 75%	Atresia with fistula of distal segment	1st day of life	Excessive salivation and coughing, choking and cyanosis	Pneumonia, dehydration, starvation
III 2 to 3%	Atresia with fistula of proximal segment or of both	1st day of life	Coughing, choking and cyanosis, no excessive salivation	Pneumonia, asphyxia
IV 2 to 4%	Fistula without atresia	Early or late, depending on size of fistula	Episodic coughing, choking and cyanosis	None or all of the above
V 13%	Stenosis	Early or late, depending on degree of stenosis	Partial regurgitation and dysphagia	Failure to gain weight

[a]Aspiration pneumonia, regardless of the presence of a fistula, is an ever-present danger when regurgitation is frequent.

should be done only in selected patients. The optimal time for surgery depends on the infant's general medical condition:

1. *Immediate primary repair* is indicated if the infant is in good physiologic condition (i.e., cardiopulmonary condition) and is not extremely premature.
2. *Delayed primary repair* is indicated when the infant requires stabilization of a cardiac (e.g., congestive heart failure) or pulmonary (e.g., pneumonia) condition or if the upper pouch needs to be stretched to allow for a primary anastomosis. The delay can be up to several weeks in duration. During this time the infant is alimented parenterally, and nursing care must be meticulous to prevent aspiration via the fistula.
3. *Staged repair* is indicated if the infant is extremely premature (less than 1200 g) or has serious cardiopulmonary disease. In this situation a gastrostomy tube is placed, and the fistula is divided and ligated. The infant can then be alimented by gastrostomy feeding. The repair is done when the infant has gained sufficient weight or

when the cardiopulmonary condition has been adequately treated (93).

EDITORIAL COMMENT

Most surgeons have had bad results with staged repair of premature babies with tracheoesophageal fistula and have abandoned a thoracotomy with simple division of the fistula without anastomosis. Either they will attempt stretching of the proximal pouch with suction on the pouch intermittently and feeding by gastrostomy, or they will carry out a formal thoracotomy even in the small baby and divide the fistula and carry out the anastomosis even though the incidence of leakage from the anastomosis is higher. In such babies, most surgeons would prefer a gastrostomy to allow enteral feeding during healing and also to decrease the chance of gastroesophageal reflux of activated gastric juice, which might cause the breakdown of a tenuous esophageal anastomosis (JAH/CNP).

Radiology		Endoscopy		Differential Diagnosis	Treatment	
Plain Film	Lipidol	Broncho-	Esophago-			
Lungs clear, no air in gastrointestinal tract	Blind pouch	Normal	No	Stenosis, obstruction from extrinsic pressure	1. Gastrostomy and construction of artificial esophagus 2. Gastrostomy, mobilization of stomach and end-to-end anastomosis 3. (Gastrostomy and end-to-end anastomosis	
Pneumonia, air in gastrointestinal tract	Blind pouch	May or may not visualize fistula	No	None	Gastrostomy, end-to-end anastomosis and closure of fistula	
Pneumonia, air may be in gastrointestinal tract	Lipidol in bronchial tree	May or may not visualize fistula	May or may not pass into trachea	None	As in 11	
Pneumonia present or absent	Lipidol may or may not reach bronchial tree	May or may not visualize fistula		None	Closure of fistula	
Lungs clear, no air in gastrointestinal tract	Stenosis visible, proximal segment dilated	Normal	May or may not pass stenosis	Atresia, achalasia, esophagitis, hiatal hernia, obstruction from extrinsic pressure	1. Dilation 2. Resection and end-to-end anastomosis	

All would agree, however, that the optimum time for surgery is when the infant is in the best condition. We feel that this should be the factor uppermost in the surgeon's mind. Too often, delay represents indecision rather than caution, and precipitousness marks impatience rather than wisdom.

Stretching of the Upper Pouch.

The distance between the blind upper pouch and the lower segment of the esophagus may be too great to perform an end-to-end anastomosis after ligation of the fistula. In 1963 Howard and Myers (94) in Australia successfully elongated the upper pouch by passing a mercury-loaded bougie by mouth into the pouch, leaving it in for 10 min a day for about a month. At the end of this period, an end-to-end anastomosis was possible and was performed successfully (Fig. 3.18). Others have also had success with this procedure (95, 96). There is evidence that the distal segment is capable of similar elongation (97).

Additional length on the upper pouch can be achieved by performing one or more circular esophagomyotomies, as described by Livaditis et al (98, 99), experimentally and clinically. Others have also reported good results when using both of these techniques to achieve adequate length for a primary end-to-end repair (100, 101).

Although these methods are time consuming and require gastrostomy feeding, the results are probably preferred to those of esophageal reconstruction.

Esophageal Reconstruction.

In rare cases the esophageal defect is such that an end-to-end anastomosis is impossible. In such infants a substitute esophagus must be constructed so that they are able to eat and drink as normal individuals.

A number of methods have been tried in past years, but of these, no one can say which is the best. Plastic prostheses, skin tubes, and grafts from stomach, jejunum, and colon have all been used, the last three with the greatest success.

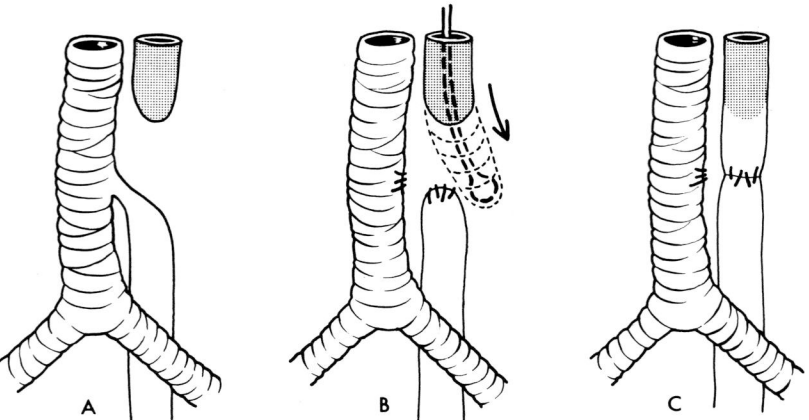

Figure 3.18. Technique of stretching the upper esophageal pouch in cases of tracheal fistula from the lower esophageal segment. **A**, The upper pouch is too short to anastomose with lower segment. **B**, Procedure for stimulating the upper pouch to elongate gradually. **C**, Anastomosis of upper and lower segments after diversion and ligation of the fistula.

Remember:

1. Be sure not to overlook the hiding upper pouch fistula (in reality, babies have upper and lower fistulae), which is difficult to diagnose in patients. The only way to be sure is to conduct a detailed, careful dissection of all upper pouches or to obtain a dilute barium (1-cc) upper "pouch-o-gram" on all patients. Upper pouch fistulae can also be detected by preoperative branchoscopy in all patients. Such a recognition is essential to avoid any further aspiration pneumonitis, which can be a major complication in a baby with recent esophageal anastomosis and thoracotomy

2. Esophageal atresia without fistula has a peculiar topographic anatomy:
   a. For all practical purposes the esophagus is absent.
   b. The proximal segment is represented by a high and short segment.
   c. The distal segment is short, "barely reaching above the diaphragm" (87).

The H-tracheoesophageal fistula is located in the cervical area of the second thoracic vertebra or the thoracic area. It originates from the posterior membranous tracheal wall. This type of fistula is very short with a diameter of approximtely 1 cm. It is best diagnosed by a careful esophagogram or bronchoscopy.

From Tables 3.7 and 3.8, one learns that current survival rates of these anomalies are 91 to 100% for categories A and B and 43% for category C. Overall survival is about 83 to 85%.

The Waterston classification (102) has been used in the past to guide surgical therapy and to compare survival data between different series of patients. This classification is based on the patient's weight and the presence or absence of pneumonia and/or congenital anomalies. The Waterston Risk Categories are as follows:

A. Birth weight over 5.5 lb and otherwise well
B. Birth weight 4 to 5.5 lb and well or higher birth weight

Table 3.7.
Esophageal Anomalies, Children's Hospital National Medical Center, 1966–1983[a]

Defects	Patients (N)	Survivors	Surviving (%)
Esophageal atresia with lower segment tracheoesophageal fistula	87[b]	72	83
Isolated esophageal atresia	10	9	90
Isolated tracheoesophageal fistula (H type)	7	7	100
Esophageal web/stenosis	3	3	100
TOTALS	107	91	85

[a]From Randolph JG, Esophageal atresia and congenital stenosis. In: Welch KT, Randolph JG, Ravitch MM, O'Neill JA Jr. Rowe MI, eds. Pediatric surgery, 4th ed. Chicago: Year Book Medical Publishers, 1986.
[b]Includes two patients with fistula in both upper and lower esophageal segments.

Table 3.8.
Operative Results in Esophageal Atresia with Tracheoesophageal Fistula (Vogt-Gross Type C), 1966–1983, Children's Hospital National Medical Center[a]

Waterston Risk Category	Operation	Patients (N)	Surviving (N)	%
A	Immediate repair	34	34	100
B	Delayed primary repair	32	29	91
C		21[b]	9	43
	1. Immediate repair	(1)	(0)	
	2. Delayed primary repair	(11)	(2)	
	3. Staged repair	(9)	(7)	
TOTALS		87	72	83

[a]From Randolph JG, Esophageal atresia and congenital stenosis. In: Welch KT, Randolph JG, Ravitch MM, O'Neill JA Jr. Rowe MI, eds. Pediatric surgery, 4th ed. Chicago: Year Book Medical Publishers, 1986.
[b]Of these 21 patients, eight had congenital anomalies incompatible with life, such as left incomplete heart, single ventricle, trisomy 13, and bilateral renal agenesis.

but moderate pneumonia and other congenital anomalies

C. Birth weight under 4 lb or higher birth weight but severe pneumonia and severe congenital anomalies

With modern day surgical, anesthetic, and neonatal care, birth weight per se and other associated nonlethal anomalies are no longer significant in determining survival and therefore should not be used to guide surgical therapy. Randolph et al. (93) propose a management scheme based solely on the physiologic status of the infant, regardless of birth weight, early gestational age, or the presence of co-existing anomalies.

In Randolph's study, group I patients had stable cardiac and respiratory status and underwent immediate primary repair. Group II patients had unstable physiologic status and underwent either delayed or staged repair. The results of treatment, along with the corresponding Waterston Classification is shown in Table 3.9.

MORTALITY

Mortality from esophageal atresia, with or without tracheoesophageal fistula, was 100% before 1939. By 1952 Leven and his colleagues reported a 55% survival rate among patients treated in St. Paul (103). By 1958 Swenson (104) was able to report only 18 postoperative deaths among 78 operations. The mortality has declined every decade since then. A 1983 report found the overall survival to be 85 to 90% (105), and in 1985 Martin and Alexander (106) reported the current survival on esophageal atresia to be almost 100%, not including infants with associated fatal malformations.

Three factors affect the prognosis: size of the infant, presence and nature of associated anomalies, and the presence and severity of dehydration or pneumonia. Dehydration is usually proportional to the delay in diagnosis. An infant weighing over 6 lb and who has no other anomalies is a good surgical risk. A premature infant with a severe associated anomaly is a very poor risk. Of the severe associated anomalies, imperforate anus has a better prognosis than have anomalies of the heart and genitourinary system (30). Pulmonary complications or associated anomalies accounted for 338 out of 353 deaths of patients with esophageal atresia and distal tracheal fistula in Holder's series of 1058 cases (30). An anastomatic leak was responsible for 73 deaths.

EDITORIAL COMMENT

Death from an anastomotic leak is extremely rare now that most repairs are carried out in the extrapleural space. With this dissection, any leak which does occur is localized in the mediastinum and can be drained with mediastinal chest tube. Prior to the recognition of this technique, empyema resulted from transpleural division and esophageal anastomosis and thus a very high mortality from sepsis. Practically all mortality is now associated with prematurity and/or major congenital heart abnormalities. The former can usually be overcome with intravenous hyperalimentation and good neonatal care until the baby is mature enough for successful staged operative correction. The severity of the congenital heart abnormality will be the ultimate determinant of survival (JAH/CNP).

Azizkhan (107) stated that more than 90% of the infants with esophageal atresia and distal tracheoesophageal fistula survive. Death, however, is related to associated anomalies or extreme prematurity.

Laryngotracheoesophageal Cleft

HISTORY

In 1792 Richter (108) reported a child with common channel, but an autopsy was not performed. The second well-documented case was reported by Finlay in 1949 (109), and Roth et al. (110) reported 85 cases in 1983.

EMBRYOLOGY

Arrest of the proximal segment of the tracheoesophageal septum occurs when the cricoid lamina fails to fuse with extension of the cleft into the larynx. For all practical purposes, this is a large H-type tracheoesophageal fistula with extention to the larynx resulting because the embryonic foregut is not separated into trachea and esophagus (111–113). If the defect is large, a common channel is formed between trachea, esophagus, and posterior wall of the larynx involving the cricoid cartilage.

Pettersson (114) reported three types of defects: larynx only (type I), partial cleft of esophagus and trachea (type II), and cleft involving larynx with extension to tracheal carina (type III). To this classification has been added type IV, the cleft extending into the mainstream branchi.

Recently, the G syndrome was classified. In 1989 Howell and Smith (115) emphasized the association of laryngotracheoesophageal cleft with the G syndrome, which is a familial constellation of congenital anomalies such as

Table 3.9.
Treatment of Esophageal Atresia with Tracheoesophageal Fistula Associated with the Waterston Classification

Physiologic Status	Waterston Classification	Mode of Treatment	Survival (%)
Group 1	A	Primary repair	100
	B	Primary repair	100
	C	Primary repair	100
Group 2	C	Delayed repair	100
	C	Staged repair	57
Overall survival			92

(Modified from Randolph JG, Newman KD, Anderson KD. Current results in repair of esophageal atresia with tracheoesophageal fistula using physiologic status as a guide to therapy. Ann Surg 1989;209:526–531.)

distinctive facia, ocular hypertelorism, prominent occiput and forehead, short lingual frenulum, hypospadias, and cryptorchidism. Allanson (116) thinks that the G syndrome perhaps is of autosomal dominant inheritance. Other esophageal anomalies may be associated with this defect, and cases of laryngotracheoesophageal cleft have been reported in some instances (110, 117–123).

SYMPTOMS

Severe respiratory problems which are aggravated by feeding with choking, cyanosis, and pneumonia are all symptoms of a laryngotracheoesophageal cleft.

DIAGNOSIS

Diagnosis is made by contrast-enhanced studies showing barium within the esophagus and trachea. Bronchoscopy and esophagoscopy are better methods for making the diagnosis and for more clearly defining the extent of the cleft. According to Randolph (87), suspicion is the physician's best indicator.

TREATMENT

The first successful repair was reported by Pettersson in 1955 (114). Surgery and closure of the defect is the treatment of choice. Donahoe and Gee (120) and Myer et al (124) clearly defined the surgical steps necessary to deal with this highly complex and potentially lethal anomaly.

Membranous Atresia and Stenosis of the Esophagus (Esophageal Webs)

ATRESIA

Esophageal atresia usually occurs in the form of an aplastic segment, but membranous diaphragmatic atresias may be encountered. Such diaphragms are similar to those found in the intestines. They may be located in midesophagus, associated with a tracheoesophageal fistula (125) (Fig. 3.8, E), or found in an otherwise normal esophagus (Fig. 3.8, D). Both a segmental atresia and a membranous diaphragm have been found in the same patient (126). A membranous atresia of the distal esophagus has also been reported (127) (Fig. 3.19). Conversion of the esophagus above such a diaphragm into an apparent duplicated segment is discussed elsewhere in this text.

In a few cases the esophageal atresia is accompanied by a duodenal atresia. VACTERL association defects also are present (128).

The diaphragms usually involve only the mucosa. Muscle fibers seem to stem from the muscularis mucosae rather than from the muscularis externa. Although these are similar to membranous diaphragms found elsewhere in the alimentary tract, their symptoms are identical to those of segmental esophageal atresia. Treatment is by

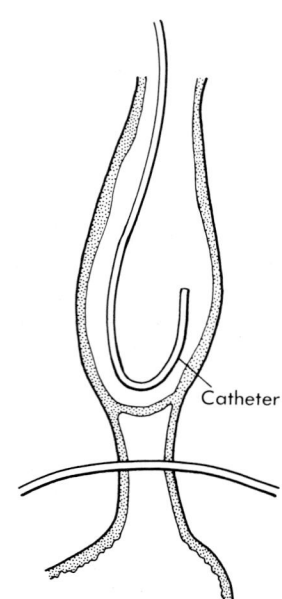

Figure 3.19. Membranous atresia of the lower esophagus with catheter in place. (After Schwartz SI. Congenital membranous obstruction of esophagus. Arch Surg, 1962;85:480–482.)

excision of the membrane, leaving a polyethylene nasogastric tube in place. Feeding by gastrostomy for several days is recommended.

STENOSIS

Esophageal webs, partially occluding the passageway, have been considered to be congenital in some cases (91, 129). The symptoms are identical to those of true stenosis, but they show a characteristic shelf-like picture on radiography. They are little more than mucosal redundancies, and other parts of the esophageal wall are not involved. A shelf-like occlusion in the diaphragm is sometimes referred to as "Schatzki's ring." It was first described in 1944 by Templeton (130) from its radiographic appearance; subsequently, an anatomic ring at the same location was reported (131). Most symptomatic cases have been found in middle-aged men (132) (Fig. 3.20). The ring is probably acquired (133), but in a few cases it may represent a perforated congenital diaphragm such as is occasionally found at the pylorus.

In a study of 32 patients, Jamieson et al. (134) concluded that esophageal stricture and Schatzki's ring are separate entities. There is no evidence that either is of congenital origin. This ring appears to be formed by repeated ingestion of quinidine, potassium chloride, tetracycline, aspirin, vitamin C, and phenytoin, which are known to injure the epithelium.

Webb et al. (135) reported that 4.8% of patients with dysphagia secondary to benign process had esophageal

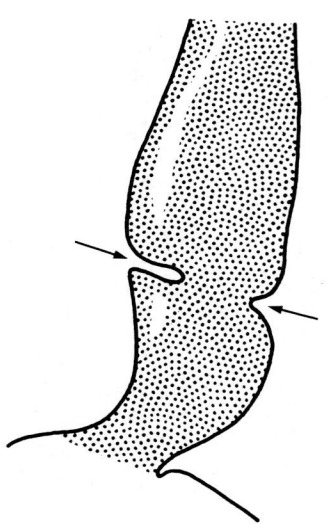

Figure 3.20. Drawing from a radiograph of a barium-filled esophagus, showing Schatzki's ring. In some cases this may represent perforation of a diaphragm, such as that shown in Figure 3.15. (After Trinkle JK. Lower esophageal ring. Ann Surg 1962;*155*:207–211.)

webs. Nosher et al. (136) reported that 5.5% of patients with possible esophageal disorders are found to have webs by cineradiographic studies.

Devitt (137) reported that, according to Elwood and Pitman (138) and Clements et al. (139), the incidence of webs in a normal population varies from 1 to 8% and most likely is asymptomatic.

EMBRYOGENESIS

In 1950 Ladd (140) stated that true congenital webs are developmental anomalies from a failure of coalescence of esophageal vacuoles, which may produce atresia or segmental stricture. Congenital webs are rare, according to Devitt (137), and fewer than 30 cases are reported in the literature (141–143).

In 1982 Shearman and Finlayson (144) reported that the rare hereditary disorder epidermolysis bulosa dystrophica has been associated with esophageal webs. Congenital webs are usually located in the midesophagus and are present in childhood, according to Devitt (137), who quotes Greenough (145), Bluestone et al. (146), and Liebman and Samloff (147). Sharma et al. (20) reported congenital intraluminal esophageal diaphragm at the lower end of the esophagus which, according to the authors, is probably the first report about this in English literature.

Tubular Duplications of the Esophagus

The reader should note that we describe duplication and cysts of the esophagus together, but we also present a separate discussion entitled "Dorsal Enteric Remnants in the Thorax" since organs below the diaphragm, such as the stomach and small intestines, participate in the production of these anomalies. Duplications located at the posterior mediastinum are the most common type of foregut duplication which presents as a cyst with epithelial mucosa within the muscular wall of the esophagus. Duplication of the alimentary tract is a very rare congenital anomaly. According to Nehme and Rabiah (148) and Whitaker et al (149), esophageal duplications represent 10 to 20% of these anomalies. Triplication was reported by Milson and colleagues (150) in 1985.

According to Game (151), Kirwan et al. (152) present other theories of duplication, such as the split notochord syndrome (153–155), tracheobronchial foregut duplication (156), and mucosal disorder syndrome, including the dysvascularization theory (157).

ANATOMY AND HISTORY

It is convenient to separate esophageal duplications that are tubular or cystic parallel channels, usually communicating with the normal esophagus or stomach, from cystic duplications that lie in the mediastinum without alimentary communication.

In 1674 Blasius (158) described doubling of the middle half of the esophagus. No other cases seem to have been noted until 1907 when Kathe (159) reported an accessory channel in the wall of the normal esophagus. Seven more were found over 10 years of careful autopsy by Ciechanowski and Glinski (160). Most of these duplications opened into the main esophageal channel at both ends. Usually they were situated in the submucosa, but sometimes they were found between muscle layers or even outside the muscularis. Most probably were asymptomatic.

In 1957 Maier (161) described a duplication extending from the level of T2 to 4 cm below the azygos vein in a 54-year-old woman. Symptoms, probably brought on by inflammation, had existed for only 6 years. A long incision dividing the partition between the channels was made. The muscularis was not involved and the cut edges of the partition retracted spontaneously.

Frank and Paul (162) reviewed the literature in 1949 and described a case in which two unequal channels running for 13 cm were seen radiographically in a patient asymptomatic before age 5 years (Fig. 3.21). Episodes of complete dysphagia then appeared, which were controlled by diet. No operation was performed, and the patient was free of symptoms at 17 years of age.

Carcinoma in an esophageal duplication was fatal in a 39-year-old man (163). The duplication ended blindly near the pharynx and opened into the stomach, communicating as well with the normal esophagus. There was a common muscular wall between the normal esophagus on the left and the duplication on the right. The duplication was lined with gastric mucosa having parietal cells.

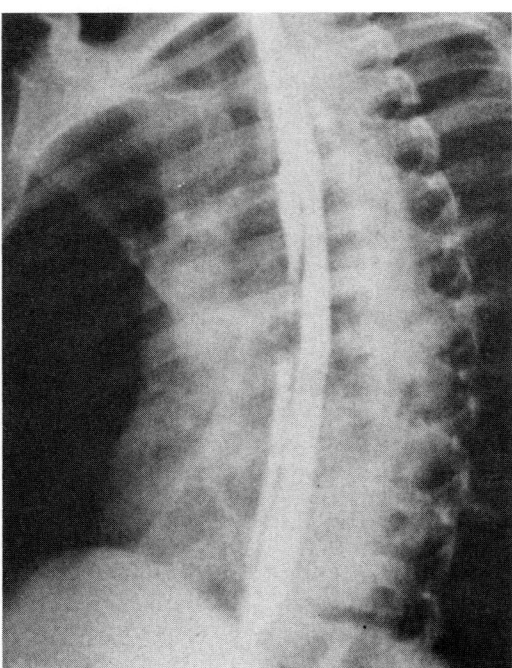

Figure 3.21. Oblique view of an almost completely duplicated esophagus in a child. The break in the barium shadow is an artifact resulting from incomplete filling at the moment of exposure. (From Frank RC, Paul LW. Congenital reduplication of the esophagus: report of a case. Radiology 1949;*53*:417.

Duplications of both stomach and esophagus are described in Chapter 5, "The Stomach."

EMBRYOGENESIS

The intramural duplications are probably true examples of faulty recanalization of the esophageal lumen, as described by Bremer (164). They represent fused longitudinal folds of mucosa.

SYMPTOMS AND INCIDENCE

Dysphagia is the only reported symptom. In one case the duplication existed for 5 years and in another for 48 years without symptoms, implying the possibility of a greater frequency than is clinically apparent. In the absence of an esophageal inflammation, it is probable that such a doubling would remain silent and undiagnosed. Symptoms of cysts of the esophagus are presented in Table 3.10.

DIFFERENTIAL DIAGNOSIS

Figure 3.22 presents a breakdown of location of mediastinal cysts and tumors of the posterior mediastinum. Note that in cases of mediastinal cysts, 20% have a spinal component.

We agree with King and Smith's breakdown of the types of mediastinal masses (165). According to their findings, of all tumors of the mediastinum, neurogenic

Table 3.10.
Symptoms of Esophageal Cysts[a]

Common	Less Common
Respiratory	Hemorrhage
Dyspnea	
Wheeze	Perforation
Dry cough	
Pneumonia	Chest pain 2 degrees to distension
Progressive respiratory distress	
Cyanosis	Cardiac arrhythmias
Nocturnal aspiration	
	Central nervous system—spinal cord signs
Gastrointestinal tract	
Regurgitation	
Dysphagia	Malignancy
Vomiting	
Failure to thrive	
Anorexia	
Epigastric pains	
Pyrosis	

Adapted from Game PA. Cysts and duplications of the oesophagus. In: Jamieson GG, ed. Surgery of the oesophagus. New York: Churchill Livingstone, 1988;887–892.

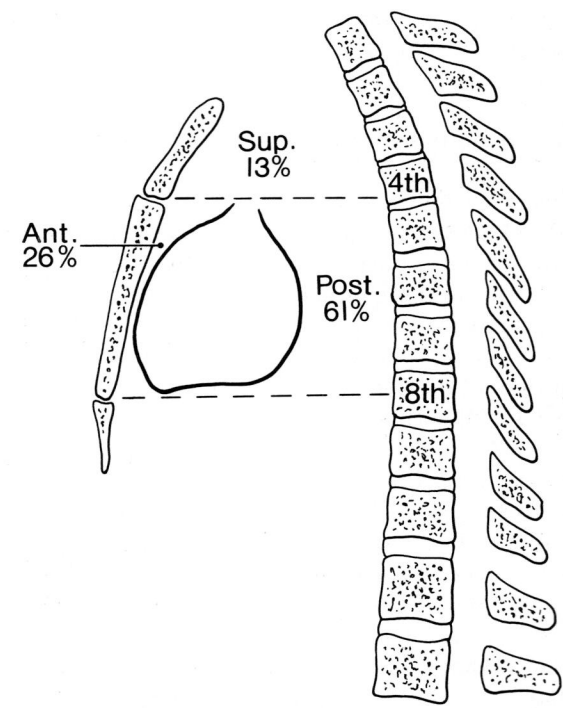

Figure 3.22. Location and frequency of mediastinal cysts and tumors in infants and children. Percentages represent approximate figures that have been rounded for clarity of presentation. (Adapted from Ravitch MM. Mediastinal cysts and tumors. In: Welch KF, Randolph JG, Ravitch MM, O'Neill JA, Rowe MI, (eds). Pediatric surgery, 4th ed, Vol 1. Chicago: Year Book Medical Publishers, 1986:602–618.)

tumors, located in the posterior mediastinum, are the most common in both children and adults. The most common malignant tumor in children and adults is the malignant lymphoma, which is located in the anterior mediastinum. In adults, the second most common malignant tumor is the thymoma, but in children it is the neuroblastoma, a malignant tumor originating from the sympathetic chain.

Other lesions which produce diagnostic problems are lipomas (166); intrathoracic hygromas (167–168); liposarcoma (169); histoplasmosis (170), and neurogenic tumors such as neuroblastoma.

The thymus is located at the superior anterior mediastinum, but occasionally thymic cysts extend posteriorly, producing a diagnostic enigma.

Kuster and Foroozan (171), reporting that Barrett's esophagus is found in 10 to 20% of patients undergoing endoscopy for esophagitis, believe that Barrett's esophagus with adenocarcinoma has a better prognosis if treated early with wide excisions.

Altorki et al. (172) documented that, in patients with high-grade dysplasia in a columnar-lined esophagus, esophagectomy is indicated because carcinoma is discovered in 45% of these patients.

Seabrook et al. (173) reported on observations on the diagnosis and management of the mystery of Barrett's esophagus. The preceding authors agree that this is secondary to reflux of gastric contents. Several other authors disagree. The etiologic factors remain uncertain, and perhaps the continuation of the McCallum study (174) will resolve the question of whether the disorder is congenital or acquired, as well as reveal a treatment.

DIAGNOSIS

In the face of so many differential diagnoses, Snyder and associates (175) are correct to discuss diagnostic dilemmas. Table 3.11 outlines diagnostic procedures for esophageal duplication.

Figure 3.23 shows an esophageal duplication cyst displacing the barium-filled esophagus laterally.

TREATMENT

Surgery should be performed after diagnosis to avoid complications (176). Surgical procedures are excision, enucleation, marsupialization, internal drainage, cauterization of mucosa, needle aspiration, and division of the septum. The esophageal duplication cyst is often encompassed within the muscle layer of the esophagus. In this case the mucosa of the cyst is removed from the muscular layer, leaving enough muscle to close over the esophagus without narrowing the lumen (Fig. 3.24).

The possible anatomic complications occur in the vagus nerve, the left recurrent nerve, and injuries related to the trachea.

Table 3.11.
Diagnostic Procedures of Esophageal Duplication

Procedure	Disorder	Author
Incidental chest x-rays	Deviation of trachea	Stringel et al., 1985[a]
	Retrocardiac mass	Milson, 1985[b]
	Occasional calcification	Maroko et al., 1984[c]
Upper gastrointestinal series filling defect	Rule out leiomyoma or a sarcoma with cystic degenerations	Gray et al., 1961[d]; Hover et al., 1982[e]; Whitaker et al., 1980[f]
	Thickened mucosal folds	Granelli et al., 1983[g]
	Communication: less than 10%	Game, 1988[h]
Computed tomography scan: adherant to the esophagus	Solid or cystic	Weiss et al., 1983[i]
Esophagoscopy and bronchoscopy	No help	
Biopsy	Not recommended	Game, 1988[h]
[99m]TC = sulfur colloid	Gastric mucosa	
Spiral x-rays to rule out spina bifida	Klippel-Feil syndrome	Anderson and Pluth, 1974[j]
Myelogram	Radiculopathy, myelopathy	

[a]Stringel G, Mercer S, Briggs V. Esophageal duplication cyst containing a foreign body. Can Med Assoc J 1985;132(5):529–531.
[b]Milson J, Unger S, Alford BA, Rodgers BM. Triplication of the esophagus with gastric duplication. Surgery 1985;98:121–125.
[c]Maroko I, Hirsch M, Sharon N, Benharroch D. Calcified mediastinal enterogenous cyst. Gastrointest Radiol 1984;9(2):105–106.
[d]Gray SW, Skandalakis JE, Shepard D. Smooth muscle tumors of the esophagus. Surgery 1961;113:205–220.
[e]Hover AR, Brade CE, Williams JR, Stewart DL, Christian C. Multiple retention cysts of the lower esophagus. J Clin Gastroenterol 1982;4:209–212.
[f]Whitaker JA, Deffenbach LD, Cooke AR. Esophageal duplication cyst. Am J Gastroenterol 1980;73:329–332.
[g]Granelli P, Angelini GP, Tambussi AM, Nicolini A, Celli L. Tubular duplication of the oesophagus in a child: clinical, radiologic and endoscopic features. Endoscopy 1983;15(4):263–265.
[h]Game PA: Cysts and duplications of the oesophagus. In: Jamieson GG, ed. Surgery of the oesophagus. New York: Churchill Livingstone, 1988:887–892.
[i]Weiss LM, Fagelman D, Warhit JM. CT demonstration of an esophageal duplication cyst. J Comput Assist Tomogr 1983;7(4):716–718.
[j]Anderson HA, Pluth JR. Benign tumours, cysts, and duplications of the esophagus. In: Payne WS, Olsen AM. The esophagus. Philadelphia:Lea & Febiger, 1974:115–237.

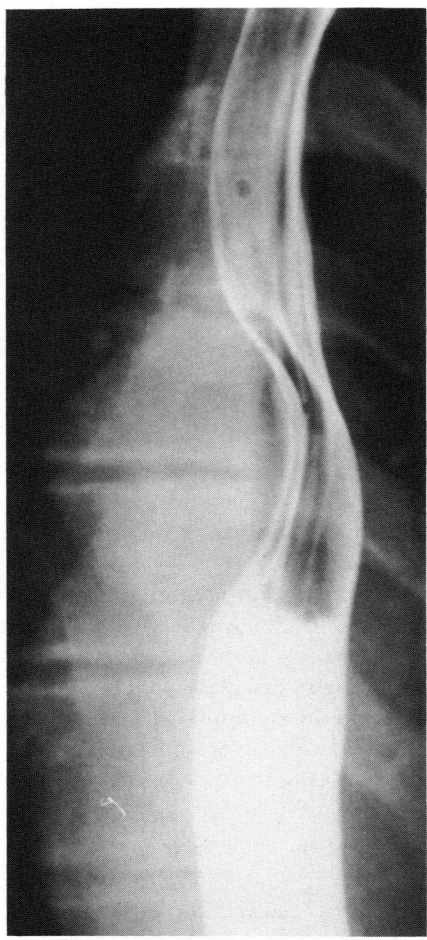

Figure 3.23. Esophageal duplication cyst.

SPLIT NOTOCHORD SYNDROME

During the third week of gestation, the notochord appears and at the same time begins its separation from the endoderm. During the separation, a gap sometimes appears in the notochord. Through this gap, a diverticulum from the foregut can herniate, and the genesis of several anomalies begins. The vertebral bodies are not united and are malformed, and the gut forms several long or short diverticula. Vertebral anomalies such as spina bifida occulta may take place, and according to Bower et al (177), vertebral column anomalies are associated with gastrointestinal duplications in 5 to 15% of cases. Duplications or cysts are found most frequently in the posterior mediastinum due to caudal movements toward the thoracic cavities of the remnants. Gastrointestinal mucosa in the lining of the duplication, the cyst, or occasionally the epithelium is ciliated.

For a complete discussion of the notochord syndrome, see the discussion of "Dorsal Enteric Remnants in the Thorax."

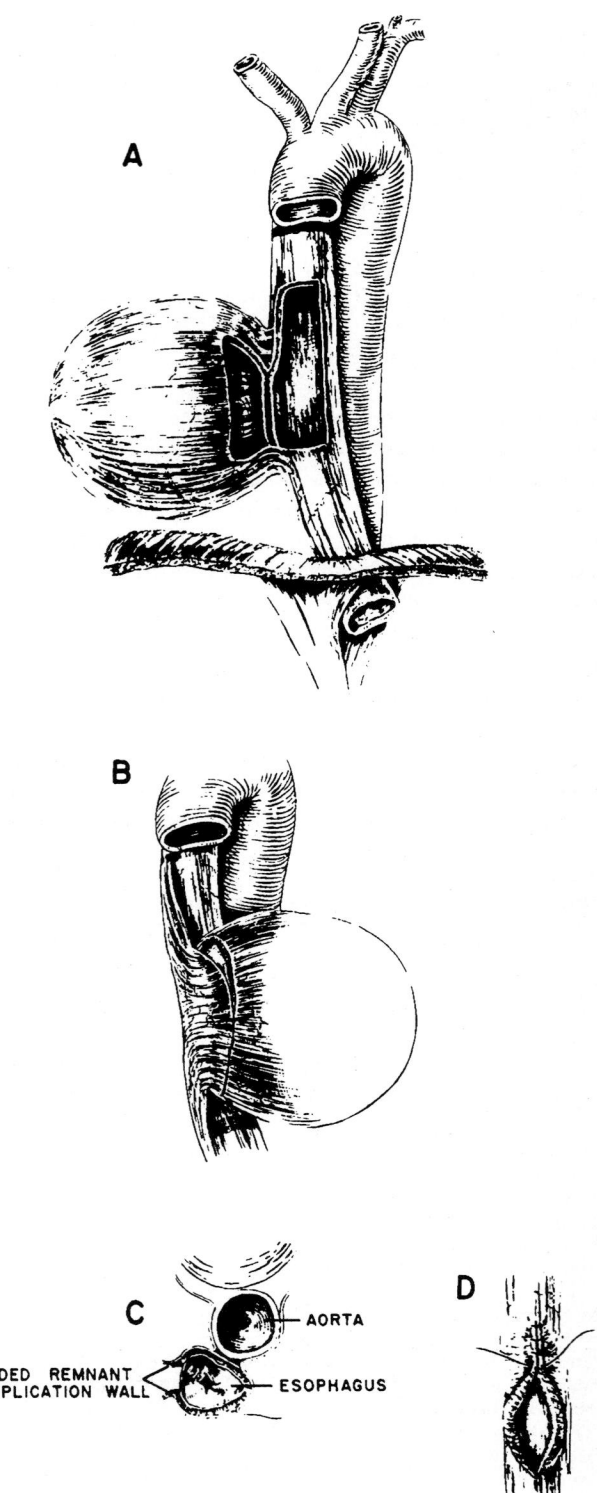

Figure 3.24. The most common form of enteric duplication within the mediastinum is ths type of cystic lesion encompassed within the muscle layers of the esophagus. Only the mucosa is removed in the portion of the cyst adjacent to the esophagus. Enough muscle is left to close over the esophageal mucosa. (From Raffensperger JG, ed. Swenson's pediatric surgery, 5th ed. Chicago: Appleton & Lange, 1990.)

Tracheobronchial Foregut Duplications. During the fourth to ninth week of gestation, the foregut separates from the tracheobronchial bud. Incomplete separation produces a congenital fistula between the respiratory tree and the foregut or a duplication which is lined by ciliated epithelium. A cyst may be formed due to complete separation from both the foregut and the respiratory tree.

Mucosal Disorders Syndrome. This is a faulty recanalization perhaps caused by residual vacuoles that remain and form duplicate or intramural esophageal cysts (178).

Dorsal Enteric Remnants in the Thorax

ANATOMY

Two types of anomalous alimentary tract structures may be found in the thorax. One is cystic and lies in the posterior mediastinum in close association with the esophagus. The other arises from the intestines and enters the thorax through the diaphragm. They differ widely in appearance but have a similar embryogenesis.

Mediastinal Cysts of Foregut Origin. A wide variety of masses may appear in the mediastinum. Among these, three are congenital and of embryonic origin: bronchogenic cysts, celomic (pericardial) cysts, and enteric (foregut) cysts. The first two are discussed elsewhere in this book; only the enteric cysts are considered here.

Enteric cysts originate from the foregut at an early stage of development and are found in the prevertebral portion of the superior mediastinum or in the posterior mediastinum. They have been variously designated as "duplications of the esophagus," "gastric cysts," "gastrocystomas," and "enterogenous cysts." We prefer the expression "dorsal enteric cyst" (179), as it is the most accurate and inclusive term. Because these cysts originate before the esophagus and trachea become separate structures, we prefer to relate them to the primitive foregut rather than to the esophagus.

Much of the confusion in terminology springs from the fact that these anomalous structures may be lined with almost any type of epithelium derived from the alimentary canal or respiratory tract. Two or three mucosal types frequently exist in different parts of the same cyst. Ware and Conrad (180) found gastric mucosa alone or in combination among 55.6% of their cases, esophageal mucosa in 33.3%, small intestinal mucosa in 21.0%, pancreatic mucosa in 5%, ciliated respiratory epithelium in 3.7%, and colonic mucosa in 2.5%. A particularly remarkable cyst was found to have three layers of muscle, hyaline cartilage, pseudostratified ciliated epithelium, stratified squamous epithelium, and intestinal epithelium. Its wall was continuous with the longitudinal musculature, and radiographically it resembled a benign smooth muscle tumor of the esophagus (181). Despite the cartilage, this and similar cysts (182) in the posterior mediastinum are

enteric and not bronchogeneic in origin. (See Table 13.15 for distinction between these cysts.)

Ciliated epithelium in these cysts is often called "respiratory epithelium," thus suggesting a tracheal rather than an esophageal origin. It should be remembered, however, that the prenatal esophagus as well as the trachea has a ciliated epithelium.

Dorsal enteric cysts in the thorax are usually associated with the middle and lower thirds of the esophagus. Their walls are reasonably similar to the wall of the gastrointestinal tract, and myenteric and submucosal ganglion cells may be present. In some cases the muscularis may be continuous with that of the normal esophagus; in others there may be a cleavage plane between the cyst and the esophagus. Rarely is there a primary fistulous connection with the esophagus although ulceration and perforation may subsequently establish a communication (183). The cysts vary in size from 1 cm in diameter to structures that fill the entire hemithorax. Bilocular cysts are known (184).

In general, dorsal enteric cysts lie posterior to the esophagus, whereas true bronchogenic cysts lie lateral to the trachea. The distinction is not always clear because the esophagus lies so close to the vertebral bodies that a cyst of any size must expand to one side or the other and, hence, become partly retropleural rather than mediastinal.

Intestinal Duplication Extending into the Thorax. In addition to the closed cysts of the posterior mediastinum, a small group of enterogenous defects occur in which the anomalous structure is immense, arising in the abdominal cavity, penetrating the diaphragm, and occupying a large portion of the thorax. These "thoracic duplications of the intestine," although rare, are exceedingly striking. Most arise from the duodenum or jejunum although the connection is not always patent: They are anchored cranially to the cervical vertebrae. Similar structures may arise from almost any portion of the abdominal intestines or even from the stomach (185). All show traces of an anchorage to the spinal cord or vertebral column at a level much higher than that of their origin from the intestines. One such duplication traversed the entire thorax, exhibiting a lining with components that ranged from salivary glands to intestinal mucosa with Brunner's glands. The subdiaphragmatic portion was a solid cord and extensive vertebral defects were present (183). Another duplication consisted of a mediastinal cyst attached to the sixth thoracic vertebra and a long thoracoabdominal cyst passing through the diaphragm and ending behind the peritoneum, with no intestinal connection (186). Still other such anomalous structures have a patent communication with the gut through which intestinal contents readily pass into the thoracic portion (27, 187). Figure 3.25 illustrates four of these striking anomalies.

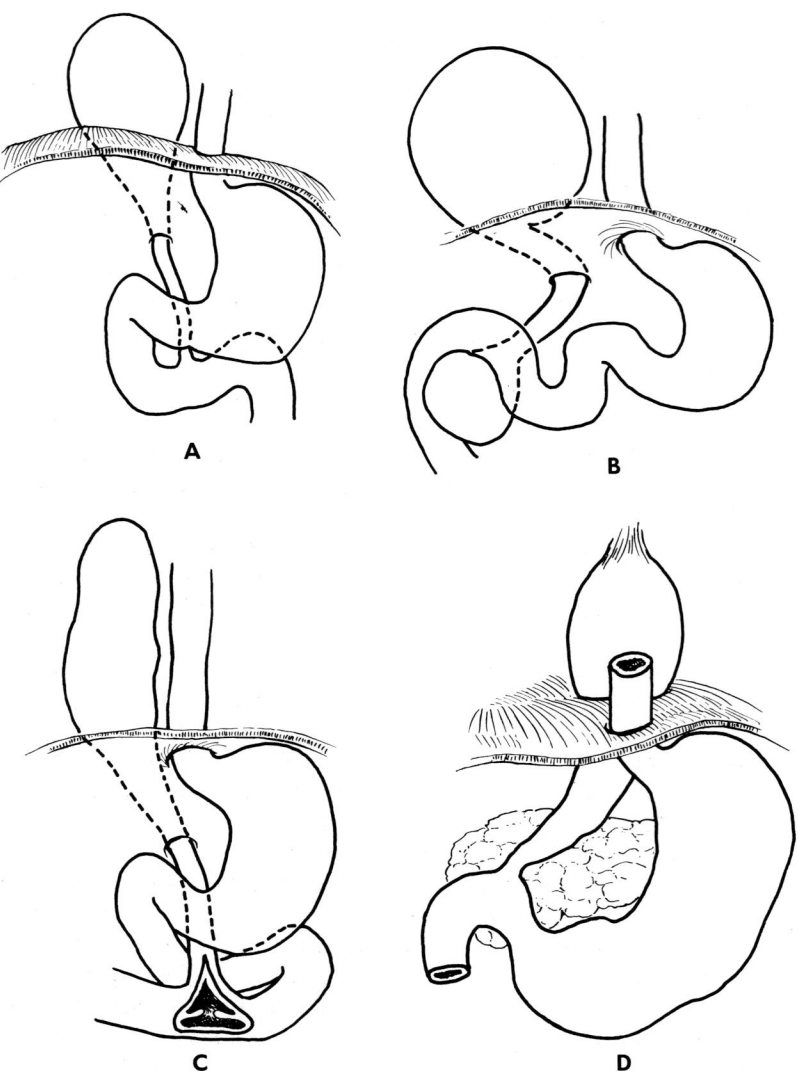

Figure 3.25. **A** to **D**, Four examples of abdominothoracic diverticula, which arise from the jejunum or duodenum, penetrate the diaphragm and occupy the right thorax. They usually terminate on cervical vertebrae. (**A**, From Spear HC, Daughtry DC, Chesney JG. Intestinal duplication cyst of abdominal origin presenting in thorax. J Thorac Surg 1959;37:810–814; **B**, from Beardmore HE, Wiglesworth FW. Vertebral anomalies and alimentary duplications. Pediatr Clin North Am 1958;5:457–474; **C**, from Gross RE. The surgery of infancy and childhood. Philadelphia: WB Saunders, 1953; **D**, from McLetchie NGB, Purves JK, Saunders RL deC H. Genesis of gastric and certain intestinal diverticula and entrogenous cysts. Surg Gynecol Obstet 1954;99:135–141.)

Alrabeeah et al. (188) reported seven cases of neurenteric cysts with additional anomalies. Three patients had mediastinal masses connected to lower cervical and upper thoracic vertebrae with intraspinal extension, and one of them had a intrapancreatic intestinal duplication cyst.

Wolf et al. (189) reported thoracoabdominal enteric duplication with meningocele, skeletal anomalies, and dextrocardia in an infant.

EMBRYOGENESIS

Earlier theories, advanced to explain duplications of various parts of the alimentary tract, were based on the formation of persisting alternative channels from the vacuolated epithelial stage or on the persistence of embryonic mucosal diverticula. Intramural communicating duplications and some diverticula may arise in these ways, but they do not explain the duplications considered here.

A third explanation, relating certain dorsal intestinal tract fistulae to the primitive and transient neurenteric canal, was suggested by many earlier embryologists and has been put forward most recently by Bremer (190) and Astley (191). While the hypotheses may be applicable to some inferior spinal defects, this canal is not involved in defects of the cervical or upper thoracic levels. A review of these theories may be found in Botha's paper (13).

The fundamental developmental error underlying the formation of these cysts occurs during formation of the notochord (18th or 19th day, stage 8) before the foregut itself is indicated. At this stage the notochord is growing cephalad from the primitive knot between the ectoderm and endoderm of the two-layered embryonic disc. The notochord at first is in intimate association with the endodermal cells, but normally it later separates from them. Cephalic growth of the ectoderm and notochord mesoderm is now greater than that of the endoderm, resulting in a shearing movement between the tissues. If the notochord fails to detach itself from the endoderm, cells of the latter will be dragged forward and upward as the tissues separate. Such endodermal cells, detached from the roof of the developing gut, round up to form a cyst. If they remain attached to the notochord, they may also act as a local barrier to the later anterior fusion of the vertebral mesoderm, resulting in anterior spina bifida. Thus, depending on the distribution of cells along the line of shear, an endodermal cyst may be attached to the esophagus, to the vertebrae, or to neither. Very occasionally, only a vertebral defect remains. Fallon and his collaborators (192) have given a good description of the process.

Beardmore and Wiglesworth (193) and McLetchie et al. (194) suggest that adhesion of endoderm and ectoderm, even prior to the appearance of the notochord, may produce the same result. The developing notochord must pass to one side of the adhesion or split to pass on both sides. Traction pulls neural tube cells downward and endoderm cells upward. This accounts for the neural connections occasionally found in enteric remnants (195, 196).

The earlier these anomalous adhesions occur, the greater is the distance between their two ends. The huge duplications arising from the duodenum and inserting on the cervical vertebrae are the result of early and extensive adhesion of notochord and archenteron. The smaller mediastinal cysts result from adhesion toward the end of differential growth and involve a smaller number of displaced cells. The variety of mucosal types found in these cysts confirms their origin from undifferentiated archenteric endoderm. Only about 25% contains epithelium normal to parts of the digestive tube arising caudal to the anterior intestinal portal, thus arguing for a relatively anterior position of the primary defect on the embryonic disc.

ASSOCIATED ANOMALIES

The most frequent anomaly found in the presence of posterior mediastinal cysts is a defect of the vertebral bodies of lower cervical and upper thoracic vertebrae. About 50% of patients with cysts have vertebral body defects eventually leading to scoliosis (197).

These defective vertebrae are the result of the intimate relationship of the superior end of the cyst, or duplication, with the spinal cord, its meninges, or the vertebral bodies. They are not incidental but are part of the process by which the cysts are formed. In extreme cases a cyst may exist in the neural canal (198). One such cyst had gastric, esophageal, and ciliated epithelium surrounded by smooth muscle, as well as a mass of central nervous system tissue at one pole (195). In another case a duplication arising from the jejunum, which passed through the diaphragm and terminated as a tube, had stratified squamous epithelium ventrally and nervous tissue dorsally. The pia mater of the cord was continuous with the connective tissue of the duplication through a defect in T2 (195). More frequently, there is only a fibrous attachment of the cyst to the defective vertebrae.

The second associated anomaly is a duplication of the small intestine. In Fallon's series (192) of 65 mediastinal cysts, there were 29 vertebral lesions and eight abdominal duplications of the intestine. Beardmore and Wiglesworth (193) suggest the existence of a triad of vertebral anomaly, posterior mediastinal cyst, and intestinal duplication. Bentley and Smith (155) propose the name "split notochord syndrome." A number of other associated anomalies are listed by Ware and Conrad (180), but they seem to be coincidental.

HISTORY AND INCIDENCE

First reported in Germany in 1909 by Staehelin-Burckhardt (199), dorsal enteric cysts were for a time considered rarities. Mixter and Clifford (200) are said to have reported the first case in the United States in 1929 although some earlier reports of dermoid cysts and teratomata in the posterior mediastinum may well have been examples of foregut cysts. Laipply (201) collected 25 cases by 1945, and Ware and Conrad (180) reported 81 cases in the English language literature by 1953.

In 1952 Veeneklaas (154) was among the first to call attention to the significance of the spinal defects frequently associated with enterogenous cysts and duplications. At least 17 patients with giant duplications passing through the diaphragm and occupying both the thoracic and abdominal cavities have been described. In some of these, the lumen communicated with that of the small intestine, usually the jejunum (202), whereas others had no connection with the alimentary tract (193). They projected into the right hemithorax about three times more frequently than into the left. Fallon et al. (192) consider them to be more common in women.

SYMPTOMS

Symptoms of mediastinal enteric cysts may derive from pain from a rise in intrinsic pressure of the cyst; ulceration and perforation from gastric secretions in the cyst;

or pressure on surrounding structures. The most common symptoms are dyspnea, cyanosis, cough, vomiting, and failure to gain weight. Less common are dysphagia, chest pain, and repeated bouts of pneumonia. Occasionally, hemoptysis, hematemesis, abdominal pain, and hoarseness are also seen. Symptoms of peptic ulcer occur when gastric epithelium with parietal cells lines the cyst. Ware and Conrad (180) mention ulceration in 14 of 45 cysts with gastric lining. Communication with the bronchial tree as a result of ulceration and erosion of adjacent tissue is known.

An unknown number of cystic lesions are completely asymptomatic for many years. They may be discovered on routine x-ray examination or autopsy or because they become symptomatic when the patient is at an advanced age.

DIAGNOSIS

The specific diagnostic sign of an enteric cyst is the radiologic appearance of a spheric or ovoid mass having smooth, clearly defined boundaries, which is located toward the right side in the posterior mediastinum, often together with developmental defects of cervical or thoracic vertebrae. Not all cysts, however, are accompanied by vertebral defects.

Rarely, when duplications have intestinal connections, peristaltic gurgling sounds may suggest the diagnosis. This should be confirmed by plain x-ray examination, which may show gas in the tubular duplication, and by barium studies, which outline the duplication. It is often extremely difficult to distinguish this condition from a diaphragmatic defect hernia.

Aspiration of the contents of the cystic tumor has frequently been undertaken, but many authors feel that it has not often led to correct diagnosis (180, 203). It should be remembered that, even when gastric mucosa is present, parietal cells may not occur and hence, the cystic contents may be neutral.

DIFFERENTIAL DIAGNOSIS

At least 13 types of tumors, in addition to enteric cysts, have been described in the "clinical" posterior mediastinum, and a few others might be included (Table 3.12). The most common tumors lying behind the esophagus are those of neurogenic origin. Neuroblastomas are usually encountered in children, ganglioneuromas in youths, and neurofibromas in adults. Erosion of the vertebrae with resulting scoliosis may accompany these tumors, but such erosion rarely simulates the developmental defects associated with enterogenous cysts. Pressure symptoms may be present, and nerve involvement usually leads to pain.

In the absence of vertebral defects and other symptoms, it is probably impossible to distinguish radiologi-

Table 3.12.
Abnormal Masses Found in the Posterior Mediastinum

Of embryonic origin	
Bronchogenic cysts	Relatively common
Dorsal enteric cysts	Rare
Pericardial cysts	Relatively common
Of neoplastic origin	
Neurogenic tumors	Relativey common (85% benign)
Lymphomas	Rare
Fibromas	Rare
Hemangiomas	Rare
Myxomas	Very rare
Intrathoracic meningoceles	Very rare
Xanthomas	Very rare
Myelomas	Very rare
Chordomas	Very rare
Fibrosarcomas	Very rare
Pleural effusion	Very rare

cally a laterally displaced enteric cyst from a bronchogenic cyst in the posterior mediastinum. The latter is more likely to be silent and to be discovered accidentally on routine x-ray examinations later in life. The similarity in appearance of both bronchogenic and enterogenous cysts to neurogenic tumors, even though such tumors are 85% benign, usually calls for their removal when any doubt exists.

TREATMENT

The impossibility of exact diagnosis in many cases, together with the possible malignant nature of a posterior mediastinal mass, makes removal of such cysts the procedure of choice. As Peabody et al. (203) asked, "Where else in the body could a large mass appear and conservative treatment be advised?"

Destruction of the cyst by marsupialization and repeated curettage to destroy the epithelium has been abandoned in favor of excision whenever possible. Should islands of epithelium remain undestroyed, regeneration of the cyst may take place. The deep pits of the gastric mucosa found frequently in such cysts makes complete extirpation especially difficult and makes a transpleural approach the treatment of choice. Rarely is the pleura adherent unless the cyst itself has perforated, in which case pulmonary lobectomy may be necessary. There may or may not be a cleavage plane between the muscular walls of the cyst and the esophagus. If the structures are inseparable in the area of contact, the musuclar wall of the cyst should be allowed to remain, but the mucosal layer must be stripped away entirely.

Treatment of those enterogenous structures that pass through the diaphragm is designed on an individual basis. Gross (28) suggests that, if gastric epithelium is absent and the symptoms are those of pressure only, the abdominal portion may safely be allowed to remain. If gastric mucosa is present and there has been bleeding, all of the anomalous tract should be removed. If an abdominal extension remains, it should be watched carefully because absence of gastric tissue above the diaphragm does not preclude its existence below. Several such large duplications have no patent connection with the intestinal tract and thus are still capable of ulceration and perforation in the abdomen. Borrie (187) has described great difficulties with the leaking stump of such a duplication resected at the level of the diaphragm.

MORTALITY

When gastric mucosa is present, ulceration and perforation may occur. In their review, Ware and Conrad (180) stated that there were 11 deaths among 63 patients (18.3%) operated on for mediastinal cysts of enterogenous origin.

Diverticula of the Esophagus

ANATOMY AND EMBRYOGENESIS

Outpouchings of the esophagus at various levels are not uncommon. They may be divided into "true" diverticula, which are covered with all the layers of the esophageal wall, and "false" diverticula, which are covered only with mucosa and submucosa. The latter are hernial rather than diverticular in nature.

Proximal Diverticula. Miskovitz and Steinberg (204) support the ideas that diverticula of the esophagus arise from the posterior wall of the cervical or upper thoracic esophagus and that, practically, they have the same embryologic origin as a duplication.

Midthoracic Diverticula. Diverticula in this area arise on the right anterolateral border of the esophagus (205) and occasionally contain gastric colonic or pancreatic epithelium. Several authors (206–209) believe that the majority of diverticula of the midthoracic division are secondary to dysmotility of the esophagus and are pulsion-type diverticula. After manometric study of 34 patients with this type of diverticula, Rivkin et al. (210) believes most cases have motor abnormalities. A right aortic arch with a retroesophageal diverticulum was reported by Spiridonov et al. (211).

Diverticulitis with erosion of the esophageal wall, bleeding, and perforation (212) has been reported. Neoplastic changes and arteriovenous fistulae have also been reported with esophageal diverticulitis.

Distal Diverticula. Hurwitz et al. (213) and Duranceau (205) believe most diverticula are of the pulsion type, and they suggest that incoordination of the lower esophageal sphincter may be the etiological or pathogenic factor in relaxation and premature closure.

Congenital True Diverticula. These are exceedingly rare. The first unquestionable case was described by Jackson and Shallow (214) in 1926. Nelson (215) subsequently reported a case of true diverticulum in a 2-year-old infant originating at the level of T1 and compressing the trachea anteriorly. The pouch was 3 cm in diameter and contained stratified squamous epithelium and all the usual esophageal layers; in addition, some striated muscle fibers were present in the muscularis. Nelson (215) searched the literature up to 1957 and concluded that the case of Jackson and Shallow (214) was the only other authentic case.

In 1959 Grant and Arneil (216) reported diverticula of the upper third of the esophagus in a newborn infant and in a 10-month-old child.

The embryonic origin of these structures may be assigned either to persistent embryonic mucosal diverticula, such as described in pig embryos by Lewis and Thyng (217), or to the presence of small, blind duplications that have subsequently become enlarged in the same manner as acquired pulsion diverticula but which are the result of intraluminal swallowing pressures and retention of food.

Pulsion Diverticula. Pulsion diverticula are herniations of the mucosa through defects in the muscular wall of the esophagus. The muscular defects may be of embryonic origin; the subsequent herniation, however, is acquired. Most appear anteriorly.

All regions of the esophagus are susceptible to the appearance of these diverticula. Lerche (218) found 150 cases in the literature, of which 22 were in the upper third, 53 in the middle third, and 75 in the lower third of the esophagus. Law and Overstreet (219) emphasized their occurrence in the midesophagus. They tend to appear in men over 50 years of age.

Diverticula of this type in the lower third of the esophagus have been called epiphrenic. They were first described in 1833, but only eight cases had been found by 1900. Goodman and Parnes (220) collected 126 acceptable cases through 1949. These diverticula are often associated with achalasia or hiatal hernia (221), and they may be asymptomatic (222). A familial tendency has been suggested (223).

The location of these diverticula is accounted for by the arrangement of the esophageal musculature, as described over a century ago by Laimer (224). The longitudinal fibers of the median anterior wall may not completely cover the underlying circular fibers, thus predisposing the patient to anterior herniation. In the lower third of the esophagus, the inner layer of fibers is spiral and is composed in part of a meshwork of fascicles rather than being a compact layer. Spaces between these fascicles may be great enough to permit herniation of the mucosa. Significantly, the majority of spontaneous ruptures of the esophagus take place in this region (225).

Surgical correction is desirable when these diverticula

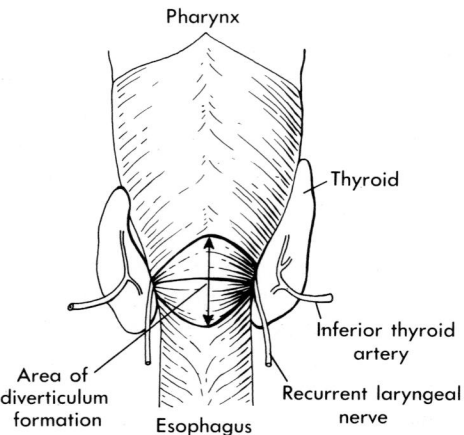

Figure 3.26. Posterior aspect of the pharyngeoesophageal junction showing the area in which "false" pulsion diverticula are formed. (After Lahey FH, Warren KW. Esophageal diverticula. Surg Gynecol Obstet 1954;*98*:1–28.

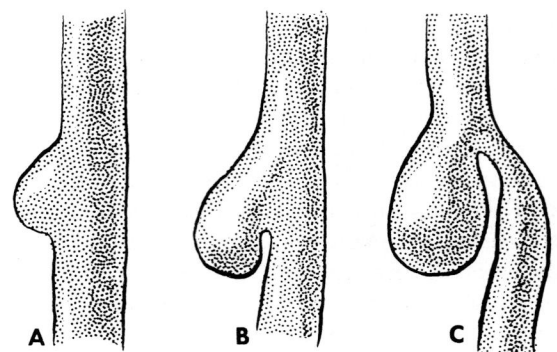

Figure 3.27. Progressive stages in the formation of pulsion esophageal diverticulum. When the diverticulum becomes dependent (**C**), it fills readily with food and compresses the esophagus distal to it. (After Lahey FH, Warren KW. Esophageal diverticula. Surg Gynecol Obstet 1954;*98*:1–28.)

become large enough to interfere with deglutition, produce pain by pressure on nerves, ulcerate, or undergo malignant degeneration. Forty-three operations with four deaths have been reported (220).

Pulsion diverticula at the junction of the pharynx and esophagus are termed *cricopharyngeal,* or Zenker's diverticula. The triangular area of the posterior wall (pharyngeal dimple) between the oblique and circular (cricopharyngeal) portions of the inferior constrictor muscle is the point of weakness through which the herniation takes place (Fig. 3.26). Congenital weakness of the esophageal wall or functional incoordination of the fibers of the inferior constrictor muscles (226) have been assigned as causes. One case was reported in which the herniation was present at birth (227). Lahey and Warren (228) reviewed the surgery of these pulsion diverticula from 1830.

The chief symptom, dysphagia, does not appear until the herniated mucosa and submucosa have formed a sac, which becomes directed downward as it enlarges. Retention of food in this sac eventually compresses the esophagus between the trachea and the sac (Fig. 3.27).

Traction Diverticula. These result from adhesions producing external traction on the esophagus. They have large mouths and are not pendant; hence, they do not enlarge with age. They are not usually embryonic in origin although it has been suggested that some in the midesophagus may be produced by a fibrous band, the atretic remnant of a tracheoesophageal fistula that closed before birth (221) (Fig. 3.28).

Symptoms of Distal Division. The primary symptom of distal diverticula is dysphagia from food entrapment (229).

DIAGNOSIS

Pulsion diverticula are best demonstrated radiographically, using thin barium mixtures. Lahey and Warren

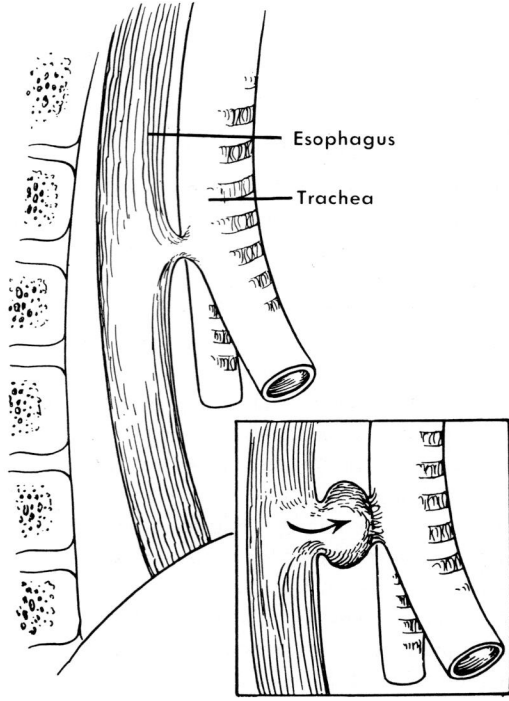

Figure 3.28. Possible origin of traction diverticula of the esophagus by adhesions. (From Cross FS, Johnson GF, Gerein AN. Esophageal diverticula. Arch Surg 1961;*83*:525–533.

(228) emphasize the need for semilateral views to confirm the diagnosis and to distinguish the pharyngoesophageal diverticulum from the dilation above an esophageal web. Malignant lesions within the sac must be kept in mind.

Bougienage is dangerous because the tip of the bougie may pass into the diverticulum, especially during the later developmental stages, and perforate the blind end of the sac. Any instrument should be passed only on a swallowed ring.

Debas et al. (229) conducted a series of good radiologic evaluations. They found 65 patients with distal division: 53 with single division, 10 with two divisions, and 2 with multiple divisions. Hiatal hernia and motor disorders are associated with epiphrenic division.

DIFFERENTIAL DIAGNOSIS

Cricopharyngeal diverticula may be diagnosed by their location. True congenital diverticula occurring elsewhere are probably indistinguishable radiologically from the pulsion type. Traction diverticula usually have a wide orifice and are directed upward, in contrast to the pendant, narrow-mouthed form of the pulsion type. There is usually a history of thoracic inflammation or, in some cases, a leiomyoma may be present (230).

TREATMENT

DeBakey et al. (231) reviewed the history of the surgical treatment of these diverticula, beginning with the first successful excision in 1886.

External fistula, diverticulopexy, inversion, and extirpation have all been employed in treating diverticula, but surgical extirpation is the method of choice at present. Lahey and Warren (228) recommend that extirpation of cricopharyngeal herniae be done in two stages 7 days apart, whereas others (231) prefer a single-stage method. The recent trend seems to favor the one-stage procedure. Even when detected early, these diverticula should be allowed to develop until a definite neck has been established so that adequate tissue is available for surgical repair.

For the epiphrenic group of diverticula, anastomosis between sac and stomach, inversion, diverticulopexy, esophageal resection, and excision have been used. Excision has been most strongly advocated for some time (232) although resection of part of the esophagus may be necessary because of the presence of a stricture.

Excision, esophagomyotomy, or both is the treatment of choice for distal diverticula. Resection and esophageal myotomy in symptomatic cases of midthoracic diverticula is the treatment of choice.

MORTALITY

Lahey and Warren (228) recorded two postoperative deaths in 365 pulsion diverticula treated surgically. There were 12 recurrences among 250 resections carried out by a two-stage procedure. Without operation, the eventual fate of a patient with a developing cricopharyngeal diverticulum is death either from rupture and mediastinitis or from starvation. Diverticula situated lower in the esophagus also eventually rupture.

Functional Disturbances of the Lower Esophagus

A variety of disturbances of normal esophageal function in both infants and adults can be related to the lower esophagus and the esophagocardiac orifice (Table 3.13). It is not always evident whether there are anatomic bases for such disturbances, but in several of the conditions, embryonic defects appear to underlie dysfunction. We consider the following here: heterotopic mucosa in the esophagus; congenital short esophagus; achalasia with or without megaesophagus; and chalasia.

The origin of these lesions is further obscured because often there is little agreement between the anatomist, radiologist, physiologist, and surgeon concerning the details of normal esophageal function (Fig. 3.29).

The radiologist has tended to consider the closure of the esophageal orifice as resulting from the constrictor cardiae muscles, the obliquity with which the esophagus enters the stomach, and the "pinchcock" action of the diaphragm.

Some anatomists and surgeons, such as Lerche (218) and Poppel et al. (233), have denied the pinchcock action of the diaphragm and have described an "inferior esophageal sphincter" that anatomically and physiologically divides the lower end of the esophagus (the phrenic ampulla) from the "gastro-esophageal vestibule" (218) or "cardiac antrum" (234). In the normal individual, the vestibule makes up the abdominal portion of the esophagus, ending at the constrictor cardiae (Fig. 3.29). Together, the "phrenic ampulla" and the vestibule are usually considered the "ampulla" by radiologists (235) and were called the "gastro-esophageal segment of expulsion" by Evans (236). Friedland et al. (129) and Berridge et al. (133) reviewed the evidence and concluded that the inferior esophageal sphincter is physiologically independent of the rest of the esophagus, but that it is anatomically indistinguishable when relaxed. Its contraction is coincident with shortening of the vestibule.

The terminology used for this region is not rendered less obscure when we attempt to define the limits of the esophagus by the nature of the mucosa rather than by gross appearance. Palmer (237) marked the mucosal function with silver clips located by esophagoscopy and biopsy and reported a wide range of movement under normal physiologic conditions as visualized by radiography. In the full stomach, the mucosal boundary was near the level of the constrictor cardiae, whereas in the empty organ, the boundary appeared to be well up into the vestibule. Palmer interpreted these findings to mean that the mucosa was mobile over the deeper layers in the region of the cardia. Lacau et al. (238) reported seven cases of dysphagia in oculopharyngeal myopathy with normal upper sphincter.

In a recent symposium about esophageal reflux in children, Ament (239) stated that the infant has a lower esophageal sphincter pressure, that the length of the lower esophageal sphincter increases with time, and that perhaps the central nervous system has some effect on the lower esophageal sphincter and gastric motility.

Table 3.13.
Anomalies and Related Lesions of the Lower Esophageal Segment and the Cardiac Orifice

Anomaly	Pathology	Onset of Symptoms	Symptoms		Radiology	Endoscopy	Treatment
			Early	Late			
Heterotopic mucosa	Patches of gastric mucosa in esophagus		None	Esophagitis?	Rarely visible	May or may not be visible	None
Congenital short esophagus	Failure of stomach to descend completely; enlarged hiatus; normal left gastric artery; no periotneal sac	Infancy to adulthood	Dysphagia, regurgitation; may be asymptomatic	Esophagitis and stricture; bleeding, anemia and failure to gain weight	Retrograde filling of distal esophagus; shortened esophagus early in disease	Normal, or redness, erosion, edema, stricture	Mobilization of esophagus to bring stomach down; repair of hiatus
Hiatal hernia	Enlarged hiatus; long left gastric artery; peritoneal sac present	Chiefly after middle age	Pain, dysphagia, regurgitation; pain may simulate coronary disease; may be asymptomatic and is usually so in children	Ulceration and stricture; anemia	Retrograde filling of distal esophagus; shortened esophagus late in disease	Normal, or redness, erosion, edema, stricture	*Conservative:* weight reduction. *Surgical:* phrenic nerve interruption; reduction of hernia; repair of hiatus
Achalasia	Deficiency of ganglion cells of myenteric plexus	1st few wk of life to adulthood	Dysphagia and regurgitation, especially with solid food and cold liquid	Megaesophagus	Dilated esophagus	Normal	*Mild cases:* careful chewing, avoidance of cold liquids, dilatation. Surgical: Heller myotomy
Chalasia	?	1st wk of life	Passive reflux regurgitation	None	Large esophagus, atonic and flaccid; lax cardial opening	Normal	Feeding in upright position
Abnormal idiopathic congenital reflux	?	1st wk of life	Vomitus aspiration	Esophagitis	Motility emptying and rule out other pathology	Confirm previous diagnosis	Surgery

HETEROTOPIC GASTRIC MUCOSA IN THE ESOPHAGUS

The lining of the embryonic foregut produces three main types of adult epithelium: stratified squamous in the esophagus; pseudostratified ciliated in the trachea and bronchi; and glandular columnar in the stomach. It is by no means surprising that misplaced epithelial patches occur.

In the course of development, the esophagus is lined first with columnar, later with ciliated columnar, and finally with stratified squamous epithelium. In addition, patches of esophageal mucosa may differentiate into the glandular columnar epithelium typical of the stomach.

Areas of ciliated epithelium may remain in the esophagus until birth. Rector and Connerley (8) found patches of ciliated esophageal epithelium in 25 male and 17 female subjects among single random sections of esophagus from 1000 autopsied children. All those with ciliated epithelium were born prematurely. Such epithelium probably does not long survive the onset of swallowing.

The presence of gastric mucosa in the esophagus, first described in 1805, is more common and more persistent. Its incidence has been variously reported as from 0.7% to as much as 70%. Schridde (239) reported islets from 1 to 2 cm in diameter to microscopic areas in 70% of the cadavers he examined. The greater number of these islets have been found in the upper portion of the esophagus. Among 57 males and 32 females, Rector and Connerley (8) found only 8% in the lower esophagus (Fig. 3.30). In about 33% of these, parietal cells were present. Intestinal metaplasia of such heterotopic gastric mucosa has also been reported (241).

In spite of the presence of large areas of gastric mucosa, some islands of stratified squamous epithelium

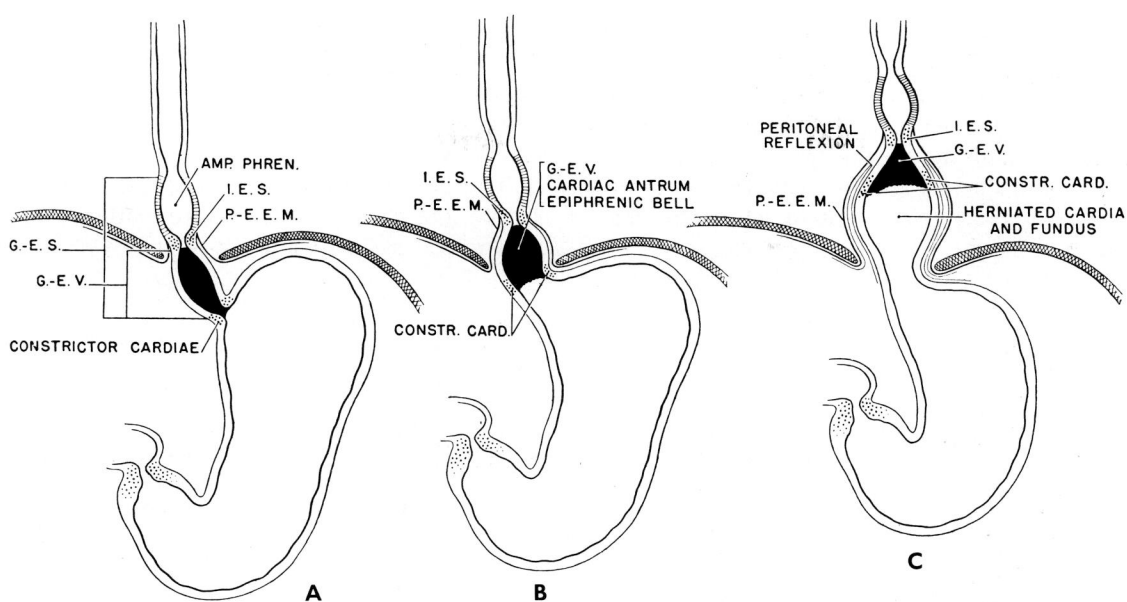

Figure 3.29. **A,** Relationships of structures in normal hiatus. *Black segment* of esophagus represents the gastroesophageal vestibule or cardiac antrum *(G.-E.V.).* **B,** Relationships of structures in so-called hiatal insufficiency. The *black segment* of esophagus lying partially in and partially above the hiatus represents the distended gastroesophageal vestibule (of Lerche), cardiac antrum (of Luschka), or so-called epephrenic bell (of Anders and Bahrmann). It is this arrangement that is the most difficult to interpret during roentgen examination and must be differentiated from a small sliding hernia. Frequently this is possible only by demonstrating, during the roentgenoscopic phase of the examination, the integrity or incompetence of the cardiac sphincter. **C,** Diagram of sliding hiatus hernia in frontal plane, showing the relationships of the various structures. *G-E.S.,* Gastroesophageal segment of expulsion; *I.E.S.,* inferior esophageal sphincter (Lerche); *Constr. Card.,* constrictor cardiac; *P.-E.E.M.,* phrenoesophageal elastic membrane (Laimer); *Amp. Phren.,* phrenic ampulla (Hasse and Strecker). (From Evans JA. Sliding hiatus hernia. AJR 1952;68:754–763.

usually remain, mucous glands are present in the submucosa, and there is no peritoneal covering. These characteristics indicate that the organ is the esophagus and not a thoracic stomach.

Several pathologic conditions have been associated with these heterotopic patches. They have been considered to be sites predisposing to carcinoma (242). However, the male/female ratio of esophageal carcinoma is 9:1, whereas heterotopic gastric mucosal islets show a ratio of less than 2:1. These areas have been said to give rise to pulsion diverticula, but there is no evidence that the local strength of the mucosa has any real effect on the strength of the esophageal wall.

Chronic peptic ulcers of the esophagus may be related to these heterotopic patches of gastric mucosa, but such ulcers do not occur in the postcricoid region where islets of gastric tissue are most numerous. However, ulcers have been found in such islets elsewhere. Barrett (243) believed that chronic peptic ulcers exist only concomitantly with congenital short esophagus. Allison (244) suggested that reflux esophagitis may produce an invasion of gastric mucosa that replaces the normal esophageal stratified squamous epithelium, but no evidence exists to support this view. In experimental lesions in dogs, esophageal stratified squamous epithelium regenerated,

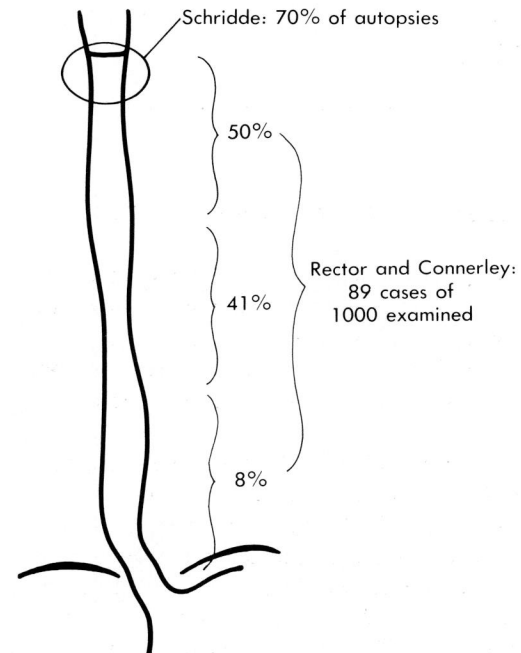

Figure 3.30. Relative frequency of heterotopic gastric mucosa in the esophagus. Curiously, more examples are in the upper end than in the lower.

whereas gastric mucosa at the lower border of the wound did not grow upward (245).

Lell (246) found an incidence of less than 4% in 5000 esophagoscopies. Fifty percent of the cases produced symptoms in individuals before the age of 5 years.

Whale (247) and Porto (248) described patients with heterotopic thyroid tissue forming an intraluminal tumor in the esophagus.

CONGENITAL SHORT ESOPHAGUS WITH THORACIC STOMACH

Columnar epithelium of congenital origin or metaplasia of squamous epithelium are due to chemical injury caused by acid.

The presence of a portion of the stomach above the diaphragm may result from three different developmental anomalies. Confusion among them is caused partly by

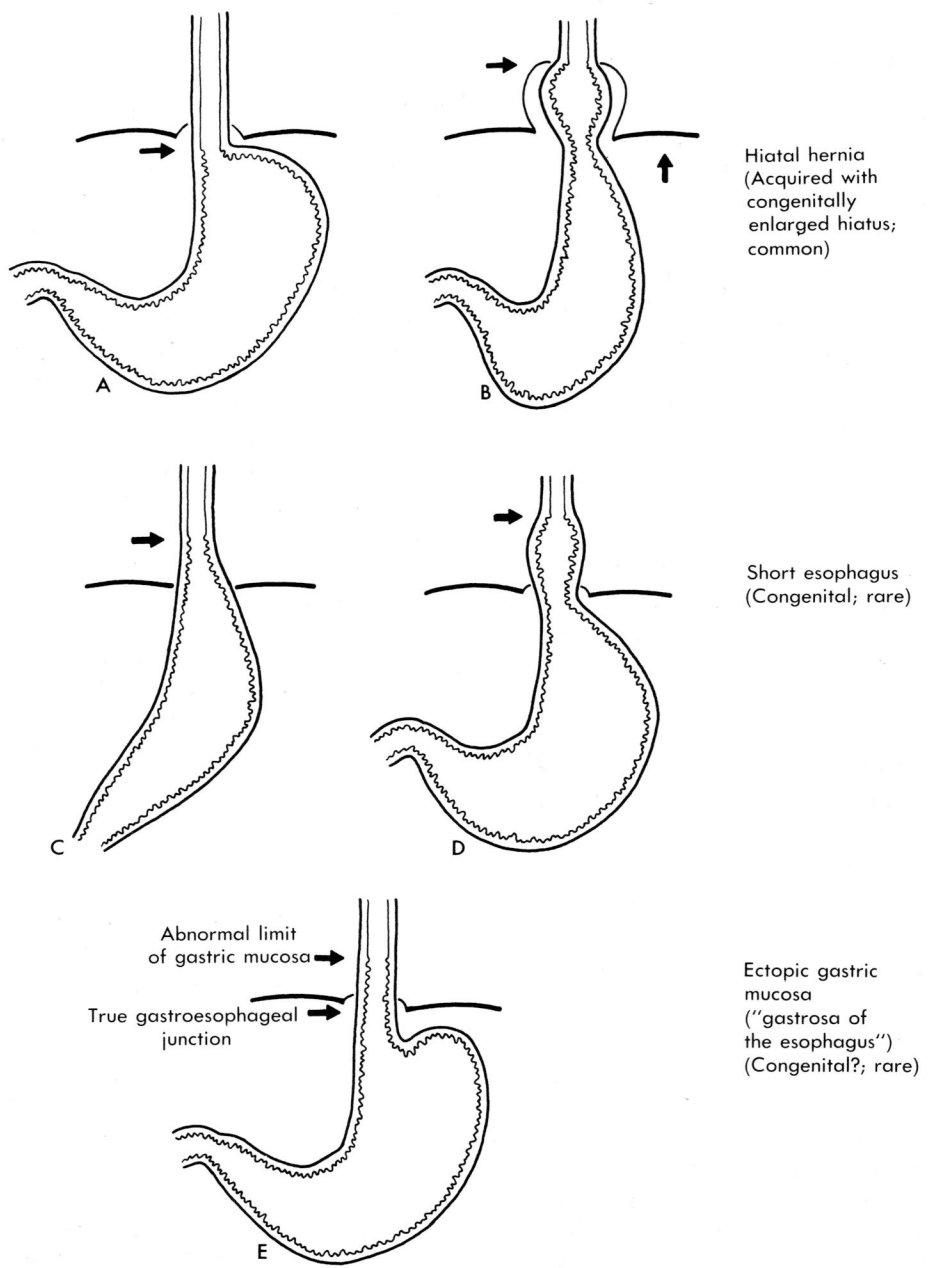

Hiatal hernia
(Acquired with
congenitally
enlarged hiatus;
common)

Short esophagus
(Congenital; rare)

Abnormal limit
of gastric mucosa ➡

True gastroesophageal
junction ➡

Ectopic gastric
mucosa
("gastrosa of
the esophagus")
(Congenital?; rare)

Figure 3.31. The three possible origins of "partial thoracic stomach." **A**, Normal relations of stomach, diaphragm, and esophagus. **B**, Hiatal hernia. **C**, Incomplete "descent" of fetal stomach resulting in either **D**, congenital short esophagus, or **E**, ectopic gastric mucosa in the esophagus. *Horizontal arrow* indicates the gastroesophageal junction.

anatomic similarities and partly by problems of terminology. Regardless of the specific terms used to describe them, the conditions are as follows:

Group 1: A grossly normal esophagus, the lower portion of which is lined with gastric mucosa (Fig. 3.31, *E*), also termed *heterotopic mucosa*. This condition is commonly referred to as "Barrett's esophagus."

Group 2: A partially supradiaphragmatic true stomach:
a. A stomach that has failed to descend completely as a result of insufficient esophageal elongation (Fig. 3.31, *C* and *D*)—"congenital short esophagus" (This classification is attractive but also is entirely hypothetical.)
b. A stomach that has secondarily herniated into the thorax through an abnormally large diaphragmatic esophageal hiatus (Fig. 3-31, B), called "hiatal hernia"

We cannot agree with those who apply the name "short esophagus" to group 1 lesions. The term has been preempted to describe the conditions listed under group 2a. We have more sympathy with those who include hiatal hernia with short esophagus. In many patients, especially in infancy, it is difficult to distinguish between the two.

EDITORIAL COMMENT

A major reason for the confusion in terminology associated with "short esophagus" was the very common clinical situation described in the past several decades in which gastroesophageal reflux in infants and young children resulted in chronic esophagitis and stricture formation which truly shortened the esophagus. These children clearly did not have a short esophagus, but an acquired shortening due to inflammation and stricture formation. In the recent past this complication of gastroesophageal reflux has been reported much less frequently because the diagnosis of gastroesophageal reflux is made much earlier and most pediatricians and family physicians are aware of this major complication if the gastroesophageal reflux is not controlled. It is extremely uncommon to see hiatus hernia and the associated "sliding esophageal hiatal hernia" in infants and children. This is a condition which takes years to develop and therefore is most commonly seen in adults. The vast majority of infants and children with significant gastroesophageal reflux do not have an anatomic hiatal defect or hernia.

True congenital short esophagus is very rare. The proposed definition that there be associated anatomic evidence that the stomach developed above the diaphragm is the only secure way to make this diagnosis. Blood vessels coming from the thoracic aorta to the stomach above the diaphragm are very rarely seen and thus true short esophagus almost never occurs. Incidentally, in those children with shortened esophagus associated with chronic esophagitis and gastroesophageal reflux, the anatomic relationship of the abdominal peritoneal lining is the same as for sliding

hiatal hernia, and all of these children, following dilation of the stricture, can have the esophagogastric junction in its normal relationship to the diaphragm during the operative correction. The best treatment for gastroesophageal reflux without a stricture and for sliding esophageal hiatal hernia in children is the fundoplication operation first proposed by Nissen (JAH/CNP).

Anatomy. The thoracic stomach associated with a congenitally short esophagus is present at birth. The supradiaphragmatic portion of the stomach is supplied by segmental arteries from the aorta. The left gastric artery does not extend above the diaphragm, and there is no associated peritoneal sac in the mediastinum (Fig. 3.32).

In theory, the condition should be recognizable by an esophagus that is too short to permit the stomach to be placed in its proper position in the abdomen. In practice, the esophagus in long-standing hiatal hernia has usually shortened so that it becomes indistinguishable from a congenitally short esophagus. The diaphragmatic esophageal hiatus is enlarged in both conditions. While an abnormally short esophagus is relatively common, we have seen a report of only one case of excessive elongation, in which an adult patient had 5 cm of abdominal esophagus, which entered the stomach low on the lesser curvature. The anomaly greatly facilitated the total gastrectomy required by carcinoma of the stomach (249) (Fig. 3.33).

A condition of inflammation and ulceration of the distal esophagus was described by Barrett (250). The lesion, beginning with columnar epithelium in the lower esophagus, may undergo metaplasia and rarely will progress to carcinoma. Barrett originally thought the lesion was congenital but subsequently accepted its acquired origin (251). The lesion is now called Barrett's esophagus (252)

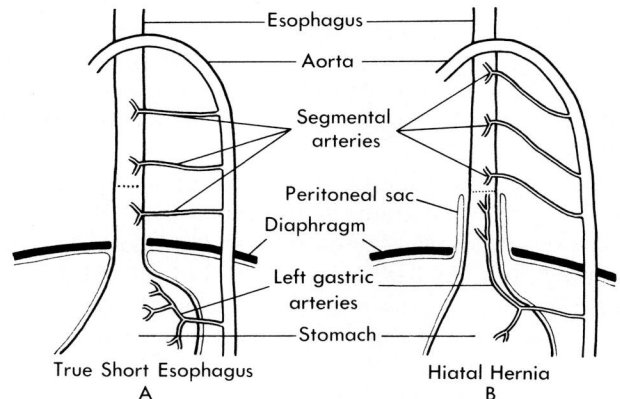

Figure 3.32. Differences between true short esophagus (**A**) and hiatal hernia (**B**). The *dotted line* represents the gastroesophageal junction. A peritoneal sac extending into the thorax may be found in hiatus hernia but not in short esophagus. (After Barrett NR. Hiatus hernia: a review of some controversial points. Br J Surg 1954;*42*:231–243.)

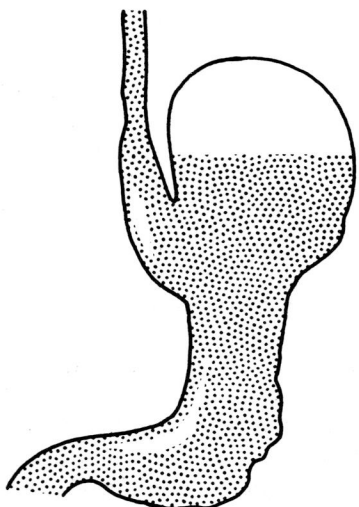

Figure 3.33. Congenitally long esophagus. (Based on a radiograph from Kirklin BR. Roentgenologic demonstration of an anomalous prolongation of the esophagus below the diaphragm, facilitating total gastrectomy. Am J Surg 1932;16:12–13.)

and usually is associated with gastroesophageal reflux, but why only a small percentage of patients with gastroesophageal reflux develop Barrett's esophagus is not known.

EDITORIAL COMMENT

In children, a Barrett's esophagus is never found without significant gastroesophageal reflux. It therefore seems likely that this is a cause-and-effect relationship, although the exact mechanism of the development of this ectopic mucosa in the distal esophagus has not been clearly defined (JAH/CNP).

In 1990 DeMeester et al. (253) reported 76 patients with Barrett's esophagus cared for over a 10-year period: 56 patients (74%) presented with complications of the disease such as stricture (20 patients), giant ulcers (7 patients), dysplasia (11 patients), or carcinoma (29 patients).

Embryogenesis. Elongation of the esophagus, resulting in "descent" of the stomach, is complete at about the end of the seventh week of gestation. At this time, the cardial opening normally lies below the level of the diaphragm. Cessation of elongation before the stomach has reached the proper level results in a portion of the stomach remaining in the thorax.

Dahms and Rothstein (254) believe that, in children, the distal columnar-lined esophagus results from chronic gastroesophageal reflux and is not a congenital anomaly. Stadelmann et al. (255) believe that certain forms of "endobrachy esophagus" appear to represent a congenital anomaly.

History. A congenitally short esophagus was often invoked during the 19th century to explain the occasional cases of thoracic stomach that came to light at autopsy, although almost all must have been the result of acquired hiatal hernia. It was unfortunate for our understanding of the esophageal hiatus that the first thoroughly described case of thoracic stomach, by Bright in 1836 (256), should have been in a 19-year-old girl who had a long history of gastric and respiratory distress. Her hiatal hernia certainly occurred early in life, perhaps before birth, but it was not a case of congenital short esophagus as the author thought.

In 1918 Bund (257) described a short esophagus with other anomalies in an 11-month-old boy. Only eight or nine cases of true short esophagus were known by 1929; however, with increased attention being given to thoracic stomach, many more are now recognized.

The association of Barrett's esophagus and carcinoma was reported from time to time. Oka et al. (258) believe that patients with Barrett's esophagus developed cancer of the esophagus at a higher rate than the general population. They hypothesized that immunosuppression perhaps plays a role in the genesis of malignancy. Li et al. (259) reported that, in 500 patients who underwent esophagectomy for carcinoma, 51 patients had an associated Barrett's esophagus.

Incidence. Most cases of thoracic stomach are acquired by herniation of the stomach through the diaphragm. Olsen and Harrington (260) found only 9 of 220 cases of short esophagus that could be considered congenital. Swyer (261) found 1 in 180 cases, Allison and Johnstone (262) found 1 in 204 cases, and Sweet (232) found 5 in 111 cases. Despite Allison and Johnson's series, the general experience is that 4 to 5% of clinical cases can be considered to be of congenital origin. Terrocol and Sweet (263), considering it to be familial, state that it is more common in males than females (the reverse of true hiatal hernia). It has been seen associated with pyloric stenosis, malrotation of intestines, short colon, and harelip.

Symptoms, Diagnosis, and Treatment. Because the clinical picture of thoracic stomach is the same regardless of the origin of the lesion, it is discussed with hiatal hernia in Chapter 15, "The Diaphragm."

ACHALASIA (CARDIOSPASM) AND MEGAESOPHAGUS

Description. Achalasia refers to a difficulty in swallowing in which the cardial end of the esophagus fails to relax enough to allow swallowed food to enter the stomach in the normal manner. It may be chronic or episodic and mild or severe, and it is accompanied by dysphagia and regurgitation. The etiology is by no means clear. It may be produced in adults by trauma; in some cases it may be psychosomatic; in a few instances it may have a congenital origin.

The relationship of megaesophagus to congenital achalasia is equally obscure. Whether it is the functional result of prolonged achalasia, a concomitant disease entity resulting from myenteric plexus deficiency, or a totally independent condition remains to be settled. In adults, the condition has been blamed on inflammatory changes in the myenteric plexus, with fibrosis and eventual disappearance of ganglion cells.

Pathogenesis. A few writers consider achalasia in adults to be of psychic origin (264, 265), but its appearance in the first few weeks of life would seem to indicate an organic etiology. Lendrum (266) believed that, as in the case of megacolon, there is a defect in myenteric plexus ganglion cells. In 200 specimens of 1-cm esophageal segments from unaffected infants, he found an average of 1250 ganglion cells per segment, whereas among specimens from 13 patients with achalasia, he found a total of only 74 ganglion cells in 233 such segments. Such aganglionosis is not present in all cases, however, and a satisfactory etiology remains to be demonstrated (267).

In areas of South America where infections with *Trypanosoma cruzi* (Chagas' disease) are frequent, achalasia that is indistinguishable from the congenital idiopathic form may result from destruction of the myenteric ganglion cells by the parasite. Megacolon and megaduodenum may be similarly caused (268).

Vagal paralysis has been suggested as an etiologic factor (222). Achalasia, produced experimentally in cats by vagal section, subsequently has been relieved by celiac sympathectomy (269). This evidence cannot be considered to conflict with the myenteric plexus theory of the origin of achalasia.

Megaesophagus may or may not accompany achalasia (270), and it is impossible to say at present whether the changes are a separate entity or the result of the esophageal constriction. Terracol and Sweet (263) described two types of megaesophagus (Fig. 3.34). One gives a sigmoid appearance on radiographs, with an apparent redundance of esophagus; this type is found in 70% of patients with megaesophagus. The second type shows a spindle-shaped or fusiform enlargement without increase in length; it appears in 30% of cases. Neither type appears to be a precursor of the other. Megaesophagus has been reported in two children with familial dysautonomy (271).

In 1986 Hill (272) stated that achalasia "almost never occurs in siblings." However, Raffensperger (273) found in the literature that diagnosis was made in infancy and the anomaly has been reported in siblings.

Achalasia in childhood accounts for only 5% of the total cases; yet most of the familial cases occur in childhood. It is also associated with familial dysautonomia, thus suggesting a congenital origin in some cases (274).

Associated Anomalies. Achalasia is occasionally associated with distal esophageal pulsion diverticula (222) and with pylorospasm (275). In Brazil, Etzel (270) found frequent association of megaesophagus with megacolon and megaureter, which he attributed to vitamin B deficiency. He produced similar microscopic alterations in Auerbach's plexus in pigeons on a vitamin B–deficient diet. Except for these associations, few major anomalies seem to occur in conjunction with achalasia. In 1988 Khalifa (276) reported two brothers with mental retardation, microcephaly, and achalasia.

The striking absence of other anomalies has helped to cast doubt on the embryonic origin of the lesion; yet the familial cases definitely imply a congenital (genetic) component in some instances.

History. In 1679 Willis (277) described symptoms and treatment in a case of persistent achalasia. He provided his patient with a whalebone rod with a sponge at its tip. The patient used this after each meal for 15 years with good results. The description of the case is quoted in Schiebel (265). In 1733 Hoffman described the exacerbating effects of cold liquids and was the first to suggest the psychosomatic aspects of the disease (275). Megaesophagus was described in 1821 by Purton (278), who observed a case of 20 years' standing. He suggested a traumatic origin of the achalasia; his patient eventually died of inanition. A similar case was described by Hannay (279) in 1833.

Mikulicz (280), demonstrating achalasia by means of the esophagoscope in 1882, introduced the term *cardiospasm*. In 1897 Rümpel (281) used bismuth to visualize the condition by the newly discovered x-rays. In 1927 Rake (282) demonstrated the absence of ganglion cells in the lower esophagus of patients with achalasia.

In 1900 Neumann (283) collected 70 cases, and by 1921 Thieding (284) found 345 cases in the world literature. Gray and Skinner (285) found 1200 cases in 1940.

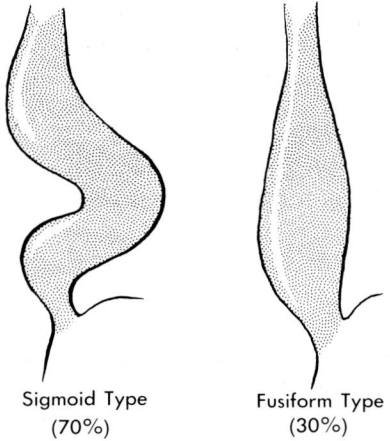

Sigmoid Type
(70%)

Fusiform Type
(30%)

Figure 3.34. Two types of megaesophagus. (After Terracol J, Sweet RH. Diseases of the esophagus. Philadelphia: WB Saunders, 1958.)

The history of surgical repair is given in detail by Steichen et al. (275). Until 1897, when Jaffé (286) proposed longitudinal excision, dilators of one sort or another were used with considerable success in mild cases. In 1914 in Germany Heller (287) described an anterior and posterior cardiomyotomy. After 45 years of neglect, this technique, with some modification, was reintroduced by Heller and is being increasingly employed (275). The basic principle of repair now is an anterior longitudinal esophagomyotomy via a left transthoracic or upper abdominal approach with or without a concomitant antireflux procedure.

EDITORIAL COMMENT

Because of the very high incidence of gastroesophageal reflux following successful Heller cardiomyotomy for achalasia, practically all pediatric surgeons recommend an antireflux procedure such as a Nissen fundoplication. Since these children will probably live a long time, their follow-up has indicated the very high likelihood of esophagitis from reflux. Thus, in children and young adults, it is probably wise to carry out an antireflux procedure. In older patients, particularly those older than 60 or 70 years of age, this may not be necessary, because the gastroesophageal reflux will not be symptomatic (JAH/CNP).

Incidence. It has been estimated that 18% of all esophageal lesions are due to achalasia (288). This can be little more than an educated guess because the condition shows such great variation in severity. When exhausted or overheated, even normal persons may have some difficulty in swallowing iced liquids.

Fish and Harrison (289) found 69 cases over a period of 11 years in a single hospital at Galveston, Texas. Males and females were equally affected, and both black and white races were represented. Ages ranged from 10 years to 82 years. Psychogenic, traumatic, and idiopathic cases were not separated.

Mayberry and Rhodes (290) from England and Erlam et al. (291) from Rochester, Minnesota, estimated that achalasia occurs in four to six cases per million per year.

Symptoms. Dysphagia is the complaint in almost all cases. Regurgitation is usually present, and pain is not uncommon. Frequently a history of weight loss is seen in adults, or a failure to gain weight occurs in infants, which results from a disinclination or an actual inability to eat. Dysphagia with both solids and liquids was described by DiMarino and Cohen (291).

Diagnosis. Occasional vomiting of undigested food particles, low food intake, and chronic cough may be the only complaints in children. The cough may be investigated by a chest x-ray film from which esophageal abnormality may be suspected. A barium esophagram will then provide evidence for diagnosis (293). A massive esophagus with evidence of spasm or stricture is highly suggestive of achalasia, although a reflux stricture can look the same. The diagnosis must be confirmed by esophageal manometry, which shows (a) elevated resting lower esophageal sphincter (LES) pressure; (b) incomplete relaxation of the LES on swallowing; and (c) aperistalsis of the body or the esophagus (274).

Projection of the enlarged esophagus is usually to the right, in extreme cases reaching the right thoracic wall. Fluid may appear, or only air may be present. Pulmonary changes such as bronchiectasis, pneumonitis, or fibrosis may be visible. Serial films show prolonged barium retention.

Treatment. Dilation by bougies or hydrostatic pressure, forceful enough to tear some fibers of the muscularis while leaving the mucosa uninjured, is effective in many cases. The operator is in effect performing a Heller myotomy without surgery. Although there is real danger of rupturing the esophagus by too great a pressure (104), too little pressure produces no improvement. Bougienage, even when satisfactory results are obtained, may need to be repeated at 3- to 6-month intervals (294).

When this method is ineffective, surgery is necessary. Most children do not respond to bougienage and require surgery. A wide variety of procedures have been employed for the condition; they are shown in Figure 3.35.

When surgery is required, the Heller extramural myotomy gives the best results. Among 474 patients treated by this procedure between 1940 and 1960, good results were obtained in 88%. Esophagogastrostomy and cardioplasty, which were performed in 238 patients from 1946 to 1960, produced good results in only 50% of cases (289).

Bonavina et al. (295) reported 206 patients treated with transabdominal Heller myotomy and anterior fundoplication by the Dor technique with very good results. Rosato et al. (296) reported good results with transabdominal esophagomyotomy and partial fundoplication in 22 patients. Stipa et al. (297) compared Heller myotomy plus Belsey repair or Nissen fundoplication in the treatment of achalasia and found that the former technique fared slightly better than the latter, with good to excellent long-term results being obtained in 87.1 and 83% of the patients, respectively.

Mortality. No adequate mortality figures are available. Schiebel (265) reported that, among 805 patients treated by dilation, 9 died from tears of the esophagus in the hospital, 12 died at home from unknown causes, and 2 died of starvation. Nutritional deficiency probably reduces longevity in many cases. Among patients treated by Heller's myotomy, there were 4 deaths in 474 operations.

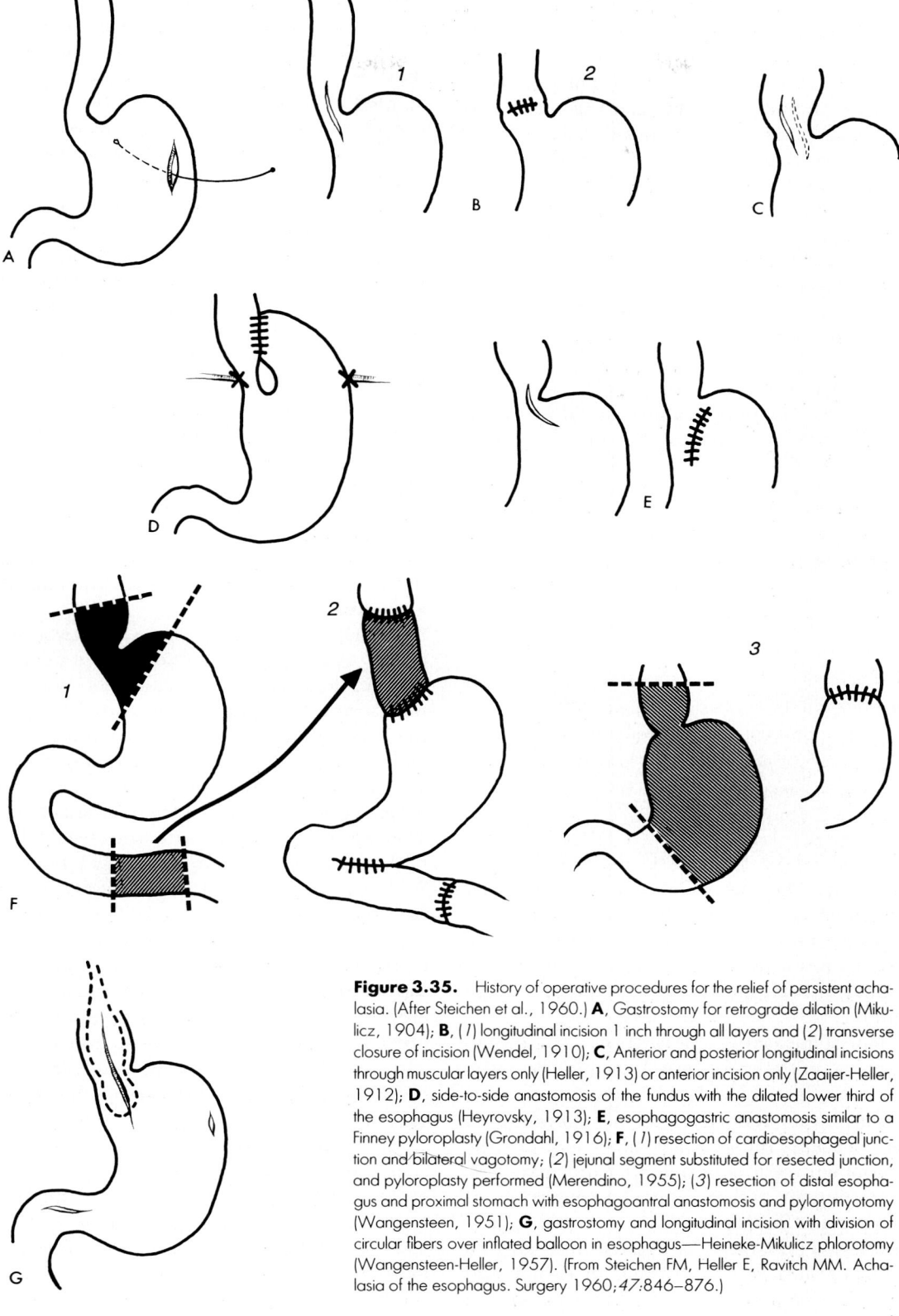

Figure 3.35. History of operative procedures for the relief of persistent achalasia. (After Steichen et al., 1960.) **A**, Gastrostomy for retrograde dilation (Mikulicz, 1904); **B**, (*1*) longitudinal incision 1 inch through all layers and (*2*) transverse closure of incision (Wendel, 1910); **C**, Anterior and posterior longitudinal incisions through muscular layers only (Heller, 1913) or anterior incision only (Zaaijer-Heller, 1912); **D**, side-to-side anastomosis of the fundus with the dilated lower third of the esophagus (Heyrovsky, 1913); **E**, esophagogastric anastomosis similar to a Finney pyloroplasty (Grondahl, 1916); **F**, (*1*) resection of cardioesophageal junction and bilateral vagotomy; (*2*) jejunal segment substituted for resected junction, and pyloroplasty performed (Merendino, 1955); (*3*) resection of distal esophagus and proximal stomach with esophagoantral anastomosis and pyloromyotomy (Wangensteen, 1951); **G**, gastrostomy and longitudinal incision with division of circular fibers over inflated balloon in esophagus—Heineke-Mikulicz phlorotomy (Wangensteen-Heller, 1957). (From Steichen FM, Heller E, Ravitch MM. Achalasia of the esophagus. Surgery 1960;*47*:846–876.)

CHALASIA

Effortless regurgitation in a newborn infant due to relaxation of the esophagocardial opening was described by Neuhauser and Berenberg (298). It usually begins in the first week of life and is equally common in males and females. Neuhauser and Berenberg considered the defect to be a failure of the diaphragmatic pinchcock action. It is more probable, however, that the failure results from a delay in the development of neuromuscular control of the lower esophagus. Manometric studies by Strawczynski and his colleagues (299) suggest that the tone of the so-called esophageal sphincter is low during the first 2 weeks of life, increasing subsequently to adult levels. This finding has been confirmed by Gryboski (300). Chalasia may represent nothing more than a delay in the development of nervous control of the lower esophagus.

The condition does not require surgical intervention, and it improves spontaneously by the time the child reaches the age of 2 to 3 years. Weight loss and the increased possibility of aspiration pneumonitis from frequent vomiting are the chief dangers from this condition.

EDITORIAL COMMENT

Indeed, it is very unwise to consider an operative antireflux procedure in a child under 1 year of age who has chalasia or frequent regurgitation unless (a) there is clear objective evidence of severe esophagitis and/or (b) the child has recurrent episodes of vomiting and aspiration which are life threatening. The vast majority of children with episodes of gastroesophageal reflux under 1 year of age "grow out" of this dysfunction because the lower esophageal sphincter has simply not matured enough to be competent (JAH/CNP).

ABNORMAL IDIOPATHIC CONGENITAL REFLUX

Is this just chalasia? The authors are not 100% sure that this is a congenital anomaly; however, if there is not a local pathology such as hiatal hernia or a remote one such as a brain lesion, one must accept that something is wrong with the esophageal wall, specifically with the LES (high-pressure zone).

Development of intraganglionic neurons was shown to be more advanced in the esophagus, less in the rectosigmoid, and least in the ileocecal area according to Vaos (301). The same author reported than any alterations in the fetal gut microenvironment may affect seriously the normal development of a multipotential precursor cell population, resulting in various congenital anomalies of the myenteric plexus. If this concept is correct, then perhaps the esophageal mucosa which has had resistance to gastric content to start with, according to Kiriluk and Merendino (302), becomes more secondary to unknown factors, perhaps with a small and weak rosette-like mucosal configuration (weak valve).

If the anatomic entities of the diaphragmatic esophageal hiatus are within normal limits (230) and if no systemic disease directly or indirectly acts on the LES (if there is one), then the distal segment of the esophagus and, to be more specific, the neuromuscular component is perhaps not equipped to face the antireflux barrier. If we accept this highly hypothetic concept, we must accept that there is a type of gastroesophageal reflex of congenital origin, and it should be grouped together with other entities such as chalasia and achalasia.

Is the LES the only antireflux barrier, or is there something still unknown responsible for the gastroesophageal reflux? Though there is a lack of consensus in answer to this question, the authors have classified a part of this reflux as idiopathic and congenital. This is just a hypothesis, which perhaps will stimulate investigations for further study of this problem.

Is the Lieberman-Meffert "muscle" congenitally hypofunctional, or is the LES, if present, also congenitally hypofunctional? We do not know. When everything is normal, and the baby has continuous devastation and gastroesophageal reflex, there must be an etiologic factor which is not "anatomical and functional, static and dynamic," to quote Boix-Ochoa, who named some of the antireflux barriers (303).

Perhaps we go too far, since the newborn needs ample time to develop tone, function, and muscular mass to face this problem. There is a maturation period for the LES with regard to length and pressure (257). The length of the LES is about 1 cm in infants of less than 1 week of age and increases to about 3 cm in infants 6 months of age. The pressure in the LES is 4 to 6 mm Hg at birth and increases to 10 to 15 mm Hg in infants 6 months of age. This maturation period correlates well with the clinical findings of regurgitation in normal infants with chalasia. Both the clinical findings and the x-ray examinations normalize in most infants as the LES matures.

Both Boix-Ochoa (303) and DeMeester et al. (304) consider the intraabdominal esophageal segment to play a great role in the antireflux mechanism. If the abdominal esophagus is small, is this a congenital anomaly? We do not know. If so, then there are anatomic reasons, and the gastroesophageal reflux is not congenital. It is not within the scope of this chapter to present the physiology of closure and opening of the gastroesophageal junction.

Clinically, gastroesophageal reflux, congenital or acquired, presents the same clinical picture: vomitus, esophagitis, aspiration, and failure to thrive.

Diagnosis. The following should be used: (a) the upper gastrointestinal series (esophagogram) which, despite its false-negative results, is a must for a diagnosis; (b) 99m Tc-sulphur colloid for reflux documentation, esophageal clearance, gastric emptying, and pulmonary aspirations, which is highly recommended by Jona et al. (305); (c) esophagoscopy with or without biopsy; (*d*) manometry to study esophageal motility; (*e*) the Johnson-DeMeester test; and (*f*) the 24-liter pH probe, which is currently the most widely used test (after UGI) to document "pathologic" versus "physiologic" gastroesophageal reflux (chalasia). The number of reflux episodes per 24 hrs., the percentage of time the pH is less than 4, and the clearance time (of the esophagus) are used to determine the need for medical and/or surgical therapy.

Treatment. Medical treatment consisting of small, frequent feedings, thickened feeds, and upright positioning (prone) is tried first; the majority of infants respond. If not, medications which increase the LES pressure and gastric emptying (e.g., metaclopromide) are instituted along with antacids. Antireflux surgery is reserved for those few patients (10 to 15%) who fail to respond to medical treatment, for those with reflux strictures, and for those with "near-miss" sudden infant death syndome

(SIDS). Surgery is usually required in patients with central nervous system derangements.

St-Cyr et al. (306) recommend fundoplication for patients 2 years of age or less who have a persistent pulmonary problem attributed to gastroesophageal reflux that does not respond to medical treatment.

Boix-Ochoa et al. (307) advise restoring the length of intraabdominal esophagus, tightening the hiatus and anchoring the esophagus to it, and restoring the angle of His. Tunell (308) and Johnson and Jolly (309) provide recent reviews on the medical and surgical management of gastroesophagus reflux in children.

Glassman et al. (310) reported perioperative evaluation and intraoperative management of gastroesophageal reflux in neurologically impaired children.

Jolley (311) presented an algorithm for the selection of antireflux procedures. (Fig. 3.36)

Dysphagia Caused by Vascular Compression of the Esophagus

Dysphagia that radiologically reveals a stenotic segment at the level of the aortic arch may be caused by constriction of the esophagus by anomalous blood vessels. Signs of tracheal compression may also be present.

The following anomalies are those which most frequently cause dysphagia: (*a*) trachea and esophagus encircled by a double aortic arch, (*b*) trachea and esophagus encircled by a right aortic arch and ligamentum arteriosum, or (*c*) esophagus compressed by an aberrant right subclavian artery arising on the left and passing posterior to the trachea or retroesophageal right subclavian.

EDITORIAL COMMENT

The first two aortic arch anomalies, double aortic arch and right aortic arch with ligamentum arteriosus, are frequently etiologies of dysphagia lusoria. Very rarely indeed is there a significant esophageal dysfunction associated with an aberrant retroesophageal right subclavian artery. In their large experience with management of tetralogy of Fallot, Blalock and Taussig brought down the subclavian artery to the pulmonary artery for the so-called Blalock-Taussig shunt; 12% of these patients were found to have an anomalous retroesophageal subclavian artery, but practically none had any swallowing difficulty. This seems convincing evidence that the presence of a retroesophageal subclavian vessel is not an adequate explanation for esophageal dysfunction if there is an associated arch anomaly. Particularly, if there is scarring following a mediastinal operative procedure such as tracheoesophageal fistula repair, then there may be constriction of the esophagus by the aberrant vessel. Otherwise, it is the unlikely cause for dysphagia, and another etiology should be suspected (JAH/CNP).

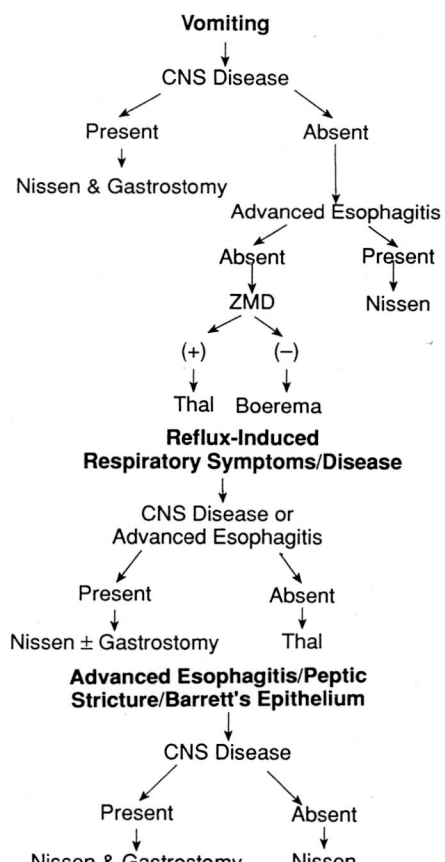

Figure 3.36. A general algorithm for the selection of antireflux operation in infants and children based on the complication of gastroesophageal reflux disease *(GERD)*, associated central nervous system *(CNS)* disease, and the prolonged (+) or normal (−) value for the mean duration of acid reflux episodes during sleep *(ZMD)* derived from extended esophageal pH monitoring. (From Jolley SG. Current surgical considerations in gastroesophageal reflux disease in infancy and childhood. Surg Clin North Am 1992;72(6):1365–1392.)

Vascular compression may be distinguished from other lesions affecting the esophagus by the following criteria: (*a*) Dysphagia is usually overshadowed by the respiratory embarrassment; (*b*) if compression is from an abnormal arch, the site of the defect, as determined by radiography, is at the level of the aortic arch; and (*c*) the defect is strikingly slanted or winding if compression is from an aberrant right subclavian artery.

After studying 204 cases of vascular ring anomalies, Idriss (312) divides the vascular ring anomalies into three groups. Group I, consisting of those with true complete vascular rings, is subdivided into double aortic arch (61 cases) and right aortic arch with left ligamentum from descending aorta (52 cases). Group II is comprised of 82 cases of left arch rings. Nine cases of pulmonary artery sling make up group III. Galizzi et al. (313) presented three cases which were diagnosed by x-ray examination, arteriography, and endoscopy, and two similar cases were presented by Cherri et al. (314).

The embryogenesis, diagnosis, and treatment of these anomalies are discussed in Chapter 28, "Thoracic and Abdominal Aorta."

REFERENCES

1. Rosenthal, AH. Congenital atresia of the esophagus with tracheo-esophageal fistula. Arch Pathol 1931;12:756–772.
2. Bossy J, Gaillard deCollogny L, Katz J. Dévelopment et croissance en longeur de l'oesophage. J Fr Otol Rhinol Laryngol 1964;13:765–778.
3. Hillemeier C. Development of the esophagus. In: Lebenthal E, ed. Human gastrointestinal development. New York: Raven Press, 1989:242.
4. Borisov AV, Shipulin AN. Development of the lymphatic bed of the human esophageal wall. Arkh Anat Gistol Embriol 1979;77:33–34.
5. Kreuter E. Die angeborenen Verschliessungen und Verengerungen des Darmkanals im Lichte der Entwicklungsgeschichte. Deutsch Z Chir 1905;79:1–89.
6. Forssner H. Die angeborenen Darm-und Oesophagusatresien. Anat Hefte 1907;34:1–163.
7. Schridde H. Über die Epithelproliferationen in der embryonalen menschlichen Speiseröhre. Virchow Arch Pathol Anat 1908;191:179–192.
8. Rector LE, Connerley ML. Aberrant mucosa in the esophagus in infants and in children. Arch Pathol 1941;31:285–294.
9. Piekarsky DH, Stephens FD. The association and embryogenesis of T-E and anorectal anomalies. Prog Pediatr Surg 1976;9:63.
10. Wesson DE, Muraji I, Kent G, Filler RM, Almachi T. The effect of intrauterine esophageal ligation on growth of fetal rabbits. J Pediatr Surg 1984;19(4):398–399.
11. Johnson FP. The development of the mucous membrane of the esophagus, stomach and small intestine in the human embryo. Am J Anat 1910;10:521–561.
12. Johns BAE. Developmental changes in the esophageal epithelium in man. J Anat 1952;86:431–442.
13. Botha GSM. Organogenesis and growth of the gastroesophageal region in man. Anat Rec 1959;133:219–239.
14. Sadler TW. Langman's medical embryology. 6th ed. Baltimore: Williams & Wilkins, 1991.
15. Zachary RB, Emery JL. Failure of separation of larynx and trachea from the esophagus: persistent esophagotrachea. Surgery 1961;49:525–529.
16. Griscom NT. Persistent esophagotrachea: the most severe degree of laryngotracheo-esophageal cleft. Am J Roentgenol 1966;97:211–215.
17. Echstein HB, Somasundaram K. Multiple tracheoesophageal fistulas without atresia: report of a case. J Pedatr Surg 1966;1:381–383.
18. Marek JJ. Congenital deformity of trachea. Ohio Med J 1940;36:1308.
19. Milles G, Dorsey DB. Intra-uterine respiration-like movements in relation to development of the fetal vascular system: discussion of intra-uterine physiology based upon cases of congenital absence of the trachea, abnormal vascular development, and other anomalies. Am J Pathol 1950;26:411–425.
20. Sharma AK, Sharma KK, Sharma CS, Chandra S, Udwat M. Congenital esophageal obstruction by intraluminal mucosal diaphragm. J Pediatr Surg 1991;26(2):213–215.
21. Wiersema JS. Partial reduplication of the oesophagus with oesophageal atresia and oesophago-tracheal fistula. Arch Chir Neerl 1965;8:97–101.
22. Dafoe CS, Ross CA. Tracheo-esophageal fistula and esophageal atresia. Dis Chest 1960;37:42–51.
23. Yahr WS, Azzoni AA, Santulli TV. Congenital atresia of the esophagus with tracheoesophageal fistula: an unusual variant. Surgery 1962;52:937–941.
24. Minnis JF, Jr, Burko H, Brevetti G. Segmental duplication of the esophagus associated with esophageal atresia and tracheo-esophageal fistula. Ann Surg 1962;156:271–275.
25. Wolf RY, Duncan L, Pate JW. Tracheoesophageal fistula associated with esophageal duplication. Surgery 1965;58:728–730.
26. Ohkuma R. Congenital esophageal atresia with tracheoesophageal fistula in identical twins. J Pediatr Surg 1978;13(4):361–362.
27. Frater RWM, Dowdle, EB. Congenital esophagobronchial fistula: report of a case and review of literature. Arch Surg 1964;89:949–954.
28. Gross RE. The surgery of infancy and childhood. Philadelphia: WB Saunders, 1953.
29. Stephens CA, Mustard WT, Simpson JS, Jr. Congenital atresia of the esophagus with tracheo-esophageal fistula. Surg Clin North Am 1956;36:1465–1478.
30. Holder TM, Cloud DT, Lewis JE, Jr, Pilling GP, IV. Esophageal atresia and tracheoesophageal fistula: a survey of its members by the surgical section of the American Academy of Pediatrics. Pediatrics 1964;34:542–549.
31. Rehbein F. Oesophageal atresia with double tracheo-oesophageal fistula. Arch Dis Child 1964;39:138–142.
32. Kluth D. Atlas of esophageal atresia. J Pediatr Surg 1976;11(6):901–916.
33. Reeves E. Osteochondroma of the esophagus removed perorally with the aid of a speculum. Arch Otolaryngol 1939;151–158.
34. Stout AP, Lattes R. Tumors of the esophagus. Washington, DC, Armed Forces Institute of Pathology, 1957.
35. Kumar R. A case of congenital oesophageal stricture due to a cartilaginous ring. Br J Surg 1935;49:533–534.
36. Beltz L. The pathogenesis of congenital stenosis of the esophagus, atresia of the esophagus and tracheoesophageal fistulas. Zentralbl Allg Pathol 1962;104:49–58.
37. Paulino F, Roselli A, Aprigliano F. Congenital esophageal stricture due to tracheobronchial remnants. 1963;53:547–550.
38. Zausch P. Ein fall von Oesophagus-Atresie und Oesophago-Trachealfistel. Virchow Arch Pathol Anat 1921;234:94.

39. Ingalls TH, Prindle RA. Esophageal atresia with tracheoesophageal fistula: epidemiologic and teratologic implications. N Engl J Med 1949;240:987–995.

40. Fluss Z, Poppen KJ. Embryogenesis of tracheoesophageal fistula and esophageal atresia: a hypothesis based on associated vascular anomalies. Arch Pathol 1951;52:168.

41. Keith A. Three cases of malformation of the tracheoesophageal septum. J Anat Physiol 1906;41:52–55.

42. Kalter H. Congenital malformations induced by riboflavin deficiency in strains of inbred mice. Pediatrics 1959;23:222–230.

43. Warkany J, Roth CB, Wilson JG. Multiple congenital malformations: a consideration of etiologic factors. Pediatrics 1948;I:462–471.

44. deLorimier AA, Harrison MR. Esophageal atresia: embryogenesis and management. World J Surg 1985;9:250–257.

45. Chittmittrapap S, Spitz L, Kiely EM, Brereton RJ. Oesophageal atresia and associated anomalies. Arch Dis Child 1989;64:364–368.

46. Rabinowitz, JG, Moseley JE, Mitty HA, Hirschhorn K. Trisomy 18, esophageal atresia, anomalies of the radius, and congenital hypoplastic thrombocytopenia. Radiology 1967;89:488–491.

47. Scott JS, Wilson JK. Hydramnios as early sign of esophageal atresia. Lancet 1957;2:569–572.

48. Carvalho O. Hidrâmnio e atresia esophágica congênita. An Acad Bras Cienc 1954;38:137–141.

49. de Snoo K. Das trinkende Kind in Uterus. Mschr Geburtsh Gyn 1937;105:88.

50. Greenwood RD, Rosenthal A. Cardiovascular malformations associated with tracheoesophageal fistula and esophageal atresia. Pediatrics 1976;57:87.

51. Andrassy RJ, Mahour H. Gastrointestinal anomalies associated with esophageal atresia or tracheoesophageal fistula. Arch Surg 1979;114:1125–1128.

52. Bond-Taylor W, Starer F, Atwell JD. Vertebral anomalies associated with esophageal atresia and tracheoesophageal fistula with reference to initial operative mortality. J Pediatr Surg 1973;8:9.

53. Schiffmann JH, Rehder H, Speer CP. Tracheal agenesis, a rare cause of respiratory insufficiency in newborn infants. Universitats-Kinderklinik Gottingen 1991;139(2):102–104.

54. Quan L, Smith DW. VATER association. J Pediatr 1973;82:104–107.

55. Quan L, Smith DW. The VATER association: vertebral defects, anal atresia, tracheoesophageal fistula with esophageal atresia, radial dysplasia. New York: The National Foundation–March of Dimes (Original Article Series) 1972;8:75–78.

56. Temtamy SA, Miller JD. Extending the scope of the VATER association: definition of the VATER syndrome. J Pediatr 1974;85(3):345–349.

57. Fernbach SK. Urethral abnormalities in male neonates with VATER association. AJR 1991;156:137–140.

58. Barry JE, Auldist AW. The VATER association: one end of a spectrum of anomalies. Am J Dis Child 1974;128:769–771.

59. Czeizel A, Lud'anyi I. An aetiological study of the VACTERL. Eur J Pediatr 1985;144:331–337.

60. Weber TR, Smith W, Grosfeld JL. Surgical experience in infants with the VATER association. J Pediatr Surg 1980;15:849–854.

61. Ashcraft KW, Holder TM. The story of esophageal atresia and tracheoesophageal fistula. Surgery 1969;65:332.

62. Myers NA. The history of oesophageal atresia and tracheo-oesophageal fistula, 1670–1684. Prog Pediatr Surg 1986;20:106–157.

63. Durston W. A narrative of monstrous birth in Plymouth, October 22, 1670, together with the anatomical observations taken thereupon by William Durston, doctor in physick, and communication to Dr. Tim Clerk. Philos Trans R Soc Lond 1670;V:2096.

64. Gibson T. The anatomy of human bodies epitomized. London: T. Flesher, 1696.

65. Mackenzie M. Malformations of oesophagus. Arch Laryngol 1880;I:301–315.

66. Lanman TH. Congenital atresia of the esophagus. Arch Surg 1940;41:1060–1083.

67. Lamb DS. A fatal case of congenital tracheoesophageal fistula. Phila Med Times 1873;3:705.

68. Steele C. Case of deficient oesophagus. Lancet 1888;2:764.

69. Plass ED. Congenital atresia of the esophagus with tracheo-esophageal fistula: associated with fused kidney: a case report and survey of the literature on congenital anomalies of the esophagus. Johns Hopkins Hosp Rep 1919;18:259–286.

70. Leven NL. Congenital atresia of the esophagus with tracheo-esophageal fistula; report of successful extrapleural ligation of fistulous communication and cervical esophagostomy. J Thorac Surg 1941;10:648.

71. Ladd WE. The surgical treatment of esophageal atresia and tracheoesophageal fistulas. N Engl J Med 1944;230:625.

72. Haight C, Towsley HA. Congenital atresia of the esophagus with tracheoesophageal fistula. Surg Gynecol Obstet 1943;76:672–688.

73. Brown RK, Brown EC. Congenital esophageal anomalies: review of twenty-four cases and report of three. Surg Gynecol Obstet 1950;91:545–550.

74. Knox G. Secular pattern of congenital oesophageal atresia. Br J Prev Soc Med 1959;13:222–226.

75. Wooley MM, Chinnock RF, Paul RH. Premature twins with esophageal atresia and tracheoesophageal fistula. Acta Paediatr Uppsala 1961;50:423–440.

76. Blank RH, Prillaman PE, Minor GR. Congenital esophageal atresia with tracheoesophageal fistula occurring in identical twins. J Thorac Cardiovasc Surg 1967;53:192–196.

77. Hansmann PF, Close AS, Williams LP. Occurrence of tracheoesophageal fistula in three consecutive siblings. Surg Gynecol Obstet 1957;41:542.

78. Haight C. Some observations of esophageal atresia and tracheoesophageal fistula of congenital origin. J Thorac Surg 1957;34:141–172.

79. Engel MA, Vos LJM, de Vries JA, Kuijjer PJ. Esophageal atresia with tracheoesophageal fistula in mother and child. J Pediatr Surg 1970;5:564–565.

80. German JC, Mahour GH, Wooley MM. The twin and esophageal atresia. J Pediatr Surg 1979;14:432–435.

81. David TJ, O'Callaghan SE. Twinning and esophageal atresia. Arch Dis Child 1974;49:660.

82. King SL, Ladda RL, Shochat SJ. Case report: monozygotic twins concordant for tracheoesophageal fistula and discordant for the VATER association. Acta Pediatr Scand 1977;66:783.

83. Chen H, Goei GS, Hertzler JH. Family studies on congenital esophageal atresia with or without tracheoesophageal fistula. Birth Defects 1979;15(5C):117–144.

84. Kiesewetter WB. Tracheoesophageal fistula in parent and offspring: a rare occurrence. Am J Dis Child 1980;134:896.

85. Ozimek GD, Grimson RC, Aylsworth AS. An epidemiologic study of tracheoesophageal fistulae and esophageal atresia in North Carolina. Teratology 1989;25:53–59.

86. Dennis NR, Nicholas JC, Kuvar I. Esophageal atresia: three cases in two generations. Dis Arch Child 1983;48:980.

87. Randolph JG. Esophageal atresia and congenital stenosis: esophageal atresia and associated malformations, including laryngo-

tracheoesophageal cleft. In: Welch KJ, Randolph JG, Ravitch MM, O'Neill JA Jr, Rowe MI, eds. Pediatric surgery. Vol I. Chicago: Year Book Medical Publishers, 1986:683.

88. Imperatori CJ. Congenital tracheoesophageal fistula without atresia of esophagus: report of a case with plastic closure and cure. Arch Otolaryngol 1939;30:352.

89. Haight C. Congenital tracheoesophageal fistula without esophageal atresia. J Thorac Surg 1948;17:600.

90. Le Roux BT, Williams MA. Congenital oesophagobronchial fistula with presentation in adult life. Br J Surg 1969;55:306–308.

91. Holinger PH, Johnston KC, Potts WJ. Congenital anomalies of the esophagus. Ann Otol 1951;60:707.

92. Richardson WR, Brown IH, Williams GR. Congenital atresia of the esophagus. Am Surg 1963;29:166–178.

93. Randolph JG, Newman KD, Anderson KD. Current results in repair of esophageal atresia with tracheoesophageal fistula using physiologic status as a guide to therapy. Ann Surg 1989;209:526–531.

94. Howard R, Myers NA. Esophageal atresia: a technique for elongating the upper pouch. Surgery 1965;58:725–727.

95. Johnston PW. Elongation of the upper segment in esophageal atresia: a report of a case. Surgery 1965;58:741–744.

96. Hays DM, Woolley MM, Snyder WH. Esophageal atresia and tracheoesophageal fistula: management of the uncommon types. J Pediatr Surg 1966;I:240–252.

97. Lafer DJ, Boley SJ. Primary repair in esophageal atresia with elongation of the lower segment. J Pediatr Surg 1966;I:585–587.

98. Livaditis A. Esophageal atresia: a method of overbridging large segmental gaps. Z Kinderchir 1973;13:298–306.

99. Livaditis A, Radberg L, Odensjo G. Esophageal end-to-end anastomosis; reduction of anastomotic tension by circular myotomy. Scand J Cardiovasc Surg 1972;6:206–214.

100. Ricketts RR, Luck SR, Raffensperger JG. Circular esophagomyotomy for primary repair of long-gap esophageal atresia. J Pediatr Surg 1981;16(3):365–369.

101. deLorimier AA, Harrison MR. Long gap esophageal atresia: primary anastomosis after esophageal elongation by bougienage and esophagomyotomy. J Thorac Cardiovasc Surg 1980;79:138–141.

102. Waterston D, Carter R, Aberdeen E. Oesophageal atresia: tracheoesophageal fistula—a study of survival in 218 infants. Lancet 1962;1:819–822.

103. Leven NL, Varco RL, Lanning BG, Tongen LA. Surgical management of congenital atresia of esophagus and tracheoesophageal fistula. Ann Surg 1952;136:701–719.

104. Swenson O. Pediatric surgery. New York: Appleton-Century-Crofts, 1958.

105. Louhimo I, Lindahl H. Esophageal atresia: primary results of 500 consecutive treated patients. J Pediatr Surg 1983;18:217.

106. Martin LW, Alexander F. Esophageal atresia. Surg Clin North Am 1985;65(5):1099–1113.

107. Azizkhan RG. Esophageal atresia and distal tracheoesophageal fistula in a neonate. Postgrad Gen Surg 1992;4:1–4.

108. Richter CF. Dissertatio medico de infanticido in artis obstetricae [Thesis]. Leipzig, Germany, 1792.

109. Finlay HVL. Familial congenital stridor. Arch Dis Child 1949;78:516–522.

110. Roth B et al. Laryngotracheoesophageal cleft: clinical features, diagnosis and therapy. Eur J Pediatr 1983;140:41.

111. O'Rahilly R, Tucker JA. Early development of the larynx in staged human embryos. Ann Otol Rhinol Cardiovasc Surg 1973;82:1–27.

112. Blumberg JB et al. Laryngotracheoesophageal cleft, the embryologic complications: review of the literature. Surgery 1965;57:559.

113. Delahunty JE, Cherry J. Congenital laryngeal cleft. Ann Otolaryngol 1969;78:96–106.

114. Pettersson G. Inhibited separation of larynx and the upper part of the trachea from the esophagus in a newborn report of a case successfully operated upon. Act Chir Scand 1955;110:250–259.

115. Howell L, Smith JD. G syndrome and its otolaryngologic manifestations. Ann Otol Rhinol Laryngol 1989;98(3):185–190.

116. Allanson JE. G syndrome: an unusual family. Am J Med Genet 1988;31(3):637–642.

117. Mahour GH, Cohen SR, Wooley MM. Laryngotracheoesophageal cleft associated with esophageal atresia and multiple tracheoesophageal fistulas in twins. J Thorac Cardiovasc Surg 1973;65:223.

118. Donahoe PK, Hendren WH: The surgical management of laryngotracheoesophageal cleft with tracheoesophageal fistulae and esophageal atresia. Surgery 1972;71:363–368.

119. Hendren WH. Repair of laryngoesophageal cleft using interposition of a strap muscle. J Pediatr Surg 1976;11:425.

120. Donahoe PK, Gee PE. Complete laryngotracheal cleft: management and repair. J Pediatr Surg 1984;19:143–147.

121. Burroughs N, Leape LL. Laryngotracheoesophageal cleft: report of a case successfully treated and review of the literature. Pediatrics 1974;53:516–522.

122. Bell JW et al. Laryngotracheoesophageal cleft: the anterior approach. Ann Otol Rhinol Laryngol 1977;86:616–622.

123. Imbrie JD, Doyle PJ. Laryngotracheoesophageal cleft: report of a case and review of the literature. Laryngoscope 1969;79:1252–1274.

124. Myer CM III, Cotton RT, Holmes DK, Jackson RK. Laryngeal and laryngotracheoesophageal clefts: role of early surgical repair. Ann Otol Rhinol Laryngol 1990;99:98–104.

125. Schwartz SI, Dale WA. Unusual tracheoesophageal fistula with membranous obstruction of esophagus and postoperative hypertrophic pyloric stenosis. Ann Surg 1955;42:1002–1006.

126. Overton RC, Creech O. Unusual esophageal atresia with distant membranous obstruction of the esophagus. J Thorac Surg 1958;35:674–677.

127. Schwartz SI. Congenital membranous obstruction of esophagus. Arch Surg 1962;85:480–482.

128. Mandell MJ, Bowen A, Shaw MD, Wood BP. Radiological case of the month: coexisting duodenal and esophageal atresia without tracheoesophageal fistula. Am J Dis Child 1988;142(8):891–892.

129. Friedland GW, Melcher DW, Berridge FR, Gresham GA. Debatable points in the anatomy of the lower esophagus. Thorax 1966;21:487–498.

130. Templeton FE. X-ray examination of the stomach: a description of roentgenologic anatomy, physiology and pathology of the esophagus, stomach and duodenum. Chicago: University of Chicago Press, 1944.

131. MacMahon HE, Schatzki R, Gary JE. Pathology of a lower esophageal ring. N Engl J Med 1958;259:1–8.

132. Trinkle JK. Lower esophageal ring. Ann Surg 1962;155:207–211.

133. Berridge FR, Friedland GW, Tagart REB. Radiological landmarks at the oesophago-gastric junction. Thorax 1966;21:499–510.

134. Jamieson J, Hinder RA, DeMeester TR, Litchfield D, Barlow A, Bailey RT Jr. Analysis of thirty-two patients with Schatzki's Ring. Am J Surg 1989;158:563–566.

135. Webb WA, McDaniel L, Jones L. Endoscopic evaluation of dysphagia in two hundred and ninety-three patients with benign disease. Surg Gynecol Obstet 1984;158:152–156.

136. Nosher JL, Cambell WL, Seaman WB. The clinical significance of cervical esophageal and hypopharyngeal webs. Radiology 1975;117:45–47.

137. Devitt PG. Oesophageal webs. In: Jamieson GG, ed. Surgery of the oesophagus. New York: Churchill Livingstone, 1988:515–518.

138. Elwood PC, Pitman RG. Observer error in the radiological diagnosis of Paterson-Kelly webs. Br J Radiol 1966;39:587–589.

139. Clements JL, Cox GW, Torres WE, Weens HS. Cervical esophageal webs: a roentgen-anatomic correlation—observations on the pharyngoesophagus. AJR 1974;121:221–231.

140. Ladd WE. Congenital anomalies of the esophagus. Pediatrics 1950;6:9–19.

141. Tedesco FJ, Moreton WJ. Lower esophageal webs. Am J Dig Dis 1975;20(1–6):381–383.

142. Postlethwait RW. Surgery of the esophagus. New York: Appleton-Century-Crofts, 1979:40–76.

143. Longstreth GF, Wolochow DA, Tu RT. Double congenital mid-esophageal webs in adults. Dig Dis Sci 1971;24:162–165.

144. Shearman DJC, Finlayson NDC. Diseases of the gastrointestinal tract and liver. Edinburgh: Churchill Livingstone, 1982:114.

145. Greenough WG. Congenital oesophageal strictures. AJR 1964;92:994–999.

146. Bluestone CD, Kerry R, Sieber WK. Congenital esophageal stenosis. Laryngoscope 1969;79(6–8):1095–1104.

147. Liebman WM, Samloff IM. Congenital membranous stenosis of the midesophagus. Clin Pediatr 1973;12:660–662.

148. Nehme AE, Rabiah F. Ciliated epithelial esophageal cyst: case report and review of the literature. Am Surg 1977;43:114–118.

149. Whitaker JA, Deffenbaugh LD, Cooke AR. Esophageal duplication cyst. Am J Gastroenterol 1980;73:329–332.

150. Milson J, Unger S, Alford BA, Rodgers BM. Triplication of the esophagus with gastric duplication surgery 1985;98(1):121–125.

151. Game PA. Cysts and duplications of the oesophagus. In: Jamieson GG, ed. Surgery of the oesophagus. New York: Churchill Livingstone, 1988:887–892.

152. Kirwan WO, Walbaum PR, McCormack RJM. Cystic intrathoracic derivatives of the foregut and their complications. Thorax 1973;28:424–428.

153. Stoeckel KH. Uber einen fall von intrathorakeler entodermcyste in mediastinum posterias bei einem neugeborenen. Zentralbl Gynakol 1935;59:2178.

154. Vaneeklas GMH. Pathogenesis of intrathoracic gastrogenic cysts. Am J Dis Child 1952;83:500.

155. Bentley JFR, Smith JR. Developmental posterior enteric remnants and spinal malformations: the split notochord syndrome. Arch Dis Child 1960;35:76–86.

156. Vaage S. Knutrud O. Congenital duplications of the alimentary tract with special regard to their embryogenesis. In: Rickham PP, ed. Progress in pediatric surgery. Baltimore: Urban & Schwarzenberg, 1974:103–123.

157. Bremer JL. Diverticula and duplications of the intestinal tract. Arch Pathol 1944;38:132–140.

158. Blasius G. Observata anatomica in homine, simia equo. Amsterdam (Amstelodam):Gassbeeck, 1674.

159. Kathe H. Partielle verdoppelung der speiser:ohre. Virchows Arch [A] 1907;190:78–92.

160. Ciechanowski S, Glinski LK. Fistulae oesophageo-oesophageales congenitae. Virchow Arch [A] 1910;199:420.

161. Maier HC. Intramural duplication of the esophagus. Ann Surg 1957;145:395.

162. Frank RC, Paul LW. Congenital reduplication of the esophagus: report of a case. Radiology 1949;53:417.

163. Boivin Y, Cholette JP, Lefebvre R. Accessory esophagus compli-

cated by an adenocarcinoma. Can Med Assoc J 1964;90:1414–1417.

164. Bremer JL. Congenital anomalies of the viscera. Cambridge: Harvard University Press, 1957.

165. King TC, Smith CR. Chest wall, pleura, lung, and mediastinum. In: Schwartz SI, Shires GT, Spencer FC, eds. Principles of surgery, 5th ed. New York: McGraw Hill, 1989:627–771.

166. Kleinhaus S, Ducharme JC. Mediastinal lipoma in children: case report. Surgery 1969;66:490.

167. Bratu M, Brown M, Carter M, Lawson JP. Cystic hygroma of the mediastinum in children. Arch Dis Child 1985;119:348.

168. Moore T, Cobo J. Massive symptomatic cystic hygroma confined to the thorax in early childhood. J Thorac Cardiovasc Surg 1985;89:459.

169. Wilson JR, Bartley TD. Liposarcoma of the mediastinum. J Thorac Cardiovasc Surg 1964;48:486.

170. Zajtchuk R, Strevey TE, Heydorn WH, Treasure RL. Mediastinal histoplasmosis. J Thorac Cardiovasc Surg 1973;66:300.

171. Kuster GGR, Foroozan P. Early diagnosis of adenocarcinoma developing in Barrett's esophagus. Arch Surg 1989;124:925.

172. Altorki NK, Sunagawa M, Little AG, Skinner DB. High grade dysplasia in the columnar-lined esophagus. Am J Surg 1991;161:97–100.

173. Seabrook M, Holt S, Gilrane T. Barrett's esophagus: observations on diagnosis and management. South Med J 1992;3:280–288.

174. McCallum RW. Progress report on ACG Barrett's esophagus study. Proceedings of the American College of Gastroenterology, San Francisco, October 1990.

175. Snyder M, Luck S, Hernandez R, et al. Diagnostic dilemmas of mediastinal cysts. J Pediatr Surg 1985;20:810.

176. Arboya JL, Fazzi, JGF, Mayhoral J. Congenital esophageal cysts: case report and review of the literature. Am J Gastroenterol 1984;79:177–182.

177. Bower RJ, Kiesewetter WB. Mediastinal masses in infants and children. Arch Surg 1977;112:1003.

178. Bremer JFR, Smith JR. Development posterior enteric remnants and spinal malformations: the split notochord syndrome. Arch Dis Child 1960;35:76–86.

179. Smith JR. Accessory enteric formations: classification and nomenclature. Arch Dis Child 1960;35:87–89.

180. Ware GW, Conrad HA. Thoracic duplication of alimentary tract. Am J Surg 1953:86:264–272.

181. Schnoor EE, Connolly JE. Paraesophageal bronchiogenic cyst. Am J Surg 1958;96:107.

182. Roddie RK. Retropharyngeal cyst of foregut origin associated with a vertebral abnormality. Br J Surg 1960;47:401–405.

183. Hutchison J, Thomson JD. Congenital archenteric cysts. Br J Surg 1953;41:15–20.

184. Matheson A, Cruickshank G, Matheson WJ. Gastric cysts of the mediastinum with a report of two cases. Arch Dis Child 1952;27:533–538.

185. Thorbjarnarson B, Haynes LL. Duplication of the stomach: a report of two cases. Surgery 1958;44:585–590.

186. Shepherd MP. Thoracic, thoraco-abdominal and abdominal duplication. Thorax 1965;20:82–86.

187. Borrie J. Duplication of the oesophagus: review and description of two cases. Br J Surg 1961;48:611–618.

188. Alrabeeah A, Gillis DA, Giacomantonia M, Lau H. Neurenteric cysts: a spectrum. J Pediatr Surg 1988;23(8)752–754.

189. Wolf YG, Merlob P, Horev G, Litwin A, Katz S. Thoraco-abdominal enteric duplication with meningocele, skeletal anomalies and dextrocardia. Eur J Pediatr 1990;149(11)786–788.

190. Bremer JL. Dorsal intestinal fistula; accessory neurenteric canal; diastematomyelia. Arch Pathol 1952;54:132–138.
191. Astley R. Duplication of the foregut and related conditions. Acta Chir Belg 1960;59:149–159.
192. Fallon M, Gordon ARG, Lendrum AC. Mediastinal cysts of foregut origin associated with vertebral abnormalities. Br J Surg 1954;41:520–533.
193. Beardmore HE, Wiglesworth FW. Vertebral anomalies and alimentary duplications. Pediatr Clin North Am 1958;5:457–474.
194. McLetchie NGB, Purves JK, Saunders RL, deC H. Genesis of gastric and certain intestinal diverticula and enterogenous cysts. Surg Gynecol Obstet 1954;99:135–141.
195. Knight G, Griffiths T, Williams I. Gastrocystoma of the spinal cord. Br J Surg 1955;42:635–638.
196. Elwood JS. Mediastinal duplication of the gut. Arch Dis Child 1959;34:474–479.
197. Pedersen H. Mediastinal enterogenous cyst with spinal malformations: case report. Acta Paediatr Scand 1965;54:392–396.
198. Rhaney K, Barclay GPT. Enterogenous cysts and congenital diverticula of the alimentary canal with abnormalities of the vertebral column and spinal cord. J Pathol Bact 1959;77:457–471.
199. Staehelin-Burckhardt A. Uber eine mit Magenschleimhaut versehene Cyste des Oesophagus. Arch Verdauungskr 1909;15:584–603.
200. Mixter CG, Clifford SH. Congenital mediastinal cysts of gastrogenic and bronchogenic origin. Ann Surg 1929;90:714.
201. Laipply TC. Cysts and cystic tumors of the mediastinum. Arch Pathol 1945;39:153.
202. Davis JE, Barnes WA. Intrathoracic duplications of the alimentary tract communicating with the small intestine. Ann Surg 1952;136:287–295.
203. Peabody JW, Sturg LH, River JD. Mediastinal tumors, survey of modern concepts in diagnosis and management. Arch Intern Med 1954;93:875–893.
204. Miskovitz PF, Steinberg H. Diverticula of the gastrointestinal tract. Disease-A-Month. Chicago: Year Book Medical Publishers, 1982.
205. Duranceau AC. Diverticula of the oesophageal body. In: Jamieson GG, ed. Surgery of the oesophagus. New York: Churchill Livingstone, 1988:489.
206. Jordan PH. Dysphagia and esophagea diverticula. Postgrad Med 1977;61:155–161.
207. Dodds WJ et al. Radial distribution of esophageal peristaltic pressure in normal subjects and patients with esophageal diverticulum. Gastroenterology 1975;69:584–590.
208. Reynolds JC, Ouyang A, Cohen S. Recent advances in diagnosis and treatment of esophageal disease. Geriatrics 1982;37:91–104.
209. Borrie J, Wilson RLK. Oesophageal diverticula: principles of management and appraisal of classification. Thorax 1980;35:759–767.
210. Rivkin L, Bremner CG, Bremner CH. Pathophysiology of midoesophageal and epiphrenic diverticula of the oesophagus. S Afr Med J 1984;66:127–129.
211. Spiridonov AA, Ivanitskii AV, Besedin SN, Petrova NN. Right aortic arch with a retro-esophageal diverticulum (embryology, anatomy, classification, clinical picture, diagnosis and surgical treatment). Grudn Khir 1991; Feb(2):9–14.
212. Balthazar EM. Esophagobronchial fistula secondary to ruptured traction diverticulum. Gastrointest Radiol 1977;2:119–121.
213. Hurwitz AL, Way LW, Haddad JK. Epiphrenic diverticulum in association with an unusual motility disturbance: report of surgical correction. Gastroenterology 1975;68:795–798.
214. Jackson C, Shallow TA. Diverticula of the esophagus: pulsion, traction, malignant and congenital. Ann Surg 1926;83:1.
215. Nelson AR. Congenital true esophageal diverticulum: report of a case unassociated with other esophagotracheal abnormality. Ann Surg 1957;145:258.
216. Grant JC, Arneil GC. Congenital diverticulum of the esophagus: a report of two cases. Surgery 1959;46:966.
217. Lewis FT, Thyng FW. The regular occurrence of intestinal diverticula in embryos of the pig, rabbit and man. Am J Anat 1907;7:505–519.
218. Lerche W. The esophagus and pharynx in action: a study of structure in relation to function. Springfield, IL: Charles C Thomas, 1950.
219. Law SW, Overstreet JW. Pulsion diverticula of the midthoracic esophagus. J Thorac Cardiovas Surg 1964;48:855–860.
220. Goodman HI, Parnes IH. Epiphrenic diverticula of the esophagus. J Thorac Surg 1952;23:145–159.
221. Cross FS, Johnson GF, Gerein AN. Esophageal diverticula. Arch Surg 1961;83:525–533.
222. Hurst AF. Two cases of diverticula from the lower end of the esophagus. Guy Hosp Rep 1925;75:361–366.
223. Hird WE, Hortenstine CB. Familial esophageal epiphrenal diverticula. JAMA 1959;171:1924–1927.
224. Laimer E. Beitrag zur Anatomie des Oesophagus. Med Jahrb Wien 1883;333–338.
225. Skandalakis JE. Spontaneous idiopathic rupture of the healthy esophagus. Acad Med (Greece) 1954;173:1–40.
226. Negus VE. Pharyngeal diverticula: observations on their evolution and treatment. Br J Surg 1950;38:129.
227. Rush LV, Stingily CR. Congenital diverticulum of the esophagus: case report. South Med J 1929;22:546.
228. Lahey FH, Warren KW. Esophageal diverticula. Surg Gynecol Obstet 1954;98:1–28.
229. Debas HT, Payne WS, Cameron AJ, Carlson HC. Physiopathology of lower esophageal diverticulum and its implications for treatment. Surg Gynecol Obstet 1980;151:593–600.
230. Gray SW, Skandalakis JE, Shepard D. Smooth muscle tumors of the esophagus. Surgery 1961;113:205–220.
231. DeBakey ME, Heaney JP, Creech O. Surgical considerations in diverticula of the esophagus. JAMA 1952;150:1076–1082.
232. Sweet RH. Excision of diverticulum of the pharyngoesophageal junction and lower esophagus by means of a one stage procedure. Ann Surg 1956;143:433–438.
233. Poppel MH, Lentino W, Zaino C, Jacobson H. Closing mechanism of lower esophagus in man: radiological study of 500 unselected patients. JAMA 1956;161:196–198.
234. Luschka H. Antrum cardiacum des menschlichen magens. Virchow Arch [A] 1857;11:427–434.
235. Inglefinger FJ, Kramer P, Sanchez GC. Gastroesophageal vestibule, its normal function and its role in cardiospasm and gastroesophageal reflux. Am J Med Sci 1954;228:417–425.
236. Evans JA. Sliding hiatus hernia. AJR 1952;68:754–763.
237. Palmer ED. An attempt to localize the normal esophagogastric junction. Radiology 1953;60:825–831.
238. Lacau St Guily J, Baril P, Tome F, Chaussade S, Ponsot P. Dysphagia in oculopharyngeal myopathies: report of 7 cases. Ann Otolaryngol Chir Cervicofac 1990;107(8):542–546.
239. Ament. Esophageal reflux in children. Contemp Surg 1991;39:43–55.
240. Schridde H. Uber Magenschleimhaut-insein vom Bau der Cardialdrüsenzone und Fundus-drüsen-region und den unteren, oesophagealen Cardialdrüsen gleichende Drüsen im obersten Oesophagusabschnitt. Virchow Arch [A] 1904;175:1–16.
241. Abrams L, Heth D. Lower oesophagus with intestinal and gastric epithelium. Thorax 1965;20:66–72.
242. Armstrong RA, Blalock JB, Carrera GM. Adenocarcinoma of the

middle third of the esophagus arising from ectopic gastric mucosa. J Thorac Surg 1959;37:398–403.

243. Barrett NR. Hiatus hernia: a review of some controversial points. Br J Surg 1954;42:231–243.

244. Allison OR. Reflux esophagitis sliding hiatal hernia and the anatomy repair. Surg Gynecol Obstet 1951;92:419–431.

245. Van de Kerckhof J, Gahagan T. Regeneration of the mucosal lining of the esophagus. Henry Ford Hosp Med Bull 1963;11:129–134.

246. Lell WA. Is congenitally short esophagus truly a rare entity? Ann Otol 1966;69:1114–1126.

247. Whale HL. Oesophageal tumor of thyroid tissue. Br Med J 1921;2:987.

248. Porto G. Esophageal nodule of thyroid tissue. Laryngoscope 1960;70:1336.

249. Kirklin BR. Roentgenologic demonstration of an anomalous prolongation of the esophagus below the diaphragm, facilitating total gastrectomy. Am J Surg 1932;16:12–13.

250. Barrett NR. Chronic peptic ulcer of the oesophagus and "oesophagitis." Br J Surg 1950;38:175–182.

251. Barrett NR. The lower oesophagus lined by columnar epithelium. Surgery 1957;41:881–894.

252. Wilson SE, Arnstein D. Barrett's esophagus, challenges and controversies. Postgrad Med 1989;85(2):65–73.

253. DeMeester TR, Attwood SEA, Sonyik TC, Therkildsen DH, Hinder RA. Surgical therapy in Barrett's esophagus. Ann Surg 1990;212:528–542.

254. Dahms BB, Rothstein FC. Barrett's esophagus in children: a consequence of chronic gastroesophageal reflux. Gastroenterology 1984;86(2)318–323.

255. Stadelmann O, Elster K, Kuhn HA. Columnar-lined oesophagus (Barrett's syndrome)—congenital or acquired? Endoscopy 1981;13(4):140–147.

256. Bright R. Account of a remarkable misplacement of the stomach. Guy Hosp Rep 1836;1:598.

257. Bund R. Ein Fall von rechtsseitiger Hernia diaphragmatica mit Austritt des Magens in den persistierenden Rezessus pneumatoentericus dexter. Frankfurt Z Pathol 1918;21:243.

258. Oka M, Attwood SE, Kaul B, Smyrk TC, DeMeester TR. Immunosuppression in patients with Barrett's esophagus. Surgery 1992;112(1):11–17.

259. Li H, Walsh TN, Hennessy TPJ. Carcinoma arising in Barrett's esophagus. Surg Gynecol Obstet 1992;175:167–172.

260. Olsen AM, Harrington SW. Esophageal hiatal hernias of the short esophagus type: etiologic and therapeutic considerations. J Thorac Surg 1948;17:189–207.

261. Swyer PR. Partial thoracic stomach and esophageal hiatus hernia in infancy and childhood. Am J Dis Child 1955;90:421–451.

262. Allison OR, Johnsone AS. The oesophagus lined with gastric mucous membrane. Thorax 1953;8:87–101.

263. Terracol J, Sweet RH. Diseases of the esophagus. Philadelphia: WB Saunders, 1958.

264. Effler DB. Surgical treatment of achalasia of the esophagus and mega-esophagus. In: Mulholland JH, Ellison EH, Friesen SR, eds. Current surgical management. Philadelphia: WB Saunders, 1957.

265. Schiebel HM. Treatment of esophageal achalasia or cardiospasm: report of four patients treated surgically. Surgery 1946;20:558.

266. Lendrum FC. Anatomic features of the cardiac orifice of the stomach: with special reference to cardiospasm. Arch Intern Med 1937;59:474–511.

267. Rickham PP. Rupture of exomphalos and gastroschisis. Arch Dis Child 1963;38:138–141.

268. Scherb J, Arias IM. Achalasia of the esophagus and Chagas' disease. Gastroenterology 1962;43:212–215.

269. Knight GC. Sympathectomy in the treatment of achalasia of the cardia. Br J Surg 1935;22:864.

270. Etzel E. Megaoesophagus and its neuropathology: a clinical and anatomo-pathological research. Guy Hosp Rep 1937;87:158.

271. Joseph R, Job JC. Familial dysautonomy and megaesophagus. Arch Fr Pediat 1963;20:25–33.

272. Hill JL. Neuromotor esophogeal disorders. In: Welch KJ, Randolph JG, Ravitch MM, O'Neill JA Jr, Rowe MI, eds. Pediatric surgery, Vol I. Chicago: Year Book Medical Publishers, 1986:720–725.

273. Raffensperger JG. Achalasia. In: Raffensperger JG, ed. Swenson's pediatric surgery, 5th ed. Chicago: Appleton & Lange, 1990:771,823–826.

274. Nihoul-Fekete C, Bawab F, Lortat-Jacob S, Arhan P, Pellerin D. Achalasia of the esophagus in childhood: surgical treatment in 35 cases with special reference to familial cases and glucocorticoid deficiency association. J Pediatr Surg 1989;24:1060–1063.

275. Steichen FM, Heller E, Ravitch MM. Achalasia of the esophagus. Surgery 1960;47:846–876.

276. Khalifa MM. Familial achalasia, microcephaly and mental retardation. Clin Pediatr 1988;27:509–512.

277. Willis T. In pharmaceutice rationalis. London: Dring, Harper, & Leight, 1679.

278. Purton T. An extraordinary case of distention of the oesophagus, forming a sac, extending from two inches below the pharynx to the cardiac orifice of the stomach. Med Physiol J Lond 1921;46:540.

279. Hannay AJ. An extraordinary dilatation (with hypertrophy) of all the thoracic portion of the oesophagus, causing dysphagia. Edin Med Surg J 1833;40:65.

280. Mikulicz J. Ueber Gastroskopie und Oesophagoskopie, mit Demonstration am Lebenden. Verh Duetsch Ges Chir 11 Congress 1822;30.

281. Rümpel T. Die klinische Diagnose der spindelförmigen Speiseröhrenerweiterung. München Med Wschr 1897;44:383.

282. Rake GW. Pathology of achalasia of cardia. Guy Hosp Rep 1927;77:141–150.

283. Neumann A. Ueber die einfach Gleichmässige ("spindelförmige") Erweiterung der Speiseröhre. Zentralbl Grenzgeb Med Chir 1900;3:166.

284. Thieding F. Ueber Kardiospasmus, Atonie und "idiopathische" Dilatation der Speiseröhre. Beitr Klin Chir 1921;121:237.

285. Gray HK, Skinner IC. The operative treatment of cardiospasm. J Thorac Surg 1940;10:220–235.

286. Jaffé K. Ueber idiopathische Oesophaguserweiterungen. Munchen Med Wschr 1897;44:386.

287. Heller E. Extramuköse Kardioplastik beim chronischen Kardiospasmus mit Dilatation des Oesophagus. Mitt Grenzgeb Med Chir 1914;27:141–149.

288. Walton AJ. The surgical treatment of cardiospasm. Br J Surg 1925;12:701.

289. Fish J, Harrison AW. Achalasia of the esophagus: a review. Ann Surg 1962;28:545–552.

290. Mayberry JF, Rhodes J. Achalasia in the city of Cardiff from 1926 to 1977. Digestion 1980;20:248.

291. Erlam RJ, Ellis FH, Nobrega FT. Achalasia of the esophagus in a small urban community. Mayo Clin Proc 1969;44:478.

292. DiMarino PJ, Cohen L. Characteristics of lower esophogeal sphincter function in symptomatic diffuse esophageal spasm. Gastroenterology 1974;66:1.

293. Adams HD. Amyenteric achalasia of the esophagus. Surg Gynecol Obstet 1964;119:251.

294. Benedict EB. Bougienage, forceful dilatation, and surgery in treatment of achalasia. JAMA 1964;188:355–357.

295. Bonavina L, Nosadini A, Bardini R, Baessato M, Peracchia A. Pri-

mary treatment of esophageal achalasia: long-term results of myotomy and dor fundoplication. Arch Surg 1992;127(2):222–226.

296. Rosato EF, Acker M, Curcillo PG, II, Reilly R, Reynolds J. Transabdominal esophagomyotomy and partial fundoplication for treatment of achalasia. Surgery Gynecol Obstet 1991;173:137–141.

297. Stipa S et al. Heller-Belsey and Heller-Nissen operations for achalasia of the esophagus. Surg Gynecol Obstet 1990;170:212–216.

298. Neuhauser EB, Berenberg W. Cardio-esophageal relaxation as a cause of vomiting in infants. Radiology 1947;48:480.

299. Strawczynski H, McKenna RD, Nickerson GH. The behavior of the lower esophageal sphincter in infants and its relationship to gastroesophageal regurgitation. J Pediatr 1964;64:17–23.

300. Gryboski JD. The swallowing mechanism of the neonate. I. Esophageal and gastric motility. Pediatrics 1965;35:445–452.

301. Vaos GC. Quantitative assessment of the stage of neuronal maturation in the developing human fetal gut: a new dimension in the pathogenesis of developmental anomalies of the mesenteric plexus. J Pediatr Surg 1989;24(9):920–925.

302. Kiriluk LB, Merendino KA. Comparative sensitivity of mucosa of different segments of alimentary tract in dog to acid peptic action. Surgery 1954;35:547–556.

303. Boix-Ochoa J. Gastroesophageal reflux. In: Welch RJ, Randolph JG, Ravitch MM, O'Neill JA Jr, Rowe MI, eds. Pediatric surgery, Vol I. Chicago: Year Book Medical Publishers, 1986:712–720.

304. DeMeester TR et al. Clinical and in vitro analysis of determinants of gastroesophageal competence: a study of principles of antireflux surgery. Am J Surg 1979:137:39.

305. Jona JZ, Sty JR, Glicklich M. Simplified radioisotope technique for assessing gastroesophageal reflux in children. J Pediatr Surg 1981;16:114.

306. St-Cyr JA et al. Treatment of pulmonary manifestations of gastroesophageal reflux in children two years of age or less. Am J Surg 1989;157(4):400–403.

307. Boix-Ochoa J, Casasa JM, Gil-Vernet JM. Une chirurgie physiologique pour les anomalies du secteur cardiohiatal. Chir Pediatr 1983;24:117.

308. Tunell WP. Gastroesophageal reflux in childhood: implications for surgical treatment. Pediatr Ann 1989;18(3):192–196.

309. Johnson DG, Jolly SG. Gastroesophageal reflux in infants and children: recognition and treatment. Surg Clin North Am 1981;61(5):1101–1115.

310. Glassman MS, Dozer AJ, Newman LJ. Gastroesophageal reflux in neurologically impaired children: perioperative evaluation and management. South Med J 1992;3:289–292.

311. Jolley SG. Current surgical considerations in gastroesophageal reflux disease in infancy and childhood. Surg Clin North Am 1992; 72:1365–1392.

312. Idriss FS. Vascular ring. In: Raffensperger JG, ed. Swenson's pediatric surgery, 5th ed. Chicago: Appleton & Lange, 1990:689–696.

313. Galizzi JM et al. Dysphagia lusoria: apropos of 3 cases. Acta Gastroenterol Latinoam 1983;13(4):727–731.

314. Cherri J et al. Surgical treatment of dysphagia lusoria. Arg Bras Cardiol 1991;56:51–55.

CHAPTER 4

THE PERITONEUM

John Elias Skandalakis / Stephen Wood Gray / Rickard Ricketts / Daniel Dale Richardson

. . . because it stretches over the organs within it [it was
given the name peritoneum].
—GALEN

DEFINITION AND HISTORY

The peritoneum is the largest serous smooth membrane of the human body with a surface area of 22,000 cm², the approximate surface area of the skin. Two names are connected with this complex anatomic entity: Ebers (1), whose archeologic studies include the first description of the peritoneum in a 3500-year-old papyrus, and James Douglas of Edinburgh, who published a detailed description in 1730 that is still considered the best to date (2). Three tables which illustrate terminology claims for omental function and ancient omental anatomy provide a good historical overview of the omentum (Tables 4.1 to 4.3).

EMBRYOLOGY

The embryogenesis of the peritoneum has been discussed in detail elsewhere in this book in the chapters concerning such topics as the pericardium, pleural cavities, and gastrointestinal tract. However, in this section we present briefly the embryogenesis of the organ for the sake of clarity.

Around the third week of embryonic life, the intraembryonic mesoderm is responsible for differentiation causing the formation of the lateral plate, the intermediate mesoderm, and the paraxial mesoderm. The lateral plate is divided into layers by further differentiation of the somatic and splanchnic mesoderms. Between them is the intraembryonic celom on each side of the midline. The next step is the union of the right and left intraembryonic celom to a large single cavity that later will subdivide to pleural, pericardial and peritoneal cavities, and the tunica vaginalis.

By further differentiation, the mesodermal cells lining the intraembryonic cavity change to mesothelial cells and produce the parietal and visceral layers of the serous membranes. The formation of the omenta, mesenteries, and ligaments is the result of several embryogenetic steps.

To start with, the gastrointestinal tract is closed, associated, and fixed with the dorsal and ventral mesentery.

In a highly diagrammatic way, this may be presented as an open book facing down (Fig. 4.1).

ANATOMY

The peritoneum is composed of two layers: the parietal, which lines the abdominal wall and is thus its innermost layer; and the visceral, which almost entirely covers the abdominal viscera. The space between the parietal and visceral peritoneum is the peritoneal cavity.

The scope of this chapter does not include discussion of the detailed anatomy of this organ. However, a systematic classification of the several peritoneal formations may help the reader understand not only the complexities of this anatomic entity but also the derivatives that spring from the longest membrane of the human body.

The peritoneum forms four kinds of anatomic entities: the omentum, mesenteries, ligaments, and fossae. Each of these is subdivided (Table 4.4). The chapter follows this structure to present the possible congenital anomalies. Further taxonomy is virtually impossible.

Jones (3) offers the following definitions of the peritoneal derivatives: The *omentum* is a particular fold of peritoneum passing between the stomach and other abdominal viscera. *Mesentery* is a fold of peritoneum passing between a portion of intestine and the posterior abdominal wall. A *ligament* is a fold of peritoneum that connects a viscus, which is not part of the intestine, to the abdominal or pelvic parietes or viscera of any kind, to each other or to the diaphragm. *Fossae,* or recesses, are small or deep pockets. However, these types of definitions are not always accurate; for instance, the anatomist and surgeon frequently use the word ligament liberally.

The discussion of fossae leads into a presentation of internal herniae.

Compartments

The peritoneal cavity may be divided into two major compartments by an imaginary cross-sectional plane that

Table 4.1.
Commonly Used Historical and Modern Terms in Medical Literature, and Their Meaning[a]

Term	Root	Meaning	Reflects Character of	Language
Dertron	Derma	Skin	Membrane	Greek
	Dero	To flay	Membrane	Greek
Epiploon	Eplma	Sole of the root	Cover	Greek
	Plein	Floating, drifting on	Cover	Greek
Omentum	Operimentum	Cover (of intestines)	Cover	Latin
	Opimus	Fat	Fat	Latin
	Ovimentum	Induo = I clothe or I cover	Cover	Latin
Rete	Reticulum	Net (of a fisherman)	Membrane	Latin
Mappa ventris	Mappa	Napkin (of the abdomen)	Cover	Latin
Cupeus	Clipeus	Shield	Cover	Latin
Zirbus	Tharb	Fat	Fat	German
Coefe	Coiffe	Lace bonnet	Membrane	French
Crépine	—	Sieve or riddle	Membrane	French
Caul	—	Hair net	Membrane	French
Guedel	—	Sac	Sac	German
Gidel	—	Sac	Sac	German
Mirach	—	Greasy hood of meat	Cover	German

[a]From Liebermann-Moffert D. Historical images and ideas about the greater omentum. In: Goldsmith HS, ed. The omentum: research and clinical applications. New York: Springer-Verlag, 1990.

Table 4.2.
Claims for Omental Function from Classical to Recent Times[a,b]

Claim	Year	Author
Prevents conception in obese by pressing on and occluding the uterus	450	Hippocrates
Inflow of ingested fat after compression of the gravid uterus on stomach into omentum; from there it ascends to the breast and turns into milk	200	Aristotle
Warmth of fat accelerates digestion, fat content lubricates peritoneum	200	Galen
Fat storage, heat exchanger	1300	Mondeville
Heat compensator for hairless human skin		
Receptacle for waste products of stomach, liver, and spleen	1619	Ab Acqua Pendente
Ruler of the whole abdomen	1620	Riolan
Fat transport via omental lymph vessels to distant body regions	1659	Wharton, Bartholin (1660), Boerhaave (1743), Haller (1747)
Production of pus and serous fluid	1666	Vesling
Fat transport via adipose omental ducts	1687	Malpighi
Lubricant production to smooth peristatic	1727	Petit
Nourishes the body, adds fat to the bile	1741	Culmus
Ability to enclose foreign bodies	1840	Robert; Renzi (1903)
Protection against infection	1874	Ravier, Roger (1898), Renzi (1903), Morison (1906)
Peritoneal absorption	1882	Maffucci; Muscatello (1895)
Active migration	1899	Milian, Heger (1903), Morison (1906)
Revascularization	1910	Boljarski

[a]From Liebermann-Meffert D. Historical images and ideas about the greater omentum. In: Goldsmith HS, ed. The omentum: research and clinical applications. New York: Springer-Verlag, 1990.
[b]Speculations about the functions of the omentum were mostly erroneous until they were followed by experiments in the late 19th century.

passes through the transverse mesocolon. This defines a supracolic and an infracolic compartment (Fig. 4.2). Within the supracolic compartment, the liver determines a right and left suprahepatic (subdiaphragmatic) space and a right and left intrahepatic space.

The infracolic compartment is divided by the mesentery of the small bowel into a right infracolic (supramesenteric) compartment, a left intracolic (inframesenteric) compartment, and a pelvic cavity. In addition, there exist the right and left paravertebral gutters. The left gutter is infracolic only, being interrupted by the phrenocolic ligament. The right gutter extends upward into the supracolic compartment. There is no right phrenocolic ligament.

The pelvic cavity is divided into right and left spaces by the sigmoid colon and the rectum. It is further subdivided in the female into anterior and posterior spaces by the broad ligament, uterine tubes, and uterus.

Table 4.3.
Knowledge of Omental Anatomy from Classical to Recent Times[a,b]

Claim	Year	Author
Warm fatty material	200	Aristotle
Attachment to stomach		
Membrane	50	Pliny
Peritoneal purse, delicate membrane, arteries, veins	200	Galen
	1000	Avicenna
	1267	Theodoric
Attachment to diaphragm, stomach, spleen, colon	1300	Mondino Da Luzzi
Life-like picture	1500	Leonardo Da Vinci
"Bird catcher's sac," two layers, tributaries to the portal vein, "glands excreting liquid" individual fat amount, first accurate picture of anatomy	1543	Vesalius
Comprehensive description, vessels, no glands	1632	Van Den Spieghel
Lymph vessels	1659	Wharton, Bartholin 1660
Adipose ducts or vessels	1687	Malpighi
Vascularity (by wax injection) confirms Spieghel: membranes have no perforation = no net	1702	Ruysch
Reflections, opening into the omentum	1732	Winslow
Tâches laiteuses (milky spots)	1874	Ranvier

[a]From Liebermann-Meffert D. Historical images and ideas about the greater omentum. In: Goldsmith HS, ed. The omentum: research and clinical applications. New York: Springer-Verlag, 1990.
[b]Poor knowledge of omental anatomy progressed slowly from classical times to the 19th century.

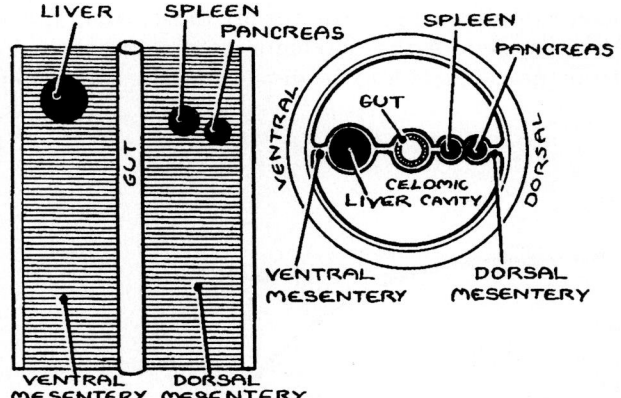

Figure 4.1. Relationship of various organs with the embryonic ventral and dorsal mesenteries. (From Brantigan OC. Clinical anatomy. New York: McGraw-Hill, 1963.)

Table 4.4.
Parts of the Peritoneum

Omenta	Great omentum
	Lesser omentum
Mesenteries	Mesentery of the small bowel
	Mesoappendix
	Transverse mesocolon
	Pelvic mesocolon
Ligaments	Of liver
	Of urinary bladder
	Of uterus
Fossae	Duodena
	Cecal
	Intersigmoid

Early in development there is a dorsal and ventral mesentery. Subsequently, all of the ventral mesentery (cranial part) disappears except that of the foregut. The persisting ventral mesentery extends from the umbilicus to the abdominal esophagus.

Two organs, the liver and the stomach (together with the first inch of the duodenum), are involved in the ventral mesentery. The liver divides the mesentery into two parts, forming anteriorly the falciform ligament and posteriorly the lesser omentum.

The falciform ligament begins at the umbilicus and passes obliquely to the superior surface of the left lobe of the liver, where it forms an excellent landmark that separates the lateral and medial segments of the left lobe. The free edge of the falciform ligament contains the cord-like round ligament (ligamentum teres) of the liver. This is the remnant of the left umbilical vein. The right umbil-

ical vein disappears early in development; the left vein carries placental blood to the fetus and closes at birth. This vascular remnant is often patent for much of its length (4). Its intrahepatic portion becomes the ligamentum venosum, which connects the left branch of the portal vein with the left hepatic vein. The falciform ligament is thus the mesentery of the umbilical vein.

We have seen two cases in which the falciform ligament was not attached to the anterior abdominal wall. Through this hiatus a loop of intestine could well have passed, producing partial or complete small bowel obstruction.

The lesser omentum usually is divided for convenience into the hepatogastric ligament and the hepatoduodenal ligament (Fig. 4.3). The hepatogastric ligament extends from the porta hepatus to the lesser curvature of the stomach and the abdominal esophagus. The ligament encloses the gastroesophageal junction on the right, and the two leaves rejoin on the left as the gastrosplenic ligament, a portion of the embryonic dorsal mesentery. The posterior leaf does not reach the gastroesophageal junc-

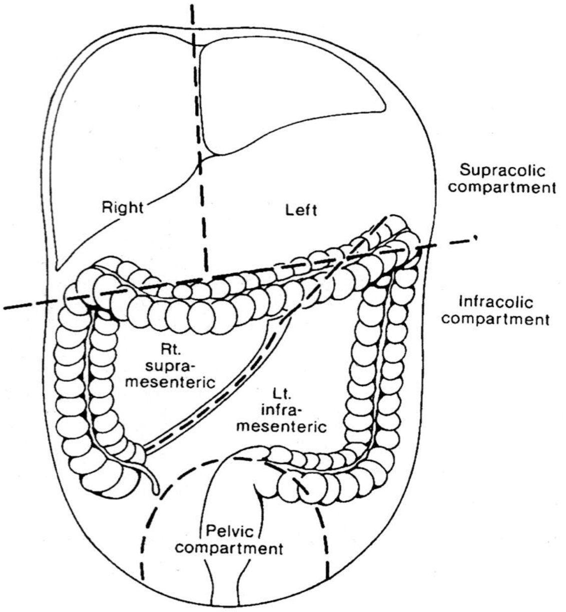

Figure 4.2. Diagram of the arbitrary compartments of the abdominal cavity. The pelvic compartment in the female may be further divided into anterior and posterior portions by the uterus and broad ligament. (From Skandalakis JE, Gray SW, Rowe JS Jr. Anatomical complications in general surgery. New York: McGraw-Hill, 1983:303.)

tion, so there is a small bare area on the posterior wall of the stomach that lies on the left crus of the diaphragm and is related to the left adrenal gland and the left gastric artery and vein (5).

The hepatogastric ligament contains the left gastric artery and vein and the hepatic division of the left vagal trunk. Occasionally, it may contain the right gastric artery and vein and both vagal trunks. In about one-fourth of subjects, it contains the left hepatic artery, which arises from the left gastric artery (6).

The hepatoduodenal ligament extends between the liver and the first portion of the duodenum at the right border of the hepatogastric ligament. It contains the common bile duct, the hepatic artery, and the portal vein. This ligament may be considered to be the mesentery of the portal triad. It is also the anterior boundary of the epiploic foramen of Winslow.

Also, there are four unusual and not constant peritoneal folds that most likely belong to the ventral mesentery (Fig. 4.4): (*a*) cholecystocolic (from the gallbladder to the hepatic flexure), (*b*) cholecystoduodenal (from the gallbladder to the first posterior or proximal area of the second posterior of the duodenum), (*c*) cholecystogastric (from the gallbladder to the distal stomach), and (*d*) hepa-

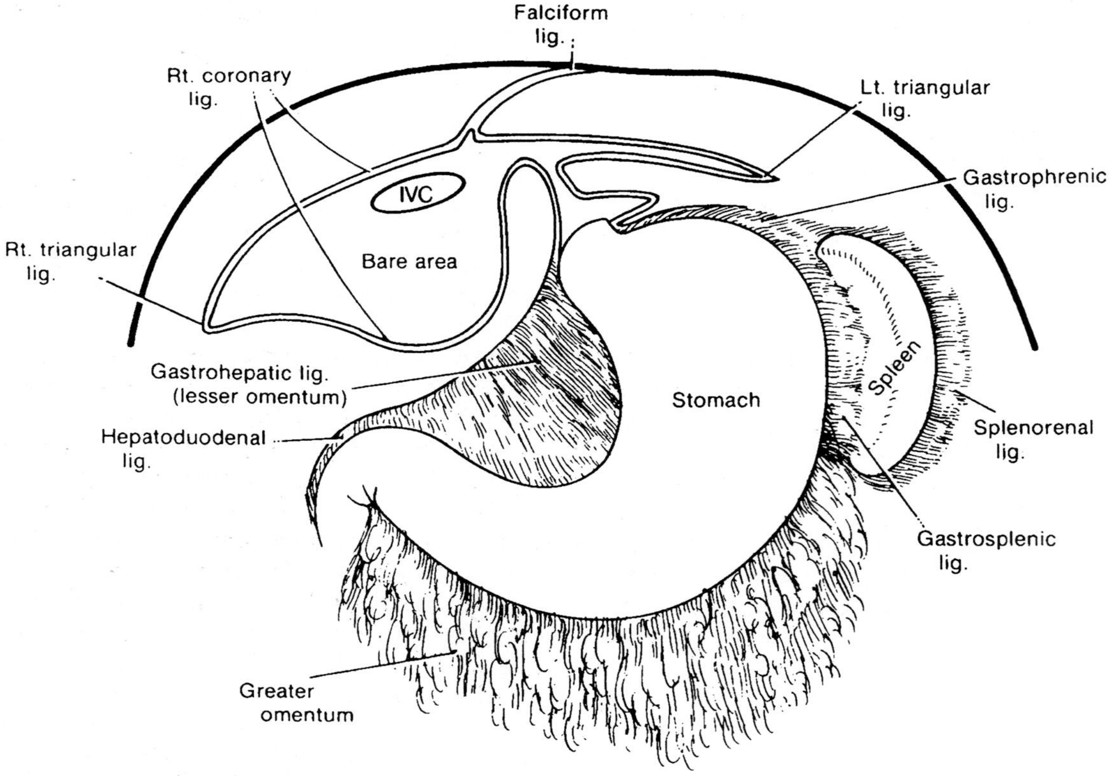

Figure 4.3. The mesenteries of the stomach. *Above* and on the *left* of the illustration, the falciform, coronary, and gastrohepatic ligaments are derivatives of the primitive ventral mesogastrium. On the *right* of the illustration, the greater omentum and the gastrophrenic ligament are derivatives of the dorsal mesogastrium. (From Skandalakis JE, Gray SW, Rowe JS Jr. Anatomical complications in general surgery: New York: McGraw-Hill, 1983:304.)

tocolic ligament (from the right lobe inferior surface to the hepatic flexure).

The coronary ligaments also are remnants of the embryonic ventral mesentery. Their outer surface is peritoneum, whereas their inner surface forms the boundary of the bare area. The right and left lateral extremities of the coronary ligaments are the triangular ligaments. They are not in line—the right is more posterior and lateral; the left is more superior and medial (Fig. 4.5).

Supracolic Ligament (Ventral Mesogastrium)

There is no question that the supracolic compartment is the most difficult area of the abdomen from a technical standpoint. Our description is based on the work of Livingston (7), Ochsner and Graves (8), Mitchell (9), Autio (10), Boyd (11), Myers (12), Harley (13), and Whalen (14).

Supracolic Compartment (Dorsal Mesogastrium and Greater Omentum)

The primitive dorsal mesentery, unlike the ventral mesentery, persists in the adult. In the supracolic compartment it forms the greater omentum and the common mesentery. Originally, the dorsal mesentery extended from the dorsal border of the stomach to the midline of the dorsal (posterior) body wall (Fig. 4.6). This simple relationship becomes altered by the counterclockwise rotation of the stomach through 90 degrees and by the developing spleen.

For all practical purposes, the embryonic dorsal mesogastrium is the adult greater omentum. It may be divided into three parts: upper, the gastrophrenic ligament; middle, the gastrosplenic ligament; and lower, the gastrocolic ligament (see Fig. 4.3).

The gastrophrenic ligament extends from the proximal greater curvature of the stomach, the gastroesopha-

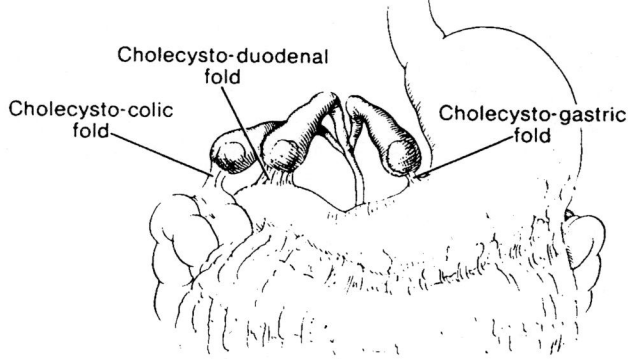

Figure 4.4. Inconstant peritoneal folds of the gallbladder to the duodenum, colon, or stomach (in order of frequency). Their presence is often associated with biliary fistulae. (From Skandalakis LJ, Gray SW, Colborn GL, Skandalakis JE. Surgical anatomy of the liver and associated extrahepatic structures. Contemp Surg 1987;31(1):30.)

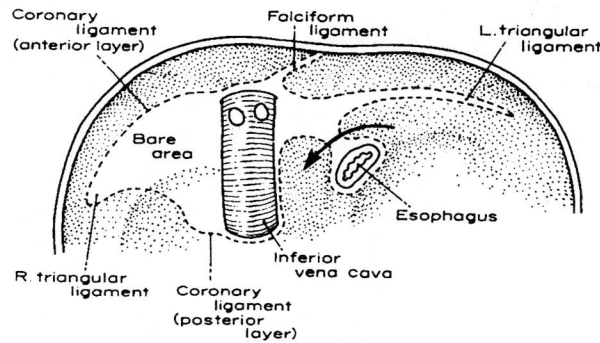

Figure 4.5. The peritoneal reflections of the diaphragm showing the bare area and the coronary, triangular, and falciform ligaments. (From Skandalakis JE, Gray SW, Rowe JS Jr. Anatomical complications in general surgery. New York: McGraw-Hill, 1983:305.)

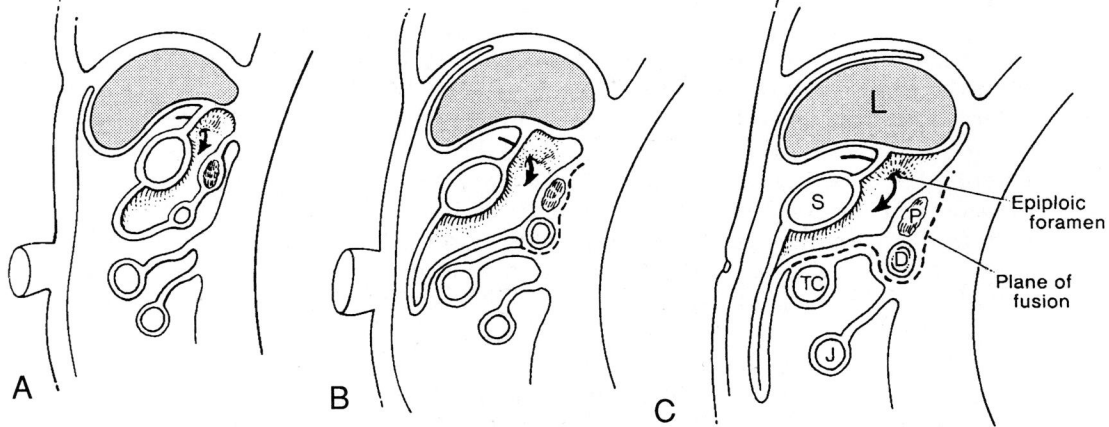

Figure 4.6. The development of the omentum and the lesser sac. **A**, At 2 months. The duodenum *(D)* and pancreas *(P)* are contained in the dorsal mesogastrium. **B**, At 4 months. The duodenum and pancreas are retroperitoneal; the greater omentum is elongating. **C**, Adult configuration. The cavity of the greater omentum is obliterated; the posterior wall has fused with the transverse colon *(TC)* and the transverse mesocolon. The *arrow* indicates the opening of the epiploic foramen into the lesser sac, and the *dashed line* indicates the plane of fusion. (From Skandalakis JE, Gray SW, Rowe JS Jr. Anatomical complications in general surgery. New York: McGraw-Hill, 1983:305.)

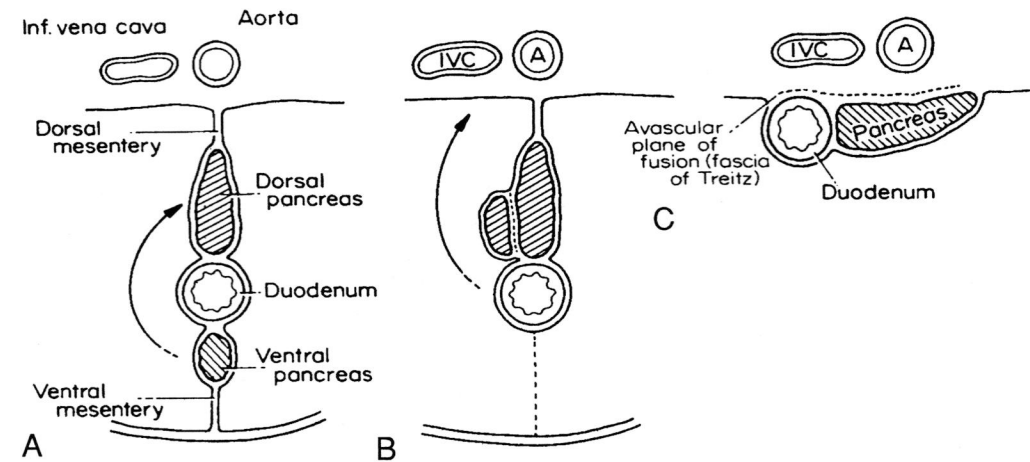

Figure 4.7.   Diagram of the changing relations of the duodenum, pancreas, and posterior body wall in the developing embryo.
(From Skandalakis et al. Anatomical complications in general surgery, New York: McGraw Hill, 1983:306.)

geal junction, and the abdominal esophagus to the diaphragm. The upper part is avascular; the lower part contains some short gastric vessels and lymph nodes.

The middle portion of the dorsal mesentery is interrupted by the spleen to form a posterior splenorenal ligament and a more anterior gastrosplenic ligament, plus several other ligaments related directly or indirectly to the spleen. Together these form the splenic pedicle. The splenorenal ligament contains the splenic artery and vein and the tail of the pancreas. The gastrosplenic ligament contains the short gastric and left gastroepiploic vessels.

The gastrocolic ligament is the part of the dorsal mesogastrium between the greater curvature of the stomach and the transverse colon. At its earliest appearance, the mesogastrium includes the duodenum and the pancreas; it attaches to the posterior body wall (Fig. 4.6, *A*). By the fourth month of gestation, the duodenum and pancreas become retroperitoneal (Fig. 4.7), and the future omentum forms a sac, the omental bursa, that extends in front of the transverse colon (Fig. 4.6, *B*). Fusion of the anterior and posterior walls of the dependent portion of the omental bursa obliterates most of the lower recess of the bursa, leaving only the superior portion of the cavity behind the stomach and in front of the colon (Fig. 4.6, C). A complete examination of the development of the omentum from birth through adulthood is presented in Table 4.5.

The anterior wall of the sac in the adult remains free; the posterior layer fuses with the transverse colon and mesocolon. Only with this fusion does it become entitled to the name *gastrocolic ligament*. The size and extent of the omental bursa depends on the degree of fusion of the two walls of the sac below, as well as the fusion of the posterior wall of the sac with the transverse mesocolon. The right portion, which arises from the antrum of the stomach, is frequently fused with the anterior surface of the head of the pancreas. The omentum should be freed from the pancreas from left to right (15).

Where two peritoneal layers of the posterior wall of the bursa fuse with two peritoneal layers of the transverse mesocolon, at first there are four peritoneal layers. Only the two outer layers, above and below, are found in the adult mesocolon.

There is considerable variation in the length of the omentum. Anson and colleagues (16) examined 125 cadavers and found that the omentum was not visible in 19%, was a "mere fringe" in 2%, and extended from 14 to 19.5 cm below the xiphisternal joint in 8%. In the remaining 71%, the omentum extended 20 to 36 cm below the xiphisternal articulation.

The Lesser Sac (Omental Bursa)

The lesser sac may be divided into a vestibule and the bursa proper. The vestibule, beginning at the epiploic foramen, is formed by the pancreaticogastric fold, which contains the left gastric artery from the retroperitoneal space to the lesser curvature of the stomach. It creates a bridge between the aorta close to the esophageal hiatus of the diaphragm and the gastrohepatic ligaments. A fingerbreadth below this fold is the pancreaticoduodenal fold, which contains the hepatic artery as it passes from the retroperitoneal space to the hepatoduodenal ligament just below the pylorus and the first part of the duodenum. The opening of the vestibule into the bursa proper has been called the *second epiploic foramen*.

The bursa proper, when considered in midsagittal section (Fig. 4.6, *C*) is bound anteriorly by the lesser omentum, stomach, and the gastrocolic ligament, and posteriorly by the retroperitoneal space. The roof is formed by the caudate lobe of the liver, the coronary ligament on the right, and the abdominal esophagus on the left. The floor is formed by the transverse colon and mesocolon.

Table 4.5.
Development of the Greater Omentum from Birth to Adulthood[a]

Age	Premature Newborn	Mature Newborn	3 to 4 mo	1 to 5 yr	5 to 10 yr	Adult
Attachments	Attached to the transverse colon but does not reach the colonic flexures	Further attachment but does not reach the colonic flexures	Distal to the transverse colon	Extends beyond the colonic flexures; some attachments to the ascending and descending colon	Resembles the adult omentum; insertion on the ascending colon and occasionally on the cecum	Width, 20 to 46 cm
Downward length	Just below the colon	Covering approx. ½ of small bowel	Covering ⅔ of small bowel	Most of the intestines are covered by the omentum	More downward extension	7 to 10 cm or 14 to 35 cm
Network	Fatless thin vascular membrane	Fatless thin vascular membrane	Fat around the vessels	More fat; occasionally some lymph nodes	More fat	Volume depends on body weight; may be fat or lean
Vascularization	Vascular pattern can be seen	Vascular pattern can be seen	Vascular pattern can be seen	Vascular pattern can be seen	Vascular pattern can be more obviously seen	Wider range of varieties; no standard pattern; unpredictable
Observations	Omentum is rudimentary fringe and extends upward toward the spleen. Its two posterior layers fused to the transverse colon and transverse mesocolon	Splenic ligaments developed; omentum reaches the diaphragm	Splenic ligaments, especially gastrosplenic and splenorenal, are better developed; better formation of omentum	Omentum well formed	Omentum and omental derivation almost with normal limits	Typical omental formation, fat or lean, voluminous or not, according to body weight; all parts well differentiated; artery, veins, and lymph nodes may be seen
Diagram						

[a]Waldschmidt J. Pathological conditions, specific investigations, and therapy. In Liebermann-Meffert D, White H, eds. Diseases of the omentum: congenital abnormalities and pediatric disease. New York: Springer-Verlag, 1983.

When considered in cross-section, the bursa is bound anteriorly by the gastroduodenal ligament and the hepatic triad: the gastrohepatic ligament, the gastrosplenic ligament, and the stomach. Posteriorly the bursa is bound by the splenorenal ligament and the pancreas. On the right is the epiploic foramen; on the left, in front, is the distal part of the gastrosplenic ligament and behind is the distal part of the splenorenal ligament.

Remember the following:

1. The greater omentum is simply a double-layered evagination of the part of the dorsal mesogastrium located between the common hepatic artery and the left gastric artery (occurring at the fifth week).
2. The stomach grows, bends, rotates, and finally forms a large portion of the anterior wall of the lesser sac. The greater omentum, by definition, attaches to the greater curvature of the stomach, which represents the original dorsal surface of the stomach.
3. By continuous growth, the omental apron forms a double-layered sac.
4. The sac of the greater omentum is attached to the greater curvature of the stomach and is closely related to the transverse mesocolon. The transverse mesocolon of the adult is a fusion between the embryonic transverse mesocolon and the portion of the dorsal mesogastrium attaching to the posterior abdominal wall.
5. The embryonic greater omentum is the product of the dorsal mesogastrium and, for all practical purposes, is the home of the spleen, pancreas, and all branches related to splenic artery and vein.

6. The ventral mesentery is present only above the umbilicus; around the fifth week, because of the formation of the liver, it divides into two sections: the peritoneal ligaments of the liver (falciform, coronary, and triangular) and the lesser omentum.
7. The dorsal mesentery is responsible for the genesis of the greater omentum. After the formation of the omental bursa (lesser sac), the dorsal mesentery elongates downward, forming its inferior recess. This is a four-layered anatomic entity: the greater omentum or fat apron.
8. Also keep in mind the relations of the greater omentum to the greater curvature of the stomach, to the transverse colon, and the formation of the several other ligaments.

Controversies exist regarding the development of the omentum. Swaen (17) in 1896 and 1897 and Broman (18) in 1905 and 1938 supported the opinion that the lesser sac was formed as an independent area (a cleft or recess). Liebermann-Meffert (19) believed that organs do not rotate and that the omentum develops independently in close relation to the spleen and not as a fold of the dorsal mesogastrium. Krutsiak and Voitiv (20) stated that the lesser peritoneal sac develops in three sections: vestibulum bursae omentalis, bursa omentalis proper, and cavity omentum majus. We believe that this process is neither connected with the development of separate organs or structures nor with independent growth, but with the total process of development of the upper abdominal cavity.

CONGENITAL ANOMALIES OF THE GREATER OMENTA

Congenital anomalies of the greater omenta are rare. Cases are reported sporadically; therefore the investigator may have difficulty understanding these malformations and their sequelae from either an embryologic and anatomic standpoint or from a clinical one.

These anomalies sometimes occur alone as well as in association with other malformations. Therefore we will postulate and hypothesize. We report our findings with the hope that someone will be able to use this information to conduct more detailed analyses.

Agenesis

Absence of the greater omentum and of all or part of the ligaments and folds related to it is rarely described in the literature. Kimura et al. (21) present an autopsy case with multiple anomalies and absence of the omentum. Waldschmidt (22) stated that agenesis and aplasia of the omentum are not satisfactorily documented and that the observations of Broman (23), Otto et al. (24), and Maegraith (25) are unsupported by personal observations. We agree.

Hypoplasia

Kiuchi et al. (26) present a case of sudden death of an infant due to asplenia syndrome with multiple other anomalies and "hypoplasia of the greater omentum."

Waldschmidt (22) presents a case of gastroschisis and states that a rudimentary fringe of omentum always is present along the greater curvature of the stomach that envelopes the gastroepiploic vessels and the spleen.

In a personal communication to Waldschmidt (22), Juskiewenski reported a failure of omental development or its absence in cases of gut atresia.

Dysplasia

We question Aschwanden and Schmid's (27) case of a 73-year-old man who underwent surgery for an aneurysm of an artery of the greater omentum secondary to fibromuscular dysplasia. We are not convinced this was a congenital anomaly.

Hyperplasia

In the laboratory as well as the operating room, we have seen omenta gigantic not only in length and breadth but also in thickness.

Castlemen's disease is characterized by large lymph node hyperplasia and is usually located in the mediastinum (70 to 75% of cases) (28,29). We recall a case in which a lymph node the size of a small egg was located at the ileocecal mesentery. The 9-year-old male suffered the signs and symptoms of acute appendicitis. Whether Castleman's disease is congenital or acquired is unknown.

Long omentum in association with atresia of the transverse colon was reported by Waldschmidt (22). The omentum was floating in the peritoneal cavity.

Duplication

Waldschmidt (22) reported that Juskiewenski, in a personal communication, mentioned duplication of the omentum.

Abnormal Attachment

Bands occur from the distal ascending colon to the proximal transverse colon and from the proximal descending colon to the distal transverse colon (Payr's membrane) (30). Perhaps this is an omental malfusion.

Occasionally, the right side of the omentum produces some peculiar attachments to the ascending colon, to the cecum, or to both. These pathologic presentations should be differentiated from the pericolic membrane of Jackson (31) and the presence of a common ileocecal mesentery with mobile cecum as reported by Nicole (32) and Skan-

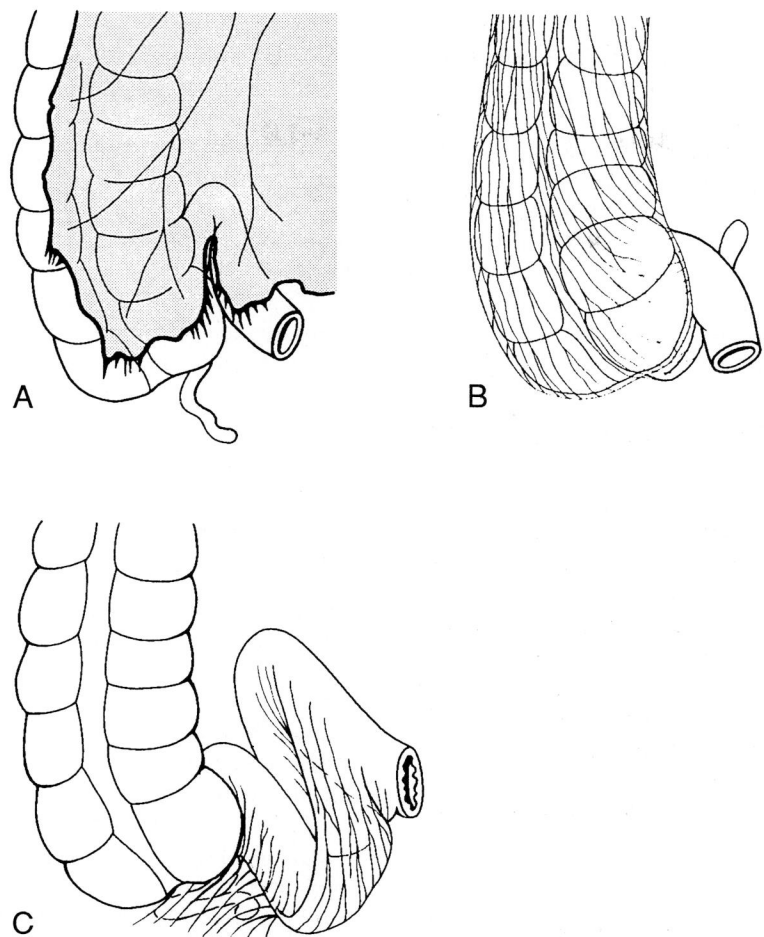

Figure 4.8. Diagrams illustrating (**A**) attachment of the omentum to the cecum, (**B**) pericolic membrane of Jackson, and (**C**) common ventral ileocecal mesentery. (Waldschmidt J. Pathological conditions, specific investigations, and therapy. In Liebermann-Meffert D, White H, eds. The greater omentum. New York: Springer-Verlag, 1983:112.)

dalakis (33) (Fig. 4.8). In Skandalakis' thesis, he observed mobile cecum in 13.19%, common ileocecal mesentery in 1.15%, and ascending colon with mesentery in 6.9% of patients studied.

FAILURE TO ATTACH

The greater omentum may partially or totally fail to attach to the greater curvature or to the gastrocolic ligament. Derivatives of the omentum also may fail to attach to their expected areas and produce some type of failure.

According to Waldschmidt (22), in coloptosis the gastrocolic ligament is often abnormally long and the omental apron short. He observed that rare cases of gastrocolic separation are characterized by caudal omental margin attachment to the transverse colon without accompanying malrotation of the gut and usually are associated with other congenital anomalies. Typically, the colon and the stomach are connected by a broad mesenteric sheath (Fig. 4.9).

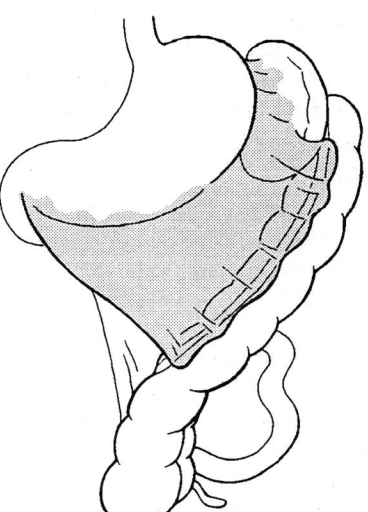

Figure 4.9. Gastrocolic separation. (Waldschmidt J. Pathological conditions, specific investigations, and therapy. In Liebermann-Meffert D, White H, eds. The greater omentum. New York: Springer-Verlag, 1983:112.)

Waldschmidt (22) also reports sigmoid atresia when the greater omentum is not attached to the normal transverse colon. In these cases it is extremely difficult to correlate the shortness of the omental apron and the long gastrocolic ligament with other modifications or anomalies. Perhaps the dorsal mesogastrium played a part in the formation of these anatomic entities. Here again, differentiation between dysplasia (abnormal tissue development), hypoplasia (underdevelopment due to a decrease of the number of cells), and atrophy (destruction) of some of the omental elements is very difficult.

In the operating room, the omentum can be fat or thin, long or short, narrow or wide, or merely absent (agenesis). It is practically impossible for the surgeon or the pathologist to be 100% scientific when categorizing these phenomena as congenital anomalies or as conditions secondary to disease.

When malrotation of the intestine occurs, faulty attachments to one flexure only, to the right colon, and to other anatomic areas occur (Fig. 4.10).

Bifid Omentum

Bifid omentum may occur, but we were unable to locate any cases in the literature.

Nontraumatic Omental Defects

We have seen congenital omental defects at the omenta, most of them asymptomatic. Occasionally, if a loop of small bowel passes through, the clinical picture of internal obstruction may be produced. We have seen asymptomatic defects at the lesser omentum and symptomatic defects at the greater omentum.

Waldschmidt (22) observed large defects in the gastrocolic ligament and internal herniation into the omental bursa. Usually these defects are located between the descending arteries of the greater omentum (34) or between the hepatic triad and the lesser curvature of the lesser omentum.

We agree with White and Waldschmidt (35) that the association of omentum in an atresia is incidental.

In 1976 Leissner (36) reported transomental strangulation, and collected 36 cases from the literature.

Congenital Adhesions

All authors agree that congenital adhesions are rare entities occurring between the omentum and several other organs or between the omentum and the anterior or posterior lateral abdominal wall. However, more congenital adhesions can be observed if other congenital anomalies such as internal and external herniae and intestinal malrotation are present. Intrauterine accidents may produce a plethora of adhesions.

We agree with Ellis (37) that adhesions are seldom congenital; however, we have seen stillborn fetuses with peculiar adhesions. These adhesions cannot be differentiated from other peritoneal adhesions or described as omental. Perhaps both the omentum and peritoneum attempt to correct embryologic defects by forming adhesions to secure the colon to the retroperitoneum or to close internal defects such as diaphragmatic herniae.

Wrzesinski et al (38) demonstrated that omental adhesions in deer developed sooner than adhesions of any other organ. Presidente et al. (39) produced diffused experimental adhesions in deer by inoculation with metacercariae of *Fasciola hepatica*. In several organs, including the omentum, widespread adhesions were observed.

Infarction and Torsion

We have seen one case of idiopathic segmental infarction (40). The lesion involved the right lower border. The pathogenesis is obscure and perhaps the etiology is of embryologic origin.

Of course, when torsion is present, the infarction is no longer idiopathic, but secondary to torsion and involvement of the blood supply (41). The causes of torsion, for all practical purposes, are unknown.

Torsion is no longer considered rare. Since Oberst (42) reported the first case in 1882, numerous reports appeared in the literature with or without infarction (Fig. 4.11). Omental torsion with or without infarction, and infarction without torsion produce an acute abdomen.

Vascular Anomalies

Nikolaeva et al. (43) observed a decrease of the efficiency of mental microcirculation with congenital heart disease.

Tumors and Cysts

Despite the many benign solid tumors described in children, the idea that perhaps some of them are of congenital origin is difficult to support. According to Gloor and Torhorst (44), 250 primary benign soft tissue tumors of the omentum have been described. All of them arose from tissues that compose the greater omentum (fat; connective tissue with possibility of bone and cartilage metaplasia; nerve; and others). Peculiar milky spots participate also in the genesis of these soft tissue tumors (22).

Benign cysts, however, may be congenital or acquired. Waldschmidt (22) collected data on 122 benign omental cysts in children and presented three cases on his own (Fig. 4.12). These cysts may be divided into two categories: true cysts (lined with endothelium or epithelium); and false cysts (pseudocysts without the lining of true cysts).

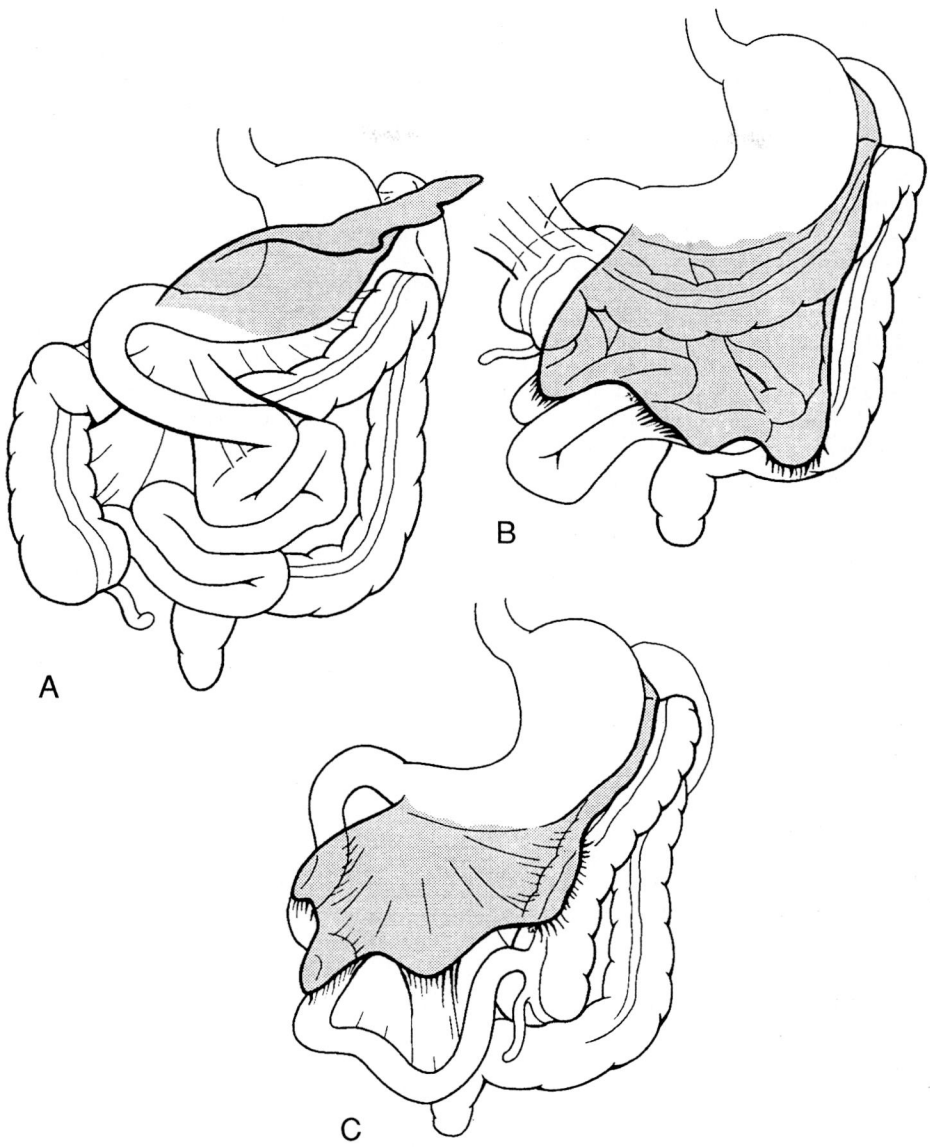

Figure 4.10. Malrotation of the intestine. **A**, Freely floating omentum. **B**, Omentum fixed to the small bowel and sigmoid colon. Ladd's membrane can be seen attaching the cecum to the lateral abdominal wall. **C**, Omentum attached to the mobile ascending colon and small bowel. (Waldschmidt J. Pathological conditions, specific investigations, and therapy. In Liebermann-Meffert D, White H, eds. The greater omentum. New York: Springer-Verlag, 1983:116.)

There are several theories and suggestions concerning the pathogenesis of the benign cysts. Some authors (45–47) believe that cysts with endothelium or mesothelium are of lymphatic origin and that cysts with epithelium, such as dermoids and teratomas, are the result of tissue displacement, this later theory was supported by Walker and Putnam (48).

According to Walsh and Williams (49), who collected data on 272 malignant tumors, only 2.9% were primary.

SIGNS, SYMPTOMS, DIAGNOSIS, TREATMENT

Patients with malignant or benign omental tumors and cysts may be asymptomatic or may present acute abdo-

men. If large, they may be palpable; if pedunculated, they may produce torsion, necrosis, or hemorrhage. Usually they are mobile. Abdominal discomfort and pain are the usual complaints when malignancy is present. Occasionally ascites is present. Diagnosis is confirmed by gastro-intestinal small bowel radiographic series and barium enema. Computed tomography (CT) is of great help, and finally, laparoscopy and diagnostic laparoscopies can assist in the diagnosis. We do not advise the use of laparoscopic biopsy, not only because of the fear of anaphylactic reaction (if this is a parasitic cyst), but also because of spread of malignant cells if the tumor is malignant. Surgery is the only treatment of choice.

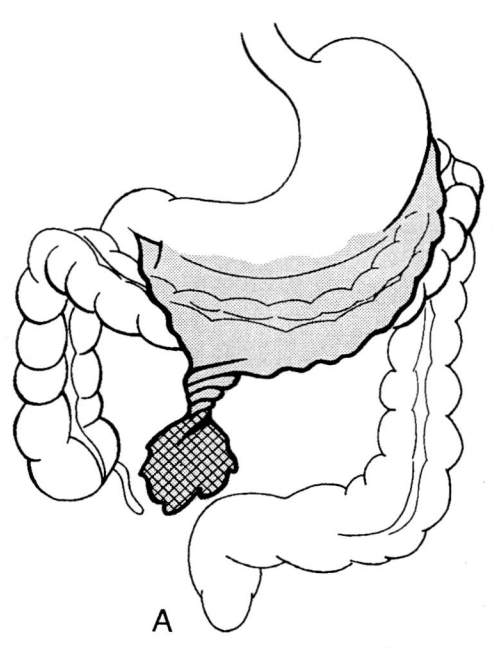

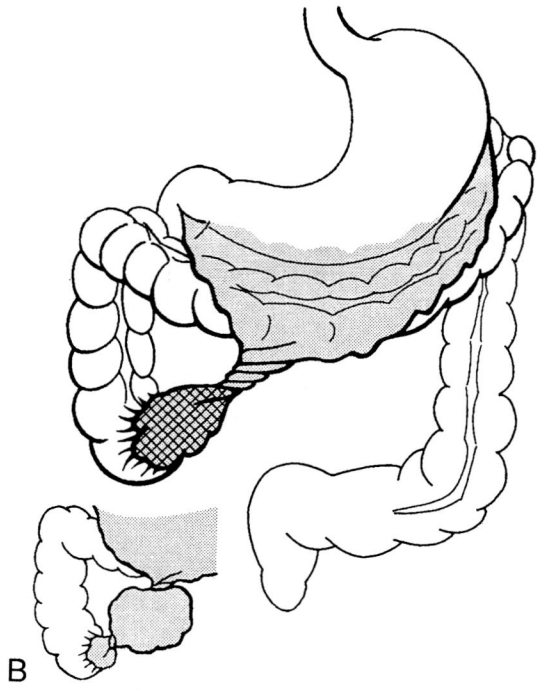

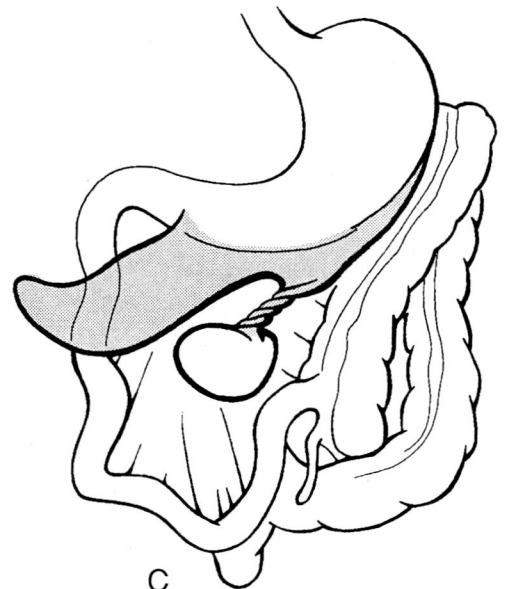

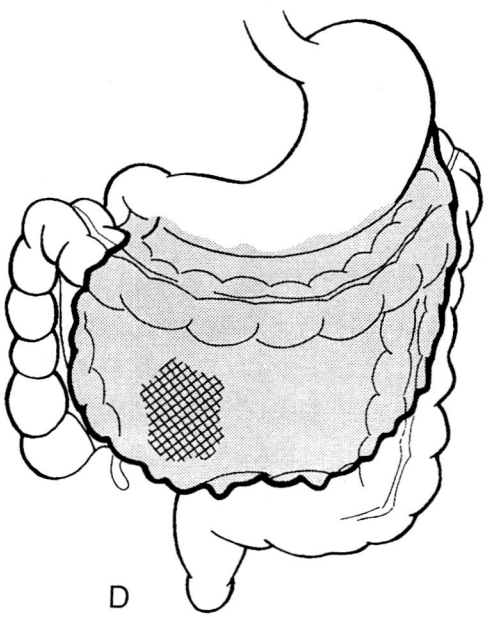

Figure 4.11.   **A**, Primary omental torsion. **B**, Secondary omental torsion. **C**, Secondary torsion of omentum and spleen in nonrotation and failure of omental attachment. **D**, Omental infarction without torsion. (From Tondelli P. Torsion and infarction. In: Liebermann-Meffert D, White H, eds. The greater omentum. New York: Springer-Verlag, 1983:144.)

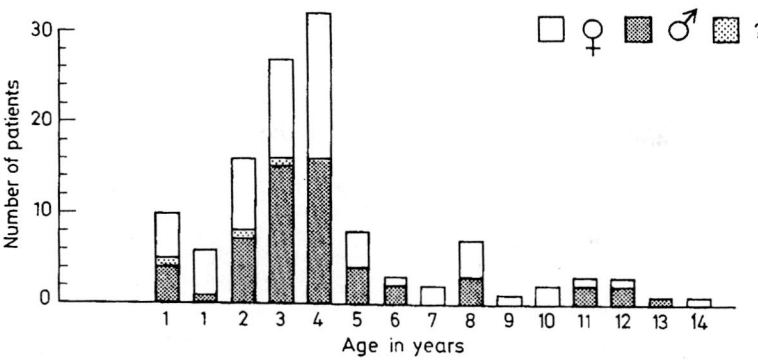

Figure 4.12. Age and sex distribution of 122 children with omental cysts. Reviewed by Waldschmidt from the literature and three cases. Sixty-three of the 122 children were female, 56 were male, and in three cases the sex was unre-corded. (From Waldschmidt J. Pathological conditions, specific investigations, and therapy. In: Liebermann-Meffert D, White H, eds. The greater omentum. New York: Springer-Verlag, 1983:154.)

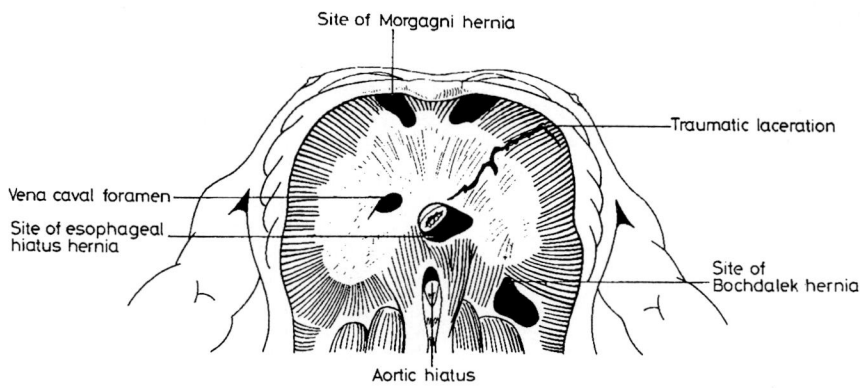

Figure 4.13. Locations of congenital weakness of the diaphragm and the most common site for traumatic laceration. (From Waldschmidt J. Pathological con-ditions, specific investigations, and therapy. In: Liebermann-Meffert D, White H, eds. The greater omentum. New York: Springer-Verlag, 1983.)

Omental Teratoma

Spurney and McCormak (50) reported a case of immature omental teratoma, a very rare condition. These authors discussed the neuroectodermal association. Boehner et al. (51) also reported a solid ovarian teratoma with metastasis to the omentum.

Accessory Spleens

Accessory spleens in the omentum, as well as omental pregnancies, have been reported (52).

Associated Anomalies

Congenital herniae in newborns and children, such as indirect inguinal, diaphragmatic, and several others, play host for the occasional visitor, the omentum (Figs. 4.13 to 4.15).

Herniation within the pericardium has been described by Haider (53).

CONGENITAL ANOMALIES OF THE LESSER OMENTUM

Embryology and Anatomy

The ventral mesentery is responsible for the genesis of the lesser omentum. Because of tremendous hepatic growth, the ventral mesentery is divided, forcing the lesser omentum between the ventral part of the stomach and the liver, and the falciform ligament, which is a remnant of the ventral mesogastrium between the liver and umbilicus. The ventral mesentery disappears below the umbilicus.

The lower omentum envelops the hepatic triad at its free margin and also constitutes the upper margin of the epiploic foramen of Winslow. The falciform ligament contains the left umbilical vein, which is nothing more than the round ligament of the liver.

Anomalies of the lesser omentum are very rare. There are several variations; however, these rare deformities are extremely difficult to classify. On rare occasions we have seen wide as well as narrow holes in the lesser omentum,

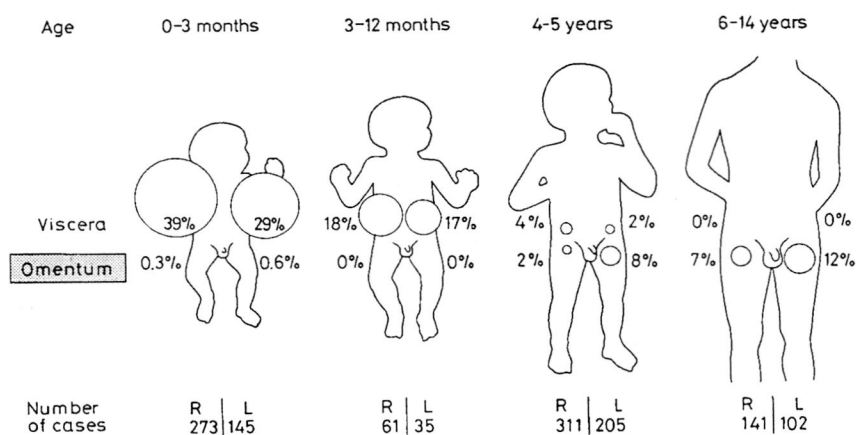

Figure 4.14. Visceral and omental herniae in children. (From Waldschmidt J. Pathological conditions, specific investigations, and therapy. In: Liebermann- Meffert D, White H, eds. The greater omentum. New York: Springer-Verlag, 1983:121.)

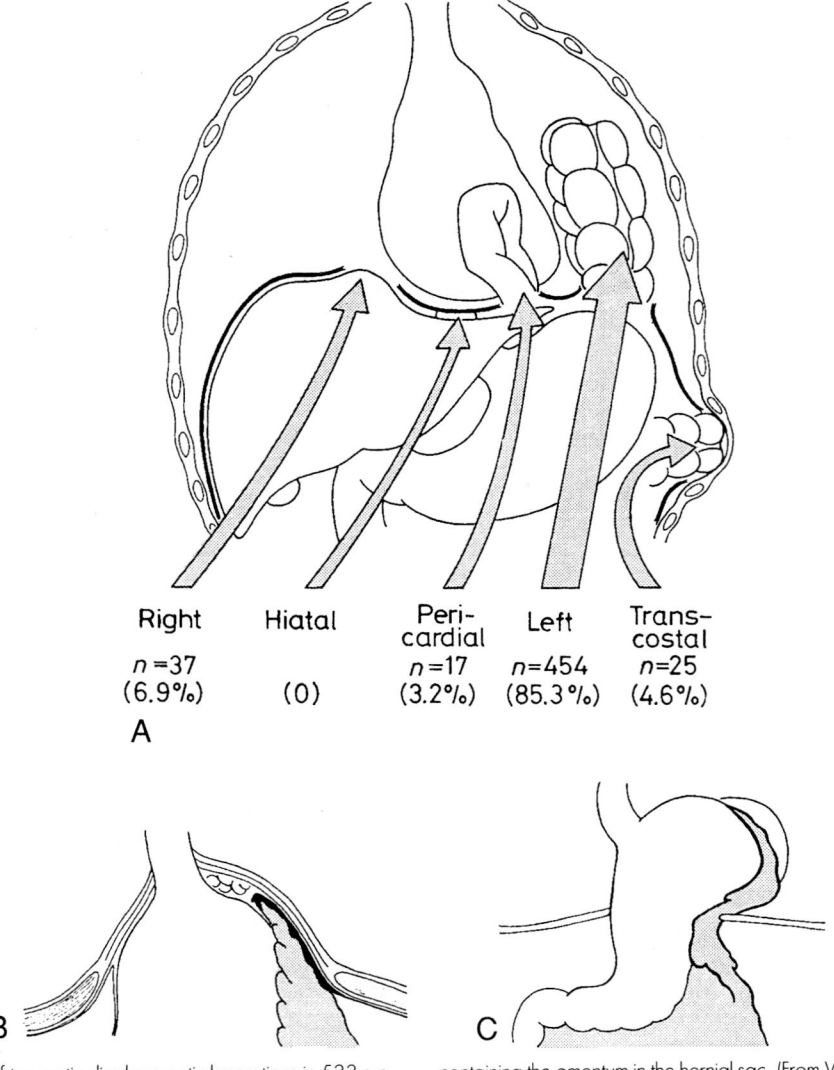

Figure 4.15. **A**, Location of traumatic diaphragmatic lacerations in 533 ruptures reviewed from the literature. Most are caused by blunt accidents (67.4%) and only 0.3% occur spontaneously. **B** and **C**, The two types of hiatal hernia containing the omentum in the hernial sac. (From Waldschmidt J. Pathological conditions, specific investigations, and therapy. In: Liebermann-Meffert D, White H, eds. The greater omentum. New York: Springer-Verlag, 1983:123.)

but making comments about this terra incognita is not within the scope of this book.

Absence of the Lesser Omentum

Hodach et al. (54) presented a case of absence of the lesser omentum with several other anomalies in a male infant.

CONGENITAL ANOMALIES OF THE MESENTERIES

For a presentation of derivatives of the mesentery, see Figure 4.16.

Mesentery of the Small Bowel

The 6-inch long mesentery, which is fused to the retroperitoneal space, extends from the left upper quadrant (first or second vertebra) to the right sacroiliac fossa. For all practical purposes, two congenital anomalies can occur here: failure of fusion or a typical defect with a hole formation, both permitting loops of small bowel to enter and producing a symptomatic or asymptomatic internal herniae. The nonfusion deformity of the mesentery of the small bowel produces a hernia of Waldeyer, as well as several other herniae in combination with nonfusion of colonic mesentery.

Jejunal atresia with agenesis of the dorsal mesentery has been reported by several authors (55–57). This pathologic entity is called "apple peel syndrome," "Christmas tree deformity," or "maypole atresia."

That the disorder is an autosomal inherited familial disease was suggested by Blythe and Dickson (58) and Mishalang and Najjar (59). But Zerella and Martin (60) assert the disease is not always inherited. They cite several cases of twin brothers. One set of twin brothers was normal; but, in the second set of identical twins, only one had the condition. Another theory is a thrombotic phenomenon of the superior mesenteric artery distal to the origin of the right colic artery with ischemic necrosis of the mesentery and part of the small bowel.

Mesoappendix

In general, the appendix and the cecum do not have any mesentery. The presence of cecal mesentery is an anomaly; the presence of appendiceal mesentery is a necessity. This mesentery is merely a continuation of the right lower part of the mesentery of the small bowel. It passes behind the terminal ileum in the form of one or two folds, extends to the appendix and, frequently, to the cecum. The artery of the appendix is located at the free edge of the appendiceal mesentery. Occasionally there is a second artery that springs from the posterior cecal artery. The appendiceal mesentery may be short or long, wide, narrow, and thick because of adipose tissue, or very thin and transparent. All these possibilities depend on the location and length of the appendix and its fixation or mobility.

We discuss the formation of the fossae in the ileocecal region later.

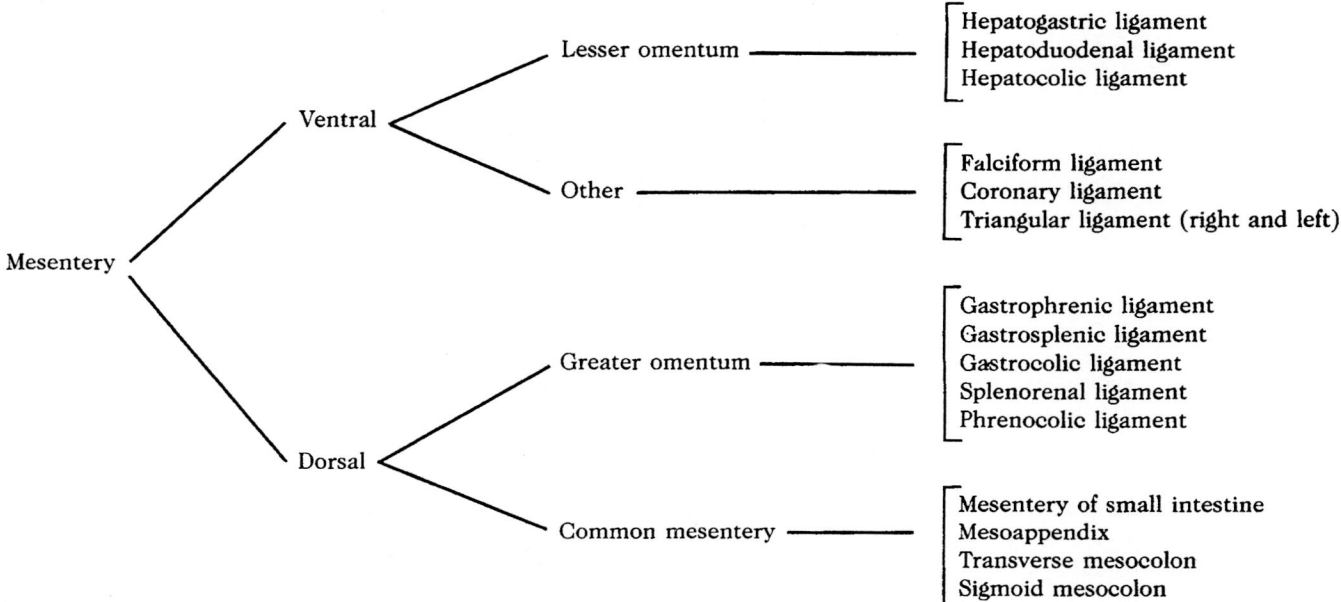

Figure 4.16. Derivatives of the mesentery. (From Skandalakis JE et al. Hernia: surgical anatomy and technique. New York: McGraw-Hill, 1989:271.)

Transverse Mesocolon

Normally, the transverse mesocolon is attached to the second part of the duodenum, the anterior border of the pancreas, and the lower pole of the left kidney. Failure to attach or any other defect producing a hole are potential causes of internal hernia.

Pelvic Mesocolon

The pelvic mesocolon occupies the space from the left pelvic wall to S3, forming a Greek λ. Here is located the intersigmoid fossa, which may be the host of an internal hernia; however, such a hernia may occur at any part of the sigmoid mesocolon. Any defect large or small may be present and the cause of an internal hernia.

Mesenteric Cysts

"Cysts of the mesentery are among the surgical rarities" (Lord Moynihan, 1897).

In a paper published in 1955, Skandalakis (61) recorded the following history of the mesenteric cyst:

The first description of a mesenteric cyst was by the great Florentine physician Antonio Benevieni (62), the so-called "father of pathologic anatomy," in 1507 at the autopsy of an 8-year-old boy. In 1842, Rokitansky (63) noted at autopsy a chylous cyst. Tillaux (62) in 1880 seems to be the first surgeon who operated upon one of these tumors. Three years later (1883), Pean, (64) using marsupialization, treated with success a mesenteric cyst. In 1890 Carson (64) reported the first case in the USA. In 1900 Dowd (65) presented another classification, and from this period to the present, many classifications have been advocated (64, 66–71).

Even though mesenteric cysts continue to be rare, they are well known today to the surgical profession. In 1948 Vaughn et al. (72) presented a good historical overview of the subject, and Caropreso (73) later presented an excellent review of mesenteric cysts. We dare to add a new period to his table (Table 4.6) about the historical periods of mesenteric cysts.

CLASSIFICATION

Although location, symptoms, and treatment of the various mesenteric cysts frequently are similar, they differ by origin. This fact, together with the frequently inadequate description and the use of a location-based terminology, has made them difficult to understand. A more detailed account of earlier attempts to classify these cysts has been published elsewhere (61), but suffice it to say that they are intelligible only when their origin is considered.

Table 4.6.
Four Historical Periods of Mesenteric Cysts[a]

Period	Date	Characteristics
1	1570–1850	The lesion was found only at autopsy.
2	1850–1880	Occasional operations were performed, but usually on an incorrect preoperative diagnosis, and none of the patients is reported to have survived.
3	1880–1974	Operations for this lesion were followed by a few recoveries. The condition was admirably described by Dowd, and surgeons took cognizance of such an entity and diagnosed several cases preoperatively.
4	1974–1990	The triumph of surgery permitted surgeons to perform more ideal procedures after good evaluation.

[a]From Caropreso PR. Mesenteric cysts: a review. Arch Surg 1974;108:243.

Table 4.7.
Classification of Cysts[a]

A. Simple
  1. Serous
  2. Chylous
  3. Irregular
B. Neoplastic
  1. From ectoderm (dermoid)
  2. From mesoderm (lymphangioma)
  3. From entoderm (enterocystoma)
  4. From fetal inclusions (teratoma)

[a]From Caropreso P. Mesenteric cysts: a review. Arch Surg 1974;108:242–246.

They may be divided thus:

A. Congenital cysts
  1. Cysts of endodermal origin
     Enteric cysts (cystic intestinal duplications)
  2. Cysts of multiple origin
     Retroperitoneal teratomata
  3. Cysts of mesodermal origin
    a. Lymphatic cysts
    b. Retroperitoneal cysts of urogenital origin
B. Acquired cysts
  1. Neoplastic
  2. Infectious
  3. Traumatic

Only the cysts in group A concern us. Because of their varied embryonic origin, congenital cysts are discussed with other lesions of similar origin. Enteric cysts are described in this chapter; lymphatic cysts in Chapter 24, and nephrogenic cysts in Chapter 17.

For historical perspective we present the tables of Caropreso (73) (Table 4.6) and Ford (74) (Table 4.7). For a

Table 4.8.
Classification[a]

I. Embryonal cysts
  A. Arising from embryonic remnants and sequestrated tissue
    1. Serous
    2. Chylous
    3. Sanguineous
    4. Dermoid
  B. Arising by sequestration from the bowel
    1. Including Meckel's diverticulum
  C. Of urogenital origin
II. Pseudocysts
  A. Of infective origin
    1. Hydatids
    2. Cystic degeneration of tuberculous nodes
  B. Cystic malignant disease
III. Embryonic and developmental cysts
  A. Enteric
  B. Urogenital
  C. Lymphoid
  D. Dermoid
  E. Embryonic defects in early formation of lymphatic vessels, lymph nodes, etc.
IV. Traumatic or acquired cysts (cyst wall composed of fibrous tissue without a lining membrane)
  A. Those caused by injury
    1. Hemorrhage causing sanguineous cysts
    2. Rupture of lacteals
    3. Extravasation of chyle into surrounding tissue
V. Neoplastic cysts
  A. Benign cysts
    1. Hyperplastic lymph of vessels resolving in lymphangiomata
  B. Malignant cysts
    1. Lymphangioendothelioma
VI. Infective and degenerative cysts
  A. Mycotic
  B. Parasitic
  C. Tuberculous
  D. Cystic degeneration of lymph nodes and other tissue

[a]From Caropreso P. Mesenteric cysts: a review. Arch Surg 1974;108:242–246.

Table 4.9.
Theories on the Etiology of Mesenteric Cysts

Name	Theory
Rokitansky	Degeneration of lymph nodes
Carson	Degeneration of lymph nodes
Hill	Congenital malformation of the lymphatic vessels
Godel	Neoplasia in the presence of lymph vessel hyperplasia
Handfield-Johes	Developmental anomalies
Arzella	Developmental anomalies
Lee	Traumatic origin
Ewing	Traumatic origin
Guthrie-Wakefield	Embryologic origin from true diverticula of the small intestine which grew into the mesentery and became pinched off
Gross-Ladd	"Misplaced bits of lymphatic tissue which proliferate and they accumulate fluid because they do not possess communications which allow them to drain properly into the remainder of the lymphatic system."
Beahrs et al.	"It is felt that chylous cysts do not have a common mode of origin but may come from several sources."

From Skandalakis JE. Mesenteric cyst: a report of three cases. J Med Assoc GA 1955;44(2).

complete historical account of classification by symptoms, see Table 4.8.

According to Skandalakis (61), the following sampling of terms have been mentioned in the literature to designate these cysts: *hematoma of the mesentery, lymphangioma, apoplexy of the mesentery, mesenteric enterocystoma, chylangioma of the mesentery,* and *hemorrhagic cyst of the mesentery.*

He also documents the advent of the term *mesenteric cyst.*

ETIOLOGY

Skandalakis (61) comments on the etiology of these cysts:

> Hadly, according to Beahrs et al. (64), believes that the only way to determine the nature of a cystic tumor is by a study of its life history, its location, the structure of its wall and the character of its content.
>
> But who can explain the case of Gerkin (75), who mentions "a chylous cyst of the mesentery that formed around a piece of gauze left at operation?"

See Tables 4.9 and 4.10 for further etiologic theories.

ANATOMY (Figure 4.17)

In his aforementioned collective review, Caropreso (73) presents the locations of mesenteric cysts (Table 4.11). Of the cases he collected, he also reports the clinical history (Table 4.12). Colodny (76) reported similar findings.

Mesenteric cysts with protein loss have been presented by Leonidas (77).

DIFFERENTIAL DIAGNOSIS

An abbreviated version of a table by Skandalakis (61) presents the difference between mesenteric and enteric cysts under gross and microscopic evaluation (Table 4.13).

Ultrasonography as a diagnostic modality was discussed by Haller et al. (78) and Mittelstaedt (79).

TREATMENT

The mode of treatment and results are discussed by Colodny in 1986. For a report of his results, see Tables 4.14, 4.15, 4.16.

CONGENITAL ANOMALIES OF THE LIGAMENTS

A complete discussion of all ligaments in the peritoneal area is not within the scope of this book. We present only the falciform and the broad ligaments; since anomalies of these ligaments are well known. Ligaments of the liver, urinary bladder, and uterus are discussed in the appropriate chapters.

Table 4.10.
Classifications of Mesenteric Cysts

Names	Year	Classification
Moynihan	1897	(1) Serous cysts (unilocular or multilocular); (2) chylous cysts (unilocular or multilocular); (3) hydatid cysts; (4) blood cysts; (5) dermoid cysts; (6) cystic malignant disease
Dowd	1900	(1) Embryonic; (2) hydatid; (3) cystic malignant disease
Nye-Wilkinson	1900	(1) Blood cysts; (2) dermoid cyst; (3) chyle cysts; (4) hydatid cysts; (5) cystic malignant diseases; (6) serous cysts
Niosi	1907	(1) Cysts of intestinal origin: (a) by sequestration from the bowel during development and (b) from Meckel's diverticulum; (2) dermoids; (3) cysts arising from retroperitoneal organs (germinal epithelium, ovary, wolffian body, müllerian duct).
Carter	1921	(1) True mesenteric cysts: (a) embryocystomata, (b) enterocystomata, and (c) obstructive, possible; (2) dermoids; (3) cystic malignant disease; (4) parasitic
Hueper	1926	(1) Cystic lymphangiomas (serous + chylous); (2) enterocystomas; (3) cysts being derived from the wolffian duct; (4) dermoid cysts; (5) teratomas; (6) fetal inclusions; (7) teratoid mixed tumors
Lahey-Ekerson	1934	(1) Wolffian; (2) lymphatic or chylous; (3) dermoid; (4) mesocolic; (5) parasitic and inflamatory; (6) traumatic hemorrhagic cysts
Roller	1935	
Peterson	1940	(A) Embryonic: (1) arising from embryonic remnants and sequestrated tissue (serous + chylous + sanguineous + dermoid), (2) intestinal origin (sequestration of the bowel and diverticula), (3) arising from urogenital organs (germinal epithelium + ovary + wolfian body + müllerian duct) (B) Pseudocysts: (1) infective origin (hydatid + degenerated tuberculus nodes), (2) cystic malignant diseases
Ewing	1940	True chylangiomata due to congenital or acquired obstruction of lacteals
Beahrs et al.	1950	(1) Embryonic and developmental; (2) traumatic or acquired cysts; (3) neoplastic cysts; (4) infective and degenerative cysts
Gross-Ladd	1953	(1) True mesenteric (lymphatic) cysts; (2) enteric cysts (duplications)
Frazier (modification of one used by Moynihan)		(1) Serous (lymphatic dilation or hemorrhages between the layers of mesentery); (2) chylous (dilation of some of the lacteals or chyliferous vessels or possibly to an effusion of chyle into preexisting cyst); (3) hydatid; (4) dermoid; (5) sanguinous

From Skandalakis JE. Mesenteric cyst: a report of three cases. J Med Assoc GA 1955;44(2).

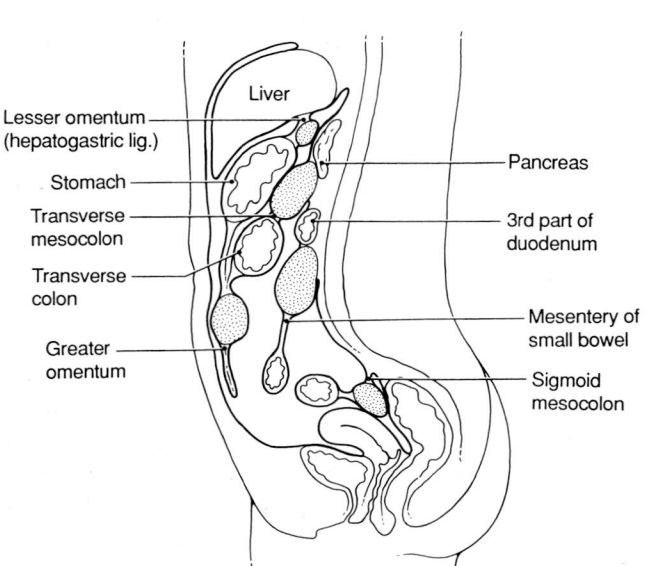

Figure 4.17. Topographical anatomy of location of omental and mesentery cysts.

Table 4.11.
Location of Cysts[a]

Location	N	%
Mesentery of small bowel	93	46.5
Mesentery of sigmoid	30	15.0
Mesocolon	22	11.0
Mesentery of cecum	16	8.0
Mesentery of descending colon	5	2.5
Mesentery of appendix	3	1.5
Omentum	4	2.0
Gastrohepatic mesentery	1	0.5
Duodenum	1	0.5
Retroperitoneum	10	5.0
Unknown	15	7.5

[a]From Caropreso P. Mesenteric cysts: a review. Arch Surg 1974;108:242–246.

Falciform Ligaments

We have seen only nontorsion hernias at the falciform ligament to the anterior abdominal wall with a defect permissive of interior hernia formation (34).

Broad Ligament

The broad ligament is the mesentery of the uterus, ovaries, and tubes that extends from the lateral pelvic wall to the lateral uterine side. It continues medially to envelope

Table 4.12.
History Obtained[a]

Symptom of Finding	N	%
Pain of some nature	58	81.5
Nausea and vomiting	32	45.0
Constipation	19	27.0
Diarrhea	4	5.5
Palpable mass	41	58.0

[a]From Caropreso P. Mesenteric cysts: a review. Arch Surg 1974;108:242–246.

Table 4.13.
Mesenteric and Enteric Cysts[a]

	Mesenteric	Enteric
Wall of cyst	Thin; "Rarely more than 1-2 mm; it consists of connective tissue"	
Serous coat		Yes
Muscle coat	No	Yes; 2 layers of smooth muscle
Mucous membrane	No; smooth inner surface	Yes
Blood supply	Between cyst and intestine "there is line of cleavage"	The same of the adjacent gut
Fluid	Serous or chylous	Clear or hemorrhagic or murky and sometimes succus entericus or fecal material
Size and shape	Orange or grapefruit	Vary tremendously in shape and vary greatly in size
Operation	(1) Resection and primary anastomosis; (2) marsupialization; (3) dissection	Resection and direct anastomosis or Mikulitz procedure
Symptoms	Enlarging abdomen; abdominal pains; intestinal obstruction	Obstruction; pain; necrosis, sloughing bleeding; hemorrhage

[a]From Skandalakis JE. Mesenteric cyst: a report of three cases. J Med Assoc Ga 1955;44(2):75–80.

Table 4.14.
Operative Treatment[a]

	Mesenteric (N = 28)	Omental (N = 14)
Excision	10	13
Partial excision	1	1
Intestinal resection	15	0
Reduction of volvulus	2	0

[a]From Colodny AH. Mesenteric and omental cysts. In: Welch KJ et al. eds. Pediatric surgery, Vol II. Chicago: Year Book Medical Publishers, 1986:924.

Table 4.15.
Postoperative Deaths and Complications[a,b]

Deaths (none since 1940)		
Intestinal infarction	2	
Peritonitis	1	
Complications		
Ileoileal intussusception	1	
Adhesive obstruction	2 (1 patient)	

[a]From Colodney AH. Mesenteric and omental cysts. In: Welch KJ et al., eds. Pediatric surgery, Vol II. Chicago: Year Book Medical Publishers, 1986.
[b]N = 42 patients.

Table 4.16.
Pathologic Findings[a]

Location	N	Serous	Chylous
Omentum	14	13	1
Mesentery			
Jejunal	11	5	6
Ileal	11	6	5
Colonic	6	6	0
TOTAL	42	30	12

[a]From Colodney AH. Mesenteric and omental cysts. In: Welch KJ et al., eds. Pediatric surgery, Vol II. Chicago: Year Book Medical Publishers, 1986.

Table 4.17.
The Five Paraduodenal Fossae[a]

Name	Direction of Hernia if Present	Relative Incidence (%)
Superior duodenal fossa of Treitz	Right	30-50
Paraduodenal fossa of Landzert	Left	2
Inferior duodenal fossa of Treitz	Right	50-75
Intermesocolic fossa of Bröesike	Right	Rare
Mesentericoparietal fossa of Waldeyer	Right	1

[a]From Skandalakis JE, et al. Hernia: Surgical anatomy and technique. New York: McGraw-Hill. 1989:283.

the uterus and inserts into the opposite pelvic wall. It is thin and practically avascular; a defect such as an internal hernia may be produced through it.

CONGENITAL ANOMALIES OF THE FOSSAE

Paraduodenal Fossae

In conjunction with the abdominal organs, the peritoneum lining of the abdominal cavity forms several spaces, folds, and fossae. Some are deep, some smaller, and some large or narrow, but all are located in the posterior abdominal wall in a very unpredictable way. Moynihan (80) described nine such fossae. We consider only five of these to be constant enough for study. Perhaps they have some clinical importance in the production of paraduodenal herniae (Table 4.17 and Fig. 4.18).

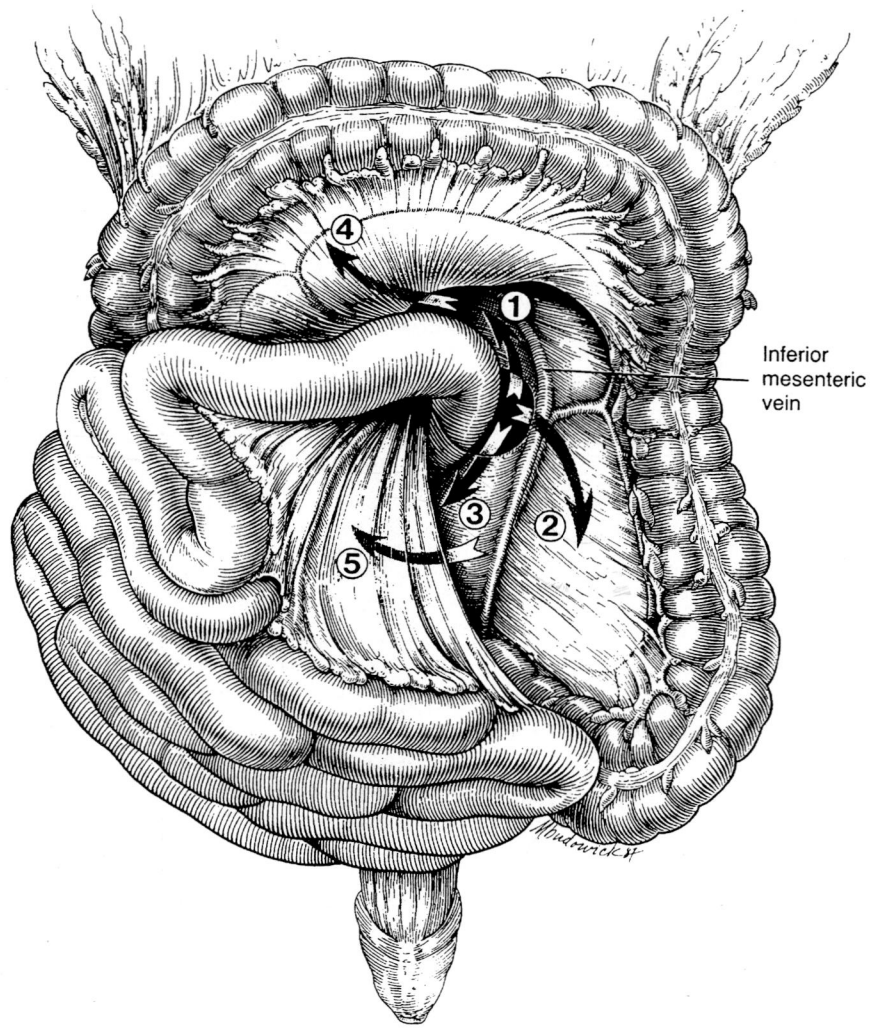

Inferior
mesenteric
vein

Figure 4.18. The five major paraduodenal fossae. The transverse colon has been reflected upward and the duodenum has been reflected to the right to reveal the paraduodenal fossae. (In Skandalakis JE et al. Hernia: surgical anatomy and technique. New York: McGraw-Hill, 1989:283.)

Each fossa has a typical location and is named by the original investigator. When an internal herniation takes place, the sac is directed to the left or to the right; therefore, we speak about right or left paraduodenal hernia.

For us, the battle of whether the fossae are acquired or congenital is over. We believe that the origin of these fossae is congenital with the protagonists being the peritoneum and the duodenojejular junction. On their way back to the abdomen, around the 10th week, the mesenteries of the ascending and descending colon fuse to the retroperitoneal space; perhaps paraduodenal fossae formed during this period. A congenital hernia may be produced when the fossae are formed; or an acquired hernia may take place later on.

It is extremely difficult to present the anatomic boundaries of these fossae. Size, length, depth, and direction play a great role in naming the anatomic entities related to each of the five fossae. Decker and Du Plessis (81) in the excellent book of McGregor, presented some anatomic boundaries.

The authors (83) will reproduce here a detailed anatomy of the right and left paraduodenal herniae since previous descriptions of boundaries are not consistent.

INCARCERATED RIGHT PARADUODENAL HERNIA

The mouth of the sac lies behind the superior mesenteric artery or the ileocolic artery at the base of the mesentery of the small intestine (mesentericoparietal fossa of Waldeyer) (Fig. 4.19). The mouth opens to the left. The sac is directed to the right and usually lies in the retroperitoneal space behind the right mesocolon or transverse mesocolon. The boundaries are thus: superior, the duodenum; anterior, the superior mesenteric artery or ileocolic artery; and posterior, the lumbar vertebrae.

To avoid vascular injury the incision must be in the lower part of the mouth. If vascular damage appears inevitable, the surgeon should open the mesentery and decompress the proximal intestinal loop before attempting reduction.

INCARCERATED LEFT PARADUODENAL HERNIA

The mouth of the sac usually lies behind the inferior mesenteric vein and the left colic artery, at the left of the fourth part of the duodenum, at the duodenojejunal flexure (Fig. 4.19). The mouth opens to the right. The sac is directed to the left and usually lies in the retroperitoneal space behind the left mesocolon. The boundaries are thus: superior, the duodenojejunal flexure or the beginning of the jejunum, pancreas, and renal vessels; anterior, the inferior mesenteric vein and left colic artery; right, the aorta; and left, the left kidney.

The incision should be made in the lower part of the mouth. McNair (83) advises division of the inferior mesenteric vein. A downward incision of the mouth avoids this sacrifice.

Skandalakis and his associates (82, 84–85) published several articles about paraduodenal hernia.

Cecal Fossae

Because the peritoneal folds and the prolongation of the left lower portion of the mesentery of the small bowel forming the mesoappendix, two fossae are observed: one above the ileum (the superior ileocecal fossa) and one below (the inferior ileocecal fossa).

The boundaries of the superior ileocecal fossa are thus: anterior, the ileocolic fold and ileocecal artery; pos-terior, the mesentery of terminal ileum and lateral right (ascending colon); and medial, below the terminal ileum.

The boundaries of the inferior ileocecal fossa are thus: anterior, the ileocecal fold; posterior, the mesoappendix; inferior, the median continuation of the ileocecal fold; and superior, the terminal ileum and mesentery.

Occasionally there is a third fossa, the retrocecal or subcecal, the boundaries of which depend on its depth and its medial and lateral expansion. It is located between the right colic gutter and the posterior surface of the cecum at the ileocecal fossa. With mobile cecum, the fossa does not exist. We have seen a herniation of the terminal ileum behind the cecum.

Intersigmoidal Fossa

At the level of the iliac crest, the descending colon becomes the sigmoid colon and acquires a mesentery. The attachment of the mesosigmoid to the body wall shows much variation (86). In most individuals, the attachment starts in the left iliac fossa and extends diagonally downward and to the right. In others, the attachment is sinuous, C, S, or inverted–U shaped. The average length of the attachment in 140 autopsies was 7.9 cm (87) (Fig. 4.20, *A*). The breadth of the mesentery was said to average 5.6 cm in 100 autopsies in New York to 15.2 cm in 40 autopsies in Iran. Whether this difference is racial or the result of diet is not clear. The left ureter passes through the base of the sigmoid mesocolon through the intersigmoid recess (Fig. 4.20, *B*).

The mouth of the fossa is directed downward and to the left, and the anatomic entities created are the left ureter and the exterior iliac vessels.

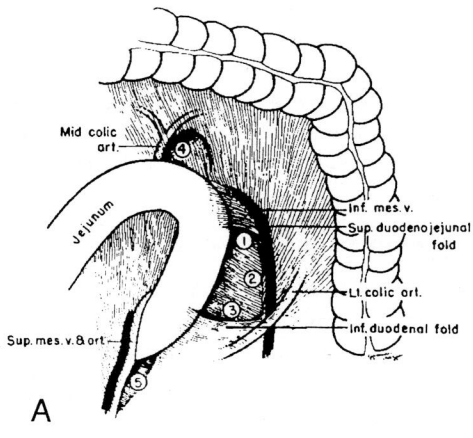

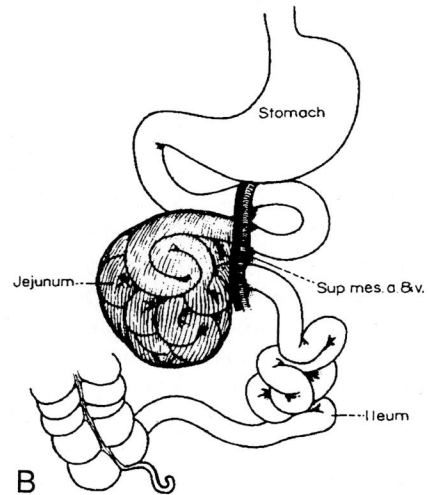

Figure 4.19. Paraduodenal herniae. **A**, The five most constant sites of paraduodenal herniae: *1, 3, 4,* and *5* are right paraduodenal hernias; *2* is a left paraduodenal hernia. The jejunum has been turned to the right. **B**, A right parad- uodenal hernia into the (mesentericoparietal) fossa of Waldeyer (site *5* in **A**). (**A** reproduced from Sims WG et al. Right paraduodenal hernia into the fossa of Waldeyer. J Med Assoc GA 1971;60:105–108. Used with permission.)

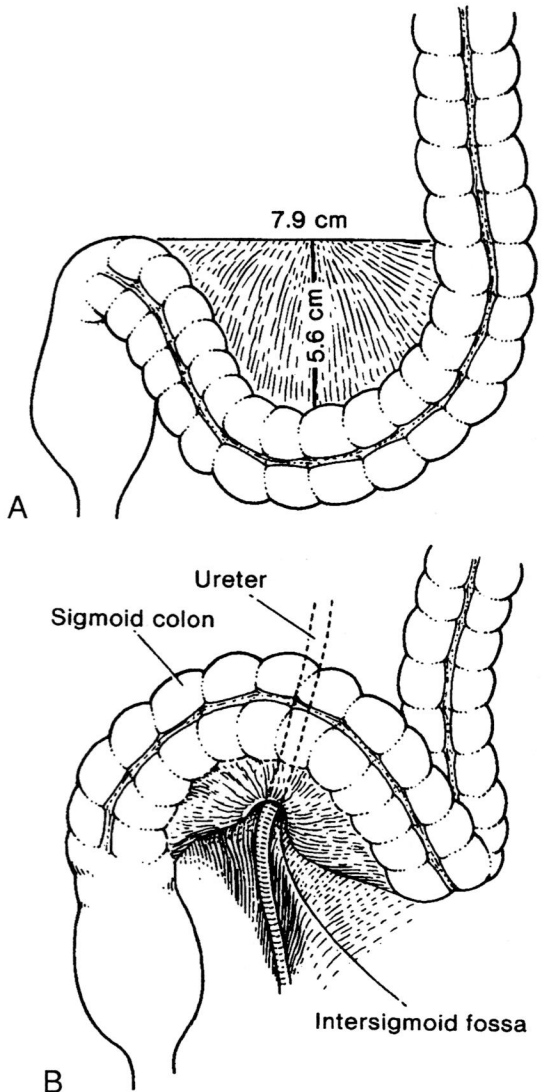

Figure 4.20. **A**, Average measurements of the sigmoid mesocolon. **B**, The relation of the base of the sigmoid mesocolon to the left ureter. (**A**, Data from Vaez-Zadeh K, Dutz W. Ileosigmoid knotting. Ann Surg 1970;172:1027.)

INTERNAL HERNIAE

Presenting a classification of congenital herniae is extremely difficult. They can be internal and external. Possible locations include the anterior or posterior abdominal wall and the respirator or pelvic diaphragm. In this chapter we present herniae related to the peritoneum only, and we describe others in appropriate chapters.

Etiology

Nonfusion of the mesentery and of right and left colon and duodenum produces fossae and pouches which,

depending on the diameter and depth of the defect, may produce spaces for an internal herniation. Obviously, malrotation as well as mesenteric fusion play great roles in the formation of herniae in the peritoneal cavity, there is another phenomenon at work: defective areas of herniation that vary in dimension from the size of a dime to several centimeters of the stoma (opening) as well as in depth. We have seen both: nonfixation of the mesentery with some malrotation of the intestine as well as folds, recesses, and fossae which are present without any other abnormality. Such fossae with good mesenteric fusion are the paraduodenal, the paracecal, and the intersigmoid.

The stoma and the depth produce a potential space for internal herniation. Some of them have a peritoneal sac; some do not. Therefore we have to consider fission and malrotation as the primary causes for the formation of an internal hernia and the deep peritoneal recesses with normal rotation and normal mesenteric fixation as the secondary cause.

Classification

Through peritoneal fossae or formina, there are five possible defects: epiploic foramen, paraduodenal, paracecal, intersigmoidal, and internal supravesical. Through peritoneal derivatives, there are mesenteric, omental, falciform, and broad ligament herniae.

Internal herniae may be asymptomatic or may produce chronic or acute intestinal obstruction with incarceration or strangulation and all their sequelae.

Diagnosis

The diagnosis of internal obstructions can be done easily with a physical examination and radiologic studies, and exploratory laparoscopy is performed as soon as the diagnosis is made—if, of course, the patient is willing to undergo the procedure.

To discuss extensively all these herniae would require an entire book, thus we briefly illustrate each of them without lengthy comments (Figs. 4.21 through 4.31).

Foramen of Winslow (Fig. 4.32)

This normal aperture is open and occasionally permits loops of small bowel to enter into the lesser sac and to produce a chronic, perhaps asymptomatic, internal hernia or an acute, incarcerated, or strangulated one.

The anatomic boundaries are thus: superior, the caudate process of the liver and the inferior layer of the right coronary ligament with rare extension to the left coronary ligament, if and only if such anomaly exists; inferior, the first part of the duodenum and the transverse part of

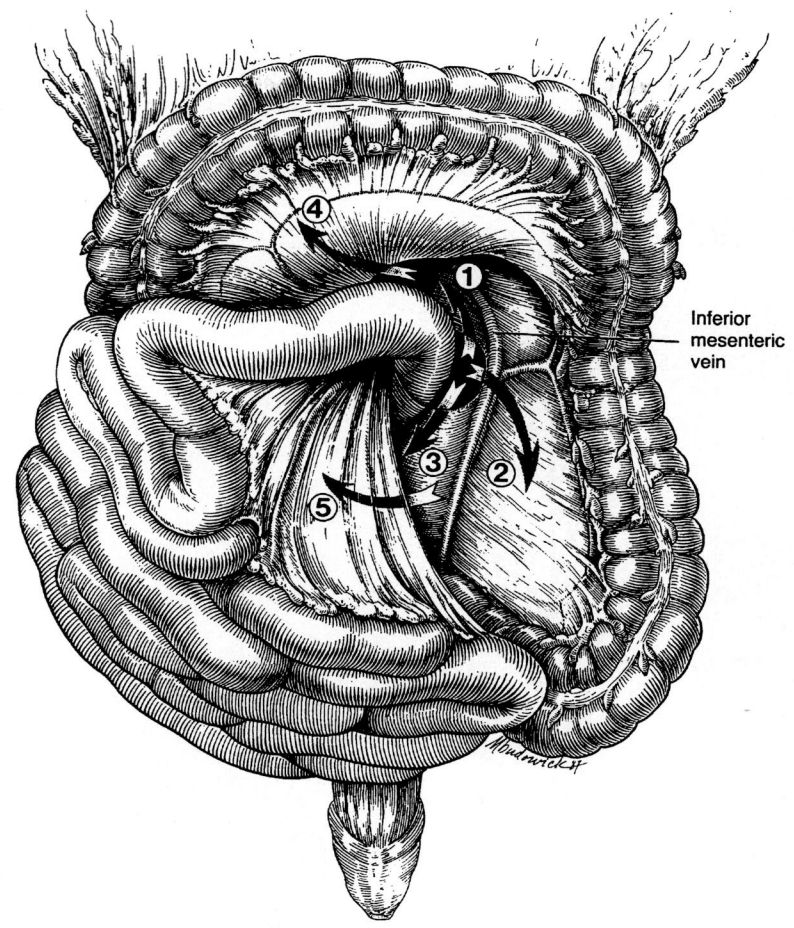

Inferior
mesenteric
vein

Figure 4.21. The paraduodenal hernia. (From Skandalakis JE et al. Hernia: surgical anatomy and technique. New York: McGraw-Hill, 1989:283–285.)

the hepatic artery; anterior, hepatoduodenal ligament and the hepatic triad (common bile duct, portal vein, and hepatic artery); and posterior, the inferior vena cava.

CONGENITAL INTERNAL HERNIAE THROUGH PERITONEAL DEFECTS

Classification

There are a number of intraperitoneal fossae and apertures through which peritoneal contents may protrude. These internal herniae account for less than 1% of intestinal obstructions; of these paraduodenal herniae account for more than 50% (88).

Anatomy

In 1899 Moynihan (80) described nine paraduodenal peritoneal pockets or fossae located near the fourth part of the duodenum. These fossae are inconstant, and any or none may be present in a given individual. Their significance lies in the fact that they are occasionally the sites of intestinal herniation, which may produce intestinal obstruction requiring surgical intervention. These are designated *right paraduodenal hernia,* if the herniated loops pass to the right, and *left paraduodenal hernia,* if they pass to the left, without reference to the midline of the body and regardless of the location of the fossa concerned.

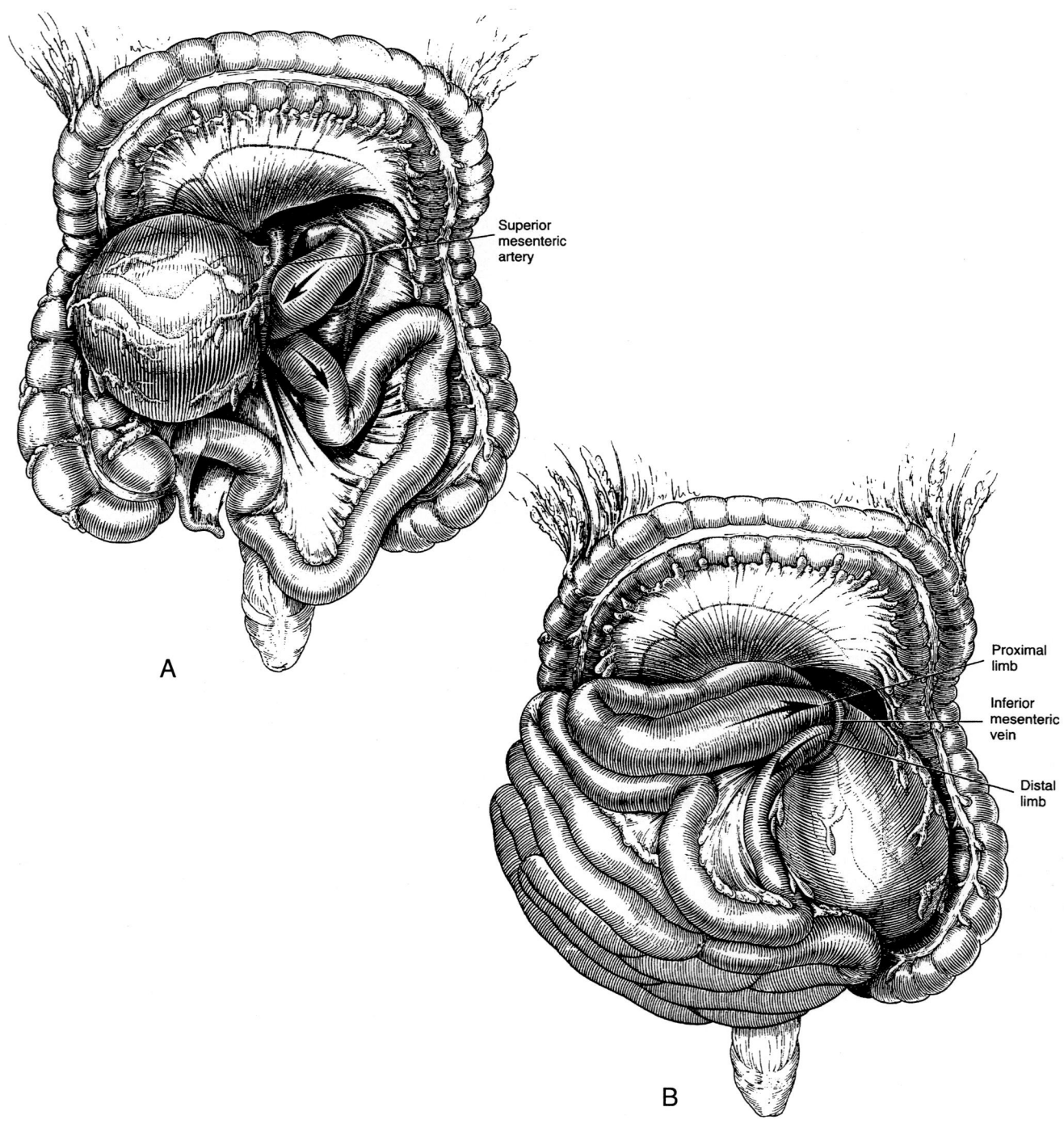

Figure 4.22. **A**, Right paraduodenal hernia. **B**, Left paraduodenal hernia. (From Skandalakis JE et al. Hernia: surgical anatomy and technique. New York: McGraw-Hill, 1989:286, 287.)

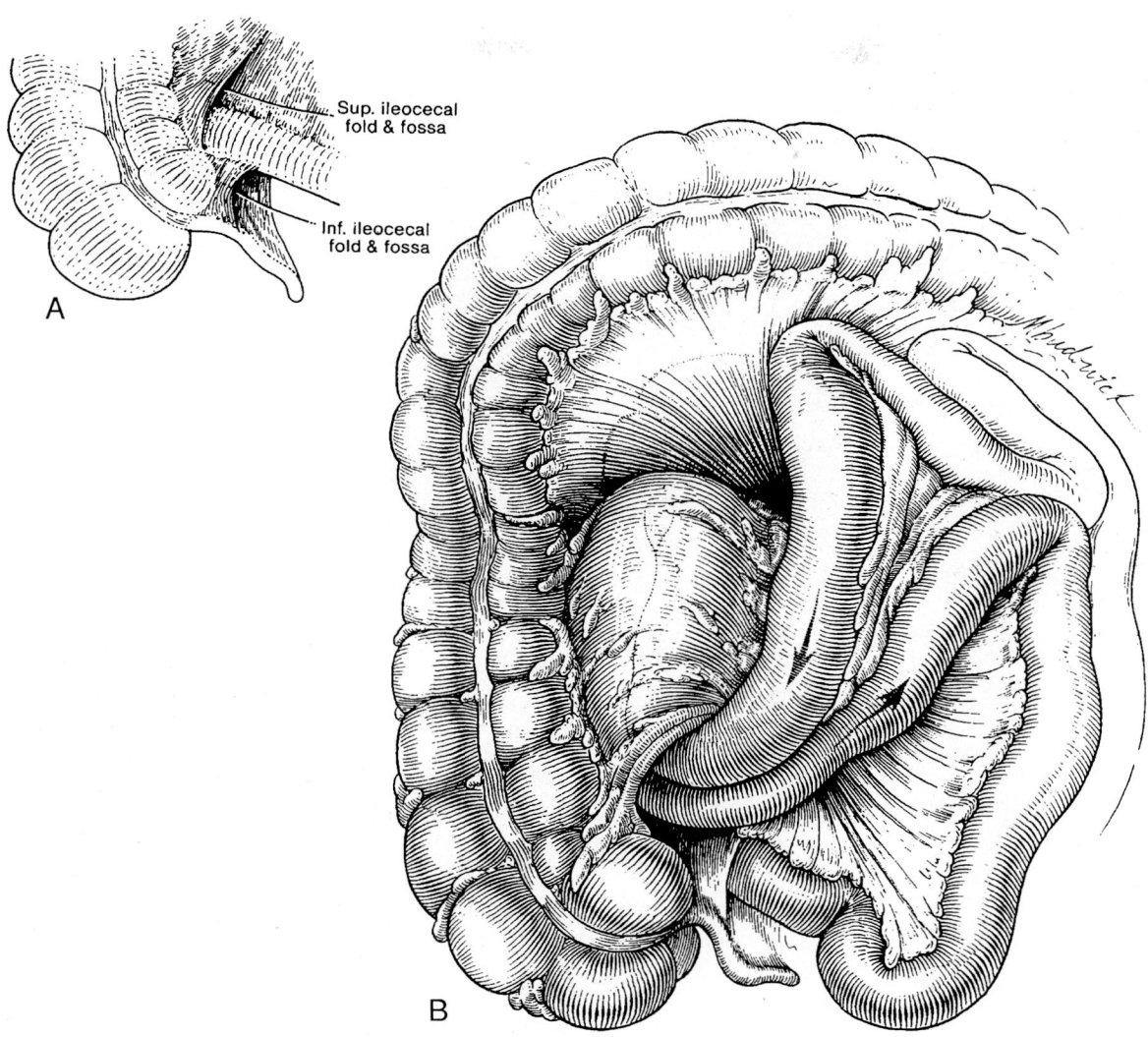

Figure 4.23. Ileocecal herniae (paracecal). **A**, Superior and inferior ileocecal folds forming paracecal fossa. **B**, The intestinal loop has been trapped by the right mesocolon during the fusion with the peritoneum of the body wall. (**A**, from Skandalakis JE, Gray SW, Rowe JS Jr. Anatomical complications in general surgery. New York: McGraw-Hill, 1983:225, **B**, from Skandalakis JE, Gray SW, Mansberger AR Jr, Colborn GL, Skandalakis LS, Hernia. New York: McGraw-Hill, 1989:288.)

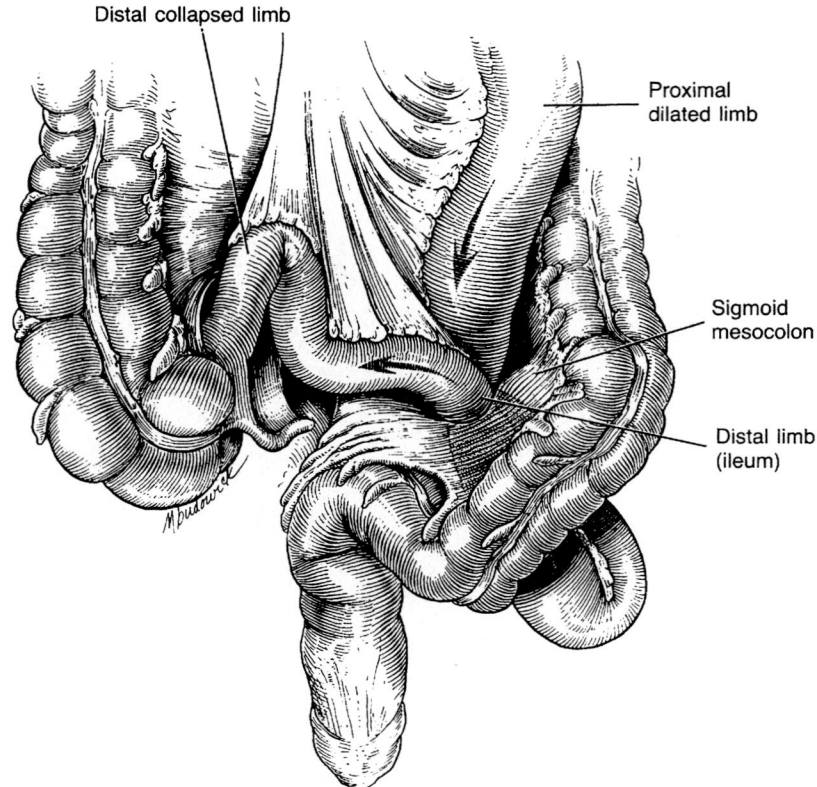

Figure 4.24. Intersigmoid fossa. Since the ring is located at the upper corner of the λ, the Greek letter "L," of the intersigmoidal fossa or at the sigmoid mesocolon, it is extremely difficult to name the boundary. There is no sac if the defect is in the mesentery, but if the hernia is intersigmoidal, there is a sac, and the sac may be traveling in different directions. (From Skandalakis JE et al. Hernia: surgical anatomy and technique. New York: McGraw-Hill, 1989:277.)

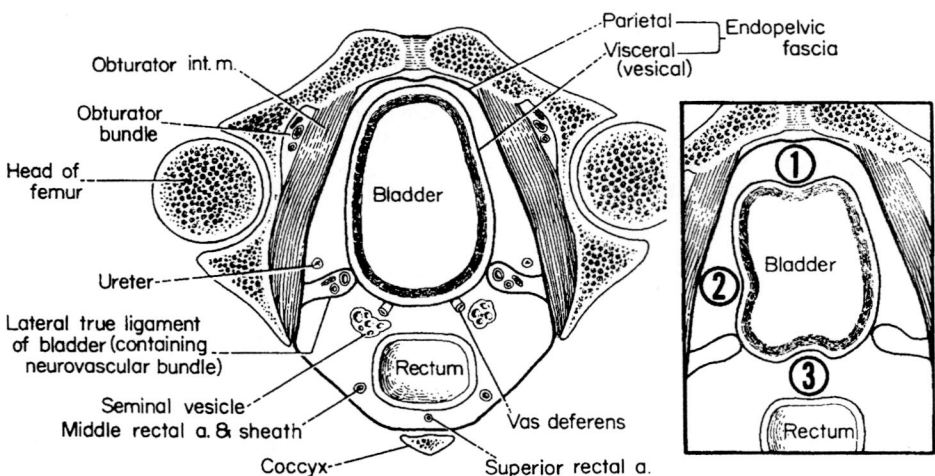

Figure 4.25. Internal supravesical hernia. Again, describing the boundaries is not the scope of this book, but the reader will appreciate the formation of this hernia by studying Figures 4.25 through 4.27. (From Skandalakis et al. Hernia: surgical anatomy and technique. New York: McGraw-Hill, 1989:296.)

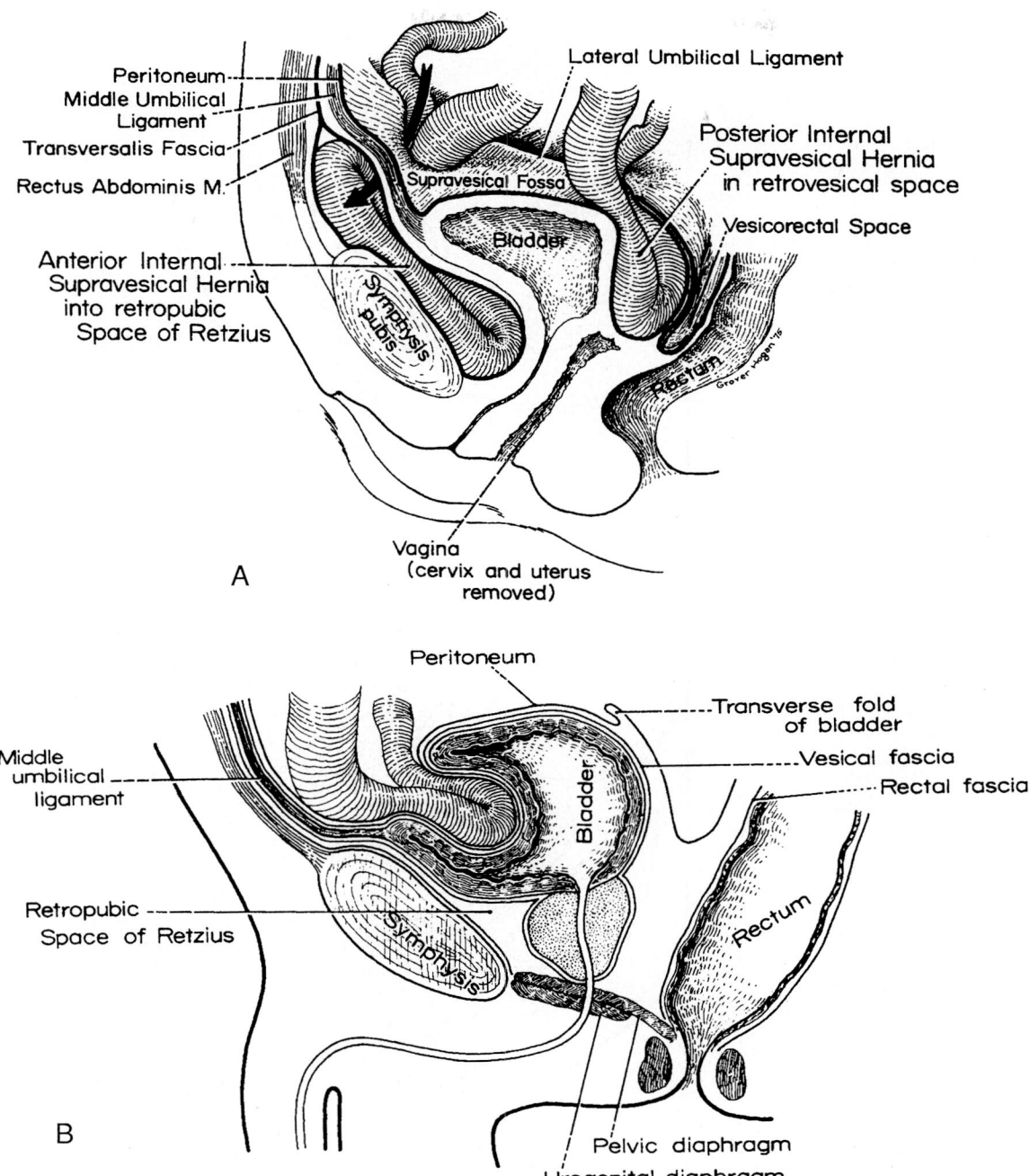

Figure 4.26. **A**, Comparison of anterior and posterior internal supravesical herniae. **B**, Invaginating type of anterior internal supravesical hernia. (From Skandalakis JE et al. Hernia: surgical anatomy and technique. New York: McGraw-Hill, 1989:297.)

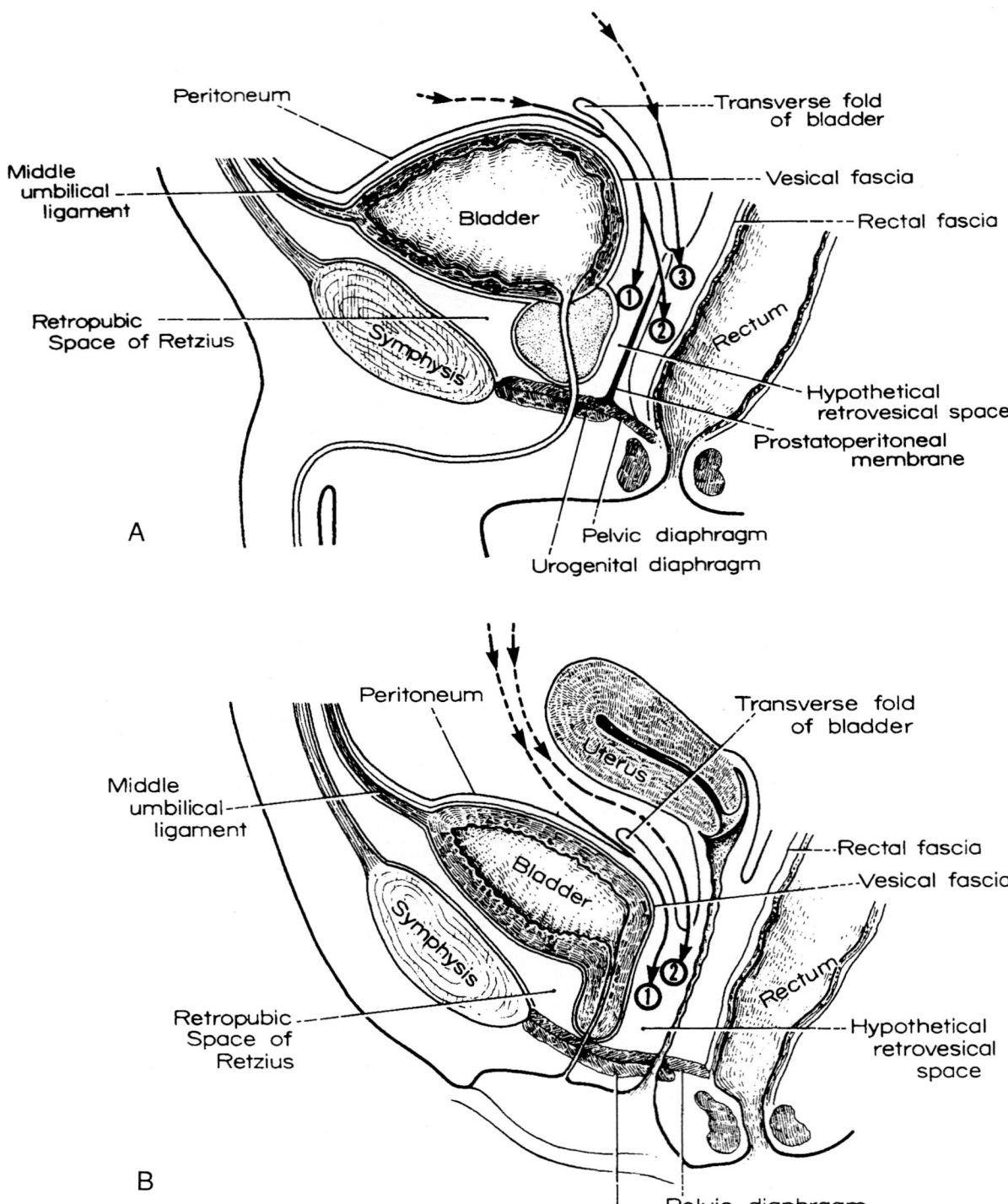

Figure 4.27.   Possible pathways of posterior internal supravesical herniae in **A**, the male, and **B**, the female. (From Skandalakis
JE et al. Hernia: surgical anatomy and technique. New York: McGraw-Hill, 1989:298.)

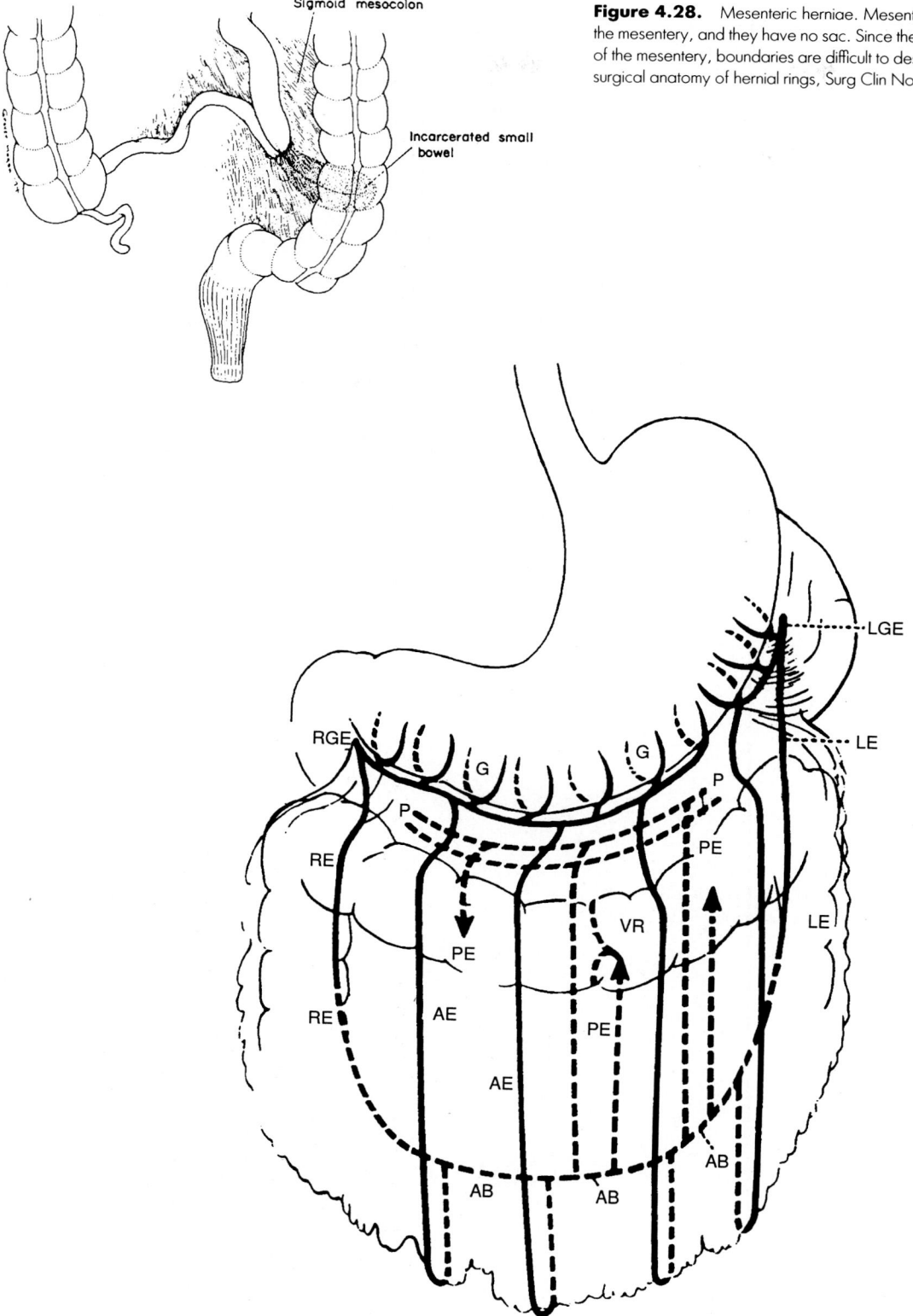

Figure 4.28. Mesenteric herniae. Mesenteric herniae can be in any part of the mesentery, and they have no sac. Since the defect can be located in any part of the mesentery, boundaries are difficult to describe. (From Skandalakis et al. The surgical anatomy of hernial rings, Surg Clin North Am 1974;54(6):1241.)

Figure 4.29. Omental hernia. Arterial supply to the greater omentum. *REG,* Right gastroepiploic a.; *LGE,* left gastroepiploic a.; *RE,* right epiploic a.; *LE,* left epiploic a.; *AB,* arc of Barkow; *G,* gastric branches; *AE,* anterior epiploic branches; *PE,* posterior epiploic branches; *P,* pancreatic a.; *VR,* vasa recta of mid-

colic a. Herniation can occur between any of these descending arteries. (From Griffith CA. Anatomy. In: Nyhus LM, Wastell C. eds. Surgery of the stomach and duodenum, 4th ed. Boston: Little, Brown, 1986.)

Figure 4.30. Falciform ligament herniae. This is not a fixation of the ligament in the anterior abdominal wall. We have seen two cases. (Skandalakis JE et al. Hernia surgical anatomy and technique. New York: McGraw-Hill, 1989:279.)

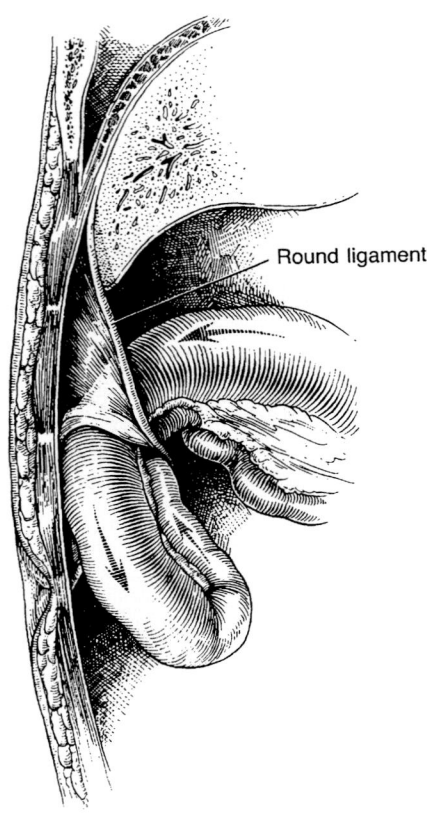

Round ligament

Figure 4.31. Broad ligament herniae. Herniae occur very rarely through the broad ligament, and loops of small bowel can pass through the defect anteriorly or posteriorly. They have no sac.

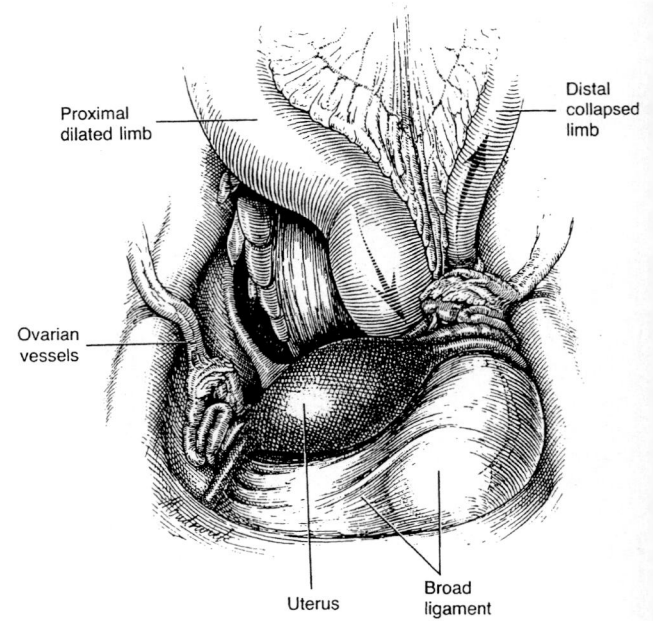

Proximal
dilated limb

Distal
collapsed
limb

Ovarian
vessels

Uterus

Broad
ligament

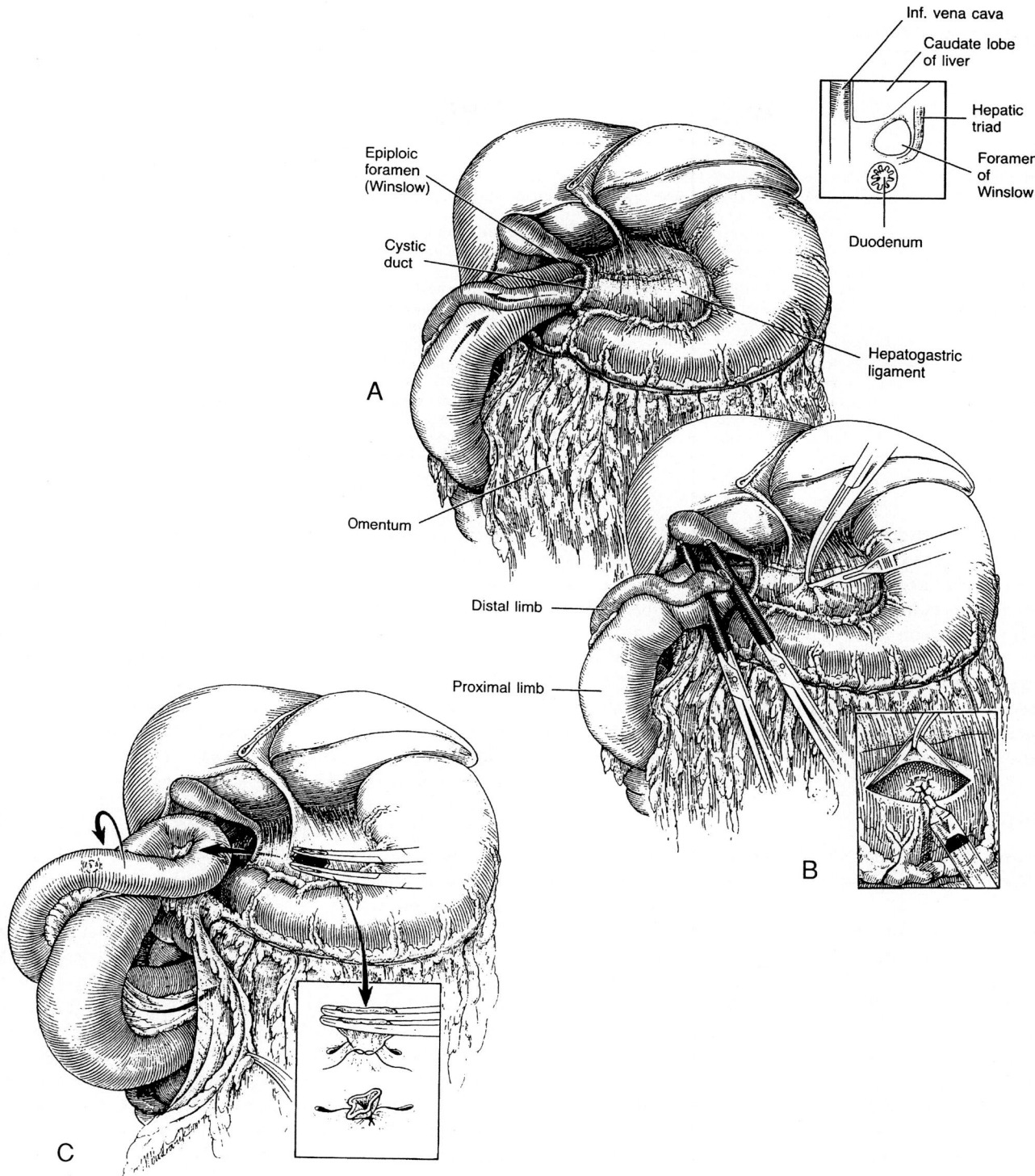

Figure 4.32. Epiploic foramen repair. **A,** A loop of small intestine has entered the epiploic foramen and is visible beneath the hepatogastric ligament containing the portal vein, hepatic artery, and common bile duct. The cystic duct forms the free edge of the hernial ring. Under no circumstance should the neck of the ring be incised. **B,** Step 1. Open the hepatogastric ligament and decompress the stran-gulated intestine. *Inset:* Close the aspiration site with a purse-string suture. **C,** Step 2. The herniated loop is released. *Inset,* close the defect in the hepatogastric lig-ament with 00 silk. (From Skandalakis JE et al. Hernia surgical anatomy and tech-nique, New York: McGraw-Hill, 1989:281–282.)

Table 4.18.
The Paraduodenal Fossae

Fossa and Eponym	Anatomic Boundaries	Incidence (%)	Surgical Significance
Superior fossa of Treitz	Behind the superior duodenal fold at the left of the fourth part of the duodenum; the cavity extends upward, approaching the pancreas	50	May contain a right paraduodenal hernia
Inferior fossa of Treitz	Behind the inferior duodenal fold at the left of the fourth part of the duodenum; a thumb-like cavity extending downward, parallel to the duodenum	75	May contain a right paraduodenal hernia
Mesentericoparietal fossa of Waldeyer	At the base of the mesentery of the first part of the jejunum, behind the superior mesenteric artery and below the duodenum; more common in fetuses than in adults	1 (Parsons, 1953)	May contain a right paraduodenal hernia
Intermesocolic fossa of Brösike	At the base of the transverse mesocolon which together with the pancreas forms the upper wall of the fossa; the lower wall is formed by the duodenojejunal junction and fourth part of the duodenum; the anterior wall is formed by a peritoneal fold between the transverse mesocolon and mesentery of the upper jejunum; the middle colic artery lies to the right of the orifice	Rare	May contain a right paraduodenal hernia
Paraduodenal fossa of Landzert	Under the fold, bridging the left end of the superior and inferior fossae (Treitz); the fold contains the inferior mesenteric vein and left colic artery; psoas muscle and hilum of left kidney lie posterior	2 (Parsons, 1953)	May contain a left paraduodenal hernia

The terminology and differentiation of these fossae are confusing. Several of those named by Moynihan seem to be merely variations of one another. We agree with Jones and his colleagues (89) that there are only five with which the surgeon need be concerned. These fossae and their boundaries are summarized in Table 4.18 and in Figures 4.33 through 4.37.

Because of the complex and often obscure anatomy of these rare herniae, some of them are discussed in a highly diagrammatic way.

Embryogenesis

The early writers, such as Moynihan (80), believed that the fossae were congenital and that the intestines herniated into them. Subsequent evidence indicates that the herniae as well as the fossae are of congenital origin. The congenital hernial sacs open at the sites of the fossae, but there is no evidence that a congenital fossa becomes a hernial sac later in life. A paraduodenal fossa is not the site of a potential acquired hernia, but instead marks the location where a congenital hernia might have occurred but failed to do so.

Both the ascending and descending limbs of the colon have mesenteries when the intestines return from the umbilical cord to the abdomen in the 10th week. These mesenteries subsequently come into contact with the posterior peritoneal wall and fuse with it, fixing the position of the colon by the fifth month. Internal herniae appear to be formed during this period of fixation of the ascending and descending mesocolon.

In the left paraduodenal hernia, the intestinal loop enters a pocket of the as yet unfused descending mesocolon, between its attachment and the inferior mesenteric vein. With subsequent fusion of the mesocolon, the pocket containing the intestinal loop, or sometimes the whole of the small intestine, becomes the hernial sac, the mouth of which lies at the site of the paraduodenal fossa of Landzert.

A right paraduodenal hernia represents a similar pocket formed in the same manner under the ascending mesocolon. The opening of the pocket may lie at the site of the mesentericoparietal fossa of Waldeyer, at the superior or inferior horns of the fossa of Treitz, or at the intermesocolic fossa of Brösike. This interpretation of events (events that have not been observed while they were occurring in the fetus) was developed by Andrews (90) and by Callander and his associates (91). It has been accepted, though not without reservation, by most subsequent writers.

Allen and his colleagues (92) suggested that the hernial sac is not formed by the mesocolon but represents the lining of the extraembryonic celom, which envelops the intestinal loops while they are in the umbilical cord and which entered the abdomen with them. This avascular celomic sac secondarily fused with the ascending or descending mesocolon to form a right or left paraduodenal hernia. In some cases such fusion does not take place and the anomalous sac remains more evident. This condition has been called *internal omphalocele*.

Incidence

Left paraduodenal herniae occur about three times more frequently than right ones, and both are more frequent in males than in females (93). Although they are congenital, they may manifest themselves by intestinal obstruction at any age, usually in adulthood.

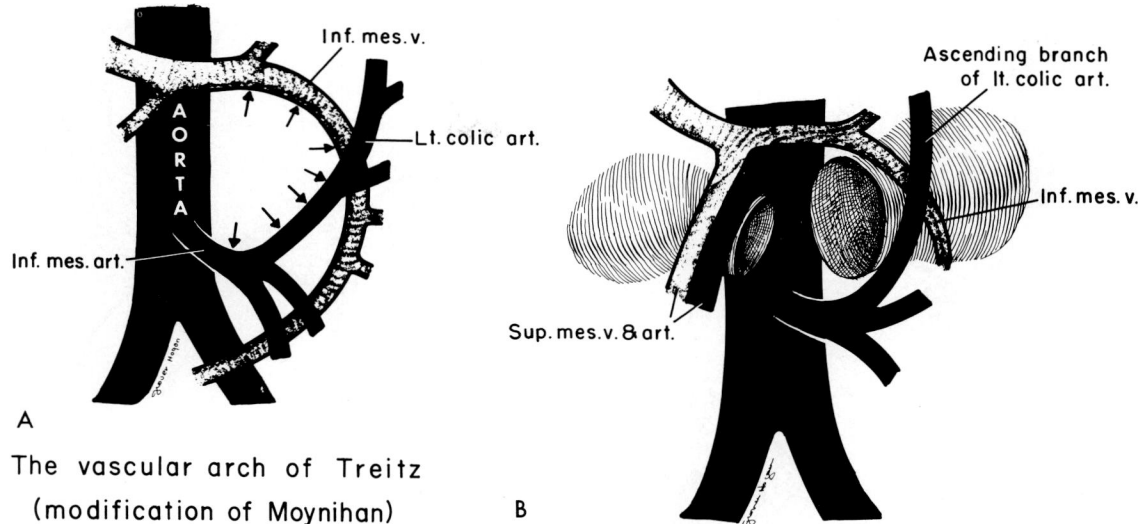

The vascular arch of Treitz (modification of Moynihan)

Figure 4.33. **A**, The vascular arch of Treitz. **B**, The relationship of the duodenum and upper jejunum to the surrounding blood vessels.

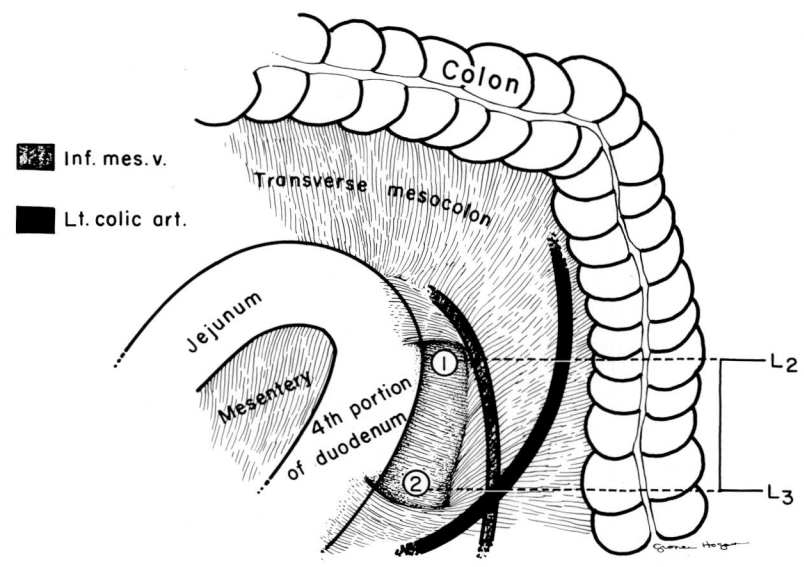

Fossa of Treitz

① Superior duodenal horn (50% present)
② Inferior duodenal horn (75% present)

Figure 4.34. The duodenal fossae of Treitz.

Symptoms

Signs and symptoms of hernia into a paraduodenal fossa are those of chronic or acute and partial or complete intestinal obstruction (nausea, vomiting, pain, distension, and dehydration). The obstruction may be high or low in the intestine. If strangulation occurs, the symptoms are even more marked.

Diagnosis

Diagnosis is based on the triad of (*a*) cramping abdominal pain, (*b*) vomiting, and (*c*) obstipation (neither feces nor gas pass).

Distension may be slight at first, with the first signs appearing in the upper abdomen. Visible peristaltic waves may be present. The pain is characteristically

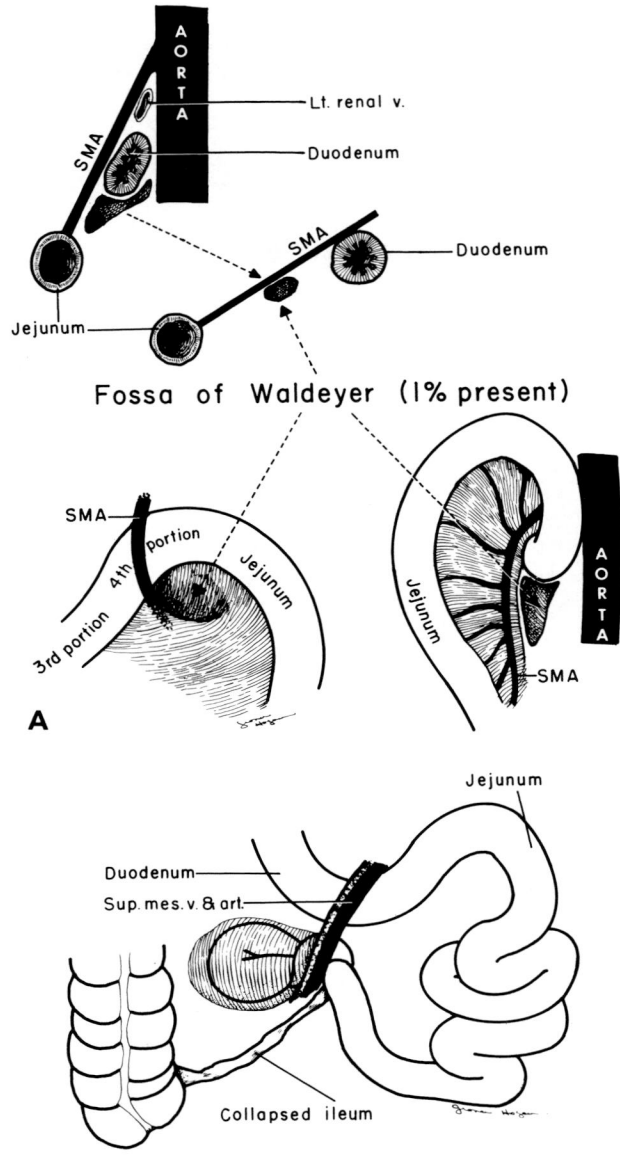

A

Fossa of Waldeyer (1% present)

B   Mesentericoparietal fossa (hernia)

Figure 4.35.   The fossa of Waldeyer: Relationships among the fossa, the superior mesenteric artery (SMA), the duodenum, and the jejunum.

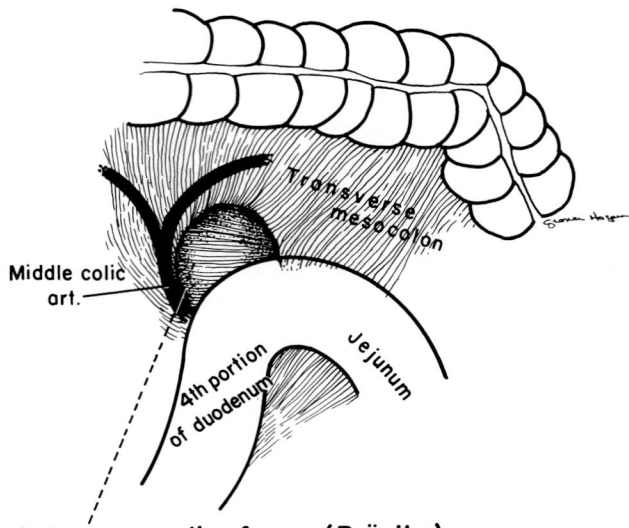

Intermesocolic fossa (Brösike)

Figure 4.36.   The intermesocolic fossa of Brösike. Relationships among the fossa, the middle colic artery, the duodenum, and the jejunum.

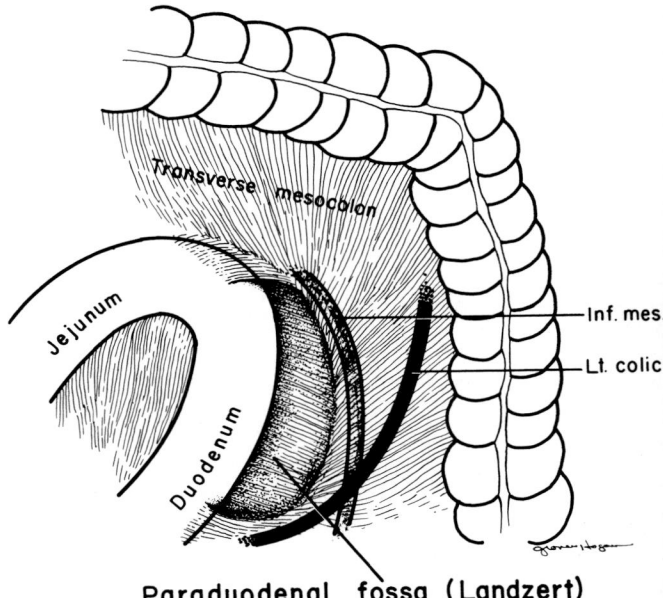

Paraduodenal fossa (Landzert)

Figure 4.37.   The paraduodenal fossa of Landzert. The jejunum has been turned to the right to show the relationships among the fossa, the blood vessels, and the duodenum.

located above the umbilicus and is worse after eating. Clinical or radiologic diagnosis of paraduodenal hernia as the cause of the obstruction must be made by exclusion of other more common causes.

The radiographic picture is not constant, but the following appearances have been described:

1. The intestines appear in a circumscribed mass as if in a bag; they cannot be displaced by manipulation nor by change in the patient's position. There is no small bowel in the pelvis.

2. Right paraduodenal hernia: No clear space can be seen between the stomach and intestinal mass. Left paraduodenal hernia: a clear space is seen between stomach and intestinal mass.

3. The ascending colon lies behind the intestinal mass in right paraduodenal hernia.

The first preoperative diagnosis was made in 1906 by Sherren (94).

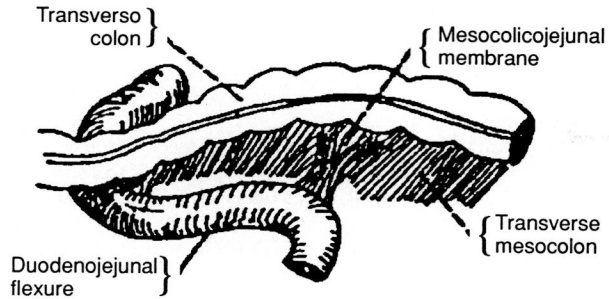

Figure 4.38. The mesocolicojejunal membrane. (From McGregor AL, DuPlessis DJ, eds. A synopsis of surgical anatomy. Baltimore: Williams & Wilkins, 1969:78.)

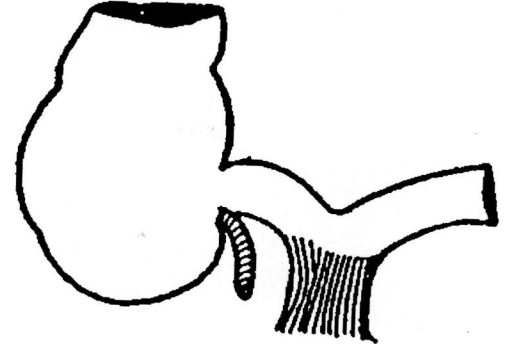

Figure 4.39. The ileal band. (From McGregor AL, DuPlessis DJ, eds. A synopsis of surgical anatomy. Baltimore: Williams & Wilkins, 1969:77.)

Treatment and Mortality

Surgery is necessary as soon as dehydration is corrected and urinary function returns. The procedure consists of reduction of the hernia and closure of the defect. The following rules should be kept in mind:

1. A paraduodenal hernia found incidentally on exploration for another cause should be left alone.
2. Any attempt to transect the mouth of the sac risks possible injury to large blood vessels.
3. The decision of whether resection is necessary must be based on the apparent viability of the herniated loop of the intestine.

The first successful operation was performed in 1898 by Neumann. Mortality is still high, but it has dropped below 20%. Nathan (95) reported only one death among thirteen operations. No recurrences of paraduodenal herniae have been reported (89).

ANOMALIES, VARIATIONS, PECULIARITIES, CURIOSITIES, AND RARITIES OF PERITONEAL FOLDS

Variations can be found in the gallbladder area at the duodenojejunal flexure, ascending and descending colon, sigmoid colon, spleen, terminal ileum, and perhaps in other areas of the peritoneal cavity.

Occasionally in the operating and the dissecting rooms, we have seen several inconstant or anomalous peritoneal folds related to the lesser omentum. In order of frequency, they run from the gallbladder to the duodenum; from the gallbladder to the hepatic flexure, or distal to it; or from the gallbladder to the stomach (Fig. 4.4).

If there is any relation between these folds and the corresponding fistulae tracts in gallstone ileus, they predispose to fistulae.

Occasionally, a fold connects the undersurface of the transverse mesocolon to the antimesenteric border of the proximal part of the jejunum (Fig. 4.38).

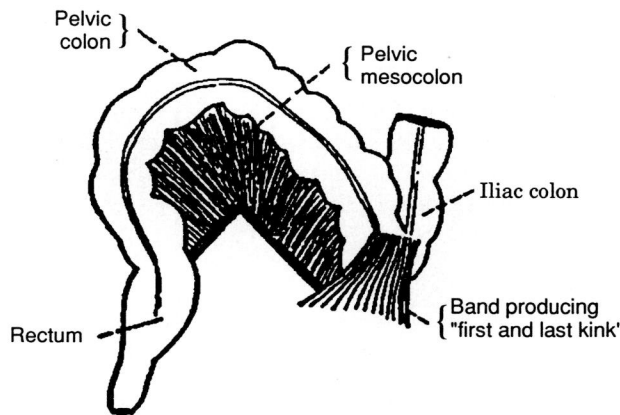

Figure 4.40. Showing Lane's "first and last kink" and the method of its production. (From McGregor AL, DuPlessis DJ, eds. A synopsis of surgical anatomy. Baltimore: Williams & Wilkins, 1969:78.)

Gray (96) mentions a band at the level of the iliac crest connecting the lateral abdominal wall to the ascending colon (sustentaculum hepatis).

Several folds or bands are reported in the literature as follows:

1. Folds also may connect the ascending colon to the right lateral paracolic gutter, forming several small fossae.
2. A fibrous band may connect the proximal and distal ends of the sigmoid colon.
3. A band extending from the terminal ileus to the posterior abdominal wall has been observed. (Fig. 4.39).
4. A band extending from the proximal sigmoid colon to the posterior abdominal wall also occasionally is present.
5. The genitomesenteric fold of Douglas Reid extends from the terminal mesenteries of the small bowel on the right to the junction of the second to third part of the duodenum by way of the suspensory ligament of ovary or testis as well as of the appendix.
6. A band may be observed from the pelvic colon to the pelvic brim (mesosigmoid membrane) (Fig. 4.40).

The membrane of Jackson is a peculiar thin network of tissue extending from the right colon to the posterior

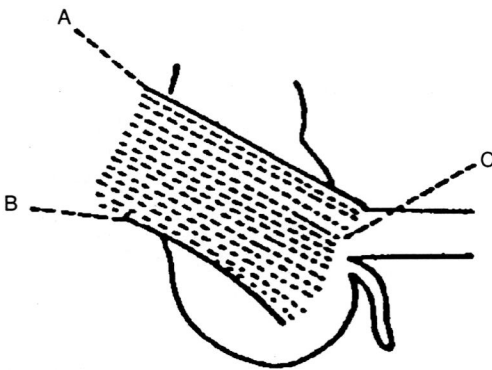

Figure 4.41. *Jackson's membrane. The membrane lies between the thick lines A and B. The lines between (C) represent the parallel, fine blood vessels so characteristic of this membrane. (From McGregor AL, DuPlessis DJ, eds. A synopsis of surgical anatomy. Baltimore: Williams & Wilkins, 1969:91.)*

abdominal wall (Fig. 4.41). Sometimes it extends upward, reaching the hepatic flexure, sometimes it extends downward, medially, covering the cecum and ileocecal valve. It is rich with blood vessels; therefore electrocoagulation or ligation should be used.

REFERENCES

1. Ebers GE. The Ebers papyrus (1500 BC).
2. Douglas J. Description of the peritoneum, and of that part of the membrana cellularis which lies on its outside: with an account of the true situation of all abdominal viscera, in respect of these two membranes. London: J Roberts, 1730.
3. Jones FW, ed. Buchanan's manual of anatomy, 8th ed. Baltimore: Williams & Wilkins, 1953.
4. Silva YJ. In vivo use of human umbilical vessels and the ductus venosus Arantii. Surg Gynecol Obstet 1979;148:595.
5. Michels NA. Blood supply and anatomy of the upper abdominal organs. Philadelphia: JB Lippincott, 1955.
6. Gray SW, Rowe JS, Jr, Skandalakis JE. Surgical anatomy of the gastroesophageal junction. Am Surg 1979;45:575.
7. Livingstone EM. A clinical study of the peritoneum. New York: Hoeber, 1933.
8. Ochsner A, Graves AM. Subphrenic abscess: an analysis of 3,372 collected and personal cases. Ann Surg 1933;98:961.
9. Mitchell GAG. The spread of acute intraperitoneal effusions. Br J Surg 1940;28:291.
10. Autio V. The spread of intraperitoneal infection. Acta Chir Scand 1964;321:5.
11. Boyd DP. The subphrenic spaces and the emperor's new robes. N Engl J Med 1966;275:911.
12. Meyers MA. Dynamic radiology of the abdomen: normal and pathologic anatomy. New York: Springer-Verlag, 1976.
13. Harley HRS. Subphrenic abscess. In: Maingot R, ed. Abdominal operations, 7th ed. New York; Appleton-Century-Crofts, 1980.
14. Whalen JP. Radiology of the abdomen: anatomic basis. Philadelphia: Lea & Febiger, 1976.
15. Alday ES, Goldsmith HD. Surgical technique for omental lengthening based on arterial anatomy. Surg Gynecol Obstet 1972;135:103.
16. Ansom BJ, Lyman RY, Lander HH. The abdominal viscera in situ: a study of 125 consecutive cadavers. Anat Rec 1936;67:17.
17. Swaen A. Recherches sur le développement du foie, du tube diges-tif, du péritoine et du mésentère. J Anat (Paris) 1897;33:32–99, 222–258, 523–585.
18. Broman I. Warum wird die Entwicklung der bursa omentalis in Lehrbüchern fort während unrichtig beschrieben? Anat Anz 1938;86:195–204.
19. Liebermann-Meffert D, White H. Development and appearance. In: Liebermann-Meffert D, White H, eds. The greater omentum: anatomy, physiology, pathology, surgery with an historical survey. New York: Springer-Verlag, 1983:13.
20. Krutsiak VN, Voitiv II. Spatial organization of the lesser peritoneal sac during the early stages of human ontogeny. Arkh Anat Gistol Embriol, 1984;87(12):46–54.
21. Kimura A et al. Sympus monopus accompanied by nephroblastoma: a case report. Acta Pathol Jpn 1975;25(3):375–84.
22. Waldschmidt J. Pathological conditions, specific investigations, and therapy. In: Liebermann-Meffert D, White H, eds. The greater omentum. New York: Springer-Verlag, 1983:111–118.
23. Broman I. Anatomie des Bauchfells. In: Von Bardeleben E, ed. Handbuch der Anatomie des Menschen, Vol 6/3. Jena, Germany: Fischer, 1914:76–112.
24. Otto HF, Wanke M, Zeitlhofer J. Darm und peritoneum. In: Dorr W, Weifert G, Uehlinger E, eds. Spezielle pathologische Anatomie, Vol 2, Part 2. New York: Springer-Verlag, 1976.
25. Maegraith B. Pathological processes in malaria. Trans R Soc Trop Med Hyg 1948;41:687–699.
26. Kiuchi M, Kawachi Y, Kimura Y. Sudden infant death due to asplenia syndrome. Am J Forensic Med Pathol 1988;9:102–104.
27. Aschwanden M, Schmid P. Ruptured aneurysm of the greater omentum in fibromuscular dysplasia. Vasa 1989;18(2):157–161.
28. Ballow M, Park BH, Dupont B. Benign giant lymphoid hyperplasia of the mediastinum with associated abnormalities of the immune system. J Pediatr 1974;84:418.
29. Keller AR, Hochholzer L, Castleman B. Hyaline-vascular and plasma-cell types of giant lymph node hyperplasia of the mediastinum and other locations. Cancer 1972;29:670.
30. McGregor AL, DuPlessis DJ. A synopsis of surgical anatomy. Baltimore: Williams & Wilkins, 1969:78.
31. Jackson JN. Membranous pericolitis and allied conditions of the ileocaecal region. Ann Surg 1913;57:374–401.
32. Nicole R. Das Coecum-mobile-Syndrom. Praxis 1967;1:869–872.
33. Skandalakis JE. Contribution to the study of the pathology and treatment of volvulus of the cecum [Thesis]. Atlanta, Georgia: Emory University, 1949.
34. Skandalakis JE, Gray SW, Mansburger AR, Colborn GL, Skandalakis LJ. Hernia: surgical anatomy and technique. New York: McGraw Hill, 1989:274.
35. White H, Waldschmidt. Hernias. In: Liebermann-Meffert D, White H, eds. The greater omentum. New York: Springer-Verlag, 1983:120.
36. Leissner KH. Transomental strangulation: a rare case of an internal hernia. Acta Chir Scand 1976;142(6):483–485.
37. Ellis H. The peritoneum. In: Goldsmith HD, Byrne JJ, eds. General surgery, 3rd ed. Thomaston, CT: Practice of Surgery Ltd, 1987:1–39.
38. Wrzesinski JT, Firestone SD, Walske BR. Primary idiopathic segmental infarction of the omentum: a report of two cases. Surgery 1956;39:663–668.
39. Presidente PJ, McCraw BM, Lumsden JH. Experimentally induced *Fasciola hepatica* infection in white-tailed deer. II. Pathological features. Can J Comp Med 1975;39(2):166–177.
40. Skandalakis JE. Idiopathic hemorrhagic infarction of the greater omentum (trans). Surg Rev (Greece) 1954;15:2–7.
41. Singhabhandhu B, Ritz C, Gray SW, Vohman MO, Skandalakis JE. Lesions of the omentum. J Med Assoc Ga 1972;61:9–13.
42. Oberst M. Zur Kasuistik des Bruchschnittes nebst einigen Bemer-

kungen uber Netzeinklemmungen. Zentralbl Chir 1882;9:441–447.

43. Nikolaeva TN, Spivak EM, Spivak LA. Pathology of microhemocirculatory vessels in congenital heart defects with left-to-right shunt. Arkh Pathol 1986;48(6):8–14.

44. Gloor F, Torhorst J. Pathological conditions, specific investigations, and therapy: diseases of the omentum—tumors. In: Liebermann-Meffert D, White H, eds. The greater omentum. New York: Springer-Verlag, 1983.

45. Martischnig E, Mair M. Ein beitrag zum lymphangioma cysticum. Wien Klin Wochenschr 1969;81:938–940.

46. Nafissi A, Vakili K. Lymphangiome kystigque du grand epiploon. Chirurgie 1976;102:198–200.

47. Vaittinen E. Lymphangiomatous omental cyst. Acta Chir Scand 1974;140:429.

48. Walker AR, Putnam TC. Omental, mesenteric, and retroperitoneal cysts: a clinical study of 33 new cases. Ann Surg 1973;178:13–19.

49. Walsh DB, Williams G. Surgical biopsy studies of omental and peritoneal nodules. Br J Surg 1971;58:428–433.

50. Spurney RF, McCormack KM. Immature omental teratoma. Arch Pathol Lab Med 1987;3:762–764.

51. Boehner JF et al. Solid ovarian teratoma with neurological metastases to periaortic lymph nodes and omentum. South Med J 1987;5:649–652.

52. Liebermann-Meffert D, Gloor F. Pathological conditions, specific investigations, and therapy: tissue deposits. In: Liebermann-Meffert D, White H, eds. The greater omentum. New York: Springer-Verlag, 1983.

53. Haider R et al. Congenital pericardio-peritoneal communication with herniation of omentum into the pericardium: a rare cause of cardiomegaly. Br Heart J 1973;35(9):981–984.

54. Hodach RJ et al. Studies of malformation syndromes in man. XXXVI: the Pfeiffer syndrome, association with kleeblattschadel and multiple visceral anomalies, Z Kinderheilkd 1975;119(2):87–103.

55. Weitzman JJ, Vanderhoof RS. Jejunal atresia with agenesis of the dorsal mesentery with "Christmas tree" deformity of the small intestine. Am J Surg 1966;111:443.

56. Zerella JT, Martin LW. Jejunal atresia with absent mesentery and a helical ileum. Surgery 1976;80:550.

57. Zwiren GT, Andrews HG, Ahmann P. Jejunal atresia with agenesis of the dorsal mesentery ("apple-peel small bowel"). J Pediatr Surg 1972;7:414.

58. Blythe H, Dickson JHS. Apple-peel syndrome (congenital intestinal atresia): a family study of 7 index patients. J Med Genet 1969;6:275.

59. Mishalang HG, Najjar F. Familial jejunal atresia: three cases in one family. J Pediatr Surg 1968;73:753.

60. Zerella JZ, Martin LW. Jejunal atresia with absent mesentery and a helical ileum. Surgery 1976;80:550.

61. Skandalakis JE. Mesenteric cyst: a report of three cases. J Med Assoc Ga 1955;44(2):75–80.

62. Oberhelman HA, Condon JB. Hemorrhagic cyst of the mesentery of the ileum. Arch of Surg 1948;57:301–306.

63. Slocum MA. Surgical treatment of chylous mesenteric cysts by marsupialization. Am J Surg 1938;41:464–473.

64. Beahrs OH, Judd ES Jr, Dockerty MB. Chylous cysts of the abdomen. Surg Clin North Am 1950;Aug:1081–1096.

65. Dowd CN. Mesenteric cysts. Ann Surg 1900;32:515.

66. Nye GC, Wilkinson AI. Mesenteric cysts. Ann Surg 1911;54:115.

67. Carter RM. Cysts of the mesentery. Surg Gynecol Obstet 1921;33:544.

68. Hueper WC. Mesenteric enterocystoma. J Lab Clin Med 1926;12:427.

69. Lahey FH, Eckerson EB. Retroperitoneal cysts. Ann Surg 1934;100:231.

70. Roller CS. Mesenteric cysts. Surg Gynecol Obstet 1935;60:1128.

71. Peterson EW. Mesenteric and omental cysts. Ann Surg 1932;96:340; and Cysts of mesentery. Ann Surg 1940;112:80–86.

72. Vaughn AM, Lees WM, Henry JW. Mesenteric cysts. Surgery 1948;23:306.

73. Caropreso P. Mesenteric cysts a review. Arch Surg 1974;108:242–246.

74. Ford JR. Mesenteric cyst: review of the literature with a report of an unusual case. Am J Surg 1960;99:878–883.

75. Thorek M. Surgical efforts and safeguards. Philadelphia: JB Lippincott, 1943:76.

76. Colodny AH. Mesenteric and omental cysts. In: Welch KJ et al., eds. Pediatric surgery, Vol 2. Chicago: Year Book Medical Publishers, 1986.

77. Leonidas JC et al. Mesenteric cyst associated with protein loss in the gastrointestinal tract. AJR 1971;112:150.

78. Haller JA et al. Sonographic evaluation of mesenteric and omental masses in children. AJR 1978;130:269.

79. Mittelstaedt C. Ultrasonic diagnosis of omental cysts. Radiology 1975;117:673.

80. Moynihan BGA. Retro-peritoneal hernia. London: Bailliere, 1889.

81. Decker GAG, Du Plessis DJ (eds). Lee McGregor's synopsis of surgical anatomy, 12th ed. Bristol: Bath Press, 1986.

82. Skandalakis JE, Gray SW, Harlaftis M, Collier HS. Hernia into the fossa of Waldeyer: three cases of right paraduodenal hernia with emphasis on surgical anatomy. In: Pontidas EJ, ed. In honour of Thomas Doxiadis. Athens, Greece: Hospital Evangelismos, 1976.

83. McNair TJ. Hamilton Bailey's emergency surgery, 2nd ed. Baltimore, Williams & Wilkins, 1972.

84. Sims WG, Skandalakis JE, Gray SW. Right paraduodenal hernia into the fossa of Waldeyer. J Med Assoc GA 1971;60(4):105–108.

85. Gray SW, Skandalakis JE. Paraduodenal hernia. Contemp Surg 1978;12:26–39.

86. Anson BJ. An atlas of human anatomy, 2nd ed. Philadelphia: WB Saunders, 1963.

87. Vaez-Zadeh K, Dutz W. Ileosigmoid knotting. Ann Surg 1970;172:1027.

88. Sawyer KC. Acute intestinal obstruction. Rocky Mount Med J 1953;50:639–645.

89. Jones TW, Nyhees LM, Harkins HN. Hernia. Philadelphia: JB Lippincott, 1964.

90. Andrews E. Duodenal hernia: a misnomer. Surg Gynecol Obstet 1923;37:740–750.

91. Callander CL, Reesk GY, Nemir A. Mechanism, symptoms, and treatment of hernia into the descending mesocolon (left duodenal hernia): a plea for a change in nomenclature. Surg Gynecol Obstet 1935;60:1052–1071.

92. Laslie M, Durden C, Allen L. Concealed umbilical hernia: Papez's concept of so-called paraduodenal hernia. Anat Rec 1966;155:145–150.

93. Hansmann GH, Morton SA. Intra-abdominal hernia: report of a case and review of the literature. Arch Surg 1939;39:973–986.

94. Sherren J. A case of strangulate left duodenal hernia. Trans Clin Soc Lond 1906;39:98–99.

95. Nathan H. Internal hernia. J Int Coll Surg 1960;34:563–572.

96. Warwick R, Williams PL, eds. Gray's anatomy, 35th ed. (British). Philadelphia: WB Saunders, 1973.

CHAPTER 5

THE STOMACH

John Elias Skandalakis / Stephen Wood Gray / Richard Ricketts

It must occur to everyone who becomes acquainted for the first time with our
investigations upon the secretion of gastric juice,
that while the main stomach during digestion is filled in the ordinary way,
the miniature stomach remains constantly
empty of food.
—*J. P. PAVLOV, "THE WORK OF THE DIGESTIVE GLANDS"*
THE CLASSICS OF MEDICINE LIBRARY (BIRMINGHAM, 1982)

DEVELOPMENT

The embryonic foregut is, at first, largely pharyngeal; however, as the embryo grows, the foregut elongates to form the primordia of the esophagus and stomach cranial to the anterior intestinal portal. Dilation in the region of the future stomach appears during the fifth week, when the embryo is 4 to 5 mm long. Blechschmidt (1) indicates no dilation in the region of the stomach until after the tracheal diverticulum has appeared, but Botha (2) considers the stomach to be demarcated before the tracheal anlage. Description of the subsequent development of the stomach is based largely on the work of Botha (2), Johnson (3), Lewis (4), and Salenius (5).

The gastric dilation is at the level of segments C3 to C5 at its first appearance. The entire cranial region of the embryo grows rapidly, and subsequently, foregut elongation will take place in what later becomes the esophagus, leaving the gastric region near its origin, just cranial to the anterior intestinal portal. This growth of other structures cephalad results in the "descent" of the stomach so that at 10 mm it lies after the level of T5 to T10 and at 17.5 mm (i.e., at the end of the seventh week) it lies between T11 and L4 (Fig. 5.1). Later growth of the trunk will restore the stomach to its final position between T10 and L3.

Lateral flattening of the gastric lumen becomes visible at the 6.3-mm stage during the sixth week. During the sixth and seventh weeks, the greater and lesser curvatures become established. Most writers state that the dorsal border grows faster than the ventral border and moves to the left to become the greater curvature (Fig. 5.2, *A*).

The fact of this rotation has been denied, and it has been stated that the left side, not the dorsal surface, becomes the greater curvature (Fig. 5.2, *B*) (6). In this view the ventral border becomes the lesser curvature and the greater curvature is a new formation (Figs. 5.3 and 5.4).

Around the sixth week a 90-degree clockwise rotation takes place, perhaps due to differential growth patterns (7, 8).

The lesser curvature becomes increasingly concave up to the fourth fetal month and then straightens again before birth. The fundic outgrowth does not appear until the eighth or ninth week. It later becomes partially absorbed into the greater curvature (9). The abdominal esophagus is as long as the lesser curvature and bends almost 90 degrees during the fourth month to enter the stomach by a funnel-shaped expansion (2) (Fig. 5.5). All of these modeling processes appear to be intrinsic to the endoderm and perhaps the mesoderm of the foregut, rather than being the result of external forces.

The rugae are identifiable microscopically by the 16-mm stage and grossly by the eighth week. At this time the circular component of the muscularis is faintly indicated. The longitudinal layer appears between weeks 8 and 10, and the oblique layer between weeks 12 and 14. The muscularis mucosa is visible by the fourth month.

The pyloric ring is well developed between the fourth and fifth months of gestation (10).

The right and left vagal trunks reach the stomach by 4½ weeks, and the sympathetic join the vagi approximately 1 week later (11, 12). The left vagus nerve becomes the anterior vagus nerve on the stomach, while the right becomes the posterior nerve on the stomach. The anatomy of the vagus nerve was reported in several papers by Skandalakis et al. (13–15).

Despite that muscular and neurogenic development in fetal human gastric motility is not well known, remember that amniotic fluid was observed in the small bowel the fourth to fifth month of gestation according to Windle (15).

The first glandular pits appear on the lesser curvature at 6 to 9 weeks. They are present throughout the body of the stomach by 8 to 9 weeks and in the pylorus by week 10

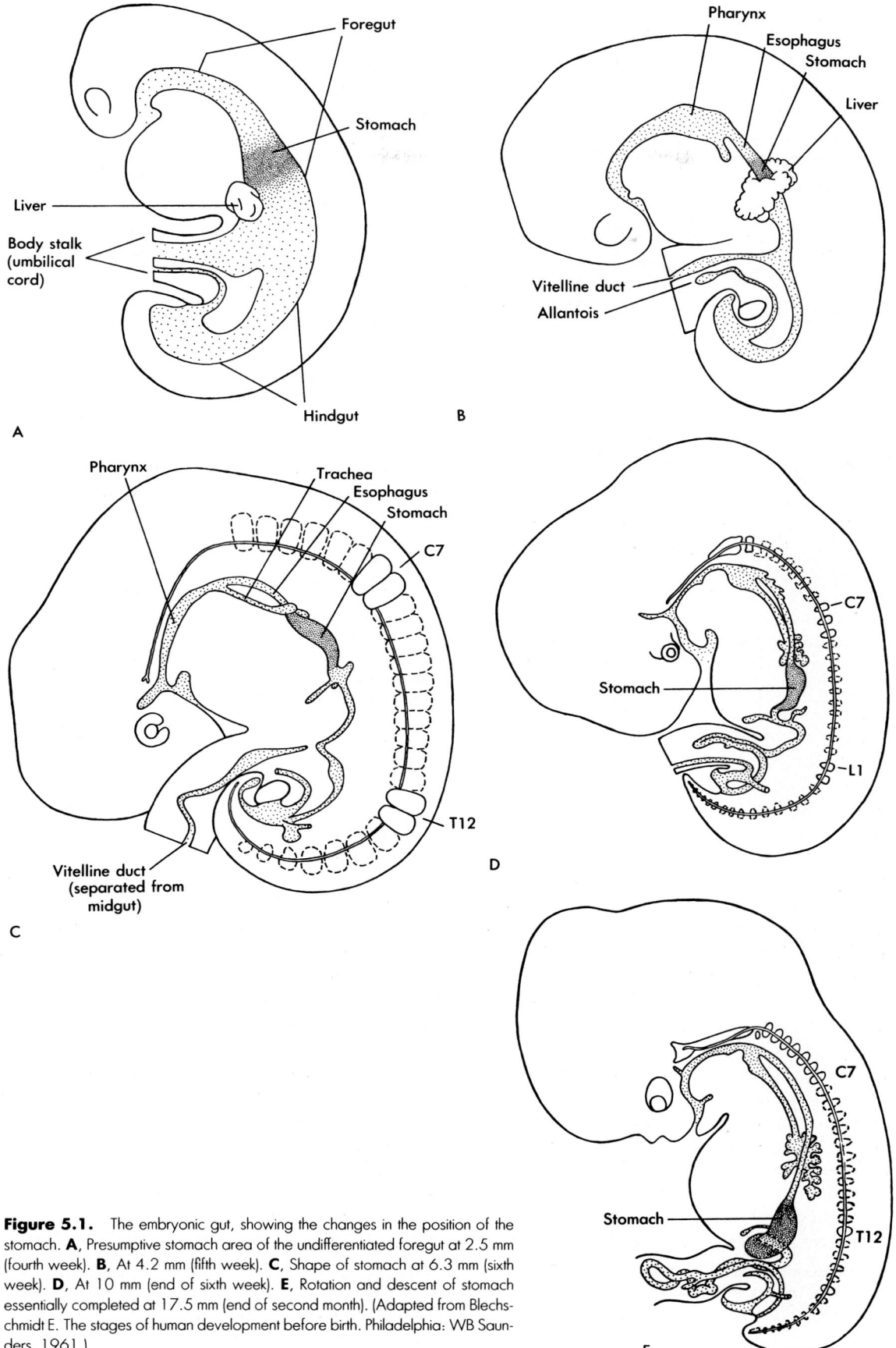

Figure 5.1. The embryonic gut, showing the changes in the position of the stomach. **A**, Presumptive stomach area of the undifferentiated foregut at 2.5 mm (fourth week). **B**, At 4.2 mm (fifth week). **C**, Shape of stomach at 6.3 mm (sixth week). **D**, At 10 mm (end of sixth week). **E**, Rotation and descent of stomach essentially completed at 17.5 mm (end of second month). (Adapted from Blechschmidt E. The stages of human development before birth. Philadelphia: WB Saunders, 1961.)

151

(Fig. 5.6). The epithelium of the stomach at this time is pseudostratified columnar (5).

New gastric pits are formed by the splitting of the original pits by upgrowth of mesoderm. Glands appear first as solid buds from the bottom of the pits (4). Both gastric

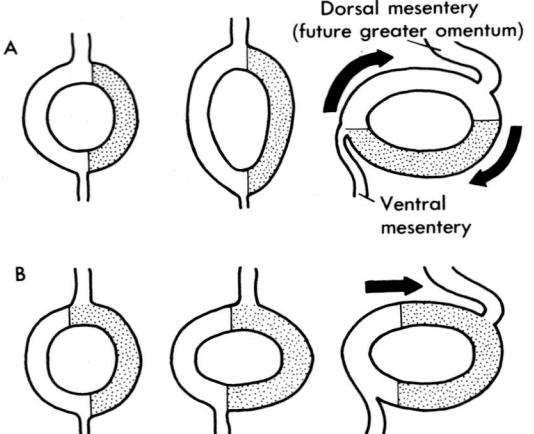

Figure 5.2. Cross sectional diagrams through the embryonic stomach during the seventh week, illustrating two hypotheses for the rotation of the stomach. **A,** Classic view, in which the dorsal border rotates to the left to become the greater curvature. **B,** View of Dankmeijer and Miete (1959), in which the left side becomes the greater curvature as a result only of increased growth—that is, no actual rotation occurs. Dankmeijer J, Miete M. Le développement précoce de l'estomac chez l'embryo humain. C R Ass Anat 1959;103:341–344.

pits and glands increase faster in length than in diameter, and new pits and glands are formed to the end of the second postnatal year. Scott (17) counted about 32 pits and 78 glands per square millimeter of gastric mucosa by the end of the eighth fetal month. At birth there are about 50 pits and 122 glands, making an estimated total of 204,000 pits and 489,000 glands in the entire newborn infant's stomach. The number of pits reaches about 66 per square millimeter of mucosa, but the number of glands decreases slightly during adult life.

Parietal cells are recognizable at about 11 weeks, but succinic dehydrogenase activity appears earlier. Chief cells appear about the twelfth week, but no pepsinogen can be identified in them until after birth. Mucous neck cells appear at about the same time. Differentiation of surface epithelial cells starts at 11 weeks in the pyloric and cardiac regions and spreads first to the lesser curvature and later to the greater curvature (Fig. 5.6). In both the pyloric and cardiac regions, epithelial cells with a striated

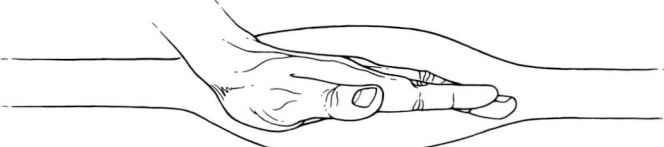

Figure 5.3. Location of the left hand at the embryonic foregut (beginning of dilated stomach).

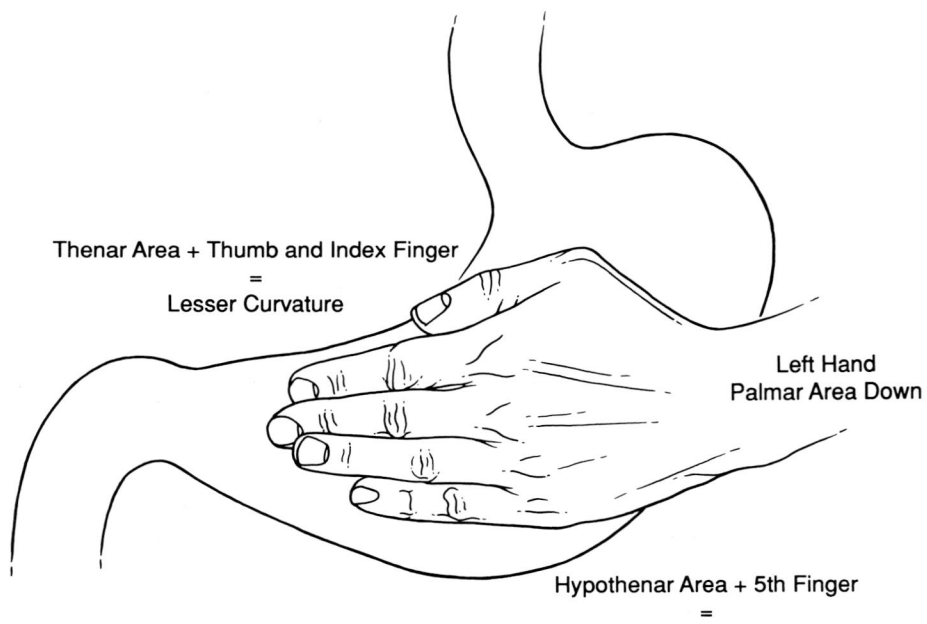

Thenar Area + Thumb and Index Finger
=
Lesser Curvature

Left Hand
Palmar Area Down

Hypothenar Area + 5th Finger
=
Greater Curvature

Figure 5.4. Use the left hand. Hypothenar and fifth finger touch the epigastrium vertically. If the same hand now turns and the fifth finger and the hypothenar touch in a transverse way, the epigastrium and the palm in toto touch the epigastrium, then: the fifth finger and hypothenar represent the thenar, the thumb and index the lesser curvature.

border and goblet cells are abundant up to the age of 20 weeks and may be found in decreasing amounts up to and even after birth (5).

Pepsin is present in the mucosa by the last half of the sixth month, but neither pepsin nor hydrochloric acid appears in the gastric contents until near term. The stomach contents are nearly neutral at birth, but gastric acid increases within a few hours (18). This increase takes place in the absence of food (19) and may be the result of increased oxygen tension of the blood acting on the parietal cells.

It is not within the scope of this book to give details on fetal physiology nor to discuss ontogeny and phylogeny; however, we wish to include in the form of a table the ontogeny of the gastrointestinal peptides from the excellent chapter of Leung and Lebenthal (20). This shows the approximate time of appearance of the peptides in various tissues of the human fetus (Table 5.1).

The infant's stomach at birth contains a gray mucous material composed of gastric secretions and desqua-

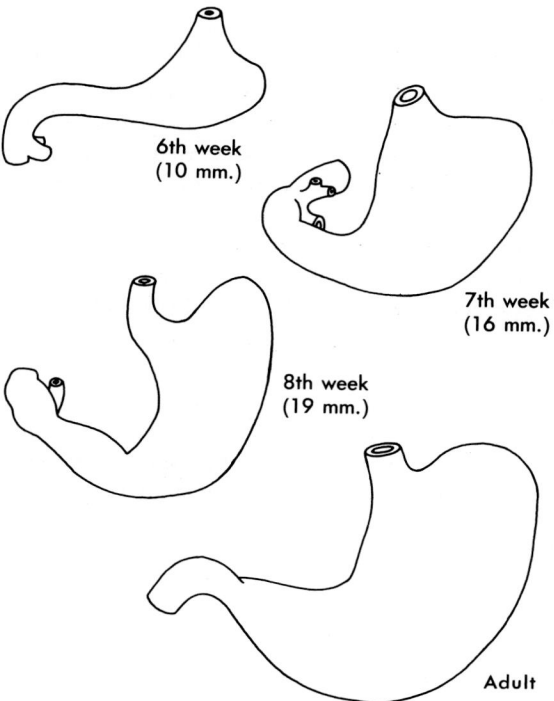

Figure 5.5. The shape of the stomach in prenatal stages and in the adult. (Redrawn from Lewis FT. The development of the stomach. In: Keibel WP, Mall FP, eds. Manual of human embryology. Philadelphia: JB Lippincott, 1912.)

Table 5.1.
Ontogeny of the Gastrointestinal Peptides

Peptide	Age of Earliest Appearance (Weeks)
Glucagon	6 (pancreas)
Insulin	10 (pancreas)
Somatostatin	8 (pancreas)
Somatostatin	9–11 (intestine)
Pancreatic polypeptide	8–9 (pancreas)
Gastrin	10–11 (duodenum)
Cholecystokinin	10 (duodenum)
Secretin	8 (duodenum)
GIP	8–10 (duodenum and jejunum)
VIP	8–9 (fundus and duodenum)
VIP	10 (VIP-nerve fibers)
Neurotensin	12 (jejunum, ileum, colon)
Motilin	8–11 (duodenum, jejunum)
Substance P	18–25 (brainstem)
Bombesin	12 (bronchus)

From Leung K-Y, Lebenthal E. Gastrointestinal peptides. In: Lebenthal E, ed. Human gastrointestinal development. NY: Raven Press, 1989:42.

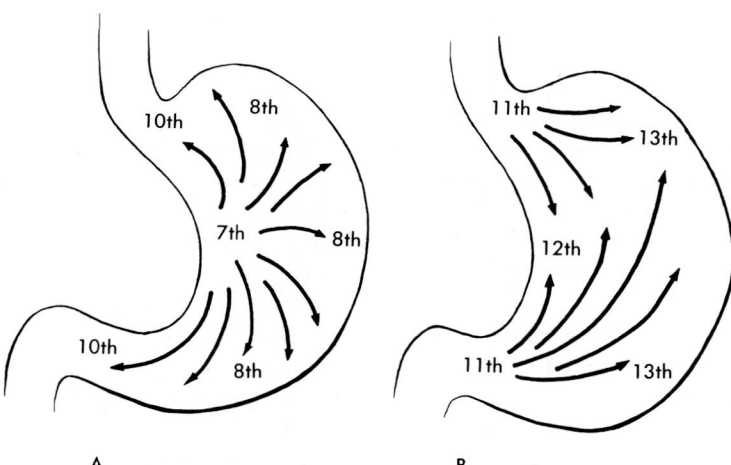

Figure 5.6. **A,** Pattern of appearance of gastric pits by weeks of embryonic development. **B,** Pattern of maturation of gastric surface epithelium by weeks of development. (Data from Salenius P. On the ontogenesis of the human gastric epithelial cells: a histologic and histochemical study. Acta Anat (Basil) 1952; 50(Suppl 46):1–76.)

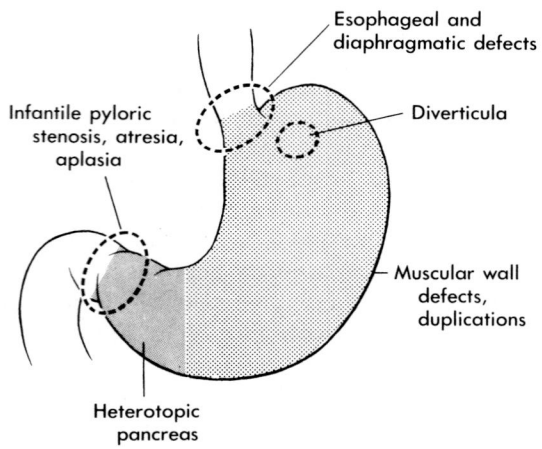

Figure 5.7. Chief locations of congenital anomalies of the stomach.

mated cells mixed with amniotic fluid. Potter (21) pointed out that maternal blood, swallowed during parturition, may be sufficient to give a positive test for occult blood during the first few days of life.

Critical Events in Development

Unlike the esophagus, the stomach undergoes little alteration in form during development. None of the malformations to which the stomach is subject are common, and the only frequent, serious gastric disorder of infancy—hypertrophic pyloric stenosis—is not of embryonic origin (Fig. 5.7).

ANOMALIES OF THE STOMACH (TABLE 5.2)

Microgastria and Agastria

The stomach is never completely absent, except in nonviable monsters, and rarely is it grossly hypoplastic.

Microgastria was reported in the necropsy of a child in one of the earliest descriptions of congenital pyloric stenosis by Blair in 1717 (22). Another child, described by Hoyt (23), had a stomach with a capacity about one-tenth that of the norm. Although this was discovered radiographically in life, it is interesting to note that the finding was dismissed as poor radiologic technique until it was proved at autopsy.

Caffey (24) described the anomalous stomach of a 6-month-old infant, which lay in the midline. The curvatures were not developed, and there was no differentiation into regions. The gastroesophageal junction was incompetent, and the esophagus was dilated. The child suffered from secondary anemia and weight loss.

Tubular stomachs have been reported in association with agenesis of the spleen (25) and splenogonadal fusion

as well as with a number of somatic anomalies (26, 27). One such infant lived for 2½ years.

HISTORY

In 1894 Dide reported a case in which the stomach was abnormally small and abnormally oriented (28). Gerbeaux et al. (29) reported a case of gastric absence (agastria).

EMBRYOGENESIS AND ASSOCIATED ANOMALIES

Microgastria and agastria represent very rare congenital anomalies of the proximal foregut involving not only the stomach but also the esophagus. Gastric malposition also was reported with other associated anomalies, such as nonrotation of the midgut with duodenal obstruction, ileal duplication, hiatal hernia with reflux, cardiac defects, and partial situs inversus. Schultz and Neiman (30) reported a case with absence of the gallbladder.

SYMPTOMS

Vomiting, diarrhea, aspiration pneumonitis, dumping syndrome, gastroesophageal reflux, and perhaps rapid gastric emptying are separately or collectively present in the obvious picture of these unfortunate babies. The result is malnutrition, failure to thrive, and developmental delay.

DIAGNOSIS AND DIFFERENTIAL DIAGNOSIS

Microgastria and the associated gastroesophageal reflux may be diagnosed through a gastrointestinal radiographic series (Fig. 5.8), as can the associated gastroesophageal reflux.

TREATMENT

Total parenteral nutrition or continuous nasogastric feedings represent conservative treatment. Gastrojejunostomy with good results was reported by Blank and Chisholm (31).

Jejunal reservoir was reported by Gerbeaux (29) and Neifeld et al. (32).

The surgeon should not forget to look for and correct associated anomalies or, when performing a gastrojejunostomy, the possible formation of a marginal ulcer. The blind loop syndrome could be avoided with meticulous technique.

Velasco et al. (33) reported on four new cases of congenital microgastria bringing the total number of cases reported to 26. Three of these cases were successfully treated with a Hunt-Lawrence pouch; the fourth died from associated severe congenital heart disease. The outcome of most other cases reported in the literature has been severe malnutrition or death.

Tubular stomachs have been associated with asplenia,

Table 5.2.
Anomalies of the Stomach

Anomaly	Origin	First Appearance	Sex Chiefly Affected	Relative Frequency	Remarks
Agastria and microgastria	Week 4	Infancy	?	Very rare	Many associated gastrointestinal tract and splenic anomalies
Malposition	Week 10	Any age	Males	Rare	May be associated with diaphragmatic eventration or hernia
Atresia and stenosis	?	Infancy to adulthood	?	Rare	Maternal hydramnios familial occurrence (?)— autosomal recessive associated with epidemiologic bullosa
Membranous partial		Infancy to adulthood			
Membranous entire	?	Infancy to adulthood			
Complete (solid)	Weeks 6–7				
Gastroduodenal discontinuity	?				
Luminal with microscopic canal	?				
Typical stenosis with perforated membrane(s)					
Hourglass stomach	?	Any age	?	Rare	Usually not congenital
Congenital pyloric stenosis	Postnatal week 2	2–4 Weeks	Male	Very common	Not a true anomaly
Infantile					
Adult					
Congenital muscular defect	Weeks 8–10	Infancy	?	Rare	May not be congenital
Diverticula	?	40–70 yr	Equal	Rare	May not be congenital
Duplication—double pylorus	Week 3	Any age	Female	Rare	Faulty separation of endoderm and notochordal plate
Mucosal heterotopia from other organs to the stomach	Weeks 4–5				Adhesion or metaplasia (endodermal transformations) cellular translocation
Pancreas					
Small bowel					
Others					
From stomach to other organs					
Partially all over gastrointestinal tract					
Congenital arteriovenous malformations	?	Adult	Male	Rare	May not be congenital
Teratoma		Infancy to adulthood	Male	Rare	Benign (usually)
Gastroduodenal adhesions	?	?	?	?	?

peromelia, micrognathia, cardiac defects, and partial situs inversus (25, 27). All of these defects, except cardiac anomalies, were presented in one patient as reported by Mandel (26). Multiple accessory spleens and splenogonadal fusion also were present.

Atresia and Stenosis of the Stomach

ANATOMY

Congenital atresia is less common in the stomach than in other portions of the alimentary tract and when present is limited to the antrum and the pyloric region.

Gastric atresia is usually produced by a membranous diaphragm in which only the mucosa is involved (Fig. 5.9, A and B). In a few cases there is a more extensive oblit-

eration of the lumen (34) (Fig. 5.9, C and D). Complete aplasia of all parts of the pyloric region has been reported (35, 36) (Fig. 5.9, E). One patient had two membranes a short distance apart (37).

If the occluding membrane is thin, it may perforate from the pressure of the gastric contents and form an annular stenosis, which will cause symptoms only later in life. Such stenoses in older infants and adults are not all of congenital origin. Rhind (38) described seven perforated diaphragms in adults. He concluded that, in five patients, the lesions were produced by alternate healing and expansion of ulcers. Where ulcer scarring is present, the stenoses are probably acquired.

Epidermolysis bullosa occasionally is associated with congenital gastric outlet obstruction (39). All types of

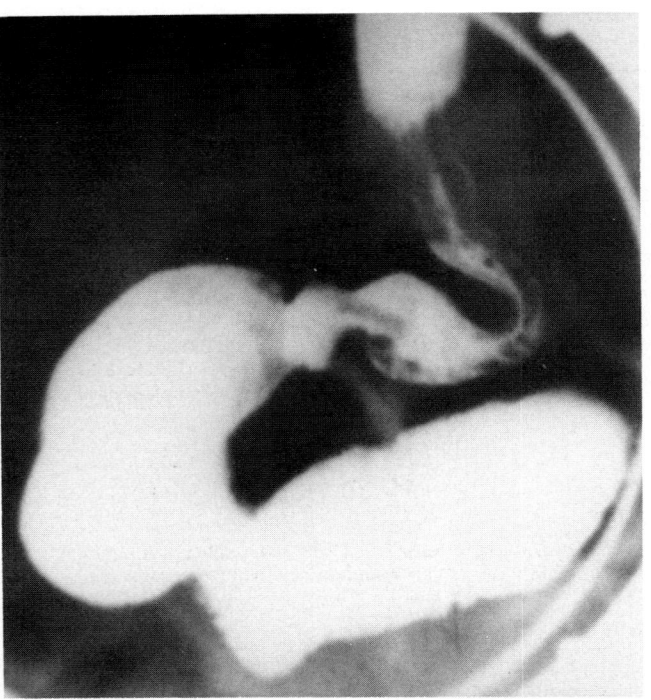

Figure 5.8.   Microgastria with associated jejunal stenosis.

atresia and stenosis may be described under the term *congenital gastric outlet obstruction.*

EMBRYOGENESIS

The origin of gastric atresia is as uncertain as that of atresia elsewhere in the gut. Failure of recanalization is not a factor here since there is no epithelial perforation in the stomach comparable to that in the esophagus or duodenum.

It is possible that a local redundancy of the endodermal tube may be the origin of the membrane diaphragm (Fig. 5.10, *A*). Longer zones of atresia probably result from a local attenuation of the endodermal tube during formation of mesochymal elements of the pylorus (Fig. 5.10, *B*). If the tube becomes discontinuous before the appearance of the musculature, complete segmental aplasia would result. If the break occurred later, there would be an interruption of the mucosa and its lumen, but the external coats would be continuous.

It is the accepted belief that membranous atresia in the stomach and in the intestines may perforate soon after birth, leaving only mild stenosis. The presence of very small perforations in adults who had obstructive symptoms for only a few months suggests that the perforation

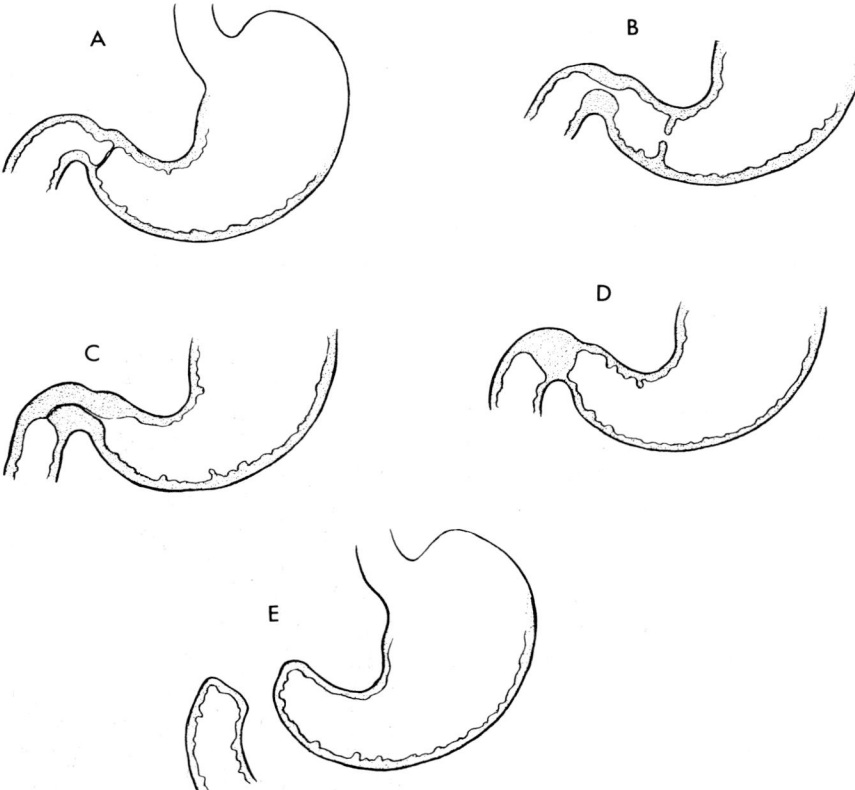

Figure 5.9.   Five types of gastric atresia. **A**, Membranous atresia. **B**, Perforated membrane (stenosis). **C**, Luminal atresia with a microscopic endodermal canal. **D**, Complete, solid atresia. **E**, Complete atresia with discontinuity.

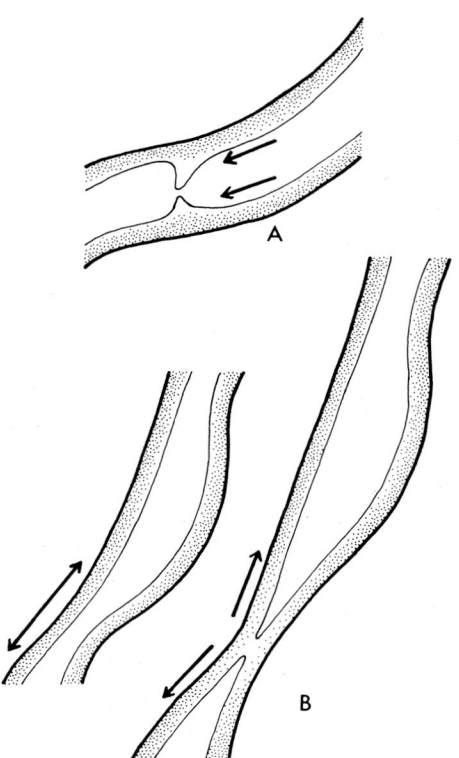

Figure 5.10. Two explanations of gastric atresia. **A**, Redundant endodermal lining. Caudal slippage of endoderm forms a circular fold, which may or may not retain a central opening. **B**, Attenuation of endoderm. Proliferation of endoderm fails to keep up with elongating foregut. Atresia or even complete discontinuity results.

may become progressively smaller with age (40–42). It is not easy to believe that these small apertures sufficed, allowing for more or less normal functioning for many years, only to produce symptoms late in life. We conclude that mucosal diaphragms in adults are probably not congenital (43). If the diaphragms present perforation with congenital diaphragmatic atresia, a subsequent stenosis must have occurred. In the absence of scarring, either increasing stenosis by local proliferation or concrescent slipping of the mucosa must be postulated. In one case the gastric surface of the stenosing diaphragm was covered with stratified squamous epithelium (44). Whether this represented heterotopia or metaplasia is not clear.

Familial occurrence was reported by Malheur et al. (45) who described pyloric and duodenal (first part) atresia in seven children from three families. Some authors (46–51) suggest an autosomal recessive mode of inheritance.

HISTORY

The first reported case of luminal occlusion was that of Crooks (52) in 1828. Wuensche (53) in 1875 and Neale (35) in 1884 described complete segmental aplasia.

The complete diaphragmatic form of atresia was first described by Bennett (54) in 1937. Pyloroplasty was performed, but the infant died 36 hours later. An imperforated diaphragm proximal to the pyloric junction was found at autopsy. Touroff and Sussman (55) successfully removed such a diaphragm, and Metz with his colleagues (56) incised one, each reporting successful operations. In both procedures the membranes were incised and the patients recovered.

INCIDENCE

Twenty-eight cases of complete gastric atresia were collected by Wolf and Zweymüeller up to 1963 (57), and at least nine more have appeared since.

Until 1970, 18 cases of congenital perforated prepyloric membranes were described in older infants, children, and adults. In none of these was there ulcerative scarring at the site of the perforated membranes.

The membranous form of atresia is the most common. Segmental atresia was reported in two cases and complete aplasia in four.

Since the incidence of Down's syndrome among patients with esophageal atresia (11% in the authors' experience) and with duodenal atresia (about 25%) is quite high, it is surprising that gastric atresia and Down's syndrome are not more frequently associated.

SYMPTOMS

The three cardinal signs of gastric atresia in infants are (*a*) persistent, bile-free vomiting after the first feeding, (*b*) distension of the upper abdomen but not of the lower, and (*c*) stools decreasing in quantity. On x-ray examination the stomach shows air and fluid levels, but no air is seen in the intestines (Figs. 5.11 and 5.12).

In adults with perforate diaphragms, the symptoms are

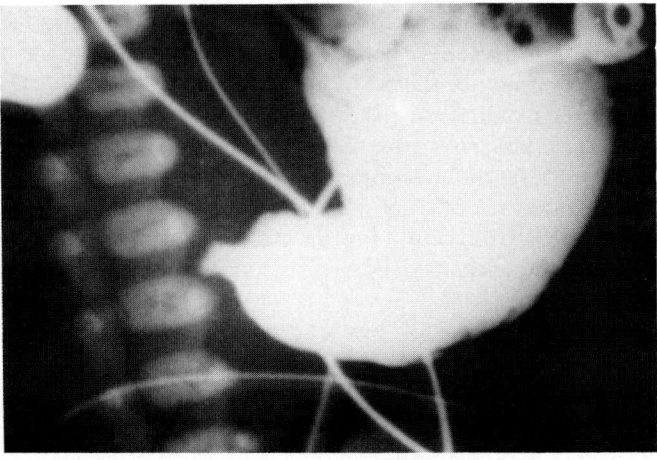

Figure 5.11. Upper gastrointestinal radiologic series demonstrating pyloric atresia.

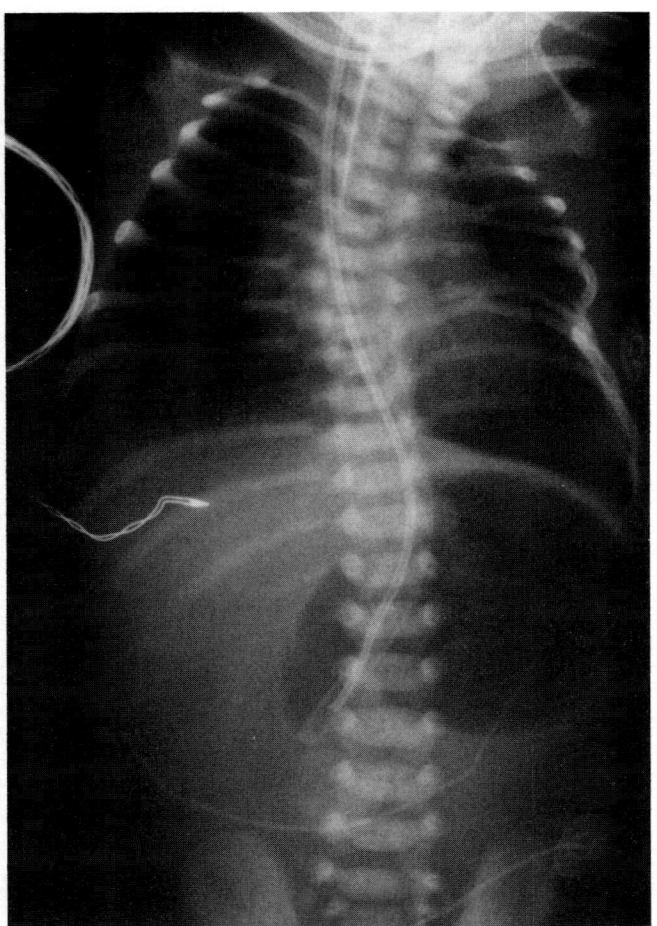

Figure 5.12. Upright x-ray films (kidneys, ureters, and bladder) demonstrating pyloric atresia.

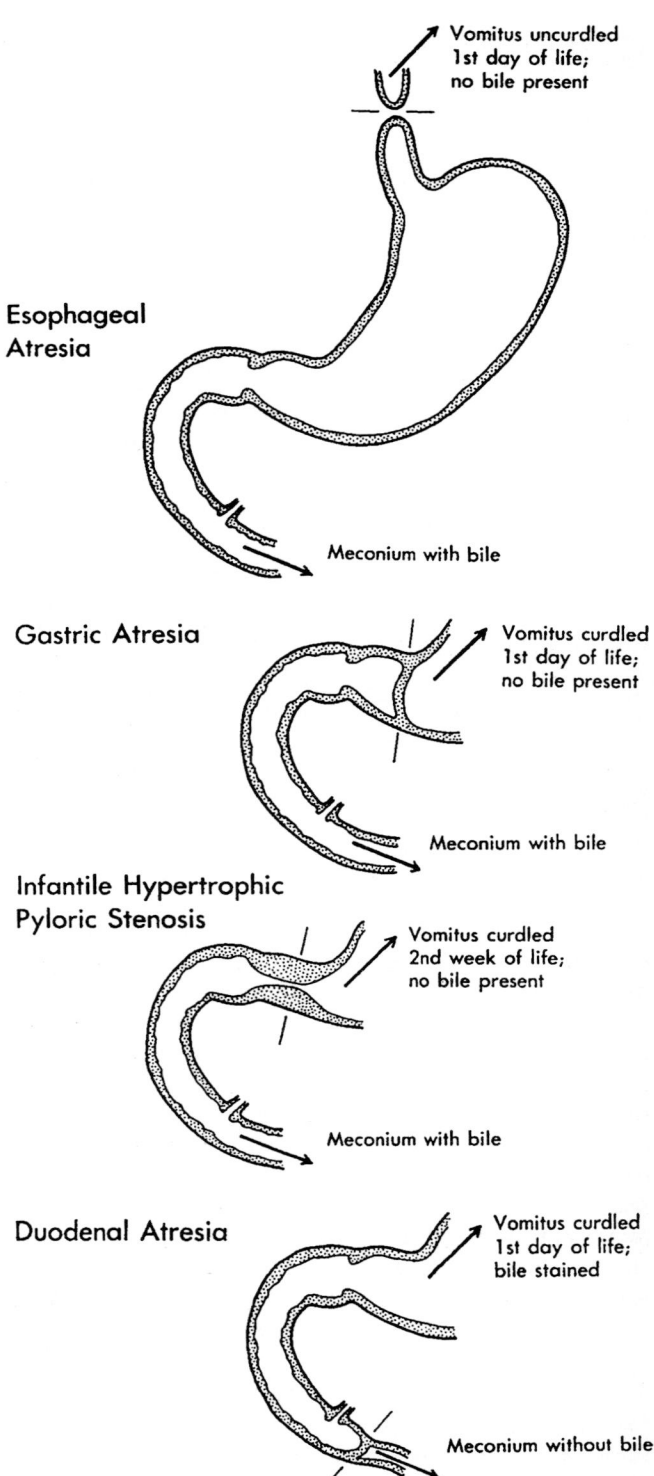

Figure 5.13. The differential diagnosis of high alimentary tract obstructions. Observation of both vomitus and feces is necessary.

usually mild and their onset is late. Epigastric pain, weight loss, nausea, and vomiting are the chief symptoms of this condition. One patient who was 52 years of age complained of loss of appetite, dyspepsia, and vomiting for only 4 months (58). Another patient who was 74 years of age had a membrane with an aperture of 4 mm, yet his symptoms had been present for only 8 years. Barium retention was 25% after 24 hours, but in other patients retention was much higher (40). An even smaller aperture was found in a 53-year-old woman whose gastric symptoms dated from only a few months (41). Death from inanition was barely averted by surgical intervention.

DIAGNOSIS

The onset of bile-free vomiting in infants immediately after birth distinguishes prepyloric atresia from hypertrophic pyloric stenosis, which rarely begins before the second week (Fig. 5.13). A catheter passed successfully into the stomach is proof against a diagnosis of esophageal atresia. The presence of meconium in the stool and its

absence in the vomitus places the obstruction above the papilla of Vater.

Polyhydramnios was present in at least 50% of reported cases of newborn infants with prepyloric atresia;

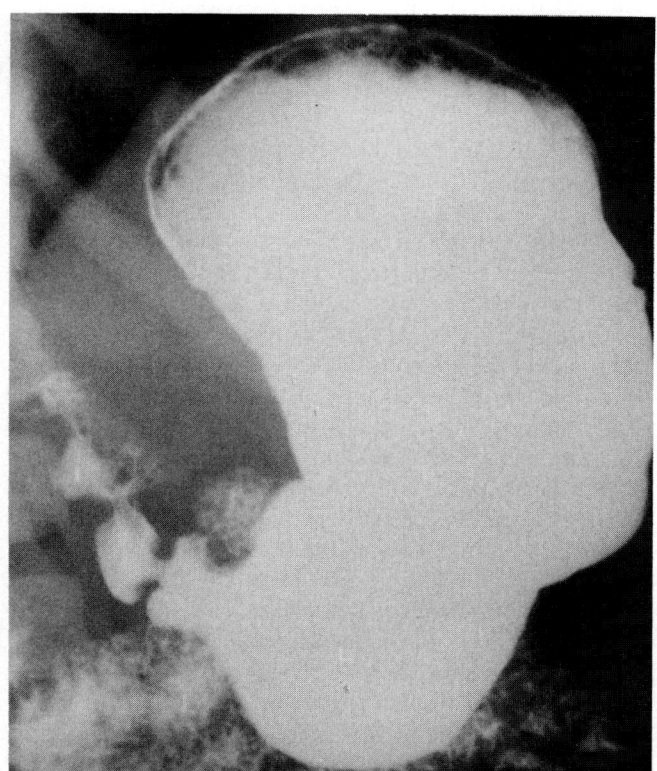

Figure 5.14. Upper gastrointestinal radiologic series demonstrating control webb.

these infants frequently were premature. As in esophageal atresia, normal swallowing and absorption of amniotic fluid is prevented by the obstruction.

In adults the clinical picture usually resembles carcinoma, benign ulcer, or gastritis with pylorospasm. Preoperative diagnosis is not to be expected; the surgeon can only keep the possibility in mind during surgery. In only one case (59) was there any indication of the defect in the external stomach wall. Campbell (60) stated that aspiration of the gastric contents, injection of the same amount of air without barium, but using radiographic "films taken in various positions may be needed to establish the correct diagnosis." Dilute barium may be required (Fig. 5.14).

TREATMENT

Prompt surgical intervention is the only hope for survival for an infant with atresia of the stomach.

In theory, with an accurate diagnosis, excision of the obstructing membrane is the treatment of choice through a generous proximal gastrostomy as recommended by Talwalker (61). Among six patients so treated, however, four required a second operation because of obstructing edema (62). In two patients (34, 63) a polyethylene tube was introduced through the gastrostomy and into the duodenum to ensure patency following excision of the

occluding diaphragm. If there is a solid atresia or atresia with a gap, gastroduodenostomy is the procedure of choice. The use of temporary gastrostomy is up to the surgeon.

The alternative to excision of the membrane is a shunt operation, such as a Heinke-Mikulicz or Finney pyloroplasty. Gastrojejunostomy should not be performed in infants because of the possibility of marginal ulceration. Vagotomy should not be performed on children.

All the successful operations have been performed before the 10th day of life. In several cases a second or third operation was required (64).

Regardless of the procedure employed, the surgeon should take time to inspect the remainder of the gut to be certain no other areas of obstruction exist in the upper gastrointestinal tract.

EDITORIAL COMMENT

A case in point was reported by Haller and associates in 1967 in which a newborn infant was found to have duodenal atresia that was corrected by a duodenoduonostomy only to find continued obstruction of the gastric outlet following several days of observation. Reexploration revealed a prepyloric or antral diaphragm which required excision to relieve the obstruction. The only way to prevent this error in management is to carry out a gastrostomy and pass a tube from the stomach through the duodenum into the jejunum to make certain there are not multiple obstructions. This baby fortunately recovered from both operative procedures (65a) (JAH).

MORTALITY

Among 22 patients operated upon, only five failed to survive. There have been no recent deaths. In addition, only one adult died following surgery for a perforated diaphragm. Unexplained mortality is reported by Campbell (60) in children with familial occurrence. Pyloric atresia with epidermolysis, however, is practically always fatal (65b).

In 1977 we presented a case and reviewed the literature of antral and pyloric diaphragm in adults (66). Parts of this paper are presented with the hope that it will stimulate investigators for a collective review.

Hourglass Stomach

Division of the stomach into two chambers by a constricting ring has been called, from its appearance, "hourglass stomach." Such annular constrictions from local hypertrophy of the musculature usually result from corrosive poison (67) or from ulcerative, neoplastic, or syphilitic lesions. In a few instances no evidence of such lesions in the stomach wall or in the patient's history can be found.

In 1851 Struther (68) suggested that, in at least some cases, the constriction was a congenital deformity. Hirsch

(69) reviewed the literature and concluded that all cases were congenital. The present viewpoint—that all such cases are sequelae to ulcer—originated with Moynihan (70) and was restated by Rowlands (71). Occasionally, an hourglass stomach showing no trace of ulceration or ulcer scarring is reported, and the question of congenital origin is revived (72).

ABNORMAL DEVELOPMENT OR INTRAUTERINE ULCERATION PROCESS?

Associated anomalies have been reported. Sager and Jenkins (73) reported esophageal stenosis in an hourglass stomach in 1935.

Infantile Hypertrophic Pyloric Stenosis (Congenital Pyloric Stenosis)

For a long time this entity was considered to be a developmental defect of the pyloric musculature. Hirschsprung (74), who first recognized it as a clinical entity in 1888, believed that it represented the failure of a normal process of involution of the fetal pylorus. His term *angeborener Pylorusstenose* (congenital pyloric stenosis) has persisted. Although "infantile hypertrophic pyloric stenosis" is more exact, it has not yet replaced the older term. The failure to find pyloric hypertrophy regularly in premature, stillborn infants has removed it from consideration as a normal prenatal condition. Furthermore, its disappearance in the course of time is contrary to the usual behavior of developmental defects. Because of its appearance early in postnatal life, however, it behaves clinically, if not developmentally, as a congenital anomaly, and for this reason it will be considered here.

ANATOMY

Hypertrophy and hyperplasia of the muscularis of the pyloric canal, especially of the circular coat, produces a thickening of the wall and a reduction in the size of the lumen. Elastic tissue of the submucosa and muscularis also is involved. With time the affected region increases in length as well as in thickness. The swelling passes through a stage of increasing tension, producing a pylorus of hard, solid consistency which reaches its greatest development at 4 to 9 weeks. Eventually, if the infant survives, the swelling relaxes and becomes softer and smaller, with complete healing after several months. The reader should consult the excellent review of Hayes and Goldenberg (75) for further details and references.

PATHOGENESIS

No longer considered a true congenital defect, pyloric stenosis remains essentially unexplained. Wallgren (76) could find no abnormal radiologic appearance in living children immediately after birth. In premature infants the symptoms may start before the date of normal birth. The disease is more frequent in first-born children. Symptoms appear later in children born in the hospital than in those born at home (77, 78); and symptoms appear later in children fed at 4-hour intervals than in those fed at 3-hour intervals (79). The specific environmental factors still elude detection.

Stringer and Brereton (80) stated that approximately 5% of the sons of affected fathers will be born with hypertrophic pyloric stenosis.

Lynn (81) believes that the pyloric mucosa and submucosa become edematous secondary to milk curds propelled by the muscular wall of the stomach with a final hypertrophy of the musculature of the canal. Spitz and Zail (82) suggest that gastrin perhaps plays a role, but Rogers et al. (83) stated that it is more reasonable to hypothesize that the early pyloric baby has a significantly higher acidity than a normal baby.

However, the search for an anatomic basis of the hypertrophy continues. Especially attractive is the view that there may be an underlying defect of the myenteric plexus, such as is the case with congenital megacolon (84). In 1961 Rintoul and Kirkman (85) stated that the myenteric plexuses of the pyloric muscular ring do not contain argyrophil neurons. Friesen et al. (86) thought that the ganglion cells were immature in patients with pyloric stenosis; Zuelzer (87) failed, however, to confirm these results. Using electron microscopic observation, Jona (88) could find no degenerative changes or immaturity of the ganglion cells.

Recent biochemical studies have implicated lack of or diminished amounts of nitric oxide (NO) as the culprit in the etiology of pyloric stenosis. This neurotransmitter triggers relaxation in the gut. Lacking NO, the gut cannot relax and thus peristalsis is ineffective (89, 90).

At present interest has shifted to the genetics of the disease. A larger proportion of both children and siblings of female patients are affected than are those of male patients, and more relatives of patients of either sex are affected than would be expected. The increased incidence over the normal rate of their sex is greater among female relatives of affected patients. The data collected by Carter (91) is shown in Figure 5.15.

Among 1120 affected patients in Detroit, 32 had other affected siblings (92). Three affected children were found in each of four families, and four children with this condition occurred in another family. The disease has been seen also in three consecutive generations of the same family (Akin J. Personal communication, 1969).

Carter (91) postulated the presence of a dominant gene, plus a sex-modified (but not sex-linked) (93) multifactor background, which varies around a mean. Only individuals at one extreme of this background are affected. In general, one may say that the risk for the chil-

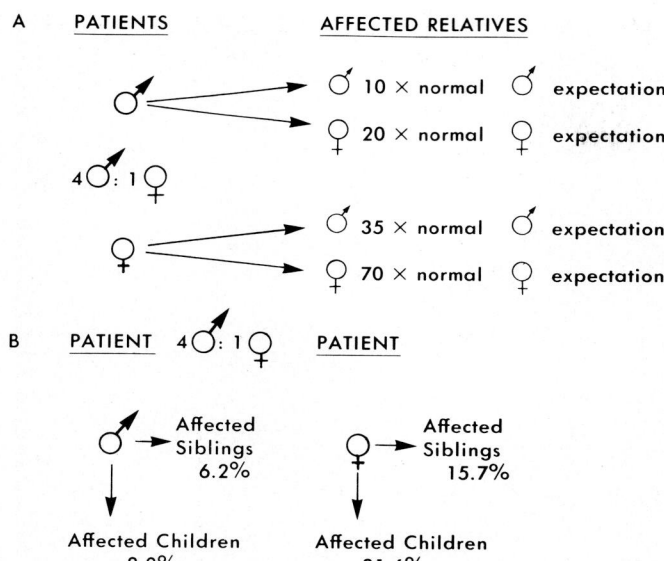

Figure 5.15. Familial incidence of hypertrophic pyloric stenosis. **A,** Increased expectation of hypertrophic pyloric stenosis among relatives of affected patients, by sex. **B,** Percentage of siblings and offspring of affected patients expected to have the disease. (Data from Carter CO. The inheritance of congenital pyloric stenosis. Br Med Bull 1961;17:251–253.)

dren of individuals who have had pyloric stenosis is proportional to, or slightly greater than, the incidence of the disease in his or her siblings.

HISTORY

In 1646 Hildanus (94) mentioned a child who had what appears to have been congenital pyloric stenosis. The child was treated by dietary regimen and recovered. Basing his speculation on the facts (*a*) that Hildanus only reported one such case among his many pediatric observations and (*b*) that his work was well known both then and in the succeeding century, Kellett (95) questions whether the paucity of reports prior to the latter half of the 19th century may not indicate a true rarity of the disease until comparatively recent times. Blair in 1717 (96) first specifically described the disease. In the United States, a description by Beardsley appeared in 1788 (97) in the earliest U.S. medical journal published. Despite these earlier reports, the publication of the description by Hirschsprung (74) in 1888 marked the first recognition of the disease as an entity. The inimitable Mark Ravitch (98) gave a thorough and entertaining history of the disease, including its surgical treatment.

INCIDENCE

Incidence of infantile pyloric stenosis varies widely. One of the highest rates (0.4%) was found in Sweden in 1960, although this reportedly has been halved since that time (99). In Pittsburgh between 1945 and 1955, Laron and

Horne (100) found an incidence of 0.12% among white infants and 0.04% among black infants. Comparable values have been reported for Israel and Scotland (0.15%); in England, however, the values have been nearer 0.3% (100–101).

In general, northern Europeans are more frequently afflicted than are southern Europeans or white Americans. The disease is even less common in black Americans, Africans, and Asians (102). Griffiths (103), studying the disease in South African Bantus, concluded that its incidence is increasing with urbanization.

The victims of pyloric stenosis are predominantly male. In large series they compose from 78% (92) to 90% (102) of subjects. About 50% of identical co-twins are affected. Because this is more than would be expected by chance, it can be concluded that the disease has a genetic basis; on the other hand, because the incidence is less than 100%, we can conclude that there must also be an environmental factor.

SYMPTOMS AND DIAGNOSIS

Vomiting, usually beginning in the second week of life, becomes increasingly severe, but neither fever nor loss of appetite is seen. Weight loss is progressive and is usually associated with increasing dehydration and scantiness of stools. The delayed onset distinguishes this condition from pyloric atresia, in which vomiting begins at birth, and the lack of fever distinguishes it from infectious vomiting, in which fever is present.

Infantile hypertrophic pyloric stenosis is among the few gastrointestinal disorders with a distinctive set of signs and symptoms that are useful in diagnosis.

Vomiting. Vomitus is curdled, but not bile stained; blood may occasionally be present. In a few cases vomiting may start at birth, but usually it begins between the second and sixth weeks of life. It begins as simple regurgitation, but the vomiting becomes more forceful, until it may be called projectile; it follows immediately on all feedings.

Peristaltic Waves. Though varying in degree, these are universally present. They move from left to right and have been likened to "the slow passage of a tangerine under the abdominal wall" (102).

Palpable Mass. If sufficient care is taken, the enlarged pylorus may usually be palpated, especially after weight loss has become marked. It is most easily felt immediately after emesis.

Dehydration, Alkalosis, and Weight Loss. These are inevitable sequelae to the continued obstruction of the pylorus.

Radiographic Signs. Abnormal barium retention in the stomach (lasting for more than 3 hours), an elongated, thread-like pylorus, and an enlarged and distended stomach are the pathognomonic signs (Fig. 5.14). Benson

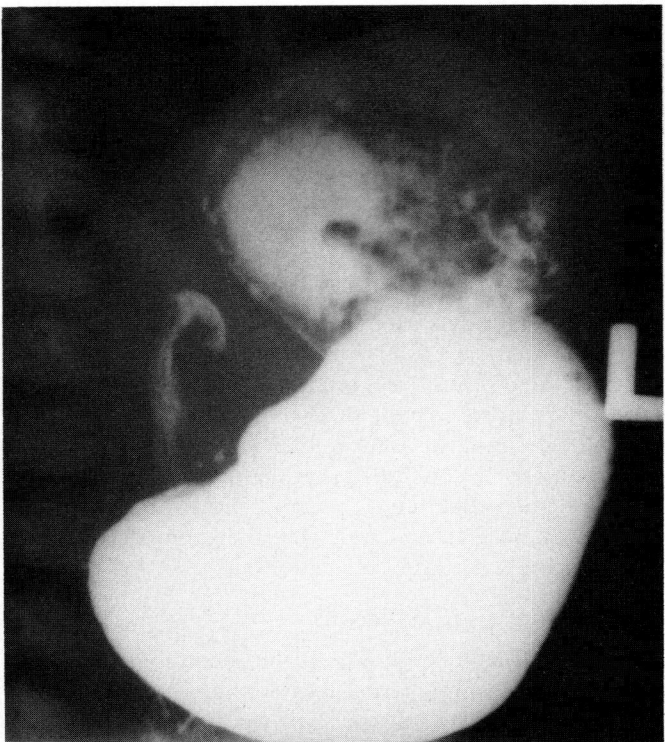

Figure 5.16. Upper gastrointestinal radiologic series demonstrating pyloric stenosis.

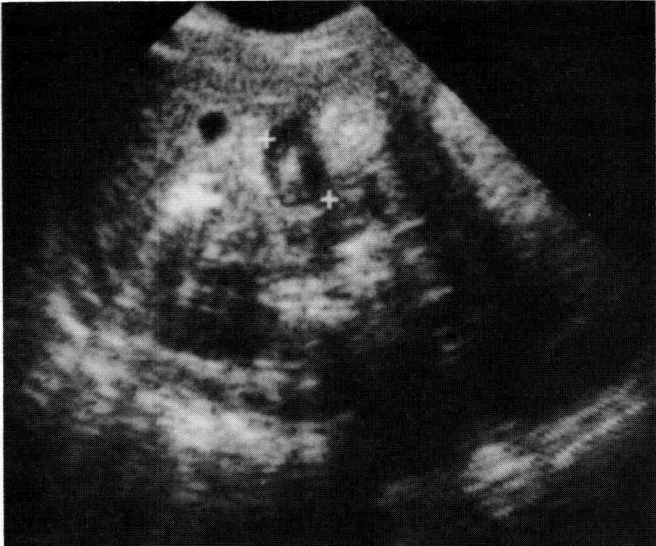

Figure 5.17. Pyloric stenosis diagnosed by ultrasound.

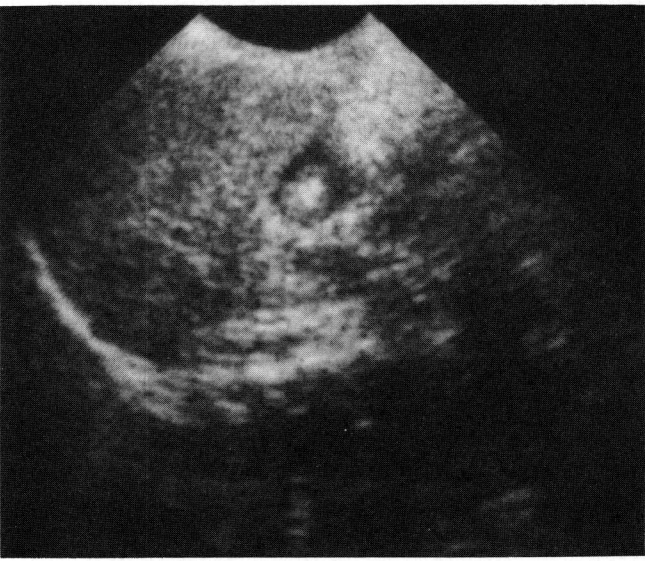

Figure 5.18. Pyloric stenosis diagnosed by ultrasound.

(104) reminds us that gastric retention of barium is not always the correct answer since other conditions may produce the same clinical picture. Ultrasound is now frequently used to confidently make the diagnosis and spare the infant the risk of aspirating barium from an upper gastrointestinal radiographic series (Figs. 5.16 to 5.18).

DIFFERENTIAL DIAGNOSIS

Esophageal Atresia. Vomiting begins with birth; the vomitus is uncurdled and not bile stained (Fig. 5.13).

Infectious Vomiting. Vomiting is accompanied by fever and by the signs of infective disease.

Chalasia and Achalasia. Regurgitation, rather than projectile vomiting, is the usual complaint in chalasia. In achalasia, the vomiting is not as unrelenting as in pyloric stenosis and is usually accompanied by a cough.

Pyloric and High Duodenal Atresia. Vomiting starts at birth; no pyloric mass is palpable. Differentiation is made by barium upper gastrointestinal radiologic series.

The pediatrician and pediatric surgeon should keep in mind all possible causes of disorders of gastric emptying. It is not within the scope of this chapter to discuss experimental work of impairment of gastric emptying. We refer the reader to the excellent book, *Human Gastrointestinal Development,* by Lebenthal (105). However, we present a table from that book so physicians will have a chart of possible disorders (Table 5.3). We believe that more causes will be added to this list with future research.

TREATMENT

Surgical Treatment. Pyloromyotomy (Ramstedt's operation) is the operation of choice. Dufour and Fredet (106) in France in 1907 and Weber (107) in Germany in 1908 originated the procedure, which was popularized by Ramstedt (108) in 1912.

Table 5.3.
Disorders of Gastric Emptying in the Newborn[a]

Obstruction
  Pyloric stenosis
  "Pylorospasm"
  Gastric atresia
  Antral web
  Gastric duplications
  Stomach volvulus
Disorders of motility associated with delayed gastric emptying
  Systemic disease
    Respiratory distress syndrome
    Congenital heart disease with congestive heart failure and/or
      failure to thrive
    Protein-calorie malnutrition
  Familial disautonomia
  Abnormal motility associated with GE reflux
Disorder associated with rapid gastric emptying
  Cystic fibrosis associated with pancreatic insufficiency

[a]From Siegel M, Lebenthal E. Development of gastrointestinal motility and gastric emptying during the fetal and newborn periods. In: Lebenthal E (ed). Human gastrointestinal development. New York: Raven Press, 1989, p. 286.

The operation is a simple longitudinal incision of the pyloric musculature down to the submucosa, leaving the mucosa intact. Both length and depth of the incision are important. If the incision is too short or too shallow, the obstruction will not be relieved. On the other hand, if the incision is too deep, the mucosa will be perforated. This latter risk is greater at the duodenal end where the wall is thinner. Immediate recognition of an accidental perforation is essential to prevent mortality. Simple closure of the perforation and delaying postoperative feeding for 48 hours alleviates this complication. In a properly made incision, the mucosa bulges up to the level of the incised muscular coat (Fig. 5.19).

Postoperatively, vomiting may continue for 2 or 3 days. If it persists for more than a week, the operation was inadequate.

Conservative Treatment. Before the introduction of the Ramstedt pyloromyotomy, treatment was largely conservative. Feedings of material with thick, paste-like consistency, a carefully adjusted feeding schedule, and the use of atropine-like drugs will produce good results in many cases (109, 110). Regardless of the occasional success of purely medical treatment, it entails a higher morbidity and mortality than does surgical treatment and thus is no longer considered the treatment of choice for pyloric stenosis.

MORTALITY

In recent years the mortality following pyloromyotomy has become essentially zero. Benson and Lloyd (92) reported only six deaths among 1119 patients (0.54%) operated on between 1940 and 1963. More recently,

Benson (104) reported no death in 1155 infants to undergo a pyloromyotomy.

Hypertrophic Pyloric Stenosis in Adults

Hypertrophy of the pyloric musculature in adults usually results from duodenal or gastric ulceration, yet a few cases occur in which there is no evidence of ulceration or neoplasm.

Nielsen (111) reviewed studies undertaken to determine if pyloric stenosis in adults might be a sequel to infantile pyloric stenosis. Among patients who had been treated medically for the infantile form of the disease, he found subjective evidence of gastritis and peptic ulceration in later life, more often than would be expected by chance. He concluded that in a few cases adult pyloric stenosis stems from the infantile disease; however, the rarity of the adult form indicates that such a relationship is unusual.

Approaching the problem retrospectively, Christiansen and Grantham (112) reviewed the histories of 122 adults with pyloric stenosis and concluded that a subclinical hypertrophy had existed in infancy and remained latent until later in life. However, this conclusion cannot be accepted without further evidence. Experience with patients in the eighth and ninth decades of life does not substantiate this view (Akin J. Personal communication, 1969).

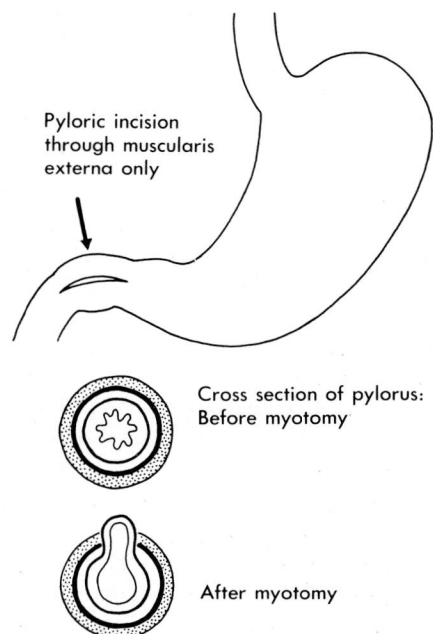

Figure 5.19. Ramstedt pyloromyotomy for infantile pyloric stenosis. The muscularis must be incised without injury to the mucosa. The incision is not sutured.

Diverticula of the Stomach (Congenital True Diverticula)

ANATOMY

Gastric diverticula may be congenital or acquired. In either group, there may be "true" diverticula (involving all layers of the stomach wall) or "false" diverticula (mucosal herniations through gaps in the muscularis externa).

Congenital True Diverticula. All the layers of the gastric wall are present, but there is no evidence of organic disease.

Acquired True Diverticula. All layers of the gastric wall are present, but evidence of disease does occur.

Congenital True Diverticula. Mucosal herniation occurs through congenitally aplastic areas of the muscularis in the newborn infant. Congenital true diverticula, which lead to early rupture of the stomach, are discussed in the section on "Congenital Defects of the Gastric Musculature."

Acquired False Diverticula. Only congenital true diverticula (group A) are of concern here. Mucosal herniation occurs through a diseased gastric wall or fistulous tract of large tumors.

The great majority of congenital true diverticula arise at a specific location on the posterior gastric wall, about 2 cm below the junction of the esophagus and stomach and about 3 cm from the lesser curvature. Palmer (113), in reviewing the reported cases up to 1951, found that 259 of 342 diverticula originated at this site. Over 50% of the remainder originated in the antrum and pylorus; the others were distributed over the rest of the stomach (Fig. 5.20). About 75% of the diverticula were less than 4 cm in length; the largest was 11 cm long. It may be difficult to distinguish these larger diverticula from communicating duplications, such as those described by Lewis and his colleagues (114).

A congenital true diverticulum of the stomach may be associated with aberrant pancreatic tissue, hiatal hernia, hourglass stomach, or diverticula in other parts of the alimentary tract.

EMBRYOGENESIS

True diverticula have been explained as persistence of the embryonic diverticula described by Lewis and Thyng (115). While a few gastric diverticula may originate in this manner, the larger number found on the posterior wall of the cardia cannot be accounted for with this hypothesis. Local muscle weakness at this point has not been shown, but even if it did exist, we would expect herniation of the mucosa and submucosa to form false rather than true diverticula.

The behavior of certain diverticula, such as the one found by Hartley (116), which descended with filling until

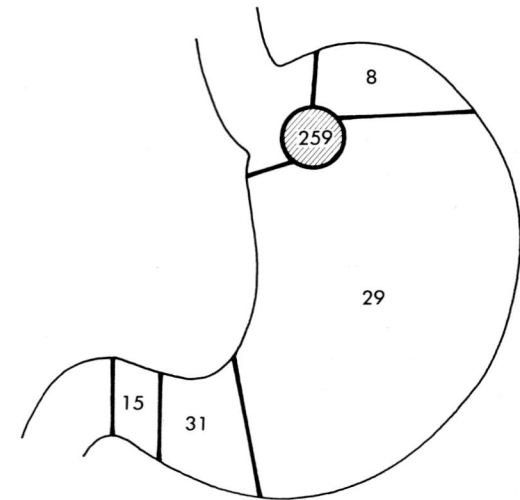

Figure 5.20. Locations of 342 diverticula of the stomach. Most are located on the *posterior wall* of the upper part of the stomach. (Data from Palmer ED. Gastric diverticula. Surg Obstet Gynecol 1951;43:432–443.)

it entered an inguinal hernial sac and retracted out of sight during emptying of the stomach, suggests an abnormality of elastic tissue rather than of muscle. Occasional reports have mentioned similar diverticula seen radiographically in the full stomach (117), but these were not found in the empty organ at operation.

Gastric diverticula occur normally in some mammals, but all appear to be species adaptations that are without phylogenetic significance. No claim for atavism is tenable.

At present, true gastric diverticula that show no evidence of local inflammation must be considered to be of embryonic origin, but only for lack of other rational etiologies. This is a negative—and by no means a convincing—argument.

HISTORY

The first true gastric diverticulum was described in 1793 by Baillie (118), who found at autopsy a gastric pouch containing five halfpence. This was a peculiar example of an acquired pulsion diverticulum. No further case appears to have been described until 1895. The case Helmont described in 1804 is an error perpetuated by recopying (119).

Zahn (120) in 1899 first observed a diverticular stoma by gastroscopy and thus probably made the first ante mortem diagnosis. The first radiographic diagnosis appears to have been made by Brown (121) in 1916.

Martin (119), reviewing the literature in 1936, found 92 cases. Palmer (113) found 412 cases by 1951, and Sommer and Goodrich (122) collected 449 cases in 1953. Interestingly, there was a period between 1915 and 1930 when many European writers denied the existence of gastric diverticula (119).

INCIDENCE

Palmer (113), using the figures available in 1951, found an incidence of 0.0043% in hospital admissions, 0.020% in routine autopsies, 0.043% in routine barium radiographic series, 0.089% in stomach operations, and 0.30% in gastroscopic examinations.

Sommer and Goodrich (122) observed an increase in the rate of discovery of diverticula with increasing interest in hiatal hernia. Examination of patients in various positions, with frequent reexamination, revealed nine cases among 5110 gastric examinations in 1952, while only eight cases had been found in 44,870 examinations during the preceding 10 years. This increase in incidence—from 0.018% to 0.18%—makes it obvious that many gastric diverticula go undetected.

Diverticula are rarer in the stomach than elsewhere in the alimentary tract. About 3% of all diverticula are gastric, 9% are esophageal, and about 68% are colonic; the remainder occur in the small intestines.

Sex. Palmer (113) found 174 males (56.5%) among 318 cases in which sex was given.

Age. Diverticula are most frequently seen in the fifth decade of life; 66% occur between the ages of 40 and 70 years. Only 10 patients under 10 years of age were reported before 1951 (113); two were embryos (119). A diverticulum of the greater curvature has been reported in an 11-week-old infant (123), and an intussuscepted, perforated diverticulum was found in a newborn infant (124). In both of these patients all layers of the stomach wall appeared to be present in the diverticula. Another report of perforated diverticulum in a newborn infant appears to have been of the false type (125).

SYMPTOMS

From 66 (122) to 85% (126) of gastric diverticula give no symptoms, being found incidentally on examination for other diseases or at autopsy. When symptoms are present, the patient may have epigastric or lower chest pain with or without vomiting or so-called indigestion.

DIAGNOSIS

Since no unequivocal clinical symptoms appear, the diagnosis of a gastric diverticulum depends on the radiologist. Roentgenograms taken with the patient in a variety of positions often are necessary. The appearance is that of a smoothly rounded, sharply defined, mobile pouch, frequently containing an air bubble above the barium. Emptying is usually but not always delayed (116). Radiologically visible diverticula have occasionally been impossible to find at surgery, and conversely, some found at surgery had never been visible on x-ray examination, probably because of food retained in the sac.

Fiberoptic endoscopy reveals a round hole with sharp edges, and active contractions of the diverticular mouth have been seen. There usually is no local alteration in the pattern of rugae.

Differential Diagnosis. A congenital true diverticulum must be distinguished from an ulcer niche, a covered perforation of gastric ulcer, advanced cystic degeneration of a gastric smooth muscle tumor (acquired false diverticulum, type D, [127]), ulceration of carcinoma, hiatal hernia, and hypertrophic gastric folds.

It is probably impossible to distinguish radiologically between congenital and acquired true diverticula (types A and B). Congenital false diverticula (type C) occur in newborn infants and usually are seen only after perforation has taken place.

Although ulcers frequently are found in diverticula, there appears to be no unusual association with gastric disease. An apparent relationship may be observed because diverticula frequently are found during an examination of the stomach for other diseases. This also seems to be true when diverticula of the duodenum or colon are found (128). Malignancy is sometimes associated with diverticula at the pylorus but not at the cardia.

TREATMENT

If one is sure that the symptoms of the patient are attributable to the diverticulum and not to any other clinical entity, then the treatment, if necessary, must be surgical. A diverticulum of the distal stomach, even if asymptomatic, should be considered a surgical problem because of the malignant changes occasionally seen with such diverticula.

The search for cardinal diverticula involves Walters' procedure of dividing the gastrocolic omentum and turning the fundus upward and medially through the incision to expose the posterior surface (129). The decision for amputation, invagination, or segmental gastric resection is up to the surgeon.

MORTALITY

The greatest danger is that of perforation of a diverticulum. Spontaneous rupture of a congenital true diverticulum is extremely rare: Palmer (113) was able to find only three cases in the literature. In contrast, false diverticula perforate readily. In either case—indeed, in any perforation of the stomach—the outlook is grave and immediate surgical repair is indicated.

Duplication of the Stomach

Duplications of the alimentary tract are named for the structures with which they are associated rather than for the mucosal lining within them. Thus a superior mediastinal cyst containing gastric mucosa must be considered a duplication of the esophagus and not of the stomach. This system is convenient because more than one mucosal type may be present and because pressure atrophy may have destroyed the epithelium. It is also embryologically sound since the duplication usually is formed before differentiation of the epithelium into characteristic adult types. Duplications of the stomach are thus parallel to, contiguous with, or even in communication with the normal stomach.

ANATOMY

Duplications of the stomach vary from the unique case of Gjörup (130), in which there was doubling of the entire esophagus and stomach, to the presence of small intramural cysts beneath the muscularis externa of the stomach wall. Between these extremes are those duplications that are larger or smaller than the normal stomach and share a common wall with it and which may or may not have a communicating opening (131).

The great majority of gastric duplications are located on the greater curvature or on the anterior or posterior walls. Among 54 duplications, Lewis and his colleagues (114) and Bartels (132) found only five associated with the lesser curvature. In two of the cases connections occurred at each end of the duplication (Fig. 5.21) (133, 134). Almost certainly, these smaller duplications on the lesser curvature (primitive ventral surface) were the original main foregut channel, and the functional stomach represents the true duplication on the greater curvature (primitive dorsal surface).

When present, a communication may open below the stomach into the duodenum (133, 135), into Meckel's diverticulum (136), or directly into the stomach (131). One remarkable duplication opened into the gastric antrum and received multiple ducts from the pancreas, to which the duplication was attached. The original diagnosis was pancreatic pseudocyst (137). Communication between the duplication and the normal stomach is not the rule; the majority of gastric duplications are spheric or ovoid closed cysts.

The mucosal lining is usually gastric, but pseudostratified respiratory epithelium has been found (138). In these instances (114, 139, 140), pancreatic tissue was present in the wall of the duplication. In closed cystic duplications, the epithelial lining is often atrophic or completely destroyed by pressure.

Most gastric duplications are less than 12 cm in their largest diameter; about 25% are larger. They occur singly, although associated esophageal intestinal duplications are not rare (132). In only three cases have vertebral anomalies, commonly seen with esophageal duplications, been reported (141). Dressler et al. (142) described complete foregut duplication (complete esophageal and gastric duplication) in a 53-year-old male who was practically asymptomatic.

EMBRYOGENESIS

Only the small gastric cysts lying within the submucosa or the muscularis can be explained by Bremer's theory (143) of persistent vacuoles within the primitive foregut epithelium. A few larger intramural cystic duplications, especially those located on the lesser curvature, may result from the persistent embryonic diverticula seen by Lewis and Thyng (115). Larger duplications—and certainly all those lying outside the normal stomach wall—are the result of faulty separation of endoderm and notochord early in development, such as described by McLetchie and his colleagues (144) and others. When the amount of endodermal tissue detached from the main endodermal sheet is large, the displaced tissue may organize itself into a more or less complete simulacrum of normal esophagus and stomach.

Other foregut duplications are discussed in Chapter 3 (duplications of the esophagus), and a more extensive consideration of endodermal duplication in general is given in Chapter 6 (duplications of the small intestines).

HISTORY

The first case described was that of a 30-year-old woman, reported by Wendel (145) in 1911. No more were discovered until those of Pancotto (146) in 1927 and Cabot (147) in 1928. Dornier (148) in 1959 could find only four European cases. Lewis and his colleagues (114) and Bartels (132) reviewed the literature. The latter considered his case to be the 55th reported. That this anomaly was not noted before the present century and occurs so rarely in the European literature is most remarkable. There must be few such striking defects with not a single case being reported in *Virchows Archiv*.

Bower et al. (149) reported five gastric duplications out of 62 cases. Kalongi and Steiner (150) described duplication in adults, and Orr and Edwards (151) described the development of carcinoma in a gastric duplication. Cystocolic fistula is reported by Izant (152). Gastric duplication not attached to the stomach but attached to other organs and contained in gastric mucosa was reported by Curran et al. (153), Gonzalez and Martinez (154), and Hélardot (155).

Perforation of duplication as well as bleeding was reported by Kleinhaus et al. (156).

Several papers (157–162) have emphasized the association of congenital gastric duplications with pulmonary sequestration. Communication between the two pathologies is not a rare phenomenon. We, however, wonder if these are real duplications of the stomach or bronchogenic cysts that communicate with the stomach. We believe that a cyst attached to the stomach, lesser omentum, or gastrocolic ligament is most likely gastric duplication or perhaps a mesenteric cyst.

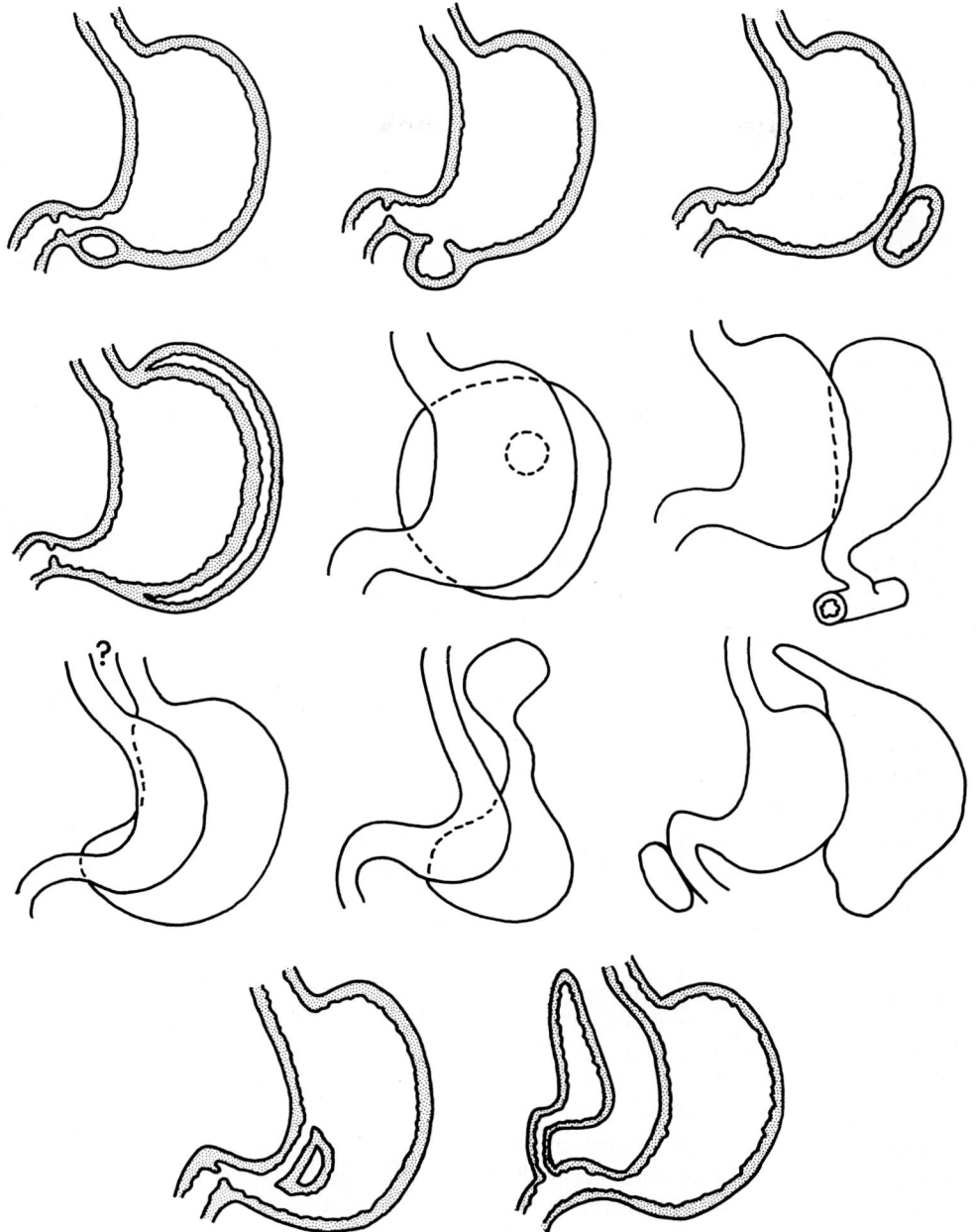

Figure 5.21. Duplication of the stomach. These rare lesions differ widely, so that few generalizations are possible. Those in the *top row* are probably more common.

INCIDENCE

As with diverticula, duplications of the stomach are less frequent than duplications of other segments of the alimentary tract. In a series of admissions ranging over more than 20 years at the Children's Hospital in Boston, Gross (163) found 68 duplications of the gut, of which two were in the stomach. In a similar series at the Children's Hospital in Pittsburgh, four gastric duplications were seen among 25 gastrointestinal tract duplications (164).

Nearly twice as many females as males are affected. The majority of cases are recognized in the first year of life, but many have not been diagnosed until maturity. One of the youngest patients, treated by hemigastrectomy for duplication of the stomach, was 5 weeks of age; this patient has since developed normally. The oldest patient was 67 years of age (165). Recently, Luks et al. (166) presented a case in a 23-year-old man of gastric duplication, not communicating with the stomach but heavily fixed to the greater curvature. The lining of this cyst was pancreatic ductal epithelium.

SYMPTOMS

The clinical picture produced by gastric duplication depends on the size, location, and presence or absence of communication with the rest of the alimentary tract.

In infants a palpable mass is usually present and is accompanied by vomiting and weight loss or failure to thrive. Infantile pyloric stenosis may be diagnosed when the duplication lies near the pylorus (167).

In older patients epigastric pain, a sensation of fullness, melena, and weight loss are frequent findings. Shaw's (165) 67-year-old patient had symptoms for only 4 months, and many other patients show symptoms only late in life. In view of this, undetected and undiagnosed cases undoubtedly exist. Bleeding is usually from a peptic ulcer in the duplication. One case of carcinoma in a gastric duplication has been reported (168).

DIAGNOSIS

When communication exists, the duplication may be visualized radiologically with barium. If there is no communication, the compression produced by the duplication may be detected. An ultrasound examination may disclose the cystic nature of the duplication causing the compression on the greater curvature of the stomach. The radiologic picture may mimic that of congenital pyloric stenosis and a palpable epigastric mass may be present (131, 167). One infant had congenital pyloric stenosis as well as a small pyloric duplication cyst, which complicated the picture (169). Though it is rare, duplication should be included in the differential diagnosis of disease caused by compression of the upper gastrointestinal tract.

Among older patients, primary benign or malignant neoplasms of the stomach, liver, or duodenum are usually the first lesions to be suspected. Anas and Miller (170) stated that a pyloric duplication could masquerade as hypertrophic pyloric stenosis. An ulcerated gastric diverticulum may rupture and communicate with the abdominal wall, pancreas, and lungs (171–173). The most useful diagnostic study is sonography, but if in doubt, a computed tomogram (CT) of the abdomen should be the next step. Koltun (174) was the first to diagnose a gastric duplication cyst by endoscopy.

TREATMENT

Removal of the entire duplication is the ideal treatment. However, the presence of a common muscular wall between the diverticulum and the normal stomach may

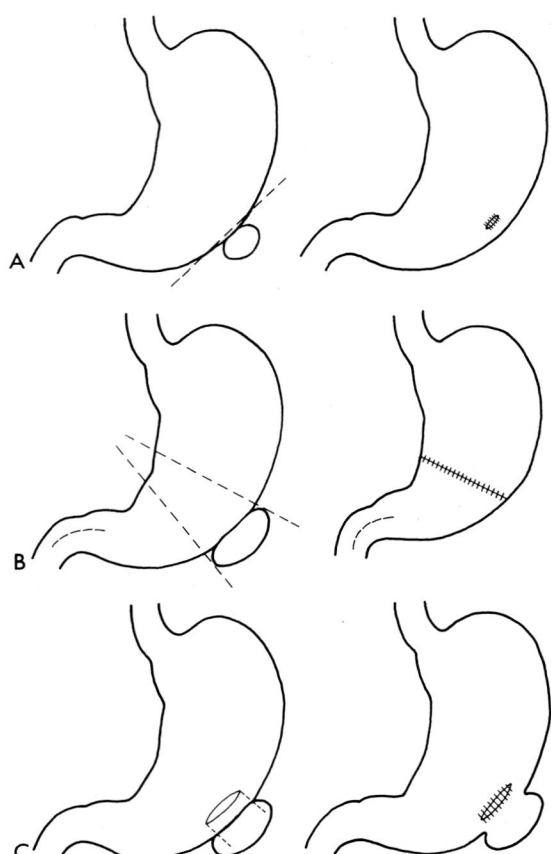

Figure 5.22. Three procedures for treatment of small gastric duplications. **A,** Excision of the duplication and closure of the gastric wall. **B,** Partial gastrectomy and pyloroplasty. **C,** Gastrotomy with cystogastrostomy with or without mucosal striping.

make this unfeasible. When complete excision is not practical, the following alternatives are available:

1. If the area of common gastric wall is small, the entire duplication may be removed, together with a portion of normal gastric wall. The resulting defect in the stomach may be treated as a gastrostomy and closed as such (Fig. 5.22, A).
2. If the defect is too large, a partial gastrectomy (Fig. 5.22, B) or stripping of the mucosa, as advocated by White and Morgan (175), may be indicated.
3. Excision of the common wall between the duplication and the normal stomach (cystogastrostomy) may be successful, especially if an opening is already present or if accumulated pressure within the diverticulum has not injured its mucosa (Fig. 5.22, C).

EDITORIAL COMMENT

Whatever the specific etiology of gastric perforation, it is mandatory that the diagnosis be made as quickly as possible because the mortality is directly related to the delay in diagnosis and definitive treatment. Mortality is associated with overwhelming sepsis and this can be prevented by early diagnosis and proper treatment. In most cases following closure of the gastric perforation, a gastrostomy is useful to be sure the stomach has not become distended and resulted in leakage of the closed gastric perforation. In a few instances, a nasogastric tube may be an appropriate alternative to gastrostomy but the tube should be a soft plastic material and carefully positioned because stiffer nasogastric tubes have been implicated in the primary gastric perforation (JAH/CNP)!

4. Where resection is impractical, marsupialization may be mandatory (141). However distasteful it is to the surgeon, this may be a life-saving procedure.

Among the 54 cases reviewed by Bartels (132), 15 were treated by excision of the cyst, 9 by excision and removal of a margin of normal stomach, and 10 by partial gastric resection. Six patients underwent cystogastrostomy, and in five, marsupialization was performed. There were four deaths among the 54 operations.

Congenital Defects of the Gastric Musculature

ANATOMY
Insufficiency of the musculature of the stomach wall may be expressed as a general thinning of all muscle coats (176) or, more frequently, as areas of complete absence of the muscularis externa, which is of normal thickness elsewhere over the stomach. In such areas the wall consists of only the mucosa, submucosa, and serosa, and the muscle coat ends abruptly at the margin of the defect (177). Such muscular defects lead to spontaneous rupture of the stomach shortly after birth.

Sixty-six percent of these defects have been found on the greater curvature of the stomach; most of the remainder occur on the anterior or posterior wall. Two have been found on the lesser curvature. Multiple perforations through separate defects have also been seen (178) (Fig. 5.23).

EMBRYOGENESIS
The muscular defects of the stomach appear to result from failure of myoblast formation to keep pace with the enlarging endodermal tube during differentiation of the muscularis in the third month or later. As might be expected, it is the greater curvature—the region of fastest growth—that is most frequently affected. Some authors state that the longitudinal muscle coat in this region has not completed its development at birth (179). Many of the affected infants are premature, and it is possible that, if rupture through the defect does not occur soon after birth, the muscularis eventually covers the weak area and the danger of rupture disappears.

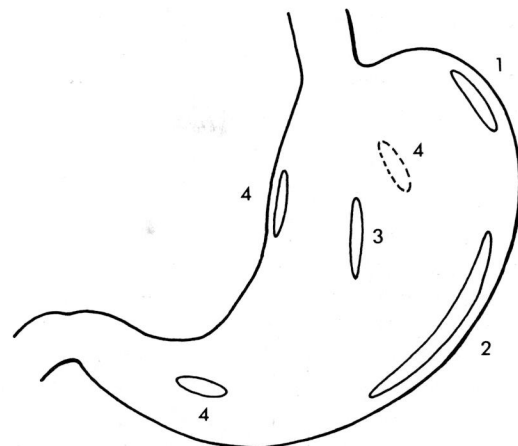

Figure 5.23. Location of spontaneous rupture through congenital defects of the gastric musculature. *Numbers* indicate the order of frequency; over half occur on the greater curvature.

Increased intragastric pressure caused by a distal congenital obstruction of the gastrointestinal tract may cause rupture of an already weakened gastric wall in a few patients (178). However, none of the associated embryonic defects suggest a generalized smooth muscle deficiency.

Shaw and his colleagues (180) denied the existence of congenital muscular defects. On the basis of experimental distension of the stomach in puppies and in human infant cadavers, they believe that distension spreads the muscle bundles and that retraction of the muscularis after rupture gives a false appearance of a muscular defect. The potential weak points between muscle bundles actually are normal, and rupture is the result of excessive stretching of the wall. The questions remain of whether this a congenital defect or bacterial colonization of the gastrointestinal tract and whether it is a mechanical phenomenon of severe gastric distention or just a trauma occurring during delivery or ischemic necrosis? The authors do not have the answers. Gastric perforation in the newborn could represent a localized "necrosed enterocolitis" caused by ischemic necrosis and/or bacterial colonization or a mechanical phenomenon resulting from compression of a full stomach during delivery (181, 182).

HISTORY AND INCIDENCE
Perforation of the stomach was first mentioned in 1825 by von Siebold (183), and Brody (184) in 1940 first described the congenital muscular defect. Vargas and his associates (117) reviewed the subject in 1955, and by 1964 Inouye and Evans (178) were able to collect 143 cases of neonatal gastric perforation, of which they considered 34 to be the result of muscular defects.

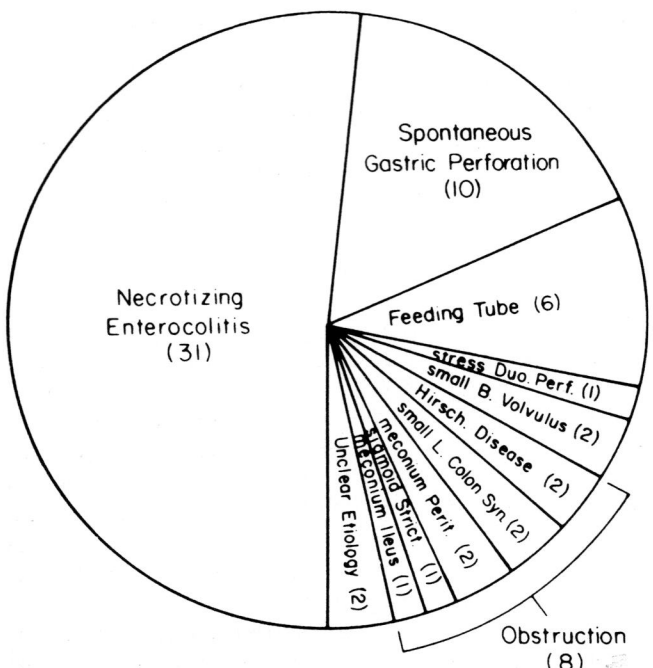

Figure 5.24. Various causes of neonatal gastrointestinal tract perforation. (Reprinted by permission from Bell MJ. Perforation of the gastrointestinal tract and peritonitis in the neonate. Surg Gynecol Obstet 1985;160(1):20–26.)

Muscle wall defects account for about 25% of perinatal gastric perforations. Ulcers, trauma by catheter, and distal obstruction account for about 33%. However, in another 33% of reported cases, no cause could be found at either operation or necropsy (178).

More males than females are affected, and patients frequently were premature. More cases have been reported among blacks than among whites (183). There is a high percentage of cases among twins, but usually only one member is affected (178). One report mentioned rupture of the stomach in two siblings of the same family (186).

In 1969 Lloyd (187) selected 315 cases from the world literature concerning perforation of the gastrointestinal tract in newborn babies. All were ischemic lesions (187). In 1985 Bell (188, 189) studied 60 neonates with perforations of the gastrointestinal tract. Ten of them had gastric spontaneous perforations (Figs. 5.24 and 5.25). Steves and Ricketts (190) reported three cases of gastric perforation among 53 infants presenting with pneumoperitoneum (6%). Excluding necrotizing enterocolitis, gastric perforation accounted for 25% of the patients with perforation treated at Cook County Hospital and Children's Memorial Hospital in Chicago (182). Holgersen (191) stated that gastric perforation is caused by over-

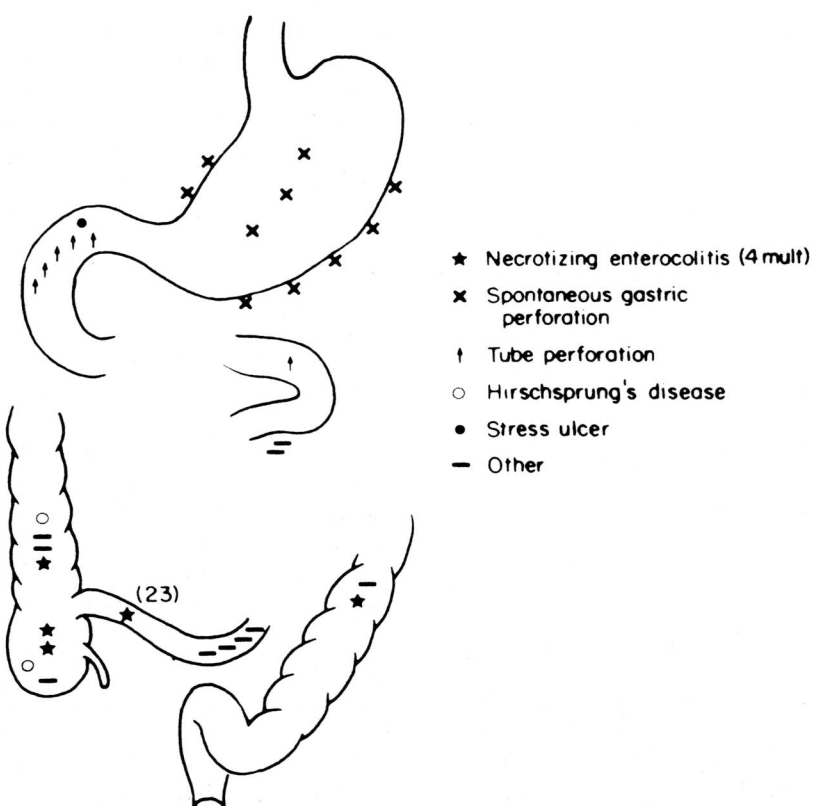

Figure 5.25. Sites of perforation in the neonate. (Reprinted by permission from Bell MJ. Perforation of the gastrointestinal tract and peritonitis in the neonate. Surg Gynecol Obstet 1985;160(1):20–26.)

distension. A predominance of the defect in black infants was reported by Rosser et al. (193).

SYMPTOMS

Rupture may occur from 12 hours to 12 days after birth; most take place between the third and fifth days.

Sudden abdominal distension, with or without vomiting, marks the onset of rupture of the stomach. The abdomen is tense but soft; there is no liver dullness and no bowel sounds. Nasogastric suction does not relieve the distension. Limitation of diaphragmatic excursion as a result of the distension may produce dyspnea and cyanosis and lead to rapid respiratory compromise unless the abdomen is decompressed.

DIAGNOSIS

The chief diagnostic sign of gastric perforation is the presence of massive air and fluid in the abdomen, which is demonstrated by plain erect and supine radiographics of gastric perforation (Figs. 5.26 and 5.27). Since death usually results from respiratory failure or peritonitis rather than from the surgical repair, the best prognosis follows when early diagnosis and decompression is accomplished followed by definitive surgical correction.

TREATMENT

The first attempt at repair was unsuccessful (193), but Selinger (194) repaired a perforated stomach in a 3-month-old infant in 1932 and Légar and his colleagues saved a newborn child in 1950. Thirty-nine survivals were reported up to 1964 (178).

Repair of the perforation and cleaning of the peritoneum should be undertaken as soon as the diagnosis has been made. If no perforation can be found on the anterior wall of the stomach, the surgeon must be prepared to open the lesser sac and examine the posterior wall. Multiple perforation must also be considered.

The repaired stomach should be filled with saline solution by catheter to test for leakage and possible distal obstruction. Isolated gastric perforations promptly treated by surgery and antibiotic therapy have better prognoses than perforations of the small bowel and colon.

Malposition of the Stomach

The most dramatic form of malposition of the stomach is found in situs inversus viscerum. Here, the stomach appears normal but completely reversed right to left. In examining x-ray films, the surgeon should be careful not to immediately turn the film over as soon as he or she sees a barium-filled stomach on the right side without checking the markings. In rare cases only the stomach is involved in malposition (196), but usually all the abdominal viscera are affected.

Inversion of the stomach, in which the cardia is lower than the pylorus, may occur, with eventration of the left side of the diaphragm (197–199). A few cases of inversion without diaphragmatic anomaly have been described

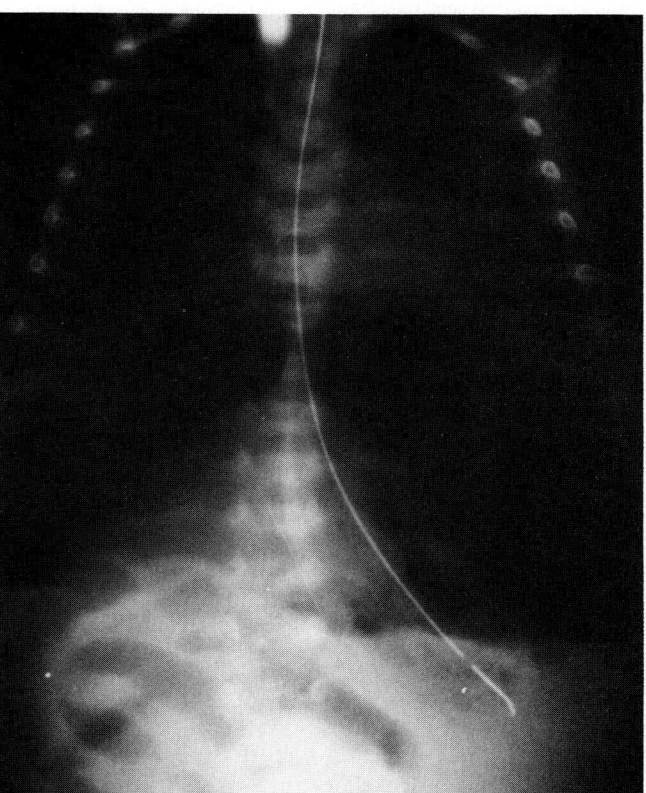

Figure 5.27. Upright (kidney, ureter, and bladder) x-ray film with gastric perforation and free intraperitoneal air.

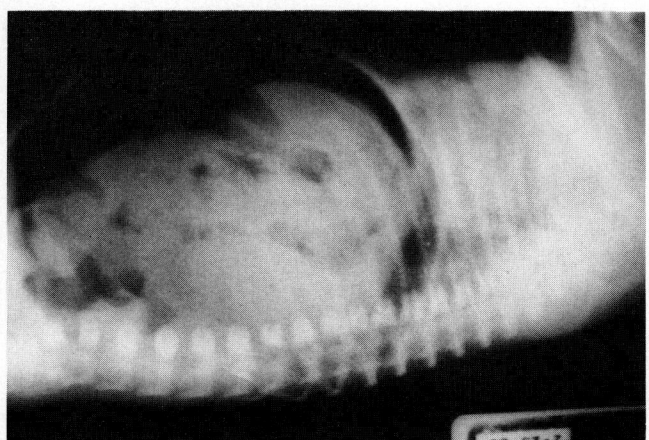

Figure 5.26. Lateral x-ray film showing massive pneumoperiforams section to gastric performation.

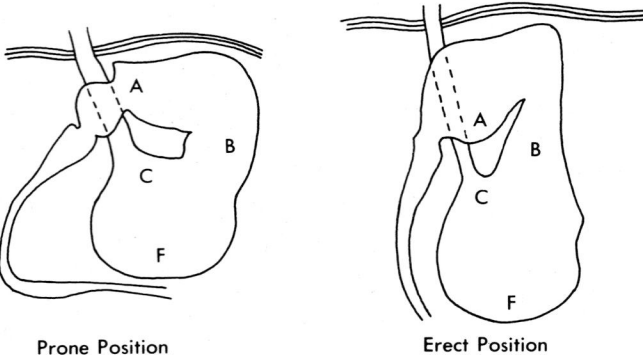

Prone Position   **Erect Position**

Figure 5.28. Inversion of the stomach. Tracings from radiographs of a 65-year-old woman. **A**, Antrum. **B**, Body. **C**, Cardia. **F**, Fundus. (From Rhinehart BA, Rhinehart DA. Congenital abnormalities of the stomach. Radiology 1926;7:492–497.)

(200) (Fig. 5.28). One was recognized radiographically at Piedmont Hospital, Atlanta, in a 16-year-old girl with a history of intermittent upper abdominal pain and emesis since infancy (Akin J. Personal communication, 1969). The congenital nature of these cases is probable but not certain.

Variations in the normal *position* of the stomach were discussed by Moody and his colleagues in 1929 (201); these are not true congenital anomalies. Gastric volvulus can occur when there is laxity or absence of the normal stomach attachment (gastrophrenic and gastrocolic ligament, etc.) (Fig. 5.29). The volvulus can be either organoaxial, along its long axis (Fig. 5.30), or mesenterioaxial (Fig. 5.31), around a vertical line that is at a right angle to the line joining the gastric cardia to the pylorus. The diagnosis is made by plain abdominal radiographs and upper gastrointestinal radiographic series (Fig. 5.32). *Gastric volvulus is a surgical emergency.* The stomach should be decompressed, the volvulus should be reduced, and the stomach fixed to the anterior wall by a gastrostomy or gastrorrhaphy (181). Although rare, Senocak et al. (202) described 21 children treated for gastric volvulus between 1977 and 1987.

Chaudhuri (203) and Hewlett (204) reported dextrogastria.

Gastric Mucosal Heterotopia

The stomach is the donor as well as the receiver. As an immigrant, the gastric mucosa may build its nest in any part of the gastrointestinal tract, and the gastric wall itself welcomes travelers from other organs. The heterotopic tissue has all the histologic characteristics of the mother-donor organ and, physiologically as well as pathologically, follows the tissues of its origin. Both the ectopic gland and the gland of origin will share the same pathology.

We agree, therefore, with Simstein (205) that these congenital abnormalities, from other organs to the stom-

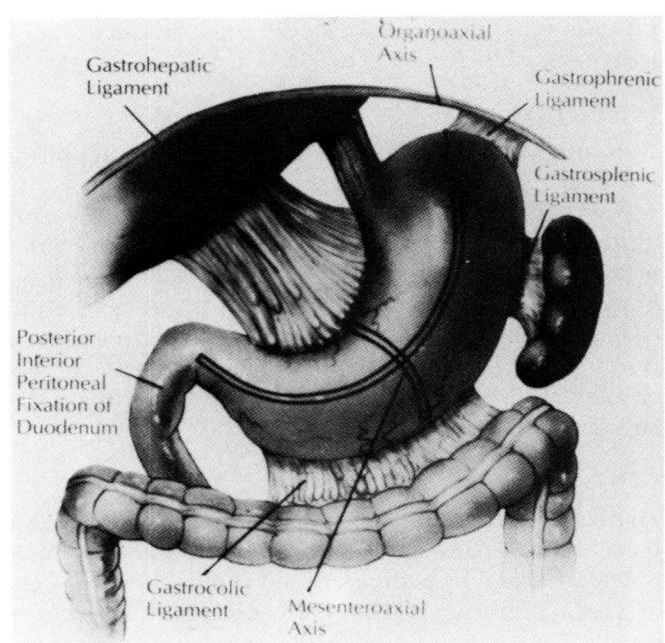

Figure 5.29. Ligamental attachments of the stomach include the gastrophrenic, gastrohepatic, gastrocolic, and gastrosplenic. Inferiorly, the stomach is anchored by the second portion of the duodenum. Axes of the stomach include the mesenteroaxial (short) and the organoaxial (long). (From Miller DL, Pasquale MD, Seneca RP, Hodin E. Gastric volvulus in the pediatric population. Arch Surg 1991;126:1148.)

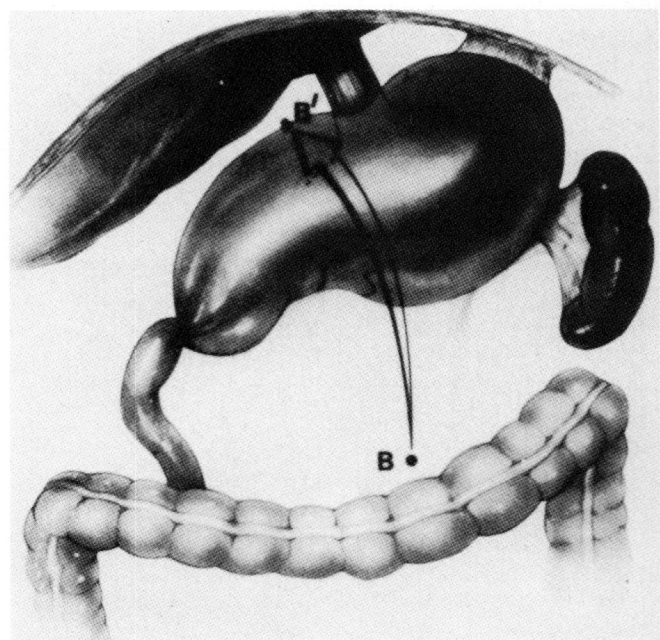

Figure 5.30. Diagram of an organoaxial volvulus. Rotation (*B* to *B'*) occurs about the long axis of the stomach. (From Miller DL, Pasquale MD, Seneca RP, Hodin E. Gastric volvulus in the pediatric population. Arch Surg 1991;126:1148.)

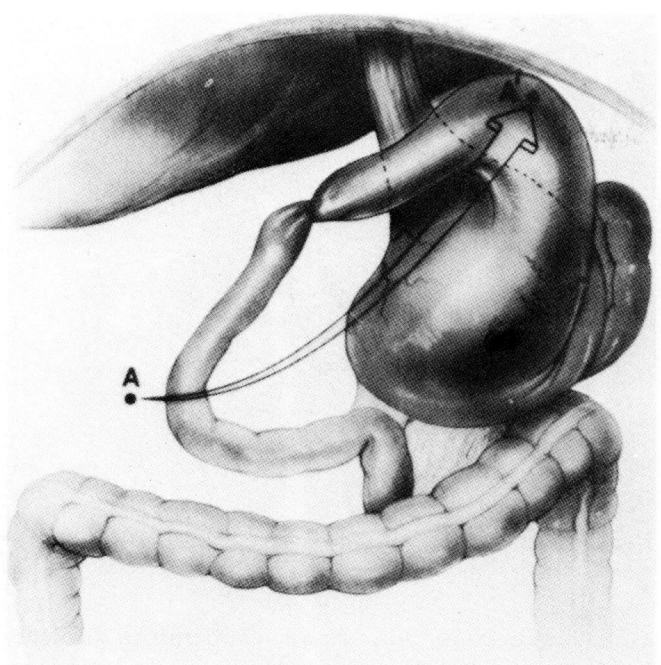

Figure 5.31. Diagram of gastric mesenteroaxial volvulus. Rotation (A to A') occurs about the short axis of the stomach. (From Miller DL, Pasquale MD, Seneca RP, Hodin E. Gastric volvulus in the pediatric population. Arch Surg 1991;126:1147.)

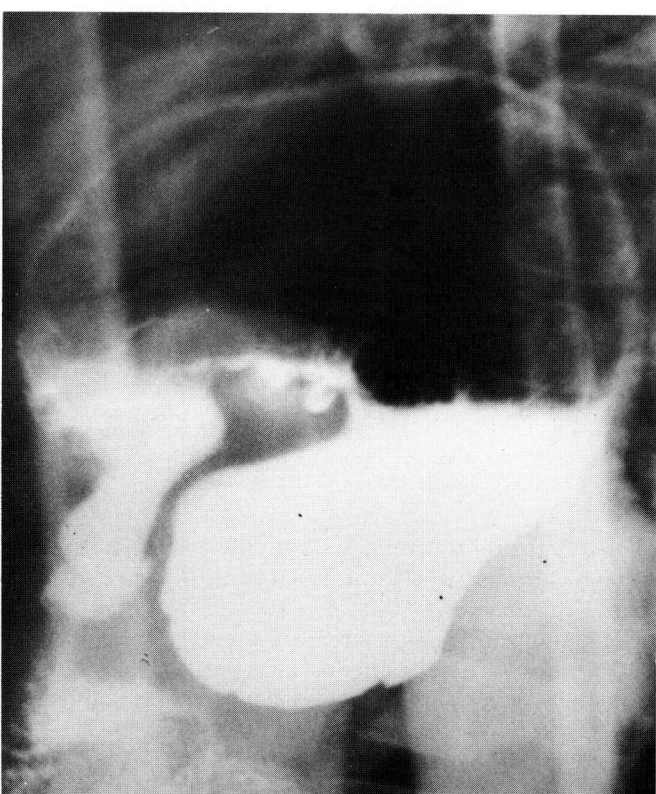

Figure 5.32. Upper gastrointestinal radiographic series demonstrating gastric volvulus.

ach and from the stomach to other organs, involve two distinct entities under the one name. Gastric mucosal heterotopia is a very common anomaly, if not the most common.

FROM OTHER ORGANS TO THE STOMACH

The most common heterotopic tissue in the gastric wall is from the pancreas. Duodenal and jejunal mucosa are occasionally present in the normal stomach as well as in gastric duplications. Gastric heterotopic pancreas was reported by Barrocas et al. (206).

Anatomy. Glandular structures with or without a duct system are often encountered in the stomach wall. Variously designated as "aberrant pancreas," "heterotopic pancreas," "adenomyoma," "Brunner's adenoma," or "myoepithelial hamartoma," all may be considered potentially pancreatic in origin. These structures have been divided by Clarke (207) into three historic types:

1. Aberrant pancreas with true pancreatic acini; possible presence of islet cells (208, 209)
2. Incompletely differentiated aberrant pancreas with some pancreatic acini; other acini of Brunner's glands or undifferentiated tissue
3. Adenomyoma with Brunner's glands only or with undifferentiated glandular tissue; heterotopic duodenal mucosa (210)

All are of the same origin, and the first two may have more or less extensive duct systems. In a few cases only duct tissue may be present. Debard and colleagues (211) reported unusual locations of pancreatic tissue in the stomach with multiple foci.

Heterotopic masses vary in size from less than 1 mm to 5 cm in diameter. The majority are between 0.6 and 3 cm (212). More than one such formation may be present.

Symptomatic pancreatic heterotopias are usually 1 to 2 cm in diameter. They may be spheric, ovoid, lenticular, or disc shaped. A navel-like area of gastric mucosa marks the location of the heterotopic tissue. The margins may be elevated, and the central depression, which is the orifice of the duct, may be large enough to be termed a *pseudodiverticulum.* Although heterotopias may be found throughout the stomach, the bulk of them occur in the distal half (Fig. 5.33).

About 75% are submucosal; 15% occur in the muscularis and 10% in the subserosa. Submucosal masses often form conical, polypoid, or nipple-like projections of the gastric wall. One or more ducts may form a grossly visible opening on the summit of these projections, although occasionally the opening may be at a distance from the body of glandular tissue. Lauche (213) used the term

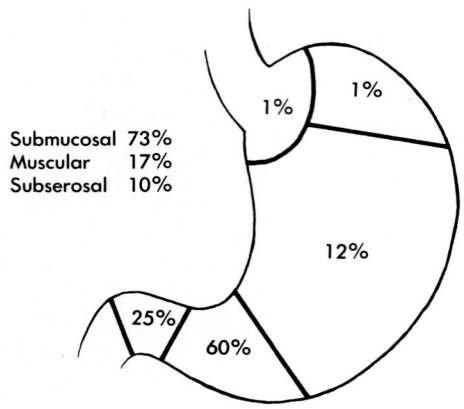

Figure 5.33. Distribution of heterotopic pancreas tissue in the stomach. (Data from Palmer ED. Benign intramural tumors of the stomach: a review with special reference to gross pathology. Medicine 1951;30:81–86.)

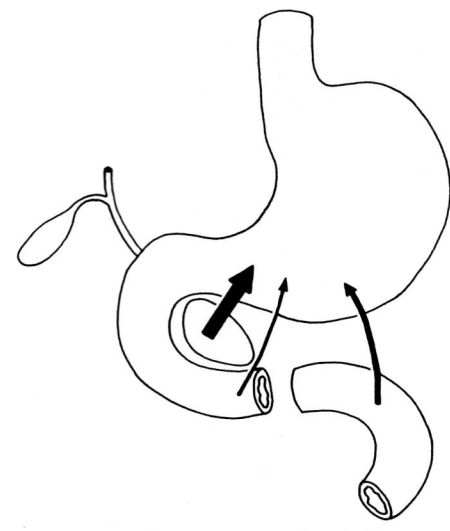

Figure 5.34. Sources of heterotopic tisues found in the stomach. Thickness of *arrows* indicates relative frequency.

organoids for those connected with the gastric lumen by a duct and *chorista* for those isolated in the wall. In rare cases cysts may form.

Histologically, the pancreatic tissue is normal, though a larger proportion of duct tissue is present than is usual in the pancreas itself. Islets are present in only about 33% of heterotopias examined.

A peculiar form of diffuse cystic disease affecting nearly half of the gastric wall has been reported (214, 215). Some of the cysts resemble Brunner's glands, but pancreatic acini are absent. This may possibly represent a true duodenal heterotopia of the stomach (Fig. 5.34).

Embryogenesis. Translocation of embryonic pancreas cells and metaplasia in situ have both been postulated to explain heterotopic pancreatic structures in the stomach. Details of these theories are discussed in Chapter 11.

Heterotopic intestinal epithelium—that is, columnar epithelial cells having a striated border and interspersed with goblet cells—are certainly of metaplastic origin. Such metaplasia has been attributed to chronic irritation from gastritis by Magnus (216), partly because he considered them to be present in adults only. Salenius (5) found such cells to be abundant in the pylorus and cardia of fetuses and found them present occasionally even after birth. The metaplasia, therefore, is similar to a primitive epithelial type widespread in the embryonic gut rather than like specific intestinal epithelium.

Associated Anomalies. Areas of aberrant pancreas may be associated with gastric diverticula. Palmer (212) observed that 9% of gastric pancreatic tissue is found in diverticula and that 11% of all gastric diverticula contain pancreatic tissue. In only one instance has a cardiac diverticulum been so affected. Bolognesi (217) produced diverticula experimentally in dogs, using subserous transplants of pancreatic tissue. Gruhn et al. (218) reported a nonpancreatic gastric hamartoma in the stomach.

History. The first histologically confirmed case of pancreatic tissue in the stomach was described in Vienna by

Klob (219) in 1959, although a similar lesion in the ileum had been reported about 125 years earlier. In 1903 Magnus-Alsleben (220) described the gradation of epithelial elements from undifferentiated tissue to mature pancreatic acini. Impressed with the proliferation of smooth muscle, he designated the formations *adenomyomata*.

Barbosa and his colleagues (221) reported 125 cases up to 1944; Busard and Walters (222) in 1950 brought the number to 149; Palmer (212) in 1951 found 215 cases in the world literature; and Nelson and Scott (223) collected 40 more by 1958.

Incidence. After the duodenum, the stomach is the most common site of pancreatic heterotopia. Barbosa and his colleagues (221) estimated that this condition may be found twice in every 1000 upper abdominal operations (0.2%) and that it is clinically significant in about 60% of such patients. The frequency with which it is reported from autopsies varies with the diligence with which it is sought, but it appears to be present in about 2% or more of individuals examined. If we combine these estimates, we can conclude that only 10 of 100 existing pancreatic heterotopias are seen at surgery, and only six of these are clinically symptomatic.

EDITORIAL COMMENT

Ectopic gastric mucosa in a Meckel's diverticulum is very important clinically because it is the secretion of gastric juice from the ectopic mucosa that is responsible for two of the three major complications of Meckel's diverticulum, mainly, perforation and massive bleeding. Meckel's diverticulitis is probably due to infection in the diverticulum and therefore not related to the ectopic gastric mucosa. Ulceration and perforation nearly always occur opposite the ectopic gastric mucosa as though the acid secretion is touching the opposite mucosa and causes a direct digestion and perforation.

Ulceration with bleeding is also usually "kissing" the ectopic gastric mucosa. These two complications, perforation and bleeding, are not seen in the absence of ectopic gastric mucosa (JAH/CNP).

Rarely reported in children (224), gastric pancreatic heterotopia is usually asymptomatic until the fourth or fifth decade of life. Among Palmer's collected cases (212), 62% of patients were between 30 and 50 years of age. About 66% were male.

Symptoms. Epigastric pain is the presenting complaint in 75% of symptomatic cases. It may arise from pylorospasm resulting from the passage of food, from the ulceration caused by pancreatic enzymes, from infection, or from actual obstruction (225). Lucaya and Ochoa (226) agree that the most frequent complaint is epigastric pain. Vomiting and weight loss over a long period of time has been reported (227). Rarely, the presenting symptom is massive upper gastrointestinal hemorrhage secondary to ulceration of the ectopic pancreatic tissue. Gastric bleeding was reported by Carcassone and Dau (228). Gastric obstruction and delayed emptying were reported by Armstrong et al. (229) and by French (230).

Martinez and his colleagues (231) tabulated detailed symptoms in 51 surgical cases from the Mayo Clinic. They divided their patients into a "clinically significant" group (55%), whose symptoms could be referred to the heterotopic pancreatic mass; a "coincidental" group (14%), in whom other lesions present in the stomach contributed to the indications for surgery; and an "incidental" group (31%), in whom the pancreatic mass was unsuspected at surgery and was incidental to other pathologic conditions.

Diagnosis. Preoperative diagnosis is entirely within the province of the radiologist and endoscopist. In theory, all submucosal masses should be identifiable by radiography. Among the cases collected up to 1951 by Palmer (212), 56 of 71 were visualized radiologically. The stoma of the excretory duct frequently is visible as a barium spot within a halo of barium. The central duct may also fill with barium and be visualized (232). These visualized ducts may be distinguished from the deep ulceration of leiomyomas or leiomyosarcomas by the size of the mass. The smooth muscle tumors do not show excavation until they are much larger than pancreatic masses usually become (127, 233, 234). Littner and Kirsh (234) listed several diagnostic radiographic features to seek:

1. A nodular prominence producing a filling defect 1 to 2 cm in diameter, with a sharp margin
2. A central depression, usually regular
3. Mucosa over the mass, stretched and thin and hence, smooth in appearance
4. No evidence of local muscular spasm, and no interference with peristaltic waves
5. No significant barium residue

Treatment. The frequency of pancreatic tissue in the stomach, found incidentally on autopsy or during surgery for other conditions, indicates that most cases safely remain untreated or can be managed medically with relative success.

Surgical treatment, when necessary, should be conservative since the lesions are benign. Martinez and his colleagues (231) suggest gastrotomy and mucosal inspection for duct openings, to avoid unnecessary radical procedure. In the case of obstruction or massive hemorrhage, wedge or segmental resection is indicated. Local excision of the incidentally discovered tumor was advised by Condon (235).

Mortality. Only one death from untreated heterotopic pancreatic tissue seems to have been reported. The lesion was in the duodenum, and infection, along with extensive erosion, was present (227).

FROM THE STOMACH TO OTHER ORGANS

Gastric mucosa is the most peripatetic fellow of the gastrointestinal tract. Ectopic gastric mucosa has been reported in the tongue (236), submandibular gland (237), esophagus (238, 239), gallbladder (240), common bile duct (241), cystic duct (242), pancreas (243), small bowel (244, 245), Meckel's diverticulum (246), appendix (247), colon (248–250), and rectum (251).

Distribution. Gastric mucosa may be found in the esophagus, intestine, Meckel's diverticulum, and in many esophageal, gastric, and intestinal duplications and diverticula. A few instances of gastric mucosa in the biliary tract have also been recorded (Fig. 5.35). It has also been associated with pancreatic tissue in the colon (249) and in the colonic ulcer (250).

Three definite cases of heterotopic tissue in the rectum have been recorded. In one, fundic glands produced an ulcer (252); in another, the gastric tissue was in an anterior diverticulum (253); and in a third, gastric mucosa was reported on a rectal polyp (251).

Embryogenesis. Three views of the origin of such seemingly displaced tissue have been advanced. Earlier embryologists leaned toward the view that these heterotopic areas represent the physical displacement of cells during embryonic development. There is considerable evidence that, in some cases, this does take place, especially on a gross scale. Ectopic and heterotopic organs and tissues are common in the body. This argument, however, will not serve to explain the presence of gastric mucosa in such places as the rectum.

A second hypothesis put forth the idea of invasive migration, which has been used chiefly to explain gastric mucosa in the lower esophagus (254). While it is not unreasonable when applied to heterotopia in this location, this explanation will not apply to gastric heterotopia in general.

The third view holds that gastric heterotopia is the

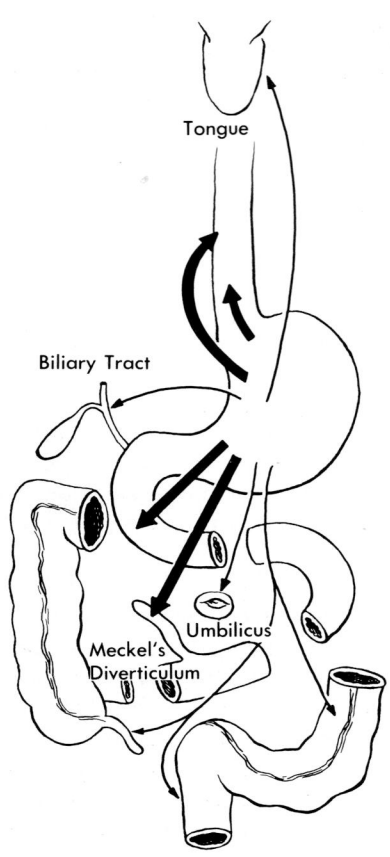

Figure 5.35. Location of heterotopic gastric mucosa in other organs of the body. Thickness of *arrows* indicates relative frequency.

result of local differentiation or metaplasia of cells already present (250, 255). Except for vague references to inflammation (256), speculations on the nature of the stimulus for such metaplasia have not been forthcoming. Burne (249) argued that, while gastric epithelial cells might arise by metaplasia, entire fundic glands with both chief and parietal cells could arise only by displacement. This may well be true if metaplasia is considered to take place in the adult; however, if the usual fate of relatively undifferentiated cells of the embryonic gut is altered, the formation of appropriate glandular structures is not surprising.

Evidence from the behavior of gastric and intestinal duplications indicates that endoderm cells from any portion of the primitive gut may form epithelium characteristic of any other portion. Even the cells of the vitelline duct, if preserved from their normal atrophic fate, may form a variety of differentiated epithelia, including gastric glands. What the specific organizers of these tissues are is unknown. In general, the potentiality of a given tissue to differentiate into a particular structure is not geographically limited, but it decreases with increasing distance from the normal site and with increasing time after

the normal period of development. What factors permit some cells to escape from the system remains one of the major problems of embryology.

There is a hierarchy among heterotopic tissue of the gut. Gastric mucosa is the most frequently displaced into other organs, into Meckel's diverticulum, and into esophageal or intestinal duplications.

Artigas et al. (257) support this hierarchy. In their presentation, one-third of Meckel's diverticula studied were without any gastric mucosa. The remaining two-thirds contained gastric mucosa, pancreatic tissue, or both; however, gastric mucosa was the most frequently found heterotopic tissue.

Heterotopic pancreatic tissue follows gastric mucosa in frequency. Jejunal, ileal, and colonic mucosa are only rarely migratory. Of the endodermal derivatives, only liver tissue seems almost never to be heterotopic within the alimentary tract.

With our present knowledge, it would be unreasonable to deny that local pathologic change may stimulate latent differentiation of tissue into cell types normally found elsewhere in the body. Such changes, if they occur, may account for the rare appearance of gastric mucosa in the postvitelline gut.

Gastroduodenal Adhesions

Gastroduodenal adhesions may be congenital or acquired. Sometimes adhesions of the first portion of the duodenum produce obstruction; however, gastric adhesions never cause any symptoms indicating a need for surgery. Thin filament-like adhesions may be cut or separated by blunt dissection, but thick cord-like adhesions should be divided and ligated. These adhesions produce occasional obstructions of the first part of the duodenum.

Gastric Teratoma

Gastric teratomas are very rare, benign lesions. In a series of 65 teratomas in children, five (8%) were in the stomach (258). DeAngelis (259) stated in 1969 that all reported cases of gastric teratoma involve male patients. Subsequent cases have involved females (260–262). Excision or subtotal gastrectomy is the treatment of choice (263).

Gastric Angiodysplasia (Telangiectasia, Angiomata, Aneurysms, Arteriovenous Malformation, Dieulafoy's Disease, Vascular Ectasia)

Gastric angiodysplasia is a rare cause of upper gastrointestinal tract bleeding due to an abnormal artery in the submucosa of the stomach. The anomalous artery is much larger (2 to 5 mm) than a normal submucosal vessel, is tortuous, and has the structure of large muscular arteries

(264). It is enlarged over its entire length and, hence, cannot be called an aneurysm. The lesion is typically located high in the fundus close to the lesser curvature but may be anywhere in the gastric wall. Similar lesions are found in the wall of the duodenum, small intestine, and colon. They are usually found in elderly males (265) but are not unknown in women and young adults (266). For all practical purposes this is an abnormality of the wall of the vessels. It may be a genetic disorder or an autosomal dominant trait like Osler-Render-Weber syndrome. A hereditary etiology has been mentioned, and of course the debate continues over whether this is a congenital or acquired phenomenon. If it is congenital, perhaps it is the result of an arrest during the development of circulation at the period of undifferentiated capillary network. Later on, when arteries and veins are well differentiated, persistent anomalous communication may persist and progress to form dilated minute arteries and veins in the mucosa and submucosa of the stomach.

Fiddian-Green (267) thinks that angiodysplasia is an acquired disease and not congenital.

Is Dieulafoy's disease a synonym or just a member of the same family? Condon (235) thinks that chronic gastritis is a predisposing factor to vascular dysplasia "which leads to thrombosis and necrosis of the arterial wall." Juler (268) reported that Dieulafoy's gastritis occurs in about 1.3% of patients who undergo an operation for massive gastric bleeding.

The frequency with which the malformed arteries occurs is unknown. Among 406 patients admitted to the hospital with gastrointestinal bleeding, only nine had arterial malformation (263). The malformations are completely silent until erosion injures them and massive intractable hemorrhage occurs. The absence of consistent degenerative changes in the malformed artery and the association of angiodysplasia with Meckel's diverticulum (270) and aortic valve disease (271) have suggested a congenital rather than an acquired origin. Why such lesions usually remain dormant until late in life remains an unanswered question (265). Multiple lesions in the stomach and duodenum have been reported (272).

CLASSIFICATION

Moretó et al. (273), with experience with 47 cases, suggested the endoscopic classifications detailed in Table 5.4.

According to Marwick and Kerlin (274) the lesions were multiple in one-third of patients and were predominantly situated in the proximal stomach.

DIAGNOSIS

Steer and Silen (275) evaluated the available diagnostic procedures: endoscopy, radionuclide imaging, vis-

Table 5.4.
Endoscopic Classifications of Gastric Angiodysplasia

Pattern	Classification
I	Flat or slightly protruded bright red lesions with frond-like margins; most common form
II	Telangiectatic form
III	Submucosal nodular

Table 5.5.
Diagnostic Steps

PTH
Nasogastric tube; connect to lower suction
Hematologic studies and blood urea nitrogen study
Fiberoptic esophagoscopy; gastroscopy; duodenoscopy
99m Tc-sulfur colloid scanning
Selective angiography
Gastrointestinal radiographic series if bleeding ceased

ceral angiography, contrast-enhanced radiography, and exploratory surgery. Perhaps because of better endoscopic, arteriographic, and ultrasound appreciation of the gastric mucosa, the diagnosis of this rare entity was made easier. The literature is filled with reports and cases. This rare pathologic entity is no longer a *terra incognita*, but a clinical entity that should be considered always in patients with chronic anemia or upper gastrointestinal bleeding, especially if upper gastrointestinal radiologic series findings are negative. Transendoscopic Doppler ultrasound was used by Rutgeerts et al. (276) with good diagnostic success (99m Tc-sulfur colloid scanning). Despite that all the above mentioned diagnostic procedures occasionally fail to give an answer, diagnostic laparotomy will be the final step (Table 5.5).

If the upper endoscopy is not successful, abdominal scintigraphy ("bleeding scan" using labeled red blood cells) will be helpful for detecting any sites of bleeding. The next step is emergency selective arteriography. If again this diagnostic procedure is unsuccessful, laparotomy will be the answer. The bleeding source, when located, will require surgery.

TREATMENT

Treatment consists of the following:

1. Endoscopic electrocoagulation
2. Injection sclerotherapy
3. Selective arterial embolization
4. Surgery (The segmental resection should be generous, after detailed study of the angiogram, to ensure that all malformed angiodysplastic areas are removed. Lewis et al. [277] advised excision of the vascular lesions removing only the involved walls.)
5. No treatment if no bleeding or chronic anemia present
6. Vasoconstrictor infusion and laser coagulation

Gastric Artery Aneurysm

Fatal gastric artery aneurysm rupture was reported recently by Witte et al. (278). According to these authors, gastric artery aneurysms are rare (approximately 50 cases reported in the literature) and account for fewer than 5% of all splanchnic arteries. Intramural location is more common than extragastric. Gallard (279) reported the first case of gastric artery aneurysm.

Hematemesis or intraperitoneal bleeding with their sequelae are the signs and symptoms of this rare clinical entity.

We reported an aneurysm of the splenic artery involving the posterior gastric artery (280).

REFERENCES

1. Blechschmidt E. The stages of human development before birth. Philadelphia: WB Saunders, 1961.
2. Botha GSM. Organogenesis and growth of the gastroesophageal region in man. Anat Rec 1959;133:219–239.
3. Johnson FP. The development of the mucous membrane of the esophagus, stomach, and small intestine in the human embryo. Am J Anat 1910;10:521–561.
4. Lewis FT. The development of the stomach. In: Keibel WP, Mall FP, eds. Manual of human embryology. Philadelphia: JB Lippincott, 1912.
5. Salenius P. On the ontogenesis of the human gastric epithelial cells: a histologic and histochemical study. Acta Anat (Basel) 1962;50(Suppl 46):1–76.
6. Dankmeijer J, Meite M. Le développement précoce de l'estomac chez l'embryo humain. C R Assoc Anat 1959;103:341–344.
7. Arey LB. Developmental anatomy. Philadelphia: WB Saunders, 1974:245–262.
8. Grand RJ, Watkins JB, Torte FM. Development of the human gastrointestinal tract. Gastroenterology 1976;70:790–810.
9. Keith A, Jones FW. A note on the development of the fundus of the human stomach. J Anat Physiol 1902;36:34.
10. Bremmer CG. Studies of the pyloric muscle. S Afr J Surg 1968;6:79–85.
11. Indir J. The development of the nerve supply of the human esophagus and stomach. J Anat Soc India 1955;4:55–68.
12. McGeady TA, Sack WO. The development of vagal innervation in the bovine stomach. Am J Anat 1967;121:121–130.
13. Skandalakis JE, Rowe JS Jr, Gray SW, Androulakis JA. Identification of vagal structures at the esophageal hiatus. Surgery 1974;75:233–237.
14. Skandalakis JE, Gray SW, Soria RE, Sorg JL, Rowe JS Jr. Distribution of the vagus nerve to the stomach. Am Surg 1980;46:130–139.
15. Skandalakis LJ, Gray SW, Skandalakis JE. The history and surgical anatomy of the vagus nerve. Surg Gynecol Obstet 1986;162:75–85.
16. Windle WF. Physiology of the fetus. Philadelphia: WB Saunders, 1940:99–111.
17. Scott GH. Growth of crypts and glands of the human stomach. Am J Dis Child 1925;30:147–173.
18. Huhtikangas H. Untersuchugen über die Readtion des Mageninhalts bei Neugeborenen. Acta Soc Med Fenn 1936;24:1.
19. Shohl AT. Gastric analysis in newborn infants. Am J Dis Child 1925;30:144.
20. Leung K-Y, Lebenthal E. Gastrointestinal peptides: physiology, oncology, and clinical significance. In: E Lebenthal, ed. Human gastrointestinal development. New York: Raven Press, 1989.
21. Potter EL. Pathology of the fetus and the newborn. Chicago: Year Book Medical Publishers, 1952.
22. Blair P. An account of the dissection of a child, communicated in a letter to Dr. Brook Taylor. R Soc Secr Phil Trans Roy Soc Lond 1717;30:631–632.
23. Hoyt RL. Micro-gastria. Med J Rec 1924;119:338–340.
24. Caffey J. Pediatric x-ray diagnosis, 3rd ed. Chicago: Year Book Medical Publishers, 1956.
25. Kessler H, Schulewicz JJ. Microgastria associated with agenesis of the spleen. Radiology 1973;107(2):393–396.
26. Mandell GA, Heyman S, Alavi A, Ziegler MM. A case of microgastria in association with splenic-gonadal fusion. Pediatr Radiol 1983;13(2):95–98.
27. Putschar WGJ, Manion WC. Congenital absence of the spleen and associated anomalies. Am J Clin Pathol 1956;26:429–470.
28. Dide M. Sur un estomac d'adulte à type foetal. Bull Soc Ant 1896;69:669.
29. Gerbeaux J et al. Absence congenital d'estomac. Ann Pediatr 1971;18:349.
30. Schultz RD, Neiman F. Kongenitale microgastria in Verbidung mit Skelettmissbildungen: in nervus syndrome. Helv Paediat Acta 1971;26:185.
31. Blank E, Chisholm AJ. Congenital microgastria: a case report with a 26-year follow-up. Pediatrics 1973;51:1037.
32. Neifeld JP et al. Management of congenital microgastria with a jejunal reservoir pouch. J Pediatr Surg 1980;15:882.
33. Velasco AL, Wolcomb GW III, Templeton JM Jr, Ziegler MM. Management of congenital microgastria. J Pediatr Surg 1990;25:192–197.
34. Brown RP, Hertzler JH. Congenital prepyloric gastric atresia: a report of two cases. Am J Dis Child 1959;97:857–862.
35. Neale AJ. Case of malformations of stomach. Lancet 1884;1:1957.
36. Holladay LJ. Case report of congenital aplasia of the pylorus. J Indiana Med Assoc 1946;39:350.
37. Metz AR, Householder R, DePree JF. Obstruction of the stomach due to congenital double septum with cyst formation. Trans West Surg Assoc 1941;50:242.
38. Rhind JA. Mucosal stenosis of the pylorus. Br Surg 1959;46:534–540.
39. Spitz L, Zail SS. Serum gastrin levels in congenital hypertrophic pyloric stenosis. J Pediatr Surg 1976;11:33.
40. Rota AN. Pyloric obstruction due to mucosal diaphragm. Arch Pathol 1953;55:223.
41. Young HB. Addisonian pigmentation due to extreme pyloric stenosis by a mucosal diaphragm. Br J Surg 1961;49:104–107.
42. Browning RW. Prepyloric antral mucosal diaphragm or "webb." Am Surg 1964;30:73–76.
43. Gray SW, Johnson HC, Skandalakis JE. Antral and pyloric mucosal diaphragm in adults. J Med Assoc Ga 1977;66:544–548.
44. Liechti RE, Mikkelsen WP, Snyder WH Jr. Prepyloric stenosis caused by congenital squamous epithelial diaphragm. Surgery 1963;53:670–673.
45. Malheur RE et al. Pyloroduodenal atresia: a report of three families with several similarly affected children. Pediatr Radiol 1975;3:1.
46. Bar-Maor JA, Nissan S, Nevo S. Pyloric atresia: a hereditary congenital anomaly with autosomal recessive transmission. J Med Genet 1972;9:70.
47. Benson CD, Coury JJ. Congenital intrinsic obstruction of stomach and duodenum in the newborn. Arch Surg 1951;62:856.
48. Bronsther B, Nadeau MR, Abrams MW. Congenital pyloric atre-

sia: a report of three cases and a review of the literature. Surgery 1971;69:130.
49. Keramidas DC, Voyatzis N. Pyloric atresia: report of a second occurrence in the same family. J Pediatr Surg 1972;7:445.
50. Olson L, Grotte G. Congenital pyloric atresia: report of a familial occurrence. J Pediatr Surg 1976;11:181.
51. Thompson NW et al. Congenital pyloric atresia. Arch Surg 1968;97:792.
52. Crooks. Estomac se terminant en cul-de-sac. Arch Gén Méd 1828;17:264.
53. Wuensche R. Ein Falle von angeborenen Verschluss des pylorus. Jahrb Kinderh 1875;8:367.
54. Bennett RJ. Atresia of the pylorus. Am J Dig Dis 1937;4:44.
55. Touroff ASW, Sussman RM. Congenital prepyloric membranous obstruction in a premature infant. Surgery 1940;8:739–755.
56. Metz AR, Householder R, DePree JF. Obstruction of the stomach due to congenital double septum with cyst formation. Trans West Surg Assoc 1941;50:242.
57. Wolf HG, Zweymüeller E. Angeborener kompletter Pylorusverschluss. Jahrb Kinderh 1963;88:516–530.
58. Bariéty M, Poulet J, Courtois-Suffit M. Diaphragme muqueux prépylorique et cancer bronchique primitif. Presse Med 1957;65:785.
59. Sames CP. Case of partial atresia of the pyloric antrum due to mucosal diaphragm of doubtful origin. Br J Surg 1949;37:244–246.
60. Campbell JR. Other conditions of the stomach. In: Welch KJ, et al. (eds). Pediatric surgery, 4th ed. Chicago: Year Book Medical Publishers, Inc. 1986;821–822.
61. Talwalker VC. Pyloric atresia: a case report. J Pediatr Surg 1967;2:458.
62. Davis DA, Douglas KR. Congenital pyloric atresia: a rare anomaly. Ann Surg 1961;153:418–422.
63. Becker JM, Schneider KM, Fischer AE. Pyloric atresia. Arch Surg 1963;87:71–74.
64. Wurtenberger H. Gastric atresia. Arch Dis Child 1961;36:161–163.
65a. Haller JA Jr, Cahill JL. Combined congenital gastric and duodenal obstruction: Pitfalls in diagnosis and treatment. Surgery 1968;63:3.
65b. El-Shafie M, Stidham GL. Pyloric atresia and epidermolysis bullosa lethalis: a lethal combination in two premature newborn siblings. J Pediatr Surg 1979;14:446.
66. Gray SW, Johnson HC, Skandalakis JE. Antral and pyloric mucosal diaphragm in adults. J Med Assoc Ga 1977;66:544–548.
67. Gandhi RD, Robarts FH. Hour-glass stricture of the stomach and pyloric stenosis due to ferrous sulphate poisoning. Br J Surg 1962;49:613–617.
68. Struther J. Case of double stomach. Month J Med Sci 1951;12:121–126.
69. Hirsch K. Ueber sanduhrmagen. Virchow Arch [A] 1895;140:459–480.
70. Moynihan BGA. Remarks on hourglass stomachs. Br Med J 1904;1:413–416.
71. Rowlands RD. A clinical lecture on hourglass contraction of the stomach. Br Med J 1931;2:50–52.
72. Schroeder CM. Hourglass stomach caused by annular muscular hypertrophy: report of a case. Ann Surg 1949;130:1905.
73. Sager WW, Jenkins WH. Hourglass stomach is associated with esophageal stenosis. Ann Surg 1935;101:969.
74. Hirschsprung H. Fälle von angeborener Pylorusstenose, boebachtet bei Säuglingen. Jahrb Kinderh 1888;28:61–68.
75. Hayes MA, Goldenberg IS. The problems of infantile pyloric stenosis (collective review). Int Abstr Surg 1957;104:105–138.
76. Wallgren A. Preclinical stage of infantile hypertrophic pyloric stenosis. Am J Dis Child 1946;72:371.
77. Ford N, Brown A, McCreary JF. Evidence of monozygosity and disturbance of growth in twins with pyloric stenosis. Am J Dis Child 1941;61:41.
78. McKeown T, MacMahon B, Record RG, Evidence of postnatal environmental influence in the aetiology of infantile pyloric stenosis. Arch Dis Child 1952;27:386–390.
79. Gerrad JW, Waterhouse JAH, Maurice DG. Infantile pyloric stenosis. Arch Dis Child 1955;30:493–496.
80. Stringer MD, Brereton RJ. Current management of infantile hypertrophic pyloric stenosis. Br J Hosp Med 1990;43:266.
81. Lynn H. The mechanism of pyloric stenosis and its relationship to preoperative procedures. Arch Surg 1960;81:453.
82. Spitz L, Zail SS. Serum gastrin levels in congenital hypertrophic pyloric stenosis. J Pediatr Surg 1976;11:33.
83. Rogers IM et al. Plasma gastrin in congenital hypertrophic pyloric stenosis. Arch Dis Child 1975;50:467.
84. Friesen SR, Pearse AG. Congenital pyloric stenosis. Surgery 1963;53:604–608.
85. Rintoul JR, Kirkman NF. The myenteric plexus in infantile hypertrophic pyloric stenosis. Arch Dis Child 1961;36:474–480.
86. Friesen SR, Boley JO, Miller DR. The myenteric plexus of the pylorus: its early normal development and changes in hypertrophic pyloric stenosis. Surgery 1956;39:21.
87. Zuelzer W. Infantile hypertrophic pyloric stenosis. In: Welch KJ Randolph JG, Rauitch MM, O'Neill JA Jr, Rowe MI, eds. Pediatric surgery, 4th ed. Chicago: Year Book Medical Publishers, 1986.
88. Jona JZ. Electron microscopic observation in infantile hypertrophic pyloric stenosis (IHPS). J Pediatr Surg 1978;13:17.
89. Culotta E, Koshland DE Jr. No news is good news. Science 1992;258:1862–1865.
90. Vanderwinder JM. Nitric oxide synthase activity in infantile hypertrophic pyloric stenosis. NEJM 1992;327:511–515.
91. Carter CO. The inheritance of congenital pyloric stenosis. Br Med Bull 1961;17:251–253.
92. Benson CD, Lloyd JR. Infantile pyloric stenosis: a review of 1,120 cases. Am J Surg 1964;107:429–433.
93. Knox G. On the nature of the determinants of congenital pyloric stenosis. Br J Prev Soc Med 1958;12:188.
94. Hildanus F. Opera ominia. Frankfort: Joh. Bejerus, 1646.
95. Kellett CE. On the incidence of congenital hypertrophic pyloric stenosis in the 17th and 18th centuries. Arch Dis Child 1933;8:323.
96. Blair P. An account of the dissection of a child, communicated in a letter to Dr. Brook Taylor, R Soc Secr Phila. Trans R Soc Lond 1717;30:631–632.
97. Beardsley HK. Cases and observations by the medical society of New Haven County. New Haven 1788;1:81.
98. Ravitch MM. The story of pyloric stenosis. Surgery 1960;48:1117–1143.
99. Wallgren A. Is the rate of hypertrophic pyloric stenosis declining? Acta Paediatr (Uppsala) 1960;49:530–535.
100. Laron Z, Horne LM. The incidence of infantile pyloric stenosis. Am J Dis Child 1957;94:151.
101. Smith IMcD. Incidence of intussusception and congenital hypertrophic pyloric stenosis in Edinburgh children. Br Med J 1960;1:551.
102. Hayes MA, Goldenberg IS. The problems of infantile pyloric stenosis (collective review). Int Abstr Surg 1957;104:105–138.
103. Griffiths J. Hypertrophic pyloric stenosis in the South African Bantus. Hum Biol 1956;28:414–419.
104. Benson CD. Infantile hypertrophic pyloric stenosis. In: Welch KJ,

Randolph JG, Rauitch MM, O'Neill JA Jr, Rowe MI, eds. Pediatric surgery, 4th ed. Chicago: Year Book Medical Publishers, 1986.

105. Lebenthal E, ed. Human gastrointestinal development. New York: Raven Press, 1989.

106. Dufour H, Fredet P. La stenose hypertrophique du pylore chex le nourisson et son traitment chirurgical. Rev Chir 1908;37:208.

107. Weber W. Ueber eine technische Neuerung bei der operation der pylorusstenose de Säuglings. Berlin Klin Wschr 1910;47:763.

108. Rammstedt C. Zur operation der angeborenen Pylorus-stenose. Med Klin 1912;8:1702.

109. Svensgaard E. The medical treatment of congenital pyloric stenosis. Arch Dis Child 1935;10:443.

110. Malmberg N. Hypertrophic pyloric stenosis: a survey of 136 successive cases with special reference to treatment with Scopyl. Acta Paediatr (Uppsala) 1949;38:472.

111. Nielsen OS. Congenital pyloric stenosis as a factor predisposing to the ulcer syndrome. Acta Paediatr (Uppsala) 1954;43:432–443.

112. Christiansen KH, Grantham A. Idiopathic hypertrophic pyloric stenosis in the adult. Arch Surg 1962;85:207–214.

113. Palmer ED. Gastric diverticula. Surg Obstet Gynecol 1951;92:417–428.

114. Lewis PL, Holder T, Feldman M. Duplication of the stomach. Arch Surg 1961;82:634–640.

115. Lewis FT, Thyng FW. Regular occurrence of intestinal diverticula in embryos of the pig, rabbit, and man. Am J Anat 1907;7:505.

116. Hartley JB. Diverticulum of the stomach found to enter left inguinal hernial sac. Br J Radiol 1945;18:231–232.

117. Vargas LL, Leven SM, Santulli TV. Rupture of the stomach in the newborn infant. Surg Gynecol Obstet 1955;101:417–424.

118. Baillie M. The morbid anatomy of some of the most important parts of the human body. London: J Johnson Publishers, 1793.

119. Martin L. Diverticula of the stomach. Ann Intern Med 1936;10:447.

120. Zahn G. Ein Beitrag zur pathologischen Anatomie der Magendivertikel. Deutsch Arch Klin Med 1899;63:359–367.

121. Brown GE. An unusual stomach case with roentgenographic findings. JAMA 1916;66:1918.

122. Sommer AW, Goodrich WA. Gastric diverticula. JAMA 1953;153:1424–1428.

123. Roth SR, Kern MJ, Diverticulum of the stomach: case report. J Newark Beth Israel Hosp 1950;1:219–222.

124. Ogur GL, Kolarsick AJ. Gastric diverticula in infancy. J Pediatr 1951;39:723–729.

125. Brody H. Ruptured diverticulum of the stomach in a newborn infant, associated with congenital membrane occluding the duodenum. Arch Pathol 1940;29:125–128.

126. Lungmuss F. Zur Klinik und Differentialdiagnose des Magendivertikels. Chir 1950;21:457.

127. Skandalakis JE, Gray SW. Smooth muscle tumors of the alimentary tract. Springfield, IL: Charles C Thomas, 1962.

128. Moses WR. Diverticula of the stomach. Arch Surg 1946;52:59.

129. Walters W. Diverticulum of the stomach. JAMA 1946;131:954–956.

130. Gjörup E. Un cas d' oesophage double et estomac double. Acta Paediatr 1933;15:90–98.

131. Abrami G, Dennison WM. Duplication of the stomach. Surgery 1961;49:794–801.

132. Bartels RJ. Duplication of the stomach: case report and review of the literature. Am Surg 1967;33:747–752.

133. Cashion WA. Supernumerary stomach with duodenal bulb associated with diaphragmatic hernia. Med Bull Vet Admin 1934;11:61–62.

134. Høyer A, Andersen I. Cardio-duodenal duct: anomaly of the stomach previously not observed. J Oslo City Hosp 1951;225–230.

135. Young GB. Duplication of the stomach. Br J Radiol 1965;38:853–856.

136. McCutcheon GT, Josey RB. Reduplication of the stomach. J Pediatr 1951;39:216–220.

137. Katz W, Annessa G, Read RC. Gastric duplication with pancreatic communication presenting as pancreatitis. Minn Med 1967;50:1175–1180.

138. Dwing SB, Roessel CW, Olmstead EV. Enterogenous cyst of the stomach wall: a rare benign lesion—case report. Ann Surg 1956;143:131–135.

139. Ellis WB. Duplication of the alimentary tract: review of the literature and report of case. Surgery 1953;34:140.

140. Nissan S. Duplication of the stomach. Am J Surg 1960;100:59–63.

141. Goon CD. Duplication of the stomach with extension into the chest. Am Surg 1953;19:721–727.

142. Dresler CM, Patterson GA, Taylor BR, Moote DJ. Complete foregut duplication. Ann Thorac Surg 1990;50(2):306–308.

143. Bremer JL. Congenital anomalies of the viscera. Cambridge, MA: Harvard University Press, 1957.

144. McLetchie NGB, Purves JK, Saunders RL de CH. Genesis of gastric and certain intestinal diverticula and enterogenous cysts. Surg Gynecol Obstet 1954;99:135–141.

145. Wendel W. Beschreibung eines operatin entfernten congenitalen Nebenmazens. Arch Klin Chir 1911;45:895–898.

146. Pancotto E. Contributo alla conoscenza delle cisti dello stomaco. Pathologica 1927;19:521.

147. Cabot RC. Case records of the Massachusetts General Hospital: case 14,242, hysteria versus obstruction. N Engl J Med 1928;199:236.

148. Dornier R. Les duplications gastriques. Arch Mal Appar Dig 1959;48:658–671.

149. Bower RJ, Sieber WK, Kiesewetter WB. Alimentary tract duplications in children. Ann Surg 1978;188:669.

150. Kalongi T, Steiner P. Les duplications gastriques à propos d'un cas observé chez l'adulte. Ann Chir 1974;28:43.

151. Orr MM, Edwards AJ. Neoplastic change in duplications of the alimentary tract. Br J Surg 1975;62:269.

152. Kremer RM, Lepoff RB, Izant RJ Jr. Duplication of the stomach. J Pediatr Surg 1970;5:360.

153. Curran JP et al. Ectopic gastric duplication cyst in an infant. Clin Pediatr 1984;23:50.

154. Gonzalez BGC, Martinez JC. A propósito de un caso de reduplicación gástrica y pancreática. Rev Esp Enf Ap Dig 1978;53:671.

155. Hélardot PG et al. Les duplication gastriques séparées de l'éstomac et en relation avec le pancréas. Chir Pediatr 1982;23:363.

156. Kleinhaus S, Boley SJ, Winslow P. Occult bleeding from a perforated gastric duplication in an infant. Arch Surg 1981;116:122.

157. Braffman B, Keller R, Gendal ES, Finkel SI. Subdiaphragmatic bronchogenic cyst with gastric communication. Gastrointest Radiol 1988;13(4):309–311.

158. Keohane ME, Schwartz I, Freed J, Dische R. Subdiaphragmatic bronchogenic cyst with communication to the stomach: a case report. Hum Pathol 1988;19(7):868–871.

159. Stanley P, Vachon L, Gilsanz V. Pulmonary sequestration with congenital gastroesophageal communication: report of two cases. Pediatr Radiol 1985;15(5):343–345.

160. Thornhill BA, Cho KC, Morehouse HT. Gastric duplication associated with pulmonary sequestration: CT manifestations. AJR 1982;138(6):1168–1171.

161. McClelland RR, Kapsner AL, Uecker JH. Pulmonary sequestration associated with a gastric duplication cyst. Radiology 1977;124(1):13–14.

162. Mahour GH, Woolley MM, Payne VC Jr. Association of pulmo-

nary sequestration and duplication of the stomach. Int Surg 1971;56(4):224–227.

163. Gross RE. The surgery of infancy and childhood. Philadelphia: WB Saunders, 1953.

164. Sieber WK. Alimentary tract duplications. Arch Surg 1956;73:383–392.

165. Shaw RC. Cyst formation in relation to stomach and esophagus. Br J Surg 1951;39:254–257.

166. Luks FI, Shah MN, Bulavitan MC, LoPresti PA, Pizzi WF. Adult foregut duplication. Surgery 1990;108(1):101–104.

167. Thorbjarnarson B, Haynes LL. Duplication of the stomach: a report of two cases in infants. Surgery 1958;44:585–590.

168. Mayo HW Jr, McKee EE, Anderson RM. Carcinoma arising in reduplication of stomach (gastrogenous cyst). Ann Surg 1955;141:550–555.

169. Artaud P, Gallerand R. Myome pylorique avec kyste. Pediatrie 1958;13:813–814.

170. Anas P, Miller RC. Pyloric duplication masquerading as hypertrophic pyloric stenosis: case reports. J Pediatr Surg 1971;6:664.

171. Cloutier R. Pseudocyst of the pancreas secondary to gastric duplication: case reports. J Pediatr Surg 1973;8:67.

172. Parker BC, Guthrie J, France NE, Atwell JD. Gastric duplications in infancy. J Pediatr Surg 1972;7:294.

173. Shochast SJ, Strand RD, Fellows KE, Folkman J. Perforated gastric duplication with pulmonary communications: a case report. Surgery 1971;70:370.

174. Koltun WA. Gastric duplication cyst: endoscopic presentation as an ulcerated antral mass. Am Surg 1991;57(7):468–473.

175. White JJ, Morgan WW. Improved operative technique for gastric duplication. Surgery 1970;67:522.

176. MacGillivray PC, Stewart AM, MacFarlane A. Rupture of stomach in newborn due to congenital defects in gastric musculature. Arch Dis Child 1956;31:56–58.

177. Braunstein H. Congenital defect of the gastric musculature with spontaneous perforation. J Pediatr 1954;44:55–63.

178. Inouye WY, Evans G. Neonatal gastric perforation: a report of six cases and a review of 143 cases. Arch Surg 1964;88:451–485.

179. Scammon RE. Summary of the anatomy of the infant and child. In: Abt IA, ed. Pediatrics. Philadelphia: WB Saunders, 1923.

180. Shaw A, Blanc WA, Santulli TV, Kaiser G. Spontaneous rupture of the stomach in the newborn: a clinical and experimental study. Surgery 1965;58:561–571.

181. Holder TM, Ashcraft KW. Pediatric surgery, 2nd ed. Philadelphia: WB Saunders, 1993.

182. Raffensperger JG. Gastrointestinal perforation. In: Raffensperger JG, ed. Swenson's pediatric surgery, 5th ed. Appleton & Lange, 1990.

183. von Siebold AE. Uber geschwuersbildungen des Gastro-duodenal-tractus im Kindersalter. Erg Inn Med Kinderh 1919 (1825);16:302–383.

184. Brody H. Ruptured diverticulum of the stomach in a newborn infant, associated with congenital membrane occluding the duodenum. Arch Pathol 1940;29:125–128.

185. Meyer JL III. Congenital defect in the musculature of the stomach resulting in spontaneous gastric perforation in the neonatal period. J Pediatr 1957;51:416–421.

186. Ozkaragoz K, Stewart CS. Spontaneous rupture of the stomach in two premature newborn siblings. Texas J Med 1959;55:305–307.

187. Lloyd JR. The etiology of gastrointestinal perforation in the newborn. J Pediatr Surg 1969;4:77.

188. Bell MJ. Peritonitis in the newborn: current concepts. Pediatr Clin North Am 1985;32(5):1181–1201.

189. Bell MJ. Perforation of the gastrointestinal tract and peritonitis in the neonate. Surg Gynecol Obstet 1985;160(1):20–26.

190. Steves M, Ricketts RR. Pneumoperitoneum in the newborn. Am Surg 1987;53:226–230.

191. Holgersen LO. The etiology of spontaneous gastric perforation of the newborn: a re-evaluation. J Pediatr Surg 1981;16:608.

192. Rosser S, Clark C, Elenchi E. Spontaneous neonatal gastric perforation. J Pediatr Surg 1985;17:390.

193. Stern MA, Perkins EL, Nessa NS. Perforated gastric ulcer in two-day-old infant. Lancet 1929;49:492–494.

194. Selinger J. Peptic ulcer in infants under one year of age. Ann Surg 1932;96:204–209.

195. Légar JL, Ricard PM, Léonard C, Piette J. Ulcère gastroque perforé chez un nouveau-né avec survie. Un Med Can 1950;79:1277–1280.

196. Johnson JR. Situs inversus with associated abnormalities: review of literature and report of 3 cases. Arch Surg 1949;58:149–162.

197. Rosenfeld DH. Unusual type of inversion of stomach associated with diaphragmatic eventration and other anomalies. Am J Roentgenol Rad Ther 1944;52:607–610.

198. Fichardt T. Eventration of diaphragm associated with inversion of stomach. Clin Proc 1946;5:328–331.

199. Peck GA, Weber GW. Inversion of the stomach with eventration of the diaphragm. Am J Radiol 1952;67:63–67.

200. Rhinehart BA, Rhinehart DA. Congenital abnormalities of the stomach. Radiology 1926;7:492–497.

201. Moody HP, Van Nuys RG, Kidder CH. The form and position of the empty stomach in healthy young adults as shown in roentgenograms. Anat Rec 1929;43:359–379.

202. Senocak ME, Buyukpamukcu N, Hicsonmez A. Chronic gastric volvulus in children—a ten-year experience. Z Kinderchir 1990;45:159–163.

203. Chaudhuri TK. False-positive liver scan caused by dextrogastria [Letter]. J Nucl Med 1976;17:1109.

204. Hewlett PM. Isolated dextrogastria. Br J Radiol 1982;55:678–681.

205. Simstein NL. Congenital gastric anomalies. Am Surg 1985;52:264–268.

206. Barrocas A, Fontenelle LJ, Williams MJ. Gastric heterotopic pancreas. Ann Surg 1973;39:361–365.

207. Clarke BE. Myoepithelial hamartoma of the gastrointestinal tract: report of 8 cases with comment concerning genesis and nomenclature. Arch Pathol 1940;30:143–152.

208. Strelinger A. Ectopic pancreatic tissue in stomach wall with unusual symptomatology. Gastroenterology 1957;33:493–498.

209. Denson JW. Aberrant pancreatic tissue in gastric wall: report of four cases simulating peptic ulcer. Am Surg 1957;23:568–576.

210. Berant M, Aviad I, Jacobs J. Heterotopic duodenal mucosa in the stomach. Am J Dis Child 1965;110:566–569.

211. Debard JR, Mazarakis JA, Nyhus LM. An unusual case of heterotopic pancreas of the stomach. Am J Surg 1981;141:269.

212. Palmer ED. Benign intramural tumors of the stomach: a review with special reference to gross pathology. Medicine 1951;30:81–96.

213. Lauche A. Die Heterotopien der ortsgehörigen Epithels im Bereich des Verdauungskanals. Virchow Arch [A] 1924;252:39–88.

214. Scott HW Jr, Payne TPB. Diffuse congenital cystic hyperplasia of stomach clinically stimulating carcinoma: report of a case. Bull Johns Hopkins Hosp 1947;81:448.

215. Oberman HA, Lodmell JG, Sower ND. Diffuse heterotopic and cystic malformation of the stomach. N Engl J Med 1963;269:909–911.

216. Magnus HA. Observations on the presence of intestinal epithelium in the gastric mucosa. J Pathol Bact 1937;44:389–398.

217. Bolognesi G. Le pancréas accessoire: contribution clinique. Arch Mal Appar Dig 1933;23:708–745.

218. Gruhn P, Blake K, Saracco T. Gastric heterotopia. Am J Surg 1950;100:396.

219. Klob J. Pancreatic Anomalien. Z K K Gesellsch Aerzte Wien 1859;15:732.

220. Mangus-Alsleben E. Adenomyome des pylorus. Virchow Arch [A] 1903;173:137–156.

221. Barbosa JJ de C, Dockerty MB, Waugh JM. Pancreatic heterotopia. Surg Gynecol Obstet 1946;82:527–542.

222. Busard JM, Walters W. Heterotopic pancreatic tissue: a report of a case presenting symptoms of ulcer and review of the recent literature. Arch Surg 1950;60:674–682.

223. Nelson RS, Scott NM Jr. Heterotopic pancreatic tissue in the stomach: gastroscopic features. Gastroenterology 1958;34:452–459.

224. Rutledge RH, Neil WH. Symptomatic aberrant pancreas in the stomach of a two-year-old boy. South Med J 1962;55:287–289.

225. Copleman B. Aberrant pancreas in the gastric wall. Radiology 1963;81:107.

226. Lucaya J, Ochoa JB. Ectopic pancreas in the stomach. J Pediatr Surg 1976;11:101–102.

227. Kalfayan B. Duodenitis with diverticulum and ectopic pancreatic tissue. Arch Pathol 1946;42:228–231.

228. Carcassone M, Dau N. Gastric bleeding and accessory pancreas in children. Chir Pediatr 1980;21:357.

229. Armstrong CP, King PM, Dixon JM, Macleod IB. The clinical significance of heterotopic pancreas in the gastrointestinal tract. Br J Surg 1981;68:384.

230. French WE. Pancreatic tissue in antral wall. Am J Surg 1967;114:956.

231. Martinez NS, Morlock CG, Dockerty MB, Waugh JM, Weber HM. Heterotopic pancreatic tissue involving the stomach. Ann Surg 1958;147:1.

232. Lapidari M. Pancreas accessorio dello stomaco o metaplasia eterotopica a tipo pancreatico della mucosa gastria? Arch Ital Chir 1937;47:432–452.

233. Skandalakis JE, Gray SW, Shepard D. Smooth muscle tumors of the stomach. Surg Gynecol Obstet 1960;110:209–226.

234. Littner M, Kirsch I. Aberrant pancreatic tissue in gastric antrum: report of 7 cases. Radiology 1952;59:201–211.

235. Condon RE. Disorders of the stomach and duodenum. In: Nyhus LM, Wastrell C, eds. Surgery of the stomach and duodenum. Boston: Little, Brown, 1986.

236. Gorlin RJ, Kalnins V, Izant RJ Jr. Occurrence of heterotopic gastric mucosa in the tongue. J Pediatr 1964;64:604–606.

237. Dauffman SL, Stout AP. Tumors of the major salivary glands in children. Cancer 1963;16:1317.

238. Schridde H. Über Magenschleimhaut-insen vom bau der cardialdrüsenzone und Fundus-drüsen-region und den unteren, oesophagealen cardialdrüsen gleichende drüsen im obersten Oesophagusabschnitt. Virchow Arch [A] 1904;175:1–16.

239. Rector LE, Connerley ML. Aberrant mucosa in the esophagus in infants and in children. Arch Pathol 1941;31:285–294.

240. Curtis LE, Sheahan DG. Heterotopic tissues in the gall bladder. Arch Pathol 1969;88:677–683.

241. Evans MM, Nagorney DM, Pernicone PJ, Perrault J. Heterotopic gastric mucosa in the common bile duct. Surgery 1990;108:96–100.

242. Kerimidas DE, Sknodros C, Anagnostou D, Doulas N. Gastric heterotopia in the gallbladder. J Pediatr Surg 1977;12:759–762.

243. Lyon DC. Recurrent pancreatitis caused by peptic ulceration in an intra-pancreatic gastric reduplication cyst. Br J Clin Pract 1969;23:425–427.

244. Briggs FLF, Moore JP. Heterotopic gastric mucosa of the small bowel with perforated ulcer. Am Surg 1979;45:413–417.

245. Douberneck RC, Deane WM, Antoine ME. Ectopic gastric mucosa in the ileum: a case of intussusception. J Pediatr Surg 1976;11:99–100.

246. Androvlakis JA, Gray SW, Lionakis B, Skandalakis JE. The sex ratio of Meckel's diverticulum. Am Surg 1969;35:455–460.

247. Draga BW, Levine S, Baker JJ. Heterotopic gastric and esophageal tissue in the vermiform appendix. Am J Clin Pathol 1963;40:190–193.

248. Dublilier LD, Caffrey PR, Hyde GL. Multifocal gastric heterotopia in a malformation of the colon presenting as a megacolon. Am J Clin Pathol 1969;51:646–653.

249. Burne JC. Pancreatic and gastric heterotopia in a diverticulum of the transverse colon. J Pathol Bact 1958;75:470.

250. Nicholson GW. Heteromorphoses (metaplasia) of the alimentary tract. J Pathol Bact 1923;23:399–417.

251. Goldfarb WB, Schaefer R. Gastric heterotopia in the rectum: report of a case. Ann Surg 1961;154:133–136.

252. Breton P, Larget P, Isidor P. Ulcère peptique du rectum. Hétérotopie de type gastrique (fundique) de la muqueuse rectal. Arch Mal Appar Dig 1955;44:1153–1161.

253. Stockman JM, Young VT, Jenkins AL. Duplication of the rectum containing gastric mucosa. JAMA 1960;173:1223–1225.

254. Allison PR, Johnstone AS. The esophagus lined with gastric mucous membrane. Thorax 1953;8:87–101.

255. Taylor AL. The epithelial heterotopias of the alimentary tract. J Pathol Bact 1927;30:415–449.

256. King ESJ, MacCallum P. Pancreatic tissue in the wall of the stomach. Arch Surg 1934;28:125.

257. Artigas V, Calabuig R, Badia F, Rius X, Allende L, Jover J. Meckel's diverticulum: valve of ectopic tissue. Am J Surg 1986;151:631–634.

258. Basa AK, Chatterjee SK. Teratoma in children under 7 years of age: analysis of 65 cases. Pediatr Surg Int 1989;4:199–201.

259. DeAngelis VR. Gastric teratoma in a newborn infant: total gastrectomy with survival. Surgery 1969;66:794.

260. Azpiroz JAC et al. Gastric teratoma in infants: case report. Am J Surg 1974;128:429.

261. Nandy AD et al. Teratoma of the stomach. J Pediatr Surg 1974;9:563.

262. Cairo M, Grosfeld J, Weetman R. Gastric teratoma: unusual cause for bleeding of the upper gastrointestinal tract in the newborn. Pediatrics 1981;67:721.

263. Skandalakis JE, Gray SW, Brown BC, Mullins JD. Nonepithelial tumors of the stomach and duodenum. In: Nyhus LM, Wastell C, eds. Surgery of the stomach and duodenum, 4th ed. Boston: Little, Brown, 1986.

264. Teng PK, Cho S. Massive gastric hemorrhage from the rupture of an arterial malformation. NY State J Med 1985;85:112–113.

265. Goldman RL. Submucosal arterial malformation (aneurysm) of the stomach with fatal hemorrhage. Gastroenterology 1964;46:589–594.

266. deVirgilio C et al. Dieulafoy's lesion associated with truncus arteriosus type IV; an unusual cause of upper gastrointestinal hemorrhage. Am J Gastroenterol 1988;83:865–867.

267. Fiddian-Green RG. Vascular diseases. In: Kelley WN, ed. Textbook of internal medicine, Vol 1. Philadelphia: JB Lippincott, 1989.

268. Juler GL, Lavitzke HG, Lamb R, Allen R. The pathogenesis of Dieulafoy's gastric erosion. Am J Gastroenterol 1984;79:195.

269. Monk JE, Smith BA, O'Leary JP. Arteriovenous malformations of the small intestine. South Med J 1989;82:18–22.

270. Hemingway AP, Allison DJ. Angiodysplasia and Meckel's diverticulum: a congenital association? Br J Surg 1982;69:493–496.

271. Weaver GA, Alpern HD, Davis JS, Ramsey WH, Reichelderfer M.

Gastrointestinal angiodysplasia associated with aortic valve disease: part of a spectrum of angiodysplasia of the gut. Gastroenterology 1979;77:1–11.

272. Gunnlaugsson O. Angiodysplasia of the stomach and duodenum. Gastrointest Endosc 1985;31:251–254.

273. Moretó M, Figa M, Ojembarrena E, Zaballa M. Vascular malformations of the stomach and the duodenum: an endoscopic classification. Endoscopy 1986;18:227–229.

274. Marwick T, Kerlin P. Angiodysplasia of the upper gastrointestinal tract: clinical spectrum in 41 cases. J Clin Gastroenterol 1986;8:404–407.

275. Steer ML, Silen W. Diagnostic procedures in gastrointestinal hemorrhage. N Engl J Med 1983;309:646–650.

276. Rugeerts P, Vantrappen G, D'Heygere F, Broeckaert L. Transendoscopic Doppler ultrasound: usefulness for diagnosis and treatment of vascular malformations. Endoscopy 1988;20:99–101.

277. Lewis JW, Mason EE, Jochimsen PR. Vascular malformations of the stomach and duodenum. Surg Gynecol Obstet 1981;153:225–228.

278. Witte JT, Hasson JE, Harms BA, Corrigan TE, Love RB. Fatal gastric artery dissection and rupture occurring as a paraesophageal mass: a case and literature review. Surgery 1990;107:590–594.

279. Gallard T. Aneurysmes millaires de l'estomac, donnant lieu à des hematemesis mortelles. Bull Soc Med Hosp Paris 1884;1:84.

280. Lumsden AB, Ricey JD, Skandalakis JE. Splenic artery aneurysms. Probl Gen Surg 1990;7:113–121.

CHAPTER 6

THE SMALL INTESTINES

John Elias Skandalakis / Stephen Wood Gray / Richard Ricketts / Daniel Dale Richardson

*[a]It is less dangerous to leap from the Clifton Suspension Bridge than to suffer from
acute intestinal obstruction and decline operation.*
—SIR FREDERICK TREVES (1899)

DEVELOPMENT

At the beginning of the third week of development, the archenteron or primitive gut of the human embryo already is demarcated into three regions. Anteriorly in the head fold lies the foregut from which will develop the pharynx, esophagus, and stomach. Posteriorly in the small tail fold lies the hindgut with its ventral allantoic outgrowth. From the hindgut will be derived the terminal colon and rectum. At this stage the midgut opens ventrally into the yolk sac between these two portions. It should be remembered that the "midgut" to the embryologist is the portion of the primitive gut that is open ventrally into the yolk sac (Fig. 6.1, *A*). It contrasts with the foregut and hindgut, which are contained within the head and tail folds. Later in development, and in the adult, the term *midgut* applies to that portion of the intestines supplied by the superior mesenteric artery (extending from the duodenum to the middle of the transverse colon). (Fig. 6.1, *B*).

Forming the anterior boundary of the open embryonic midgut is the transverse septum. Into its substance the primordium of the liver will grow by proliferation of the endoderm of the terminal foregut. Dorsally, within the mesentery, will grow the pancreas. These structures mark the site of the future duodenum.

During the third and fourth weeks, the embryo grows rapidly, whereas the yolk sac and open midgut do not. By the fifth week, the connection with the yolk sac is no larger in diameter than that of the gut itself. It is referred to as the yolk stalk, the vitelline duct, or the omphalomesenteric duct. At this time a ventral swelling just posterior to the yolk stalk marks the beginning of the cecum and hence of the boundary between large and small intestines.

Elongation of the midgut, especially of its cranial limb between the duodenum and the yolk stalk, now proceeds

faster than does elongation of the embryonic body. According to Scammon and Kittelson (1), the small intestine at birth is six times the length of the colon and approximately three times the length of the infant. The result of this discrepancy between growth of the intestine and growth of the body is a series of remarkable intestinal movements which culminate in the final position of the large and small intestines in the abdomen. These movements may be divided into three stages (Fig. 6.2).

Stages of Development

THE FIRST STAGE: HERNIATION

The middle portion of the growing intestine buckles ventrally and begins to push out into the celom of the body stalk during the sixth week (10 mm). The apex of the entering loop is marked by the yolk stalk (omphalomesenteric duct), and its axis by the superior mesenteric artery, which is the proximal portion of the primitive blood supply to the yolk sac (vitelline artery). As this initial loop pushes into the body stalk, it undergoes a counterclockwise twist of 90 degrees, so that the cranial half, called "prearterial" in relation to the superior mesenteric artery, lies cranial to the caudal ("postarterial") half.

Continued elongation of the herniated loop is confined largely to the prearterial segment. Thus, while the postarterial limb, most of which will form the colon, remains relatively straight, the prearterial limb forms some six primary loops. Keibel and Mall believed that these primary loops maintain their identity in the adult (2).

THE SECOND STAGE: RETURN TO THE ABDOMEN

Herniation of the embryonic intestines was observed and recognized as a normal process by Meckel (3) in 1817. Not until 1897, however, did Mall (4) mark the time of their return to the abdomen, noting that the process must be rapid since embryos of about the same size—that is, 40 mm in length (10th week)—had intestines either in the cord or in the abdomen. Two years later, Mall (5) found

[a]Intestinal Obstruction, It's Varieties, with Their Pathology, Diagnosis and Treatment. The Jacksonian Prize Essay of the Royal College of Surgeons of England. From the Rise of Surgery by Wangensteen and Wangensteen, p. 106 and 611.

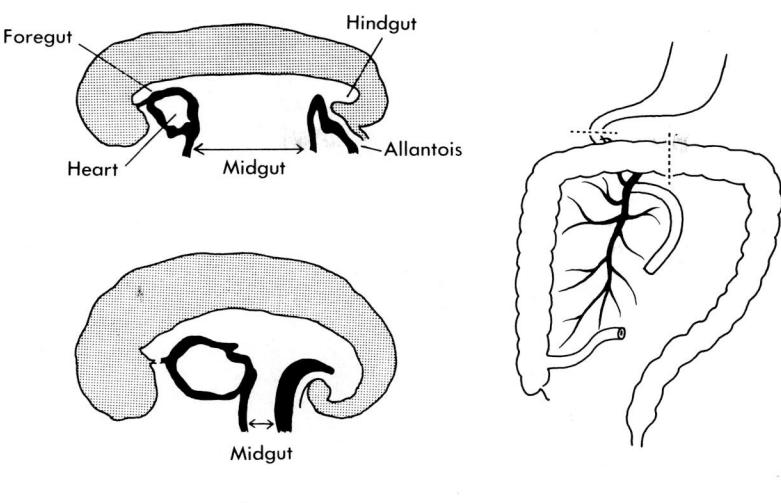

Figure 6.1. The ''midgut'' of the embryologist and of the surgeon. **A.** To the embryologist, the midgut is the central portion of the primitive gut, which is open to the yolk sac ventrad. Its extent decreases rapidly with embryonic growth. **B,** To the surgeon, the midgut is that part of the adult alimentary tract supplied by the superior mesenteric artery. It extends from the second part of the duodenum to the junction of middle and left thirds of transverse colon.

an embryo in which the intestines were ''in the act of returning from the coelom of the cord to the peritoneal cavity.''

The forces involved in this sudden return are still unknown. Herniation occurs because there is no room in the abdomen for the growing gut; later, as the liver decreases in relative size, more space is available. The actual return, however, is too rapid to be accounted for by growth forces alone although there may be some traction on the gut. The movement resembles one produced by external pressure, which builds up until resistance is overcome and finally pops the intestinal mass through the umbilical ring into the abdomen. In the course of this return, there is a further anticlockwise rotation of 180 degrees, which, added to the previous rotation, makes a total of 270 degrees.

The precise manner in which the coils of intestine return to the abdomen in this short time determines the position which they will occupy in the adult. Considerable debate about the details has taken place. The interested reader is referred to Estrada's monograph (6) for discussion and references.

The prearterial limb leaves the cord, first entering the abdomen to the right of the superior mesenteric artery. The abdominal portion of the colon is pushed to the left. The herniated colon now enters the abdomen, with the cecum and the terminal prearterial segment entering last. The colon lies in front of the superior mesenteric artery, and the cecum is at the level of the iliac crest. The transverse colon is still slightly lower than in the adult because of the size of the liver. It is during this stage that most of the anomalous arrangements occur.

THE THIRD STAGE: FIXATION

From the 12th week to well after birth, the final rearrangement of the colon takes place, and the mesenteries of the ascending and descending portions become adherent to the parietal peritoneum. Fixation may be arrested in various stages of completion. The cecum remains in its original position, whereas the colon is still elongating with the growing abdomen. The increasing distance between liver and the iliac fossa is occupied by the lengthening ascending colon. ''Descent'' of the cecum thus is accomplished by ''ascent'' of the hepatic flexure. Treitz (7) in 1857 explained fixation of the ascending and descending colon as the result of the enlarging viscus spreading the leaves of the mesentery until it was obliterated by the fusion of the intestine with the abdominal wall. In 1879 Toldt (8), from a study of a large number of embryos and infants, concluded that certain areas of mesentery undergo ''physiological fusion'' upon coming into contact with parietal peritoneum.

Prior to herniation, there is little difference between the endodermal lining of the various portions of the gut. The duodenum has grown faster and is larger than the more caudal portions. In keeping with the general cranial-to-caudal developmental gradient of the embryo, changes in the duodenum usually precede changes in more caudal segments.

The histogenesis of the intestinal tract was described in detail by Lewis (9) in Keibel and Mall's 1910 *Manual of Human Embryology*. To this fundamental work has been added the studies of Johnson (10), Lineback (11), Kanagasuntheram (12), Daikoku et al. (13), Orlic and Lev (14), Moxey and Trier (15), and others.

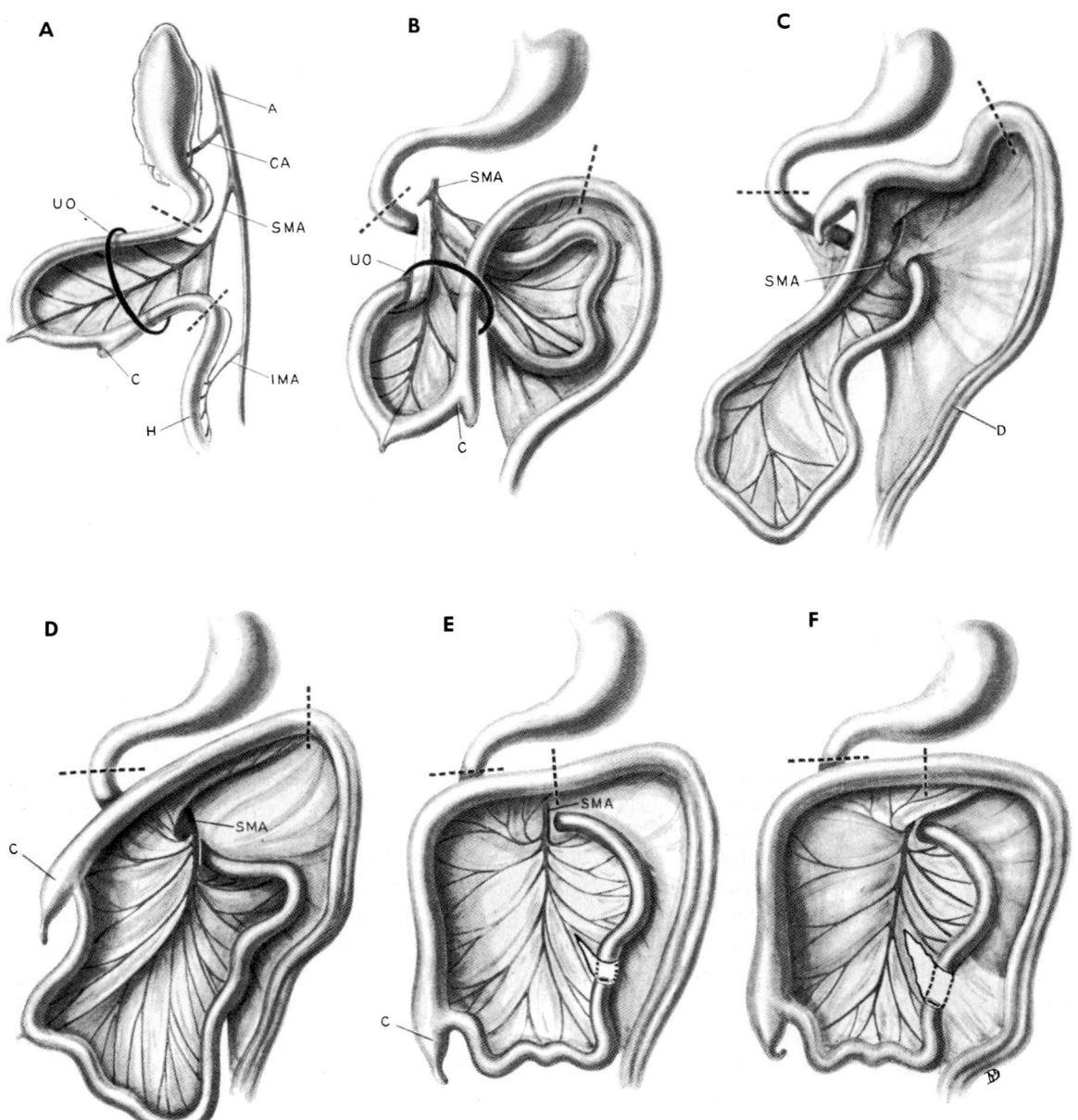

Figure 6.2. Schematic drawing of normal development, rotation, and attachment of the midgut. The midgut in each sketch is that part included between the *dashed lines* and represents that portion of the alimentary tract from the duodenum to midtransverse colon which is supplied by the superior mesenteric artery. **A**, Fifth week of fetal life (lateral view). The foregut, midgut, and hindgut with their respective blood supplies are indicated. Most of the midgut is extruded into the base of the umbilical cord, where it normally resides from about the fifth to the tenth week. **B**, Tenth week of fetal life. The intestine is elongating and the hindgut is displaced to the left side of the abdomen. The developing, intraabdominal intestines come to lie behind the superior mesenteric artery. A portion of the midgut still protrudes through the umbilical orifice into the base of the cord. **C**, Eleventh week of fetal life. All of the alimentary tract is withdrawn into the abdomen. The cecum lies in the epigastrium, beneath the stomach. **D**, Late 11th week of fetal life. The colon is rotating; the cecum lies in the right upper quadrant of the abdomen. **E**, Rotation of the colon is complete, and the cecum lies in its final position. There is a common mesentery—the mesocolon of the ascending colon is continuous with the mesentery of the ileum. There is no posterior attachment of this common mesentery except at the origin of the superior mesenteric artery. **F**, Final stage in attachment of the mesenteries. The ascending and descending mesocolons become fused to the posterior abdominal wall; thereby, the mesentery of the jejunum and ileum gain a posterior attachment from the origin of the superior mesenteric artery obliquely downward to the cecum. (From Gross RE. The surgery of infancy and childhood. Philadelphia: WB Saunders, 1953.)

As early as the 4-mm stage (stage 12), the duodenal mucosa begins to proliferate, especially along the right wall near the origin of the hepatic diverticulum, which arises from the ventral wall during this stage. By 14 mm (stage 16), only a few luminal clefts remain in the epithelium. Moutsouris (16) examined 70 embryos between 7 and 40 mm and observed the epithelial proliferation, although he rejected the terms *occluded* and *solid* state. The lumen is completely restored by the 18-mm stage and has become almost entirely single-layered by 37 mm (10th week).

Although the hepatic bud arises ventrally, the bile duct enters the left wall of the duodenum during the period of epithelial proliferation. Kanagasuntheram (12) believes the orifice of the duct migrates in the thick epithelium and that there is no true rotation of the duodenum. He assigns the change in the mesenteric attachment to extension of the celom rather than to rotation.

Around the turn of the 19th century, the hypothesis that the lumina of both the esophagus and the duodenum were occluded by proliferating epithelium was more or less accepted. To this occlusion was subsequently ascribed the formation of diverticula, duplications, and atresias, as the result of recanalization—or its failure—of the epithelial plug (17, 18). Complete occlusion of the esophagus has since been denied. The situation in the lower gut has been somewhat clarified by the studies of Lynn and Espinas (19), who found occlusion in various portions of the gut in 40% of embryos during the fifth and eighth weeks. Occlusion is probably the incidental result of epithelial proliferation rather than a definite, necessary stage in gut development. It seems unquestionable that intramural duplication and small diverticula present in some individuals may result from this occlusion, such as was described by Bremer (17).

During this same period, the exuberant proliferation of the epithelium produces bulges into the antimesenteric mesenchyme to form the bud-like diverticula described by Lewis and Thyng (20), Johnson (10), and Guthrie and Wakefield (21). These diverticula appear in large numbers in embryos between 16 and 30 mm (sixth to eighth weeks). Over 40 have been counted in a single embryo. They are more frequent in the duodenum and in the ileum than in the jejunum. After the 30-mm stage (eighth week), they are normally absorbed into the wall of the rapidly growing gut. That they are not always resorbed is evident from Carter's report (22) of their presence in a newborn infant.

Another characteristic phenomenon, reported by Lacroix et al. (23), is the early organogenesis of the small bowel. This takes place at the eighth to tenth week of gestation when the luminal surface of the entire length of the small intestine is covered by stratified epithelium four-layers thick.

Villus formation is first observable in the duodenum at 19 mm (eighth week) by the extension of mesodermal cords into the epithelium. The first sign of villi on the mucosal surface is in the lower duodenum and upper jejunum, at about 23 mm. In some portions of the jejunum and ileum, Johnson (10) observed longitudinal mucosal folds, which subsequently fragmented to form longitudinal rows of villi, between which new villi formed as the diameter of the gut increased. It is not until the fourth month (130 mm) that the whole of the small intestine is provided with villi.

By approximately 12 weeks, the small intestine in toto is covered with villi as demonstrated by the reports of Daikoku et al. (13) and Orlic and Lev (14).

Touloukian and Hastings (24) reported villus hypertrophy on both the proximal and the distal segment of 19 newborn infants with jejunoileal atresia. Does Mother Nature want to compensate the intestinal loss with that? These authors speculated, and we agree with them.

Crypts first appear as solid knobs on the mesenchymal side of the epithelium at 55 mm. A few Brunner's glands are seen in the upper duodenum as early as 78 mm (third month), before the muscularis mucosae is present. By 120 mm (fourth month), they extend throughout the duodenum. By the fifth month, they appear to be secretory (25). Circular folds (plicae) appear at 73 mm (third month) in the upper ileum and spread craniad and caudad until the 240-mm stage (seventh month).

Goblet cells appear in the villous epithelium by the third month. They are said to arise from chief cells, which during the third and fourth months are rich in glycogen. The striated border is present by the third month. Paneth cells appear in the crypts in the fifth month and reach their adult concentration by the ninth month (25). However, Moxey and Trier (15) reported formation of crypts 1 week after the appearance of the villi with the Paneth cells at their base, columnar epithelium at their apex, and (approximately around the ninth week) undifferentiated goblet cells all over the stratified epithelium.

Menard (26) also stated that at 8 to 9 weeks, villi are present at the duodenum and proximal ileum, and 2 to 3 weeks later, the entire small intestinal mucosa is lined by villi which are covered by simple columnar epithelium. Crypts are formed between the 10th to 12th weeks, and by 16 weeks, morphologically, the small bowel is similar to that of the adult (Fig. 6.3).

Enterochromaffin (argentaffin) cells, which secrete serotonin, were once assumed to migrate into the gut from the neural crest. Chick embryo experiments by Andrew (27) seem to suggest a local origin. This view is supported by observations in the human embryo (28). Chromaffin cells appear in the duodenum by the 39-mm stage and in the colon by 65 mm. They reach their greatest concentration in the fifth month (28, 29) and also are

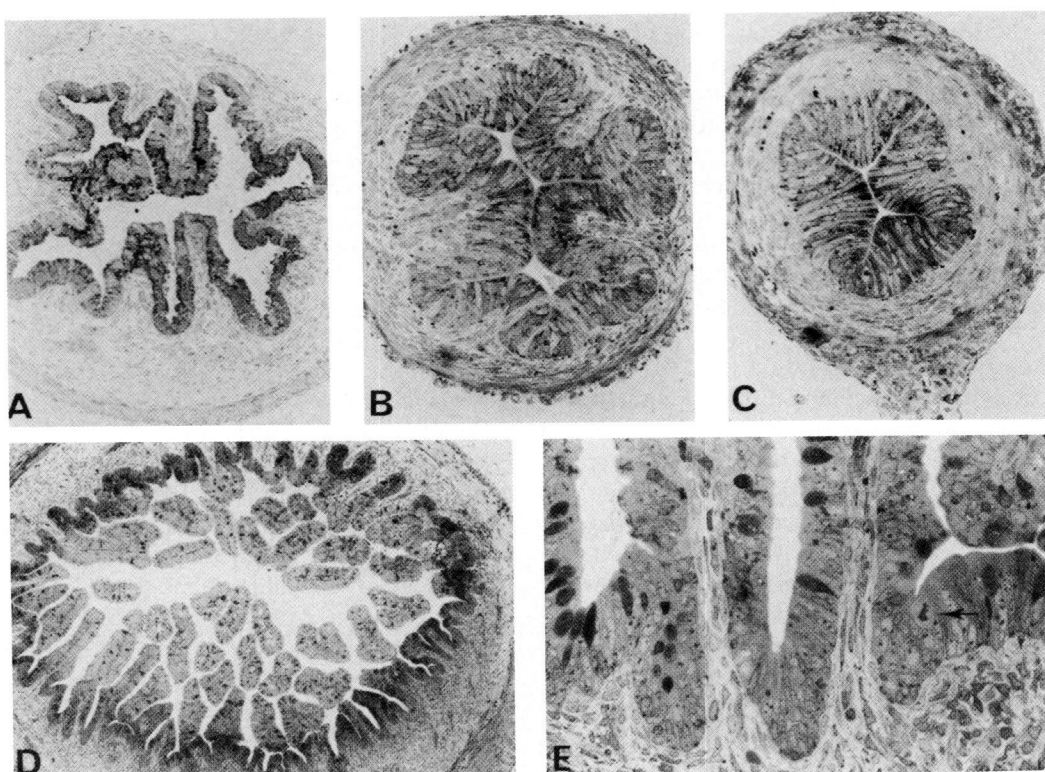

Figure 6.3. Epoxy sections (1 μ thick) of developing human small intestine stained with a mixture of 1% methylene blue, 1% azure II, and 1% borax. **A** to **C**, Morphogenesis of villi in a 9-week-old fetus in the proximal jejunum (**A**, ×25), proximal ileum (**B**, ×40), and distal ileum (**C**, ×40). **D**, This section from a 16- week fetus illustrates the presence of well-defined villi and crypts (×16). **E**, High magnification of the crypt region with undifferentiated cells and mitosis *(arrow)* (×100). (From Lebenthal E, ed. Human gastrointestinal development. New York: Raven Press, 1989:124.)

present in aganglionic colons (27). The origin of endocrine cells of the small bowel is unknown, according to Seidman and Walker (30). However, the research of Bryant et al. (31) in the development of intestinal regulatory peptides is very promising.

The circular muscle may be identified in the duodenum as early as the 10-mm stage (late fifth week); it is differentiated from the mesenchyme at the ileocecal junction by the end of the sixth week. Longitudinal muscle appears in the third month and the muscularis mucosae by late in the fifth month. Lymphoid tissue appears at the seventh month (12).

The neuroblasts of the myenteric plexus follow the vagus down the gut before the longitudinal muscle layer forms (32). Okamoto and Ueda (33) found neuroblasts at the esophagus in the sixth week and throughout the cranial loop of the gut in the seventh week. Sympathetic fibers without neuroblasts also are present. By the eighth week, neuroblasts are present in all but the distal half of the colon. Innervation of the gut and of the base of the bladder is complete by the 12th week. The ganglion cells of the submucosal plexus appear to arise from the myenteric plexus by migration.

Gabella (34) counted ganglion cells of Auerbach's plexus in the rat. There are seven times as many cells per square centimeter of intestine at birth than at maturity. As the surface area of the intestine increases 28 times, the number of ganglion cells increased four times between birth and maturity. Specific details of development of the colon and rectum are described in Chapter 7, The Colon and Rectum.

There are new concepts in gastrointestinal development. The scope of this book is the etiology and morphology of normal and abnormal anatomic entities. However, we refer the interested reader to the 1989 edition of *Human Gastrointestinal Development* by Lebenthal (35), which presents in a beautiful way the interactions of his four concepts: genetic endowment, developmental clock, regulatory mechanism, and environmental influences (Fig. 6.4 and Table 6.1). Lebenthal thinks "there is light in the long tunnel ahead," but much work must be done to understand the pathophysiology of selected diseases of the gastrointestinal tract.

Haffen et al. (36) stated in 1989 that there is no question that theoretical changes involving the fundamental role of intestinal mesenchyme "in promoting intrinsic

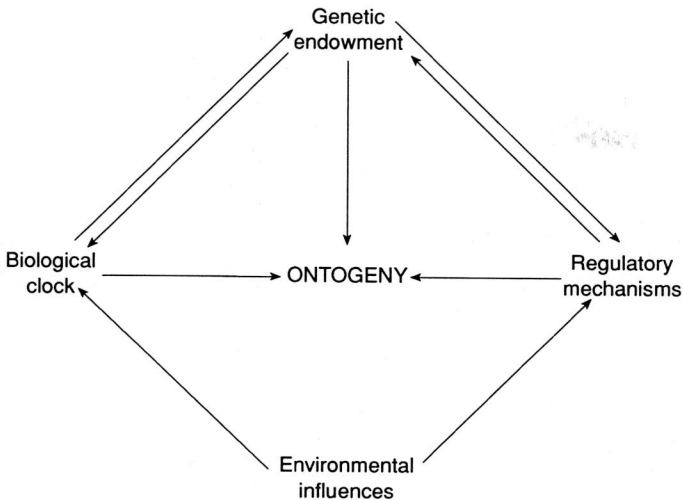

Figure 6.4. Interaction of determinants in the ontogeny of the gastrointestinal tract. (From Lebenthal E, ed. Human gastrointestinal development. New York: Raven Press, 1989:4.)

developmental capacities of endodermal and crypt cells through permissive inductive effects," and the role of intestinal endoderm in smooth muscle morphogenesis are currently evolving.

A peculiar phenomenon is the concentration of cholecystokinin (CCK). The concentration is highest in the duodenum but has the largest mass in the jejunum. Perhaps this is because CCK localizes in endocrine cells at the duodenum. In contrast, CCK is localized in nerves in the distal gut, as reported by Leung and Lebenthal (37). The overall ontogeny of the gastrointestinal hormones was mentioned previously, but Table 6.2 should be studied for the approximate time of the several peptides in several anatomic entities.

Saxena et al. (38), after experimental work in rats, suggested that epithelial cell migration occurs before proliferation during regeneration of the epithelium of the ileum after surgery. They further suggest that perhaps epidermal growth factor of endogenous origin may be responsible in intestinal regeneration.

In summary, the stages in development of the human small intestine are presented very well in the following table from Seidman and Walker (28) (Table 6.3).

Critical Events in Development

The greatest number of intestinal malformations are related to three developmental events:

1. Separation of the notochord from the endoderm of the archenteron roof during the third week. Failure of separation results in a variety of duplications of the intestines.
2. Regression of the vitelline stalk during the fifth week. Failure of regression causes Meckel's diverticulum or other less common vestiges.

Table 6.1.
Temporal Sequence of Development of the Gastrointestinal Tract in Human Fetus[a]

Anatomic Development	Week
Esophagus	
Superficial glands develop	20
Squamous cells appear	28
Stomach	
Gastric glands form	14
Pylorus and fundus defined	14
Pancreas	
Differentiation of endocrine and exocrine tissue	14
Liver	
Lobules form	11
Small intestine	
Crypt-villi develop	14
Lymph nodes appear	14
Colon	
Diameter increases	20
Villi disappear	20

Functional Development	
Suckling and swallowing	
Only mouthing	28
Immature suck-swallow	33–36
Stomach	
Gastric motility and secretion	20
Pancreas	
Zymogen granules	20
Liver	
Bile metabolism	11
Bile secretion	22
Small intestine	
Active transport of amino acids	14
Glucose transport	18
Fatty acids absorption	24
Enzymes	
α-Glucosidases	10
Dipeptidases	10
Lactase	10
Enterokinase	26

[a]From Lebenthal E. Human gastrointestinal development. New York: Raven Press, 1989:6.

Table 6.2.
Ontogeny of the Gastrointestinal Peptides[a]

Peptide	Age of Earliest Appearance (wk)
Glucagon	6 (pancreas)
Insulin	10 (pancreas)
Somatostatin	8 (pancreas)
Somatostatin	9–11 (intestine)
Pancreatic polypeptide	8–9 (pancreas)
Gastrin	10–11 (duodenum)
Cholecystokinin	10 (duodenum)
Secretin	8 (duodenum)
Gastric inhibitory polypeptide	8–10 (duodenum and jejunum)
Vasoactive intestinal polypeptide	8–9 (fundus and duodenum)
Vasoactive intestinal polypeptide	10 (VIP-nerve fibers)
Neurotensin	12 (jejunum, ileum, colon)
Motilin	8–11 (duodenum, jejunum)
Substance P	18–25 (brainstem)
Bombesin	12 (bronchus)

[a]Leung YK, Lebenthal E. Gastrointestinal peptides: physiology, ontogeny, and clinical significance. In Lebenthal E, ed. Human gastrointestinal development. New York: Raven Press, 1989:42.

Table 6.3.
Stages in Development of the Human Small Intestine[a]

Age (wk)	Length (Crown-Rump) (mm)	Structural	Cellular	Functional	Immune
2.5	1.5	Gut not distinct			
4	5	Foregut, midgut, hindgut distinguishable			
6	12				
7	17	Intestine herniates into umbilical cord	Epithelium stratified		Intraepithelial and lymph node lymphocytes
8	23	Villi appear (duodenum) Circular muscle layer		Gut neuroendocrine peptides appear	
9	30	Crypts appear Longitudinal muscle layer Auberbach's plexus appears	Goblet cells Blood vessels develop Meconium corpuscles appear		
10	40	Intestine returns to abdominal cavity	Crypts of Lieberkuhn present Paneth cells (crypt base) Columnar cells line villi Microvilli and glycocalyx		T cells have surface recognition
12	50	Villi to distal ileum		Active glucose transport Peristalsis present	Lymphocytes PHA responsive
14		Meissner's plexus		Dipeptidases Pepsin	Lymphocyte-mediated cytotoxity to PHA
16				L-Alanine specific transport Trypsinogen	GVH capability
20	160	Muscularis mucosae appears		α-Glucosidases Pancreatic amylase	Peyer's patches (ileum) and M cells
26			Absorptive cell maturity	Lingual lipase	
34	280			Pancreatic lipase	Few Ig-containing cells
38–40	350			Lactase 2–4 × (N)	Suppressor T cells predominate

[a]From Seidman EG, Walker WA. Development of the small intestines. In: Anderson CM, Burke V, Gracey M, ed. Paediatric gastroenterology. Melbourne, Australia: Blackwell Scientific Publications, 1987:118–136.

3. Return of the intestines to the abdomen in the 10th week. Malrotations, omphalocele, and anomalies of the mesenteries arise from failure of proper return to the abdomen.

ANOMALIES OF THE SMALL INTESTINES (TABLE 6.4 AND FIG. 6.5)

Anomalies of Intestinal Rotation and Fixation (Table 6.5)

Much of the growth and development of the intestinal tract takes place outside the abdomen. During the 10th week, the intestines are rapidly repacked into the abdominal cavity. This repacking may result in anomalies of rotation or fixation.

The formation of most but not all of these anomalies is easily deduced from their appearance in the infant or adult. However, we must keep in mind that developmental stages have not been observed directly. Our theories of maldevelopment during the third stage and formation of "internal herniae" must remain open to reinterpretation from experimental data.

It is convenient to group these intestinal anomalies according to the developmental stages during which they may occur. These are:

1. *First stage:* Herniation (10 to 40 mm, sixth to tenth week); the rapidly elongating gut pushes out of the abdomen into the body stalk.
2. *Second stage:* Return to the abdomen (40 mm, 10th week); the gut reenters the abdominal cavity, and the loops assume their definitive positions.
3. *Third stage:* Fixation (50 mm, 11th week until well after birth); portions of the mesentery fuse with the parietal peritoneum, and the cecum descends to its adult position.

Table 6.4.
Anomalies of the Small Intestines

Anomaly	Origin of Defect	First Appearance	Sex Chiefly Affected	Relative Frequency	Remarks
Nonrotation and malrotation	10th week	At any age	Male	Common	
Atresia: Primary	6th to 7th week (failure of recanalization)	At birth	Equal	Rare	
Extensive intestinal atresia, "apple peel"	10th week	At birth	Equal	Rare	
Secondary	10th week: (umbilical snaring): 4th month or later (volvulus or intussusception)	First few days of life	Equal	Common	
Stenosis	6th to 7th week	Infancy	Equal	Uncommon	May accompany annular pancreas
Patent omphalomesenteric duct	5th week	At birth	Male	Rare	Symtomatic early in life if gastric mucosa is present
Meckel's diverticulum	5th week	Childhood or later	Male	Common	
Nonmeckelian diverticulum	4th week or later	Middle age	Equal	Rare	
Cystic and tubular duplication	4th week	At any age	Equal	Uncommon	
Preduodenal portal vein	4th week	Infancy	?	Rare	May be asymptomatic
Superior mesenteric artery syndrome	?	Middle age	Female	Rare	Not certainly of congenital origin
Arteriovenous malformation	Unknown	Any age	Equal	Rare	

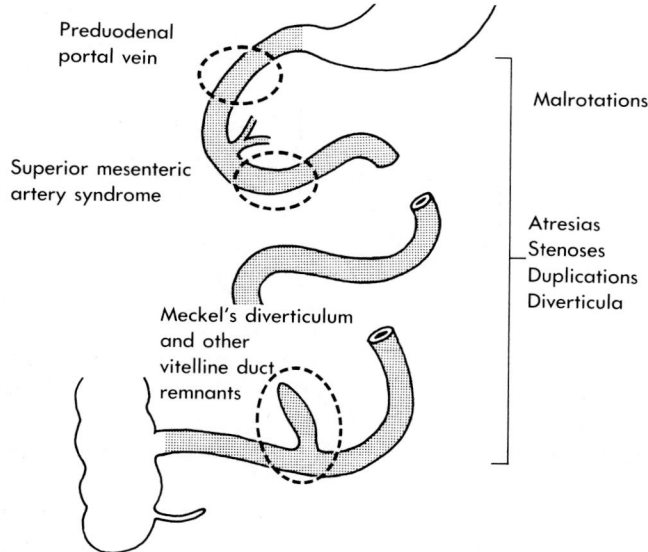

Figure 6.5. The congenital anomalies of the small intestines.

ANATOMY

Maldevelopment During the First Stage.

Malrotation of the Duodenum.

The duodenum rotates 90 degrees to reach the region of the superior mesenteric artery before the return of the intestines. It may become prematurely fixed by adhesions before completing its rotation. Subsequent rotation of the returning intestines is not affected (39). Very few cases have been observed.

Exomphalos.

Exomphalos, as well as many umbilical herniae, represents a developmental arrest at the end of the first stage of intestinal development. The intestines fail to return to the abdomen (Fig. 6.6).

In such patients the abdomen at birth is too small to contain the ectopic intestines. This has led some authors to believe that failure to return is the result of inadequate development of the body wall (40). We believe that the undersized cavity is secondary to the failure of intestinal return. The bulk of the contents determines the size of the abdomen. Regardless of the cause, the surgical problem centers on the abdominal wall. Exomphalos and related conditions are discussed in Chapter 16, The Anterior Body Wall.

Adams et al. (41) reported that conservative treatment of major exomphalos has less local and systemic complication.

Maldevelopment During the Second Stage. The normal rotation of the midgut around the superior mesenteric artery axis is 90 degrees counterclockwise to the observer during the first stage. During the second stage, a further rotation of 180 degrees takes place. While some rotational errors may originate in the first stage, it is convenient to consider them together here.

Table 6.5.
Synopsis of Anomalies of Intestinal Rotation and Fixation

Condition	Incidence	Symptoms and Diagnosis
Nonrotation	Common; more frequent in males	Asymptomatic, or may result in volvulus
Mixed rotation	Common	Volvulus often present in first few days of life; twisted barium column in duodenum; signs of duodenal obstruction
Reversed rotation	Rare; more frequent in males	Ileocecal volvulus eventually develops; attacks become progressive
Hyperrotation	Rare	Asymptomatic
Undescended subhepatic cecum	Common; more frequent in males	Asymptomatic
Inverted cecum	Rare	Asymptomatic
Mobile cecum	Common; more frequent in males	Volvulus of right colon: recurrent right lower quadrant attacks: barium enema fails to fill ascending colon
		Volvulus of small intestine: recurrent lower or left lower quadrant attacks since childhood; hypertrophy of jejunum; variation in position of cecum
Anomalous fixation of cecum	Rare; sexes equally affected	Volvulus of small intestine: cecum constantly on left; barium meal may show duodenal dilation and gastric retention; intermittent attacks
Retroperitoneal cecum	Common	Asymptomatic
Paraduodenal herniae	Rare; more frequent in males; 3 to 6 times as frequent on left	Asymptomatic or with trivial symptoms until obstruction takes place; abdominal examination useful only during attacks; radiography shows intestines confined to oval or spherical zone, from which they cannot be displaced

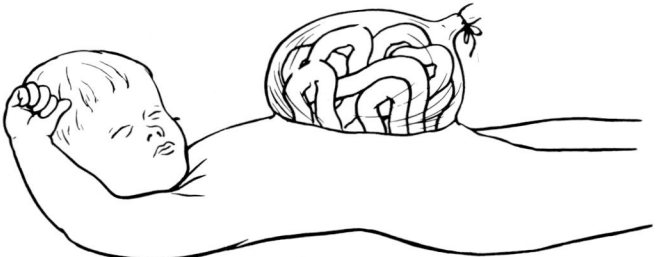

Figure 6.6. Exomphalos. The intestines have failed to return to the abdomen in the first stage of intestinal rotation and fixation.

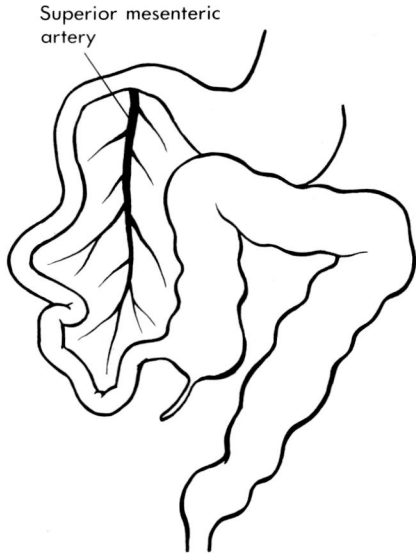

Figure 6.7. Nonrotation. Return of the postarterial segment leaves the whole of the colon on the left and the small intestine on the right.

Nonrotation.

In this condition, the gut is rotated only 180 degrees instead of the normal 270 degrees. The postarterial (colonic) limb reenters the abdomen first instead of last; thus the colon lies on the left, the cecum is in the midline, and the small intestine is on the right (Fig. 6.7). This condition is said to be found in 0.5% of autopsies and seems to be twice as frequent in males as in females. Hadley (42) suggests a familial occurrence. Volvulus as a result of local clockwise rotation frequently accompanies nonrotation.

Mixed Rotation.

A rotation of only 180 degrees takes place, and the terminal ileum enters the abdomen first.

The cecum is subpyloric and fixed to the abdominal wall, binding down the duodenum (Fig. 6.8). There may or may not be a clockwise rotation of the rest of the small intestine. As with nonrotation, volvulus is frequently present as a complication and constitutes the usual "obstruction due to malrotation" in infancy. Among Gross's patients (40), 18% had other anomalies.

Reversed Rotation.

A rotation of 90 degrees counterclockwise takes place during the first stage, followed by a rotation of 180 degrees clockwise in the second stage.

1. If the postarterial segment reenters the abdomen first, the colon lies behind the superior mesenteric artery and the small intestine is ventral to colon and artery (Fig. 6.9).

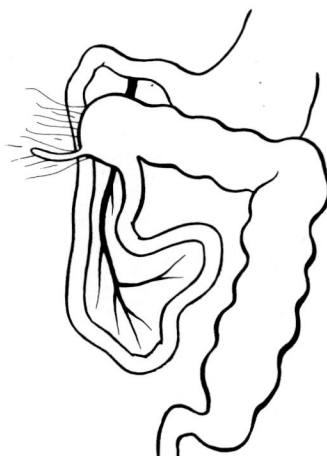

Figure 6.8. Mixed rotation. The prearterial segment has failed to rotate. The cecum becomes fixed to the abdominal wall and lies anterior to the second portion of the duodenum which may be compressed by the cecum.

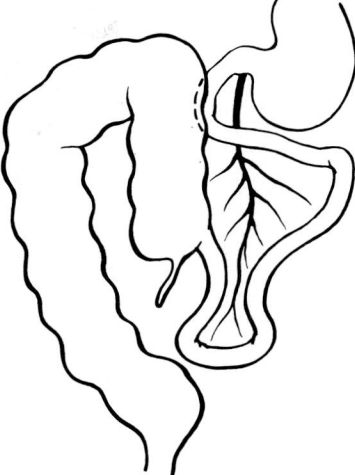

Figure 6.10. Reversed rotation. The colon occupies the right half of the abdomen, while the small intestine occupies the left half.

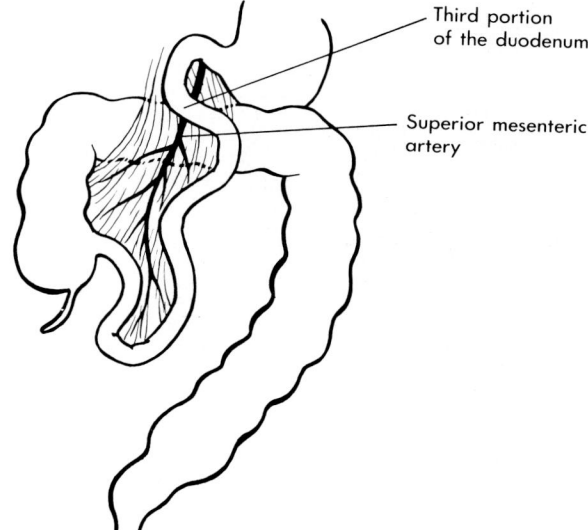

Figure 6.9. Reversed rotation. The third portion of the duodenum is anterior to the superior mesenteric artery, which in turn is anterior to the transverse colon. The postarterial segment has entered the abdodmen ahead of the prearterial segment.

Some 30 cases have been described since 1883. About 66% of them were males.

2. If the prearterial segment reenters first, the small intestine lies in front of the artery and fills the left side of the abdomen, while the colon lies to the right, with the cecum in the midline (Fig. 6.10). Only about six cases are known, two of them with situs inversus viscerum.

Hyperrotation (Hyperdescent of the Cecum).
The general intestinal pattern is normal, but the cecum continues to descend into the pelvis during the first few

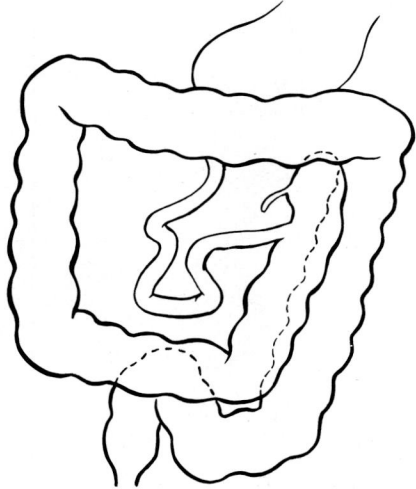

Figure 6.11. Hyperrotation. The colon is longer than normal, and the cecum has reached the splenic flexure instead of remaining in the right lower quadrant. (From Low FN, Hildermann WC. A case of hyperrotation of the colon. Anat Rec 1940;77:27–30.)

months of life (43). In one patient the cecum reascended to a position medial to the descending colon and posterior to the small intestine, ending near the splenic flexure and thus achieving a rotation of 495 degrees (44) (Fig. 6.11).

Encapsulated Small Intestine (Internal Omphalocele).
This is a rare condition in which the whole of the small intestine lies within an avascular sac that has no communication with the abdominal cavity proper (Figs. 6.12 and 6.13). The enclosed intestines may be normal, or they may be malrotated. The sac is not mesenteric in origin; it is the lining of the extraembryonic celom that has entered the

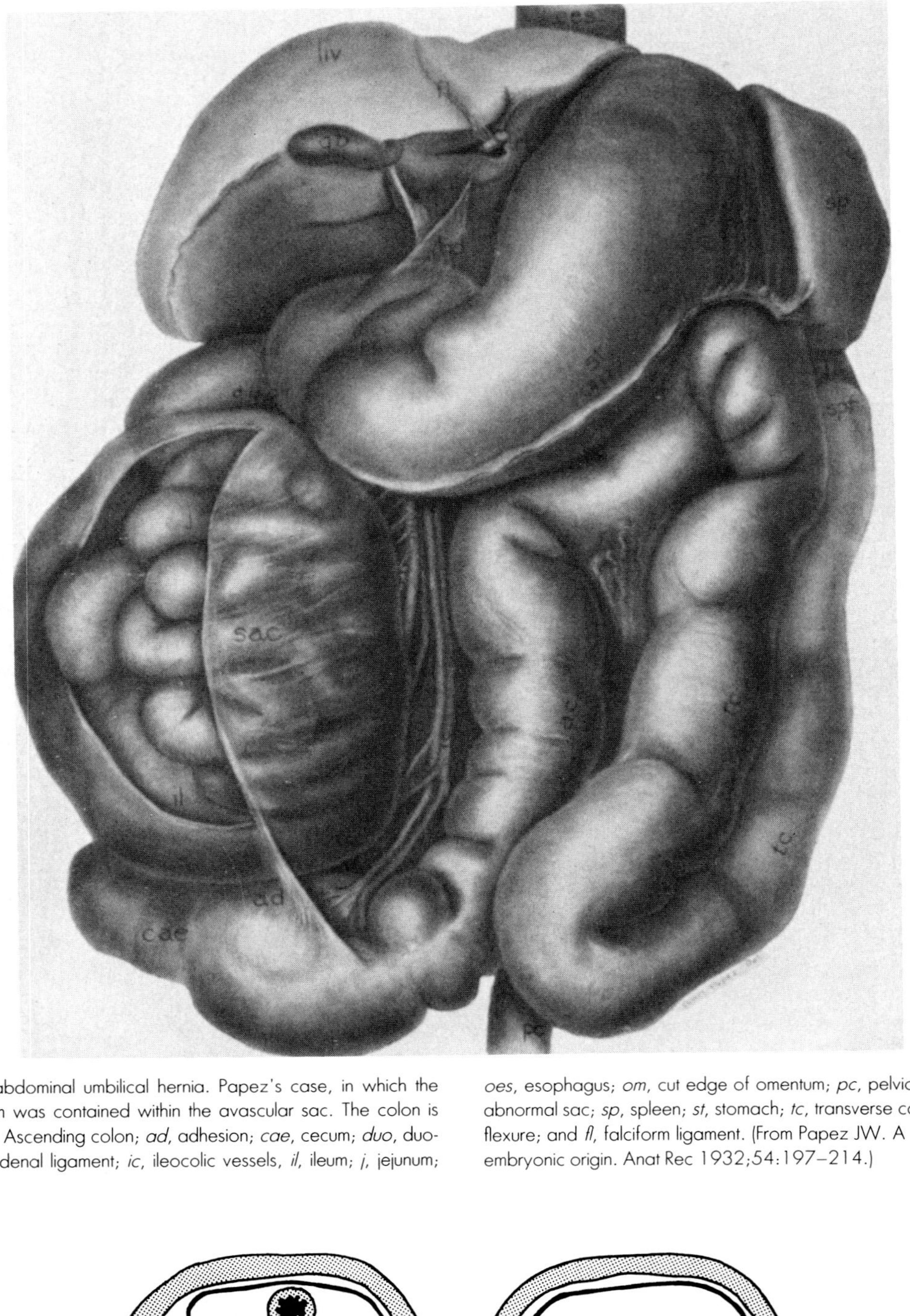

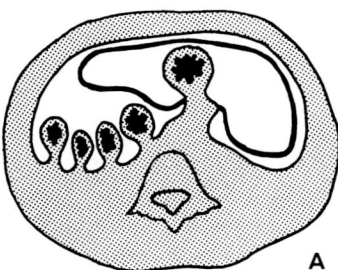

Figure 6.12.   Intraabdominal umbilical hernia. Papez's case, in which the entire ileum and jejunum was contained within the avascular sac. The colon is abnormally placed. *ac*, Ascending colon; *ad*, adhesion; *cae*, cecum; *duo*, duodenum; *hd*, hepatoduodenal ligament; *ic*, ileocolic vessels, *il*, ileum; *j*, jejunum; *oes*, esophagus; *om*, cut edge of omentum; *pc*, pelvic colon; *py*, pylorus; *sac*, abnormal sac; *sp*, spleen; *st*, stomach; *tc*, transverse colon; *liv*, liver; *spf*, splenic flexure; and *fl*, falciform ligament. (From Papez JW. A rare intestinal anomaly of embryonic origin. Anat Rec 1932;54:197–214.)

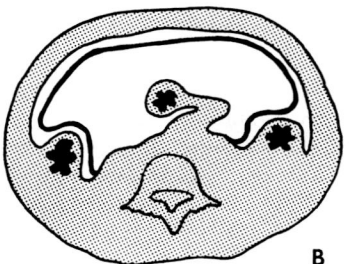

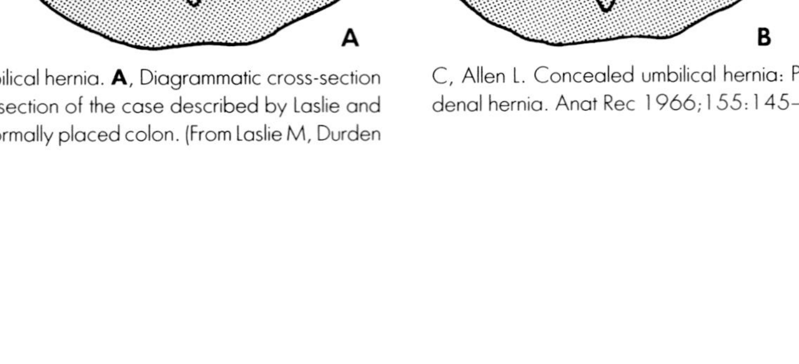

Figure 6.13.   Intraabdominal umbilical hernia. **A**, Diagrammatic cross-section of the hernia. **B**, Diagrammatic cross-section of the case described by Laslie and his colleagues, in which there was a normally placed colon. (From Laslie M, Durden C, Allen L. Concealed umbilical hernia: Papez's concept of so-called paraduodenal hernia. Anat Rec 1966;155:145–150.) Compare with Figure 6.12.

abdomen with the intestines instead of remaining in the base of the umbilical cord. The explanation for this bizarre anomaly was first proposed by Papez (45) and supported subsequently by Batson (46) and Laslie and his colleagues (47). This is not the same as "paraduodenal hernia."

No symptoms are produced by this anomaly, nor can it be diagnosed radiographically. Several examples have been found on dissection in elderly patients who had no known history of intestinal complaints.

Maldevelopment During the Third Stage.
Undescended Cecum.

Strictly speaking, this is a misnomer. Failure of the colon to elongate permits the cecum to move upward with the liver as the abdomen enlarges prior to fixation of the cecum (Fig. 6.14). More common in males than in females, this condition is present in about 6% of individuals. Some elongation of the colon occurs after birth, since the incidence of undescended cecum is higher at birth than it is at the age of 18 months (43).

Inverted Cecum.

Cecal inversion, a condition that is rare and asymptomatic, results from early fixation of the cecum in the subhepatic position. Subsequent elongation of the transverse colon causes the cecum to point upward (Fig. 6.15).

Mobile Cecum.

Mobile cecum results from incomplete fixation of the ascending colon. The cecum alone may be free, or there may be an ascending mesocolon. All gradations occur (48). In 5.6% of 194 cadavers examined, the cecum was completely fixed; in 11.2%, it was free enough to twist and hence to produce volvulus. From other series reviewed, it appears that in about 10% of adults the cecum is free to undergo volvulus (49). In the newborn infant the incidence is higher than in the adult. Fixation may proceed up to 6 months of age.

A persistent ascending mesocolon may or may not be associated with a mobile cecum, and the cecum may be secondarily anchored. In many cases part of the mesocolon is a pseudomesentery pulled out from the parietal peritoneum to equalize the strain resulting from partial obliteration of the true mesentery (50).

Retroperitoneal Cecum.

The normally lateral parietal peritoneal attachment of the cecum is on the posterior and lateral colonic surface. A revolution of the cecum around its long axis after fixation may cause the cecum to roll partly under its lateral attachment (Fig. 6.16). The terms *Jackson's membrane* or *pericolic hyperfixation* (43) have been used.

Persistent Descending Mesocolon.

Failure of fixation may extend to other parts of the colon. A persistent left mesocolon may permit the colon to lie in the midline, where it may become secondarily fixed. The situation precedes left paraduodenal hernia. When the mesocolon persists into adult life, no true hernia exists although loops of the small intestine may be trapped behind the descending colon (51).

Persistent Ventral Mesentery.

We have seen a single report of a ventral sigmoid mesentery that included the uterus and bladder (Fig. 6.17). It was found incidentally to pelvic surgery (52). The anterior free edge from the bladder to the abdominal wall appeared to include the urachal remnant. Vesicorectal folds associated with double uterus also represent the ventral mesentery.

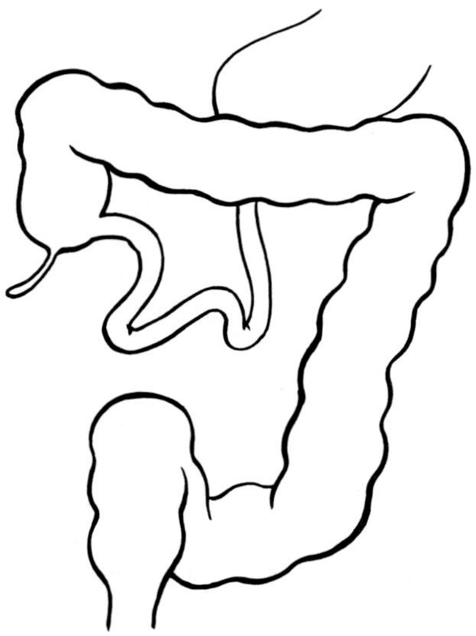

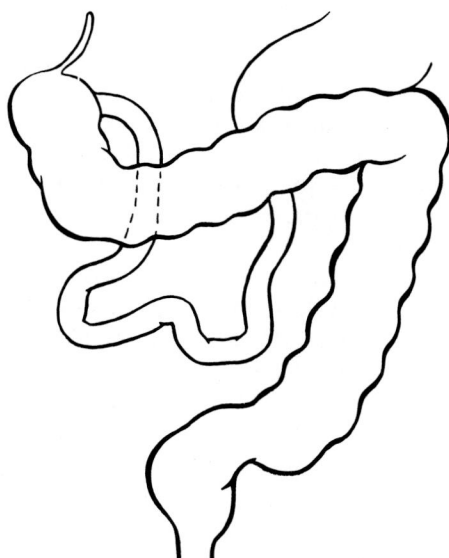

Figure 6.14. Undescended cecum. An arrest of colonic growth has occurred, so that the infantile position of the cecum is retained.

Figure 6.15. Inverted cecum. Early fixation, before elongation of the colon ceases, forces the cecum into this position.

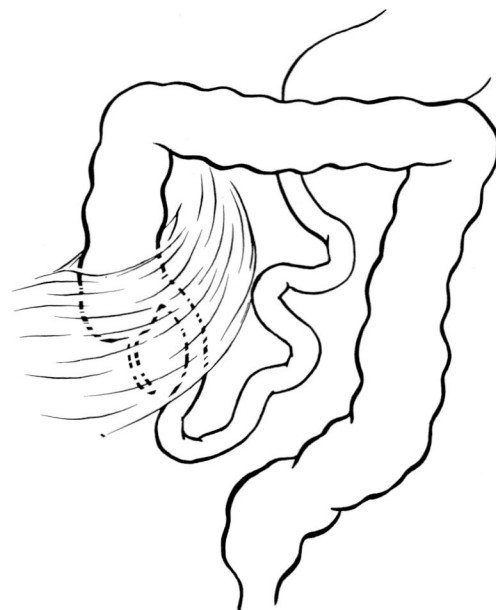

Figure 6.16. Retroperitoneal cecum. The cecum, appendix, and part of the ascending colon lie beneath a peritoneal membrane (Jackson's membrane).

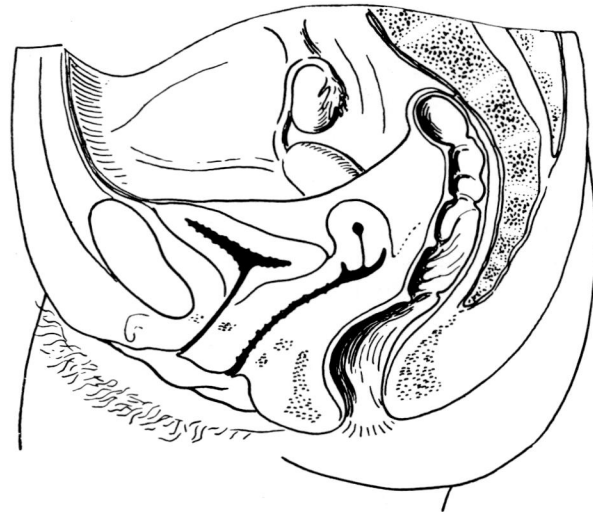

Figure 6.17. Persistent ventral mesentery extending from the colon to the bicornuate uterus and ending at the urachal remnant and dome of the bladder. (From Guillemin A, Dollander A. Persistance du septum cloacal sous forme d'un meso-vesico-utero-recto-sigmoide, chez une femme porteuse d'un uterus bicorne unicervical. Bull Fed Gynecol Obstet Franc [Suppl] 1961;13:505–507.

In summary, the abnormal anatomy presented is the result of failure of rotation and failure of fusion:

1. Failure of rotation of the duodenojejunal loop (Because of this failure, the duodenum is not behind but in front of the superior mesenteric vessels.)
2. The failure of the ileocolic loop to rotate and locate in front of the vessels or the small bowel mesentery
3. The failure of fusion of the mesentery of the small bowel (hernia of Waldyer) and transverse mesocolon

There are several degrees of fixation abnormalities of the intestines and their mesenteries. A special note should be made about the extrinsic obstruction of the duodenum by the membranes or folds of Ladd. There are folds starting from the abnormally high-positioned cecum to the posterior abdominal wall and across the second portion of the duodenum, producing a partial or total duodenal obstruction with the occasional participation of the cecum.

The double set of these retroperitoneal attachments are illustrated beautifully by Ford et al. (53) (Fig. 6.18).

Remember, congenital folds or membranes may be present in the duodenal vicinity without producing obstruction of a normally rotated or located duodenum. Another example is the formation of bands or folds between the terminal ileum and the proximal jejunum, in which the mesenteries are not fixed; a volvulus of one or several twists may be produced. Because several authors such as Willwerth et al. (54) questioned the lack of fixation of the mesocolon and mesentery of the small bowel, especially with the formation of paraduodenal herniae

(Fig. 6.19), we discuss this with the peritoneal defects in Chapter 4, The Peritoneum.

However, classification of clinical pictures of rotation of the loops of the midgut, with or without both fixation of the mesentery and the formation of folds or peritoneal bands, is very difficult. Rotation can stop anywhere, nonfixation can be of few centimeters or more, and bands may produce complete obstruction or just be innocent bystanders. The Smith classification is acceptable to us (Table 6.6).

Rescorla et al. (55), reporting in 1990, analyzed 447 cases with anomalies of rotation and fixation. They divided the cases into four groups:

1. Acute midgut volvulus
2. Duodenal obstruction or intermittent volvulus
3. Malrotation observed incidentally at exploration
4. Malrotation associated with diaphragmatic hernia or abdominal wall defects

Ford et al. (53) stated that the associated congenital malformations are very common and most of them have a gastrointestinal origin (Table 6.7).

HISTORY

Although a case of reversed rotation was described by Morgagni in 1761 (56), understanding of the arrangement of the intestines proceeded slowly. The extraembryonic growth of the intestines was known by Meckel (3) in 1817, but their return to the abdomen was not observed until 1899 (5) by Mall.

The work of Frazer and Robbins (57) in 1915 and especially that of Dott (58) in 1923 clarified the normal

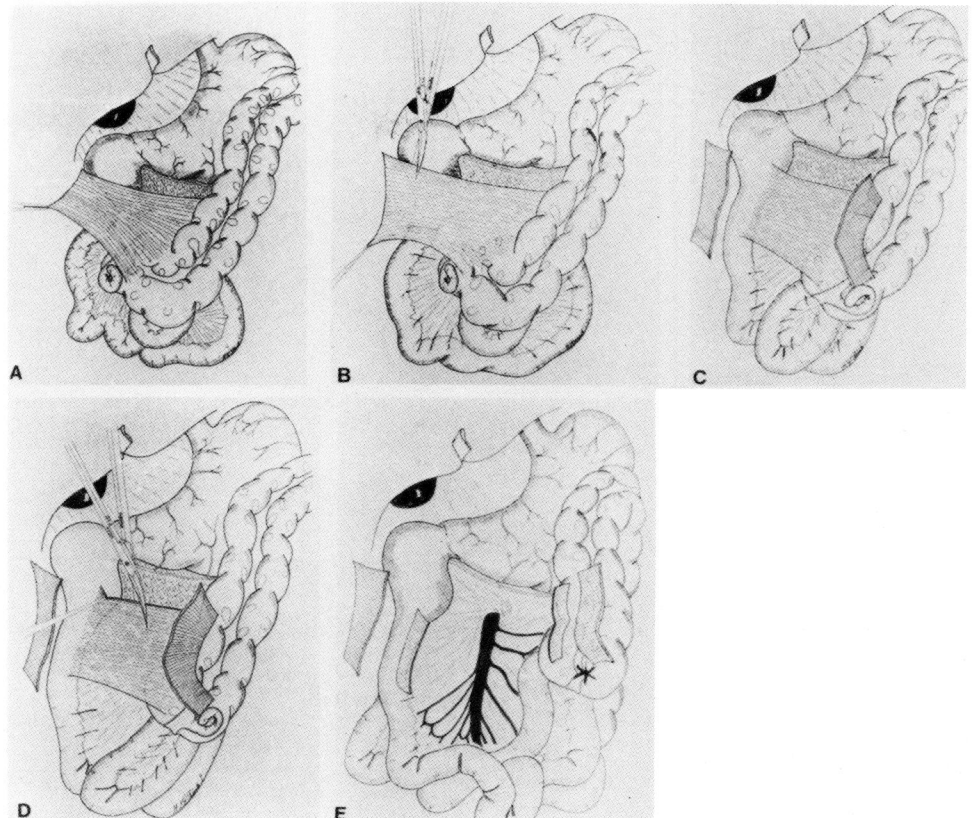

Figure 6.18. Operative repair of malrotation of the intestine. **A,** Ladds' bands traverse the duodenum, producing duodenal obstruction. **B,** Ladds' bands are incised along the anterior or anterolateral surface of the duodenum to relieve the duodenal obstruction. **C,** Division of Ladds' bands does not completely release the colon from its attachment to the duodenum. The ω shape is retained by a second set of attachments from the medial portion of the duodenum to the colon. **D,** The duodenocolic attachments are incised to completely release the colon from the duodenum. Caution must be taken during this step because the superior mesenteric artery and vascular arcades of the small intestine lie directly beneath these bands. **E,** Division of both sets of retroperitoneal attachments allows the cecum to be moved entirely to the left side of the abdomen. The malrotation repair is complete when the duodenum lies right of the midline and traverses directly caudad, and the cecum and large bowel lie completely left of the midline. The superior mesenteric artery and its arcades are clearly visible when the mesentery is unfolded. (From Ford EG, Senac MO Jr, Srikanth MS, Weitzman JJ. Malrotation of the intestine in children. Ann Surg 1992;215:172–178.)

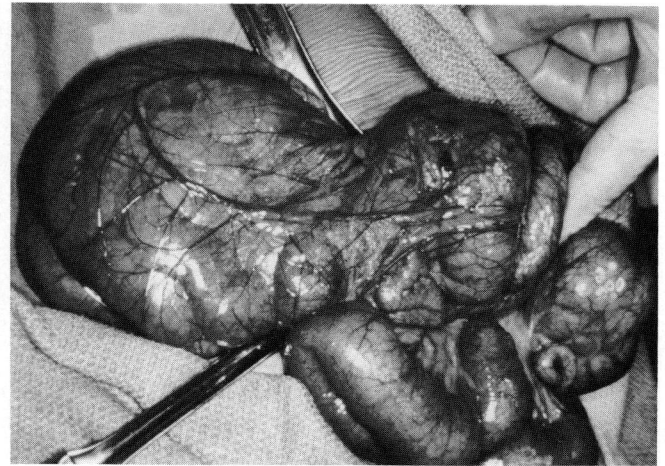

Figure 6.19. Paraduodenal hernia.

Table 6.6.
Classification of Abnormalities of Intestinal Rotation and Fixation[a]

Stage	Embryologic	Clinical
I. Nonrotation	Midgut lengthens on superior mesenteric artery	Midgut volvulus
II. Incomplete rotation	Return prearterial and postarterial loops and rotation	Midgut volvulus; duodenal obstruction; reverse rotation (internal hernia)
III. Incomplete fixation	Descent of cecum; fixation of mesenteries	Internal hernia; cecal volvulus

[a]From Smith EI. Malrotation of the intestine. In: Welch KJ, Randolph JG, Ravitch MM, O'Neill JA, Rowe MI, ed. Pediatric surgery. Chicago: Year Book Medical Publishers, 1986:882–895.

Table 6.7.
Congenital Gastrointestinal Anomalies Associated with Malrotation

Congenital Anomaly	Patients (N)
Omphalocele	9
Gastroschisis	6
Duodenal atresia/stenosis/web	6
Meckel's diverticulum	7
Gastroesophageal reflux	6
Other intestinal atresia/web	6
Biliary atresia	4
Imperforate anus	3
Annular pancreas	2
Rectovaginal fistula	2
Colon duplication	1
Microcolon	1
Tracheoesophageal fistula	1

[a]From Ford EG, Senac MO, Jr, Srikanth MS, Weitzman JJ. Malrotation of the intestine in children. Ann Surg 1992;215:172–178.

Table 6.8.
Some Milestones in the History of Malrotation

Name	Year	Studies
Mall[a]	1898	Embryology of rotation and fixation
Dott[b]	1923	Embryology and clinical problems
Waugh[c]	1928	Volvulus due to nonrotation
Haymond and Dragstedt[d]	1931	Embryology and internal hernia
Gardener and Hart[e]	1934	Classification of 104 cases
Ladd[f]	1932 and 1936	Treatment of malrotation
Gross[g]	1953	Review of 156 cases
Snyder and Chaffin[h]	1954	Gratitude of students received by explaining the rotation with a board, a rope, and a wire
Estrada[i]	1958	Anomalies of intestinal rotation and fixation

[a]Mall FP. Development of the human intestine and its position in the adult. Bull Johns Hopkins Hosp 1898;9:197–208.
[b]Dott NM. Anomalies of intestinal rotation: their embryology and surgical spects, with report of 5 cases. Br J Surg 1923;11:251–286.
[c]Waugh GE. Congenital malformation of the mesentery: a clinical entity. Br J Surg 1928;15:438–449.
[d]Haymond HE, Dragstedt LR. Anomalies of intestinal rotation. Surg Gynecol Obstet 1931;53:316–329.
[e]Gardner CE, Hart D. Anomalies of intestinal rotation as a cause of intestinal obstruction. Arch Surg 1934;29:942–981.
[f]Ladd WE. Congenital obstruction of the duodenum in children. N Engl J Med 1932;206:277–283.
[g]Gross RE. The surgery of infancy and childhood. Philadelphia: WB Saunders, 1953.
[h]Snyder WH, Chaffin L. Embryology and pathology of the intestinal tract: presentation of 48 cases of malrotation. Ann Surg 1954;140:368–380.
[i]Estrada RL. Anomalies of intestinal rotation and fixation. Springfield, IL: Charles C Thomas, 1958.

Table 6.9.
Neonatal Intestinal Obstruction[a]

Atresia	80%
Esophagus	30%
Anorectal	30%
Small intestine	20%
Hirschsprung's disease	10%
Malrotation	6%
Meconium ileus	2%
Others	2%

[a]From Rickham PP, Soper RT, Stauffer UG. Synopsis of pediatric surgery. Stuttgart, Germany: George Thieme, 1975;61.

sequence of events and established the present classification of errors of rotation and fixation. Dott reviewed 45 cases of malrotation. His illustrations of their development are still widely copied. Most of the remaining problems have been clarified by subsequent workers (5, 59, 60). Manson (61) reviewed the literature in the mid–1950s. (See Table 6.8 for milestones in the history of malrotation.)

INCIDENCE

The incidence of rotational defects is not easily estimated because innumerable minor deviations from the normal occur, as well as deviations that are major but asymptomatic.

Smith et al. (62) found malrotation in three among 1252 cases of mechanical obstruction. Of his total cases, roughly 121 appear to be of congenital origin. Among 58 cases of obstruction seen over a period of 12 years in the series of Waldron and Hampton (63), there were seven cases of rotational defects.

In our own experience in Atlanta (64), there were five cases of malrotation among 43 infants with obstruction. Three of the five were associated with intestinal stenosis or atresia which was the primary cause of obstruction.

Rickham et al. (65) estimate that about 6% of neonatal intestinal obstructions are caused by a rotational anomaly (Table 6.9).

Relative Incidence. Nonrotation and mixed rotation are relatively common; other types are rare. Nonrotation is estimated to be present in 0.5% of autopsies, according to Estrada (6), but its clinical incidence is far less. It may produce symptoms at any age, or it may remain asymptomatic. Mixed rotation, on the other hand, always produces symptoms during the first few days of life (6). Of the cases requiring surgery, 10 to 20% are classified as

nonrotation, 70 to 80% as incomplete rotation, less than 5% as reversed rotation, and 5 to 10% as paraduodenal herniae.

Thirty-six cases of reversed rotation have been described, all of which eventually had obstruction from volvulus of the free ileocecal segment.

Hyperdescent of the cecum into the pelvis occurs in 10

to 20% of individuals. True hyperrotation, with reascent of the cecum on the left, is very rare.

Undescended subhepatic cecum, inverted or normal, is asymptomatic. Its discovery during abdominal surgery suggests an incidence of about 6% (6).

Mobile cecum with an ascending mesocolon has been found in 32% of autopsies and 13% of surgical cases.

Sex and Age. All the defects of rotation and fixation are more frequent in males than in females. Mobile cecum, however, appears to occur more often in females although males are more susceptible to the volvulus that may result.

Rotational defects may produce symptoms at any age, but most symptomatic cases manifest themselves in infancy. Among 44 cases reported by Kiesewetter and Smith (66), 24 were discovered in the first week of life. Twenty-four cases in adults have been reviewed by Findlay and Humphreys (67).

Symptoms. Many cases of anomalous rotation and fixation are without symptoms. Estrada (6) estimated an incidence of 1:200 in anatomic specimens and a clinical incidence of 1:25,000 admissions. In one clinical series, 82 cases of malrotation were reported from radiographic examination; only 31 were symptomatic.

Nonrotation or malrotation is symptomatic only when obstruction takes place. In the absence of volvulus or kinking, these defects are of surgical importance only when appendicitis or other intestinal disease requires surgical intervention. In these cases prior knowledge of the condition may prevent needless delay.

Obstruction of the intestine in infants results in vomiting, abdominal distension, and dehydration. The vomitus is usually bile-stained. Fever may be present.

In adults, there is usually a history of chronic or intermittent intestinal complaints since childhood. Diagnosis may be made accidentally from radiographs taken for other purposes. In a few adult patients, an acute episode may occur without previous history of intestinal complaints.

EDITORIAL COMMENT

The diagnosis of high intestinal obstruction in a newborn infant, usually indicated by bilious vomiting, is the only absolute indication for emergency surgery due to intestinal obstruction. This is not because the obstruction results from malrotation and possible bands across the duodenum but because the associated midgut volvulus may be present with the impending ischemic necrosis of the entire midgut. This requires the neonatologist and surgeon to seek immediate radiologic verification that this is not abnormal rotation if the decision is made to wait until the next regular operative schedule. If there is documented malrotation, the potential lethal complication of strangulation necrosis of the volvulated small intestine requires immediate operative intervention (JAH/CNP).

DIAGNOSIS

Radiologic Findings. An upper gastrointestinal radiographic series is the most effective means of recognizing anomalous rotation. Some of the features of the upper gastrointestinal series in a patient with malrotation include a spiral (corkscrew) duodenum (Fig. 6.20), extrinsic duodenal compression, jejunal loops on the right side of the abdomen (Fig. 6.21), edematous jejunal loops, and abnormal location of the ligament of Trietz.

Simpson et al. (68) made a correct diagnosis of malrotation in 22 of 23 patients with upper gastrointestinal radiographic series. Also, Berdon et al. (69) reported the problem of interpreting barium enema radiographs if the ascending colon is shifted medially. If barium enters the terminal ileum, localization of the cecum will be difficult.

When asymptomatic rotational and fixation anomalies present only at operation for real or suspected appendicitis, Estrada (6) has suggested the following guidelines:

1. If only the ileum appears at the incision, consider undescended hepatic cecum or anomalous fixation of cecum.
2. If only the jejunum appears, consider nonrotation.
3. If a freely movable colon appears attached superiorly, consider inverted cecum.

EDITORIAL COMMENT

Traditionally, the first approach to radiologic diagnosis of abnormal rotation with potential midgut volvulus has been a barium enema radiograph because abnormal position of the cecum is the diagnostic evidence of abnormal rotation and potential midgut lat-

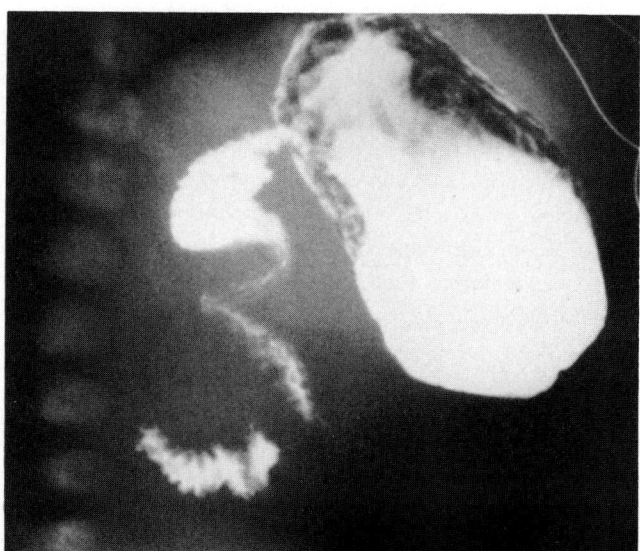

Figure 6.20. Upper gastrointestinal radiographic series of an infant with malrotation and midgut volvulus. Note the absence of the normal duodenal C loop and the corkscrewing of the proximal small bowel.

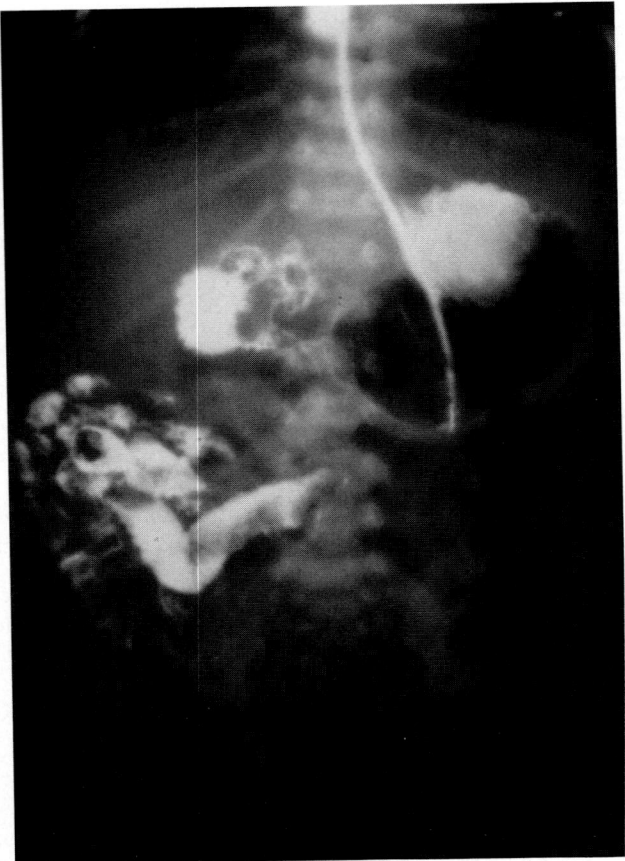

Figure 6.21. Upper gastrointestinal radiographic series of an infant with malrotation. Note all the small bowel on the right side of the abdomen.

eralis. More recently, pediatric radiologists have preferred an upper gastrointestinal series, usually using thin barium or water-soluble contrast medium because they believe they can identify the exact site of the intestinal obstruction and locate the position of the ligament of Treitz. In this way, a definitive diagnosis of midgut volvulus can be made rather than the generic diagnosis of abnormal rotation which can be made with the sequel displacement. Since it is the midgut volvulus that requires emergent operative intervention, an upper gastrointestinal radiographic study in experienced hands is more definitive than is the barium enema radiographic series (JAH/CNP).

TREATMENT

Surgery is indicated whenever malrotation is diagnosed. Although midgut volvulus occurs infrequently, the consequences are life threatening. The procedure of choice is the Ladd's procedure without fixation of the bowel. No attempt should be made to replace the intestinal loops in the "normal" location.

Schmelling and Ross (70) strongly advised passing a catheter in the duodenum during surgery to rule out duo-

denal web, since such a congenital anomaly is present in approximately 15% of malrotations with midgut volvulus.

Results. Stewart et al. (71) report that all 21 infants who underwent surgery for simple malrotation in their study survived. With other associated anomalies and gangrene of the bowel, however, the same author presents fatalities.

The mortality for rotational anomalies currently is 5 to 15%; almost all deaths are attributable to midgut volvulus with bowel infarction. It is for that reason that an elective Ladd's procedure is indicated whenever the diagnosis of malrotation is made.

In our 10-year personal experience with 26 cases of malrotation (excluding those associated with gastroschisis, omphalocele, and congenital diaphragmatic hernia), 13 (50%) had midgut volvulus. Of these, two had infarcted bowel; both died (8% overall mortality).

Ford et al. (53) reported 102 cases of intestinal malrotation treated surgically with a mortality of 2.9%.

Intestinal Stenosis and Atresia

ANATOMY

Defects of the continuity of the intestinal lumen may take several forms and show varying degrees of severity. They may be divided into stenoses and atresias on a functional basis, but the morphologic picture is more complex.

Stenosis. A narrowing of the intestinal lumen is rare and usually associated with annular pancreas or aberrant pancreatic tissue in the duodenal wall. The muscularis is often irregular and the submucosa thickened.

Stenosis also may result from a perforated diaphragmatic atresia. The perforation may be primary but usually represents postnatal rupture under pressure. In some cases the aperture is so small that functional atresia develops in adult life (72). Sixteen proven cases of such perforated diaphragms have been reported in adults (73). Similar atresias are known in the stomach and more rarely in the esophagus (see Chapter 5, The Stomach, and Chapter 3, The Esophagus).

Atresia.

Type I.

In this form of atresia, obstruction is produced by a diaphragm or membrane formed of mucosa and submucosa; the muscularis is not interrupted (Figs. 6.22, *A*, 6.23, *A*, and 6.24).

The diaphragm, whether perforated or not, forms an inverted dome across the intestinal lumen. Pressure on it may produce a slight external indentation at its site of attachment. The perforation, when present, is usually off center and may be from 2 to 10 mm in diameter. Because of its shape under proximal pressure, the diaphragm usually appears to be situated more distally than is actually

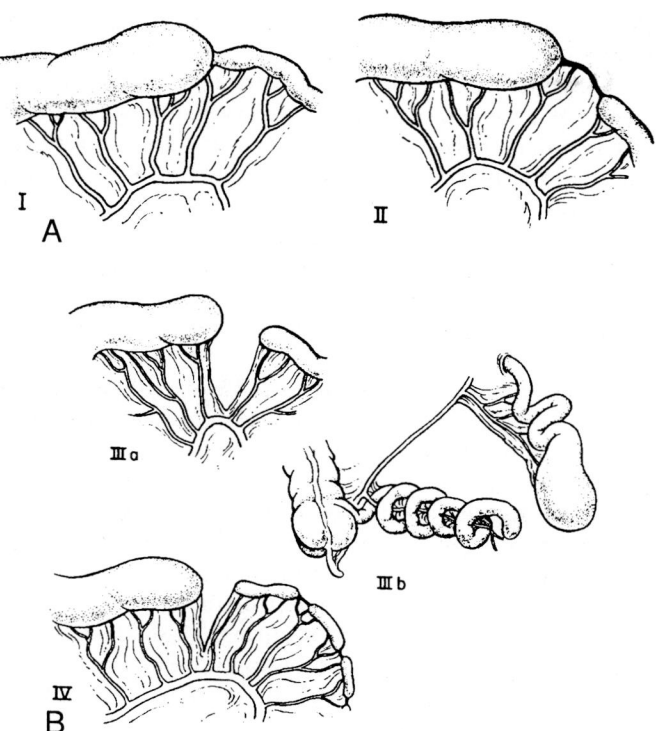

Figure 6.22. Classification of intestinal atresia. Type I: mucosal (membranous) atresia with intact bowel wall and mesentery. Type II: blind ends are separated by a fibrous cord. Type IIIa: blind ends are separated by a V-shaped (gap) mesenteric defect. Type IIIb: "apple peel" atresia. Type IV: multiple atresias ("string of sausages"). (From Grosfeld JK. Jejunoileal atresia and stenosis, In: Welch KJ, Randolph JG, Ravitch MM, O'Neill JA, Rowe MI, eds. Pediatric surgery. Chicago: Year Book Medical Publishers, 1986:843.)

the case. When the perforation is not central, an intraluminal diverticulum may form from the fundus of the diaphragm (74). McClenathan and Okada (75) in 1989 reported seven such cases in adults.

In a few cases the lumen is obliterated over an appreciable distance, forming a plug rather than a diaphragm. The muscle coats are unaffected.

Type II.
Two blind ends of intestine are connected by a short length of fibrous cord lying along the edge of the intact mesentery (Figs. 6.22 and 6.23, *B*).

Type III.
The intestine ends blindly proximal and distal to the atresia, similar to type II. However, there is no connecting fibrous cord and the mesentery between the blind ends of the intestine is absent (Figs. 6.22 and 6.23, *C*).

In all three types, the intestinal segment proximal to the highest atresia is dilated and the distal segment is completely unexpanded.

These types of atresias are sometimes called "conventional." Including the duodenum, type II is most common; type III is the next most common.

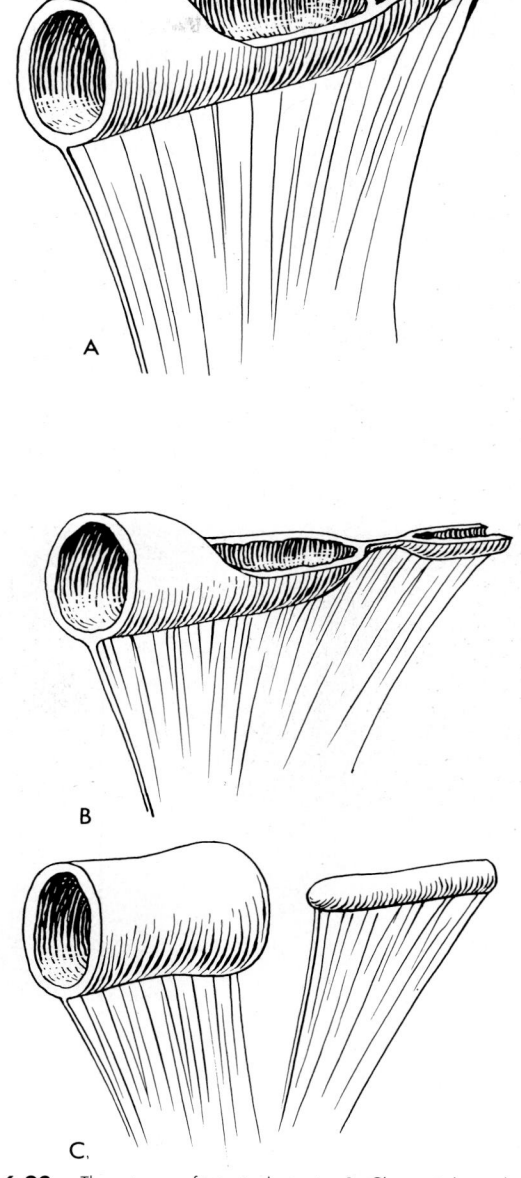

Figure 6.23. Three types of intestinal atresia. **A**, Closure is by a diaphragm of mucosa. **B**, A segment of the intestine is reduced to a solid cord without a lumen. **C**, There is complete segmental absence of a portion of the intestine and of the associated mesentery. In all types, the proximal normal segment is dilated, and the distal normal segment is unexpanded.

LOCATION AND INCIDENCE

The most frequent sites of stenosis and atresia are the duodenum and the ileum above Meckel's diverticulum. The least frequent site is the colon. Louw (76) classified 138 cases of stenosis or atresia by both type and location (Table 6.10 and Fig. 6.25).

In Louw's series, atresias were three times as frequent

as stenoses. In older series, stenosis was even less frequently reported (77–78).

Multiple atresias of types II and III are not rare; frequencies as high as 22% have been reported (79). As many as 12 atresias have been found in a single patient (80). All three types of atresia have occurred in one individual (81). The intestine is dilated proximal to the first atresia only. Additional atretic areas, especially of the diaphragmatic type (type I), are thus easily overlooked.

Atresia in the first part of the duodenum is rare (82), but it is common at the level of the papilla of Vater. Garvin (83) found 19 of 97 atresias there, and Madden and McCann (84) found 27 of 76 diaphragms at this level. There may be an associated common duct atresia (85).

Ileal atresias and stenoses usually occur in the proximal portion. They also may occur at the ileocecal valve

(40, 86). Double stenoses are known to occur at this location (87).

Feingold and Shulman (88) described an infant with atresia of a portion of the intestine just below the pylorus. The segment distal to the atresia was 34-cm long and ended normally at the ileocecal junction. In addition, there was a portion of intestine 45-cm long and blind at both ends. As the combined length of the two segments was still far short of the length of the normal intestine (250 cm), it seems evident that there had been multiple atresias with complete resorption of a considerable portion of intestine.

More remarkable is the case of a 32-year-old woman in whom Douglas (89) found the ileum to pass abruptly into a normal but short colon by a stenosis 0.75 inches in length and 0.25 inches in diameter. There was no terminal ileum, appendix, or ascending or proximal transverse colon. The author believed that the stenosis represented the undeveloped and undifferentiated postarterial link of the midgut loop. It seems equally probable that strangulation and amputation of a normal loop could have occurred at the umbilicus, and a spontaneous anastomosis of the remaining portion occurred. Carcinoma of the

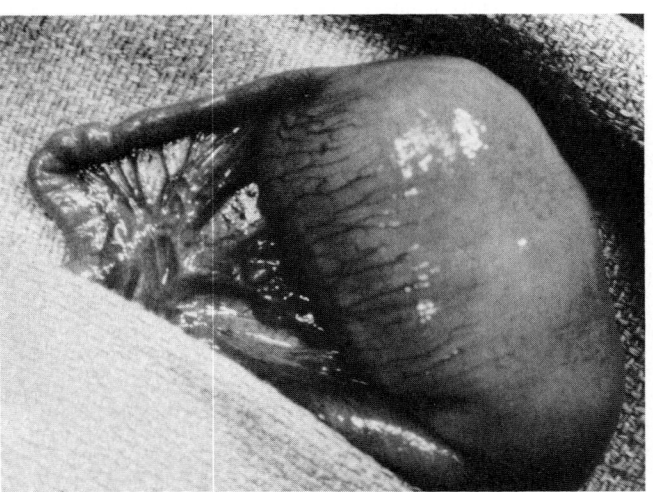

Figure 6.24. Type I jejunal atresia.

Table 6.10.
Type and Site of 138 Intestinal Stenoses and Atresias[a]

| Site | Stenoses | Types of Atresia | | | TOTAL |
		I	II	III	
Duodenum	24	19	12	—	55
Jejunum	2	3	7	9	21
Ileum	6	2	10	17	35
Colon	—	1	1	4	6
Multiple sites	—	—	13	8	21
TOTAL	32	25	43	38	138

[a]From Louw JH. Jejunoileal atresia and stenosis. J Pediatr Surg 1966;1:8–23.

STENOSES   ATRESIAS

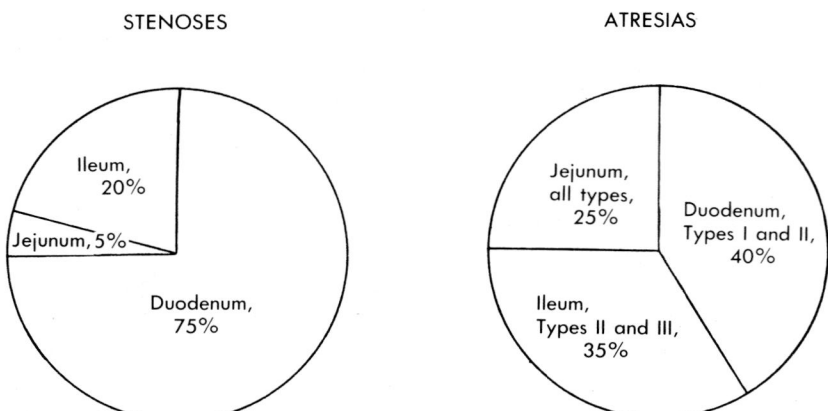

Figure 6.25. Proportionate frequency of stenoses and atresias in the duodenum and small intestine.

existing transverse portion of the colon was found. Both stenosis and tumor were resected, further shortening the colon. Two similar cases were reported by Royster (90).

We agree with Raffensperger (91) that a gap in the mesentery is not just a defect but an intrauterine vascular accident when atresias are present.

In 1966 Weitzman and Vanderhoof (92) presented jejunal atresia with mesentery agenesis and named this pathological entity "Christmas tree" deformity. (Raffensperger (91) used the word "picturesque," when describing both "Christmas tree" and "apple peel" small bowel.) Zerella and Martin (93) 10 years later reported a similar case with helical ileum.

Seven similar cases were reported (93) in 1976, and earlier, Santulli and Blanc (81) reported three cases of jejunal atresia with a peculiar attachment of a small distal bowel; the attachment they called "apple peel." Since then, several more cases have been reported (Table 6.11).

EDITORIAL COMMENT

We believe the term "apple peel" is far more descriptive than "Christmas tree" because the coiled small intestine around the single short vessel closely resembles an apple peel which has been pared from an apple with a pocket knife. The only resemblance to a Christmas tree is that the mass effect may resemble some form of a tree but hardly one that we usually see at Christmas time (JAH/CNP)!

Familial Jejunal Atresia, Extensive Intestinal Atresia, "Apple Peel" Atresia. In 1987 Seashore et al. (94) collected 57 cases of "apple peel" jejunal atresia and added three of their own. The syndrome consists of proximal intestinal atresia, absence of the distal superior mesenteric artery and the dorsal mesentary, and a retrograde blood supply to the surviving distal small intestine from the right colic vessels. The authors estimate that this anomaly accounts for less than 5% of all intestinal atresias. Two patients were from the same family. Concurrent defects in this collected series were: prematurity, 70%; malrotation, 54%; short gut, 74%; multiple atresias, 15%; complications, 68%; and mortality, 54%. All three of Seashore's patients survived to 3½ years or longer.

In 1985, Puri and associates (95) reported multiple atresias in three consecutive siblings. The atresias started in the prepyloric area of the stomach and continued to the rectum. Intraluminal calcification was visible on plain radiographs. Each lumen was surrounded by a normal mucosa and muscularis mucosae, but a single layer of muscularis externa often surrounded more than one lumen.

A third example of extensive small intestine loss

Table 6.11.
Jejunal Atresia

Year	Author	Cases Reported
1961	Jiminez and Reiner[a]	Reported one case of jejunal atresia with unattached ileum
1961	Santulli and Blanc[b]	Reported three cases of jejunal atresia with "apple peel" attachment of very small distal bowel
1966	Weitzman and Vanderhoof[c]	Introduced term *Christmas tree deformity,* as suggested by Swenson, and reported four cases
1968	Mishalany and Najjar[d]	Reported three cases with jejunal atresia in one family
1968	Spencer[e]	Reported five patients with mesenteric defect; one had multiple ileal atresias distal to the mesenteric gap
1969	Blyth and Dickson[f]	Reported eight cases in seven families, inherited as an autosomal recessive condition in six of them
1969	Benson and Lloyd[e]	Reported two cases
1970	Dickson[f]	Reported seven cases
1971	Zwiren, Andrews, and Ahmann[g]	Reported five patients
1974	Thomas and Carter[h]	Reported one case

[a]Ziminez FA, Reiner L. Arteriographic findings in congenital abnormalities of the mesentery and intestines. Surg Gynecol Obstet 1961;113:346.
[b]Santulli TV, Blanc WS. Congenital atresia of the intestine. Ann Surg 1961;154:939.
[c]Weitzman JJ, Vanderhoof RS. Jejunal atresia with agenesis of the dorsal mesentery. Am J Surg 1966;111:443.
[d]Mishalany HG, Najjar F. Familial jejunal atresia: three cases in one family. J Pediatr 1968;73:753.
[e]Spencer R. The various patterns of intestinal atresia. Surgery 1968;64:661.
[f]Blyth, Dickson JAS. Apple peel syndrome, Med Genet 1969;6:275.
[g]Benson CD, Lloyd JR. Atresia and stenosis of the jejunum and ileum. In: Mustard WT et al., eds. Pediatric surgery. Chicago: Year Book Medical Publishers, 1969:850.
[h]Dickson JAS. Apple peel small bowel: an uncommon variant of duodenal and jejunal atresia. J Pediatr Surg 1970;5:595.
[i]Zwiren GT, Andrews HG, Ahmann P. Jejunal atresia with agenesis of the dorsal mesentery ("apple peel small bowel"). J Pediatr Surg 1972;7:414.
[j]Thomas CG, Carter JM. Small intestinal atresia. Ann Surg 1974;179:663.

appears to be the response to the presence of a chromosome aberration, the deletion of the long arm of chromosome 13 (13 q syndrome). This case appears to be the first of its kind recorded (96).

EMBRYOGENESIS

A variety of explanations for intestinal atresia and stenosis have been suggested. They may be collected under the following three main headings.

Developmental Defects. Excessive resorption of the vitelline duct, together with adjacent ileum, may occur (Fig. 6.26, A). This was suggested by Bland-Sutton (97) in 1889. It may account for some ileal atresias at the site of the vitelline duct.

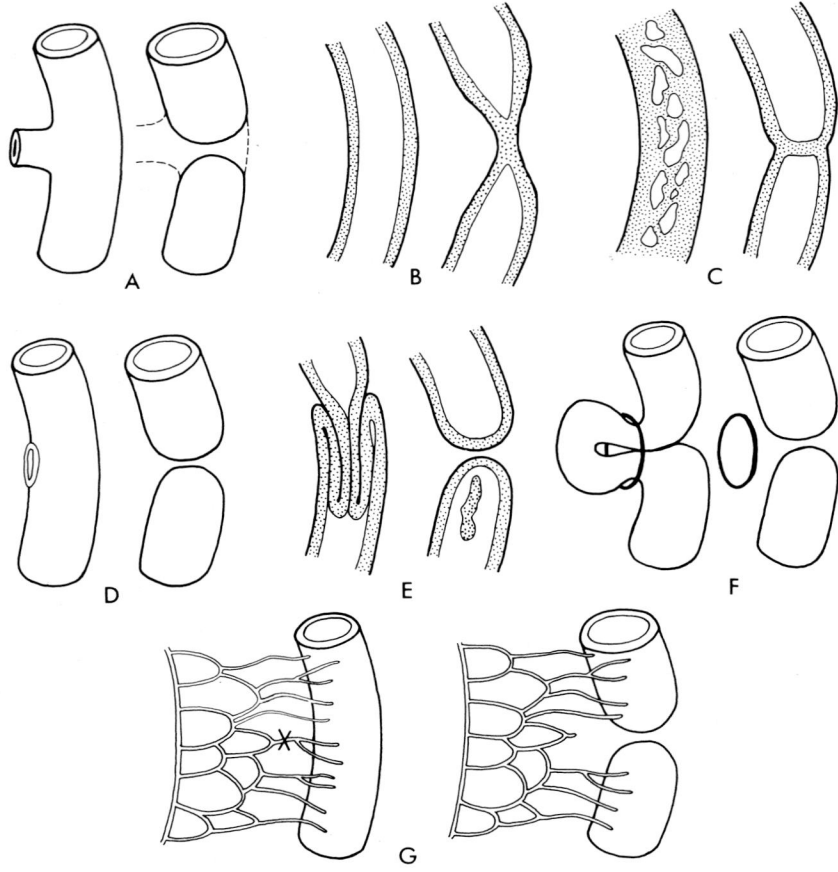

Figure 6.26. Seven possible causes of intestinal atresia. **A**, Excessive resorption of Meckel's diverticulum. **B**, Attenuation of intestine where cell proliferation has failed to keep up with elongation. **C**, Failure of complete recanalization following partial occlusion of the lumen by epithelial proliferation. **D**, Intestinal perforation in utero, followed by local necrosis and repair, leaving an atretic zone. **E**, Intussusception in utero, with necrosis and atresia. **F**, Snaring of an intestinal loop in the umbilical ring, with resorption of the snared loop. **G**, Thrombosis of vascular supply, with local necrosis and closure of distal and proximal ends.

Disproportionate growth of body and gut may take place (Fig. 6.26, *B*). Politzer (98) has suggested that inadequate endodermal proliferation may result in attenuation of the embryonic gut to the point of atresia.

Failure of recanalization after epithelial occlusion during development, an explanation put forward by Tandler (99), has received considerable support (Fig. 6.26, *C*).

Inflammatory Changes. This explanation, offered first by Theremin (100) in 1877, is representative of the period in which intrauterine inflammation was considered to be a major cause of congenital malformations of all types. The inflammation theory was revived by Bernstein et al. (101), who suggested that some atresias result from scar formation following perforation produced by meconium ileus (Fig. 6.26, *D*).

Fetal Accidents. Intussusception, which Chiari (102) in 1888 found in the intestine distal to an atresia of type II or III, may be involved (Fig. 6.26, *E*). Several similar cases have been reported (101, 103, 104).

An intestinal loop may become snared in the umbilical ring, causing a type III atresia in the jejunum or ileum (Fig. 6.25, *F*). This was first suggested by Spriggs (86) in 1912.

Volvulus, perforation, strangulation through mesenteric apertures, and constriction by mesenteric bands, as well as infarction or other interruption of local blood supply, can and do produce atresia of the intestine in the fetus (105, 106) (Fig. 6.26, *G*).

Failure of recanalization after a temporary solid state of the intestine has found the greatest favor as an explanation, less from definite evidence than from the obvious limitations of other hypotheses. Tandler (99, 107) observed epithelial occlusion of the duodenum during the sixth and seventh weeks of gestation and concluded that membranous atresia might result from failure to complete recanalization. Forssner (77) suggested that such occlusion might occur throughout the small intestine. The facts were not seriously examined until Lynn and Espinas (19) sectioned 68 human embryos between 7 and 23 mm (5 to 8 weeks) and found occlusion or vascular indications of earlier occlusion present in 27. Of these, the duodenum was occluded in 20; the ileum and jeju-

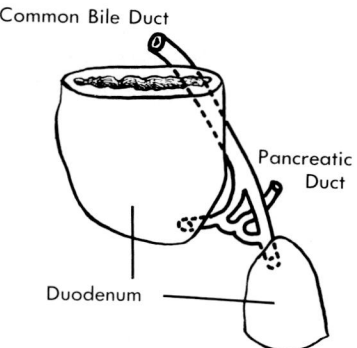

Figure 6.27. Atresia of the duodenum at the papilla of Vater. Both the bile and pancreatic ducts divide to enter the duodenum above and below the atresia. (Redrawn from Boyden EA, Cope JG, Bill AH. Anatomy and embryology of congenital intrinsic obstruction of the duodenum. Am J Surg 1967;114:190–202.)

num in 4; duodenum, ileum, and jejunum segments in 1; and ileum, jejunum, and colon in 2. In 41 embryos, there was no evidence of occlusion. Thus occlusion is not always present, but it is not unusual. If the occluding epithelial plug persists long enough, it becomes replaced by connective tissue and true atresia results. Duodenal occlusion has been examined in some detail by Schwegler and Boyden (108, 109). As the occluding epithelial proliferation begins to break up at the 15-mm stage of development (stage 17), vacuoles coalesce to form two channels, and two openings develop in the hepatopancreatic duct at its junction with the duodenum. The two openings communicate separately with the two duodenal channels. This situation is normally transitory, but atresia at the level of the papilla is not unusual. Persistence of the two channels is evidenced by cases in which atresia has occurred at the site of the papilla of Vater, leaving a forked common bile duct entering both proximal and distal segments of the duodenum (109, 111) (Fig. 6.27). Among 83 cases of duodenal atresia collected by Boyden and his colleagues (109), 69 were at or close to the site of the papilla. In a few cases errors of canalization at this location may result in a membranous atresia with an intraluminal diverticulum (74).

EDITORIAL COMMENT

We believe that most evidence now points toward a true genetic developmental etiology for duodenal atresia since it is so frequently associated with other genetic defects including the various trisomies. Atresia of the jejunum and ileum, on the other hand, results almost exclusively from some type of vascular accident that occurs in utero to otherwise normally formed intestine. Thus duodenal atresia is a true congenital abnormality in the genetic sense, whereas jejunal and ileal atresia are "acquired defects" in utero (JAH/CNP).

The fetal accident hypothesis appears to account for most jejunal and ileal atresias of types II and III. Santulli and Blanc (81) observed bile and swallowed squamous cell debris in the intestine distal to the atresia, indicating that the obstruction could not have been present before the fourth month. They noted also that the intestines in infants with type III atresias are often shorter than in normal infants. As early as 1922 Davis and Poynter (112) suggested that vascular disease might be responsible for atresias of types II and III. Louw and Barnard, together (113) and later separately (114, 115), reported experimental interference with the blood supply to intestinal segments in puppies in utero. After 10 days, the infarcted segment was represented by a fibrous strand. They produced stenosis and all types of atresias in their animals.

In 1959 Courtois (116), using fetal rabbits, performed a variety of experiments and concluded that perforation of the fetal intestine: (*a*) may heal without trace and without evidence of meconium peritonitis; (*b*) may heal with residual stenosis; or (*c*) may heal with a residual atresia (type II). Isolation of an intestinal loop results in resorption of the loop if the vascularization is poor or in persistence of the loop if vascularization is good. Dickinson (106) presented a case of intrauterine volvulus resulting in atresia, which illustrates partial resorption of an isolated loop.

There is no correlation between atresia or stenosis and parental age, parental disease, or birth rank of infant (117). This is contrary to the findings of Ingalls and Prindle (118) for tracheoesophageal defects. It supports the view that intestinal atresia is often a fetal accident rather than a true developmental defect, such as the esophageal anomaly.

Duodenal atresia may be membranous (Fig. 6.23, *A*) or segmental (Fig. 6.23, *B* and *C*), the former being the more common. Membranous atresia, complete or perforated, has been called intraluminal duodenal diverticulum (119). While this is not incorrect, it does not reflect the origin of the lesion from an atresia. In all forms of duodenal atresia, the proximal duodenum is dilated and the distal duodenum is completely unexpanded; obstruction is complete. Three-fourths of all intestinal stenoses and 40% of intestinal atresias are found in the duodenum. Multiple atresias are not unknown; in such cases only the proximal one will have a dilated proximal segment, according to Gray et al. in 1989 (120).

In summary, atresias of the gut may be divided into primary types (true malformations), which may be represented by esophageal and duodenal atresias, and secondary types (fetal accidents), which are represented by most nonmembranous jejunal and ileal atresias. The precise assignment of cause to specific atresias may not always be easy, and the origins of membranous atresias (type I) at all locations remains obscure.

Rittenhouse et al. (121) presented a case of an infant with multiple septa of jejunum and ileum who exhibited severe diarrhea without oral feedings and did not respond to any kind of treatment. According to the authors, septal atresia is the least common of all types of multiple atresias. Because severe proximal distal inflammatory processes were present at surgery and finally autopsy, the authors speculated that the septa were formed prenatally.

ASSOCIATED ANOMALIES

Evans (117), analyzing the literature up to 1951, found the following anomalies associated with intestinal atresia with figures higher than would be expected to occur by chance:

Omphalocele or fistula	3.67%
Annular pancreas	2.14%
Imperforate anus	1.67%
Malformation of bile ducts	1.54%
Esophageal atresia	1.00%

In our own experience in Atlanta, other anomalies were found in 11 of 23 cases of atresia and in 5 of 9 cases of stenosis. Nine patients had two or more additional anomalies (122).

A high incidence of Down's syndrome is associated with intestinal atresia and stenosis. In our own series, 8 among 32 patients (25%) had this condition. Botseas et al. (123) found a 12% incidence in a smaller series. Down's syndrome has been said to be especially associated with duodenal atresia (85, 124, 125). Maternal polyhydramnios is present in about 50% of infants born with duodenal or high jejunal obstruction (126). Gardener et al. (127) reported ileal atresia with Hirschsprung's disease.

EDITORIAL COMMENT

The consensus clearly supports a genetic etiology for duodenal atresias and an acquired or accidental vascular injury as causative for jejunal and ileal atresia. It is therefore not surprising that duodenal atresia is more frequently associated with all other systemic anomalies, whereas it is extremely rare to find other organ abnormalities associated with jejunal and ileal atresia. It is true that jejunal and ileal atresia may be associated with gastroschisis but that is because the bowel has been exposed to amniotic fluid and has become mechanically injured as a result of this exposure. The other major abdominal wall defect—namely, omphalocele—is not associated with a high frequency of jejunal or ileal atresia (JAH/CNP).

HISTORY

In 1673 Binninger (128) described a newborn infant who was found at necropsy to have total atresia of the colon. Almost 125 years later in 1797 Osiander (129) described a case of ileal atresia. In 1804 Voisin (130) performed an enterostomy for intestinal obstruction in an infant, and in 1894 Wanitschek (131) attempted the first resection and anastomosis. In the United States, Jacobi (128) observed the absence of squamous amniotic cells in the meconium and made the first clinical diagnosis in 1861.

In 1812 Meckel (133) reviewed the literature of intestinal atresia and speculated on its etiology. In 1877 Theremin (100) made the first thorough study of a series of cases in Vienna and St. Petersburg. In 1889 Bland-Sutton (97) suggested the classification that is still in use today.

Although the condition was more or less understood, none of the 73 enterostomies and 9 anastomoses that were performed between 1804 and 1911 resulted in a survival of longer than 15 days. This long series of failures prompted Clogg (134) to suggest in 1904 the abandonment of surgical procedures. In his 1912 monograph on the subject, Spriggs (86) counseled persistence. Even as the monograph was in press, Fockens (135) in Germany reported the first successful repair of an ileal atresia. In 1916 Ernst (136) in England performed successful surgery on duodenal atresia.

Despite these successes, O'Neill and his colleagues (137) were able to find only 36 cases of survival following surgery for intestinal atresia by 1948. It remained for Ladd and Gross (138) in Boston to develop the techniques that finally brought mortality below 50% since 1940. Experimental production of these lesions starting in 1955 has begun to shed new light on their pathogenesis.

INCIDENCE

Estimates of incidence of intestinal atresia range from 1 in 20,000 births (139) to 1 in 1500 births (117). There were about 1500 published cases by 1951 (117). Atresia and stenosis account for between 16% (117) and 34% (80) of infantile intestinal obstructions, depending on how the figures are computed. Waldron and Hampton (63) found that atresia and stenosis accounted for 4.06% of obstruction in persons of all ages in Houston, Texas. If adhesions, mostly postoperative, are eliminated from this series, atresia and stenosis are responsible for 6.83% of all obstructions.

Age and Sex. Atresias manifest themselves in the first few days of life; 66% of cases are found in full-term infants. Stenoses, on the other hand, are not usually apparent so soon. Of 71 patients seen by Gross (40), only 31 were hospitalized in the first week of life. Eight were over 1 year of age when diagnosis was made. Walker and his colleagues (140) collected 11 cases of duodenal stenosis in adults, the oldest of whom was 72 years of age. All but one had obstruction of a perforated diaphragm; four had no related symptoms. Fifteen cases of duodenal diaphragms in adults have been reported (141). Similar cases are known in connection with the stomach (see Chapter 5, The Stomach).

DeLorimier et al. (142) as well as Shafie and Rickham (143) reported multiple atresias from 6 to 22%, and Martin and Zerella (144) reported an incidence in the United States of 10 to 12%. No gender difference has been reported in the incidence of either atresia or stenosis. There is no familial tendency although affected twins have been reported (145, 146), and a few cases of affected siblings are known (147, 148).

EDITORIAL COMMENT

It is not surprising that there are multiple atresias in approximately 10% of patients with ileal and jejunal atresia because these result from vascular accidents in utero. As a matter of fact, the patterns of ileal and jejunal atresia clearly reflect the vascular insufficiency etiology because some atresias are quite extensive where there has been volvulus or intussusception, whereas others are quite isolated and short, suggesting a local twist of the loop of the intestine or even an embolus to that single vessel. Multiple duodenal atresias, on the other hand, are quite uncommon because this represents a genetically determined abnormality rather than multiple vascular insults (JAH/CNP).

SYMPTOMS

Abdominal Distension. About 80% of infants with obstruction show distension. If the obstruction is high, the distension is limited to the upper abdomen. Tenderness is not present unless there has been perforation.

Vomiting. Nearly all patients with intestinal obstruction vomit. Vomitus is green when the obstruction is distal to the ampulla of Vater. In general, the higher the obstruction, the earlier the onset of vomiting.

Stools. Stools are usually absent or scanty. When present, they may be bile stained even though the atresia is below the entrance of the bile duct (81). The obstruction may have arisen after the beginning of the fourth month of gestation, when meconium begins to appear. When the obstruction in the duodenum is below the ampulla, accessory bile ducts may nevertheless empty below the obstruction (149).

Pain. Pain is not usually present among infants with atresia unless perforation has occurred. On the other hand, of nine patients with stenosis whom we have seen, eight had pain. Partial functioning seems to be more painful than complete occlusion.

Temperature. A slightly elevated temperature was found in 66% of our patients with atresia. This may be caused by dehydration. A temperature above 103° F usually indicates that perforation has occurred.

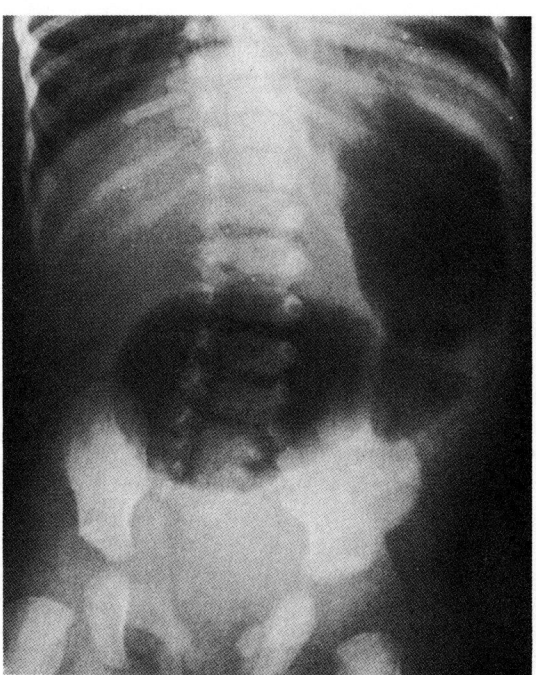

Figure 6.28. Duodenal atresia. The markedly dilated stomach and duodenal cap are filled with air. The absence of other gas-filled intestinal loops indicates a duodenal obstruction.

DIAGNOSIS

Atresia. The diagnosis of intestinal obstruction can and must be made in the first few hours after onset. Whether the obstruction is extrinsic or intrinsic is of academic interest at this stage. There are no criteria for preoperative identification of the cause of the blockage.

The demonstration of air in the gastrointestinal tract on x-ray examination is often pathognomonic. Air reaches the stomach on the first breath, the duodenum within a few minutes, and the cecum in 3 to 8 hours (150). When the obstruction is duodenal, a double–air bubble shows on the film (Fig. 6.28). On the left, the stomach contains air; on the right, there is a smaller bubble in the dilated duodenum above the obstruction. If air is present in the intestinal loops, a barium enema may be required to distinguish low, small intestinal obstruction from colonic obstruction. A narrow colonic lumen is highly suggestive of obstruction above. Hirschsprung's disease may be ruled out, malrotation may be recognized, and patency of the colon may be demonstrated. That another atresia may frequently be found below the primary obstruction must be kept in mind.

A catheter should be passed to rule out atresia of the esophagus because air may reach the stomach or intestines through a tracheoesophageal fistula.

Stenosis. If the stenosis is narrow, most of the symptoms of atresia will be present immediately after birth.

Large openings may produce no symptoms until adulthood, and still larger openings may be only incidental
findings at autopsy (151). Persistent vomiting and failure
to gain weight may be the only findings in cases in which
the lumen is moderately occluded. Dietary regulation
may, in fact, relieve all symptoms and the stenosis may go
undiscovered for many years. Bill and Pope (152) have
described the cases of two infants in whom three operations each were performed before the existence of perforated duodenal diaphragms were recognized. Extrinsic
bands were initially blamed for the obstruction, but these
were not the actual cause.

In adults, the diagnosis of stenosis is usually not considered when symptoms are limited to abdominal pain. A
patient described by Reid (87) suffered from lower
abdominal pain since the age of 14 years. He underwent
surgery for appendicitis when he was 27 years of age and
for enlarged cecum when he was 32 years of age; his right
colon was removed when he was 41 years of age. Three
months after the last operation, the terminal ileum was
removed. It had a diaphragmatic stenosis with a 0.25 inch
opening 2 inches above the ileocecal junction, and a second diaphragm a few inches above the first.

Vomiting and weight loss, dysphagia with gastroesophageal reflux, and an enlarged stomach and proximal duodenum are the usual symptoms in adults. That these

symptoms have not been present since childhood does
not eliminate the possibility of a diaphragmatic stenosis
(72, 73).

Differential Diagnosis. The differential diagnosis of intestinal atresia and stenosis is a long one. It is useful to characterize the obstruction as "high" or "low," occuring
proximal or distal to the ligament of Treitz, respectively
(153). High intestinal obstructions include pyloric atresia
(extremely rare), pyloric stenosis, duodenal atresia or stenosis, duodenal web, annular pancreas, malrotation with
obstructing Ladd's bands, and duodenal duplication cysts
(very rare). Pyloric stenosis is characterized by nonbilious
vomiting and presents at between 3 to 6 weeks of age. The
others generally present in the newborn period with bilious vomiting. The "double–bubble" abdominal radiograph (Fig. 6.29) is characteristic of a complete high
intestinal obstruction from duodenal atresia, obstructing
Ladd's bands, or annular pancreas. An upper gastrointestinal radiographic series for an incomplete high intestinal obstruction will demonstrate duodenal stenosis or
web, partially obstructing annular pancreas, or malrotation with midgut volvulus (Fig. 6.20).

Low intestinal obstructions include jejunoileal atresia
or stenosis, meconium ileus, meconium peritonitis, meconium plug syndrome or small left colon syndrome,
Hirschsprung's disease, and anorectal agenesis. All these

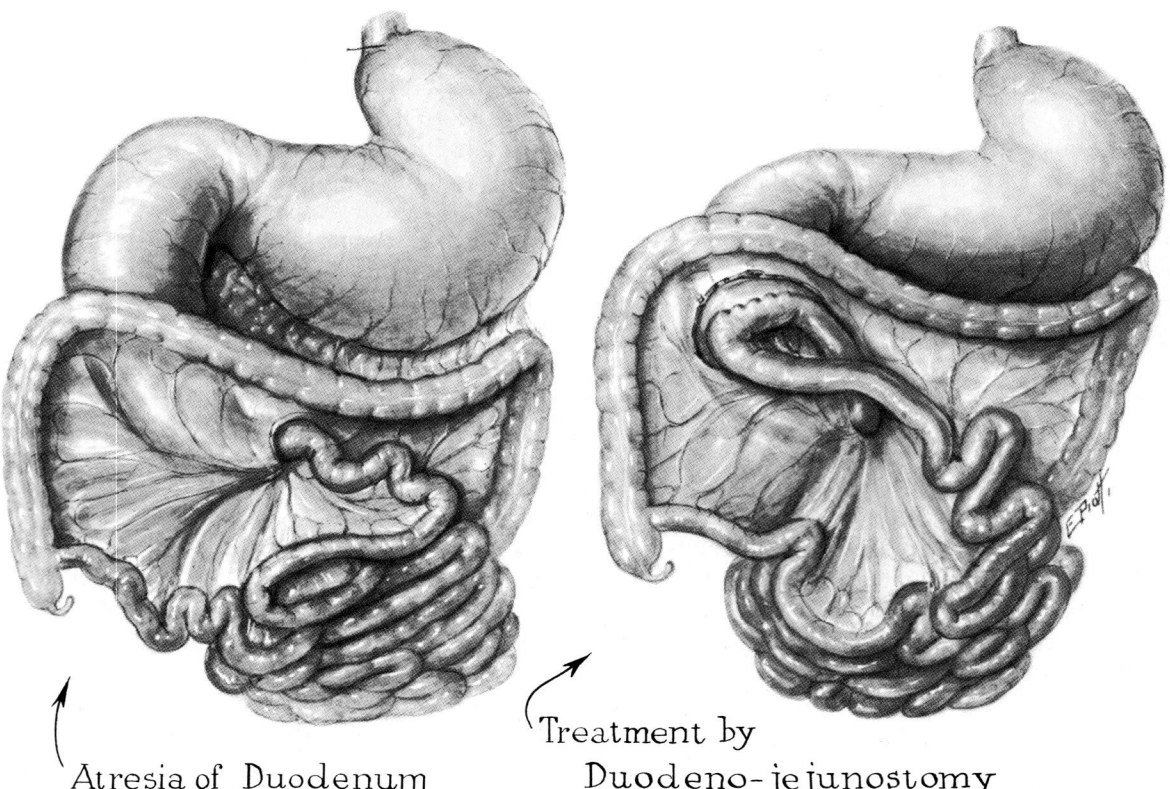

Figure 6.29. Duodenal atresia and its repair by duodeno-jejunostomy. (From Gross RE. An Atlas of children's surgery. Philadelphia: WB Saunders, 1970.)

are characterized by bilious vomiting, abdominal distension, and failure to pass meconium stool. Anorectal agenesis is diagnosed by physical examination. Meconium peritonitis is characterized by the presence of calcifications on the abdominal radiograph. The remaining diagnoses are established by barium enema radiographs and/or rectal biopsy. A microcolon ("unused" colon) characterizes atresias, stenoses, and meconium ileus (cystic fibrosis), whereas a normal or enlarged colon characterizes meconium plug syndrome, small left colon syndrome, or Hirschsprung's disease. The latter is definitively diagnosed with a rectal suction mucosal biopsy.

TREATMENT

Restoration of the continuity of the alimentary tract is the aim of treatment for patients with stenoses or atresias. All procedures involve at least four steps:

1. Reestablishment of water and electrolyte balance in the usually dehydrated infant
2. Decompression of the proximal segment, which is usually distended by food or air
3. Resection of the atretic segment and anastomosis of the ends of healthy intestine
4. Examination of the distal intestine for the presence of other atresias or stenoses

EDITORIAL COMMENT

The best evidence of adequate replacement of water and electrolytes toward normal volemia is the establishment of adequate urinary output. Thus careful monitoring of renal function during resuscitation of babies with intestinal obstruction is critical to the decision regarding operative intervention. The basic principle is simply to restore adequate intravascular volume so there will not be signs and symptoms of hypovolemia during induction of anesthesia and/or the operative procedure (JAH/CNP).

A number of operative procedures have been employed to correct these anomalies (Figs. 6.30 and 6.31). All have given good results under the proper circumstances and in the proper hands.

Excision of the Occluding Membrane. This procedure, although it seems to be the simplest and most direct, is not always satisfactory since it may leave a stenosis at the site. For some surgeons, the results have been completely successful (154).

Resection of the Atretic Segment and Anastomosis. This is the method of choice for all atresias except those of the upper part of the duodenum. A number of anastomotic procedures have been employed.

Side-to-Side Anastomosis.

This method avoids the problem caused by the disparity

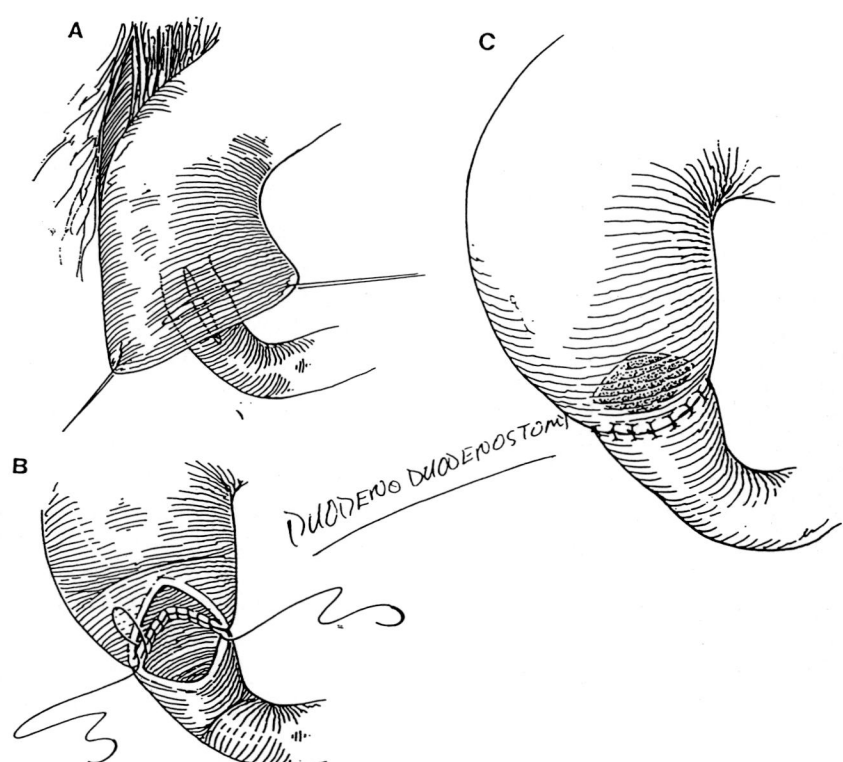

Figure 6.30. Diamond-shaped anastomosis. (From Kimura K et al. Diamond-shaped anastomosis for duodenal atresia: an experience with 44 patients over 15 years. J Pediatr Surg 1990 25(9):978.)

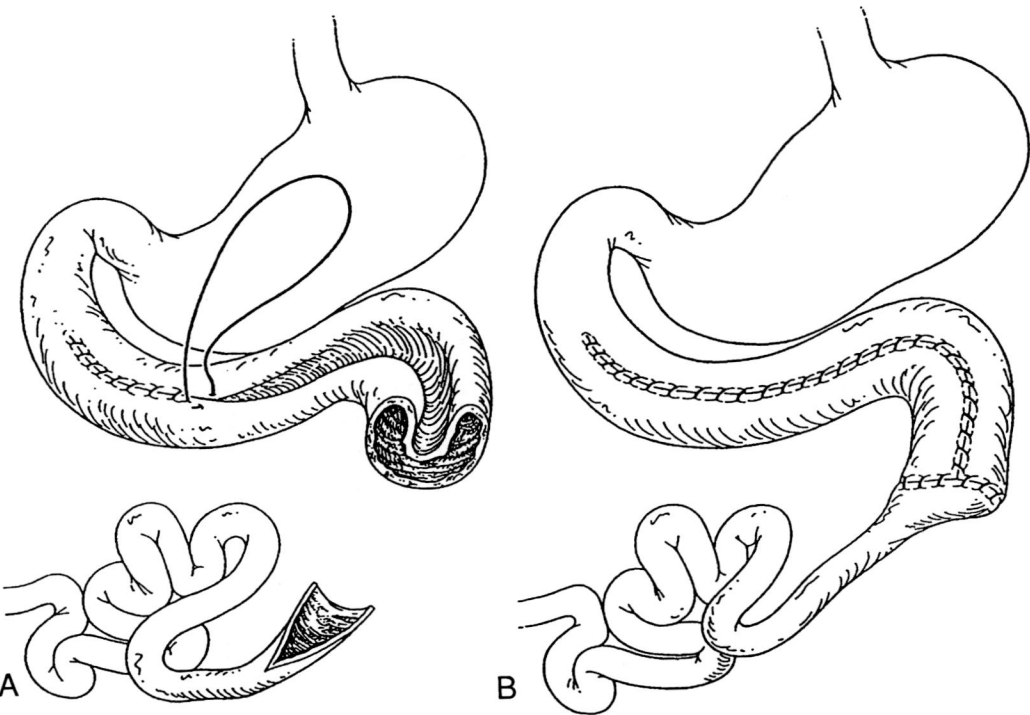

Figure 6.31. **A**, The proximal dilated bowel is opened at the tip and tapered with a continuous suture back to near normal sized intestine. **B**, After tapering the proximal bowel and spatulating the distal intestine, an end-to-end anastomosis can be carried out. The junction of the two suture lines should be reinforced with an additional suture. (From Raffensperger JG, ed. Jejunoileal atresia and stenosis. In: Swenson's pediatric surgery, 5th ed. Norwalk, CT: Appleton & Lange. 1990:530.)

in size between the distended proximal segment and the unexpanded distal segment. However, this may lead to development of the blind-loop syndrome and therefore is no longer recommended (Fig. 6.32).

End-to-End Anastomosis.
Swenson and Fisher (155) recommended dilation of the distal segment by saline injection and resection of the distended bulbous end of the proximal segment, after which the two ends are more nearly equal in caliber and may be joined end to end. Louw (115) advocates resection of the blind ends prior to rejoining them. The blind ends probably have an inadequate blood supply (Fig. 6.33).

EDITORIAL COMMENT

It is not surprising that the blind ends do not function well because they not only have inadequate blood supply but the adjacent bowel has had chronic ischemia which has also affected the integrity of the bowel wall. Experimental studies have shown that the blind ends have abnormal muscular tissue and may have absence of ganglion cells. In a sense, this tissue barely escaped ischemic necrosis (JAH/CNP)!

Mikulicz Exteriorization.
In this procedure, the blind ends are stitched together and brought outside the abdominal wall. Opening the ends allows decompression of the proximal segment and permits gradual distension of the distal segment by administration of fluids. The adjacent walls of the two segments are destroyed by crushing. After a suitable healing period, the single opening thus created is closed. The intestine is then returned to the abdomen and the abdomen closed. This procedure reduces the danger of sepsis from a leaking anastomosis. However, it is rarely performed today.

End-to-Side Anastomosis.
Santulli and Blanc (81) have modified the exteriorization procedure so that the end of the proximal segment only is brought to the outside, the end of the distal segment being attached to the side of the proximal segment within the abdomen. Control of the enterostomy is obtained by the use of an indwelling catheter (into the distal segment) and a Pott's clamp. After the anastomosis becomes functional, the proximal segment is resected back to the anastomosis and the abdomen closed. This procedure may be used in an infant with meconium ileus (e.g., cystic fibrosis) but is no longer used for the treatment of intestinal atresia.

EDITORIAL COMMENT

After many years of trial and error, it is now quite clear that the best technique of anastomosis for jejunal and ileal atresia is some

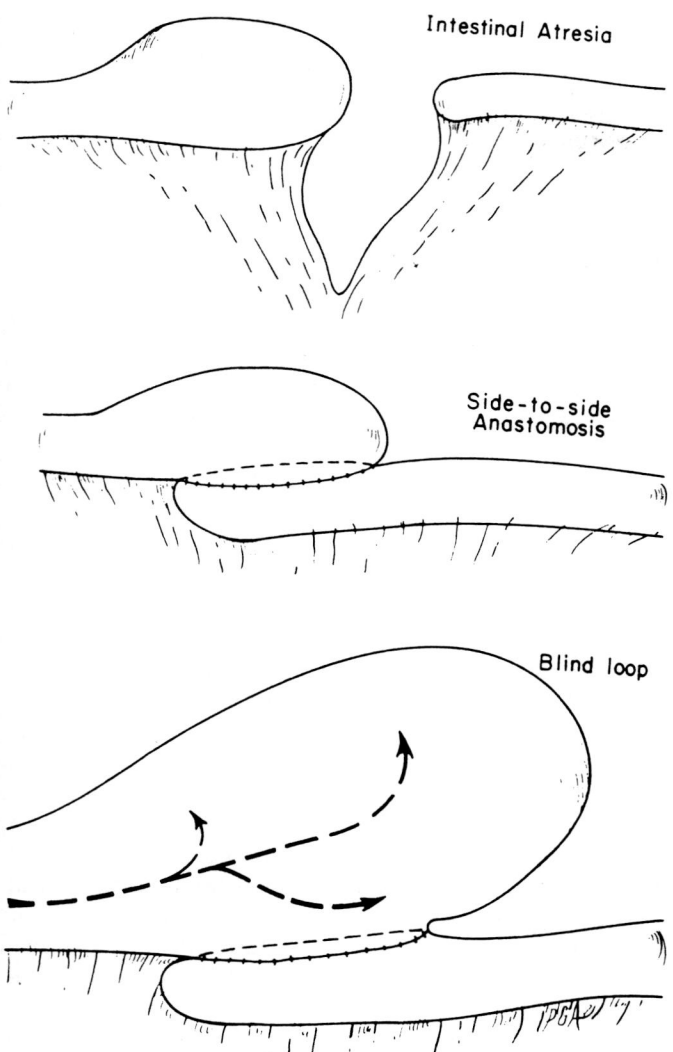

Intestinal Atresia

Side-to-side Anastomosis

Blind loop

Figure 6.32. Blind loop syndrome which can result from side-to-side anastomosis in small bowel. (From Hendren WH III, Kim SH. Abdominal surgical emergencies of the newborn. Surg Clin North Am 1974;54(3):495.)

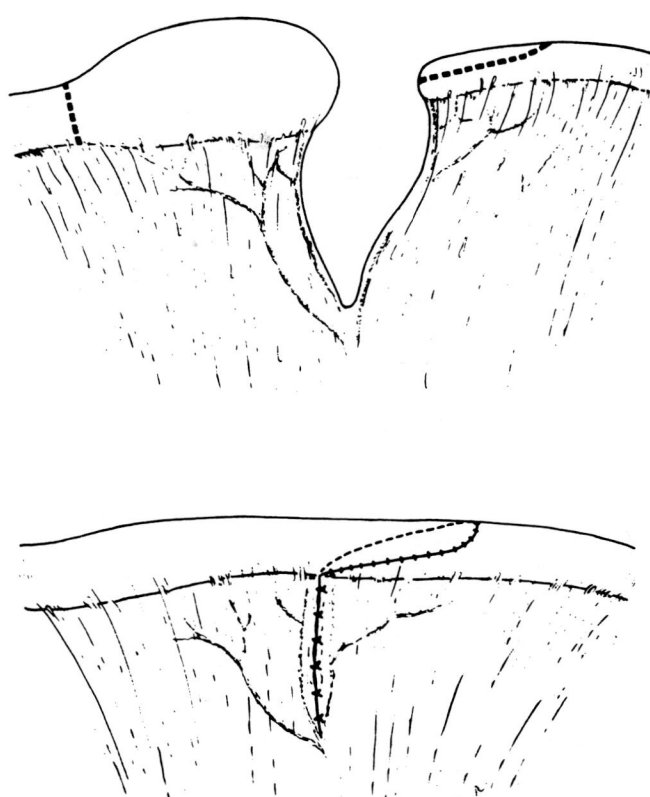

Figure 6.33. Preferred management in most cases of jejunoileal atresia. Hendren and Kim prefer a one-layer anastomosis. (From Hendren WH III, Kim SH. Abdominal surgical emergencies of the newborn. Surg Clin North Am 1974;54(3):496.)

form of end-to-end anastomosis. Because of discrepancy in size of the lumina, a proximal end-to-distal back anastomosis is what most pediatric surgeons use. This is carried out by opening the antimesenteric side of the distal unused small intestine large enough to accommodate the end of the resected dilated atretic segment. A single-layer anastomosis using interrupted suture material is preferred because it allows for growth of the anastomosis and avoids folding in extra tissue which occurs if a double-layer anastomosis is used. In older children and adults with stenoses rather than atresia, a double-layer anastomosis may be appropriate (JAH/CNP).

Special Procedures for Duodenal Atresias.
Gastroenterostomy.
Atresias in the first part of the duodenum may be bypassed by retrocolic gastrojejunostomy. The risk for marginal ulceration is great; thus most surgeons now favor a duodenoduodenostomy.

Billroth II Gastric Resection.
In certain adults with high duodenal stenosis, partial gastrectomy with gastroenterostomy has been recommended over gastroenterostomy alone (156).

Duodenojejunostomy.
The procedure of choice for duodenal atresia is a duodenoduodenostomy or a retrocolic duodenojejunostomy.

Tapering Enteroplasty.
In special cases, a tapering enteroplasty is advised (Fig. 6.31).

Special Procedure for Atresia of the Ascending Colon. The terminal ileum may be anastomosed to the distal colon and the proximal distended colon removed (158).

In all cases the distal intestine must be examined for other atresias and stenoses. Air or saline is usually used, but Berman and Lalonde (159) have recommended passing a catheter because a perforated diaphragm may permit passage of enough air or fluid to mislead the surgeon into thinking that the intestine was fully patent.

Del Pin et al. (160) reported a 6-month survival rate after surgery in 48 cases, from 37 to 100%.

MORTALITY

The mean survival time of untreated infants with intestinal atresia is less than 6 days (117) (Table 6.12). Until 1951 only 139 patients with atresia or stenosis had been treated successfully. Most affected infants were not treated at all, and before 1940 the mortality for treated patients approached 80%. At the Boston Children's Hospital, 52 infants underwent surgery prior to 1940, and 7 lived (40). Survival rates of 75% and more have been reported (81, 125, 155). Louw (115) reported a survival rate of over 90%.

According to Harmon and Holcomb (161), most of the infants with isolated jejunoileal atresia have low mortality and morbidity and an excellent prognosis when diagnosed early.

If the atresia or stenosis is recognized at once, the prospects for survival are good. Louw (115) divided patients with atresia into three groups with increasing operative risk:

1. Weight over 5.5 lb with no other anomaly
2. Weight 4 to 5.5 lb with no other anomaly, or weight over 5.5 lb with a moderately severe associated anomaly
3. Weight under 4 lb with no other anomaly; weight 4 to 5.5 lb with a moderately severe associated anomaly; or weight over 5.5 lb with a severe associated anomaly

Louw (115) obtained a 80% survival rate in group-3 patients.

Raffensperger (91) reports that his current survival rate for 75 infants with jejunoileal atresias is 92%.

Table 6.12.
Percentage Survival in Jejunoileal Atresia[a]

Researcher	Jejunal	Midbowel	Ileal	All Cases
deLorimier et al. (1960)[a]	58	—	75	68
Nixon and Tawes (1971)[b]	33	65	77	62
Louw (1967)[c]	Locations not specified			94
Grosfeld, Riley Hospital (1976)[d]	92	—	92	92
Martin and Zerella (1976)[e]	—	—	—	—

[a]From Grosfeld JL. Jejunoileal atresia and stenosis. In: Welch KJ et al., eds. Pediatric surgery. Chicago: Year Book Medical Publishers, 1986:846.
[b]deLorimier AA, Fonkalsrud EW, Hays DM. Congenital atresia and stenosis of the jejunum and ileum. Surgery 1969;65:819.
[c]Nixon HH, Tawes R. Etiology and treatment of small intestinal atresia: analysis of a series of 127 jejunoileal atresias and comparison with 62 duodenal atresias. Surgery 1971;69:41.
[d]Louw JH. Resection and end-to-end anastomosis in the management of atresia and stenosis of the small bowel. Surgery 1967;62:940.
[e]Grosfeld JL. Jejunoileal atresia and stenosis. In: Welch et al., eds. Pediatric surgery. Chicago: Year Book Medical Publishers, 1986:846.
[f]Martin LW, Zerella JT. Jejunoileal atresia: proposed classification. J Pediatr Surg 1976;11:399.

Remember that the prognosis after small bowel resection depends on the length. Good health and development was reported with 31 cm of small bowel in situ by Raffensperger (91) in 1990 and with 26 cm of bowel by Rickham et al. (162).

Topographic Anatomy of the Small Intestine

LENGTH OF INTESTINE

The alimentary tract length in humans has proved surprisingly difficult to measure. In cadavers the length of the small intestine was reported to be anywhere from 10 to 40 feet, according to a 1924 literature review by Bryant (163), who himself recorded an average length of 20.5 feet (624.8 cm). From his tables, an average of 20 to 22 feet has been widely quoted in textbooks.

That these figures bear no relation to the intestine in the living patient was apparent in 1924 when Reis and Schembra (164) measured the intestine in living dogs and remeasured it at various intervals after death. In the first 10 min, the intestines elongated 23 to 25%. Four hours after death, the increase in length reached 135%. This occurs because tonus of the longitudinal muscle is lost much faster than that of the circular muscle. Alvarez (165) offers an interesting discussion of the problems of measurement of intestinal length.

Blankenhorn et al. (166) intubated eight patients and obtained calculated average lengths of the duodenum, 22 cm (8.5 inches); jejunoileum, 258 cm (8 feet, 6 inches); and colon, 110 cm (3 feet, 7 inches). The overall nose-to-anus length averaged 452 cm (14 feet, 10 inches). There is some evidence that intestinal length is greater in obese individuals (167).

The surgeon is more concerned with the length of intestine remaining after a resection than with the amount resected. In the earlier literature are lists of operations in which 4 to 5 m or more of intestine were removed with survival of the patient (168). Undoubtedly the resected segment was measured only after the resection was completed and the abdomen closed. Elongation of the specimen was by then well under way. Accurate measurements should be made before the intestine is removed and with the least manipulation possible. We cannot explain why earlier measurements are still widely accepted.

Dimensions of the Mesentery

Shackleford (169) states that the length of the mesentery measured between the attachment to the intestine and the root of the mesentery usually does not exceed 20 to 25 cm. This length permits a loop of intestine to slide down into an inguinal hernia, especially if the mesentery is slightly relaxed at its extraperitoneal attachment. Sim-

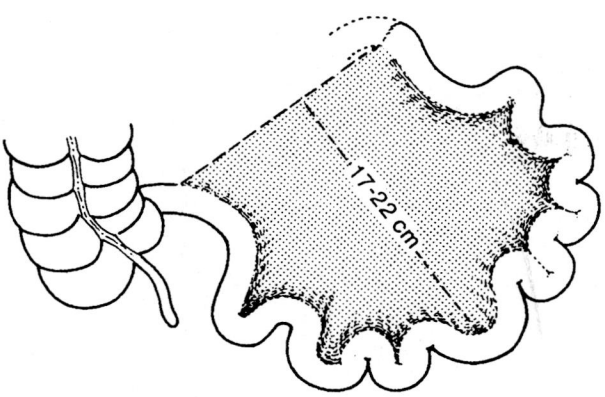

Figure 6.34. The breadth of the mesentery. It is usually long enough to reach the internal inguinal ring. (Data from Vaez-Zadeh K, Dutz W. Ileosigmoid knotting. Ann Surg 1970;172:1027.)

ilarly, it is usually long enough to permit the surgeon to bring a loop up to form an esophagojejunostomy.

There is considerable variation in the breadth of the small bowel mesentery and the sigmoid mesentery. In patients with volvulus and intestinal knots, the breadth of the affected mesentery is greater than that found in healthy patients (170) (Fig. 6.34). That there may be a racial difference needs confirmation.

Diverticula and Duplications of the Intestines

Adjacent or attached to the small and large intestines may be found a variety of anomalous structures designated by such names as "duplications," "reduplications," "diverticula," "giant diverticula," and "enteric cysts," as well as other less commonly used expressions. Although the names are confusing, the variety of the structures themselves is even more so. When is a long diverticulum a short reduplication, and how elongated may an enteric cyst be before it is a duplication? We deplore use of the term *reduplication* because it connotes a doubling back, but it connotes equally well a second doubling or four-folding.

To further confuse the subject, various authors use adjectives such as "gastric" or "ileal" to refer with great impartiality to (*a*) the site of the origin, (*b*) the type of mucosa contained, and (*c*) the normal organ that is actually paralleled by the duplication.

No classification of these anomalies can satisfy entirely the considerations of embryonic origin, anatomy, symptoms, and surgical procedure in a single set of terms. We suggest the following nomenclature, examples of which (except for cystic remnants of the tailgut) are illustrated by Figure 6.35.

   I. Diverticula
     A. Meckel's diverticulum (antimesenteric)
     B. Nonmeckelian true diverticula (antimesenteric)
     C. Primary false (acquired) diverticula (usually mesen-

teric in small intestine or between the teniae in the colon)
     D. Dorsal enteric remnants (mesenteric)
  II. Duplications
     E. Dorsal enteric remnants (cystic or tubular)
     F. Cystic remnants of the tailgut (presacral cysts)
     G. Bilateral duplication of the colon

Because of the pluripotency of the endoderm cells, the mucosa of these structures may resemble that of the esophagus, stomach, or any portion of the intestines. More than one mucosal type often is present. For this reason, the diverticula are best named for the segment from which they arise, and the duplications for the segment to which they lie adjacent.

MECKEL'S DIVERTICULUM AND OTHER REMNANTS OF THE VITELLINE DUCT

The most common anomaly of the gastrointestinal tract is a persistent diverticulum arising from the antimesenteric border of the terminal ileum, which represents the remains of the vitelline (omphalomesenteric) duct or embryonic yolk stalk. Although an ileal diverticulum (Meckel's diverticulum) is the most frequently encountered remnant of the vitelline duct, other vestigial forms of this structure may be found.

Evans (117) illustrated 24 variations of persistent vitelline duct anomalies, and others could perhaps be added. For convenience, these can be reduced to six major types:

  1. Omphaloilial fistula: A patent tube connecting the ileum with the umbilicus
  2. Meckel's diverticulum
     a. Tip attached to body wall or other structure
     b. Tip unattached (common form)
  3. Umbilical mucosal remnant: Umbilical sinus or umbilical "polyp"
  4. Cystic remnant of vitelline duct
     a. In body wall
     b. In abdominal cavity
  5. Solid cord from ileum to umbilicus
  6. Remnants of the vitelline blood vessels attached to the umbilicus

Of these varieties, Meckel's diverticulum is by far the most frequent. The incidence of the other varieties is variable, and Table 6.13 shows the frequency of the varieties in two large series.

Anatomy.

Omphaloilial Fistula (Patent Meckel's Diverticulum).
Kittle and his colleagues (171) reviewed 131 cases of fistula from 1834 to 1937, and Söderlund (172) estimated that 180 cases had been reported by 1958. Males predominated by more than 5:1. The fistula may be simple, or it may be associated with a protruding umbilical polyp several centimeters in length. Gastric mucosa was present in 33% of Söderlund's cases of complete fistula. In a curious

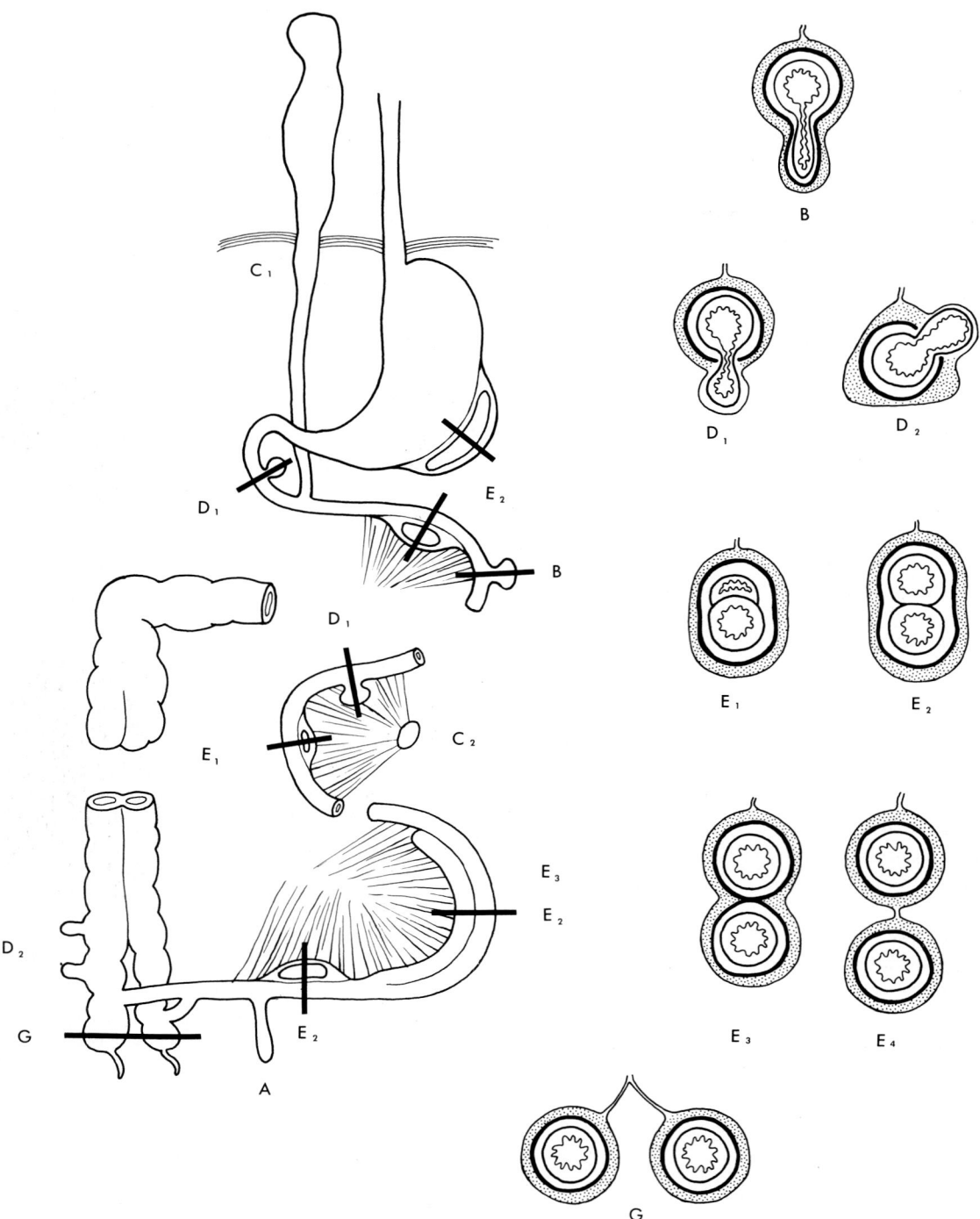

Figure 6.35. Various types of duplications and diverticula encountered in the gastrointestinal tract. **A**, Meckel's diverticulum (antimesenteric). **B**, True, antimesenteric, nonmeckelian diverticulum. **C₁**, Giant abdominothoracic enterogenous diverticulum. **C₂**, Small mesenteric enterogenous cyst. **D₁** and **D₂**, False diverticula, not containing all of the normal intestinal coats. **E₁** to **E₄**, Duplications of the gut with varying degrees of separation. All are on the mesenteric side of the normal gut. **G**, Bilateral duplication of the gut. Each member of the pair may have its own mesentery or the two may be partially fused side by side.

case reported in an adult, a pilonidal abscess at the umbilicus eroded into the tip of an attached Meckel's diverticulum, producing an acquired patency (173).

In 20% of the 131 cases of Kittle et al. (171) prolapse of the vitelline duct or of the ileum occurred in infancy or childhood. Before 1947 only two such patients had survived. Since then, successful treatment has been reported more frequently (174–177). Prolapse of the duct starts as an umbilical protrusion with enteric mucosa both inside and out. As prolapse continues and involves the ileum, the protrusion becomes Y or T shaped with two openings, the upper one leading to the proximal ileum and the lower one to the distal ileum. Symptoms of complete intestinal obstruction occur, and leakage is from the upper opening only. Prolapse must never be mistaken for an umbilical polyp (Fig. 6.36); an unwitting ligation of the prolapsed loop might easily be catastrophic (174).

Meckel's Diverticulum.

Meckel's diverticulum is a "true" diverticulum, containing all layers of the gut wall. It arises antimesenterically and is supplied by a continuation of the superior mesenteric artery, which is itself the persistent proximal portion of the embryonic right omphalomesenteric artery. In about 25% of cases the diverticulum is attached to the umbilicus or to another portion of the body wall by a fibrous cord. In the remainder the tip of the diverticulum is free (Fig. 6.37).

Table 6.13.
Relative Frequency of Vitelline Duct Remnants

Type	Moses (1947) 1605 cases (%)	Söderlund (1959) 413 cases (%)
Omphalo-ileal fistula	6	2.4
Meckel's diverticulum	82	96.0
(Tip attached)		[22.2]
(Tip unattached)		[73.8]
Umbilical remnant		1.2
Cystic remnant	1	0.24
Solid cord	10	—

Typically, Meckel's diverticulum arises about 40 cm from the ileocecal valve in infants and about 50 cm from it in adults (Fig. 6.38). It is 3 to 6 cm in length and approximately 2 cm in diameter. All of these measurements are variable. Jay et al. (178) found 4% within 15 cm of the cecum, 24% from 15 to 46 cm, 44% from 46 to 91 cm,

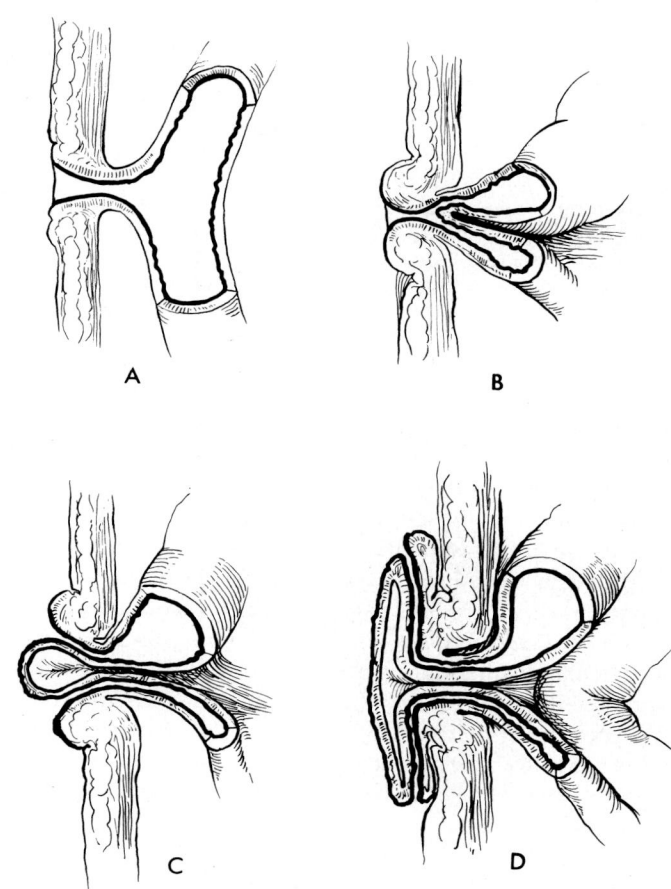

Figure 6.36. **A,** Patent vitelline duct (patent Meckel's diverticulum). **B** to **D,** Stages of prolapse of the ileum through the patent duct. Note that the mucosal surfaces are on the outside.

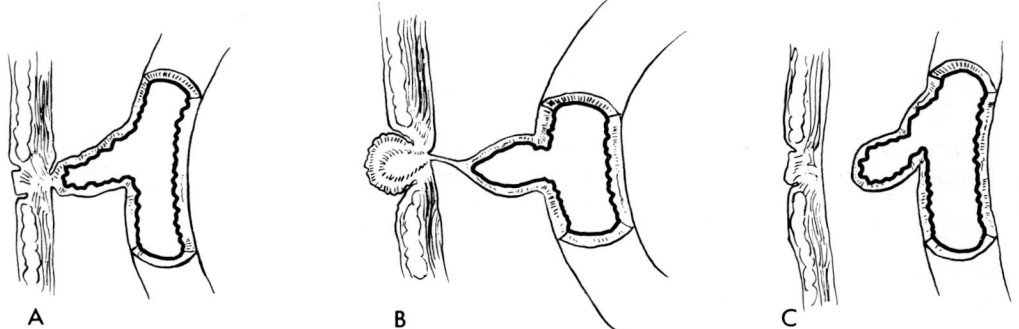

Figure 6.37. Varieties of Meckel's diverticulum. **A** and **B,** Tip is attached to body wall. **C,** Tip is free.

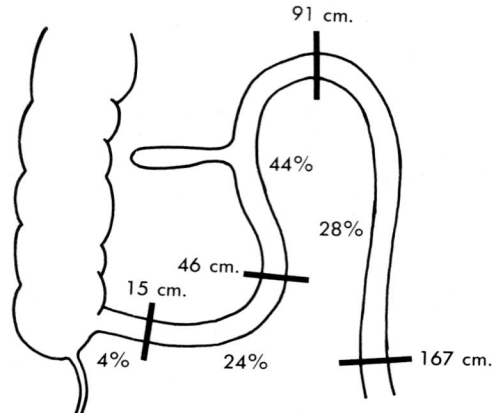

Figure 6.38. *Distribution of Meckel's diverticulum on the distal ileum. Distances are measured from the ileocecal valve. (Data from Jay GD III, Margulis RR, McGraw AB, Northrip RR. Meckel's diverticulum: a survey of one hundred and three cases. Arch Surg 1950;61:158–169.)*

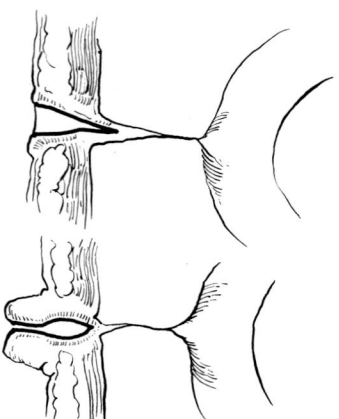

Figure 6.39. *Umbilical sinuses formed by unclosed distal vitelline duct.*

and 28% more than 91 cm from the ileocecal valve. The most distant was 167 cm from the cecum. Not less than 5 feet of ileum should be examined to not miss a Meckel's diverticulum. Our own experience suggests that the distance between the diverticulum and the ileocecal valve is proportionate to the length of the small intestine, but we have no quantitative confirmation for this hypothesis.

Although variations do occur in the position of this structure, there are limits beyond which diverticula cannot be considered to be of vitelline origin. Some jejunal diverticula may be Meckelian (179), but most diverticula cranial to the ileum are not (171). Neither diverticula arising from the appendix (180) nor those arising from the colon (181) are acceptable. We also are unable to credit a report of two Meckel's diverticula arising from the same ileum (182).

In length, Meckel's diverticulum may be as short as 1 cm or as long as 26 cm (183). Seventy-five percent are from 1 to 5 cm; the remainder are longer.

Most very long ileal diverticula are not Meckelian but belong to the group of "giant diverticula." One long structure (90 cm) that was probably vitelline was described by Pollard (184) in 1896. Arising only 60 cm from the pylorus, it reached the umbilicus and continued into the umbilical cord. It represented the entire yolk stalk rather than merely the proximal end, which forms the usual Meckel's diverticulum.

Because of its ventral origin, Meckel's diverticulum is antimesenteric. Although a rotation in the position of the diverticulum by the pull of fibrosed omphalomesenteric arteries has been postulated (185), we cannot accept a diverticulum arising on the mesenteric border as meckelian. Somers (186) has described an ileal diverticulum lying within the leaves of the mesentery as Meckel's diverticulum. The diverticulum contained gastric mucosa and

was at the proper distance from the cecum. There are other, similar cases (187). Such diverticula, of whatever length, are remnants of traction between endoderm and ectoderm at an early stage and belong to the class of dorsal enteric remnants.

True Meckel's diverticula may arise at the antimesenteric border, curl around the ileum, and become adherent to the mesentery. Moll (185) described a 54-cm diverticulum of this type. As in Pollard's case (184) it may have represented the whole of the yolk stalk. Not only may the diverticulum itself turn toward the mesenteric side, but it may have a fibrous termination free from the umbilicus and secondarily attached to mesentery, omentum, or serosal surface of the gut (188).

The mucosa lining of Meckel's diverticulum is chiefly ileal, as would be expected, but gastric, pancreatic, duodenal, and colonic mucosa in various combinations are frequent. Bile duct mucosa has been reported in a few cases (189, 190). Alleged salivary gland tissue in a diverticulum (191) was probably pancreatic. Berman et al. (192) believe that one could find gastric mucosa in every Meckel's diverticulum sectioned serially, but 81% is the highest incidence we have seen reported (190). Söderlund (172), who searched carefully, found gastric mucosa in 43% and pancreatic mucosa in 3.2% of Meckel's diverticula. Gross (40) found gastric mucosa in 54% and pancreatic in 5.4% of 130 diverticula. Duodenal mucosa was present in four cases and colonic mucosa in seven. Where gastric mucosa exists, fundic glands (hydrochloric acid producing) are present in about 85% of the cases. Pyloric glands only are found in the remainder.

Umbilical Mucosal Remnants.
Corresponding to Meckel's diverticulum at the ileal end of the vitelline tract is the umbilical sinus or umbilical "polyp" at the distal end (Fig. 6.39). The sinus projects inward to end blindly a variable distance from the surface, while the umbilical polyp (umbilical adenoma) extends

out from the body wall. A Meckel's diverticulum also may be present, only the middle of the vitelline tract having undergone normal atresia (172). Umbilical sinuses are not common. Aschner and Karelitz (193) reviewed 23 cases up to 1930.

Histologically, the mucosa of these umbilical sinuses and polyps may be ileal or gastric. There are three reports of pancreatic tissue at this location (194). Only a few such structures seem to have been thoroughly examined. Curd (191) reported that four of ten examples of gastric mucosa at the umbilicus contained parietal cells.

Vitelline Cysts.
When involution of the vitelline tract occurs at the umbilical and at the ileal ends, a middle portion may fail to close and remain as a cystic structure connected with the ileum and the body wall by fibrous bands (Fig. 6.40). Although such structures have been called *enterocystomas,* this term is too broad since it has been applied also to cystic duplications of the gut. Relatively few cases have been reported. Fox (175) reported four, and Söderlund (172) found only one in his 413 cases of vitelline duct remnants.

These cysts resemble duplication cysts of the mesenteric border of the intestine: They have all the layers of the normal gut. Degenerative changes may make the mucosa impossible to recognize. Unlike mesenteric duplication cysts, vitelline cysts may be removed without endangering the blood supply to the normal gut.

Persistent Solid Cords.
The vitelline duct itself, or the omphalomesenteric vessels, may persist as fibrous cords extending from the ileum to the umbilicus (195) (Fig. 6.41). Although they are not common, their significance lies in their ability to produce intestinal obstruction (177). Hoffert and Strachman (196) described obstruction of a loop of ileum, transverse colon, and duodenum in an infant by a persistent (and patent) umbilical vein extending from the umbilicus to the hilus of the liver. Three similar cases, two associated with malrotation of the gut (197, 198) and one producing chylous ascites (199), have been reported (Fig. 6.42).

Anomalies Associated with Vitelline Remnants. In spite of their proximity at the umbilicus, the vitelline duct and urachus (allantois stalk) regress independently of one another. Cullen (195) was able to find only one authentic case of a persistent fistula in both structures in the same individual. Since then, eight cases have been reported (200–202).

Among autopsied infants, a large percentage of those with Meckel's diverticulum have other defects. In the largest series reported, 21 of 63 had other anomalies, chiefly of the central nervous and cardiovascular systems (203). Death in the majority of these infants was from a cause unrelated to Meckel's diverticulum.

On the other hand, living patients with disease resulting from the presence of Meckel's diverticulum are much less frequently affected with other anomalies. In a series of 68 of our own patients, only three had other severe defects (4.4%). There is no evidence that patients presenting with Meckel's diverticulum disease need be suspected of harboring an undue share of other anomalies.

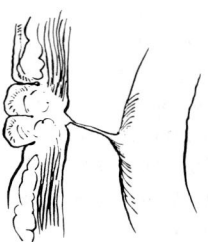

Figure 6.41. Vitelline duct reduced to a solid cord attaching to the ileum to the body wall.

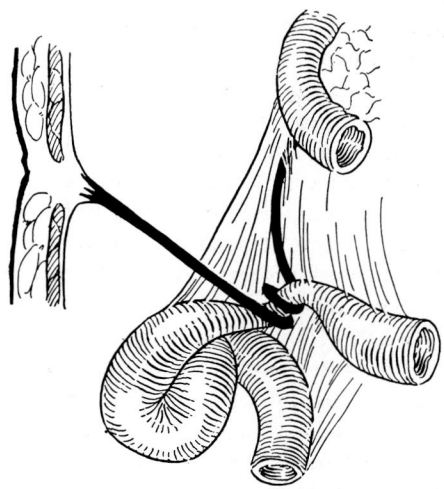

Figure 6.42. A persistent right vitelline vein forming a strangulating loop around the intestine. (From Hollinshead 1956; after Buchanan JS, Wapshaw H. Remnants of the vitelline vascular system as a cause of intestinal obstruction. Br J Surg 1940;27:533–539.)

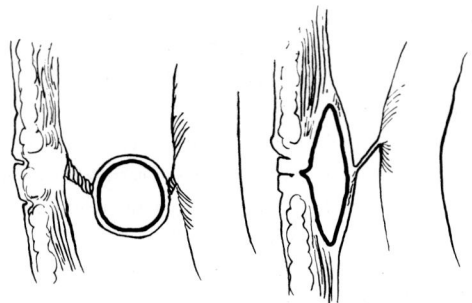

Figure 6.40. Vitelline cysts formed by unclosed midportion of the vitelline duct.

History. Meckel's diverticulum was unknown to both Galen and Vesalius; it is said to have been first mentioned in 1598 by Fabricius Hildanus (204) and later in 1672 by Lavater (205). Ruysch (206), who coined the word "epithelium," illustrated the anomaly in 1701. At about the same time, Littré (207) described a hernia containing Meckel's diverticulum (Littré's hernia). In 1769 Morgagni (De Sedibus XXXIV: 16, 17) recognized the structure to be of congenital origin.

In his 1809 report and in later publications Meckel (208) devoted serious attention to the structure and established its embryonic origin from the yolk sac. The clue to its origin had been provided by Cuvier's work on avian development. Meckel saw fistulous and fibrous cord types, as well as the more usual forms. It remained for Brun (209) in 1834 to describe persistent mucosa at the umbilicus.

Patent fistulous vitelline ducts have been known from antiquity. The escape of roundworms through such fistulae was often the presenting complaint. Cullen (195) gives credit to Brun, working in Dupuytren's clinic, for good descriptions of three cases of such umbilical fecal fistulae.

The presence of pancreatic tissue in the diverticulum was reported by Zenker (210) in 1861. Gastric tissue was not recognized until 1883 when Tillmanns (211) detected it in an umbilical polyp. Common as is gastric mucosa, there was no mention of it before 1900 (191).

In 1916 Cullen (195) reviewed the literature in his book on the umbilicus; he seems, however, to have been unaware or unconvinced of the existence of gastric mucosa in Meckel's diverticulum. A comprehensive review was attempted by Moses (212), who in 1947 reported on 1605 cases in the literature. In 1959 Söderlund (172) examined 413 cases, the largest individual series to date. In 1962 Weinstein et al. (213) reviewed 722 cases from the Mayo Clinic.

Embryogenesis. The yolk sac, from the roof of which arises the primitive gut, ceases growing when the embryo is about 3.5 mm long. The stalk between it and the embryonic gut—the vitelline duct—becomes increasingly smaller until the attenuated connection breaks; sometime during the fifth week, it separates from the intestine. Blechschmidt (214) indicates separation by the 6.2-mm stage. It has been found to be patent as late as the 12.5-mm stage (35th day) and solid as early as the 4.5-mm stage (48th day) (195). Just prior to separation, the epithelium of the yolk sac forms short, sometimes branched tubules suggestive of the earliest stages of gastric pit formation in the stomach, which appear during the sixth week. Mucous granules are evident in the epithelial cells (215, 217).

It is at this stage that the fate of Meckel's diverticulum is determined. That portion of the vitelline duct that does not become completely atretic renews its growth and keeps pace with the gut itself; most diverticula are only slightly smaller than the ileum to which they are attached. Whether the end will be blind or a fistula will occur is determined by the length of the unclosed tract and the extent to which it is withdrawn from the cord during the 10th week. If the tip remains in the cord, there will be a fistula; if the whole of the patent portion is withdrawn, there will be a blind diverticulum. Very rarely, a stenosis of the ileum occurs at the site of the diverticulum, which suggests excessive involution of the vitelline duct (218).

Distal to the tip of the diverticulum there may be a solid cord representing either the yolk stalk, the vitelline vessels, or both. It may remain attached to the umbilical region, or its free end may attach to serosal surfaces elsewhere. It is often long enough to form one or more coils (188).

The vitelline (omphalomesenteric) arteries form from a vascular plexus arising from the paired aortae. With the fusion of the latter during the fourth week, the paired vitelline arteries fuse to form a single blood supply to the yolk sac. The proximal portion of this vessel becomes the superior mesenteric artery. Where Meckel's diverticulum persists, the artery continues beyond the ileum to serve it. The vitelline veins draining the yolk sac are the first blood vessels to appear in the embryo. Originally paired, only the left normally persists beyond the 7-mm stage. After birth, the central portion persists as the portal vein.

Incidence. The frequency of Meckel's diverticulum is 2%. The range reported in a number of large series is as follows: those found at autopsy, 1.1 to 2.5% (in four series) (66, 178, 203, 219, 220) and those found during appendectomy, 2 to 4.5% (in four series) (172, 221–223).

The largest series represents 50,000 appendectomies, in which 1019 Meckel's diverticula were found (223).

Sex.

Reports may indicate that males are affected with disease of Meckel's diverticulum about three times as frequently as are females; however, this does not reflect the true incidence. When Meckel's diverticulum is found incidentally at surgery or at autopsy, the sex ratio is approximately equal. This is usually overlooked because most reports of Meckel's diverticulum include only cases of diverticular disease. An exception is the series of 650 incidental diverticula from the Mayo Clinic reported by Weinstein and his colleagues (213), in which both sexes were equally represented.

Most of the apparent "gender differences" in the group of diseased diverticula is accounted for by the frequency with which they cause intussusception in young males. Meckel's diverticulum formed the leading point of intussusception in 36.5% of our own cases of diverticular disease (224). Eighty-five percent were in young males (Fig. 6.43).

Even with intussusception excluded, ulceration,

omphaloileal fistula, and neoplasms are more frequent in males (225, 226). Only in the patients with inflammatory disease does the sex ratio appear reasonably equal.

Age.

From 33 to 50% of operative cases are in patients under 2 years of age, and 80% of surgical patients are under age 10 years. A few cases are found among older patients, such as a 77-year-old man with obstruction from torsion caused by Meckel's diverticulum (227). Veith and Botsford (228) have discussed 20 symptomatic cases in adults.

Familial Tendency.

It is not surprising that so common an anomaly should occasionally be found in siblings; as a matter of fact, this should be expected to occur once in about 2500 families. More curious is the case of the family reported by Lewenstein and Levenson (229) in which two sisters, their mother, and a niece were affected. In another family, two brothers, their mother, and the mother's sister were affected (230). The preponderance of females in these lines suggests that some families may show a predisposition to Meckel's diverticulum.

Clinical Classification and Diagnosis. Vitelline duct remnants may produce a pathologic abdominal condition, or they may remain silent. The frequency with which they produce disease has been placed at 22% of 722 cases at the Mayo Clinic (213) and at 34% of 413 cases in Sweden reported by Söderlund (172). These figures are, of course, high since silent Meckel's diverticula may remain undiscovered throughout life. In general, those diverticula that give rise to disease are more likely to contain heterotopic gastric mucosa. Jay et al. (178) found gastric mucosa in 62% of patients with diverticulitis, in 22% of patients in whom the diverticula were found incidental to other surgery, and in only 17% of autopsy cases.

Leijonmarck et al. (231) reported on 260 diverticula found at laparotomy; 112 were symptomatic and 148 were silent. The authors concluded that an incidentally discovered, symptomless Meckel's diverticulum should be left in place. Cornacchia et al. (232) used the phrase, "great imitator" in describing Meckel's diverticulum, and it is a good one.

The clinical manifestations produced by Meckel's diverticula and related anomalies may be divided into the major groups listed in Table 6.14.

The Peptic Ulcer Group.

Peptic ulceration of Meckel's diverticulum was not recognized until 1913 (233) and indeed was not widely accepted as an entity until 1925 when the frequency with which gastric mucosa could be found in diverticula was demonstrated (234). Not all gastric mucosa produces ulceration. In 6% of diverticula and 30% of fistulae and umbilical "polyps," the gastric mucosa contained only pyloric glands without parietal cells (191).

The pain is ulcer-like, but, unlike that from peptic ulcers of the duodenum, it is not relieved by food or by antacids. It is rarely localized. Hemorrhage, massive or intermittent, usually accompanies ulceration, and anemia may be severe. Unexplained rectal bleeding in young boys (boys are much more frequently affected than are girls)

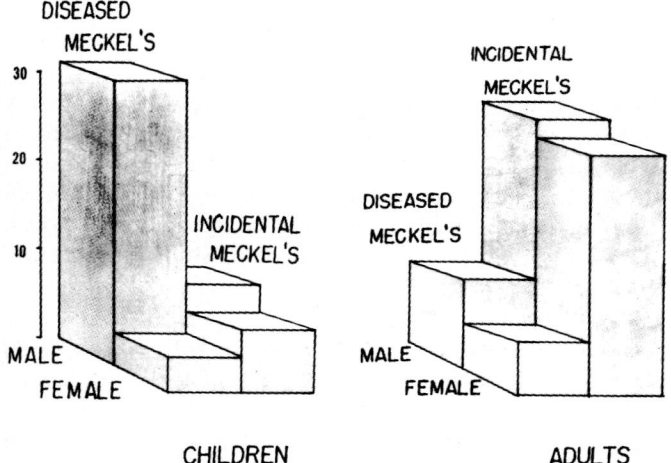

Figure 6.43. The proportions of Meckel's diverticulum and Meckel's diverticulum disease by age and sex. The disproportion of affected male children is evident. (From Androulakis JA, Gray SW, Lionakis B, Skandalakis JE. The sex ratio of Meckel's diverticulum. Am Surg 1969;25:455–460.)

Table 6.14.
Meckel's Diverticula: Clinical Manifestations and Related Anomalies[a]

Symptoms Group and Frequency	Onset of Symptoms	Symptoms	Complications
I. Ulcerating (40%)	Infancy or childhood	Pain, melena	Perforation
II. Obstructing (32%)	Any age, but usually childhood	Symptoms of low obstruction	Volvulus or intussusception, gangrene, and perforation
III. Inflammatory (17%)	Infancy or childhood	Appendicitis-like, acute or chronic	Perforation
IV. Umbilical (5%)	First few weeks of life	Weeping or leakage at umbilicus	Infection, prolapse, and obstruction
V. Neoplastic (6%)	Middle life	As intestinal neoplasm	Perforation or obstruction

[a]The percentages have been computed from several large series and are only approximations.

always should suggest peptic ulcer of Meckel's diverticulum. Cobb (235) mapped the location of ulcers in 45 diverticula; the greatest number are in the ileal mucosa at the neck of the diverticulum.

Perforation of these ulcers is common and may be accompanied by nausea and vomiting. The pain is said to be less acute than that from perforation of duodenal ulcers (172).

The Obstruction Group.

Intussusception, hernia, incarceration, and volvulus may all result from the presence of a Meckel's diverticulum. The first two complications are associated with diverticula not connected to the abdominal wall, whereas the second two usually occur when diverticula are connected by a fibrous band to the body wall. Obstruction is the most frequent symptom, accounting for about a third of symptomatic cases (236).

Intussusception is associated with Meckel's diverticula in 5 to 10% of cases, and from 5 to 10% of all intussusceptions contain diverticula. Intussusception accounts for about 25% of the obstructive symptoms.

According to Amoury (237), in three series totaling 183 cases (40, 172, 238), intussusception was the cause of internal obstruction in 47% and herniation, bands, kinking, and volvulus in 53%.

In our own experience, 13 of 136 intussusceptions in infants and children could be referred to as Meckel's diverticulum (64). The clinical picture of intussusception caused by Meckel's diverticulum does not differ from that produced by other causes although 80% are in males. Older children and adults are affected more frequently than are infants (239).

Pain and the presence of a palpable mass are the usual symptoms. Rarely does the apex pass beyond the hepatic flexure, and fewer than 50% of patients have blood in their stools. In spite of the tendency toward milder attacks in these patients, the incidence of irreducibility and gangrene is nearly twice as high as in nonmeckelian intussusception. Invagination of the diverticulum precedes actual intussusception, and the condition is occasionally recognized at this stage (172).

The presence of Meckel's diverticulum in a hernial sac (Littré's hernia) accounts for about 15% of the obstructive group. About 50% of these are found in inguinal herniae, the remainder being umbilical or femoral (240). As Littré (207) noted over 150 years ago, incarceration of Meckel's diverticulum produces the toxemia of intestinal hernia but not the abdominal distension. Fecal fistula at the site of these herniae is common (241). Wollgast and Hilz (240) have discussed some unusual hernial sites.

Whereas intussusception may be produced by diverticula unattached at the tip, diverticula attached to the umbilicus or elsewhere by fibrous bands produce

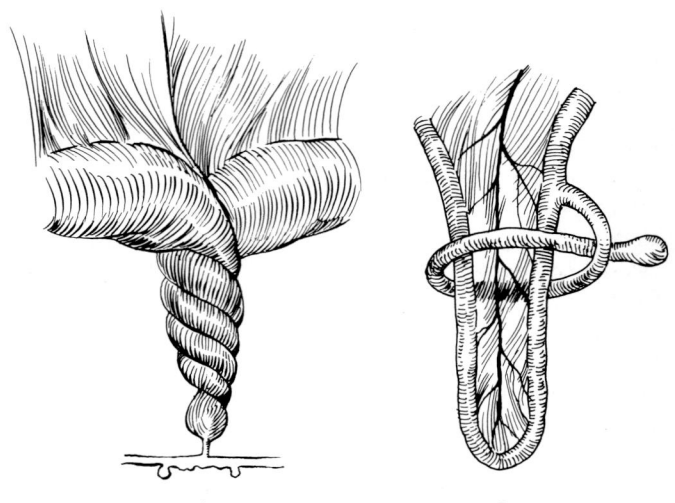

Figure 6.44. Two examples of intestinal obstruction produced by vitelline duct remnants. **A,** Volvulus around a fibrous cord attached to the body wall. **B,** Intestinal loop caught in a half hitch of a long, unattached Meckel's diverticulum. (**A,** From Aitken J. Remnants of the vitello-intestinal duct: a clinical analysis of 88 cases. Arch Dis Child 1953;28:1–7; **B,** from Dowse JL. Meckel's diverticulum. Br J Surg 1961;48:392–399.)

obstruction by incarceration of an intestinal loop or by volvulus (242). Rarely, a long, free diverticulum may form a half hitch about a loop of intestine (243, 244). Various types of obstruction are shown in Figure 6.44. Abdominal pain, vomiting, and constipation are the chief symptoms, and abdominal tenderness and distension are the chief physical signs.

The Inflammatory Group.

Chronic or acute inflammation of Meckel's diverticulum is difficult to distinguish from appendicitis and is usually diagnosed as the latter. In appendicitis, pain and tenderness settle in the right lower quadrant, whereas the pain from diverticulitis may be located elsewhere (40), frequently near the umbilicus (245). Absence of pathologic changes in the appendix at operation should direct attention toward a diverticulum.

In about 15% of cases in this group, inflammation and perforation are results of a foreign body in the diverticulum. Moses (212) reported 32 cases up to 1947, and Dowse (243) found 30 in children by 1961. Alhadeff (245) considered that 10% of perforations were caused by foreign bodies. Fish bones were the most common offenders, and fibrous vegetable remains were next. Boldero (246) reported a patient with diverticulitis from gallstones.

The Umbilical Group.

Ectopic mucosa must be distinguished from ordinary granulation tissue at the umbilicus. The former is bright red instead of pink; its discharge is mucous instead of serous or purulent; it shows no sign of healing and persists until removed. The mucosa has frequently been reported to increase its secretion after meals and after mechanical stimulation (193, 195). Ligation of polypoid forms is often effective, but sinus formations require complete destruction of the mucosa if they are not to recur.

If there is doubt about the extent of an umbilical sinus in the absence of fecal leakage, opaque material should be injected at the umbilicus to visualize the tract radiographically.

The Neoplastic Group.

Skandalakis, Gray, and their colleagues (225, 247) collected six cases of leiomyoma and 16 cases of leiomyosarcoma in Meckel's diverticulum. Weinstein et al. (220) collected 26 cases of benign tumors and 80 cases of malignant tumors. About 75% occurred in males. Among benign tumors, leiomyomas predominate; in the malignant group, carcinoid tumors are the most frequent (248), followed by leiomyosarcomas and adenocarcinomas. There are probably more such tumors than the published cases indicate, as Moses (212) found 27 neoplasms among 1810 Meckel's diverticula. Considering the size of the structure and the infrequency of its occurrence, Meckel's diverticulum is more subject to neoplasms than is any other portion of the intestines.

Treatment.

Uncomplicated Meckel's Diverticulum.

Meckel's diverticulum may be found during surgery for appendicitis or for other abdominal disease. In most cases there is nothing pathologic about the diverticulum. Stewart and Story (190) introduced an additional class— called "indeterminate"—to include those cases with abdominal symptoms but without visible pathologic disease of the diverticulum or of other abdominal organs. It is our conviction that all Meckel's diverticula should be removed when found, whether or not pathologic changes are evident. The potentialities of the most healthy diverticulum for intussusception, obstruction, or neoplastic change are sufficient to warrant this procedure.

Soltero and Bill (249) disagree. In these uncomplicated cases a simple diverticulectomy may be performed (Fig. 6.45, *A* and *B*). We prefer a V-shaped excision of the ileum, including the diverticulum, but not reaching the mesenteric border of the ileum.

Meckel's Diverticulum with Complications.

Resection of the ileum above and below the diverticulum with end-to-end anastomosis may be necessary when ulceration, perforation, or obstruction is present (Fig. 6.45, *C*). The surgeon should remember that peptic ulceration from ectopic gastric mucosa occurs in the adjacent mucosa, usually in the ileum below the diverticulum (Fig. 6.45, *D* and *E*). After sectioning obstructing bands or

reducing intussusception, the surgeon must examine the ileum for edema and gangrene, the presence of which will determine the extent of resection necessary.

A more radical resection is necessary when neoplasm appears in the diverticulum (Fig. 6.45, *F*). The ileum should be resected at least 10 cm above the site of the diverticulum, and a typical right colectomy should be performed.

Umbilical Polyps and Sinuses.

Excision of umbilical polyps and sinus tracts should be undertaken as soon as they are identified to prevent recurrent infection (Fig. 6.45, *G*).

Omphaloileal Fistula (Patent Meckel's Diverticulum).

Once a fistula has been diagnosed, it should be treated without delay. Ileal prolapse progresses very rapidly and reduction is difficult (Fig. 6.36). Such prolapse through the umbilicus should be considered a surgical emergency (250).

NON–MECKELIAN ANTIMESENTERIC TRUE DIVERTICULA

These diverticula are extremely rare and are not always easily explained. Carter (22) has described eight antimesenteric diverticula less than 1 cm long in the upper jejunum of a 2-day-old infant who had multiple congenital anomalies. Carter believes, as does Moynihan (251), that these diverticula represent rudimentary pancreatic diverticula that were not suppressed by the formation of the definitive pancreatic diverticula. There is no evidence for, and little against, this theory.

An unusual diverticulum with gastric mucosa was reported in the anterior wall of the rectum of a 4-year-old girl who had no other abnormalities (252). The anterior location precludes the diagnosis of dorsal enteric remnant, and the caudal position makes its identification with Meckel's diverticulum impossible. The presence of gastric mucosa below the midgut is equally difficult to explain (see Chapter 5, The Stomach).

PRIMARY, FALSE DIVERTICULA

These diverticula are called "primary" because they are not the result of local disease, and they are "false" because they are not covered with the muscular coats of the intestine. They are, however, true herniations through defects of the gut wall. The actual herniations are acquired; developmental defects in the musculature are the predisposing cause.

According to Gray et al. (120) in 1989, false diverticula of the duodenum are usually found on the concave wall of the second and third parts of the duodenum, often close to the duodenal papillae. More than two-thirds of duodenal diverticula are located within 2 cm of the vicinity of the ampulla of Vater (253). Although they usually

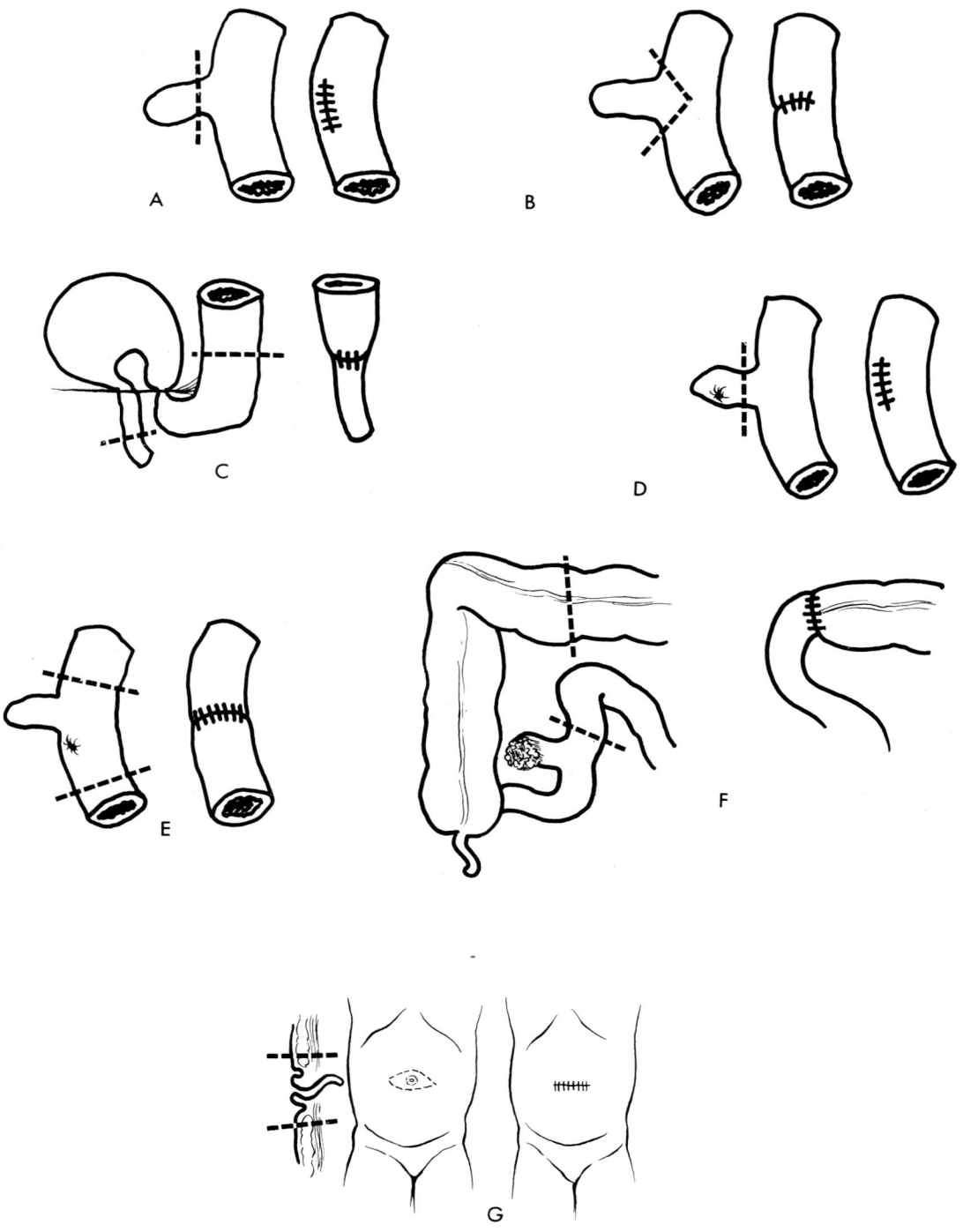

Figure 6.45. Procedures for treating vitelline duct remnants: **A** and **B**, Simple excision of Meckel's diverticulum. **C**, Resection of an ileal loop strangulated by a cord-like vitelline remnant. **D** and **E**, Excision of ulcerated Meckel's diverticulum. **F**, Resection of terminal ileum, diverticulum, and right colon after diagnosis of neoplasm in the diverticulum. **G**, Infraumbilical incision for excision of vitelline sinus; the umbilicus is spared.

reveal themselves only in adult life, many such lesions originate before birth. They are usually solitary and asymptomatic, and we agree with Eiseman et al. (254) that it is best to leave them alone. A diverticulum near the papilla may present difficulties for the endoscopist.

Gray et al. (120) further state that cystic intramural duplications of the alimentary tract are uncommon, but 20% of all such lesions are found in the duodenum.

Duodenal Diverticula.

Anatomy.

About 75% of duodenal diverticula are in the second part of the duodenum, and most of the remainder are in the third part (255). The great majority are on the concave (pancreatic) side, although the few found on the convex side are said to be the largest (256) (Fig. 6.46).

Most duodenal diverticula are globular, but they may be conical or tubular. They are usually solitary; in 5 to 30% of patients they are multiple, depending on the series. Dean (257) described a patient with five duodenal diverticula.

Intraluminal diverticula in the duodenum that arise from a membranous diaphragm are complications of atresia, not diverticula in the sense used in this section (Fig. 6.47).

Etiology.

The usual view is that diverticula form where a duct or a blood vessel pierces the duodenal wall, with a consequent hiatus in the musculature. Spriggs and Marxer (258) observed that they occur where they are least likely to be produced by pressure if the duodenum were of uniform strength throughout. Beer (259) showed that water pressure in the duodenum of the living animal produced pulsion diverticula on the antimesenteric (convex) border; whereas in the cadaver—10 hr or more after death—such diverticula appeared on the mesenteric (concave) border. There is no reason, however, to believe that the diverticula encountered clinically are the result of sudden high duodenal pressure; they are more likely produced by long, continued, moderate elevations of pressure, which distend the wall at some weakened point.

Linsmayer (260) suggested that small areas of aberrant pancreatic tissue often interrupt the regularity of the muscularis fibers and hence might create areas susceptible to diverticulum formation. On the other hand, many authors have pointed to the transitory embryonic diverticula first observed by Lewis and Thyng (20). Guthrie and Wakefield (21) described these diverticula in guinea pig embryos. They found 76 diverticula in 36 of 53 embryos between 6 and 34 mm in length. These may be the origin of the congenital true diverticula mentioned previously, as well as of some of the intramural cystic duplications described later in this chapter.

Definite developmental gaps in the musculature, such as those encountered in the stomach (see Chapter 5, The Stomach), seem to be rare in the duodenum.

History.

Chomel (261) in 1710 described a duodenal pouch which contained 22 stones, probably gallstones, in an 80-year-old woman. The stones did not cause the diverticulum, but they must have contributed to its enlargement. Morgagni and a few other 18th century writers reported instances of the lesion. In spite of these cases, Cruveilhier (262) in 1849 stated that diverticula did not occur between the esophagus and colon.

Fewer than 100 cases appeared in the literature up to 1912, when Case made the first x-ray demonstration (263, 264). In 1916 Forsell and Key (265) made the first preopertive diagnosis and successfully removed a duodenal diverticulum. In 1943 Ackermann (266) systemati-

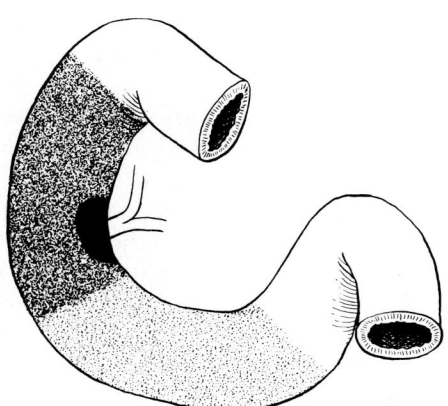

Figure 6.46. Relative incidence of primary false diverticula of the duodenum. The most common location is near the papilla of Vater.

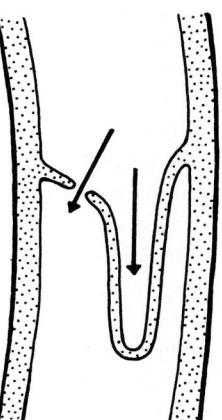

Figure 6.47. An internal intestinal diverticulum formed in a perforated membranous atresia. Such a mucosal pocket will continue to enlarge until it forms an obstruction. (Redrawn from Heilbrun N, Boyden EA. Intraluminal duodenal diverticula. Radiology 1964;82:887–894.)

cally examined 50 cadavers and found 11 with diverticula, suggesting that the condition was far more common than had been supposed. The best reviews of the condition are those of Edwards (267), Hollender et al. (256), and Jones and Merendino (255).

Incidence.

Estimates from autopsies have varied from 2.7% (268) to 14.5%, the highest reported frequency (260). The incidence reported depends both on the technique used in the search (plaster of Paris injection, water pressure, air pressure, or simple inspection) and (particularly) on the age distribution of the group examined. Grant (269) found only 3.9% among individuals 52 years of age and younger, and 15.8% among older patients. Duodenal diverticula are rare below the age of 40 years.

In radiologic studies the incidence has been variously reported as from 0.016 to 5.19% (255). This difference between radiologic and autopsy incidence reflects the number of asymptomatic diverticula as well as the difficulties encountered in detecting them.

Slightly more females than males are affected, although the difference may not be significant. Moreno and DeLandazuri (270) found that affected patients under 40 years of age were predominantly women, whereas older patients more often were men.

Symptoms.

Only about 75% of duodenal diverticula seen radiographically and only 10 to 15% of those found at autopsy produce symptoms (271). Those that do so, however, simulate a variety of intestinal disorders.

Pain is present in about 50% of patients. It may be epigastric, umbilical, interscapular, at the costovertebral angle, or in the right upper quadrant. Hollender et al. (256) consider that central pain indicates a lesion of the third part of the duodenum, whereas pain to the left of the midline indicates involvement of the second part. The pain varies with posture and may be brought on or worsened by a meal. Constipation, eructation, nausea, and vomiting may all be present. Weight loss is said to be rare, but it occurred in 12 of 39 patients reported by Moreno and DeLandazuri (270). Jaundice may occur if the diverticulum exerts pressure on the bile duct.

The symptoms may be classified according to their cause: (*a*) mechanical obstruction of the duodenum itself or of the pancreatic or common bile duct; (*b*) inflammation; (*c*) diverticulitis; (*d*) ulceration; (*e*) perforation; and (*f*) neoplastic changes.

The obstructive changes cause the greatest diagnostic problems; the inflammatory changes usually are recognized even if the existence of the diverticulum is not suspected.

Associated Pathologic Conditions.

At least 23 perforations, with 12 deaths, have been reported in the literature (272), and six malignancies are known to have been associated (256). Morrison and Feldman (273) have described a case of primary carcinoma in a duodenal diverticulum.

Diagnosis.

Identification of a duodenal diverticulum is largely in the province of the radiologist. In addition to films taken in erect and recumbent positions, radiographs should be taken with the patient lying on the left side, especially if this position is the one that produces discomfort. Other lesions may give a diverticulum-like picture on radiography. The most frequently found are ulcer and traction diverticula and pseudodiverticula.

Ulcer diverticula, which usually occur in the first part of the duodenum, have all coats of the intestinal wall. They result from scar tissue puckering of the duodenum.

Traction diverticula may result from inflammatory adhesions or from contraction of the bile duct following fibrosis of the gall bladder.

Pseudodiverticula may result from central necrosis of large smooth muscle tumors in any part of the intestine (225).

Treatment.

Surgery is advised for symptomatic diverticula if conservative treatment fails. Fewer than 2% of cases in which duodenal diverticula are visualized on roentgenograms should require surgical treatment (274). Zinninger (275) suggests surgery only for large, symptomatic diverticula that retain barium for more than 24 hr.

Excision and closure, with inversion of the neck of the sac, are most frequently employed. Roux-en-Y diverticulojejunostomy and end-to-end duodenojejunostomy have been advocated. A long T-tube and duodenostomy for safe dissection of perivaterian diverticula is advised. The complications of duodenal diverticula have been discussed by Neill and Thompson (276).

Jejunal and Ileal Diverticula.

Anatomy.

Diverticula of the jejunum and ileum are similar in structure and pathogenesis to those of the duodenum. They tend to be multiple. In the Mayo Clinic series (277), 54% of patients had more than two diverticula. As many as 400 in one patient have been reported (278).

History.

Primary false intestinal diverticula were first observed by Sömmering (279) in 1794 and were illustrated by Cooper (280) in 1807. Case (264) found 17 reported between 1854 and 1920. By 1941 Kozinn and Jennings (281) found 220 reports of diverticula in the jejunum alone.

Diverticular disease of the jejunum was reported recently by Ross et al. (282), who presented four cases in adults of the mesenteric side of the intestine with several complications. The diverticular disease was referred to as an "acquired condition."

Incidence.

Diverticula are more frequent in the jejunum than in the ileum. Noer (268) found 10 jejunal, 2 ileal, and 6 duodenal diverticula among 218 autopsies, during which the intestines were examined while inflated with water. This incidence of 8.3% must be contrasted with the 0.19% found by the same author among nearly 30,000 autopsies performed without special procedures. As in the duodenum, the incidence of diverticula in the intestine seems to depend on how carefully the search is made.

Diverticula of the small intestine, like those of the duodenum, rarely are found in children or young adults. Only seven patients under 10 years of age had been reported up to 1943 (227). Jejunal diverticulitis was reported in a 2-year-old girl; this was probably a true congenital diverticulum (281).

The greatest frequency among clinical cases is in patients from 60 to 69 years of age. Thirty-one percent of the cases from the Mayo Clinic from 1909 to 1942 occurred in patients in this age range. Among autopsy cases, Noer (268) found 50% of the diverticula in patients over age 75 years although they constituted only 25% of the autopsies. About twice as many men as women were affected.

Symptoms.

The great majority, perhaps 90%, produce few symptoms and require no treatment (283). When symptoms are present, they are often those of obstruction, volvulus, intussusception, perforation, or hemorrhage. Thorek and Manzanilla (278) found only 15 cases of perforation between 1922 and 1954. This is surprising in view of the nature of the diverticular wall. Considerable elasticity of the submucosa must protect against rupture. Hemorrhage is equally rare, with only 24 reports found in the literature (283). The microcytic anemia accompanying continuous blood loss should be distinguished from the macrocytic anemia of reduced intestinal absorption. It is not surprising that idiopathic intestinal bleeding frequently has been ascribed to undetected intestinal diverticula.

Concomitant Occurrence of Diverticula.

Anatomy.

Among 85 patients with jejunal or ileal diverticula seen by Benson and his colleagues (277), 49 had diverticula elsewhere. There were 30 colonic, 22 duodenal, and 2 esophageal diverticula; bladder diverticula were present in 10. Chitambar (284) found that 31% of patients with duodenal diverticula had diverticula at other sites in the gastrointestinal tract. It is possible that a quantitative study might show that the gut musculature in some individuals has a generalized deficiency, which permits herniation to occur more readily.

Diagnosis.

Radiologically, diverticula of the jejunum or ileum are much harder to visualize than are those of the duodenum. The fixed position of the latter permits the retention of barium for longer periods of time than is the case with the more mobile, distal segments of the intestine.

Treatment.

If diverticulitis is present, with perforation, abscess, bleeding, or intestinal obstruction, the only treatment is surgical. The specific operation depends on the complications. Resection, with end-to-end anastomosis, is usually required.

DORSAL ENTERIC REMNANTS (GIANT DIVERTICULA)

Although often called "reduplications," these structures could more properly be designated "accessory" or "ectopic" intestines. They differ from tubular duplications in that they do not parallel the normal gut, as do true tubular duplications (Fig. 6.35; see Fig. 3.25). They usually arise at right angles to the gut and terminate near the vertebral column some distance cranial to their origin. They are often of great length—hence, their common name—and they may arise from the mesenteric side of any part of the large or small intestine. The giant diverticula sometimes pierce the diaphragm and extend into the thoracic cavity. There is often an attachment, or a trace of one, on the anterior surface of cervical or thoracic vertebrae. At the intestinal end, the lumen is sometimes stenotic or even absent. Technically, these latter are not diverticula, but the distinction is hardly worth making. The greater number of these diverticula arise from the jejunum, ileum, or colon and are confined to the abdomen. Their mucosa is usually of more than one type, with gastric mucosa common. Normark (285) reviewed incidents of these diverticula in the small intestines prior to 1938, and Wright (286) described in detail a giant diverticulum of colonic origin. Brown (287) has demonstrated vertebral defects associated with an intraabdominal diverticulum.

These dorsal enteric remnants, whether long or short, are of similar origin. The basic defect is a failure of the endoderm of the gut to separate from the overlying neural tube or notochord. This failure is discussed in detail later in this chapter.

DORSAL ENTERIC REMNANTS (CYSTIC AND TUBULAR DUPLICATIONS)

Intestinal duplications may be classified in several ways. They may be cystic or tubular, closed, or communicating with the normal gut; they may be adjacent to the gut or completely separated from it. A formal classification of all of the possible varieties is unnecessary. For practical purposes, these structures may be divided into (a) cystic duplications, which are usually closed, and (b) tubular duplications, which usually communicate with the normal gut.

Anatomy.

Cystic Duplications.

Enteric cysts (enterocystomas) occur throughout the length of the digestive tract (Fig. 6.35). Over 66% are associated with the intestines and over 50% with the small intestine. Of all of the abdominal cystic duplications, 75% have a mucosa resembling that of the adjoining gut. They tend to occur singly although many patients with thoracic cysts have abdominal duplication as well. Egelhoff and associates (288) reported the case of an infant with esophageal, gastric, and duodenal duplications.

The distribution of cystic duplication along the digestive tube is not uniform, yet no specific pattern is suggested. The ileum is the most often affected, followed by the esophagus and duodenum. The colon is less frequently involved, and there is a gradient of decreasing frequency from cecum to rectum. However, the fewest cystic duplications are found associated with the stomach and jejunum. Dohn and Povlsen (289) reviewed the literature up to 1950 and Anderson et al. (290) from 1950 to 1959. Inouye et al. (291) reviewed duplications of the duodenum through 1962.

Duodenum.

The students of duodenal duplications, such as Inouye et al. (289) and Leenders et al. (292), agree that duodenal duplications develop at the second portion of the duodenum posterior wall.

There is confusion in the literature surrounding duodenum duplications. Are they duodenal arising from the duodenal wall? Are they pancreatic since they are practically fixed with the pancreas? Does the common bile duct participate in these duplications? Black et al. (293) presented an interesting case of recurrent pancreatitis attributable to an intestinal duplication. According to Dickinson et al. (294), 15% of duodenal duplications contain gastric mucosa. Characteristically, these duplications project into the duodenum.

Symptoms and Complications. Duodenal duplications may be totally asymptomatic or may produce bleeding, duodenal obstruction, or obstruction at the ampulla of Vater.

Treatment. The ideal advice of total extirpation is not good because of the close relation to the vaterian system.

In 1990 Raffensperger (92) advised intraoperative cholangiography to determine the topography of the cyst to the vaterian system. Raffensperger compromises with partial removal and mucosal excision.

Duplications of Ileum and Jejunum.

These may be cystic or tubular, large or small, communicating or noncommunicating with the enteric lumen, and asymptomatic or symptomatic. Rarely they have a separate mesentery. If this is the case, complete extirpation may be done as in the case of Norris et al. (295). Raffensperger (92) says that good surgical judgment and management with ingenuity in the operating room is the answer.

Intramural Cystic Duplications.

These are found in the submucosa or the muscularis of the gut and are usually small and often asymptomatic. They rarely communicate with the normal lumen, but occasionally they will do so. Wiot and Spiro (296) found in the literature 10 cases in infants and 4 cases in children. They added a case of their own of a 69-year-old woman whose first symptoms occurred at age 45 years. Presumably, many such intramural duplications remain asymptomatic and elude discovery even at autopsy. Moore and Battersby (297) described two patients in whom there were numbers of small cysts lined with cuboidal epithelium and surrounded by smooth muscle, as well as isolated epithelial cells in the submucosa of the ileum. Their appearance was suggestive of undifferentiated pancreatic tissue. Occasionally, larger cysts are found which, being beneath the muscular coat, tend to bulge toward the lumen and produce obstruction (298).

Mesenteric Cystic Duplications.

The great majority of cystic duplications of the intestines lie in the mesentery but are more or less intimately attached to the gut. There is usually a common muscular wall—often of the circular coat only—between the duplication and the normal gut. There may be little external indication of a division. These cystic duplications should not be confused with mesenteric cysts or chylous cysts of lymphoid origin. The latter may have a few smooth muscle fibers in their walls, but they have no true muscular coats and do not have alimentary tract mucosa.

The mucosa of enteric cysts is usually that of the adjoining intestine. However, in 6 of 27 such structures described by Gross (40), there was gastric mucosa as well. In one ileal duplication, ileal, gastric, and colonic mucosa were present.

These cysts range from 0.8 to 8 cm in their greatest dimension; a few larger ones have been reported (299).

Our separation of this group from the tubular type to be considered in the next section is strictly arbitrary. However, the difference may actually be real, since intermediate forms are not common. An adequate collective review of these structures is needed.

Tubular Duplications. Two unrelated types of tubular duplications occur. In one type, the duplication lies in the sagittal plane, the duplicated portion being dorsal to the normal gut. In the second type, the duplication is lateral, producing a paired structure in place of a normally single midline tube. This second type is rare and of different embryonic origin. It is discussed separately in Chapter 7, The Colon and Rectum. Only the sagittal duplications are considered here.

Tubular duplications are only about half as frequent as are cystic duplications. Unlike the latter, they usually communicate with the lumen of the normal gut at their caudal ends or, occasionally, at both ends. Strictly speaking, a communicating duplication is a diverticulum, but we feel that the use of this term obscures rather than clarifies the nature of these structures.

On both embryonic and anatomic grounds we would limit "tubular duplications" to those structures that lie adjacent and parallel to the normal gut. Similar enteric structures that diverge from the gut and course through the mesentery in a general craniodorsal direction are giant diverticula, the dorsal enteric remnants of Smith (300), discussed previously.

Tubular duplications of the intestine almost exclusively are associated with the jejunum, ileum, or colon. Almost all lie on the mesenteric side of the normal intestine. In a few cases the duplication has become the main channel of the intestine and the redundant portion is antimesenteric. Unless obstruction has produced distension, the duplication and the normal intestine are of the same diameter. The mucosa may or may not be identical to that of the adjacent intestine. Long duplications usually have gastric mucosa in some part of their length (297, 301). A short, partly intramural diverticulum of the transverse colon, having colonic, appendiceal, intestinal, gastric, and pancreatic tissue, has been reported (302). This seems to be the widest variety of mucosal types encountered in a duplication.

In one remarkable case a section of lower jejunum had a longitudinal strip of gastric mucosa 2 to 3 cm broad. Two portions of this mucosa lay within open-ended submucosal duplications, each with several openings in the dividing wall. Intestinal plicae did not cross the strip, which had its own lower and broader folds (303).

Tubular duplications usually are connected intimately with the normal ileum; the common muscularis forms the dividing partition, but all degrees of fusion may be found. The cranial end of the duplication is usually more completely separated than is the caudal end. A duplication extending from the ligament of Treitz to the ileocecal junction, reported by Wrenn (304), displayed all degrees of separation along its length. Carcinoma in a tubular duplication has been reported (305).

Long colonic duplications may have other malformations at the anus. Duplication of the rectum with both tubes ending blindly, septate anus, and rectourethral fistula from the anterior of the two tubes have been described (40, 252).

These duplications, which may originate from the ileum, usually communicate proximally and have a common external musculature. They are midline duplications with anterior and posterior channels. If an accessory anal opening occurs, it lies in the midline in front or behind the normal opening. There is no duplication of urinary or genital structures, as is usual in the paired (side-by-side) colonic duplications discussed in Chapter 7, The Colon and Rectum.

Embryogenesis. The frequency with which duplications occur has induced much speculation and produced many explanations. The review of the most reasonable theories is provided by Jelenko (306).

There is no single explanation for all forms and locations of duplications. Some are readily accounted for, whereas others remain obscure or even inexplicable. The most acceptable hypotheses are as follows:

1. Failure of normal regression of embryonic diverticula
2. Persistence of transitory intestinal diverticula
3. Median septum formation
4. Errors of recanalization of transitory epithelial plugs
5. Traction between adhering neural tube ectoderm or notochordal mesoderm and gut endoderm

Failure of Normal Regression of Embryonic Structures.
Two groups of enteric cysts are remnants of embryonic structures. First, enteric cysts that are attached to the antimesenteric side of the ileum or to the anterior body wall are remnants of the vitelline duct. These have been discussed previously. A few may be tubular rather than cystic. Second, presacral enteric cysts, which are persistent remnants of the postanal tailgut, are discussed in Chapter 7, The Colon and Rectum.

Persistence of Transitory Diverticula.
Diverticula of the digestive tract of human embryos in the sixth to eighth weeks, observed first in 1907 by Lewis and Thyng (20), have been reported since then in both human and animal embryos (21, 306, 307) and do not seem to be rare. They are usually transient in the embryo. They may occasionally remain as small cysts or diverticula in the intestinal wall or between the leaves of the mesentery. If they contain gastric mucosa, they eventually perforate (307).

Median Septum Formation.
The suggestion that flattening of the gut with subsequent adherence of opposite walls could result in doubling of the lumen was put forward by Bremer (17). This is a possible mechanism for the formation of tubular duplications, but there is no evidence that it actually occurs.

Errors of Recanalization of Epithelial Plugs.
Portions of the intestinal tract, chiefly the duodenum, undergo epithelial proliferation, which may completely occlude the lumen for a short time between the fifth and eighth weeks. Recanalization takes place through formation of vacuoles, which coalesce to form the definitive lumen. Small submucosal duplications probably result from the formation of double channels during this process.

Traction Between Gut Endoderm and Overlying Structures.
In 1952 Veeneklaas (308) called attention to the association of vertebral defects with enteric duplications. Soon afterward, Fallon et al. (309) proposed an attractive hypothesis to explain diverticula and duplications of the digestive tract. This view holds that, prior to notochord formation, the endodermal roof of the archenteron is in contact with the ectodermal neural plate. With the forward growth of the notochord during the 18th to 21st days (stages 8 to 9), the roof of the archenteron separates from the neural plate but becomes attached to the notochord. About the 24th day (2.5 to 3 mm, stage 11), the

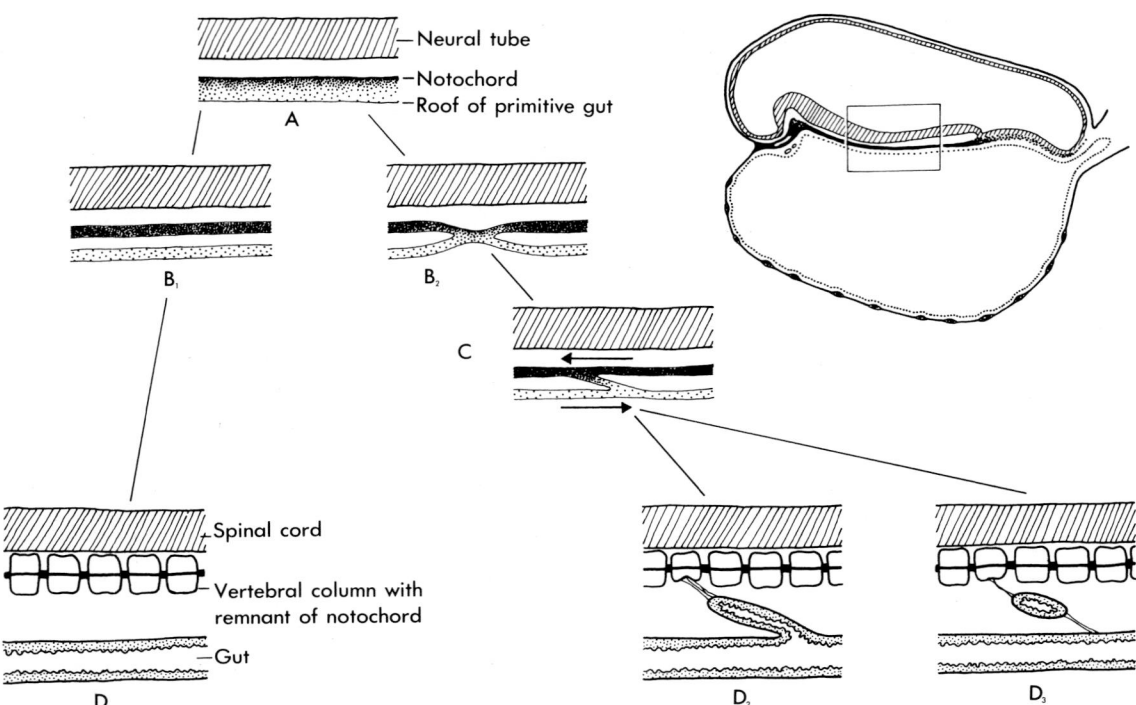

Figure 6.48. Suggested mechanism of formation of dorsal enteric duplications and diverticula. Up until the early fourth week, the notochord and the endoderm of the roof of the primitive gut are not separated (**A**). During the fourth week, the notochord separates from the gut wall (**B₁**), and normal gut and vertebral column result (**D₁**). If during stage B a portion of notochord and gut wall fail to sep-

arate (**B₂**), differences in growth between the two organs will pull a cord of endoderm cells from the gut roof (**C**). The final result will be a duplication of the gut, either a diverticulum (**D₂**) or a cyst (**D₃**). Some vertebral deformation is often present at the dorsal end of the attachment.

separation of mesodermal and endodermal elements takes place ("excalation"). During this period, anterior growth of the ectodermal and mesodermal portion of the embryo exceeds that of the endodermal portion, resulting in a shearing movement between the archenteron roof and the notochord and neural tube. If separation of archenteron and notochordal tissues is not complete, a cord of endoderm cells is pulled from the roof of the developing gut like a thread of viscous fluid. Depending on the extent of the attachment and on the amount of tissue involved, the thread may remain continuous, or it may separate as it becomes attenuated by the traction (Fig. 6.48).

Should the connection be near the midgut and the band of endoderm cells remain unbroken, it reorganizes itself into a tubular structure similar to a typical gut. The epithelium will induce from the mesenchyme the development of the appropriate connective tissue and muscular coats, to form a giant diverticulum arising from the abdominal gut, piercing the diaphragm, and reaching into the thorax to a dorsal attachment on the cervical or thoracic spine.

Should attenuation break the connection near the midpoint of the band, an endodermal remnant will remain at the notochordal end to form a mediastinal thoracic "esophageal duplication," while at the intestinal

end, another remnant persists as a dorsal diverticulum or duplication, either attached or separated from the gut.

If the connection breaks at the notochordal end, the cells will form a longer or shorter duplication attached to the intestine. If it parts at both ends, an isolated duplication in the mesentery or in the mediastinum will result.

The attachment to the notochord may interfere with the normal closing of one or more vertebral bodies, so that the site is marked by an anterior spina bifida. Beardmore and Wiglesworth (310) have considered as an entity the triad of posterior mediastinal cyst, duplication, and vertebral anomalies.

Huge duplications may result, or only a few cells may remain dissociated by the separation. Retroperitoneal enteric cysts, some mesenteric enteric cysts, and some small diverticula with complete muscle coats may be the only results.

McLetchie et al. (311) suggested that adhesion between endoderm and ectoderm before the appearance of the notochord may have similar results. The advancing notochord must pass to one side or split to pass around such an adhesion (312). As with notochordal adhesion, there will be a vertebral defect. Direct connection of a posterior enteric remnant with the neural tube has been reported (313, 314).

The most striking case of a split notochord, split spinal

cord, and anterior and posterior spina bifida with herniation of most of the gut through the defect was described by Denes et al. (314). In this case, that of an infant born alive, the split axis extended from T12 to the sacrum. The dorsal sac, into which the gut herniated, appears to have been a postvertebral dorsal enteric remnant that contained a small accessory liver. The authors were able to find only 12 cases of postvertebral cysts or protrusions of the gut through split vertebrae in the literature. None were so extensive as that of their patient.

In summarizing the ways in which duplications can form, we may conclude the following:

1. Small, cystic, intramural duplications arise from persistent embryonic diverticula or from errors of recanalization.
2. Tubular duplications lying close to the main gut and sharing a common muscular coat possibly result from the formation of a septum dividing the gut into two parallel tubes.
3. Both cystic and tubular duplications with independent muscular coats and giant diverticula are dorsal enteric remnants of an early adhesion between the gut and more dorsal structures.
4. Antimesenteric cystic duplications of the midgut are vitelline duct remnants.
5. Presacral enteric cysts are remnants of the embryonic tailgut.

History. A long, posterior enteric remnant was seen by Calder (316) in 1733. No other case appears to have been reported until 1876, when a diverticulum of the ascending colon was reported by Grawitz (317). A 13-inch diverticulum from the duodenum was described in 1879 by Fairland (318). All of these appear to have been posterior enteric remnants communicating with the intestine. The terminology during the period was confused because most writers were convinced that these structures were vitelline duct remnants.

The first cystic duplication was described by Fraenkel (319) in 1882, and 2 years later Fitz (320) originated the term *duplication* for these cysts. Sprengel (321) performed the first resection in 1900. By 1935 Hudson (322) was able to find 92 cases of duplications of the alimentary tract below the diaphragm. His report provides an excellent bibliography of the early literature.

Incidence. By 1951 Dohn and Povlsen (289) were able to collect 315 cases of cystic duplication from the literature. Of these 20 were of Meckelian origin, 62 were esophageal, 22 were duodenal, 157 were jejunal or ileal, and 36 were colonic. The remainder could not be definitely located. No collection of tubular duplications seems to have been attempted.

Duplications are not always recognized in infancy. Anderson et al. (290) collected reports of duplications in adults from the period 1950 to 1959 and found 17 cystic and 14 tubular duplications arising from stomach and

intestines. Thompson and Labow (323) estimated that 33% of patients with duodenal duplications were 20 years of age or older.

Whereas Hudson (322) in 1935 found both sexes to be equally affected, later series (290, 324, 325) indicated that twice as many males as females are affected. Only duodenal duplications are more common in females (298, 306).

Symptoms. Obstruction, pain, and bleeding are the chief symptoms associated with intestinal duplications although many are asymptomatic and found only at autopsy. A palpable mass may be present.

About 85% of cystic duplications are symptomatic, and about 66% manifest themselves in infancy and childhood. Fifteen to twenty percent produce intussusception. Among intussusceptions in infants and children in our experience, two out of 159 were caused by duplications. Both were jejunal.

Duodenum.
Partial obstruction with a palpable mass, vomiting, pain, and dehydration are the usual signs of a symptomatic duodenal duplication. Obstructive jaundice has been observed in several cases, and perforation of a duplication containing gastric mucosa has occurred (325).

Jejunum and Ileum.
When duplications occur in the small intestine below the duodenum, infants and children experience pain and vomiting. Among 12 adult cases, 6 reported pain, and 3 a palpable mass. Obstruction, vomiting, and melena each were present in 1, and in 3 cases the duplication was an incidental finding.

Bleeding usually indicates a long communicating duplication, with gastric mucosa causing ulceration of intestinal mucosa distal to it.

Colon.
Constipation may be the only symptom although acute obstruction has been reported (324). Fecal material in the urine may indicate a urethral fistula with a long tubular diverticulum communicating proximally with the normal colon (40) (see Fig. 7-7, *A*).

Associated Anomalies. Duplications of the intestine in infants are often associated with other congenital defects. Vertebral defects commonly accompany esophageal duplications and giant diverticula arising in the abdomen. They are less often associated with intestinal diverticula. In one series 14 of 29 patients with intestinal duplications had other defects. Three had anal defects, one had esophageal atresia, and one had jejunal atresia; the remainder had defects of other organ systems.

Diagnosis. The diagnosis of intestinal obstruction by an extrinsic mass is probably the best that can be done when a noncommunicating cystic duplication is present. Correct preoperative diagnosis is rare (291). When a tubular duplication communicates with the normal intestine, the duplication may be visualized with barium-enhanced radiography. Most duplications, however, are identified only at operation.

Treatment. In principle, cystic and tubular duplications should be removed. Unfortunately, they occur on the mesenteric side of the intestine, and their excision nearly always requires resection of an equal amount of the normal gut (Fig. 6.49, *A* and *B*). In some cases this is not practicable.

Duodenal Duplications.
A generous communication between the cyst and the duodenum should be established by cystoduodenostomy.

Small Intestinal Duplications.
The treatment of choice is resection of the cysts and the adjacent normal intestine, with end-to-end anastomosis (Fig. 6.50, *A*).

If resection is contraindicated, the duplication should be opened, the contents aspirated, and the mucosa carefully stripped from the wall. It is essential that all of the mucosa be destroyed to prevent recurrence.

Resection of tubular duplications may require an intolerable loss of intestine. Such duplications often communicate with the intestine at the distal end. A proximal communication can be formed, creating a double-barreled intestine (Fig. 6.50, *B*). If ulceration indicates the presence of gastric mucosa in the proximal portion of a long duplication, this area may be resected, together with

the necessary amount of normal intestine (Fig. 6.50, *C*). The remainder of the duplication may be preserved by anastomosis at both ends.

Colonic Duplications.
The cystic duplication and adjacent normal colon should be resected and the ends of the colon rejoined. Tubular duplications may be anastomosed to the normal colon at both ends. If the duplication is short and has a common wall with the normal colon, the common wall may be divided (Fig. 6.50, *D*).

Mortality. Although the first intestinal resection for a duplication was made in 1900, the surgical mortality was still 79% by 1934 (326). Dohn and Povlsen (289), in their review of 315 cystic duplications, concluded that only 25% were fatal if left untreated. A larger number of tubular duplications would probably be fatal because their gastric mucosa eventually produces ulceration.

Among 45 intestinal duplications treated by Gross (40), three died without operation and eight failed to survive surgery. Among the 38 adults reviewed by Anderson et al. (290), two, both with thoracoabdominal duplications, died.

CYSTIC REMNANTS OF THE TAILGUT

For a discussion of these defects, see Chapter 7, The Colon and Rectum.

BILATERAL DUPLICATIONS OF THE COLON

These duplications are discussed in Chapter 7, The Colon and Rectum.

Congenital Aganglionosis of Duodenum, Jejunum, and Ileum

Congenital absence of myenteric ganglion cells of the duodenum is rarely a cause of enlarged duodenum (327), and proof of aganglionosis only rarely has been obtained (328).

Mechanical obstruction, duodenal ileus, degenerative changes in the myenteric plexus, or presence of the parasite *Trypanosoma cruzi* (agent of Chagas' disease) may all produce megaduodenum. In addition to these, a hereditary form of megaduodenum often associated with megacystis has been described (329, 330). Apparently, normal duodenal ganglion cells may be present (331).

Small atonic segments of duodenum are probably asymptomatic since their contents are liquid; but, in some patients, resection of the affected segment is necessary. Gastrojejunostomy alone may fail to drain the enlarged duodenum, and a partial gastric resection, partial duodenal resection, and gastrojejunostomy may be necessary (331).

According to Grosfeld and Rescorla (332), extension of the aganglionic process to the middle or proximal small

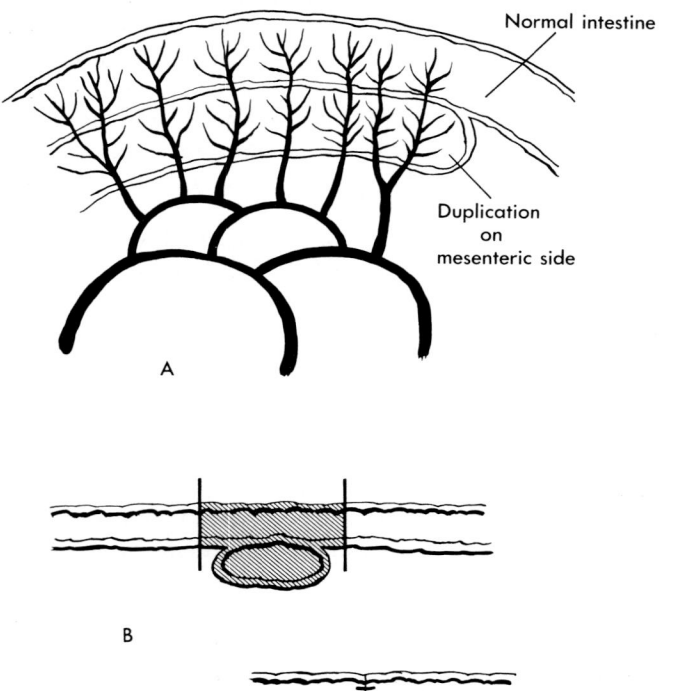

Figure 6.49. **A**, Relationship of blood vessels supplying the intestine and its duplication, which requires resection of both. **B**, Resection of a cystic duplication and a comparable portion of normal intestine, with anastomosis of the ends.

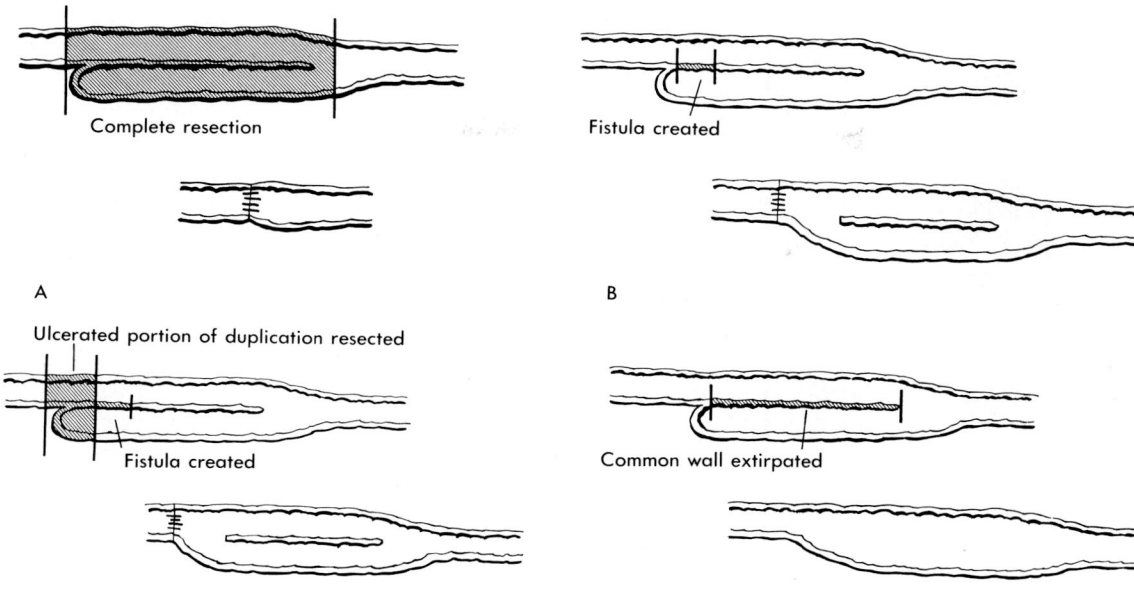

A — Complete resection

B — Fistula created

C — Ulcerated portion of duplication resected / Fistula created

D — Common wall extirpated

Figure 6.50. Repair of tubular duplications of the intestine. **A**, Resection of the duplication and normal gut. **B**, Creation of a proximal opening between the duplication and the normal gut, without loss of intestine. **C**, Combination of procedures **A** and **B**, when ulceration from gastric mucosa in the duplication has occurred. **D**, Extirpation of the septum between the duplication and the normal gut, when a common wall is present. Procedure **A** is suitable for cystic and short tubular diverticula; procedures **B** and **D** may be necessary when long duplications would otherwise require sacrifice of several feet of normal intestine.

bowel, producing a rare, short bowel syndrome, is present in about 20% of infants with total colonic aganglionosis. The same authors treated seven infants with initial simple enterostomy in the intestine with biopsy-proved ganglion cells. Later on, three of the babies underwent pull-through procedures with an antimesenteric aganglionic patch enteroplasty to improve intestinal absorption.

Congenital Absence of Intestinal Musculature

A newborn infant with extensive absence of the muscularis externa of the intestine has been reported (333). Five segments of intestine, from 2 to 50 cm in length, were affected. All other coats of the intestinal wall were normal. The infant did not survive. In a similar case involving only the duodenum, gastrojejunostomy was successful. Ganglion cells were present, but obstruction was the presenting symptom (334). A similar case was presented by Steiner et al. (335) with absence of muscle layers in multiple small segments with normal bowel within.

Megacystis-Microcolon-Intestinal Hypoperistalsis Syndrome

In 1976 Berdon et al. (336) reported five infants with what is now termed the "megacystic-microcolon-intestinal hypoperistalsis syndrome." This syndrome almost always occurs in females and is characterized by intestinal malrotation, reduced small bowel length, a microcolon, a morbidly dilated bladder, and no anatomic obstruction of the intestinal or urinary tract. An imbalance between several kinds of gut peptides and/or decreased autonomic inhibiting input to the smooth muscle cells or the intestine may be the cause of hypoperistalsis (337, 338). Ganglion cells are present and normal. At least 36 additional cases with this syndrome have been reported; all but 5 of the reported 41 patients have died (237, 339–365).

Preduodenal Portal Vein

ANATOMY

The hepatic portal vein normally lies posterior to the first part of the duodenum, but in some instances it is known to lie anterior to the duodenum. In this position it may sometimes compress the duodenum to the point of obstruction (Fig. 6.51).

EMBRYOGENESIS

The development of the portal vein belongs to the history of the vitelline veins, the primitive paired vessels that arise on the surface of the yolk sac and pass up the body stalk to enter the primordium of the heart. They appear, reach their greatest development, and begin to decline during the fourth week. By the end of this week there are three cross-connections between them. The cranial crossing lies within the liver, anterior (ventral) to the foregut. Out-

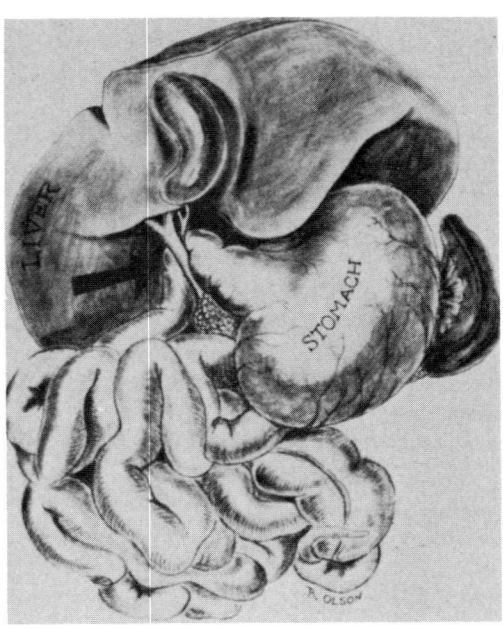

Figure 6.51. Preduodenal portal vein. In this patient, the vein has angulated and compressed the duodenum. Malrotation is also present. (From Boles, ET, Jr, Smith B. Preduodenal portal vein. Pediatrics 1961;28:805–809.)

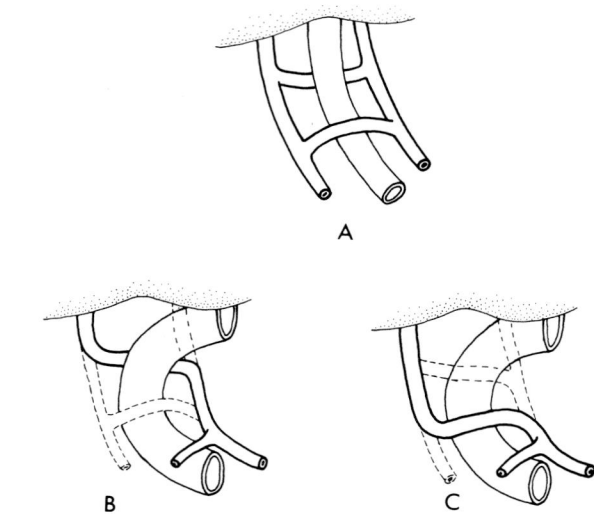

Figure 6.52. Origin of the preduodenal portal vein. **A**, The two extrahepatic communications between the vitelline veins, which are present early in the sixth week. **B**, Normal development. The cranial, postduodenal communicating vein is incorporated into the portal vein. **C**, Anomalous development. The caudal, preduodenal communicating vein becomes the portal vein.

side the liver, the middle anastomosis passes posterior (dorsal) to the gut, and the caudal anastomosis passes anterior (ventral) to it. Of these vessels the caudal left vitelline vein, the middle (dorsal) anastomosis, and the cranial right vitelline vein persist to form the portal vein. The other pathways atrophy (Fig. 6.52).

A preduodenal portal vein arises from the persistence of the caudal (ventral) anastomosis instead of the middle (dorsal) one.

ASSOCIATED ANOMALIES

The portal vein anomaly seems to be secondary to a variety of serious malformations. Malrotation, complete or partial situs inversus viscerum, annular pancreas, duodenal atresia, cardiac anomalies, and biliary anomalies are among those usually encountered (366).

HISTORY AND INCIDENCE

Block and Zikria (367) were able to find only nine reports of preduodenal portal vein in the literature up to 1961. They added one case, and Boles and Smith (366) added four more in 1961. The earliest case we have seen is that reported by Knight (368) in 1921, who found an apparently asymptomatic preduodenal portal vein in the cadaver of a 60-year-old male who had no other anomalies.

SYMPTOMS AND DIAGNOSIS

Block and Zikria found compression of the duodenum by the anomalous vein produced obstruction in three of

fourteen patients. In two others, intrinsic duodenal obstruction was present (366). One patient was 10 years old; the others were infants. Preoperative diagnosis was merely "duodenal obstruction."

A preduodenal portal vein that does not produce obstruction may be a hazard during surgery on the duodenum or the biliary tract. Ligation without identification, or inadvertent transection, would be serious if not fatal.

TREATMENT

If other anomalies are not too severe, the obstruction of the duodenum by the portal vein can be bypassed by a duodenostomy or a gastroenterostomy. The former operation was successfully performed in a 10-year-old child by Block and Zikria (367).

Superior Mesenteric Artery Syndrome

ANATOMY

This condition—which also has been called duodenal stasis, duodenal compression, arteriomesenteric occlusion, mesenteric root obstruction, duodenal ileus, and Wilkie's disease—is the result of compression of the duodenum by the superior mesenteric artery. The third, or transverse, portion of the duodenum is compressed by this vessel against the aorta and the vertebral column at the level of the second or third lumbar vertebra. The resulting obstruction may be chronic or acute, intermittent, partial, or complete (Fig. 6.53).

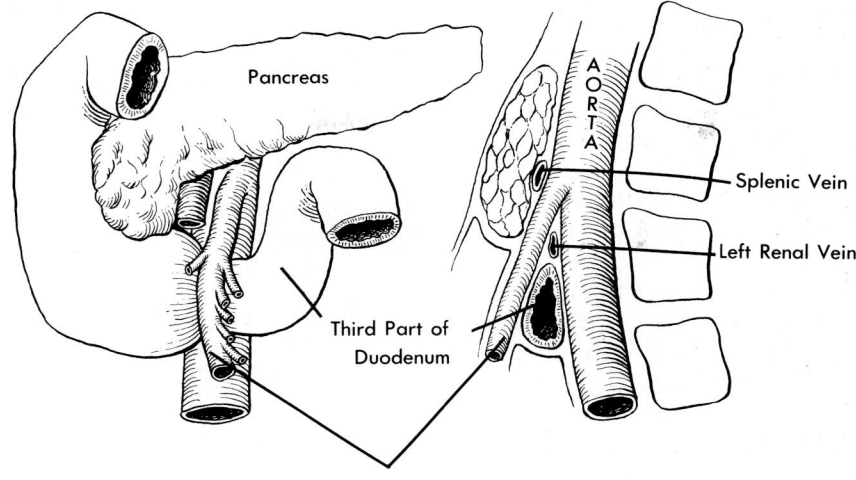

Figure 6.53. Relationship between the superior mesenteric artery and the duodenum. Compression of the duodenum between the artery and the aorta may produce the obstruction characteristic of the superior mesenteric artery syndrome.

PATHOGENESIS

While the mechanics of the obstruction are clear, the contributing events are not. A number of congenital factors that predispose the patient to duodenal compression by the artery have been suggested.

1. Congenitally short mesentery of the intestine
2. Aberrant superior mesenteric artery or anomalous branches
3. Excessive mobility of the right colon
4. Malrotation of the intestines
5. Abnormally high fixation of the suspensory muscle of the duodenum

The last two are easily recognized, but they are not present in many cases of the syndrome. The first three are difficult to evaluate anatomically and impossible to prove embryologically.

In addition to these, acquired factors such as obesity, excessive weight loss, changes in spinal curvature, the presence of a body cast (369) ("cast syndrome"), or anything that might unfavorably alter the angle of mesenteric traction can contribute to the effect.

In very few cases can a specific anomaly be demonstrated. All degrees of duodenal compression may be found, and clinical obstruction may only appear when other factors, minor in themselves, are added.

Haley et al. (370, 371) studied the suspensory muscle or ligament of Treitz and described its variations. In 11% of cadavers, no definite structure could be found. In the remainder, the suspensory fibers attached to the duodenojejunal flexure only in about 5%, to the flexure and the third and fourth parts of the duodenum in 61%, and to the third and fourth parts in 16%. The shortest attachments were those to the flexure only. These investigators did not relate their findings to the position of the duodenum in the arterial angle, but the variations suggest that some congenital arrangements may predispose patients to obstruction more than do others. In about 70% of cadavers, muscle fibers were present in the duodenal suspension. Hypertonicity of these fibers in life may hold the duodenum more snugly in the arterial angle.

HISTORY

The first description appears to be that of Boener (372) in 1754, but Rokitansky (373) in 1861 was the first to suggest the etiology. Stavely (374) has been credited with performing the first successful duodenojejunostomy for the condition in 1908. In 1921 Wilkie (375) made the most thorough study published up to that time—hence, the eponym "Wilkie's syndrome." Pool et al. (376) collected 300 cases in 1933. Between 1920 and 1930 the condition was considered common, and there is reason to believe that its frequency resulted as much from the zeal of the radiologist as from the shortness of the artery. Since then, some writers have entertained doubt about the existence of the syndrome (327, 377). Lontok and Taber (378) and Kaiser et al. (379) discussed the syndrome in adults; Rabinovitch et al. (380) reviewed the cases in infants and children, and Barner and Sherman (381) analyzed 281 selected cases from the literature.

INCIDENCE

Commonly encountered in adults, superior mesenteric artery syndrome has occasionally been reported in children and even in infants. Because of the difficulty of diagnosis and the loose terminology, it is impossible to estimate the frequency of its occurrence. Three times as many women as men are affected, usually in the fourth decade of life. The victims are frequently of asthenic habitus; attacks often follow emotional strain or fatigue. The syndrome tends to appear in patients confined to bed in the supine position for a long time.

SYMPTOMS

Symptoms may be long standing and relatively mild, or they may appear suddenly, with no previous history of gastrointestinal discomfort.

In the chronic form, pain is the usual complaint; nausea and vomiting and a feeling of fullness are not uncommon. The pain localizes slightly above and to the left of the umbilicus. Firm hand pressure tends to relieve the pain, as does changing to the prone position. Walking and standing increase discomfort. Attacks may be episodic, from 4 to 5 weeks apart. There is usually a long history of gradually worsening "stomach trouble."

In the acute form, all of the symptoms of upper intestinal obstruction appear, often with tremendous distension of the stomach and duodenum.

DIAGNOSIS

Gaseous distension of the stomach and duodenum, seen on plain radiographs, may provide the diagnosis. When visualized with barium-enhanced radiographs in the erect position, the stomach and duodenum are large, and the obstruction appears as a straight line across the duodenum. A to-and-fro churning of the barium before it passes the point of partial obstruction may be observed. Placing the patient in the prone position often helps the barium to pass the obstruction. There may be a delay in stomach emptying time of 5 to 7 hr.

Distinguishing this disease from pancreatitis, hiatal hernia, peptic ulcer, and gallbladder disease in adults and from peritoneal bands or adhesions, annular pancreas, duodenal stenosis, intestinal duplication, volvulus, and malrotation in children often is difficult.

TREATMENT

Correction of malnutrition, posture therapy, and antispasmodic agents should be tried before intervening surgically in adults. When the disease appears in infants, conservative measures are usually ineffective.

Duodenojejunostomy is the effective surgical procedure. Wilkie (375) performed the operation on 64 of his patients. Most of the infants and children were immediately or eventually operated on. The high incidence of surgical cures is perhaps more apparent than real; there are probably many spontaneous cures. In the absence of surgery, the disease can rarely be absolutely established.

Another approach has been to sever the muscle of Treitz to displace the duodenum downward and away from the apex of the angle between the superior mesenteric artery and aorta (382).

Heterotopic Mucosa of the Intestine

Gastric and pancreatic mucosa are occasionally present in the normal intestine, as well as in intestinal duplications. Gastric mucosa is common in Meckel's diverticulum but rare elsewhere in the intestine. Accessory pancreatic tissue is relatively frequent in the stomach and duodenum. See Chapter 5, The Stomach, for a discussion of heterotopic gastric mucosa and Chapter 11, The Pancreas, for pancreatic heterotopia.

REFERENCES

1. Scammon RE, Kittelson JA. The growth of the gastrointestinal tract of the human fetus. Proc Soc Exp Biol Med 1926;24:303–307.
2. Keibel F, Mall FP, eds. Manual of human embryology. Philadelphia: JB Lippincott, 1910.
3. Meckel JF. Bildungsgeschichte des darmkanals der saughthiere und namentlich des menschen. Deutsch Arch Phys 1817;3:1–84.
4. Mall FP. Ueber die entwickelung des menschlichen darms und seiner lage beim erwachsenen. Arch Anat Entw [Suppl] 1897:403–434.
5. Mall FP. Supplementary note on the development of the human intestine. Anat Anz 1899;16:492–495.
6. Estrada RL. Anomalies of intestinal rotation and fixation. Springfield, IL: Charles C Thomas, 1958.
7. Treitz W. Hernia retroperitonealis. Prague, 1857.
8. Toldt C. Bau und wachsthumsveranderungen des gekrose des menschlichen darmkanales. Denkschr Math Naturw Cl Akad Wissensch Wien, 1897;41.
9. Lewis FT. The development of the digestive tract and of the organs of respiration: the development of the small intestine. In: Keibel F, Mall FP, eds. Manual of human embryology. Philadelphia: JB Lippincott, 1910.
10. Johnson FP. The development of the mucous membrane of the oesophagus, stomach, and small intestine in the human embryo. Am J Anat 1910;10:521–561.
11. Lineback PE. Studies on the longitudinal muscle of the human colon, with special reference to the development of the taeniae. Contrib Embryol Carnegie Inst Wash 1920;11:33–44.
12. Kanagasuntheram R. Some observations on the development of the human duodenum. J Anat 1960;94:231–240.
13. Daikoku S, Ikeuchi C, Miki S. Electron microscopic studies on developing intramural ganglia of the small intestine in human and rabbit fetuses. Acta Anat (Basel) 1975;91:429–454.
14. Orlic D, Lev R. An electron microscopic study of intraepithelial lymphocytes in human fetal small intestine. Lab Invest 1977;37:554–561.
15. Moxey PC, Trier JS. Specialized cell types in the human fetal small intestine. Anat Rec 1978;191:269–286.
16. Moutsouris C. The "solid stage" and congenital intestinal atresia. J Pediatr Surg 1966;1:446–450.
17. Bremer JL. Diverticula and duplications of the intestinal tract. Arch Pathol 1944;38:133–140.
18. Bremer JL. Congenital anomalies of viscera. Cambridge, MA: Harvard University Press, 1957.
19. Lynn HB, Espinas EE. Intestinal atresia: an attempt to relate location to embryologic processes. Arch Surg 1959;79:357–361.
20. Lewis FT, Thyng FW. The regular occurrence of intestinal diverticula in embryos if the pig, rabbit and man. Am J Anat 1907;7:505–519.
21. Guthrie RF, Wakefield EG. Mesenteric cysts. Proc Mayo Clin 1943;18:52–58.

22. Carter RA. Multiple congenital diverticula of the jejunum. Br J Surg 1959;46:586–588.

23. Lacroix B, Kedinger M, Simon-Assmann P, Haffen K. Early organogenesis of human small intestine: scanning electron microscopy and brush border enzymology. Gut 1984;25:925–930.

24. Touloukian RJ, Hastings KW. Intrauterine villus hypertrophy with jejunoileal atresia. J Pediatr Surg 1973;8:799.

25. Nagakawa T. Histogenetic and cytological studies on the duodenal mucous membrane in human foetuses. Arch Histol 1959;16:495–522.

26. Menard D. Growth-promoting factors and the development of the human gut. In: Lebenthal E, ed. Human gastrointestinal development. New York: Raven Press, 1989:129.

27. Andrew A. A study of the developmental relationship between enterochromaffin cells and neural crest. J Embryol Exp Morphol 1963;11:307–324.

28. Singh I. The prenatal development of enterochromaffin cells in the human gastro-intestinal tract. J Anat 1963;97:377–387.

29. Cole JW, McKalen A. Argentaffin cells in the intestinal epithelium of human embryos. Nature 1962;193:198.

30. Seidman EG, Walker WA. Part I: development of the small intestine. In: Anderson CM, Burke V, Gracey M, ed. Paediatric gastroenterology, 2nd ed. Melbourne, Australia: Blackwell Scientific Publications, 1987:118–136.

31. Bryant MG, Buchan AMJ, Gregor M, Ghatel MA, Polak JM, Bloom SR. Development of intestinal regulatory peptides in the human fetus. Gastroenterology 1982;82:47–54.

32. Yntema CL, Hammond WS. Depletions and abnormalities in the cervical sympathetic system of the chick following extirpation of neural crest. J Exp Zool 1945;100:237.

33. Okamoto E, Ueda T. Embryogenesis of intramural ganglia of the gut and its relation to Hirschsprung's disease. J Pediatr Surg 1967;1:437–443.

34. Gabella G. Nombre et disposition des neurones du plexus d'auerbach au cours du developpement. C R Assoc Anat 1966;135:406–409.

35. Lebenthal E, ed. Human gastrointestinal development. New York: Raven Press, 1989:1–824.

36. Haffen K, Kedinger M, Simon-Assmann P. Cell contact dependent regulation of enterocytic differentiation. In: Lebenthal E, ed. Human gastrointestinal development. New York: Raven Press, 1989:19–39.

37. Leung YK, Lebenthal E. Gastrointestinal peptides: physiology, ontogeny, and clinical significance. In: Lebenthal E, ed. Human gastrointestinal development. New York: Raven Press, 1989:55.

38. Saxena SK, Thompson JS, Sharp JG. Role of epidermal growth factor in intestinal regeneration. Surg 1992;3:318–325.

39. Lewis E. Partial duodenal obstruction with incomplete duodenal rotation. J Pediatr Surg 1966;1:47–53.

40. Gross RE. The surgery of infancy and childhood. Philadelphia: WB Saunders, 1953.

41. Adams AS, Corbally MT, Fitzgerld RJ. Evaluation of conservative therapy for exomphalos. Surg Gynecol Obstet 1991;172:394–396.

42. Hadley HG. Non-rotation of the colon. Br J Radiol 1940;13:35–36.

43. Harvey SC. Congenital variations in the peritoneal relation of the ascending colon, caecum, appendix, and terminal ileum. Ann Surg 1918;67:641–686.

44. Low FN, Hildermann WC. A case of hyperrotation of the colon. Anat Rec 1940;77:27–30.

45. Papez JW. A rare intestinal anomaly of embryonic origin. Anat Rec 1932;54:197–214.

46. Batson OV. Anatomic variations in the abdomen. Surg Clin North Am 1955;36:1527–1537.

47. Laslie M, Durden C, Allen L. Concealed umbilical hernia: Papez's concept of so-called paraduodenal hernia. Anat Rec 1966;155:145–150.

48. Wolfer JA, Beaton LE, Anson BJ. Volvulus of the caecum: anatomical factors in its etiology—report of a case. Surg Gynecol Obstet 1942;74:882–894.

49. Skandalakis JE. Contribution to the study of the pathogenesis and treatment of volvulus of the cecum [Dissertation]. University of Athens Medical School: Athens, Greece, 1949.

50. Waugh GE. The morbid consequences of a mobile ascending colon, with a record of 180 operations. Br J Surg 1920;7:343–383.

51. Morgenstern L. Persistent descending mesocolon. Surg Gynecol Obstet 1960;110:197–202.

52. Guillemin A, Dollander A. Persistance du septum cloacal sous forme d'un meso-vesico-utero-recto-sigmoide, chez une femme porteuse d'un uterus bicorne unicervical. Bull Fed Gynecol Obstet Franc [Suppl] 1961;13:505–507.

53. Ford EG, Senae MO Jr, Srikanth MS, Weitzman JJ. Malrotation of the intestine in children. Ann Surg 1992;2:172–178.

54. Willwerth BM, Zollinger RM, Izant RJ. Congenital mesocolic (paraduodenal hernia) embryological basis of repair. Am J Surg 1974;128:358.

55. Recorla FJ, Shedd FJ, Grosfeld JL, Vane DW, West KW. Anomalies of intestinal rotation in childhood: analysis of 447 cases. Surgery 1990;108(4):710–716.

56. Morgagni JB. The seats and causes of disease investigated by anatomy. Alexander B. (transl). New York: Hafner, 1960.

57. Frazer JE, Robbins RH. On the factors concerned in causing rotation of the intestine in man. J Anat Physiol 1915;50:75–110.

58. Dott NM. Anomalies of intestinal rotation: Their embryological and surgical aspects, with report of five cases. Br J Surg 1923;11:251–286.

59. Haymond HE, Dragstedt LR. Anomalies of intestinal rotation: review of literature with report of 2 cases. Surg Gynecol Obstet 1931;53:316–329.

60. McIntosh R, Donovan EJ. Disturbances of rotation of intestinal tract: clinical picture based on observations of 20 cases. Am J Dis Child 1939;47:116–166.

61. Manson G. Anomalies of intestinal rotation and mesenteric fixation. J Pediatr 1954;45:214–233.

62. Smith GA, Perry JF, Yonehiro EG. Mechanical intestinal obstruction: a study of 1252 cases. Surg Gynecol Obstet 1955;100:651–660.

63. Waldron GW, Hampton JM. Intestinal obstruction: a half century comparative analysis. Ann Surg 1961;153:839–850.

64. Lionakis B, Gray SW, Skandalakis JE, Akin JT, Jr. Intussusception in infants and children. South Med J 1960;53:1226–1235.

65. Rickham PP, Soper RT, Stauffer UG. Synopsis of pediatric surgery. Stuttgart, Germany: George Thieme, 1975:61.

66. Kiesewetter WB, Smith JW. Malrotation of midgut in infancy and childhood. Arch Surg 1958;483–491.

67. Findlay CW, Jr, Humphreys GH. II: Congenital anomalies of intestinal rotation in the adult. Int Abstr Surg 1956;103:417–438.

68. Simpson AJ, Leonidas JC, Krasna IH, Becker JM, Schneider KM. Roentgen diagnosis of midgut malformation: value of upper gastrointestinal radiographic study. J Pediatr Surg 1972;7:243–252.

69. Berdon WE, Baker DH, Bull S, Santulli T. Midgut malrotation and volvulus (which films are most helpful?). Radiology 1970;69:375.

70. Schmeling DJ, Ross AJ, III. Malrotation with midgut volvulus: a review of rotational anomalies of the intestinal tract. Postgrad Gen Surg 1992;1:20–25.

71. Stewart DR, Colodny AL, Taggett WC. Malrotation of the bowel in infants and children: a 15 year review. Surgery 1976;19:716.

72. Hudson CN. Congenital diaphragm of the duodenum causing intestinal obstruction in an adult. Br J Surg 1961;49:234–236.
73. Johnston GW, Stevenson HM. Reflux oesophagitis secondary to duodenal diaphragm in an adult. Thorax 1966;21:65–67.
74. Heilbrun N, Boyden EA. Intraluminal duodenal diverticula. Radiology 1964;82:887–894.
75. McClenathan JH, Okada F. Primary neurilemoma of the diaphragm. Ann Thorac Surg 1989;48(1):126–128.
76. Louw JH. Investigations into the etiology of congenital atresia of the colon. Dis Colon Rectum 1964;471–478.
77. Forssner H. Die angeborenen darm und oesophagusatresien. Anat Hefte 1907;34:1–163.
78. Morley J. Congenital occlusion of the ileum. Br J Surg 1921;9:103–110.
79. Smith GH, Glasson M. Intestinal atresia: factors affecting survival. Aust NZ J Surg 1989;59(2)151–156.
80. Santulli TV. Intestinal obstruction in newborn infants. J Pediatr 1954;44:317–337.
81. Santulli TV, Blanc WA. Congenital atresia of the intestine. Ann Surg 1961;154:939.
82. Goldhahn WE. Congenital duodenal stenosis. Deutsch Gesundh 1963;18:1483–1488.
83. Garvin JA. Congenital occlusion of duodenum by a complete diaphragm. Am J Dis Child 1928;35:109–112.
84. Madden JL, McCann WJ. Congenital diaphragmatic occlusion of the duodenum with a report of three cases. Int Abstr Surg 1956;103:1–15.
85. Mackenzie WC, Lang A, Friedman MHW, Calder J. Congenital atresia of the second portion of the duodenum with associated obstruction of the biliary tract. Surg Gynecol Obstet 1960;110:755–758.
86. Spriggs NI. Congenital intestinal occlusion. Guy Hosp Rep 1912;66:143–218.
87. Reid DK. Congenital obstruction of the colon in an adult. Br J Surg 1948;36:52–54.
88. Feingold BJ, Shulman AG. Isolated segment of intestine associated with duodenal atresia. Am J Dis Child 1942;63:541–545.
89. Douglas KM. Congenital absence of part of the colon associated with carcinoma of the colon. Br J Surg 1954;41:373–375.
90. Royster HA. Appendicitis. New York: Appleton, 1927.
91. Raffensperger JG, ed. Swenson's pediatric surgery. Norwalk, CT: Appleton & Lange, 1990:531.
92. Weitzman JJ, Vanderhoof RS. Jejunal atresia with agenesis of the dorsal mesentery. Am J Surg 1966;3(3):443–449.
93. Zerella JT, Martin LW. Jejunal atresia with absent mesentery and a helical ileum. Surgery 1976;80(5):550–553.
94. Seashore JH, Collins FS, Markowtiz RI, Seashore MR. Familial apple peel jejunal atresia: surgical, genetic, and radiographic aspects. Pediatrics 1987;80(4):540–544.
95. Puri P, Guiney EJ, Carroll R. Multiple gastrointestinal atresias in three consecutive siblings: observations on pathogenesis. J Pediatr Surg 1985;20(1):22–24.
96. Nishikawa A et al. A 13 q− syndrome with extensive intestinal atresia. Acta Paediatr Scand 1985;74(2):305–308.
97. Bland-Sutton J. Imperforate ileum. Am J Med Sci 1889;98:457–462.
98. Politzer G. Die formale genese der kongitalen atresie des darmes beim menschen. Roux Arch Entwicklungsmech 1954;147:119.
99. Tandler J. Zur entwicklungsgeschichte des menschlichen darmarterien. Anat Anz 1903;23:132–134.
100. Théremin E. Ueber kongenitale occlusionen des duenndarms. Deutsch Z Chir 1877;8:34–71.
101. Bernstein J, Vawter G, Harris GBC, Young V, Hillman LS. The occurrence of intestinal atresia in newborns with meconium ileus. Am J Dis Child 1960;99:804–818.
102. Chiari H. Euber eine intrauterin entstandare und un darmatresie gefolgte intussusception des ileums. Prag Med Wschr 1888;13:399–401.
103. Parkkulainen KV. Intrauterine intussusception as a cause of intestinal atresia. Surgery 1958;44:1106–1111.
104. Gherardi GJ, Fisher TH. Atresia of the small intestine produced by intussusception in utero. N Engl J Med 1961;264:229–231.
105. Rosenman LD, Gropper AN. Small intestine stenosis caused by infarction: an unusual sequel of mesenteric artery embolism. Ann Surg 1955;141:254–262.
106. Dickinson SJ. Origin of intestinal atresia of newborn. JAMA 1964;190:119–121.
107. Tandler J. Zur entwicklungsgeschichte des menschlichen duodenum in frühen embryonalstadien. Morph Jahrb 1900;29:187–216.
108. Schwegler RA, Boyden EA. The development of the pars intestinalis of the common bile duct in the human fetus with special reference to the origin of the ampulla of Vater and the sphincter of Oddi. I. The involution of the ampulla. Anat Red 1937;67:441–467.
109. Boyden EA, Cope JG, Bill AH. Anatomy and embryology of congenital intrinsic obstruction of the duodenum. Am J Surg 1967;114:190–202.
110. Karpa P. Zwei falle von dünndarmatresie. Virchow Arch Pathol Anat 1906;185:208–226.
111. Katz K. Atresie des Duodenums mit Verdoppelung des Ductus choledochus und pancreaticus. Virchow Arch Pathol Anat 1930;278:290–294.
112. Davis DL, Poynter CWM. Congenital occlusions of the intestines with report of a case of multiple atresia of the jejunum. Surg Gynecol Obstet 1922;34:35–41.
113. Louw JH, Barnard CN. Congenital intestinal atresia: observations on its origin. Lancet 1955;2:1065–1067.
114. Barnard CN. The genesis of intestinal atresia. Surg Forum 1956;7:393–396.
115. Louw JH. Jejunoileal atresia and stenosis. J Pediatr Surg 1966;1:8–23.
116. Courtois B. Les origines foetales des occlusions congenitales du grele dites par atresie. J Chir (Paris) 1959;78:405–426.
117. Evans CH. Atresias of the gastrointestinal tract: collective review. Int Abstr Surg 1951;92:1–8.
118. Ingalls TH, Prindle RA. Esophageal atresia with tracheoesophageal fistula: Epidemiologic and teratologic implications. N Engl J Med 1949;240:987–995.
119. Abdel-Hafiz AA, Birkett DH, Ahmed MS. Congenital duodenal diverticula: a report of three cases and a review of the literature. Surgery 1988;104:74–78.
120. Gray SW, Pemberton LB, Skandalakis LJ, Colborn GL, Skandalakis JE. Surgical anatomy of the duodenum. Am Surg 1989;55:15–16.
121. Rittenhouse EA, Beckwith JB, Chappel JS, Bill AH. Multiple septa of the small bowel: description of an unusual case, with review of the literature and consideration of etiology. Surgery 1972;71(3):371–379.
122. Gray SW, Lionakis B, Skandalakis JE. Congenital intestinal obstruction. J Med Assoc Ga 1960;49:228–232.
123. Botseas DS, Crystal DK, Johnson W. Intestinal atresia and stenosis in infancy: a review of 34 cases including three with multiple atresias. West J Surg 1961;69:236–241.
124. Aitken J. Congenital intrinsic duodenal obstruction in infancy: a series of 30 cases treated over a 6 year period. J Pediatr Surg 1966;1:546–558.
125. Dykstra G, Sieber WK, Kiesewetter WB. Intestinal atresia. Arch Surg 1968;97:175–182.

126. Clatworthy HW, LLoyd JR. Intestinal obstruction of congenital origin. Arch Surg 1957;75:880–890.

127. Gardener M, Rothstein F, Izant R. Ileal atresia with long segment Hirschspring's disease in a neonate. J Pediatr Surg 1984;19:15.

128. Binninger JN. Observationum et curationum medicinialium, centuriae quinque. Montbelgardi: Hypianis, 1673.

129. Osiander FB. Neue Denkwurdigkeiten fuer Aerzte und Geburtshelfer. Gottingen: JG Rosenbusch, 1797.

130. Voisin F. Observation sur une imperforation extraordinaire de l'anus chez un nouveau-né, auquel, en pratiquant l'opération iléon de Littré, un ouvrit l'intestin iléon au lieu du cólon, qui manquoit aines: que les deux autres gros intestins. J Gen Med Chir Soc Med Paris 1804;21:353–364.

131. Wanitscheck E. Ein Fall von congenitaler Dünndarm-occlusion. Prager Med Woch 1898;23:429.

132. Jacobi A. Defective development of the intestine. Am Med Month NY 1861;16:30–32.

133. Meckel JF. Handbuch der pathologischen Anatomie. Leipzig, 1812.

134. Clogg HS. Congenital intestinal atresia. Lancet 1904;2:1770–1774.

135. Fockens P. Ein operativ geheilter Fall von kongenitaler Duenndarmatresie. Zentralbl Chir 1911;38:532–535.

136. Ernst NP. A case of congenital atresia of the duodenum treated successfully by operation. Br Med J 1916;1:644–645.

137. O'Neill JF, Anderson K, Bradshaw HH, Lawson RB, Hightower F. Congenital atresia of the small intestine in the newborn. Am J Dis Child 1948;75:214–237.

138. Ladd WE, Gross RE. Abdominal surgery of infancy and childhood. Philadelphia: WB Saunders, 1941.

139. Webb CH, Wangensteen OH. Congenital intestinal atresia. Am J Dis Child 1931;41:262–284.

140. Walker WF, Dewar DAE, Stephen SA. Congenital intrinsic duodenal stenosis presenting after infancy. Br J Surg 1958;46:28–32.

141. Kazmers N. Duodenal diaphragm in the adult: a case report. Am J Gastroenterol 1966;45:342–347.

142. DeLorimier AA, Fonkalsrud EW, Hays DM. Congenital atresia and stenosis of the jejunum and ileum. Surgery 1969;65:819.

143. Shafie ME, Rickham PP. Multiple intestinal atresias. J Pediatr Surg 1970;5:655.

144. Martin LW, Zerella JT. Jejunoileal atresia, a proposed classification. J Pediatr Surg 1976;11(3):399–402.

145. Denny ES, Sloan LH. Congenital intestinal malformation in identical twins. Surg Clin North Am 1932;12:227–240.

146. Olson LM, Flom LS, Kierney CM, Shermeta DW. Identical twins with malrotation and type IV jejunal atresia. J Pediatr Surg 1987;11:1015–1016.

147. Pequet AR, Watson EH. Duodenal atresia occurring in siblings. Univ Mich Med Bull 1959;25:363–370.

148. Gibson MF. Familial multiple jejunal atresia with malrotation. J Pediatr Surg 1987;22(11):1013–1014.

149. Saunders JB deCH, Lindner HH. Congenital anomalies of the duodenum. Ann Surg 1940;112:321–338.

150. Wasch MG, Marck A. Radiographic appearance of the gastrointestinal tract during the first day of life. J Pediatr 1948;32:479–489.

151. Krieg EG. Duodenal diaphragm. Ann Surg 1937;106:33–41.

152. Bill AH, Jr. Pope WM. Congenital duodenal diaphragm: report of 2 cases. Surgery 1954;35:482–486.

153. Raffensperger J, Johnson FR, Greengard J. Nonmechanical conditions simulating obstructive lesions of the intestinal tract in newborn infant. Surgery 1961;49:696–700.

154. McGarity WC, Akin JT Jr. Excision of congenital diaphragm of the jejunum with report of a successful case. Surgery 1953;33:425–430.

155. Swenson O, Fisher JH. Small bowel atresia: treatment by resection and primary aseptic anastomosis [12 cases]. Surgery 1960;47:823–835.

156. Threadgill FD, Hagelstein A. Duodenal diaphragm in the adult. Arch Surg 1961;83:878–882.

157. Weber TR, Vane DW, Grosfeld JL. Tapering enteroplasty in infants with bowel atresia and short gut. Arch Surg 1982;117:684–688.

158. Harbour MJ, Altman DH, Gilbert M. Congenital atresia of the colon. Radiology 1965;84:19–23.

159. Berman EJ, Lalonde AH. An important step in management of intestinal atresia. Arch Surg 1962;85:348–350.

160. Del Pin CA, Czyrko C, Ziegler MM, Scanlin TF, Bishop HC. Management and survival of meconium ileus. Ann Surg 1992;2:179–185.

161. Harmon CM, Holcomb GW. Jejunoileal atresia. Postgrad Gen Surg 1992;1:26–31.

162. Rickham PB, Irving I, Smerling DH. Long-term results following extensive small intestinal resection in the neonatal period. Prog Pediatr Surg 1977;10:65.

163. Bryant J. Observations upon the growth and length of the human intestine. Am J Med Sci 1924;167:499.

164. Reis van der V, Schembra FW. Lange und lage des verdauungsrohres beim lebenden. Z Ges Exp Med 1924;43:94.

165. Alvarez WC. An introduction to gastroenterology. New York: Hoeber, 1940.

166. Blankenhorn DH, Hirsch J, Ahrens EH Jr. Transintestinal intubation: technique for measurement of gut length and physiologic sampling at known loci. Proc Soc Exp Biol Med 1955;88:356.

167. Backman L, Hallberg D. Small-intestinal length. Acta Chir Scand 1974;140:57.

168. Flint JM. The effect of extensive resections of the small intestine. Johns Hopkins Hosp Bull 1912;23:127.

169. Shackleford RT. Surgery of the alimentary tract. Philadelphia: WB Saunders, 1955.

170. Vaez-Zadeh K, Dutz W. Ileosigmoid knotting. Ann Surg 1970;172:1027.

171. Kittle CF, Jenkins HP, Dragstedt LR. Patent omphalomesenteric duct and its relation to the diverticulum of Meckel. Arch Surg 1947;54:10–36.

172. Söderlund S. Meckel's diverticulum: a clinical and histological study. Acta Chir Scand [Suppl] 1959;118:1–233.

173. Steck WD, Helwig EB. Umbilical granulomas, pilonidal disease, and the urachus. Surg Gynecol Obstet 1965;120:1043–1057.

174. Arnheim EE. Surgical complications of congenital anomalies of the umbilical region. Surg Gynecol Obstet 1950;91:71–80.

175. Fox PF. Uncommon umbilical anomalies in children. Surg Gynecol Obstet 1951;92:95–100.

176. Lowman RM, Waters LL, Stanley HW. The roentgen aspects of the congenital anomalies in the umbilical region. AJR 1953;70:883–910.

177. Moore TC. Omphalomesenteric duct anomalies. Surg Gynecol Obstet 1956;103:569–580.

178. Jay GD, III, Margulis RR, McGraw AB, Northrip RR. Meckel's diverticulum: a survey of one hundred and three cases. Arch Surg 1950;61:158–169.

179. Benson CD. Meckel's diverticulum. Arch Surg 1948;56:718–724.

180. Merritt WH, Rabe MA. Meckel's diverticulum: review of the literature and report of an unusual case. Arch Surg 1950;61:1083–1095.

181. McMurrich JP, Tisdall FF. A remarkable ileal diverticulum. Anat Rec 1928;39:325–332.

182. Carlson LE. Duplication of a Meckel's diverticulum with other congenital anomalies. Arch Pathol 1935;20:245–246.

183. Wansbrough RM, Thomson S, Leckey RG. Meckel's diverticulum:

a 42-year review of 273 cases at the hospital for sick children, Toronto, Canada. J Surg 1957;1;15–21.

184. Pollard B. A diverticulum ileum of unusual length and position. Trans Pathol Soc Lond 1896;47:47–48.

185. Moll HH. Giant Meckel's diverticulum (33-and-one-half inches long). Br J Surg 1926;14:176–179.

186. Somers LA. Meckel's diverticulum: an unusual position. Surgery 1961;49:331–333.

187. Roberg OT. Result after empiric gastric resection for massive hemmorrhage from concealed Meckel's diverticulum. Am J Surg 1966;111:712–714.

188. Aitken J. Remnants of the vitello-intestinal duct: a clinical analysis of 88 cases. Arch Dis Child 1953;28:1–7.

189. Greenblatt RB, Pund ER, Chaney RH. Meckel's diverticulum: an analysis of eighteen cases with report of one tumor. Am J Surg 1936;31:285–293.

190. Stewart JH, Storey CF. Meckel's diverticulum: a study of 141 cases. South Med J 1962;55:16–28.

191. Curd H. Histologic study of Meckel's diverticulum with special reference to heterotopic tissues. Arch Surg 1936;32:506–523.

192. Berman EJ, Schneider A, Potts WJ. Importance of gastric mucosa in Meckel's diverticulum. JAMA 1957;156:6–14.

193. Aschner PW, Karelitz I. Peptic ulcer of Meckel's diverticulum and ileum. Ann Surg 1930;91:573–582.

194. Harris LE, Wenzl JE. Heterotopic pancreatic tissue and intestinal mucosa in the umbilical cord: report of a case. N Engl J Med 1963;268, 721–722.

195. Cullen TS. Embryology, anatomy, and diseases of the umbilicus, together with diseases of the urachus. Philadelphia: WB Saunders, 1916.

196. Hoffert PW, Strachman J. Intestinal obstruction due to aberrant umbilical vein and hypertrophic pyloric stenosis. Arch Surg 1960;81:890–892.

197. Ternberg JL, Winters K. Intestinal obstruction caused by persistence of the umbilical vein as a transperitoneal structure. Am J Surg 1961;102:473–474.

198. Buchanan JS, Wapshaw H. Remnants of the vitelline vascular system as a cause of intestinal obstruction. Br J Surg 1940;27:533–539.

199. Gross JI, Goldenberg VE, Humphries EM. Venous remnants producing neonatal chylous ascites. Pediatrics 1961;27:408–414.

200. Davis HH, Niehaus FW. Persistent omphalomesenteric duct and urachus in the same case. JAMA 1926;86:685–687.

201. Nix JT, Menville JG, Albert M, Wendt DL. Congenital patent urachus. J Urol 1958;79:264–273.

202. Moutzouris C, Wielandt J. Ductus omphaloentericus et urachus persistens. Acta Paediatr (Uppsala) 1963;52:313–318.

203. Christie A. Meckel's diverticulum: a pathologic study of sixty-three cases. Am J Dis Child 1931;42:544–553.

204. Fabricius Hildanus. Opera observationum et curationum medico—chururgicarum, quae extant omnia, etc. Francof, J. Beyeri, 1646.

205. Lavater JH. De Εντεροπεριστολη seu intestinorum compressione. Basilae, 1672.

206. Ruysch F. Thesaurus anatomicus. Amsterdam, 1701.

207. Littré A. Observation sur une nouvelle espèce de hernie. Mem Acad R Sci 1700:300.

208. Meckel JF. Ueber die Divertikel am Darmkanal. Arch Physiol 1809;9:421.

209. Brun LA. Sur une espèce particulière de tumeur fistuleuse stercorale de l'ombilic. Thèse de Paris, No. 238, 1834.

210. Zenker FA. Nebenpancreas in des Darmwand. Virchow Arch Pathol Anat 1861;21:369–376.

211. Tillmanns H. Über angeborenen Prolaps von Magenschleimhaut durch den Nabelring (Ectopia Ventriculi) und über sonstige Geschwülste und Fisteln des Nabels. Deutsch Z Chir 1883;18:161–202.

212. Moses WR. Meckel's diverticulum: a report of 2 unusual cases. N Engl J Med 1947;237:118–122.

213. Weinstein EC, Cain JC, ReMine WH. Meckel's diverticulum. JAMA 1962;182, 251–253.

214. Blechschmidt E. The stages of human development before birth. Philadelphia: WB Saunders 1961.

215. von Spee F. Zur Demonstration uber die Entwickelung der Drüsen des Menschlichen Dottersacks. Anat Anz 1896;12:76–79.

216. Jordan HE. A microscopic study of the umbilical vesicle of a 13 mm human embryo. Anat Anz 1910;37:12–32.

217. Meyer A. On the structure of the human umbilical vesicle. Am J Anat 1904;3:155–166.

218. Taylor S. Symptoms due to Meckel's diverticulum. Lancet 1947;2:786–789.

219. Mitchell LJ. Notes on a series of thirty-nine cases of Meckel's diverticulum. J Anat Physiol 1898;32:675–678.

220. McParland FA, Kiesewetter WB. Meckel's diverticulum in childhood. Surg Gynecol Obstet 1958;106:11–14.

221. Gross GW. Das Meckelsche Divertikel als klinish bedeutsame Gefahrenguelle. Beitr Klin Chir 1953;187:409–419.

222. Rosenfeld W. Über die Haufigkeit des Meckelschen Divertikels. Zbl Chir 1955;80:2024–2026.

223. Collins DC. A study of 50,000 specimens of the human vermiform appendix. Surg Gynecol Obstet 1955;101:437–445.

224. Androulakis JA, Gray SW, Lionakis B, Skandalakis JE. The sex ratio of Meckel's diverticulum. Am Surg 1969;35:455–460.

225. Skandalakis JE, Gray SW, Shepard D, Bourne GH. Smooth muscle tumors of the alimentary tract. Springfield, IL: Charles C Thomas, 1962.

226. Weinstein EC, Dockerty MB, Waugh JM. Neoplasms of Meckel's diverticulum. Int Abstr Surg 1963;116:103–111.

227. Haber JH. Meckel's diverticulum: a review of literature and analytical study of 23 cases with particular emphasis on bowel obstruction. Am J Surg 1947;73:468–485.

228. Veith FJ, Botsford TW. Disease of Meckel's diverticulum in adults. Am Surg 1962;28:674–677.

229. Lewenstein HJ, Levenson SS. Familial occurrence of Meckel's diverticulum. N Engl J Med 1963;268:311–312.

230. Michel ML, Field RJ, Ogden WW Jr. Meckel's diverticulum: an analysis of 100 cases and the report of a giant diverticulum and of four cases occurring within the same immediate family. Ann Surg 1955;141:819–829.

231. Leijonmarck CE, Bonman-Sandelin K, Frisell J, Rof L. Meckel's diverticulum in the adult. Br J Surg 1986;73:146–149.

232. Cornacchia LG, Virden CP, Wahlstrom HE. Meckel's diverticulum: another "great imitator." Hosp Pract Off 1991;26:65–68.

233. Hübschmann. Spätperforation eines Meckelschen Divertikels nach Trauma. Med Wschr 1913;11:2051–2053.

234. Shaetz G. Beiträge zur Morphologie des Meckelschen Divertikels (Ortsfremde Epithelformationen in Meckel). Beitr Pathol Anat 1925;74:115.

235. Cobb DB. Meckel's diverticulum with peptic ulcer. Ann Surg 1936;103:747–768.

236. Mackey WC, Dineen P. A fifty year experience with Meckel's diverticulum. Surg Gynecol Obstet 1983;156(1)56–64.

237. Amoury RA et al. Megacystis-microcolon-intestinal hypoperistalsis syndrome: a cause of intestinal obstruction in the newborn period. J Pediatr Surg 1977;12(6):1063–1065.

238. Seagram CGF et al. Meckel's diverticulum: a 10-year review of 218 cases. Can J Surg 1968;11:369–373.

239. Leconte D et al. A rare cause of neonatal occlusion by a palpable abdominal mass: Meckel's diverticulum. Chir Pediatr 1988;29(4):216–218.

240. Wollgast GF, Hilz JM. Littré's hernia: strangulation of Meckel's diverticulum in a femoral hernia and inguinal hernia. Amer Surg 1962;28:741–744.

241. Weinstein BM. Strangulated Littré's femoral hernia with spontaneous fecal fistula: case report with a review of the literature. Ann Surg 1938;108:1076–1082.

242. Moore GP, Burkle FM Jr. Isolated axial volvulus of a Meckel's diverticulum. Am J Emerg Med 1988;6(2):137–142.

243. Dowse JL. Meckel's diverticulum. Br J Surg 1961;48:392–399.

244. Brocklehurst G, Cran IM. An unusual complication of a Meckel's diverticulum. Br J Surg 1962;49:604–605.

245. Alhadeff R. Perforation of Meckel's diverticulum by foreign body and review of the literature. Br J Surg 1955;42:527–530.

246. Boldero JL. Calculi in a Meckel's diverticulum. Clin Radiol 1958;9:157–160.

247. Skandalakis JE, Gray SW. Smooth muscle tumors of the alimentary tract. In: Ariel IM, ed. Progress in clinical cancer, Vol. 1. New York: Grune & Stratton, 1965.

248. Doyle JL, Severance AO. Carcinoid tumors of Meckel's diverticulum. Cancer 1966;19:1591–1593.

249. Soltero MJ, Bill AH. The natural history of Meckel's diverticulum and its relation to incidental removal. Am J Surg 1976;132:168–173.

250. Kling S. Patent omphalomesenteric duct: a surgical emergency. Arch Surg 1968;96:545–548.

251. Moynihan BGA. Retro-peritoneal hernia. London: Bailliere, 1899.

252. Stockman JM, Young VT, Jenkins AL. Duplication of the rectum containing gastric mucosa. JAMA 1960;173:1223–1225.

253. Eggert A, Teichmann W, Whitmann DH. The pathologic implication of duodenal diverticula. Surg Gynecol Obstet 1982;154:62–64.

254. Eiseman B, Moore EE, Dunn EL. En passant abdominal operations. In: Delaney JP, Varco RL, eds. Controversies in surgery. Philadelphia: JB Lippincott, 1983.

255. Jones TW, Merendino KA. The perplexing duodenal diverticulum. Surgery 1960;48:1068–1084.

256. Hollender L, Adloff M, Grenier J. Les diverticules duoduodenum [4 cases]. Arch Mal Appar Dig 1959;48:1060–1091.

257. Dean ACB. An abnormality of the pancreas, with diverticula of the duodenum and jejunum. Br J Surg 1959;46:549–551.

258. Spriggs EI, Marxer OA. Intestinal diverticula. Q J Med 1925;19:1–34.

259. Beer E. Some pathological and clinical aspects of acquired (false) diverticula of the intestine. Am J Med Sci 1917;128:135–145.

260. Linsmayer H. Euber duodenaldivertikel. Verh Deutsch Ges Pathol 1914;17:445–455.

261. Chomel JBL. Histoire de l'académie Royale. Paris, 1710.

262. Cruveilhier J. Traite d'anatomie pathologique générale. Paris, JB Baillière et fils, 1849–1864.

263. Perry EC, Shaw LE. On diseases of the duodenum. Guy Hosp Rep 1893;50:171–308.

264. Case JT. Diverticula of small intestine other than Meckel's diverticulum. JAMA 1920;75:1463–1470.

265. Forsell G, Key E. Ein Divertikel an der Pars descendons duodeni mittels Röntgenuntersuchung diagnosziert und operative entfernt. Fortschr Roentgenstr 1916–1917;24:48–57.

266. Ackermann W. Diverticula and variations of the duodenum. Ann Surg 1943;117:403–411.

267. Edwards HC. Diverticula of the duodenum. Surg Gynecol Obstet 1935;60:946–965.

268. Noer T. Non-meckelian diverticula of the small bowel: the incidence in an autopsy material. Acta Chir Scand 1960;120:175–179.

269. Grant JCB. On the frequency and age incidence of duodenal diverticula. Can Med Assoc J 1935;33:258–262.

270. Moreno FG, DeLandazuri EO. Diverticules de l'intestin grele. Arch Mal Appar Dig 1959;48:1436–1442.

271. Mahorner H, Kisner W. Diverticula of the duodenum and jejunum, with a report of a new technical procedure to facilitate their removal and a discussion of their surgical significance. Surg Gynecol Obstet 1947;85:607–622.

272. Zeifer, HD, Goersch H. Duodenal diverticulitis with perforation. Arch Surg 1961;82:746–754.

273. Morrison TH, Feldman M. Gallbladder visualization by oral administration of tetraiodophenol phthalein. Trans Am Gastroenterol Assoc 1927;29:259–276.

274. Waugh JM, Johnston EV. Primary diverticula of the duodenum. Ann Surg 1955;141:193–200.

275. Zinninger MM. Diverticula of the duodenum: indications for and technique of surgical treatment. Arch Surg 1953;66:846–856.

276. Neill SA, Thompson NW. The complications of duodenal diverticula and their management. Surg Gynecol Obstet 1965;120:1251–1258.

277. Benson RE, Dixon CF, Waugh JM. Nonmeckelian diverticula of the jejunum and ileum. Ann Surg 1943;118:377–393.

278. Thorek M, Manzanilla MA Jr. Perforated jejunal diverticula: review of the literature and report of a case. J Int Coll Surg 1954;21:409–418.

279. Sömmering ST. Anat d krankhaften baues, [etc]. Aus dem englischen mit zusätzen von ST sömmering. Berlin, 1794.

280. Cooper A. Anatomy and surgical treatment of crural and umbilical hernia. London: Longman, 1807.

281. Kozinn PJ, Jennings KG. Jejunal diverticulitis: its occurrence in a two year old girl. Am J Dis Child 1941;62:620–623.

282. Ross CB et al. Diverticular disease of the jejunum and its complications. Am Surg 1990;56(5):319–324.

283. Shackelford RT, Marcus WY. Jejunal diverticula: a cause of gastro-intestinal hemorrhage—report of 3 cases and review of literature. Ann Surg 1960;151:930–938.

284. Chitambar A. Duodenal diverticula. Surgery 1953;33:768–791.

285. Normark A. Klinische manifestationen bei intramesenterialem dünndarmdivertikel. Acta Paediat (Stockholm) 1938;20:475–496.

286. Wright G. Congenital diverticulum of the colon. Proc R Soc Med 1920;13:119–128.

287. Brown WG. Duplication of the ileum with associated vertebral defect. Can Med Assoc J 1961;84:789–790.

288. Egelhoff JC, Bisset GS III, Strife JL. Multiple enteric duplications in an infant. Pediatr Radiol 1986;16(2):160–161.

289. Dohn K, Povlsen O. Enterocystomae: report of six cases. Acta Chir Scand 1951;102:21–35.

290. Anderson MC, Siblerman WW, Shields TW. Duplications of the alimentary tract in the adult. Arch Surg 1962;85:94–108.

291. Inouye WY, Farrell C, Fitts WT Jr, Triston TA. Duodenal duplications case report and review. Ann Surg 1965;162:910–916.

292. Leenders EL, Osman MZ, Sukarochana K. Treatment of duodenal duplications with international review. Am Surg 1970;36:368.

293. Black P, Welch K, Eraklis A. Juxtapancreatic intestinal duplications with pancreatic ductal communication: a cause of pancreatitis and recurrent abdominal pain in childhood. Pediatr Surg 1986;21:257.

294. Dickinson WE, Weinberg SM, Vellios F. Perforating ulcer in a duodenal duplication. Am J Surg 1971;122:418.

295. Norris R, Brereton R, Wright V, Gudmore R. A new surgical approach to duplications of the intestine. J Pediatr Surg 1986;21:167.

296. Wiot JF, Spiro E. Intraluminal diverticulum: a form of duplication. Radiology 1963;80:46–49.

297. Moore TC, Battersby JS. Congenital duplication of the small intestine: report of 11 cases. Surg Gynecol Obstet 1952;95:557–567.

298. Kirtley JA, Matuska RA. Enterogenous cysts of the duodenum. Ann Surg 1957;145:265–268.

299. Evans A. Developmental enterogenous cysts and diverticula. Br J Surg 1929;17:34–83.

300. Smith JR. Accessory enteric formations: a classification and nomenclature. Arch Dis Child 1960;35:87–89.

301. Jewitt TC Jr. Duplication of the entire small intestine with massive melena. Ann Surg 1958;147:239–244.

302. Burne JC. Pancreatic and gastric heterotopia in a diverticulum of the transverse colon. J Pathol Bact 1958;75:470–471.

303. Pugh RJ, Feather DB, Goldie W. Duplication of small intestine: report of a case. Br J Surg 1958;46:83–86.

304. Wrenn EL Jr. Tubular duplication of small intestine. Surgery 1962;52:494–498.

305. Micolonghi T, Meissner GF. Gastric-type carcinoma arising in duplication of the small intestine. Ann Surg 1958;147:124–127.

306. Jelenko C. Duplication of the duodenum: a review and report of a case. Am Surg 1962;28:120–132.

307. Lasher EP. Small diverticular duplications of the intestine with peptic ulceration. Am Surg 1967;33:550–554.

308. Veeneklaas GMH. Pathogenesis of intrathoracic gastrogenic cysts. Am J Dis Child 1952;83:500–507.

309. Fallon M, Gordon ARG, Lendrum AC. Mediastinal cysts of foregut origin associated with vertebral anomalies. Br J Surg 1954;41:520–533.

310. Beardmore HE, Wiglesworth FW. Vertebral anomalies and alimentary duplications. Pediatr Clin North Am 1958;5:457–474.

311. McKletchie NGB, Purves JK, Saunders RL deCH. Genesis of gastric and certain intestinal diverticula and enterogenous cysts. Surg Gynecol Obstet 1954;99:135–141.

312. Bentley JFR, Smith JR. Developmental posterior enteric remnants and spinal malformations: the split notochord syndrome. Arch Dis Child 1960;35:76–86.

313. Knight G, Griffiths T, Williams I. Gastrocystoma of the spinal cord. Br J Surg 1955;42:635–638.

314. Elwood JS. Mediastinal duplication of the gut. Arch Dis Child 1959;34:474–479.

315. Denes J, Honti J, Leb J. Dorsal herniation of the gut: a rare manifestation of the split notochord syndrome. J Pediatr Surg 1967;2:359–363.

316. Calder J Jr. Two examples of children born with preternatural conformations of the guts. Med Essays Observ (Edinburgh) 1733;1:203–206.

317. Grawitz P. Ueber den bildungsmechanismus eines grossen dickdarmdivertikel. Virchow Arch Pathol Anat 1876;68:506–518.

318. Fairland E. Congenital malformation of bowel: Amussat's operation. Br Med J 1879;1:851.

319. Fraenkel E. Ueber cysten im darmkanal. Virchow Arch Pathol Anat 1882;87:275–285.

320. Fitz RH. Persistent omphalo-mesenteric remains: their importance in the causation of intestinal duplication, cyst formation and obstruction. Am J Med Sci 1884;88:30–57.

321. Sprengel C. Ein angeborene cyste des darmwand als ursach des invagination. Verh Deutsch Ges Chir 1900;24:537–552.

322. Hudson HW. Giant diverticula of reduplications of the intestinal tract: report of 3 cases. N Engl J Med 1935;213:1123–1131.

323. Thompson NW, Labow SS. Duplication of the duodenum in the adult. Arch Surg 1967;94:301–306.

324. Mellish RW, Koop CE. Clinical manifestations of duplication of the bowel. Pediatrics 1961;27:397–407.

325. Basu R, Forshall I, Rickham PP. Duplications of the alimentary tract. Br J Surg 1960;47:477–484.

226. Hughes-Jones WEA. Enterogenous cysts. Br J Surg 1934;22:134–141.

327. Fischer HW. The big duodenum. AJR 1960;83:861–875.

328. Barnett WO, Wall L. Megaduodenum resulting from absence of the parasympathetic ganglion cells in Auerbach's plexus: review of the literature and report of a case. Ann Surg 1955;141:527–535.

329. Weiss W. Zur ätiologie des megaduodenums. Deutsch Z Chir 1938;251:317–330.

330. Law DH, Ten Eyck EA. Familial megaduodenum and megacystis. Am J Med 1962;33:991–922.

331. Newton WT. Radical enterectomy for hereditary megaduodenum. Arch Surg 1968;96:549–553.

332. Grosfield JL, Rescorla FJ. Short-bowel syndrome in infants. In: Nelson RL, Nyhus, LM. Surgery of the small intestine. Norwalk, CT: Appleton & Lange, 1987;117–125.

333. Emanuel B, Gault J, Sanson J. Neonatal intestinal obstruction due to absence of intestinal musculature: a new entity. J Pediatr Surg 1967;2:332–335.

334. Handelsman JC, Bloodwell R, Bender H, Hartmann W. An unusual cause of neonatal intestinal obstruction: congenital absence of the duodenal musculature. Surgery 1965;58:1022–1026.

335. Steiner DH, Maxwell JG, Rasmussen BL, Jones R. Segmental absence of intestinal musculature: an unusual cause of intestinal obstruction in the neonate. Am J Surg 1969;118:964–967.

336. Berdon WE, Baker DH, Blanc WA, Bay B, Santulli TV. Megacystis-microcolon-intestinal hypoperistalsis syndrome: a new cause of intestinal obstruction in the newborn—report of radiologic findings in five newborns. AJR 1976;126(5):957–964.

337. Taguchi T et al. Autonomic innervation of the intestine from a baby with megacystis microcolon intestinal hypoperistalsis syndrome. I. Immunohistochemical study. J Pediatr Surg 1989;24(12):1264–1267.

338. Kubota M, Ikeda K, Ito Y. Autonomic innervation of the intestine from a baby with megacystis microcolon intestinal hypoperistalsis syndrome. II. Electrophysiological study. J Pediatr Surg 1989;24:1267–1270.

339. Wisewell TE, Rawlings JS, Wilson JL, Pettett G. Megacystis-microcolon-intestinal hypoperistalsis syndrome. Pediatrics 1979;63(5):803–808.

340. Vezina WC, Morin FR, Winsberg F. Megacystis-microcolon-intestinal hypoperistalsis syndrome: antenatal ultrasound appearance. AJR 1979;133(4):749–750.

341. Patel R, Carty H. Megacystis-microcolon-intestinal hypoperistalsis syndrome: a rare cause of obstruction in the newborn. Br J Radiol 1980;53(627):249–252.

342. Krook PM. Megacystis-microcolon-intestinal hypoperistalsis syndrome in a male infant. Radiology 1980;136(3):649–650.

343. Hoehn W, Thomas GG, Mearadji M. Urologic evaluation of megacystis-microcolon-intestinal hypoperistalsis syndrome. Urology 1981;17(5):465–466.

344. Young LW, Yunis EJ, Girdany BR, Sieber WK. Megacystis-microcolon-intestinal hypoperistalsis syndrome: additional clinical, radiologic, surgical, and histopathologic aspects. AJR 1981;137(4):749–755.

345. Jona JZ, Werlin SL. The megacystis microcolon intestinal hypoperistalsis syndrome: report of a case. J Pediatr Surg 1981;16(5):749–751.

346. Oesch I, Jann X, Bettex M. Ultrasonographic antenatal detection of obstructed bladder. Kinderchir 1982;35(3):109–111.

347. Nelson LH, Reiff RH. Megacystis-microcolon-intestinal hypoperistalsis syndrome and anechoic areas in the fetal abdomen. Am J Obstet Gynecol 1982;144(4):464–467.

348. Shalev J et al. Antenatal ultrasound appearance of megacystis

microcolon intestinal hypoperistalsis syndrome. Isr J Med Sci 1983;19(1):76–78.

349. Puri P, Lake BD, Gorman F, Odonnell B, Nixon HH. Megacystis-microcolon-intestinal hypoperistalsis syndrome: a visceral myopathy. J Pediatr Surg 1983;18(1):64–69.

350. Oliviera G, Boechat MT, Ferreira MA. Megacystis-microcolon-intestinal hypoperistalsis syndrome in a newborn girl whose brother had prune belly syndrome: common pathogenesis? Pediatr Radiol 1983;13(5):294–296.

351. Vinograd I, Mogle P, Kernau OZ, Nissan S. Megacystis-microcolon-intestinal hypoperistalsis syndrome. Arch Dis Child 1984;59(2):169–171.

352. Redman JF, Jimenez JF, Golladay ES, Siebert JJ. Megacystis-microcolon-intestinal hypoperistalsis syndrome: case report and review of the literature. J Urol 1984;131(5):981–983.

353. Kirtane J, Talwalker V, Dastur DK. Megacystis-microcolon-intestinal hypoperistalsis syndrome: possible pathogenesis. J Pediatr Surg 1984;19(2):206–208.

354. Manco LG, Osterdahl P. The antenatal sonographic features of megacystis-microcolon-intestinal hypoperistalsis syndrome. Clin Ultrasound 1984;12(9):595–598.

355. Alexacos L, Skoutell H, Sofatzis J, Nacopoulou L. Megacystis-microcolon-intestinal hypoperistalsis syndrome: a functional intestinal obstruction in the female newborn. Z Kinderchir 1985;40(1):53–59.

356. Tomomasa T, Itoh Z, Koizumi T, Kitamura T, Suzuki N. Manometric study on the intestinal motility in a case of megacystis-microcolon-intestinal hypoperistalsis syndrome. J Pediatr Gastroenterol Nutr 1985;4(2):307–310.

357. Gillis DA, Grantmyre EB. Megacytsis-microcolon-intestinal hypoperistalsis syndrome: survival of a male infant. J Pediatr Surg 1985;20(3):279–281.

358. Bulut M, Kalayoglu M, Altin MA, Gursoy MH, Kale G. The megacystis-microcolon-intestinal hypoperistalsis syndrome: a case report. Turk J Pediatr 1985;27(3):169–176.

359. Tokuda Y et al. Copper deficiency in an infant on prolonged total parenteral nutrition. Parenteral Enteral Nutr 1986;10(2):242–244.

360. Willard DA, Gabriele OF. Megacystis-microcolon-intestinal hypoperistalsis syndrome in a male infant. Ultrasound 1986;14(6):481–485.

361. Winter RM, Knowles SA. Megacystis-microcolon-intestinal hypoperistalsis syndrome: confirmation of autosomal recessive inheritance. J Med Genet 1986;23(4):360–362.

362. Vintzileos AM et al. Megacystis-microcolon-intestinal hypo-peristalsis syndrome: prenatal sonographic findings and review of the literature. Am J Perinatol 1986;3(4):297–302.

363. Deutinger J, Bernaschek G, Gherardini G, Schatten O. Fetal megacystis prenatal diagnosis and attempt at therapy. Z Geburt-shilfe Perinatol 1986;190(4):168–171.

364. Dogruyol H, Gunay U, Esmer A, Kahveci R. Megacystis-microcolon-intestinal hypoperistalsis syndrome in a newborn after clomiphene ingestion during pregnancy. Z Kinderchir 1987;42(5):321–323.

365. Farrell SA. Intrauterine death in megacystis-microcolon-intestinal hypoperistalsis syndrome. J Med Genet 1988;25(5):350–351.

366. Boles ET Jr, Smith B. Preduodenal portal vein. Pediatr 1961;28:805–809.

367. Block MA, Zikria EA. Preduodenal portal vein causing duodenal obstruction associated with pneumatosis cystoides intestinalis. Ann Surg 1961;153:407–408.

368. Knight HO. An anomalous portal vein with its surgical dangers. Ann Surg 1921;74:697–699.

369. Kauffman RR, Gerbode F. Arteriomesenteric duodenal ileus. Stanford Med Bull 1951;9:262–272.

370. Haley JC, Peden JK. The suspensory muscle of the duodenum. Am J Surg 1943;59:546–550.

371. Haley JC, Perry JH. Further study of the suspensory muscle of the duodenum. Am J Surg 1949;77:590–595.

372. Boener F. Acta nat curios. Norimb 1974;10:225 (appendix).

373. Rokitansky C. Lehrbuch der pathologischen anatomie, 3rd ed, Vol 3. Wien: W Braunmuller, 1861.

374. Stavely AL. Acute and chronic gastro-mesenteric ileus with cure in a chronic case by duodeno-jejunostomy. Bull Johns Hopkins Hosp 1908;19:252–255.

375. Wilkie DPD. Chronic duodenal ileus. Br J Surg 1921;9:204:214.

376. Pool EH, Niles WL, Martin KA. Duodenal stasis: duodenojejunostomy. Ann Surg 1933;98:587–618.

377. Thieme ET, Postmus R. Superior mesenteric artery syndrome. Ann Surg [Suppl] 1961;154:139–143.

378. Lontok RM, Taber KW. Arterio-mesenteric duodenal occlusion (report of 8 proven cases). Penn Med J 1959;62:1529–1533.

379. Kaiser GC, McKain JM, Shumacker HB Jr. The superior mesenteric artery syndrome. Surg Gynecol Obstet 1960;110:133–140.

380. Rabinovitch J, Pines B, Felton M. Superior mesenteric artery syndrome. JAMA 1962;179:257–263.

381. Barner HB, Sherman CD. Vascular compression of the duodenum. Int Abstr Surg 1963;117:103–118.

381. Martorell R, Guest M. Operative treatment of the superior mesenteric artery syndrome. Am Surg 1961;27:681–685.

CHAPTER 7

THE COLON AND RECTUM

John Elias Skandalakis/Stephen Wood Gray/Richard Ricketts

"The surgeon who has some knowledge of embryology, however imperfect or controversial, will be better prepared to understand the relationship of the anus and rectum to surrounding structures and to the fistulas that so frequently connect the rectum to the genitourinary system."
—RAFFENSPERGER (1)

DEVELOPMENT

The early development of the whole gut and the specific development of the small intestine is discussed in Chapter 6. Here we are concerned with the development of that portion of the embryonic midgut caudal to the ileocecal valve, as well as the hindgut and the dorsal cloaca.

Colon

Growth of the postarterial limb of the intestine lags behind that of the prearterial limb, so that in the 10th week, when the intestines return to the abdomen, the "large" intestine is actually smaller than the "small" intestine (see Chapter 6). Early writers reported no solid epithelial state of the colon, but Lynn and Espinas (2) found complete but transitory occlusion in two embryos among a sample examined during the fifth to eighth weeks.

Goblet cells and the striated border of the epithelial cells may be recognized by the 11th week. During the third month, villi and glands appear in the colon. The villi reach their maximum development in the fourth month and gradually shorten and disappear as the colon enlarges during the seventh and eighth months. Villi are also transitory in the appendix during the fourth month.

Circular muscle of the hindgut appears at the caudal end by the 30-mm stage (ninth week) and spreads over the whole colon by 42 mm (10th week). Ganglion cells of the myenteric plexus reach the colon in the seventh week, and innervation appears to be complete by the 12th week (3). At the 40-mm stage (early 10th week), the first longitudinal muscle fibers are present at the anal canal, and by 46 mm (late 10th week), they have reached the region of the sigmoid colon. Above this level, the long fibers extend only along the mesenteric side of the colon, reaching the cecum by 50 mm (11th week). By 90 mm (early fourth month), the longitudinal layer has encircled the colon but is still thickened along the mesentery. Local thickening of the muscle fibers results in the appearance of the two antimesenteric teniae by 105 mm (fourth month). Sacculations resulting from attachment of circular fibers to the longitudinal teniae appear by 150 mm. Meconium gradually fills the colon and lower ileum from 125 mm (late fourth month) to birth.

The vascular anatomy of the intestinal circulation is not well known. In their excellent presentation Nowicki and Oh (4) stated that ontogeny of intestinal vascular anatomy during ante- and postnatal development has not been investigated.

These authors raise several points, such as:

1. Changes of the vascularity during development need to be examined.
2. Further investigation is required of extrinsic neural regulation such as the role of nonadrenergic femoral factors.
3. Additional studies are necessary to clarify the developmental physiology of intrinsic vascular regulation.

Cloacal Region

The hindgut becomes established very early as that part of the archenteron that extends into the tail fold of the developing embryo. From it, at about the 13th day, develops a ventral diverticulum, the allantois. The junction of the allantoic stalk with the hindgut will subsequently become the cloacal region. The postallantoic gut (tailgut) remains small and disappears during the sixth week (10-mm stage).

During the fifth week, the cloaca appears triangular from the side, with the hindgut, tailgut, and allantois forming the apices. A definite closing plate, the cloacal membrane, occupies the curve formed between the tail and the body stalk. It is composed of two layers—endoderm and ectoderm—in contact. By the end of this week, the cranial portion of the cloaca receives the paired mesonephric (wolffian) ducts, which have formed their ureteric buds just before they enter the cloaca.

Table 7.1.
Anomalies of the Colon, Rectum and Appendix

Anomaly	Origin of Defect	First Appearance	Sex Chiefly Affected	Relative Frequency	Remarks
Bilateral duplication of the colon	Early 3rd week	At birth	Female	Very rare	
Cystic remnants of the tailgut	6th week	Any age	Female	Rare	
Hirschsprung's congenital megacolon	7th to 8th weeks	Infancy	Male	Uncommon	May extend into small intestine
Anal stenosis	6th to 8th weeks				
Membranous anal atresia	8th week				
Anal ectopia	6th to 9th weeks	At birth or early infancy	Male	Common	
Anorectal agenesis	6th week				
High rectal atresia	6th to 7th weeks				
Colonic agenesis	10th week?	At birth (agenesis)	Female	Very rare	
Appendiceal anomalies	8th week	None	Equal	Rare	Found only incidentally at surgery
Small left colon syndrome	?	At birth	Equal	Rare	Associated with maternal diabetes

The urorectal septum is that wedge of mesoderm lying ventral to the hindgut, and dorsal to the proximal portion of the cloaca. This wedge appears to move caudally toward the cloacal membrane. Its movement is the result of progressively caudal fusion of lateral ridges growing inward from the sides of the cloaca (5–7). By about 16 mm (middle of the seventh week), the septum has reached the cloacal membrane and united with it. It now forms the perineal body, dividing the cloacal membrane into a caudal anal membrane, and a larger ventral urogenital membrane. The cloaca itself now is divided into the dorsal rectum and the ventral urogenital sinus (Fig. 7.1).

The anal membrane is slightly depressed below the surface of the body, forming the proctodeum, or anal dimple. The pectinate line in the anal canal of the adult indicates its level. Rupture of the anal membrane usually occurs during the eighth week (at about 30 mm) or earlier.

According to Potter (8) adult colonic function is different from fetal and newborn colonic function. Patients with total colectomy experience a healthy life despite the absence of the colon and limited conservation of water and electrolytes. Perhaps the terminal ileum plays a role by absorbing more water and salt. The fetal and newborn colon resembles the small bowel, having villi, disaccharides, and active transport of glucose (8). Therefore, with so many functions, the colon of the newborn baby plays an important role in nutrition.

In 1913 Johnson (9) presented his work on the development of colonic mucosa. Longitudinal folds, villi, and glands exist in intrauterine life, but when the baby is born villi does not exist. The scientific work of several investigators using electromicroscopy and other techniques report that the human colon and the small bowel have many similarities in fetal human development.

The colon is involved in several functions and mechanisms, such as sodium conservation, bile acid resistance, and transport of ions, and contributes to nutrition. Therefore the past dictum that the colon is useless (since human beings can tolerate a total colectomy) is superseded by a new philosophy that the colon is useful and contributes much to the developmental nutrition of the newborn infant.

The villous differentiation of the human colon is supported by the electromicroscopic studies of Bell and Williams (12).

In the female the fused müllerian ducts that will form the uterus and vagina move down the urorectal septum to reach the urogenital sinus about the 16th week. In the male the site of the urogenital membrane will be obliterated by the fusion of the genital folds, and the sinus itself will become incorporated into the urethra.

The embryonic rectum at the time of its separation from the cloaca shows two enlargements; the upper will form the rectal ampulla of the adult; the lower will form the anal canal.

The anus is more than the external orifice of the rectum. The embryonic musculature of the region forms around the whole of the cloacal region, and subsequently the most dorsal portion forms a pair of anal tubercles on either side of the most dorsal portion of the cloacal membrane. These swellings fuse dorsally to form a horseshoe-

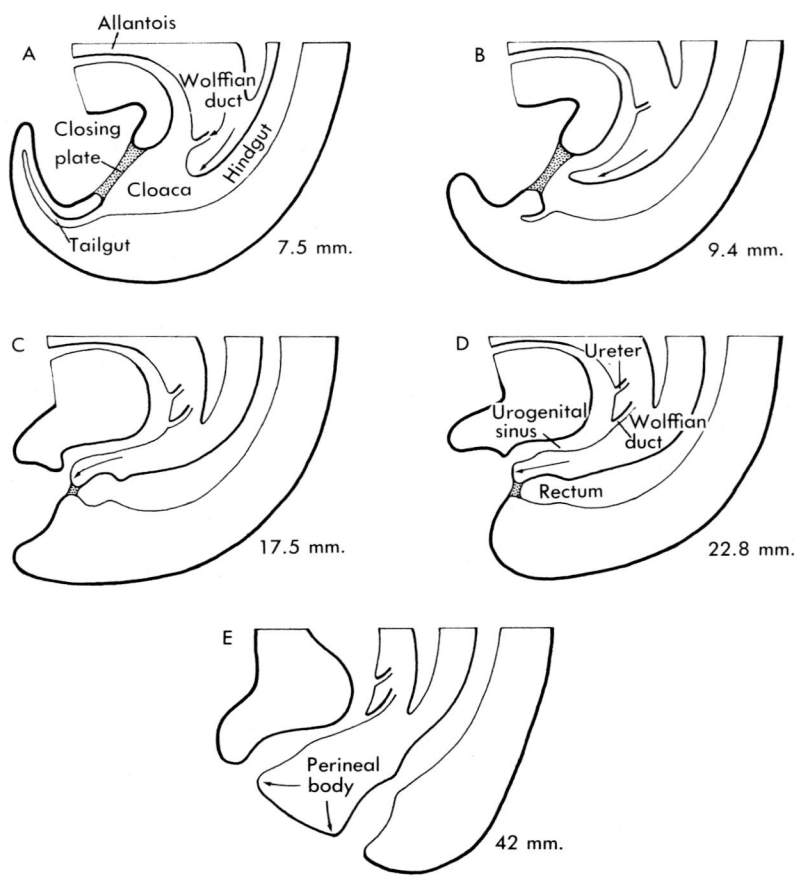

Figure 7.1. Five stages in the normal division of the cloacal region by the descent of the urorectal septum (indicated by *arrows*). (**A, B, D,** and **E,** Redrawn from Ladd WE, Gross RE. Congenital malformations of the anus and rectum: report of 162 cases. Am J Surg 1934;23:167; **C,** redrawn from Blechschmidt E. The stages of human development before birth. Philadelphia: WB Saunders, 1961.)

shaped structure, the ventral tips of which fuse with the perineal body during the 10th week (11) (See Fig. 21–7, *B*).

This musculature forms the external anal sphincter of striated muscle at the normal location of the anus, even when the rectum ends blindly, or at another site. Smith and Gross (12) found external sphincter fibers present in all but one of sixteen serially sectioned specimens of imperforate anus from infants. The exception was a case of exstrophy of the bladder, with widespread malformation of the lower abdominal musculature.

In contrast, the internal anal sphincter of smooth muscle forms as the most caudal part of the rectal muscularis, and hence surrounds the actual orifice, even when it is in an abnormal location.

Cecum and Appendix

The cecum is visible as a ventral enlargement of the hindgut during the fifth week (6.3 mm) (13). A transitory protuberance appears on this cecal enlargement during the sixth week, only to disappear by the end of the following

week. The significance of this structure is not clear, but it is not the definitive appendix. Kelly and Hurdon (14) recognized it in eight of ten fetuses between 6 ½ and 8 weeks of age. The appendix itself is visible about the eighth week. The usual intepretation is that the appendix is the terminal portion of the cecum, which becomes visible by its failure to keep pace with the growth of the proximal portion. Growth does not cease, but the appendix continues to lag behind the cecum even in postnatal life. At birth the diameter of the colon is 4.5 times that of the appendix; at maturity, it is 8.6 times larger (15) (Fig. 7.2).

During fetal life, the appendix projects from the apex of the cecum, but subsequent faster growth of the right terminal haustrum displaces the appendix medially toward the ileocecal valve. The teniae of the longitudinal muscle coating the colon originate at the base of the appendix and show the same displacement.

The section of the appendix is circular in cross-section up to about the 12th week, after which it assumes its typically lobed appearance. Villi are present during the fourth and fifth months but disappear before birth. A few lymph nodules are visible by the seventh month. Lym-

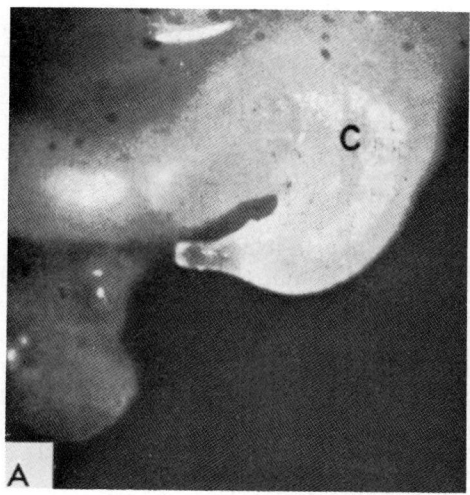
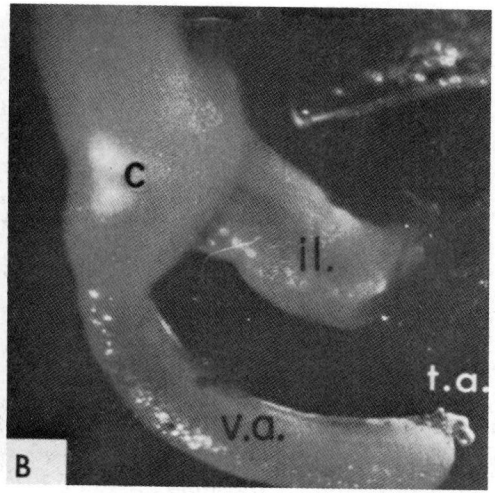

Figure 7.2. Shape of the developing cecum and appendix in the human embryo. **A**, At 20mm. **B**, At 32 mm. *V.a.*, vermiform appendix; *t.a.*, transitory appendix; *C*, cecum; *il.*, ileum. (From Maisel H. The shape of the human cecum during fetal life. Acta Anat 1963;52:252–259.)

phoid tissue increases up to puberty, then slowly decreases. Obliteration of lumen is common in the elderly.

Criticial Events in Development

Most of the anorectal defects arise from a slight posterior shift in the position of the urorectal septum as it divides the cloaca during the sixth to eighth weeks or result from excessive resorption of the tailgut at about the same time.

During the same period, arrest in the migration of ganglion cells down the developing gut produces colonic aganglionosis.

ANOMALIES OF THE COLON, RECTUM, AND APPENDIX (TABLE 7.1 AND FIG. 7.3)

Agenesis and Aplasia of the Colon

In agenesis of the colon, the gut ends blindly and part or all of the colon is absent. In aplasia, the continuity of the gut from pylorus to anus is uninterrupted, but no differentiation into the colon has occurred. Both conditions appear to be very rare.

Several cases of agenesis of the left half of the colon, imperforate anus, and dilation of the remaining colon have been reported. A vesical or vaginal fistula was present in some. Most of these patients have other serious malformations. Teratoma; duplication of the ileum, appendix, or uterus; hypospadias; urinary tract malformations; bifid aorta; and syndactyly have all been described. Trusler and his colleagues (16) reported seven cases in 1959. A few other single case reports have also appeared (17, 18).

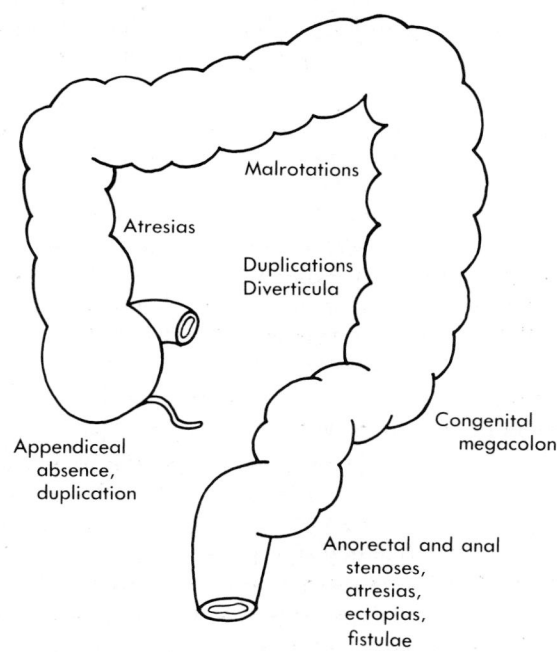

Figure 7.3. Anomalies of the colon.

In one case of congenital absence of the colon reported by Kleinfelter (19), the colon was replaced by a band and 1 cm of the anus was present.

Blunt and Rich (20) reported on a female infant with congenital absence of the colon just above the cecum onwards. The left kidney, ureter, left tube, and ovary were also absent.

Resection of the dilated colon with ileostomy or colostomy has been successful in a few cases (16, 18). The enlarged colon does not decrease in size after colostomy, and it has little or no motor function.

The defect is not a primary endodermal deficiency because the urogenital sinus and the allantois form normally or nearly so. It appears to be a secondary loss of much or all of the postarterial intestinal loop between the sixth and eighth weeks of embryonic life. Such loss is a type III intestinal atresia, perhaps of vascular origin (pages 203–205).

Aplasia of the colon is even less common. In one case (21) there was no evidence of a cecum or large intestine, although the mucosa was not examined histologically. In a similar, more recent case (22) only 75 cm of gut of uniform caliber extended from pylorus to anus. The mucosa was that of the small intestine, without ileocecal valve, cecum, appendix, or teniae coli. The first 60 cm were supplied by the superior mesenteric artery. Failure of both differentiation and elongation of the hindgut must be assumed.

Douglas (23) described an adult with a continuous intestinal lumen; the ileum joined the distal half of the colon through a stenotic segment, which the author believed to be the aplastic proximal colon. Two similar cases have been mentioned by Royster (24).

Atresia of the Colon

Atresias of the colon are similar to those of the small intestine (see Chapter 6). There may be a mucosal diaphragm (type 1), two blind ends connected by a fibrous cord in the mesentery (type II), or two blind ends with a corresponding gap in the mesentery (type III). The frequency of colonic atresias has been estimated to be as high as 11.7% of all intestinal atresias (5) and as low as 4.6% (26). Sturim and Ternberg (27) found nearly equal numbers of the three types. In their study, more type I atresias occurred in the ascending and sigmoid colon, and more type III atresias occurred in the transverse colon. One type II and four type III atresias were long, some involving more than half of the total length of the colon.

Apparently both sexes are equally affected. Other congenital anomalies are present in about 20% of the cases. More than one atresia occasionally is present.

Colonic atresia, according to Powell (28), is the least common form of congenital atresia, perhaps comprising 5 to 15% of reported cases.

Pohlson et al. (29) agree, advising that colonic atresia comprises less than 10% of neonatal intestinal obstruction. They report 11 patients who underwent surgical repair. Five of the patients were premature, and two had associated gastroschisis.

In his review Powell (28) reported 23 cases: 14 occurred in the ascending, 1 in the transverse, and 8 in the descending colon. In 12 of these cases, there was a V-shaped defect of the mesentery. The pathology was located in the ascending colon, and the colon was absent up to the splenic flexure or descending colon.

Moore (30) reported splenic flexure atresia with absence of the distal colon. Jackman and Brereton (31) reported distal ileal atresia and atresia of the sigmoid colon in a female infant.

Powell (28) reported several associated anomalies such as ophthalmic defects, bladder exstrophy, and duodenal atresia. Hyde and Delorimier (32) reported atresia associated with Hirschsprung's disease.

Bilious vomiting, tremendous abdominal distension, and no bowel movement or minimal passage of meconium are signs of colonic atresia.

Peck and his colleagues (33) reviewed 12 cases of successfully treated colonic atresias, and Hartman and his associates (34) reviewed 12 cases with two deaths. Sturim and Ternberg (27) found a total of 49 cases in the literature (Fig. 7.4).

Benson and his colleagues (35) recommend end-to-end primary anastomosis for atresias proximal to the splenic flexure and colostomy with subsequent resection and end-to-end anastomosis 10 to 12 months later for atresias of the distal colon (Fig. 7.5).

A barium enema radiograph will locate the obstruction, and sometimes the "windsock sign" may be present (36). Surgery should be performed as soon as possible to avoid necrosis, perforation, and generalized peritonitis.

COLONIC MALPOSITIONS

Colonic malposition not related to the abnormal presence of its mesentery is a peculiar phenomenon. The most characteristic representation is the so-called Chilaiditi's

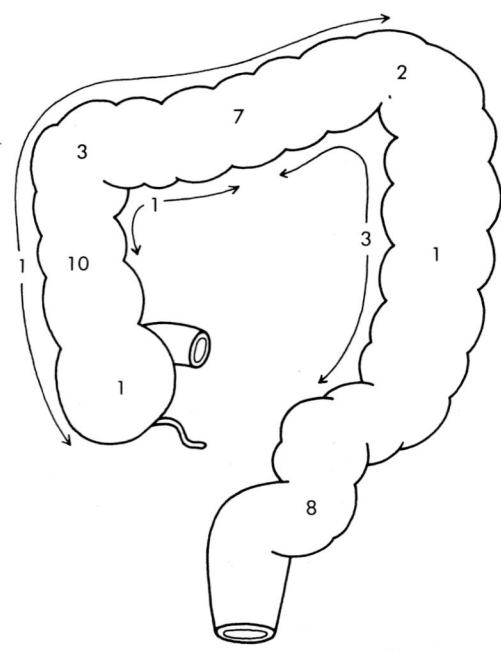

Figure 7.4. The location of 37 colonic atresias successfully treated. (Data from Sturim HS, Ternberg JL. Congenital atresia of the colon. Surgery 1966;59:458–464.)

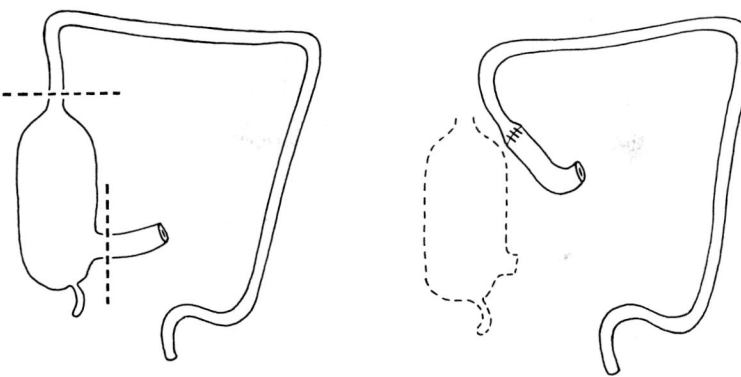

Figure 7.5. Procedure for repair of colonic atresia near the ileocecal valve. The terminal ileum is anastomosed to the unexpanded colon distal to the atresia.

syndrome. Chilaiditi (37) described a syndrome in which the hepatic flexure is situated between the liver and the diaphragm. Since that description Jackson and Hodson (38) and Werner (39) reported that this syndrome is a phenomenon secondary to an anomaly of the hepatic ligament which occurs in about 1:50,000 adults.

SMALL LEFT COLON SYNDROME

In this syndrome the left colon is small in caliber but the rectum is normal. The small left colon syndrome is specific to the newborn and associated with maternal diabetes. The obstruction is caused by a meconium plug at the splenic flexure, and therefore some people use this term synonymously with *meconium plug syndrome*. Both usually are diagnosed and treated successfully with a barium enema. The small left colon in the small left colon syndrome often persists throughout childhood. It is not the same microcolon, which merely refers to an unused colon that otherwise is normal. Microcolons occur with proximal atresias. After the atresia is repaired, the colon quickly assumes its normal caliber (40, 41).

Diverticula of the Colon

Although true diverticula—those having all layers of the colon wall—have been reported, false diverticula are far more common. True diverticula are limited largely to the cecum and ascending colon, whereas false diverticula are more frequent in the transverse and descending colon. The greatest concentration is in the sigmoid colon.

False diverticula of the colon, like those of the small intestine, appear at weak points in the wall. The incomplete longitudinal musculature of the colon provides areas of weakness between the teniae that are not true muscular defects. In only a few cases is there evidence of a congenital abnormality (42).

Sikirov (43) supports the theory that the sitting posture is perhaps responsible for the etiology and pathogenesis of diverticula.

In most discussions of colonic diverticula, no effort is made to distinguish congenital from acquired forms. In many cases inflammation has so distorted the anatomy that the origin of the diverticulum cannot be determined. According to Fischer (44) congenital diverticula are located on the right colon and involve all the layers plus the muscle. Wagner and Zollinger (47) observe that diverticula of the left colon become more frequent with age, whereas those of the right colon do not (Fig. 7.6). Presumably, more of the latter are congenital. Colonic diverticula of either kind are rarely reported in infants (42, 46) and are only occasionally found in adults under 30 years of age (47). Diverticula of the left colon occur twice as frequently in men as in women.

As we stated earlier it is difficult, because of the severe inflammatory process secondary to diverticula, to confidently use the terms *congenital* and *acquired* when referring to colonic diverticula. The literature is also confusing about this subject.

Do patients under 30 or 40 years of age belong to a mixed group which have both types of diverticula? Perhaps the two patients of Bova et al. (48) who were under the age of 40 years had congenital diverticula. Norfray et al. (49) reported that in the age group under 30 years old, 24 to 50% of patients have "cecal" diverticulitis. Early diagnosis is discussed by Chodak et al. (50).

Other questions arise when considering diverticulitis. For instance, why in Japan does 77.4% of diverticulitis occur in the right colon (51), when in the non–Asiatic population only 1.3 to 13% of diverticular disease occurs in that location (52). The same approximate results were reported by Tan et al. (53). Sardi et al (54) reported that 3.6% of diverticula occur in the right colon in a patient population ranging from 7 to 87 years of age. Perhaps some of these cases have a congenital etiology.

Andricopoulos and Christopoulos (55) presented a case of a 4-year-old boy with a large inflamed diverticulum of the sigmoid colon. Since the pathologist found all

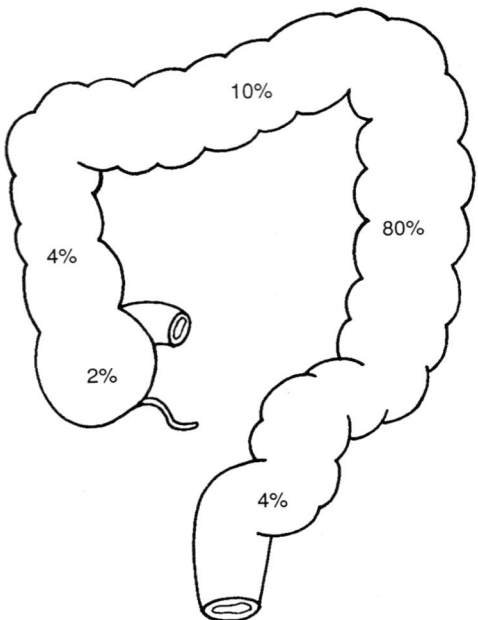

Figure 7.6. Diverticulosis is more frequent in the left colon with age, in comparison to that in the right colon. (After Wagner DE, Zollinger RW. Diverticulitis of the cecum and ascending colon. Arch Surg 1961;83:436–443.)

the layers of the colon present, this diverticulitis must have been of congenital origin.

Rectal bleeding with right-sided colonic diverticula was reported by Casarella et al. (56). In 1987 Wilkinson (57) presented a case of acute solitary diverticulitis of the transverse colon in a 13-year-old girl. In 1983 Halata et al. (58) reported 12 cases of diverticulitis in patients under 21 years of age in a search of the literature of the past 50 years. In the same year, Ouriel and Schwartz (59) found only 1 of 4673 cases of diverticulitis occurred in a patient under 20 years of age. Omojola and Mangete (60) reported colonic diverticula in three Nigerian siblings. Schippers and Dittler (61) reported the case of a 16-year-old boy with perforation of sigmoid diverticula and multiple other anomalies.

The great majority of inflamed diverticula of the cecum and right colon are diagnosed as appendicitis. Mann (62) considers a correct diagnosis of diverticulitis to be possible only if the appendix is known to have been removed.

If diverticulitis can be diagnosed, it may be treated conservatively with bland diet and antibiotic therapy. Surgical intervention becomes necessary if (a) repeated episodes of diverticulitis occur, (b) there are signs of intestinal obstruction, or (c) there are signs of ulceration or perforation.

In most cases a cecal diverticulum may be recognized on inspection of the cecum. In these cases excision of the lesion is all that is required. In other cases the diverticu-

lum is small, hidden in the cecal wall, and represented on the outer surface of the cecum by an inflammatory mass. The diverticulum cannot always be identified at surgery, and the diagnosis is often that of carcinoma. Unless this diagnosis can be ruled out at once, the surgeon is obliged to perform a right colectomy.

Duplications of the Colon

Duplications of the colon may be cystic or tubular with normal colonic epithelium, in comparison with other duplications of the small bowel in which islands of gastric or pancreatic mucosa may be present. Therefore, according to Raffensperger (1), the cardinal symptoms may be constipation and obstruction but not bleeding.

However, Stockman et al. (63) reported a case of an anterior rectal "diverticulum" containing gastric mucosa. Explanation of this phenomenon is practically impossible from an embryologic and topographicoanatomic standpoint since the duplication was reached by the finger at the surgical anal canal (the distal 4 cm below the insertion of the pelvic diaphragm and the formation of the puborectal muscle or just above the canal, perhaps 6 cm above the puborectal muscle). Also, this is a rare location since most of the rectal duplications are located posteriorly.

Paddock and Arensman (64) reported a polysplenia syndrome with duplications. Bower et al. (65) reported seven cystic duplications of the colon and two of the rectum. Malignant changes in colonic duplications are reported by Orr and Edwards (66).

The authors divide these congenital anomalies into three groups: midline duplications, bilateral duplications of the colon and rectum, and cystic remnants of the tailgut.

Midline Duplications of the Colon

Cystic duplications lie posterior to the rectum and usually have a common wall with it (Fig. 7.7). Removal may require excision of the posterior rectal wall, with subsequent repair. Thirty-two such cystic duplications were collected by Kraft (67). A cystic duplication lying anterior to the rectum is illustrated without explanation by Martorell and Murphey (68). Many of these cysts are remnants of the embryonic tailgut, the embryogenesis of which is discussed in a later section.

Midline tubular duplications are rare. Septate anal canals have been described by Gross (26) (Fig. 7.7, C) and Stockman and his colleagues (69). An apparently unique case—in which the subject had a normal rectum and anus, as well as a second perineal anal orifice leading to a sinus 12 cm long that ended blindly at the wall of the normal rectum—was reported by Batchelor and Grieve (70).

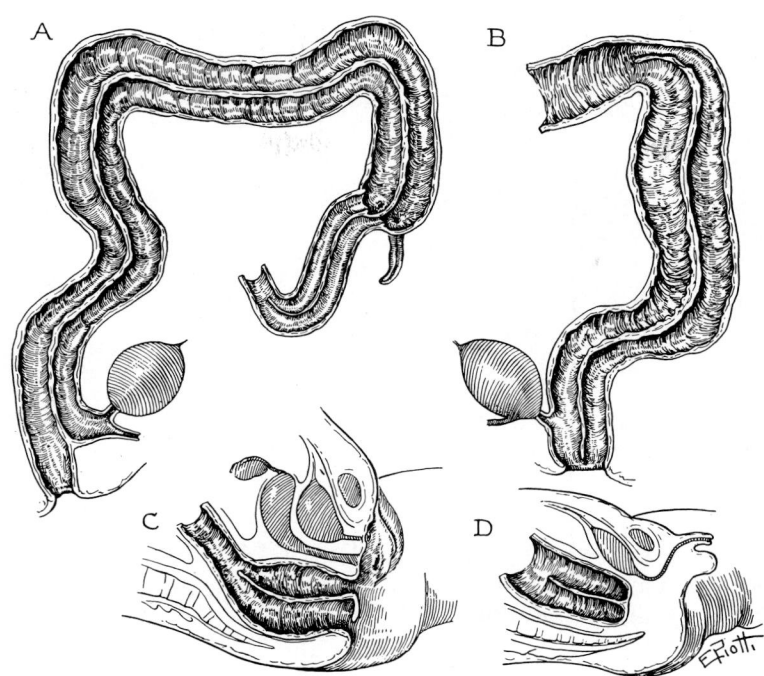

Figure 7.7. Examples of tubular duplications of the intestine. **A**, Duplication from ileum to rectum. One canal ends at a normal anus, the other in a fistula to the urethra. **B**, Duplication of the descending colon with double anus and a fistula to the urethra. **C**, Short duplication of the rectum, with two anal openings. **D**, Dupli- cation of the rectum with both canals ending blindly (more frequently the cranial end of the duplication is blind). (From Gross RE. The surgery of infancy and child- hood. Philadelphia: WB Saunders, 1958.)

Bilateral Duplications of the Colon and Rectum

In addition to the cystic and tubular duplications that are similar in structure and embryogenesis to those in the small intestine and which are discussed with them (page 225), a special type of tubular duplication is encountered in the colon. This is a side-by-side rather than an over-and-under doubling. Such pairing of the colon often is accompanied by pairing of other midline structures of the posterior part of the body.

ANATOMY

In its fully developed form, the duplication begins at the level of Meckel's diverticulum, and all caudal intestinal structures are duplicated and separate, ending in separate anal openings. In females, there are also two vaginae which communicate with two unicornate uteri and open into separate vulvae. Two bladders, each supplied with one ureter, empty through two urethrae into separate orifices. The lumbar or even the thoracic vertebral column, together with the sacrum, are sometimes doubled or bifid. This complete duplication is most nearly approximated in only a few cases (71) (Fig. 7.8).

Most of the cases show less than complete doubling. Beach and his colleagues (72), reviewing the reported cases, found the following anal conditions:

Double rectums, each ending in a patent anus	8 cases
Double rectums, one anus, one blind-ending rectum	4 cases
Double rectums, one anus, one rectum ending in a fistula (urethral or vaginal)	5 cases
Double rectums, each ending blindly	1 case
Double rectums, each ending in a fistula	3 cases

In addition to the cases of hindgut duplication described previously, two cases are known in which three colons were present (73, 74).

In one of these cases the vagina and external genitalia were absent, the müllerian tubes were unfused, and the bladder was exstrophic. Hydronephrosis was present, and the pubic bones were separated. All three colonic passages were open at the cecum, which was not doubled, and two opened into the single anus. The third extended nearly to the anus but ended blindly and was greatly distended. The circular muscle coats were separate, but there was a single longitudinal muscle coat without teniae (75).

Because failure of urogenital fusion was present in both cases we believe that they represent a combination of paired, lateral duplication and an additional dorsal tubular duplication that formed the third structure. If this hypothesis is correct, it should be possible to have a four-barreled colon, with each of the paired colons having its own dorsal duplication.

Besides the urogenital and skeletal anomalies men-

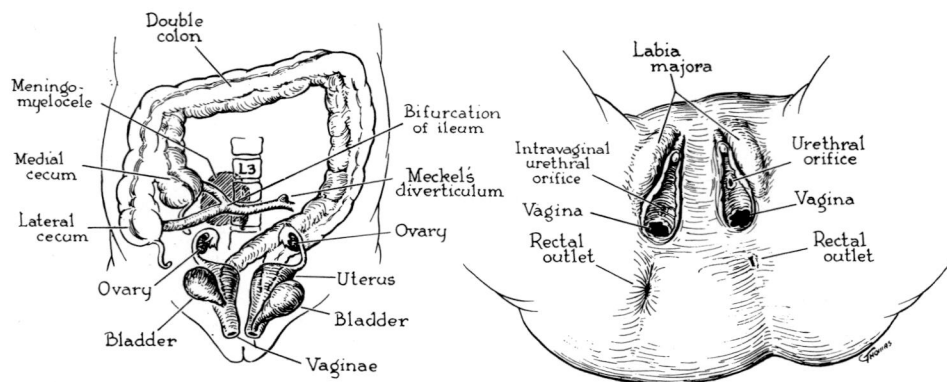

Figure 7.8. Bilateral duplication of colon, uterus and bladder in a 4-month-old female. The terminal ileum and all distal intestinal structures are duplicated. Hemiuteri and hemibladders are present. Anal, vaginal, and urethral orifices are doubled. (From Beach PD et al. Duplication of the primitive hindgut of the human being. Surgery 1961;49:779.)

tioned, malrotation (75), horseshoe kidney (76), absence of kidney (77), and clubfoot (72) have been associated with colonic duplication. The urogenital duplications are discussed elsewhere.

EMBRYOGENESIS

The term *partial twinning* has been used to express the defect involved in this type of duplication, but it is misleading because only axial structures are duplicated. The separated lateral halves each form a more or less complete normal organ. The condition is not to be confused with dipygus twinning, which is the result of anterior fusion of two separate embryonic individuals.

In one case a hypoplastic median iliac bone with a rudimentary limb represented the suppressed portion of the duplication (78). In spite of this case we believe that all these malformed infants represent single individuals in which the cranial end of the primitive streak became split to form two blastopores. From these arose two notochords, slightly separated at their caudal ends, which subsequently fused into one during their cranial elongation.

No early human embryos showing the development of this defect are known, and we can only speculate about the process. The splitting might occur as early as Streeter's presomite stage 9 and certainly before the completion of the hindgut at stage 11. Notochordal splitting is obvious in some cases and less so in others although it probably existed, if only temporarily, in all cases. Common to all of these cases is evidence of a divided proctodeum and urogenital sinus; possibly the allantois was divided as well. The failure of müllerian and wolffian structures to fuse is thus secondary to the primary splitting of the hindgut and the cloacal membrane. There are no reports of duplicated umbilical veins or arteries that might be expected to accompany a duplicated allantois.

HISTORY AND INCIDENCE

It is surprising that so extensive an anomaly, having such striking external manifestations, was not described earlier; the first case seems to be one reported in the "Ephemerides" of the Leopoldine Academy at Frankfurt for 1712 to 1717 (79). Calder in 1733 (80) mentioned a similar case, but the earliest full description is that of Suppiger in 1876 (81). Since then 37 cases have been collected by Beach and his colleagues (72). A few more have been reported since. In at least 15 of these, the bladder also was duplicated. These latter cases are the only ones that certainly belong to the group of paired doubling of the colon (82) (Fig. 7.9). In some cases the description is too inadequate to decide which type of duplication was encountered. The reported cases have been reviewed by Van Zwalenburg (83), Ravitch (84), Van Velzer and his colleagues (85), and Beach and his colleagues (72). Similar anomalies are known in dogs and rats (86).

About twice as many affected patients are female as are male. In the latter, bifid penis and scrotum replace double vaginae when the urogenital system is involved (76, 87).

The majority of these anomalies found were in infants, most of whom died. One male lived to age 35 years (87); a woman, reported by Hinckle (71), was 62 years old and had been pregnant. In another case (78) the patient was alive and healthy 2 years after birth.

SIGNS AND SYMPTOMS

Most of these paired colonic abnormalities manifest at birth because of the doubling of anal and urogenital orifices. When both colonic lumina are patent, no physiologic difficulties arise (71, 78, 88). When one lumen ends blindly (73) or has a fistulous opening into the bladder (76), the normal colon becomes compressed by the dilation of the occluded portion. In one patient (77), hema-

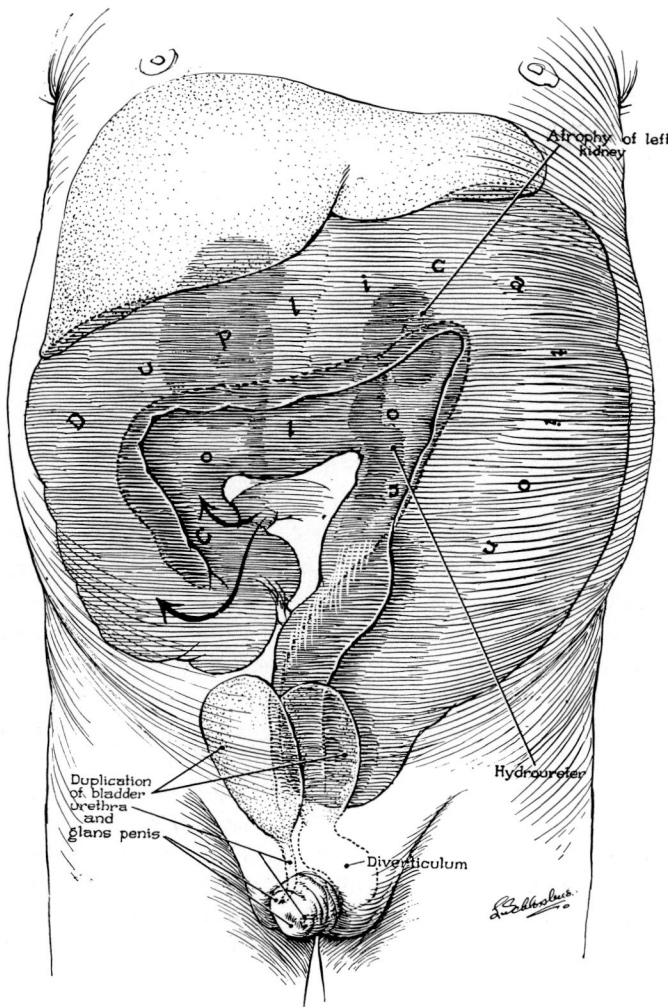

Figure 7.9. Bilateral duplication of colon and bladder in a 4½-year-old male. There is one terminal ileum and only one vermiform appendix, but the normal colon at the cecum is continuous with an enormously dilated and hypertrophied duplication, which parallels the colon and is densely adherent to it as far as the very depth of the pelvis where it ends blindly. The right kidney and ureter are normal. The left kidney is atrophic, and there is a hydroureter on the left. Two bladders of about equal size are present, the right bladder emptying by its own urethra through the meatus in the glans. There is a large diverticulum in the urethra leading from the left bladder and a very small meatus almost in the prepuce. (From Ravitch MM, Scott WW. Duplication of the entire colon, bladder, and urethra. Surgery 1953;34:843–858.)

tocolpos developed because the vagina had no external orifice, the extra rectum having been considered to be the vagina.

DIAGNOSIS

When two anal orifices are present, barium may be used to outline each colonic channel. Where but one is present, the colon may fill with barium yet leave loops of intes-

tine containing feces but no barium. The situation is difficult to diagnose prior to surgery. In the patient of Ravitch and Scott (82), the distended abdomen and the hypertrophic blind duplication suggested a preoperative diagnosis of Hirschsprung's disease (Fig. 7.9).

TREATMENT

As restoration of the normal condition is not feasible, treatment must be directed toward establishing functional organ systems. Intestinal obstruction is the usual cause of death in untreated cases.

Blind duplications have been treated by forming a distal communication with the normal colon after repair of rectovaginal or rectourethral fistulae. Excision of the septum between rectal orifices has been successfully performed. Ravitch and Scott (82) were able to remove most of the duplication and to save some of the normal colon in their patient. Their paper discusses in detail operative procedures in their own and earlier cases.

Cystic Remnants of the Tailgut

ANATOMY

Cystic tumors containing alimentary tract mucosa are occasionally found lying between the coccyx or the sacrum and the rectum. They are similar in structure to cystic duplications arising elsewhere in the gut. Many are duplications of the rectum and originate in the same way as do other cystic duplications. Some, however, are cystic remnants of the transitory embryonic tailgut and, hence, represent the persistence of a normal embryonic structure rather than being true duplications.

EMBRYOGENESIS

The cloacal membrane of the embryo is formed not at the caudal tip of the hindgut but on its ventral surface, slightly proximal to the tip. The portion of primitive archenteron extending caudal to the cloaca is the tailgut. In this region the tapering ends of the neural tube, the notochord, and the gut lie in close proximity within the tissues of the pointed embryonic tail.

The tailgut reaches its greatest development during the early sixth week and shortly thereafter regresses. The terminal portion persists longer than does the proximal portion. Mucosal glands are present, but distinct muscle coats do not develop. By the seventh week, no trace is normally present, although Peyron (89) demonstrated cystic remnants of the tailgut in sheep and pig fetuses near term.

An early embryonic structure in this region, the neuroenteric canal, has sometimes been considered to be the source of presacral cysts. The neuroenteric canal is a transitory opening between ectoderm and endoderm at the anterior end of the primitive streak (Henson's node) and the posterior end of the neural tube. It persists up to the beginning of the somite formation (early fourth week) and perhaps later. To this hypothetical, continued persistence has been attributed at one time or another almost all dorsal midline defects, including pilonidal sinuses. We agree with Peyron (89) that there is no way of recognizing possible derivations of this transitory structure. Until further proof is available, we prefer to relate enteric cystic structures in this region to the tailgut.

HISTORY AND INCIDENCE

The earliest description of a tailgut remnant is that of Middeldorpf in 1885 (90). Middeldorpf's tumor was described as having intestinal epithelium; some authors considered it to have been a teratoma. For this reason, presacral teratomata and, by extension, all presacral masses are often mistakenly called Middeldorpf tumors.

Perry and Merritt (91) collected 10 cases of enterogenous cysts derived from the tailgut and added a case of their own. Nine of the eleven cases were in females, four were in infants, and seven were in adults between the ages of 26 and 48 years.

SYMPTOMS

The symptoms associated with presacral tumors provide no help in distinguishing their origin. Pain or a sense of pressure in the rectum are usual in adults. Signs of obstruction are present in infants. In two of the cases reviewed by Perry and Merritt (91), the enterogenous cysts were found on routine examination and apparently produced no symptoms.

DIFFERENTIAL DIAGNOSIS

Chordomas, which are more common in males, usually produce symptoms after the age of 50 years. Teratomata are usually large and present at birth; they chiefly affect females. Diagnosis must rest on the histologic examination (92).

The potential sources of tumors in the sacrococcygeal region are summarized in Table 7.2.

Table 7.2.
Potential Sources of Tumors in the Sacrococcygeal Region

Germ Layer	Normal Structure	Tumor
Ectoderm	Epidermis	Pilonidal cyst
	Neuroectoderm	Neuroblastoma
Mesoderm	Meninges	Meningocele
	Notochord	Chordoma
	Smooth muscle	Leiomyoma, leiomyosarcoma
	Coccygeal gland?	Paraganglioma
Endoderm	Postanal gut (embryonic)	Enteric cyst

TREATMENT

Complete excision of the tumor, with removal of the coccyx and as much of the sacrum as is necessary, should always be performed. The great majority of tumors in this region have malignant potentialities, and even the apparently benign enterogenous cysts are known to harbor carcinoma (93).

Other Dorsal Cloacal Remnants.
A perineal cyst lined with stratified columnar ciliated epithelium was described by Gius and Stout (94). From its location and the absence of intestinal glands in its wall, they considered it to be derived from the cloaca. A sacrococcygeal cyst was present in the same patient.

EDITORIAL COMMENTS

Dr. J. J. White and associates have reported a patient with a "tail," which represents a part of the dorsal remnant but is not attached to or derived from the mucosa of the developing cloaca since there is no lumen and no mucosa present. This did not represent a true sacrococcygeal tumor because there was no evidence of cellular hyperplasia. These "tails" need to be considered embryologic abnormalities but, fortunately, are rarely associated with other skeletal or cloacal anomalies. (JAH and CNP).

Unusually large or supernumerary anal glands have been considered to be cloacal remnants. Gius and Stout (94) described two suggestive cases. Tucker and Hellwig (95) described the embryology of these glands and concluded that they are derived from the cloacal wall at the same time as the prostate and the paraurethral ducts.

Congenital Aganglionic Megacolon (Hirschsprung's Disease)

ANATOMY

Hirschsprung's disease manifests as nearly complete constipation from birth, with no demonstrable physical obstruction. With time there is a secondary dilation and hypertrophy of the colon above a narrowed distal portion of variable length. It is one of the most distressing of nonlethal anomalies and, until recently, one of the most misunderstood. The actual defect is the absence of ganglion cells or Auerbach's plexus (myenteric), Henle's plexus (deep submucosal), and Meissner's plexus (submucosal) of the colon below the dilated segment. Dilation is the result of failure of the distal segment musculature to move the colonic contents onward. The dilated colon has normal ganglion cells. A physiologic obstruction, more insidious than an anatomic atresia, blocks the free passage to the anus.

The dilated proximal segment ends in a funnel-shaped annular or constricted transition zone, which joins it to the narrowed distal segment. Occasionally, the "narrowed" segment is normal in diameter although it is

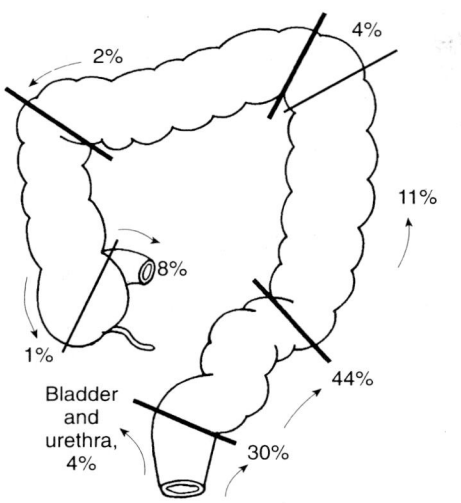

Figure 7.10. The frequency of aganglionic segments of varying length. The lesion extends proximal to the splenic flexure in only 4% of patients.

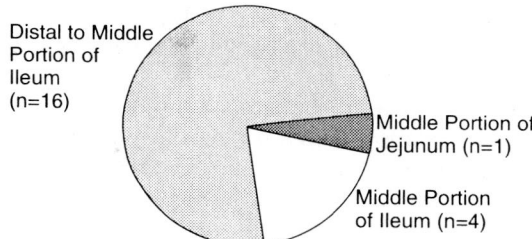

Figure 7.11. Anatomical site of the transition zone from ganglionic to aganglionic bowel in 21 patients with long-segment Hirschsprung's disease. (From Bickler SW et al. Long segment Hirschsprung's disease. Arch Surg 1992;1270:1047–1051.)

smaller than the dilated segment above. It must be kept in mind that the action of the dilated portion has filled the most proximal part of the aganglionic segment, and thus the transition zone belongs to the aganglionic segment, not to the normal segment.

The extent of the aganglionosis is variable. The internal sphincter is involved in all cases, and the whole of the rectum in most. The rectosigmoid segment is included in about half of the cases. In addition, to these "short aganglionic segments," about 15% of patients have aganglionosis extending to the splenic flexure or to the hepatic flexure or even involving the entire colon (Fig. 7.10). Stone and his colleagues (96) reviewed 55 cases involving the entire colon. In 24 of these a short ileal segment also was affected, and in 10 cases nearly the entire small intestine as well as the colon was without ganglion cells. In one case the whole of the intestinal tract from the pylorus to the anus was affected (97). Bickler et al. (98) reported 21 children with long-segment Hirschsprung's disease with extension proximal to the ileocecal valve (Fig 7.11). It should be noted that, when the aganglionosis begins above the ileocecal valve, there will be not a "megacolon" but a "megaileum" or "megajejunum." In such circumstances the entire colon may be smaller than normal.

In a few patients (99, 100) the aganglionic portion is said to be discontinuous, providing a "skip area" that has normal ganglion cells and normal function between two aganglionic segments. The existence of such discontinuities has been doubted by other authors (101). Recent studies have tended to support the validity of such skip segments (102, 103).

ASSOCIATED ANOMALIES

Serious anomalies associated with Hirschsprung's disease are rare. Swenson (104) found increased bladder capacity in about 50% of his patients, and in 4% there was megaureter and megacystis with some ganglion cell deficiency. Three to four percent of patients with Hirschsprung's disease have Down's syndrome (105–107).

Aganglionosis cannot be recognized grossly at autopsy in the newborn because dilation and hypertrophy have not yet developed. Its possible association with other lethal malformations is therefore unknown. Prematurity is not associated with aganglionosis.

EMBRYOGENESIS

The neurenteric ganglion cells migrate from the neural crest to the upper end of the alimentary tract, then follow vagal fibers caudad (108–110). An in situ origin of the ganglion cells has been suggested (109, 111) probably to explain the occurrence of segmental aganglionosis with normal colon distal to it. However, the existence of such skip segments has not been confirmed.

Why the migrating ganglion cells stop before they reach the rectum is unknown. The answer does not lie in the failure of vagal fibers to prepare the way. Unmyelinated fibers can be demonstrated between the muscle layers of the aganglionic segment of the colon. These are postganglionic fibers from normal ganglia proximal to the affected segment and preganglionic parasympathetic (vagal) fibers that have failed to connect with ganglion cells and continued to elongate (101, 112, 113).

Ehrenpreis and his colleagues (114) suggest that aganglionosis may result from vascular disturbances and that adrenergic neurons may be absent—whereas cholinergic neurons are normal—in the effected segments. A transitory "megacolon" has been produced in dogs by clamping the blood supply to the colon for several hours (115). We cannot accept this suggestion as an explanation of Hirschsprung's megacolon. Such vascular obstruction would result in many cases of aganglionic segments followed by normal colon. If they exist at all, lesions of this type are very rare.

Not all patients with megacolon can be said to have Hirschsprung's disease. It is now recognized that several anomalies of the myenteric plexus may produce the same clinical picture as Hirschsprung's disease. These lesions have been called "idiopathic megacolon." They include areas of neuronal loss, abnormal neurons, and neuronal dysplasia.

Siegel and Lebenthal (116) state that Hirschsprung's disease is the most common motility disorder of the colon. They present all disorders of intestinal motility in the newborn in Table 7.3.

Munakata (117) presented six cases with hypoganglionosis in which small numbers of ganglia and absent or poor formation of plexus in the affected segment was present. The same author reported a baby with immature ganglion cells involving both small and large intestines, but plexus and the number of cells were normal. This functional obstruction of the intestine also was reported by Burghaighis and Emery (118). Tanner et al. (119) reported functional intestinal obstruction due to neuronal abnormality.

Absence of intestinal musculature or muscle defects of the intestinal wall are responsible for neonatal intestinal obstruction (120, 121).

Tam and Lister (122) examined the pylorus, ileum, and colon in 28 human fetuses at 9 to 12 weeks of gestation using immunohistochemical localization of neuron-specific enolase, a specific neuronal marker indicative of differentiation. The authors suggest a dual gradient of neuronal development with the most highly developed cells in the pylorus, less in the colon, and least in the ileum. This is in contrast to the earlier view that differentiation and migration follow the vagus nerve in a simple craniocaudal gradient (123).

NEUROPATHOPHYSIOLOGY

The absence of ganglion cells is a useful anatomic marker for the neuropathophysiologic abnormalities which result in the functional obstruction in Hirschsprung's disease. The normal colon receives extrinsic innervation via the parasympathetic (cholinergic) and sympathetic (adrenergic) nervous systems. The parasympathetic system is excitatory to the colon and inhibitory to the internal sphincter, whereas the sympathetic system is inhibitory to the colon and excitatory to the internal sphincter. In addition, the normal colon receives intrinsic innervation via the purinergic (adenosine triphosphate as the mediator), serotonergic (serotonin as the mediator), and peptidergic (vasoactive intestinal polypeptide (VIP) and substance P as mediators) systems.

These systems form what is collectively called the "nonadrenergic inhibitory fibers" (124). Ganglion cells receive impulses from the cholinergic fibers but mainly from the intrinsic nonadrenergic inhibitory fibers. In Hirschsprung's disease, extrinsic innervation is preserved and, in fact, enhanced with an increase in cholinergic and adrenergic fibers which can be demonstrated histochemically. However, intrinsic innervation is absent.

Histochemical studies have demonstrated absence of the purinergic fibers, serotonergic fibers, and peptidergic fibers. Because of the absence of the intrinsic nervous system (nonadrenergic inhibitory fibers) in Hirschsprung's disease, the wave of relaxation which normally proceeds each propulsive contraction does not occur. The reflux relaxation of the internal sphincter following rectal distension also does not occur. Therefore a functional obstruction results. The ganglion cells act to "coordinate" the intrinsic and extrinsic impulses on the muscle wall and internal sphincter (125). Aganglionosis therefore results in a total breakdown of both systems' regulation of intestinal motility. The result is a failure of relaxation of the bowel wall and the internal sphincter, resulting in a profound functional obstruction. It is thus the absence of the intrinsic nervous system which is the basic neuropathophysiologic abnormality in Hirschsprung's disease.

HISTORY

In 1888 Hirschsprung (126) described the autopsies of two infants who died from congenital megacolon. His name promptly became attached to the condition. So serious a disease had, of course, been seen before. The earliest recognizable case in an adult was described by Parry in 1825 and the earliest infant case by Billard in 1829 (127). Some two dozen other cases were reported before 1888.

Hirschsprung's description contained complete clinical as well as postmortem findings in the two patients. He emphasized the congenital nature of the dilation and hypertrophy and unfortunately directed attention to the dilated segment as the seat of the disease. Lee and Bebb (97) observed that Treves (128) very nearly solved the problem of megacolon in the following decade. A poorly functioning colostomy in a patient led to a resection of the distal segment, with relief of symptoms. Treves failed

Table 7.3.
Disorders of Intestinal Motility in the Newborn[a]

Systemic Disease	Developmental Defects
Decreased motility	Decreased motility
Sepsis	Unknown cause
Necrotizing enterocolitis	Gastroschisis
Respiratory distress syndrome	Neurologic defects
Adrenal insufficiency	Hirschsprung's disease
Hypokalemia	Hypoganglionosis
Hypothyroidism	Immature ganglion cells
Increased motility	Combined hypoganglionosis
Hyperthyroidism	and aganglionosis
Jaundiced infants receiving	Deficiency of argyrophil
phototherapy	neurons
	Muscle defects in segments of
	small intestine
	Unknown cause
	Decreased motility

[a]From Lebenthal E. Human gastrointestinal development. New York: Raven Press, 1989:290.

to preserve the anal sphincter, hence the operative results were considered unsuccessful and the true site of the lesion remained unrecognized.

In 1908 Finney (127) listed no fewer than nine theories concerning possible causes of this condition, ranging from abnormally long mesentery to congenital valves. Among these theories he mentioned the idea of "neuropathic" dilation of a segment with consequent inability to expel the contents. This had been proposed the previous year by Hawkins (129). The first clue appeared even earlier: Tittel in 1901 (130) mentioned abnormalities of ganglion cells in the large intestine of an infant of 15 months who had megacolon.

The myenteric ganglion cells were observed by Finney, (127) but he examined only the dilated segment. The Italian investigator Dalla Valle (131) deserves the credit for directing attention in 1920 to the distal, apparently normal segment for which he reported the absence of ganglion cells in Auerbach's plexus. Cameron (132) compared megacolon with megaesophagus (cardiospasm) and described the aganglionic state of the rectum. These observations were made again in the next decade by Perrot and Danon (133) in France, Etzel (134) in Argentina, and Robertson and Kernohand (135), at the Mayo Clinic.

The result of these reports—and of the denervation experiments in cats by Adamson and Aird (136)—was the theory that the stasis in the aganglionic segment was caused by deficient parasympathetic innervation. A number of attempts were made, therefore, to correct the condition by sympathectomy without achieving marked success (137).

Bodian and his colleagues (138) showed that aganglionosis was not the result of failure of development of the extrinsic parasympathetic innervation but was itself the primary lesion; therefore there was no "autonomic imbalance" to be corrected by sympathectomy.

It remained for Swenson and his colleagues (139–142) to design the operation for removal of the aganglionic segment while preserving the anal sphincter. This operation, based on rational physiologic principles, has proved to be safe and effective. Modifications of this procedure include the Duhamel, Soave, and Boley procedures (142–144). Procedures for dealing with total colonic aganglionosis include that described by Martin (145) and Kimura (146).

INCIDENCE

Hautau (147) found five cases of Hirschsprung's disease among the 205,791 children born in Michigan in 1958. This is an incidence of 1:41,200, about half the incidence estimated by Bodian and his colleagues in 1951 (112). As the disease is not immediately apparent at birth, the Michigan figures are probably too low.

More recently, it has been thought that the incidence should be placed at greater than 1:5000. Richardson and

Brown (148) considered the disorder second to pyloric stenosis as a cause of intestinal obstruction in infants.

Age and Sex.

The disease is more common in males by a ratio of 4:1 (106, 149). Bodian and his associates (138) found 12 females among 73 patients with congenital megacolon (16.4%), whereas Keefer and Mokrohisky (99) found 4 among 18 (22.2%) and Richardson and Brown (148) found only 1 female among 18 (5.6%).

The disease is present at birth, but its severity is governed by the length of the aganglionic segment. Hence, while most patients reach surgery before they are 1 year of age, many are older and a few are adults before being treated (150). A patient of 54 years of age has been treated (151).

Familial Tendency.

Richardson and Brown (148) found 57 cases in 21 families in the literature and described a family in whom 5 of 6 sons of the same mother, but of 3 different fathers, had Hirschsprung's disease. Bodian and his associates (112) estimated the probability of producing a second male sibling with the disease to be 20%.

Klein (152) believes that males and females are equally affected with long aganglionic segments, but that more males have short aganglionic segments. He estimates the probability of a second child with a short segment to be 5% if the child is male and less than 1% if female. The risk for either sex following birth of a child with a long defect is 12.5%. Bielschovsky and Schofield (153) described inheritance of aganglionic megacolon in a strain of piebald mice.

We agree with Swenson (141, 142) and Raffensperger (1) that the disease appears to be an autosomal recessive and sex-linked trait.

SYMPTOMS

Infants.

The usual signs of low intestinal obstruction appear at birth or within the first few weeks of life. Nearly 50% of the patients are diagnosed within the first month of life, 75% within the first 3 months, and 80% by the end of the first year of life (107). Vomiting with progressive distension, which is partially relieved by enema, is the usual pattern. Some patients may display alternate constipation and diarrhea.

Children.

Increasingly severe attacks of vomiting, distension, and diarrhea may appear with age. These attacks may be followed by a relatively long period of freedom from symptoms with gradually increasing tendency toward constipation. The constipation is handled easily at first with laxatives, but it becomes less tractable as the child becomes older.

Chronic distension will eventually result in an enlarged abdomen with a high diaphragm and a deep and wide chest with flared costal margins. Such children show lags in weight and height, are undernourished (as judged by the appearance of the extremities), and often are anemic. Growth may make a dramatic spurt following correction of the megacolon (96).

DIAGNOSIS

The chief diagnostic features of Hirschsprung's disease are:

1. A history of constipation since birth
2. No fecal incontinence
3. Abdominal distension, with palpable fecal masses
4. Radiographic evidence of a distal "narrowed segment" and a proximal distended segment of colon
5. Histologic evidence of absence of ganglion cells
6. Anorectal manometry showing failure of relaxation of the internal sphincter in response to rectal distension

Radiological Diagnosis.

Colonic distension; fluid levels in the colon; an empty, air-filled rectum; and fecal mottling on plain radiographic films are all suggestive of Hirschsprung's disease. Small bowel obstruction can rarely be ruled out of these films because of the difficulty in identifying the loops showing distension.

An enema of barium or other contrast medium is required for a more definite diagnosis. The technique described by Neuhauser, working with Swenson and Pickett (140), is the safest and most effective. Following evacuation of the colon by saline enemas, the contrast medium is introduced under fluoroscopy by catheter. As soon as the transition from narrowed to dilated lumen is visualized, the enema should be stopped (Figs. 7.12 and 7.13). Filling the dilated segment does not contribute to the diagnosis and actually is dangerous since subsequent evacuation of barium may be difficult. Once the patency of the lumen to the dilated segment has been established and mechanical obstruction can be ruled out, diagnosis can be made. Spot radiographs in several positions should be made when the transition zone has been visualized.

Swenson (104) noted four circumstances that may render radiologic diagnosis difficult:

1. The narrowed segment may be very short and confined to the rectum.
2. The entire colon may be aganglionic, and the proximal dilation is in the ileum.
3. In the newborn or in the infant under 6 months of age, dilation and hypertrophy may not have developed sufficiently to demonstrate a transition zone.
4. After a year or more following colostomy, the distal colon may be uniformly narrow and show no transition zone. In most cases when barium enema fails to suggest aganglionosis, the cause is either the second or third item (154).

Histologic Diagnosis.

The absence of myenteric ganglion cells is the only positive confirmation of the lesion and should always be used to establish a positive diagnosis.

In an infant a section mucosal biopsy taken 2 cm above

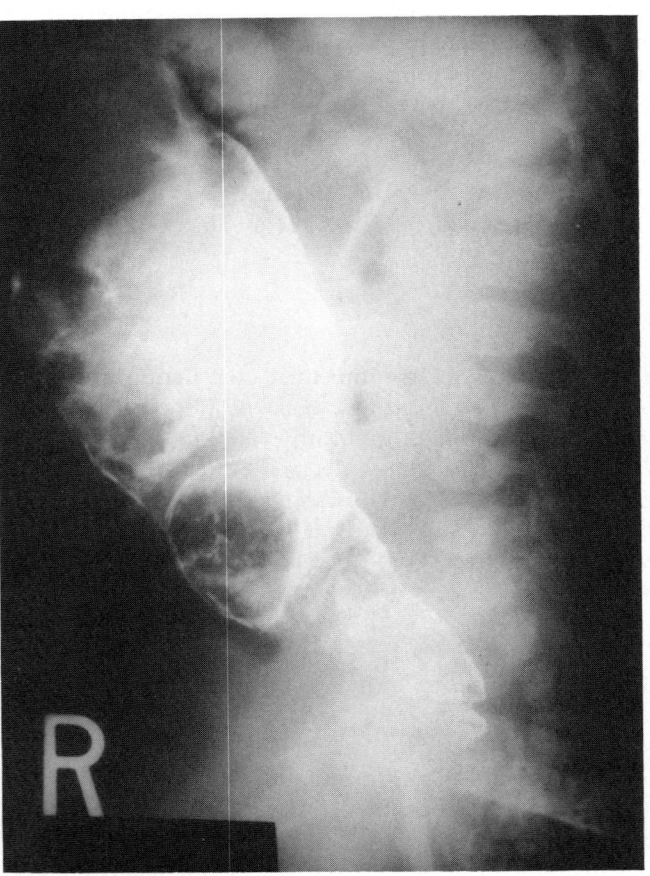

Figure 7.12. Barium enema in newborn with Hirschsprung's disease.

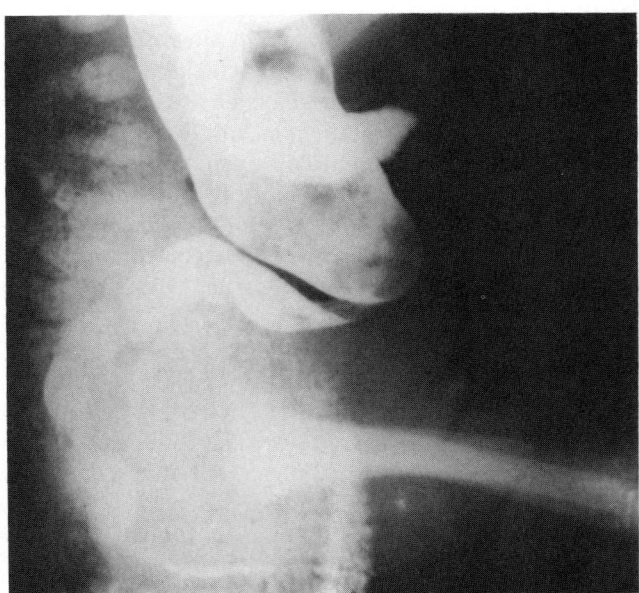

Figure 7.13. Barium enema in infant with Hirschsprung's disease.

the mucocutaneous junction provides sufficient tissue for diagnosis (155). In the older child or adult, a full-thickness biopsy specimen should be taken from the lateral wall, 2 to 3 cm above the mucocutaneous border. Swenson's transmucosal approach (104) seems to be the most effective although other approaches have been successful (156). The specimen must contain both circular and longitudinal muscle layers and should have some mucosa as well. A number of sections must be examined for an adequate evaluation. Routine hematoxylin and cosin staining is all that is required (Fig. 7.14).

Differential Diagnosis.

Not every megacolon is the result of congenital aganglionosis. A number of conditions may closely simulate the picture although the ganglion cells are normal (Fig. 7.15).

Psychogenic Constipation (Pseudo-Hirschsprung's Disease). More common than Hirschsprung's disease, this condition arises in the third to fourth year. The patient does not have a history of early constipation. In contrast to organic disease, the rectal ampulla rarely is empty, and incontinence is frequent. Ravitch (157) discussed the symptoms and the effective treatment.

Megacolon Resulting from Anal Obstruction. Following surgical repair of imperforate anus, fecal retention may result in colonic dilation. This may have a psychologic basis, or it may be due to surgical interference with the normal innervation of the rectum.

A few cases of anal stenosis have been diagnosed as aganglionic megacolon, and conversely, the megacolon occasionally has been erroneously assigned to anal stricture (158).

Megacolon in Mentally Defective Children. Cerebral defects are known to produce chronic constipation and hypertrophy of the colon (157).

Megacolon in Cretinism. Congenital cretinism may produce megacolon from a very early age, and the intestinal symptoms may be the presenting complaint. The

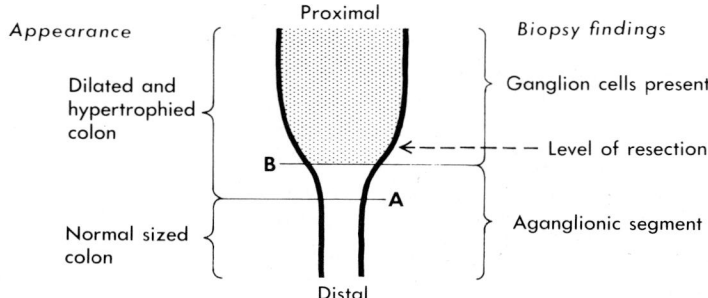

Figure 7.14. Relationship between the gross appearance on the colon and biopsy findings. Note the *line A,* dividing enlarged and normal sized colon, does not coincide with *line B,* dividing the ganglionic from the aganglionic segments. Resection must be made well into the ganglionic segment. *Lines A* and *B* are from 1 to 5 cm apart.

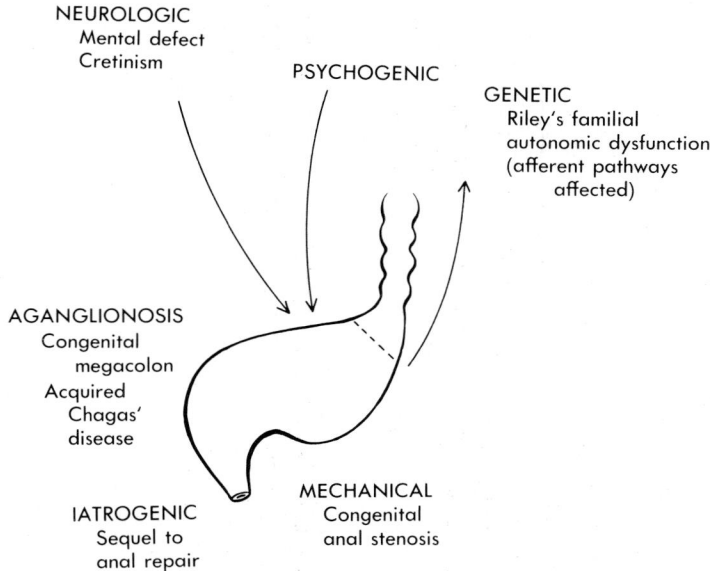

Figure 7.15. Diagram of the possible causes of megacolon, which must be considered in diagnosis.

condition responds readily to treatment with thyroid extract.

Familial Autonomic Dysfunction (Riley's Syndrome). Grossman and his colleagues (159) reported a case of megacolon in a patient with deficient lacrimation, excessive perspiration, motor incoordination, indifference to pain, and emotional instability. The authors consider that failure to receive signals from the colon produced the condition.

Chagas' Disease. Jung (160) commented on the geographic coincidence of megacolon and Chagas' disease in Brazil. The megacolon is aganglionic and toxins from *Trypanosoma cruzi* are thought to destroy the ganglion cells of the lower esophagus and rectum, as well as produce the characteristic cardiac bundle branch block. This parasite is not unknown in the southern United States.

TREATMENT

Acute obstruction of the colon in the infant requires immediate relief by colostomy. The colostomy must be in the normal colon to be effective. It should be placed just above the aganglionic segment, as determined by intraoperative biopsy examined by rapid frozen sections.

The definitive operation on infants should be performed within a year. The objectives are to remove the entire aganglionic portion of the colon and to anastomose, without tension, the normal colon to the last 1 or 2 cm of the rectum. In older children some of the grossly hypertrophied colon above the aganglionic segment may have to be excised.

Three operations are widely used with success: Swenson's "pull-through" procedure (139), Duhamel's subsequent modification (161), and the modification by Soave and Boley (143, 144) (Fig. 7.16). Since these classic operations were first described, there have been many modifications (162), but these improve the procedure

rather than alter its fundamental rationale, which is to resect the aganglionic colon.

In summary, for any procedure to be successful (a) colostomy must be done in the normal (ganglionic) colon and (b) the normal colon must be anastomosed to the rectal cuff just above the mucocutaneous junction.

MORTALITY AND PROGNOSIS

The mortality in untreated cases of aganglionic megacolon is unknown. Certainly an appreciable number of individuals having only short affected segments learn to adjust their diets and live with their constipation. Prognosis improves after the first few years of life if acute obstruction, on the one hand, and electrolyte imbalance, on the other, can be avoided.

Operative mortality has declined from 50% at the Mayo Clinic between 1909 and 1919 to 4% between 1941 and 1945 (163). Swenson (104) reported six deaths among 200 patients treated and later (106) a 1.25% per year mortality during the last 20 years. Benson and Lloyd (162) reported a mortality of 4.3% in 660 Swenson operations at the Children's Hospital of Michigan. Ehrenpreis and his colleagues (114) reported two deaths among 135 children undergoing the Duhamel procedure (1.48%). Enterocolitis remains the greatest danger to life.

Very long aganglionic segments have the poorest prognosis, owing largely to the difficulty of diagnosis. Mortality was 73% as late as 1960 (165). Among two series (148, 165), three of six fatal cases had lesions involving the whole colon and the terminal ileum. Two patients with aganglionosis of the entire colon reached 13 years of age without correction of their condition. One eventually underwent complete colectomy (98), and in the other an ileosigmoid anastomosis without resection was performed (166). Ileorectal anastomoses have been successful in some cases (162). Ratta and his colleagues (167)

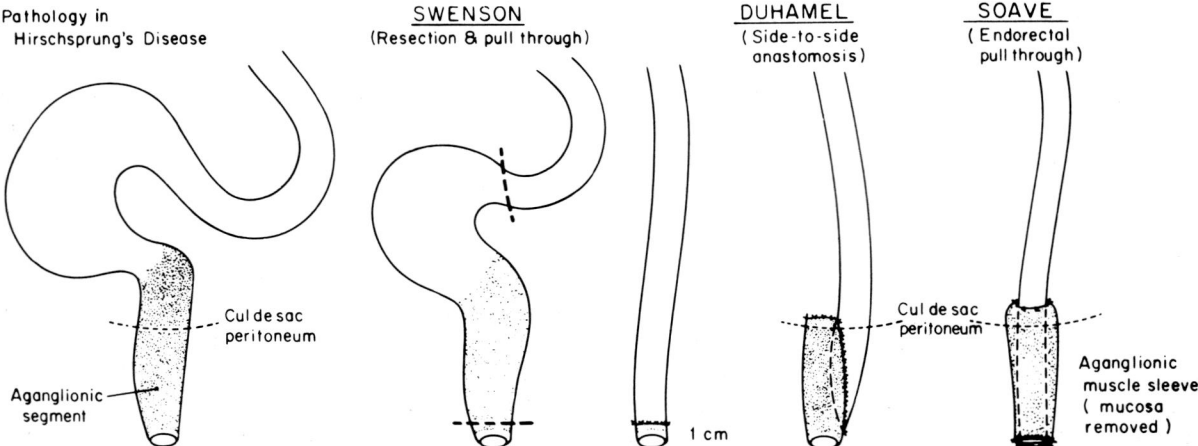

Figure 7.16. Surgical treatment of Hirschsprung's disease. Swenson: colectomy with abdominoperineal pull-through. Duhamel: retrorectal transanal pull-through. Soave: endorectal pull-through. (From Hendren WH, Kein SH. Abdominal surgical emergencies of the newborn. Surg Clin NA 1974;54:489–527.)

reviewed the results of treating patients with total colonic aganglionosis at the Great Ormond Street Hospital for Sick Children between 1978 and 1987. Of the 40 patients, 8 (20%) died. However, the mortality of the patients treated between 1983 and 1987 was only 6%. Good functional results may not always be obtained. An appreciable number of patients have constipation, diarrhea, or anal incontinence following either the Duhamel, Soave, or Swenson procedures.

In the longest follow-up study thus far reported, Sherman et al. (107) reported normal bowel habits in 90% of patients followed for 5 years or more and in 94% of patients followed for 20 years or more. In this study of 880 Swenson procedures performed around the world, only 1.3% of patients had a permanent ileostomy or colostomy. Greater than 95% of patients had no soiling and greater than 95% had only one to three bowel movements per day.

EDITORIAL COMMENTS

Sherman's series noted above was contributed by a very select group of pediatric surgeons with senior experience who had either been trained by Dr. Swenson himself or who were closely associated with his trainees. No other series has reported nearly such a long follow-up nor such outstanding results. Most surgeons find the Boley modification of the Soave procedure to be technically easier than the classical Swenson procedure, and it seems to accomplish about the same results. This was reported in a comparative follow-up from a large number of centers by Dr. Alexander Holschneider from Germany. The important principle is that all of the aganglionic segment be removed. If any of the muscle fibers are left behind, they are essentially nonfunctional and represent only a thin sleeve through which ganglion containing colon is pulled to the anus and anastomosed. Using this principle, which is the Swenson contribution, good results are to be expected, especially if the child is operated upon before 2 years of age (JAH and CNP).

ANORECTAL ANOMALIES

Defects of the anus and rectum resemble those of the esophagus in that they consist of stenoses, atresias, and fistulae to other systems of the body. Interestingly, anal and rectal anomalies are associated with esophageal anomalies rather more frequently than would be expected by chance.

CLASSIFICATION (FIG. 7.17)

In 1908 Keith (168) made the first attempt to classify the anomalies previously lumped together as "imperforate anus," but he had insufficient material for the task. In 1934 Ladd and Gross (169) proposed a system that is still in wide use in the United States. It is convenient and simple, but it cannot indicate the complex relationships now

known to occur. Gough (171, 172) in England and Santulli and his colleagues (172) in the United States proposed more complete classifications, basing them on whether the rectum terminates above or below the puborectalis sling.

Stephens and Smith (173) organized an international workshop at the Wingspread Convention Center in Wisconsin in 1984, and a new classification was presented which is much better from a surgical and topographicoanatomic standpoint. At this meeting, the anomalies were grouped as high, intermediate, low cloacal, and rare (Table 7.4).

In the high lesions, the rectum ends above the pelvic diaphragm (supralevator) and may or may not have a fistula to the genitourinary tract. In males there is usually a fistula to the prostatic urethra, and in females there is usually a rectovaginal pelvic diaphragm (partially translevator). There also is usually a fistula extending from the rectum through the pelvic diaphragm to the distal genitourinary tract. In males this results in a rectobulbourethral fistula; and in females, a rectovestibular fistula or a low rectovaginal fistula. Occasionally a fistula may not be present. In the low lesions the rectum has penetrated the pelvic diaphragm (fully translevator) but has not penetrated the skin at the normal anal location. In males this results in an anocutaneous fistula with the fistula opening anywhere along the median raphe. In females, an anocutaneous fistula also can be present anywhere along the midline of the perineum up to the level of the vestibule, in which case an anovestibular fistula is present. A cloacal anomaly is a rare condition found only in female infants, in which the rectum, urethra, and vagina have joined to form a common channel which empties through a single perineal orifice. These are complex anomalies and may be associated with other serious genitourinary tract anomalies such as a hydrometrocolpos.

The most important point, from a surgical point of view, is to distinguish true low anomalies from those which have not penetrated the pubo-rectalis sling—i.e., "high." The low anomalies can be treated with a perineal anoplasty in the newborn period. All other lesions—or if there is any doubt about the type of lesion with which one is dealing—require a diverting colostomy as the initial treatment followed by a subsequent pull-through procedure at a later date.

ANATOMY

The anatomy of the abnormal pelvis associated with anorectal congenital anomalies is not well known. There are very few dissections of babies with these defects.

Peña (174) was correct when he stated that evaluations from a clinical and functional standpoint are observed after the repair of the congenital anomaly and not before.

Peña presents the following general characteristics. (*a*) The striated mass distal to the defect is practically a mid-

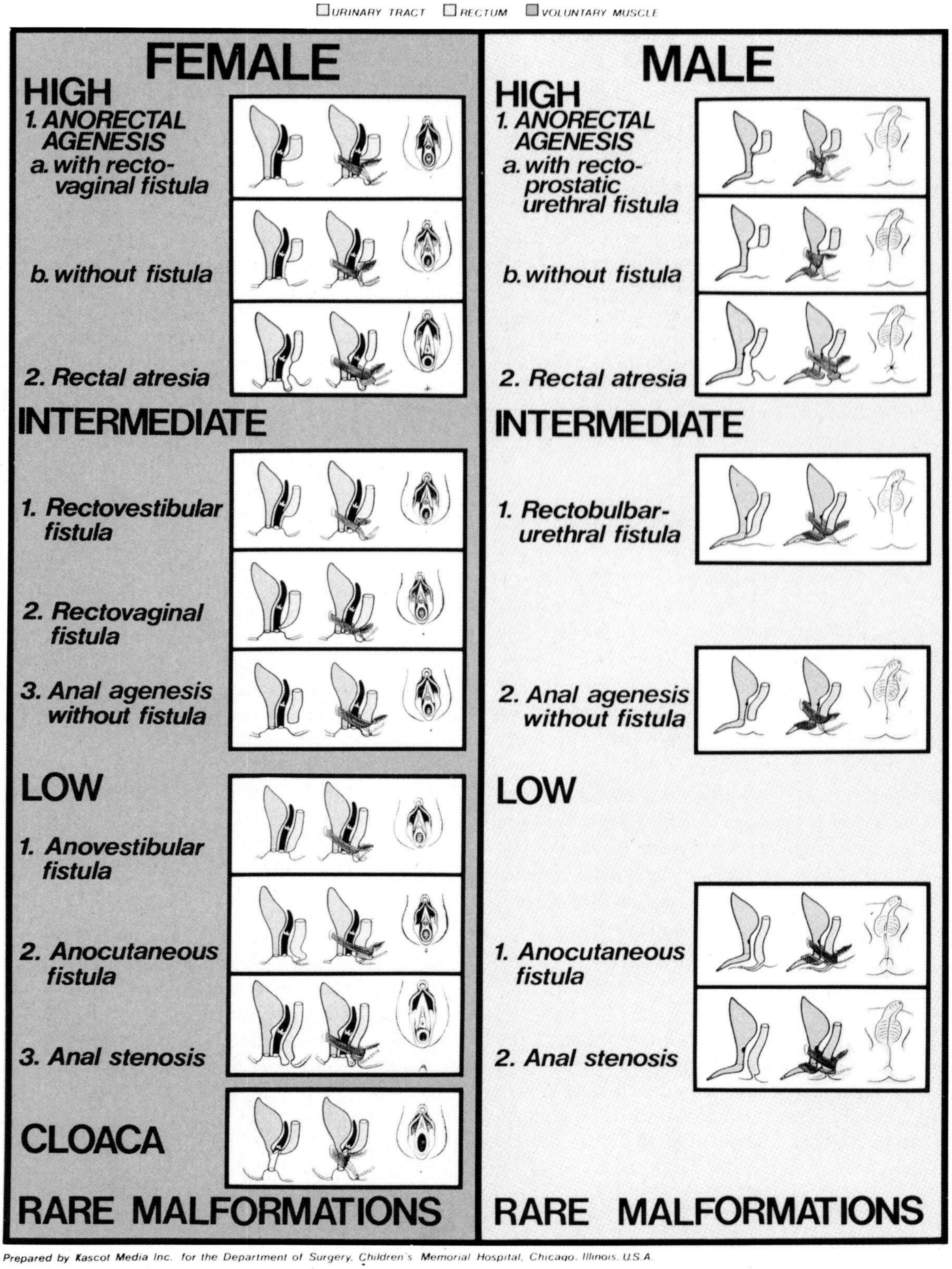

Figure 7.17. Classification of anorectal malformations—1984. (From Raffensperger JG, ed. Swenson's pediatric surgery, 5th ed. Norwalk, CT: Appleton & Lange, 1990. Prepared by Kascot Media, Inc., for the Department of Surgery, Children's Memorial Hospital, Chicago, IL.)

Table 7.4.
Anatomical Classification of Anorectal Malformations[a]

Female	Male
High	High
Anorectal agenesis	Anorectal agenesis
With rectovaginal fistula	With rectoprostatic urethral fistula[b]
Without fistula	Without fistula
Rectal atresia	Rectal atresia
Intermediate	Intermediate
Rectovestibular fistula	Rectobulbar urethral fistula
Rectovaginal fistula	Anal agenesis without fistula
Anal agenesis without fistula	
Low	Low
Anovestibular fistula[b]	Anocutaneous fistula[b]
Anocutaneous fistula[b,c]	Anal stenosis[b,d]
Anal stenosis[d]	
Cloacal malformations[e]	
Rare malformations	Rare malformations

[a]From Templeton, O'Neill. In: Swenson's pediatric surgery, 1990.
[b]Relatively common lesion.
[c]Includes fistulae occurring at the posterior junction of the labia minora often called "fourchette fistulae" or "vulvar fistulae."
[d]Previously called "covered anus."
[e]Previously called "rectocloacal fistulae." Entry of the rectal fistula into the cloaca may be high or intermediate, depending on the length of the cloacal canal.

line solid mass, thin laterally, with its length depending up to high or low defect. High defects have poor muscular development. Lambrecht and Lierse (175) stated that the internal sphincter is present. (*b*) Blood supply as well as sensory innervation are terra incognita.

Anal Defects.
In these patients the defect is confined to the anal canal. The rectum passes through the puborectalis sling and the pelvic floor.

Anal Stenosis (Fig. 7.18, A). Some slight stricture of the rectum is present in 25 to 33% of newborn infants. Brown and Schoen (176) found a stricture on digital examination in 39% of infants examined. Only about 25% of these showed any evidence of interference with normal evacuation. In all but one of their patients, the stricture dilated spontaneously between 3 and 6 months of age. Greater stricture results in constant unrelieved difficulties in evacuation: The stricture does not spontaneously dilate. Browne (177) described the most extreme form, in which the opening is so small that only an occasional small drop of meconium marks the orifice. The presence of such an opening, however small, indicates that a normal sphincter mechanism exists. Bill and his colleagues (178) suggest that some cases of Hirschsprung's disease have been confused with the colonic distension resulting from moderate stenosis of the anus.

Membranous Atresia (Covered Anus) (Fig. 7.18, B).
A membrane of skin separates the blind end of the anal canal from the surface. The membrane is thin enough to bulge on straining, and it appears blue from the presence of meconium behind it. This defect is very rare: Browne (177) and Bill and his associates (178) have denied its existence.

Most of the defects usually classified here have a perineal opening and are discussed with the "covered anus" group.

Anal Agenesis.
This group includes defects of Ladd and Gross type 3 (169), in which the rectum extends below the puborectalis sling (Fig. 7.18 *C* and *D*). It may end blindly, but more often there is an ectopic opening or fistula to the perineum anterior to the location of the normal anus, to the vulva of the female, or to the urethra of the male. The perineal fistula may be visible just beneath the skin as a blue line extending anteriorly from the covered anus. The sphincter is present at the normal site, regardless of the location of the ectopic orifice.

By definition, in anal agenesis the end of the bowel passes through the puborectalis sling. The sling itself may be higher than in a normal individual although it does not lie above the pubococcygeal line. Kiesewetter and Nixon (179) observed that there is usually a gap of as much as 2 or 3 cm between the sling and the external sphincter in patients with anal agenesis.

Anorectal Defects. These anomalies, in which the colon ends above the puborectalis sling, were also included in type 3 defects of Ladd and Gross. The fistula in the female extends below the sling.

Anorectal Agenesis (Fig. 7.19, A to C).
In this, the most common type of "imperforate anus," the anus is represented by a dimple and the rectum ends well above the surface. The anal sphincter is normal. The rectal ending may be blind, but in most cases a fistula or a fibrous remnant of a fistula extends to the urethra in the male or to the vagina or posterior vaginal fornix in the female. More males than females are affected.

Anorectal agenesis with rectovestibular fistula (Fig. 7.19, *B*) must be distinguished from ectopic vulvar anus. In the former, the rectum ends above the puborectalis sling and the fistula follows the posterior vaginal wall to open in the vestibule. In anovulvar ectopia, the rectum passes through the sling to the end closer to the surface. The fistula passes anteriorly to reach its ectopic opening (Figs. 7.19).

Rectal Atresia ("High Atresia").
In rectal atresia, both the anal canal and the rectum are present but are separated from each other by an atretic portion (Figs. 7.20). While clinically associated with the other anorectal defects, these atresias belong embryologically with other atresias of the large intestine (page 246). They are the most caudal of the hindgut atresias.

Persistent Cloaca. This is a rare condition found in female infants in which the rectum, urethra, and vagina have a common opening to the outside (Fig. 7.21, *B*). The anorectal defect resembles anal ectopia to the vagina, but the anomaly is much more extensive and represents an additional malformation of the urogenital sinus that began at an earlier stage. Other severe anomalies usually are present (180–182).

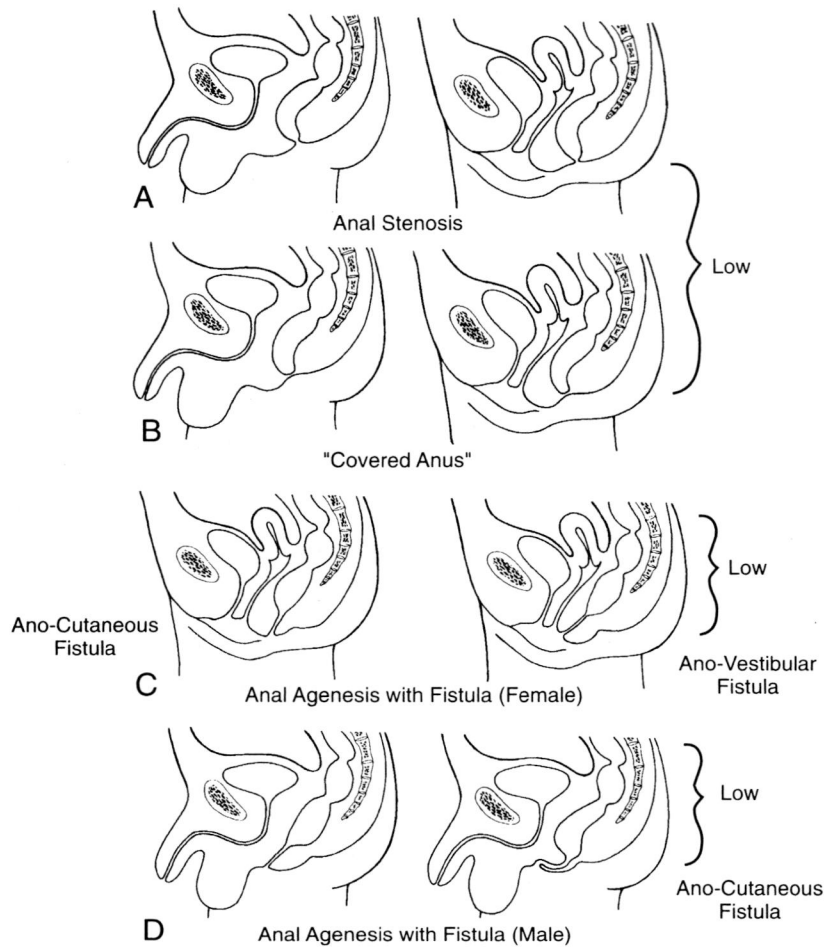

Figure 7.18. Types of anal ("low") defects.

RELATIVE INCIDENCE

Anal and anorectal defects occur in roughly the proportions given in Table 7.5. The incidence of anal stenosis probably is grossly underestimated. Few cases come to the attention of the surgeon; most mild cases are treated in the office or at home by simple dilation.

Anal agenesis and anorectal agenesis are not easily separated in a series based on the Ladd and Gross scheme. Where separation is possible, anal agenesis accounts for 46% and anorectal agenesis for 54% of the combined total. Over 80% of the anomalies in females are in the ectopic anus group, and 75% of those in males are anorectal agenesis.

ASSOCIATED ANOMALIES

In some series of patients with anal and anorectal anomalies, as many as 70% have other malformations (183, 184). Most frequently the skeleton and urinary tract are affected. Gross malformations of the lumbar and sacral vertebrae as well as varying degrees of sacral dysplasia and aplasia are frequently associated with functional distur-

bances of the bladder and ureter. Kidneys may be seriously damaged by vesicoureteral reflux, even at birth. Unilateral renal agenesis and crossed renal ectopias are sometimes found.

These defects are most frequently found in patients with "high" anorectal defects. When they occur in patients with "low" anal defects, it is usually in males. Females with low malformations usually are not affected (172, 185, 186).

Fleming and colleagues (187) evaluated 162 female patients with imperforate anus. In 79% there was a communicating anomaly of the anus or rectum; in 21% there was no such communication. Associated anatomic anomalies were distributed in the following percentages:

Lower urinary tract	15%
Upper urinary tract	25%
Lower genital tract	27%
Upper genital tract	35%
Other	51%

Twenty-six (16%) patients died, nineteen from associated malformations rather than from the basic anomaly.

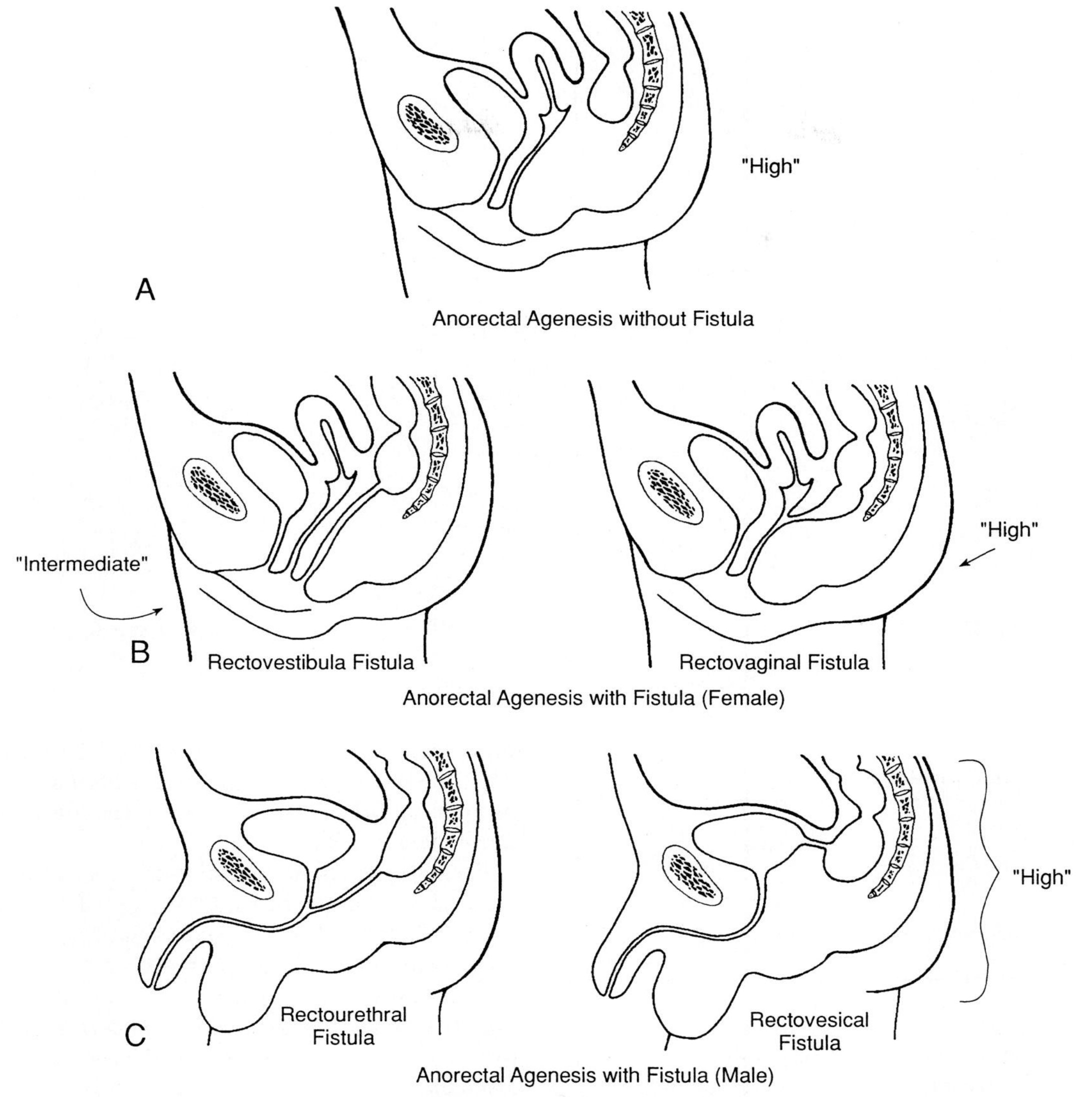

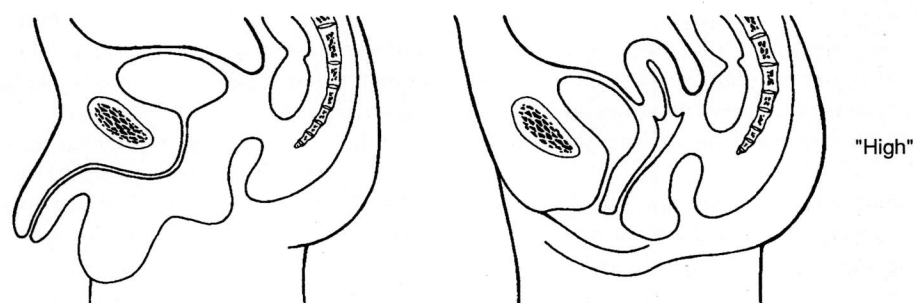

"High"

A

Anorectal Agenesis without Fistula

"Intermediate"

B Rectovestibula Fistula

"High"

Rectovaginal Fistula

Anorectal Agenesis with Fistula (Female)

C Rectourethral Fistula

Rectovesical Fistula

"High"

Anorectal Agenesis with Fistula (Male)

Figure 7.19. Types of anorectal (''high'') defects.

"High"

Figure 7.20. High rectal atresia. These forms do not arise from abnormal partition of the cloaca; they are related to other intestinal atresias.

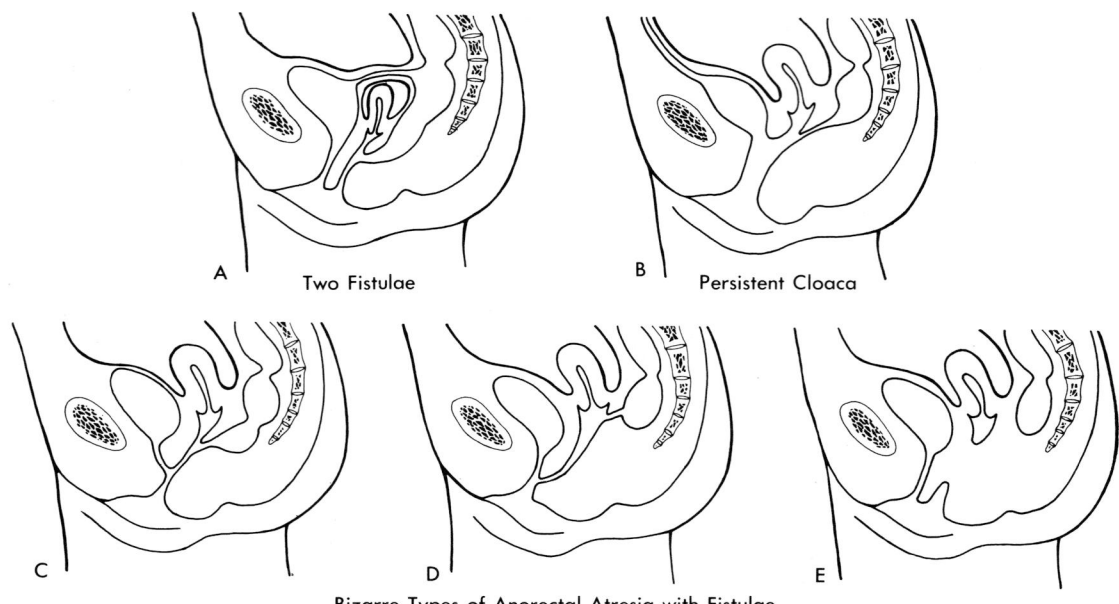

Bizarre Types of Anorectal Atresia with Fistulae

Figure 7.21.   Bizarre combinations of developmental arrests, atresias, and fistulae. All are rare. **A**, Rare. **B**, Cloaca. **C**, Cloaca. **D**, Rare. **E**, Rare.

Table 7.5.
Occurrence of Anal and Anorectal Defects

Defect	Percentage	Sex Ratio (Male/Female)
Anal stenosis	7	2.7:1
Membranous atresia	11	4.7:1
Anal agenesis and anorectal agenesis	78	1.5:1
Rectal atresia	4	3.4:1

Bowel, urinary, and renal functions were normal or nearly so in 85% of patients 13 years of age or older.

RELATIVE INCIDENCE

A review of 1142 children treated by members of the Surgical Section of the American Academy of Pediatrics for the years 1965 to 1969 revealed that 50% of males had supralevator lesions in contrast to 19% of females. Fistulae of various forms were identified in 72% of the males and in 90% of the females (188). Thus, as a general rule, females have a higher incidence of "low" anomalies, whereas males have a higher incidence of "high" anomalies. Fistulae are present in almost all cases although they may be difficult to demonstrate during the initial workup.

Cardiac, alimentary tract, and abdominal wall defects are also common. Tracheoesophageal fistula or esophageal stenosis occur in about 10% of patients with anorectal defects.

The frequent presence of other severe anomalies greatly increases the mortality among patients with imperforate anus. Among Moore and Lawrence's cases (184), 23 deaths of 50 were the result of a combination of anomalies, and in Gross's (26) series of 198 with other anomalies, 42 died.

Prematurity is not commonly associated with these anomalies. Only eight of 120 cases of Moore and Lawrence (184) were born prematurely, despite the presence of other anomalies in 86 patients.

The frequent association of *v*ertebral, *a*norectal, *ca*rdiac, *t*racheoesophageal, *r*enal, and *l*imb anomalies has given rise to the VACTERL syndrome (189, 190). These anomalies occur coincidentally more frequently than would be expected by chance alone. Thus, when an anomaly of one of these systems is present, a search must be made for anomalies in all of the other potentially affected systems (see Chapter 3, "The Esophagus").

EMBRYOGENESIS

It has been suggested that all of the anal and rectal anomalies can be traced to developmental arrest at various stages of normal maturation (191). This view explains some types of these malformations, but it cannot explain the entire series.

Duhamel (192) suggested that there is a "syndrome of caudal regression," with anorectal malformations as the mildest expression and sirenoid monsters as the most extreme. The high incidence of spinal, sacral, and lower limb defects associated with these malformations lends support to this view. At least two cases of anal stenosis have been attributed to thalidomide (193), but the relationship may be spurious.

Van Gelder and Kloepfer (194) have marshaled the evidence for familial occurrence of anorectal defects. Multiple occurrence has been reported in six family lines, one of which included a pair of identical twins. The risk in a family of a second occurrence of some form of imperforate anus has been estimated at 50 times the normal (195). This estimate is based on little evidence and is probably too high.

Anal Defects.

Anal Stenosis (Fig. 7.22, A).
Division of the cloacal closing plate into an anterior urogenital plate and a posterior anal plate by the descending

urorectal septum during the sixth to eighth weeks of fetal life normally leaves an anal plate of adequate size. A slight posterior shift in the position of the septum will reduce the size of the anal opening. Stenosis also has been attributed to excessive fusion of the anal tubercles (171); this seems to be a less probable explanation.

Membranous Atresia (Fig. 7.22, B).
Most cases of membranous atresia occur in males and probably represent excessive posterior closure of the urogenital folds (170). In some cases a band of tissue extends across the anal orifice, leaving an opening on one or both sides (196). In one case such a band crossed the

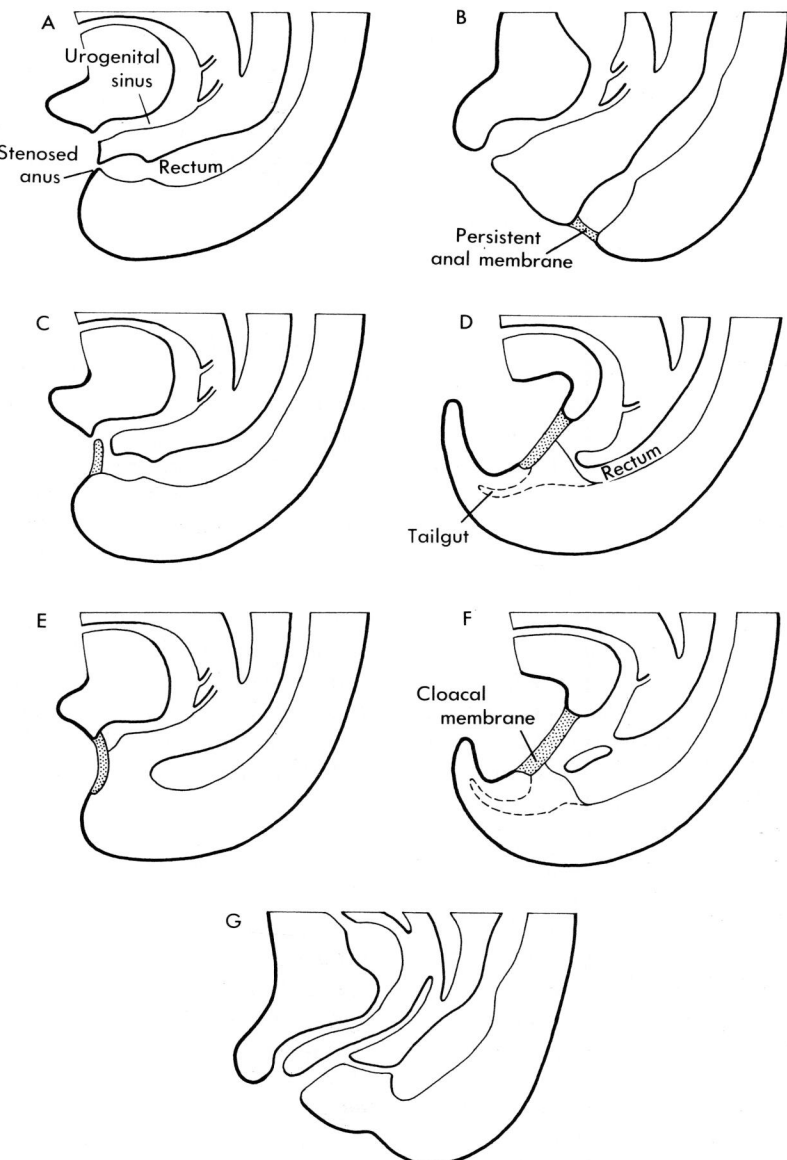

Figure 7.22. Embryogenesis of anal and anorectal defects. **A**, Anal stenosis resulting from disproportionately small anal portion of the cloacal membrane. **B**, Membranous atresia from persistent anal closing plate. **C**, Covered anus. The perineal body has not fused with the persistent cloacal plate, and a perineal fistula is present. **D** and **E**, Anorectal agenesis with and without arrested descent of the urorectal septum. **E**, Anal agenesis with failure of midline fusion of the folds forming the urorectal septum, leaving two fistulous openings. **G**, Anal agenesis with rectovaginal fistula.

dimple of an imperforate anus. Bill and Johnson (197) reviewed these cases of "congenital median bands" and suggested that the bands result from fusion of the transitory anal tubercles.

This type of atresia also has been attributed to the failure of the anal closing plate to perforate in the eighth week. If the descending urorectal septum stops just short of contact with the cloacal membrane, a fistula just beneath the skin will remain (Fig. 7.22, *C*). This is the only explanation for covered anus in the female.

Anal Agenesis with Fistula.

Anal ectopia results from arrest of growth of the urorectal septum just short of completion (Fig. 7.22, *F*). Bill et al. (198) have shown a complete series of cases with openings into the lower vagina, the fossa navicularis, and at all locations on the perineum, from near the vulva or scrotum to the normal position. All of these represent more or less retardation of perineal development during the eighth and ninth weeks. Gans and Friedman (191) emphasized the term *ectopic* and reject the term *fistula* for this opening. It is the true anus although it is displaced and often hypoplastic. In some cases its lining is normal anal epithelium (199).

Anorectal Defects.
Anorectal Agenesis.

Anorectal agenesis has been explained as the result of excessive obliteration of the embryonic tailgut and the adjacent dorsal portion of the cloaca. The descending urorectal septum reaches the dorsal wall of the diminished cloaca, leaving a blindly ending colon above and an isolated rectal membrane below (Fig. 7.22, *D* and *E*).

The fistulae associated with this malformation are of different origin from those that form an ectopic anus. The urorectal septum forms by progressive caudal fusion of two lateral ridges of the cloaca (5, 6). Fistulae represent areas in the septum where these lateral ridges have joined but failed to unite although more caudal union is complete (Fig. 7.22, *F*). The opening may be primary, or it may be a secondary rupture, resulting from pressure within the blindly ending gut after initial closure. We favor the latter view since fistulae do not occur in otherwise normal anorectal genesis. In the male these fistulae remain between rectum and urethra; in the female the descending and fusing müllerian ducts "capture" the fistula, which then becomes rectovaginal (Fig. 7.22, *G*).

High and low fistulae are thus separate defects. Vaginal and urethral fistulae with anorectal agenesis originate as early as the sixth or seventh weeks, whereas the perineal fistulae of anal ectopia arise in the eighth or ninth weeks of fetal life.

Any of the fistulae may become reduced to fibrous strands or may remain patent. In the latter case, they may be of microscopic caliber, or they may be adequate enough to empty the infant colon. Gross (28) found 50%

of fistulae present in his patients too small to prevent complete obstruction from taking place. The presence of obstruction must not be considered as evidence of the absence of fistula.

Rectal Atresia.

The position of high atresia, from 1 to 3 cm above the anal opening, has suggested to some observers that there is a proctodeal segment that forms the anal canal and that the atresia is at the site of the anal portion of the cloacal plate. The weight of evidence supports the contentions that the proctodeal contribution is no more than the anal dimple and that rectal atresia is simply a caudal colonic atresia, such as is found elsewhere in the intestinal tract.

Persistent Cloaca (Figs. 7.23 and 7.24).

In these cases development has been arrested at about the 10-mm stage, with total failure of the urorectal septum to descend. In some patients the vaginal and uterine portions of the müllerian ducts fail to develop, and the uterine tubes themselves open into the cloaca (180). We agree with Raffensperger (1) about the variations and complexity of this problem.

HISTORY

Aristotle (200) mentions imperforate anus with a rectourethral fistula in a cow (IV:4). Paul of Aegina (201), a seventh century Byzantine physician, usually is credited with having successfully incised the perineum of an infant without an anus, but we have not traced the source of this story. In his own writings, Paul speaks of rupturing an anal membrane with the fingers. His remark implies that this was already a recognized procedure.

Morgagni (202) mentions a number of 16th and 17th century cases, including rectovaginal and rectourethral fistulae. He describes several unsuccessful operations—and at least one successful one—on infants with true imperforate anus. The first recorded U.S. operation was performed in Flemingsburg, Kentucky, in 1899 by Campbell (203). The defect was an anorectal atresia without fistula, and the child was living 3 months after the operation.

Although a number of successful operations for this condition were performed in the 18th century, the first real progress took place in 1835 when Amussat (204) emphasized the necessity of mucosal continuity with the skin and described dissection of the perineum, mobilization of the end of the rectum, and suture of the mucosa to the skin without tension. If the rectum could not be brought down, Amussat resected the coccyx to bring the skin up.

Until radiography became available, the greatest problem was still that discussed by Morgagni (202): How far from the perineum is the blind end of the rectum? Chassaignac in 1856 inserted a sound through a colostomy to

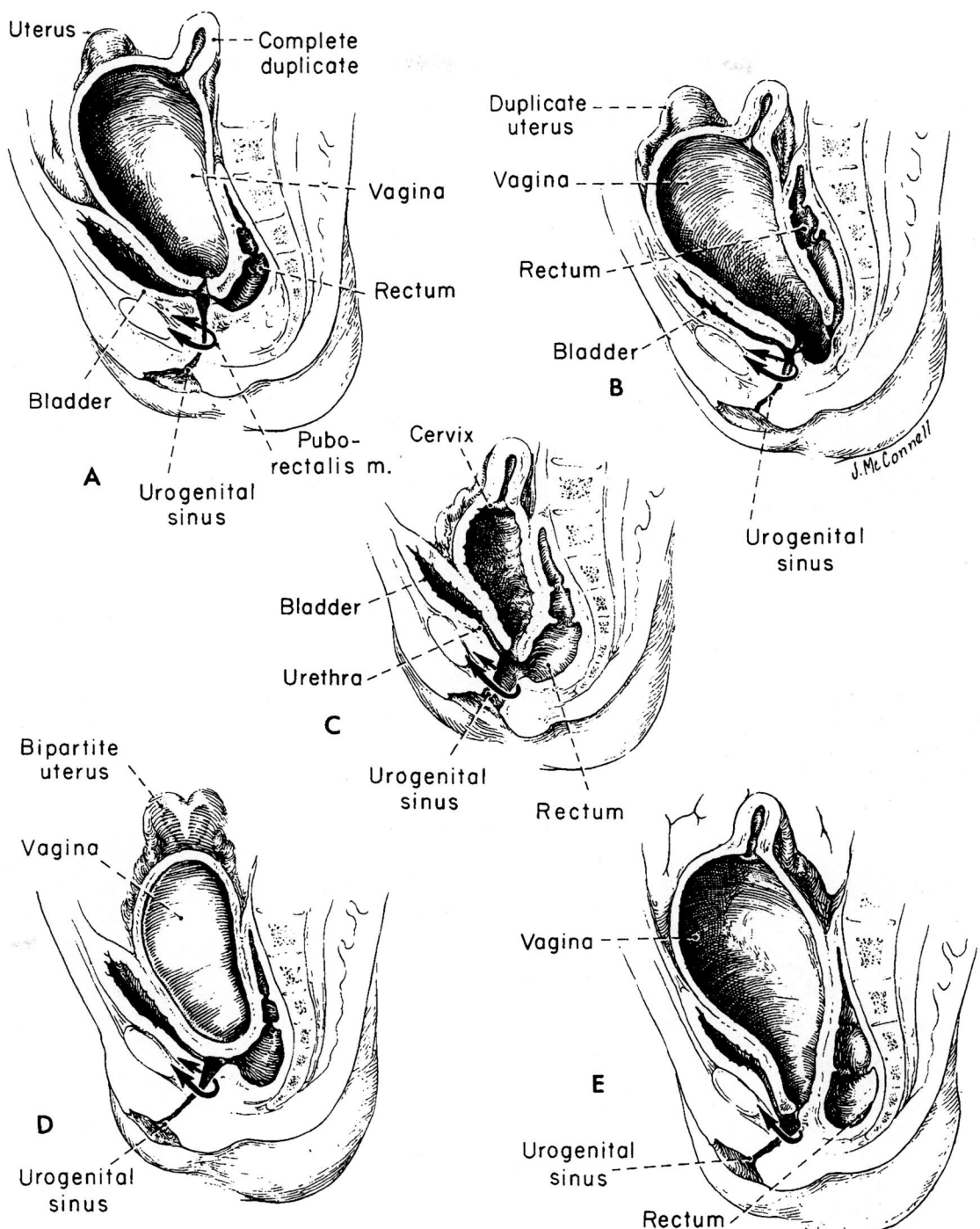

Figure 7.23. **A** through **E**, Five cloacal anomalies that vary in the height of the insertion of the rectum into the vagina (also called urogenital sinus). In each of these defects the puborectalis surrounds the urogenital sinus. The vagina is invari-ably septate with either bipartite or duplicate uterus. (From Raffensperger JG, ed. Swenson's pediatric surgery, 5th ed. Norwalk, CT: Appleton & Lange, 1990.)

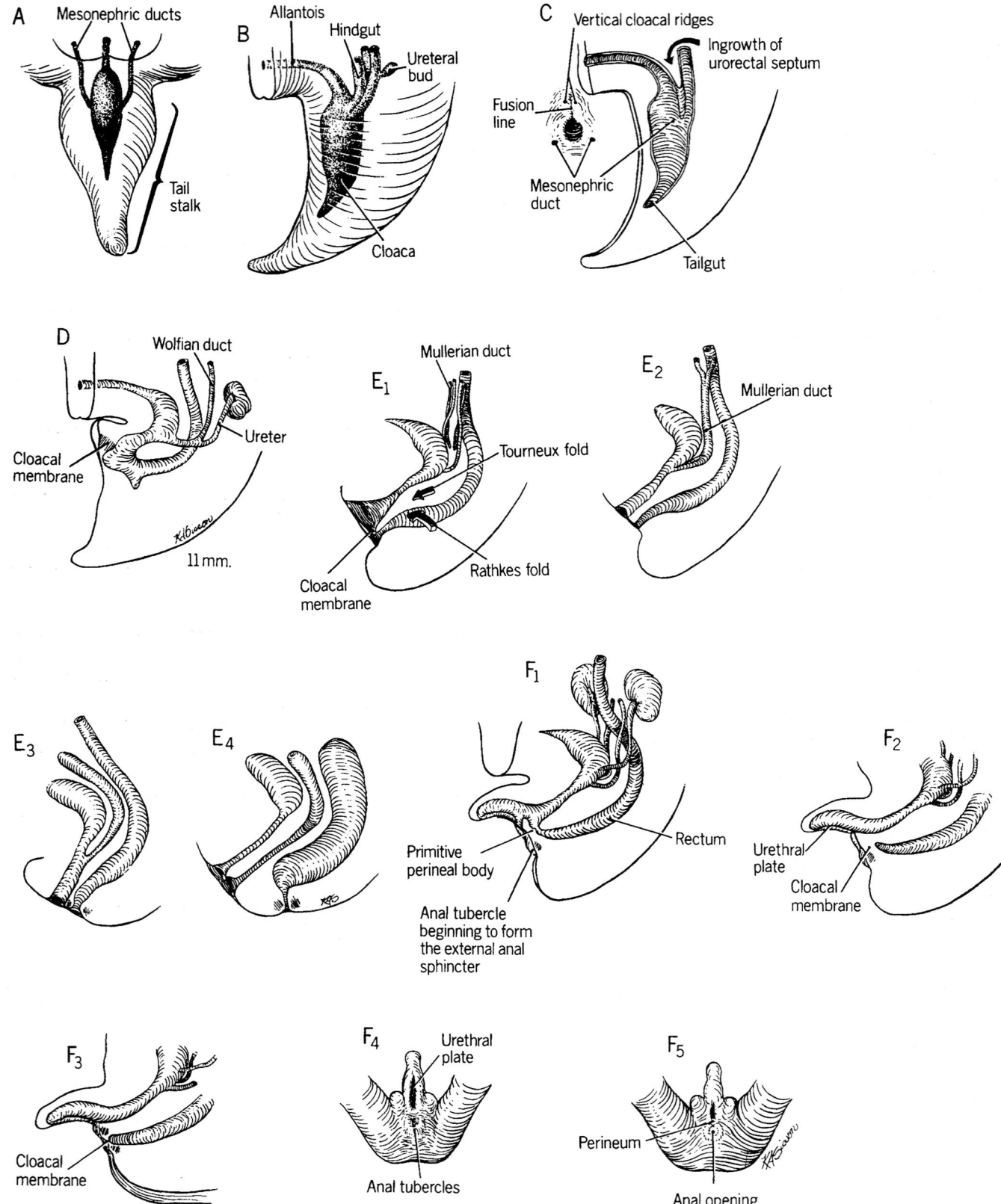

Figure 7.24. Normal anorectal embryology, illustrating the separation of the cloaca into the urogenital system and the rectum. The anus forms on the perineum from the anal tubercles. (From Raffensperger JG, ed. Swenson's pediatric surgery, 5th ed. Norwalk, CT: Appleton & Lange, 1990.)

locate the blind end and to hold it against the perineum (205).

Bodenhamer (206) in 1860 collected 287 cases of anorectal defects; he provided the first classification. He was able to record 87 relatively successful operations up to 1855. Matas (205) wrote the first thorough paper in the U.S. literature in 1897, advocating the Amussat procedure in treatment.

INCIDENCE

Anorectal defects are easily recognized and show symptoms soon after birth, hence their incidence is well documented. However, the figures obtained usually exclude the anal stenosis group, which is large, and the persistent cloaca group, which is negligible.

Reported Series	Total Births
Liverpool, 1923–1932 (207)	1:3575
Indianapolis (184)	1:4500
Pennsylvania 1951–1955 (208)	1:9630
Michigan, 1958 (147)	1:4780
New York (209)	1:3500
	Hospital Admissions
Boston, 1908–1932 (169)	1:7500
Pittsburgh, 1946–1956 (210)	1:1000

With the exception of the low incidence in Ivy's Pennsylvania series, most of the values indicate a frequency of from 0.02 to 0.03% of births.

Santulli et al. (188) reviewed 1142 children for the years 1965 to 1969 with the following analysis:

661 males—328, or 50%, had high lesions; 72% with fistulae
481 females—90, or 19%, had low lesions, 90% with fistulae

Remember, this paper was presented prior to the newly accepted classification which was reported in 1986 by Stephens and Smith (172).

Recently, Raffensperger (1) presented the frequency of anorectal anomalies in Table 7.6.

Table 7.6.
Anorectal Anomalies: Children's Memorial Hospital, 1970—1986[a]

Males		Females	
Low	53	Low	49
Intermediate	6	Intermediate	14
High	73	High	7
		Cloaca	14
Total	132		
		Total	84

[a]From Raffensperger JG, ed. Swenson's pediatric surgery. Norwalk, CT: Appleton & Lange, 1990.

Hasse (211) gave the incidence of associated anomalies with anorectal malformations (Table 7.7). Belman and King (212) gave the incidence of urinary tract anomalies associated with imperforate anus (Table 7.8).

SIGNS AND SYMPTOMS

Symptoms are those of partial or complete obstruction. Meconium may be present in urine or vagina. Distension appears within the first day, followed by vomiting; the vomitus becomes bile stained. Respiratory embarrassment may be produced by the distension.

DIAGNOSIS AND TREATMENT

The diagnosis of any anorectal anomaly is simply made by inspecting the perineum and performing a digital rectal examination. A digital examination is necessary to diagnose rectal atresia where a normal-appearing anal opening will be present. The critical element in diagnosis is determining which type of anomaly—"high," "intermediate," or "low"—is present. This is critical since the initial treatment depends on the precise diagnosis of the level of the lesion. Hence, diagnosis and treatment go hand in hand.

Peña (174) provides a decision-making algorithm for the management of anorectal malformations in males (Fig. 7.25) and in females (Fig. 7.26). Remember that the essential aspect of diagnosis is to determine whether the lesion is low, intermediate, or high. A low lesion can be treated in the newborn period with some type of anoplasty without the need for a colostomy; all other lesions require an initial diverting colostomy.

In most cases involving males (Fig. 7.25) careful perineal inspection and a urinalysis will determine whether the lesion is low, intermediate, or high. If the patient has a perineal fistula, a bucket-handle deformity, a fistula to the perineum, or an anal membrane, the diagnosis is that

Table 7.7.
Incidence of Associated Anomalies in 1420 Patients with Anorectal Malformations[a]

Type or Location of Defect	Number of Patients	Percentage
Urogenital	278	19.7
Extremities and spine	188	13.1
Cardiovascular	113	7.9
Gastrointestinal	89	6.0
Esophageal atresia and esophagotracheal fistula	65	5.6
Abdominal wall	28	1.9
Hare lip and cleft palate	23	1.5
Mongolism	22	1.5
Meningomyelocele	7	0.4
Others	114	8.2

[a]From Hasse W. Associated malformations with anal and rectal atresia. Prog Pediatr Surg 1976;9:100.

Table 7.8.
Anomalies Associated with Anorectal Malformations at Children's Memorial Hospital, 1970–1977[a]

Type and Number of Malformations	Associated Anomalies and Number of Patients	Type and Number of Malformations	Associated Anomalies and Number of Patients
Male		Female	
Low lesions (1)	Inguinal hernia (2)	Low (13)	Duplication of genitalia, absent kidney (1)
	Hypospadius (2)		Duplication of genitalia, epispadias (1)
	Bilateral ureteral reflex (1)		TEF (1)
Intermediate (4)	Prune belly, megaurethra, open urachus (1)		Aganglionosis, distal bowel (1)
	Severe gastroesophageal reflux, ureteral reflux (1)		VSD, subaortic stenosis (1)
High (29)	Ureteral reflux (3)		Hemisacrum, neurogenic bladder (1)
	Bilateral renal dysplasia (1)	Intermediate (8)	Ureteral reflux (unilateral) (1)
	Dysplasia with pelvic kidney (1)		Hydronephrosis, neurogenic bladder, esotropia (1)
	Absent kidney (1)		PDA (1)
	Absent kidney, VSD, bilateral clubfeet (1)	High (rectovaginal) (3)	Bicornuate uterus (1)
	Ureteral reflux, TEF, VSD, clubhand (1)		Absent kidney (1)
			Absent kidney, hemisacrum (1)
	TEF (1)	Cloacal (7)	Pseudotruncus absent radius (1)
	Dislocated hips (1)		Absent kidney (1)
H type (1)	Urethral stricture (1)		Ureterouterine fistula (1)
			Bilateral ureteral reflux (1)
			Unilateral ureteral reflux (1)

[a]Belman AB, King LR. Urinary tract abnormalities associated with imperforate anus, J Urol 1972;108:823. Reprinted in Raffensperger JG, ed. Swenson's pediatric surgery, 5th ed. Norwalk, CT: Appleton & Lange, 1990.
PDA, patent ductus arteriosus; *TEF*, tracheoesophageal fistula; *VSD*, ventricular septal defect.

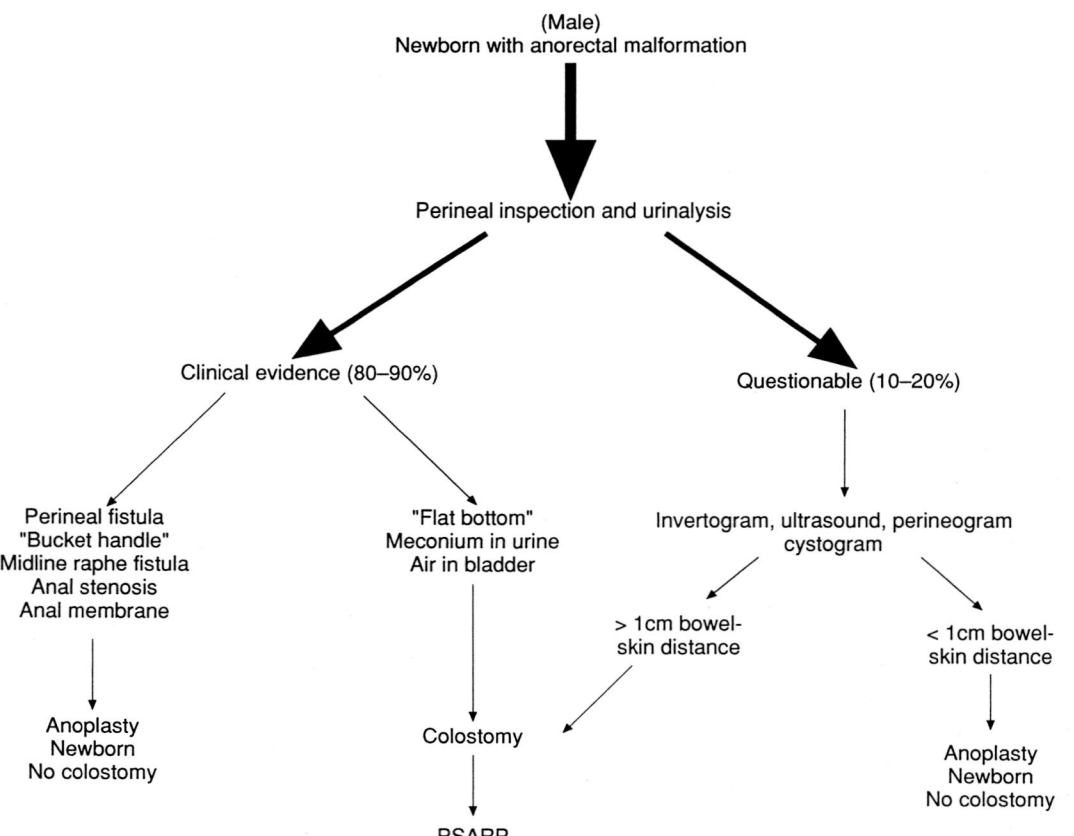

Figure 7.25. Decision-making algorithm for the management of male patients. (Adapted from Peña A. Atlas of surgical management of anorectal malformations. New York: Springer-Verlag, 1990.)

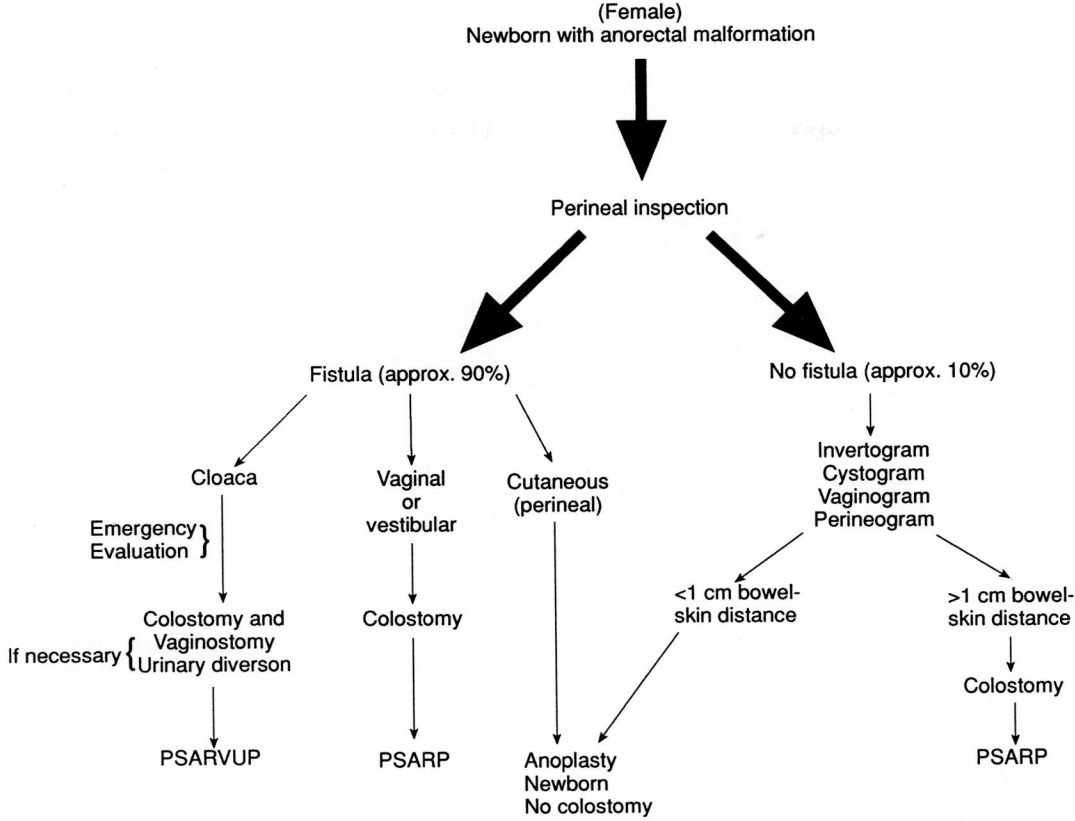

(Female)
Newborn with anorectal malformation

Perineal inspection

Fistula (approx. 90%)

No fistula (approx. 10%)

Cloaca

Vaginal
or
vestibular

Cutaneous
(perineal)

Invertogram
Cystogram
Vaginogram
Perineogram

Emergency
Evaluation }

<1 cm bowel-
skin distance

>1 cm bowel-
skin distance

If necessary { Colostomy and
Vaginostomy
Urinary diverson

Colostomy

Colostomy

PSARVUP

PSARP

Anoplasty
Newborn
No colostomy

PSARP

Figure 7.26. Decision-making algorithm for the management of female patients. (Adapted from Peña A. Atlas of surgical management of anorectal malformations. New York: Springer-Verlag, 1990.)

of a low lesion which can be treated with a perineal anoplasty. If there is no gluteal crease or if there is meconium or air in the urine or bladder, then a rectourethral fistula must exist, and therefore the patient has an intermediate or high anomaly and is treated initially with a colostomy. If careful clinical examination and the urinalysis do not differentiate between a high and low lesion, then various radiologic examinations—such as the invertogram (Fig. 7.27) (213), ultrasound, or direct injection of the rectal pouch through the perineum—can be performed (Figs. 7.28 and 7.29). If these evaluations reveal a low lesion, then an anoplasty is performed; if the lesion is anything other than a low lesion, then a colostomy is performed. At a later date the definitive pull-through procedure (posterior sagittal anorectoplasty) is performed (see description to follow).

In females (Fig. 7.26) careful perineal inspection will usually locate a fistula which then will determine which type of initial treatment is appropriate. If a cloaca is present (single perineal orifice) or if the rectal fistula goes to the vagina or vestibule, a colostomy is performed. If the fistula opens out onto the perineum, then an anoplasty can be performed. If no fistula is present, then an invertogram, cystogram, vaginogram, or perineogram can be

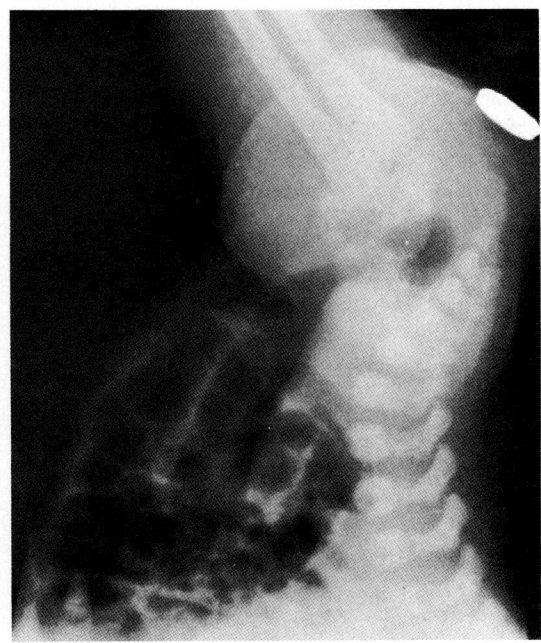

Figure 7.27. Anorectal atresia. The film was made with the infant held upside down. A metallic marker indicates the normal site of the anus. Air outlines the distal end of the colon.

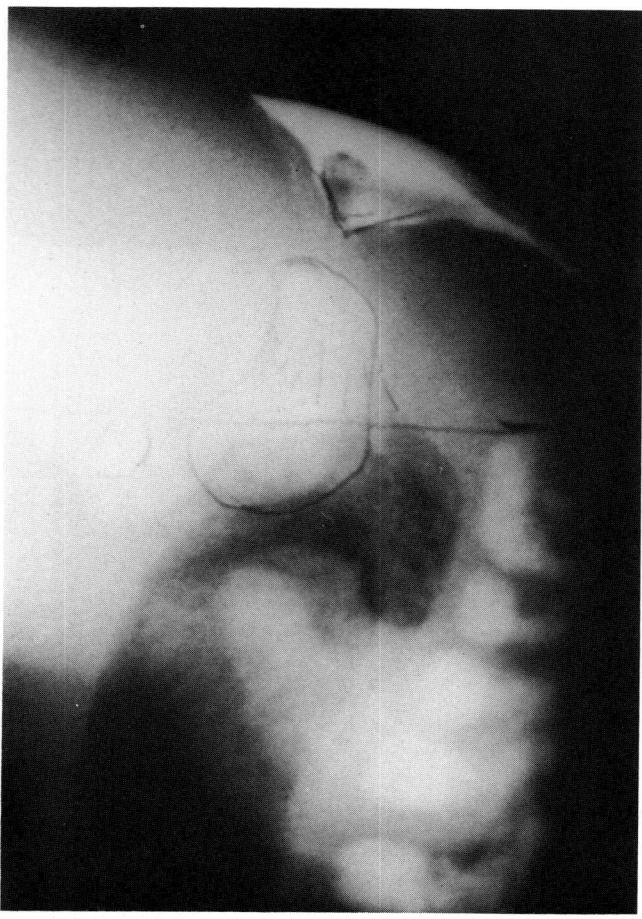

Figure 7.28. Wangensteen-Rice invertogram demonstrating a "high" anorectal malformation.

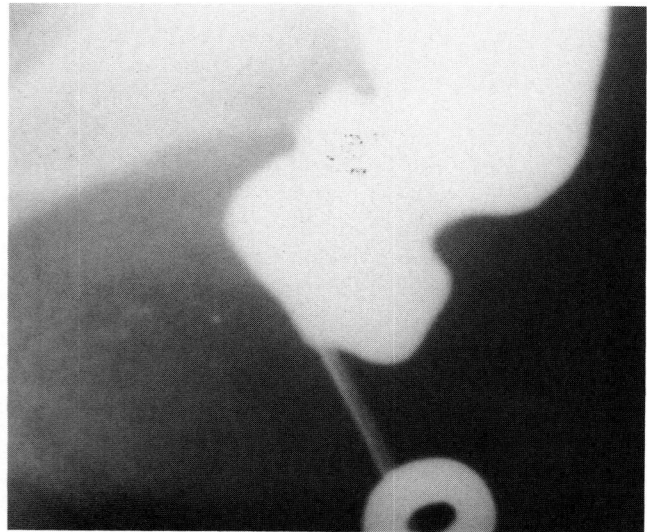

Figure 7.29. Direct rectal pouch injection with contrast material, demonstrating a "low" anorectal malformation.

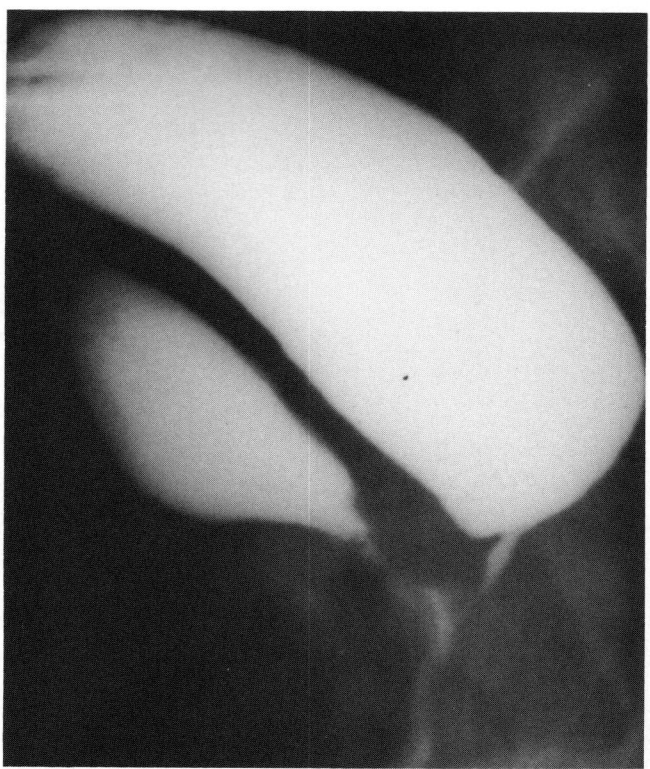

Figure 7.30. Voiding cystourethrogram demonstrating "high" anorectal malformation in a male with a rectourethral fistula.

performed and the appropriate treatment decided upon according to the findings therefrom.

Coincident with the diagnosis of the anorectal malformation, a search for other co-existing anomalies must ensue. An oral gastric tube should be passed to rule out tracheoesophageal anomalies. A renal ultrasound should be performed to evaluate the status of the upper urinary tracts, to look for ectopic kidneys, or to document renal agenesis. Voiding cystourethrograms are performed to further evaluate the genitourinary tract and to help localize any rectourethral fistula which may be present (Figs. 7.30 and 7.31). Radiographic films of the entire spine, particularly the lumbosacral spine, are indicated to discover vertebral abnormalities. Abnormalities of the sacrum, including lateral deviation, absence of sacral vertebrae, and complete sacral dysgenesis, are prognostic with respect to future continence of stool. If more than three segments are missing, it is unlikely that the patient will ever obtain voluntary control of his or her bowel movement.

TREATMENT

The surgical treatment of anal and anorectal defects is one of the most demanding operations the pediatric surgeon is called upon to perform. To preserve life, it is

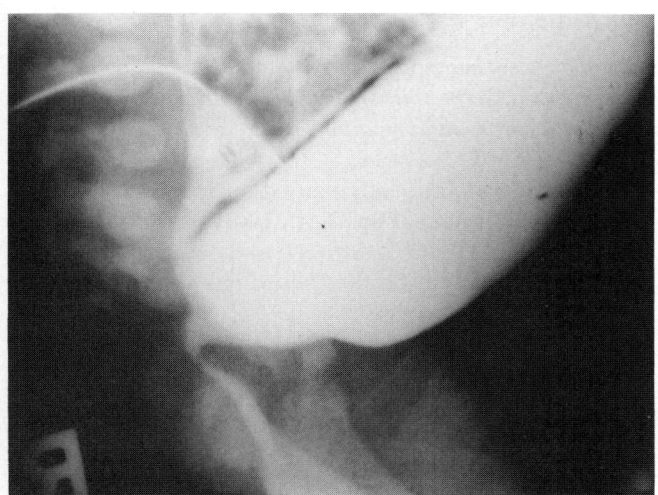

Figure 7.31. Voiding cystourethrogram demonstrating "high" anorectal malformation with a rectovesical fistula and agenesis of the sacrum.

often necessary to establish normal evacuation. To ensure that the life saved will not be one of continuous misery, it is always necessary to establish normal control of evacuation. Further increasing the surgeon's responsibility is the axiom that the first operation is the most important for producing satisfactory results. Even the best procedure will have less satisfactory results if it follows earlier, inadequate surgery. Fortunately, colostomy can be used to relieve the obstruction while definitive surgery is planned.

Control of evacuation is not yet fully understood. Many of the sensory endings appear to lie in the wall of the anal canal in precisely the region that is absent in most patients with anorectal defects (214, 215). Duthie and his colleagues (216, 217) have shown the importance of endings in the anal skin and rectal wall. Kiesewetter and Nixon (179) stated that there may be sensory endings in the puborectalis sling. These findings suggest that the nerves of the pelvic region, especially those of the blind end of the bowel and the anal skin, must be disturbed as little as possible during surgical repair procedures.

Anal stenosis can be treated by dilation of the anal canal using Hegar dilators. The caretaker can be taught to do this at home. Other types of "low" anomalies can be treated by a cut-back anoplasty (Fig. 7.25) or by the anal transposition technique (Fig. 7.26).

"Intermediate" or "high" lesions are treated by the posterior sagittal anorectoplasty or, in the case of the cloaca, by the posterior sagittal anorectovaginourethroplasty as described by Peña and deVries (174, 218). The details of these procedures are beyond the scope of this text; the interested reader is referred to the atlas by Peña for the technical details involved (174). The essential features of these procedures is the use of electrical stimulation to identify the levator mechanism and the "striated muscle complex" (the fusion of the fibers of the external sphincter layers and the levator muscles); midsagittal skin incision which goes down to and through the anterior margin of the anus; tapering of the ectatic blind-ending rectum so that it will fit within the striated muscle complex; and precise reconstruction of the muscle complex and levator muscles around and posterior to (respectively) the pulled-through rectum. The resultant anal canal is very narrow and requires several months of dilation to achieve an adequate size to allow for the passage of stool after closure of the colostomy. The anal dilations are performed initially in the office and subsequently by the caretakers at home.

The essential steps in the posterior sagittal anorectoplasty may be found in Peña's 1990 Atlas of Surgical Management of Anorectal Malformations (174). In the 91st Annual Convention and Exhibition of the American Society of Colon and Rectal Surgeons (June 1992), Peña (219) advised a posterior sagittal approach for correction of anorectal anomalies. Peña and deVries (220) question the presence of the puborectalis sling, something which is accepted universally, especially after the work of Shafik (220–223).

RESULTS

The results in treating patients with anorectal abnormalities are graded according to the level of continence achieved. "Good" indicates continence most of the time with only occasional soiling; "fair" refers to occasional soiling but with a socially acceptable level of continence; and "poor" refers to frank incontinence. Utilizing these criteria, results of low anorectal anomalies are good in 70 to 90% of patients, fair in 10 to 23%, and poor in 0 to 7%, depending on the method of assessment (224). Utilizing the Wingspread grades of "clean," "smearing," "intermittent soiling," and "constant soiling," the results are 32, 44, 21, and 3%, respectively (224).

With respect to "intermediate" or "high" anorectal malformations, the results are good in 20 to 30% of patients, fair in 40 to 50%, and poor in 20 to 30%, depending on the scoring method used (225).

In reports published since 1960, Stephens and Smith quote a combined mortality for patients with anorectal anomalies varying from 11.1 to 34.7% (226). The cause of death in these patients is virtually always related to their associated congenital anomalies. In general, males have a mortality twice that of females for both "high" and "low" lesions. A more recent report by Raffensperger (1) cites a mortality of 5% in 216 patients treated between 1970 and 1986. Ten of the 12 deaths occurred during the neonatal period secondary to associated congenital malformations.

MORTALITY

The frequency of other severe anomalies makes mortality from anorectal defects difficult to evaluate. When the rectum lies below the pelvic floor, operative mortality is of the order of 5%. High atresia, with its greater number of associated anomalies, has a mortality of 25 to 30%.

Untreated rectal anomalies usually result in death within 8 to 10 days, although a few patients with large rectovaginal fistulae have survived to adulthood.

Cozzi and Wilkinson (227), using the following classification for neonatal patients, cite a mortality of 3.8% in group A, 3.7% in group B, and 55% in group C.

Group A: Weight over 5.5 lb with no other anomaly
Group B: Weight 5 to 5.5 lb with no other anomaly, or weight over 5.5 lb with a moderately severe associated anomaly
Group C: Weight under 4 lb with no other anomaly, or weight 4 to 5.5 lb with a severe associated anomaly

EDITIORIAL COMMENTS

The rediscovery of the posterior sagittal anorectoplasty by Peña, after some preliminary observations by Devries, has added the most recent and most helpful chapter in the management of anorectal anomalies. The bottom line is that careful identification of the pelvic structures and pull-through of the end of the rectum with division of the fistula will give the best possible anatomic and, subsequently, functional result. Nevertheless, if there is abnormal or absent innervation, or if there is missing muscular tissue, or both, then the eventual results will be compomised in function even though the anatomic relationships have been restored as nearly as possible. To paraphrase an old dictum, ''You cannot make a silk purse out of a sow's ear—unless you have a silk sow!'' (JAH and CNP).

The Appendix

"It is the duty of every physician to be mindful that, for all practical purposes, perityphlitis, perityphlitic tumor, and perityphlitic abcess mean inflammation of the vermiform appendix" (228).

Sir Frederick Treves explained appendiceal positions in the form of a clock (Figs. 7.32, 7.33 and 7.34). Wakeley (229) analyzed 10,000 postmortem cases for locations of the appendix and found the following locations and their frequency of occurrence:

Rectocecal	65.28%
Pelvic	31.01%
Subcecal	2.26%
Preileal	1.00%
Right pericolic and postileal	0.40%

Polukhin and Kuzmenko (230) reported perforative appendix in an intramesenteric location.

Kalker et al. (231) reported a 7-month-old girl with multiple anomalies and a small hymenal appendix. Morozov and Khvorostof (232) reported an appendix within the ileal mesentery.

Retroperitoneal cecum and appendix is reported by Repin and Svitich (233), and a similar case is reported by Slipchenko (234). Budd and Fouty (235) presented a family pedigree containing 16 individuals with acute appendicitis. All but one had a retrocecal appendix. Perhaps this is, according to the authors, a predisposing factor inherited as a simple dominant.

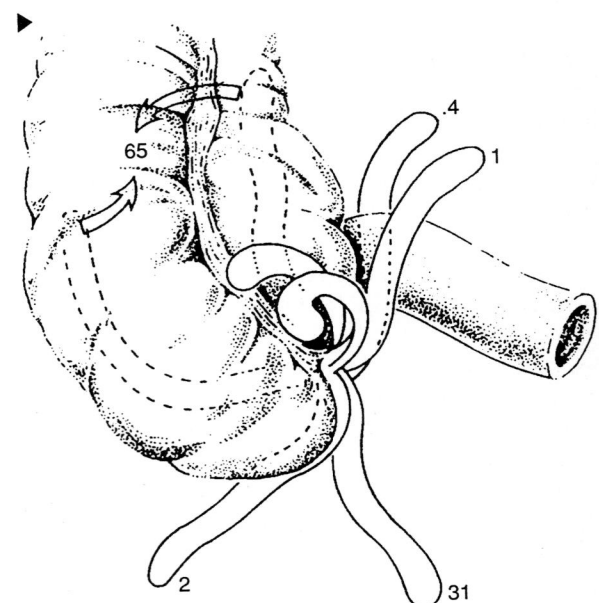

Figure 7.33. Positions of vermiform appendix. The diagram illustrates the positions the appendix may occupy in relation to the cecum and ileum, with frequencies of occurrence (%). (From Wakeley CPG. The position of the vermiform appendix as ascertained by an analysis of 10,000 cases. J Anat Physiol 1933;67:277–283.)

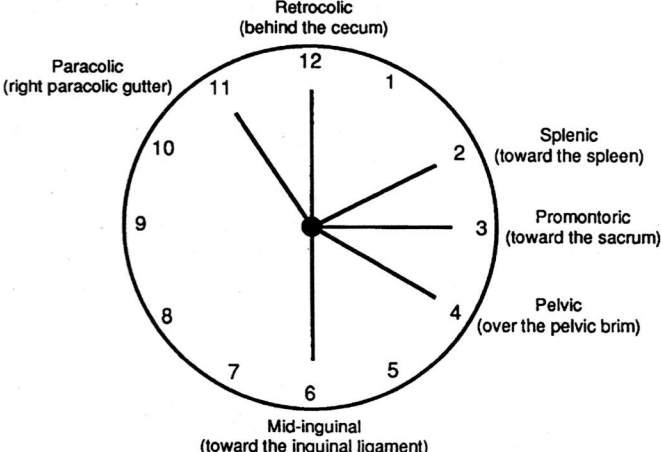

Figure 7.32. Graphic illustration of appendeceal position. (Adapted from McGregor AL, Du Plessis DJ. Synopsis of surgical anatomy, 12th ed. Baltimore: Williams & Wilkins, 1986.)

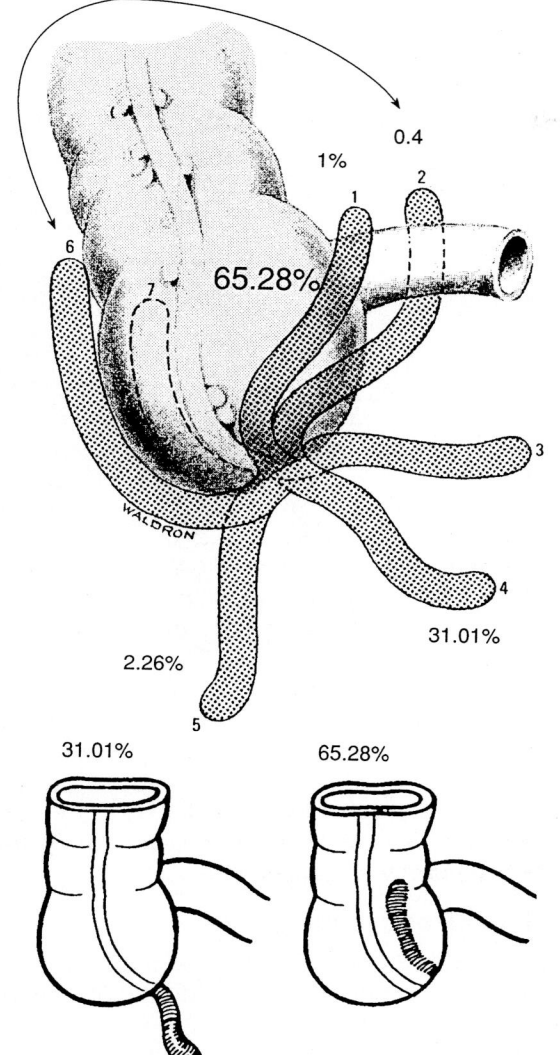

Figure 7.34. Various positions the appendix can occupy: *1*, preileal; *2*, postileal; *3*, promontoric; *4*, pelvic; *5*, subcecal; *6*, paracolic or prececal; and *7*, retrocecal. (From Maingot R. Abdominal operations, 6th ed. New York: Appleton-Century-Crofts, 1974.)

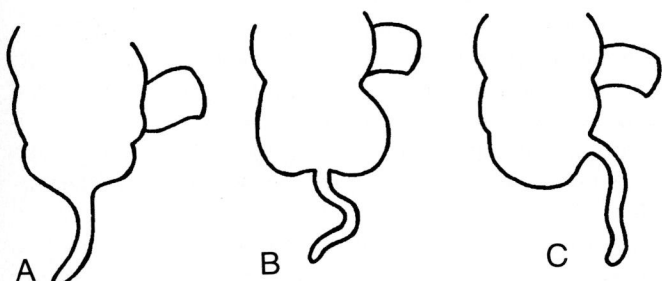

Figure 7.35. Three configurations of the appendix and cecum. **A**, and **B**, Infantile forms, which when present in an adult must be considered to be mild cases of developmental arrest. **C**, The completely mature condition and by far the most common.

VARIATIONS OF THE APPENDIX

Variations of the shape and location of the appendix were first discussed in 1827 by Melier (236). Treves in 1885 (237) described in detail the relationships among the ileum, the cecum, and the appendix. Three types of appendices are found (238) (Fig. 7.35):

1. The appendix is funnel shaped and situated at the apex of the cecum.
2. The appendix is completely demarcated and of a constant diameter, but it is still situated apically.
3. The appendix is of the adult type, situated posteromedially on the cecum, toward the ileum.

The third group included 85 to 95% of appendices encountered.

Variations in length from 0.3 to 33 cm have been reported. About 66% of appendices are between 6 and 9 cm in length; the appendix averages a few millimeters longer in the male than the female.

ABSENCE OF THE APPENDIX

Morgagni in 1719 (202) was the first and Hunter in 1762 (239) was the second to report cases of appendix absence, yet in 1895 Berry (240) denied that the condition existed, and Dorland in 1925 (241) was able to find but 34 authentic cases, exclusive of those in which the whole of the cecum was absent. Collins (242), in his series of 50,000 persons, found appendices absent in only four; he states in his thesis that there were 46 cases in the literature up to 1931. Robinson (243) found 69 cases by 1952. In spite of the apparent rarity, seven cases were reported in 1963 alone (244, 245).

Absence may result from failure of the appendix to develop during the eighth week or from failure of the appendix to lag behind the cecum in its growth. In the latter case the appendix is present without demarcation from the cecum. Schridde (246) suggested that this was the case when the cecum was composed of more than four haustra.

Absence of the appendix and cecum together is known in a few cases, such as that reported by Douglas (23), in which the entire right colon was absent. Three earlier cases are cited by Gladstone (247). Valla et al. (248) reported the absence of the appendix in a 16-year-old-female. Piquet et al, (249) stated that the frequency is about 1:100,000. Similar cases were presented by Shperber et al. (250), Shand and Bremner (251), Host et al. (252), and Piquet et al. (249).

DUPLICATION OF THE APPENDIX

Three types of appendiceal duplication have been described (253):

1. Double-barreled appendix, with a common muscularis and often a distal communication between the lumina

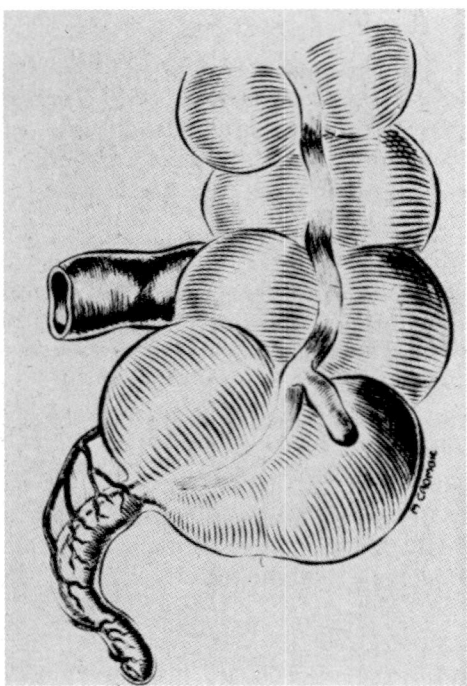

Figure 7.36. Posterolateral view of a type 3 duplication of the appendix. The supernumarary appendix arises on a tenia. (From Waugh TR. Appendix vermiformis duplex. Arch Surg 1941;42:311–320.).

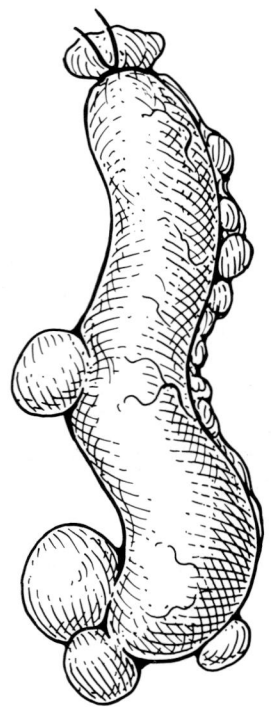

Figure 7.37. Diverticulosis of the appendix.

2. Bird-type paired appendix, in which the structures are symmetrically placed on either side of the ileocecal valve. (All such cases have been found in newborn infants who had other severe defects.)
3. Tenia coli type, with a normal appendix at the usual site and another smaller one on a tenia (Fig. 7.36)

The double-barreled type probably represents a tubular duplication similar to those found elsewhere in the large and small intestine. The paired type may represent the mildest possible case of hindgut twinning, described on page 248. The third type has been considered by Waugh (253) and Cave (252) to represent the persistence and development of the transient cecal protuberance of the sixth embryonic week, as described by Kelly and Hurdon (16). Pseudoduplication results when autoamputation following infection leaves the tip adherent to the cecum in a new location (255).

In at least three cases, Meckel's diverticulum has been stated to originate from the appendix (page 213). In one case it was histologically an appendix and almost certainly a duplication or a diverticulum (256).

In spite of the large number of appendices examined, duplication is rare. Collins (15) mentioned only five cases in 1932, and only 31 had been collected by 1945 (257). This does not include cases of duplications of the colon with double cecum, each with an appendix (page 248).

Double appendix was reported by Bonk (258). One of the appendices was in normal position, and a rudimentary one was also present.

APPENDICEAL DIVERTICULA

The appendix, like the rest of the intestine, is subject to diverticulum formation (Fig. 7.37). Stout (259) cites estimates of incidence between 0.3 and 2.2%. Diverticula are small (3 to 5 mm), may be multiple, and are usually found in adults. Almost all are primary false herniations of the mucosa through gaps in the musculature, perhaps around the entrance of blood vessels.

Royster (24) recognized seven cases of true congenital appendiceal diverticula, illustrating the case of Maloney (260). There is the possibility that in a few cases such diverticula are meckelian in origin.

Wetzig (261) presented a case, and in a 10-year study the incidence was 0.65%. Wetzig stated that he was able to collect only 43 cases of congenital origin. He advised appendicectomy when the diagnosis of diverticulosis is made since the perforation rate of an inflamed appendix with diverticula (27%) is higher than one without diverticula (6.6%).

Piattoev (262) presented a case in a 13-year-old girl, Balsano and Reynolds (263) presented a case of rupture of a true congenital diverticulum without associated appendicitis. Favara (264) reported a case with multiple diverticula.

Heterotopic Mucosa in the Appendix

Pancreatic tissue is occasionally present in the appendix (235), and there has been a single report (265) of an appendix lined distally with esophageal mucosa, having two polyps covered with gastric mucosa containing parietal cells. Unless these appendices are actually displaced Meckel's diverticula, their heterotopic mucosa is as inexplicable as is that occasionally found in the colon.

REFERENCES

1. Raffensperger JG, ed. Swenson's pediatric surgery, 5th ed. Norwalk, CT: Appleton & Lange, 1990.
2. Lynn HB, Espinas EE. Intestinal atresia: an attempt to relate location to embryologic processes. Arch Surg 1959;79:357–361.
3. Okamoto E, Ueda T. Embryogenesis of intramural ganglia of the gut and its relation to Hirschsprung's disease. J Pediatr Surg 1967;2:437–443.
4. Nowicki PT, Oh W. Perinatal intestinal circulation. In: Lebenthal E. Human gastrointestinal development. New York: Raven Press, 1989:169–182.
5. Retterer E. Sur l'origin et de l'evolution de la région ano-génitale des mammifères. J Anat Physiol 1890;26:126.
6. Stephens FD. Malformations of the anus. Aust N Z J Surg 1953;23:9–24.
7. Pegum JM, Loly PCM, Falkiner NM. Development and classification of anorectal anomalies. Arch Surg 1964;89:481–484.
8. Potter GD. Development of colonic function. In: Lebenthal E. Human gastrointestinal development. New York: Raven Press, 1989:545–560.
9. Johnson FP. The development of the mucous membrane of the large intestine and vermiform process in the human embryo. Am J Anat 1913;14:187–233.
10. Bell L, Williams L. A scanning and transmission electron microscopical study of the morphogenesis of human colonic villi. Anat Embryol 1988;165:437–455.
11. Tench EM. Development of the anus in the human embryo. Am J Anat 1936;59:333–345.
12. Smith EI, Gross RE. The external anal sphincter in cases of imperforate anus: a pathologic study. Surgery 1961;49:807–812.
13. Blechschmidt E. The stages of human development before birth. Philadelphia: WB Saunders, 1961.
14. Kelly HA, Hurdon E. The vermiform appendix and its diseases. Philadelphia: WB Saunders, 1905.
15. Collins DC. The chronic inflammatory and obliterative reactions of the appendix, in 3 volumes [Thesis]. Minneapolis: University of Minnesota, 1932.
16. Trusler GA, Mestel AL, Stephens CA. Colon malformation with imperforate anus. Surgery 1959;45:328–334.
17. Zaidi ZH. Congenital absence of most of colon. Am J Dis Child 1959;98:385–387.
18. Ashcraft KW, Holder TM. Congenital megaileocolon (basketball bowel) with teratoma. J Pediatr Surg 1966;1:178–183.
19. Kleinfelter EW. Congenital absence of the colon. Arch Dis Child 1935;50:454.
20. Blunt A, Rich GF. Congenital absence of the colon and rectum. Am J Dis Child 1967;114:405–406.
21. Morton J. Congenital absence of the colon. Br Med J 1912;1:1118–1119.
22. Bennington JL, Haber SL. The embryologic significance of an undifferentiated intestinal tract. J Pediatr 1964;64:735–739.
23. Douglas K. Congenital absence of part of the colon associated with carcinoma of colon. Br J Surg 1954;41:373.
24. Royster HA. Appendicitis. New York: Appleton, 1927.
25. Davis DL, Poynter CWM. Congenital occlusions of the intestine. Surg Gynecol Obstet 1922;34:35.
26. Gross RE. The surgery of infancy and childhood. Philadelphia: WB Saunders, 1958.
27. Sturim HS, Ternberg JL. Congenital atresia of the colon. Surgery 1966;59:458–464.
28. Powell RW. Colon atresia. In: Raffensperger JG, ed. Swenson's pediatric surgery. Norwalk, CT: Appleton & Lange, 1982.
29. Pohlson EC, Hatch EI, Jr, Glick PL, Tapper D. Individualized management of colonic atresia. Am J Surg 1988;155:6909–6912.
30. Moore TC. Atresia of the colon at the splenic flexure with absence of the distal colon and ischemic destruction of the proximal colon. J Pediatr Surg 1978;13:89.
31. Jackman S, Brereton RJ. A lesson in intestinal atresias. J Pediatr Surg 1988;23:852–853.
32. Hyde GA Jr, Delorimier AA. Colon atresia and Hirschsprung's disease. Surg 1968;69:976.
33. Peck DA, Lynn HB, Harris LE. Congenital atresia and stenosis of the colon. Arch Surg 1963;87:428–439.
34. Hartman SW, Kincannon WN, Greaney EM, Jr. Congenital atresia of the colon. Am Surg 1963;29:699–702.
35. Benson CD, Lofti MW, Brough AJ. Congenital atresia and stenosis of the colon. J Pediatr Surg 1968;3:253–257.
36. Blank E et al. "Windsock sign" of congenital membranes atresia of the colon. Am J Roentogenol Radium Therm Nucl Med 1974;120:330.
37. Chilaiditi D. Zur Frage der Hepatoptose und Ptose im allgemeinem im anschluss an drei Fälle von temporären, partieller Leberverlagerunz. Fortschr Rontgenstr Berl 1910;16:173–208.
38. Jackson ADM, Hodson CJ. Interposition of the colon between liver and diaphragm (Chilaiditi's syndrome) in children. Arch Dis Child 1957;32:151–158.
39. Werner E. Hepatic diaphragmatic interposition: Chilaiditi syndrome. Z Erkr Atmungsorgane 1984;163:198–199.
40. Davis WS, Campbell JB. Neonatal small left colon syndrome. Am J Dis Child 1975;129:1024–1027.
41. Davis WS, Allen RP, Favara BE, Slovis TC. Neonatal small left colon syndrome. Am J Roentgenol Radium Therm Nucl Med 1974;120:322.
42. Andersen DH. Pathology of cystic fibrosis. Ann NY Acad Sci 1962;93:500–517.
43. Sikirov BA. Etiology and pathogenesis of diverticulosis coli: a new approach. Med Hypotheses 1988;26:17–20.
44. Fischer JE. Segmental resection for acute and chronic diverticulitis. In: Nyhus LM, Baker RJ, eds. Mastery of surgery, 2nd ed, Vol 2. Boston: Little, Brown, 1992.
45. Wagner DE, Zollinger RW. Diverticulitis of the cecum and ascending colon. Arch Surg 1961;83:436–443.
46. Fischer AE. Fetal peritonitis. Am J Dis Child 1928;36:774–784.
47. Greaney EM, Snyder NH. Acute diverticulitis of the cecum encountered at emergency surgery. Am J Surg 1957;94:270–281.
48. Bova JG, Hopens TA, Goldstein HM. Diverticulitis of the right colon. Dig Dis Sci 1984;29:150–156.
49. Norfray JF, Givens JD, Sparberg MS, Dwyer RM. Cecal diverticulitis in young patients. Gastrointest Radiol 1980;5:379–382.
50. Chodak GW, Rangel DM, Passaro E, Jr. Colonic diverticulitis in patients under age 40: need for earlier diagnosis. Am J Surg 1981;141:699–702.
51. Mukuboh Y et al. Presentation to the International Society of Colon Rectal Surgeons. Munich, May 1982.
52. Beranbaum SL, Zausner J, Lane B. Diverticular disease of the right colon. AJR 1972;115:334–348.
53. Tan EC, Tung KH, Tan L, Wee A. Diverticulitis of caecum and

ascending colon in Singapore. J R Coll Surg Edinb 1984;29:373–376.

54. Sardi A, Gokli A, Singer JA. Diverticular disease of the cecum and ascending colon: a review of 881 cases. Am Surg 1987;53:41–45.

55. Andricopoulos PC, Christopoulos D. Congenital diverticula of the sigmoid colon. J R Coll Surg Edinb 1986;31:249–250.

56. Casarella WJ, Kanter IE, Seaman WB. Right-sided colonic diverticula as a cause of acute rectal hemorrhage. N Engl J Med 1972;286:450–453.

57. Wilkinson S. Acute solitary diverticulitis of the transverse colon in a child. Dis Colon Rectum 1988;31:574–576.

58. Halata MS, Newman LJ, Easton LB, Dove D, Stone RK. Diverticulitis in an adolescent. Clin Pediatr 1983;22:716–718.

59. Ouriel K, Schwartz SI. Diverticular disease in the young patient. Surg Gynecol Obstet 1983;156:1–5.

60. Omojola MF, Mangete E. Diverticula of the colon in three Nigerian siblings. Trop Geogr Med 1988;40:54–57.

61. Schippers E, Dittler HJ. Multiple hollow organ dysplasia in Ehlers-Danlos syndrome. J Pediatr Surg 1989;24:1181–1183.

62. Mann RW. Solitary cecal diverticulitis. Arch Surg 1958;76:527–529.

63. Stockman JM, Young VT, Jenkins AL. Duplication of the rectum containing gastric mucosa. JAMA 1960;173:1223.

64. Paddock RJ, Arensman RM. Polysplenia syndrome: spectrum of gastrointestinal congenital anomalies. J Pediatr Surg 1982;17:563.

65. Bower RJ, Sieber WK, Kiesewetter WB. Alimentary tract duplications in children. Ann Surg 1978;188:669.

66. Orr MM, Edwards AJ. Neoplastic change in duplications of the alimentary tract. Br J Surg 1975;62:269.

67. Kraft RE. Duplication anomalies of the rectum. Ann Surg 1962;155:230.

68. Martorell RA, Murphey DR. Duplications of the rectum. Am Surg 1967;33:462–466.

69. Stockman JM, Young VT, Sholes DM. Duplication of the rectum. Dis Colon Rectum 1960;3:223–229.

70. Batchelor ADR, Grieve J. Duplication of the rectum. Scott Med J 1962;7:316–318.

71. Hinckle WA. Case of double anus, vagina and uterus. JAMA 1928;90:455–456.

72. Beach PD, Brascho DJ, Hein WR, Nichol WW, Gappert LJ. Duplication of the primitive hindgut of the human being. Surgery 1961;49:779.

73. Gray AW. Triplication of the large intestine. Arch Pathol 1940;30:1215–1222.

74. Léon-Diaz. In: Ravitch MM, Scott WW. Duplication of the entire colon, bladder, and urethra. Surgery 1953;34:843–858.

75. Bornstein FP. Duplication of large intestine associated with multiple malformations. Arch Pathol 1957;75:379–380.

76. Volpe M. Dell'asta doppia. Policlinico [Chir] 1903;10:46–52.

77. Cook WH, Singer B, Frank LJ, Jr. Duplication of distal colon. Arch Surg 1960;80:650–654.

78. Montagnani CA, Pampaloni L. A case report of a posterior incomplete double monster with duplication of the spine, colon, bladder and urethra in male newborn baby. Z Kinderchir 1967;4:304–317.

79. Gould GM, Pyle WL. Anomalies and curiosities of medicine. London: Rebman Publishing, 1897.

80. Calder J. Medical essays and observations, Vol 1. Edinburgh, 1733:302.

81. Suppiger J. Bildungsfehler der weiblichen Beckenorgane. Schweiz Med Wochenschr 1876;6:418–419.

82. Ravitch MM, Scott WW. Duplication of the entire colon, bladder, and urethra. Surgery 1953;34:843–858.

83. Van Zwalenburg BR. Double colon: differentiation of cases into two groups. AJR 1952;68:22–27.

84. Ravitch MM. Hindgut duplication: doubling of colon and genital urinary tracts. Ann Surg 1953;137:588–601.

85. Van Velzer DA, Barrick CW, Jenkinson EL. Duplication of the colon: a case presentation. AJR 1956;75:349–353.

86. Mainland D. Posterior duplicity in dog with reference to mammalian teratology in general. J Anat 1929;63:473–495.

87. Bruni C. Seltene Anomalie des urogenital Organe, doppelter Penis. Z Urol 1927;21:193–195.

88. Lesbre, FX. Traité de teratologie. Paris: Vigot Fréres, 1927.

89. Peyron A. Les vestiges embryonnaires de la région sacro-coccygienne et leur rôle dans la production des kystes ou tumeurs d'origine congénitale. Bull Assoc Franç Cancer 1928;17:613–632.

90. Middeldorpf K. Zur Kenntniss der Angebornen Sacralgeschwülste. Virchow Arch [A] 1885;101:37.

91. Perry CL, Merritt JW Jr. Presacral enterogenous cyst. Ann Surg 1949;129:881–889.

92. Gwinn JL, Dockerty MB, Kennedy RLJ. Presacral teratomas in infancy and childhood. Pediatrics 1955;16:239–249.

93. Ballantyne EN. Sacrococcygeal tumors. Arch Pathol 1932;14:1.

94. Gius JA, Stout AP. Perianal cysts of vestigial origin. Arch Surg 1938;37:268–287.

95. Tucker CC, Hellwig CA. Anal ducts: comparative developmental histology. Arch Surg 1935;31:521.

96. Stone WD, Hendrix TR, Schuster MM. Aganglionosis of the entire colon in an adolescent. Gastroenterology 1965;48:636–641.

97. Lee CM, Jr, Bebb KC. The pathogenesis and clinical management of megacolon with emphasis on the fallacy of the term "idiopathic." Surgery 1951;30:1026–1048.

98. Bickler SW, Harrison MW, Campbell TJ, Campbell JR. Long segment Hirschsprung's disease. Arch Surg 1992;127:1047–1051.

99. Keefer GP, Mokrohisky JF. Congenital megacolon (Hirschsprung's disease). Radiology 1954;63:157–175.

100. Sprinz H, Cohen A, Heaton LD. Hirschsprung's disease with skip area. Ann Surg 1961;153:143–148.

101. Nixon HH. Hirschsprung's disease. Arch Dis Child 1964;39:109–115.

102. Anderson KD, Chandra R. Segmental aganglionosis of the appendix. J Pediatr Surg 1986;21:852–854.

103. Seldenrijk CA et al. Zonal aganglionosis: an enzyme and immunohistochemical study of two cases. Virchows Arch 1986;410:75–81.

104. Swenson O. Pediatric surgery. New York: Appleton-Century-Crofts, 1958.

105. Graivier L, Sieber WK. Hirschsprung's disease and mongolism. Surgery 1966;60:458–461.

106. Sherman JO et al. A 40-year multinational retrospective study of 880 Swenson procedures. J Pediatr Surg 1989;24:833–838.

107. Ikeda K, Goto S. Diagnosis and treatment of Hirschsprung's disease in Japan: an analysis of 1628 patients. Ann Surg 1984;199:400–405.

108. Dereymaeker A. Recherches expérimentales sur l'origine du systéme nerveux entérique chez l'embryon de poulet. Arch Biol (Paris) 1943;54:359–375.

109. Van Campenhout E. The epithelioneural bodies. Q Rev Biol 1946;21:327–347.

110. Yntema CL, Hammond WS. The development of the automatic nervous system. Biol Rev 1947;22:344–359.

111. Weber A. Recherches sur l'origine du plexus sympathetique de la région gastroduodenale chez l'embryon de poulet. Bull Histol Tech Micr 1940;17:149–171.

112. Bodian M, Carter CO, Ward BCH. Hirschsprung's disease (with radiological observations). Lancet 1951;1:302–309.

113. Kamijo K, Hiatt RB, Koelle GB. Congenital megacolon: a comparison of the spastic and hypertrophied segments with respect to cholinesterase activities and sensitivities to acetylcholine, DFP, and the barium ion. Gastroenterology 1953;24:173.

114. Ehrenpreis T, Livaditis A, Okmian L. Results of Duhamel's operation for Hirschsprung's disease. J Pediatr Surg 1966;1:40–46.

115. Hukuhara T, Kotani S, Sato G. Effects of destruction of intramural ganglion cells on colon motility: possible genesis of congenital megacolon. Jpn J Physiol 1961;11:635–640.

116. Siegel M, Lebenthal E. Development of gastrointestinal motility and gastric emptying during the fetal and newborn periods. In: Lebenthal E. Human gastrointestinal development. New York: Raven Press, 1989.

117. Munakata K, Okabe I, Morita K. Histologic studies of rectocolic aganglionosis and allied disease. J Pediatr Surg 1978;13:67–75.

118. Burghaighis AC, Emery JL. Functional obstruction of the intestine due to neurological immaturity. Prog Pediatr Surg 1971;3:37–52.

119. Tanner MS, Smith B, Lloyd JK. Functional intestinal obstruction due to deficiency of argyrophic neurons in the mesenteric plaxus. Arch Dis Child 1976;51:837–41.

120. Emanuel B, Gault J, Sanson J. Neonatal intestinal obstruction due to the absence of intestinal musculature: a new entity. J Pediatr Surg 1967;2:332–335.

121. Steiner DH, Maxwell JG, Rasmussen BL, Jones R. Segmental absence of intestinal musculature: an unusual cause of intestinal obstruction in the neonate. Am J Surg 1969;118:964–967.

122. Tam PK, Lister J. Development profile of neuron-specific enolase in human gut and its implications in Hirschsprung's disease. Gastroenterology 1986;90:1901–1906.

123. Okamoto E, Ueda T. Embryogenesis of intramural ganglia of the gut and its relation to Hirschsprung's disease. J Pediatr Surg 1967;2:437–443.

124. Nirasawa Y et al. Hirschsprung's disease: catacholamine content, alpha-adrenoceptors, and the effect of electrical stimulation in aganglionic colon. J Pediatr Surg 1986;21:136–142.

125. Touloukian RJ, Aghajanian G, Roth RH. Adrenergic hyperactivity of the aganglionic colon. J Pediatr Surg 1973;8:191–195.

126. Hirschsprung H. Fälle von angeborener Pylorusstenose beobachtet bei Säuglingen. Jahrb Kinderh 1988;27:61.

127. Finney JMT. Congenital idiopathic dilatation of the colon. Surg Gynecol Obstet 1908;6:624–643.

128. Treves F. Idiopathic dilatation of the colon. Lancet 1898;1:276–279.

129. Hawkins HP. Remarks on idiopathic dilatation of the colon. Br Med J 1907;1:477–483.

130. Tittel K. Uber eine angeborene Missbildung des Dickdarmes. Wien Klin Wochenschr 1901;14:903–907.

131. Dalla Valle A. Richerche istologiche su di un caso di megacolon congenito. Pediatrica 1920;28:740–752.

132. Cameron JAM. On the aetiology of Hirschsprung's disease. Arch Dis Child 1928;3:210–211.

133. Perrot A, Danon L. Obstruction intestinale de cause rare, chez un nourrisson. Ann Anat Pathol (Paris) 1935;12:157–165.

134. Etzel E. La dilatation del esofago frente a las lesiones del plexo de Auerbach en el megaesophago. Bol Trab Soc Cir Buenos Aires 1937;21:131–148.

135. Robertson HE, Kernohan JW. The myenteric plexus in congenital megacolon. Proc Mayo Clin 1938;13:123–125.

136. Whitehouse FR, Kernohan IW. Myenteric plexus in congenital megacolon. Arch Int Med 1948;82:75–90.

137. Scott WJM, Morton JJ. Sympathetic inhibition in the large intestine in Hirschsprung's disease. J Clin Invest 1930;9:247–262.

138. Bodian M, Stephens FD, Ward BCH. Hirschsprung's disease and idiopathic megacolon. Lancet 1949;1:6–11.

139. Swenson O, Bill HA, Jr. Resection of the rectum and rectosigmoid with preservation of the sphincter for benign spastic lesions producing megacolon. Surgery 1948;24:212–220.

140. Swenson O, Neuhauser EBD, Pickett LK. New concepts of the etiology, diagnosis, and treatment of congenital megacolon (Hirschsprung's disease). Pediatrics 1949;4:201–209.

141. Swenson O. A new surgical treatment for Hirschsprung's disease. Surgery 1950;28:371.

142. Duhamel B. A new operation for the treatment of Hirschsprung's disease. Arch Dis Child 1960;35:38–39.

143. Soave F. Hirschsprung's disease: a new surgical technique. Arch Dis Child 1964;39:116.

144. Boley SJ. New modification of the surgical treatment of Hirschsprung's disease. Surgery 1964;56:1015.

145. Martin LW. Surgical management of total colonic aganglionosis. Ann Surg 1972;176:343–346.

146. Kimura K et al. A new surgical approach to extensive aganglionosis. J Pediatr Surg 1981;16:840–843.

147. Hautau ER. Congenital malformations in infants born to Michigan residents in 1958. Mich Med 1960;59:1833–1836.

148. Richardson WR, Brown IH. Hirschsprung's disease in infants and children. Am Surg 1962;28:149–164.

149. Kleinhaus S, Boley SJ, Sheran M, Sieber WK. Hirschsprung's disease: a survey of the members of the surgical section of the American Academy of Pediatrics. J Pediatr Surg 1979;14:588, 597.

150. Ricketts RR, Pettitt BJ. Management of Hirschsprung's disease in adolescents. Am Surg 1989;55:219–225.

151. Rosin JD, Bargen JA, Waugh JM. Congenital megacolon of a man 54 years of age: report of a case. Proc Mayo Clin 1950;25:710–715.

152. Klein D. Un nouveau pas franchi dans le pronostic génétique do la maladie de Hirschsprung (mégacôlon congénital). J Genet Hum 1964;13:233–235.

153. Bielschovsky M, Schofield GC. Studies on megacolon in piebald mice. Aust J Exp Biol Med Sci 1962;40:395–403.

154. Soper RT, Miller FE. Congenital aganglionic megacolon (Hirschsprung's disease): diagnosis, management, and complications. Arch Surg 1968;96:554–562.

155. Campbell P, Noblet H. Experience with the rectal suction biopsy in the diagnosis of Hirschsprung's disease. J Pediatr Surg 1969;4:510.

156. Bill AH Jr, Creighton SA, Stevenson JK. The selection of infants and children for the surgical treatment of Hirschsprung's disease. Surg Gynecol Obstet 1957;104:151–156.

157. Ravitch MM. Pseudo Hirschsprung's disease. Ann Surg 1958;147:781–795.

158. Bill AH, Jr. Congenital abnormalities of colon, rectum and anus. Surg Clin North Am 1959;39:1165.

159. Grossman HJ, Limosani MA, Shore M. Megacolon as a manifestation of familial autonomic dysfunction. J Pediatr 1956;49:289–296.

160. Jung RC. Chagas' disease: possible cause of megaesophagus and megacolon. Am J Gastroenterol 1959;32:311.

161. Duhamel B. Technique chirurgicale infantile. Paris: Masson et Cie, 1957.

162. Benson CD, Lloyd JR. An evaluation of the surgical treatment of Hirschsprung's disease. Surg Clin North Am 1964;44:1495–1508.

163. Dixon CF, Judd DB. The surgical treatment of congenital megacolon. Surg Clin North Am 1948;28:889–901.

164. Edelman S, Strauss L, Becker JM, Arnheim E. Universal aganglionosis of the colon. Surgery 1960;47:667–677.

165. Hallenbeck GA, Brown PM, Waugh JM, Stickler GB. Surgical treatment of Hirschsprung's disease. Arch Surg 1961;83:928–933.

166. Gerald B. Aganglionosis of the colon and terminal ileum. AJR 1965;95:231–234.

167. Ratta BS, Kiely EM, Spitz L, Brereton RJ. Improvements in the management of total colonic aganglionosis. Pediatr Surg Int 1990;5:30–36.

168. Keith A. Malformations of the hind end of the body. Br Med J 1908;2:1736–1740.

169. Ladd WE, Gross RE. Congenital malformations of the anus and rectum: report of 162 cases. Am J Surg 1934;23:167.

170. Gough MH. Congenital abnormalities of the anus and rectum. Arch Dis Child 1961;36:146–151.

171. Partridge JP, Gough MH. Congenital abnormalities of the anus and rectum. Br J Surg 1961;49:37–50.

172. Santulli TV, Schullinger JN, Amoury RA. Malformations of the anus and rectum. Surg Clin North Am 1965;45:1253–1271.

173. Stephens FD, Smith DE. Classification, identification and assessment of surgical treatment of anorectal anomalies. Pediatr Surg Int 1986;1:200–205.

174. Peña A. Atlas of surgical management of anorectal malformations. New York: Springer-Verlag, 1990.

175. Lambrecht W, Lierse W. The internal sphincter in anorectal malformations: morphologic investigations in neonatal pigs. J Pediatr Surg 1987;22:1160–1168.

176. Brown SS, Schoen AH. Congenital anorectal stricture. J Pediatr 1950;36:746.

177. Browne D. Congenital deformities of the anus and rectum. Arch Dis Child 1955;30:42.

178. Bill AH, Jr, Johnson RJ. Failure of migration of the rectal opening as the cause for most cases of imperforate anus. Surg Gynecol Obstet 1958;106:643–651.

179. Kiesewetter WB, Nixon HH. Imperforate anus. I. Its surgical anatomy. J Pediatr Surg 1967;2:60–68.

180. Gough MH. Anorectal agenesis with persistence of cloaca. Proc R Soc Med 1959;52:886–889.

181. Stephens FD. Congenital malformations of the rectum and anus in female children. Aust N Z J Surg 1961;31:90–104.

182. Snyder WH. Some unusual forms of imperforate anus in female infants. Am J Surg 1966;111:319–325.

183. Lee MJ Jr. Congenital anomalies of the lower part of the rectum. Am J Dis Child 1944;68:182–189.

184. Moore TC, Lawrence EA. Congenital malformations of rectum and anus. II. Associated anomalies encountered in a series of 120 cases. Surg Gynecol Obstet 1952;95:281.

185. Berdon WE, Hochberg B, Baker DH, Grossman H, Santulli TV. The association of lumbosacral spine and genitourinary anomalies with imperforate anus. AJR 1966;98:181–191.

186. Pellerin D, Bertin P. Genito-urinary malformation and vertebral anomalies in anorectal malformations. Z Kinderchir 1967;4:375–383.

187. Fleming SE, Hall R, Gysler M, McLorie GA. Imperforate anus in females: frequency of genital tract involvement, incidence of associated anomalies, and functional outcome. J Pediatr Surg 1986;21:146–150.

188. Santulli TV, Schullinger JN, Kiesewetter WB, Bill A. Imperforate anus: a survey of the members of the surgical section of the American Academy of Pediatrics. J Pediatr Surg 1971;6:484.

189. Weaver DD, Mapstone CL, Yu P. The VATER association: analysis of 46 patients. Am J Dis Child 1986;140:225–229.

190. deLorimier AA, Harrison MR. Esophageal atresia: embryogenesis and management. World J Surg 1985;9:250–257.

191. Gans SL, Friedman NB. Some new concepts in the embryology, anatomy physiology and surgical correction of imperforate anus. West J Surg 1961;69:34.

192. Duhamel B. From the mermaid to anal imperforation: the syndrome of caudal regression. Arch Dis Child 1961;36:152–155.

193. Ives EJ. Thalidomide and anal abnormalities. Can Med Assoc J 1962;87:670–672.

194. Van Gelder DW, Kloepfer HW. Familial anorectal anomalies. Pediatrics 1961;27:334–336.

195. Anderson RC, Reed SC. The likelihood of congenital malformations. Lancet 1954;74:175.

196. Perry EG. Congenital median band of the anus. Aust N Z J Surg 1963;32:292–294.

197. Bill AH, Jr, Johnson RJ. Congenital median band of the anus. Surg Gynecol Obstet 1953;97:307–311.

198. Bill AH Jr, Johnson RJ, Foster RA. Anteriorly placed rectal opening in perineum, "ectopic anus": a report of 30 cases. Ann Surg 1958;147:173.

199. Scott JES. The microscopic anatomy of the terminal intestinal canal in ectopic vulval anus. J Pediatr Surg 1966;1:441–445.

200. Aristotle. Generation of animals. AC Peck (trans). Cambridge: Harvard Univ Press (The Loeb Classical Library), 1943.

201. Paul of Aegina. The Seven Books of Paulus Aegineta. Adam F (trans). London: Sydenham Society, 1846.

202. Morgagni JB. The seats and causes of disease investigated by anatomy. Alexander LB (trans). New York: Hafner Publishing, 1960.

203. Campbell JP. Case of imperforate anus. Med Repository 1802;1802:45–46.

204. Amussat JZ. Histoire d'une opération d'anus artificiel pratiquée avec succés par un nouveau procédé dans un cas d'absence congénitale de l'anus suivie de quelques réflexions sur l'obliteration du rectum. Gaz Med Paris 1935;Nov;1835.

205. Matas R. The surgical treatment of congenital anorectal imperforation considered in the light of modern operative procedure. Trans Am Surg Assoc 1897;15:453–553.

206. Bodenhamer W. A practical treatise on the aetiology, pathology and treatment of the congenital malformation of the rectum and anus. New York: SS & W Wood, 1860.

207. Malpas P. The incidence of human malformations and the significance of changes in the maternal environment in their causation. J Obstet Gynaecol Br Commw 1937;44:434–454.

208. Ivy RH. Congenital abnormalities. Plast Reconstr Surg 1957;20:400–411.

209. Davis DA. Malformations of the anus and rectum. In: Turell R, ed. Diseases of the colon and anorectum. Philadelphia: WB Saunders, 1959.

210. Kiesewetter WB. Imperforate anus. Surg Clin North Am 1956;36:1531–1544.

211. Hasse W. Associated malformations with anal and rectal atresia. Prog Pediatr Surg 1976;9:100.

212. Belman AB, King LR. Urinary tract abnormalities associated with imperforate anus. J Urol 1972;108:823.

213. Wangensteen OH, Rice CO. Imperforate anus: a method of determining the surgical approach. Ann Surg 1930;92:77.

214. Gaston EA. The physiology of fecal continence. Surg Gynecol Obstet 1948a;87:280.

215. Gaston EA. Fecal continence following resections of various portions of the rectum with preservation of the anal sphincters. Surg Gynecol Obstet 1948b;87:669–678.

216. Duthie HL, Gairns FW. Sensory nerve endings and sensation in the anal region of man. Br J Surg 1960;47:585.

217. Duthie HL, Watts JM. Contribution of the external anal sphincter to the pressure zone in the anal canal. Gut 1965;6:64.

218. deVries PA, Peña A. Posterior sagittal anorectoplasty. J Pediatr Surg 1982;17:638–643.

219. Verderese C, ed. Peña describes success, rationale for posterior sagittal approach. ASCRS Meeting Reporter, Highlights Issue. Patterson, NY: Caduceus Medical Publishers, 1992.

220. Peña A, de Vries PA. Posterior sagittal anorectoplasty: important technical considerations and new applications. J Pediatr Surg 1982;17:796–811.

221. Shafik A. A new concept of the anatomy of the anal sphincter mechanism and the physiology of defecation, the external sphincter: a triple loop mechanism. Invest Urol 1975;12:415.

222. Shafik A. A new concept of the anatomy of the anal sphincter mechanism and the physiology of defecation: III. The longitudinal anal muscle: anatomy and role in anal sphincter mechanism. Invest Urol 1976;13:271.

223. Shafik A. A new concept of the anatomy of the anal sphincter mechanism and the physiology of defecation: IV. Anatomy of the perianal spaces. Invest Urol 1976;13:424.

224. Ong NT, Beasley SW. Long-term functional results after perineal surgery for low anorectal anomalies. Pediatr Surg Int 1990;5:238–240.

225. Ong NT, Beasley SW. Comparison of clinical methods for the assessment of continence after repair of high anorectal anomalies. Pediatr Aurg Int 1990;5:233–237.

226. Stephens FD, Smith ED. Anorectal malformations in children. Chicago: Year Book Medical Publishers, 1971.

227. Cozzi F, Wilkinson AW. Congenital abnormalities of anus and rectum: mortality and function. Br Med J 1968;1:144–147.

228. Fitz R. Persistant omphalo-mesenteric remains: their importance in the causation of intestinal duplication, cyst-formation and obstruction. Am J Med Sci 1884;88:30–57.

229. Wakeley CPG. The position of the vermiform appendix as ascertained by an analysis of 10,000 cases. J Anat Physiol 1933;67:277–283.

230. Polukhin SI, Kuzmenko LM. Perforative appendicitis complicated by diffuse peritonitis in an intramesenteric location of the appendix. Vestn Khir 1988;141:39–40.

231. Kalker U, Gabriel M, Jacobi G. Van der Woude syndrome in combination with ring chromosome 18. Somatsschr Kinderheilkd 1988;136:95–98.

232. Morozov SA, Khvorostov ED. A case of location of the appendix in the ileal mesentery. Klin Khir 1989;4:54.

233. Repin NA, Svitich IUM. Acute phlegmonous appendicitis in retroperitoneal location of the cecum and the appendix. Klin Khir 1983;5:49–50.

234. Slipchenko GI. Acute destructive appendicitis with retroperitoneal position of the cecum and vermiform appendix. Klin Khir 1976;10:71.

235. Budd DC, Fouty WJ. Familial retrocecal appendicitis. Am J Surg 1977;133:670–671.

236. Melier F. Mémoire et observations sur quelques maladies de l'appendice caecale. J Gén Med Chir Pharm Paris 1827;100:317–345.

237. Treves F. The anatomy of the intestinal canal and peritoneum in man. Br Med J 1885;1:415–419, 470–474, 527–530, 580–583.

238. May EA. Chronic appendicitis; its roentgen diagnosis. J Med Soc 1937;34:91.

239. Hunter W. Medical commentaries. London, 1762.

240. Berry RJA. The anatomy of the vermiform appendix. Anat Anz 1895;10:761–769.

241. Dorland WAN. Congenital absence of the vermiform appendix. Int Clin 1925;4:44–54.

242. Collins DC. A study of 50,000 specimens of the human vermiform appendix. Surg Gynecol Obstet 1955;101:437–445.

243. Robinson JO. Congenital absence of vermiform appendix. Br J Surg 1952;39:344.

244. Dhawan R. Congenital absence of the vermiform appendix: report of 4 cases. Indian J Surg 1963;25:302–303.

245. Endo M, Tokuda M, Hayano S, Ito H. Three cases of congenital absence of vermiform appendix. Arch Jpn Chir 1963;32:713–716.

246. Schridde H. Über den angeborenen Mangel des Processus vermiformis. Virchow Arch [A] 1904;177:150–166.

247. Gladstone RJ. Congenital absence of the appendix of the cecum. J Anat Physiol 1915;49:414–417.

248. Valla JS, el Gharbi N, Baoud N, Grinda A. Ileo-caeco-appendicular agenesis, 1 case. Chir Pediatr 1989;30:288–289.

249. Piquet F, Elmale C, Elhdad A. Absence of the appendix. J Chir 1986;123:117–118.

250. Shperber J, Halevy A, Sayfan J, Oland J. Congenital absence of the vermiform appendix. Isr J Med Sci 1983;19:214–215.

251. Shand JE, Bremner DN. Agenesis of the vermiform appendix in a thalidomide child. Br J Surg 1977;67:203–204.

252. Host WH, Rush B, Lazaro EJ. Congenital absence of the vermiform appendix. Am Surg 1972;38:355–356.

253. Waugh TR. Appendix vermiformis duplex. Arch Surg 1941;42:311–320.

254. Cave AJE. Appendix vermiformis duplex. J Anat 1936;70:283.

255. Goldschmidt W. Vergetauschter doppelter Wurmfortsatz. Zentralbl Chir 1930;57:3123–3125.

256. Walthard B. Über die Kombination von Nabelfistel und Verdoppelung des Wurmfortsatzes. Dtsch Z Chir 1931;230:413–423.

257. Menten MJ, Denny HE. Duplication of the vermiform appendix, the large intestine and the urinary bladder. Arch Pathol 1945;40:345.

258. Bonk U. Double appendix. Pathol Res Pract 1980;167:400–401.

259. Stout AP. A study of diverticulum formation in the appendix. Arch Surg 1923;6:793–829.

260. Maloney JJ. The "ligation and drop" treatment of the appendectomy stump: results of 3500 cases. Ann Surg 1925;82:260.

261. Wetzig NR. Diverticulosis of the vermiform appendix. Med J Aust 1986;145:464–465.

262. Piattoev IuG. Congenital diverticulosis of the appendix in a 13-year-old girl. Vestn Khir 1982;129:122–123.

263. Balsano NA, Reynolds BM. Ruptured true congenital diverticulum of vermiform appendix without associated appendicitis. NY State J Med 1971;71;2877–2878.

264. Favara BE. Multiple congenital diverticula of the vermiform appendix. Am J Clin Pathol 1968;49:60–64.

265. Droga BW, Levine S, Baber JJ. Heterotopic gastric and esophageal tissue in the vermiform appendix. Am J Clin Pathol 1963;40:190.

CHAPTER 8

THE LIVER

John Elias Skandalakis / Stephen Wood Gray / Richard Ricketts / Lee John Skandalakis

"For the King of Babylon stood at the parting of the way, at the head of the
two ways, to use divination; he made his arrows bright, he consulted with images,
he looked in the liver."
—EZEKIEL 21:21

DEVELOPMENT

The primordium of the liver is first visible as a flat plate of endoderm cells on the ventral surface of the anterior intestinal portal early in the fourth week. The plate projects ventrally, and the cells lie close to the endothelial lining of the heart in the transverse septum (1). The septum already contains the vitelline veins and the lateral umbilical vessels (Fig. 8.1).

From evidence supplied by the chick embryo, differentiation of the components of the liver begins long before the appearance of the endodermal primordium. Croisille and Le Douarin (2) postulated two separate inductions acting on the endoderm. The first occurs when the splanchnic mesoderm migrates anteriorly and the lateral portions join beneath the embryonic pharynx. This tissue, termed the *hepatocardiac mesoderm,* induces differentiation of the endodermal cells at the anterior intestinal portal during the 5 to 6 somite stage although the hepatic bud will not begin to grow until the embryo has 20 to 22 somites (around day 25 to 26).

By the time the hepatic bud begins to grow into the mesoderm, the hepatic and cardiac areas have become segregated, and the former may be considered the hepatic mesoderm. At this stage a second induction takes place by which the hepatic mesoderm stimulates the developing endodermal cords to form hepatic cells. At the same time the mesoderm cells, stimulated by the endodermal hepatocytes, differentiate into the endothelial cells of the liver sinusoids. These relationships can be seen in Figure 8.2, modified from Le Douarin (3).

The original diverticulum arises from the ventral side of the archenteron, but as the midgut narrows and the duodenum is formed, rotation of the latter to the right brings the original diverticulum to a dorsal location by the 7-mm stage (34 days). Recent studies of the duodenum have suggested that the orifice of the liver diverticulum migrates in the multilayered epithelium at this stage and that the duodenum itself does not rotate (4). The diverticulum itself produces two outpockets. One, near its junction with the gut, becomes the ventral anlage of the pancreas (see Fig. 11.1), while the other, which is more distal, forms the cystic duct and gallbladder (see Fig. 9.1). The unexpanded terminal portion of the diverticulum becomes the extrahepatic portion of the hepatic duct. From this terminal portion, continued cell proliferation produces masses of cells that further invade the transverse septum. These cellular masses constitute the primordium of the liver parenchyma. Further discussion of the extrahepatic ducts is found in Chapter 9.

The formation of the human liver parenchyma has been the subject of considerable discussion. There is evidence that the process varies in detail from one mammalian group to another (5); the following description is based largely on the work of Lewis (6), Lipp (7), and Elias (5).

The septum transversum at this time consists of mesenchyme surrounding, at first, the vitelline veins and, by the 5-mm stage (32 days), the umbilical veins (Table 8.1 and Fig. 8.3). Two processes, separate in humans but not in all animals, take place. The veins break up into a plexus of branches and by invading the endoderm cells occupy the spaces around and between them. Minot (8) believed that the division of the veins was produced by the endodermal cells, a process termed *intercrescence.* Although this process appears to occur in the pig (5) and the mouse (9), vascular subdivision precedes invasion in humans (7). Invasion in humans is not by continuous, well-defined cords of cells, but by cell migration in an irregular mass. Individual endoderm cells do not remain in contact with each other but mingle freely with mesenchymal cells.

Elias (5, 10) describes a second source of liver parenchyma from mesodermal celomic lining cells, which invade the transverse septum in the same manner as do the endodermal cells and which become indistinguishable from them at the beginning of the fifth week (28-somite stage). The existence of this mesodermal component has been confirmed by some (9), but it is not universally accepted.

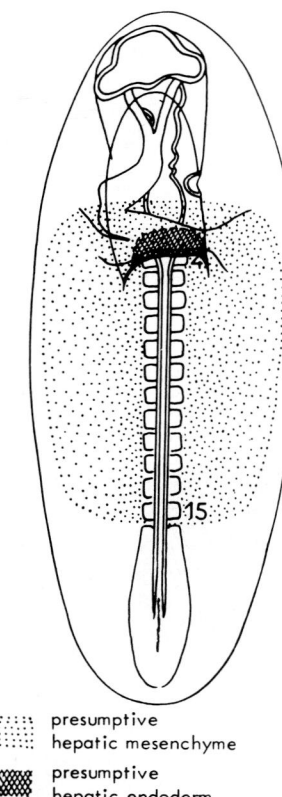

:::::: presumptive
:::::: hepatic mesenchyme

▓▓ presumptive
▓▓ hepatic endoderm

Figure 8.1. Distribution of the hepatic endodermal and mesodermal areas in the 15-somite chick embryo. The presumptive hepatic endoderm is localized in the anterior intestinal portal. (From Croisille Y and Le Douarin NM. Development and regeneration of the liver. In: DeHaan RL and Urspung H (eds). Organogenesis. New York: Holt, Rinehart & Winston, 1965.)

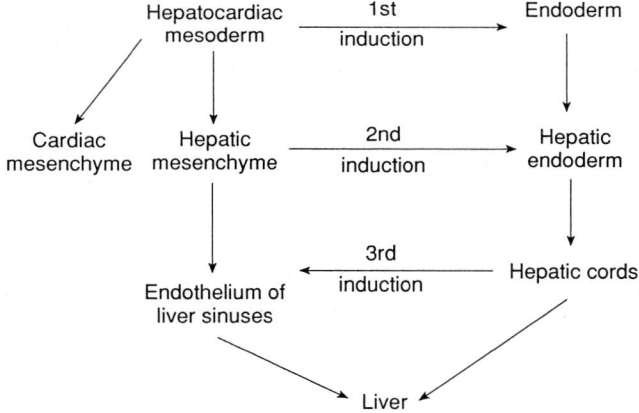

Figure 8.2. Embryogenesis of hepatic tissue.

Bennett (11) emphasized three sets of events:

1. Cell multiplication
2. New and differentiated cells from the undifferentiated zygote
3. New and differentiated cells with specific histology, function, and physiologic destiny

Table 8.1.
Development of Blood Vessels of the Liver

Week	Vessels Involved
4th	Paired vitelline and umbilical veins, not yet involved with liver primordium.
Early 5th	Vitelline veins completely invaded by liver; some branches from umbilical veins are involved.
Late 5th	Extrahepatic anastomoses of vitelline veins occur; superior (dorsal) left-to-right anastomosis forms portal vein; intrahepatic channel of left umbilical vein is dominant (ductus venosus); all placental blood passes through liver.
6th	*Portal branches in liver:* Right branch from portal vein, left branch joins left umbilical to form ductus venosus; distal left vitelline vein arises from left umbilical vein. *Hepatic branches:* Proximal right vitelline vein persists as hepatic vein, joined by ductus venosus.

Bennett thinks that embryonic differentiation is the result of different gene activities, different proteins, and different cell functions. Endodermal cells differentiate to produce the liver diverticulum from which the liver cells arise. Molecules at the cell surface are responsible for development and differentiation.

Sherer (12) also believes that the development of the hepatic parenchyma depends on interaction of its epithelial and mesenchymal tissues, that is, by the combination of endoderm and mesenchyme of mesodermal origin. The epithelium most likely originates from ectoderm or endoderm and, by mesenchymal (endoderm) stimulation, forms the hepatic parenchyma. Sherer maintains that the hepatic capillary bed is formed by two mechanisms: angioplastic (vasculogenesis) and angiotrophic (angiogenesis), the first one being responsible for the in situ differentiation of the mesenchymal intrinsic cells to vascular endothelium and the second one for the growth and migration of the extrinsic endothelium.

By the 6-mm stage, nearly the entire flow from the umbilical veins has been diverted to the expanding liver. The invading cells have united to invest completely the venous channels that will become the sinusoids. The investing parenchyma is at first three to five cells thick, becoming reduced to a single layer with growth of the blood vessels.

During this period of growth, the liver begins to bulge out of the transverse septum and becomes a true abdominal organ lying within the mesentery. The bare area of the liver and diaphragm remains as a trace of its origin within the transverse septum.

Although intrahepatic ducts have been said to form from extensions of extrahepatic duct epithelium (13), the present view is that they differentiate from hepatic cells and subsequently join the extrahepatic duct system

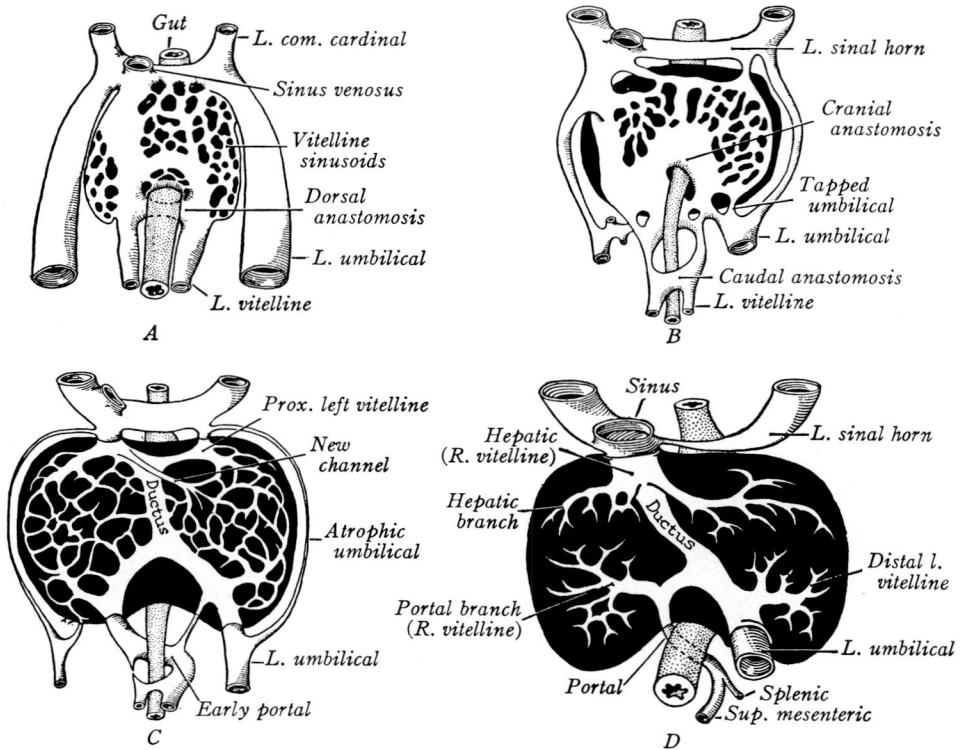

Figure 8.3. Relationships of the developing liver to the omphalomesenteric (vitelline) and the umbilical veins and the formation of the portal vein and ductus venosus. **A**, Fifth week (4.5 mm). **B**, Late fifth week (5 mm). **C**, Early sixth week (6 mm). **D**, Later sixth week (9 mm). The liver substance is shown in *black*. (From Arey LB. Developmental Anatomy, ed 7. Philadelphia: WB Saunders Co., 1965.)

(5, 14). Intrahepatic ducts begin to appear in the region of the hilus and spread peripherally. The duct system is essentially complete by the 10th week. Short segments that fail to connect with the rest of the hepatic tree may remain as sources of hepatic cysts in later life. (See Table 8.1 for a synopsis of the development of the blood vessels serving the liver.)

Tubular structures bounded by four or more hepatic cells with microvilli have been considered the earliest traces of bile canaliculi (6, 15); other authors (9) consider them to be developing cholangioles and small bile ducts. True bile canaliculi probably arise in situ and connect secondarily with the developing duct system. Bile may appear as early as the third month and often is visible in the intestine by the fifth month.

By the ninth week, the liver represents 10% of body volume. It subsequently decreases in relative size, especially during the last 2 months of gestation, until at birth it represents only 5% of body volume.

The hemopoietic tissue of the fetal liver is formed by the transverse septum mesenchyme, which lies between the developing liver cords and the endothelial cells of the blood vessels. It is this tissue that contributes to the relatively large size of the fetal liver. According to Zimniak and Lester (16) in 1989, the metabolism of bile acids in the fetus and newborn is still largely uncharted territory.

Remodeling of the liver occurs during the sixth to eighth weeks. The right lobe increases in size at the expense of the left, which undergoes peripheral degeneration after the ninth week (17) (Fig. 8.4). It is well known that, in the early development of the fetus, the liver constitutes 10% of the body weight. In a later stage of fetal development the weight drops to 5%.

Without further explanation, the modern intrahepatic anatomy is outlined in Table 8.2.

Critical Events in Development

The liver undergoes few dramatic changes during development. The most serious lesion is considered to be intrahepatic biliary atresia, but the time of its appearance is unknown and even its status as a developmental anomaly is in doubt. Biliary atresia is most likely an acquired defect rather than a developmental one.

EDITORIAL COMMENT

The best evidence that biliary atresia is an acquired defect is the observation that a stillborn infant has never been documented with intrahepatic biliary atresia. Thus, it seems likely that some infection or other toxic influence occurs in the perinatal period which is ultimately responsible for the development of biliary atresia (JAH/CNP).

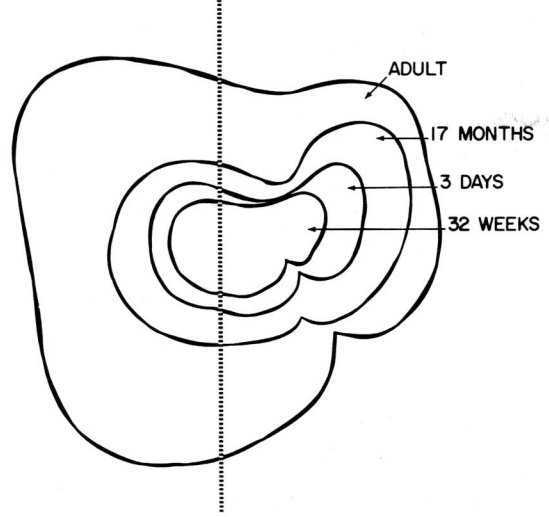

Figure 8.4. The relative sizes of the left and right lobes of the liver in the fetus at 32 weeks; in the infant at 3 days and at 17 months; and in the adult. The *dotted line* represents the location of the main lobar fissure. (From Healey JE Jr and Sterling JA. Segmental anatomy of the newborn liver. Ann NY Acad Sci 111:25–36, 1963.)

ANOMALIES OF THE LIVER (TABLE 8.3 AND FIG. 8.5)

Anomalies of Liver Lobulation.

Although the exterior of the liver is demarcated into obvious "lobes," neither the internal structure nor the embryonic development supports this division. An arbitrary division into right, left, and central lobes was proposed by Rex (18), Cantlie (19), and Bradley (20) early in this century. More recent studies of the intrahepatic biliary and vascular architecture suggest that there are true right and left lobes. This division was proposed by the above authors and supported by the work of McNee (21), Healey and his colleagues (17, 22, 23), Coinaud (24), Platzer and Maurer (25), and the surgeons of today performing hepatic resection.

The line between right and left lobes passes through the fossa of the vena cava, splits the caudate "lobe" (23, 24) or passes to left of it (25), and passes through the fossa of the gallbladder. On the parietal surface, it parallels the attachment of the falciform ligament, but no fissure

Table 8.2.
Relations of Resections to Vascular and Ductal Structures[a]

Resection	Line of Incision	Vascular and Ductal Structures Divided	Vascular and Ductal Structures Preserved
Right hepatic lobectomy (segments V, VI, VII, VIII)	Gallbladder fossa to IVC	Right hepatic vein; right branch of hepatic pedicle Branches entering middle hepatic vein from right; accessory veins from segments VI and VII	Middle and left hepatic veins; left branch hepatic pedicle
Extended right hepatic lobectomy (segments IV, V, VI, VII, VIII)	1 cm to right of portoumbilical fissure	Right and middle hepatic veins; right branch of hepatic pedicle and branches of left hepatic pedicle to segment IV	Left hepatic vein; left branch hepatic pedicle, including branches to segments II and III
Right lateral lobectomy (segments VI and VII)	Right fissure	Right hepatic vein, posterior division; right hepatic pedicle	Middle and left hepatic veins, anterior division; right hepatic pedicle
Left hepatic lobectomy (segments II, III, IV)	I cm to left of median fissure	Left hepatic vein and tributaries entering middle hepatic vein from left; left branch hepatic pedicle	Middle hepatic vein
Left lateral lobectomy (segments II and III)	1 cm to left of portoumbilical fissure	Left hepatic vein before junction with the middle hepatic vein; branches of hepatic pedicle to segments II and III	Middle hepatic vein; left branch of hepatic pedicle, including branches to segment IV
Mesohepatectomy/ median hepatectomy (segments IV, V, VIII)	1 cm to right of portoumbilical fissure, 1 cm to left of right fissure; inferiorly obliquely to hilum, leftward to 1 cm from portoumbilical fissure, to anterior margin of liver	Middle hepatic vein, branches joining left side of right hepatic vein, anterior division; right branch hepatic pedicle, left branch hepatic pedicle to segment IV, cystic duct, and artery	Right and left hepatic veins, posterior division; right branch hepatic pedicle, left branch hepatic pedicle

[a]From Ger R. Relations of resections to vascular and ductal structures: surgical anatomy of the liver. Surg Clin North Am 1989;69(2):179–192.

Table 8.3.
Anomalies of the Liver

Anomaly	Origin of Defect	First Appearance	Sex Chiefly Affected	Frequency	Remarks
Anomalous lobes:					
Riedel's lobe	Unknown	None; unexplained mass present in adult	Female	Probably rare	—
Supradiaphragmatic lobe	4th–5th week	None	?	Very rare	—
Cysts:					
Solitary	Unknown	Adulthood	Female	Rare	May not be congenital
Polycystic disease	Unknown	None	?	Uncommon	Associated with polycystic kidney
Intrahepatic biliary atresia	Unknown	1st mo of life	Female	Rare	May not be of embryonic origin

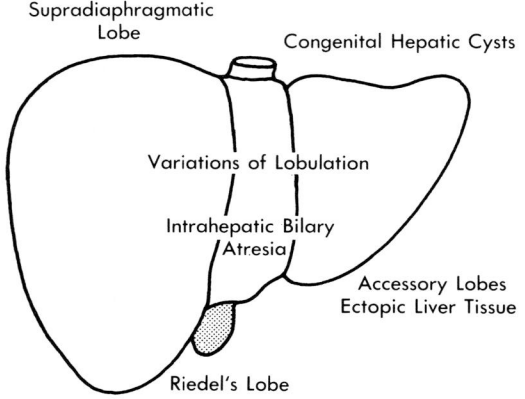

Figure 8.5.   Sites of the major anomalies of the liver.

marks its course. The two main lobes may be further subdivided into medial and lateral segments on the left and into anterior and posterior segments on the right (Fig. 8.6A–H). Additional subdivision of these segments, based on biliary drainage (23) or on portal vein branches (25), is possible, but the lobulations thus obtained vary among individuals in both boundaries and actual number (Fig. 8.7).

Minor variations in the size of the various portions of the liver are not uncommon and do not affect function. The most common variations are diminution of the left lobe (26) or increased size of the quadrate lobe. Morgenstern and Mazur (27) reviewed a rare case of hypoplasia of the right lobe.

Agenesis of the right lobe of the liver with hypertrophy of the left and caudate lobes and supra- or retrohepatic gallbladder was reported by Demirci et al. (28) in 1990. Another case was also reported by Collay et al. (29). According to them, these cases are rare and can be diagnosed by ultrasound or computed tomography. Meyers and Jacobson (30) have discussed visceral displacement resulting from anomalous lobulation. Watanabe et al. reported diagnosis of hepatic lobe atrophy by laparoscopy (31).

True anomalies of the form of the liver, on the other hand, are extremely rare. Accessory liver lobes were seen and recognized by hepatoscopists (practitioners of divination) from prehistoric times until the Middle Ages. However, because of the nature of their profession, such findings were rarely recorded.

RIEDEL'S LOBE

In 1888 Riedel (32) described 10 female patients who had an elongated tongue of liver tissue extending from the right lobe to, or below, the level of the umbilicus. This projection has since been referred to as Riedel's lobe (Fig. 8.8). Among 31 cases reported at the Mayo Clinic by Reitemeier et al., through 1956, all but one were in women, and all were discovered when the patients were between the ages of 31 and 77 years (33).

The tissue is normal, sometimes adherent to the hepatic flexure of the colon. In one case this adhesion produced a partial obstruction (34). A number of these patients suffer from cholecystitis. Riedel stated that the accessory lobe tends to disappear after cholecystectomy.

Dick (35) and van der Reis et al. (36) described a similar tongue-shaped projection from the left instead of the right lobe (Fig. 8.9). The right lobe was diminished and the left was enlarged. The fact that the gallbladder was in the normal position seemed to exclude situs inversus.

In another case Chiba et al. (37) reported a tongue-like projection of the left lobe in an adult female which originated from a medioinferior portion of the left lobe. Splenorenal venous shunt and intrahepatic arterial anastomosis were noted.

The chief significance of this accessory lobe is that it usually presents as an unexplained abdominal mass. The possibility of its presence must be kept in mind. The use of a liver scan will identify such areas of abnormally located liver tissue (38).

SUPRADIAPHRAGMATIC LOBES

There are three reported cases of portions of liver tissue lying in the right thoracic cavity (39–41). In each case, the

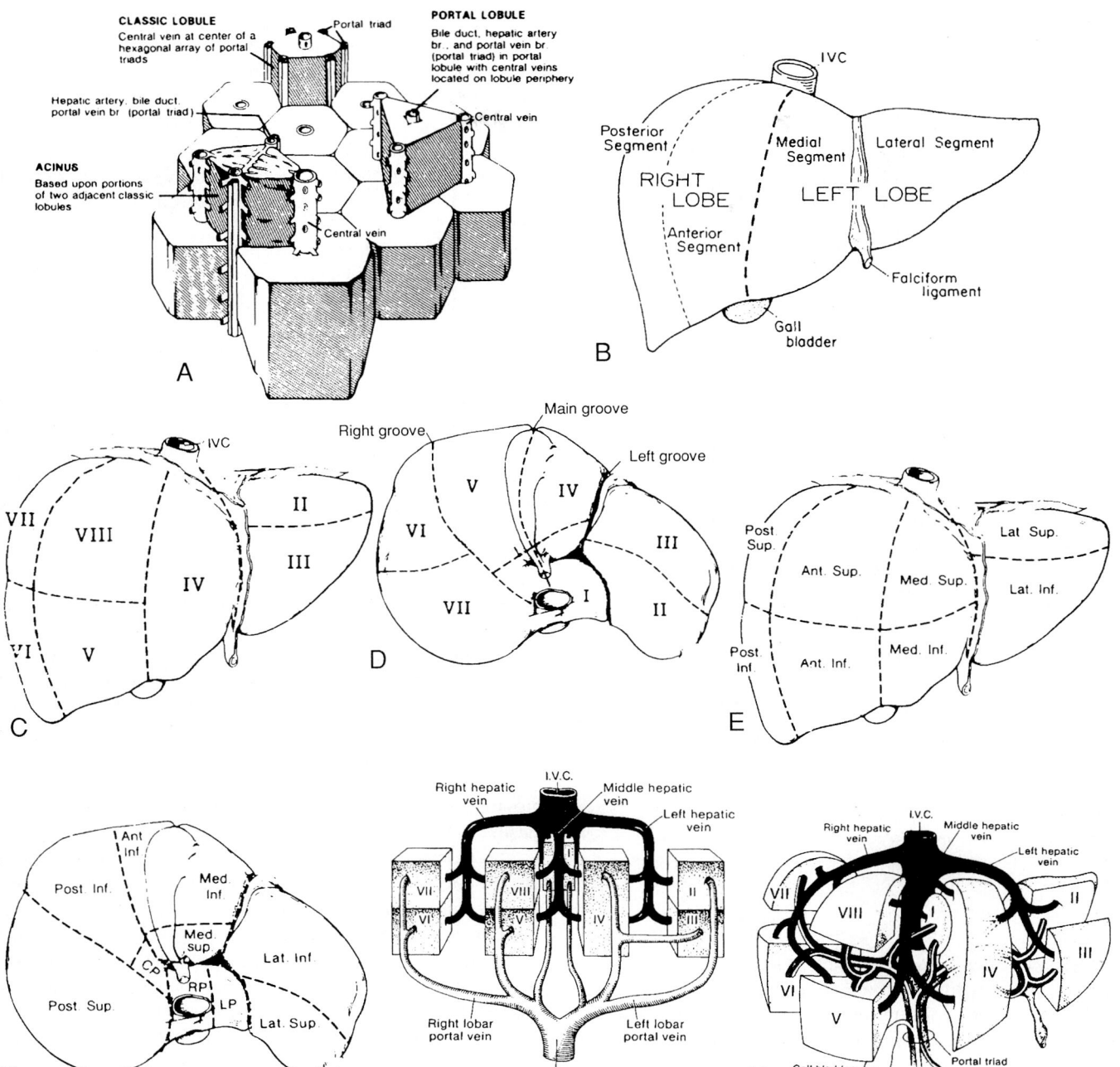

Figure 8.6. **A**, Three concepts of the liver lobule. The "classic" lobule, with central veins and peripheral hepatic triads; the "portal" lobule, centered on the hepatic triads; and the hepatic acinus. Both the central vein and the hepatic triads are peripheral. It is the concept of the acinus that has proved to be the most useful for understanding liver functions. **B**, Modern concept of the lobes and segments of the human liver. **C** to **F**, Projection of liver lobes and segments based on the distribution of intrahepatic ducts and blood vessels. **C** and **D**, Terminology of Couinaud (1954). **E** and **F**, Terminology of Healey and Schroy (1953). (*CP*, caudate process; *RP* and *LP*, right and left portions of the caudate lobe). **G**, Highly diagrammatic presentation of the segmental functional anatomy of the liver emphasizing portal distribution and hepatic veins. **H**, Exploded segmental view of the liver emphasizing the intrahepatic anatomy and hepatic veins.

ectopic lobe was connected to the liver by a pedicle that passed through a small defect in the diaphragm. These cases are congenital and are not to be confused with liver tissue secondarily herniated into the thorax through a congenital diaphragmatic defect.

Strangely enough, we have seen no autopsy reports of

this condition. All three of the cases were found accidentally on radiography in adults; all were asymptomatic. In addition, the histology was normal; artery, vein, and bile duct passed through the pedicle (Fig. 8.10). The smallest of these accessory structures was 4.4 cm in its greatest diameter. Katz and Williams (42) reviewed instances of

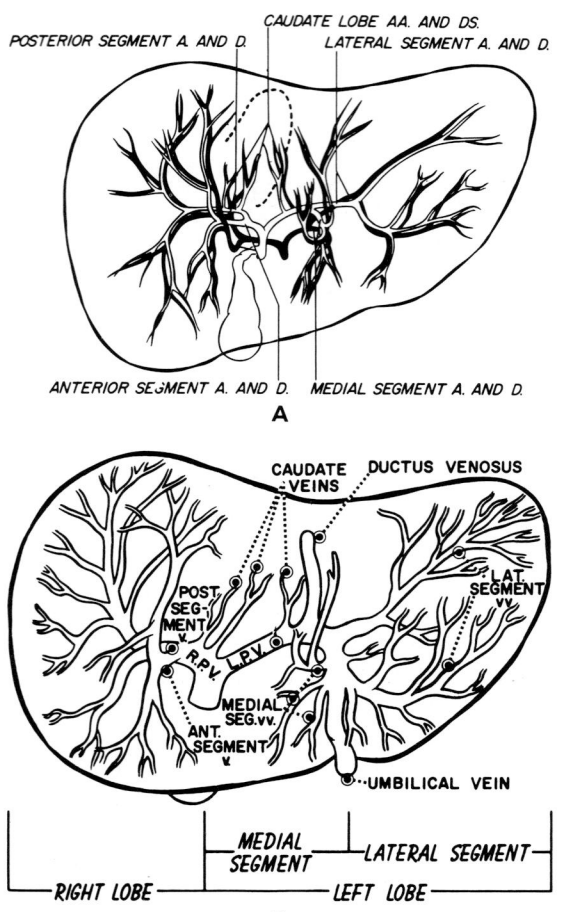

Figure 8.7. **A,** The prevailing pattern of branching of the hepatic artery *(dark)* and the bile ducts *(light)* in the newborn liver. **B,** The pattern of branching of the portal vein in the newborn liver. *R.P.V.,* Right portal vein; *L.P.V.,* left portal vein. (From Healey JE Jr and Sterling JA. Segmental anatomy of the newborn liver. Ann NY Acad Sci 1963;111:25–36.)

abnormal lobes lying beneath the diaphragm, which appear on x-ray films to be thoracic.

A much more anomalous case was reported by Mulla and Weintraub (43) in which the intestines had herniated through a diaphragmatic defect into the right thorax. In addition, there was an accessory liver lobe in the thorax, and the right lung was absent. The right pulmonary artery served as the hepatic artery to this tissue. The accessory lobe was joined to the abdominal liver by a narrow isthmus.

In a personal communication, Gauderer (1990) reported two infants with intrapericardial hepatic herniation and absence of the central portion of the diaphragm. According to the author, only nine infants with intrapericardial herniation were reported, and seven of the herniations contained liver (Figs. 8.11 and 8.12). It is difficult to explain this phenomenon. Hypothetically and

speculatively, this is the rupture of the central tendon together with the adjacent part of the pericardium with an upward spearheading of the liver through the septum transversum. Ake et al. (44) described a similar herniation of a portion of the liver into the pericardium in association with a right-sided congenital diaphragmatic hernia. Shapiro and Metlay (45) pointed out that severe cardiac anomalies may accompany a heterotopic supradiaphragmatic liver.

Since the liver forms within the transverse septum, it is surprising that portions of liver are not trapped above the diaphragm more often.

OTHER ANOMALOUS LOBES AND HETEROTOPIC LIVER TISSUE

Small accessory lobes attached to the liver by pedicles or by mesentery are occasionally reported. Liver nodules have been found on the surface of the gallbladder (46) and in its wall (47). Davies (48) found liver tissue associated with the pancreas; the bile duct of the heterotopic tissue entered the pancreatic duct. Cullen (34) reported ectopic liver tissue in the adrenal gland of a child. Heid and von Haam (49) found liver tissue in the splenic capsule. Liver cell cords without canaliculi were present; bile ducts were seen, but their drainage was not determined. An accessory liver lobe arising from the anterosuperior border of the left liver has been reported as herniated through the upper abdominal wall (50). In two cases ectopic liver tissue was found in an omphalocele (51). In one there was a rudimentary gallbladder. This case suggested a duplication of hepatic diverticulum distal to the normal site. We have found no other report of a similar case.

Accessory lobes attached to the liver have been related to the presence of extra branches of the developing embryonic veins (52) or to excessive connective tissue development, which constricts the liver tissue (53). More probably, the gap between the accessory lobule and the liver represents groups of primary liver cells that are slightly displaced during the proliferative stage.

Tejada and Danielson (54) reported a hepatic nodule on the gallbladder wall, which had its own $11 \times 6 \times 4$-cm mesentery and which was not connected with the liver. Recently, Ger (55) studied the surgical anatomy of the liver. Table 8.2 summarizes his work and, coupled with ultrasonography, provides the surgeon with the necessary tools to perform a sound operation.

Nonparasitic Cysts of the Liver

SOLITARY CYSTS OF THE LIVER

Solitary, nonparasitic hepatic cysts are rare structures of doubtful etiology which were first described by Bristowe in 1857 (56). Thirty-eight cases were reported in children

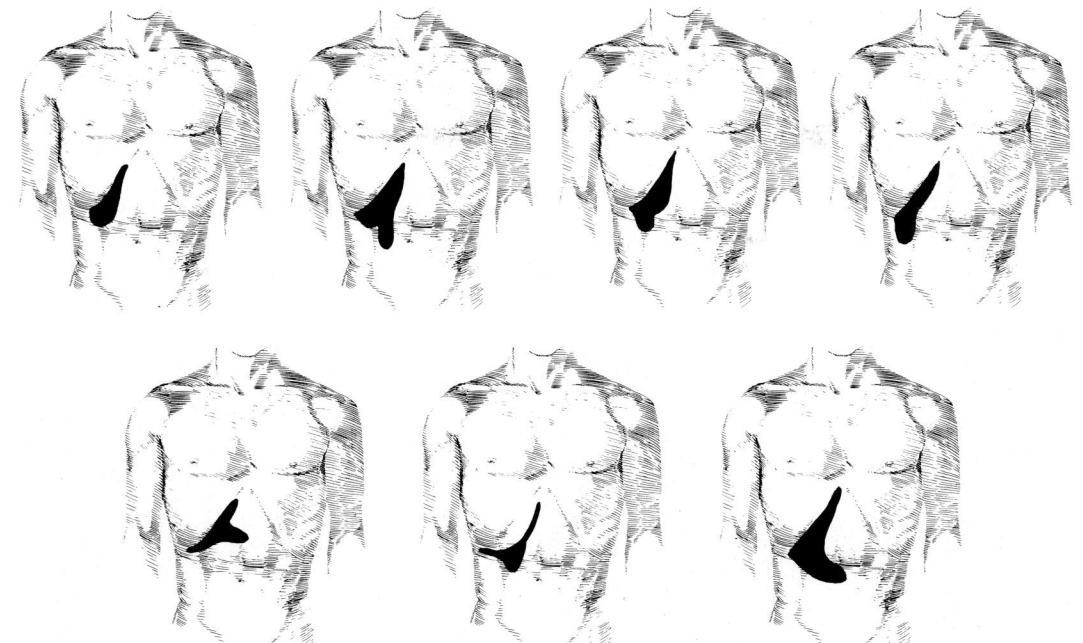

Figure 8.8. Examples of Riedel's lobe of the liver (Redrawn from Dick J. Riedel's lobe and related partial hepatic enlargements. Guy Hosp Rep 1951;100:270–277.)

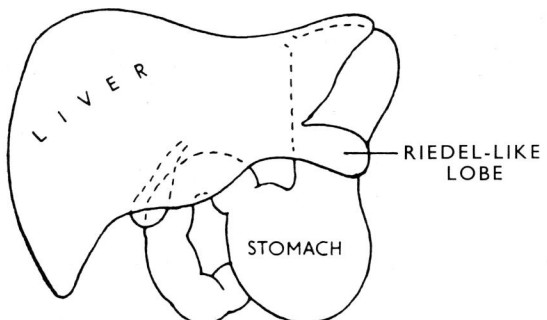

Figure 8.9. An anomalous lobe on the left side of the liver resembling Riedel's lobe on the right side. (From Dick J. Riedel's lobe and related partial hepatic enlargements. Guy Hosp Rep 1951;100:270–277).

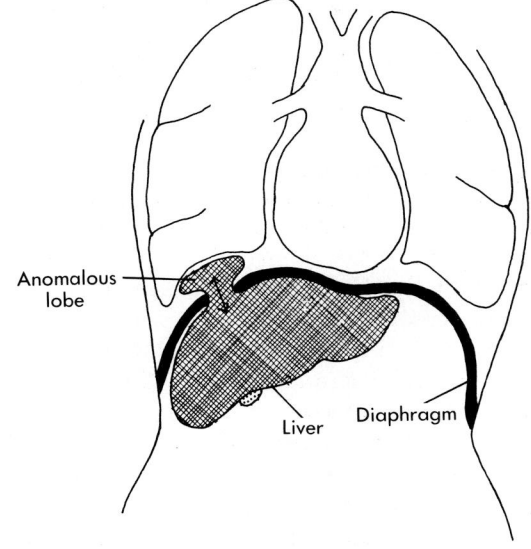

Figure 8.10. Anomalous supradiaphragmatic lobe of the liver with a pedicle passing through the diaphragm, carrying an artery, a vein, and a bile duct.

up to 1956 (57), and some 250 cases have been described in adults (58). Eliason and Smith (59) found 28 cases among 20,000 autopsies. Women are more frequently affected.

The cysts are usually pedunculated, arising from the undersurface of the right lobe of the liver. About 10% are multilocular. The epithelium varies from columnar to squamous and may be ciliated. Clear or hemorrhagic fluid, but not bile, is usually contained in the cysts.

That their origin is congenital is a reasonable assumption, but it has not been proved, although one case was found in a 3-day-old infant (60). Improper fusion of developing bile ducts is the only suggested developmental mechanism (59).

Symptoms are usually only those of abdominal distension with displacement of viscera, although pain (61) and jaundice (62) occasionally are present. The cysts are usually small and may be loculated, but they have been known to reach a capacity of 700 cc (58). Carcinoma has been reported in two cases (63).

Unlike parasitic cysts, which are under high pressure and hence may be palpated, these nonparasitic solitary

Figure 8.11. **A**, X-ray film of Baby A showing intrapericardiac diaphragmatic hernia. There is massive opacification of the chest. **B**, Autopsy examination of intrapericardiac diaphragmatic hernia in Baby A. This picture shows the stretched pericardium, the thymus, the compressed heart, and the large intrapericardiac portion of liver. The liver has been retracted to show the anatomy. (Courtesy Dr Michael WL Gauderer, Rainbow Babies and Childrens Hospital, Cleveland, Ohio.)

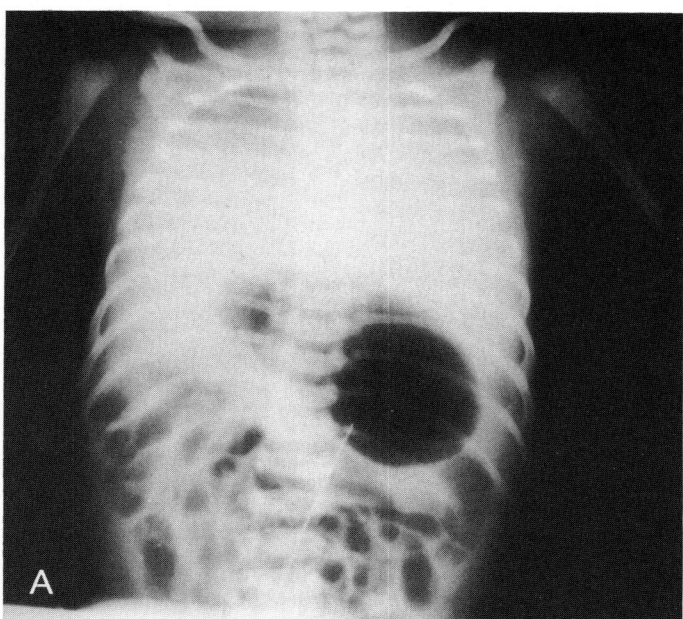

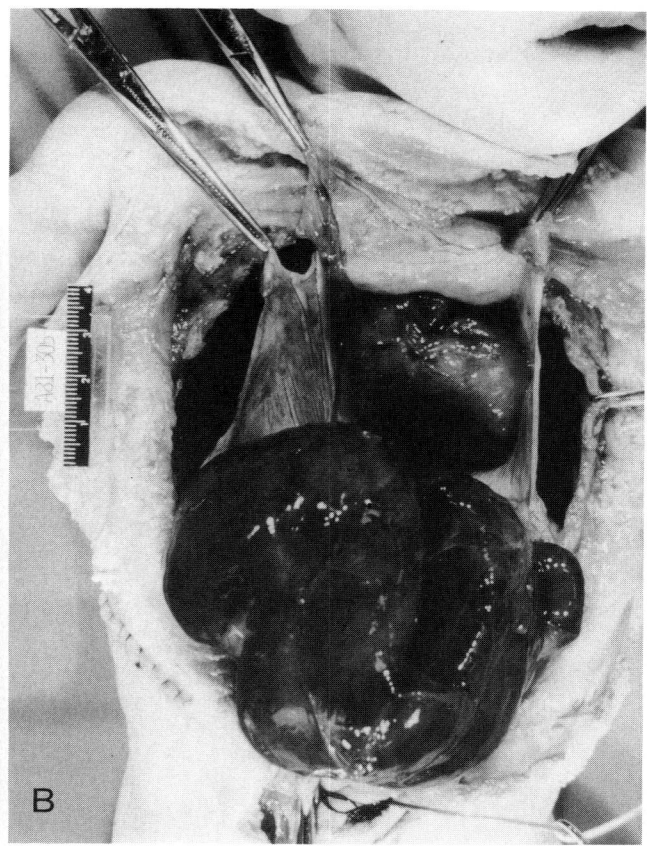

cysts are flaccid and not easily palpable. Parasitic cysts may show calcifications; nonparasitic cysts do not. It is not surprising that only three cases have been diagnosed prior to surgery.

The cyst should be excised whenever possible. Any portion not removed must be cauterized. Marsupialization with drainage has been employed, but it is a slow process (64). With this method, however, the cyst collapses and can be removed entirely at a later operation. Greig and Stinson (65) found enucleation feasible in their three cases. Manheimer (66) suggested anastomosing the cyst to the stomach to provide drainage.

According to Benhamou and Menu (67) in 1988, the hepatic cyst is a localized process of a congenital anomaly which is transmitted as an autosomal dominant trait.

POLYCYSTIC DISEASE OF THE LIVER

Three views have been held about the origin of polycystic liver disease: (*a*) Virchow (68) considered it to be the result of inflammatory stricture of the hepatic ducts; (*b*) for a time, many thought it to be of neoplastic origin; and (*c*) it has been held to result from congenital defects of development. This last view was established by a review of 91 cases by Moschcowitz in 1906 (69). In 1918 von Mey-

enburg (70) described groups of supernumerary intrahepatic bile ducts that failed to disappear with development of the liver. These, by gradual cystic dilation, produced the condition. The absence of bile in the cysts was evidence that the ducts had not formed a connection with true bile capillaries.

The cysts usually are numerous and measure from 1 to 3 cm in diameter although they are known to reach 10 to 12 cm. They are lined with cuboidal or squamous epithelium, depending on the distension; the content is nearly always clear. The total mass of cysts may reach 70 cm or more in diameter.

In many cases the cysts produce no liver dysfunction, and they are rarely diagnosed in life. In at least 50% of patients, polycystic disease of the kidney is present as well (71, 72). Ten of Melnick's 70 cases had diverticula of the esophagus, jejunum, colon, or bladder, and four had cerebral aneurysms as well as polycystic kidneys (72). Bigelow (73) and Poutasse and his associates (74) noted that cerebral aneurysms are often associated with polycystic kidney disease. Campbell (75) found polycystic livers in 20 of 186 patients with polycystic kidneys.

The disease manifests itself late in life. Melnick (72) found only three patients in 70 who were under the age

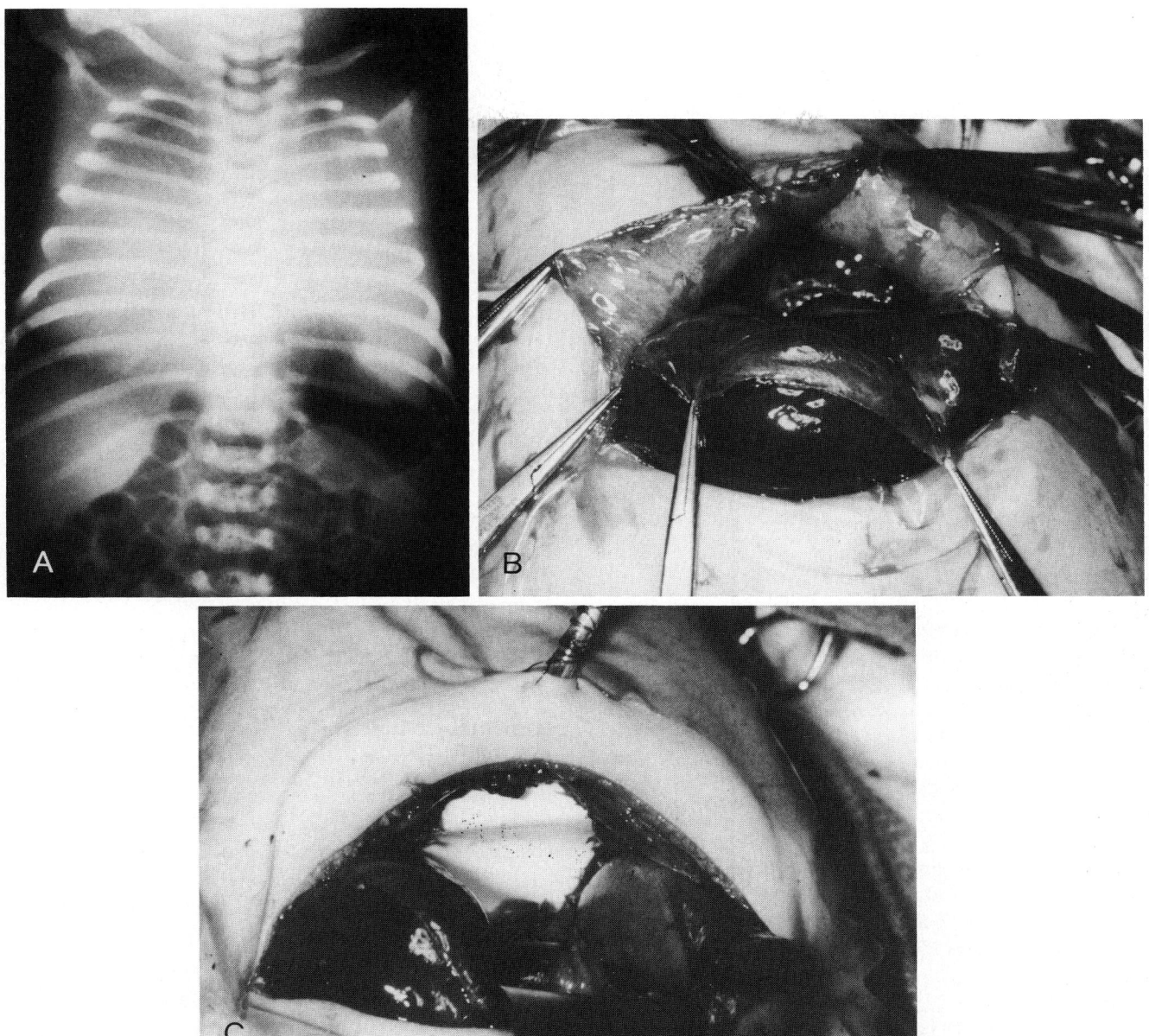

Figure 8.12. **A**, X-ray film of Baby B on first day of life showing intrapericardiac diaphragmatic hernia. This x-ray film is similar to Baby A, although a portion of the liver is still seen below the diaphragm on the right side. **B**, Operative approach of the intrapericardiac diaphragmatic hernia. The displaced heart can be seen. The liver has been pulled out and retracted. **C**, The completed repair. A Gore Tex patch measuring 4.2 × 3.6 cm is in place. The chest tube is positioned in the massively stretched pericardiac cavity. This child survived and was doing well at 8 months of age. (Courtesy Dr Michael WL Gauderer, Rainbow Babies and Childrens Hospital, Cleveland, Ohio.)

of 30 years. Davis (76) collected 499 cases from the literature up to 1937. Melnick estimated that polycystic livers were found in one of 687 autopsies in Los Angeles.

Symptoms are usually those of abdominal distension only. These liver cysts alone probably do not shorten life, but the prognosis depends on the progress of the associated cystic kidney disease.

Excision of the entire cystic area or lobe of the liver is the only operative procedure that is effective. The presence of polycystic kidneys or ascites is a contraindication to surgery. In the absence of these complications, the surgeon must weigh the severity of the disease against the risk of operation. Note that this is not to be confused with Caroli's syndrome, which is described elsewhere and for which, according to Tandon et al. (77), fewer than 150 cases have been reported.

Intrahepatic Biliary Atresia

ANATOMY

This condition is characterized by the absence of interlobular bile ducts in the infant liver. Bile canaliculi are present, and the extrahepatic ducts may be either atretic or present and patent. Fibrosis occurs, most markedly in the left lobe.

PATHOGENESIS

The origin of intrahepatic biliary atresia is unknown. The following views have been expressed (78).

Congenital Origin. Two main theories exist: (*a*) The condition is an extension of extrahepatic biliary atresia, with the entire biliary tree being of common origin; and (*b*) the condition is distinct from extrahepatic atresia, with the two groups of ducts being of separate embryonic origin.

Acquired Origin. The condition arises secondarily to extrahepatic biliary atresia or hepatitis and is probably a disuse atrophy or a postinflammatory atresia (78). In addition, it can be produced experimentally by ligating the hepatic artery (79).

The arguments in favor of a congenital malformation origin rest on the condition's appearance early in life and its obvious analogy to extrahepatic biliary atresia. The argument in favor of an acquired origin rests on the associated fibrosis. No abnormal chromosome picture has been found (80). Altman suggests that the cause is infectious or immunologic (81).

HISTORY

Ahrens and his colleagues first distinguished the disease in 1951 (82). Haas and Dobbs (83) reviewed 10 cases in 1958, and Brent (78) collected cases from the experience of 10 pediatricians in 1962.

INCIDENCE

Krovetz (84) found 14 cases of intrahepatic biliary atresia and 109 cases of extrahepatic atresia in the same period of time. There was a preponderance of females among these cases.

SYMPTOMS

Jaundice is the presenting symptom. Xanthomatous cutaneous lesions, preceded by pruritis, often appear months or even years later.

DIAGNOSIS

Persistent jaundice, with rising serum conjugated bilirubin, is indicative of the disease. Stools are never completely acholic. Stools to be tested should be taken from the rectum to avoid contamination with urinary bile pigments. A liver biopsy will confirm the absence of interlob-

ular bile ducts or the presence of infection and necrosis from hepatitis (85).

TREATMENT

Supportive and symptomatic treatment are all that is presently possible. No means of reducing the hypercholesterolemia has been effective. The forming of artificial ducts or anastomosing the cut edge of the liver (Longmire procedure) does not appear to be successful. Suruga (86) observed that ducts, if present at all, will be larger in the right than in the left lobe. Any anastomotic procedure should take this into account. He recommends transplantation of the thoracic duct to the sublingual part of the oral cavity to prevent progressive cirrhosis. In spite of the possibility of some successful anastomoses (see the discussion on the Kasai procedure in Chapter 9, pages 303–306), liver transplantation offers the greatest hope for the future treatment of intrahepatic biliary atresia.

PROGNOSIS

Most patients die before the age of 4 years, but a few have lived as long as 12 (83) or 13 years (84). Survival is better when extrahepatic biliary ducts are patent. Longmire (87) believes that there may be varying degrees of hypoplasia. If atresia were absolute, such long survival with some biliary excretion would be difficult to explain.

EDITORIAL COMMENT

The best current theory of etiology for intrahepatic and extrahepatic biliary atresia is progressive fibrosis and destruction of the epithelial elements by either a viral, toxic, or immunologic mechanism. That there is great variation in the patterns of biliary atresia can be explained by this theory in that the etiologic agent presents with different degrees of severity. Giant cell hepatitis has certainly been documented as an early process in the newborn liver, which can progress to destruction of bile ducts and the histologic and clinical picture of biliary atresia. It is unlikely that this is the only cause of atresia, but it does represent one cause, and others may be closely related to this destructive and inflammatory process which may lead to fetal biliary obstruction. Further evidence for this ongoing acquired disease process is the fact that the number of children following successful operative relief of obstruction for biliary atresia (the various forms of the Kasai operation) eventually have further episodes of hepatitis with further destruction of epithelial elements and ultimately die of liver failure due to progressive biliary fibrosis and more extensive biliary atresia.

Because of this progression of the disease process following relief of obstruction due to biliary atresia, liver transplantation is the ultimate solution to extensive biliary atresia because in this way a normal liver is substituted for the diseased organ and presumably will not be attacked by the same process responsible for biliary atresia in the native liver. Not enough follow-up is yet available for long term results following liver transplantation for biliary atresia, but no cases have been reported with the development of secondary biliary atresia in the transplanted normal liver unless there is extensive ischemic necrosis and/or secondary viral hepatitis (JAH/CNP).

Other Hepatic Anomalies

Bands of fibrous tissue with linear and circular degeneration, lined with bile duct epithelium as a simple entity but usually associated with pancreatic or renal anomalies, was reported by Murray-Lyon et al. (88) as congenital hepatic fibrosis. Annand et al. (89) presented this anomaly associated with polycystic renal disease.

Watson and Miller (90) introduced the term *arteriohepatic dysplasia* when a heterogenous liver disease is associated with congenital hypoplasia and stenosis of the pulmonary arteries. Greenwood et al. (91) presented similar anomalies. Intrahepatic bile duct hypoplasia with facial abnormalities was described by Alagille et al. (92).

Congenital Hepatic Hemangioma, Hemangioendothelioma, and Lymphangioma

Congenital vascular malformation of the liver ranging from solitary hemangiomas to multiple hemangioendotheliomas are now being discovered with increased frequency because of the widespread use of prenatal and neonatal ultrasound. The hemangiomas tend to be of the cavernous type and measure less than 5 cm in diameter (93). The hemangioendotheliomas may be single or multiple, are not well encapsulated, and are characterized by vascular spaces lined by plump endothelium (93–95). Both are characterized by the clinical syndrome of progressive hepatomegaly, cutaneous hemangiomas, and congestive heart failure (96). Both follow the natural history of cutaneous hemangiomas with progressive enlargement during infancy, stabilization, and regression by the age of 2 to 3 years (97). If progressive congestive heart failure ensues, however, the overall mortality is greater than 50% (96).

EDITORIAL COMMENT

Very frequently, sonographic evidence of cavernous hemangiomas of the liver are entirely without clinical symptoms. These probably undergo progressive maturation with obliteration of the epithelial spaces and fibrosis. Rarely, as noted above, due to large shunting and, occasionally, arteriovenous components, there can be congestive heart failure on the basis of the hemodynamic abnormality. Another major complication associated with large cavernous hemangiomas of the liver is sequestration of platelets leading to a consumptive coagulopathy. This syndrome also is associated with widespread subcutaneous ecchymoses and soft tissue hemorrhage, and may be the earliest evidence of impending death. Occasionally, this syndrome can be reversed with steroids in large doses, and rarely, the hemodynamic instability can be altered by direct embolization into the tumor mass (JAH/CNP).

Treatment involves supporting the infant's cardiovascular system with diuretics and digitalis until spontaneous regression occurs (94, 98–100). If these measures are unsuccessful, steroids, hepatic artery ligation or embolization, and/or radiation are used with variable degrees of success (94, 101). Hepatic resection should be reserved for those patients who do not respond to the above measures or in whom the lesion fails to regress (102).

Hepatic lymphangioma is a very rare disease. According to Gorenstein et al. (103), it may involve only the liver or the involvement may be part of the generalized process that includes other organs (lymphangiomatosis). Multiple, smooth-walled cysts with serous fluid and blood, separated by thin walls which are lined by flattened endothelium, constitute the gross and microscopic pathology. No treatment of lymphangiomatosis is necessary if the patient is asymptomatic. If it is a localized process, liver resection is recommended. Miller et al. reported orthotopic liver transplantation for massive lymphangiomatosis (104).

REFERENCES

1. Severn CB. The morphological development of the hepatic diverticulum in staged human embryos. Anat Rec 1968;160:427.
2. Croisille Y, Le Douarin NM. Development and regeneration of the liver. In: DeHaan RL, Urspung H, eds. Organogenesis. New York: Holt, Rinehart & Winston, 1965.
3. Le Douarin N. Isolement expérimental du mésenchyme propre du foie et rôle morphogène de la composante mésodermique dans l'organogènese hépatique. J Embryol Exp Morphol 1964;12:141–160.
4. Kanagasuntheram R. Some observations on the development of the human duodenum. J Anat 1960;94:231–240.
5. Elias H. Origin and early development of the liver in various vertebrates. Acta Hepat 1955;3:1–56.
6. Lewis FT. The development of the liver. In: Keibel F, Mall FP, eds. Human embryology. Philadelphia: JB Lippincott, 1912.
7. Lipp W. Die Entwicklung der Parenchymarchitektur der Leber. Verh Anat Ges 1952;50:241–249.
8. Minot SS. On a hitherto unrecognized form of blood circulation without capillaries in the organs of vertebrata. Proc Boston Soc Nat Hist 1900;29:185–215.
9. Wilson JW, Groat CS, Leduc EH. Histogenesis of the liver. Ann NY Acad Sci 1963;111:8–24.
10. Elias H. Appositional growth of the embryonic liver. Rev Int Hepat 1964;14:317–322.
11. Bennett D. Modern views of embryonic development and differentiation. In: Javitt NB, ed. Neonatal hepatitis and biliary atresia: an international workshop. Bethesda: National Institutes of Health, March 21–23, 1977.
12. Sherer GK. Vasculogenic mechanisms and epithelio-mesenchymal specificity in endodermal organs. In: Feinberg RN, Sherer GK, Auerbach R, ed. The development of the vascular system. Basel: Karger, 1991.

13. Bloom W. The embryogenesis of human bile capillaries and ducts. Am J Anat 1926;36:451–465.

14. Horstmann E. Entwicklung und entwicklungsbedingungen des intrahepatischen Gallengangsystems. Arch Entwicklungsmech Organ 1939;139:363–392.

15. Wood RL. Observations on the fine structure of developing bile canaliculi in the rat. Anat Rec 1963;145:302.

16. Zimniak P and Lester R. Bile acid metabolism in the perinatal period. In: Lebenthal E, ed. Human gastrointestinal development. New York: Raven Press, 1989:561.

17. Healey JE, Jr, Sterling JA. Segmental anatomy of the newborn liver. Ann NY Acad Sci 1963;111:25–36.

18. Rex H. Beitrage sur Morphologie der Saugerleber. Morph Jahrb 1888;14:517.

19. Cantlie J. On a new arrangement of the right and left lobes of the liver. J Anat 1897;32:4–6.

20. Bradley OC. A contribution to the morphology and development of the mammalian liver. J Anat Physiol 1909;43:1–42.

21. McNee JW. Croonian lectures on liver and spleen: their clinical and pathological associations. Br Med J 1932;1:1068.

22. Healey JE, Jr, Schroy PC. Anatomy of the biliary ducts within the human liver: analysis of the prevailing pattern of branchings and the major variations of the biliary ducts. Arch Surg 1953;66:599.

23. Healey JE, Jr, Schroy PC, Sorensen RJ. The intrahepatic distribution of the hepatic artery in man. J Int Coll Surg 1953;20:133.

24. Coinaud C. Le foie. Paris: Masson et Cie, 1957.

25. Platzer W, Maurer H. Zur Segmenteinteilung der Leber. Acta Anat 1966;63:8–31.

26. Merrill GG. Complete absence of the left lobe of the liver in man. Arch Pathol 1946;42:232–233.

27. Morgenstern L, Mazur M. Hypoplasia of the right hepatic lobe (1 case). Am J Surg 1959;98:628–630.

28. Demirci A, Diren HB, Selcuk MB. Computed tomography in agenesis of the right lobe of the liver. Acta Radiol 1990;31(1):105–106.

29. Collay R, Anne F, deVanssay-deBlavous P, Gazel-de-la-Contrie D. Agenesie du lobe hepatique droit: a propos d'une observation. Ann Radiol 1990;33:108–113.

30. Meyers HI, Jacobson G. Displacements of stomach and duodenum by anomalous lobes of the liver. AJR 1958;79:789–792.

31. Watanabe M et al. Laparoscopic observation of hepatic lobe atrophy. Endoscopy 1989;21:234–236.

32. Riedel I. Über den zungenförmigen Fortsatz des rechten Leberlappens und seine pathognostische Bedeutung für die Erkrankung der Gallenblase nebst Bemerkungen über Gallensteinoperationen. Berl Klin Wschr 1888;25:577, 602.

33. Rietemeier RJ, Butt HR, Bagenstoss AH. Riedel's lobe of the liver. Gastroenterology 1958;34:1090.

34. Cullen TS. Accessory lobes of the liver. Arch Surg 1925;11:718–764.

35. Dick J. Riedel's lobe and related partial hepatic enlargements. Guy Hosp Rep 1951;100:270–277.

36. van der Reis L, Clark AG, McPhee VG. Congenital hepatomegaly. California Med 1956;85:41–42.

37. Chiba S, Suzuki T, Kasai T. A tongue-like projection of the left lobe in human liver, accompanied with lienorenal venous shunt and intrahepatic arterial anastomosis. Okajimas Folia Anat Jpn 1991;68:51–66.

38. Feist JH, Lasser EC. Identification of uncommon liver lobulation. JAMA 1959;169:1859–1862.

39. Hansbrough ET, Lipin RJ. Intrathoracic accessory lobe of the liver. Ann Surg 1957;145:564–567.

40. Kaufman SA, Madoff IM. Intrathoracic accessory lobe of the liver (1 case). Ann Intern Med 1960;53:403–407.

41. LeRoux BT. Heterotopic intrathoracic liver. Thorax 1961;16:68–69.

42. Katz HJ, Williams AJ. Accessory lobes of the liver: significance in roentgen diagnosis. Ann Intern Med 1952;36:880–883.

43. Mulla N, Weintraub S. Accessory liver with double gallbladder. Arch Surg 1955;71:202–204.

44. Ake E, Fouron JC, Lessard M, Boisvert J, Grignon A, van Doesburg NH. In utero sonographic diagnosis of diaphragmatic hernia with hepatic protrusion into the pericardium mimicking an intrapericardial tumor. Prenat Diagn 1991;11:719–724.

45. Shapiro JL, Metlay LA. Heterotopic supradiaphragmatic liver formation in association with congenital cardiac anomalies. Arch Pathol Lab Med 1991;115:238–240.

46. Bassis ML, Izenstark JL. Ectopic liver: its occurrence in the gallbladder. Arch Surg 1956;73:204–206.

47. Horányi J, Füsy F. Nebenpankreas in der Gallenblasenwand. Zentralbl Chir 1963;88:1414–1418.

48. Davies JNP. Accessory liver in Africans. Br Med J 1946;2:736–737.

49. Heid GJ, von Haam E. Hepatic heterology in the splenic capsule. Arch Pathol 1948;46:377–379.

50. Johnstone G. Accessory lobe of liver presenting through a congenital deficiency of anterior abdominal wall. Arch Dis Child 1965;40:541–544.

51. Foch G. Ectopic liver in omphalocele. Acta Paediatr 1963;52:288–292.

52. Chouke KS. A note on anomalous lobe of the liver. Anat Rec 1932;53:177–180.

53. Potter EL. Pathology of the fetus and the newborn. Chicago: Year Book Medical Publishers, 1952.

54. Tejada E, Danielson C. Ectopic or heterotopic liver (choristoma) associated with the gallbladder. Arch Pathol Lab Med 1989;113(8):950–952.

55. Ger R. Surgical anatomy of the liver. Surg Clin North Am 1989;69(2):179–192.

56. Bristowe JS. On the connection between abscess of the liver and gastro-intestinal ulceration. Trans Pathol Soc Lond 1857;10:241.

57. Desser PL, Smith S. Nonparasitic liver cysts in children. J Pediatr 1956;49:297.

58. David CE Jr, Rydeen JO. Massive congenital solitary cyst of the liver in infants. Surgery 1961;49:265–270.

59. Eliason EL, Smith DC. Solitary nonparasitic cyst of the liver. Clinics 1944;3:607.

60. Chaffin L. Congenital cystic disease of the liver. West J Surg 1948;56:193.

61. Henson SW Jr, Gray HK, Dockerty MB. Benign tumors of the liver. III. Solitary cysts. Surg Gynecol Obstet 1956;103:607–612.

62. Caravati CM, Watts TD, Hopkins JE, Kelly FR. Benign solitary non-parasitic cyst of the liver. Gastroenterology 1950;14:317.

63. Richmond HG. Carcinoma arising in congenital cysts of the liver. J Pathol Bact 1956;72:680.

64. Maingot R. Solitary nonparasitic cyst of the liver: report of a case. Br Med J 1940;2:867.

65. Greig GWV, Stinson R. Solitary nonparasitic cysts of the liver. Br J Surg 1961;48:457–460.

66. Manheimer LH. Solitary nonparasitic cyst of the liver. Ann Surg 1953;137:410–415.

67. Benhamou JP, Menu Y. Nonparasitic cystic diseases of the liver and intrahepatic biliary tree. In: Blumgart LH, ed. Surgery of the liver and biliary tract. New York: Churchill Livingstone, 1988;1013–1024.

68. Virchow R. Historisches, Kritisches und Positives zur Lehre der Unterleibsaffektionen. Virchow Arch [A] 1853;5:281.

69. Moschcowitz E. Non-parasitic cysts (congenital) of the liver, with a study of aberrant bile ducts. Am J Med Sci 1906;131:674.

70. von Meyenburg H. Über die Cystenleber. Beitr Pathol Anat 1918;64:477–532.

71. Comfort MW, Gray HK, Dahlin DC, Whitesell FB Jr. Polycystic disease of the liver: a study of 24 cases. Gastroenterology 1952;20:60.

72. Melnick PJ. Polycystic liver. Arch Pathol 1955;59:162–172.

73. Bigelow NH. The association of polycystic kidneys with intracranial aneurysms and other related disorders. Am J Med Sci 1953;225:485–494.

74. Poutasse EF, Gardner WJ, McCormack LJ. Polycystic kidney disease and intracranial aneurysm. JAMA 1954;154:741.

75. Campbell M. Urology. Philadelphia: WB Saunders, 1954.

76. Davis CR. Non-parasitic cysts of liver. Am J Surg 1937;35:590.

77. Tandon RK, Grewal H, Anand AC, Vashisht S. Caroli's syndrome: a heterogeneous entity. Am J Gastroenterol 1990;85:170–173.

78. Brent RL. Persistent jaundice in infancy. J Pediatr 1962;61:111–144.

79. Morgan WW, Rosenkrantz JG, Hill RB. Hepatic arterial interruption in the fetus: an attempt to simulate biliary atresia. J Pediatr Surg 1966;1:342–346.

80. Sterling JA, Smith KD. Normal karyotype in biliary atresia. J Einstein Med Center 1964;12:121–125.

81. Altman RP. Infantile obstructive jaundice. In: Schiller M, ed. Pediatric surgery of the liver, pancreas, and spleen. Philadelphia: WB Saunders, 1991:62.

82. Ahrens EH Jr, Harris RC, MacMahon HE. Atresia of the intrahepatic bile ducts. Pediatrics 1951;8:628.

83. Haas L, Dobbs RH. Congenital absence of the intrahepatic bile ducts. Arch Dis Child 1958;33:396–402.

84. Krovetz LJ. Intrahepatic biliary atresia. Lancet 1959;79:228–235.

85. Congenital atresia of the bile ducts [Editorial]. Lancet 1963;179–181.

86. Suruga K. A clinical and pathological study of congenital biliary atresia. J Pediatr Surg 1967;2:558–564.

87. Longmire WP. Congenital biliary hypoplasia. Ann Surg 1964;159:335–343.

88. Murray-Lyon IM, Ochendan BG, Williams R. Congenital hepatic fibrosis: is it a single clinical entity? Gastroenterology 1973;64:653–656.

89. Annand SK, Chan JG, Liberman E. Polycystic disease and hepatic fibrosis in children. Am J Dis Child 1975;129:810–825.

90. Watson GH, Miller V. Arterio-hepatic dysplasia. Arch Dis Child 1973;48:459–466.

91. Greenwood RD, Rosenthal A, Crocker AC, Nadas AS. Syndrome of intrahepatic biliary dysgenesis and cardiovascular malformations. Pediatrics 1976;58:243–254.

92. Alagille D, Odievre M, Gautier M, Dommergues JP. Hepatic ductular hypoplasia associated with characteristic facial, vertebral malformations, retarded physical mental and skeletal development and cardiac murmur. J Pediatr 1975;86(1):63–71.

93. Clift DAL, Campbell PE, Matthews JP, Yuen K. Primary liver tumors in children in Victoria: incidence and pathology. Pediatr Surg Int 1988;3:382–395.

94. Becker JM, Heitler MS. Hepatic hemangioendotheliomas in infancy. Surg Gynecol Obstet 1989;168:189–200.

95. Dehner LP, Ishak KG. Vascular tumors in the liver in infants and children. Arch Pathol 1971;92:101–111.

96. Ricketts RR, Stryker S, Raffensperger JG. Ventral fasciotomy in the management of hepatic hemangioendothelioma. J Pediatr Surg 1982;17:187–188.

97. deLorimier AA, Simpson EB, Baum RS, Carlsson E. Hepatic-artery ligation for hepatic hemangiomatosis. N Engl J Med 1967;277:333–336.

98. Berman B, Lim HWP. Concurrent cutaneous and hepatic hemangiomata in infancy: report of a case and review of the literature. J Dermatol Surg Oncol 1978;4:869–873.

99. Rocchini AP, Rosenthal A, Issenberg HJ, Nadas AS. Hepatic hemangioendothelioma: hemodynamic observations and treatment. Pediatrics 1976;57:131–135.

100. Weber TR, Connors RH, Tracy TF, Jr, Bailey PV. Complex hemangiomas of infants and children: individualized management in 22 cases. Arch Surg 1990;125:1017–1021.

101. Rotman M, John M, Stowe S, Inamdar S. Radiation treatment of pediatric hepatic hemangiomatosis and coexisting cardiac failure. N Engl J Med 1980;302:852.

102. Raffensperger JG, ed. Swenson's pediatric surgery, 5th ed. Norwalk CT: Appleton & Lange, 1990:371–373.

103. Gorenstein A, Abu-Dalu K, Schiller M. Vascular lesions. In: Schiller M, ed. Pediatric surgery of the liver, pancreas, and spleen. Philadelphia: WB Saunders, 1991:11–17.

104. Miller C et al. Orthotopic liver transplantation for massive hepatic lymphangiomatosis. Surgery 1988;103:490–495.

THE EXTRAHEPATIC BILIARY DUCTS AND THE GALLBLADDER

John Elias Skandalakis / Stephen Wood Gray / Richard Ricketts / Lee John Skandalakis / Thomas Dodson

"Gladstone's first article—an attack on science—caused such a flow of bile that I have been the better for it ever since."
—*LETTER OF THOMAS HUXLEY* (1825–1895) *TO SIR JOHN SKELTON*
JANUARY 21, 1886

DEVELOPMENT

The extrahepatic biliary duct system and the gallbladder as well as the ventral anlage of the pancreas arise from the hepatic diverticulum, the distal portion of which also gives rise to the biliary system of the liver. By late in the fourth week (23 somites), the cystic duct and gallbladder primordium is visible as a bud from the side of the diverticulum. By the beginning of the fifth week, the gallbladder, cystic duct, hepatic ducts, common bile duct, and the pancreatic duct are all demarcated (Fig. 9.1). During the fifth week, the proximal portion of the liver diverticulum elongates but does not increase greatly in diameter, in contrast to the tremendous growth of the distal end, which forms the liver cords within the septum transversum. During this stage of elongation, the future duct system becomes, like the duodenum itself, a solid cord of cells.

Toward the end of this week, growth of the duodenum, apparently limited to the left side of its wall, initiates a shift of the base of the liver diverticulum, together with the ventral pancreatic anlage, to their eventual position on the dorsal side just below the origin of the dorsal pancreatic diverticulum (Fig. 9.1 *C* and *D*).

Reestablishment of the lumina of the ducts starts in the sixth week with the common duct and progresses slowly distad. The lumen extends into the cystic duct by the seventh week; but, the gallbladder remains solid until the 12th week. Recanalization of a duct frequently results in the temporary appearance of two or three lumina, which will eventually coalesce. Two or more openings of the duct into the duodenum are frequent. The lower one usually is suppressed, but occasionally both may persist, leaving a bifurcated common bile duct (1). The solid stage and recanalization of the biliary system parallel the changes in

the duodenum itself, but strangely, no solid stage seems to occur in the pancreatic ducts.

Rudimentary accessory hepatic ducts are found at this stage, emptying into the hepatic or cystic ducts. One or more of these may occasionally persist, with a connection to a small portion of the liver (2). At the junction of the hepatic, cystic, and common ducts, a dilated region—the antrum—may be present. In 1926 Boyden (3) interpreted it as the residual hepatic diverticulum, which vanishes as the ducts elongate.

Indications of the muscular coats of the gallbladder appear during the ninth week and develop progressively from the gallbladder toward the duodenum.

An unconfirmed report (4) stated that the gallbladder becomes completely enveloped by the liver during the second month and arrives at its final position by subsequent atrophy of the overlying tissue. In cases of intrahepatic gallbladder, which may produce diagnostic problems for the operating surgeon, this report holds true. If a gallbladder series or sonography are positive for gall stones and if the gallbladder is not visible during open or laparoscopic procedures, the surgeon must entertain the possibility that there is an intrahepatic gallbladder and act accordingly. Whether or not this report is always true, the cystic fossa appears to form independently of the gallbladder and frequently is present when the gallbladder is absent.

The proximal portion of the hepatic diverticulum is usually absorbed by the intestinal wall so that the common duct and the pancreatic duct enter the duodenum side by side. This arrangement will persist in about 25% of adults. In the remainder, the septum will withdraw between the ducts to the level of the submucosa during the eighth week (1). In Boyden's view (3) the muscle fibers of the sphincter of Oddi are derived directly from the

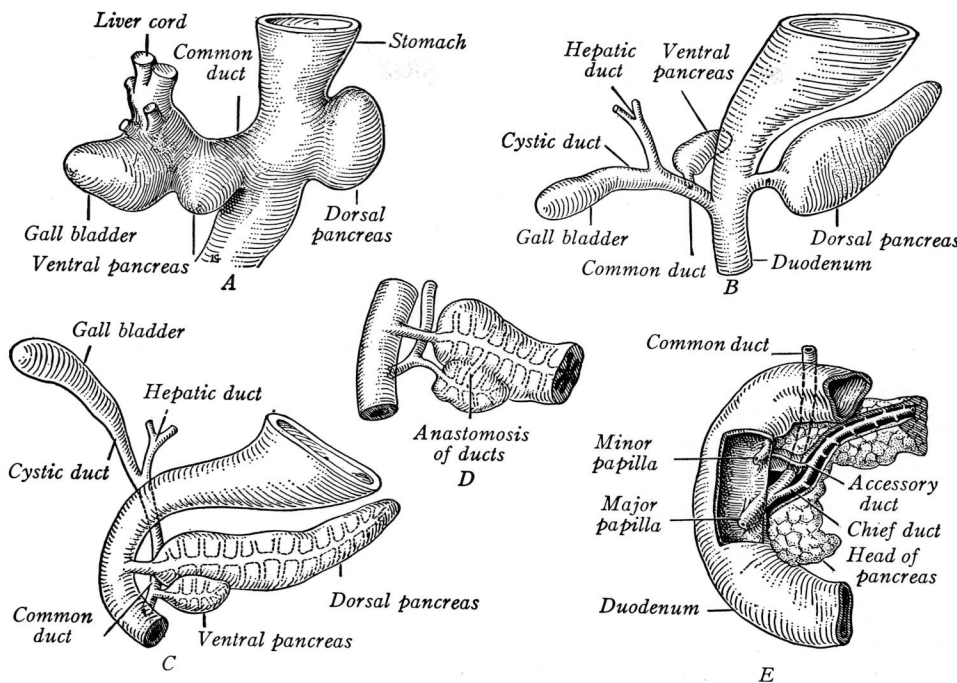

Figure 9.1. Development of the gallbladder, pancreas and biliary tract. **A**, At five weeks (6 mm). **B**, Sixth week (8 mm). **C**, At the end of the sixth week (12 mm). **D**, At the end of the seventh week (16 mm). **E**, At birth. NOTE: Right-to-left migration of the common bile duct and the ventral pancreatic primordium. (From Arey LB. Developmental anatomy, 7th ed. Philadelphia: WB Saunders, 1965.)

mesenchyme around the common duct during the 11th week.

Critical Events in Development

Failure of the liver or the pancreas to develop from this system of endodermal diverticula rarely if ever occurs. The important source of anomalies lies in the failure of the embryonic connections between the liver and the gut to develop into patent tubes. Although the extrahepatic biliary tract is probably an unnecessary structure before birth, absence of its component segments may be fatal in postnatal life. Structural variations, although physiologically compatible with life, may result in operative catastrophes if these are unrecognized later in life when surgical intervention is required.

To be more specific, despite the fact that the Kasai procedure is one of the triumphs of surgery, in biliary atresia the overall results are very poor. Perhaps transplantation will be the answer in the future.

Most of these anomalies occur in the fourth to sixth weeks of development. Biliary atresia, on the other hand, is considered to be an acquired defect rather than a congenital one.

ANOMALIES OF THE EXTRAHEPATIC DUCTS AND THE GALLBLADDER (TABLE 9.1)

For an illustration of possible sites of malformations in the biliary tract, see Figure 9.2. For a complete presentation of the characteristics of these anomalies, see Table 9.2.

Extrahepatic Biliary Atresia

Biliary atresia is the most serious of the anomalies of the extrahepatic biliary system and the most difficult to treat.

ANATOMY

Extrahepatic biliary atresia may involve a short segment of a duct, an entire duct, or the entire system. Except for the complete type, few cases are alike. Thompson (5) and Holmes (6) illustrated large numbers of the varieties encountered.

The defective duct may be stenosed; it may be present but solid; or it may be reduced to a fibrous band that is easily overlooked. In the latter case it is often considered to be absent. On developmental grounds, when the liver is present, agenesis of structures other than the cystic duct and gallbladder is hard to imagine; we prefer the term *atresia* even when no remnant of the duct can be identified. Rarely, the ducts may be hypoplastic (7).

Table 9.1.
Anomalies of the Extrahepatic Biliary Ducts and the Gallbladder

Anomaly	Origin of Defect	First Appearance	Sex Chiefly Affected	Relative Frequency	Remarks
Extrahepatic biliary atresia	Acquired	Soon after birth	Equal	Rare	Most likely infectious or environmental; not genetic or congenital
Variation of the hepatic ducts	5th week	None	Equal	Very common	
Accessory hepatic duct	4th week?	None	Equal	Common	
Duplication of common hepatic duct	4th week?	None	?	?	
Subvesicular and hepatocystic ducts	6th week	None	?	Rare	Anomaly not well established
Variations of the common bile duct	4th week	None	?	Common	
Cystic dilations of common bile duct	Unknown	Any age	Female	Rare (most common in Japanese)	
Duplication of common bile duct	4th–5th week	None	?	Very rare	
Absence of gallbladder	4th week	Adulthood, if ever	Female	Rare	
Duplication of gallbladder	4th week	None	Equal	Rare	
Deformation of gallbladder	6th week	None	Equal	Uncommon	
Left-sided gallbladder	4th week?	None	?	Very rare	
Intrahepatic gallbladder	2nd month	None	?	Rare	
Mobile gallbladder	2nd month	Late adulthood, if ever	Female	Rare	Symptoms result from torsion
Heterotopic mucosa in gallbladder	4th week?	None	?	Very rare	
Adenomyoma of gallbladder	6th week?	Late adulthood, if ever	Female	Rare	
Anomalies of cystic duct	5th week	None	?	Common	

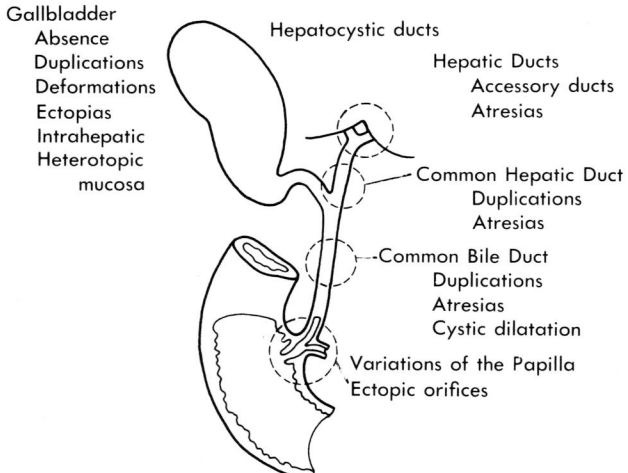

Figure 9.2. Sites of potential malformations in the biliary tract.

Extrahepatic biliary atresias may be grouped roughly into seven types, as illustrated in Figure 9.3. However, one may classify these anomalies in three common anatomic groups (Fig. 9.4).

The changes in the liver secondary to atresia become increasingly marked with time. Cirrhosis and bile stasis appear, together with increasing disruption of the normal lobular pattern of the liver. Bile duct proliferation in the portal spaces occurs. In addition, the hepatic arteries are enlarged and have thicker walls than usual. These secondary features led earlier writers (8) to consider the cirrhosis to be primary. They attributed the disease to maternal poisons producing fetal cirrhosis and cholangitis, which resulted in stenosis and atresia of the extrahepatic ducts.

EMBRYOGENESIS

The presence of the liver indicates that the primordium of the common bile duct and the hepatic ducts appeared normally. However, complete agenesis of the cystic diverticulum is possible, and the resulting condition is a true agenesis rather than an atresia of the cystic duct and gallbladder.

Elongation of the future common bile duct and hepatic ducts takes place during the fifth week; at the same time, epithelial proliferation fills their lumina. Yllpö (9) in 1913 explained the atresia as a failure of recanali-

Table 9.2.
Symptoms, Diagnosis, and Treatment of Anomalies of the Biliary Tract

Anomaly	Pathology	Symptoms	Diagnosis	Treatment	Remarks
Extrahepatic biliary atresia		Early: Persistent progressive jaundice Late: Enlarging abdomen; white stools	Elevated serum bilirubin; biopsy to confirm presence of intrahepatic ducts; operative cholangiogram	Anastomosis where possible: Hepatocholedochostomy; Choledochoduodenostomy; Cholecystoduodenostomy or Kasai portoenterostomy (various modifications)	80% will ultimately require liver transplant
Variations of hepatic ducts		Asymptomatic	Incidental radiographic or surgical finding	None required	
Accessory hepatic duct		Asymptomatic	Incidental radiographic or surgical finding	None required	
Duplication of common hepatic duct		Asymptomatic	Incidental radiographic or surgical finding		
Subvesicular and hepatocystic ducts		Abdominal distension	Identified only at autopsy		Possible souce of hepatic cysts
Variations of common bile duct		Asymptomatic	Incidental radiographic or surgical finding		
Cystic dilation of common bile duct		Early: jaundice	IV cholangiogram, abdominal ultrasound; ERCP	Cystectomy with Roux-en-Y; common hepaticojejunostomy	Source of malignancy if not totally resected

Table 9.2—*continued.*
Symptoms, Diagnosis, and Treatment of Anomalies of the Biliary Tract

Anomaly	Pathology	Symptoms	Diagnosis	Treatment	Remarks
Duplication of common bile duct		Asymptomatic	Incidental radiographic or surgical finding		
Ectopic orifice of common bile duct		Asymptomatic	Usually at surgery or autopsy		
Absence of gallbladder		Asymptomatic	Absence on x-ray film not diagnostic; preoperative diagnosis not possible		
Duplication of gallbladder		Asymptomatic	Recognizable on radiography		
Deformations of gallbladder		Asymptomatic	May be recognized on radiography		May be result of cholecystitis and not of congenital origin
Abnormal positions of gallbladder					
Left sided		Asymptomatic	May be outside the radiographic field, hence not visualized		
Intrahepatic		Asymptomatic	Visualized radiopgrahically; apparently absent at operation		
Mobile		Symptoms of torsion or strangulation	At surgery		
Absence of cystic duct (sessile gallbladder)		Asymptomatic	Incidental radiographic or surgical finding		

Table 9.2—*continued.*
Symptoms, Diagnosis, and Treatment of Anomalies of the Biliary Tract

Anomaly	Pathology	Symptoms	Diagnosis	Treatment	Remarks
Anomalies of junction of cystic and common bile ducts	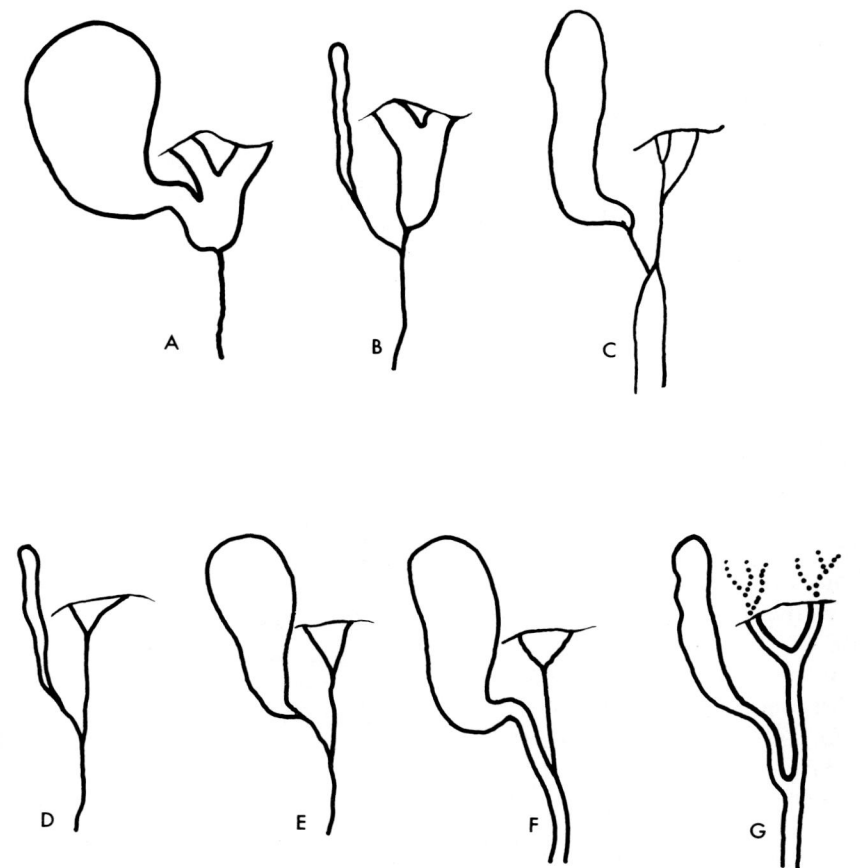	Asymptomatic	Incidental finding at surgery		May predispose to lithiasis

Figure 9.3. Atresias of the biliary tract. **A** to **F**, Extrahepatic biliary atresia. **G**, Intrahepatic atresia with normal extrahepatic structures. Defects **A**, **B**, and **C** are "correctable"; **D**, **E**, **F**, and **G** are "noncorrectable" atresias. Types **D** and **E** are the most common.

zation of the solid epithelial cords, together with an arrest in growth in diameter of the ducts; this view has been widely accepted (10). That the entire extrahepatic system frequently is present only as fibrous cords agrees with this explanation. The developmental arrest can be assigned to the sixth week.

There is a second possibility: The growth of the epithelium fails to keep up with elongation during the fifth week, and the duct becomes attenuated and finally breaks, resulting in a complete gap in continuity. In such cases no fibrous cord would remain.

In 1956 it was suggested that the atresia may result from liver disease late in prenatal life or even after birth (11); a decade later Holder and Ashcraft (12) pointed out that some children do not manifest jaundice in the first 2 weeks of life, and a few have been found to have atresia even though earlier cholangiography indicated the ducts were patent.

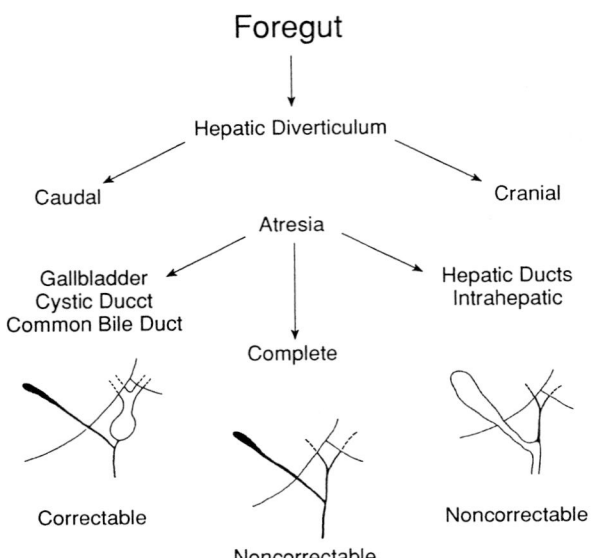

Figure 9.4. Development of the three most common anatomic expressions of biliary atresia. (Modified from Lilly J. Biliary atresia: the jaundiced infant. In: Welch KJ, Randolph JG, Ravitch MM, O'Neill JA, Rowe MI, ed. Pediatric Surgery, 4th ed., Vol 2. Chicago: Year Book Medical Publishers, 1986:1047–1056 and Karrer FM, Raffensperger JG. Biliary atresia. In: Raffensperger JG, ed. Swenson's pediatric surgery, 5th ed. New York: Appleton & Lange, 1990:649–660.)

ETIOLOGY

Injury to the blood supply of ducts was reported by Picket and Briggs (13) who experimentally produced biliary obstruction with vascular ligation in fetal sheep. Abnormal bile acids were reported by Okamoto et al. (14) and McSherry et al. (15) who produced biliary atresia by devascularization of the common bile duct and by administration of bile acids to the mother at late pregnancy or to the newborn animal.

Infection. This is the most probable etiologic factor because progressive disease is a characteristic of biliary atresia. Congenital rubella syndrome, neonatal viral hepatitis (non–A and B), cytomegalovirus, and *reovirus* type 3 all have been mentioned by several authors as responsible for the genesis of biliary atresia. Morecki et al. (16) reported that 17 of 85 babies with biliary atresia had *reovirus* type 3 antibodies and concluded that there is a suggestion of causal relation of biliary atresia to *reovirus* type 3.

Using a model of common bile duct obstruction in the newborn rat in their experimental studies, Tracy et al. (17) reported that altered liver gene expression is of viral etiology in some neonatal cholestatic syndromes.

At present we agree with Raffensperger (18) that biliary atresia is not a single embryologic event but is most likely an inflammatory or infectious disease perhaps starting in fetal life or immediately after birth. *Reovirus* type 3 was suggested as an etiologic factor for the development of biliary atresia by Bangaru et al. (19) and Glaser et al. (20). Three theories of atresia are presented in Figure

9.5. For historical perspective, we retained the congenital theories.

ASSOCIATED ANOMALIES

Biliary atresia is not usually accompanied by other malformations. Absence or hypoplasia of the kidney, imperforate anus, ileal stenosis, situs inversus, and tetralogy of Fallot were reported in five of 31 cases in Moore's series (21). In 1936 Gross (22) found two patients with biliary atresia among 148 with complete situs inversus.

According to Lilly and Chandra (23), 10 to 15% of patients with biliary atresia have associated anomalies of the inferior vena cava (absence), portal vein (preduodenal portal vein), intestine (intestinal malrotation), and spleen (polysplenia).

HISTORY

The history of extrahepatic biliary atresia begins with the review and illustration of 50 cases collected from the literature by Thompson (5) in 1891 and 1892. Although he traced the lesion back to a description by Home (24) in 1813 and Holmes (6) was able to find a case report in 1795, little attention had been paid to these isolated reports. Beneke (25) added 24 cases in 1907. In 1916 Holmes (6) was able to collect 119 cases, many of which he illustrated, and he republished Thompson's illustrations.

In 1916 Holmes (6) stated, "In at least 16% of all cases yet reported the anatomical relations are such that operative relief is theoretically possible." Twelve years later, Ladd (26) performed the first successful repair of biliary atresia. One of the patients was alive and well 37 years later, according to Lou et al. (27) in 1972. By 1960 about 500 cases were to be found in the literature (28).

The most monumental advance in the understanding and treatment of biliary atresia occurred in 1957 when Kasai (29) described the treatment of "noncorrectable" cases of biliary atresia by a hepatic portoenterostomy. This work, published in Japanese, was largely ignored in the Western world until 1968 when Kasai (30) reported in the English literature his results in treating 92 patients with biliary atresia. These contributions revolutionized the treatment for biliary atresia which, until the "Kasai procedure," was a uniformly fatal disease. Current management of patients with biliary atresia is based on the principles initially outlined by Kasai. However, in the last decade in certain cases, liver transplantation is becoming a viable treatment modality.

EDITORIAL COMMENT

As pointed out in the editorial comment in the chapter on the liver under the discussion of intrahepatic biliary atresia, the best evidence currently supports an acquired etiology, possibly viral, for both intrahepatic and extrahepatic biliary atresia. The data clearly indicates that abortuses have never been documented to have

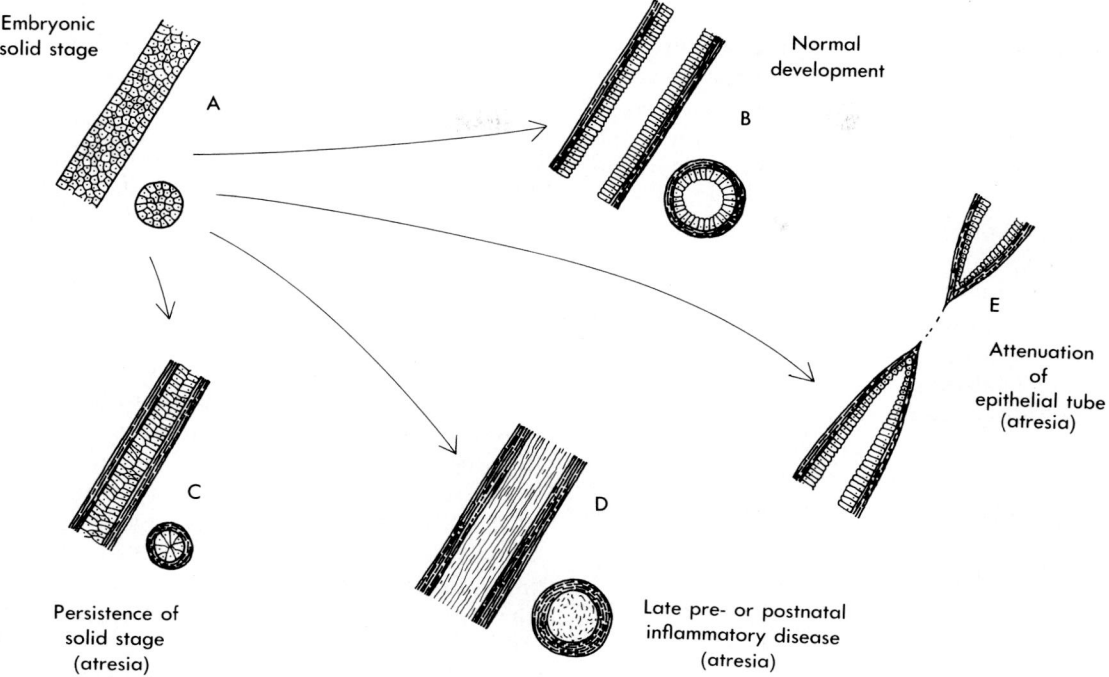

Figure 9.5. Three possible mechanisms for formation of biliary atresia. **A**, Solid stage of biliary tract before the sixth week. **B**, Normal recanalization of the ducts to form a patent tube. **C**, Failure of recanalization, leaving a minute epithelial strand without a functional lumen. **D**, Postinflammatory fibrosis late in fetal life producing atresia. **E**, Attenuation and loss of continuity of a biliary duct during elongation in the fifth week.

either form of biliary atresia and only in rare instances is biliary atresia present in stillborn infants.

One of the most remarkable aspects of the Kasai operation for "noncorrectable" biliary atresia is the anastomosis. This anastomosis is carried out between the portal parenchyma and the Roux-en-Y loop of jejunum. This is the only example of an enteric anastomosis in which there is not a mucosa-to-mucosa switcher-line. Exactly why this anastomosis works when there is no continuity of epithelium is unclear. One would expect the anastomosis to become fibrotic and obstructed, and yet a large percentage of these anastomoses are successful, apparently because the epithelium of the intrahepatic ducts and the mucosa of the jejunum migrate toward each other and eventually cover the area of absent epithelium in the area of the connection.

Further evidence of the acquired nature of biliary atresia, however, is demonstrated by the fact that the majority of patients with "successful" Kasai anastomoses will eventually go on to develop liver failure secondary to progressive hepatitis and biliary cirrhosis. Some of this failure is due to recurring episodes of cholangitis but many seem to result from a smoldering hepatitis, which probably was the primary etiology (JAH/CNP).

INCIDENCE

In 1953 Moore (21) estimated the incidence of congenital extrahepatic biliary atresia at 1:20,000 to 1:30,000 births, basing this conclusion on his experience that it occurred only one-fourth as often as did imperforate anus. On the other hand, Stowens (31) concluded from 10,000 autopsy reports of infants and children that biliary atresia occurred more than twice as frequently as imperforate anus and three times as frequently as Down's syndrome. He found no race or gender difference and no evidence of a familial tendency.

Alternatively, the presence of 13 cases in five families has been offered as evidence of a familial tendency by Krauss (32). There seems to be no clinical nor pathologic difference between these cases and others.

Hassall and Guna-Sekaran (personal communication, 1991) reported two children with extrahepatic biliary atresia. They were born of the same father but different mothers. The authors raised the question of whether a genetic factor might cause the development of the atresia. Perhaps this is the case. However, Elsas (personal communication, 1991) postulated that the father's "sensitivity" genes were perhaps involved in the embryologic development of the hepatopancreatic complex during the fifth week of gestation. We agree.

The incidence of biliary atresia currently is estimated to be between 1:10,000 to 1:20,000 live births without apparent racial or genetic predilection but with a female predominance of 1.4 to 1 (33). The increase in incidence is four- to fivefold in populations of the Pacific and Indian Ocean areas, and there seems to be female predominance in Asians (34).

SYMPTOMS

Persistent, progressive jaundice starting at birth or shortly afterward is the cardinal sign of biliary atresia. It is, at first, indistinguishable from the normal physiologic jaundice of the newborn infant. Absence of color in the meconium is probably the first sign that should alert the physician.

In contrast to the picture of icterus neonatorum, the skin color deepens daily and the abdomen begins to enlarge; the infant does not appear ill and has a good appetite and good disposition. The urine is dark and the stools are white; although, they may be colored from intestinal bleeding later in the course of the disease. The liver and spleen are enlarged; and, rarely, there is ascitic fluid in the abdomen.

Although initial growth is good, weight gain decreases and physical retardation with signs of malnutrition are present in the later stages. The untreated patient usually succumbs in less than a year. Occasionally, an infant may survive longer.

DIAGNOSIS

On physical examination the infant will be markedly icteric and have hepatosplenomegaly. The liver is hard when palpated, distinguishing it from neonatal hepatitis when the liver is generally softer. Laboratory studies reveal a direct hyperbilirubinemia, marked elevation of the alkaline phosphatase, moderate elevation of the liver enzymes, positive results for urine bilirubin, and negative results for urine urobilinogen. Radionuclide hepatobiliary imaging utilizing 99ᵐTC-sulfur colloid–labeled derivatives of diethyl-imino-diacetic acid are useful in distinguishing biliary atresia from neonatal hepatitis (35). In neonatal hepatitis, the nuclide will be excreted into the gastrointestinal tract, whereas in biliary atresia it will not. An ultrasonogram is useful in distinguishing biliary atresia from a choledochal cyst, both of which can result in neonatal jaundice. The ultrasound examination also is useful in demonstrating other causes of neonatal jaundice such as idiopathic perforation of the common bile duct and inspissated bile duct syndrome.

Liver biopsy and operative cholangiography are the only methods by which biliary atresia can be diagnosed with certainty. In most cases surgical exploration of the extrahepatic biliary tree will reveal a small gallbladder, with or without a lumen, and fibrous obliteration of the ductal system. If a gallbladder lumen is present, an operative cholangiogram is performed which will confirm the diagnosis and reveal the type of extrahepatic ductal obstruction present. If the entire extrahepatic biliary system is patent but diminutive in size ("biliary hypoplasia"), the Kasai procedure is not indicated. An open liver biopsy completes the diagnostic workup. Bile deposition in the periphery of the lobules, portal fibrosis, bile duct prolif-

eration in portal areas, and enlarged and thickened hepatic arteries constitute the histologic picture.

DIFFERENTIAL DIAGNOSIS

Intrahepatic Biliary Atresia. The presence of perilobular bile ducts in the biopsy specimen will indicate whether or not intrahepatic atresia is present. The presence of one form of atresia does not preclude the presence of others.

Icterus Neonatorum. The normal jaundice of the newborn decreases rather than progresses with time, disappearing after the first month. Stools and urine are normal in color, and there is no liver enlargement.

Erythroblastosis Fetalis. Jaundice due to erythroblastosis appears early and is intermittent; the stools are colored. Blood typing of both parents and infant and tests for anti-Rh agglutinins will confirm or eliminate this diagnosis.

Infections. If there is a history of hepatitis in the family or if the mother has received a blood transfusion, the investigator may suspect infection. Giant cells in the liver biopsy are not conclusive since they have been reported with both intrahepatic and extrahepatic biliary atresia (36).

Rutenburg and colleagues (37) proposed using a serum leucine aminopeptidase (LAP) assay to differentiate biliary atresia and obstructive jaundice from acute hepatitis and icterus neonatorum. In their study, the LAP levels were consistently high in the former group and unaltered in the latter group.

The possibility of syphilis must be considered and eliminated by serologic examination and radiography of the long bones. Fever and lymphocytosis may indicate other infectious disease, which may be confirmed by blood cultures.

TREATMENT

Successful treatment of biliary atresia requires prompt diagnosis and early operative intervention to achieve bile drainage. Kasai (38) observed that bile excretion was obtained in 89% of patients operated on before 60 days of age; the 10-year survival rate for these patients was 74%. In patients operated on after 90 days of age, only 41% obtained bile drainage and only 19% experienced a 10-year survival rate.

EDITORIAL COMMENT

The obvious reason for poor results in patients undergoing surgery after 90 days of age is the progression of biliary cirrhosis which has taken place. For this reason, it is imperative that an earlier diagnosis be made and that babies with biliary atresia be explored before they are 30 days of age to decrease the progressive development of biliary cirrhosis (JAH).

The operative treatment begins with exploration of the porta, operative cholangiography, and open liver biopsy.

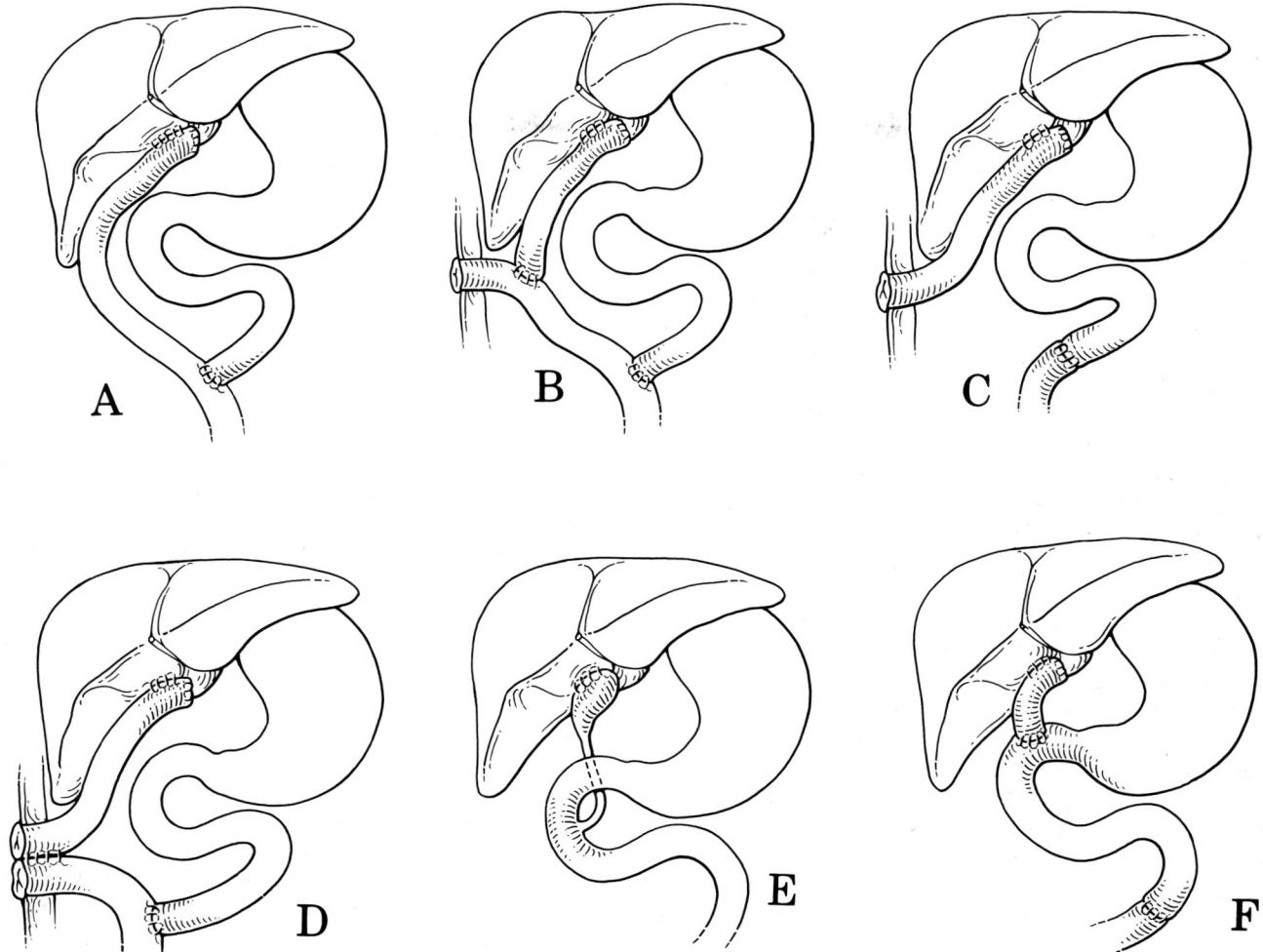

Figure 9.6. Variations of the Kasai portoenterostomy. **A**, Original Kasai procedure. **B**, Double Roux-en-Y portoenterostomy ("Kasai II"). **C**, Sawaguchi procedure. **D**, Roux-en-Y portoenterostomy with Mickulicy exteriorization. **E**, Por- tocholecystostomy ("gallbladder Kasai"). **F**, Jejunal interposition portoduoden- ostomy. (Modified from Karrer FM et al. Biliary atresia registry, 1976–1989. J Pediatr Surg 1990;25:1076–1081.)

A surgeon performing this portion of the procedure should be capable of proceeding to the definitive surgical procedure of portoenterostomy as described by Kasai. If the cholangiogram shows patency of the gallbladder and common bile duct into the duodenum with obliteration of the proximal biliary tree, a hepatic portocholecystostomy can be performed (39). In all other cases a portoenter- ostomy, as described by Kasai, or one of its modifications is performed (30, 40–44). In many of these modifications, the intestinal conduit from the porta is externalized in an attempt to prevent ascending cholangitis and to quanti- tate the amount of bile flow achieved. In these cases the bile is re-fed to the infant either by mouth or through the distal limb of the externalized conduit. Some procedures incorporate a "valve" to help prevent ascending cholan- gitis (33). For operative procedure illustrations, see Fig- ure 9.6.

EDITORIAL COMMENT

We strongly recommend that the bile drainage conduit in the Kasai procedure be kept internal and not brought out as an ostomy. There is a natural reluctance to do this because the bile drainage cannot be documented as coming from an ostomy site. Neverthe- less, the ostomy will often be the site of the formation of very large portal vein collaterals. Progressive biliary cirrhosis and bleeding, which can be massive, may occur from these collaterals. In addi- tion, the external stoma greatly complicates liver transplantation subsequently because of the associated scarring and increased collateral circulation around the stoma. If the surgeon wishes to document bile drainage following the anastomosis he or she can insert a percutaneous silastic drainage catheter through the wall of the Roux-en-Y loop and both irrigate and drain the contents of the jejunal limb to verify the function of the new anastomosis. This eliminates an external stoma and avoids some of the complications of collateral circulation (JAH/CNP).

The main complications in patients with biliary atresia even after the Kasai procedure are cholangitis, progressive liver fibrosis, liver cirrhosis with portal hypertension, and deficiency of fat-soluble vitamin absorption. These complications lead to the eventual need for a liver transplant in approximately 80% of long-term survivors following the Kasai procedure for biliary atresia (33).

Starzl (45) first performed liver transplantation in 1963 on a 3-year-old male with biliary atresia. The patient's overall condition was poor with a preoperative weight of 9 kg. He had hepatosplenomegaly, jaundice (bilirubin of 21 mg%), and ascites. He bled to death on the operating table, 4 hr after revascularization of the homograft. After five consecutive deaths, Starzl returned to the laboratory for several years before resuming transplantation in humans. In 1976 he (46) was able to report the results of orthotopic liver transplantation in 93 patients, and one year later Calne (47) reported his first 60 patients. These initial results were poor; but, they did note a gradual improvement over time.

In 1980 Starzl (48) reported a series of 23 liver transplant patients with only a 26% 1-year survival rate, clearly a disappointing result after 17 years of effort. That same year, however, cyclosporine became available for clinical trials. One year later the first report of liver transplantation using cyclosporine was announced (49). In that series of 14 patients, two patients died during operation, but of the 12 patients who survived surgery, 10 (83%) were still alive 8 to 14 months after the operation. With the NIH Consensus Conference Statement (50) in June of 1983 that transplantation of the liver was a "therapeutic modality" and with the release of cyclosporine in the United States in November of that same year, the modern era of liver transplantation began.

More than half of pediatric patients who undergo orthotopic liver transplantation have biliary atresia, with inborn errors of metabolism making up the second but smaller category of disorders (51). Approximately 250 infants with biliary atresia will be born in this country each year (52). If a decision is made that transplantation of the liver is the appropriate treatment for these 250 infants, the majority of these patients will require transplantation during the first 2 years of life. This premise is based on the previously noted data that the majority of untreated patients with biliary atresia will live only 1½ years.

Although recent studies (53) have noted an overall 80% survival rate in pediatric patients, two studies (54, 55) that dealt specifically with patients of less than 1 year of age showed a 1-year survival of 60 to 65%. Thus, if early transplantation were elected for all patients with biliary atresia, the expected survival rate would be less than might be expected if the patients were older and somewhat larger.

To take advantage of the fact that about one-quarter to one-third of patients undergoing a hepatic portoenterostomy will ultimately do well, it seems important to look at the Kasai procedure and orthotopic liver transplantation as "complementary rather than competitive" procedures (56).

This approach was adopted by investigators from the University of California–Los Angeles and Harvard with salutary results. In 1988 Millis and colleagues (57) reported that, of 45 patients with biliary atresia, 36 underwent liver transplantation, 28 of whom had had a previous portoenterostomy. They could detect no differences in blood loss, technical complications, or survival rates in children with or without previous Kasai procedures.

In 1990 Vacanti et al. (58) reported on a series of 28 infants who underwent Kasai portoenterostomy as a primary surgical procedure. Nine of these infants ultimately underwent liver transplantation, and, at the date of the report, 25 of 28 infants were alive. With nearly 90% of their patients alive 1 to 8 years during this study, these investigators noted that they would continue to offer a surgical approach combining the two procedures.

What does the future hold? The major barrier to liver transplantation (and other organs as well) as the sole treatment of patients with biliary atresia is the lack of acceptable cadaver donors. An estimated 20,000 individuals could be organ donors in the United States each year, but only 20% of those individuals actually donate their organs (59). Pediatric donors are particularly difficult to identify, and in response to that problem, liver transplant centers have increasingly turned to "reduced-size" liver transplants (60–63). Otte and his colleagues (64) from Brussels also have reported on the use of two livers for four patients. They suggested that this technique can be useful in "urgent" liver transplantation.

The management of organ donors after they have been declared "brain dead" also has come under scrutiny (65). With attention to hemodynamics, fluids, electrolytes, ventilation, oxygenation, temperature, and other factors, the supply of functional organs for transplantation can potentially be increased.

An experimental method currently under investigation to increase the donor pool is the use of a living related donor (66). The ethics of this method have been discussed by the liver transplant team at the University of Chicago, which is in the process of evaluating 20 liver transplants with living donors (63).

If the donor problem can be solved by a combination of education, "split liver" procedures, and perhaps occasional use of living donors, the next most pressing prob-

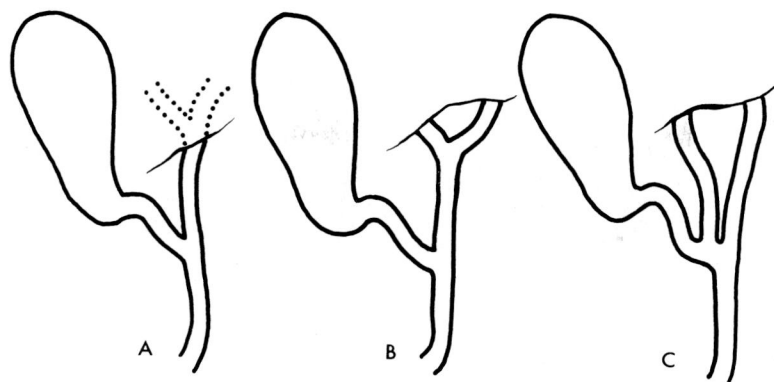

Figure 9.7. Variations of the hepatic ducts. **A**, Intrahepatic union of right and left hepatic ducts. **B**, Extrahepatic union of right and left hepatic ducts. **C**, Distal union of hepatic ducts resulting in absence of the common hepatic duct.

lem is the improvement of results from the present day standards of approximately a 70% 1-year survival in adult patients and 80% 1-year survival in pediatric patients. Better immunosuppressive agents seem to be the key to such improvement. One new drug, FK-506, already is undergoing clinical trials in both Europe and North America (68, 69), and other agents are on the drawing board.

With these new developments, it can be seen that the future of patients with biliary atresia is not static. As of 1991, a combination of portoenterostomy and liver transplantation is the standard method of therapy. In the days to come, liver transplantation alone may be the treatment of choice in the management of patients with obstruction, destruction, or absence of the extrahepatic bile ducts. It must be noted that previous anatomic boundaries have fallen to diligent surgical investigators using techniques undreamed of in years past (70). Is it too much to wonder that perhaps one day we may be able to detect such congenital anomalies and that their repair will lie not with the scalpel but with the gene and the cell?

Anomalies of the Hepatic Ducts

VARIATIONS OF THE HEPATIC DUCTS

The right and left hepatic ducts unite outside the liver in about 90% of cases and within the liver substance in 10% (71) (Fig. 9.7 A and B). The common hepatic duct, which may be as long as 7.5 cm, extends from this point of union to the junction of the cystic duct. If the cystic duct inserts at the junction of the right and left hepatic ducts, however, the common hepatic duct may be absent (72) (Fig. 9.7, C). The duct is usually about 4 cm in length, but the variations in length and the angle between the right and left hepatic ducts is such that Michels (72) stated, "The mode of formation of the hepatic duct by the extrahepatic bile ducts varies to such an extent that no two patterns are ever exactly the same."

ABSENCE OF THE COMMON HEPATIC DUCT

So-called absence of the common hepatic duct must not be confused with atresia. Absence produces no loss of continuity in the biliary tract, and no surgical correction is required.

The common hepatic duct may be absent because the right and left hepatic ducts join at the insertion of the cystic duct (Fig. 9.7, C). Occasionally, however, there is no common duct because the right and left hepatic ducts fail to join. The right hepatic duct receives the cystic duct, whereas the left hepatic duct enters the duodenum independently (73) (Fig. 9.14). This condition is more accurately called duplication of the common bile duct; it arises early as a split in the hepatic diverticulum.

The unpredictable variability of the left hepatic duct was studied recently by Couinaud (74) and Russell et al. (75).

ACCESSORY HEPATIC DUCTS

Accessory, anomalous, or supernumerary hepatic ducts are not rare. Michels (72) compiled the reports of 12 investigators who found 184 accessory ducts among 1162 individuals (15.8%). Dowdy and colleagues (76) found one or more accessory ducts in 24 of 100 autopsies. Almost always found on the right side, these accessory ducts may join the common duct along with the usual left and right hepatic ducts (Fig. 9.8, A), at the insertion of the cystic duct (Fig. 9.8, B), or anywhere in between. They also may enter the cystic duct directly (77) (Fig. 9.8, C). Left accessory hepatic ducts are unusual, but they do occur (72, 78). They represent union of the medial and lateral segmental ducts outside the liver.

DUPLICATION OF THE COMMON HEPATIC DUCT

Michels (72) described a shunt that arose from the common hepatic duct just below the junction of the right and left hepatic ducts (Fig. 9.9, A). It passed behind the cystic duct and entered the common bile duct. In another case

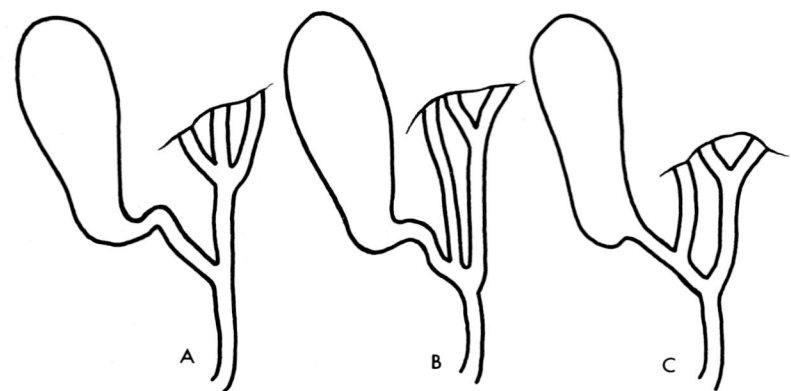

Figure 9.8. Accessory hepatic ducts. Usually the accessory duct is on the right, but left accessory ducts are known.

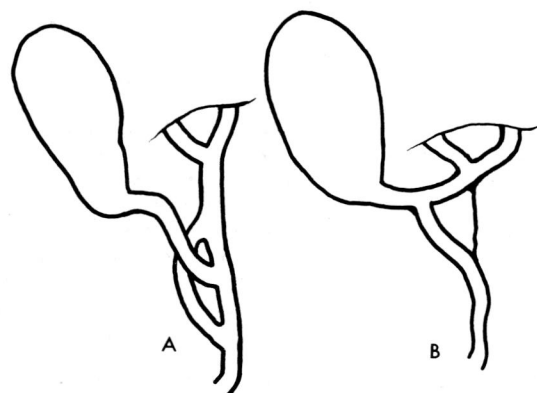

Figure 9.9. Duplications of the common hepatic duct. **A**, Case described by Michels **B**, Case described by Nygren and Barnes. The duplication is patent, while the normal duct is atretic. (**A**, From Michels NA. Blood supply and anatomy of the upper abdominal organ with a descriptive atlas. Philadelphia: JB Lippincott, 1955; **B**, from Nygren EJ, Barnes WA. Atresia of the common hepatic duct with shunt via an accessory duct. Arch Surg 1954;68:337.)

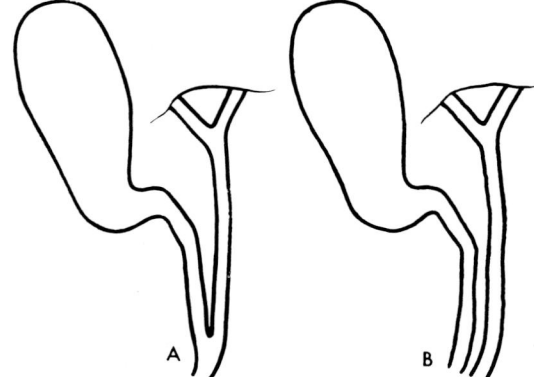

Figure 9.10. Variations of the common bile duct. **A**, Absence of the supraduodenal common bile duct (low insertion of the cystic duct). **B**, Absence of the entire common bile duct (separate entrance of the common hepatic duct and the cystic duct into the duodenum).

a shunt passed from the cranial end of the common hepatic duct to the neck of the gallbladder. The normal common duct was atretic (79) (Fig. 9.9, *B*).

SUBVESICULAR AND HEPATOCYSTIC DUCTS

Supernumerary hepatic ducts formed during development of the liver may occasionally persist (3). In some cases they fail to connect with the true bile capillaries and may then become a source of polycystic disease. In other cases they persist as accessory hepatic ducts that open directly into the gallbladder (Fig. 9.8).

Mentzer (80) found these hepatocystic ducts present in eight of 96 autopsies. Other workers (81) warned against the danger of bile peritonitis from leakage of these vessels following removal of the gallbladder. For this reason, we believe a Jackson-Pratt drain after cholecystectomy is up to the surgeon.

Michels (72), in 500 dissections, found none of these

ducts and questioned whether they actually enter the gallbladder. He found branches of the ramus subvesicularis from the right hepatic duct in the gallbladder bed, but saw no evidence that they communicated with the gallbladder. These subvesicular ducts may cause postoperative bile leakage if they are injured.

Anomalies of the Common Bile Duct

VARIATIONS OF THE COMMON BILE DUCT

The common bile duct is 5 to 15 cm long and is customarily divided into four segments called the supraduodenal, retroduodenal, intrapancreatic, and transduodenal portions.

Supraduodenal Portion. This section extends from the junction of the common hepatic and cystic ducts to the upper free border of the duodenum. In 14 to 20% of individuals, the cystic duct inserts so low that the supraduodenal portion is absent (Fig. 9.10, *A*). In rare cases, the cystic duct enters the duodenum independently, resulting in a true absence of the entire common bile duct (Fig. 9.10, *B*).

Retroduodenal Portion. This extends from the upper free border of the duodenum to the pancreatic capsule. Atresia of this segment, bypassed by an accessory duct, has been reported (82).

Intrapancreatic Portion. The variations in the relationship of the common bile duct to the head of the pancreas are of no functional significance, but they are of importance to the surgeon.

Beginning with von Wyss in 1870 (83), a number of workers studied these variations, including Smanio (84) who examined 200 cadavers and divided them into five groups based on the extent to which the common duct was covered by the pancreas, as viewed from the posterior surface. A modification of his division is given here:

1. A part of the duct is covered by a fold of pancreatic tissue (lingula) arising inferior to the duct (42.5%) (Fig. 9.11, *A* and *B*).
2. The entire pancreatic portion of the duct is covered by a similar fold (30%) (Fig. 9.11, *C*).
3. The duct lies free on the pancreatic surface or in a shallow groove (16.5%) (Fig. 9.11, *D*).

4. The entire duct is covered by two folds of pancreatic tissue arising above and below the duct (9%) (Fig. 9.11, *E*).
5. Rare variations not included in the other groups (2%).

In groups 3 and 4 and part of group 1, the common duct is easily accessible, being either free or covered by a thin flap of pancreatic tissue that has an easily separated cleavage plane. In the remaining cases the covering flap of tissue is thick and the cleavage plane difficult to find. Surgically, if not anatomically, these must be considered intrapancreatic. In three of Smanio's cadavers, some pancreatic tissue had to be cut to free the duct, and in one, the duct lay in a groove on the anterior face of the pancreas. No gender or race differences were found (84).

Transduodenal Portion. The common bile duct and the pancreatic duct (derived from the ventral pancreatic anlage) arise from a common embryonic diverticulum of the foregut and, hence, at first have a common entrance (which forms the ampulla of Vater) into the posterior medial wall of the second part of the duodenum. Abnormal locations of the orifice are discussed later in this chapter. Growth of the duodenum tends to absorb some of the proximal portion of the ampulla, so that among

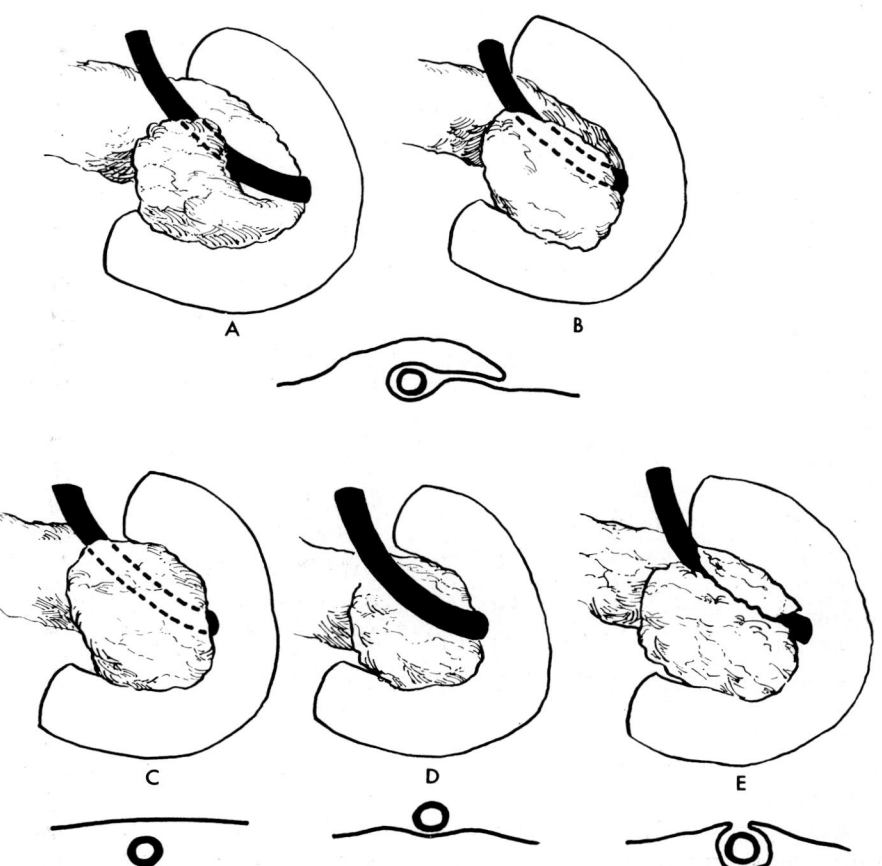

Figure 9.11. Variations of the intrapancreatic portion of the common bile duct. See text for explanation. (From Smanio T. Varying relations of the common bile duct with the posterior face of the pancreas in negroes and white persons. J Int Coll Surg 1954;22:150–173.)

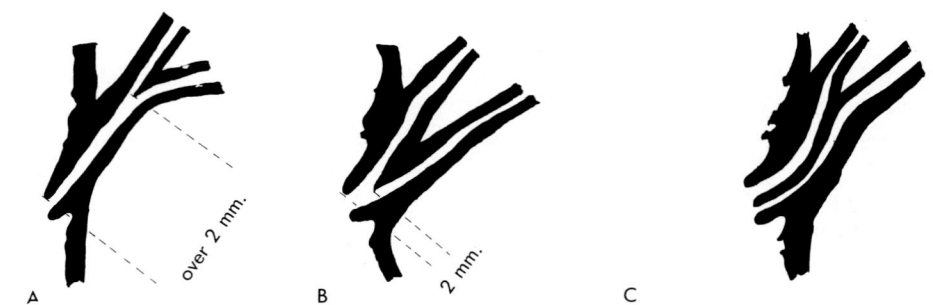

Figure 9.12.   Variations in the ampulla of Vater. **A**, The ampulla is over 2 mm long. **B**, The ampulla is at least 2 mm long. **C**, The common bile duct and the pancreatic duct have separate openings on the papilla; no ampulla is present.

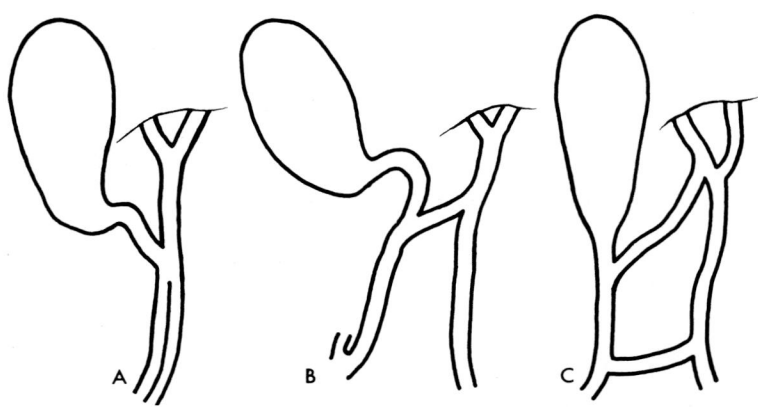

Figure 9.13.   Duplications of the common bile duct. **A**, Double and parallel lumina of the common bile duct. **B**, **X** type of anastomosis between duplicated bile ducts. **C**, **X** and **H** types of anastomosis between duplicated bile ducts.

adults there is considerable variation in this region. The primitive condition is represented by a long ampulla (the longest, 14 mm, was found by Rienhoff and Pickrell in 1945 [85]) (Fig. 9.12, *A*), whereas maximum resorption is represented by the absence of an ampulla with completely separate orifices for the two ducts (Fig. 9.12, *C*).

Measurements of the ampullary pattern have been made by a number of investigators (85–88). Reinhoff and Pickrell (85) found the septum dividing the ducts to be more than 2 mm behind the duodenal orifice in about 33% of their cases (Fig. 9.12, *A*). In the remainder the tip of the septum reached or nearly reached the orifice, so that little or no ampulla existed (Fig. 9.12, *B* and *C*). In two cases in Dardinski's (88) series, resorption had proceeded further, and two completely separate orifices were present. The pancreatic duct was atretic in 2 to 4% of cases. Pancreatic drainage was evidently taking place entirely through the accessory duct of Santorini.

The significance of these variations lies in the possibility that a gallstone obstructing the duodenal orifice of a long ampulla might permit reflux of bile up the pancreatic duct. Obstruction of this type has been said to cause 4 to 10% of cases of acute pancreatitis (89, 90).

EDITORIAL COMMENT

The original description of obstruction of the ampulla of Vater with stones by Professor Opie at Johns Hopkins resulted in the theory of the common pathway obstruction which is a very real etiology for both pancreatitis and cholangitis, setting up the possibility of flow of bile into the pancreatic duct and vice versa. We believe, from the historic standpoint, that Opie's work should be mentioned and emphasized at this point.

It must be stated, however, that the mechanism of acute pancreatitis has no sound etiology.

DUPLICATION AND ECTOPIA OF THE COMMON BILE DUCT

Anatomy.
Duplication.

A common bile duct containing two lumina, but appearing single externally, is not rare (Fig. 9.13, *A*). More unusual is the presence of two sometimes widely separated ducts with separate orifices into the gastrointestinal tract.

True doubled ducts may separate at any level, but typically separation is above the junction with the cystic duct.

Rarely are the right and left hepatic ducts, the common hepatic duct, and the common bile ducts entirely duplicated. When the double ducts are parallel, there may be one or more cross-connections. These may be divided into broad, short, X-type anastomoses (Fig. 9.13, *B*) and long, right angle H types (Fig. 9.13, *C*), but the reported varieties go far beyond such a simple classification. The orifices of the two ducts may be adjacent or separated by several centimeters. In certain cases the arrangement could be interpreted as a cystic duct paralleling the common duct and opening independently into the duodenum (91) (Fig. 9.10, *B*). In other cases the right hepatic duct joins the cystic duct to form a common duct, while the left hepatic duct enters the duodenum independently, without cross-anastomoses (73, 92) (Fig. 9.14). Duplicated common bile ducts may rejoin one another and have a single duodenal orifice (93).

Ectopic Orifices.

An otherwise normal common bile duct or an accessory bile duct may open into the gut far enough from the normal site to be described as ectopic.

At least seven cases of a common bile duct opening into the stomach have been reported (94, 95). In several the ectopic duct was the only one present; it represented a duplication, with the duct at the normal location secondarily obliterated. In other cases a duct was present in the normal as well as in an abnormal location.

A duodenal opening of the duct above or below the normal site of the papilla of Vater need not be associated with duplication. Cases of proximal shift of the orifice were collected by Boyden (94), whereas Wood (96) reported 20 cases of an opening in the third part of the duodenum. This distal displacement has been reported in 8% of Soviet necropsies (97).

Reports from the early literature of accessory bile ducts that open into the transverse colon refer to acquired secondary fistulae. The prenatal location of the colon is such that an embryonic connection with the biliary system is precluded.

Embryogenesis.

Septation Duplication.

This condition has been seen in several embryos (94). The double-barreled state may, in fact, be a normal stage of the recanalization process (Fig. 9.13, *A*). Presence of the double lumen in later life thus would represent developmental arrest during the sixth week.

Bifurcation Duplication.

Separation of the common bile duct into two parts occurs at, or before, formation of the diverticulum late in the fourth week. An abnormally long area of differentiating cells of the foregut will produce a liver diverticulum which, during the elongation in the fifth week, could result in two cellular strands (instead of one) connecting the duodenum to the liver cords growing in the transverse septum. Boyden (94) illustrated such an elongated primordium in a 24-somite embryo. When the duplications are several centimeters apart, it is possible that two liver primordia may have arisen on the ventral wall of the foregut. The rapid elongation of the foregut would be sufficient to carry the site of the cranial primordium away from that of the normally placed one and into the region destined to become the stomach. That this "captured" primordium is the accessory and not the main primordium is evidenced by the normal position of the pancreas, part of which is derived from the liver diverticulum.

At least two cases are known in which a duodenal atresia occurred at the site of the origin of the common bile duct early enough to divide the duct into two branches, one joining the proximal and the other joining the distal segment (98, 99) (see Fig. 6.27).

History and Incidence. Although accessory bile ducts with ectopic insertion into the gastrointestinal tract are extremely rare, their existence has long been known. Indeed, the idea that there were two ducts from the liver, one to the duodenum and one to the stomach, was held in antiquity and persisted for many centuries. In 1522 DaCarpi (100) stated, "The other duct according to some goes to the pylorus of the stomach. . . . Some deny the existence of this duct." Galen is said to have believed in its existence at one time and to have influenced the Arabs in the same belief. This idea survived long enough for Vesalius (101) in 1543 to deny it; although, he states that he found a branch of the bile duct passing to the fundus of the stomach in the body of an "oarsman of a Pontifical trireme," who had no history of digestive disease (Fig. 9.15, *A*). Fallopius (102) in 1606 also denied its existence although he said he had seen double openings into the duodenum two or three times. Altogether, 12 cases of accessory common bile ducts were reported before 1800.

With such a start, it is remarkable that only four cases of ectopia were reported in the 19th century; and, Boy-

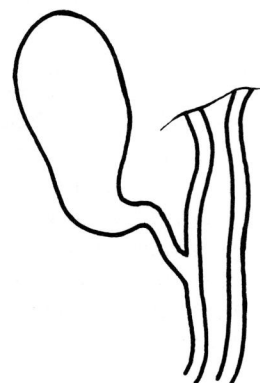

Figure 9.14. Duplication of the common bile duct. This may also be described as absence of the common hepatic duct.

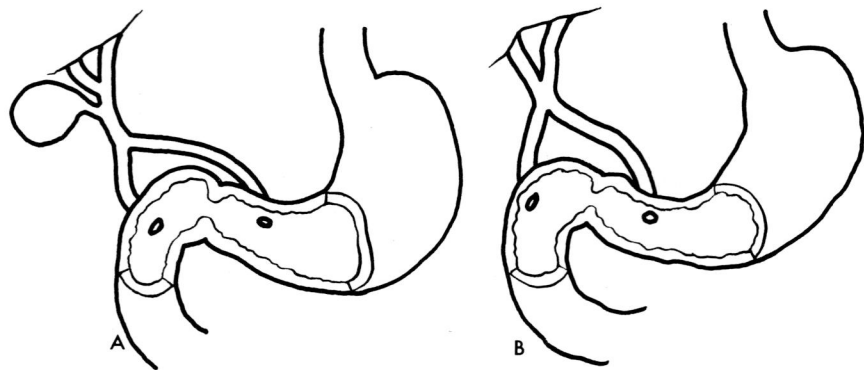

Figure 9.15. Ectopic opening of the common bile duct into the stomach. **A,** Case of Vesalius **B,** Case of Everett and Macumber in which the gallbladder and cystic duct were absent. (**A,** From Vesalius A. De humani corporis fabrica. Basil [Basileae]: J Oporinus, 1543; **B,** from Everett C, Macumber HE. Anomalous distribution of the extrahepatic biliary ducts. Ann Surg 1942;115:472–474.)

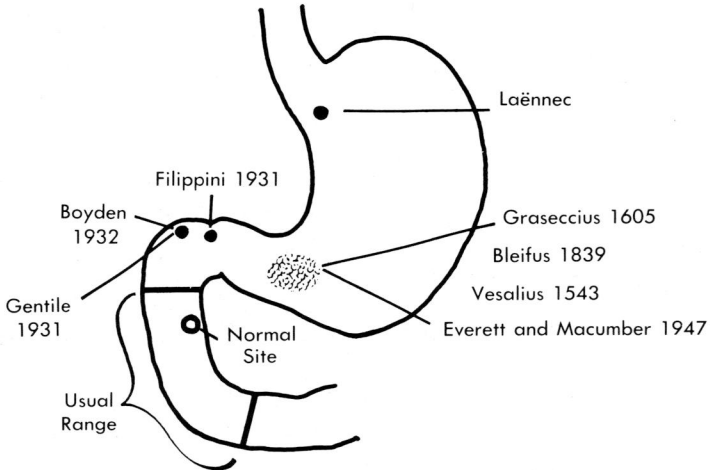

Figure 9.16. Sites of ectopic openings of the common bile duct. Note that most openings into the stomach have been into the pyloric antrum. (From Boyden EA. The problem of the double ductus choledochus: an interpretation of an accessory bile duct found attached to the pars superior of the duodenum. Anat Rec 1932;55:71–94.)

den (94) was able to find but eight more from 1900 to 1932. In five cases the ectopic duct was the only one found. The locations of some of these ectopias are shown in Figure 9.16. Unlike duplications of the gallbladder, duplication of the common bile duct has not been found in domestic animals (94).

Symptoms and Diagnosis. These anomalies produce no symptoms and are encountered only at surgery for gallbladder disease or at autopsy.

CONGENITAL CYSTIC DILATION OF THE COMMON BILE DUCT

Anatomy. In congenital idiopathic dilation of the common bile duct, a localized, balloon-like expansion forms, in contrast to the cylindric enlargement resulting from bile duct obstruction. Neither the gallbladder nor the remainder of the common duct is enlarged.

Classification. In 1959 Alonso-Lej et al. (103) developed the first classification system of choledochal cysts. He described three categories: ductal dilation, diverticular dilation, and choledochocele.

Simple Ductal Dilation (Fig. 9.17, A).
The common duct dilation may be immense: Alonso-Lej et al. (103) found eight cases in which it contained over 4500 cc. The largest reached the incredible capacity of over 13 liters (104). Perhaps because of slow accumulation of the contents, the wall becomes thickened rather than thinned. Dense connective tissue with smooth muscle is present, but the epithelium rarely is preserved. Inflammation is common, but in only seven cases were stones present. Malignant degeneration has been reported occasionally, and in one patient, carcinoma of the intrahepatic ducts existed (105). Ascarids were present in two cases (106). Daughter cysts may be present in

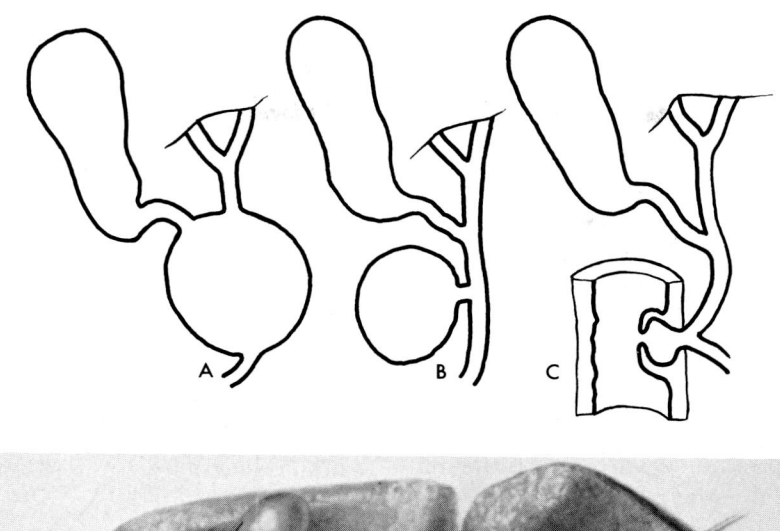

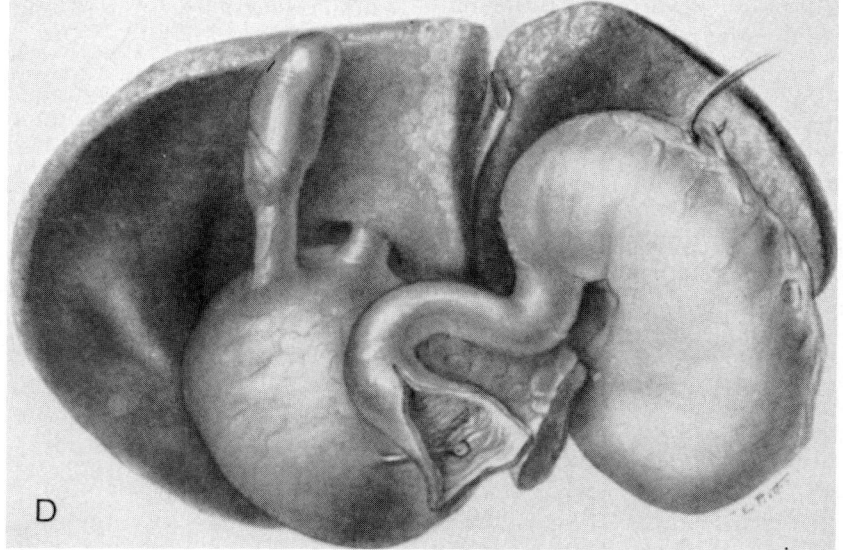

Figure 9.17. Types of congenital cystic dilation of the common bile duct. **A**, Simple ductal dilation. **B**, Diverticular dilation. **C**, Choledochocele. **D**, Cystic dilation of type A from a 3-year-old girl. Cystic and hepatic ducts are dilated; the common duct distal to the dilation is normal. The dilated portion measured 7 × 12 cm. (**D**, From Gross RE. The surgery of infancy and childhood. Philadelphia: WB Saunders, 1953.)

the triangle of Calot, and the surgeon should be well aware of these (107).

Diverticular Dilation (Fig. 9.17, B).
Several cases of dilated congenital diverticulum have been recognized. In two (108, 109), the diverticulum could be accounted for by assuming a local weakness of the bile duct wall. In one case (110) a long pedicle existed between the common duct and the dilated portion. Although no lumen was detected in the pedicle, the dilation was filled with bile. This structure could hardly have been a pulsion diverticulum and must represent a developmental anomaly. Two other cases are mentioned by Alonso-Lej and his colleagues (103).

Choledochocele (Fig. 9.17, C).
In this condition the dilated portion of the duct is intramural; and its structure has been likened to that of a ure-

terocele. It also has been designated a cyst of the ampulla of Vater.

Alonso-Lej et al. (103) found only four examples in the literature. We are inclined to view them as a variety of cystic dilation of the common duct, essentially similar to those found elsewhere in the duct.

Using Alonso-Lej's system, in combination with the work of Caroli (111), Todani et al. (112) developed what is generally considered to be the current standard classification (Fig. 9.18). A breakdown of the prevalence of each type based on a limited literature review (113) is presented in Table 9.3.

The authors wonder about a type II choledochocele. Is this a real diverticulum or a second gallbladder? If no acute changes are present, the histology of the wall will help the pathologist to make a correct diagnosis because

CHOLEDOCHAL CYSTS
'Todani Classification'

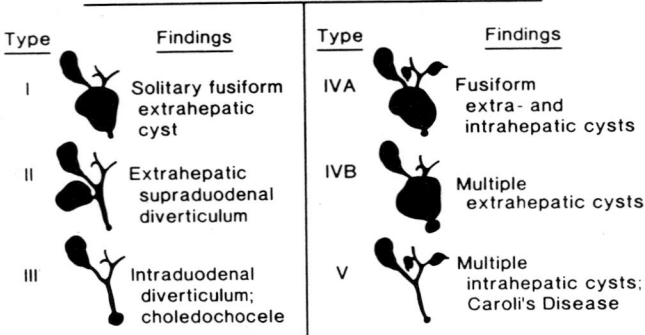

Figure 9.18. Classification of choledochal cyst. (From Nagorney DM. Choledochal cysts in adult life. In: Blumgart LH, ed. Surgery of the liver and biliary tract, Vol 2. New York: Churchill Livingstone, 1988.)

Table 9.3.
Distribution of Bile Duct Cysts by Type (Todani Classification)[a,b]

	I	II	III	IV	V
Alonso Lej et al.[c,d]	86	4	4	?	—
Lee et al.[c,e]	86	2	5	?	—
Flannigan[b,f]	659	23	42	19	?
Powell et al.[b,g]	255	7	13	60	?
Nunez-Hoy[h]	6	1	1	6	1
Rattner et al.[i]	4	—	—	5	—
Nagorney et al.[j]	22	1	2	4	—
Ono et al.[k]	21	—	—	1	—
Todani et al.[l]	—	—	—	38	—
TOTAL	1139	38	67	133	11
Percentage	82	3	5	9	<1

[a] From Nagorney DM. Choledochal cysts in adult life. In: Blumgart LH, ed. Surgery of the liver and biliary tract, Vol 2. New York: Churchill Livingstone, 1988.
[b] Multiple cysts not subclassified.
[c] Multiple cysts not included in classification scheme.
[d] Alonso-Lej F, Rever WB, Pessagno DJ. Congenital choledochal cyst, with a report of 2, and an analysis of 94, cases. Arch Surg 1982;117:611–616.
[e] Lee SS, Min PC, Kim GW, Hong PW. Choledochal cyst. Arch Surg 1969;99:19.
[f] Flanigan DP. Biliary cysts. Ann Surg 1975;182:635–643.
[g] Powell CS, Sawyers JL, Reynolds VH. Management of adult choledochal cysts. Ann Surg 1981;193:666–676.
[h] Nunez-Hoy M, Lees CD, Hermann RD. Bile duct cysts: experience with 15 patients. Am J Surg 1982;144:295–299.
[i] Rattner DW, Schapiro RH, Warshaw AL. Abnormalities of the pancreatic and biliary ducts in adult patients with choledochal cysts. Arch Surg 1983;118:1068–1073.
[j] Nagorney DM, LeSage GD, Charboneau JW, McGough PF. Cystadenoma of the proximal common hepatic duct: the use of abdominal ultrasonography and transhepatic cholangiography in diagnosis. Mayo Clin Proc 1984b;59:118–121.
[k] Ono J, Sakoda K, Akita H. Surgical aspect of cystic dilatation of the bile duct: an anomalous junction of the pancreatobiliary tract in adults. Ann Surg 1982;195:203–208.
[l] Todani T et al. Congenital choledochal cyst with intrahepatic involvement. Arch Surg 1983;119:1038–1043.

the wall is thick and fibrotic, with or without mucosa, in cases of cystic dilation of the gallbladder duct.

The authors feel that the type II of Longmire et al. (114) is controversial. Are there any histologic studies of the duct of this "diverticulum"? The wall of both normal gallbladder and of a noninfected choledochal cyst is lined by columnar epithelium, and the histology is practically the same. We treated a type II choledochal cyst and described it histologically as follows: "The wall of the cyst is composed of fibrous tissue and granulation tissue and is lined by cuboidal epithelium showing squamous metaplasia. These features are those of a diverticulum" (Ricketts, unpublished data).

For some reason, congenital dilation of the gallbladder duct in Asia is not rare. Several publications from Japan (112, 115–117) support the congenital origin of this phenomenon and report that an abnormal choledochopancreatic duct junction is present practically always, something which was reported by Babbitt (118).

Okada et al. (117) reported 100 cases of congenital dilation of the bile duct. Their cases are associated with an anomalous junction of the pancreatic biliary ductal system. They divide the cases in two groups: 77 of cystic type and 23 cylindric type. Characteristically, in patients of more than 1 year of age, the disease was of either the cystic or cylindric type; in patients of less than 1 year of age, the disease was of the cystic type.

There are several questions that must be answered:

1. Why are there so many cases in Asia? Perhaps the environment plays a role.
2. Do Asians living in the United States have a higher incidence of this condition?
3. Why is there not dilation of the bile ducts in some cases with abnormal extra vaterian pancreatobiliary ductal junction?
4. Since the sphincteric apparatus of Boyden does not exist in an abnormal junction and since pancreatic juice most

likely enters into the bile ducts because of the higher pressure within the pancreatic duct, why is there no clinical picture of pancreatitis and histologic changes in the pancreas after the first month of life?

5. Is type II cyst a real congenital dilation or a double gallbladder?
6. How can we explain the formation of dilation in the biliary tree after a normal cholangiogram? Is this an acquired problem?

Associated Anomalies. Few other major anomalies have been reported in patients with congenital cystic dilation of the bile duct. In one case there was a double common duct with dilation of one (92); in another the gallbladder was double (119); and in a third it was absent (120). Associated kidney anomalies have been reported (121). Heterotopic gastric mucosa in the common bile duct was reported by Evans et al. (122).

Pathogenesis. The etiology of cystic dilation of the common bile duct is obscure. Early writers considered it to be acquired as a complication of pregnancy, abdominal trauma, or stenosis of the intramural portion of the bile duct resulting from infection (compare Madding [123]). While there are cases which, taken by themselves, would favor these explanations, most cannot be accounted for by such factors. Experimental incomplete stricture of the common duct in dogs raises the pressure in the common duct but produces dilation of the entire biliary tract rather than only cystic dilation (124). Dilation following a congenital malformation of the common duct at its junction with the duodenum or an abnormal valvular mechanism at the ampulla has been suggested, but this seems improbable.

In 1936 Yotuyanagi (125) suggested that excessive proliferation of the epithelium during the solid stage of development of the ductus choledochus would account for the dilation. Why the overgrowth is always at the same location was not explained.

Still another view, first advanced by Rolleston (126) in 1905 and later supported by Weber (127) in 1934 and Saltz and Glaser (128) in 1956, is that there exists a neurologic dysfunction similar to that found in megacolon or megaesophagus; but, there is little evidence to support this view. The term *megacholedochus* was proposed by Saltz and Glaser.

Congenital weakness of the wall, coupled with obstruction was suggested by Gross (129) and accepted by many. Subsequent reviewers (103, 130, 131) have all favored the idea of a congenitally weakened wall. This could arise through local thinning of the duct wall during the period of recanalization of the solid stage of the common bile duct. Against this explanation is the fact that the epithelium is not usually a source of strength in the wall of a hollow viscus. The fibrous and muscular coats of the wall must in some way be implicated.

Ravitch and Snyder (132) felt that obstruction, even during intrauterine life, plays no part in the dilation and that the expanded portion develops anomalously without the influence of pressure. They consider obstruction, when present, to be the result of the cyst and not the cause of it.

In spite of the difficulty in assigning a specific cause, the high percentage of very young patients, including one newborn infant and one fetus (103), indicates a congenital origin. The relatively high incidence in Japan and the differences between the gender distribution in Caucasians and Japanese suggest a genetic basis, which otherwise remains unconfirmed.

History. Vater (133) has been credited with reporting the first case in 1723; although its congenital nature has been denied. A similar case was reported by Todd (134) in 1818. Douglas (135) in 1852 described the first unequivocal case. In 1894 Swain (136) performed the first successful operation, a cholecystojejunostomy. By 1909 Laverson (137) collected 28 cases. The first preoperative diagnosis was made in 1924 by Neugebauer (138). Shallow and his colleagues (130) found 175 cases by

1943, and Tsardakas and Robnett (131) reviewed 242 cases in 1956. Alonso-Lej et al. (103) brought the number to 403 in 1959. Japanese cases were reviewed in 1954 by Hatano and Imoto (139).

Incidence. Tsardakas and Robnett (131) listed three series of hospital admissions totaling 976,027, among which were five cases. These rather unsatisfactory figures indicate an incidence of 1:200,000 hospital admissions.

About 33% of reported cases have been in Japanese patients with the gender ratio nearly equal. Among Caucasians, however, over five times as many women as men are affected (22, 103, 131).

Of the 92 cases analyzed by Alonso-Lej et al. (103), 18% were under 1 year of age; 45% were under 10 years of age; 82% were under 30 years of age. Gross (22) mentions a case in a fetus.

The incidence of cancer in a choledochal cyst is well known. Voyles et al. (140) reported 67 cases of choledochal cyst with cancer. The same authors reported that 14.3% of patients with choledochal cyst developed cancer; in contrast, only 0.7% of patients younger than 10 years of age were found to have cancer.

Coyle and Bradley (141) reported cholangiocarcinoma which developed after the removal of a type II choledochal cyst. They collected 1823 cases of choledochal cyst. Cholangiocarcinoma developed in 106 patients (5.8%). The authors hypothesized that adenomatous hyperplasia may be an early phase of malignant degeneration suggesting the need for radical surgical procedures.

Symptoms. Jaundice, right upper quadrant pain, and abdominal mass are the predominant symptoms. While all three were present in 63% of the cases reviewed by Tsardakas and Robnett [131], Alonso Lej and his co-workers (103) observed that the simultaneous presence of all three had decreased to 21% by 1959. They suggested that this indicates earlier diagnosis. Fever, nausea, and vomiting were present in about 25% of cases.

Tran et al. (106), reviewing 110 cases among Vietnamese, suggested that either a palpable mass or jaundice appears first in infants. Both of these are present usually in children up to age 10 years; pain, mass, and jaundice are present in older children and adults.

All the symptoms are at first intermittent and may resemble cholecystitis attacks. The history of these attacks often may be traced back to infancy. In infants, the symptoms may be those of obstructive jaundice due to biliary atresia (142). Severity of symptoms is not related to the size of the mass.

In long-standing cases cirrhosis of the liver, ascites, and splenomegaly may be present, and infection is common. Rupture of the cyst may result from infection and perforation or from trauma (143).

Diagnosis. Only one correct preoperative diagnosis was made among 64 cases before 1928. By 1943 the correct diagnosis had been at least suspected in 22 of 175 cases

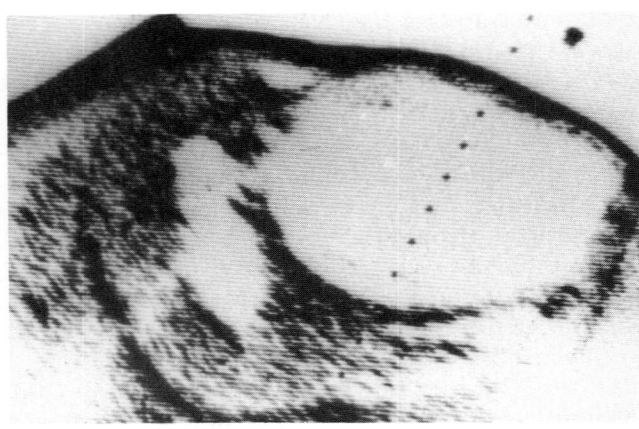

Figure 9.19. Ultrasound of a choledochal cyst (*C*) showing its relationship to the gallbladder (*GB*).

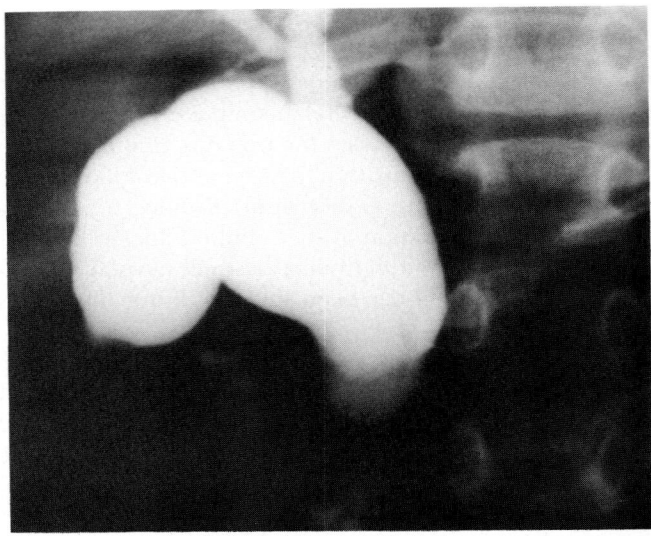

Figure 9.21. Operative cholangiogram reviewing a large type I choledochal cyst with slight enlargement of the common hepatic duct and minimal flow of contrast material into the duodenum.

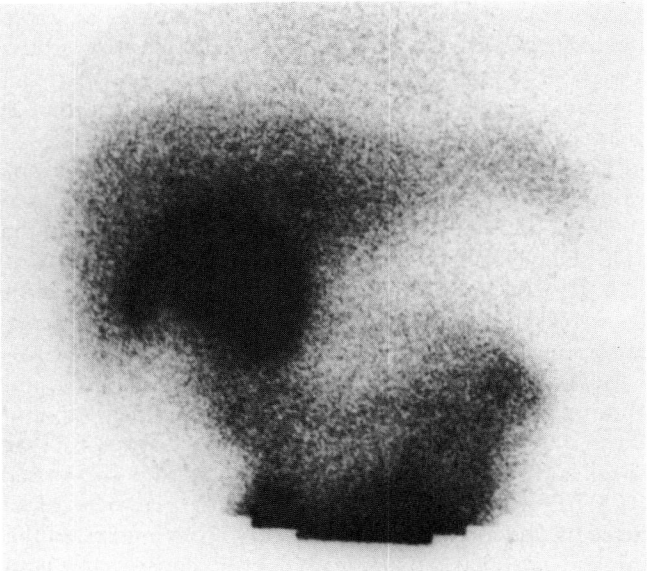

Figure 9.20. HIDA scan of a choledochal cyst showing uptake of the radionuclide within the cyst and gallbladder with some excretion into the gastrointestinal tract.

(131). In 94 cases since then and up to 1959, the diagnosis was correctly made in 11 and suggested in 17 cases (30%) (103).

Plain abdominal roentgenograms and contrast-enhanced studies of the gastrointestinal tract may show displacement of structures in the right upper quadrant. Abdominal ultrasound will show a large cyst in the portal region (Fig. 9.19). A radionuclide scan (PIPIDA, DIS-IDA, or HIDA) will demonstrate the biliary tract origin of the cyst since the radionuclide will be detected within the cyst (Fig. 9.20). Intravenous cholangiography will visualize the cyst if jaundice is not present. An operative cholangiogram is essential in all cases prior to the definitive surgical procedure (Fig. 9.21).

Differential Diagnosis. Several criteria may be helpful in distinguishing among pathologic conditions:

1. Cholelithiasis may be eliminated if there is a long history of symptoms from childhood.
2. *Echinococcus* cysts are rare among North Americans. Progressive enlargement of the mass, rather than an intermittent appearance, is usual.
3. Congenital biliary atresia manifests itself earlier and exhibits progressive jaundice, but exceptions are known.
4. Neoplasms—retroperitoneal, of the liver, or of the head of the pancreas—are rapidly progressive.
5. Pancreatic cysts usually displace the duodenum to the right and expand the duodenal curvature.

Treatment. The only effective treatment is surgical. When conservative treatment has been used, 21 of 22 patients died within 1 month (144).

The aim of surgery is to resect the cyst and to restore adequate bile drainage. Anything less than this leads to an unacceptably high complication rate from recurrent cholangitis, stricture, and malignant transformation (145, 146). Lilly (147) described an operative procedure in which a small portion of the cyst wall adjacent to the portal vein is left intact, but the entire mucosal lining of the cyst is removed. This procedure minimizes damage to the portal vein, which in the past resulted in a high surgical morbidity and mortality. Biliary tract reconstruction usually is accomplished with Roux-en-Y hepaticojejunostomy or with a hepaticojejunoduodenostomy as described by Oweida and Ricketts (148–151) (Fig. 9.22). Cosentino and her collegues (152) reported 21 patients with choledochal duct cyst who underwent resection and

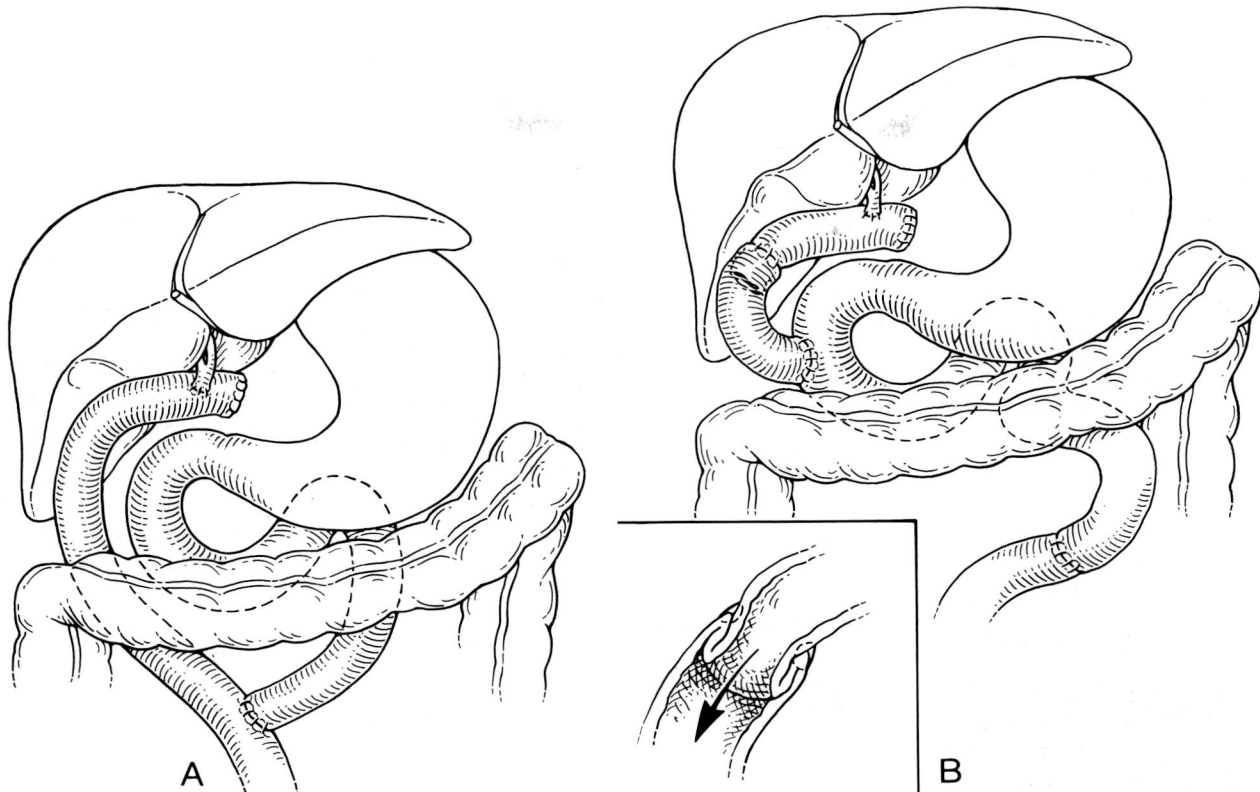

Figure 9.22.   Reconstruction following excision of a choledochal cyst. **A**, Roux-en-Y hepaticojejunostomy. **B**, Valved hepatico-jejunoduodenostomy. (From Okada A et al. Surgical treatment of congenital dilatation of bile duct (choledochal cyst) with technical considerations. Surgery 1987;101:238–243.)

reconstruction by valved jejunal interposition hepatico-duodenostomy with excellent results.

Lopez et al. (153) reported 23 patients treated by cystectomy, choledochojejunostomy, and endoscopic incision and drainage according to type and local pathologic anatomy. Karrer et al. (154) recently reviewed congenital biliary tract disease, including choledochal cyst, and emphasized the importance of complete mucosal excision of the lesions.

Mortality. Although congenital cystic dilation of the common duct may remain asymptomatic until adulthood, it appears to be uniformly fatal if left untreated after symptoms of obstruction appear. Mortality from surgical treatment has steadily decreased: 83% in 1927, 51% in 1943, 12% in 1959 (103), and 2% in 1965 (155).

Anomalies of the Gallbladder and Cystic Duct

The gallbladder, in contrast to the liver itself, is subject to a number of anomalous conditions. It may be absent, vestigial, duplicated, or bilobed. It may be misplaced and deformed and may suffer intrusion of mucosa from other parts of the digestive tract. Any of these conditions may be associated with atresia of part or all of the extrahepatic

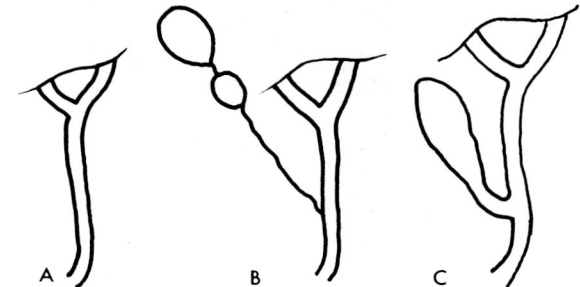

Figure 9.23.   Anomalies of the gallbladder. **A**, Complete absence of gallbladder and cystic duct. **B**, Vestigial cystic structures representing the gallbladder. **C**, Cystic duct without gallbladder.

biliary ducts. While these defects are all rare and none by itself is fatal, they confuse the radiologic picture and sometimes baffle the unwary surgeon.

ABSENCE OF THE GALLBLADDER

Anatomy.   In most cases of this anomaly, both gallbladder and cystic duct are absent, and the common bile duct often is dilated (Fig. 9.23, *A*). In about 20%, the entire extrahepatic duct system is atretic (Fig. 9.3). In 1928 Bower (156) reported an extreme case in which the gall-

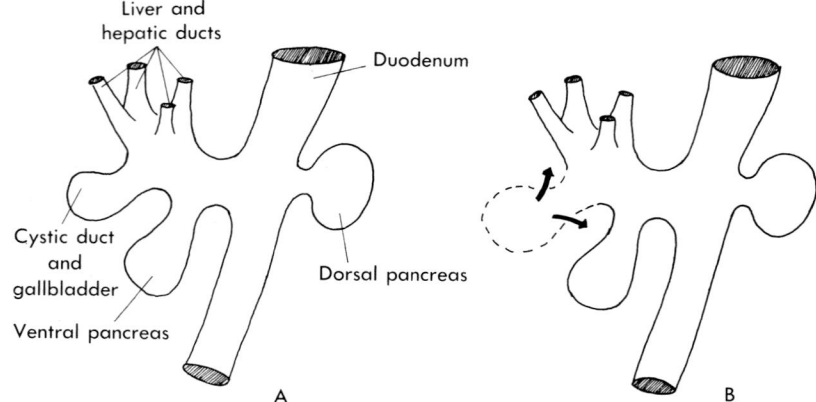

Figure 9.24. **A,** The four primordia of the hepaticopancreatic complex in the fifth week. **B,** Of these, only the cystic primordium is occasionally absent, having been absorbed into the hepatic or pancreatic primordium.

bladder, the cystic and common ducts, and the left lobe of the liver all were absent. Absence of the duct system is said to be incompatible with life; yet the average survival of these infants is about 2 months, and some have lived as long as 7 months.

Although the head of the pancreas is derived from the ventral pancreatic primordium formed at the base of the hepatic diverticulum, we have seen only one report in which the head of the pancreas as well as the gallbladder was absent (152). However, some embryologists believe that only the uncinate process originates from the ventral pancreatic primordium and that the head, body, and tail originate from the dorsal diverticulum (Weidman and Gest, personal communication, 1991). The implication is that the pancreatic and cystic diverticula, though in close proximity, form under the influence of different organizers.

The cystic fossa, which marks the boundary between the quadrate and the right lobe of the liver, may be present even with congenital absence of the gallbladder (158). Vestigial or hypoplastic gallbladders are rare. Small cystic structures that are not connected with the remainder of the biliary tract have been reported (159) (Fig. 9.23, *B*), and dilated stumps of the cystic duct have been seen (160) (Fig. 9.23, *C*). These cases represent relative rather than complete failure of development of the cystic anlage. In 1916 Holmes (6) found in the earlier literature a number of cases in which only remnants of the gallbladder were present. Remember, however, there is the possibility of an intrahepatic gallbladder if the gallbladder is "absent."

Embryogenesis. Failure of the cystic bud from the hepatic diverticulum to form during the fourth week accounts for the agenesis of the gallbladder and cystic duct. However, when agenesis is more extensive, another explanation must be sought.

The liver arises from the tip of the hepatic diverticulum, and the ventral pancreas arises as a bud from its

base. These two structures are never absent although the derivatives of the middle portion of the diverticulum, the gallbladder, and extrahepatic ducts frequently are missing or defective (Fig. 9.24). We must suppose that the proximal portion of the diverticulum is wholly absorbed into the pancreatic anlage, whereas the distal portion becomes attenuated by excessive conversion into liver cords. Such agenesis must occur in the fifth week or later.

Associated Anomalies. Among infants, other severe anomalies may accompany agenesis of the gallbladder. Tracheoesophageal fistula, imperforate anus, cleft palate, and cardiac and genitourinary malformations have been reported (161–163).

History. Aristotle mentioned the absence of the gallbladder in animals (164). In 1522 Jacopo DaCarpi (100) said, "Sometimes a man lacks a gallbladder; he is then of infirm health and shorter life." The first definite case seems to be that of Bergman (156) in 1701. Some six other cases were reported in the 18th century, including one by Littré in 1705 (156) and one by Morgagni in 1769 (II, 48:55) (165). By 1968 there were about 200 cases in the literature.

Frey et al. (163) accepts only 56 confirmed cases of congenital absence of the gallbladder without complete biliary atresia reported in the English language literature. Thirteen of these were confirmed at operation and 43 at autopsy. These workers list 25 other probable cases, 45 possible cases, and 16 questionable reports.

Incidence. Estimates of frequency range from 1:1530 autopsies (0.065%) (166) to 1:2403 autopsies (0.042%) (167) and 1:7480 autopsies (0.013%), according to a 1959 survey of the experience of 799 pathologists and 1,352,000 autopsies (168). McIlrath et al. (162) found 10 among 26,531 autopsies at the Mayo Clinic (0.04%). These estimates were considered to be too high by Frey et al. (163).

As late as 1947, 66% of cases reported were found at

autopsy (169), but by 1961 only 18% were first discovered in this manner (161).

Among autopsy cases the gender ratio is nearly equal, but among clinical cases females are more frequently seen than are males. Among 31 surgical patients reported in the literature between 1937 and 1954, Flannery and Caster (170) found only eight men. Other estimates have yielded closer to twice as many females as males (168).

Nearly 50% of patients reported are treated within the first year of life, but in many others the condition is recognized only at an advanced age (171). Eight of the 55 patients in Gerwig's review (161) were 70 years old or older. In 1989 Petromilli et al. (172) reported a case.

Clinical Picture. See discussion on page 323.

HYDROPS OF THE GALLBLADDER

Scobie and Bentley (171) reported a case of hydrops of the gallbladder in a newborn infant.

DUPLICATION OF THE GALLBLADDER (SEPTATE AND BILOBED GALLBLADDER)

There have been more than 200 cases reported of duplication of the gallbladder (173). Several degrees of dupli-

cation may be found. We believe they are best described by the five types arising by either of two distinct embryonic processes (174).

Anatomy. The mildest form of duplication of the gallbladder is that in which the septum divides an otherwise normal gallbladder into longitudinal chambers (Fig. 9.25, *A*). There may or may not be an external cleft at the tip of the fundus. In a more developed form of the condition, separate fundi enter a common neck and common cystic duct (175) (Fig. 9.25, *B*).

In complete duplication, the gallbladders are separate. The cystic ducts may join one another before entering the common duct (Y type) (Fig. 9.25, *C*), or each cystic duct may enter separately (H type) (Fig. 9.25, *D*). One gallbladder may arise directly from the hepatic or the common duct without a cystic duct, while the other may be normally arranged (18). Two cystic arteries are usually present. The two bladders may lie side by side, or they may be on opposite sides of the common duct (Fig. 9.25, *F*). If they lie side by side, they may be separate or have a common serosa. One, usually the left, may be larger than the other (81).

In rare cases one gallbladder may open into the right

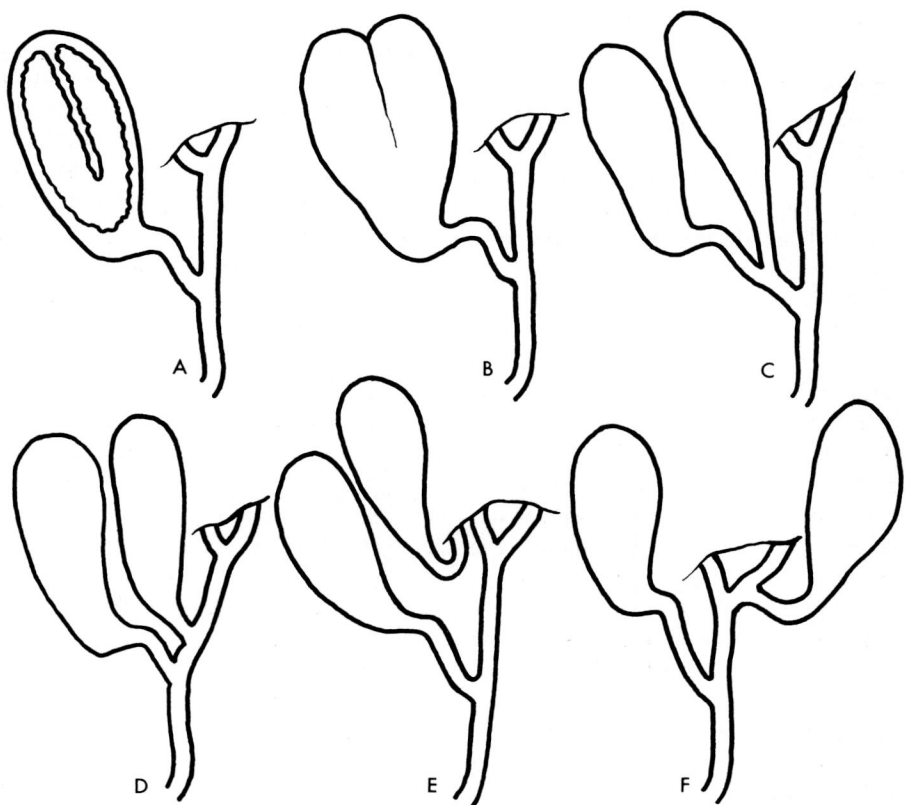

Figure 9.25. Duplication of the gallbladder. **A,** Septate gallbladder without external separation. **B,** External duplication of the fundus only. **C,** Y type of double gallbladder with a common cystic duct. **D,** Complete duplication (H type) of gall-bladder and cystic duct. **E,** Double gallbladder, one normal and one with cystic duct entering the liver by accessory hepatic duct. **F,** "Bilateral" gallbladders with separate cystic ducts.

or left hepatic duct or into an accessory hepatic duct (82). Occasionally, the cystic duct of one of the two gallbladders enters the substance of the liver while that of the other enters the common duct (128, 176) (Fig. 9.25, *E*).

One case of triple gallbladder and cystic duct has been reported. All three organs lay in a common fossa with a common serosa, and all cystic ducts entered the common bile duct separately but close together (177).

Embryogenesis. Several conditions may lead to total or partial duplication. In the most extreme, or H-type, duplication, the two cystic buds have grown from the common duct (Fig. 9.25, *D*). While suggestions have been made that this represents an original pairing of the structures and hence a primitive condition, there is no embryologic or phylogenetic basis for this view.

If a single cystic bud bifurcates after it has begun to grow, the Y-type anomaly is produced (Fig. 9.25, *C*). If the division occurs near the origin, two confluent cystic ducts with separate gallbladders are formed; if the division takes place a little later in development, only a bilobed gallbladder will result. A single cystic artery usually arises from the hepatic artery.

The septate form, like the phrygian cap variety discussed below, originates still later when the solid cystic anlage becomes hollow during the 12th week. The septum remains between two areas of vacuolization (94).

Split Primordium Group.

Type I. A septate gallbladder is divided into two chambers by a partial or complete longitudinal septum. There is usually no external indication of the internal division.

Type II. Bilobed (V type), which has two gallbladders, separate at the fundus but join at the neck.

Type III. A Y-type duplication has two separate gallbladders, each with a cystic duct. The two ducts join to form a common cystic duct before entering the common bile duct.

These three types of duplication arise by a splitting of the cystic primordium, which elongates in the fifth or early in the sixth week of gestation. A growth irregularity of the tip results in two tips, each competent to form a complete gallbladder. The degree of duplication depends on the time at which the bifurcation occurs; the earlier the bifurcation, the more complete the duplication.

Accessory Gallbladder Group.

Type IV. These duplications have two or more cystic ducts opening independently into the biliary tract ("ductular" or H types). Hurst and Mayo (178) reported a case in which the two cystic ducts entered the duodenum separately. The two gallbladders may be equal, or one may be smaller than normal. The one nearest the liver is considered to be the accessory organ. The two may lie together, covered with a common peritoneal coat, but they usually lie in separate but adjacent fossae. This is the most com-

mon type of multiple gallbladder, accounting for nearly half of all duplications.

Type V. This is the so-called trabecular accessory gallbladder in which the superior cystic duct may enter the right hepatic duct within the substance of the liver.

These duplications arise from two separate primordia on the biliary tree, one at the usual level and one higher. The developing liver cords also have the potential to form a gallbladder—hence, the term *trabecular* type of duplication.

MISCELLANEOUS ANOMALIES

The gallbladder may be single but drained by a double-cystic duct. In one patient, a cystic duct entered the left hepatic duct, producing a "left" gallbladder under the left lobe of the liver in addition to the normal organ (179).

Eight cases of triple gallbladder have been reported up to 1972 (100). The relative incidence of multiple gallbladders is shown in Table 9.4.

Like many anomalies, the healthy double gallbladder is asymptomatic. We believe that the increasing number of healthy double gallbladders seen by cholecystography implies that they are not more disposed to disease than are single organs.

Multiple gallbladders are often a surprise to the surgeon. There is no reason why two gallbladders should not be visualized as readily as one, but such is the case (Table 9.5). We ourselves have operated on three patients with totally unexpected double gallbladders (181).

History. Pliny the Elder recorded the occurrence of double gallbladder in ritually sacrificed animals, as did Aristotle.

Boyden (3) quoted the Talmudic laws, or terefah, that

Table 9.4.
Relative Frequency of Anatomic Types Among 242 Multiple Gallbladders[a]

Type	Number	Percentage
Split primordium		
Septate	16	
V type (bilobed)	12	
Y type	36	
Triple	2	
SUBTOTAL	66	46.5
Accessory gallbladder		
H type (ductular)	67	
Trabecular	3	
Triple	4	
SUBTOTAL	74	52.1
Mixed		
Triple	2	
SUBTOTAL	2	1.4
TOTAL	142	

[a]From Harlaftis N, Gray SW, Skandalakis JE. Multiple gallbladders. Surgery 1977;145:928–934.

Table 9.5.
Diagnosis in 200 Cases of Multiple Gallbladder

Diagnostic Method	Diagnosed (N)	Total Cases	Percentages
Radiology		105	52.5
Confirmed at surgery	23		
Unconfirmed (no operation)	82		
Surgery		79	39.5
Negative radiographic findings	37		
Equivocal radiographic findings	2		
No radiograph reported	40		
Autopsy		16	8.0
TOTAL		200	100.0

*a*From Harlaftis N, Gray SW, Skandalakis JE. Multiple gallbladders. Surgery 1977;145:928–934.

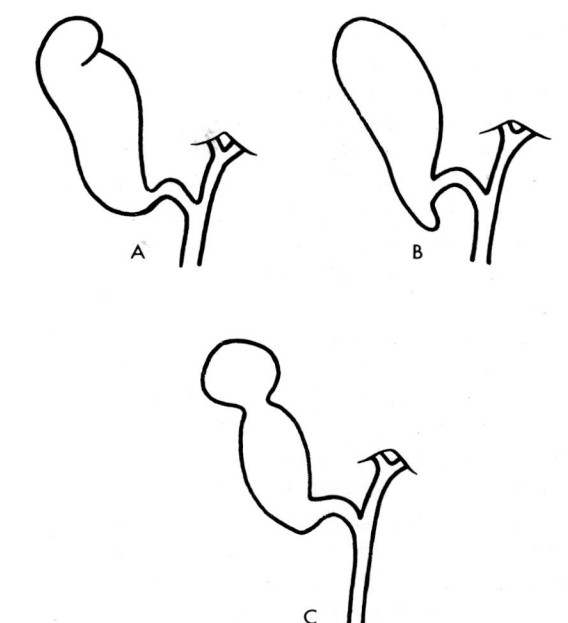

Figure 9.26. Deformities of the gallbladder. **A**, Phrygian cap deformity. **B**, Hartmann's pouch. **C**, Hourglass gallbladder.

pertain to disease or abnormalities of ritually clean animals. By the 16th century, codifications of the law recognized absence of the gallbladder, septate and V-shaped, bilobed gallbladders, and double gallbladders of both Y and H types. The regular absence of the structure in pigeons and deer also was recognized.

The earliest case reported in a human was that of Blasius in 1676 (181). His drawing is reproduced in Boyden's 1926 paper (3). Corcoran and Wallace (81) collected 49 cases up to 1954, and Skielboe (177) estimated that there were 122 cases by 1958.

Incidence. Double gallbladder is rarer in human beings than in most domestic animals. Boyden (3), examining over 10,000 domestic animals, found a marked tendency toward duplication (including both bilobed and true double organ) in some species. The incidence was thus: cats, 1:8; calves, 1:28; sheep, 1:85; pigs, 1:198; and humans, 1:3000 to 1:4000. Among the ungulates, duplication tended to be by diverticulum formation; in cats, by cleft or septate gallbladder; and in humans, by secondary outgrowth of the cystic or common duct to form complete duplication.

There are no differences in incidence between the sexes, and most cases are found in adults, incidental to cholecystectomy or at autopsy. The partial form is rarer than the complete form.

Clinical Picture. See discussion on page 323.

Our experience with multiple gallbladders has been presented in several papers (174, 180, 182).

DEFORMATIONS OF THE GALLBLADDER

Hourglass Gallbladder (Fig. 9.26, C). In this deformity, there is a partial transverse septum across the organ, which is not always marked by an external sulcus. Either or both cavities may be inflamed or contain stones. Flannery and Caster (170) discussed the clinical and radiologic pictures.

Embryologically, the hourglass shape may represent an incipient degenerative state. Holmes (6) reported a patient whose gallbladder was reduced to a pair of small connecting vesicles with an atretic cystic duct. He noted three other cases in which the vestigial gallbladder was reduced to two cysts arranged in tandem. Morgagni in 1769 mentioned a similar type of gallbladder (xxix:18) (165).

Phrygian Cap Deformity (Fig. 9.26, A). This deformation is produced by a folding over of the tip of the fundus, resulting from presence of a partial transverse septum. The name derives from that of the "liberty cap," the widely used symbol of the French Revolution. Named and described by Bartel in 1916, it is the most common of the deformations (183). Of gallbladders examined, 2 to 6% show a phrygian cap shape, and Flannery and Caster (184) believe these are more prone to lithiasis than are normally shaped organs. The deformation may be externally visible as a serosal cleft, or it may be concealed by a smooth surface. Boyden (185) suggested that the fold represents a persistent embryonic bend formed at the time the lumen is reestablished.

Hartmann's Pouch (Fig. 9.26, B). Hartmann's pouch is probably an acquired deformation resulting from dilation of the infundibulum, produced by long-continued resistance to gallbladder emptying. It often occurs when there is an acute angle between the fundus and neck and between the neck and the cystic duct. Such a "siphon form" predisposes the patient to inflammation and lithiasis. Kaiser (186) considers this shape to be a normal constitutional variation, associated with a short, stocky (pyknic) habitus.

Diverticula of the Gallbladder. These deformities were first seen by Morgagni in 1769 (165). Flannery and Caster collected 10 cases between 1936 and 1953 (184). The mechanism of diverticulum formation has been related to dilation of the Rokitansky-Aschoff sinuses; but, this has not been proved. Robertson and Ferguson (187) considered the condition to be acquired.

Diverticula at the cervical end of the bladder have been thought to be related to the persistence of the embryonic cystohepatic ducts (true ducts of Luschka). With such an origin, diverticula should develop only on the hepatic side of the gallbladder; but, they are found on the serosal side as well (81). It is hard to believe that they are congenital.

Fundic diverticula are incompletely expanded portions of the original gallbladder primordium and represent arrested rather than excessive development.

Clinical Picture.
See discussion on page 323.

ABNORMAL POSITION OF THE GALLBLADDER

The gallbladder has been found in a number of unusual positions. Among the most striking locations reported have been the falciform ligament (188), the abdominal wall (189), the inferior surface of the right lobe of the liver (18, 190), and outside the peritoneum (191). In addition to these unusual locations, there are three other conditions of specific surgical interest.

In 1988 Feldman and Venta (192) reported a case of retrohepatic gallbladder, and in that same year Hopper (193) reported a case of liver inversion with anterior suprahepatic midline gallbladder.

Left-Sided Gallbladder (Fig. 9.27). Up to 1953, 16 cases in which the gallbladder lies on the inferior surface of the left lobe of the liver were known (194). In this position the gallbladder may be outside the area covered by the routine cholecystography film. No unusual functional disorders are associated with this anomaly.

Left-sided gallbladder is not to be confused with situs inversus in which all the viscera, including the liver and gallbladder, are reversed right for left. In these cases the surgeon should be aware of the visceral inversion and should expect to find the gallbladder on the left. In one case (195) situs inversus appeared to be limited to the liver and gallbladder with other viscera in their normal positions.

Intrahepatic Gallbladder. In 1903 Dévé (4) first called attention to a condition in which the gallbladder is completely submerged in the liver substance. In 1913 Kehr (196) gave the first clinical reports of three cases in adults. By 1935 McNamee (197) collected 14 cases in infants and 13 in adults. It is obvious that such cases may easily be mistaken for absence of the gallbladder at either autopsy

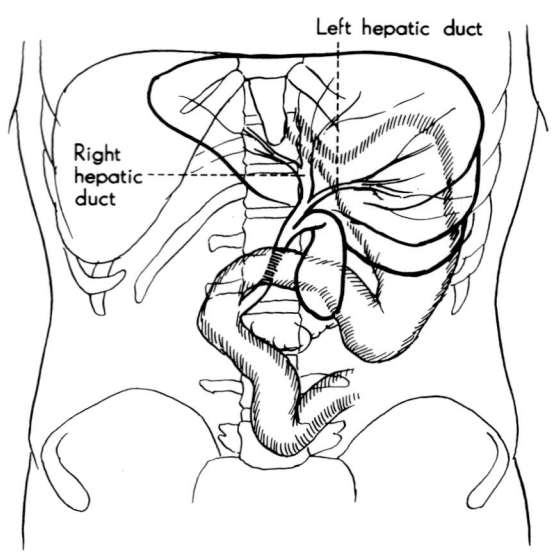

Figure 9.27. Left-sided gallbladder and liver without situs inversus. (From Large AM. Left-sided gallbladder and liver without situs inversus. Arch Surg 1963;87:982–985.)

or surgery, yet on cholecystography the condition may not be suspected. In some cases failure to find the gallbladder has led to closure of the abdomen and subsequent reoperation for further search. A high percentage of lithiasis is associated with the condition, perhaps because the submerged organ cannot readily empty itself. Location and removal of an imbedded gallbladder presents a considerable surgical problem. Incision of the liver substance is accompanied by hemorrhage, which can be difficult to control.

Mobile Gallbladder Resulting in Torsion. The mobile gallbladder, free or attached to the liver by a mesentery, represents the opposite extreme from the intrahepatic location. How frequently such a loose connection exists is not known, but in over 100 cases torsion and strangulation have been reported. Most of the patients are between 55 and 75 years of age; women are affected twice as often as men. The etiology is unknown, but cholecystitis seems not to be a factor (184). Morgagni (xxiv:16) (165) may have been the first to see this anomaly. In 1988 De Weerd and Frima (198) reported two cases of torsion of the gallbladder.

HETEROTOPIC MUCOSA IN THE GALLBLADDER

The presence of gastric mucosa in the biliary tract is not uncommon in cattle but is very rare in humans (199). Fundic mucosa with both chief and parietal cells has been found in the wall of the gallbladder (200), and a few nodular papillomas with gastric, pancreatic, or intestinal mucosa have been found in the antrum (201).

Pancreatic mucosa has been found in the gallbladder

in six cases (200). In at least one case islets as well as acini were found (202). In view of the formation of the ventral pancreas from the liver diverticulum, it is strange that more such cases do not occur.

A duplication cyst with gastric mucosa, lying at the junction of the cystic and common ducts, has been reported by Lee (203). However, this appears to be a cystic duplication of the duodenum rather than of a biliary duct.

Tejada and Danielson in 1989 reported a case of an ectopic hepatic nodule which was not associated with the liver and which was fixed at the gallbladder wall, having a short 11 × 6 × 4 mesentery (204).

ADENOMYOMA OF THE GALLBLADDER

Spaces lined with epithelium and surrounded by smooth muscle in the gallbladder wall are encountered in about 1% of gallbladders removed at operation. Designated "adenomyomas" by Shepard and his associates (205), these spaces are lined with typical gallbladder epithelium. They have been considered to be of congenital origin, either as persisting vestiges of hepatocystic ducts or as hamartomas (206).

Adenomyomas occur chiefly in women and in middle-aged persons, the latter fact arguing against a congenital origin. Intramural abscesses and, occasionally, gallstones may form in these cysts and tubules. Symptoms seem to be the result of inflammation and are similar to those of cholecystic disease.

CLINICAL PICTURE OF GALLBLADDER ANOMALIES

Signs and Symptoms. None of the anomalies of the gallbladder alone, including its absence, gives rise to any characteristic symptoms. While some of the defects predispose an individual to attacks of cholecystitis, the attacks themselves have no unusual aspects, and the symptoms only serve to call attention to the anomaly. The patients present with the usual picture of chronic subacute, or acute gallbladder disease. Gallbladder radiographs and intravenous cholangiograms may assist in the recognition of some of the anomalies and may help the operator avoid a surgical catastrophe. The surgeon must be familiar with the possible abnormalities which may be encountered in this region, where great variation occurs. He or she must especially keep in mind that more than one gallbladder may exist and that a seemingly absent gallbladder may be actually present intrahepatically or even on the left side.

Diagnosis. A radiographic report of "no visualization of the gallbladder" in the presence of right upper quadrant symptoms is not an adequate indication of absence of the gallbladder. Apparently, there have been no reports of correct preoperative diagnosis of this condi-

tion. Dilation of the biliary ducts commonly occurs with gallbladder agenesis, and this sign may prepare the surgeon for an anomalous finding.

The intrahepatic gallbladder that is buried beneath the liver surface may lead to a mistaken diagnosis of congenital absence. If radiographic visualization was good, there is no diagnostic problem although there may be a surgical problem. When the gallbladder is neither visualized radiographically nor apparent on gross inspection, the surgeon must be prepared to consider the possibility of a diseased, nonfunctioning gallbladder embedded in the liver substance before concluding that the structure is absent. As the intrahepatic gallbladder will probably contain stones, the surgeon should palpate the cystic fossa if it is present. Aspiration may be necessary to aid in localization. Cholecystostomy is the preferred procedure since bleeding is the major complication in the removal of an intrahepatic gallbladder. In addition, exploration of the common bile duct is mandatory since the duct frequently is filled with stones.

A left-sided gallbladder also may give rise to a suspicion of agenesis because, even if it is functioning, it may lie outside the field of the usual cholecystographic plate.

The diagnosis of double and bilobed gallbladders is usually obvious from radiographic visualization. It should be remembered that stones and inflammation may exist in one portion but not in the other (160).

Septate duplication, diverticula, and phrygian cap deformities may or may not be visualized before operation, but their presence will not affect surgical procedure. Note that infection or lithiasis may affect only one loculus.

Treatment. With anomalous gallbladders, the surgeon's art is involved chiefly in diagnosis. Except for the intrahepatic gallbladder discussed above, the treatment of the diseased gallbladder, once it is located, is determined without regard for its anomalies. While few of these are pathologic in themselves, most show an increased propensity for lithiasis and obstruction. The treatment of choice is cholecystectomy of "all gallbladders present," but in a few cases the decision for cholecystostomy represents a more mature surgical judgment. The operator should take special care to identify and isolate the cystic artery and the cystic duct when gallbladder structure is unusual since arterial anomalies commonly accompany biliary tract anomalies.

The surgeon should be extremely careful during laparoscopic cholecystectomy. We recently entered the new era of laparoscopic surgery; and because of the ease with which a gallbladder can be removed laparoscopically, almost all gallbladder surgery done today is through the laparoscope. There appears to be a tendency among surgeons doing this procedure to not perform intraoperative cholangiograms. That controversy is for another dis-

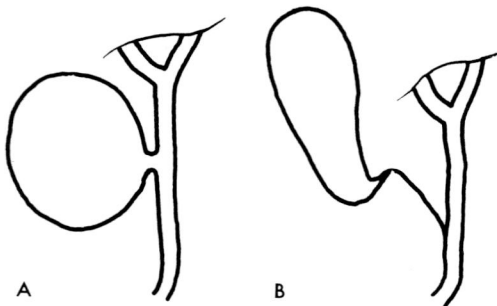

Figure 9.28. **A**, Absence of the cystic duct, with sessile gallbladder. **B**, Atresia of the cystic duct, with preservation of the gallbladder.

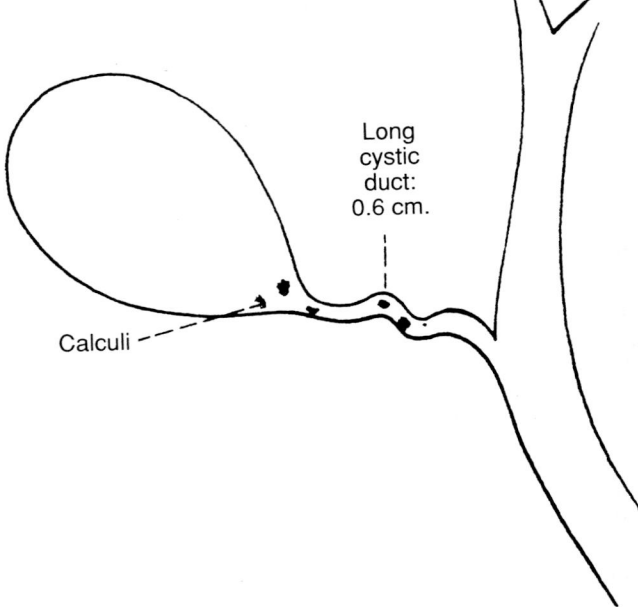

Figure 9.29. The long cystic duct. The danger lies in leaving part of the cystic duct with calculi. (From Furste W, Solt R. The surgical significance of the external length of the cystic duct. Surg Gynecol Obstet 1961;112:126.)

cussion. However, whenever the anatomy of this region appears abnormal, the safe approach is to obtain an intraoperative cholangiogram, thus defining the anatomy of the biliary system and exposing any variations.

Variations and Anomalies of the Cystic Duct

When the cystic primordium from the liver diverticulum fails to form, both the gallbladder and the cystic duct will be absent.

Among the cases collected by Latimer et al. (169), there were six in which at least part of the cystic duct was present without a gallbladder. Excluding the possibility that a fibrotic, atrophic gallbladder was overlooked, these cases represent a failure of the tip of the cystic diverticulum to differentiate. In one case the duct was small and contained a gallstone (207). In another the duct was short and dilated (166). Interestingly, in none of the six cases were biliary symptoms present.

The cystic duct also may be said to be absent when the gallbladder empties directly into the common duct (Fig. 9.28, A). Rabinovitch et al. (160) illustrated such a case, and Gross reported a case in which a normal gallbladder and cystic duct were accompanied by an accessory gallbladder without cystic duct, which was sessile on the main hepatic duct (18).

In a few instances the gallbladder is present even though the cystic duct appears to be absent or to be represented only by a fibrous band (6) (Fig. 9.28, B). These cases result from a secondary atresia of the cystic duct similar to those found elsewhere in the biliary tract, rather than a failure of the anlage to form. In most cases the common duct is atretic as well. These defects arise from failure of canalization of the cystic duct in the 12th week. Milder irregularities of canalization may result in dilation or strictures of the cystic duct with obvious potentialities for eventual obstruction.

Furste and Solt (208) reported several variations in the length of the cystic duct, from 0.6 to 5.6 cm (Figs. 9.29 and 9.30).

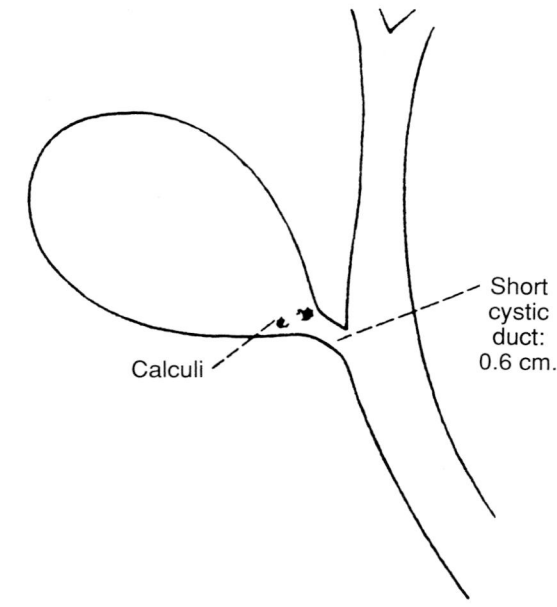

Figure 9.30. The short cystic duct. The danger lies in excising part of common duct or stenosis of duct with suture. (From Furste W, Solt R. The surgical significance of the external length of the cystic duct. Surg Gynecol Obstet 1961;112:126.)

Double cystic ducts are known to drain a single, nonseptate gallbladder (Fig. 9.31, A to C). The supernumerary duct may join the system at the common bile duct or at the right hepatic duct (209). An apparently single duct may consist of two epithelial tubes within a single mus-

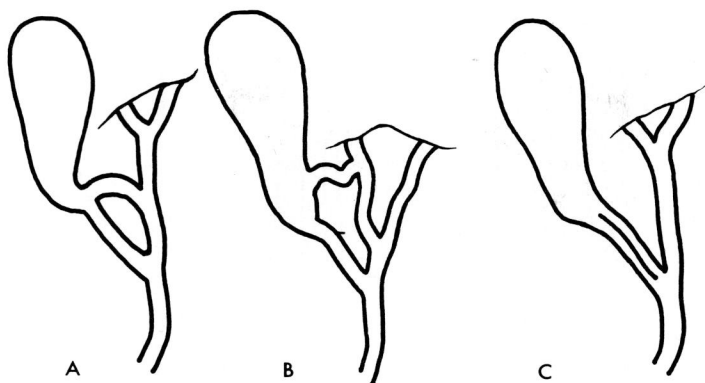

Figure 9.31. Duplication of the cystic duct with single gallbladder. **A**, Both cystic ducts entering the common hepatic duct. **B**, Accessory cystic duct opening into the right hepatic duct. **C**, Double-barreled duplication of the cystic duct.

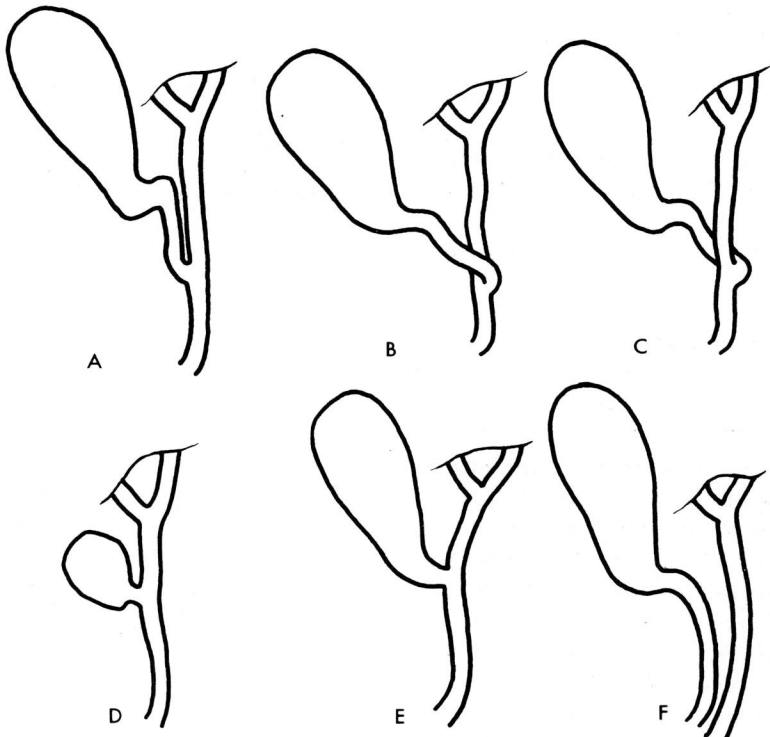

Figure 9.32. Variations of the cystic duct. **A**, Junction of cystic and common hepatic ducts at an unusually small angle. **B** and **C**, Entrance of the cystic duct on the left side of the common hepatic duct. **D** and **E**, Short cystic ducts. **F**, Long cystic duct. This may be equally well termed *absence of the common bile duct.*

cularis: These were formed when epithelial vacuoles failed to coalesce during recanalization.

In about 75% of individuals, the cystic duct joins the common duct at an angle of about 40 degrees. In 17%, it may parallel the bile duct for a shorter or longer distance, or it may even reach the duodenum independently (Fig. 9.32, *A*).

Two cases have been reported in which the cystic duct opened into an accessory right hepatic duct (2, 82).

None of these variations in the course of cystic duct is of significance in itself. Any tortuosity may, however, increase the likelihood of obstruction from gallstones. When surgery is required, it becomes important to know that, in a large number of cases, the situation encountered differs greatly from the textbook pattern. In 1918 Eisendrath (210) was among the first in the United States to illustrate these variations and emphasize the frequency of their occurrence.

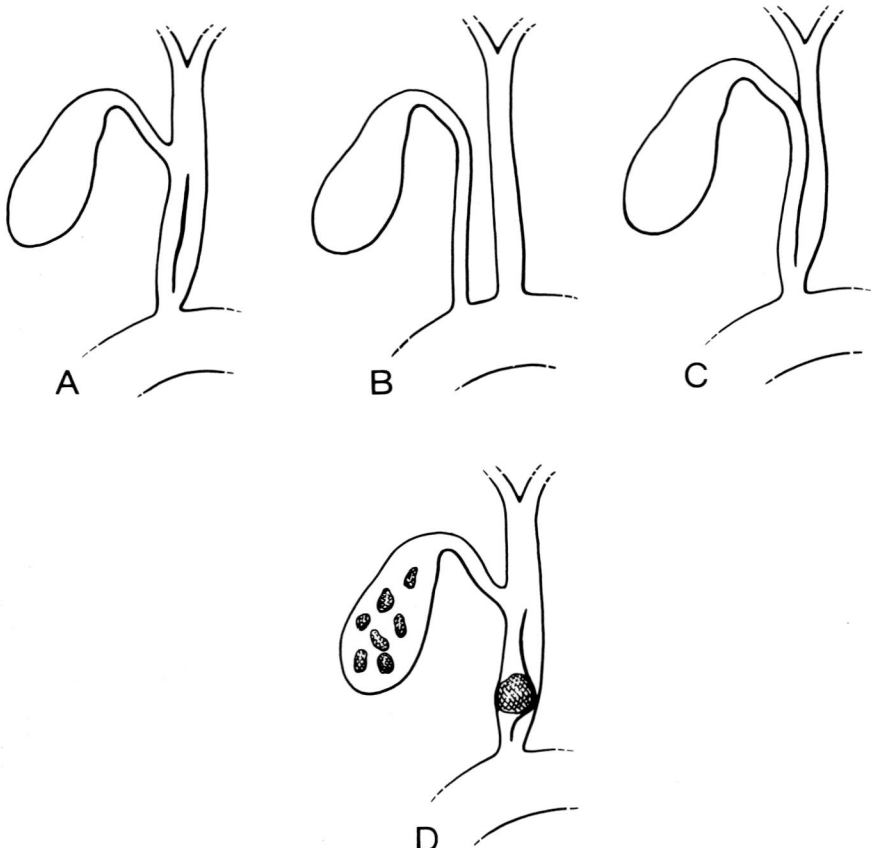

Figure 9.33. **A**, Common bile duct with septum. **B**, Long cystic duct draining the gallbladder independently into the duodenum. **C**, Long septum of the common bile duct incorporating the cystic and common hepatic duct union. **D**, Mirizzi's pathology and presentation of the syndrome.

Variations in length of the cystic duct are not unusual, but extremes deserve surgical consideration. Dowdy and his colleagues (76) found the cystic duct to vary from 0.4 to 6.0 cm in length among 100 cadavers. A very short duct, one that is only a few millimeters or less in length, requires careful manipulation to prevent injury to the hepatic and common duct (Fig. 9.32, *D* and *E*). If a very long duct is allowed to remain after cholecystectomy, it may be responsible for recurrence of symptoms (the "cystic duct remnant" syndrome) (Fig. 9.32, *F*, and Fig. 9.10, *A* and *B*).

MIRIZZI'S SYNDROME (SINDROME DEL CONDUCTO HEPATICO)

In 1948 P.L. Mirizzi (211) first reported this syndrome characterized by a long cystic duct with an impacted stone which produces extrinsic obstruction in the common hepatic duct with symptoms and signs of obstructive biliary duct disease. It is marked by mild or severe obstructive jaundice with or without cholecystitis. In 1989 Roullet-Audy et al. (212) presented six cases of Mirizzi's syndrome, and Didlake and Haick (213) and Dewar et al.

(214) discussed the operative strategy in this syndrome. There is a long cystic duct, parallel to the common hepatic duct, with a low opening into the hepatic duct (absence of the supraduodenal common duct) or separate entrance of the common hepatic duct and cystic duct in the duodenum (Fig. 9.33).

Variations of the Hepatic and Cystic Arteries

THE HEPATIC ARTERY (FIG. 9.34)

The right hepatic artery passed posterior to the common hepatic duct in 64% of individuals examined by Grant (215). It passed anterior to the duct in 24%. In the remaining 12%, the right hepatic artery arose from the superior mesenteric artery and lay to the right of and parallel to the common hepatic duct, passing posterior to the cystic duct.

THE CYSTIC ARTERIES (FIG. 9.35)

In 76% of individuals, the cystic artery arises from the right hepatic artery to the right of the common hepatic duct. In 24%, it arises to the left of the common hepatic

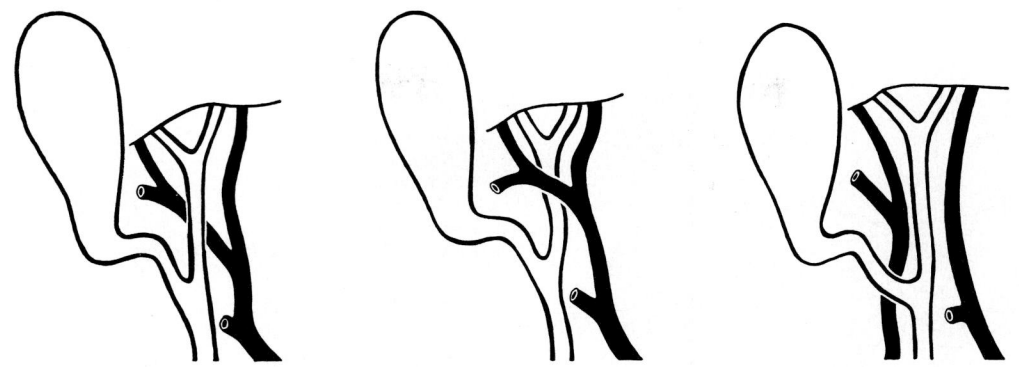

Figure 9.34. *Variation of the hepatic arteries. (After Grant JCB. Grant's atlas of anatomy. Baltimore: Williams & Wilkins, 1962.)*

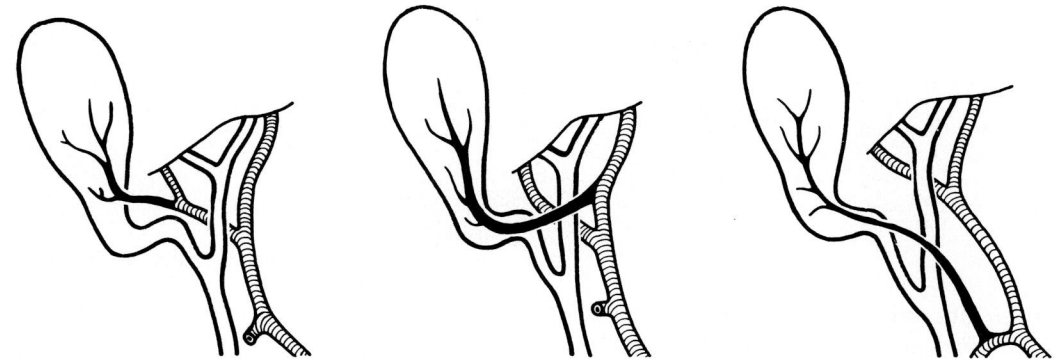

Figure 9.35. *Variation in origin of the cystic arteries. (After Grant JCB. Grant's atlas of anatomy. Baltimore: Williams & Wilkins, 1962.)*

duct—from the left hepatic artery, the proximal right hepatic artery, the hepatic artery, or the gastroduodenal artery. In these cases the cystic artery passes anterior to the duct (210, 216). Two or more cystic arteries may occur, or the artery may branch before reaching the gallbladder (76). Very rarely, the cystic artery is recurrent, reaching the gallbladder at the fundus and branching toward the neck (78, 217) (Fig. 9.36).

Identification of the right hepatic and the cystic arteries while exposing the operative field will prevent the surgeon from accidentally severing them.

Variations in the Cholecystohepatic Triangle

The cholecystohepatic triangle is formed by the cystic duct and gallbladder below, the right lobe of the liver above, and the common hepatic duct medially (Fig. 9.37). Within the boundaries of the triangle are a number of structures that must be identified before they are ligated or sectioned.

Over the years the triangle, described originally by Calot in 1891, has enlarged. For Calot, the upper bound-

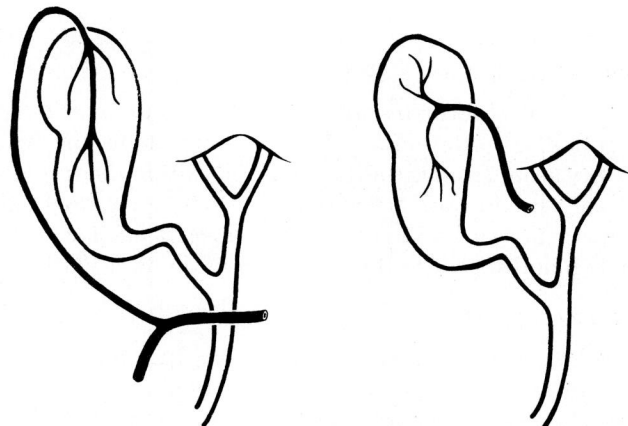

Figure 9.36. *Recurrent cystic arteries. (After Nikolic V. Artère cystique récurrente. Bull Assoc Anat 1967;136:739–744.*

ary was the cystic artery; it is now the lower border of the right lobe of the liver (218).

RIGHT HEPATIC ARTERY

The right hepatic artery enters the triangle posterior to the common hepatic duct (87%) or anterior to it (13%). It

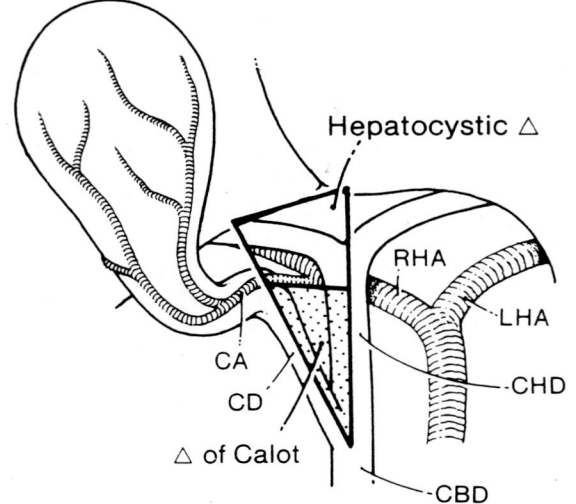

Figure 9.37. The hepatocystic triangle and the triangle of Calot. The upper boundary of the former is the margin of the liver; that of the latter is the cystic artery. The triangle of Calot is stippled. *CA*, cystic artery; *CD*, cystic duct; *CHD*, common hepatic duct; *CBD*, common bile duct; *LHA/RHA*, left and right hepatic arteries. (From Skandalakis JE, Gray SW, Rowe JS, Jr. Anatomical complications in general surgery. New York: McGraw-Hill Book, 1983.)

parallels the cystic duct for a short distance before turning superiorly to reach the liver. In 20% of the cadavers examined by Moosman (219), the artery lay within 1 cm of the duct and might have been mistaken for the cystic artery. As a rule of thumb, any artery of more than 3 mm in diameter within the triangle will probably not be a cystic artery.

ABERRANT RIGHT HEPATIC ARTERY

In 18% of Moosman's specimens, there was an aberrant right hepatic artery. In 83% of these specimens, the cystic artery arose from the aberrant artery within the triangle. In 4%, the aberrant artery was accessory to a normal right hepatic artery, and in 14%, it was a replacing artery, the only blood supply to the right lobe of the liver (219).

CYSTIC ARTERY

The cystic artery arises usually from the normal right hepatic artery or an aberrant right hepatic artery within the cholecystohepatic triangle. At the neck of the gallbladder, the cystic artery divides into a superficial branch to the serosal surface and a deep branch to the hepatic surface of the gallbladder. This pattern is found in 61 to 87% of individuals (219, 220).

In a few cases the cystic artery arises from the right hepatic artery to the left of the common hepatic duct and enters the triangle of Calot by passing anterior to the duct. The same course is followed by a cystic artery arising from the left hepatic artery (3%). Where the origin is from

Table 9.6.
Origin of the Cystic Artery[a]

Origin	Percentage	
Right hepatic artery		
Normal	61.4	
Aberrant (accessory)	10.2	
Aberrant (replacing)	3.1	
Left hepatic artery	5.9	
Bifurcation of common hepatic artery	11.5	
		92.1
Common hepatic artery	3.8	
		95.9
Gastroduodenal artery	2.5	
Superior pancreaticoduodenal artery	0.15	
Right gastric artery	0.15	
Celiac trunk	0.3	
Superior mesenteric artery	0.9	
Right gastroepiploic artery	Rare	
Aorta	Rare	
		99.9

[a]From Anson BJ. Anatomical considerations in surgery of gallbladder. Q Bull Northwest Univ Med Sch 1956;30:250.

Table 9.7.
Segments of the Biliary Tract and the Frequency of Arteries Lying Anterior to Them[a]

Segment	Artery Anterior	Percentage Frequency
Right and left hepatic ducts	Right hepatic artery	12–15
	Cystic artery	<5
Common hepatic duct	Cystic artery	15–24
	Right hepatic artery	11–19
	Common hepatic artery	<5
Supraduodenal common bile duct (CBD)	Anterior artery to CBD	50
	Posterosuperior pancreaticoduodenal artery	12.5
	Gastroduodenal artery	5.7–20[b]
	Right gastric artery	<5
	Common hepatic artery	<5
	Cystic artery	<5
	Right hepatic artery	<5
Retroduodenal common bile duct	Posterosuperior pancreaticoduodenal artery	76–87.5
	Supraduodenal artery	11.4

[a]From Johnston EV, Anson BJ. Variations in the formation and vascular relationships of the bile ducts. Surg Gynecol Obstet 1952;94:669.
[b]In another 36%, the gastroduodenal artery lay on the left border of the common bile duct. (From Maingot R. Abdominal operations, Vol 1. New York: Appleton-Century-Crofts, 1974.)

a common hepatic artery (5%) or a gastroduodenal artery (2%), the cystic artery enters the triangle from below.

In 96% of individuals, the cystic artery arises from the right, left, or common hepatic artery. In the remainder, a number of other sites occur (Table 9.6). In all cases in which the origin of the cystic artery lies to the left of the common hepatic duct, the artery crosses anterior to the duct. Among 482 cadavers studied by Moosman, the cystic artery arose in or traversed the cholecystohepatic triangle in 96% (219).

Duplication of the cystic artery is found in as many as 25% of individuals (221). These two vessels may arise from adjacent or separate sites. This duplication usually represents separation of the superficial and deep branches.

ABERRANT (ACCESSORY) BILE DUCTS

In 16% of 250 subjects studied by Moosman and Coller (222), there were aberrant (accessory) bile ducts within the hepatocystic triangle. These entered the cystic or common hepatic ducts. Many were multiple, and all were small enough to be overlooked (2 to 3 mm), yet large enough to cause bile to leak into the abdominal cavity.

Variations in the Vascular Relations of the Extrahepatic Biliary Tract

In general, the major blood vessels in the neighborhood of the biliary tree are posterior to the ducts, but they may lie anterior. The surgeon must recognize and preserve these arteries. Table 9.7 shows the frequency with which specific arteries are found anterior to segments of the biliary tract.

Couinard (223) studied the parabiliary venous system, and reported several findings:

1. The parabiliary venous system is most likely embryologically independent of the portal vein. It develops with the bile ducts and the hepatic artery.
2. Part of the cystic veins were anastomosed with the parabiliary system in 46.5% of the specimens studied.

REFERENCES

1. Schwegler RA, Boyden EA. The development of the pars intestinalis of the common bile duct in the human fetus, with special reference to the origin of the ampulla of Vater and the sphincter of Oddi I: the involution of the ampulla. Anat Rec 1937;67:441–468.
2. Mueller GF. Anomalous biliary duct. Minn Med 1960;43:253.
3. Boyden EA. The accessory gallbladder: an embryological and comparative study of aberrant biliary vesicles occurring in man and the domestic animals. Am J Anat 1926;38:177–231.
4. Dévé F. De quelques particularites anatomiques et anomalies de la vésicule biliaire. Bull Mém Soc Anat Paris 1903;78:261–270.
5. Thompson J. On congenital obliteration of the bile ducts. Edinb Med J 1891–1892;37:523, 604, 724.
6. Holmes JB. Congenital obliteration of the bile ducts: diagnosis and suggestions for treatment. Am J Dis Child 1916;11:405–431.
7. Longmire WP. Congenital biliary hypoplasia. Ann Surg 1964;159:335–343.
8. Rolleston HD, Hayne LB. A case of congenital hepatic cirrhosis with obliterative cholangitis. Br Med J 1901;1:758–760.
9. Yllpö A. Zwei falle von Kongenitalen gallengangsverschluss: fett-

und bilirubin-stoffwechselversuch bei einem derselben. K Kinderheilk 1913;9:913.
10. Bremer JL. Diverticula and duplication of the intestinal tract. Arch Pathol 1944;38:132.
11. Myers RL, Baggenstoss AH, Logan GB, Hallenbeck GA. Congenital atresia of the extrahepatic biliary tract: a clinical and pathological study. Pediatrics 1956;18:767–781.
12. Holder TM, Ashcraft KW. The effects of bile duct ligation and inflammation in the fetus. J Pediatr Surg 1967;2:35–40.
13. Picket LK, Briggs HC. Biliary obstruction secondary to hepatic vascular ligation in fetal sheep. J Pediatr Surg 1969;4:95–101.
14. Okamoto E, Okasora T, Toyosaka A. An experimental study on the etiology of congenital biliary atresia. In: Kasai M, Shiraki K, ed. Cholestasis in infancy. Baltimore: University Park Press, 1980
15. McSherry CK, Morrissey KP, Swarm RL, May PS, Niemann WH. Chenodeoxycholic acid-induced liver injury in pregnant and neonatal baboons. Ann Surg 1976;184:490–499.
16. Morecki R, Glaser JH, Horwitz MS. Etiology of biliary atresia: the role of reo 3 virus. In: Daum F, Fisher SE, eds. Extrahepatic biliary atresia. New York: Marcel Dekker, 1983:5.
17. Tracy TF, Jr, et al. Delayed bile duct proliferation in newborn cholestatic liver injury: correlations between morphology and liver gene expression. Surg Forum 1991;42:582–584.
18. Raffensperger JG, ed. Swenson's pediatric surgery. Norwalk, CT: Appleton & Lange, 1990:650.
19. Bangaru B et al. Comparative studies of biliary atresia in the human newborn and reovirus-induced cholangitis in weanling mice. Lab Invest 1980;43:456.
20. Glaser J, Balistravi W, Morecki R. Role of reovirus type 3 in persistent infantile cholestasis. J Pediatr 1984;105:912.
21. Moore TC. Annular pancreas: a review of the literature and report of 2 infant cases. Surgery 1953;33:138.
22. Gross RE: Congenital anomalies of the gallbladder: a review of 148 cases, with report of a double gallbladder. Arch Surg 1936;32:131–162.
23. Lilly JR, Chandra RS. Surgical hazards of co-existing anomalies in biliary atresia. Surg Gynecol Obstet 1974;139:49.
24. Home E. On the formation of fat in the intestines of living animals. Phil Trans R Soc Lond 1813;103:146–158.
25. Beneke R. Die entstehung der kongenitalen atresie der grossen gallengänge nebst bemerkungen über den begriff der abschnürung. Marbury NG, Elwert, 1907.
26. Ladd W. Congenital atresia and stenosis of the bile ducts. JAMA 1928;91:1082.
27. Lou MA, Schmutzer KJ, Regan JF. Congenital extrahepatic biliary atresia. Arch Surg 1972;105:771.
28. Krovetz LJ. Congenital biliary atresia. I. Analysis of thirty cases with particular reference to diagnosis. II. Analysis of the therapeutic problem. Surgery 1960;47:453–489.
29. Kasai M, Watanabe K, Wamagata A, Takamura U. Surgical treatment of biliary atresia. Nihonijishinpo 1957;1730:15.
30. Kasai M et al. Surgical treatment of biliary atresia. J Pediatr Surg 1968;3:665–675.
31. Stowens D. Pediatric pathology. Baltimore: Williams & Wilkins, 1959.
32. Krauss AN. Familial extrahepatic biliary atresia. J Pediatr 1964;65:933–937.
33. Karrer FM, Hall RJ, Stewart BA, Lilly JR. Congenital biliary tract disease. Surg Clin North Am 1990;70:1403–1418.
34. Alagille D. Extrahepatic biliary atresia. Hepatology 1984;4:7S–10S.
35. Peters H et al. The diagnostic significance of cholescintigraphy and ultrasound examination in cholestatic syndromes in infancy. Pediatr Surg Int 1988;3:37–42.

36. Silverberg M, Craig J, Gellis SS. Problems in the diagnosis of biliary atresia. Am J Dis Child 1960;99:574–584.

37. Rutenberg AM et al. Differential test for infant jaundice. Am J Dis Child 1962;103:47–54.

38. Kasai M et al. Surgical limitations for biliary atresia: indication for liver transplantation. J Pediatr Surg 1989;24:851–854.

39. Lilly JR. Hepatic portocholecystostomy for biliary atresia. J Pediatr Surg 1979;14:301–304.

40. Lilly JR et al. The surgery of biliary atresia. Ann Surg 1989;210:289–296.

41. Kaufman BH, Luck SR, Raffensperger JG. The evolution of a valved hepatoduodenal intestinal conduit. J Pediatr Surg 1981;16:279–283.

42. Freund H, Berlatzky Y, Schiller M. The ileocecal segment: an antireflux conduit for hepatic portoenterostomy. J Pediatr Surg 1979;14:169–171.

43. Canty TG. Encouraging results with a modified Sawaguchi hepatoportoenterostomy for biliary atresia. Am J Surg 1987;54:19–26.

44. Altman PR. The portoenterostomy procedure for biliary atresia: a 5 year experience. Ann Surg 1978;188:351–362.

45. Starzl TE et al. Homotransplantation of the liver in humans. Surg Gynecol Obstet 1963;117(6):659–676.

46. Starzl TE et al. Orthotopic liver transplantation in ninety-three patients. Surg Gynecol Obstet 1976;142:487–505.

47. Calne RY, Williams R. Orthotopic liver transplantation: the first 60 patients. Br Med J 1977;1:471–476.

48. Starzl TE et al. Decline in survival after liver transplantation. Arch Surg 1980;115:815–819.

49. Starzl TE, Klintmalm GBG, Porter KA, Iwatsuki S, Schröter GPJ. Liver transplantation with use of cyclosporin A and prednisone. N Engl J Med 1981;305(5):266–269.

50. National Institutes of Health. Consensus development conference statement: liver transplantation, June 20–23, 1983. Hepatology 1984;4(1)107S–110S.

51. Starzl TE, Demetris AJ, Thiel DV. Liver transplantation. N Engl J Med 1989;(I)321(15):1014–1022, (II)321(16):1092–1099.

52. Lilly JR, Hall RJ, Altman RP. Liver transplantation and Kasai operation in the first year of life: therapeutic dilemma in biliary atresia [Editorial]. J Pediatr 1987;110(4)561–562.

53. Busuttil RW, Seu P, Millis JM. Liver transplantation in children. Ann Surg 1991;213(1):48–57.

54. Esquivel CO et al. Liver transplantation before 1 year of age. J Pediatr 1987;110(4):545–548.

55. Sokal EM et al. Liver transplantation in children less than one year of age. J Pediatr 1990;117(2), (I):205–210.

56. Wood RP et al. Optimal therapy for patients with biliary atresia: portoenterostomy ("Kasai" procedures) versus primary transplantation. J Pediatr Surg 1990;25(1):153–162.

57. Millis JM et al. Orthotopic liver transplantation for biliary atresia: evolution of management. Arch Surg 1988;123:1237–1239.

58. Vacanti JP, Shamberger RC, Eraklis A, Lillehei CW. The therapy of biliary atresia combining the Kasai portoenterostomy with liver transplantation: a single center experience. J Pediatr Surg 1990;25(1):149–152.

59. Monaco AP. Transplantation: the state of the art. Transplant Proc 1990;22(3):896–901.

60. Otte JB et al. Size reduction of the donor liver is a safe way to alleviate the shortage of size-matched organs in pediatric liver transplantation. Ann Surg 1990;211(2):146–157.

61. Kalayoglu M et al. Experience with reduced-size liver transplantation. Surg Gynecol Obstet 1990;171:139–147.

62. Broelsch CE, Whitington PF, Emond JC. Evolution and future perspectives for reduced-size hepatic transplantation. Surg Gynecol Obstet 1990;171:353–360.

63. Superina RA, Strasberg SM, Greig PD, Langer B. Early experience with reduced-sized liver transplants. J Pediatr Surg 1990;25(11):1157–1161.

64. Otte JB, deVille deGoyet J, Alberti D, Balladur P, deHemptinne B. The concept and technique of the split liver in clinical transplantation. Surgery 1990;107(6):605–612.

65. Darby JM, Stein K, Grenvik A, Stuart SA. Approach to management of the heartbeating "brain dead" organ donor. JAMA 1989;261(15):2222–2228.

66. Strong et al. Successful liver transplantation from a living donor to her son. N Engl J Med 1990;322(21):1505–1508.

67. Singer PA et al. Ethics of liver transplantation with living donors. 1989;321(9):620–622.

68. Starzl TE et al. FK 506 for liver, kidney, and pancreas transplantation. Lancet 1989; 8670:1000–1004.

69. Macleod AM, Thomson AW. FK 506: an immunosuppressant for the 1990s. Lancet 1991;337:25–27.

70. Harrison MR et al. Successful repair in utero of a fetal diaphragmatic hernia after removal of herniated viscera from the left thorax. N Engl J Med 1990;322(22):1582–1584.

71. Thompson IM. On the arteries and ducts in the hepatic pedicle: a study in statistical human anatomy. Univ Calif Publ Anat 1933;1:55.

72. Michels NA. Blood supply and anatomy of the upper abdominal organ with a descriptive atlas. Philadelphia: JB Lippincott, 1955.

73. Rabinovitch J, Rabinovitch P, Zisk HJ. Rare anomalies of the extra-hepatic bile ducts. Ann Surg 1956;144:93–98.

74. Couinaud C. Exposure of the left hepatic duct through the hilum or in the umbilical of the liver: anatomic limitations. Surgery 1989;105(1):21–27.

75. Russell E et al. Left hepatic duct anatomy: implications. Radiology 1990;174(2):353–356.

76. Dowdy GS, Waldron GW, Brown WG. Surgical anatomy of the pancreatobiliary ductal system. Arch Surg 1962;84:93–110.

77. Norman O. Studies of the hepatic ducts in cholangiography. Acta Radiol 1951;84(Suppl):1–81.

78. Healey JE, Schroy PC. Anatomy of the biliary ducts within the human liver: analysis of the prevailing pattern of branchings and the major variations of the biliary ducts. Arch Surg 1953;66:599–616.

79. Nygren EJ, Barnes WA. Atresia of the common hepatic duct with shunt via an accessory duct. Arch Surg 1954;68:337.

80. Mentzer SH. Anomalous bile ducts in man. JAMA 1929;93:1273–1277.

81. Corcoran DB, Wallace KK. Congenital anomalies of the gallbladder. Am Surg 1954;20:709–725.

82. Stauber R. Ein seltener Fall von angeborener Missbildung des Choledochus. Zentralbl Chir 1963;88:1219–1223.

83. von Wyss H. Zur Kenntnis der heterologen Flimmercysten. Virchow Arch [A] 1870;51:143–144.

84. Smanio T. Varying relations of the common bile duct with the posterior face of the pancreas in negroes and white persons. J Int Coll Surg 1954;22:150–173.

85. Reinhoff WF, Jr, Pickrell KL. Pancreatitis: an anatomic study of pancreatic and extrahepatic biliary systems. Arch Surg 1945;51:205.

86. Mann FC, Giordano AS. The bile factor in pancreatitis. Arch Surg 1923;6:1.

87. Cameron AL, Noble JF. Reflux of bile up the duct of Wirsung caused by an impacted biliary calculus. JAMA 1924;82:1410.

88. Dardinski VJ. The anatomy of the major duodenal papilla of man, with special reference to its musculature. J Anat 1935;69:469–478.

89. Dragstedt LR, Haymond HE, Ellis JC. Pathogenesis of acute pancreatis (acute pancreatic necrosis). Arch Surg 1934;28:232.

90. Colp R, Gerber IE, Doubilet H. Acute cholecystitis associated with pancreatic reflux. Ann Surg 1936;103:67.

91. Gentile A. A unique anomaly of the biliary tract: communication between cystic and hepatic ducts with occlusion of common duct and separate entrance into the duodenum. Am J Med Sci 1931;182:95–99.

92. Swartley WB, Weeder SD, Choledochus cysts with a double common bile duct. Ann Surg 1935;101:912–920.

93. Sachs D. Septation of the ductus choledochus. Fortschr Roentgenstr 1963;98:363.

94. Boyden EA. The problem of the double ductus choledochus: an interpretation of an accessory bile duct found attached to the pars superior of the duodenum. Anat Rec 1932;55:71–94.

95. Everett C, Macumber HE. Anomalous distribution of the extrahepatic biliary ducts. Ann Surg 1942;115:472–474.

96. Wood M. Anomalous location of the papilla of Vater. Am J Surg 1966;111:265–268.

97. Lurje A. The topography of the extrahepatic biliary passages with reference to dangers of surgical technic. Ann Surg 1937;105:161.

98. Karpa P. Zwei Fälle von Dünndarmatresie. Virchow Arch [A] 1906;185:208–226.

99. Katz K. Atresie des Duodenums mit Verdoppelung des Ductus choledochus und pancreaticus. Virchow Arch [A] 1930;278:290–294.

100. DaCarpi JB. Isagogae Breves, 1522. (Lind LR, trans.) Chicago: University of Chicago Press, 1959.

101. Vesalius A. De humani corporis fabrica. Basil (Basileae): Oporinus J, 1543.

102. Fallopius G. Opera genuina omnia. Venice (Venetiis): JA et J deFrancisicis, 1606.

103. Alonso-Lej F, Rever WB, Pessagno DJ. Congenital choledochal cysts, with a report of 2, and an analysis of 94 cases. Int Abstr Surg 1959;108:1–30.

104. Browne HJ. Choledochal (bile duct) cysts. J Irish Med Assoc 1955;37:208.

105. Dexter D. Choledochal cyst with carcinoma of the intrahepatic bile ducts and pancreatic ducts. Br J Cancer 1957;11:18.

106. Tran NN, Pham BT, Tran SD, Nguyen TL. La dilatation kystique congénitale due cholédoque chez l'enfant: étude clinique d'après l'analyse de six cas personnels et revue de la littérature. Arch Mal Appar Dig 1964;53:1213–1239.

107. Moir CR, Scudamore CH. Emergency management of choledochal cysts in adult patients. Am J Surg 1987;153:434–438.

108. Nitsche E. Über einen Fall einer Choledochuscyste. Dtsch Z Chir 1942;255:650.

109. Dennison WM. A study of choledochus cyst in childhood. J Int Coll Surg 1954;21:113–117.

110. Egry G, Epstein O, Killner G. Gallengangcyste. Virchow Arch [A] 1957;330:119–125.

111. Caroli J, Saupault R, Kossakowski J, Placker L, Paradowska M. La dilatation polykystique congenitale des voies biliares intrahepatiques. Sem Hop Paris 1958;34:488.

112. Todani T, Watanabe Y, Narasue M, Tabuchi K, Okajima K. Congenital bile duct cysts: classification, operative procedures, and review of thirty-seven cases including cancer arising from choledochal cyst. Am J Surg 1977;134:263–269.

113. Nagorney DM. Choledochal cysts in adult life. In: Blumgart LH, ed. Surgery of the liver and biliary tract, Vol 2. New York: Churchill Livingstone, 1988;1003–1012.

114. Longmire WP, Jr, Mandiola SA, Gordon HE. Congenital cystic disease of the liver and biliary system. Ann Surg 1971;174(4):711–726.

115. Todani T et al. Anomalous arrangement of the pancreaticobiliary duct system in patients with a choledochal cyst. Am J Surg 1984;147:672.

116. Iwai N, Tokiwa K, Tsuto T, Yanagihara J, Takahashi T. Biliary manometry in choledochal cyst with abnormal choledochopancreatico ductal junction. J Pediatr Surg 1986;21(10):873–876.

117. Okada A et al. Congenital dilatation of the bile duct in 100 instances and its relationships with anomalous junction. Surg Gynecol Obstet 1990;171:291–298.

118. Babbitt DP. Congenital choledochal cyst: new etiological concept based on anomalous relationships of common bile duct and pancreatic bulb. Ann Radiol 1969;12:231.

119. Kázar G. Kettös epehólyag és choledochyscysta. Magy Sebész 1950;3:298–301.

120. Rheinlander HE, Bowens OL, Jr. Congenital absence of the gallbladder with cystic dilatation of the common bile duct. N Engl J Med 1957;256:557–559.

121. Böttger H. Zur ätiologie der Choledochuszysten. Zentralbl Allg Pathol 1951;87:407.

122. Evans MM et al. Heterotopic gastric mucosa in the common bile duct. Surgery 1990;108(1):96–100.

123. Madding GF. Congenital cystic dilatation of the common bile duct. Ann Surg 1961;154:288–294.

124. Pikula JV, Dunphy JE. Some effects of stenosis of the terminal common bile duct on the biliary tract and liver. N Engl J Med 1959;260:315–318.

125. Yotuyanagi S. Contributions to aetiology and pathogeny of idiopathic cystic dilatation of common bile duct with report of 3 cases. Gann 1936;30:601–650.

126. Rolleston HD. Diseases of the liver, gallbladder, and bile ducts. Philadelphia: WB Saunders, 1905.

127. Weber FP. Cystic dilatation of the common bile duct. Br J Child Dis 1934;31:27–36.

128. Saltz NJ, Glaser K. Congenital cystic dilatation of the common bile duct. Am J Surg 1956;91:56.

129. Gross RE. The surgery of infancy and childhood. Philadelphia: WB Saunders, 1953.

130. Shallow TA, Eger SA, Wagner FB, Jr, Sherman A. Congenital cystic dilatation of the common bile duct: case report and review of the literature. Ann Surg 1943;117:355–387.

131. Tsardakas E, Robnett AH. Congenital cystic dilatation of the common bile duct: report of 3 cases, analysis of 57 cases and review of the literature. Arch Surg 1956;72:311.

132. Ravitch MM, Snyder GB. Congenital cystic dilation of the common bile duct. Surgery 1958;44:752.

133. Vater A. Diss. de scirrhis viscerum. Wittenberg (Vitembergae), 1723.

134. Todd CH. History of a remarkable enlargement of the biliary duct. Dublin Hosp Rep 1818;1:325.

135. Douglas AH. Case of dilatation of the common bile duct. J Ment Sci 1852;14:97.

136. Swain WP. A case of cholecystenterostomy with the use of Murphy's button. Lancet 1895;1:743.

137. Laverson RS. Cysts of the common bile duct. Am J Med Sci 1909;137:563.

138. Neugebauer F. Zur Kenntnis der idiopathischen Choledochuscyste. Beitr Klin Chir 1924;131:448.

139. Hatano S, Imoto M. Congenital cystic dilatation of the common bile duct, with report of a new case. Jpn Nagasaki Igakkai Zassi 1954;29:307.

140. Voyles CR et al. Carcinoma in choledochal cysts: age related incidence. Arch Surg 1983;118:986–988.

141. Coyle KA, Bradley EL III. Cholangiocarcinoma developing after

simple excision of a type II choledochal cyst. South Med J 1992;85:540–544.

142. Fonkalsrud EW, Boles ET. Choledochal cysts in infancy and childhood. Surg Gynecol Obstet 1965;121:733–742.

143. Blocker TG, Jr, Williams H, Williams JE. Traumatic rupture of a congenital cyst of the choledochus. Arch Surg 1937;34:695–701.

144. Attar S, Obeid S. Congenital cyst of the common bile duct: a review of the literature and a report of two cases. Ann Surg 1955;142:289–295.

145. Yamaguchi M. Congenital choledochal cyst: analysis of 1,433 patients from the Japanese literature. Am J Surg 1980;140:653–657.

146. Crittenden SL, McKinley MJ. Choledochal cyst-clinical features and classification. Am J Gastroenterol 1985;80:643–647.

147. Lilly JR. The surgical treatment of choledochal cysts. Surg Gynecol Obstet 1979;149:36–42.

148. Oweida SW, Ricketts RR. Hepatico-jejuno-duodenostomy reconstruction following excision of choledochal cysts in children. Am Surg 1989;55:2–6.

149. Zhang J et al. The spur valve jejunal interposition and choledochus cystectomy: a clinical and experimental study. Chin Med J 1987;100:535–540.

150. Narasimha KL et al. Jejunal interposition hepaticoduodenostomy for choledochal cysts. Am J Gastroenterol 1987;82:1042–1045.

151. Okada A et al. Jejunal interposition hepaticoduodenostomy for congenital dilatation of the bile duct (choledochal cyst). J Pediatr Surg 1983;18:588–591.

152. Consentino CM, Luck SR, Raffensperger JG, Reynolds M. Choledochal duct cyst: resection with physiologic reconstruction. Surgery 1992;112:740–748.

153. Lopez RR, Pinson CW, Campbell JR, Harrison M, Katon RM. Variation in management based on type of choledochal cyst. Am J Surg 1991;161:612–615.

154. Karrer FM, Hall RJ, Stewart BA, Lilly JR. Congenital biliary tract disease. Surg Clin North Am 1990;70:1403–1418.

155. Holder TM. Choledochal cyst management by Rouxen-Y jejunal drainage. In: Ellison EH, Friesen SR, Mulholland JH, eds. Current surgical management, III. Philadelphia: WB Saunders, 1965.

156. Bower JO. Congenital absence of gall-bladder. Ann Surg 1928;88:80–90.

157. Theodor E. Angeborene Aplasia der Gallenwege verbunden mit Lebercirrhose, durch Operation behandelt. Arch Kinderheilk 1908;49:358–366.

158. Dixon CF, Lichtman AL. Congenital absence of gallbladder. Surgery 1945;17:11–21.

159. Banks PJ, Lawrance K. A case of vestigial gallbladder. Br Med J 1955;2:1254–1255.

160. Rabinovitch J, Rabinovitch P, Rosenblatt P, Pines B. Congenital anomalies of the gallbladder. Ann Surg 1958;148:161–168.

161. Gerwig WH, Jr, Countryman LK, Gomez AC. Congenital absence of the gallbladder and cystic duct. Ann Surg 1961;153:113–125.

162. McIlrath DC, ReMine WH, Baggenstoss AH. Congenital absence of the gallbladder and cystic duct: report of 10 cases. JAMA 1962;180:781–783.

163. Frey C, Bizer L, Ernst C. Agenesis of the gallbladder. Am J Surg 1967;114:917–926.

164. Aristotle. DeGeneratione, IV, iv, 771a.

165. Morgagni. JB. The seats and causes of disease investigated by anatomy. B. Alexander (transl). New York: Hafner Publishing, 1960.

166. Tallmadge GK. Congenital absence of gallbladder. Arch Pathol 1938;26:1060.

167. Mouzas G, Wilson A. Congenital absence of the gallbladder with stone in common bile duct. Lancet 1953;1:628.

168. Monroe SE. Congenital absence of the gallbladder. J Int Coll Surg 1959;32:369–371.

169. Latimer EO, Mendez FL, Hage WJ. Congenital absence of the gallbladder: report of 3 cases. Ann Surg 1947;126:229.

170. Flannery MG, Caster MP. Congenital hourglass gallbladder. South Med J 1957;50:1255–1258.

171. Rogers AI, Crews RD, Kalser MH. Congenital absence of the gallbladder with choledocholithiasis. Gastroenterology 1965;48:524–529.

172. Petromilli G et al. A new case of gallbladder genesis. Minerva Chir 1989;44(22):2351–2354.

173. Scobie WG, Bentley JFR. Hydrops of the GB in a newborn infant. J Pediatr Surg 1969;4:457.

174. Harlaftis N, Gray SW, Skandalakis JE. Multiple gallbladders. Surg Gynecol Obstet 1977;145:928.

175. De Arzua Zulaica E. Bilobular gallbladder. Rev Esp Enferm Apar Dig 1963;22:1105–1109.

176. Croudace WHH. Case of double gallbladder. Br Med J 1931;I:707.

177. Skielboe B. Anomalies of the gallbladder: vesica fellia triplex. Am J Clin Pathol 1958;30:252–255.

178. Hurst JM, Mayo RA. Unsuspected latent pairing of the cystic primordium, South Med J 1980;73:950.

179. Wischnewsky AW. Doppolgallenblase, während der operation aufgedeckt (ektomie der erkrankten supplementären blase). Arch Klin Chir 1925;135:779.

180. Harlaftis N, Gray SW, Olafson RP, Skandalakis JE. Three cases of unsuspected double gallbladder. Am Surg 1976;42(3):178–180.

181. Blasius G. Observata anatomica in homine, simia, equo, (etc.): accedunt extraordinaria in homine reperta praxin medicam aeque ac anatomen illustrantia. Amsterdam (Amstelodami): Gaasbeeck, 1674.

182. Gray SW, Olafson RP, Skandalakis JE, Harlaftis N. Developmental origin of the double gallbladder. Contemp Surg 1974;4(5):71–76.

183. Bartel J. Cholelithiasis und Körperkonstitution cholelithotripsie. Frankfurt. Z Pathol 1916;19:206–237.

184. Flannery MG, Caster MP. Congenital abnormalities of the gallbladder: 101 cases. Int Abstr Surg 1956;103:439–457.

185. Boyden EA. The "Phrygian cap" in cholecystography: a congenital anomaly of the gallbladder. AJR 1935;33:589.

186. Kaiser E. Congenital and acquired changes in gallbladder form. Am J Dig Dis 1961;6:938–953.

187. Robertson HE, Ferguson WJ. The diverticula (Luschka's crypts) of the gallbladder with choledocholithiasis. Gastroenterology 1945;40:312–333.

188. Nelson P, Schmitz R, Perutsea S. Anomalous position of the gallbladder within the falciform ligament. Arch Surg 1953;66:679.

189. Bullard RW, Jr. Subcutaneous or extraperitoneal gallbladder: a report of an unusual case. JAMA 1945;129:949.

190. Burke J. An anomaly in the position of the gallbladder. JAMA 1961;177:508–509.

191. Rachlin SA. Congenital anomalies of the gallbladder and ducts. Milit Surg 1951;109:20–25.

192. Feldman L, Venta L. Percutaneous cholecystostomy of an ectopic gallbladder. Gastrointest Radiol 1988;13(3):256–258.

193. Hopper KD. Hepatic inversion with an epigastric gallbladder. Gastrointest Radiol 1988;13(4):355–357.

194. Etter L. Left-sided gallbladder: necessity for film of the entire abdomen in cholecystography. AJR 1953;70:987–990.

195. Large AM. Left-sided gallbladder and liver without situs inversus. Arch Surg 1963;87:982–985.

196. Kehr H. Ueber angeborene der Gallenblase und der Atresia hepatica. Berl Klin Woch 1913;50:511.

197. McNamee EP. Intrahepatic gallbladder. AJR 1935;33:603.

198. De Weerd GJ, Frima AJ. Torsion of the gallbladder. Neth J Surg 1988, 40(2):49–50.

199. Jones TC. Analogous pathologic patterns in different animal species: approach to study of obscure lesions. Bull Int A M Museums 1950;31:24–35.

200. Williams MJ, Humm JJ. Heterotopia composed of gastric epithelium and smooth muscle in the wall of the gall bladder. Surgery 1953;34:133–139.

201. Pessel JF, Beairsto EB, Wise JS, Greeley JP, Rathmell TK. Gastrointestinal mucosa in wall of human gallbladder. Gastroenterology 1950;15:533–540.

202. Thorsness ET. Aberrant pancreatic nodule arising on the neck of the human gallbladder. Anat Rec 1940;77:319–329.

203. Lee CM. Duplication of the cystic and common hepatic ducts, lined with gastric mucosa. N Engl J Med 1957;256:927–931.

204. Tejada E, Danielson C. Ectopic or heterotopic liver (choristoma) associated with the gallbladder. Arch Pathol Lab Med 1989;113(8):950–952.

205. Shepard VD, Walters W, Dockerty MB. Benign neoplasms of gallbladder. Arch Surg 1942;45:1–18.

206. Eiserth P. Adenomyome der Gallenblase. Virchow Arch [A] 1938;302:717–723.

207. Miller JK. Congenital absence of the gallbladder. Am J Surg 1936;33:315.

208. Furste W, Solt R, Jr. The surgical significance of the external length of the cystic duct. Surg Gynecol Obstet 1961;112:124–126.

209. Perelmann H. Cystic duct reduplication. JAMA 1961;175:710–711.

210. Eisendrath DN. Anomalies of the bile ducts and blood vessels as the cause of accidents in biliary surgery. JAMA 1918;71:864.

211. Mirizzi PL. Syndrome del conducto hepatico. Bull Soc Int Chir 1948;8:731–737.

212. Roullet-Audy JC, Guivarc'h M, Mosnier H. Mirizzi's syndrome. Presse Med 1989;18(15):761–764.

213. Didlake R, Haick AJ. Mirizzi's syndrome: an uncommon cause of biliary obstruction. Am Surg 1990;56(4):268–269.

214. Dewar G, Chung SCS, Li AKC. Operative strategy in Mirizzi syndrome. Surg Gynecol Obstet 1990;171:157–159.

215. Grant JCB. Grant's atlas of anatomy. Baltimore: Williams & Wilkins, 1962.

216. Daseler EH, Anson BJ, Hambley WC, Reiman AF. The cystic artery and constituents of the hepatic pedicle: a study of 500 specimens. Surg Gynecol Obstet 1947;85:47–63.

217. Nikolic V. Artère cystique récurrente. Bull Assoc Anat 1967;136:739–744.

218. Rocko JM, Swan KG, DiGioia JM. Calot's triangle revisited. Surg Gynecol Obstet 1981;153:410.

219. Moosman DA. Where and how to find the cystic artery during cholecystectomy. Surg Gynecol Obstet 1975;141:769.

220. Anson BJ. Anatomical considerations in surgery of gallbladder. Q Bull Northwest Univ Med Sch 1956;30:250.

221. Michels NA. The hepatic, cystic, and retroduodenal arteries and their relations to the biliary ducts. Ann Surg 1951;133:503.

222. Moosman DA, Coller FA. Prevention of traumatic injury to the bile ducts. Am J Surg 1951;82:132.

223. Couinard C. The parabiliary venous system. Surg Radiol Anat 1988;10:311–316.

CHAPTER 10

THE SPLEEN

Lee John Skandalakis / Stephen Wood Gray / Richard Ricketts / John Elias Skandalakis

If you desire the spleen and will laugh yourself into stitches, follow me.
—SHAKESPEARE, TWELFTH NIGHT

DEVELOPMENT

Many of the organs that are asymmetric in the human body are of midline origin, like the stomach, or are originally bilateral with suppression of the component of one side, like the aortic arches and the venae cavae. The spleen forms an exception; it never was either midline or bilateral in origin. From time to time, workers suggest that a potential right spleen fails to develop, and at least one individual with paired, symmetric spleens has been reported (1). In spite of this case there is no evidence from ontogeny or phylogeny that there are normally bilateral splenic anlagen.

The spleen arises as a mesenchymal bulge on the left side of the dorsal mesogastrium, at the time the stomach has begun its rotation. The earliest indication is seen at the 6-mm stage; by 8 mm, the organ is definitely present (Fig. 10.1). When the spleen first appears, the celomic lining is merely the outer layer of mesenchymal cells; by the 10- to 12-mm stage it has differentiated into a true epithelium, and shortly afterward a basement membrane becomes visible. Until differentiation is complete, there is evidence that surface mesenchymal cells as well as deeper cells contribute to formation of the spleen (2).

Earliest sinusoids, in evidence by the 11-mm stage (3), have been described as mesenchymal clefts, without endothelial lining but in communication with capillaries. Splenic hemopoiesis was observed to begin in the pig embryo between the 30- to 60-mm stages and erythropoiesis is at its height by the middle of embryonic life (4). Typical splenic nodules appear only after birth.

Earlier researchers were concerned first with establishing the purely mesodermal origin of the spleen, and later investigators sought evidence to support the open or closed theories of circulation. None of the embryologic studies shed light on the formation of multiple or accessory spleens or on the mechanism by which the spleen occasionally becomes fused with the gonad.

In comparison with other organs, this enigmatic organ does not have critical events or, if there are any, they are unknown to the authors.

CONGENITAL SPLENIC ANOMALIES

Splenic anomalies and variations are many (Figs. 10.2 and 10.3). Some of them are quite benign, some are associated with other anomalies, and some produce multiple syndromes.

Classification of these anomalies is extremely difficult especially the multiply named and unnamed syndromes. In other words, polysplenia could be asymptomatic and could occur with other anomalies such as situs inversus and cardiac anomalies (Table 10.1).

Table 10.2 gives a possible classification of these anomalies. Body symmetry is discussed in Chapter 30 as partial or total situs inversus.

Splenic anomalies may be divided into six categories.

1. Anomalies of the spleen per se
2. Anomalies or variations of the splenic ligaments
3. Anomalies or variations of the extrasplenic vessels
4. Associated anomalies: the syndromes
5. Cysts and tumors
6. "Hodgepodge": inherited (genetic) disorders

It is not within the scope of this book to discuss all these categories. The purpose of this book is to present the morphologic anatomy as well as the associated anomalies from an embryologic standpoint in a broad way. We do not plan to discuss disorders of specific origin.

We do not claim that Table 10.3 is a complete one. Note in Table 10.3 that we found most common multiple anomalies associated with asplenia to be complex, such as pulmonary isomerism of the right lung type and congenital heart disease. With polysplenia we found fewer associated anomalies such as pulmonary isomerism of the left lung type and less severe congenital heart disease.

ASPLENIA AND SPLENIC HYPOPLASIA

Asplenia is autosomal recessive, whereas splenic hypoplasia is autosomal dominant.

Absence of the spleen produces a characteristic picture in the peripheral blood, as follows:

DEVELOPMENT

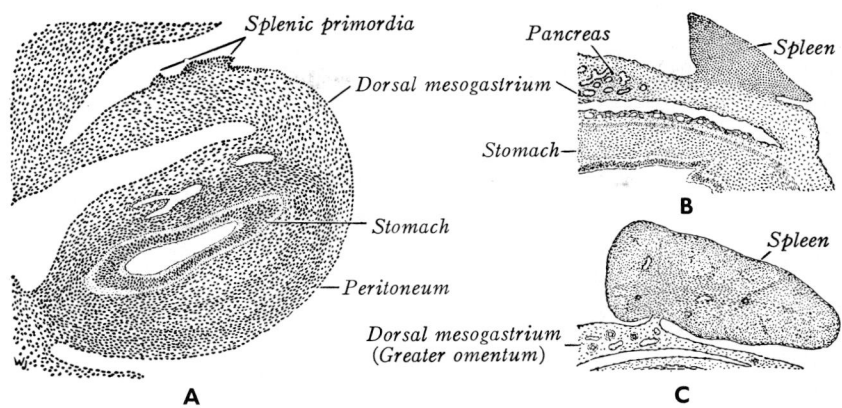

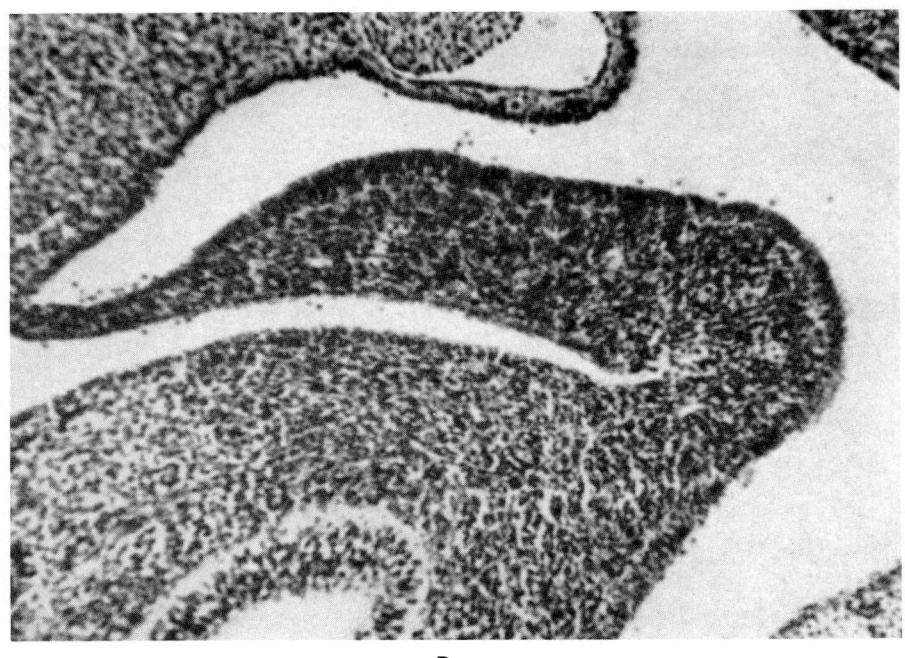

Figure 10.1. The development of the spleen. **A**, Splenic primordium on the left side of the dorsal mesogastrium at 6 weeks. **B**, At 2 months. **C**, At 4 months. **D**, Early splenic primordium. Angiogenesis is beginning. (**A** to **C**, From Arey LB. Developmental anatomy, 7th ed. Philadelphia: WB Saunders, 1965; **D**, from Ivemark BI. Implications of agenesis of the spleen on the pathogenesis of cono-truncus anomalies in children. Acta Paediatr (Uppsala) 1955;44(Suppl)104:1–110.)

1. Red blood cells (RBCs) are thinner and broader.
2. RBCs produce many target forms.
3. Because of the absence of pitting, Howel-Jolly as well as Pappenheimer bodies most likely will be present in the peripheral blood.
4. Reticulocytes and polychromic RBCs are increased.
5. White blood cell (WBC) levels are elevated.
6. Platelet levels are in the high range.

For all practical purposes, congenital asplenia, iatrogenic splenectomy, and splenic hypofunction secondary to several other diseases, such as sarcoidosis, sickle cell anemia, or splenic vascular obstruction, all produce the same picture in the peripheral blood, and they all increase the possibility of overwhelming sepsis.

According to Sills (5), many of the disorders that cause hyposplenia in adults have not been noted to do so in children. The same author advised detailed examination of the peripheral blood and, if possible, quantitation of RBC pits and radionuclide scans.

According to Stark and co-workers (6), the normal

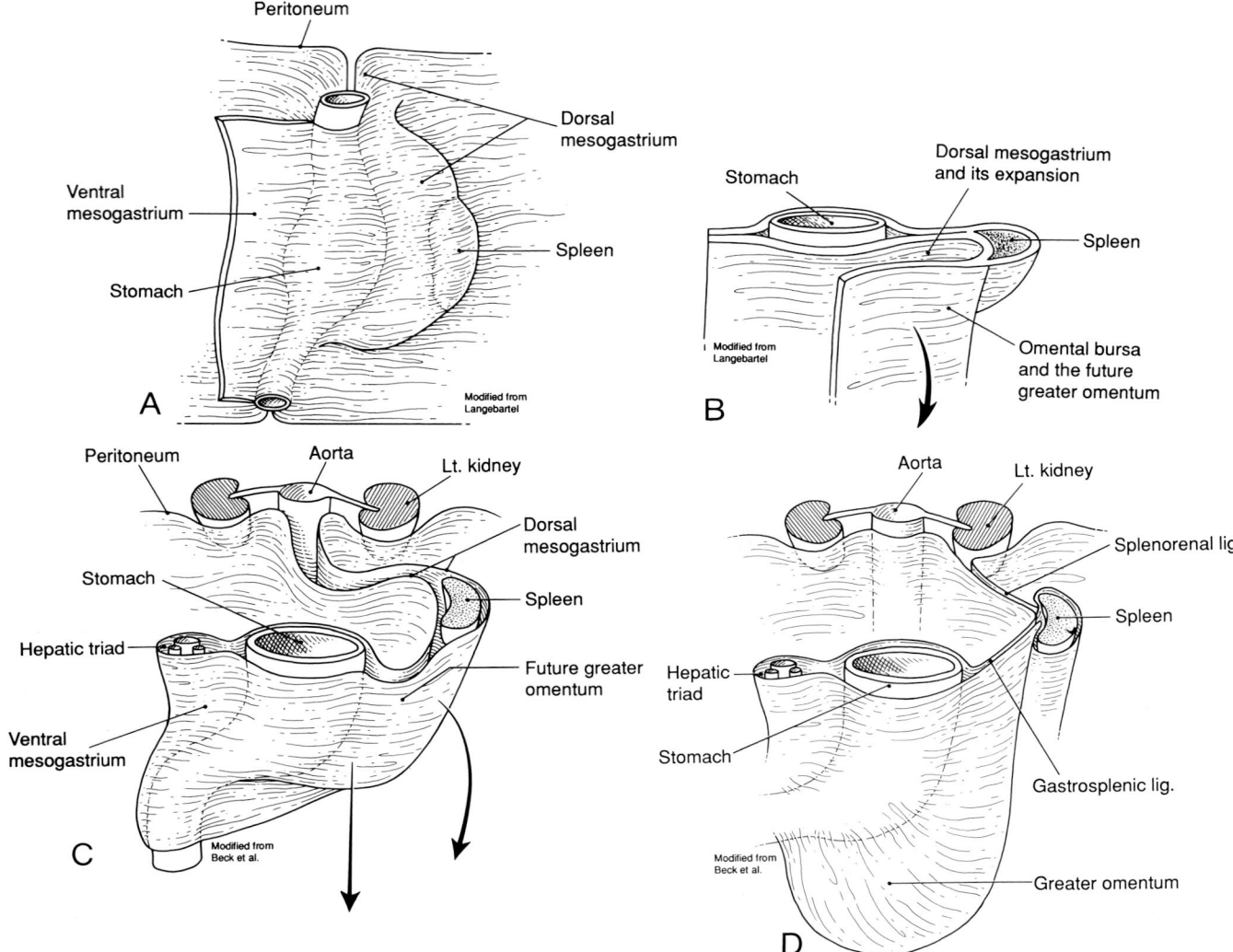

Figure 10.2. Brief summary of splenic development. **A,** Mesenchyme of the dorsal mesogastrium sixth week. The beginning of the splenic genesis. Invasion of lymphocytes into the splenic mass. **B,** Expansion of the dorsal mesogastrium. The omental bursa is formed and proceeds downward to form the greater omentum. **C,** Dorsal mesogastrium and its omental bursa keep the spleen in the left upper quadrant. **D** and **E,** The dorsal mesentery is fused to the posterior body wall and the genesis of the several splenic ligaments starts. (Reproduced with permission from Beck F, Moffat DB, Davies DP. Human embryology. London: Blackwell Scientific, 1985.)

spleen has longer T1 and T2 relaxation times than the liver or pancreas, and nuclear magnetic resonance imaging (NMRI) will not be useful for the diagnosis of splenic disorders such as metastasis or lymphoma. Boles (7) is correct when he stated that, whether the spleen is anatomically missing or functionally damaged or destroyed, trapping and destroying of bacteria and antibody production are impaired.

Malangoni and co-workers (8) reported that, after hemisplenectomies or subtotal splenectomies, the phagocytic function of the spleen correlates to the weight of the splenic remnant. These authors noticed that phagocytic function after autotransplantation remains reduced.

ACCESSORY SPLEENS

Anatomy

Accessory spleens are small nodules of splenic tissue that are present in addition to a normal spleen. The condition should be distinguished from polysplenia, in which the main spleen is divided into several roughly equal portions and which will be discussed later.

About 75% of accessory spleens are located at or near the hilus of the normal spleen, and about 20% are embedded in the tail of the pancreas. Others are distributed along the splenic artery, in the omentum, in the mesentery, or retroperitoneally. They are found occasionally in

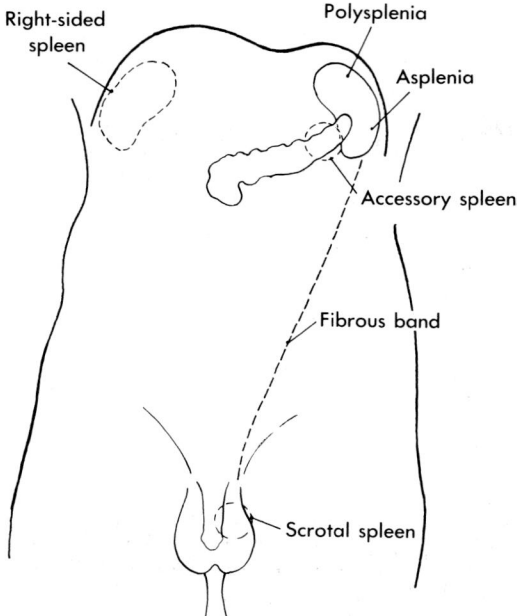

Figure 10.3. Sites of splenic anomalies.

Table 10.1.
Serious Malformations Associated with Anomalies of the Spleen

Splenic Anomaly	Associated Malformations
Absence of spleen (asplenia syndrome)	Partial situs inversus Severe cardiac anomalies Mesenteric defects Spina bifida
Right-sided spleen	Kartagener's triad: total situs inversus, bronchiectasis, malformed paranasal sinuses
Multiple spleens (polysplenia syndrome)	Partial situs inversus Severe cardiac anomalies
Splenogonadal fusion	Ectromelia Micrognathia

Table 10.2.
Anomalies of the Spleen

Anomalies per se	Asplenia Polysplenia Right-sided spleen Accessory spleen Splenogonadal fusion Splenic pregnancy

Anomalies or variations of spleen ligaments	Aplasia of ligaments
	Hypoplasia
	  Too short
	  Too narrow
	Hyperplasia (wandering)
	  Too long
	  Too wide

Anomalies or variations of spleen vessels	Arteries Veins Lymph nodes
Associated anomalies: the syndromes	Asplenia syndrome Polysplenia syndrome
Cysts and tumors	Congenital cysts and tumors
Hodgepodge inherited genetic disorders	Hereditary spherocytosis Hereditary elliptocytosis Idiopathic (immune) thrombocytopenic purpura Thalassemia Sickle cell anemia Gaucher's disease Idiopathic immune hemolytic anemia Nieman-Pick disease Thrombotic thrombocytopenic purpura Erythropoietic porphyria

Table 10.3.
Some Anomalies Associated with Asplenia and Polysplenia

Asplenia	Polysplenia
Pulmonary isomerism of right lung type	Pulmonary isomerism of left lung type
Absence of the spleen	Multiple spleens with total weight less than normal
Symmetric entry of the right and left superior venae cavae into the right and left atrial chambers, both of which have the anatomy of right atria	High frequency of interruption of the inferior vena cava with the inferior canal return via the azygos system
High frequency of extracardiac pulmonary venous connection	High frequency of symmetric partial anomalous pulmonary connection with the right pulmonary veins entering the right atrium

the scrotum. These bodies, which resemble lymph nodes covered with peritoneum, range from 0.2 to 10 cm and are usually about 1 cm in diameter. Retroperitoneal accessory spleen was reported by Miller et al. (9).

Accessory spleens rarely are found in more than two locations although there may be more than one accessory spleen at the hilus (10). Among 602 males with accessory spleens found at autopsy (11, 12), the following were found:

One accessory spleen	519 cases
Two accessory spleens	65 cases
Three accessory spleens	13 cases
Four accessory spleens	3 cases
Five accessory spleens	2 cases

Curtis and Movitz (10) found 10 accessory spleens in one patient.

Occasionally, hundreds of splenic nodules are found throughout the peritoneum and mesentery (splenosis) following traumatic rupture and removal of the spleen. These are the result of implantation of splenic tissue released into the peritoneal cavity by the rupture: The nodules are not true accessory spleens. The "splenoid" theory of von Stubenrach (13)—that the nodules arise from the development of undifferentiated tissue in situ under the stimulus of splenectomy—is not tenable.

Associated Anomalies

Even mild variations in splenic structure seem to be associated occasionally with cardiac malformation.

Embryogenesis

Accessory spleens result from a failure of separate splenic masses forming on the dorsal mesogastrium to fuse. The splenic ligaments may carry unfused masses to ectopic locations. Most are not separated far and are vascularized by branches of the splenic artery (14).

Incidence

Accessory spleen is one of the most frequently encountered anomalies in the body. Its reported incidence ranges from just over 10% (11) to 31% (10) of the population. Slightly more blacks seem to have accessory spleens than do whites. The gender ratio is unknown since almost all of the data has been obtained from male autopsies.

Symptoms

Cases of accessory spleen are nearly always asymptomatic. Brown and Dobbie (15) and Das Gupta and Busch (16) reported cases in which accessory spleens in the tail of the pancreas produced an indentation of the gastric fundus. In Das Gupta and Busch's patient, the main spleen had been removed previously and epigastric pain had been present for almost a year. The indentation produced a filling defect on radiography, which was diagnosed as a neoplasm.

Diagnosis

The diagnosis can be made only at surgery.

Clinical Implications

The accessory spleen usually shares in any pathologic changes that may occur in the main spleen. For example, in malaria, all splenic tissue is affected.

The accessory spleen also shares the function of the main spleen, and this must be considered when splenectomy for congenital hemolytic anemia or primary thrombocytic purpura is contemplated. Recurrence of the disease following splenectomy usually results from the presence of accessory spleens. Curtis and Movitz (10) reported such a recurrence in 17% of splenectomies for thrombocytic purpura.

Treatment

No treatment is required for uncomplicated accessory spleens. If splenectomy is performed for a hematologic disorder, the hilar region and the tail of the pancreas should be inspected for accessory splenic tissue, which should be removed along with the main spleen.

SPLENOGONADAL FUSION

Anatomy

The presence of splenic tissue in the left scrotum is one of the more bizarre ectopias in the body. The patient usually is convinced that he has three testicles, and the physician usually suspects a neoplasm.

The earliest description we have seen is that of Morgagni (XXXIX:42), who described a man with a large spleen in the groin. The spleen appeared to be "connected to the stomach by a kind of rope which lay hid under a part of the intestines, being two inches in thickness, made up of sanguiniferous vessels, and contained in a thickish coat like a capsula."

Successful removal of ectopic splenic tissue was not reported until 1952 (17). A complete review with abstracts of earlier cases was undertaken in 1956 by Putschar and Manion (18), and 39 cases were reported in the literature by 1961. Several more have since been reported (19).

In 1985 Gouw et al. (20) presented their own case and reviewed 84 reported cases.

Two varieties of the anomaly are recognized. In one a band of tissue connects the normally located spleen with the testis, epididymis, ovary, or mesovarium. The band may be splenic tissue or it may be fibrous with splenic nodules at more or less frequent intervals along it. Forty-seven of the reported cases were of this type. In the second type there is no band between the normal and ectopic splenic organs; 33 of the cases were of this type.

Gouw et al. (20) stated that only 6 of the 84 cases were females. Figure 10.4 represents the gender distribution among the two types of splenogonadal fusion. For the distribution of continuous and discontinuous types, see Figure 10.5.

Associated Anomalies

Gouw et al. (20) presented the congenital anomalies associated with splenogonadal fusion in the form of a table (Table 10.4).

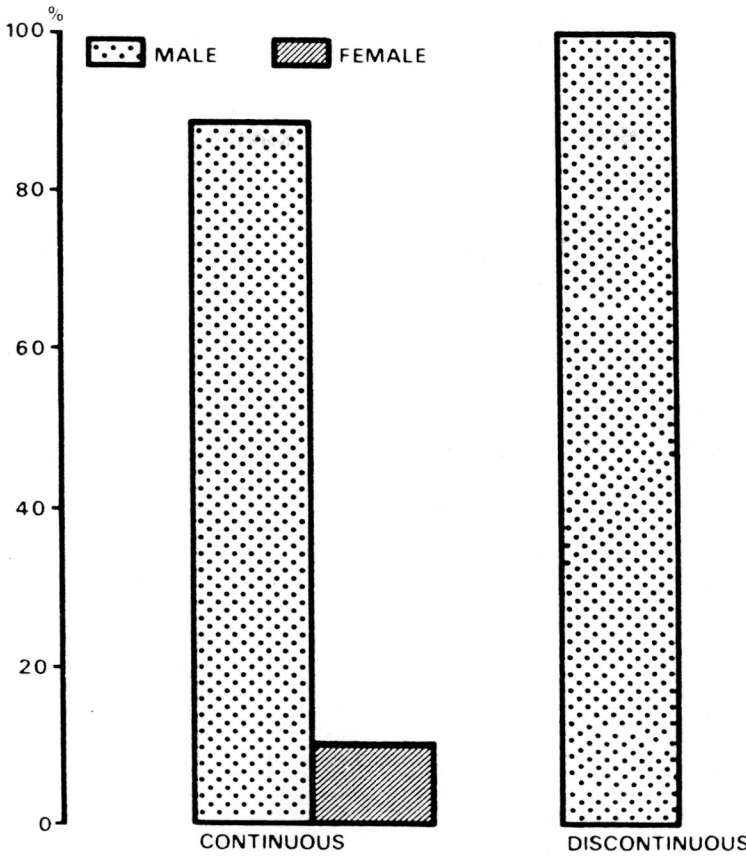

Figure 10.4. Percentages of males and females among patients with continuous and discontinuous types of splenogonadal fusion. (Reprinted with permission from Gouw ASH, Elema JD, Bink-Boelkens MTHE, deJongh HJ, ten Kate LP. The spectrum of splenogonadal fusion: case report and review of 84 reported cases. Eur J Pediatr 1985;144:318.)

As rare as the condition is, it occasionally associates with two other rare defects: ectromelia and micrognathia. In Pommer's reported case (21), all four limbs were absent, the mandible was reduced, and the anus was imperforate. In three other cases micrognathia alone was present. Only two of these patients with ectromelia survived infancy (22). In a number of cases descent of the left testis is incomplete, especially among those patients in whom bands connect the normal and ectopic spleens (Fig. 10.6).

Embryogenesis

Adherence of the splenic primordium to structures derived from the mesonephric ridge must occur near the end of the seventh or the beginning of the eighth week. Later than this, the spleen is not in contact with the mesonephric ridge. Descent of the testis seems to draw out the developing spleen into a long band in some cases and to detach a portion of the splenic primordium and carry it down with the testis in others. Willis (23) mentions the possibility that a portion of the mesonephric tissue may be induced to form spleen, but this seems improbable. In only one case (17) was there any intermingling of splenic and testicular tissue.

The coincidental occurrence of defective appendages supports the suggested timing of the defect late in the seventh week.

Abnormalities within chromosomes are most likely not responsible for this anomaly since studies have reported normal chromosomes in such cases. No familial tendency has been reported.

The cause of splenogonadal fusion–peromelia syndrome is not known. McKusick (24) believes the splenogonadal fusion with peromelia is an autosomal dominant disorder.

Symptoms

Scrotal pain, tenderness, and swelling are the usual complaints, but the mass may be entirely painless (25, 26). Pain with strenuous exercise and swelling in response to

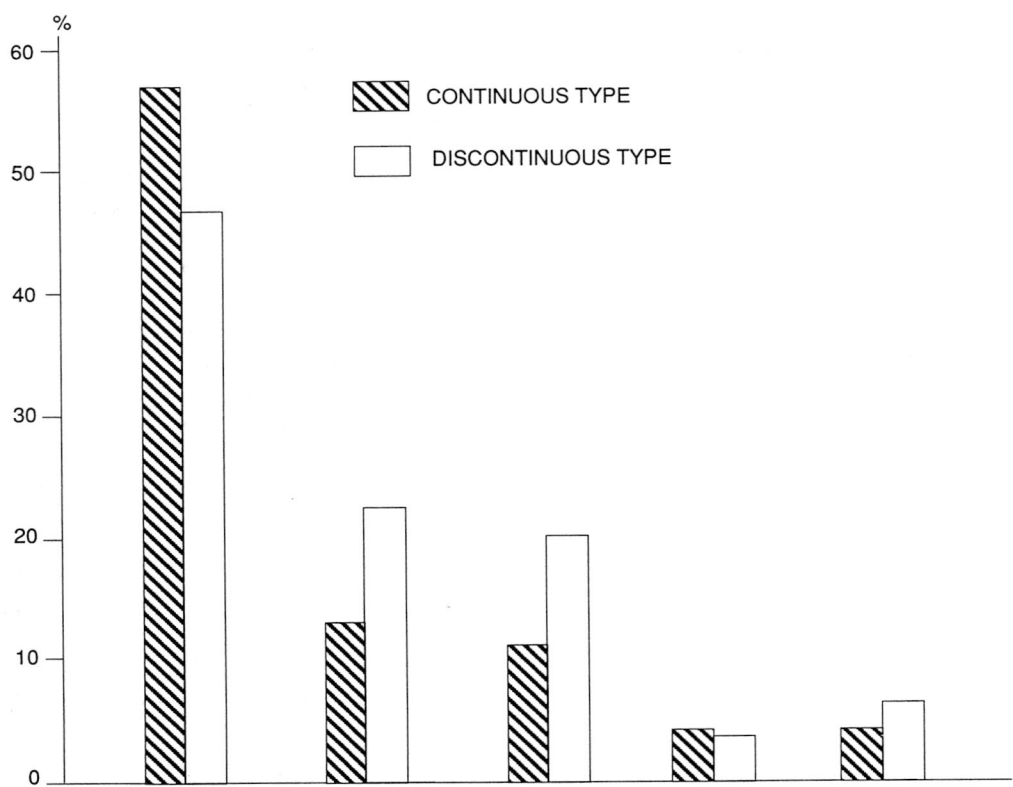

Figure 10.5.   Age distribution at detection in percentages of male and female patients with continuous and discontinuous types of splenogonadal fusion.   (Reprinted with permission from Gouw et al. The spectrum of splenogonadal fusion: case report and review of 84 cases. Eur J Pediatr 1985;144:318.)

systemic infections have both been reported. Daniel (27) describes a typical case in an adult.

Hines and Eggum (22) reported a patient in whom the connecting band caused obstruction of the transverse colon near the splenic flexure. The patient was 15 years old, and the obstruction had existed for only a week. Resection of the band relieved the obstruction. This patient is the only one with ectromelia known to have survived childhood (Fig. 10.7).

According to Gouw et al. (20), the patient with splenogonadal fusion has all the symptoms of an inguinal hernia, plus a left scrotal mass that is sometimes painless. However, in the discontinuous type there is pain in 78% of the cases and in the continuous type, in 13%.

Inguinal hernia or cryptorchidism were the symptoms in 30% of cases of the continuous type and in 12% of the discontinuous type.

Diagnosis

The splenic tissue usually is found at surgery for hernia or undescended testes or at postmortem. Preoperative diagnosis has rarely been reported, although there would be little difficulty in recognizing it were the condition not so rare (Fig. 10.8). Incredibly, Jayne and Jessiman (28) reported a patient who had two scrotal operations performed for pain and swelling, without his true condition being recognized. When peromelia is present, the doctor should consider the possibility of this syndrome.

Left scrotal mass is not only a herniation or hydrocele, therefore, a sonogram will be in order to discover the mass although not the rare splenogonadal fusion. Splenic scan will give the answer if there are indications or thoughts about such an anomaly.

Remember, there has been accidental discovery at autopsy in 38% of the continuous type and in 3% of the discontinuous type.

Treatment

Treatment may consist in merely severing the obstructive band, as in Hines and Eggum's case (22), or in removal of the scrotal spleen. If the spleen is not under the tunica albuginea, the testis can be preserved (25). If splenic and testicular tissue are fused, the testis may have to be sac-

Table 10.4.
Congenital Malformations Present in 84 Cases of Splenogonadal Fusion

Type of Malformation	All Cases		Categorized According to Presence or Absence of Connective Cord						Categorized According to Presence or Absence of Peromelia			
			Continuous Type (N = 47)		Discontinuous Type (N = 33)		Unknown (N = 4)		With Peromelia (N = 17)		Without Peromelia (N = 67)	
	n	%	n	%	n	%	n	%	n	%	n	%
Defects of limbs	16	19	16	34	1	3	—	—	17	100	0	0
Micrognathia	7	8	6	13	1	3	—	—	5	30	2	3
Asymmetric skull	2	2	2	4	—	—	—	—	2	12	—	—
Craniosynostosis	1	1	2	4	—	—	—	—	—	—	1	2
Möbius syndrome	1	1	1	2	—	—	—	—	—	—	1	2
Hypertelorism	—	—	—	—	1	3	—	—	1	6	1	2
Cleft palate	1	1	1	2	—	—	—	—	1	6	1	2
Hypoplastic lungs	1	1	1	2	—	—	—	—	—	—	1	2
Four-lobed right lung	1	1	1	2	—	—	—	—	1	6	—	—
Abnormal fissuring of the lungs	1	1	1	2	—	—	—	—	1	6	—	—
Persistent ductus arteriosus (Botallo's duct)	1	1	—	—	1	3	—	—	—	—	1	2
Ventricular septal defect	1	1	—	—	1	3	—	—	—	—	1	2
Multiple cardiac malformations	1	1	2	4	—	—	—	—	2	12	—	—
Left diaphragmatic hernia	2	2	1	2	1	3	—	—	2	12	—	—
Partial situs inversus	1	1	1	2	—	—	—	—	1	6	—	—
Meckel's diverticulum	1	1	1	2	—	—	—	—	—	—	1	2
Bilobed spleen	4	5	4	9	—	—	—	—	3	18	1	2
Hepatolienal fusion	1	1	1	2	—	—	—	—	1	6	—	—
Abnormal fissuring of the spleen	1	1	1	2	—	—	—	—	—	—	1	2
Accessory spleen	1	1	1	2	—	—	—	—	—	—	1	2
Anal malformations	3	4	1	2	—	—	—	—	3	18	—	—
Adrenogonadal fusion	1	1	—	1	3	—	—	—	—	—	1	2
Hypoplastic adrenals	1	1	1	2	—	—	—	—	1	6	—	—
Hypospadias	1	1	1	2	—	—	—	—	—	—	1	2
Spinal malformations	3	4	3	6	—	—	—	—	3	18	—	—
Double uterus	1	1	—	—	—	—	1	25	—	—	1	2

rificed. In most cases, repair of a hernial sac also is required, but not intraabdominal removal of the cord (29).

The following observations are made with references to the literature on splenogonadal fusion.

1. It was unclear whether four cases were continuous or discontinuous.
2. All reported cases were on the left side of the body except one with right scrotal swelling (30).
3. Fusion of skin and right kidney was reported (31).
4. Fusion with testicle, epididymis, or sperm cord was reported.
5. Splenic mass has been found at the upper testicular pole of both continuous and discontinuous types under the tunica vaginalis.
6. Spleen mass was located under the tunica albuginea in four cases.
7. In three cases the spleen mass was fused with the left ovary and in another three cases, with the left adnexa.
8. Intraovarian occurence of two nodules was reported by von Hochstetter (32).
9. Anaplastic seminoma in the fused testicle was reported by Falkowski and Carter (33).
10. Bilobed spleen was present in four cases.
11. Abnormal fissures were present in one case.
12. Accessory spleen was reported.
13. Hepatosplenic fusion was reported by Fritzsche (34).
14. The cord can be intraperitoneal, extraperitoneal, or combined.
15. Vascularization of the cord was from (a) left ovarian artery and nerves (32) and (b) spermatic and splenic arteries (35).
16. The cord may be fibrous but, in most cases, is continuous or interrupted normal splenic tissue.
17. The male/female ratio is 13:1 (36) (or perhaps 4:1) since discovery in males is easier than in females.
18. One-half of both types of reported cases are discovered during childhood.
19. Twenty-five percent of all continuous-type patients and only 5% of the discontinuous-type group were less than 1 year of age when the fusion was discovered.
20. Other congenital defects were found in 48% of the continuous-type cases and 9% of the discontinuous-type cases.

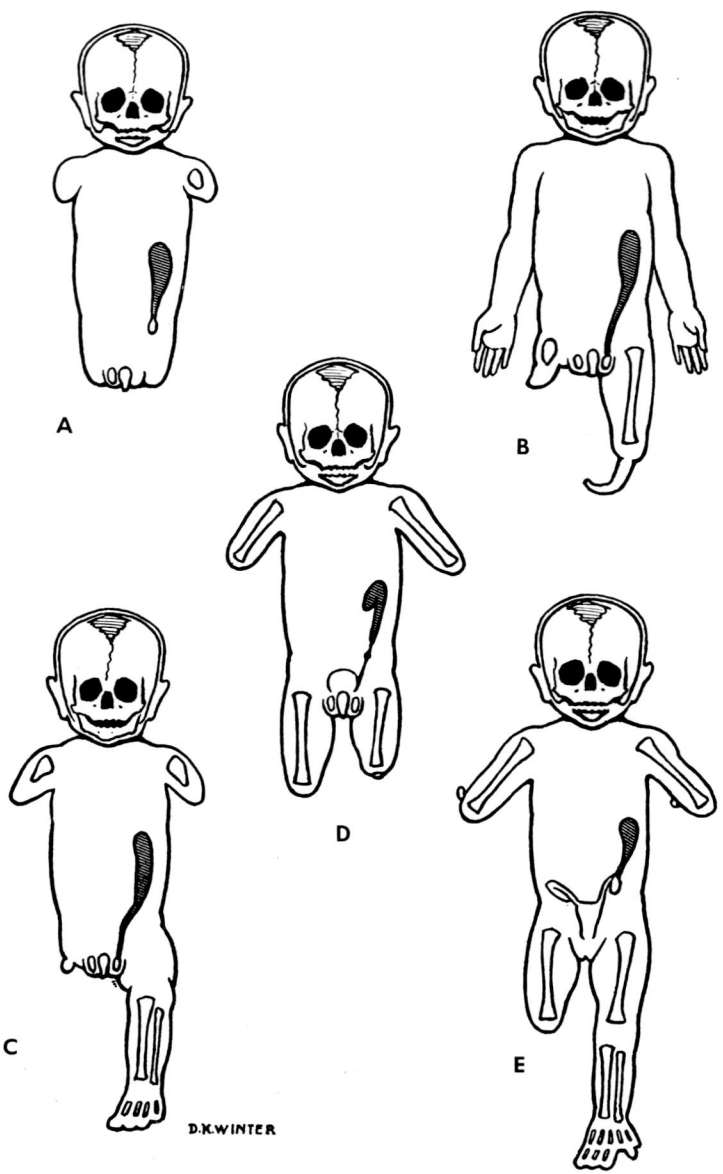

Figure 10.6. Splenogonadal fusion. Five cases with varying degrees of associated ectromelia. In **A**, **D**, and **E**, micrognathia was also present. The condition may occur in females **(E)**. (From Putschar WGJ, Manion WC. Congenital absence of the spleen and associated anomalies. Am J Clin Pathol 1956;26:429–470.)

21. A painless scrotal half was found in 78% of discontinuous and 13% of continuous cases.
22. Inguinal hernia or cryptorchism were the symptoms in 33% of continuous and in 12% of discontinuous types.
23. In 38% of continuous and 3% of discontinuous types, the condition was incidentally discovered during autopsy.
24. Of all reported cases, 33% were associated with one or more congenital anomalies. Of the 26 patients with associated malformations, 22 were of the continuous type, 3 were of the discontinuous type, and 1 case was unclear. In other words, 48% of all continuous types are associated with one or more defects, and only 9% of the discontinued type have other defects.
25. Limb defects are noted in the continuous type.
26. A continuous type fusion carries approximately a five times greater risk of associated congenital anomalies than does a discontinuous type.

Gouw et al. (20) had the following to say about splenogonal fusion:

As for the type of malformation, limb defects predominate, especially in the continuous type. They vary from a total absence of limbs to absence of parts of the lower limbs. Defects of the upper limbs unaccompanied by defects of the lower ones have not been reported. Six of the seven cases with micrognathia were found within the continuous group. Anal malformations, vertebral malformations, diphragmati-

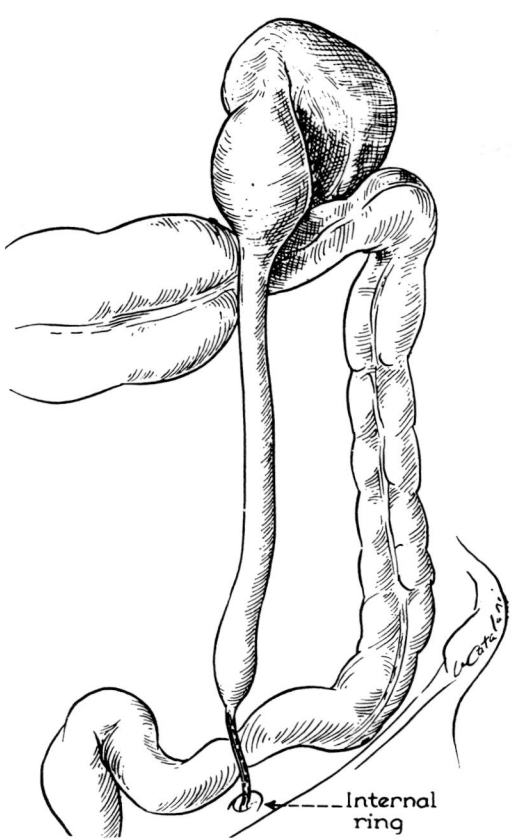

Figure 10.7. Splenogonadal fusion in a 15-year-old boy with ectromelia. The elongated spleen, connected with the testis, caused obstruction of the transverse colon near the splenic flexure. (From Hines JR, Eggum PR. Splenic gonadal fusion causing bowel obstruction. Arch Surg 1961;83:109–111.)

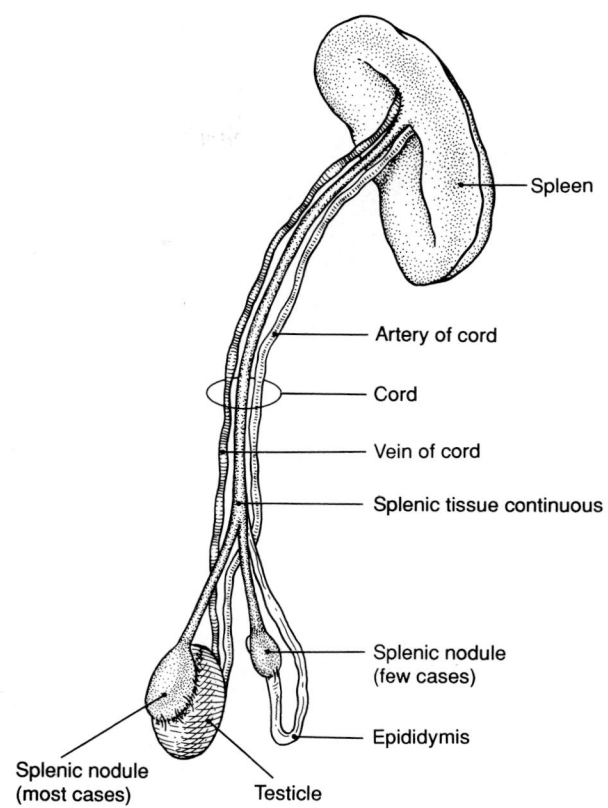

Figure 10.8. Highly diagramatic drawing of splenogonadal fusion.

cal hernia, and asymmetric skull have all been reported more than once.

The most remarkable difference between the peromelia and the non-peromelia group is the presence of other congenital defects. Of the cases in the peromelia group, 75% have at least one other congenital defect against only 15% of those without limb defects.

Splenic Pregnancy

Abdominal pregnancy is reported by Pagano (37) as 1:40,000 deliveries, by Beachman et al. (38) as 1:3000 pregnancies, and by Breen (39) as 1.4% of all ectopic pregnancies.

Abdominal pregnancies may be divided into two groups: (a) that primary group including normal tubes, normal ovaries, normal uterus, and pregnancy of less than 12 weeks and (b) that group including secondary early tubal rupture and implantation. Primary peritoneal pregnancy was studied by Studdiford (40) and Friedrich et al. (41).

Alcaly et al. (42) believes that primary splenic preg-

nancy is the rarest form of extrauterine pregnancy. There are fewer than 10 cases in the literature (43–45).

TOPOGRAPHY AND RELATIONS

The spleen is located in the left upper quadrant of the abdomen in a niche formed by the diaphragm above (posterolateral), the stomach medially (anteromedial), the left kidney and left adrenal gland posteriorly (posteromedial), the phrenologic ligament below, and the chest wall (ribs 9 to 11) externally (46).

The upper third of the spleen is related to the lower lobe of the left lung, the middle third to the left gastrophrenic sinus, and the lower third to the left pleura and gastral diaphragmatic origin (Fig. 10.9).

Skandalakis et al. (46) describe the spleen as follows.

Size

A spleen may be small or large. The extremes are 1 ounce (Storck) to 20 pounds (Schenck) as reported by Gould and Pyle (47). These extremes include both healthy and diseased spleens.

The size of the spleen may change readily, increasing with increases in blood pressure. The size increases after

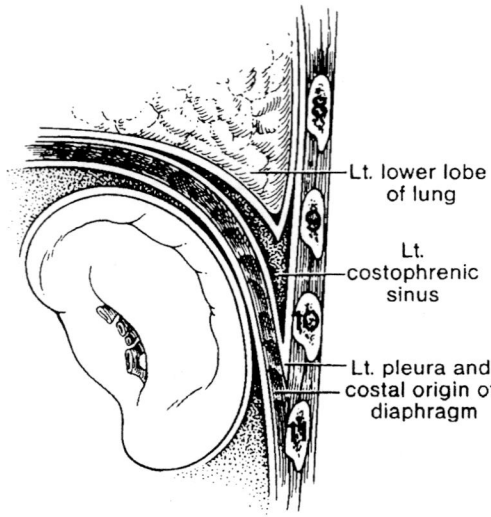

Figure 10.9.   Location of the spleen. (From Skandalakis JE et al. The surgical anatomy of the spleen. Probl Gen Surg 1990;7:1–17.)

meals. After exercise or immediately postmortem the spleen decreases in size. The lymphoid tissue of the spleen, like lymphoid tissue elsewhere in the body, undergoes diminution sometime after the patient reaches the age of 10 years (48). Sometime after he or she reaches the age of 60 years, there is some involution of the organ as a whole.

Harris's odd numbers 1, 3, 5, 7, 9, and 11, as reported by Last (49), are a good mnemonic device for remembering the average dimensions of the spleen: It measures 1 × 3 × 5 inches (2.5 × 7.5 × 12.5 cm) in size. It weighs 7 oz (20 g), and it relates to left ribs 9 through 11.

Shape

According to Michels (50), the spleen has three forms. It is wedge shaped in 44% of specimens, tetrahedral in 42%, and triangular in 14% (Fig. 10.10).

More useful is another topographic division used by Michels (50). These forms are a compact type with almost even borders and a narrow hilus in which the arterial branches are few and large (30%) and a distributed type with notched borders and a large hilus in which the arterial branches are small and numerous (70%) (Fig. 10.11). In an enlarged spleen, the notched anterior border, when present, may be palpated. Michels advises surgeons that spleens with a notched border have multiple arteries (more than two) entering the medial surface of the spleen. Polar arteries are common. A notched anterior border represents a difficult splenectomy.

Surfaces

For all practical purposes, the spleen has two surfaces—parietal and visceral. (Fig. 10.11). The convex parietal

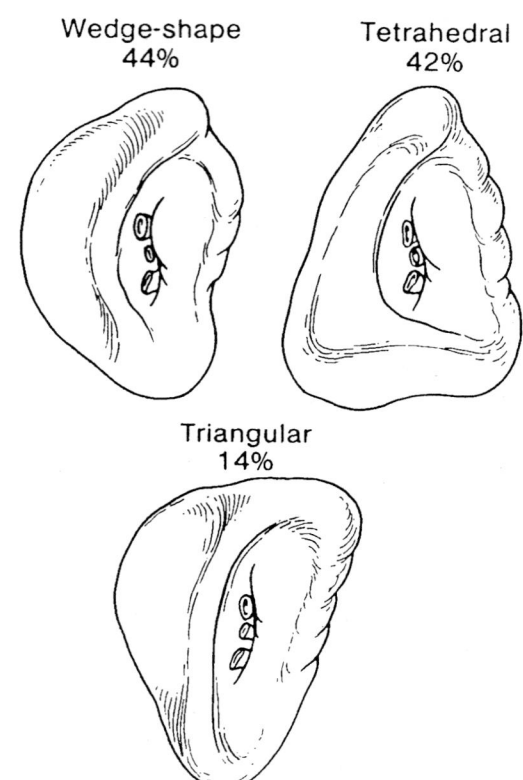

Figure 10.10.   Shapes of the spleen. (From Skandalakis JE et al. The surgical anatomy of the spleen. Probl Gen Surg 1990;7:1–17.)

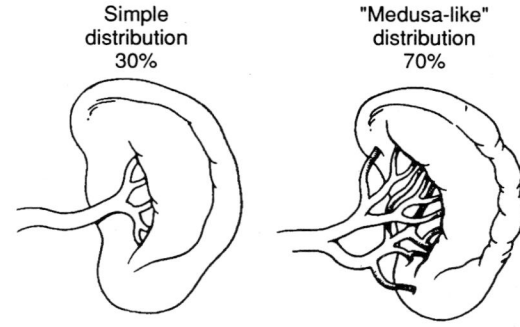

Figure 10.11.   Classification of spleen shape based on general arterial distribution. (From Skandalakis JE et al. The surgical anatomy of the spleen. Probl Gen Surg 1990;7:1–17.)

surface is related to the diaphragm, and the concave visceral surface is related to the stomach, kidney, colon, and tail of the pancreas (gastric, renal, colonic, and pancreatic). In this concave area, the entrance and exit of the splenic vessels at the splenic portae in most specimens form the letter S if one connects the upper polar, hilar, and lower polar vessels (Fig. 10.10).

Borders

The spleen has two borders—the superior or anterior and the inferior or posterior (Fig. 10.11). The superior border separates the gastric from the diaphragmatic area, and the inferior border separates the renal from the diaphragmatic area.

Segmental Anatomy

Corrosion casts of human splenic arterial trees revealed the presence of two splenic segments—a superior and an inferior—in 84% of specimens, and three segments—a superior, a middle, and an inferior—in 16% of specimens. These arterial segments are separated by avascular planes (51). The plane of separation of adjacent lobes passes transversely to the longitudinal axis of the spleen completely through the organ. The planes separating segments or subsegments are usually obliquely situated with respect to the long axis and often do not traverse the full thickness of the spleen from the visceral to the parietal surface (52). Garcia-Porrero and Lemes (53), using radiopaque injection media, found that anastomoses between splenic arterial branches, especially between secondary branches, occur in about 30.5% of specimens. In addition, they noted anastomoses of vessels supplying adjacent segments within the spleen in about 16.7% of specimens. This frequency of intrasplenic anastomoses was noted also by Mandarim-Lacerda et al. (54) in a study of 66 full-term newborn infants, in whom they also found an incidence of two lobar (segmental) branches in 68.2%, three branches in 10.6%, and four branches in 4.5%, from which the conclusion was drawn that segmental splenic resection is also possible in infants.

The separation of the spleen into lobes and segments by its arterial supply has been reported in a number of studies. Less well appreciated is the fact that the same segmental pattern can be observed, based on its venous drainage, in obvious keeping with the embryologic development of the organ, whereby the organ is formed by the fusion of vascularized, isolated mesenchymal aggregates. As reported by Dawson et al. (52) in a study of veins in unfixed, injected spleens, 71% had two lobes and 29% had three lobes. In half of the specimens, the lobes were further subdivided into two segments. The avascular lines of separation of the lobes followed those of the arteries. In more than half of the specimens, the lines of lobar separation could be equated to marginal notching of the splenic border. The veins were accessible at the hilus. Doubly injected (arterial and venous vessels) specimens confirmed that neither the arterial supply nor the venous supply to lobes or segments crossed to adjacent parenchyma. Earlier studies by Dryer and Budtz-Olsen (55) also reported apparent venous segmentation of the spleen.

Dixon et al. (56) stated that intrasplenic vessels are lobar, segmented, and generally without intersegmental communication (Fig. 10.13). They conceived the spleen as divided into three-dimensional cones with hilar, intermediate, and peripheral zones. Each zone requires a special technique for hemostasis. They advised conservative

treatment, such as with microfibrillar collagen for the peripheral zone (arteriole and venous injury) and hilar (segmental) ligation for the intermediate zone (trabecular vessels) (Fig. 10.14).

Peritoneum and Ligaments

The peritoneum covers the entire spleen in a double layer, except for the hilus (Figs. 10.15 and 10.16). The

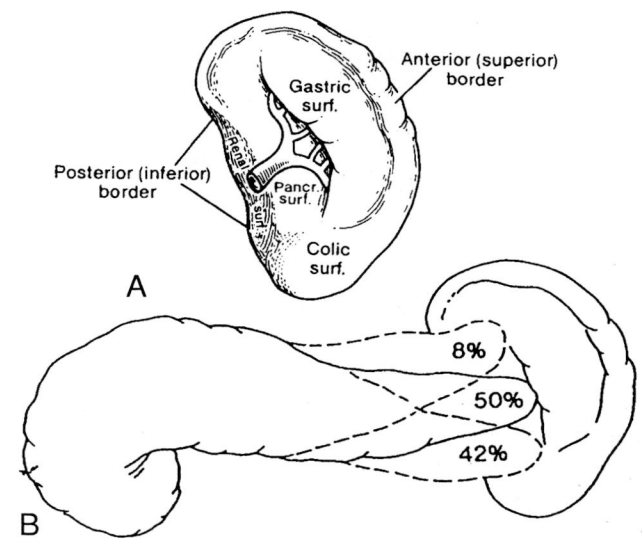

Figure 10.12. Splenic borders. **A,** Anterior and posterior borders. **B,** Relations of the tail of the pancreas to the spleen. (From Skandalakis JE et al. The surgical anatomy of the spleen. Probl Gen Surg 1990;7:1–17.)

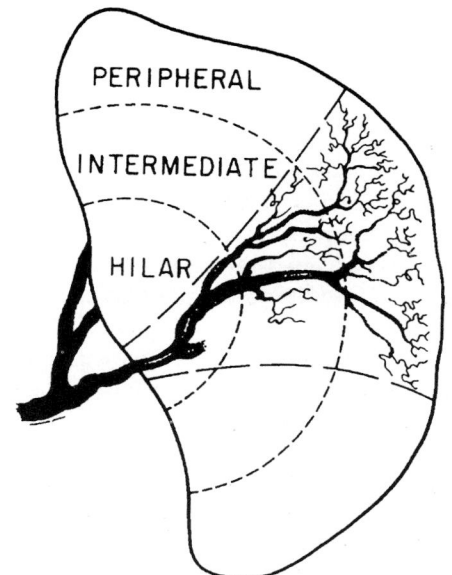

Figure 10.13. Regions indicated are shaped as a three-dimensional cone described by the length of a radius originating at the point of entrance of the major artery into the spleen. All regions contain penicilli, venules, and sinuses with the addition of larger vessels as the hilus is approached. (From Dixon JA, Miller F, McCloskey D, Siddoway J. Anatomy and techniques in segmental splenectomy. Surg Gynecol Obstet 1980;150:518.)

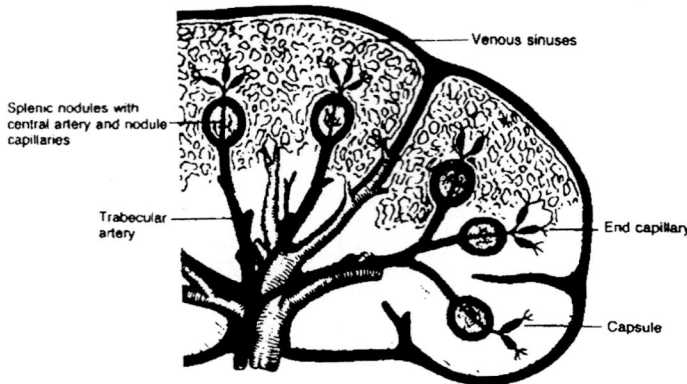

Figure 10.14. *Schematic representation of the human spleen. Arteries are in black; veins are cross-hatched. (From Bargmann W. Histologie und mikroskopische Anatomie des Menschen, 7th ed. Stuttgart: Thieme, 1977.)*

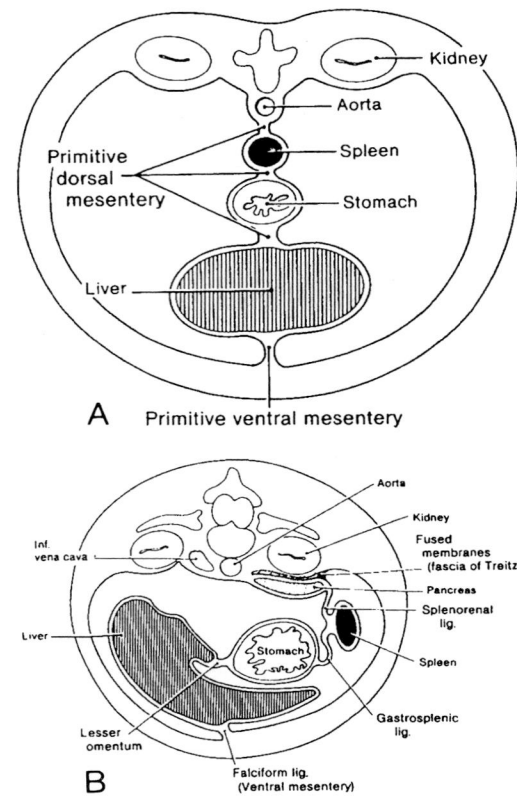

Figure 10.15. *The peritoneal reflections of the spleen are developed from the primitive dorsal mesentery. **A**, Diagram of primitive embryonic relations. **B**, Diagram of adult relations. (From Skandalakis JE, Gray SW, Rowe JS. Anatomical complications in general surgery. New York: McGraw-Hill, 1983.)*

two chief ligaments of the spleen are the gastrosplenic and the splenorenal. They are portions of the embryonic dorsal mesentery (mesogastrium, the leaves of which separate to surround the spleen) (Fig. 10.15, *B*).

At the hilus, the visceral peritoneum joins the right layer of the greater omentum and forms the gastrosplenic and the splenorenal ligaments. These two ligaments form the splenic pedicle. The capsule is formed by the visceral peritoneum, which is as friable as the spleen itself and as easily injured (Fig. 10.17).

In addition to the two chief ligaments, there are several minor splenic ligaments; their names indicate their connections (Fig. 10.18). They are the splenophrenic ligament, splenocolic ligament, pancreaticosplenic ligament, presplenic fold, phrenocolic ligament, and pancreaticocolic ligament (Figs. 10.19 to 10.21).

SPLENIC LIGAMENTS

There are eight ligaments in the associated splenic area. Six associate directly: gastrosplenic, splenophrenic, splenorenal, splenopancreatic, splenocolic, and presplenic fold. Two are in the vicinity but associate with the organ in an indirect way: pancreaticocolic and colophrenic.

The splenic ligaments are subject to variations, and can be normal, too long, too wide, too narrow, too short, or absent. The embryologist, anatomist, radiologist, pediatric surgeon, and general surgeon should be familiar with all of them. The pediatric surgeon should be especially careful since all of the ligaments except the splenogastric and splenorenal are minute and not well developed in early infancy.

Embryology

Embryologically, the splenic ligaments develop from the dorsal mesentery (mesogastrium). For all practical pur-

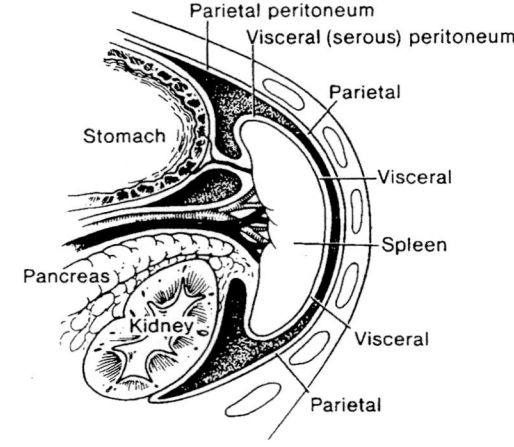

Figure 10.16. *Sagittal view of peritoneum covering the spleen. (From Skandalakis JE et al. The surgical anatomy of the spleen. Probl Gen Surg 1990;7:1–17.)*

poses, these ligaments belong to the omentum, mesenteries, and peritoneum. They form folds that sometimes are too long, sometimes absent or too short, and sometimes present but abnormally fused.

In the operating room, remember the possibility of the following: the ptotic or ectopic spleen, splenic torsion, or an avulsed capsule with bleeding.

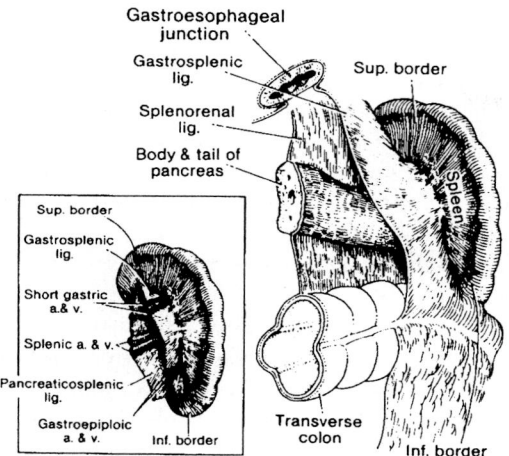

Figure 10.17. Peritoneal attachments of the spleen. *Inset:* The hilus of the spleen showing the short gastric and gastroepiploic vessels in the gastrosplenic ligament. (From Skandalakis JE, Gray SW, Rowe JS. Anatomical complications in general surgery. New York: McGraw-Hill, 1983.)

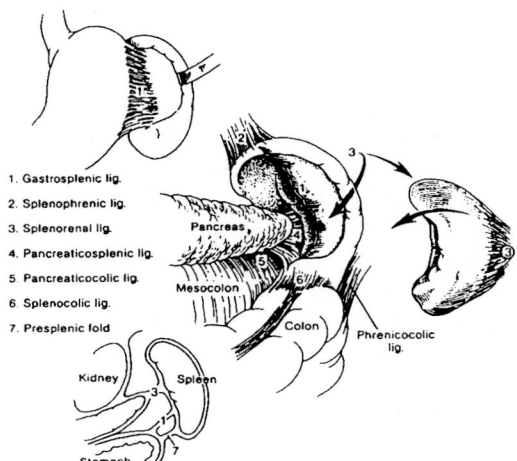

Figure 10.18. Minor splenic ligaments. (From Skandalakis JE et al. The surgical anatomy of the spleen. Probl Gen Surg 1990;7:1–17.)

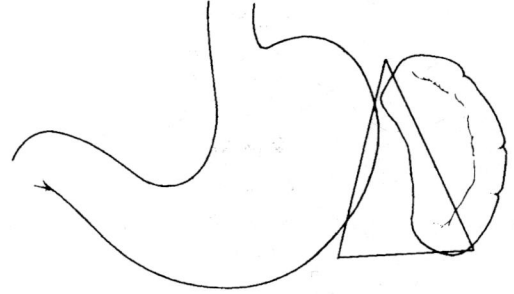

Figure 10.19. The gastrosplenic ligament connects the stomach and the spleen. The two organs may be in contact superiorly, and the ligament is short. Inferiorly, the two organs are 5 to 7 cm apart and the ligament is longer. (From Skandalakis JE, Gray SW, Rowe JS. Anatomical complications in general surgery. New York: McGraw-Hill, 1983.)

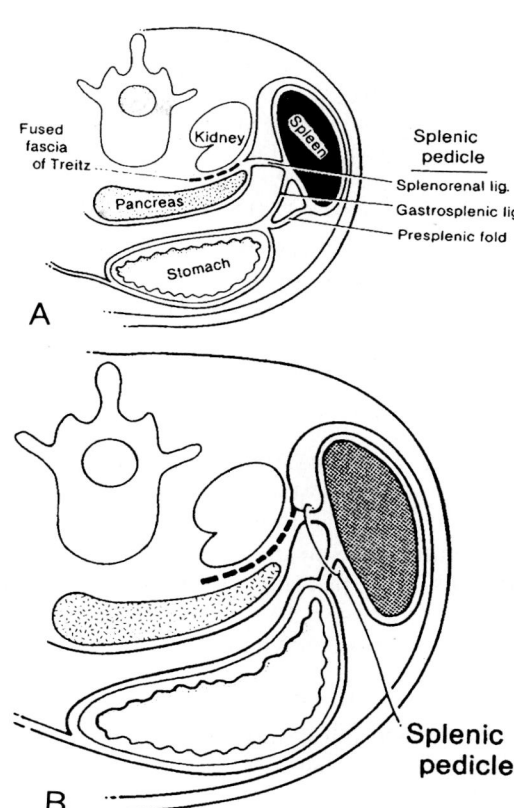

Figure 10.20. Splenic pedicle. **A,** Long pedicle with a presplenic fold. **B,** Short pedicle. (From Skandalakis JE, Gray SW, Rowe JS. Anatomical complications in general surgery. New York: McGraw-Hill, 1983.)

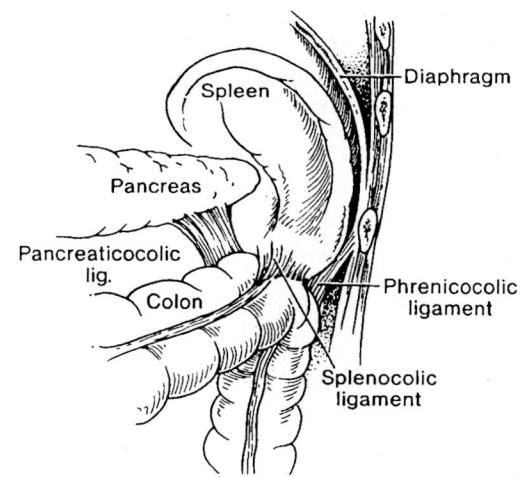

Figure 10.21. Relation of the pancreaticocolic, phrenicocolic, and splenocolic ligaments to the transverse mesocolon. (From Skandalakis JE et al. The surgical anatomy of the spleen. Probl Gen Surg 1990;7:1–17.)

We do not consider these to be embryological anomalies of the spleen per se, but omental anomalies with the above mentioned sequelae.

As we mentioned in a previous publication (46), there is a degree of ambiguity about the three "colic" liga-

ments: the pancreaticocolic, splenocolic, and phrenocolic. Do these peritoneal folds belong to the transverse
mesocolon? Most likely, the answer is yes, despite the Byzantine ambiguities that the omenta and peritoneal folds
present.

VARIATIONS OR ANOMALIES

We have seen all these variations in the laboratory from
time to time. However, we agree with Liebermann-Meffert and White (57) that omental anomalies—and therefore splenic ligament anomalies—have not been satisfactorily documented. We have seen the long, wide, narrow,
short, and absent ligaments of the spleen, but no clinical
or anatomic investigation, except of the wandering
spleen. When the splenic pedicle is narrow or wide, the
embryologic question of the absorption of the dorsal
mesentery arises, and sometimes the answer is unknown.
The investigator starts to speculate and hypothesize since
"reconstruction of the crime" is impossible. Despite our
tremendous progress, 65% of congenital anomalies in
humans are still of unknown origin.

GASTROSPLENIC LIGAMENT

The normal gastrosplenic ligament is a triangular area of
the dorsal mesentery between the greater curvature and
the medial border of the spleen. For all practical purposes, it is a left and upward continuation of the gastrocolic ligament. It is composed of anterior and posterior
leaves; the posterior leaf itself is nothing else but the anterior leaf of the splenorenal ligament.

At the apex (upper corner) of this triangle, the superior pole of the spleen lies close to the stomach, perhaps
fixed partially to it at the greater curvature or just at the
anterior or posterior gastric wall. The base of the triangle

has a length of 5 to 7 cm; therefore the lower pole of the
spleen is located away from the greater curvature. Since
this ligament contains the left gastroepiploic vessels at the
base and the short gastric vessel at the apex, it should be
incised between clamps or, preferably, cut after the vessels are ligated one by one. The surgeon should start this
approach by opening a window in the left avascular area
of the gastrocolic ligament and should proceed upward
between stomach and spleen by application of clamps
(Fig. 10.22).

Variations of Anomalies. The length of a ligament
depends on the number of short gastric vessels and the
topography or origin of the gastroepiploic vessels. A
great number of short gastric vessels require an upward
reaching of the ligament, and a low origin of the gastroepiploic vessels a downward extension toward the left
part of the gastrocolic ligament.

The opposite constitutes a short ligament. A narrow
one will bring the spleen closer to the stomach, and for all
practical purposes, the medial border of the spleen and
the lower pole are fixed to the greater curvature of the
stomach. Rarely is the spleen fixed or fused with the
greater curvature because of absence of the gastrosplenic
ligament.

If the upper pole of the spleen is away from the stomach, the medial border is away from the greater curvature
of the stomach, and the distance approaches the length
of the base of the triangle (approximately 5 to 7 cm or
more), then the gastric splenic ligament is too wide. From
time to time we have observed these anomalies in the laboratory as well as in the operating room. .

Perhaps, since the upper pole of the spleen normally is
near the medial plane (like the upper poles of the kidneys), we can call the line through the center of the upper

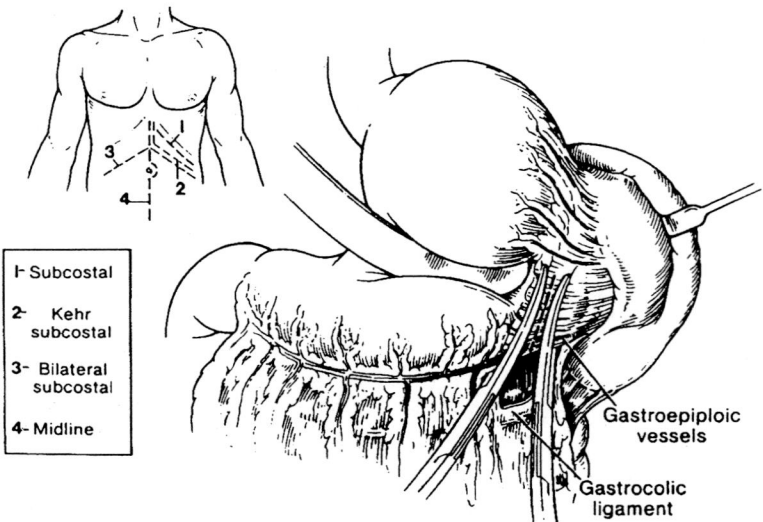

Figure 10.22.   Incision for total splenectomy by the anterior approach and access to the lesser sac. (From Pemberton LB, Skandalakis LJ. Indications for and technique of total splenectomy. Probl Gen Surg 1990;7:85–102.)

and lower pole the *splenic axis*. Perhaps, any deflection of the splenic axis suggests a ligamental anomaly or other problems in the left upper quadrant.

We believe that the width of the ligament depends on the length of the splenic vessels.

SPLENORENAL LIGAMENT

The splenorenal ligament is the posterior portion of the dorsal mesogastrium. The tail of the pancreas and the splenic vessels are enveloped between the two leaves of this avascular ligament. The outer layer of the splenorenal ligament forms the posterior layer of the gastrosplenic ligament.

The normal splenorenal ligament per se is a short ligament and occasionally is confused with the splenophrenic ligament, but we consider this ligament to be one of the principal ligaments of the spleen. It is this ligament that extends to form the splenophrenic ligament as well as the pancreaticosplenic ligament.

We think that Van Damme (58) is correct (anatomically and embryologically) to incorporate the splenic ligaments into one large structure which he calls the ligamentum splenium.

The spleen is an intraperitoneal organ covered practically in toto by peritoneum; it is fixed, however, with the peritoneum of the retroperitoneal space by these combined ligaments and especially by the splenorenal ligament.

The splenorenal and splenogastric ligaments form the splenic pedicle, which can be short or long, narrow or wide, depending on the length of the vessels as well as on the extent of dorsal mesogastrium absorption into the body wall.

Division of the splenorenal ligament will partially free the spleen, which may be held medially to be delivered outside of the peritoneal cavity. Again, remember that a short splenic artery may make it impossible to mobilize and deliver the spleen out of the abdomen.

The splenic pedicle must be handled carefully during splenic mobilization. Overenthusiastic finger and hand mobilization may produce venous or arterial bleeding from the short gastric vessels or other vessels from the pedicle.

SPLENOPHRENIC LIGAMENT

A ligament between the upper pole of the spleen close to the stomach and the inferior surface of the diaphragm, the splenophrenic ligament is an extension of the splenorenal ligament to the diaphragm and to the posterior body wall. We have seen long ligaments configured as follows: (*a*) attachment to the upper pole only; (*b*) attachment to the upper pole and anterior border; and (*c*) attachment to the upper pole and anterior border by two separated attachments.

Whitesall (59) found smooth muscle fibers in 80% of cases; in some specimens these were well developed and in others they were attenuated.

Careful traction of the spleen downward will help to appreciate the presence of this ligament, which may be divided by cautery or ligation.

On only one occasion, we observed a band from the lower splenic pole to the diaphragm in a virgin peritoneal cavity. We considered whether this was two splenophrenic ligaments—upper and lower—but it is unwise to suggest such a thing based on only one observation.

SPLENOPANCREATIC LIGAMENT

This ligament is also related to the splenorenal ligament and exists only when the tail of the pancreas does not reach the spleen. Since the location of the tail of the pancreas is not always the same (Fig. 10.18), the ligament, if any, may be related to the upper, middle, or lower splenic portas.

PANCREATICOCOLIC LIGAMENT

This ligament is the upper extension of the transverse mesocolon (Fig. 10.18).

SPLENOCOLIC LIGAMENT

The splenocolic ligament is the remnant of the extreme left end of the transverse mesocolon (Fig 10.18). Occasionally, this ligament may contain vessels such as the left gastroepiploic or perhaps aberrant inferior polar vessels. Because of this, incision of the ligament between clamps is mandatory.

PRESPLENIC FOLD

The presplenic fold is a peritoneal fold anterior to the gastrosplenic ligament (Fig. 10.18). Occasionally the presplenic fold contains the left gastroepiploic vessels. Henry (60) described this peculiar peritoneal fold in 1940, and Lord et al. (61) emphasized that it may be derived from the anterior limb of the inverted Y arrangement of some hili.

PHRENOCOLIC OR PHRENICOCOLIC LIGAMENT

In *Problems in General Surgery*, we (46) report on the phrenocolic ligament.

> The phrenocolic ligament (Fig. 10.18) develops at the region of junction of the midgut and the hindgut after the ascending colon and the descending colon become retroperitoneal. It is the rudimentary left end of the transverse mesocolon. Smooth-muscle cells migrate into the ligament from the mesocolic taeniae. The ligament fixes the splenic flexure in place. Moreover, the development of the upper abdominal organs results in a descent of the spleen and contact of the caudal pole of the spleen with the ligament. As the spleen

continues to grow, the phrenocolic ligament is deformed, forming a pocket for the spleen [62].

The phrenocolic ligament extends between the splenic flexure and the diaphragm. Although not a splenic ligament, the spleen rests upon it. While forming the "splenic floor," it is not connected to the spleen.

Only in pathologic conditions is the lower pole of the spleen fixed to the phrenocolic ligament.

Remember, the phrenocolic ligament acts as a barricade at the left gutter. In most instances it is responsible for prohibiting blood from a ruptured splenic artery or the spleen itself from traveling downward. Such blood collects at the anterior pararenal space retroperitoneally or around the spleen at the left upper quadrant by displacing the colon laterally. It is a mistake to call the phrenocolic ligament the left phrenocolic ligament because there is no right phrenocolic ligament.

This is the reason the right gutter forms a highway from the pelvis to liver, permitting an inflammatory pelvic process to communicate with the liver and right subdiaphragmatic spaces (Fitz-Hugh and Curtis syndrome, gonococcal perihepatitis). Perisplenitis with this syndrome, which is most likely secondary to liver involvement, may be present.

WANDERING SPLEEN

An unusual mobility of the spleen within the peritoneal cavity produces the wandering spleen, a clinical entity without symptoms. The spleen may be found anywhere in

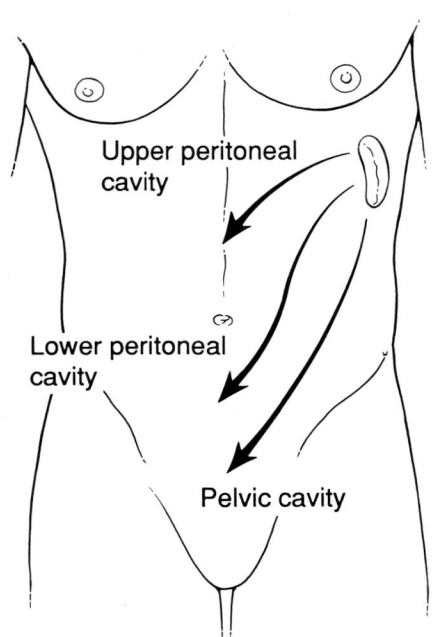

Figure 10.23.   Common sites of wandering spleen.

the peritoneal cavity except the right upper quadrant (Fig. 10.23).

Terminology

The literature has named the wandering system *displaced, ectopic, aberrant,* or *floating.* The designation "wandering spleen" is the best.

Incidence

In 1933 Abell (63) collected from the literature 97 cases of torsion of wandering spleen: 72 of them in women and, of them, 51 multiparous. In 1989 Allen and Andrews collected 35 cases (64) in children younger than 10 years of age (Table 10.5), with 63% predominance in boys. The youngest case was that of a 3-month-old girl.

Allen (65) offers the following observations about the wandering spleen.

Embryogenesis

The spleen, a mysterious and enigmatic organ, continues to give us embryological, anatomical, histological, physiological, and pathological problems.

The etiology of wandering spleen has been the topic of some debate. Considering the increased incidence in young multiparous females, abdominal laxity and the hormonal effects of pregnancy have been cited by some investigators as the cause of the anomaly (63). This theory does not, however, explain the condition in adult males, children, and nulliparous females. Splenomegaly has also been implicated; however, several investigators (66, 67) report no higher incidence of wandering spleen in populations of the world in which splenomegaly is endemic.

While the etiology may be multifactorial, the most compelling evidence points toward an error in the embryologic development of the spleen's primary supporting ligaments (Figs. 10.17 and 10.19). Embryologically, the splenic ligaments develop from the dorsal mesentery (mesogastrium) (Figs. 10.15, 10.20, 10.21, & 10.18) which is responsible for the formation of the peritoneum of the greater omentum and of the several peritoneal folds, but developmental anomalies or variations may take place. These ligaments may be normal or may be absent; they may be too long or too short and too wide or too narrow, and finally, they may be abnormally fused. When the splenic pedicle is narrow or wide, the question of the absorption or not of the dorsal mesentery arises.

Some of these anomalies do not have any clinical or surgical significance, but occasionally they can produce problems such as an abnormal mass secondary to a ptotic or ectopic spleen, an acute emergency (torsion of the

Table 10.5.
Pediatric Wandering Spleen (WS): Reports for Children Younger than 10 Years[a]

Author	Patient Age	Sex	Preoperative Diagnosis	Treatment
Southam	6 yr	M	Appendicitis	Splenectomy
Percy	10 yr	M	Appendicitis	Splenectomy
Motley	8 yr	M	Appendicitis	Splenectomy
Truesdale et al.	8 yr	F	Appendicitis	Splenectomy
DeBartolo et al.	4 yr	M	Appendicitis	Splenectomy
Shende	4 yr	F	Appendicitis	Splenectomy
Smevik et al.	1 yr	M	Torsion WS	Splenectomy
Zakaria	3 yr	M	Torsion WS	Splenectomy
Fried et al.	5 mo	M	Torsion WS	Splenectomy
Martin et al.	6 mo	M	Torsion WS	Splenectomy
Broker et al.	7 yr	M	Torsion WS	Splenectomy
Broker et al.	5 yr	M	Torsion WS	Splenectomy
Carswell	8 yr	F	Torsion WS	Splenectomy
Carswell	7 yr	M	Torsion WS	Splenectomy
Muckmel et al.	5 yr	F	Acute abdomen	Splenectomy
Carswell	5 yr	M	Acute abdomen	Splenectomy
Stringel et al.	9 yr	F	Acute abdomen	Splenectomy
Lau et al.	2 yr	F	Acute abdomen	Splenectomy
Thompson et al.	7 yr	M	WS	Observation
Gordon et al.	6 mo	M	WS	Observation
Gordon et al.	2 yr	M	WS	Observation
Barnett et al.	3 yr	F	WS	Observation
Carswell	8 yr	M	WS	Splenectomy
Carswell	7 yr	F	WS	Splenectomy
Bellmaine	3 yr	F	WS	Splenectomy
Bellmaine	2 yr	M	WS	Splenectomy
Allen et al.	6 yr	F	WS	Splenopexy
Thompson et al.	3 mo	F	WS	Splenopexy
Carswell	8 yr	M	WS	Splenopexy
van der Staak et al.	5 yr	F	WS	Splenopexy
Stringel et al.	6 mo	M	Abdominal mass	Splenopexy
Carswell	6 yr	M	Abdominal mass	Splenectomy
Pearson	1 yr	M	Abdominal mass	Splenectomy
Hall	10 yr	F	Abdominal mass	Splenectomy
Colin	2 yr	M	Abdominal mass	Splenectomy

[a]From Allen KB. Wandering spleen. Probl Gen Surg 1990;7:122–127.

spleen), or bleeding in the operating room by avulsion of the splenic capsule producing bleeding.

We agree with Waldschmidt (68) that omental anomalies—and therefore splenic ligament anomalies—have not been satisfactorily documented.

As previously stated there are six ligaments (gastrosplenic, splenorenal, splenophrenic, splenocolic, splenopancreatic, and presplenic fold) directly associated with the spleen and two others (pancreaticocolic and colophrenic) indirectly associated. Most of the literature holds the gastrosplenic, splenorenal, and colophrenic [pocket-like splenic floor] ligaments responsible for ptosis of the spleen. However, the authors believe that, from an anatomical standpoint, the other ligaments, especially the splenocolic, also participate in the development of ptosis of the spleen.

In summary, the authors conclude that the fixation of the spleen to the left upper quadrant is most likely the synergistic work of these four ligaments, perhaps in conjunction with the other aforementioned ligaments.

Splenic Mobility

Splenic mobility is discussed by Skandalakis et al. (46).

The mobility of the spleen depends on the laxity of the splenic ligaments and of the splenic blood vessels. We believe that only four of the ligaments can affect the position of the spleen.

The strength of the gastrosplenic ligament depends on the mobility of the stomach. If the left kidney is fixed without other abnormalities, the splenorenal ligament may play a small role. It is well known to radiologists that the left transverse colon and splenic flexure are not displaced by renal tumors, and it is well known to clinicians that colonic resonance is present in that area. The strength of the splenocolic ligament depends on the mobility of the transverse colon and splenic flexure. A low splenic flexure contributes to mobility of the spleen. The phrenocolic ligament limits the downward movement of the spleen.

Adkins [69] stated that splenoptosis can be congenital or acquired. The congenital type is the result of a long splenic pedicle. The acquired type is a sequel to splenomegaly and a relaxed abdominal wall.

A question arises as to when ptosis becomes ectopia. Is ptosis a normal variation, or is ectopia a pathologic entity involving several organs secondary to a named pathologic condition? Radiologists [70] suggest that the following conditions affect abdominal organs: posture (gravity), respiratory movements, tonus of abdominal wall and diaphragm, degree of distention of viscera, tonus of the organ, intrinsic movements of viscera, and pressure of adjacent viscera. If one compares the liver with the spleen, one finds that hepatoptosis does not exist. The liver is fixed by the inferior vena cava and hepatic veins, the upper portae. The fixation of the spleen to the left upper quadrant is most likely synergistic from the action of several ligaments and not by any vascular presence [69].

Traveras [71] wrote that "the spine, aorta, and the vena cava are probably the only structures that do not shift with change in position of the body. From the viewpoint of the cephalic end of the subject, all of the movable organs rotate in a counterclockwise direction when the body is turned on its left side, and vice versa when it is turned on its right side. Gravity tends to displace movable structures towards the earth" [Fig. 10.24].

Therefore, incomplete fusion of the dorsal mesogastrium during development results in increased mobility of the spleen due to the absence of these important supporting structures (72–75).

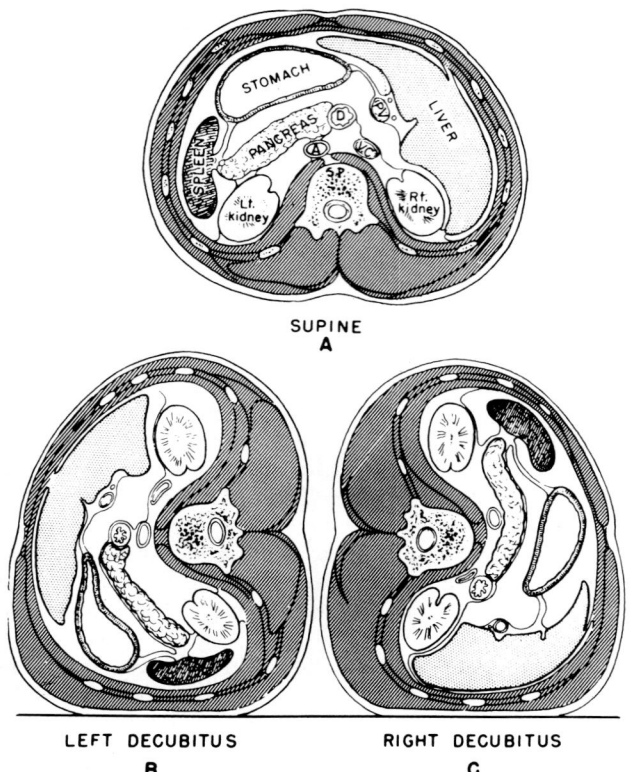

Figure 10.24. Schematic drawing of horizontal sections viewed from the head illustrates Tavera's concept of the mobility of organs caused by changes in position. **A,** With the patient in the supine position, the liver and spleen remain in a posterior position. **B,** With the patient in the left lateral decubitus position, the right kidney and descending duodenum drop forward and the left lobe of the liver extends anteriorly toward the stomach, causing a prominent indentation on the anterior surface of the stomach. **C,** With the patient in the right lateral decubitus position, the left kidney and spleen and tail of the pancreas extend forward. The descending duodenum drops laterally and posteriorly, effacing the inferior vena cava. The left lobe of the liver does not indent the anterior surface of the stomach as prominently as in the left decubitus position. (Reproduced with permission from Whalen JP. Radiology of the abdomen. Philadelphia: Lea & Febiger, 1976:101.)

Clinical Features

The clinical presentation of wandering spleen is variable (Table 10.6). Patients may be asymptomatic or have chronic vague complaints of lower abdominal and back pain. The most common presentation in children is an acute surgical abdomen secondary to splenic infarction from splenic pedicle torsion (64). Findings on physical examination that can suggest the diagnosis of wandering spleen include palpation of a firm ovoid mass with a notched edge, painful movement of the mass in any direction except towards the left upper quadrant, and resonance to percussion in the left upper quadrant. The nonspecific nature of the symptoms and the rarity of the condition makes preoperative diagnosis difficult.

Table 10.6.
Presentations of Wandering Spleen[a]

Presentation	Clinical Features
Asymptomatic	Found incidentally on physical or roentgenographic examination
Chronic	Recurrent abdominal pain, occurring over months or years, due to episodes of spontaneous torsion and detorsion
Acute	Torsion, with splenic infarction, presenting as acute abdomen

[a]From Allen KB. Wandering spleen. Probl Gen Surg 1990;7:122–127.

Diagnosis

Multiple imaging modalities can suggest or confirm the diagnosis of wandering spleen. Roentgenographically, a wandering spleen can be demonstrated on the plain x-ray film of the abdomen, but typically the plain x-ray film only suggests the presence of an abdominal mass. The intravenous pyelogram and barium enema (BE) are usually normal but the BE can suggest extrinsic sigmoid colon compression from an ectopic spleen (76).

Ultrasonography is reported by numerous investigators as the most reliable in diagnosing wandering spleen (77–82). An abdominal mass characterized as ectopic spleen and absence of splenic echos in the normally identifiable position confirms the diagnosis of wandering spleen. Furthermore, gray scale sonographic findings are specific even when vascular occlusion has occurred secondary to twisting of the splenic pedicle. Splenic infarction produces a complex sonographic mass with mixed echogenicity. Anechoic, cystic spaces may be present in association with areas of increased echogenicity. Doppler studies can confirm the presence of decreased or absent blood flow to the ectopic spleen. The noninvasive nature of ultrasound makes it particularly appealing in diagnosing this condition in the pediatric population.

Radionuclide imaging compliments ultrasonography in confirming the diagnosis of wandering spleen. The absence of splenic uptake, however, has been reported in patients who were subsequently diagnosed with torsion of a wandering spleen (77, 83). Furthermore, failure to visualize the spleen by isotopic scanning is nonspecific since there are a number of causes of acquired asplenia (84).

Angiography also is capable of demonstrating an ectopic spleen (76, 83, 85, 86). However, angiography, like isotopic scanning, relies on an intact vascular pedicle. Furthermore, its invasive nature makes it less attractive considering the availability of noninvasive diagnostic tools such as ultrasound.

CT and MRI offer valuable diagnostic aids if ultrasonography fails to make the diagnosis. CT also has the advantage of being able to determine if the pancreatic tail is involved in the pedicle of the ectopic spleen (79). Their routine use, however, is not needed to establish the diagnosis.

Treatment

In past years, splenectomy was the standard recommended treatment for wandering spleen with or without the presence of torsion. However, the increasing knowledge of the spleen's role in the reticuloendothelial system makes the casual, unnecessary removal of the noninfarcted wandering spleen, particularly in children, unwarranted. Several investigators advocate conservative watchful management when the diagnosis of wandering spleen is made in the asymptomatic child (73, 77, 81, 86). However, two-thirds of children are completely asymptomatic prior to their emergent presentation (64). Since 66% of acute cases are without symptoms prior to their abdominal catastrophe, watchful management in the asymptomatic patient is not indicated. Splenopexy is the treatment of choice.

Elective splenopexy is recommended, even in the asymptomatic patient, because of the high incidence of splenic torsion and the increased risk of trauma to an unprotected abnormally located spleen.

An embryologic anomaly—absence or laxity of some of the ligaments or failure of fusion of the mesogastrium—likely accounts for the increased mobility of the spleen. Thus the question still remains about the etiology of this clinical entity. Although based on speculation, at the present time we must accept that a congenital error is the cause of the wandering spleen since concrete reconstruction of the etiology to prove the embryological and anatomical causes is impossible. Hypothesis is in order. We recommend splenopexy in children even if the spleen is infarcted.

The interested student will find useful information in the papers of Buehner and Baker (87) and Allen and colleagues (88).

SPLENIC ARTERIES AND VEINS (FIG. 10.25)

Origin of the Splenic Artery

Vandamme and Bonte (89) reported that the splenic artery arose as one of the three main branches of the celiac trunk in 86% of their specimens.

> One of these three main celiac branches may have a separate origin, leaving a gastrosplenic trunk (6%), hepatosplenic trunk (6%), or hepatogastric trunk (none in our specimens). In an extreme arrangement, there is no celiac trunk at all because the three main branches have a separate origin [Fig. 10.26].
>
> The diameter of the splenic artery and vein were measured at the left paravertebral line on arteriograms in vivo by Haertel and Beusch [90]. The splenic artery measured 6 mm (range: 4 to 8 mm), and the splenic vein measured 10 mm (range: 7 to 13 mm). These measurements are to be reduced by 15% to 20% for roentgenographic magnification.

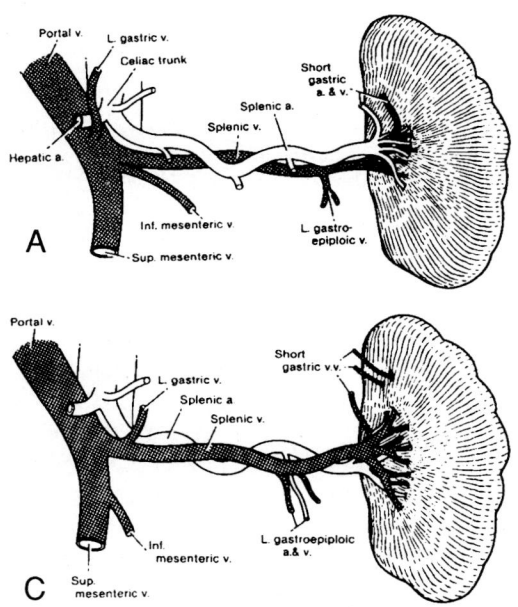
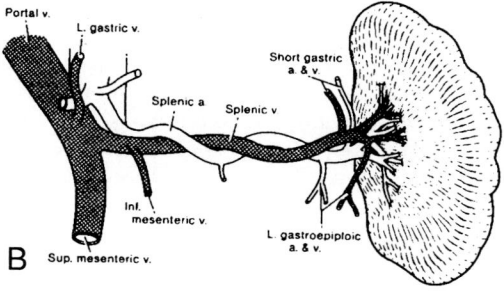

Figure 10.25. Relation of splenic artery and splenic vein. **A**, Artery anterior to vein (this is the usual pattern). **B**, Artery both anterior and posterior to vein. **C**, Artery posterior to vein (this is the least common configuration). (From Skandalakis JE, Gray SW, Rowe JS. Anatomical complications in general surgery. New York: McGraw-Hill, 1983.)

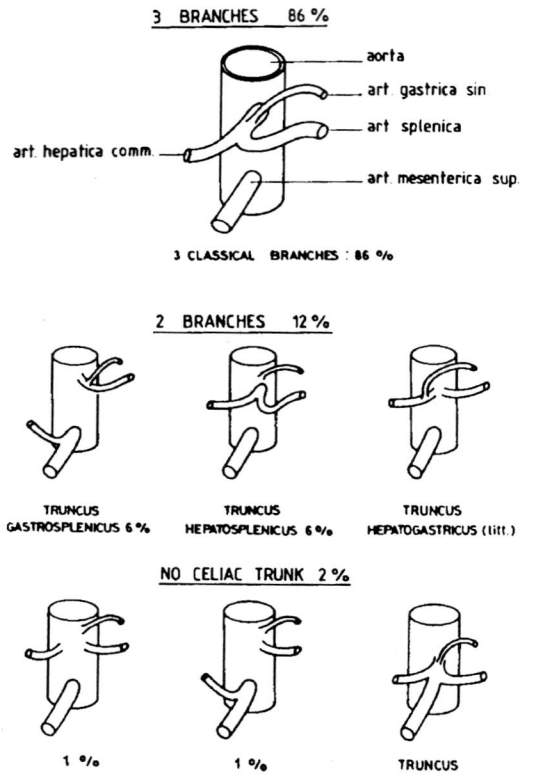

Figure 10.26. The celiac trunk and its branches. (Reproduced with permission from Van Damme J-P, Bonte MD. Arteria splenica and the blood supply of the spleen. Probl Gen Surg 1990;7:18–27.)

Course of the Splenic Artery

In adults the diameter of the splenic artery exceeds that of the hepatic artery, and the vessel usually becomes tortuous with age, although this relation to age is not as absolute as was suggested by Rossi and Cova [91]. Loss of this tortuosity on arteriograms is often an important sign of abnormalities in this area.

We follow the text from Skandalakis et al. (46):

Waizer et al. [92] reported that in 9 of 26 cadavers, the splenic artery, as soon as it emerged from the celiac artery, made a loop to the right, appearing at the border of the lesser omentum, therefore being vulnerable to iatrogenic injury during procedures on supracolic organs.

On its way to the spleen the splenic artery forms the splenic peritoneal fold and then ends in the splenorenal ligament, forming a peculiar tree, which is never the same, and reaches and enters the splenic porta.

Michels [14] found a superior polar artery 65% of the time and an inferior polar artery or arteries 82% of the time. He also called attention to the paradox of the large splenic artery supplying a relatively small organ, the

spleen, as contrasted to the narrower hepatic artery, which serves an organ five times larger.

We return to Vandamme and Bonte (89):

The division of the splenic artery [Figs. 10.27 and 10.28] is the key to the blood supply for the left hypochondrium. According to Michels [14], this division is so variable that no two are alike. . . . [We agree with Ssoson-Jaroschewitsch [93] who summarized the splenic branches well by dividing them into comb- and fan-shaped types.] Between both arrangements, several intermediate patterns are possible. The division takes place at an average of 2 to 6 cm from the hilum with extremes between 1 and 12 cm [94]. If the splenic branches arise early, there is a long pedicle, and secondary divisions take place well outside the spleen. This is the fan-shaped, horizontal Y, distributed type; it is the most frequent (70%) [14] and, fortunately for the surgeon, the most easy type for intrahilar dissections. If the splenic branches arise late, close to the spleen, the pedicle is short, like a horizontal T whose branches lie deep in the hilum. It is the condensed [95], comb-shaped type [93] found in 23% [95] to 30% [14] of specimens and that is less compliant for surgical dissection. Fortunately, the vascular arrangements within the splenic hilum are much simpler in children than in adults because secondary branches usually arise outside the splenic parenchyma [95]. The splenic artery divides into two (28% [96], 80% [14], 90% [95] of specimens), three (10% [95],

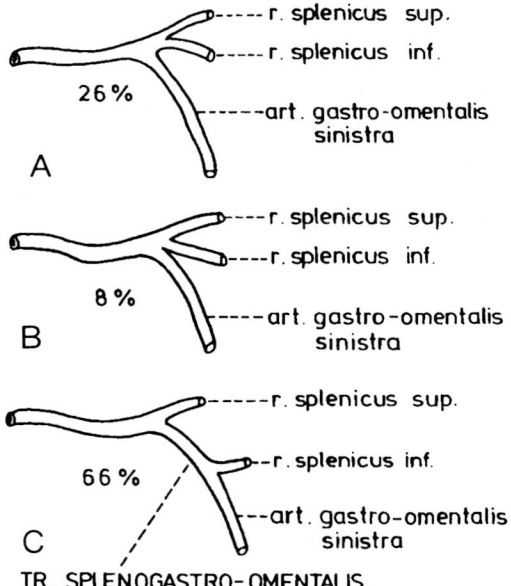

Figure 10.27. The division patterns of the splenic artery. **A**, The splenic artery divides into the two rami splenici; the left gastroomental artery is a collateral of the splenic stem. **B**, Trifurcation of the splenic artery. **C**, The left gastroomental artery and the ramus splenicus inferior have a common stem: the truncus spleno-gastroomentalis. (Reproduced with permission from Van Damme J-P, Bonte MD. Arteria splenica and the blood supply of the spleen. Probl Gen Surg 1990;7:18–27.)

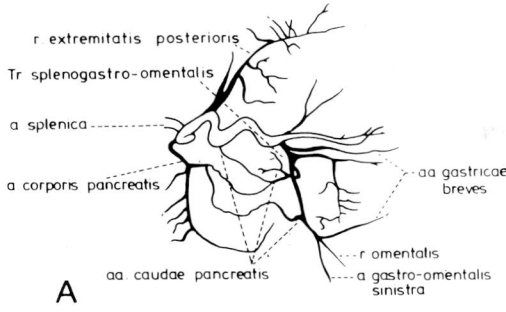

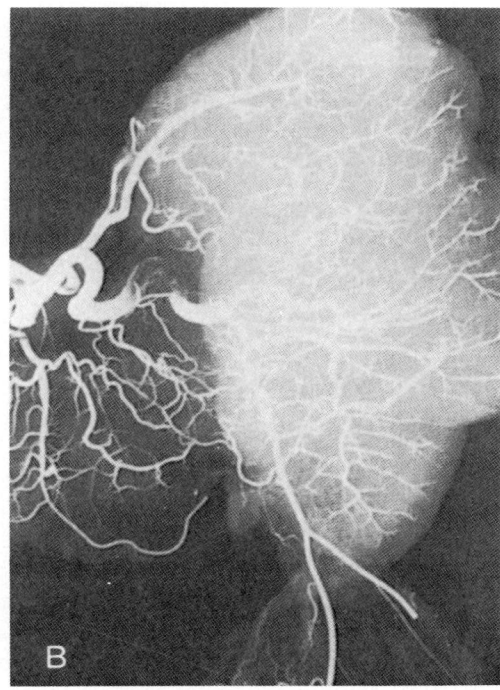

Figure 10.28. **A**, and **B**, The division of the splenic artery. (Reproduced with permission from Van Damme J-P, Bonte MD. Arteria splenica and the blood supply of the spleen. Probl Gen Surg 1990;7:18–27.)

20% [14], 33% [97], and 62% of specimens) or more (10% [96], 70% [93], 67% [97] of specimens) rami splenici arteries.

Van Damme and Bonte (89) describe the branches to the spleen as anterior and posterior, stating that the posterior vessel was found in 52% of abdominal preparations and speculating that perhaps an accessory splenic artery, as described by van Haller (98) and Michels (14), is responsible for the genesis of the vessel.

Intrasplenic Blood Supply

Van Damme and Bonte (89) describe intrasplenic blood supply as follows:

ARTERIAL BLOOD SUPPLY

The splenic branches are [thought] to be terminal arteries forming no anastomoses [99], except for some intrahilar shunts [100–102]. In some instances, we found distinct intrasplenic anastomoses even between the posterior polar and the other splenic branches. Nevertheless, the spleen is to be considered a segmented organ [102, 103]. The segments are perpendicularly superposed along the long axis of the spleen, and they are separated by poorly vascularized planes [95]. According to Cayotte et al. [95], and Simionescu et al. [104] the spleen is divided into two lobes having two segments each. The intersegmental planes are not always horizontal, and in extreme instances the mesospleen may have a longitudinal cleavage plane [95]. . . .

Venous Blood Supply

Dreyer and Budtz-Olson [105], [reported that by] venography, [some] segments . . . had their own vein. Simionescu et al. [104] believed that although the arteries are terminal, the veins are arranged in a single network with broad anastomoses situated within the organ. Dawson et al. [52] investigated the venous segmentation in corrosion casts of 14 spleens. Ten of the 14 spleens had 2 lobes and 4 had 3 lobes, giving a total of 32 lobes. Of these 16 were divided into a maximum of two segments. The relatively avascular planes between the lobes were usually approximately perpendicular to the long axis and oblique to the transverse axis of the spleen. More than half of the interlobar planes corresponded to marginal notches. In the four spleens in which arteries and veins were injected, contrary to the findings of Simionescu et al. [104], there was no overlapping, indicating that both the arterial supply and the venous drainage of a unit are intralobar or intrasegmental not interlobar or intersegmental.

Skandalakis et al. (46) continue:

Douglass et al. [106] also studied the anatomy of the splenic vein. Their findings can be summarized in [Fig. 10.29]. The patterns are highly variable, and, as in the arteries, no one vein resembles the next. Considerable variation is found in the points of the exit of the veins, their point of confluence for the formation of the main splenic vein, and their entrance into other veins at the hilus or outside it.

The single characteristic finding reported by Douglass et al. [106] was that the short gastric veins, or most of them, communicate directly with the spleen, entering the upper part of the spleen rather than entering the extrasplenic venous vessels. The left gastroepiploic venous drainage is into the splenic veins.

The splenic vein begins by the coalescence of five or six tributaries that emerge from the splenic hilus [107]. The splenic vein is of large caliber but does not possess the tortuosity of the splenic artery. The vein passes through the splenorenal ligament with the artery and the tail of the pancreas, passing to the right, usually inferior to the artery and behind the body of the pancreas, receiving tributaries from

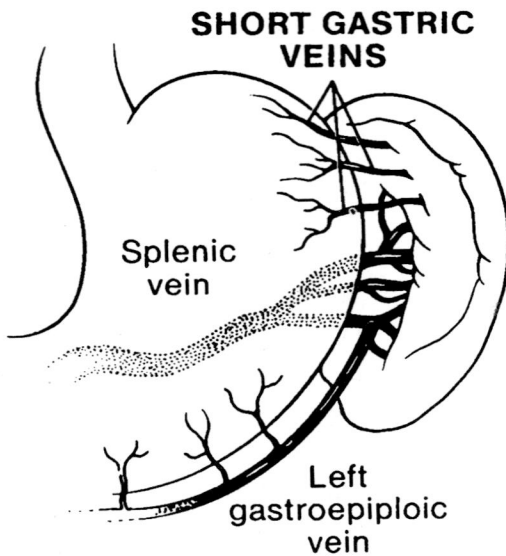

Figure 10.29. Anatomy of the splenic vein. (From Skandalakis JE et al. The surgical anatomy of the spleen. Probl Gen Surg 1990;7:1–17.)

it. It ends deep to the neck of the pancreas by joining the superior mesenteric vein to form the portal vein.

The splenic vein travels with the splenic artery. In 75 consecutive autopsies, Gerber et al. [108] found three anatomic arrangements:

1. The vein lay entirely posterior to the artery in 54% of the bodies.
2. The vein was wrapped around the artery, in part posterior to it and in part anterior in 44%.
3. The vein lay entirely anterior to the artery in 2%.

Vandamme and Bonte (89) continue:

ARTERIOVENOUS ANASTOMOSES

After arterial injection of the spleen, venous return was seen by Cayotte et al. [95], Nguyen Huu et al. [94], and us but we never saw an anastomosis or roentgenograms or corrosion casts.

Skandalakis et al. (46) add:

THE SHORT GASTRIC ARTERIES

Helm [109] wrote that the common origin of the short gastric arteries is from the left gastroepiploic artery or from proper splenic branches. Four to six short gastric arteries were found in each of our specimens. They were considered to be end arteries, not anastomosing at the greater curvature of the stomach. In our series, we counted a total of 145 short gastric arteries. These short gastric arteries anastomose with the cardiac branches of the left gastric artery [110].

COLLATERAL CIRCULATION

The splenic artery is not the only artery to supply the organ with blood. The additional blood supply comes from the inferior or transverse pancreatic artery, short gastric arteries, left gastric artery, and other pancreatic arteries.

Because the origins of the splenic branches are unpredictable, use of a preoperative arteriogram is paramount in determining the point of ligation of the splenic artery. There is no question that the spleen can tolerate ligation of the splenic artery because of the available collateral circulation. Therefore, the spleen can be saved if necessary. Surgeons should remember that ligation of the splenic artery near its origin can result in hyperamylasemia resulting from deterioration of the pancreatic blood supply [111]. Preoperative splenic arterial occlusion as an adjunct to high-risk splenectomy has been advised by Fujitani et al. [112]. According to *Gray's Anatomy*, there are no anastomoses between the smaller branches of the splenic arteries, so that obstruction leads to infarction of the spleen [113]. Dumont and Lefleur [107] suggested increased splenic arterial flow in patients with isolated obstruction of the splenic vein.

VENOUS DRAINAGE

The Splenic Vein and Its Branches. The splenic vein originates from the trabecular vein. We studied the splenic vein in 22 dissections. We found that the vein was formed by three trunks in 16 cases, four trunks in 8 cases, and in the remaining 3 cases, three trunks plus the left gastroepiploic formed the splenic vein.

AGENESIS OF THE SPLEEN AND THE ASPLENIA SYNDROME

Anatomy

Today we believe that the individual without a spleen is seriously impaired in his defense against intravascular organisms since IgM, the largest of the immune globulins and main antibody of immune process, does not exist. Also phagocytosis is very limited in infants. Neither antibody production or phagocytosis is well developed. The microcirculation of the spleen is impaired by disease.

Absence of the spleen is an unusual anomaly, which by itself is clinically unimportant, producing no symptoms and having little observable effect on life expectancy. It is its frequent association with cardiac malformations and disturbances of body symmetry that gives it significance.

Putschar and Manion (18) divided cases of splenic agenesis into five groups:

1. Agenesis of the spleen without other embryonic defects (24%)
2. Agenesis of the spleen with severe malformation of the heart and partial situs inversus viscerum (37%)
3. Agencies of the spleen with malformation of the heart only (26%)
4. Agenesis of the spleen with normal heart and partial situs inversus viscerum (8%)
5. Agenesis of the spleen with anomalies other than heart defects or situs inversus (5%)

These groups can in turn be reduced to two, probably separate, embryonic entities: (*a*) simple agenesis of the spleen (groups 1 and 5) and (*b*) agenesis of the spleen with defects of symmetry and cardiac anomalies (groups 2 to 4)—the asplenia (Polhemus-Schafer-Ivemark) syndrome. In a few cases of this syndrome the spleen is hypoplastic rather than entirely absent (2, 114, 115). Such a hypoplastic spleen may be ectopic (116).

Simple Agenesis of the Spleen

Patients without a spleen may be otherwise normal, or they may have a variety of unrelated congenital anomalies. An example is a case of gargoylism with agenesis of the spleen (117). This is certainly a coincidental expression of two rare anomalies. There have been suggestions that persons without spleens may have an increased susceptibility to infection (118, 119), but the number of undiagnosed cases of splenic agenesis makes it probable that the infections are not related. The genders in this group are equally affected.

Agenesis of the Spleen with Cardiac and Symmetric Defects (Asplenia Syndrome)

CARDIAC DEFECTS

The cardiac defects among these patients are severe and often lethal (120, 121).

Common atrioventricular canal, transposition of the great vessels, pulmonary stenosis or atresia, and persistent truncus arteriosus are the most frequent. The first three defects are found in over 50% of cases of the asplenia syndrome (122). Vascular anomalies, such as a right superior vena cava, are part of the situs inversus and should not be considered to be primary malformations. Double superior vena cava is common (123). Right isomerism of the atria—that is, with both atria resembling right atria—together with total anomalous pulmonary return, has been described in four cases by Van Mierop and Wiglesworth (124) (Fig. 10.30).

SYMMETRY DEFECTS

The stomach is most frequently transposed; the liver is either transposed or symmetric. Less often, other abdominal organs are affected. Very rarely is situs inversus complete. One such case was described by Putschar and Manion (18).

The left lung has three lobes (pulmonary isomerism) in over 50% of affected patients examined (2, 122). In a few cases both lungs had two lobes.

OTHER DEFECTS ASSOCIATED WITH ASPLENIA

In simple asplenia (group A), about 16% of affected individuals have various associated malformations. Mesen-

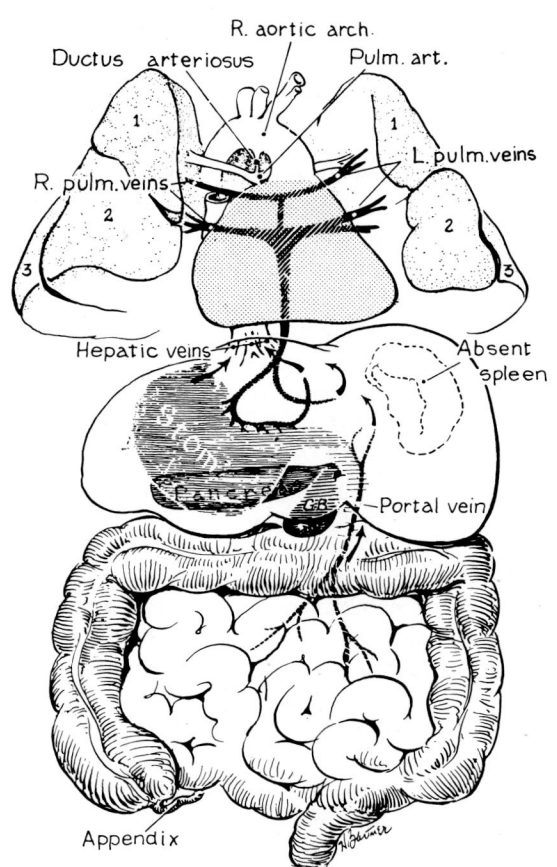

Figure 10.30. Asplenia. Partial situs inversus, symmetrically lobed lungs, and abnormal systemic and pulmonary veins. The aortic arch turns to the right. The stomach, pancreas, and liver are transposed, but the colon and appendix are normally situated although the mesenteric attachments of the small intestine were abnormal. (From Roberts WC, Berry WB, Morrow AG. The significance of asplenia in the recognition of inoperable congenital heart disease. Circulation 1962;26:1251–1253.)

teric defects are common. Absence of the omentum, persistent common mesentery of the small intestine and colon, persistent dorsal mesogastrium, and intestinal malrotation have all been reported. Anomalous abdominal arteries, spina bifida, and genitourinary defects are also known. While there is no set pattern to these defects, they are far more frequent than would be expected by chance.

Embryogenesis

The splenic primordium appears during the sixth week of gestation, at the time at which the endocardial cushions are fusing to separate the atrioventricular canals. Toward the end of this period, division of the truncus arteriosus takes place. Thus the origin of splenic and cardiac defects can be definitely determined. While rotation of the stomach also begins at this time, the underlying situs inversus has been determined much earlier in development.

Among mice, Tihen (125) and his associates in 1948 reported a strain in which situs inversus occurred, along with abnormalities of spleen and lungs. This strain had a high mortality from hydrocephalus. Partial lethality may also be present since the ratio of affected to normal among hybrid animals was less than the mendelian expectation. A mouse strain with absence of the spleen (Dh) has been described from the Jackson Laboratories, Maine. The dominant mutant gene produced skeletal and gastrointestinal anomalies lethal in the homozygous state. Cardiac and symmetry defects did not accompany splenic agenesis in these mice (126).

There is no obvious relationship between asplenia and twinning, but three double monsters having a spleen in the left body only were described early in this century (127).

History

Aristotle mentioned absence of the spleen in animals [De Generatione Animalium IV:iv:771a]. The earliest mention of the condition in man was by Schenk von Grafenburg in 1594 (128). In 1826, Martin (129) described the heart defects and visceral transpositions associated with absence of the spleen. In spite of this early recognition of the condition, only 12 cases were reported before 1900 and only 25 more before 1950. By 1958 Gilbert and his colleagues (130) were able to find 48 more cases in the literature, bringing the total to 85. They found another 27 cases without associated cardiac defects. Many more cases are now in the literature.

In 1952, Gasser and Willi (131) described the hematologic picture in these patients, and Ivemark in 1955 (3) and Putschar and Manion in 1956 (18) thoroughly reviewed the literature and analyzed the congenital cardiac defects that accompany splenic agenesis.

The splenic agenesis, cardiac defects, and partial situs inversus have been named "Ivemark's syndrome" (132). While we recognize the excellence of Ivemark's monograph, we believe a better name would be the "Polhemus-Schafer-Ivemark syndrome" (133–135). For those who dislike eponyms, the "asplenia syndrome" may be acceptable.

Incidence

Ivemark (3) found 11 cases of splenic agenesis among 352 children with congenital heart defects in a total of 7,032 autopsies of children at Boston Children's Hospital between 1920 and 1953. Muir (136) found 7 cases among 520 deaths from congenital heart disease in 22,500 autopsies in Singapore. These are the only series of cases for which incidence figures are available. A case in a dog (137) seems to be the only nonhuman example (except

the mice mentioned above) reported since Aristotle's time.

More males than females are affected. Gilbert and his colleagues (130) found 44 males and 33 females among cases in the literature. In Ivemark's collected cases (3), the relative incidence of males was even higher. This sex difference appears in those patients with cardiac and symmetric anomalies in addition to their splenic agenesis; uncomplicated absence of the spleen seems to affect both sexes equally (18).

However, a great number of people are living well with splenectomy although they are seriously impaired in their defense against intravascular organisms. It is well known that immunity has not been established in children in whom the splenic function is so immature that the infection may become overwhelming, leading to a threatening condition and possible death.

Symptoms

Agenesis of the spleen by itself produces no symptoms. The accompanying anomalies usually lead to its discovery.

Diagnosis

In 1952 Gasser and Willi (131) diagnosed splenic agenesis from hematologic evidence. Erythrocytes containing Heinz bodies had been demonstrated after splenectomy by Zadek and Burg in 1930 (138). Heinz bodies are single, round structures located near the edge of the erythrocyte and are considered to represent denatured hemoglobin rather than nuclear remnants (Fig. 10.31). They are visible with the phase-contrast microscopy, and they stain supravitally with brilliant crystal blue. Gasser and Willi considered their presence in 10% of erythrocytes to be diagnostic of splenic absence. They may appear also under conditions in which the spleen is not involved, such as in toxic hemolytic anemia produced by sulfonamides.

Some observers have failed to find Heinz bodies but have noted an increase in Howell-Jolly bodies, which are nuclear remnants made visible with Wright's stain. All agree that there is a high normoblast count.

Polhemus and Schafer (135) suggest that blood studies should be made on all infants with cyanotic heart disease. If these studies are positive, radiographic evidence of visceral transposition will confirm the presence of the asplenia syndrome.

The presence of situs inversus can usually be determined by the position of the gastric air bubble on the right. The surgeon must be sure that he or she does not unconsciously reverse the roentgenogram while examining it.

Elliott and his colleagues (139), on the basis of 14 cases of asplenia syndrome, observed by angiography that the

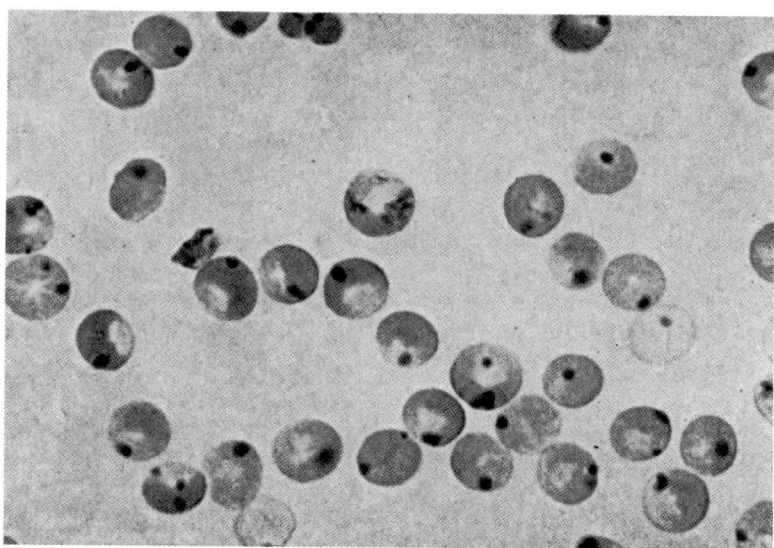

Figure 10.31. Heinz bodies in erythrocytes. A drug response, not asplenia, produced the Heinz bodies in this illustration. (From Beutler E, Dern RJ, Alving AS. The hemolytic effects of Primaguine VI. J Lab Clin Med 1955;45:40–50.)

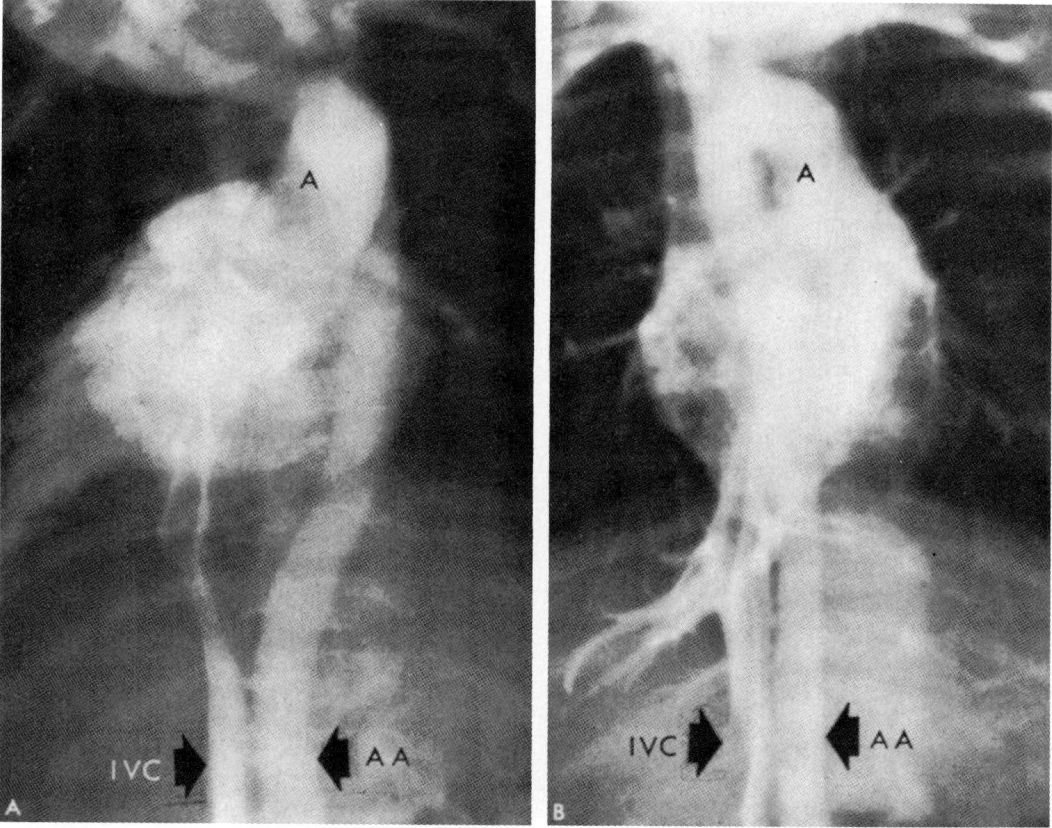

Figure 10.32. Anomalous relationships of the abdominal aorta and the inferior vena cava in patients with asplenia. **A**, The thoracic aorta descends on the opposite side of the spine from the vena cava and crosses to the same side in the abdomen. **B**, The aorta lies on the same side of the spine as the vena cava in the thorax and abdomen. (From Elliott LP, Cramer GG, Amplatz K. The anomalous relationship of the inferior vena cava and abdominal aorta as a specific angiocardiographic sign in asplenia. Radiology 1966;87:859.)

abdominal aorta and the inferior vena cava lie on the same side of the vertebral column (Fig. 10.32). In both situs solidus and situs inversus without asplenia, the vessels are separated by the vertebral column. This observation requires confirmation.

However, the pediatric surgeon should differentiate splenic agenesis from "asplenia." The first is a congenital phenomenon whereas asplenia is the asplenic state which is secondary to splenectomy, autosplenectomy (due to multiple splenic infarctions secondary to sickle cell anemia), or to splenic atrophy (due to malabsorption syndrome), or to neonatal functional anemia (in premature but normal neonates).

Treatment

Surgical treatment of patients with the asplenia syndrome is directed toward correction of their cardiac defects or palliation of the symptoms of those defects.

Mortality

Persons with simple agenesis of the spleen without other malformations may be expected to reach adulthood with few symptoms and without diagnosis. It has been suggested that absence of the spleen lowers resistance to infection (140, 141). Ivemark (3) carefully evaluated the literature and concluded that this was not the case. Gross (142) had only two deaths from subsequent infection among 58 children undergoing splenectomy for congenital hemolytic anemia.

The asplenia syndrome with its severe and often complex cardiac malformations is 90% to 95% fatal in the first year of life. So serious are the heart defects in the asplenia syndrome that Lyons and his colleagues (143) consider situs inversus and absence of the spleen to always indicate the presence of inoperable cardiac lesions. We consider this view too pessimistic, although the extent of the anomalies encountered in some cases is discouraging. As an illustration, a child with asplenia had situs inversus, hydrocephalus, cor biloulare, dextrocardia, transposition of the great vessels, pulmonary stenosis, common atrioventricular canal, anomalous drainage of the vena cava and the pulmonary veins, and meningomyelocele (144). Albert and his colleagues (145) performed corrective surgery successfully on a child with asplenia, an ostium primam atrial septal defect, absence of the inferior vena cava with hemizygous venous drainage to the superior vena cava, which itself entered the left atrium, and hepatic venous drainage to both atria. They concluded that cardiac defects associated with asplenia were not always inoperable.

THE POLYSPLENIA SYNDROME

Anatomy

An absent spleen usually is associated with situs inversus and cardiac anomalies, and a multilobate spleen or a spleen composed of from two to nine distinct and relatively equal portions often is associated with similar defects. Polysplenia must be distinguished from accessory spleens, in which a normal spleen is present, together with one or more small splenic nodules separated from the main organ (Fig. 10.33).

Associated Anomalies

Partial situs inversus and cardiovascular anomalies tend to accompany polysplenia (Fig. 10.34). Bilateral superior venae cavae occur, but less frequently than in the asplenia syndrome. Transposition of the great vessels, common atrioventricular canal, and anomalous pulmonary venous return may be found, but again the incidence is slightly less frequent than in the asplenia syndrome. In some cases polysplenia and partial situs inversus may occur without cardiovascular defects (120).

Embryogenesis

Moller and his associates (146) argued that the situs inversus associated with asplenia is a bilateral right-sidedness

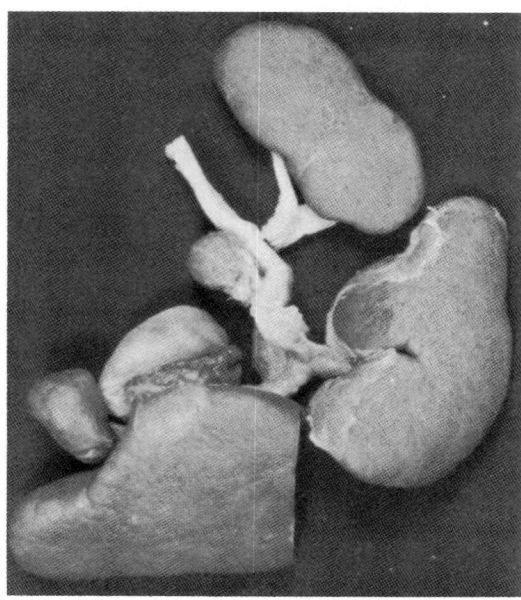

Figure 10.33. Polysplenia. Six splenic masses distributed along the splenic artery. (From Moller JH, Nakib A, Anderson RC, Edwards JE. Congenital cardiac disease associated with polysplenia: a developmental complex of bilateral left-sidedness. Circulation 1967;36:789–799.)

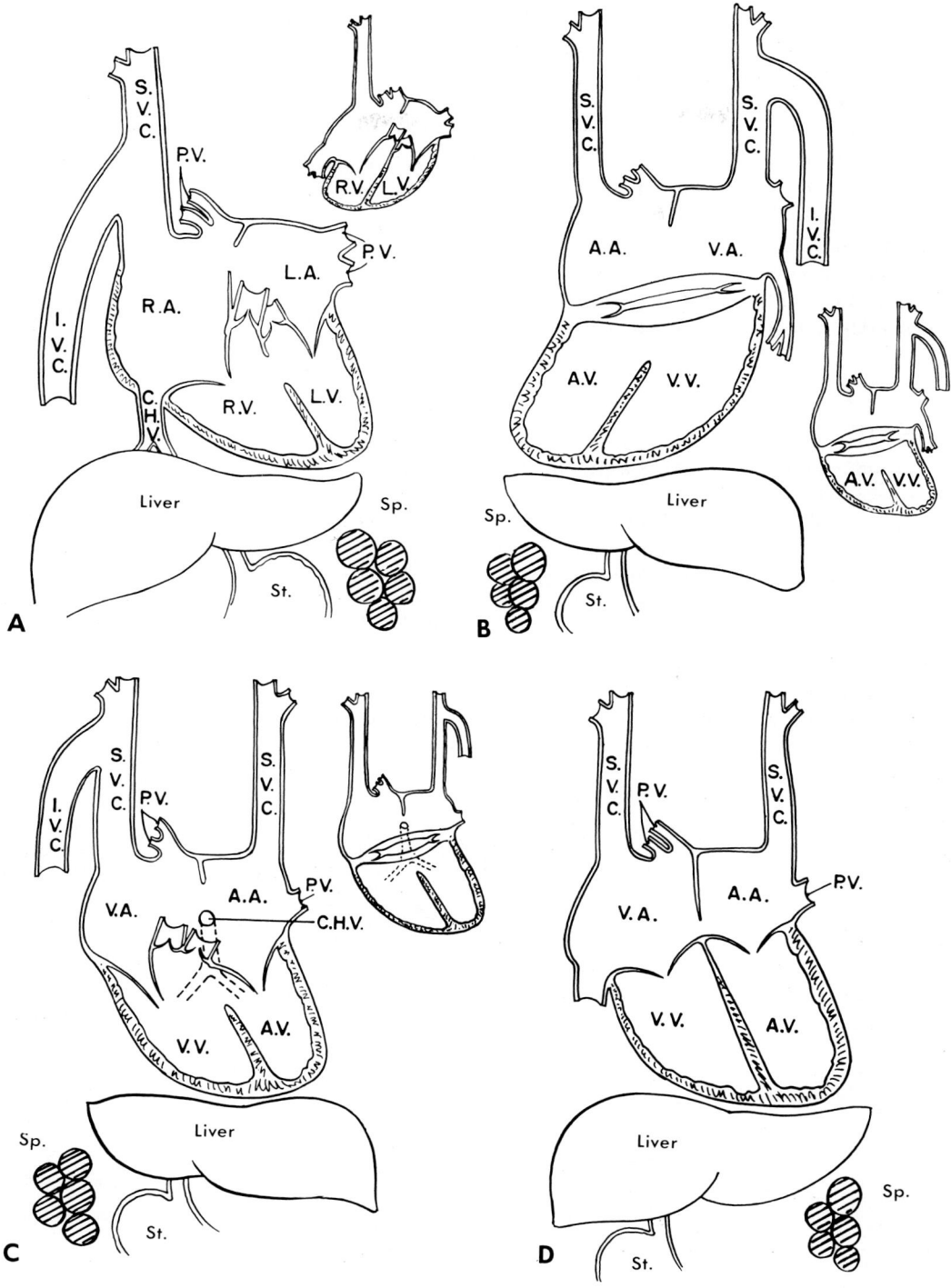

Figure 10.34. Varieties of situs in polysplenia. **A**, Situs solitus. Major lobe of liver on the right, stomach on the left; venous atrium on the right. Anomalous pulmonary veins and both atrial and ventricular septal defects are present. *Inset:* Dextroversion of situs solitus heart without inversion. **B**, Situs inversus with systemic and pulmonary vein anomalies and common atrioventricular canal. *Inset:* Levoversion of situs inversus heart. **C**, Mixed situs. Abdominal viscera inverted, heart with normal situs. Systemic and pulmonary vein anomalies as well as septal defects are present. *Inset:* A similar heart with common atrioventricular canal. **D**, Mixed situs.

Stomach and major lobe of liver on the right. Situs solitus heart with systemic and pulmonary vein anomalies. *S.V.C.,* Superior vena cava; *I.V.C.,* inferior vena cava; *A.A.,* arterial atrium; *R.V.,* right ventricle; *L.V.,* left ventricle; *V.V.,* venous ventricle; *A.V.,* arterial ventricle; *St.,* stomach; *Sp.,* spleen. (From Moller JH, Nakib A, Anderson RC, Edward JE. Congenital cardiac disease associated with polysplenia: a development complex of bilateral left-sidedness. Circulation 1967;36:789–799.)

(dextroisomerism), whereas that associated with polysplenia is a bilateral left-sidedness (levoisomerism). The strongest argument for the existence of two types of inversion lies in the anatomy of the lungs.

In many but not all patients with the asplenia syndrome, both lungs are three-lobed and both have eparterial bronchi. The left lung is thus a mirror image of the normal right lung (Fig. 10.35, *B*). In contrast, patients with polysplenia often have two-lobed lungs with hyparterial bronchi—that is, the right lung is a mirror image of the normal left lung (Fig. 10.35, *C*). This left-sidedness may also be expressed by a nearly symmetric liver without a gallbladder (146).

History and Incidence

Polysplenia was considered separately from asplenia only when the differences in the situs inversus were noted by Moller and colleagues (146). Earlier workers, such as Ivemark (3), lumped together cases of polysplenia and asplenia. If polysplenia is to be included, therefore, the eponym "Ivemark's syndrome" is better than the term "asplenia syndrome."

Brandt and Liebow (122) considered polysplenia to occur three times as frequently as asplenia. The difficulty in recognizing the syndrome, even when the nature of the cardiac defects is clear, makes any estimate of frequency very doubtful.

Symptoms

Symptoms are those springing from the associated cardiovascular defects.

Diagnosis

Polysplenia can rarely be diagnosed without surgery. The multiple spleens function normally; unlike the case with asplenia, polysplenia presents no characteristic hematologic picture.

Treatment

Only the cardiovascular components of the syndrome require treatment.

Mortality

Eighty percent of affected individuals die in the first year of life. In 1958 Brandt and Liebow (122) were able to find only one patient over 50 years of age.

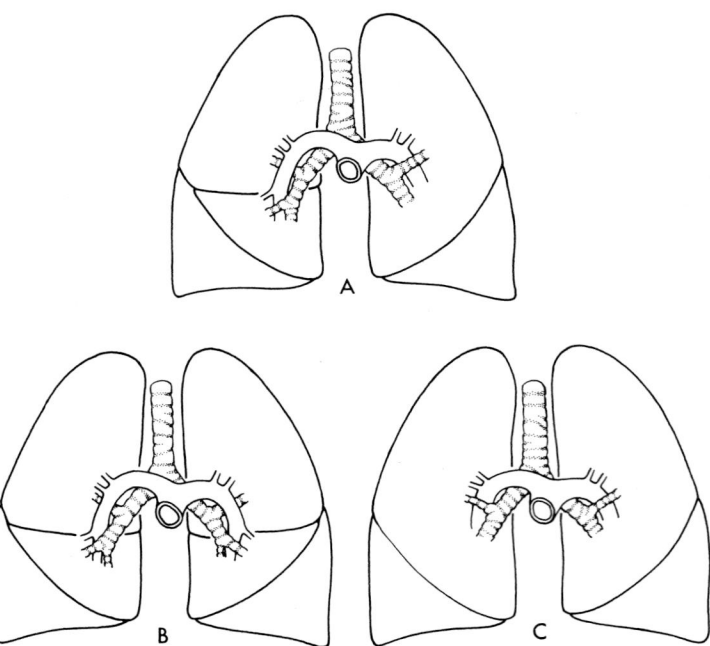

Figure 10.35. Pulmonary patterns associated with splenic anomalies. **A**, Situs solitus and normal spleen. The right lung has three lobes and the upper lobe bronchus is eparterial. The left lung has two lobes, and the upper lobe bronchus is hyparterial. In situs inversus totalis and normal spleen, the lungs form a mirror image of this pattern. **B**, Asplenia syndrome. Both lungs have three lobes and eparterial bronchi (i.e., there are two ''right lungs''). **C**, Polysplenia syndrome. Both lungs have two lobes and hyparterial bronchi (i.e., there are two ''left lungs''). (Redrawn from Moller JH, Nakib A, Anderson RC, Edward JE. Congenital cardiac disease associated with polysplenia: a development complex of bilateral left-sidedness. Circulation 1967;36:789–799.)

CONGENITAL SPLENIC CYSTS

Congenital cysts of the spleen are lined with epithelium. In 1970 Talerman and Hart (147) reported several hundred epithelial cysts. Most of these cases involved children and young adults. Panossian et al. (148) reported an epidermoid cyst of the spleen as a generalized peritonitis. The authors reviewed 159 cases, adding one of their own and advising splenectomy and an antibiotic regimen, including coverage for *Salmonella* infection.

TUMORS

Intrasplenic lipoma was reported by Easler and Dowlin (149).

REFERENCES

1. Gurich HG. Symmetrische Doppelmitz bei partiellem situs inversus der Bauchorgane. Acta Hepatosplen 1968;15:43–48.
2. Holyoke EA. The role of the primitive mesothelium in the development of the mammalian spleen. Anat Rec 1936;65:333–350.
3. Ivemark BI. Implications of agenesis of the spleen on the pathogenesis of cono-truncus anomalies in children. Acta Paediatr (Uppsala) 1955;44(Suppl)104:1–110.
4. Thiel GA, Downey H. The development of the mammalian spleen, with special reference to its hematopoitec activity. Am J Anat 1921;28:279–339.
5. Sills RH. Splenic function: physiology and splenic hypofunction. Boll Soc Ital Biol Sper 1987;63:383–390.
6. Stark DD, Moss AA, Goldberg HI. Nuclear magnetic resonance of the liver, spleen, and pancreas. Cardiovasc Intervent Radiol 1986;8:329–341.
7. Boles ET. The spleen. Pediatr Surg 1986;2:1108–1113.
8. Malangoni MA, Dawes LG, Droege EA, Rao SA, Collier BD. Splenic phagocytic function of the partial splenectomy and splenic autotransplantation. Arch Surg 1985;120:275–278.
9. Miller EJ, Nowak E, Hair L, Mouradian J. Retroperitoneal accessory spleen. Am Surg 1990;56:293–294.
10. Curtis GM, Movitz D. The surgical significance of the accessory spleen. Ann Surg 1946;123:276–298.
11. Halpert B, Alden ZA: Accessory spleens in or at the tail of the pancreas. Arch Pathol 1964;77:652–654.
12. Halpert B, Györkey F. Lesions observed in accessory spleens of 311 patients. Am J Clin Pathol 1959;32:165–168.
13. von Stubenrach K. Verlust und Regeneration der Milz beim Menschen. Beitr Z Klin Chir 1919;118, 285, 305.
14. Michels NA. The variational anatomy of the spleen and splenic artery. Am J Anat 1942;70:21–72.
15. Brown RB, Dobbie RP. Splenic indentation of gastric fundus resembling gastric neoplasm: report of two cases. AJR 1959;81:599–602.
16. Das Gupta TK, Busch RC. Accessory splenic tissue producing indentation of the gastric fundus resembling gastric neoplasm. N Engl J Med 1960;263:1360–1361.
17. Bennett-Jones ML, St Hill CA. Accessory spleen in the scrotum. Br J Surg 1952;40:259–262.
18. Putschar WGJ, Manion WC. Congenital absence of the spleen and associated anomalies. Am J Clin Pathol 1956;26:429–470.
19. Scholtmeijer RJ. An accessory spleen in the scrotum. Ned Tijdsclr Geneeskd 1966;110:90–92.
20. Gouw AS, Elema JD, Bink-Boelkens MT, de Jongh HJ, ten Kate LP. The spectrum of splenogonadal fusion: case report and review of 84 reported cases. Eur J Pediatr 1985;144:316–323.
21. Pommer G: Verwachsung des linken kryptorchischen Hodens und Nebenhodens mit der Milz in einer Missgeburt mit zalreichen Bildungsdefecten. Berl Naturw Med Ver Innsbruck 1887–1889;17–19:144–148.
22. Hines JR, Eggum PR. Splenic gonadal fusion causing bowel obstruction. Arch Surg 1961;83:109–111.
23. Willis RA. The borderland of embryology and pathology. London: Butterworth, 1958.
24. McKusick VA. Mendelian inheritance in man. 6th ed. Baltimore: Johns Hopkins University Press, 1983:491.
25. Grossman SL, Goldberg MM, Herman HB. A case report of ectopic splenic tissue in the scrotum. J Urol 1959;81:294–296.
26. Lynch JB, Kareim OA. Aberrant splenic tissue in the scrotum. Br J Surg 1962;49:546–548.
27. Daniel DS. An unusual case of ectopic splenic tissue resembling a third testicle. Ann Surg 1957;145:960–962.
28. Jayne WHW, Jessiman AG. A case of accessory spleen in the scrotum. Br J Surg 1955;42:555–556.
29. Tsignoglou S, Wilkinson AW. Splenogonadal fusion. Br J Surg 1976;63:297–298.
30. Gordeef J, Cuennant J. Rate surnuméraire à localisation scrotale. Maroc Méd 1951;30:744.
31. Rosenthal JT, Bedetti CD, Labayen RF, Christy WC, Yakulis R. Right splenogonadal fusion with associated hypersplenism. J Urol 1981;126:812–814.
32. von Hochstetter A. Milzgewebe im linken Ovarium des linken Individualteiles eines menschlichen Thoracopagus. Virchows Arch 1953;324:36–54.
33. Falkowski WS, Carter MF. Splenogonadal fusion associated with an anaplastic seminoma. J Urol 1980;124:562–564.
34. Fritzsche F. Lien caudatus mit eigenartiger implantation des oberen milzopols in die leber. Virchows Arch [A] 1956;329:35–45.
35. Sommer JR. Continuous splenic gonadal fusion with ectromelia: teratogenesis, a case report. Pediatrics 1958;22:1183–1189.
36. Watson RJ. Splenogonadal fusion. Surgery 1968;63(5):853–858.
37. Pagano R. Ectopic pregnancy: A seven-year survey. Med J Aust 1981;2:586–588.
38. Beachman WD et al. Abdominal pregnancy at Charity Hospital in New Orleans. Am J Obstet Gynecol 1982;84:1257–1270.
39. Breen JL. A 21-year survey of 654 ectopic pregnancies. Am J Obstet Gynecol 1970;106:1004–1019.
40. Studdiford WA. Primary peritoneal pregnancy. Am J Obstet Gynecol 1942;44:487–491.
41. Friedrich EG, Rankin CA. Primary pelvic peritoneal pregnancy. Obstet Gynecol 1968;31:649–653.
42. Alcalay J, Reif RM, Bogokowsky H. Primary splenic pregnancy (Heb). Harefuah 1981;100(12):577.
43. Kushner DH, Dobrzynski FA. Abdominal pregnancy with placenta attached to the spleen. Am J Obstet Gynecol 1946;52:160–161.
44. Repin AV. Abdominal pregnancy of 28 weeks with implantation of the fertilized ovum at the hilum of the spleen (Rus). Akush Ginekol 1962;2:107–108.
45. Caruso V, Hall WHJ. Primary abdominal pregnancy in the spleen: a case report. Pathology 1984;16:93–94.
46. Skandalakis JE et al. The surgical anatomy of the spleen. Probl Gen Surg 1990;7:1–17.
47. Gould GM, Pyle WL. Anomalies and curiosities of medicine, 2nd ed. New York: Bell Publishing, 1956:657.
48. Allen L. The lymphatic system and the spleen. In: Anson BJ, ed. Morris's human anatomy, 12th ed. New York: McGraw-Hill Book, 1966:907.

49. Last RJ. Anatomy: regional and applied, 5th ed. Baltimore: Williams & Wilkins, 1972:470.

50. Michels NA. Blood supply and anatomy of the upper abdominal organs, with a descriptive atlas. Philadelphia: JB Lippincott, 1955.

51. Gupta CD, Gupta SC, Aorara AK, Singh P. Vascular segments in the human spleen. J Anat 1976;121:613.

52. Dawson DL, Molina JE, Scott-Conner CEH. Venous segmentation of the human spleen. Am Surg 1986;42:253.

53. Garcia-Porrero JA, Lemes A. Arterial segmentation and subsegmentation in the human spleen. Acta Anat 1988;131:276.

54. Mandarim-Lacerda CA, Sampaio FJ, Passos MA. Segmentation vasculaire de la rate chez le nouveau-ne: support anatomique pour la resection par tielle. J Chir (Paris) 1983;120:471.

55. Dryer B, Budtz-Olsen OE. Splenic venography: demonstration of the portal circulation with diodome. Lancet 1952;1:530.

56. Dixon JA, Miller F, McCloskey D, Siddoway J. Anatomy and techniques in segmental splenectomy. Surg Gynecol Obstet 1980;150:516.

57. Liebermann-Meffert D, White H. The greater omentum. New York: Springer-Verlag, 1983.

58. Van Damme JP, Bonte J. Vascular anatomy in abdominal surgery. New York: Thieme Medical Publishers, 1990.

59. Whitesall FB. A clinical and surgical anatomic study of rupture of the spleen due to blunt trauma. Surg Gynecol Obstet 1960;110:750.

60. Henry AK. The removal of large spleens. Br J Surg 1940;107:464.

61. Lord MD, Gourevitch A. The peritoneal anatomy of the spleen, with special references to the operation of partial gastrectomy. Br J Surg 1965;52:202.

62. VanderZypen E, Revez E. Investigation of development, structure and function of the phrenicocolic and duodenal suspensory ligaments. Acta Anat (Basel) 1984;119:142.

63. Abell I. Wandering spleen with torsion of the pedicle. Ann Surg 1933;98:722–735.

64. Allen KB, Andrews G. Pediatric wandering spleen: the case for splenopexy—review of 35 reported cases in the literature. J Pediatr Surg 1989;24:432–435.

65. Allen KB. Wandering spleen. Probl Gen Surg 1990;7(1):122–127.

66. Carswell JW. Wandering spleen. Eleven cases from Uganda. Br J Surg 1974;61:495–497.

67. Pearson JB. Torsion of the spleen associated with congenital absence of the left kidney. Br J Surg 1964;51:393–395.

68. Waldschmidt J. Pathological conditions, specific investigations, and therapy. In: Liebermann-Meffert D, White H, eds. The greater omentum. New York: Springer-Verlag, 1983:11.

69. Adkins EH. Ptosed spleen with torsion of pedicle. Ann Surg 1938;107:832.

70. Hamilton WJ, Simon G, Hamilton SGI. Surface and radiological anatomy. Baltimore: Williams & Wilkins, 1976.

71. Traveras JM. Golden's diagnostic roentgenology, Vol 3. Baltimore: Williams & Wilkins, 1964.

72. Broker FHL, Fellows K, Treves S. Wandering spleen in three children. Pediatr Radiol 1978;7:211–214.

73. Thompson JS, Ross RJ, Pizzaro ST. The wandering spleen in infancy and childhood. Clin Pediatr 1980;19:221–224.

74. DeBartolo HM, van Heerden JA, Lynn HB. Torsion of the spleen: a case report. Mayo Clin Proc 1973;48:783–786.

75. Woodwards DAK. Torsion of the spleen. Am J Surg 1967;114:953–955.

76. Smulewicz JJ, Clement AR. Torsion of the wandering spleen. Dig Dis 1975;20:274–279.

77. Gordon DH, Burrell MI, Levin DC. Wandering spleen: the radiological and clinical spectrum. Radiology 1977;125:39–46.

78. Miller EI. Wandering spleen and pregnancy. J Clin Ultrasound 1975;3:281–282.

79. Parker LA, Mittelstaedt CA, Mauro MA. Torsion of a wandering spleen: CT appearance. J Comput Assist Tomogr 1984;8:1202–1204.

80. Tait NP, Young JR. The wandering spleen: an ultrasonic diagnosis. J Clin Ultrasound 1985;13:141–144.

81. Agee JH, Crepps LF, Layton M. Wandering pelvic spleen. J Clin Ultrasound 1985;13:145–146.

82. Hunter TB, Haber K. Sonographic diagnosis for a wandering spleen. Am J Radiol 1977;129:925–926.

83. Rosenthal L, Lisbona R, Banerjee K. A nucleographic and radioangiographic study of a patient with torsion of the spleen. Radiology 1974;110:427–428.

84. Spencer RP, Pearson HA, Binder JH. Identification of cases of "acquired" functional asplenia. J Nucl Med 1970;11:763–765.

85. Dublin AB, Rosenquist CJ. Diagnosis of splenic torsion: a combined radiographic approach. Br J Radiol 1976;49:1045–1046.

86. Shende A, Lanzkowsky PH, Becker J. Torsion of a visceroptosed spleen. Am J Dis Child 1976;130:88–91.

87. Buehner M, Baker MS. The wandering spleen. Surg Gynecol Obstet 1992;175(10):373–387.

88. Allen KB, Gay BB, Skandalakis JE. Wandering spleen: anatomic and radiologic considerations. South Med J 1992;85(10):976–984.

89. Vandamme J-P, Bonte MD. Arteria splenica and the blood supply of the spleen. Probl Gen Surg 1990;7:18–27.

90. Haertel M, Beusch HR. Die angiographische Normalanatomie der Milz. Fortschr Rontgenstr 1974;120:653.

91. Rossi G, Cova E. Studio morfologico delle arterie dello stomaco. Arch Ital Anat Embriol 1904;3:485.

92. Waizer A, Baniel J, Zin Y, Dintsman M. Clinical implications of anatomic variations of the splenic artery. Surg Gynecol Obstet 1989;168:57.

93. Ssoson-Jaroschewitsch A. Zur chirurgischen Anatomie des Milzhilus. Z Anat Entw Gesch 1927;84:218.

94. Nguyen Huu, Person H, Hong R, Vallée B, Hoan Vu N. Anatomical approach to the vascular segmentation of the spleen (lien) based on controlled experimental partial splenectomies. Anat Clin 1982;4:265.

95. Cayotte JL et al. Essai sur l'organisation vasculaire de la rate. C R Assoc Nat 1970;149:591.

96. Lipschutz B. A composite study of the coeliac artery. Ann Surg 1917;65:159.

97. Piquand G. Le pédicule vasculaire de la rate. Progr Progrès Méd 1910.

98. von Haller A. Icones anatomicae in quibis aliquae partes corporis humani delinatae proponuntur et anteriarum potissimum historia continetur. Göttingen: Vandenhoeck, 1756.

99. McKenzie D, Whipple A, Wintersteiner M. Studies on the microscopic anatomy and physiology of living transilluminated mammalian spleen. Am J Anat 1941;68–397.

100. Volkmann J. Anatomische und experimentelle Beiträge zur konservativen Chirurgie der Milz. Arch Klin Chir 1923;125:231.

101. Henschen C. Die chirurgische Anatomie der Milzgefässe. Schweiz Med Wochenschr 1928;58:164.

102. Clausen E. Anatomie der Milzarterie und ihrer segmentalen Äste beim Menschen. Anat Anz 1958;105:315.

103. Gutierrez Cabillos C. Segmentation of the spleen. Rev Esp Enferm Apar Dig 1969;29:341.

104. Simionescu N, Aburel V, Giobanu M, Curelaru I, Marin D. Les segments artériels de la rate chez l'homme. Arch Anat Pathol 1960;8:2.

105. Dreyer B, Budtz-Olson OE. Splenic venography: demonstration of portal circulation with diodone. Lancet 1952;1:530.

106. Douglass BE, Baggenstoss AH, Hollinhead WH. The anatomy of

the portal vein and its tributaries. Surg Gynecol Obstet 1950;91:562.

107. Dumont AE, Lefleur RS. Significance of an enlarged splenic artery in patients with splenic vein thrombosis. Am Surg 1988;54:613.

108. Gerber AB, Lev M, Goldberg SL. The surgical anatomy of the splenic vein. Am J Surg 1951;82:339.

109. Helm HM. The gastric vasa brevia. Anat Rec 1915;9:637.

110. Graves FT. Seeing operative surgery. London: William Heineman Medical Books, 1979;132.

111. Seufert RM, Mitrou PS. Surgery of the spleen. (Reber HA, trans). New York: Thieme, 1986.

112. Fujitani RM et al. Preoperative splenic artery occlusion as an adjunct for high risk splenectomy. Am Surg 1988;54:602.

113. Williams PL, Warwick R. Gray's anatomy, 36th ed. Philadelphia: WB Saunders, 1980.

114. Christiaens L, Fontaine G, Laude M, Dehaene, P. Considerations anatomo-cliniques sur le syndrome d'Ivemark. (A propos de trois cas). Arch Franc Pediatr 1962;19:1213–1232.

115. Kevy SV, Tefft M, Vawter GF. Hereditary splenic hypoplasia. Pediatrics 1968;42:752–757.

116. Layman TE, Levine MA, Amplatz K, Edwards JE. Asplenic syndrome in association with rudimentary spleen. Am J Cardiol 1967;20:136–140.

117. Stransky E, Lara RT. On congenital absence of the spleen combined with gargoylism. Philipp J Pediatr 1963;12:174–182.

118. Gilbert GJ, Phillippi PJ, Scripter LJ. Thrombotic angiitis and congenital asplenia. JAMA 1965;192:415–417.

119. Myerson RM, Koelle WA. Congenital absence of spleen in an adult. N Engl J Med 1956;254:1131–1132.

120. Roberts WC, Berry WB, Morrow AG. The significance of asplenia in the recognition of inoperable congenital heart disease. Circulation 1962;16:1251–1253.

121. Ruttenberg HD et al. Syndrome of congenital cardiac disease with asplenia: distinction from other forms of congenital cyanotic cardiac disease. Am J Cardiol 1964;13:387–406.

122. Brandt HM, Liebow AA. Right pulmonary isomerism associated with venous, splenic, and other anomalies. Lab Invest 1958;7:469–504.

123. Campbell M, Deuchar DC. Absent inferior vena cava, symmetrical liver, splenic agenesis, and situs inversus, and their embryology. Br Heart J 1967;29:268–275.

124. Van Mierop LH, Wiglesworth FW. Isomerism of cardiac atria in the asplenia syndrome. Lab Invest 1962;11:1303–1315.

125. Tihen JA, Charles DR, Sippel TO. Inherited visceral inversion in mice. J Hered 1948;39:29–31.

126. Meier H, Hoag WG. Blood proteins and immune response in mice with hereditary absence of spleen. Naturwissenchaften 1962;49:329.

127. Van Westrienen A. Die vergleichende Teratologie der Doppelbildungen. Rotterdam: WJ Van Hengel, 1911.

128. Schenk von Grafenburg J. Observationum medicarum, rararum, novarum, admirabilium et monstrosarum, liber secundus [etc.]. Freiburg: Martini Becklerii, 1594.

129. Martin MG. Observation d'une déviation organique de l'éstomac, d'une anomalie dans la situation, dans la configuration du coeur et des vaisseaux qui en partent ou qui s'y rendent. Bull Soc Anat (Paris) 1826;1:40.

130. Gilbert EF, Nishimura K, Wedum BG. Congenital malformations of the heart associated with splenic agenesis. Circulation 1958;17:72–86.

131. Gasser C, Willi H. Spontane Innenkörperbildung bei Milzagenesic. Helv Paediatr Acta 1952;7:369–382.

132. Chaptal J, Cazal R, Bonnet JH, Mandin A. Agenesie de la rate, situs inversus et cardiopathies complexes (syndrome d'Ivemark). Pediatrie 1960;15:125–134.

133. Polhemus DW, Schafer WB. Congenital absence of the spleen: syndrome with atrioventricularis and situs inversus—case reports and review of the literature. Pediatrics 1952;9:696–708.

134. Polhemus DW, Schafer WB. Congenital absence of the spleen. Pediatrics 1955;16:495–497.

135. Polhemus DW, Schafer WB. Absent spleen syndrome: hematologic findings as an aid to diagnosis. Pediatrics 1959;24:254–257.

136. Muir CS. Splenic agenesis and multilobulate spleen. Arch Dis Child 1959;34:431–435.

137. Patellani L, Moroni E. Osservazioni sopra un cane senza milza. Ann Univ Med (Milano) 1864;187:555–571.

138. Zadek I, Burg K. Innenkörperanämien. Folia Haemat 1930;41:333–355.

139. Elliott LP, Cramer GG, Amplatz K. The anomalous relationship of the inferior vena cava and abdominal aorta as a specific angiocardiographic sign in asplenia. Radiology 1966;87:859.

140. King H, Shumacker HB, Jr. Splenic studies. I. Susceptibility to infection after splenectomy performed in infancy. Ann Surg 1952;136:239–242.

141. Murphy JW, Mitchell WA. Congenital absence of the spleen. Pediatrics 1957;20:253–256.

142. Gross RE. The surgery of infancy and childhood. Philadelphia: WB Saunders, 1953.

143. Lyons WS, Hanlon DG, Helmholz HF, DuShane JW, Edwards JE. Congenital cardiac disease and asplenia: report of seven cases. Proc Mayo Clin 1957;32:277–286.

144. Duckett S. A propos d'un cas d'agenésie de la rate associée à des malformations abdominales, cardiaques et neurologiques chez l'enfant. Presse Med 1963;71:2043–2044.

145. Albert HM, Fowler RL, Glass BA, Yu S-K. Cardiac anomalies and splenic agenesis. Am Surg 1968;34:94–98.

146. Moller JH, Nakib A, Anderson RC, Edwards JE. Congenital cardiac disease associated with polysplenia: a developmental complex of bilateral left-sidedness. Circulation 1967;36:789–799.

147. Talerman A, Hart S. Epithelial cysts of the spleen. Br J Surg 1970;57:201–204.

148. Panossian DH, Wang N, Reeves CD, Weeks DA. Epidermoid cyst of the spleen presenting as a generalized peritonitis. Am Surg 1990;56:295–298.

149. Easler RE, Dawlin WM. Primary lipoma of the spleen: report of a case. Arch Pathol 1969;88:557–559.

CHAPTER 11

THE PANCREAS

John Elias Skandalakis / Stephen Wood Gray / Richard Ricketts / Lee John Skandalakis

*For me the tiger country is removal of the pancreas. The anatomy is
very complex and one encounters anomalies.*
—SIR ANDREW WATT KAY, CONTEMPORARY SURGERY, 1978;13:71

DEVELOPMENT

The liver diverticulum grows from the ventral side of the foregut, just caudal to the dilation of the stomach into the transverse septum during the fourth week. In the following week (6 mm), two more diverticula appear. One arises directly from the dorsal side of the duodenum almost opposite the liver primordium, and the other arises from the base of the liver diverticulum itself. These two diverticula are the dorsal and ventral anlagen that will fuse to form the definitive pancreas. They first were recognized in the human embryo by Phisalix (1) in 1888.

The ventral primordium is the more variable of the two. It has been found to arise directly from the duodenum. Some evidence exists that it may be transiently paired (2).

The early differentiation of the pancreas has been studied experimentally in the chick (3) and in the mouse (4). The presumptive pancreatic tissue in the mouse becomes determined as early as the 15-somite stage before condensed pancreatic mesoderm appears, although mesoderm cells appear to be necessary for epithelial growth and maturation (5). Actual outgrowth of the diverticulum in the mouse does not begin until the 22- to 25-somite stage.

According to Gittes et al. (6), their experimental work confirmed that the pancreas originates from endoderm. They suggest that a state of prodifferentiation does not exist.

In the human embryo by the sixth week, the dorsal primordium, which is the larger and grows the faster of the two primordia, has developed primary acini and extends into the dorsal mesentery. During the same period, the ventral primordium has been carried away from the duodenum by elongation of the proximal part of the liver diverticulum from which it arises. This proximal stalk may now be called the common duct. Its orifice, originally ventral, is shifted to a dorsal position by duodenal growth, which is limited to the left half of the circumference. The result of these movements is to bring the opening of the common duct to the same side and below the opening of the dorsal primordium of the pancreas (Fig. 11.1).

During the seventh week, the smaller ventral primordium fuses with the proximal part of the dorsal pancreas. The ventral primordium forms the uncinate process and part of the head of the pancreas, whereas the larger dorsal primordium forms the remainder of the organ.

Following the fusion of the two primordia, the duct systems anastomose. The duct of the ventral anlage usually persists, together with the distal portion of the duct of the dorsal anlage, to form the main pancreatic duct. On the other hand, the proximal portion of the dorsal duct may disappear or persist as the accessory pancreatic duct. By the end of the seventh week, little evidence remains of the double origin of the organ (Fig. 11.2).

Duct cells comprise 14% of the total gland in the adult human pancreas, according to Tasso et al. (7). Dawson and Langman (8) stated that the fusion of the duct systems appears to occur usually in the postnatal period because 85% of infants have patent accessory ducts as compared with 40% of adults.

Githens (9) found that, as of 1989, little was known about the development of duct cells in humans; he presented the model of pancreatic development illustrated in Figure 11.3.

The point of junction of the pancreatic and common bile ducts recedes from the common orifice with elongation of the papilla of Vater and with increasing thickness of the duodenal wall. Schwegler and Boyden (10) stated that, at term, the junction lies halfway between the end of the papilla and the muscularis externa of the duodenum. However, this is subject to much individual variation.

Acini

The secretory acini appear during the third month as clusters of cells around the ends of the ducts, from which they were derived. From their first formation the acinar cells are readily distinguishable from the terminal cells of the ducts, the centroacinar cells (11). As in organs such as the lung and the kidney, the pancreatic endodermal cells require the presence of the local mesenchyme for their growth and differentiation (12). No evidence was found

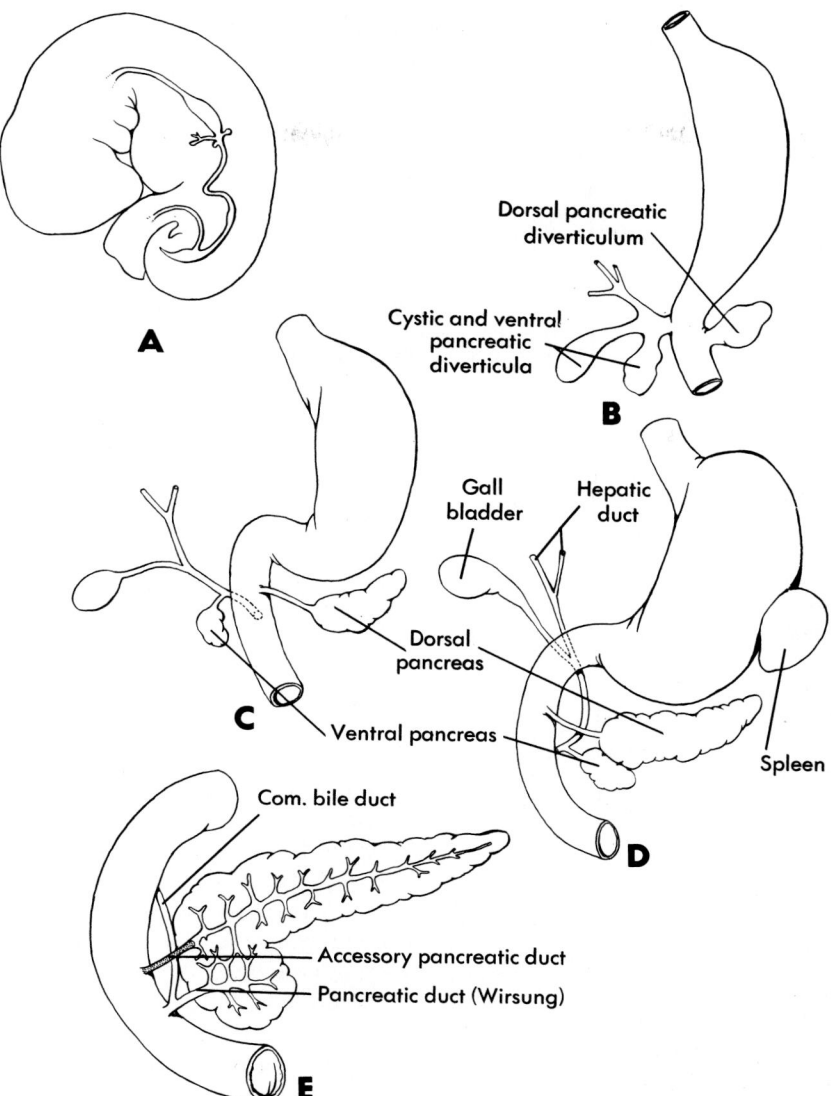

Figure 11.1. Development of the derivatives of the caudal end of the foregut. **A,** Orientation of the gut within an embryo of about 30 days. **B** to **D,** The stomach, duodenum, and pancreatic and hepatic diverticula at approximately 30, 33, and 36 days. **E,** The definitive relationships of the pancreatic and common bile ducts. (From Allan FD. Essentials of human embryology. New York: Oxford University Press, 1969.)

of secretory activity in the fetal acini, even though zymogen granules are present from the fifth month onward (13). Trypsin may appear as early as 22 weeks; lipase is present only near term (14).

The acini secrete pancreatic digestive juice containing enzymes such as trypsin, chymotrypsin, carboxypolypeptidase, ribonuclease, and deoxyribonuclease into the second part of the duodenum.

Islands of Langerhans

Acinar cells and islet cells both differentiate from duct cells of the pancreas (Fig. 11.4). Whether this differentiation is permanent or whether acinar cells may become islet cells by subsequent differentiation has not been settled. From experimental procedures, a number of authors have concluded that new islets could be formed from existing acinar cells (15, 16), but several investigators question the evidence and doubt the interchangeability of the cell types in normal embryogenesis (11, 17–19).

The existence of two generations of islets was first suggested in 1896 by Laguesse (20) and was confirmed by Liu and Potter (11), who examined 130 human embryos ranging in age from 5 weeks to term (Fig. 11.5).

The earliest islets are visible at the end of the second month (30 mm), just before the acini appear; these undergo regression after the fifth month. While a few of

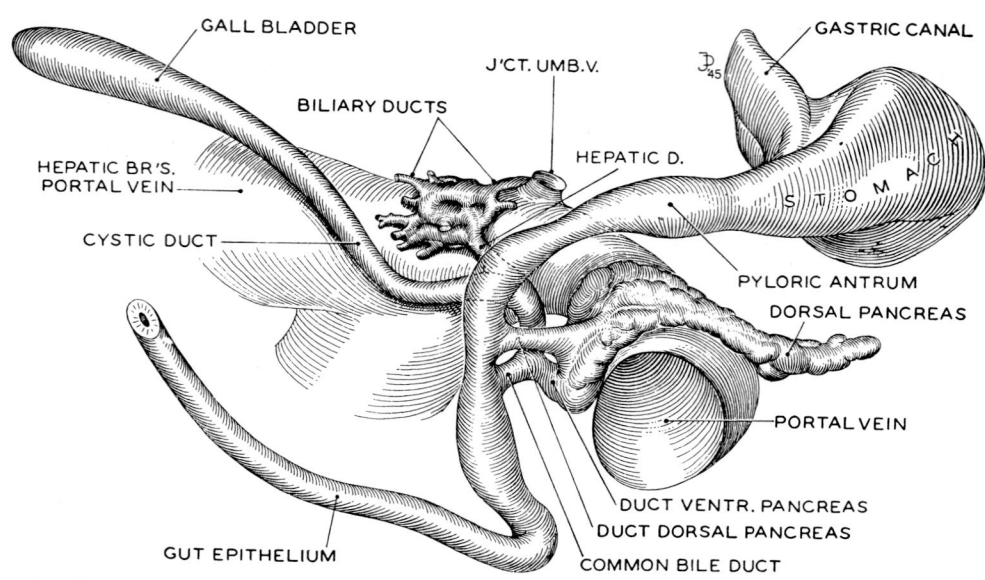

Figure 11.2. Relationship of pancreatic primordia to the duodenum and the portal vein. The dorsal primordium has fused with the ventral primordium, but the two are still identifiable. (From Streeter GL. Developmental horizons in human embryos: description of age groups XV, XVI, XVII, and XVIII. Contrib Embryol Carnegie Inst Wash 1948;32:133–204.)

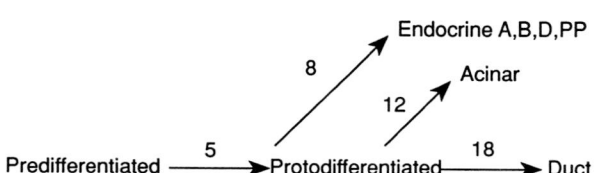

Figure 11.3. A model for human pancreatic development. The predifferentiated cells are from the region of the foregut epithelium that gives rise to the pancreatic rudiment, which consists of protodifferentiated cells committed to develop into one or more of the pancreatic cell types. The numbers associated with the *arrows* represent the earliest time that adult characteristics are first detected by immunohistochemical means. (From Githins S. Development of duct cells. In: Lebenthal E. Human gastrointestinal development. New York: Raven Press, 1989:679.)

these primary islands may remain in the pancreas of premature infants, all have degenerated by term (21). Secondary islets arise from centroacinar cells during the third month and migrate out of the acini in which they are formed, remaining connected with the end of the duct by a thin stalk (the tubule of Bensley). According to Liu and Potter (10), the primary islets are located in the interlobular connective tissue, whereas the secondary islets are found among the acini within lobules.

Histogenesis of the specific cell types has been described by Liu and Potter (11) and Conklin (13). According to Guyton, the 1 million islets of Langerhans contain four major types of cells:

α = 25% = glucagon
β = 60% = insulin
δ = 10% = somatostatin
PP = ~5% = pancreatic polypeptide

Acini appear around the third month of fetal life.

It is not the purpose of this chapter to deal with insulinomas and gastrinomas. However, their embryologic origin from the ventral and dorsal anlage is discussed by Howard et al. (22). They reported in 1990 that gastrinomas, pancreatic polypeptide-secreting tumors, and somatostatinomas are located to the right of the superior mesentery artery (SMA) 75% of the time, whereas insulinomas and glucagonomas are to the left of the SMA 75% of the time. Because of their findings, the authors suggest the possible embryologic origin of these tumors from the ventral pancreatic anlage (e.g., gastrinoma) and from the dorsal pancreatic anlage (e.g., insulimona).

Similar findings were reported by Sawicki et al. (23) with 47 cases of gastrinomas, of which 85% were located to the right of the SMA. They searched the world's literature and found 10 extrapancreatic cases with 9 of them located on the right side. These authors suggest that the pancreatic and extrapancreatic gastrinomas perhaps have a common origin.

Duodenal wall gastrinomas were reported by Delcore et al. (24). They stated that these are single, small or microscopic, submucosal, located in the proximal duodenum with rare liver metastasis. Usual treatment is by surgical excision.

Critical Events in Development

Rotation and fusion of the pancreatic primordia are the only critical morphologic events in pancreatic development. Malrotation of the ventral primordium in the fifth

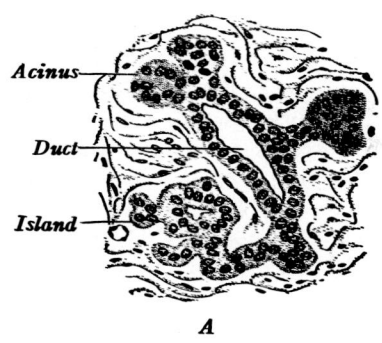
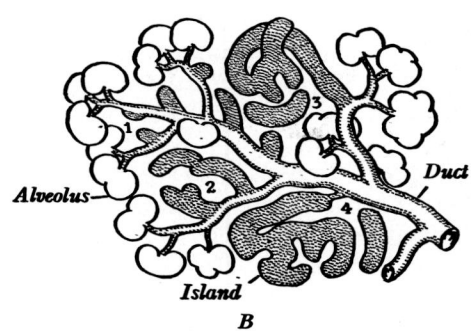

Figure 11.4. Differentiation of the human pancreas. **A**, Section, at 14 weeks, demonstrating the origin of acini and islands from ducts. **B**, Diagram showing four progressive stages (1 to 4) in the organization of islands. (**A**, from Lewis FP. The development of the liver. In: Keibel F, Mall FP, eds. Human embryology. Philadelphia: JB Lippincott, 1912; **B**, from Arey LB. Developmental anatomy. Philadelphia: WB Saunders, 1965.)

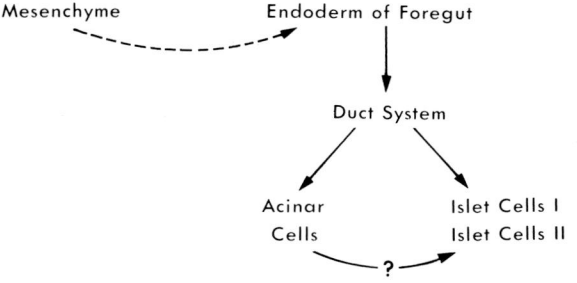

Figure 11.5. Under the influence of local mesenchyme, the foregut endoderm forms the pancreatic duct system, from which will differentiate acinar and islet cells.

week may result in annular pancreas. Variations in the duct system date from the fusion of the dorsal and ventral primordia in the seventh week.

Remember that differentiation of endocrine and exocrine pancreas takes place in early embryonic life. At birth the exocrine pancreas resembles that of the adult from a histologic standpoint. The development of pancreatic enzymes is under the influence of exogenous factors (nutrition) and endogeneous factors such as hormonal (glucocorticoid and thyroxine) and neural agents, according to Lee (25). Lee also reported that there is a hint of the existence of a hypophyseal-hypothalamic-thyroid-adrenal-pancreatic axis in the control of pancreatic exocrine development.

Another interesting study was reported by Jhappan et al. (26) from the National Institutes of Health on why transforming growth factor α (TGF = α) overexpression induces liver neoplasia and abnormal development of the mammary gland and pancreas. The authors stated that the pancreas shows progressive interstitial fibrosis and a florid acinoductular metaplasia during which acinar cells appear to degranulate, dedifferentiate, and assume characteristics of intercalated or centroacinar duct cells.

CONGENITAL ANOMALIES OF THE PANCREAS

Pancreatic anomalies are numerous, and new discoveries of syndromes of embryologic and anatomic entities are

frequent. Consequently, the student of the pancreas is faced with the ever-growing, complex body of knowledge of the pancreas and its associated structures. This abundance of information poses a cumbersome challenge in exposition. We have carefully chosen our topics and understand that some omission is inevitable.

1. Aplasia—hypoplasia
2. Hyperplasia—hypertrophy
3. Dysplasia
4. Variations and anomalies of the ducts
5. Familial pancreatitis
6. Pancreas divisum
7. Annular pancreas
8. Pancreatic gallbladder
9. Rotational anomalies
10. Accesory and heterotopic pancreas
11. Pancreatic cysts
12. Cystic fibrosis (meconium ileus)
13. Arterial, vascular, and lymphatic anomalies

Aplasia—Hypoplasia

If aplasia is failure of development and if agenesis is failure of primordia to form, then both words practically mean the same thing: No pancreatic tissue is present. The word hypoplasia is used here and elsewhere to mean incomplete development.

Total absence of the pancreas (aplasia-agenesis) is a very rare anomaly associated with growth retardation and early death. The gallbladder may be present or absent. Such cases were reported by Mehes et al. and others (27—29).

Absence of islet-cell tissue, even when the pancreas is of normal size, also is accompanied by growth retardation, according to Dodge and Laurence (30).

Wolf et al. (31) reported that maternal insulin does not pass to the fetus through the placenta; therefore, insulin deprivation results from the first trimester onward when fetal islet cell tissue is not present. This deprivation has a direct effect on fetal growth.

The ontogeny of insulin is similar to many other gastrointestinal peptides. It appears approximately at the tenth week of embryonic life and regulates pancreatic exocrine functions, which become abnormal with insulin deficiency.

More frequent than islet-cell agenesis is aplasia of acinar tissue with normal islet cells and normal ductal systems. Whitington (32) believes this defect is part of Schwachman's syndrome (pancreatic insufficiencies, bone marrow dysfunction, metaphyseal dysplasia, and other anomalies), which most likely is an autosomal recessive characteristic. Malnutrition, neutropenia, anemia, and dwarfism are the result of this anomaly. Pancreatic enzymes may help treat the malnutrition, but the bone marrow disease with resultant infections from leukopenia is eventually fatal. Is marrow transplantation of any value here? As far as we have found out, it has never been tried, so we do not know.

Hypoplasia (partial agenesis) is rare incomplete development of the pancreas. Lechner and Read (33) reported the absence of the parts formed from the dorsal primordium. Their patient was diabetic, and most likely the remaining pancreas which appeared normal was quantitatively inadequate. Two cases of partial agenesis of the pancreas in adults were reported by Gilinsky et al. (34).

In the laboratory we have seen only one case of partial pancreatic agenesis, where part of the distal one-fourth of the body, including the tail, was absent. The body of the pancreas was connected to the splenic porta of a grossly normal spleen with a cord-like formation of fibrous tissue that most likely represented the pancreaticosplenic ligament. This structure exists when the tail of the pancreas does not touch the spleen (35). We have seen variations of the uncinate process of the pancreas as follows.

On dissection of 20 cadavers (10 male and 10 female),

the uncinate process was absent in two (one male and one female). In most cases the uncinate process lies between the inferior vena cava and the aorta, covering the superior mesentery vessels superiorly and ventrally. It is the presence or absence of the uncinate process which dictates how much pancreas is removed during partial pancreatectomies.

In our 18 cadavers in which the uncinate process was well developed, the head was small or within normal limits. A big head was noted in the two cases without the uncinate process. Therefore we agree with Fry (36) that, if the uncinate process is present, a 60 to 65% pancreatectomy is done with a Whipple procedure, and with the uncinate process absent, 70 to 80% of pancreas is removed.

Landau and Schiller (37) gave a schematic representation of the approximate percentages of pancreatic resection (Fig. 11.6).

Remember: (*a*) The extent of resection is empiric. (*b*) With division of the neck most likely, 60 to 70% of the pancreas is resected. (*c*) With division at the proximal body to the left of the portal vein above and to the superior mesenteric vein below, approximately 50 to 60% of the pancreas will be resected. (*d*) With an 80% pancreatectomy, the system maintains good exocrine and endocrine activity. (*e*) The ligament of the uncinate process is located at the vicinity of the superior mesenteric vein. If such is the case, the ligament is quite dense, and it fixes the process to the superior mesenteric artery.

Hyperplasia-Hypertrophy

PANCREATIC HYPERPLASIA

This is a rare lesion which manifests itself by severe hypoglycemia caused by hyperinsulinemia immediately after birth. It is part of the general visceromegaly of the Beck-

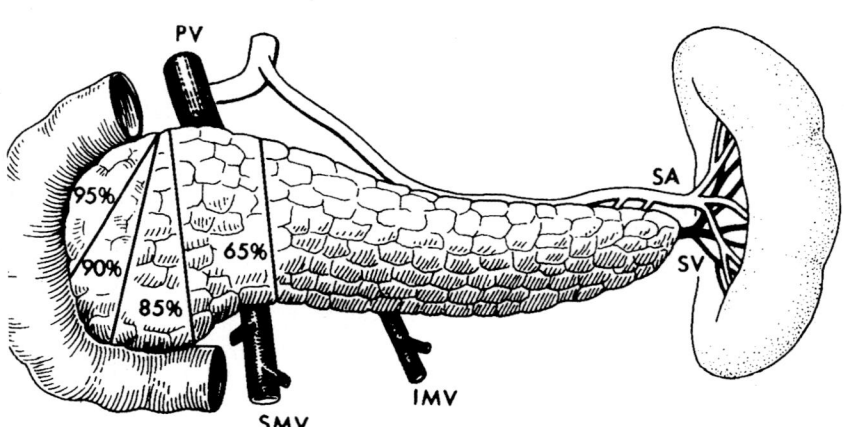

Figure 11.6. *Schematic representation of pancreatic anatomy. Note the approximate percentages of pancreatic resections. (PV, Portal vein; SMV, superior mesenteric vein; IMV, inferior mesenteric vein; SV, splenic vein; SA, splenic* artery.) (From Landau H, Schiller M. Persistent hyperinsulinemic hypoglycemia of infancy and childhood. In: Schiller M, ed. Pediatric surgery of the liver, pancreas, and spleen. Philadelphia: WB Saunders, 1991:187–201.)

with-Wiedemann syndrome and is associated with a high birth weight, enlarged tongue, and umbilical hernia. The hypoglycemia can be controlled by dietary regimen. Partial pancreatectomy may be necessary in some patients (38).

ISLET CELL DYSMATURATION SYNDROME

Islet cell dysmaturation syndrome (ICDS) encompasses the causes of infantile hyperinsulinemic hypoglycemia; histologically, it has been described as islet cell hyperplasia, pancreatic adenomatosis, nesidioblastosis, and by other terms (39, 40). It manifests itself as persistent hypoglycemia in neonates, resulting in jitteriness, lethargy, and seizures. The diagnosis is established by confirming the presence of paradoxic hyperinsulinism in a patient who is persistently hypoglycemic. Histologically, there is diffuse involvement of the pancreas with poor delineation and random scattering of the various endocrine cells into the acinar portion of the gland (41). The normal segregation of endocrine cells into islets is not present; insulin secreting β cells are present within the pancreatic ducts (42).

Emergency treatment is required to prevent the devastating effects of hypoglycemia on the central nervous system of the infant (43). A central line is placed to provide the infant with high concentrations of glucose to maintain normal glycemia as the workup is in progress. Medical treatment consists of diazoxide to a maximum of 20 mg/kg body weight/day. If this regimen fails to control the symptoms within several days, surgery is indicated (42, 43).

At the time of the operation, if a distinct adenoma is encountered, a subtotal pancreatectomy with preservation of the spleen is indicated. This condition can sometimes be found in older infants and children but is extremely rare in neonates. In patients with diffuse glandular involvement—and particularly in neonates—a near total or "95%" pancreatectomy with preservation of the spleen and the small amount of pancreatic tissue adjacent to the intrapancreatic portion of the common bile duct is performed (39–43). Anything less than this results in a high recurrence rate and the need for additional medical and/or surgical therapy. Another cause for operative failure is failure to excise ectopic pancreatic tissue containing the same abnormal histologic condition as the native gland (44).

A large pancreatic head when the uncinate process is absent should not be considered part of this syndrome but rather a compensatory phenomenon.

The authors do not know under which subdivision to classify total or partial hypertrophy or hyperplasia. It is unclear whether these "anomalies" are hyperplasia or dysplasia.

Weidenheim et al. (45) reported hyperinsulinemic hypoglycemia in five adults with islet cell hyperplasia and degranulation of exocrine cells of the pancreas. They suggest that the spectrum of islet cell hyperplasia and acinar cell change is due to neoformation of islet cells from the ducts, a factor of unknown etiology.

Pancreatic islet cell hyperplasia was reported by Murata (46) in association with bilateral nephroblastomatosis and several other anomalies. Hyperplasia of the endocrine pancreas was reported in connection with Perlman syndrome (familial renal dysplasia, Wilms' tumor, fetal gigantism, mental retardation, and multiple congenital anomalies) (47).

Dysplasia

With dysplasia, there are alterations in the size, shape, or organization of parts, resulting in defective pancreatic development.

In 1989 enlargement of the pancreatic head in patients with pancreas divisum was reported by Soulen et al. (48). Such variation could confuse the radiologist about whether a pathologic condition (carcinoma) is present in that area.

Pancreatic pseudotumor in pancreas divisum was also noted by Silverman et al. (49). Pancreatic, hepatic, and renal dysplasia were reported by Carles et al. (50), who found that the pancreas had dilated ducts, cysts, and fibrosis.

Kikuchi et al. (51) described a bifid tail of the pancreas with a gastric submucosal tumor in one of the tails. Anomalous drainage of the common bile duct into the fourth portion of the duodenum was found by Doty et al. (52) in two patients. The pancreatic duct was connected with the common bile duct by a long common channel.

The Pancreatic Ducts

The complicated anatomy and embryology of the pancreatic ducts with their anomalies and variations is examined together with the common bile duct (third and fourth parts) and the duodenum.

Embryologically, anatomically, and surgically, these three entities form an inseparable unit. Their relations and blood supply make it impossible for the surgeon to remove completely the head of the pancreas without removing the duodenum and the distal part of the common bile duct. Here embryology and anatomy conspire to produce some of the most difficult surgery of the abdominal cavity. The only alternate procedure, the so-called 95% pancreatectomy, leaves a rim of pancreas along the medial border of the duodenum to preserve the duodenal blood supply.

The common bile duct may be divided into four parts: supraduodenal, retroduodenal, pancreatic, and intramural. It is the third and fourth portions that concern us here.

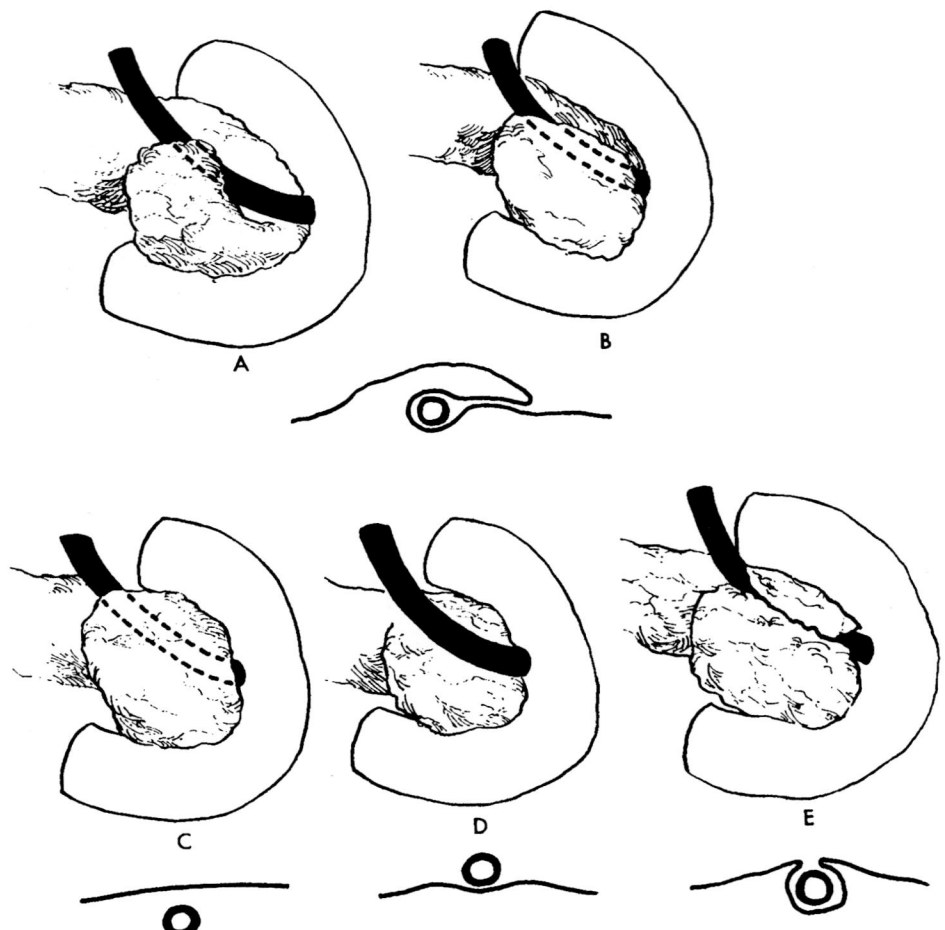

Figure 11.7. Five variations of the relation of the third part of the common bile duct to the pancreas. In the most frequently encountered condition, **A** and **B**, the bile duct is partially covered by a tongue of pancreatic tissue (44%). It is completely covered (**C**) in 30%; uncovered on the posterior surface of the pancreas (**D**) in 16.5%; and covered by two tongues of pancreas (**E**) in 9%. (From Smanio T. Varying relations of the common bile duct with the posterior face of the pancreas in negroes and white persons. J Int Coll Surg 1954;22:150.)

PANCREATIC (THIRD) PART OF THE COMMON BILE DUCT

From the upper margin of the head of the pancreas to the point of entrance into the duodenum, the course of the pancreatic portion of the common bile duct is downward and to the right, posterior to the pancreas. From a series of 200 specimens, Smanio (53) described five patterns in the relation of pancreas and common bile duct (Fig. 11.7).

1. A lingula of pancreatic tissue from the caudal side partially covers the duct (42.5%) (Fig. 11.7, *A* and *B*).
2. A lingula from the caudal side completely covers the duct (30%) (Fig. 11.7, *C*).
3. There is no covering pancreatic tissue. The duct lies in an open groove in the pancreas, covered only by a membrane derived from the primitive mesoduodenum (16.5%) (Fig. 11.7, *D*).

4. Two lingulas, one from each side, cover the duct (9%) (Fig. 11.6, *E*).
5. Other variations exist (2%).

We have seen a case in which the common bile duct was completely extrapancreatic and close to the renal vein. A prepancreatic common bile duct was reported in seven cases among 550 cadavers examined by various workers (54).

Lytle (55) has observed that the pancreatic groove or tunnel occupied by the duct may be palpated by passing the fingers of the left hand behind the second part of the duodenum after mobilization with the Kocher maneuver. The groove is located in front of the right renal vein.

The posterior superior pancreaticoduodenal artery "double crosses" the third portion of the common bile duct—first by passing ventral to the duct at the point of the origin from the gastroduodenal artery and second by passing dorsal to the duct a few millimeters above the entrance of the duct into the duodenal wall. The duct may be in intimate contact with the duodenum for 8 to 22 mm before entering the wall (56).

INTRAMURAL (FOURTH) PART OF THE COMMON BILE DUCT AND PANCREATIC DUCT

The main pancreatic duct passes obliquely through the duodenal wall together with the fourth portion of the common bile duct.

The anatomic entities in this region are the intramural portions of the common bile duct and the main pancreatic duct, major duodenal papilla, ampulla of Vater, if present, and the sphincter of Oddi. Taken together they form the *Vaterian system* of Dowdy (57). The term expresses the anatomic and surgical unity of these structures, but it has no functional significance.

As the common bile duct enters the duodenal wall, it suddenly or gradually decreases in diameter from about 10 to 5.4 mm (58). Within the wall the length averages 15 mm (59).

The main pancreatic duct enters the duodenal wall caudal to the bile duct. Dowdy (57) states that it, like the common duct, decreases in diameter as it enters the duodenal wall. He reports an average decrease from 2 to 1.4 mm in diameter.

The bile and pancreatic ducts usually lie side by side, having a common adventitia for several millimeters. The septum between them becomes reduced to a membrane of mucosa before the actual confluence of the two channels is reached.

Small pancreatic ducts entering the intrapancreatic and intraduodenal portions of the common bile duct as well as opening directly into the duodenum near the papilla have been described by Gross (60). These might be a source of pancreatic juice leakage after a 95% pancreatectomy.

MAJOR DUODENAL PAPILLA

Although this structure bears the name of Abraham Vater (61), it was first illustrated by Gottfried Bidloo (62) of the Hague in 1685 and should have been called the papilla of Bidloo.

The papilla is on the posteromedial wall of the second portion of the duodenum to the right of the second or third lumbar vertebra. Very rarely, the papilla may be in the third portion of the duodenum (63). On endoscopy the papilla lie to the right of the spine at the level of the second lumbar vertebra in 85% of the cases of Cotton (64) and 75% of the cases of Varley (65). It was at the level of the third lumbar vertebra in 57% of autopsy specimens examined by Kreel and Sandin (63). The distance from the pylorus varies from 7 to 10 cm, with extremes of 1.5 to 12 cm. In the presence of inflammation of the cap or

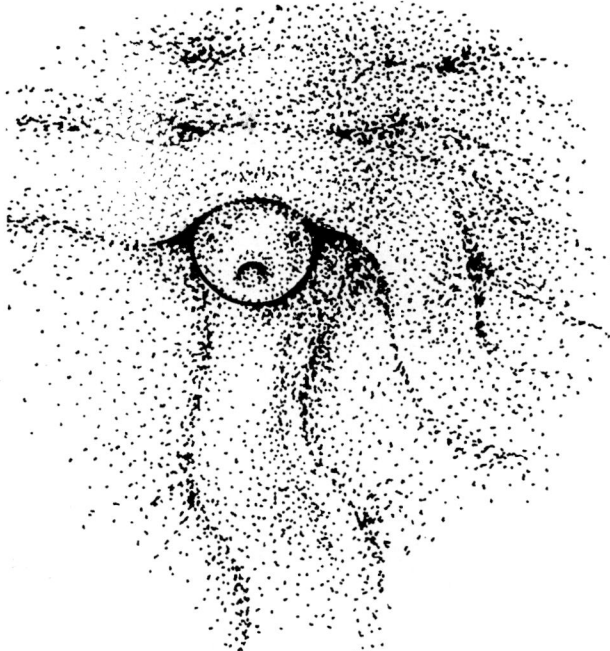

Figure 11.8. The T arrangement of duodenal mucosal folds indicating the site of the major duodenal papilla. In some cases a mucosal fold may cover the orifice of the papilla. No such arrangement marks the site of the minor papilla. The major papilla is rarely this obvious. (From Skandalakis JE, Gray SW, Rowe JS, Skandalakis LJ. Anatomical complications of pancreatic surgery. Contemp Surg 1979;15(11):35.)

the postbulbar area of the duodenum, the distance will be decreased.

Viewed from the mucosal surface of the duodenum, the papilla is found where a longitudinal mucosal fold or frenulum meets a transverse mucosal fold to form a T (Fig. 11.8). This was beautifully illustrated in a plate by Santorini (66) in 1775 and reproduced by Livingston (67). Dowdy and his colleagues (59) stated that the papilla was "prominent, easily found" in 60% of their specimens. Remember that these workers had more experience than most surgeons. There are several practical considerations:

1. Too much lateral or distal traction on the opened duodenum may erase the folds and distort the T.
2. The papilla may be covered by a transverse fold. It will be revealed by gently elevating the fold.
3. If the T is not apparent and the papilla cannot be palpated, the common bile duct must be probed from above.
4. A duodenal diverticulum may lie very close to the papilla. This can produce difficulties for the surgeon or the endoscopist.

AMPULLA (OF VATER)

The ampulla is a dilation of the common pancreaticobiliary channel within the papilla and below the junction of

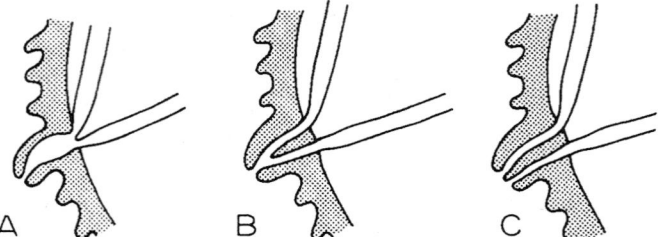

Figure 11.9. Diagram of the variations in the relation of the common bile duct and main pancreatic duct at the duodenal papilla. **A,** Minimal absorption of the ducts into the duodenal wall during embryonic development; an ampulla is present. **B,** Partial absorption of the common channel; no true ampulla is present. **C,** Maximum absorption of the ducts into the duodenum. Separate orifices are on the papilla, with no ampulla. (From Skandalakis JE, Gray SW, Rowe JS, Skandalakis LJ. Anatomical complications of pancreatic surgery. Contemp Surg 1979;15(11):36.)

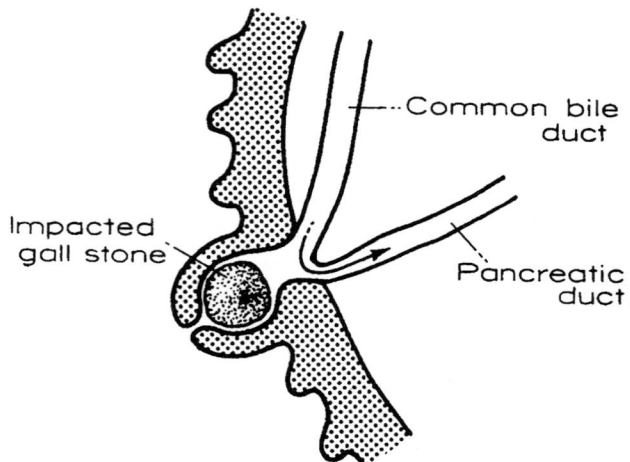

Figure 11.10. The effect of a gallstone impacted in the duodenal papilla. The *arrow* represents the reflux of bile into the pancreatic duct. (From Skandalakis JE, Gray SW, Rowe JS, Skandalakis LJ. Anatomical complications of pancreatic surgery. Contemp Surg 1979;15(11):36.)

the two ducts (Fig. 11.9, *A*). If a septum is present as far as the duodenal orifice, the ampulla does not exist (Fig. 11.9, *C*).

Michels (54) collected the findings of 25 investigators in 2500 specimens and concluded that an ampulla was present in 63%. By definition, an ampulla was said to be present if the edge of the septum between the two ducts fell short of the tip of the papilla. Actual measurements of the distance between septal edge and papillary tip range from 1 to 14 mm, with 75% being 5 mm or less (68).

Purists would require a dilation of the common channel to apply the term *ampulla*. Where the common channel is less than 5 mm long, there is little or no dilation (69). In such specimens, the presence of a true ampulla becomes a matter of opinion (Fig. 11.9, *B*). We agree with Michels (54) that the following classification is the most useful:

> *Type 1:* The pancreatic duct opens into the common bile duct at a variable distance from the opening in the major duodenal papilla. The common channel may or may not be dilated (85%).
> *Type 2:* The pancreatic and bile ducts open close to one another but separately on the major duodenal papilla (5%).
> *Type 3:* The pancreatic and bile ducts open into the duodenum at separate points (9%).

A true dilated ampulla is present in about 75% of individuals with type 1 and is absent in types 2 and 3.

This variation in the distance between the pancreaticobiliary junction and the duodenal lumen is the result of developmental processes (10). In the embryo, the main pancreatic duct arises as a branch of the common bile duct, which in turn arises from the duodenum. Growth of the duodenum absorbs the proximal bile duct up to its junction with the pancreatic duct. When the resorption is minimal, there is a long ampulla and the junction of the

ducts is high in the duodenal wall (type 1) or even extramural. With increased resorption of the terminal bile duct, the junction lies closer to the duodenal orifice and the ampulla is shortened. The maximum resorption results in separate orifices for the main pancreatic duct and the common bile duct (type 3).

PANCREATITIS AND AMPULLARY LITHIASIS

Opie (70) first expressed the idea that a gallstone impacted in the papilla at the duodenal orifice would, in the presence of a long ampulla, permit bile to back up into the pancreatic duct and produce pancreatitis (Fig. 11.10). Dragstedt and his colleagues (71) believed that as many as 10% of cases of pancreatitis were the result of such impacted gallstones. This "common channel" theory was revived by Doubilet and Mulholland (72). Spasm of the papillary sphincter (sphincter of Oddi) as well as ampullary lithiasis was implicated in biliary reflux into the pancreatic duct system.

Silen (73) questioned the frequency of this source of pancreatitis, pointing out that only 18% of patients with gallstone pancreatitis have choledocholithiasis. He also observed that pancreatic secretory pressure is usually higher than that of the liver. Although reflux pancreatitis is a real condition, the frequency of its origin from ampullary obstruction by stone or muscular spasm is still controversial.

SPHINCTER OF BOYDEN

Like the papilla of Vater, the sphincter of Oddi at the duodenal end of the pancreatic and common bile ducts is misnamed. By priority of description, it should have been named for Francis Glisson who in 1654 described annular

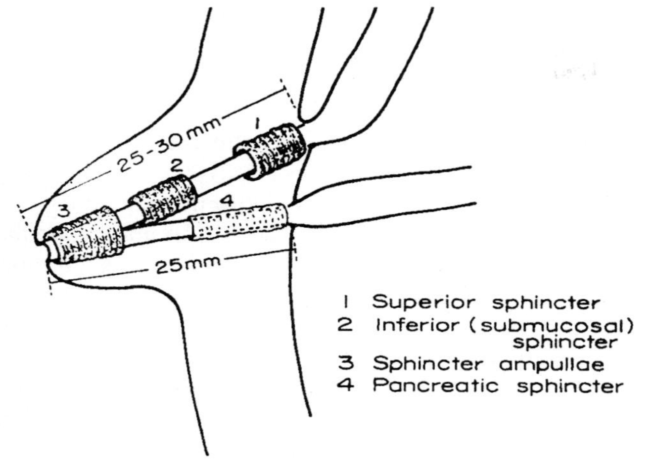

Figure 11.11. Diagrammatic representation of the four sphincters making up the sphincter of Boyden: *1*, superior choledochal sphincter; *2*, inferior choledochal sphincter; *3*, sphincter ampullae (papillae); and *4*, sphincter pancreaticus. The measurements are from White (White TT. Surgical anatomy of the pancreas. In: Carey LC, ed. The pancreas. St Louis: CV Mosby, 1973; from Skandalakis JE, Gray SW, Rowe JS, Skandalakis L J. Anatomical complications of the pancreas. Contemp Surg 1979;15(11):37.)

fibers around the whole of the intramural portion of the bile duct. He believed they guarded the opening against reflux of duodenal contents. Glisson's account of his work is found in Boyden (74). Jones (75) would call the entire sphincter complex the sphincter of Boyden, in recognition of his contributions to the anatomy of this region. We agree.

The present concept is that there is a complex of several sphincters, composed of circular or spiral smooth muscle fibers, surrounding the intramural part of the common bile duct, the main pancreatic duct, and the ampulla (if present). The sphincteric complex has a separate embryonic origin from that of the duodenal musculature, and it is functionally separate from it.

While the anatomy has been well described by Boyden (76, 77) and others, the terminology is unsettled. Boyden (76) defined three entities: sphincter choledochus, sphincter pancreaticus, and muscularis proprius ampullae. In a subsequent publication, Boyden (77) modified this classification and described four sphincteric elements (Fig. 11.11).

The total length of the sphincteric complex may be as little as 6 mm or as great as 30 mm, depending on the obliquity of the path taken by the bile and pancreatic ducts through the duodenal wall (75). In some cases the sphincter may extend beyond the duodenal wall into the pancreatic portion of the bile duct (78). This is important to know when complete destruction of the sphincteric apparatus is attempted.

Complete anatomic transection of the sphincter may not be necessary to obtain satisfactory physiologic results. Incision by 5-mm steps and testing with a suitable dilator will limit the incision to the shortest length necessary to achieve the desired results.

Fischer and McSherry (79) warned that endoscopic papillotomy to divide the sphincter of Oddi is frequently unnecessary and not without danger. The current mortality is 1.5%. They believe that papillary stenoses are much less frequent than are endoscopic papillotomies to relieve them.

MINOR DUODENAL PAPILLA

The minor duodenal papilla is located about 2 cm cranially and slightly anterior to the major papilla. It is smaller, and its site does not have the characteristic mucosal folds that mark the site of the major papilla.

Baldwin (80) found the minor papilla to be present in all of a series of 100 specimens. More recently in a sample of the same size, Dowdy et al. (59) could find no minor papilla in 18 specimens. One concludes that some papillae may be difficult to identify even if present.

An excellent landmark is the gastroduodenal artery, under which is the accessory pancreatic duct (duct of Santorini) and the minor papilla. During gastrectomy, duodenal dissection should end proximal to this artery. This becomes especially important in those few patients in whom the accessory duct carries the major drainage of the pancreas.

In many cases the minor papilla contains no duct or only a tiny, tortuous channel opening into the base of an intestinal crypt. A true sphincter (of Helly [81]) is only occasionally present, usually at the point of the entrance of the duct into the muscularis of the duodenum.

PANCREATIC DUCTS

Anatomy and Variations. The main pancreatic duct (duct of Wirsung) arises in the tail of the pancreas in the left upper quadrant at the level of the 12th thoracic vertebra. Occasionally, two small ducts arise and join to form the main duct (82). Through the tail and body of the pancreas, the duct lies midway between the superior and inferior margins and slightly more posterior than anterior. The main duct and the accessory duct lie anterior to the major pancreatic vessels. Pathologic ducts are readily palpated and opened from the anterior surface.

The main duct crosses the spine, almost always between the 12th thoracic and the second lumbar vertebrae (83–84). In more than half of subjects, the crossing is at the first lumbar vertebra (65).

In the tail and body of the pancreas, from 15 to 20 short tributaries enter the duct at almost right angles (82). The superior and inferior tributaries tend to alternate with one another. In addition, the main duct may receive a longer tributary, draining the uncinate process, and in some subjects the accessory pancreatic duct in the head empties into the main duct). Small tributary ducts in the head may open directly into the intrahepatic portion of the common bile duct, according to Gross (60).

On reaching the head of the pancreas, the main duct may or may not join the accessory duct of Santorini. The main duct turns caudally and slightly posterior. At the level of the major papilla, the duct takes a horizontal turn to join the caudal surface of the common bile duct and enters the wall of the duodenum, usually at the level of the 2nd lumbar vertebra.

The accessory pancreatic duct (duct of Santorini) may drain the anterosuperior portion of the head of the pancreas either into the duodenum at the minor papilla or into the main pancreatic duct.

Because of the developmental origin of the two pancreatic ducts, a number of variations are encountered. Some are found more frequently than others; all can be considered normal.

In Figure 11.12 are examples of persistence of the accessory duct and progressive suppression of the main duct (Fig. 11.12, B to D). The usual configuration is seen in Figures 11.12, A, and 11.13, A. The accessory duct (Santorini) is smaller than the proximal main duct (Wirsung) and opens into the duodenum on the minor papilla. Figure 11.13, B to E, shows examples of progressive suppression of the accessory duct. Figure 11.13, A to C, accounts for about 90% of cases. The absence of an accessory duct opening into the duodenum has been associated with duodenal ulcers. Reich (85) suggested that the absence of accessory ductal secretion may decrease the alkalinity of the duodenum.

In about 10% of cases (86) there is no connection between the accessory duct and the main duct (Figs. 11.12, D, and 11.13, D). This is important to remember when contrast medium is injected into the main duct.

In about 30% of individuals there is no minor papilla (Fig. 11.13, B, C and E). In some subjects having a minor papilla, the terminal portion of the accessory duct is so small and tortuous that it cannot permit the passage of any quantity of fluid. Three papillae have been seen (Fig. 11.14, A and D) (68, 87). The curious loop in the main pancreatic duct (Fig. 11.15, B) was found in 3 out of 76 specimens examined by Baldwin (80). An identical case was reported by Rienhoff and Pickrell (68).

Rare anomalous patterns have been reported (Fig. 11.15, E); Rienhoff and Pickrell (68) mention a case in which three ducts opened into separate papillae.

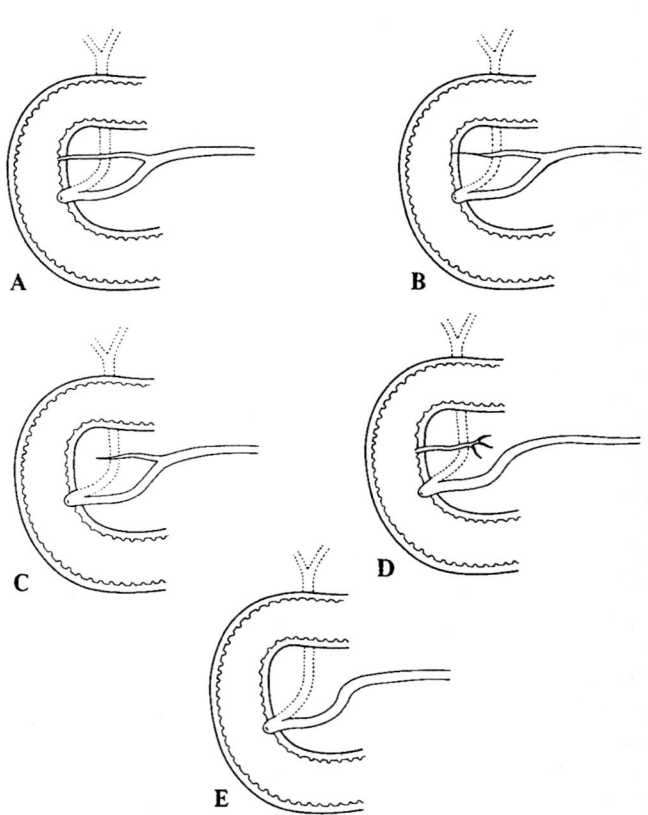

Figure 11.13. Variations of the pancreatic ducts. Degrees of suppression of the accessory duct. **A,** Both ducts open into the duodenum. **B,** The accessory duct ends blindly in the duodenal wall. **C,** The accessory duct ends blindly before reaching the duodenum. **D,** The accessory duct has no connection with the main duct. **E,** The accessory duct is absent. Type **A** is present in 60%; type **C** is present in 30%. (From Skandalakis JE, Gray SW, Rowe JS, Skandalakis L J. Anatomical complications of the pancreas. Contemp Surg 1979;15(11):27.)

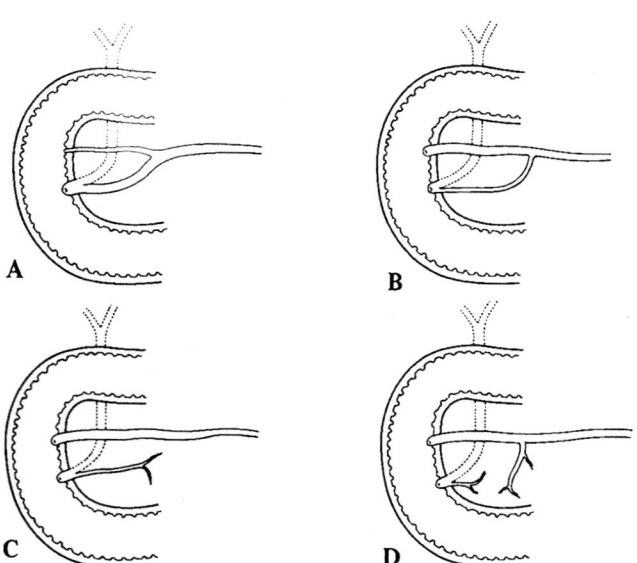

Figure 11.12. Degrees of suppression of the main duct. **A,** Both ducts open into the duodenum. **B,** The main duct is smaller than the accessory duct. **C,** The main duct has no connection with the larger accessory duct. **D,** The main duct is short or absent. The accessory duct drains almost the whole pancreas. Types **C** and **D** are present in 10%. (From Skandalakis JE, Gray SW, Rowe JS, Skandalakis L J. Surgical anatomy of the pancreas. Contemp Surg 1979;15(11):37.)

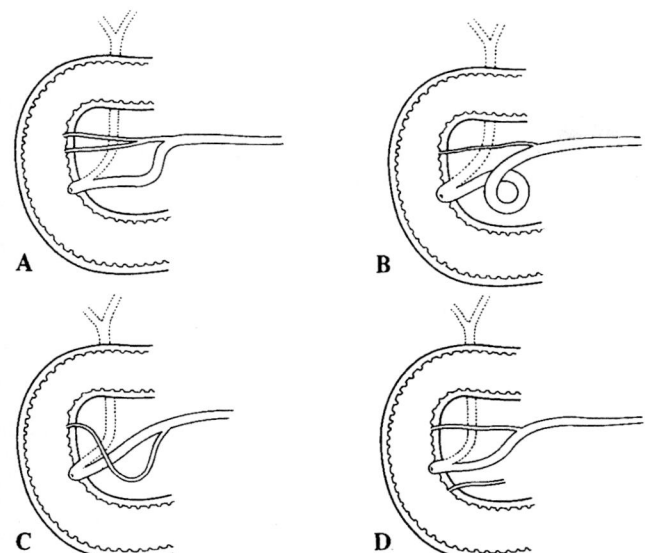

Figure 11.14. Variation of the pancreatic ducts: rare forms. **A**, Duplication of the accessory duct. **B**, Loop in the main duct. **C**, Anomalous course of accessory duct. **D**, Triple pancreatic ducts. (From Skandalakis JE, Gray SW, Rowe JS, Skandalakis L J. Anatomical complications of the pancreas. Contemp Surg 1979;15(11):40.)

In addition to the major drainage system, a number of small ducts from the head of the pancreas enter the pancreatic duct, the common bile duct, or the duodenum (whichever is closest) in the papillary region. They are frequently difficult to distinguish from ducts of Brunner's glands, which also open into the duodenal crypts. The lobules drained by these ducts often lie within the duodenal muscularis or submucosa or within the wall of the common duct. They were first observed by Opie (88) in 1903 and have been studied in detail by Loquvam and Russell (89) and Cross (90). Cross emphasized the structural identity of the pancreatic ducts with the common ducts and their tendency to receive small pancreatic ducts. The ducts emptying directly into the duodenum may be "captured" lateral branches of the pancreatic diverticulum. More probably, they may represent pancreatization of adjacent Brunner's glands.

An apparently unique anomaly has been reported by Palileo and Gallager (91) in which the pancreatic duct broke into more than 20 small ducts before entering the duodenal lumen (Fig. 11.16). Because the patient was 65 years of age, it is possible that these represented adaptation of the previously described small pancreatic ducts, following destruction of the main channel by disease.

Another anomaly currently receiving mention is the anomalous union of the pancreaticobiliary ductal system, since it is incriminated as the etiologic factor of congenital dilation of the hepatic ducts. A great number of papers on this subject are published yearly from Japan. In 1990

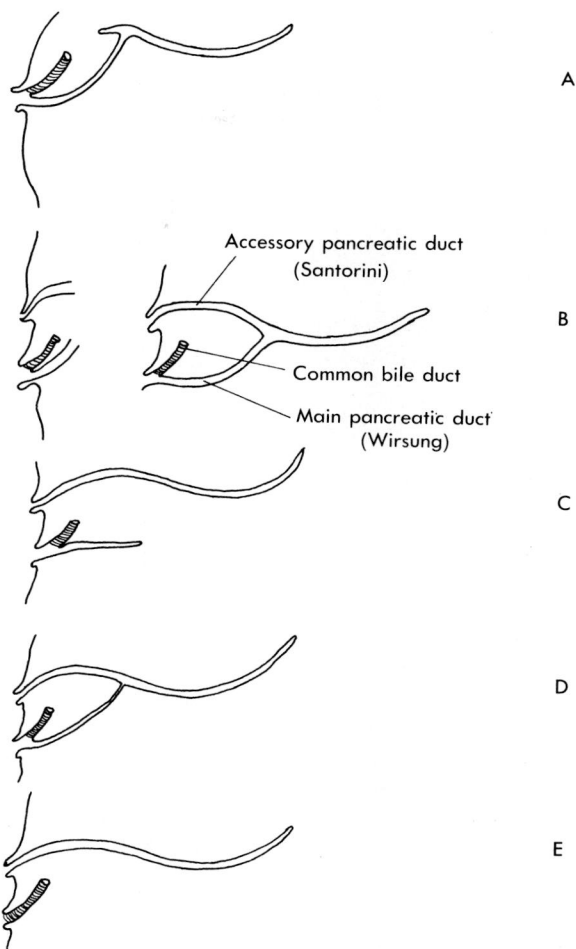

Figure 11.15. Variations of the pancreatic ducts. **A**, The dorsal duct has lost its connection with the duodenum and drains by an anastomosis into the ventral duct that joins the common bile duct as it enters the duodenum (about 20%). **B**, Persistence of the proximal portion of the dorsal duct. Its orifice may be normal or stenosed (about 70%). **C**, Persistence of the embryonic duct system with no connection between the two ducts (about 10%). **D**, Full-sized dorsal duct with hypoplastic ventral duct (rare). **E**, Absence of the ventral duct (rare).

Uetsuji et al. (92) reported a case of anomalous choledochopancreatic ductal junction with carcinoma of the gallbladder and gallbladder duct. A similar case was reported by Ohta et al. (93). Kato et al. (94) stated that congenital biliary dilation is secondary to anomalous junction of the pancreaticobiliary ductal system, which is frequently complicated by biliary tract cancer.

Dimensions: Length, Width, and Capacity of the Pancreatic Ducts. The greatest diameter of the pancreatic duct is at the head of the pancreas, just before the duct enters the duodenal wall. From this diameter, there is gradual tapering of the duct toward the tail. Like the bile duct, the pancreatic duct becomes constricted as it enters the wall of the duodenum.

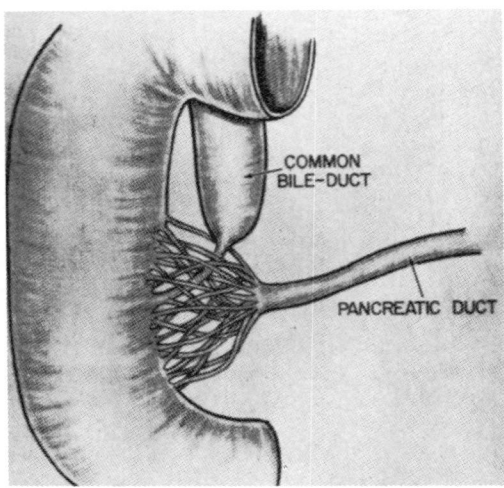

Figure 11.16. Diagrammatic representation of a unique arrangement of the structures in the papilla of Vater, as reconstructed from serial sections. (From Palileo LG, Gallager HS. Anomalous termination of pancreatic duct. Arch Pathol 1961;71:381–383.)

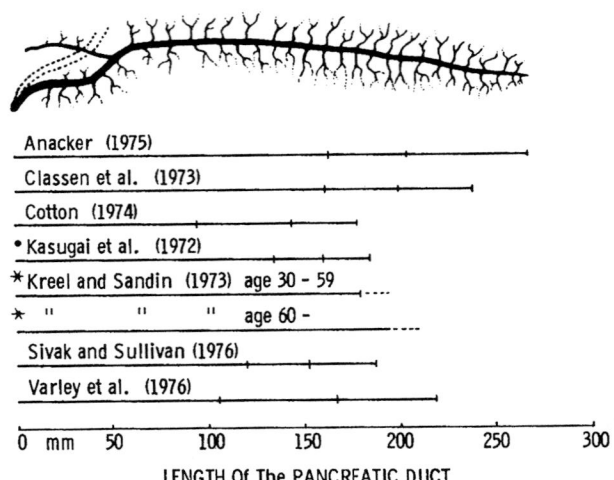

Figure 11.17. Length of the main pancreatic duct as reported by several authors (From Skandalakis JE, Gray SW, Rowe JS, Skandalakis LJ. Anatomical complications of the pancreas. Contemp Surg 1979;15(12):21.)

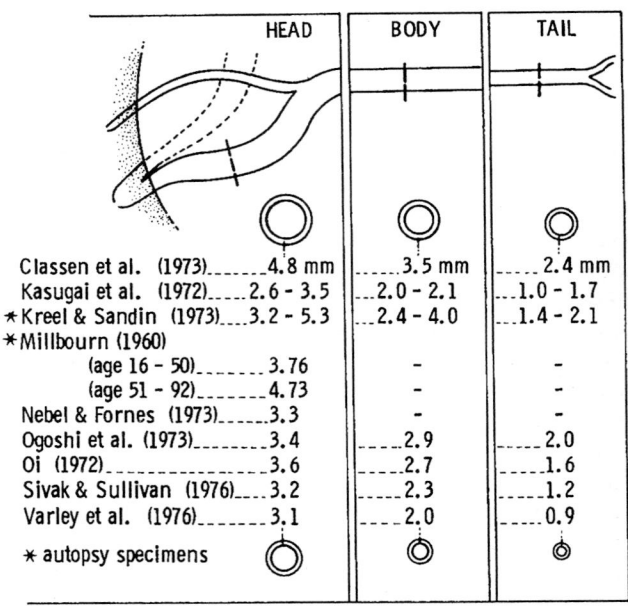

Figure 11.18. Diameter of the main pancreatic duct in the head, body, and tail as reported by several authors. (From Skandalakis JE, Gray SW, Rowe JS, Skandalakis LJ. Anatomical complications of the pancreas. Contemp Surg 1979;15(12):22.)

The use of retrograde pancreatic endoscopy has made the determination of the length, diameter, and capacity of the pancreatic duct system of considerable importance. Although the results obtained by various workers do not all agree, most of the differences are less than the range of individual differences in the same series. Some published values are shown in Figures 11.17 and 11.18. The diameter of the pancreatic duct increases with the age of the subject (95, 96), and there is no sex difference.

Kasugai and his colleagues (96) found that 2 to 3 ml of contrast medium will fill the main pancreatic duct in the living patient, and 7 to 10 ml will fill the branches and the smaller ducts. In autopsy specimens, Trapnell and Howard (97) found 0.5 to 1.0 ml sufficient to fill the duct system.

Familial Pancreatitis

Freud et al. (98) presented the third reported case in Western literature of simultaneous familial pancreatitis in 9-year-old identical twin sisters. These authors stated that the etiology and hereditary properties are not well defined, but both girls had irregular pancreatic ducts.

Makela and Aarimaa (99) reported 500 cases of pancreatitis with 100 in family members. We agree with the authors about the enigmatic etiology of the disease despite the evidence of abnormal pancreatic ducts with strictures, dilation, and chain of lakes.

Pancreas Divisum (Isolated Ventral Pancreas)

Disappearance of the ventral mesentery and rotation of the ventral pancreatic primordium result in fusion of the dorsal and ventral primordia and the rearrangement of their ducts. Persistance of the distal two-thirds of the dorsal duct and proximal portion of the ventral duct is the usual configuration. The ventral duct joins the common bile duct on the major duodenal papilla; the dorsal duct may persist to reach the minor duodenal papilla. If both ducts persist without a connection between, the configu-

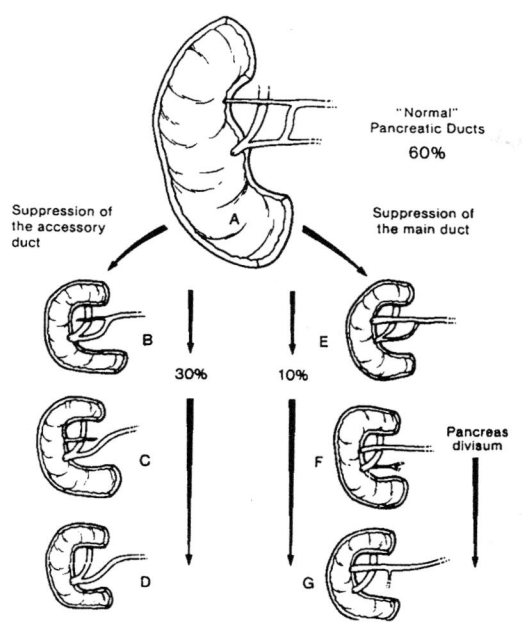

Figure 11.19. Diagram of variations of the pancreatic ducts. **A**, Usual configuration (60%). **B** to **D**, Progressive suppression of the accessory duct (30%). **E** to **G**, Progressive suppression of the main duct (10%). **F**, "Pancreas divisum." (From Skandalakis JE, Gray SW, Rowe JS, Skandalakis L J. Anatomical complications of the pancreas. Contemp Surg 1979;15:17.)

ration is the "pancreas divisum" of U.S. authors and the "isolated ventral pancreas" of British authors (Fig. 11.19, *F*). This configuration is found in from 4 to 11% of cadavers and in 3.25% of patients undergoing endoscopic retrograde cholangiopancreatography (ERCP). The 3.25% figure may be too low since the ERCP procedure does not identify total absence of the dorsal duct. However, such patients undergoing ERCP are a selected group, and it might not be right to infer this data to the general population.

Several investigators (100–103) suggested that those patients with pancreas divisum are more likely to get pancreatic disease than other patients, but this relationship was denied by Mitchell et al. (104). In their examinations of 449 patients undergoing ERCP, 21 (4.7%) were found to have an isolated ventral pancreas. Their study showed that the rate of occurrence of pancreatitis (four patients, or 19%) in the group of patients with nonfusion of the pancreatic ducts was parallel to that found in the group of patients with a normally fused duct system (116 patients, or 27%). Thus it was their opinion that nonfusion of the pancreatic ducts was not a cause of pancreatitis.

When a surgeon assumes that recurrent acute pancreatitis in patients with pancreas divisum may be the result of stenosis at the minor papilla, then sphincteroplasty to enlarge the opening should be attempted. Rusnak et al. (105) presented 11 patients with pancreas divisum and

associated pancreatitis. Nine of these patients were reported to be asymptomatic after surgical decompression of the dorsal pancreatic duct.

Madura (106) presented 30 patients diagnosed by ERCP as having pancreas divisum and advised sphincteroplasty of both major and minor ampullae plus cholecystectomy. Gregg et al. (107) performed sphincteroplasty on both papillae in 19 patients with pancreas divisum. Pancreatitis caused by congenital anomalies of the pancreatic ducts was reported by Leese et al. (108).

Agha and Williams (109) reported complete duplication of the ventral pancreatic ductal systems in two patients. Thirty cases of nonfusion of the dorsal and ventral pancreatic ducts were reported by Oi (110). Recurrent acute pancreatitis associated with pancreas divisum was reported by Reshef et al. (111).

An obstructing pseudocyst of the duct of Santorini in pancreas divisum was reported by Browder et al. (112).

Annular Pancreas

ANATOMY

An annular pancreas consists of a thin, flat band of pancreatic tissue surrounding the second part of the duodenum and continuing, usually without demarcation, into the head of the pancreas on either side (Fig. 11.20). The tissue of the annulus is histologically normal, containing both acini and islets. The pancreatic tissue may penetrate the muscularis of the duodenum (113), or it may be free enough to lift away from the duodenal surface. A large duct usually is present; it connects with the duct of Wirsung or, less often, opens either independently into the common duct or by several orifices into the duodenum (114) (Fig. 11.21).

ASSOCIATED ANOMALIES

Seventy percent of infants with annular pancreas have other anomalies (115–117). Stenosis or atresia of the duodenum at the site of the annulus is present in about 40%, and Down's syndrome is present in about 16%. Malrotation of the gut is common. Tracheoesophageal fistula has been found in 9%, and congenital heart defects in 7% (116). Among 10 patients of Gross (60), only one had no other defect.

In Raffensperger's study of 24 patients with annular pancreas (118), 18 had severe associated congenital anomalies including Down's syndrome, tracheoesophageal fistula, and cyanotic congenital heart disease. Annular pancreas also has been associated with congenital absence of the gallbladder and obstruction of the common bile duct (119).

Kirillova et al. (120) found two cases of annular pancreas with duodenal stenosis among 3307 induced abortuses of 5 to 12 weeks. This incidence is greater than the

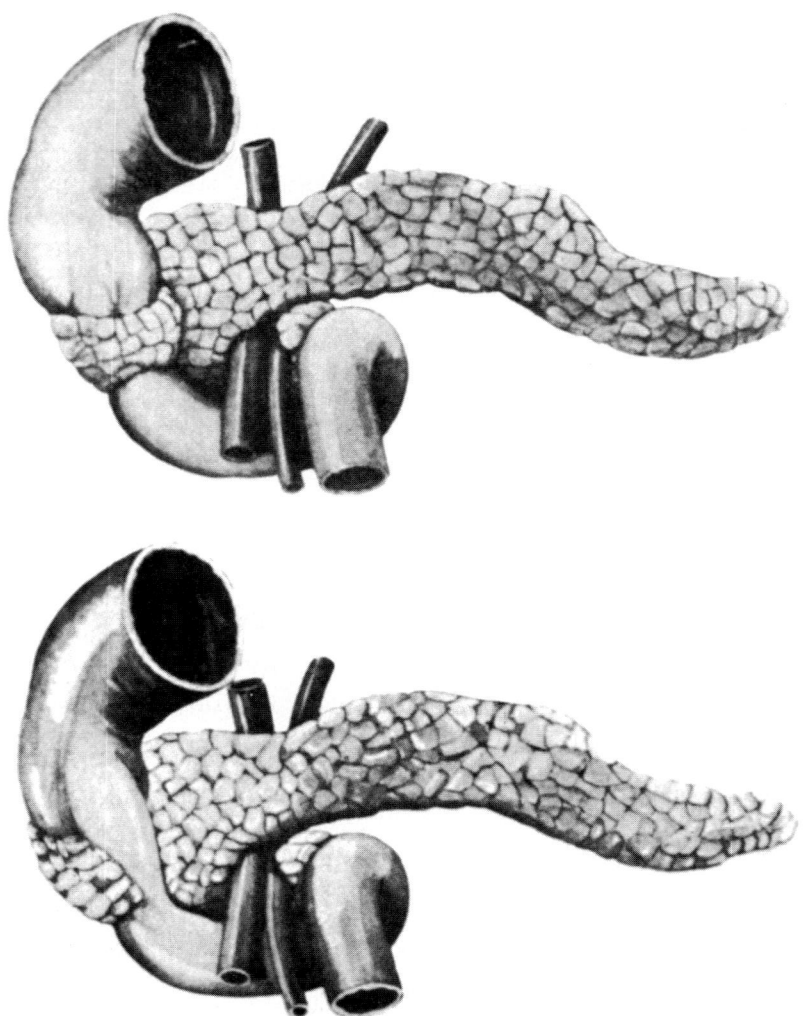

Figure 11.20. Annular pancreas. **A**, A broad ring of pancreatic tissue, continuous with the head of the pancreas, completely surrounds the second part of the duodenum. **B**, Less frequently, the annulus is incomplete. (From Théodoridès T. Pancréas annulaire. J Chir (Paris) 1964;87:445–462.)

occurrence in newborn infants. Microscopic examination revealed multiple congenital malformations in one abortus, suggesting a partial lethal agent in operation. Lin (121) reported a rare type of annular pancreas in which the tail of the annular duct was fused with the dorsal pancreatic duct. Heij and Niesen (119) presented a very rare case of annular pancreas with congenital absence of the gallbladder. Four cases of annular pancreas in adults were reported by Yogi (122) and diagnosed by ERCP.

EMBRYOGENESIS

In the normal course of development, between the 8- and 12-mm stages (sixth week), the common duct and the right portion of the ventral primordium are carried dorsally around the circumference of the duodenum to lie adjacent to the dorsal pancreas. This rotation is the result of duodenal growth in which all enlargement is from the ventral side only (Fig. 11.22, *A* and *B*).

The duct of the longer, dorsal pancreas anastomoses with that of the ventral pancreas to form the main pancreatic duct (duct of Wirsung), which opens into the common duct. If the proximal portion of the duct of the dorsal primordium persists, it forms the accessory duct (duct of Santorini). How this normal pattern is altered to produce an annular pancreas is not obvious. A number of explanations have been proposed:

1. Hypertrophy of both dorsal and ventral primordia until they fuse ventrally around the duodenum in the sixth week (123) (Fig. 11.22, *C*)
2. Fixation of the tip of the ventral primordium to the duodenal wall—before rotation during the fifth week—resulting, with subsequent growth, in fusion of this tip

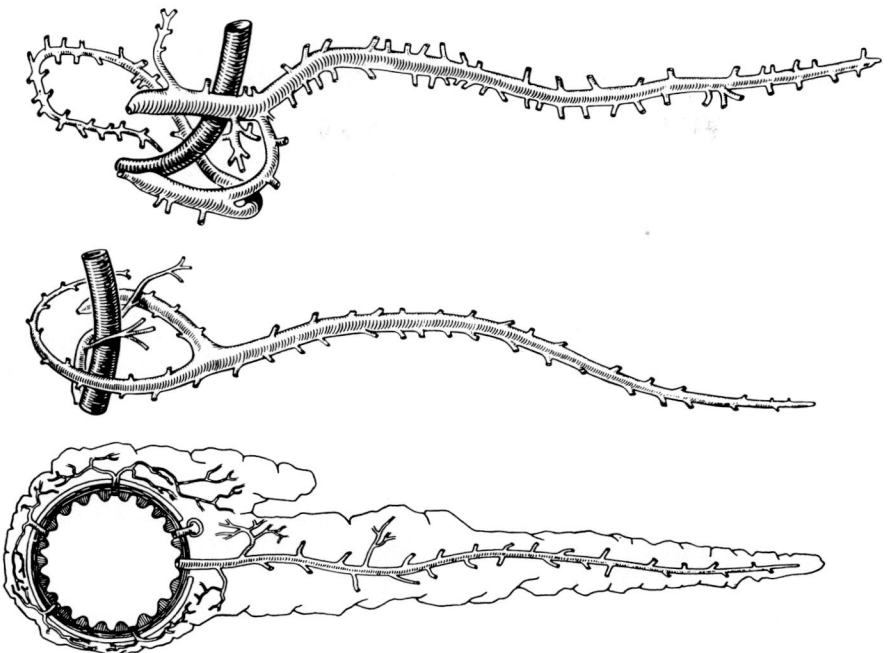

Figure 11.21 Patterns of the pancreatic ducts in annular pancreas. **A**, A branch of the ventral duct passes to the left, posterior to the duodenum: This is the usual pattern. The dorsal and ventral ducts open into the duodenum by separate orifices. **B**, The annulus is supplied by two ducts from the dorsal pancreatic duct. **C**, A possibly unique case. (From Erimoglu C. A case of pancreas annulare. Proc Kon Nederl Akad Wet [Biol Med] 55:18, 1952), in which the duct of the annulus opens into the duodenum by several orifices. The dorsal duct does not appear to be involved. (From Théodoridès T. Pancréas annulaire. J Chir (Paris) 1964;87:445–462.)

with the dorsal primordium on the far side (124) (Fig. 11.22, *D*)

3. Persistence of a hypothetic left ventral bud, which extends around the duodenum ventrally to join the dorsal primordium in the fifth week (125) (Fig. 11.22, *E*)
4. Formation of the pancreatic ring by diffuse tissue with pancreatic potential in this area of the duodenum during the third week (In this sense, the ring might be considered aberrant pancreatic tissue [126].) (Fig. 11.22, *F*)

The evidence at present seems to favor Lecco's (124) hypothesis. The duct within the ring usually passes dorsally to the right and enters the main pancreatic duct. In patients having incomplete pancreatic annuli, the gap is usually anterior (primitive left). In the 16-mm embryo described by Weissberg (127), the ring was formed by the ventral primordium.

The fourth theory seems untenable in most instances, but Erimoglu's (126) specimen was said to have four small ducts from the ring opening directly into the duodenum (128). A second, similar case is known (129). It is possible that annuli are formed in more than one way. In at least one case (130) an annular pancreas was accompanied by aberrant pancreatic nodules.

The atresias or stenoses frequently found at the site of the pancreatic ring are undoubtedly the result of duodenal constriction by the pancreas during the period of epithelial proliferation of the developing duodenum.

Removal of the encircling tissue does not always relieve the stenosis, which indicates that growth of the ring has failed to keep pace with the enlarging intestine.

HISTORY

The first description of an annular pancreas was made by Ecker (131) in 1862 in the course of a dissection. Ravitch does not accept earlier cases (132). Vidal (133) in France performed the first successful gastrojejunostomy in 1905 on a newborn infant with annular pancreas. From then to 1949 only 27 cases were reported in the literature. In 1955 Sanford (134) reviewed 35 pediatric and 38 adult cases that were treated surgically, and in 1959 Lundquist (135) was able to collect 217 cases. McNaught (136) and Kie et al. (128) reviewed the embryologic aspects.

INCIDENCE

The condition is congenital, but it may manifest itself at any age of life. Of the 73 cases from the literature examined by Sanford (134), 24 (33%) produced symptoms in the first week of life and 33 (45%) in the first year. Relatively few new cases are found in the second decade of life, but the incidence rises again after maturity. Fifteen percent of Reemtsma's patients were adults over the age of 50 years (137). The sexes are equally affected in the pediatric group, but males make up about 66% of the adult group (135, 138). Cases have been reported in cau-

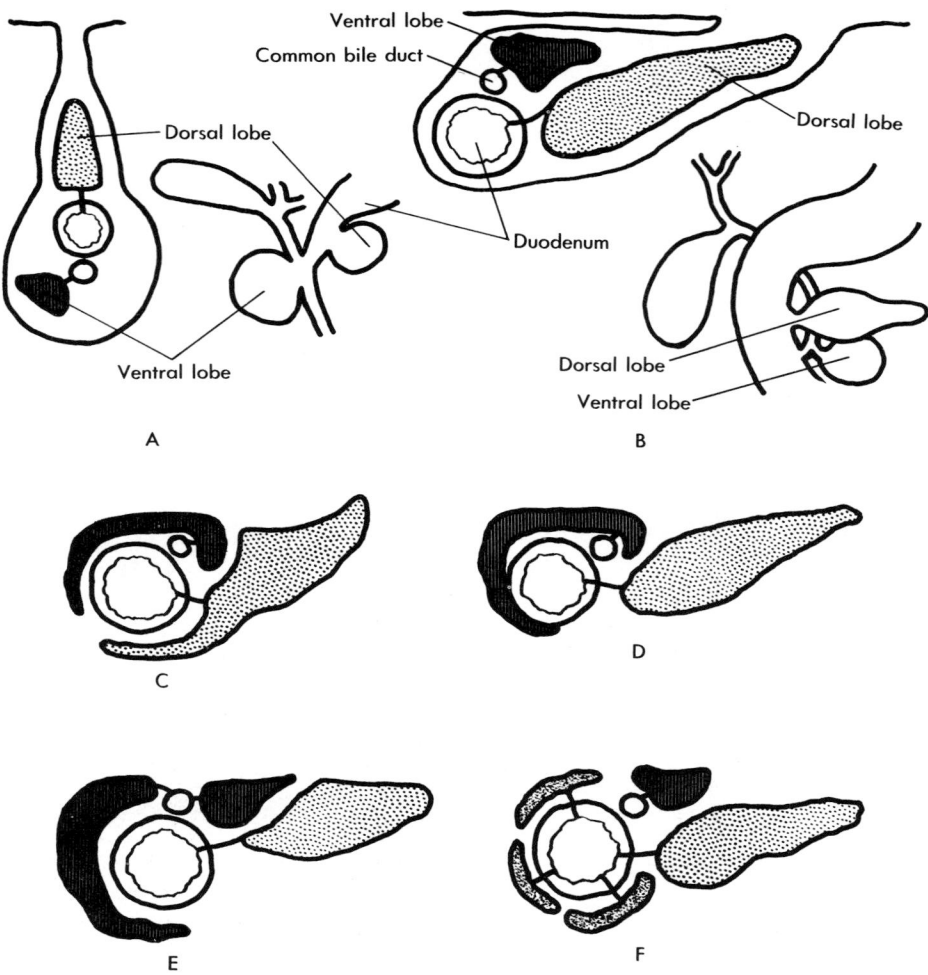

Figure 11.22. Several theories of the embryogenesis of annular pancreas. **A**, Normal relationship of dorsal and ventral pancreatic primordia at 6 weeks. **B**, At 7 weeks, just before fusion of the primordia. The ventral primordium was migrated to the left, posterior to the duodenum. **C**, Hypothetic hypertrophy of both lobes, eventually coalescing to form the annulus **D**, Hypothetic adhesion of the distal tip of the ventral primordium to the duodenal wall prior to its migration. **E**, Persistence of a hypothetical left ventral lobe, based on an assumption that the ventral lobe was originally a paired structure **F**, Formation of the annulus by fusion of aberrant pancreatic tissue from the duodenum. See text for the evaluation of these theories. (Redrawn from Anderson JR, Wapshaw H. Annular pancreas Br J Surg 1951;39:43–49; **C**, from Tieken T. Annular pancreas. Trans Chicago Pathol Soc 1899–1901;4:180; **D**, from Lecco TM. Zur Morphologie des Pankreas annulare. Sitzungsb Akad Wissensch Math Naturw Clin 1910;119:391–406; **E**, from Baldwin WM. Specimen of annular pancreas. Anat Rec 1910;4:299–304; **F** from Erimoglu C. A case of pancreas annulare. Proc Kon Nederl Akad Wet [Biol Med] 1952;55:18.)

casian, black, and Asian patients. Regan and Wren (139) estimate there is a total of about 260 cases in the literature, 65% of them reported since 1952.

SYMPTOMS

The ring of normal pancreatic tissue produces symptoms only when it obstructs the duodenum or the biliary tract (Fig. 11.23). The obstruction may be present at birth, or it may be secondary to swelling of the annulus due to pancreatitis. In many patients the condition produces no symptoms and is only found on autopsy. It has been estimated that only about 33% of the cases are symptomatic (140). Partial obstruction of the duodenum may result in

peptic ulceration from stasis (141). Biliary obstruction, on the other hand, may produce jaundice or pancreatitis. Symptoms of acute obstruction (vomiting, weight loss, alkalosis, dehydration, and jaundice) are common in infants with annular pancreas, whereas symptoms of chronic obstruction (ulceration and pancreatitis) are more usual in adults.

DIAGNOSIS

Infants. In infants, an annular pancreas generally presents with bilious vomiting since the obstruction is at or just distal to the ampulla of Vater. The infant will not be distended once the stomach is decompressed with an oro-

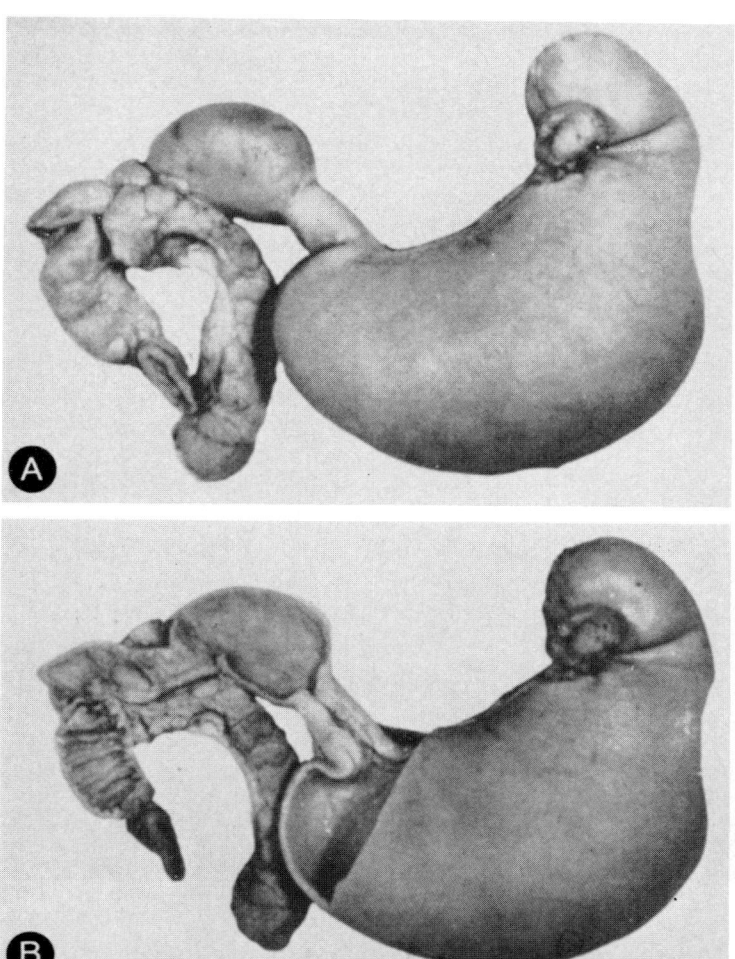

Figure 11.23. Annular pancreas. **A,** Necropsy specimen of stomach and duodenum, showing narrowing of the second part of the duodenum and dilation of the first part. **B,** Same specimen opened to show stenosis of the pylorus by muscular hypertrophy as well as the stenotic duodenal segment. (From Moore TC. Annular pancreas: review of literature and report of 2 infant cases. Surgery 1953;33–138.)

gastric tube. The abdominal radiograph will show the "double-bubble" sign with air in the distended stomach and the upper portion of the duodenum, with no air in the remaining gastrointestinal tract if the obstruction is complete (Fig. 11.24). If the obstruction is incomplete, a small amount of air may be seen in the distal gastrointestinal tract. In such cases an upper gastrointestinal radiographic series should be obtained emergently to exclude the diagnosis of malrotation with or without midgut volvulus (Fig. 11.25), according to Ricketts (142).

EDITORIAL COMMENT

Ricketts' suggestion that an upper gastrointestinal radiographic series be obtained emergently is mandatory for infants born with near complete duodenal obstruction if there is to be any delay in operative correction. The reason is that, in the differential diagnosis, midgut volvulus is a part of abnormal rotation, and this is an absolute emergency since further delay may result in ischemic necrosis of the volvulated valve. The other absolute indication for the upper gastrointestinal radiographic series might be a decision to delay treatment because of major associated anomalies; one wants to be certain of the extent of the gastrointestinal abnormality before making this type of judgment (JAH/CNP).

Adults. Pancreatitis has been observed in about 25% of adult cases, and duodenal ulceration in about 33% (136). Correct preoperative diagnosis is not common. Radiographic studies may show dilation of the first part of the duodenum, and the double-bubble sign is usually present. In one patient, auscultation of the duodenum revealed stasis and led to a correct diagnosis (143). When pancreatitis is suspected, serum amylase or serum lipase studies may confirm the diagnosis.

At surgery, mobilization of the duodenum by opening

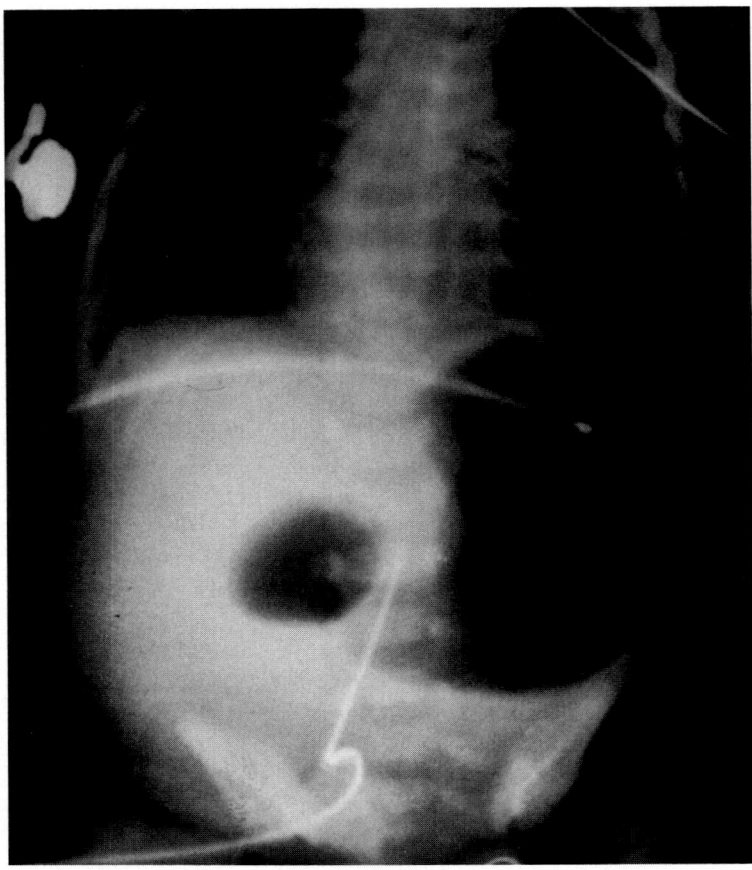

Figure 11.24.   Abdominal radiograph demonstrating a "double-bubble" in an infant with annular pancreas.

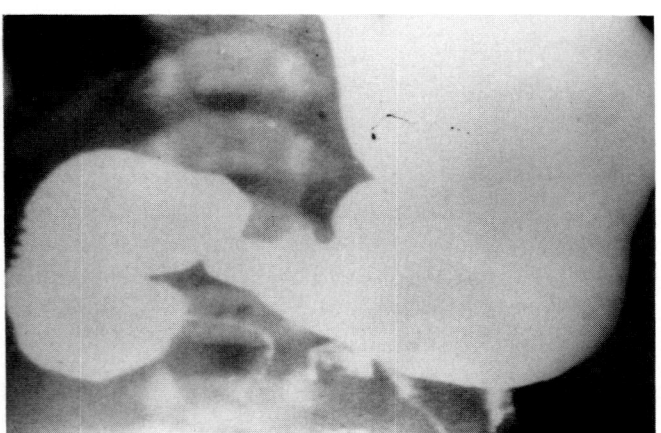

Figure 11.25.   Upper gastrointestinal radiographic series in an infant with partial high intestinal obstruction demonstrating an annular pancreas; malrotation is excluded because of the normal duodenal "C-loop."

the posterior peritoneum may be necessary to determine the exact pancreatic and duodenal relationships. Warren (144) and Sanford (134) have warned against reliance on palpation alone. Annular pancreas may be distinguished from the superior mesenteric artery syndrome (see Chap-

ter 6, "The Small Intestines") by the fact that the latter affects the third portion of the duodenum and is relieved by assumption of the knee-chest position.

TREATMENT

Surgery provides the only relief for symptoms produced by an annular pancreas. Four main procedures have been employed:

1. Division of the constricting ring of pancreatic tissue. This procedure is the most tempting because it is the simplest, but it is not recommended because of three important drawbacks.
    a. The danger of pancreatic fistula is high owing to the impossibility of visualizing the exact duct pattern in a given annulus. Fistulae occurred in five of twenty procedures of this type reviewed by Sanford (134).
    b. The duodenum at the site of the ring may be stenosed or even atretic requiring further surgery. This was the case in seven of twenty ring resections (Fig. 11.23).
    c. If the pancreatic tissue is interspersed with the muscle fibers of the duodenum, division of the ring will not relieve the stenosis (113).
2. Posterior gastrojejunostomy is the simplest of the effective bypass procedures. If peptic ulceration is present as

a result of partial obstruction and duodenal stasis, vagotomy will help avoid later ulceration at the anastomosis. Gross (60) observed that this procedure may fail to drain adequately the proximal duodenal loop.

3. Duodenojejunostomy, first proposed by Gross and Chisholm (145) in 1944, is one of the present treatments of choice (117, 128, 134, 139, 145, 146). Duodenal stasis is relieved and pancreatic fistula is avoided by this procedure.

4. Duodenoduodenostomy as described by Weitzman (147) is a more physiologic bypass procedure. However, it requires considerably more dissection because of the requirement to reflect the right colon to the left and to mobilize a greater length of duodenum by the Kocher maneuver (147, 148). This procedure avoids leaving a long defunctionalized limb of jejunum which can serve as the focus for development of the ''blind loop syndrome'' and is our preferred method.

EDITORIAL COMMENT

More severe forms of constriction of the duodenum from an annular pancreas will result in considerable dilation of the proximal duodenum and stomach at the time of operative correction. In such infants it is probably wise to carry out a concomitant gastrostomy at the same time the duodenoduodenostomy is completed because these infants may have prolonged delay in normal emptying of the stomach and duodenum due to this dilation. The gastrostomy both decompresses during the healing of the anastomosis and provides a means of monitoring the return of function which will occur in the duodenum and obstructed stomach.

A closer related option to pure gastrostomy and drainage in the management of the child requiring duodenoduodenostomy is to pass a small plastic catheter through the gastrostomy site past the new anastomosis into the distal jejunum for postoperative feeding purposes. This is particularly useful when there is extensive dilation of the proximal duodenum and stomach which may not return to normal function for several weeks. In this way the baby may be fed enternally through the small plastic catheter which is brought out alongside the gastronomy tube. In the management, suction is applied to the gastrostomy tube and feedings are instilled through the small plastic feeding catheter. This will avoid prolonged use of intravenous alimentation and thus decrease some of the complications associated with prolonged intravenous feedings (JAH/CNP).

MORTALITY

The overall mortality among 35 operative pediatric cases was 43%, and among 38 adult cases it was 13% (134). The higher mortality among infants is explained by the presence of other serious anomalies. All the deaths reported by Gross (60) occurred in patients who had other defects. One patient had tracheoesophageal fistula, imperforate anus, and a congenital heart defect in addition to annular pancreas.

Currently, deaths in infants with annular pancreas

result solely from associated congenital anomalies (149). Survival rates now approach 90 to 95% in postoperative patients, and some patients are not operated on because of other lethal anomalies (148, 150).

Pancreatic Gallbladder

Gallbladder duplication in cats was reported by Boyden (151) in 1926 as part of a study of aberrant biliary vesicles in humans and domestic animals. The accessory gallbladder arose from the ventral pancreatic bud instead of the cystic primordium. This suggested the possibility of similar accessory gallbladders in humans.

In 1971 a pancreatic bladder presenting as a double gallbladder was reported by Wrenn and Favara (152) and confirmed by Boyden (152).

The authors join Garcia and Raul in stating that pancreatic tissue in the wall of an otherwise normal gallbladder does not indicate origin from the ventral pancreatic primordium (153, 154).

Rotational Anomalies

The persistence of a dorsal mesoduodenum may cause gross misplacement of the pancreas. Wilson (155) described an unusual duodenopancreatic relationship associated with incomplete rotation of the mid-gut loop in a discussion of several cases. Rotational anomalies are rare, with some being unique.

Accessory and Heterotopic Pancreas (Aberrant Pancreas)

Pancreatic tissue has been described in a number of locations in the body. Accessory pancreas in the duodenum, pancreatic tissue in the stomach wall (see Chapter 5, ''The Stomach'') and pancreatic tissue in Meckel's diverticulum (see Chapter 6, ''The Small Intestines'') are relatively common. More unusual locations are the colon (associated with gastric mucosa) (156), appendix (157), gallbladder (158–160), and anomalous bronchoesophageal fistulae (161, 162) (Fig. 11.26) (see also Chapter 14, ''Pulmonary Circulation''). A few examples of pancreatic tissue in the omentum or the mesentery have been reported (163). In most cases the accessory pancreatic tissue is functional. Islets of Langerhans are present in about 33% of gastric pancreatic heterotopias, but only rarely are they present in pancreatic heterotopias elsewhere.

DISTRIBUTION

More than 50% of reported aberrant pancreatic structures have been found in the stomach or duodenum. Most of those in the stomach occur in the pylorus (see Chapter 5, ''The Stomach''). Busard and Walters (164) reviewed 543 cases from the literature; their findings are shown in Figure 11.26. The actual incidence of aberrant

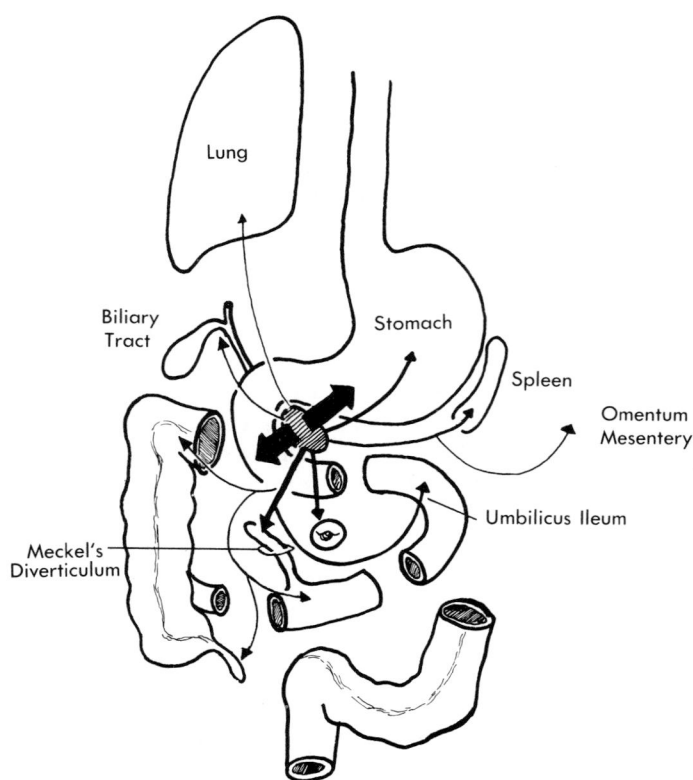

Figure 11.26.   Chief sites of heterotopic pancreatic tissue. Fifty percent of these structures occur in the duodenum or the pylorus.

pancreas in the stomach, duodenum, and jejunum is undoubtedly much higher since most of these structures are asymptomatic and can be revealed only by meticulous search.

Heterotopic pancreas obstructing the ampulla of Vater was reported by Laughlin et al. (165). Herrera et al. (166) documented gastrointestinal bleeding with ectopic pancreas in two cases.

Briceno et al. (167) reported pancreatic tissue from an anomalous bronchoesophageal fistula. Carr et al. (168) reported a mediastinal cyst with pancreatic tissue. Spence et al. (169) found accessory pancreas in a gastric duplication.

In 1990 Tsunoda et al. (170) found a heterotopic pancreas producing bile duct dilation. Burke et al. (171) reported heterotopic pancreas with pancreatitis, pancreatic pseudocyst, and gastric outlet obstruction.

EMBRYOGENESIS

Although the liver and pancreas appear in close proximity and about the same time, pancreatic cell potentiality is much more widespread. The specificity of the hepatocardiac mesenchyme as the organizer for liver cells apparently limit it to liver formation, whereas there is a less specific requirement for differentiation of pancreatic tissue.

Duodenal accessory pancreatic organs are sometimes

obviously portions of the normal pancreas that have been sequestered beneath the muscularis externa. These are merely displaced pancreatic lobes (Fig. 11.27).

In other cases the relationship of the accessory tissue to the normal pancreas is not apparent, and these must be considered errors of cell differentiation in situ instead of misplaced tissues. The submucosal glands of Brunner, rather than the pancreatic acini, are the archetypes of these aberrant "pancreatic" structures. Brunner's glands represent the primitive submucosal glandular epithelium of the distal part of the foregut. Their formation normally is suppressed above and below the limits of this segment. If the organ-forming field of the normal pancreas is weakened, submucosal glands higher or lower in the duodenum may escape from its control and proceed to differentiate into pancreatic acini. All stages of this process—from undifferentiated glandular tissue to completely developed pancreatic acini and islets—may be found (172). This view may be considered a modern expression of Zenker's idea that an aberrant duodenal pancreas arises from a normally suppressed third pancreatic anlage of the gut wall. Each Brunner's gland may be considered a suppressed pancreatic anlage.

The acini in the normal pancreas and Brunner's glands of the duodenum differentiate during the third month of fetal life, with the acinar maturation slightly preceding

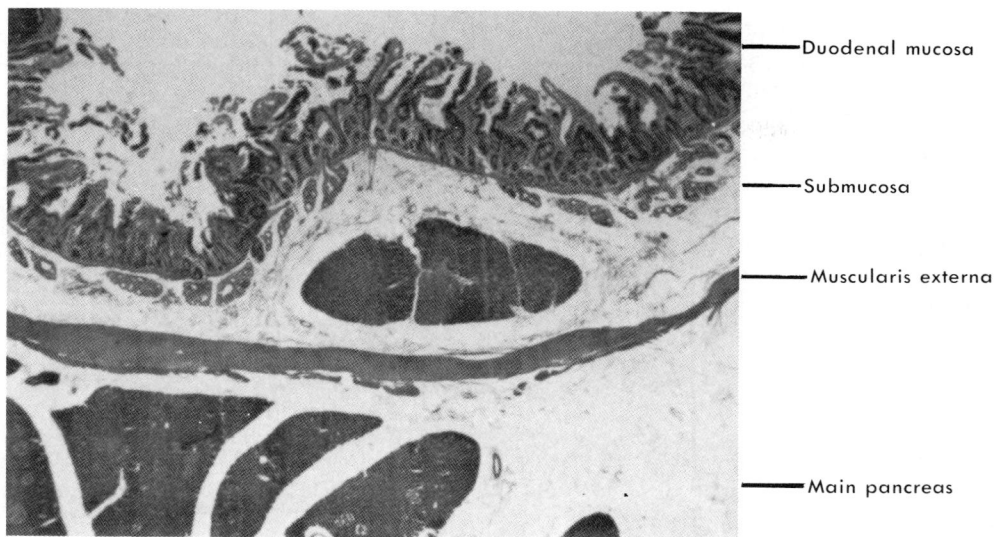

Duodenal mucosa

Submucosa

Muscularis externa

Main pancreas

Figure 11.27. Photomicrograph of ectopic pancreas sequestered in the submucosa of the duodenum. This is the mildest and most common expression of pancreatic ectopia.

that of Brunner's glands. It is probably at this stage or later that local escape of glandular cells from the dominance of the pancreatic organ-forming field takes place.

It is more difficult to account for extraduodenal pancreatic tissue. The proposed explanations fall into two groups:

1. Metaplasia
   a. Abnormal differentiation of multipotent endodermal cells in situ
   b. Differentiation of mature gastric or intestinal epithelial cells during adult life as the result of inflammation (173)
2. Transplantation
   a. Adhesion of embryonic pancreatic cells to neighboring structures during rotation of normal or abnormal pancreatic primordia (fourth to fifth weeks)

The metaplastic theories are supported by the late appearance of symptoms in most cases and by the difficulty in imagining a suitable means by which pancreatic cells could be transported to some of the locations in which they are found. The presence of both pancreatic and gastric mucosa in Meckel's diverticulum as well as in some intestinal duplications may be accounted for by the metaplasia of multipotent embryonic cells. The vitelline stalk contains endodermal cells similar to those of the foregut. Normally, these cells degenerate, but if the diverticulum persists, the mucosa differentiates into some or even all of the mature types of cells normally derived from foregut endoderm, with the striking exception of hepatic cells.

The transplantation theory adequately explains gastric, biliary, and jejunal heterotopic pancreas and also

accounts for the much rarer omental and mesenteric pancreatic structures.

The presence of varying amounts of smooth muscle associated with aberrant pancreatic tissue has been interpreted as the displacement of normal musculature invaded by pancreatic tissue, as an initial malarrangement that pinched off the pancreatic tissue, or as abnormal proliferation of muscle elements induced by the abnormal pancreatic tissue. The fact that pancreatic tissue is sometimes present in diverticula other than Meckel's has suggested that it may cause such diverticula by local disruption of muscle fibers.

HISTORY

In 1859 Klob (174) first described aberrant pancreatic tissue in the stomach and jejunum and confirmed their presence microscopically. Warthin (163) in 1904 reviewed the literature and found 47 cases to which he added two of his own. Most were in the stomach, duodenum, or jejunum. By 1934 Hunt and Bonesteel (175) found 185 cases in the literature, and in 1951 Pearson (176) collected 589 cases.

INCIDENCE

Pearson (176) estimated that aberrant pancreatic tissue could be found in 1 to 2% of autopsies if it were carefully sought. About 6% of Meckel's diverticula contain pancreatic tissue (177). The majority of these pancreatic structures are small and produce no symptoms.

SYMPTOMS AND DIAGNOSIS

Most patients with heterotopic pancreatic tissue exhibit no symptoms. When symptoms are present, they may resemble those of duodenal ulcer, gallbladder disease, or even appendicitis. Because pancreatic structures in the stomach usually occur at the pyloric end, pyloric obstruction with ulceration and bleeding may occur. In the jejunum and ileum, such complications as intussusception or perforation may develop.

In some systemic disorders, heterotopic pancreatic tissue as well as the normal pancreas is affected (178).

Barium radiography may show a filling defect of the stomach resembling that produced by a benign or malignant tumor, such as a leiomyoma or leiomyosarcoma, or there may be signs of gastric or duodenal ulceration.

TREATMENT

The treatment of heterotopic pancreas is surgical, with the procedure depending on the form and the location. In Meckel's diverticulum, removal of the whole diverticulum is necessary; in the intestine, a segmental resection is required. Pedunculated structures may simply be excised.

Congenital Cysts of the Pancreas

In an excellent, detailed chapter of his book, Howard (179) classified pancreatic cysts (Table 11.1). Despite our belief that this is a good classification of a complicated clinical entity, there is still a possibility that some of these cysts, such as teratomatous or angiomatous cysts, could be of congenital origin. We agree with Howard that the distinction is not always clear-cut, since the epithelial lining of true congenital cysts may be replaced with a lining of fibrous tissue. We do accept that the cyst described by Eha (180) and McPherson and Heersma (181) were true congenital cysts. Also, we consider as true congenital cysts the case described by Caironi et al. (182) of a 40-year-old male with a true pancreatic cyst and a case mentioned by Wolloch et al. (183) of a 50-year-old female with columnar epithelium. True pancreatic cysts were reviewed by Rheudasil et al. (184) who discussed the congenital and acquired types of these rare clinical entities lined with columnar epithelium.

SOLITARY CYSTS

Solitary cysts are differentiated from pancreatic pseudocysts by the presence of an epithelial lining. They vary in size from 0.5 cm to the 23×12-cm cyst found by Miles (185) in a newborn child. The head, body, or tail of the pancreas may be involved. The lining of the cyst is cuboidal or stratified squamous epithelium and may contain pancreatic enzymes (186) as a result of communication with the pancreatic ducts. In Miles' patient the cyst was loculated by a thin septum. Bikoff (187) reported what he believed to be a congenital cyst in ectopic pancreatic tissue in the stomach wall of an infant. While this is by no

Table 11.1.
Classification of Pancreatic Cysts.[a]

Congenital (True) Cysts
  A. Single or simple true cysts
  B. Polycystic disease
     1. Polycystic disease of the pancreas without related anomalies
     2. Pancreatic macrocysts associated with cystic fibrosis
     3. Polycystic disease of the pancreas associated with cerebellar tumors and retinal angiomata (von Hippel-Lindau disease)
     4. Pancreatic cysts associated with polycystic disease of kidneys (Osathanondh-Potter, type I or II).
  C. Enterogenous cysts
  D. Dermoid cysts
Angiomatous Cysts
  A. Simple or proliferative cysts
Proliferative Cysts
  A. Cystadenoma and cystadenocarcinoma of the pancreas
     1. Benign (microcystic) serous cystadenoma
     2. Benign and malignant mucinous (macrocystic) cystadenoma and cystadenocarcinoma
     3. Papillary-cystic epithelial neoplasm
     4. Acinar cell cystadenocarcinoma
  B. Teratomatous cysts
Acquired Cysts
  A. Retention cysts
  B. Parasitic cysts
     1. *Echinococcus* cysts
     2. Cysts caused by *Taenia solium* (tapeworm)
  C. Pseudocysts
     1. "Acute" pseudocyst or cystic necrosis of pancreas
     2. Chronic pseudocysts
Cysts of Uncertain Nature

[a]From Howard JM. Cysts of the pancreas. In: Howard JM, Jordan GL, Jr, Reber HA, eds. Surgical diseases of the pancreas. Philadelphia: Lea & Febiger, 1987: 540.

means improbable, the evidence is unconvincing. The structure was more likely an intramural enterogenous cyst of the stomach.

Pilot et al. (188) reported common bile duct obstruction by a cyst in a newborn. Iovchev (189), Pomosov et al. (190), and Assawamatiyamont and King (191) reported dermoid cysts, a rare pancreatic anomaly. Black et al. (192) reported pancreatic duplications with ductal communications and lining of gastric mucosa.

Solitary pancreatic cysts are rare. Miles (185) reviewed eight cases in infants from the literature and added one of his own. Howard and Jordan (138) described a cyst in a 56-year-old man and mentioned two other cases in adults. A few solitary pancreatic ducts have been found incidentally on autopsy.

No other anomalies are associated with these cysts although several unrelated malformations were present in one patient (186). There was also suspicion of polycystic disease in this case. The only symptoms, according to Miles (185), are those of abdominal distension with pressure on surrounding viscera.

Treatment of such cysts consists of excision. The cyst must not be ruptured before removal because of the danger of fat necrosis should the fluid contain pancreatic enzymes.

Among reported cases of infants, three have died and six have recovered. There have been no reports of recurrence.

MULTIPLE CYSTS

Even rarer than solitary cysts are multiple pancreatic cysts. Howard and Jordan (138) described one patient in which a polycystic pancreas was found at surgery, and four patients in which the disease was recognized at autopsy. Two of the latter had cysts of the kidney and one had cysts of the liver as well. In von Hippel-Lindau's disease (193), polycystic pancreas and polycystic kidneys are associated with angiomatosis of the retina and the cerebellum.

PANCREATIC PSEUDOCYSTS

These are cystic structures without epithelial lining. They contain pancreatic enzymes and usually result from pancreatitis or trauma (194). They are more common than congenital cysts but are rare in persons below the age of 30 years and are found very rarely in infants.

EDITORIAL COMMENT

With the increased interest of pediatric surgeons in the care of children with serious blunt trauma to the abdomen, the incidence of pancreatic pseudocyst has increased considerably. Any child who develops an upper abdominal mass following blunt trauma to the abdomen either accidentally induced or as a result of battered child syndrome should be considered a candidate for a pseudocyst. While this condition may disappear with decrease in the inflammation associated with the trauma, some pseudocysts persist and may require operative drainage. The simplest approach to operative drainage is through the stomach by cystogastrostomy. Occasionally it may be necessary to use the more complicated Roux-en-Y anastomosis to appropriately drain the persistent pseudocyst of the pancreas (JAH/CNP).

Cystic Fibrosis (Meconium Ileus)

Pancreatic cystic fibrosis is a congenital familial dysfunction of the pancreas and other exocrine glands. It often expresses itself as meconium ileus, an obstruction of the intestine by a thick, viscid meconium; as meconium peritonitis; and as meconium plug syndrome. Although cystic fibrosis is not a morphologic anomaly, meconium ileus is a surgical problem and hence within our purview.

Heterozygotic parents host the abnormal gene responsible for the genesis of several forms of related clinical syndromes such as meconium ileus, meconium peritonitis, and meconium plug syndrome.

However, a series of events also takes place to produce complex clinical pictures without revealing the real cause

of these syndromes. Most likely, cystic fibrosis is a secondary phenomenon of abnormal secretions of all exocrine glands. The viscosity of mucous secretions is high, and because of this, obstruction of organ passages takes place.

Pancreas, lungs, intestines, liver, mucous membranes of the nose, testicles and ovaries, and salivary glands are some of the organs affected by an obstructive phenomenon leading to fibrosis.

Roy et al. (195), in reporting the relationship between cystic fibrosis and exocrine insufficiency, emphasized the malabsorption present, a situation not yet well understood.

PATHOLOGY

No demonstrable structural changes in the pancreas precede the onset of the disease. Hurwitt and Arnheim (196) investigated the possibility of a congenital occlusion of the pancreatic ducts and concluded from an examination of a large number of human embryos that no solid stage existed in the pancreatic duct system and that congenital atresia was not an etiologic factor.

The sequence of events starts with abnormal secretion from the pancreatic acini before birth. Duct obstruction, atrophy, and fibrosis follow. In the early stages just after birth, the pancreas may appear normal. Later the ducts become dilated and filled with eosinophilic material. Blind ducts without acini are often present. Brunner's glands of the duodenum are dilated with cystic lesions, and the salivary glands may be atrophic (197). Peptic ulcers may be found in older children (198). The meconium producing the obstruction usually occupies the lower 10 to 30 cm of the ileum. Above this, the meconium is more fluid and tends to produce dilation; below this, the intestine may be empty or have small, dry pellets of meconium (Fig. 11.28).

In addition to obstruction, volvulus with eventual gangrene and perforation of the intestine may occur in as many as 33% of affected infants. Meconium ileus is the most frequent single cause of intestinal perforation during intrauterine life. Such perforation gives rise to sterile meconium peritonitis (199) and eventually to sterile necrosis of the occluded loop (200). The peritonitis will not be sterile, however, if perforation occurs more than a few hours after birth.

In the lungs, excessive mucous secretion leads to chronic respiratory disease (Fig. 11.29), whereas increased electrolyte excretion in perspiration leads to salt depletion in hot weather. The presence of elevated electrolyte levels in perspiration formed the basis for the genetic studies of Smoller and Hsia (201).

ASSOCIATED ANOMALIES

Donnell and Cleland (202) found nine patients with fibrocystic disease among 103 infants with intestinal atresia.

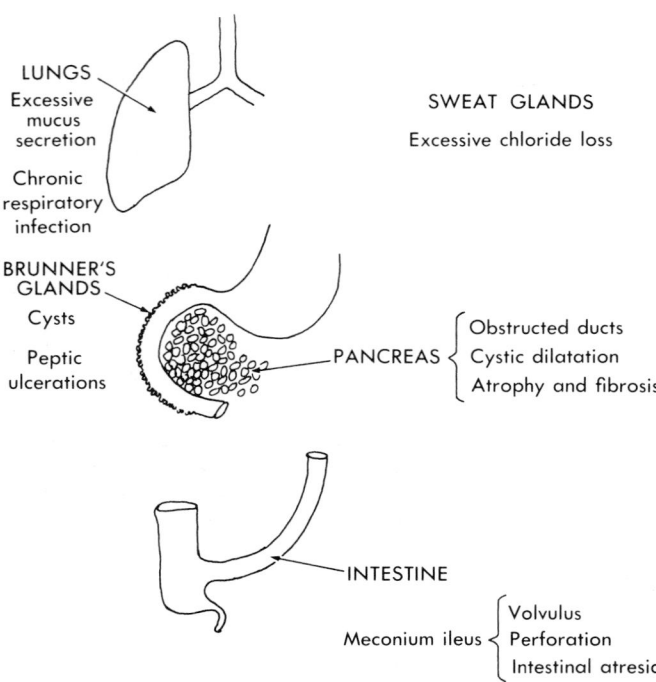

Figure 11.28. Cystic fibrosis of the pancreas. Many exocrine glands are affected, not all with equal severity in the same patient. The meconium ileus resulting from abnormal pancreatic secretion brings the disease to the attention of the surgeon.

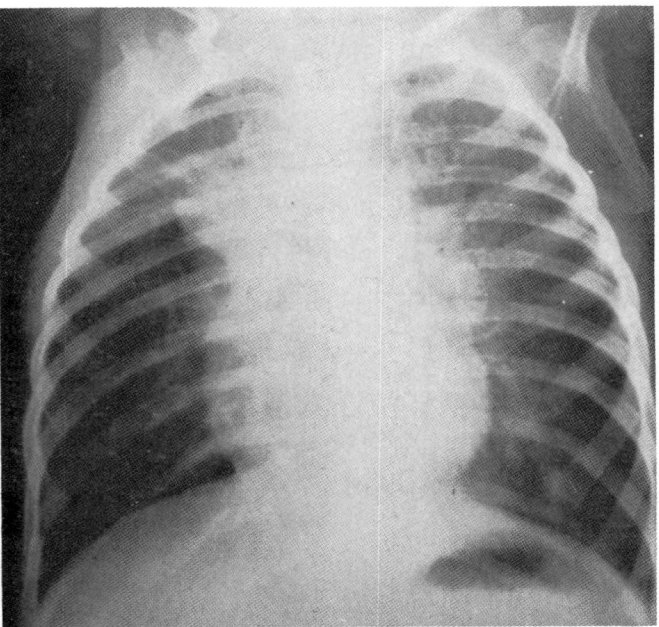

Figure 11.29. Cystic fibrosis as seen in the lungs. There are extensive inflammatory changes in both lungs. Peribronchial abscesses with extensive scarring are present. In most patients progressive pulmonary hypertension develops. In this x-ray film the central pulmonary arteries are enlarged.

This is 90 times the expected association of the two conditions if they existed independently. An even greater frequency has been reported in some series. For this reason, all infants with intestinal atresia should have a sweat chloride test to rule out the presence of cystic fibrosis.

EMBRYOGENESIS

Abnormal mucoprotein, which does not dissolve in water in the presence of trypsin, is present in the mucus secreted by the pancreas. The fluidity of the meconium in the intestine is thus reduced, and eventually plugs of insoluble mucus in the pancreatic ducts block secretion from the acini. Fibrous replacement of the acini follows (203). Presumably, a recessive gene controls the protein formed by the secretory cells. The protein involved has been considered to be a globulin, but it may be an albumin (204).

FAMILIAL INCIDENCE

The disease is a recessive lethal trait, affecting about one of four children of parents who both carry the recessive gene. It is estimated that 6% of the population carry the gene and that in 0.36% of marriages, both parents will carry it. This results in an incidence of 1:1100 births (205). It is estimated that only about 15% of these infants will exhibit the intestinal obstruction produced by abnormal meconium. Both sexes are equally affected.

HISTORY

Meconium ileus was related to a disorder of the pancreas as early as 1905 by Landsteiner (206), but the broader aspects of cystic fibrosis of the pancreas were not characterized until 1938 and 1939 studies by Anderson (207, 208). Subsequently, Farber (209) showed that all mucus-secreting glands were involved, and diSant'Agnese and his colleagues (210) observed the altered electrolyte concentration in perspiration. Andersen and Hodges (211) first presented evidence of the hereditary nature of the disease.

MECONIUM ILEUS

The current philosophy of the meconium ileus pathogenesis is that abnormal intestinal secretions and delayed passage of meconium resulting in obstruction of the lumen of the intestine. The pancreatic pathology most likely plays a secondary role, according to Thomaidis and Arey (212). Rickham and Boeckman (213) and Dolan and Touloukian (214) reported cases of meconium ileus without pancreatic cystic fibrosis.

Meconium. Amniotic fluid, cellular debris, bile, pancreatic and intestinal secretions join with other sources to form meconium. The majority of weight (74%) is water. Several enzymes also participate and concentrate in the

Table 11.2.
Cystic Fibrosis: Meconium Enzyme Concentrations[a]

Enzymes increased
    Lactase
    Sucrase
    Maltase
    Palatinase
    Alkaline phosphatase
    Mannosidase
    Glucuronidase
    Fucosidase
Enzymes decreased
    Trypsin

[a]From Heitlinger LA. Intestinal and pancreatic enzymes in amniotic fluid and meconium: content as an index of fetal maturity, well-being, or disease. In: Lebenthal E, ed. Human gastrointestinal development. New York: Raven Press, 1989: 522.

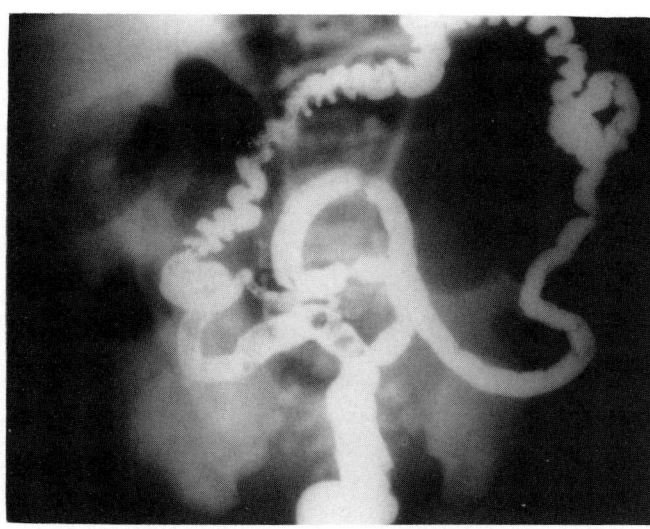

Figure 11.30. Barium enema radiograph of an infant with meconium ileus demonstrating the microcolon and pellets of inspissated meconium in the terminal ileum.

formation of meconium. Table 11.2 by Heitlinger (215) presents enzyme concentrations in meconium in infants with cystic fibrosis.

In 1980 Seeds (216) reported that the predominant pathway for amniotic fluid accumulation is by transfer of water across the placenta.

SYMPTOMS AND DIAGNOSIS

Abdominal distension is usually the first sign of meconium ileus. Vomiting appears early and becomes progressive. No meconium is passed. Palpation may reveal hard or doughy movable masses in the abdomen. If these findings are associated with a history of cystic fibrosis in other members of the family, the diagnosis is confirmed.

The plain abdominal radiograph will show distended loops of bowel without gas fluid levels since the meconium is too thick to layer out on the upright or cross-table lateral view. A barium enema should be done to evaluate for other causes of a low intestinal obstruction such as jejunoileal atresia, Hirschsprung's disease, or small left colon syndrome (142). The barium enema will demonstrate a microcolon with radiolucent pellets within the ascending and terminal ileum, representing concretions formed by the thickened, solidified meconium (Fig. 11.30). If the diagnosis is established, treatment with liquifying enemas is begun (see the section on "Treatment").

Fluid or free air in the abdominal cavity indicates that perforation has occurred, and areas of calcification on the peritoneum indicate a prenatal perforation ("meconium peritonitis"). In one of our patients, volvulus with necrosis of the intestine and meconium peritonitis was present at birth (200).

Other aspects of the disease include chronic respiratory infections resulting from abnormally viscid mucus in the respiratory passages. Atelectasis, bronchial obstruction, and sinus trouble are not unusual. The pancreatic

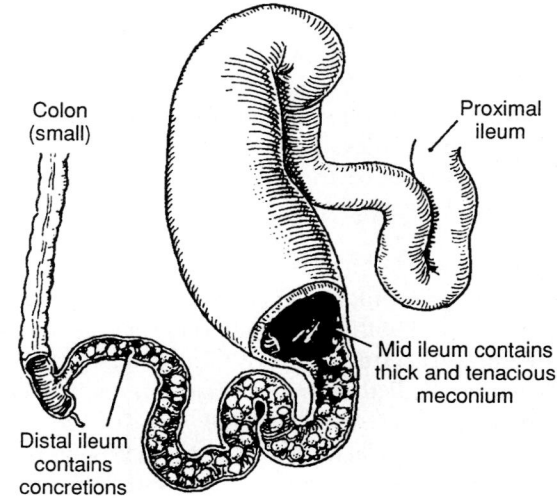

Figure 11.31. Illustration of the pathologic and anatomic abnormality in uncomplicated meconium ileus. (From Santulli TV. Meconium ileus. In: Mustard WT et al., eds. Pediatric surgery. Chicago: Year Book Medical Publishers, 1969.)

achylia leads to malnutrition from failure to metabolize carbohydrates and fat. Cirrhosis of the liver, with portal hypertension and esophageal varices, may occur. Anemia, vitamin K deficiency, and splenomegaly may appear.

TREATMENT

Uncomplicated meconium ileus due to inspissated meconium obstructing the distal ileum (Fig. 11.31) is treated with gastrografin (meglumine diatrizoate) or Mucomyst (acetylcysteine) enemas with a high degree of success, according to Raffensperger, Boyd, Rescorla, and their colleagues (150, 217, 218). Boyd reports a 67% success rate in treating patients with uncomplicated meconium ileus with repeated gastrografin enemas (217). Infants who are not treated successfully with enemas require operative decompression. This can be done through an enterotomy which is subsequently closed (150), a Bishop-Koop end-to-side enterostomy (219), or a simple T-tube enterostomy (220).

EDITORIAL COMMENT

A useful adjunct to operative decompression is to inject a 2% Mucomyst solution through the intestinal wall to allow for breakdown of the inspissated meconium into a more liquid form. This then can be extracted either through an enterostomy or can occasionally be milked more distally and evacuated through the anus. The use of Mucomyst as an adjunct has made operative treatment for meconium ileus much more satisfactory with more rapid return of intestinal function (JAH/CNP).

Approximately 50% of infants will have complications from meconium ileus, including volvulus, intestinal atresia, perforation, and meconium peritonitis. All of these patients are managed by intestinal resection with primary anastomosis or enterostomy (218).

It must be kept in mind that the infant whose meconium ileus is thus relieved is in no better position than one with cystic fibrosis of the pancreas without meconium ileus. Medical therapy must be instituted at once.

MORTALITY AND PROGNOSIS

Prior to 1945 few infants with meconium ileus survived. From 1945 to 1952 Gross (60) relieved the intestinal obstruction successfully in 22 of 47 infants. Eight of these 22 subsequently died of their disease; among the remainder, one was still alive and well at $4\frac{1}{2}$ years of age.

At present, survival at 1 year of age is 90% in patients with uncomplicated meconium ileus and 85% for those with complicated meconium ileus (218). All of these patients will eventually die from their underlying cystic fibrosis during the first two to three decades of life.

Arterial, Vascular, and Lymphatic Anomalies

ARTERIAL SYSTEM OF THE PANCREAS

The pancreas is supplied with blood from both the celiac trunk and the superior mesenteric artery. The general system is shown in Fig. 11.32, but variations are common. Differing textbook illustrations are all "correct" for at least some individual patients.

In general, it appears that the blood supply is greatest to the head of the pancreas, less to the body and tail, and least to the neck. We know of no actual measurements of blood flow to these regions that would provide a quantitative basis for this.

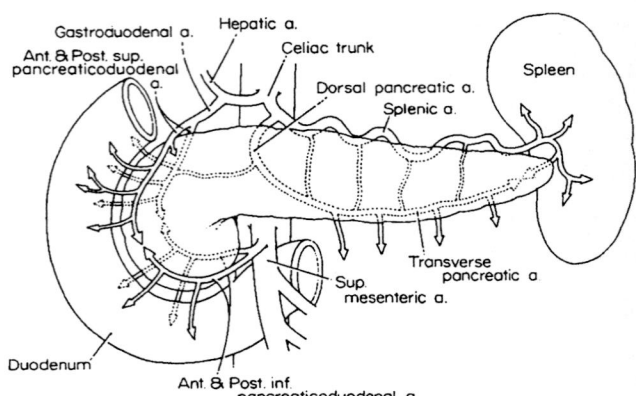

Figure 11.32. Major arterial supply to the pancreas: anterior view (left and right gastric arteries not shown). (From Skandalakis JE, Gray SW, Rowe JS, Skandalakis LJ. Anatomical complications of the pancreas. Contemp Surg 1979;15(12):33.)

The head of the pancreas and the concave surface of the duodenum are supplied by two pancreaticoduodenal arterial arcades that are always present. These are formed by a pair (anterior and posterior) of superior arteries from the celiac trunk which join a second pair of inferior arteries from the superior mesenteric artery. These vascular arcades, lying within the pancreas but also supplying the duodenal wall, are the chief obstacles to complete pancreatectomy. Ligation of both vessels will result in duodenal ischemia and necrosis. At the neck, the dorsal pancreatic artery usually arises from the splenic artery close to its origin from the celiac trunk. A right branch supplies the head of the pancreas and usually joins the posterior arcade; one or two left branches pass through the body and tail of the pancreas, often making connections with branches of the splenic artery and, at the tip of the tail, with the splenic or the left gastroepiploic artery. All major arteries lie posterior to the ducts.

Pancreatic Arcades. The gastroduodenal artery arises as the first major branch of the common hepatic branch of the celiac trunk. About 1 cm from its origin, it gives off the right gastroepiploic artery and subsequently divides to form the anterosuperior and posterosuperior pancreaticoduodenal arteries. Occasionally, all three branches arise by trifurcation of the gastroduodenal artery.

The anterosuperior pancreaticoduodenal artery lies on the surface of the pancreas giving eight to ten branches to the anterior surface of the duodenum, one to three branches to the proximal ileum, and numerous branches to the pancreas. At surgery for pancreatic resection, the duodenal branches may be sacrificed, but the jejunal branches should be preserved. The artery enters the substance of the pancreas, and on the posterior surface it joins the anteroinferior pancreaticoduodenal artery from the superior mesenteric artery. Mellière

(221) found four cases in which the anastomosis between superior and inferior vessels was narrow or absent, but he considered the condition to be pathologic or the result of transitory spasm. The superior arteries are about 2mm in diameter; the inferior arteries are usually slightly smaller (222).

Two or even more anterosuperior pancreaticoduodenal arteries may be present. One arises from the gastroduodenal artery, and another may arise from the right gastroepiploic artery. Woodburne and Olsen (223) should be consulted for the basic arterial pattern and its history. Michels (54) has provided an exhaustive description of the possible variations that may be encountered.

The anteroinferior pancreaticoduodenal artery arises from the superior mesenteric artery at, or above, the inferior margin of the pancreatic neck. It may form a common trunk with the posteroinferior artery. One or both vessels may arise from the first or second jejunal branches of the superior mesenteric artery. Ligation of the jejunal branch itself will endanger the blood supply to the fourth part of the duodenum. Even more striking are the not unusual cases in which a posteroinferior artery arises from an aberrant right hepatic artery, springing from the superior mesenteric artery. In a case described by Ziegler (224), the anteroinferior artery arose from the middle colic artery.

The posterosuperior pancreaticoduodenal artery arises from the gastroduodenal artery. Its course is visible only when the pancreas is turned upward to expose its posterior surface (Fig. 11.33). Branches may anastomose with branches of the gastroduodenal artery or with a right branch of the dorsal pancreatic artery. Other branches supply the anterior and posterior surfaces of the first part of the duodenum. The course of the posterior arcade is farther from the duodenum than is that of the anterior arcade. It passes posterior to the intrapancreatic portion of the common bile duct. Ziegler (224) illustrated two cases in which a middle colic artery arose from the gastroduodenal artery, supplying the anterior surface of the pancreas as it descended. Ligation of the gastroduodenal artery in this patient would have comprised the blood supply to the transverse colon.

Michels (54) found a cystic artery arising from the gastroduodenal or the retroduodenal artery in 4% of specimens examined. An accessory right hepatic artery may have a similar origin and may be mistaken for an aberrant cystic artery. Such arteries may or may not contribute branches to the head of the pancreas.

The posterior arcade, like the anterior, may be doubled or tripled, with the extra arcades joining the posteroinferior pancreaticoduodenal artery or the superior mesenteric artery separately. The posterior arcade may also anastomose with an aberrant right hepatic artery from the superior mesenteric artery (Fig. 11.34, C), separately or together with the anterior arcade.

Dorsal Pancreatic Artery. This is the "supreme pancreatic artery" of Kirk (225). It lies posterior to the neck of the pancreas and posterior to the splenic vein and is about 1.5 mm in diameter. Michels (54) considers it to be the most variable of the celiacomesenteric vessels. Its most common origin is from the proximal 2 cm of the splenic artery (39%), but it may arise from other arteries, including an aberrant hepatic artery (Fig. 11.35).

Occasionally, the dorsal pancreatic artery is the middle colic or accessory middle colic artery. It gives off the transverse pancreatic artery to the left and continues in

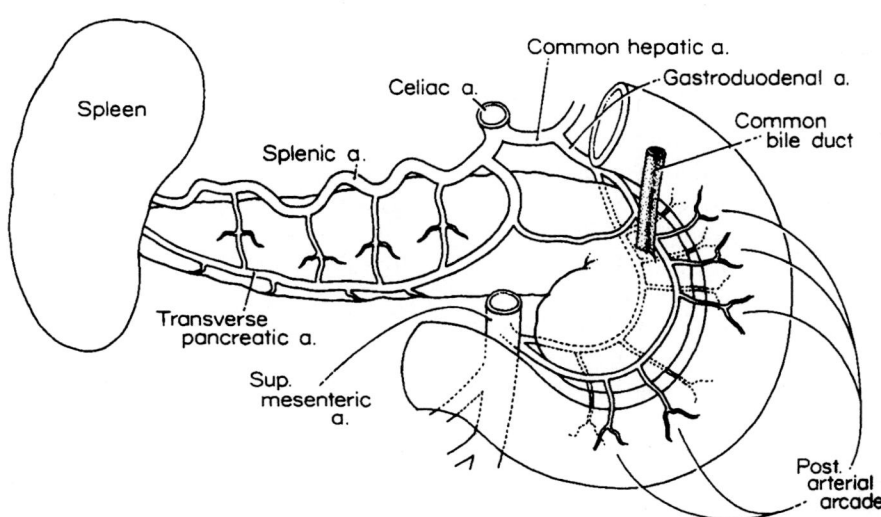

Figure 11.33. *Major arterial supply to the pancreas: posterior view (left and right gastric arteries not shown). (From Skandalakis JE, Gray SW, Rowe JS, Skandalakis LJ. Anatomical complications of the pancreas. Contemp Surg 1979;15(12):23.)*

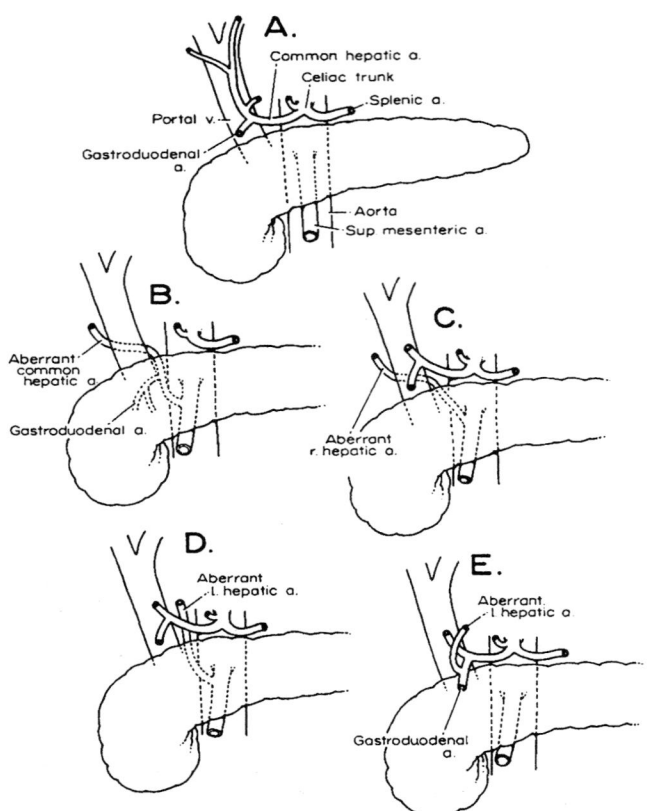

Figure 11.34. Variation of the hepatic arteries. **A**, The normal configuration; the common hepatic artery arises from the celiac trunk. **B**, An anomalous common hepatic artery arises from the superior mesenteric artery. **C**, An anomalous right hepatic artery arises from the superior mesenteric artery. **D**, An anomalous left hepatic artery arises from the superior mesenteric artery. **E**, An anomalous left hepatic artery arises from the gastroduodenal artery. The anomalous artery may be accessory to, or replacing, a normal hepatic artery. (From Skandalakis JE, Gray SW, Rowe JS, Skandalakis L J. Anatomical complications of the pancreas. Contemp Surg 1979;15(12):32.)

the transverse mesocolon. To the right it sends branches to the head and the uncinate process. Arteriography is essential for determining its course.

Transverse Pancreatic Artery. The transverse (inferior) pancreatic artery is the left branch of the dorsal pancreatic artery supplying the body and tail of the pancreas.

In about 10% of individuals, the transverse pancreatic artery arises from the gastroduodenal, the right gastroepiploic, or the superior pancreaticoduodenal arteries (54). It may also arise from the superior mesenteric artery (226). The artery may be single, double, or absent; it may or may not anastomose with the splenic arteries (221) (Fig. 11.36). If it does not, thrombosis of the artery can produce infarction and limited necrosis of the body and tail of the pancreas (227). The transverse pancreatic artery may be large enough to constitute a second splenic artery, effectively supplying that organ. Branches supply the wall of the pancreatic duct for much of its length. There are also from four to eight posterior epiploic

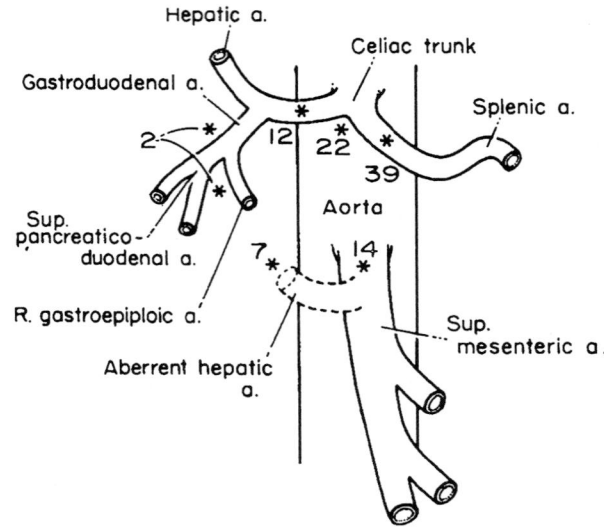

Figure 11.35. Possible sites of origin of the dorsal pancreatic artery. More than one-half arise from the proximal splenic artery or the celiac trunk. (From Skandalakis JE, Gray SW, Rowe JS, Skandalakis L J. Anatomical complications of the pancreas. Contemp Surg 1979;15(12):27. Percentages from Michels NA. Blood supply and anatomy of the upper abdominal organs. Philadelphia: JB Lippincott, 1955.)

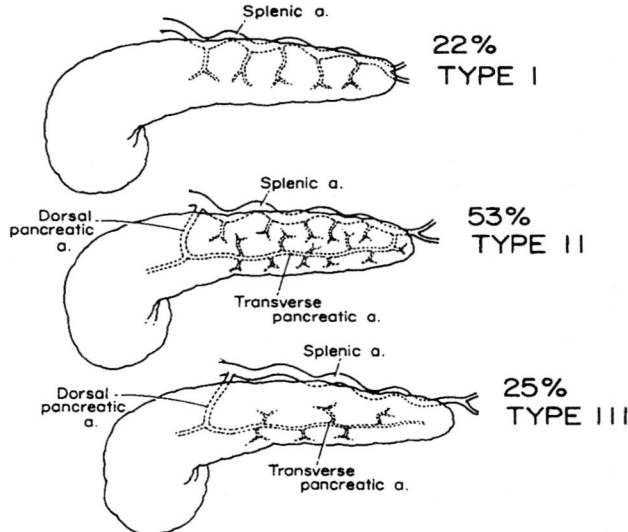

Figure 11.36. Diagram of the possible configurations of the blood supply to the distal pancreas. *Type I,* Blood supply from the splenic artery only. *Type II,* Blood supply from splenic and transverse pancreatic arteries with anastomosis in the tail of the pancreas. *Type III,* Blood supply from splenic and transverse pancreatic arteries without distal anastomoses. This type is susceptible to infarction from emboli in the transverse artery. (From Skandalakis JE, Gray SW, Rowe JS, Skandalakis L J. Anatomical complications of the pancreas. Contemp Surg 1979;15:(12):27.)

branches to the omentum. These may include a specific right epiploic artery and a colic branch to the left colic flexure. Remember that the arteries and veins lie posterior to the duct.

Branches of the Splenic Artery. The splenic artery is located on the posterior surface of the body and tail of the pancreas. In its course it loops like a snake above and below the superior margin of the organ, becoming more tortuous with increasing age of the subject. Two to ten branches of the splenic artery anastomose with the transverse pancreatic artery. The largest of these, the great pancreatic artery (of von Haller), is the main blood supply to the tail of the pancreas. Ligation of the splenic artery does not require splenectomy, but ligation of the splenic vein does.

Caudal Pancreatic Artery. This vessel arises from the left gastroepiploic artery or from a splenic branch at the hilum of the spleen. It anastomoses with branches of the great pancreatic and the transverse pancreatic arteries. The caudal pancreatic artery supplies blood to accessory splenic tissue when it is present at the hilum of the spleen.

Significant Variations of Major Arteries. The hepatic artery is usually a main branch of the celiac trunk which arises cranial to the pancreas (Fig. 11.34, *A*). An anomalous hepatic artery may, however, arise from the superior mesenteric artery or one of its branches. It may pass behind, in front of, or through the pancreas. The surgeon should always determine whether such an anomalous artery is present before proceeding with resection.

Anomalous Common Hepatic Artery. In 2 to 4.5% of individuals (228, 229), an anomalous common hepatic artery arises from the superior mesenteric artery. It is related to the head or neck of the pancreas and occasionally passes through the head of the pancreas (229) (Fig. 11.34, *B*). It subsequently passes behind the portal vein. Almost the whole blood supply of the duodenum comes from the superior mesenteric artery in such individuals. Accidental ligation of this vessel will not only result in hepatic ischemia and perhaps necrosis, but it will jeopardize the duodenum as well. Selective arteriography before pancreatic surgery is a comfort in the operating room.

Anomalous Right Hepatic Artery. The more frequent anomalous right hepatic artery also arises from the superior mesenteric artery. Its course is unpredictable, but it is related to the head and neck of the pancreas. Such an artery may pass behind the common bile duct or behind the portal vein (Fig. 11.34, *C*). An aberrant right hepatic artery was present in 26% of cadavers examined by Michels (229). It may give off the inferior pancreaticoduodenal arteries.

Anomalous Left Hepatic Artery. This vessel presents a problem in pancreatic surgery only when it arises from the right side of the superior mesenteric artery (Fig. 11.34, *C*) or from the gastroduodenal artery (Fig. 11.34, *E*). Michels (229) found an anomalous left hepatic artery in 27% of his specimens.

Anomalous Middle Colic Artery. A middle colic artery may pass through the head of the pancreas or between the

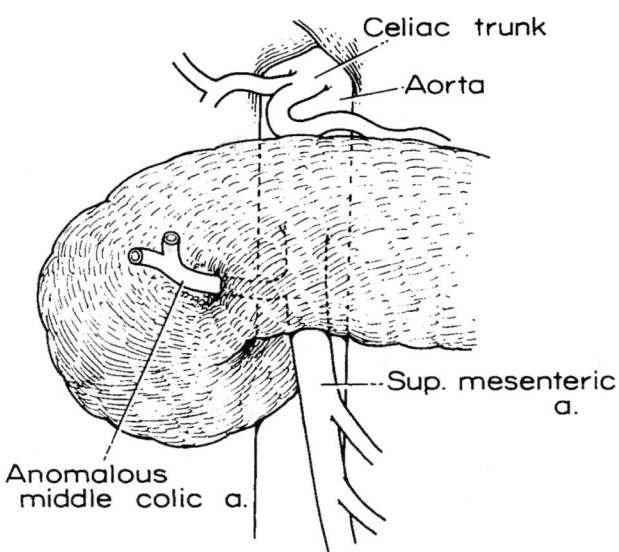

Figure 11.37. A middle colic artery may arise from the superior mesenteric artery, passing through the head of the pancreas. It may supply small branches to the pancreas. (From Skandalakis JE, Gray SW, Rowe JS, Skandalakis LJ. Anatomical complications of the pancreas. Contemp Surg 1979;15(12):32.)

head and the duodenum. It may arise from the superior mesenteric, the dorsal pancreatic, or the inferior pancreaticoduodenal arteries (Fig. 11.37).

VENOUS DRAINAGE OF THE PANCREAS

In general, the veins of the pancreas parallel the arteries and lie superficial to them. Both lie posterior to the ducts. The drainage is to the portal vein, splenic vein, and superior and inferior mesenteric veins (Figs. 11.38 and 11.39).

Veins of the Head of the Pancreas. Four pancreaticoduodenal veins form venous arcades draining the head of the pancreas and the duodenum. The anterosuperior pancreaticoduodenal vein joins the right gastroepiploic vein. This vein receives a colic vein to form a short gastrocolic vein which is a tributary to the superior mesenteric vein. The posterosuperior vein enters the portal vein above the superior margin of the pancreas. The anteroinferior and posteroinferior pancreaticoduodenal veins enter the superior mesenteric artery together or separately. Other small unnamed veins in the head and neck drain independently into the superior mesenteric vein and the right side of the portal vein (226). The surgeon must avoid traction of the head and ligate these veins carefully.

White (78), perhaps relying on the studies of Falconer and Griffiths (226), states that pancreatic tributaries do not enter the anterior surface of the portal or superior mesenteric veins. This, of course, reduces the risk of bleeding when incising the neck of the pancreas to resect the body and tail. Silen (85) warns that the superior pan-

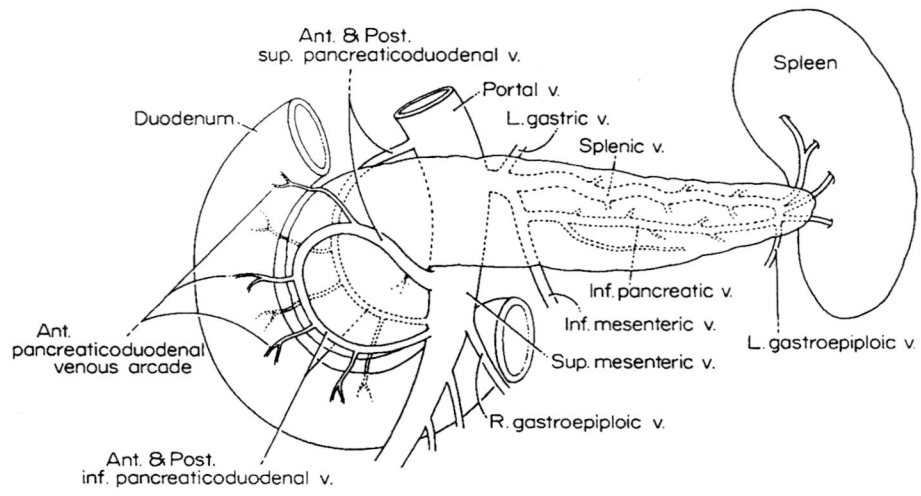

Figure 11.38. The venous drainage of the pancreas: anterior view. (From Skandalakis JE, Gray SW, Rowe JS, Skandalakis LJ. Anatomical complications of the pancreas. Contemp Surg 1979;15(12):33.)

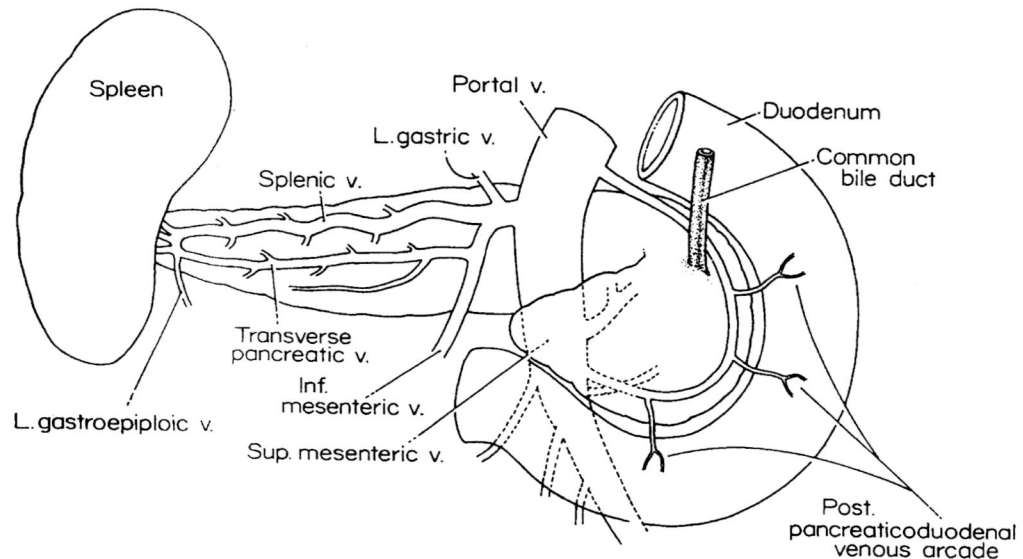

Figure 11.39. The venous drainage of the pancreas and formation of the hepatic portal vein: posterior view. (From Skandalakis JE, Gray SW, Rowe JS, Skandalakis LJ. Anatomical complications of the pancreas. Contemp Surg 1979;15:31.)

creaticoduodenal vein and the gastrocolic vein may, in some patients, enter the portal vein and the superior mesenteric vein anteriorly.

In 1986 Thomford et al. (230) advised preoperative arteriography for visualization of the anatomy of pancreatic arteries and provided a very informative table (Table 11.3). In 1989 Howard (231) reported absence of the celiac axis and replacement of the pancreaticoduodenal arcade by an anomalous prepancreatic vessel, serving both liver and spleen.

Veins of the Neck, Body, and Tail of the Pancreas. The veins of the left side of the pancreas form two large venous channels, the splenic vein above and the transverse (infe-

rior) pancreatic vein below. A smaller superior pancreatic vein may sometimes be identified.

The splenic vein receives from 3 to 13 short pancreatic branches (232). In a few cases one such pancreatic branch entered the left gastroepiploic vein in the tail of the pancreas. Since the inferior mesenteric vein terminates in the splenic vein in about 38% of individuals and the left gastric vein has a similar ending in 17%, ligation of the splenic vein distal to the entrance of these vessels is mandatory. Such ligation will require splenectomy as well.

The inferior pancreatic vein may enter the left side of the superior mesenteric vein, the inferior mesenteric vein, or occasionally the splenic or the gastrocolic veins.

Table 11.3.
Principal Arteries of the Pancreas: Origin and Arteriographic Visualization in 30 Patients[a]

Origin	Arteries						
	ASPD	PSPD	AIPD	PIPD	Dorsal	Great Pancreatic	Transverse
Gastroduodenal	29	28			1	—	5
Superior mesenteric	—	—	15	17	1	1	1
Jejunal branch	—	—	12	9	—	—	—
Hepatic	—	—	1	1	4	1	2
Splenic	1	1	—	—	20	24	6
Total	30	29	28	27	26	26	14
Percentage visualized	100	96.6	93.3	90	86.6	86.6	46.6

[a]From Thomford NR et al. Anatomic characteristics of the pancreatic arteries. Am J Surg 1986; 151:690–693.
AIPD, Anterointerior pancreaticoduodenal; *ASPD,* anterosuperior pancreaticoduodenal; *PIPD,* posterointerior pancreaticoduodenal; *PSPD,* postosuperior pancreaticoduodenal.

Portal Vein. The hepatic portal vein is formed behind the neck of the pancreas by the union of the superior mesenteric and splenic veins (Fig. 11.39). The inferior mesenteric vein entered at this junction in about one-third of specimens examined by Douglass and his colleagues (232). In another one-third, the inferior mesenteric joined the splenic vein close to the junction, and in the remainder, it joined the superior mesenteric vein.

The portal vein lies behind the pancreas and in front of the inferior vena cava, with the common bile duct to the right and the hepatic artery to the left. The portal vein and the superior mesenteric vein can be easily separated from the posterior surface of the pancreas in the absence of disease.

In the 22 subjects we dissected, the left gastric (coronary) vein entered the portal vein in 16 and entered the splenic vein in 6. Where drainage is to the portal vein, the left gastric vein lies in the gastrohepatic ligament.

Anomalies of the Hepatic Portal Vein. Four possible vascular anomalies may be present:

1. The portal vein may lie anterior to the pancreas and the duodenum (Fig. 11.40, *A*).
2. The portal vein may empty into the superior vena cava.
3. A pulmonary vein may join the portal vein (Fig. 11.40, *B*).
4. The portal vein may have congenital strictures.

The first of these is very important to the surgeon but is rare. It represents a persistence of the preduodenal rather than the postduodenal plexus of the primitive vitelline veins (Fig. 11.41). Inadvertent section of this vessel would be fatal. It is often associated with annular pancreas, malrotation, and biliary tract anomalies. It should be mentioned again that the normal portal vein receives tributaries on its lateral wall but not its anterior wall.

Preduodenal portal vein was reported by Matsusue et al. (233) in association with other multiple anomalies and carcinoma of the pancreas. Dumeige et al. (234) reported a prepancreatic but retroduodenal portal vein.

LYMPHATIC DRAINAGE OF THE PANCREAS

The position of the pancreas allows for lymphatic drainage from all areas of the organ to the nearest lymph nodes. No standard terminology for the specific lymph nodes exists although one has been proposed (235). Despite multiple efforts to characterize specific drainage areas, none has been widely accepted (236, 237). Cubilla and associates (238) have made the most recent attempt at standardization.

Their description states that the lymphatic vessels of the pancreas form an abundant, perilobar, interanastomosing network attended by channels coursing the surface of the pancreas and into the interlobular spaces along with the blood vessels. There are five main collecting trunks and lymph node groups served by these lymphatics, and these are described as follows.

Superior Nodes. From the anterior and posterior upper half of the pancreas, these collecting trunks emerge. Most will end in the suprapancreatic lymph nodes which are found at the superior border of the pancreas. The designation of superior head and superior body is appropriate for the nodes in these areas. However, there will be an occasional lymphatic that ends in the nodes of the gastropancreatic fold or in those of the hepatic chain.

Inferior Nodes. The collecting trunks of these nodes drain the anterior and posterior lower halves of the pancreas, leading into the inferior pancreatic group of lymph nodes; most of them are located along the inferior border of the head and body of the pancreas. These vessels also may extend into the superior mesenteric and left lateroaortic lymph nodes. On rare occasions, a collecting trunk terminates directly in a lumbar trunk.

Anterior Nodes. Two collecting trunks course the anterior surface of both superior and inferior portions of the head of the pancreas and extend to the infrapyloric and the anterior pancreaticoduodenal lymph nodes. It is possible they may also extend to some of the mesenteric

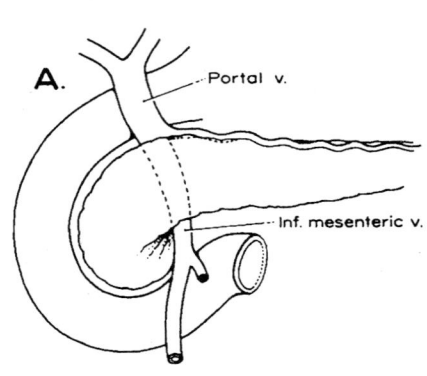

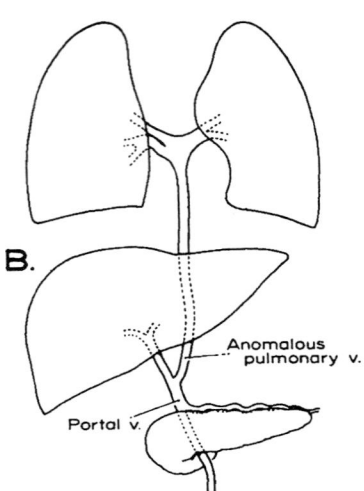

Figure 11.40. Some rare anomalies of the portal vein. **A**, The portal vein lies anterior to the duodenum. **B**, The pulmonary veins drain anomalously into the portal vein. This is one form of total anomalous pulmonary drainage. It may be asso-

ciated with severe cardiac defects. (From Skandalakis JE, Gray SW, Rowe JS, Skandalakis L J. Anatomic complications of the pancreas. Contemp Surg 1979;15(12):33.)

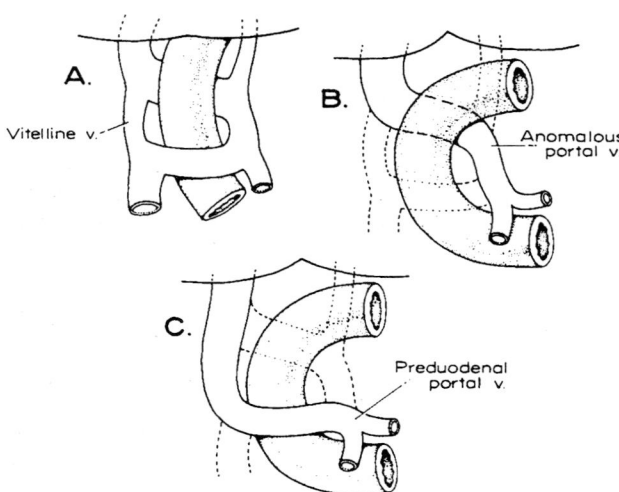

Figure 11.41. Diagrams of the embryonic origin of the preduodenal portal vein. **A**, Embryonic extrahepatic communications between the vitelline veins. **B**, Normal development. Persistent superior communicating vein forms a part of the normal, postduodenal portal vein. **C**, Anomalous persistent inferior communicating vein forms a part of an anomalous preduodenal portal vein. (From Skandalakis JE, Gray SW, Rowe JS, Skandalakis L J. Anatomic complications of the pancreas. Contemp Surg 1979;15(12):36.)

lymph nodes at the root of the mesentery of the transverse colon.

Posterior Nodes. These lymphatics run along the posterior surface of the superior and inferior portions of the head of the pancreas. They empty into the posterior pancreaticoduodenal lymph nodes as well as into the common bile duct lymph nodes, right lateroaortic lymph nodes, and some nodes at the origin of the superior mes-

enteric artery. Most of the lymphatics of the common bile duct and ampulla of Vater also terminate in the posterior pancreaticoduodenal group of lymph nodes.

Splenic nodes. Starting from the tail of the pancreas, these lymphatics drain into the following lymph nodes: those at the hilum of the spleen, the phrenolienal ligament, and the inferior and superior lymph nodes of the tail of the pancreas. Some lymphatic channels terminate in the lymph nodes superior and inferior to the body of the pancreas.

Between the pancreas and the lymph nodes of the greater and lesser curvatures of the stomach, there is no lymphatic communication. The lymphatics of the head and body of the pancreas do not drain into the tail of the pancreas or the splenic nodes although, rarely, lymph vessels from the tail of the pancreas can terminate in the superior body and inferior body subgroups of nodes.

When Cubilla et al. (238) examined surgical specimens removed during regional pancreatectomy in pancreatic and peripancreatic cancer patients, they determined the number of lymph nodes present in each of the nodal drainage areas as well as the presence of metastatic disease in them (Fig. 11.42). The average number of lymph nodes present in each lymph node group were:

Superior nodes: Seventeen superior head and thirteen superior body
Inferior group: One inferior body, one midcolic, and no inferior head
Anterior group: Three pancreaticoduodenal and three jejunal mesenteric
Posterior group: Four pancreaticoduodenal and two common bile duct
Splenic group: Ten tail of pancreas and spleen

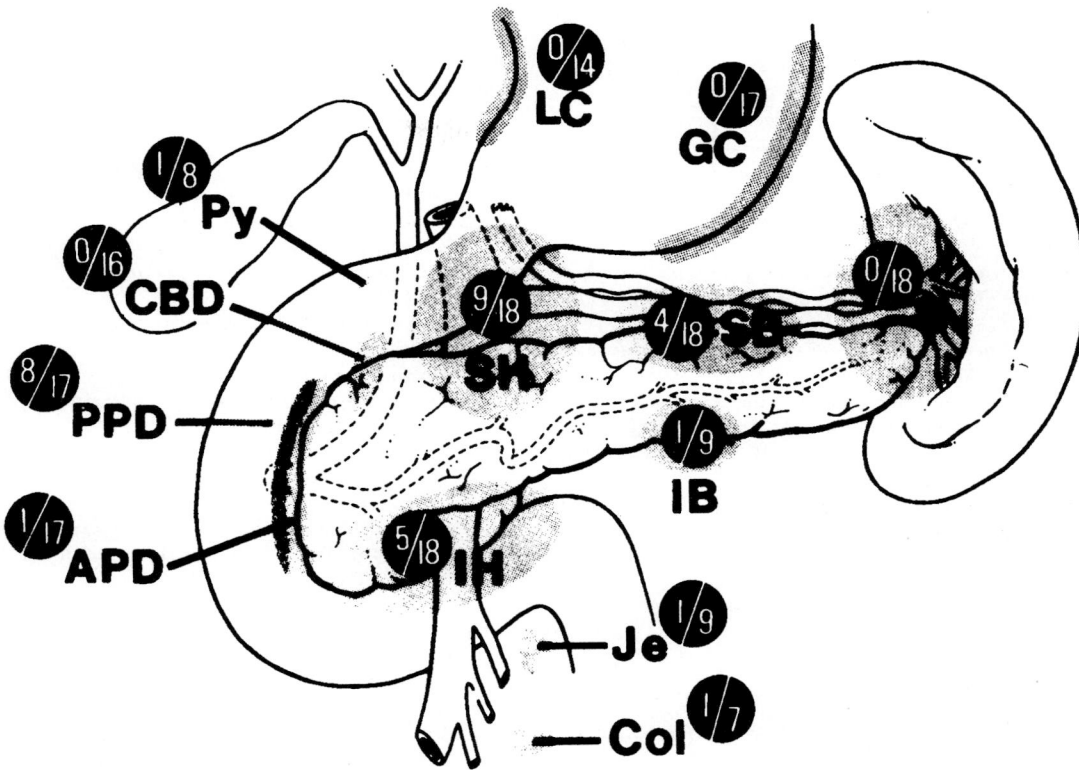

Figure 11.42. Distribution of lymph nodes in 18 pancreatectomy resection specimens. Numerator of fraction of each group indicates number of patients with metastasis in that lymph node group; denominator indicates number of patients in which group nodes were examined. Thirteen cases were pancreas duct cancer; 5 were other cancers in the head of the pancreas area. (*SH*, Superior head; *SB*, superior body; *IH*, inferior head; *IB*, inferior body; *APD*, anterior pancreaticoduodenal; *PPD*, posterior pancreaticoduodenal; *CBD*, common bile duct; *Py*, pyloric; *LC*, lesser curvature; *GC*, greater curvature; *Je*, jejunal; *Col*, midcolic.) (From Cubilla AL, Fortner J, Fitzgerald PJ. Lymph node involvement in carcinoma of the head of the pancreas area. Cancer 1978;41:880.)

According to the investigators, these numbers, derived from a study of 18 pancreatic regional pancreatectomy specimens, reflect the minimum number of lymph nodes present in each nodal group. Other lymph nodes were probably removed with the surgical specimen or overlooked during the study.

Valves in the lymphatics connecting the head of the pancreas and the wall of the duodenum are arranged so that normal flow is from pancreatic to duodenal vessels and not the reverse, according to evidence reported by Bartels in 1907 (239).

On a final note and of interest from an embryologic standpoint is a 15-case study involving the spread of pancreatic cancer in which Fujii and his co-workers (240) concluded that most of pancreas head cancers arising from a ventral pancreas involved the retropancreatic soft tissue at the early stage and that those arising from a dorsal pancreas showed an apparent tendency to spread to the epithelial linings of the main pancreatic duct.

REFERENCES

1. Phisalix C. Étude d'un embryon humain de 10 millimètres. Arch Zool Exper Gen Hist Nat Morphol Histol Evol Animaux. 1888 (Ser 2);6:279–350.

2. Lewis FP. The development of the liver. In: Keibel F, Mall FP, eds. Human embryology, Vol 2. Philadelphia: JB Lippincott, 1912.

3. Dieterlen-Lièvre F. Étude morphologique et expérimentale de la différenciation du pancréas chez l'embryon de poulet. Bull Biol Franc Belg 1965;99:3–116.

4. Wessels NK, Cohen JH. Early pancreas organogenesis: morphogenesis, tissue interactions and mass effects. Develop Biol 1967;15:237–270.

5. Rutter WJ, Wessells NK, Grobstein C. Control of specific synthesis in the developing pancreas. J Nat Cancer Inst 1964;13:51–65.

6. Gittes GK, Debas HT, Rutter WJ. Gene expression during pancreatic organogenesis. Surg Forum 1991;42.

7. Tasso F, Stemmelin N, Sarles H, Clopp J. Comparative morphometric study of the human pancreas in its normal state and in primary chronic calcifying pancreatitis. Biomedicine 1973;18:134–144.

8. Dawson W, Langman J. An anatomical-radiological study on the pancreatic duct pattern in man. Anat Rec 1961;139:59–68.

9. Githens S. Development of duct cells. In: Lebenthal E. Human gastrointestinal development. New York: Raven Press, 1989;669–683.

10. Schwegler RA Jr, Boyden EA. The development of the pars intestinalis of the common bile duct in the human fetus, with special reference to the origin of the ampulla of Vater and the sphincter of Oddi. I. The involution of the ampulla. Anat Rec 1937;67:441–468.

11. Liu HM, Potter EL. Development of the human pancreas. Arch Pathol 1962;74:439–452.

12. Golosow N, Grobstein C. Epitheliomesenchymal interaction in pancreatic morphogenesis. Develop Biol 1962;4:242–255.

13. Conklin JL. Cytogenesis of the human fetal pancreas. Am J Anat 1962;111:181–193.

14. Warkany J. Embryology as related to fibrocystic disease of the pancreas: 18th report of Ross Pediatric Research Conference. Ross Laboratories, Columbus, Ohio, 1956:13–17.

15. Adams DJ, Harrison RG. The vascularization of the rat pancreas and the effect of ischemia on the islets of Langerhans. J Anat 1953;87:257.

16. Johnson DD. Alloxan administration in the guinea pig: a study of the regenerative phase of the islands of Langerhans. Endocrinology 1950;47:393.

17. Bencosme SA. The histogenesis and cytology of the pancreatic islets in the rabbit. Am J Anat 1955;96:103.

18. Hard W. The origin and differentiation of the alpha and beta cells in the pancreatic islets of the rat. Am J Anat 1944;75:369.

19. Gomori G. Pathology of the pancreatic islets. Arch Pathol 1943;36:217.

20. Laguesse E. Recherches sur l'histogénie du pancréas chez le mouton. J Anat Physiol 1896;32:171–198.

21. Emery JL, Bury HPR. Involutionary changes in the islets of Langerhans in the fetus and newborn. Biol Neonat 1964;6:16–25.

22. Howard TJ et al. Anatomic distribution of pancreatic endocrine tumors. Am J Surg 1990;159:258–264.

23. Sawicki MP, Howard TJ, Dalton M, Stabile BE, Passaro E, Jr. The dichotomous distribution of gastrinomas. Arch Surg 1990;125:1584–1587.

24. Delcore R, Jr, Cheung LY, Friesen SR. Characteristics of duodenal wall gastrinomas. Am J Surg 1990;160:621–632.

25. Lee PC. Functional development of the exocrine pancreas. In: Lebenthal E, ed. Human gastrointestinal development. New York: Raven Press, 1989:663.

26. Jhappan C et al. TGF alpha overexpression in transgenic mice induces liver neoplasia and abnormal development of the mammary gland and pancreas. Cell 1990;61(6):1137–1146.

27. Mehes K, Vamos K, Goda M. Agenesis of pancreas and gallbladder in infant of incest. Acta Paediatr Acad Sci Hung 1976;17:175.

28. Lemons JA, Ridenour R, Orsini EN. Congenital absence of the pancreas and intrauterine growth retardation. Pediatrics 1979;64:255.

29. Dourov N, Buyl-Strovrens ML. Agenesie du pancréas. Arch Franc Pediatr 1969;26:641.

30. Dodge JA, Laurence KM. Congenital absence of islets of Langerhans. Arch Dis Child 1977;52:411.

31. Wolf H, Sabata V, Frerichs H, Stubbe P. Evidence for the impermeability of the human placenta for insulin. Horm Metab Res 1969;1:274.

32. Whitington PF. Schwachman syndrome. In: Bergsma D, ed. Birth defects compendium, 2nd ed. New York: Alan R. Liss, 1979. Cited in: Howard JM, Jordan GL, Reber HA, eds. Surgical diseases of the pancreas. Philadelphia: Lea & Febiger, 1987:39.

33. Lechner GW, Read RC. Agenesis of the dorsal pancreas in an adult diabetic presenting with duodenal ileus. Ann Surg 1966;163:311.

34. Gilinsky NH, Del-Favero G, Cotton PB, Lees WR. Congenital short pancreas: a report of two cases. Gut 1985;26(3):304–310.

35. Skandalakis JE et al. The surgical anatomy of the spleen. Probl Gen Surg 1990;7:1–17.

36. Fry WJ, Child CG. Ninety five percent distal pancreatectomy for chronic pancreatitis. Ann Surg 1965;161:543.

37. Landau H, Schiller M. Persistent hyperinsulinemic hypoglycemia of infancy and childhood. In: Schiller M, ed. Pediatric surgery of the liver, pancreas, and spleen. Philadelphia: WB Saunders, 1991:187–201.

38. Cohen MM, Jr, Ulstrom RA. Beckwith-Wiedemann syndrome. In: Bergsma D, ed. Birth defects compendium, 2nd ed. New York: Alan R. Liss, 1979.

39. Bjerke HS, Kelly RE Jr, Geffner ME, Fonkalsrud EW. Surgical management of islet cell dysmaturation syndrome in young children. Surg Gynecol Obstet 1990;171:321–325.

40. Warden MJ, German JC, Buckingham BA. The surgical management of hyperinsulinism in infancy due to nesidioblastosis. J Pediatr Surg 1988;23:462–465.

41. Kramer JL et al. Clinical histological indications for extensive pancreatic resection in nesidioblastosis. Am J Surg 1982;143:116–119.

42. Spitz L et al. Surgical treatment of nesidioblastosis. Pediatr Surg Int 1986;1:26–29.

43. Moazam R, Rodgers BM, Talbert JL, Rosenbloom AL. Near-total pancreatectomy in persistent infantile hypoglycemia. Arch Surg 1982;117:1151–1154.

44. Qualman S, Caniano D, King D, Zipf W. Ectopic pancreas and the islet cell dismaturational syndrome. Ann Clin Lab Sci 1991;21:19–25.

45. Weidenheim KM, Hinchey WW, Campbell WG, Jr. Hyperinsulinemic hypoglycemia in adults with islet-cell hyperplasia and degranulation of exocrine cells of the pancreas. Am J Clin Pathol 1983;79(1):14–24.

46. Murata T et al. Bilateral diffuse nephroblastomatosis, pancortical type: a case report with immunohistochemical investigations. Arch Pathol Lab Med 1989;113(7):729–734.

47. Neri G, Martini-Neri ME, Katz BE, Opitz JM. The Perlman syndrome: familial renal dysplasia with Wilms' tumor, fetal gigantism and multiple congenital anomalies. Am J Med Genet 1984;19(1):195–207.

48. Soulen MC et al. Enlargement of the pancreatic head in patients with pancreas divisum. Clin Imag 1989;13(1):51–57.

49. Silverman PM et al. Pancreatic pseudotumor in pancreas divisum: CT characteristics. J Comput Assist Tomogr 1989;13(1):140–141.

50. Carles D, Serville F, Dubecq JP, Gonnet JM. Renal, pancreatic and hepatic dysplasia sequence. Eur J Pediatr 1988;147(4):431–432.

51. Kikuchi K, Nomiyama T, Miwa M, Harasawa S, Miwa T. Bifid tail of the pancreas: a case presenting as a gastric submucosal tumor. Am J Gastroenterol 1983;78(1):23–27.

52. Doty J, Hassall E, Fonkalsrud EW. Anomalous drainage of the common bile duct into the fourth portion of the duodenum: clinical sequelae. Arch Surg 1985;120(9):1077–1079.

53. Smanio T. Varying relations of the common bile duct with the posterior face of the pancreas in negroes and white persons. J Int Coll Surg 1954;22:150.

54. Michels NA. Blood supply and anatomy of the upper abdominal organs. Philadelphia: JB Lippincott, 1955.

55. Lytle WJ. The common bile-duct groove in the pancreas. Br J Surg 1959;47:209.

56. Kune GA. Surgical anatomy of common bile duct. Arch Surg 1964;89:995.

57. Dowdy GS, Jr. The biliary tract. Philadelphia: Lea & Febiger, 1969.

58. Baggenstoss AH. Major duodenal papilla variations of pathologic interest and lesions of the mucosa. Arch Pathol 1938;26:853.

59. Dowdy GS Jr, Waldron GW, Brown WG. Surgical anatomy of the pancreatobiliary ductal system. Arch Surg 1962;84:229.

60. Gross RE. The surgery of infancy and childhood. Philadelphia: WB Saunders, 1953.

61. Vater A. Dissertatio anatomica, qua novum bilis diverticulum ut et valvulosam colli vesicae felleae constructionem, etc. In: Haller's Disputationum anatomicarum selectarum, Gottingen, III, 1748:259.

62. Bidloo G. Anatomia humani corporis. Amsterdam (Amstelodami), 1685.

63. Kreel L, Sandin B. Changes in pancreatic morphology associated with aging. Gut 1973;14:962.

64. Cotton PB. The normal endoscopic pancreatogram. Endoscopy 1974;6:65.

65. Varley PF, Rohrmann CA, Silvis SE, Vennes JA. The normal endoscopic pancreatogram. Radiology 1976;118:195.

66. Santorini G. Anatomici summi: septemdecim tabulae quas nunc primum edit atque explicat. Parma: Parmae ex Regia Typographia, 1775.

67. Livingston EM. A clinical study of the abdominal cavity and peritoneum. New York: Hoeber, 1932.

68. Rienhoff WF, Jr, Pickrell KL. Pancreatitis: an anatomic study of pancreatic and extra hepatic biliary systems. Arch Surg 1945;51:205.

69. Dardinski VJ. The anatomy of the major duodenal papilla of man, with special reference to its musculature. J Anat 1935;69:469.

70. Opie EL. Etiology of acute hemorrhagic pancreatitis. Bull Johns Hopkins Hosp 1901;12:182.

71. Dragstedt IR, Haymond HF, Ellis JC. Pathogenesis of acute pancreatitis (acute pancreatic necrosis). Arch Surg 1934;28;232.

72. Doubilet H, Mulholland JH. Eight years study of pancreatitis and sphincterotomy. JAMA 1956;160:521.

73. Silen W. Pancreas. In: Schwartz SI, ed. Principles of surgery, Vol 2. New York: McGraw-Hill, 1974.

74. Boyden EA. The pars intestinalis of the common bile duct, as viewed by the older anatomists (Vesalius, Glisson, Bianchi, Vater, Haller, Santorini, etc.). Anat Rec 1936;66:217.

75. Jones SA. Sphincteroplasty (not sphincterotomy) in the treatment of biliary tract disease. Surg Clin North Am 1973;53(5):1123–1137.

76. Boyden EA. The sphincter of Oddi in man and certain representative mammals. Surgery 1937;I:25.

77. Boyden EA. The anatomy of the choledochoduodenal junction in man. Surg Gynecol Obstet 1957;104:641.

78. White TT. Surgical anatomy of the pancreas. In: Carey LC, ed. The pancreas. St. Louis: Mosby, 1973.

79. Fischer MG, McSherry CK. Endoscopic papillotomy: a plea for rational restraint. Arch Surg 1979;114:991.

80. Baldwin WM. The pancreatic ducts in man, together with a study of the microscopical structure of the minor duodenal papilla. Anat Rec 1911;5:197.

81. Helly KK. Beitrag zur Anatomie des Pankreas und seiner Ausfuhrungsgange. Arch F Mikrosk Anat 1898;52:773.

82. Anacker H. Radiological anatomy of the pancreas. In: Anacker H, ed. Efficiency and limits of radiologic examination of the pancreas. Acton, MA: Theime, 1975.

83. Classen M, Koch H, Ruskin H, Pesch HJ, Demling L. Pancreatitis after endoscopic retrograde pancreatography (ERP). Gut 1973;14:431.

84. Sivak MV, Sullivan BH. Endoscopic retrograde pancreatography: analysis of the normal pancreatogram. Am J Dig Dis 1976;21:263.

85. Reich H. Relation of the duct of Santorini to the pathogenesis of duodenal ulcer. N Engl J Med 1963;269:1119.

86. Silen W. Surgical anatomy of the pancreas. Surg Clin North Am 1964;44:1253.

87. Berman LG, Prior JT, Abramow SM, Zeigler DD. A study of the pancreatic duct system in man by the use of vinyl acetate casts of postmortem preparations. Surg Gynecol Obstet 1960;110:391.

88. Opie EL. Anatomy of the pancreas. Bull Johns Hopkins Hosp 1903;14:229–232.

89. Loquvam GS, Russell WO. Accessory pancreatic ducts of the major duodenal papillae. Am J Clin Pathol 1950;20:305–313.

90. Cross KR. Accessory pancreatic ducts. Arch Pathol 1956;61:434–440.

91. Palileo LG, Gallagher HS. Anomalous termination of pancreatic duct. Arch Pathol 1961;71:381–383.

92. Uetsuji S et al. A double cancer of the gallbladder and common bile duct associated with an anomalous arrangement of the choledocho-pancreatic ductal junction: a case report and a review of the literature. Gan No Rinsho 1990;36(6):752–757.

93. Ohta T et al. Clinical experience of biliary tract carcinoma associated with anomalous union of the pancreaticobiliary ductal system. Jpn J Surg 1990;20(1):36–43.

94. Kato T et al. Pathology of anomalous junction of the pancreaticobiliary ductal system: mutagenicity of the contents of the biliary tract and nuclear atypia of the biliary epithelium. Keio J Med 1989;38(2):167–176.

95. Millbourn E. Calibre and appearance of the pancreatic ducts and relevant clinical problems. Acta Chir Scand 1960;118:286.

96. Kasugai T, Kuno N, Kobayashi S, Hattori K. Endoscopic pancreatocholangiography. I. The normal endoscopic pancreatocholangiogram. Gastroenterology 1972;63:217.

97. Trapnell JE, Howard JM. Transduodenal pancreatography: an improved technique. Surgery 1966;60:1112.

98. Freud E et al. Familiar chronic recurrent pancreatitis in identical twins: case report and review of the literature. Arch Surg 1992;127:1125–1128.

99. Makela P, Aarimaa M. Pancreatography in a family with hereditary pancreatitis. Acta Radiol Diagn 1985;26:63–66.

100. Cotton PB. Congenital anomaly of pancreas divisum as cause of obstructive pain and pancreatitis. Gut 1980;21:105.

101. Richter JM, Schapiro RH, Mulley AG, Warshaw AL. Association of pancreas divisum and pancreatitis, and its treatment by sphincteroplasty of the accessory ampulla. Gastroenterology 1981;81:1104.

102. Thompson MH, Williamson RCN, Salmon PR. The clinical relevance of isolated ventral pancreas. Br J Surg 1981;68:101.

103. Tulassay Z, Papp J. New clinical aspects of pancreas divisum. Gastrointest Endosc 1980;26:143.

104. Mitchell CJ, Lintoff DJ, Ruddell WSJ. Clinical relevance of an unfused pancreatic duct system. Gut 1979;20:1066.

105. Rusnak CH et al. Pancreatitis associated with pancreas divisum: results of surgical intervention. Am J Surg 1988;155(5):641–643.

106. Madura JA. Pancreas divisum: stenosis of the dorsally dominant pancreatic duct—a surgically correctable lesion. Am J Surg 1986;151(6):742–745.

107. Gregg JA, Monaco AP, McDermott WV. Pancreas divisum: results of surgical intervention. Am J Surg 1983;145(4):488–492.

108. Leese T, Chiche L, Bismuth H. Pancreatitis caused by congenital anomalies of the pancreatic ducts. Surgery 1989;105(2 Pt 1):125–130.

109. Agha FP, Williams KD. Pancreas divisum: incidence, detection and clinical significance. Am J Gastroenterol 1987;82(4):315–320.

110. Oi I. Non-fusion of the ventral and dorsal pancreatic ducts. Nippon Geka Gakkai Zasshi 1985;86(9):1149–1152.

111. Reshef R, Shtamler B, Novis BH. Recurrent acute pancreatitis associated with pancreas divisum. Am J Gastroenterol 1988;83(1):86–88.

112. Browder W, Gravois E, Vega P, Ertan A. Obstructing pseudocyst of the duct of Santorini in pancreas divisum. Am J Gastroenterol 1987;82(3):258–261.

113. Hyden WH. The true nature of annular pancreas. Ann Surg 1963;157:71–77.

114. Théodoridès T. Pancréas annulaire. J Chir (Paris) 1964;87:445–462.

115. Whelan TJ, Jr, Hamilton GB. Annular pancreas. Ann Surg 1957;146:252–262.
116. Jackson JM. Annular pancreas and duodenal obstruction in the neonate: a review. Arch Surg 1963;87:379–383.
117. Free EA, Gerald B. Duodenal obstruction in the newborn due to annular pancreas. AJR 1968;103:321–325.
118. Merrill JR, Raffensperger JG. Pediatric annular pancreas: twenty years experience. J Pediatr Surg 1976;11:921.
119. Heij HA, Niessen GJ. Annular pancreas associated with congenital absence of the gallbladder. J Pediatr Surg 1987;22(11):1033.
120. Kirillova IA et al. Pancreas annulare in human embryos. Acta Anat 1984;118(4):214–217.
121. Lin SZ. Annular pancreas: etiology, classification and diagnostic imaging. Chin Med J [Engl] 1989;103(5):368–372.
122. Yogi Y, Shibue T, Hashimoto S. Annular pancreas detected in adults, diagnosed by endoscopic retrograde cholangiopancreatography: report of four cases. Gastroenterol Jpn 1987;22(1):92–99.
123. Tieken T. Annular pancreas (transl). Chicago Pathol Soc 1899–1901;4:180.
124. Lecco TM. Zur Morphologie des Pankreas annulare. Sitzungsb Akad Wissensch Math Naturw Cl 1910;119:391–406.
125. Baldwin WM. Specimen of annular pancreas. Anat Rec 1910;4:299–304.
126. Erimoglu C. A case of pancreas annulare. Proc Kon Nederl Akad Wet [Biol Med] 1952;55:18.
127. Weissberg H. Ein Pancreas annulare bei einem menschlichen Embryo von 16 mm. Länge Anat Anz 1935;79:296.
128. Kie ATS, Wittebol P, Lunding J. Annular pancreas. Acta Paediatr 1961;50:72–79.
129. Boothroyd LSA. Annular pancreas. Ann Surg 1957;146:139–144.
130. Chapman JL, Mossman HW. Annular pancreas accompanied by an aberrant pancreatic nodule in the duodenum. Am J Surg 1943;60:286.
131. Ecker A. Bildungsfehler des Pancreas und des Herzens. Z Rat Med Leipz 1862;14:354–356.
132. Ravitch MM, Woods AC, Jr. Annular pancreas. Ann Surg 1950;132:1116.
133. Vidal E. Quelques cas de chirurgie pancreatique. Assoc Fran Chir 1905;18:739–747.
134. Sanford CE. Annular pancreas as a surgical problem. Arch Surg 1955;71:915–926.
135. Lundquist G. Annular pancreas: pathogenesis, clinical features, and treatment, with a report on two operation cases. Acta Chir Scand 1959;117:451–464.
136. McNaught JB. Annular pancreas: a compilation of 40 cases with a report of a new case. Am J Med Sci 1933;185:249–260.
137. Reemtsma K. Embryology and congenital anomalies of the pancreas. In: Howard JM, Jordan GL, Jr, eds. Surgical diseases of the pancreas. Philadelphia: JB Lippincott, 1960.
138. Howard JM, Jordan GL. Surgical diseases of the pancreas. Philadelphia: JP Lippincott, 1960.
139. Regan RA, Wren HB. Annular pancreas: a review with a report of eight cases treated surgically. Am Surg 1962;28:732–740.
140. Bickford B, Williamson JCFL. Annular pancreas. Br J Surg 1952;39:49–52.
141. Huebner GD, Reed PA. Annular pancreas. Am J Surg 1964;104:869–873.
142. Ricketts RR. Work-up of neonatal intestinal obstruction. Am Surg 1984;50:517–521.
143. Brant J, Hamlin HH. Annular pancreas. JAMA 1960;173:1586–1588.
144. Warren KW. Surgical treatment of uncommon lesions of the duodenum. Surg Clin North Am 1952;32:877–898.
145. Gross RE, Chisholm TC. Annular pancreas producing duodenal obstruction. Ann Surg 1944;119:759.
146. Moore TC. Annular pancreas: review of literature and report of 2 infant cases. Surgery 1953;33:138.
147. Weitzman JJ, Brennan LP. An improved technique for the correction of congenital duodenal obstruction in the neonate. J Pediatr Surg 1974;9:385–386.
148. Schnaufer L. Duodenal atresia, stenosis and annular pancreas. In: Welch KJ, Randolph JG, Ravitch MM, O'Neill JA, Rowe MI, eds. Pediatric surgery. Chicago: Yearbook Medical, 1986;829–837.
149. Akhtar J, Guiney EJ. Congenital duodenal obstruction. Br J Surg 1992;79:133–135.
150. Raffensperger JG. Pyloric and duodenal obstruction. In: Raffensperger JG, ed. Swenson's pediatric surgery. Norwalk, CT: Appleton & Lange, 1990:509–516.
151. Boyden EA. The accessory gallbladder: an embryological and comparative study of aberrant biliary vesicles occurring in man and domestic mammals. Am J Anat 1926;38:117.
152. Wrenn EL, Favara BI. Duodenal duplication (or pancreatic bladder) presenting as double gallbladder. Surgery 1971;69:858.
153. Garcia FG, Raul JJ. Pancreas aberrante en la pared vesicular con perforacion aguda. Prensa Med Argent 1971;58:1829.
154. Harlaftis N, Gray SW, Skandalakis JE. Multiple gallbladders. Surg Gynecol Obstet 1977;145:928.
155. Wilson PM. Unusual duodeno-pancreatic relationships associated with incomplete rotation of mid-gut loop. Anat Rec 1964;149:397.
156. Burne JC. Pancreatic and gastric heterotopia in a diverticulum of the transverse colon. J Pathol Bact 1958;75:470.
157. Collins DC. A study of 50,000 specimens of the human vermiform appendix. Surg Gynecol Obstet 1955;101:437.
158. Thorsness ET. Aberrant pancreatic nodule arising on the neck of the human gallbladder. Anat Rec 1940;77:319–329.
159. Jacobsen AS. Accessory pancreas in the wall of the gallbladder. Arch Pathol 1940;30:908.
160. Horányi J, Füsy F. Hepar succenturiatum in the wall of the gallbladder. Zentralbl Chir 1963;88:768–771.
161. Baar HS, d'Abreu AL. Duplications of the foregut: superior accessory lung (2 cases); epiphrenic oesophageal diverticulum; intrapericardial teratoid tumour; and oesophageal cyst. Br J Surg 1949;37:220–230.
162. Beskin CA. Intralobar enteric sequestration of the lung containing aberrant pancreas. J Thorac Cardiovasc Surg 1961;41:314–317.
163. Warthin AS. Two cases of accessory pancreas (omentum and stomach). Physician Surg (Detroit) 1904;26:337–350.
164. Busard JM, Walters W. Heterotopic pancreatic tissue: report of a case presenting symptoms of ulcer and review of the recent literature. Arch Surg 1950;60:674–682.
165. Laughlin EH, Keown ME, Jackson JE. Heterotopic pancreas obstructing the ampulla of Vater. Arch Surg 1983;118(8);979–980.
166. Herrera MN et al. Digestive hemorrhage associated with ectopic pancreas. Rev Esp Enferm Apar Dig 1989;75(1):91–94.
167. Briceno LI, Grases PJ, Gallego S. Tracheobronchial pancreatic remnants causing esophageal stenosis. J Pediatr Surg 1981;16:731.
168. Carr MJT, Deiraniya AK, Judd PA. Mediastinal cyst containing mural pancreatic tissue. Thorax 1977;32:512.
169. Spence RK, Schnaufer L, Mahboubi S. Coexistant gastric duplication and accessory pancreas: clinical manifestations, embryogenesis, and treatment. J Pediatr Surg 1986;21(1):68–70.
170. Tsunoda T et al. Heterotopic pancreas: a rare cause of bile duct dilatation—report of a case and review of the literature. Jpn J Surg 1990;20(2):217–220.

171. Burke GW et al. Heterotopic pancreas: gastric outlet obstruction secondary to pancreatitis and pancreatic pseudocyst. Am J Gastroenterol 1989;84(1):52–55.

172. Clarke BE. Myoepithelial hamartoma of gastrointestinal tract: report of eight cases with comment concerning genesis and nomenclature. Arch Pathol 1940;30:143–152.

173. King ESJ, MacCallum P. Cholecystitis glandularis proliferans (cystica). Br J Surg 1931;19:310–323.

174. Klob J. Pankreas anomalien. Z Ges Aerztl Wien 1859;15:732.

175. Hunt VC, Bonesteel HTS. Meckel's diverticulum containing aberrant pancreas. Arch Surg 1934;28:425.

176. Pearson S. Aberrant pancreas: review of the literature and report of 3 cases, one of which produced common and pancreatic duct obstruction. Arch Surg 1951;63:168–184.

177. Curd H. Histologic study of Meckel's diverticulum with special reference to heterotopic tissues. Arch Surg 1936;32:506–523.

178. Ackerman LV. Surgical pathology. St. Louis: Mosby, 1953.

179. Howard JM. Cysts of the pancreas. In: Howard JM, Jordan GL, Jr, Reber HA, eds. Surgical diseases of the pancreas. Philadelphia: Lea & Febiger, 1987:540.

180. Eha CE. Case of congenital pancreatic cyst. JAMA 1922;78:1294.

181. McPherson TC, Heersma HS. Diagnosis and treatment of pancreatic cysts in children with report of a case. J Pediatr 1948; 33:213.

182. Caironi C, Fraschini A, Ambrogi G, Canali B. Notes on pancreatic cysts in the light of three personal cases. Panminerva Med 1980;22:17.

183. Wolloch Y, Chaimoff C, Lubin E, and Dintsman M. Splenic vein thrombosis, segmental portal hypertension and bleeding esophageal varices produced by congenital pancreatic cyst. Isr J Med Sci 1974;10:670.

184. Rheudasil JM, Brown B, Gray SW, Skandalakis JE. True pancreatic cysts: a review. J Med Assoc GA 1986;75:534–537, 737.

185. Miles RM. Pancreatic cysts in the newborn. Ann Surg 1959;149:576–581.

186. de Lange C, Janssen TAE. Large solitary pancreatic cyst and other developmental errors in a premature infant. Am J Dis Child 1948;75:587.

187. Bikoff HS. Embryonal cyst of the wall of the stomach: report of a case in which symptoms of pyloric obstruction occurred. Am J Dis Child 1938;56:594–599.

188. Pilot LM, Gooselow JG, Isaackson PC. Obstruction of the CBD in the newborn infant by a pancreatic cyst. Lancet 1964;84:204.

189. Iovchev II. Suppurative dermoid cyst of the pancreas. Vestn Khir 1972;107:124.

190. Pomosov DV et al. Dermoid cyst of the pancreas in a child. Vestn Khir 1973;110:93.

191. Assawamatiyamont S, King AD, Jr. Dermoid cysts of the pancreas. Am Surg 1977;43:503.

192. Black PR, Welch KJ, Eraklis AJ. Juxtapancreatic intestinal duplications with pancreatic ductal communication: a cause of pancreatitis and recurrent abdominal pain in childhood. J Pediatr Surg 1986;21(3):257–261.

193. Lindau A. Studien über Kleinhirncysten: Bau, Pathogenese und Beziehungen zur Angiomatosis retinae. Acta Pathol Microbiol Scand (Suppl) 1926;1:1–128.

194. Eastman PF et al. Pseudocysts of the pancreas. Ann Surg 1961;154(Suppl 6):231–238.

195. Roy CC et al. Digestive and absorptive phase anomalies associated with the exocrine pancreatic insufficiency of cystic fibrosis. J Pediatr Gastroenterol Nutr 1988;7(Suppl 1):1–7.

196. Hurwitt ES, Arnheim EE. Meconium ileus associated with stenosis of the pancreatic ducts: a clinical, pathological and embryologic study. Am J Dis Child 1942;64:443.

197. Norris RF, Tyson RM. The pathogenesis of congenital polycystic lung and its correlation with polycystic disease of other epithelial organs. Am J Pathol 1947;23:1075.

198. Andersen DH. Cystic fibrosis of pancreas. J Chronic Dis 1958;7:58–90.

199. Payne RM, Nielsen AM. Meconium peritonitis. Am Surg 1962;28:224.

200. Molnar EM, Gray SW, Cale EF, Skandalakis JE. Meconium ileus with volvulus and meconium peritonitis. Am Surg 1963;29:900–904.

201. Smoller M, Hsia DY. Studies of the genetic mechanism of cystic fibrosis of the pancreas. Am J Dis Child 1959;98:277–292.

202. Donnell GN, Cleland RS. Intestinal atresia or stenosis in the newborn associated with fibrocystic disease of the pancreas. Calif Med 1961;94:165–170.

203. di Sant'Agnese PA, Dische Z, Danilczenko A. Physicochemical differences of mucoproteins in duodenal fluid of patients with cystic fibrosis of the pancreas and controls. Pediatrics 1957;19:252–260.

204. Wiser WC, Beier FR. Albumin in the meconium of infants with cystic fibrosis: a preliminary report. Pediatrics 1964;33:115.

205. Honeyman MS, Siker E. Cystic fibrosis of the pancreas: genetic review and estimate of incidence. Conn Health Bull 1961;75:275.

206. Landsteiner K. Darmverschluss durch eingedicktes Meconium Pankreatitis. Zentralbl Allg Pathol Anat 1905;16:903.

207. Andersen DH. Cystic fibrosis of the pancreas and its relation to celiac disease. Am J Dis Child 1938;56:344.

208. Andersen DH. Cystic fibrosis of the pancreas, vitamin A deficiency and bronchiectasis. J Pediatr 1939;15:763.

209. Farber S. The relation of pancreatic achylia to meconium ileus. J Pediatr 1944;24:387.

210. di Sant'Agnese PA, Darling RC, Perera GA, Shea E. Sweat electrolyte disturbances associated with childhood pancreatic disease. Am J Med 1953;15:777–784.

211. Andersen DH, Hodges RG. Celiac syndrome: genetics of cystic fibrosis of the pancreas with a consideration of etiology. Am J Dis Child 1946;72:62.

212. Thomaides TS, Arey JP. Intestinal lesions in cystic fibrosis of pancreas. J Pediatr 1963;63:444–453.

213. Rickham PP, Boeckman CR. Neonatal meconium obstruction in the absence of mucoviscidosis. Am J Surg 1965;109:173–177.

214. Dolan TF, Touloukian RJ. Familial meconium ileus not associated with cystic fibrosis. J Pediatr Surg 1974;9:821–824.

215. Heitlinger LA. Intestinal and pancreatic enzymes in amniotic fluid and meconium: content as an index of fetal maturity, well-being, or disease. In: Lebenthal E, ed. Human gastrointestinal development. New York: Raven Press, 1989:522.

216. Seeds AE. Current concepts of amniotic fluid dynamics. Am J Obstet Gynecol 1980;138:575.

217. Boyd A et al. Gastrografin enemi in meconium ileus: the persistent approach. Pediatr Surg Int 1988;3:139–140.

218. Rescorla KJ, Grosfeld JL, West KJ, Vane DW. Changing patterns of treatment and survival in neonates with meconium ileus. Arch Surg 1989;124:837–840.

219. Bishop HC, Koop CE. Management of meconium ileus: resection, Roux-en-Y anastomosis and ileostomy irrigation with pancreatic enzymes. Arch Surg 1957;145:410.

220. Harberg F, Senekjian EK, Pokorny WJ. Treatment of uncomplicated meconium ileus via T-Tube ileostomy. J Pediatr Surg 1981;16:61–63.

221. Mellière D. Variations des artères hépatiques et du carrefour pancréatique. J Chir (Paris) 1968;98:5.

222. Pierson JM. The arterial blood supply of the pancreas. Surg Gynecol Obstet 1943;77:426.

223. Woodburne RT, Olsen LL. The arteries of the pancreas. Anat Rec 1951;111:255.

224. Ziegler HR. Excision of the head of the pancreas for carcinoma with studies of its blood supply. Surg Gynecol Obstet 1942;74:137.

225. Kirk E. Untersuchungen über die gröbere and feinere topographische verteilung der arterien, venen und ausfuhrungsgange in der menschlichen bauchspeicheldrüse. Ges Anat 1931;94:822.

226. Falconer CWA, Griffiths F. Anatomy of the blood vessels in the region of the pancreas. Br J Surg 1950;37:334.

227. Jonsell G, Boutelier P. Observations during treatment of acute necrotizing pancreatis with surgical ablation. Surg Gynecol Obstet 1979;148:385.

228. Thompson IM. On the arteries and ducts in the hepatic pedicle. A study in statistical human anatomy. Univ Calif Publ Anat 1953;1:55.

229. Michels NA. The hepatic, cystic, and retroduodenal arteries and their relations to the biliary ducts. Ann Surg 1951;133:503.

230. Thomford NR, Chandnani PC, Taha AM, Chablani VN, Busnardo AC. Anatomic characteristics of the pancreatic arteries. AM J Surg 1986;151:690–693.

231. Howard JM, Woldenberg LS, Conover SV. Arterial anomaly of crucial importance in resection of head of pancreas. Pancreas 1989;4(5):606–608.

232. Douglass TC, Lounsbury BF, Cutter WW, Wetzel N. An experi-mental study of healing in the common bile duct. Surg Gynecol Obstet 1950;91:301.

233. Matsusue, S, Kashiihara S, Koizumi S. Pancreatectomy for carci-noma of the head of the pancreas associated with multiple anom-alies including the preduodenal portal vein. Jpn J Surg 1984;14(5):394–398.

234. Dumeige F, Hermieu JF, Farret O. A pre-wirsungal portal vein: apropos of a case [transl]. Chirurgie 1989;115(3):245–249.

235. Evans BP, Ochsner A. Gross anatomy of the lymphatics of the human pancreas. Surgery 1954;36:177.

236. Rouviere H. Anatomy of the human lymphatic system. Tobias MJ, transl. Ann Arbor: Edwards Brothers, 1938.

237. Healey JF Jr. A synopsis of clinical anatomy. Philadelphia: WB Saunders, 1969.

238. Cubilla AL, Fortner J, Fitzgerald PJ. Lymph node involvement in carcinoma of the head of the pancreas area. Cancer 1978;41:880.

239. Bartels P. Ueber die Lymphage faesse des Pankreas. III. Die regionaeren Drusen des Pankreas beim Menschen. Arch F Anat Entw 1907:267.

240. Fujii H, Matsumoto Y, Suda K, Aoyama H, Yamamoto M, Suga-hara K. The modes of spread of pancreas head cancer based on difference of the pancreatic anlagen. Nippon Geka Gakkai Zasshi 1989;90(3):415–422.

CHAPTER 12

THE LARYNX

Norman Wendell Todd / John Elias Skandalakis / Stephen Wood Gray

They followed Czerny's experiments on the extirpation of the larynx, after which
I succeeded, a few years ago, in removing a larynx that was affected with a
cancerous growth.
—*LETTER OF THEODORE BILLROTH TO DR. L. WITTELSHÖFER FEBRUARY 4, 1881*

DEVELOPMENT

The respiratory primordium appears in the floor of the foregut early in the fourth week. This laryngotracheal groove represents the primitive glottis.

This primitive slit-like glottis, the laryngeal aditus, lies on the pharyngeal floor between the fourth and sixth branchial arches (Fig. 12.1, *A*). Below the aditus is an epithelial plate traversed dorsally by a narrow canal, the pharyngotracheal duct, connecting the pharynx with the tracheal lumen. Rostral to the slit is the primordium of the epiglottis, which is derived from the ventral ends of the third and fourth branchial arches which Arey stated is peculiar to mammals (1). Lateral to the slit are the paired arytenoid swellings derived from the sixth branchial arches (Fig. 12.1, *B*). During the fifth and sixth weeks, medial movement of the arytenoid swellings changes the aditus from a simple slit to a T-shaped aperture (Fig. 12.1, *C* and *D*).

Wilhelm His, Sr., did monumental work in the late 1800s on the development of the gastrointestinal tract and the branchial arches (2). The main body of knowledge of laryngeal embryology was reported within 30 years of His' publication. These studies were wax-plate reconstructions from serially sectioned specimens. Yet, there are two conflicting concepts of the origin of the laryngeal cavity that remain to be resolved. One is that the entire laryngeal cavity is developed from the floor of the pharynx cephalad to the respiratory primordium (lung bud). The other concept is that the tracheal "mouth" is the glottis and that, therefore, the lumen immediately caudal must be the subglottis. Until the eighth week, the early larynx is shut except for a tiny duct dorsally that connects the pharyngeal cavity to the trachea by way of the glottis (2). The laryngeal, tracheal, and bronchial portions of the respiratory primordium develop in a proximodistal sequence, as do the components of limb buds. But in terms of recognizable morphology, the larynx acquires its characteristic complexity relatively late. One of the most detailed descriptions is that of Tucker and O'Rahilly in 1972 (3).

Before the characteristic lumen of the larynx is developed, its lining is identifiable by epithelial lamina between arytenoid swellings. Anteriorly, the epithelial lamina bifurcates into a T shape (2–4). The laryngeal vestibule of the human adult is composed of the embryonic transverse and sagittal clefts that develop in these epithelial laminae (4) (Fig. 12.2). As the laryngeal cavity is established anteriorly and caudally, the upper and lower lips of the (ventrodorsally elongated) openings of the ventricles become the false (or vestibular) and true vocal folds, respectively.

The earliest cartilages to appear are the thyroid and cricoid. While these are evident at 5 weeks, chondrification begins at the end of the seventh week. Chondrification of the arytenoid and corniculate cartilages starts toward the end of the third month. The epiglottis chondrifies during the fourth month, and the cuneiforms late in the seventh month (5).

The ventral portion of the skeleton of the second branchial arch forms the lesser horns of the hyoid bone; the dorsal portion forms the styloid process, the stapes suprastructure, and parts of the incus and malleus. The ventral third arch forms the greater horns of the hyoid bone. The ventral fourth and fifth arches fuse to form the thyroid cartilage. The cuneiform cartilage arises from the fourth arch, and the corniculate, arytenoid, and cricoid cartilages derive from the fifth arch. Identification of specific branchial arches caudal to the fourth arch in the human embryo is difficult. Cricoid chondrification occurs bilaterally from a single center in the ventral arch of a precartilaginous template that encircles the subglottic cavity, meeting dorsally to form the dorsal lamina of the cricoid (2). The laryngeal epithelium becomes ciliated by the end of the fourth month, and elastic tissue and muscles appear during the fifth month. The muscles are derivatives of the fourth and fifth arches and are innervated by the 10th cranial nerve (CN X). Myofibrils are present by the 12th week.

During fetal life and the first 3 years of postnatal life, the larynx is relatively larger and higher in the neck than it will be in adulthood. Relative growth decreases after

405

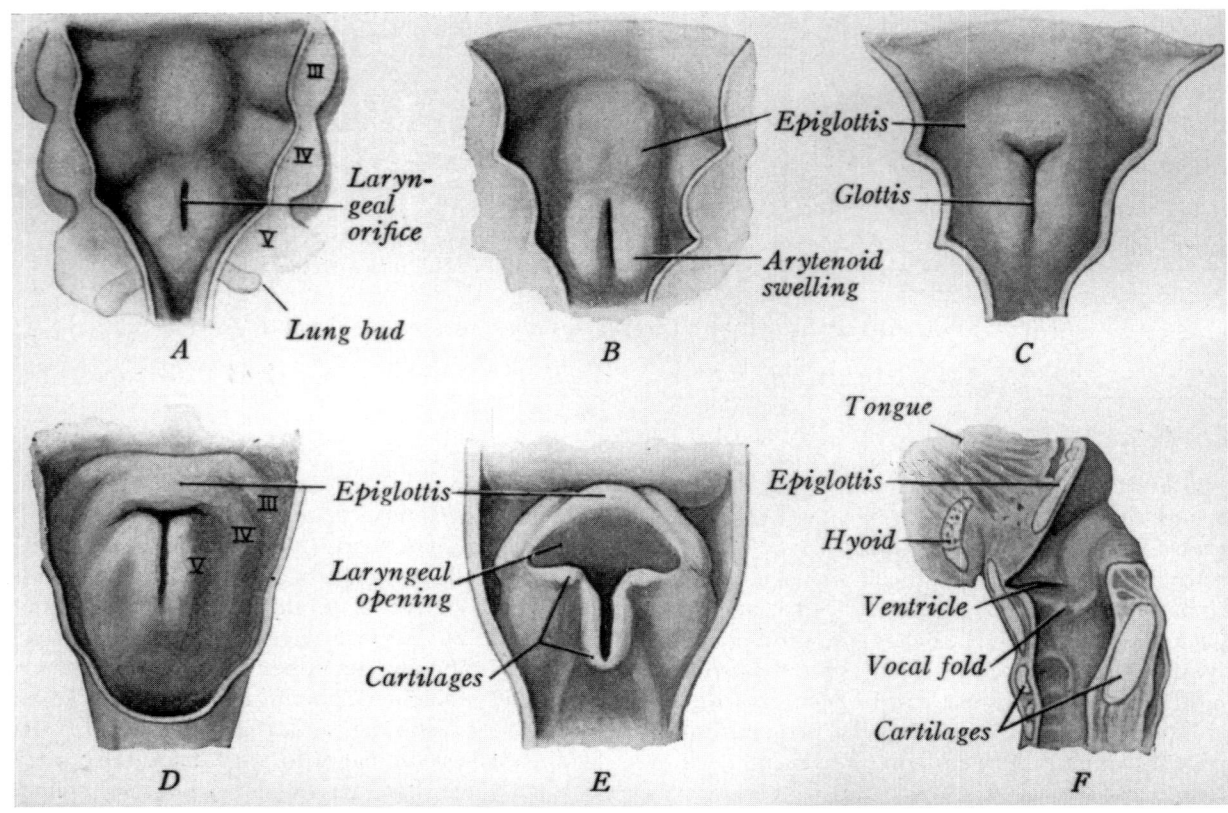

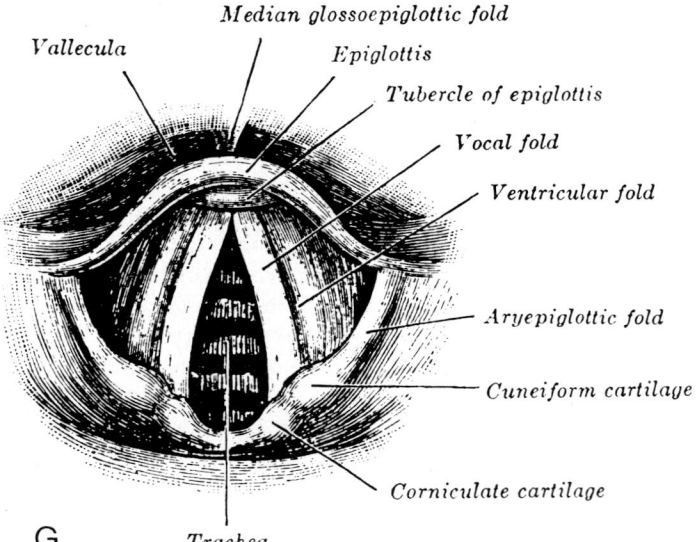

Figure 12.1. Development of the human larynx. **A**, At 5 mm. **B**, At 9 mm. **C**, At 12 mm. **D**, At 16 mm. **E**, At 40 mm (× 7). **F**, Sagittal hemisection, at birth (× 15). **G**, The vallecula is the depression on both sides of the median glossoepiglottic fold and is demonstrated here in adults, from a laryngoscopic view of the larynx. (**A** to **F**, From Arey LB. Developmental anatomy, 7th ed. Philadelphia: WB Saunders, 1974:264; **G**, from Williams PL, Warwick R, Dyson M, Bannister LH, eds. Gray's anatomy, 37th ed. Philadelphia: WB Saunders, 1989:1254.)

the third year. During puberty, under hormonal influence, further changes in shape and size occur in the male.

The tracheoesophageal septum, sometimes called the "party wall" of the trachea and esophagus, has been considered to develop from caudal to cephal, reaching the level of the fourth branchial pouches. However, there is

now agreement that the septum is present from the initial appearance of the lung bud (fourth week) (4, 6). The lung bud (and subsequently the trachea) grows caudally into the mesenchyme ventral to the foregut. This mesenchyme between the respiratory and gut tubes constitutes the tracheoesophageal septum.

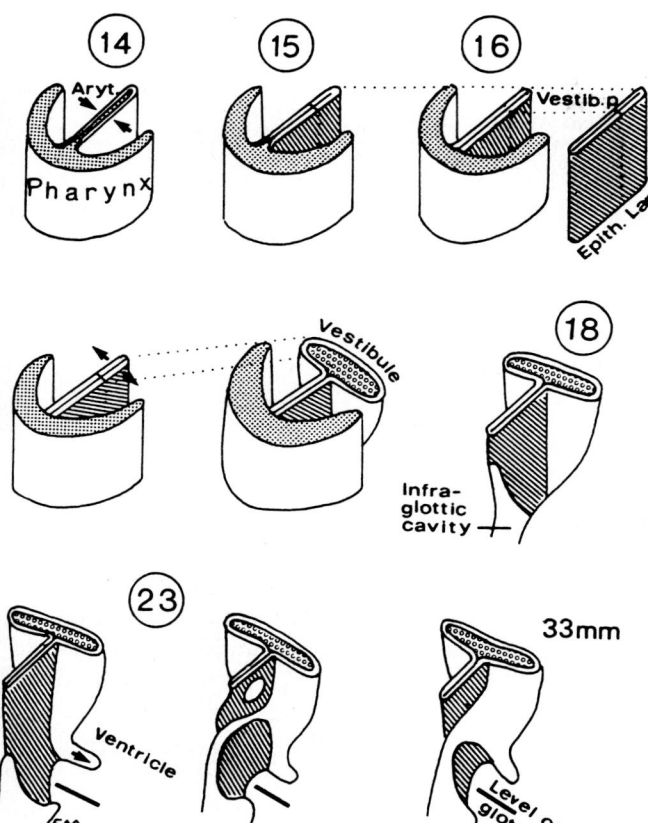

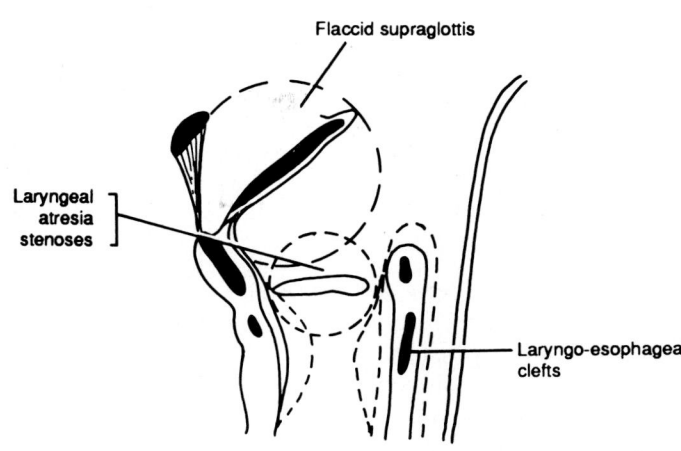

Figure 12.2. Right posterolateral views of developing pharynx and larynx from 4 weeks to beginning of fetal period. Epithelial walls between arytenoid swellings (arrows) become apposed and constitute epithelial lamina, ventral portion of which may be termed its vestibular part. Lateral expansion (arrows) of vestibular part gives rise to embryonic vestibule. Lamina then begins to disintegrate to varying degrees during remainder of embryonic and commencement of fetal period. Formation of right ventricle is also shown, and level of future glottis is indicated. (From O'Rahilly R, Müller F. Respiratory and alimentary relations in staged human embryos: new embryological data and congenital anomalies. Ann Otol Rhinol Laryngol 1984;93(5):424.)

Critical Events of Development

Most of the severe laryngeal anomalies arise from the failure of the larynx to open at the eighth week (atresia); from establishment of an abnormally shaped and sized subglottic lumen; or from abnormal dorsal fusion of cricoid chondrification (Fig. 12.3).

ANOMALIES OF THE LARYNX (TABLE 12.1 AND FIG. 12.3)

Laryngeal Atresia

ANATOMY

Laryngeal atresia is a complex anomaly which is fatal unless tracheotomy is performed immediately after birth. Smith and Bain (7) arbitrarily divided the anomaly into three types, which grade into one another (Fig. 12.4). Belmont et al. (8) reported a unilateral case.

Figure 12.3. Highly diagramatic presentation of sites of developmental anomalies of the larynx.

Type I: Panglottic Atresia. The vestibule and ventricles are absent. The normally paired intrinsic muscles are fused across the midline. The arytenoid cartilages are fused over part of their length, and the cricoid mass is conically shaped. A fine duct, less than 1 mm in diameter, passes behind the fused arytenoids and through the cricoid.

Type II: Infraglottic Atresia. The vestibule and ventricles are normal, but the glottis is a blind cleft between the vocal folds. The arytenoid cartilages are separate, but the cricoid is dome shaped. A tiny pharyngotracheal duct is dorsal to the malformed cricoid.

Type III: Glottic Atresia. The glottis is occluded. Ventrally the occlusion is by fibrosis and muscle. Dorsally the occlusion is by the fusion of the left and right arytenoid cartilages. A tiny pharyngotracheal duct is just dorsal to the arytenoids. The cricoid is normal.

EMBRYOGENESIS

Laryngeal atresia can only partially be accounted for by simple failure of epithelial recanalization to occur. Abnormal cricoid development is involved in types I and II.

INCIDENCE

Fewer than 40 cases have been reported (9).

ASSOCIATED ANOMALIES

Most reported cases have other congenital abnormalities. Characteristically, the lungs are bulky and edematous, with a marked increase in surface area and lung volume for age. Obstructed drainage of lung liquid through a pinhole laryngeal orifice is thought to account for the pulmonary findings (10).

SYMPTOMS AND DIAGNOSIS

There are active respiratory movements of the thorax, but no passage of air. Endotracheal intubation is unsuccessful. Diagnosis can be made only by laryngoscopy.

TREATMENT

Immediate tracheotomy provides the only hope for survival. Subsequent laryngeal repair may afford an adequate laryngeal airway and speech.

Incomplete Laryngeal Atresia ("Web")

ANATOMY

The true vocal folds have the appearance of being welded together, anteriorly. The web-like appearance appreciated at laryngoscopy can belie the thickness of the lesion, and the presence of subglottic extension. In general, the "webs" with the greater anteroposterior involvement have the greater subglottic extension. The findings are reminiscent of but not as severe as type III laryngeal atresia.

The upper surface of the web is stratified squamous epithelium and the lower surface is pseudostratified ciliated epithelium, typical of the lower respiratory tract. Between the surfaces is connective tissue, which may be dense fibrous tissue, striated muscle, or cartilage.

EMBRYOGENESIS

There is incomplete dissolution of the epithelial lamina.

INCIDENCE

Cohen (11) reported his experience with 51 children, seen during 32 years of practicing pediatric otolaryngology.

ASSOCIATED ANOMALIES

About half of patients have other concomitant congenital anomalies (11). Nearly one-third of the anomalies involve the head and neck.

SYMPTOMS AND DIAGNOSIS

Almost all patients have voice dysfunction, and most have stridor at least during upper respiratory tract infections. Recurrent croup, tracheobronchitis, and pneumonia are less common symptoms. Though the web can be appreciated at mirror laryngoscopy in older cooperative children, careful direct laryngoscopy is usually required to establish the diagnosis (Fig. 12.5).

TREATMENT

Tracheotomy is often required (in 22 of 51 patients in Cohen's experience). Therapy may be endolaryngeal (dilations, knife, scissors, laser) or external laryngofissure techniques. According to Cohen, "The acme of perfection of therapy is the patient with a perfect airway and an almost perfect voice" (11).

Subglottic Stenosis

ANATOMY

The subglottic space is enclosed ventrally and laterally by the elastic cone. Posteriorly the space is bound by the cricoid plate. The subglottic space extends from the plane of the true vocal folds to the plane of the caudal border of the cricoid ring. In its widest definition, now archaic, the space extends from the vocal folds down to the smallest bronchi.

EMBRYOGENESIS

Cricoid stenosis is the result of a defect in the development of the sixth branchial arch, probably during the seventh embryonic week.

INCIDENCE

Subglottic stenosis is considered to be congenital if the history does not include prolonged endotracheal intubation or other apparent cause. Most subglottic stenosis nowadays is acquired, manifesting after intraluminal trauma. The mechanism of acquiring subglottic stenosis is complex and may involve an autoimmune process (12), according to Stolovitzky and Todd in 1990.

Congenital subglottic stenosis is less common than laryngomalacia. In a 10-year period, Holinger et al. (13)

Table 12.1.
Anomalies of the Larynx

Anomaly	Origin of Defect	First Appearance	Sex Chiefly Affected	Relative Frequency	Remarks
Atresia of the larynx	6th–10th weeks	At birth	Equal	Very rare	Fatal unless tracheostomy is performed at once
Laryngeal "webs"	10th week?	At birth if large; asymptomatic if small	Equal	Uncommon	
Subglottic (cricoid) stenosis	10th week	At birth	Male	Rare	
Laryngomalacia	?	At birth	Male	Common	Symptoms usually disappear by 2nd year of life
Laryngotracheoesophageal cleft	6th week	At birth	Equal	Very rare	Familial tendency has been suggested

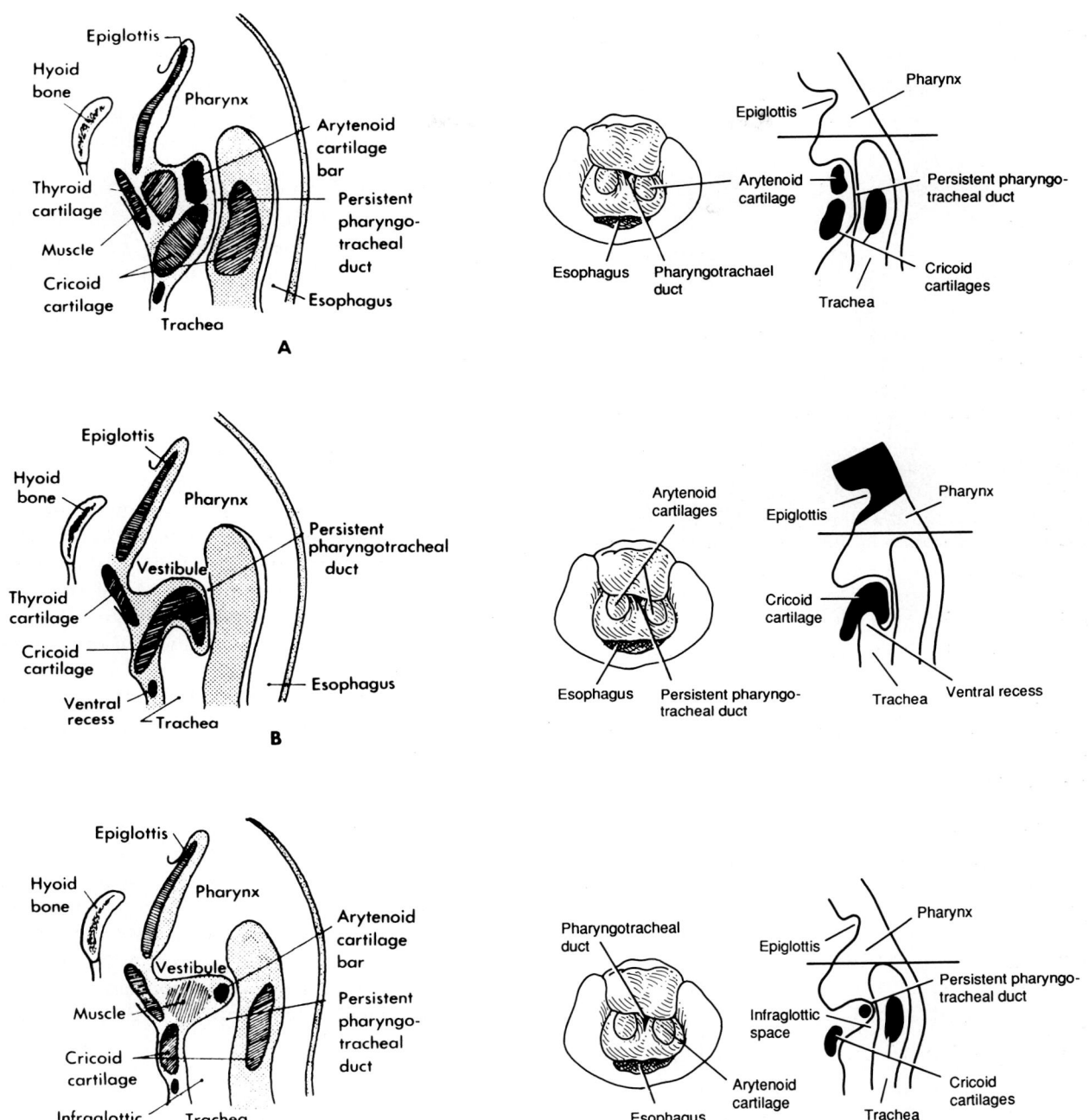

Figure 12.4. Diagrammatic sagittal sections illustrating types of congenital laryngeal atresia proposed by Smith and Bain (1965). **A**, Type I. **B**, Type II. **C**, Type III. **A1** to **C1**, adjacent to each section is the endoscopist's view. (Modified from Belmont JR, Grundfast KM, Heffner D, Hyams VJ. Laryngeal dysgenesis. Ann Otol Rhinol Laryngol 1985;604; **A** to **C**, Redrawn from Smith II, Bain AD. Congenital atresia of the larynx. Ann Otol 1965;74:338–349.)

identified 115 cases of congenital subglottic stenosis at Children's Memorial Hospital, Chicago.

ASSOCIATED ANOMALIES

Associated laryngeal and tracheobronchial pathologic findings are found in about 13% of cases of congenital subglottic stenosis. Congenital defects in other regions are also found in about 13% of cases (13).

SYMPTOMS AND DIAGNOSIS

Respiratory distress with inhalatory stridor is the hallmark. Symptoms are not always present at birth but usually become evident during the first few weeks or months of life. Endoscopic evaluation is necessary to establish the diagnosis. The finding of a lumen too small to allow easy passage of a 4- to 4.5-mm (outside diameter) bronchoscope is considered definitive. The point of greatest

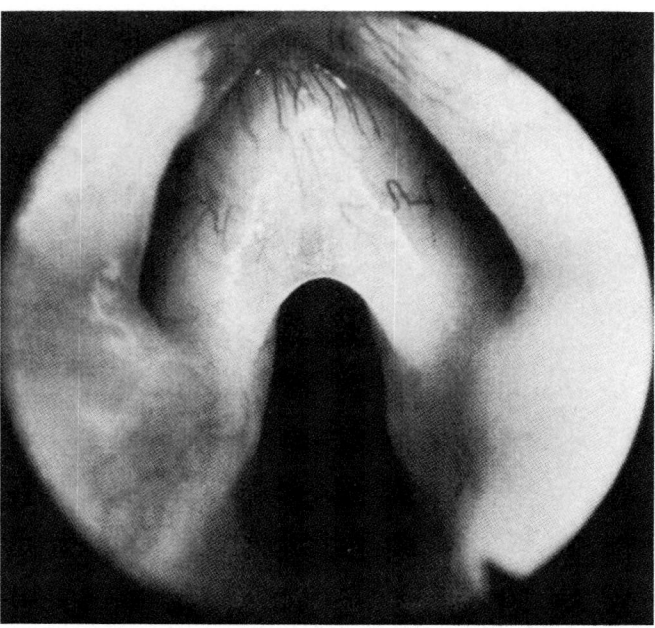

Figure 12.5. Medium-sized, thin congenital anterior glottic web in an infant with a weak cry. (From Benjamin BNP. Diagnostic laryngology: adults and children. Philadelphia: WB Saunders, 1990:92.)

obstruction is generally 2 to 3 mm caudal to the free edges of the true vocal folds (13).

TREATMENT

Many children outgrow congenital subglottic stenosis. Tracheotomy was required in nearly half the patients reported by Holinger et al. (13). Growth of the airway usually permits decannulation by 4 years of age. Laryngotracheoplasty with free graft of costal cartilage is the preferred treatment, if surgery is required.

Laryngomalacia

In laryngomalacia, the supraglottic structures collapse excessively inward during inhalation. Prior to the 1940s, the generalization "congenital laryngeal stridor" was used to describe this condition. There is no consensus that laryngomalacia is related to an embryologic anomaly of the larynx. Though laryngomalacia is a specific disease state, the pathogenesis is ill-defined (14).

ANATOMY

Present evidence does not support the notion that a cartilage deficiency or abnormality is the etiologic factor for laryngomalacia. The ω-shaped epiglottis is normal in infancy. The suggestion that a minimal interarytenoid cleft may be a factor in laryngomalacia has not been answered (15).

INCIDENCE

Laryngomalacia accounts for most (about 60%) of the congenital laryngeal anomalies that present with stridor (13). Premature infants do not have a greater incidence of laryngomalacia than do full-term infants.

ASSOCIATED ABNORMALITIES

Concurrent airway anomalies are often found in infants with laryngomalacia. Gonzales et al. (16) found that 27% of infants with laryngomalacia had an additional airway disorder.

Immature or defective neuromuscular control is often found in infants with laryngomalacia. Associations with gastroesophageal reflux, hypotonia, and central apnea have been reported (17).

SYMPTOMS AND DIAGNOSIS

Intermittent and low-pitched inhalatory stridor is characteristically found in the infant with laryngomalacia. Symptoms usually appear in the first weeks of life but may not begin until several months of age. Usually, the symptoms are at their worst by 6 months of age, then decrease gradually to disappear by age 2 or 3 years. The stridor is worse during agitation and feeding and with viral upper respiratory tract infections.

The diagnosis may be suggested in the awake child by using flexible fiberoptic laryngoscopy through the nose (with the tip of the scope just behind the uvula). Collapse of the supraglottic structures into the airway of the lumen is seen during inhalation. The most lax portions of the supraglottis may be the aryepiglottic folds or the lateral aspects or tip of the epiglottis (Fig. 12.6). The diagnosis is confirmed by direct laryngoscopy: "When the laryngoscope blade is placed behind the epiglottis on its laryngeal surface and above the vocal cords, the aryepiglottic folds and arytenoids are splinted outward, collapse of the airway is prevented, and the obstruction and stridor is immediately corrected" (18), according to Benjamin in 1990.

TREATMENT

Expectant observation is appropriate for the majority of infants with laryngomalacia. Treatment of gastroesophageal reflux and avoidance of inhalant irritants and people with "colds" is indicated. In severe cases with failure to thrive, life-threatening apnea episodes, or developing cor pulmonale, tracheotomy or endoscopic laser "supraglottoplasty" is indicated.

Laryngotracheoesophageal Cleft (Fig. 12.7)

ANATOMY

A defect in the posterior wall of the larynx through the cricoid cartilage provides a communication between the larynx and the esophagus. Such a cleft may be confined

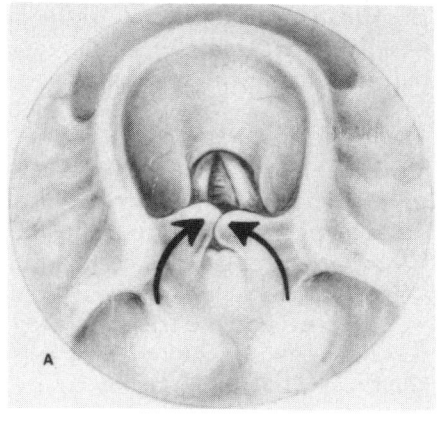
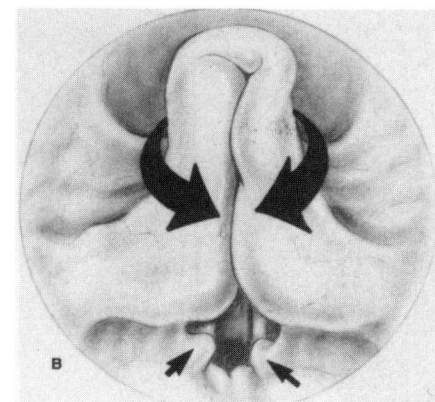
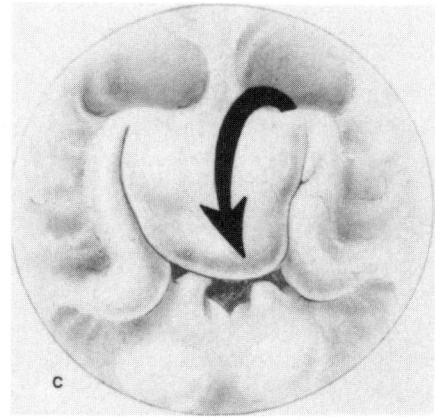

Figure 12.6. Various mechanisms of laryngomalacia. **A**, Inspiratory collapse of prominent cuneiform carilages *(arrows)* with the aryepiglottic folds. **B**, Anterior collapse of the cuneiform cartilages *(small arrows)* and arytenoids (inferiorly) often occurs in association with obstruction by an abnormal long, tubular epiglottis *(large arrows)*. **C**, Airway obstruction may occur when the epiglottis is displaced posteriorly to form a seal against the posterior pharyngeal wall or folds upon itself to be drawn to or even between the vocal cords. (From Holinger LD, Konior RJ. Surgical management of severe laryngomalacia. Laryngoscope 1989;99:139.)

to the larynx, or it may extend downward through the tracheoesophageal septum, sometimes as far caudally as into a major bronchus (Fig. 12.8).

EMBRYOGENESIS

A controversy exists about whether the respiratory primordium is initially common with the esophagus or if it is always separate from the esophagus. The former notion is classic, and the cleft deformity has been considered to be due to failure of formation of the cephalic end of the septum between the trachea and esophagus. However, Zaw-Tun (2) maintains that the septum is defined by the separate respiratory primordium, so that there is no cephalad development of such a septum. The dorsal fusion of the cricoid shelves and the demarcation of the tracheoesophageal septum appear to be independent developments (19).

The classic notion of failure of cephalad ascent of the forming tracheoesophageal septum is at odds with two clinical observations. First, tracheoesophageal fistula without laryngeal cleft is comparatively common. Second, patients with clefts do not seem to have a tissue deficiency, per se; rather, the edges of the cleft tend to approximate, and the edges often herniate into the larynx or trachea, presenting as a soft tissue mass.

HISTORY AND INCIDENCE

Cleft larynx was first described in a doctoral thesis by Richter in 1792 (20). No other cases were reported until the 20th century. At least 130 cases have been reported (19), according to Eriksen et al. in 1990. Most defects involve the larynx and cervical trachea. Familial occurrence, consistent with autosomal dominant inheritance, has been noted in three families.

ASSOCIATED ANOMALIES

Other defects are common in these babies. The incidence of tracheoesophageal fistula may be as high as 20%. Polyhydramnios and prematurity are common. Laryngotracheoesophageal cleft is included in the physical findings in G syndrome and Pallister-Hall syndrome.

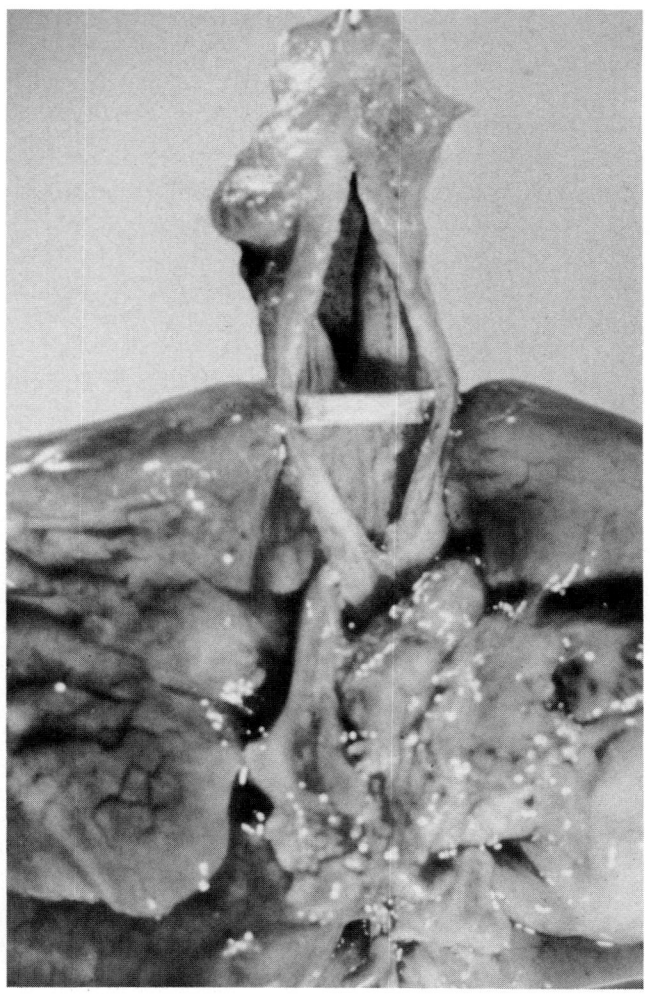

Figure 12.7. Type III laryngotracheoesophageal cleft viewed from the front; wooden peg holding anterior surface of trachea open. The cleft extends to within 1 cm of the carina.

SYMPTOMS

The chief presenting symptoms of cleft larynx are stridor, aspiration, and perhaps some voice change. Clefts involving the trachea usually have more severe symptoms. Attempts at endotracheal intubation often result in esophageal intubation, even though the tube was seen to pass through the glottis. The explanation, of course, is that the tube displaced posteriorly through the cleft larynx.

DIAGNOSIS

Cleft larynx is often extremely difficult to identify. The diagnosis is made by careful direct laryngoscopy using rigid (not flexible) technique. As the two arytenoid masses touch in the midline, they must be specifically spread apart so that the cleft can be visualized (21). While various

classifications of the extent of the defect have been proposed, more important is the total delineation of the defect and any other anomalies.

TREATMENT

Minimal clefts—that is, those that are confined to the supraglottic larynx and do not involve the cricoid—can often be managed nonsurgically. Management is similar to that for laryngomalacia, plus thickening of feeds so that aspiration is minimized.

Clefts through the cricoid and cervical trachea require surgical repair. A lateral pharyngotomy approach has been used, but the anterior laryngofissure approach is probably better. Gastrostomy is required.

EDITORIAL COMMENT

Recent experiences by pediatric otolaryngologists and pediatric surgeons indicate the clear superiority of an anterior midline laryngeal incision which gives the surgeon direct access to the posterior laryngeal defect. Under this direct observation, the esophageal component of the cleft can be easily identified and repaired, following which the posterior wall of the larynx can be freely mobilized and individually repaired, attempting to bring viable vascularized tissue between the two suture lines. Using this direct open approach, excellent results are now being reported (JAH/CNP).

Complete laryngotracheoesophageal cleft repair has resulted in long-term survival (22).

Extrinsic Laryngeal Obstruction.

Extrinsic obstruction of the larynx by a congenital lesion is extremely rare. An example of such a lesion is the external laryngocele in a 2-day-old boy, reported in 1990 by Lewis et al. (23). Laryngoceles are abnormal dilations of the appendix of the laryngeal ventricle. An external laryngocele protrudes through the thyrohyoid membrane, where the superior laryngeal neurovascular bundle enters the larynx.

Extrinsic obstruction of the tracheobronchial tree by a congenital abnormality is comparatively common. Arterial anomalies causing such problems include double aortic arch and innominate artery compression.

REFERENCES

1. Arey LB. Developmental anatomy, ed 7. Philadelphia: WB Saunders, 1974:260.
2. Zaw-Tun HA, Burdi AR. Reexamination of the origin and early development of the human larynx. Acta Anat 1985;122:163–184.
3. Tucker JA, O'Rahilly R. Observations on the embryology of the human larynx. Ann Otol Rhinol Laryngol 1972;81:520–523.
4. O'Rahilly R, Müller F. Respiratory and alimentary relations in staged human embryos: new embryological data and congenital anomalies. Ann Otol Rhinol Laryngol 1984;93:421–429.

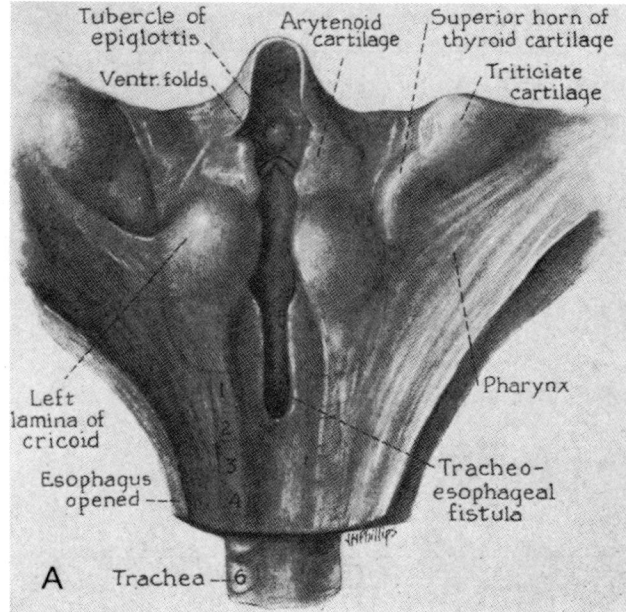
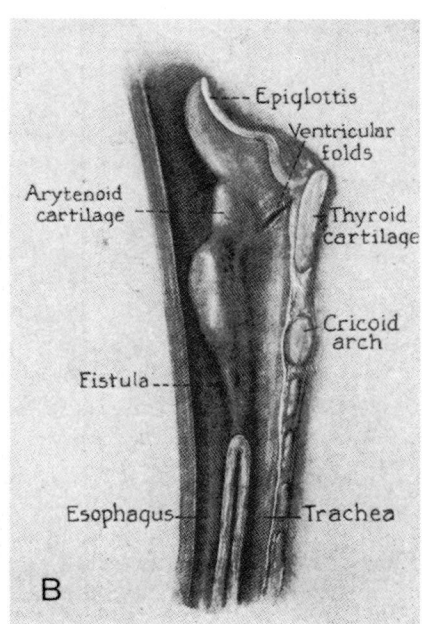

Figure 12.8. Laryngoesophageal fistula. **A**, Pharynx spread open and anomalous laryngeal defect viewed from posterior aspect. The fistula extends past the first tracheal ring. **B**, Same defect viewed from the right. (From Blumberg JB, Stevenson JK, Lemire RJ, Boyden EA. Laryngotracheoesophageal cleft, the embryologic implications: review of the literature. Surgery 1965;57:559–566.)

5. Magriples U, Laiman JT. Developmental change in the position of the fetal human larynx. Am J Phys Anthropol 1987;72:463–472.
6. Zaw-Tun HA. The tracheo-esophageal septum: fact or fancy—Origin and development of the respiratory primordium and esophagus. Acta Anat (Basel) 1982;114(1):1–21.
7. Smith II, Bain AD. Congenital atresia of the larynx. Ann Otol Rhinol Laryngol 1965;74:338–349.
8. Belmont JR, Grundfast KM, Heffner D, Hyams VJ. Laryngeal dysgenesis. Ann Otol Rhinol Laryngol 1985;94:602–606.
9. Miller RH, Cagle PT, Pitcock JK, McGavran M. Laryngeal atresia: a detailed histologic study. Int J Pediatr Otorhinolaryngol 1984;7:273–280.
10. Wigglesworth JS, Desai R, Hislop AA. Fetal lung growth in congenital laryngeal atresia. Pediatr Pathol 1987;7:515–525.
11. Cohen SR. Congenital glottic webs in children: a retrospective review of 51 patients. Ann Otol Rhinol Laryngol 1985;94(Supp 121):1–16.
12. Stolovitzky JP, Todd NW. Autoimmune hypothesis of acquired subglottic stenosis in premature infants. Laryngoscope 1990;100:227–230.
13. Holinger PH, Kutnick SL, Schild JA, Holinger LD. Subglottic stenosis in infants and children. Ann Otol Rhinol Laryngol 1976;85(5):591–599.
14. Holinger LD, Konior RJ. Surgical management of severe laryngomalacia. Laryngoscope 1989;99:136–142.
15. Zaw-Tun HIA. Development of congenital laryngeal atresias and clefts. Ann Otol Rhinol Laryngol 1988;97:353–358.
16. Gonzales C, Reilly JS, Bluestone CD. Synchronous airway lesions in infancy. Ann Otol Rhinol Laryngol 1987;96:77–80.
17. Belmont JR, Grundfast K. Congenital laryngeal stridor (laryngomalacia): etiologic factors and associated disorders. Ann Otol Rhinol Laryngol 1984;93:430–437.
18. Benjamin BNP. Diagnostic laryngology: adults and children. Philadelphia: WB Saunders, 1990.
19. Eriksen C, Zwillenberg D, Robinson N. Diagnosis and management of cleft larynx: literature review and case report. Ann Otol Rhinol Laryngol 1990;99:703–708.
20. Richter CF. Dissertation medico de infanticideo in artis obstetricae [Thesis]. Leipzig, 1792.
21. Evans JNG. Management of the cleft larynx and tracheoesophageal clefts. Ann Otol Rhinol Laryngol 1985;94:627–630.
22. Donahoe PK, Gee PE. Complete laryngotracheoesophageal cleft: management and repair. J Pediatr Surg 1984;19:143–148.
23. Lewis CA, Castillo M, Patrick E, Sybers R. Symptomatic external laryngocele in a newborn: findings on plain radiographs and CT scans. AJR 1990;11:1002.

CHAPTER 13

THE TRACHEA AND THE LUNGS

John Elias Skandalakis / Stephen Wood Gray / Panagiotis Symbas

Endotracheal anesthesia has little place in practical surgery.
—A. D. BEVAN, *1918*

When the individual receives sufficient artificial respiration simultaneously with ether anesthesia, the heart may be handled with practical impunity. It is different when the respiration is insufficient, the heart often responds to each touch with a series of irregular beats which in some hearts may lead to ventricular fibrillation and death.
—S. J. MELTZER, *1918*

DEVELOPMENT

The earliest adequate study of the adult bronchial tree was made in 1880 by Aeby (1). Seven years later His (2), using wax reconstruction, attempted a description of its development. He ascribed a regular branching pattern to the bronchi that, although oversimplified, was widely repeated in the literature. In 1919 Heiss (3) showed that Aeby's concept of an axial stem bronchus was mistaken; subsequently, Ekehorn (4) and Palmer (5) reinvestigated the embryology of the bronchial tree. The work of Wells and Boyden (6) in 1954, described the development of the bronchopulmonary segments, essentially completing our picture of the gross embryology of the lungs.

As early as the end of the third week of gestation (stage 10, 3 mm), the first indication of the laryngotracheal groove can be seen in the upper end of the embryonic foregut (7). The groove arises by a ventral enlargement of the foregut and by the formation of thickened epithelial ridges, which impinge on the lumen. The ridges become externally visible only with subsequent necrosis and resorption of the outermost cells of the wall.

Considerable discussion has been given to the question of whether the respiratory tract initially is paired or not. Hjortsjö (8) has reviewed the discussion, and concluded that much of the disagreement is semantic. The pulmonary primordium arises from the midline of the foregut and has a right and left half; hence, Hjortsjö believes it should be considered paired. Some of the discussion has resulted from attempts to fit the lung primordia into the sequence of pharyngeal structures as the eighth bronchial pouch (9).

While the laryngotracheal groove is forming, there is a proliferation of the mesenchyme of the primitive mesentery (mediastinum) by division of cells lining the celomic cavity. From this mesenchyme, the cartilage, muscle, and connective tissue of the lungs will develop.

After its first appearance, the laryngotracheal groove grows caudally, forming the primordium of the trachea. It lies ventral to and parallel with the dorsal portion of the foregut, which in this region may now be designated the esophagus. The lateral ridges separating the trachea from the esophagus advance craniad, while the esophagus itself is elongating (10) (Fig. 13.1). This separation of alimentary and respiratory structures is not always completed successfully. Faulty or incomplete separation is one of the more frequent of the serious congenital defects. These defects, as well as the subsequent normal development of the esophagus, are discussed in Chapter 3, "The Esophagus."

The backwardly growing tip of the tracheal primordium bifurcates at about the 4-mm stage (stage 13) to form the two lung buds (Fig. 13.2, *A*). Asymmetry is apparent almost from the start, with the left bud being shorter and more nearly horizontal than the right. By 7 to 8 mm (stage 15), the buds of the secondary bronchi are present, and separation of the trachea and esophagus is well under way. Separation will be complete by 11 to 14 mm (stage 17), by which time three to five orders of bronchi have appeared (Fig. 13.3).

EDITORIAL COMMENT

Since the term *lung bud* is used to identify the earliest primordium of the tracheal bronchial tree, the various anomalies associated with this structure are conveniently referred to as *bronchopulmonary lung bud abnormalities.* They include congenital lobar emphysema, bronchogenic or duplication cysts, congenital cystic adenomatoid malformations, and sequestration of the lung, among others (JAH/CNP).

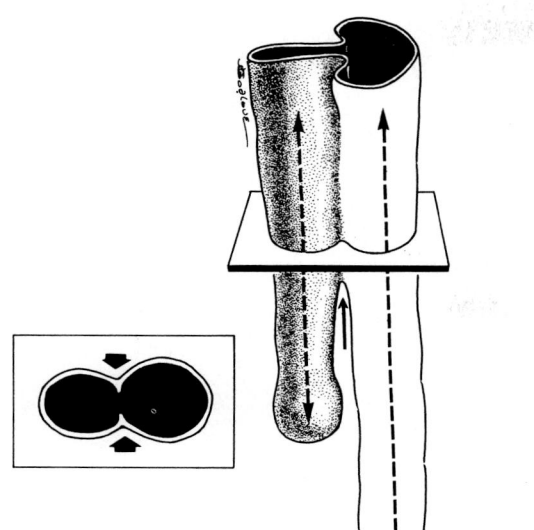

Figure 13.1. *Division of the foregut into trachea and esophagus, with stippled area showing the future tracheal portion.* Arrows *indicate the local morphogenetic movements.*

Although it was assumed for many years that the epithelial bronchial tree was self-differentiating, a few workers suspected that the mesenchyme might be responsible for epithelial development. Hjortsjö (8) discussed this view even while disagreeing with it. The first proof that mesenchyme was indispensable to the growth of the bronchial tree was provided by Rudnick (11) in 1933. Subsequently, work with cultured lung tissue by Dameron (12, 13), and Alescio and Cassini (14, 15) has shown that morphogenesis of bronchial epithelium will not take place in the absence of the pulmonary mesenchyme. Neither will mesenchyme from other regions of the embryo stimulate bronchial development.

A mathematic model of the way in which cells must divide to produce a branching tubular structure, such as the bronchial tree, was constructed by Hjortsjö (8). He concluded that there must be a shift in the plane of cell division between the formation of a bud and its subsequent elongation.

At the start the level of the tracheal bifurcation is high in the cervical region. During the next month it will descend to the level of the first thoracic vertebra. At birth it will be at the level of the fourth or fifth thoracic vertebra. At the same time the lungs, which are at first dorsal to the heart, grow laterally and ventrally to surround it. Ekehorn (4) thought the shape of the thorax molded the shape of the growing lung. However, the studies of Wells and Boyden (6) on living as well as preserved embryos have shown that the lungs do not fill the pleural sacs during the period in which the definitive bronchial tree is forming. All major bronchial buds are present before closure of the pleuroperitoneal canals (stage 21, 23 mm).

The surface of the developing lung shows definite lob-

ulations, which indicate the underlying structure. At stages 17 to 18, the elevations represent bronchopulmonary segments; at stage 19, segments and subsegments are indicated. It is usually held that the lobulations disappear and the lung surface is smooth after about the 10th week, but Wells and Boyden (6) found them still present in a living fetus of 66 mm (about 13 weeks).

Up to approximately the third month, the right lung grows faster than the left, being both larger (5) and having more generations of bronchial branching (16). This difference persists, and the right lung remains slightly larger throughout life.

Cartilage appears in the trachea and primary bronchi at approximately 10 weeks and in the segmental bronchi at 16 weeks (16). Glands appear during the 11th week and reach their full extent by the 30th week (17).

Dubreuil et al. (18, 19) suggested the division of lung development into a "glandular stage" (up to 16 weeks) and an "alveolar stage" (24 weeks to birth). During the first stage the pulmonary mesenchyme is solid, and the distal portions of the developing bronchial tree show little or no evidence of a lumen. During the second stage the distal ends of the ducts are open and alveoli are formed.

The development of the alveoli during the latter portion of gestation and the first few years of life has received much attention; however, questions still remain. There is reason to believe the details of alveolar development vary in different mammalian species. Broman (20) believed six to seven generations of bronchial branching took place after birth. Emery and Mithal (21) and Cudmore et al. (22) concluded there is only a small increase in branching after birth; but there is an increase in the length of the tree, which is more marked in the proximal than in the distal branches. In addition, they found a rapid increase in the number of alveoli up to 6 months of age, and a slower increase up to 12 years of age. Mithal and Emery (23) found no evidence of precocious development in the lungs of prematurely born infants. Dunnill (24) essentially confirmed this, adding the observation that the mean size of alveoli in the infant at birth is 150 μ and in the adult, 280 μ.

In the "alveolar stage" (after 24 weeks), there is an apparent decrease in the number of generations of bronchi due to epithelial changes in terminal bronchioles and their conversion into respiratory bronchioles (16) (Fig. 13.4). After birth a reversal occurs: respiratory bronchioles become terminal bronchioles, and new alveoli are formed. Figure 13.5 sums up the changes in the lung observed by Bucher and Reid (16, 17).

There is disagreement about the method of alveolar multiplication. Dubreuil et al. (18, 19) believed that alveolar ducts are the only respiratory portions of the tree present at birth and that alveoli were formed from them. Ham and Baldwin (25) made the interesting suggestion

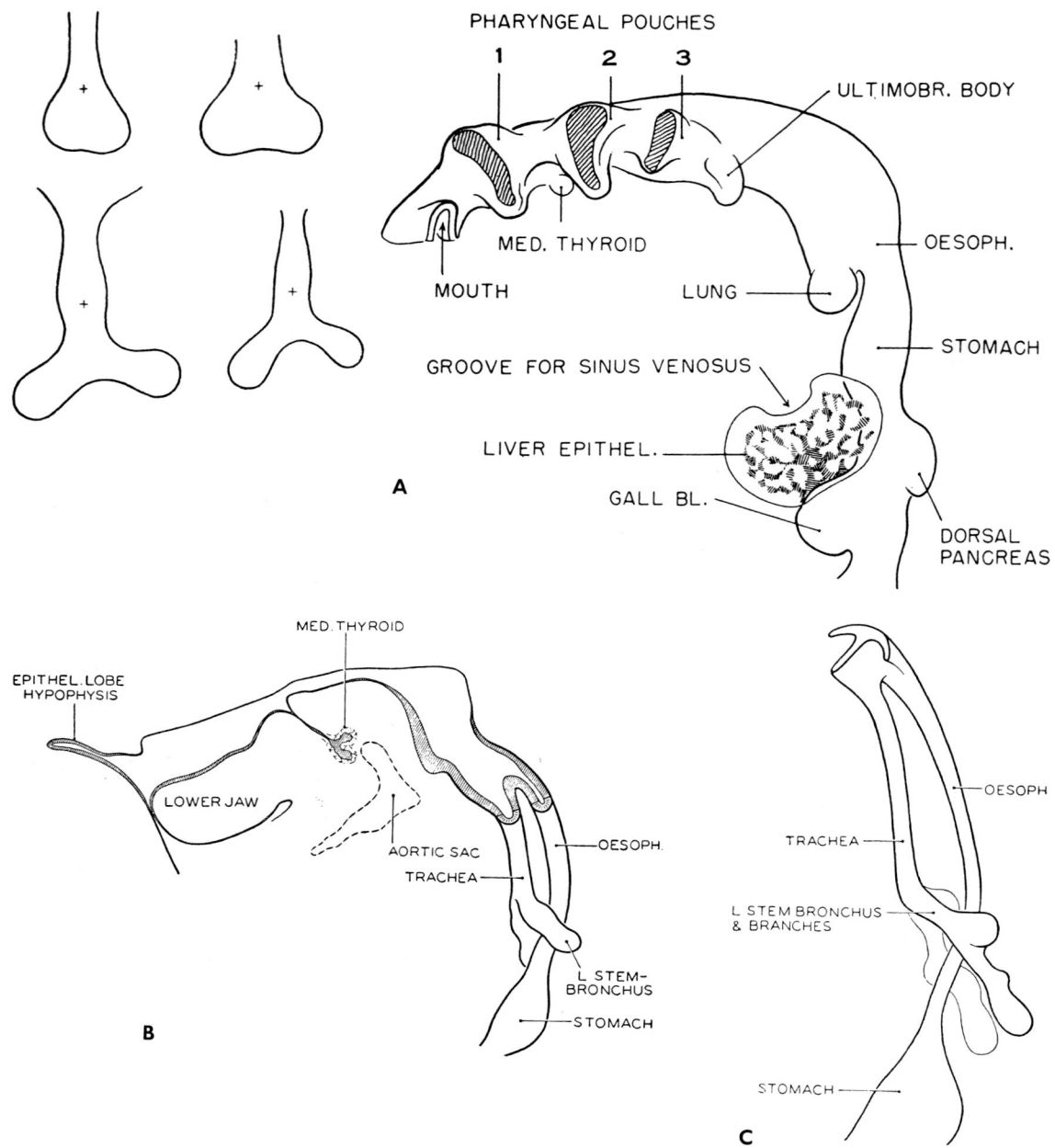

Figure 13.2.   Development of trachea and bronchi. **A**, Four anterior views and lateral view of lung buds at the end of the fifth week (horizon XIII). **B**, Lateral view at the middle of the sixth week (horizon XV). **C**, Lateral view near the end of the sixth week (horizon XVI). (From Streeter GL. Developmental horizons in human embryos: description of age group XIII, embryos about 4 or 5 millimeters long, and age group XIV, period of indentation of the lens vesicle. Contrib Embryol Carnegie Inst Wash 1945;31:27–63; and from Streeter GL. Developmental horizons in human embryos: description of age groups XV, XVI, XVII, and XVIII. Contrib Embryol Carnegie Inst Wash 1948;32:133–204.)

that new alveoli were created by splitting of the septa by air. The term *physiologic interstitial emphysema* was proposed. The more common view, however, holds that older alveoli become subdivided by the formation of new septa.

Observations by Boyden (26) support Dubreuil's view. The most distal bronchioles in the newborn infant become converted into alveolar ducts by centripetal formation of new alveoli during the first 2 months of postnatal life. Alveolarization of terminal bronchioles themselves occur up to the fourth year of life. Thus the number of branching generations of the respiratory tree does not increase and may even decrease with age.

By the age of 7 years, diverticula arising from terminal

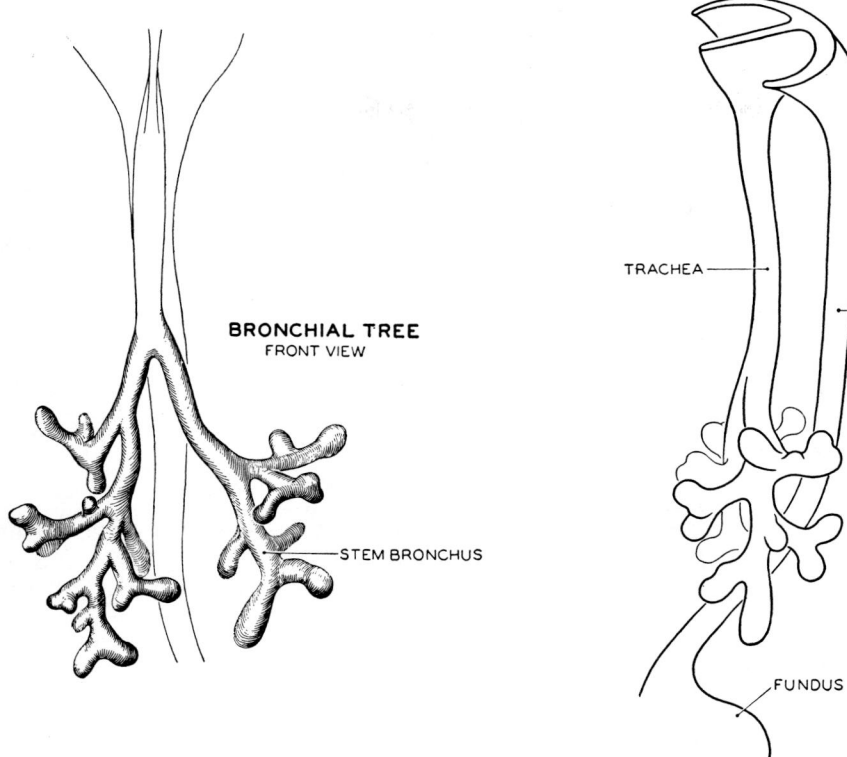

Figure 13.3. Development of trachea and bronchi. Anterior and lateral views at the beginning of the seventh week (horizon XVII). The trachea and esophagus have elongated, and five orders of bronchial branching are visible. (From Streeter GL. Development horizons in human embryos: description of age groups XV, XVI, XVII, and XVIII. Contrib Embryol Carnegie Inst Wash 1948;32:133–204.)

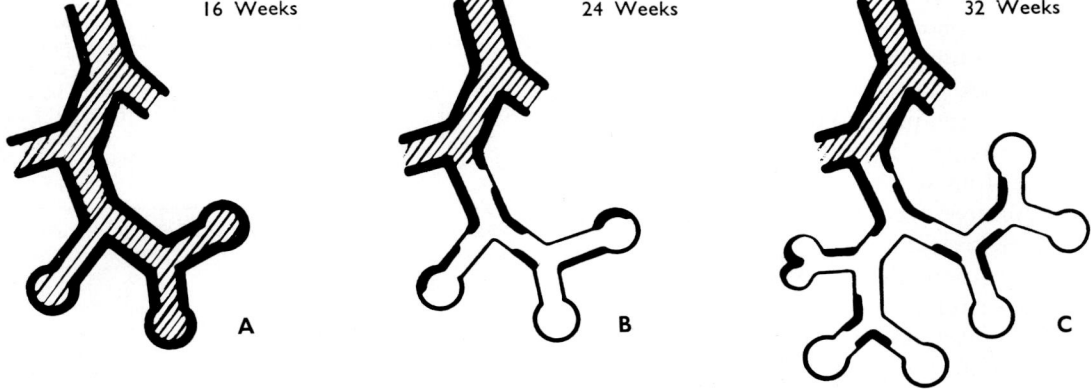

Figure 13.4. Ultimate generations of the bronchial tree at various stages of intrauterine development. **A**, Sixteen weeks, bronchial tree completely lined with epithelium. **B**, Twenth-four weeks, epithelium interrupted by ingrowth of capillaries (i.e., respiratory or alveolar part arises from transformation in the terminal branches). **C**, Thirty-two weeks, additional growth of respiratory portion of the tree. (From Bucher U, Reid L. Development of the intrasegmental bronchial tree: the pattern of branching and development of cartilage at various stages of intra-uterine life. Thorax 1961;16:207–218.)

or preterminal bronchioles reach and perforate adjacent alveoli belonging to other branches of the tree. Boyden (26) terms them *Lambert ducts*.

Dunnill (24) calculates that at birth the infant has 24×10^6 alveoli and that the adult has 296×10^6 alveoli. The number of superscript generations of airways increases from 21 to 23. Most of the increase is achieved in the first 8 years of life. These estimates have been independently confirmed by Weibel and Gomez (27) in their quantitative study of the lung. Emery (28) reports multiplication of the primitive alveoli by segmentation. Hogg et al. (29) stated that, in a full-term baby, the number of

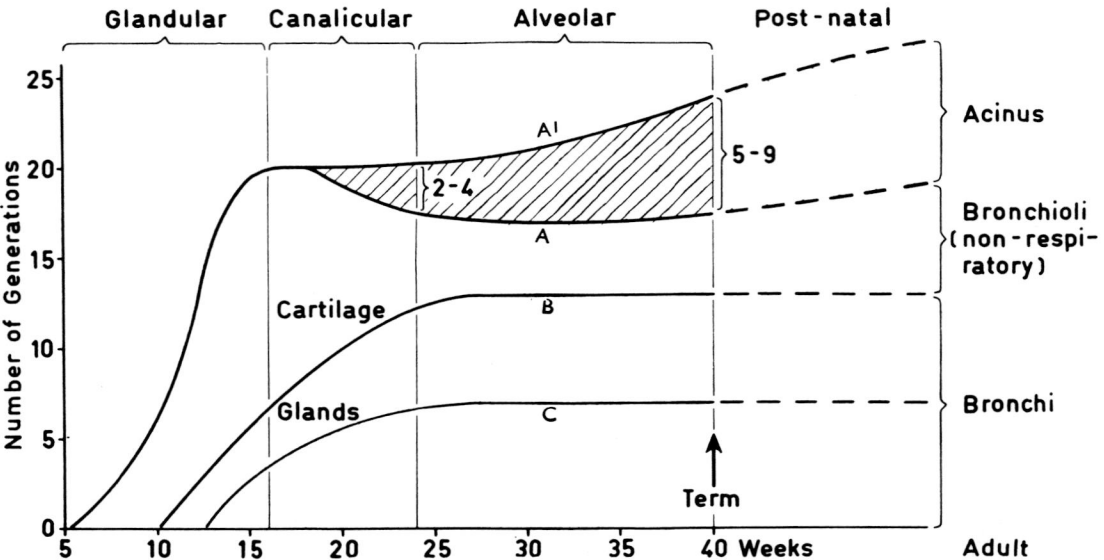

Figure 13.5. Summary of intrauterine development of the intrasegmental bronchial tree. *Line A* represents the increase in the number of bronchial generations; shaded area between *A* and *A′* represents the respiratory part of the bronchial tree, (i.e., respiratory bronchioles and alveolar ducts). *Line B* shows the extension of cartilage along the bronchial tree, and *line C*, the extension of mucous glands. The diagram includes adult values, showing the increase in total generations in the postnatal period. (From Bucher U, Reid L. Development of the intrasegmental bronchial tree: the pattern of branching and development of cartilage at various stages of intra-uterine life. Thorax 1961;16:207–218.)

primitive alveoli is approximately 8% of adult. Until the age of 8 years, the alveoli increase up to 100,000 per day, raising the total number to 300 million (3×10^{14}) approximately if the arithmetic is correct.

The influence of fetal respiratory movements on alveolar development has been debated. The older view (30) held that respiratory movements in utero were normal and indeed were necessary for normal development. Windle and his colleagues (31) agreed that such movements occurred but considered them to be responses to abnormally low fetal oxygen. Potter and Bohlender (32) observed normal alveolar development in two stillborn infants with respiratory tract obstruction, which would have prevented fetal respiration.

Two experiments strongly suggested that fluid in the prenatal lungs is secreted and not aspirated. Tracheal ligation in rabbit fetuses before term resulted in dilation of the lungs (33), and radiopaque material injected into the amnionic sac of fetuses near term could not be detected in the lungs after birth (34).

Thurlbeck (35) presented a table classifying phases of human intrauterine lung growth (Table 13.1). We recommend his excellent chapter to the interested reader. The terminology is slightly different than ours, but by all means acceptable.

Tibboel and Kluth (36) produced comparative data for the stages of embryonic development of the respiratory system (Table 13.2). O'Rahilly and Muller (37) emphasized that the respiratory primordium produces part of

Table 13.1.
Classification of Phases of Human Intrauterine Lung Growth[a]

Phase	Time of Occurrence	Significance
Embryonic	Day 26–day 52	Development of trachea and major bronchi
Pseudoglandular	Day 52–16 week	Development of remaining conducting airways
Canalicular	17 week–28 week	Development of vascular bed, framework of acinus, flattening of epithelium
Saccular	29 week–36 week	Increased complexity of saccules
Alveolar	36 week–term	Presence and development of alveoli

[a]From Thurlbeck W. Lung growth. In: Thurlbeck, WM, ed. Pathology of the lung. New York: Thieme, 1988.

the larynx, trachea, primary bronchi and, of course, lungs.

Development of the Respiratory System

Zaw-Tun (38) demonstrated that the foregut proximal to the pulmonary primordium is responsible for the formation of the supraglottic region of the larynx and not of the trachea.

Kluth et al. (39) believe the tracheoesophageal septum exists but its formation and identification has been incorrectly described. Furthermore, Kluth and colleagues

Table 13.2.
Comparative Data for the Stages of Embryonic Development of the Respiratory System[a]

Stage[b]	Number of Somites	Crown-to-Rump Length (mm)	Postovulatory Days	
9	1–3	1.5–2.5	20	Foregut appears
10	4–12	2.0–3.5	22	Pulmonary primordium
11	13–20	2.5–4.5	24	
12	21–29	3.0–5.0	26	Lung buds develop
13	30–50	4.0–6.0	28	Trachea and esophagus recognizable; lung bud separates from foregut
14		5.0–7.0	32	Lung sacs curve dorsally
15		7.0–9.0	33	Pharyngotracheal duct connects digestive and respiratory tubes; lobar buds develop

[a]From Tibboel D, Kluth D: Embryology of congenital lesions of the tracheobronchial tree. In: Lobe TE, ed. Tracheal reconstruction in infancy. Philadelphia: WB Saunders, 1991; data in this table were adapted from the study by O'Rahilly R, Muller F. Chevalier Jackson Lecture: respiratory and alimentary relations in staged human embryos—new embryological data and congenital anomalies. Ann Otol Rhinol Laryngol 1984;93:421–429.
[b]Horizons in Streeter's nomenclature.

agreed with Zaw-Tun and O'Rahilly and Muller (37) that there are lateral ridges or signs of fusions at the components of the lateral wall separating the trachea from the foregut.

Tibboel and Kluth (36) reported that an independent mesenchymal sheet develops between trachea and esophagus.

According to Tibboel and Kluth, the modern philosophy about congenital anomalies of the trachea can be conceptualized as a failure of normal growth and differentiation of the several anatomic and embryologic entities of the respiratory system. T-E fistula is therefore caused by an abnormal epithelial connection between two separated tubes.

Kluth and Habenicht (40) believe that atresias of trachea and esophagus as well as laryngotracheoesophageal clefts are defects secondary to foregut folds or defects of developmental movements of the folds.

Pulmonary hypoplasia or agenesis of the lung cannot be explained. Asplenia and polysplenia syndromes are associated with tracheoesophageal malformations.

The reader will find useful information regarding qualitative and quantitative normal and abnormal structural development in Kavlock and Crabowski (41).

In summary, the respiratory system develops from the ventral wall of the foregut during gestation around the fourth week and continues development during the first 2 years or life. The epithelium of trachea, bronchi, and alveoli originates from the endoderm, but the muscles and cartilages originate from mesoderm. The enigmatic tracheoesophageal septum is present and perhaps is even responsible for the splitting of the foregut, but embryologists and pediatric surgeons disagree. A vivid example is the explanation of the T-E fistula. In the primitive alveolus, exchange of gas may take place around the seventh month when bronchioli cells are present. Alveolar epithelial cells are present, producing fluid, mucus, and surfac-

tant. Hyaline membrane disease may develop if surfactant is absent or insufficient. During the first 2 years of life the lung growth is due to the increase of respiratory bronchioli and alveoli and not to an alveoli increase in size (42).

Critical Events in Development

The chief critical event in the formation of the respiratory system is the initial separation of the primitive foregut into the respiratory and alimentary tracts, beginning late in the third week and becoming complete by the sixth week. Failure of this process to proceed normally may result in tracheoesophageal fistula (see Chapter 3, "The Esophagus"). Asymmetry of the developing lung buds during the early part of this separation may result in the formation of a lung on one side only. Most of the anomalies of the lungs themselves occur rarely or very rarely.

ANOMALIES OF THE TRACHEA AND LUNGS (TABLE 13-3 AND FIG. 13-6)

Classification of the congenital anomalies of the tracheobronchopulmonary apparatus is extremely difficult not only from an embryologic and morphologic standpoint but from the pathologic and clinic viewpoints as well. The most vivid example is the so-called pulmonary cysts which, with their multiple facets, muddy the already unclear water in this area.

May the reader forgive possible mistakes in this section and accept with understanding a classification which is basically a summary of work from deLorimier (43) and Sieber (44).

There are cases such as tracheobronchopulmonary malformation in which the problem is not due (per se) to a primary congenital anomaly to these organs but other reasons, such as phrenic nerve agenesis and diaphrag-

Table 13.3.
Anomalies of the Trachea and Lungs[a]

Anomaly	Origin of Defect	First Appearance (or Other Diagnostic Clues)	Sex Chiefly Affected	Relative Frequency	Remarks
Tracheal atresia	Week 3–4	At birth	?	Very rare	Fatal at birth
Congenital tracheal stenosis	Week 3–4	At birth	?	Rare	Usually fatal soon after birth
Tracheobronchomegaly	Mo 5	Late childhood or later	?	Rare	
Bilateral agenesis of the lungs	Week 4	At birth	?	Very rare	Fatal at birth
Unilateral agenesis and hypoplasia of the lungs	Late week 4	Infancy and childhood	Female	Uncommon	50% die in first 5 yr
Anomalies of lobulation	Week 10	None	Male ?	Common	Asymptomatic
Pulmonary isomerism	Unknown	None	?	Uncommon	Associated with heterotaxy, asplenia and anomalous pulmonary veins
Congenital cysts of the respiratory tract:					
Bronchogenic cysts	Week 6–7	Infancy, if at all	?	Uncommon	Compression of trachea may be fatal
Pulmonary cysts	Week 24	Infancy and childhood	Male	Uncommon	Eventually fatal if untreated

[a]Pulmonary telangiectasia, see Chapter 14; accessory lung tissue, see Chapter 14.

matic amyopathia (45), congenital diaphragmatic herniae producing hypoplasia (46), or chest deformities (47).

Lung Anomalies

Lung anomalies can be listed as follows:

Trachea and bronchi
   Agenesis
   Stenosis
   Complete tracheal rings
   Tracheal bronchus
   Esophageal bronchus
   Tracheomalacia
   Bronchomalacia
   Bronchial cysts
   Hemangioma
   Lymphangioma
Pulmonary parenchyma
   Agenesis
   Unilateral
   Bilateral
   Hypoplasia
   Congenital cysts
   Bronchogenic
   Lung cysts
   Adenomatoid
   Bronchiectasis
   Sequestration
Vascular anomalies
Others
   Chest wall deformities
   Phrenic nerve agenesis

   Diaphragmatic herniae
   Congenital chylothorax

Dyon et al. (48) presented factors influencing pulmonary arrest (Table 13.4).

ANOMALIES OF THE TRACHEA AND LUNGS

Lethal Anomalies of the Trachea and Lungs

De Lorimier (43) stated in 1986 that at least eight cases of agenesis of both bronchi and lungs had been reported in the literature.

It should be noted that respiratory anomalies, however lethal, have no effect on the ability of the fetus to proceed to term. The extreme rarity of complete developmental failure is thus all the more remarkable.

BILATERAL AGENESIS OF LUNGS

Oyamada et al. (49) reported a case of pulmonary agenesis and reviewed the literature. Devi and More (50) presented total tracheopulmonary agenesis associated with multiple other anomalies.

Six cases of absence of both lungs have been recorded (51, 52). In one, a trachea with 10 rings remained connected to the esophagus throughout its length. There were neither lung buds nor pleural cavities. The pulmonary artery joined the aorta and the pulmonary veins were absent (53). Another case was slightly less extreme: the trachea was separated from the esophagus but ended blindly with only two cartilaginous rings (50). In two

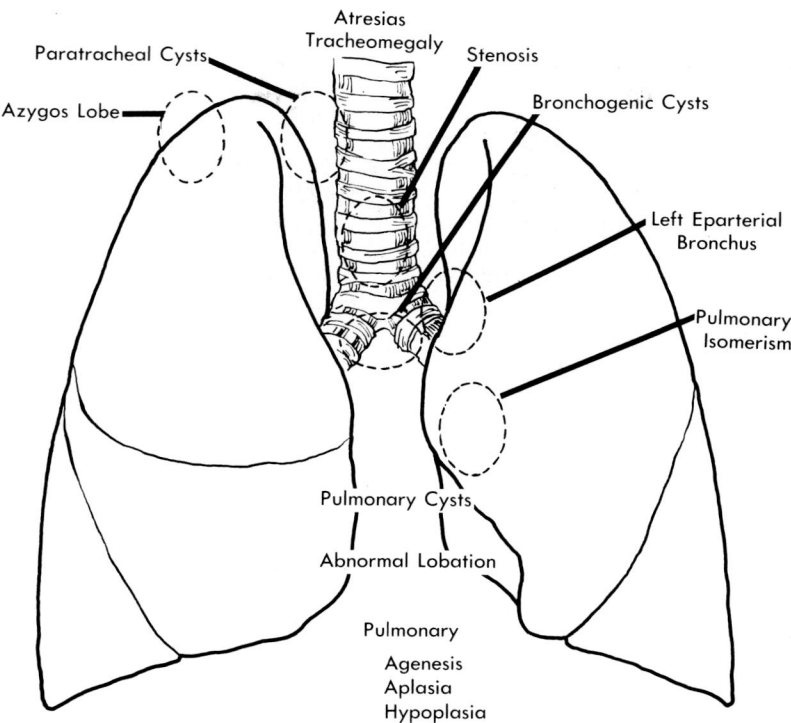

Figure 13.6. Pattern of anomalies of the trachea and lungs.

Table 13.4.
Factors Influencing Pulmonary Developmental Arrest[a]

1. Bronchial developmental fault
    → agenesis
    → aplasia
2. Pulmonary vessels developmental fault
    → harmonious lung hypoplasia
3. Extrinsic factors of lung compression
    → localized hypoplasia
4. Unknown

[a]From Dyon JF, Baudain P, Alibeu JP. Malformations of the lung mass. In: Fallis JC et al. Pediatric thoracic surgery. New York: Elsevier, 1991.

other cases the respiratory primordium had progressed to the bronchial bud stage but had formed no lung tissue (54, 55). In all cases the diaphragm lay at a higher than normal level.

Unlike tracheal atresia, this type of agenesis results from a simple arrest in development of the respiratory primordium rather than from an error in division of the foregut endoderm.

TRACHEAL AGENESIS—ATRESIA

Absence or atresia of the trachea, with normal bronchi and lungs, has been seen several times. In some cases the bronchi communicated with the esophagus (56–60), whereas in others no opening existed (61, 62). Marek's patient (58) tried to breathe. However, a catheter could not be passed and no trachea could be found when tra-

cheotomy was attempted. The trachea ended as a blind sac below the larynx. When an esophageal communication exists, the lungs may be partly expanded; and one infant seems to have lived for a short while (57). In most cases the larynx is present and normal, the atresia beginning a short distance below it.

Bronchial atresia without agenesis of the lung has been seen in an anencephalic fetus (63). Several authors have presented cases and reviewed the literature on tracheal agenesis (64–68). This is a lethal anomaly. Evans et al. (69) pointed out the associated malformation.

Embryologically, these cases are the converse of esophageal atresia. Although the tracheal primordium formed properly at both the upper end (normal larynx) and the lower end (normal lungs), the midportion of the foregut developed into esophagus only, with no endoderm being left to form a trachea (see Chapter 3, "The Esophagus").

Ashley (70) reported a case of congenital tracheal obstruction with esophageal atresia. Peison et al. (71) reported a case of atresia with T-E fistula and malformation of the larynx. Chaurasia (72) reported aplasia of the trachea in a human fetus with multiple congenital anomalies. According to Ferguson and Ferguson (73), congenital bronchial atresia is the second most common tracheobronchial malformation.

Faro et al (74) described seven types of tracheal agenesis or atresia in 39 reported cases.

1. Total agenesis of tracheobronchial tree and lungs, 8% (three patients)
2. Tracheal agenesis, but both bronchi arising from the esophagus, 10% (four patients)
3. Tracheal atresia with the right and left bronchi forming a common airway arising from the midesophagus, 56% (22 patients)
4. Tracheal atresia with cord-like formation of a fibrous band connecting the larynx to the combined main bronchi, which communicate with the esophagus, 10% (four patients)
5. Atresia of the upper trachea with intact distal trachea and tracheoesophageal fistula, 5% (two patients)
6. Atresia of the proximal trachea and an intact distal trachea without esophageal fistula, 5% (two patients)
7. Short-segment tracheal atresia with normal proximal and distal trachea, 5% (two patients)

Tracheomalacia

In a classic and excellent review Landing and Dixon (75) discussed the congenital malformations of the respiratory tract.

The congenital pathology of tracheomalacia may include segmental or total softness or fragmentation or absence of the approximately 22 tracheal rings. In most cases it is associated with other congenital malformations such as tracheoesophageal fistulae, vascular rings, and pulmonary anomalies.

Generalized tracheomalacia is an extremely rare phenomenon which was described by Levin et al. (76) and Davies and Cywes (77). Segmental tracheomalacia was reported by Benjamin et al. (78) and Glason (79). Their cases were associated with T-E fistulae. Aortopexy by fixation of the aorta to manubrium sterni was reported by Benjamin (78) et al. and Glason (79).

Tracheomalacia does not have any embryologic explanation. De Lorimier stated in 1986 that, with increasing age and growth, the severity of problems lessen (43). Filler (80) cites the abnormalities associated with tracheomalacia in Table 13.5. He also tabulates the indications for surgery (Table 13.6) and types of surgery performed in Table 13.7.

Aortopexy and splinting are the procedures of choice for treatment of this anomaly. Vallas and de Beaujeu (81)

Table 13.5.
Abnormalities Associated with 30 Cases of Tracheomalacia, 1978–1987[a]

Esophageal atresia	25[b]
Vascular ring	3[b]
None	3

[a]From Filler RM. Tracheomalacia. In: Fallis JC et al. Pediatric thoracic surgery. New York: Elsevier, 1991.
[b]One patient had both esophageal atresia and vascular ring.

presented their experience in surgical management of tracheomalacia (Table 13.8). We refer the reader to the excellent discussion of tracheomalacia in the book edited by Fallis et al. (82).

Congenital Tracheal Stenosis

ANATOMY

Stenosis of the trachea is a rare condition in which the trachea alone or both trachea and bronchi are narrowed. The degree and extent of narrowing determine the seriousness of the anomaly. Most reported cases have been fatal, and the final evidence was usually available at autopsy; however, nonlethal cases are known (83).

Two types of stenosis have been described and classified by Wolman (84):

Type A: Simple local narrowing of the trachea, usually in the lower third. The distal trachea and bronchi are of normal size (Fig. 13.7, *A*).
Type B: Progressive narrowing of the trachea toward the bifurcation. The bronchi also are narrowed (Fig. 13.7, *B*).

In both types, the tracheal rings may be complete rather than **C** shaped, or they may show various degrees of disorganization of cartilage formation. In one patient the stenosis resulted from collapse of a portion of trachea that contained no cartilaginous rings (85).

Pulmonary artery sling is a rare congenital anomaly in which the left pulmonary artery originates from the right pulmonary artery and encircles the right mainstem bron-

Table 13.6.
Indication for Surgery in 30 Cases of Tracheomalacia, 1978–1987[a]

Dying spells	14
Recurrent pneumonia	4
Intermittent respiratory obstruction	5
Inability to extubate airway	7

[a]From Filler RM: Tracheomalacia. In: Fallis JC et al. Pediatric thoracic surgery. New York: Elsevier, 1991.

Table 13.7.
Types of Surgery in 30 Patients, 1978–1987[a]

	Number of Patients	Cessation of Symptoms
Aortopexy	25	22
Aortopexy + splint	3	3[b]
Splint only	2	2

[a]From Filler RM. Tracheomalacia. In: Fallis JC et al. Pediatric thoracic surgery. New York: Elsevier, 1991.
[b]One patient required splint removal 18 months later; one patient died (see text); two patients still require tracheostomy.

Table 13.8.
Experience in Surgical Management of Tracheomalacia[a]

Case	Etiology	Associated Malformation	Age	Surgical Technique	Associated Procedure	Result	Follow up
1	Congenital	Aberrant right (retroesophageal) subclavian artery	4 mo	Pasting with Histoacryl	Section of aberrant right subclavian artery	Good	20 yr
2	Congenital	—	1 mo	Pasting with Histoacryl	—	Good	18 yr
3	Congenital	Right pulmonary hypoplasia, anomalous pulmonary venous drainage	10 mo	External splint of bone on left bronchus	Right pneumonectomy	Good	8 yr
4	Acquired	—	2 yr	External splint with Histoacryl + Surgical	Aortopexy	Good for malacia. Post-op stenosis: resection	5 yr
5	Congenital	Esophageal atresia type III, laryngeal cleft	3 mo	External splint with Histoacryl + Silastic sheet	Esophagocoloplasty (2 mo) aortopexy, esophageal reconstruction with colon	Good	5 yr

[a]From Valla JS, de Beaujeu MJ. Tracheomalacia. In: Fallis JC et al. Pediatric thoracic surgery. New York: Elsevier, 1991.

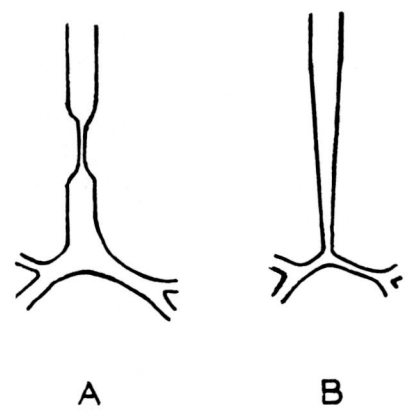

Figure 13.7. Schematic representation of the two most common types of tracheal stenosis. **A,** The constriction is limited to a short segment of the trachea. **B,** The constriction is widespread and most marked at or above the bifurcation. (From Wolman IJ. Congenital stenosis of the trachea. Ann J Dis Child 1941;61:1263.)

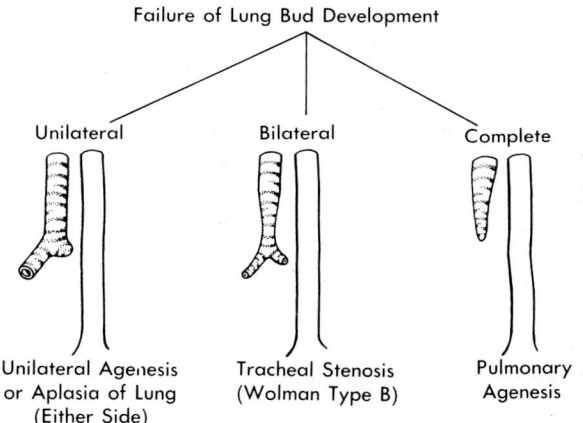

Figure 13.8. Normal separation of alimentary and respiratory structures but with arrested development of the lung buds. See Fig. 3.6. for abnormal separation of trachea and esophagus.

chus and distal trachea, causing compression of each (86–88). One must be aware of this anomaly when evaluating an infant with apparent segmental distal tracheal stenosis. Nakayama et al. (89) pointed out that tracheal stenosis can be segmented or complete.

EMBRYOGENESIS

Type A defects that have a narrowed segment represent examples in which the esophageal portion of the foregut gained tissue at the expense of the tracheal portion. In one autopsied case a dilated esophagus accompanied the stenosed trachea (85). This condition, in its most severe form, results in tracheal agenesis. It is one stage in a series of defects of tracheoesophageal separation (see Chapter 3, "The Esophagus").

Type B defects appear to represent failure of normal growth of the distal part of the trachea and the lung buds. In its more severe form, this results in bilateral agenesis of the lungs (Fig. 13.8).

In some cases the defect extends into the lungs. There may be anomalous lobulation or unilateral agenesis (90, 91). In one case only the upper lobe of each lung was said to be formed (92).

According to Lobe and Swischuk (93) the cause of the defect is not known. Perhaps a vascular accident or organogenesis may take place at a critical point in development.

ASSOCIATED ANOMALIES

Truncus arteriosus communis (92), atrial septal defects (94), ventricular septal defects, imperforate anus, and clubfoot (84, 92) have been reported (Table 13.9).

HISTORY AND INCIDENCE

No adequate collection of examples has been made. Wolman (84) cited a case reported in 1832 and listed 11 cases, including one of his own. Three were type A and eight were type B. Heikel (92) mentioned 22 cases without specifying the form.

Type A, stenosis of the trachea only, probably occurs more frequently, although it has been reported less often. Many subclinical cases probably exist. A few have been found accidentally in adults (95). Type B cases predominate in published reports because they are usually fatal and may be verified at autopsy.

Table 13.9.
Associated Anomalies in Patients with Congenital Tracheal Stenosis[a]

More Common Anomalies
Airway
  Bronchial stenosis
  Tracheal bronchus
  Tracheomalacia
  Tracheal web
  Congenital subglottic stenosis
  Laryngeal hypoplasia with complete absence of the glottic and subglottic airways
Pulmonary
  Hypoplasia of one or both lungs
  Unilateral pulmonary agenesis
  Congenital lobar emphysema
Esophageal
  H-type tracheoesophageal fistula
  Congenital stenosis of the upper esophagus
  Gastroesophageal reflux
Diaphragm
  Accessory diaphragm
  Diaphragmatic hernia
Less Often Seen Anomalies
Airway
  Laryngomalacia
Cardiovascular
  Triventricular communis
  Coarctation of the aorta
  Dextrocardia with patent ductus arteriosus
  Ventricular septal defect
Skeleton
  Hemivertebrae in the cervical, thoracic, or lumbar regions
  Hypoplasia or absence of the thumb
  Proximal radioulnar synostosis
  Widened pedicles of vertebrae L2 to L4
  Hypoplastic mandible
Genitourinary
  Imperforate anus with rectovulvar fistula
Gastrointestinal
  Extrahepatic portal hypertension

[a]From Lobe TE, Swischuk LE: Signs and symptoms of congenital tracheal stenosis: diagnostic considerations. In: Lobe TE, ed. Tracheal reconstruction in infancy. Philadelphia: WB Saunders, 1991.

Berdon et al. (96) reported complete cartilage-ring tracheal stenosis with anomalies of the left pulmonary artery. Cundy and Bergstrom (97) reported congenital subglottic stenosis. Devine et al. (98) recorded complete cartilaginous trachea in a child with Crouzon syndrome. Paparo and Symchych (99) reported postintubation subglottic stenosis and cor pulmonale. Parkin et al. (100) discussed acquired and congenital subglottic stenosis in the infant. Ratner and Whitefield (101) cited acquired subglottic stenosis in the very low birth weight infant.

SYMPTOMS

Cough, dyspnea, episodes of cyanosis, and stridor are the usual symptoms of tracheal stenosis. The stridor is both expiratory and inspiratory. Dysphagia may be present (83).

DIAGNOSIS

Stridor during both phases of breathing suggests subglottic obstruction. Laryngoscopy will eliminate laryngeal stenosis as a cause. Air tachogram obtained by an overexposed x-ray film provides significant information on the presence, site, and extent of the stenosis. Bronchoscopy and bronchography, although very helpful in diagnosing tracheal stenosis, should be used cautiously because the possible accompanying trauma and increased secretions may result in obstruction. However, according to Hirschberg and Lellei (102), they make up the most important diagnostic procedures.

TREATMENT

Tracheostomy provides temporary relief; but, it has been permanently effective in only one case (103). Wolman (83) employed an oxygen tent, achieving some relief of symptoms, but his patient later succumbed.

Gebauer (104) successfully incised the stenosed trachea and corrected the defect with skin grafts. This repair is suitable for type A anomalies (Figure 13.9).

The form of therapy for tracheal stenosis depends on the type of the stenosis. Tracheal webs can be removed bronchoscopically with biopsy forceps or laser. Balloon dilation of bronchial stenosis with excellent results was reported by Tonkin et al. (105). Messineo et al. (106) and Bagwell et al. (107) extended this form of therapy, balloon dilation, to tracheal stenosis as well. Campbell and Lilly (108) reported the case of an infant with total congenital tracheal stenosis who was treated successfully by insertion of a cartilaginous graft. Mambrino et al. (109) reported another infant with multiple anomalies treated with a costal cartilage graft. The patient died 2 months postoperatively from associated cardiac disease. At autopsy, excellent incorporation of the graft with no evidence of stenosis was documented.

Tracheal dilation is of no use when circular rings are

present. In such cases, resection of the stenotic segment with end-to-end anastomosis or tracheoplasty with the use of tissue patch or flaps can be applied successfully (110–111). This form of tracheal reconstruction should be delayed as long as possible to avoid the problems associated with anastomosis of airways of a few millimeters in size (112).

Synthetic free or pedicle graft is advised by Janik et al.

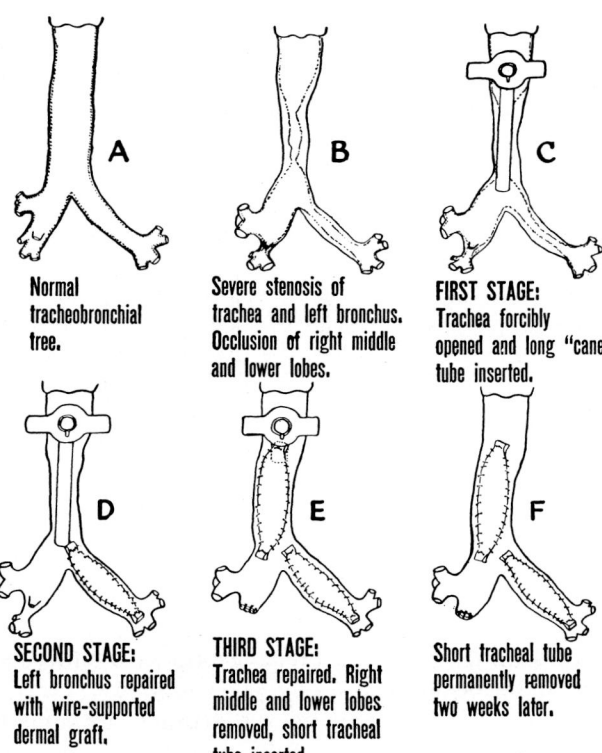

Figure 13.9. Diagrams illustrating tracheobronchial deformities and corrective procedures applied. The dermal grafts used to correct the deformities of the left bronchus and trachea were actually inserted on the posterior and posterolateral aspects of these structures but are drawn on the anterior aspect for increased clarity. (From Gebauer PW. Reconstructive tracheobronchial surgery. Surg Clin North Am 1956;36:893–911.)

(113) for the treatment of funnel-shaped stenosis. Idriss et al. (110) operated successfully on four infants with long tracheal stenosis, performing a pericardial patch tracheoplasty.

Tracheoplasty for congenital long segment intrathoracic stenosis segment in six patients was employed by Van Meter, Jr. et al. (114) in 1991 (Table 13.10).

According to Branscheid et al. (115), the treatment of choice for tracheal stenosis is segmental resection with end-to-end anastomosis if the stenotic segment is neither too long nor involved with other anatomic entities. An excellent summary of the different management options for patients with various forms of tracheobronchial obstruction is provided by de Lorimier et al. (116).

PROGNOSIS

Simple tracheal stenosis of type A defects may be mild enough to permit the patient to live a normal life (95). Patients with slightly more severe defects may be saved by prompt diagnosis and surgical intervention. When the narrowing involves the trachea and bronchi, there is at present little hope for effective therapy. Only one patient in this group has survived for more than a few months (91).

Tracheobronchomegaly

DEFINITION

Tracheobronchomegaly is a rare congenital anomaly resulting in dilation of the trachea and bronchi. The nature of the condition suggests a congenital defect of the trachealis muscle and its associated elastic tissue. No theory of origin suggesting acquired forms has been offered.

HISTORY

The disease was first reported in 1897 by Czyhlarz (117), who suggested a congenital origin. A number of cases were added by Mounier-Kuhn (118) in 1932, and 15 to 18 cases were known by 1962 (119). Tracheobronchomegaly also is known as Mounier-Kuhn syndrome.

Table 13.10.
Patient Data[a]

Patient No.	Age	Size of Lumen	Type of Patch	Result
1	2 mo	1.5	Pericardial	Death at 22 mo from tracheoplasty site occlusion (emergently trached before surgery)
2	7 weeks	1.5	Pericardial	Death at 7 days from sepsis
3	1 mo (premature)	1.0	Pericardial	Death at 10 mo from interventricular bleed
4	13 mo	1.5	Rib graft	Well at 16 mo
5	5 weeks	2.5	Rib graft	Well at 1 yr
6	3 mo (premature)	1.5	Rib graft	Well at 6 mo

[a]From Van Meter CH Jr, Lusk RM, Muntz H, Spray TL. Tracheoplasty for congenital long-segment intrathoracic tracheal stenosis. Am Surg 1991;57:168.

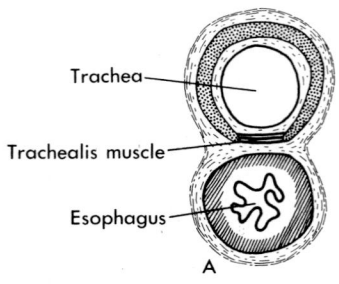

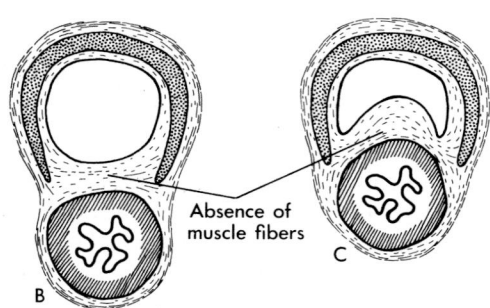

Figure 13.10. Tracheobronchomegaly. **A**, Normal trachea and esophagus. **B**, Appearance of enlarged trachea at expiration. Note absence of the trachealis muscle. **C**, Appearance at inspiration.

EMBRYOGENESIS AND PATHOLOGY

A thinning of the musculus trachealis with reduction of the longitudinal elastic fibers of the posterior tracheal wall results in an enlargement of the trachea and primary bronchi, and in a broad posterior protrusion of the unsupported tracheal mucosa (Fig. 13.10). The protrusion may be either uniform or sacculated between bands of musculus trachealis. Pulsion diverticula may form (120). The affected trachea may reach a diameter of 3.5 to 4.5 cm, and the bronchi may be from 2.5 to 3.2 cm in diameter. The normal trachea ranges from 1.3 to 2.5 cm in diameter, and normal bronchi vary from 0.9 to 2.2 cm (119). In some cases the lumen is actually reduced on inspiration by inversion of the large segment of redundant mucosa (121) (Fig. 13.10, *C*). Gay and Dee (122) think that tracheobronchomegaly is a congenital anomaly with atrophy of the muscular and elastic wall of the trachea and bronchi. Engle et al. (123) postulate that infection is not an etiologic factor, and that barotrauma may play a role in the pathophysiology of this syndrome.

ANATOMY

The tracheal length in living infants was reported by Butz (124) and presented graphically by deLorimier (43) (Table 13.11).

According to Grant and Basmajian (125), the tracheal bifurcation in cadavers and living subjects in the supine position lies as follows:

Table 13.11.
Tracheal Length in Living Infants, from Vocal Cords to Carina[a]

Age (mo)	No. Cases	Length (cm)	Range (cm)
Birth–3	25	5.7	5.0–7.5
3–6	28	6.7	5.5–8.0
6–12	35	7.2	5.0–9.0
12–18	12	8.1	7.0–9.0

[a]From deLorimier AA. Congenital malformations and neonatal problems of the respiratory tract. In: Welch KJ, Randolph JG, Ravitch MM, O'Neill JA, Rowe MI, eds. Pediatric surgery, 4th ed. Chicago: Year Book Medical Publishers, 1986:635.

Table 13.12.
Tracheal Diameters from Wood's Metal Casts[a]

Age (mo)	No. of Cases	Tracheal Diameter (mm)			
		Abt		Engel	
		Sagittal	Coronal	Sagittal	Coronal
0–1	11	3.6	5.0	5.7	6.0
1–3	35	4.6	6.1	6.5	6.8
3–6	37	5.0	5.8	7.6	7.2
6–12	25	5.6	6.2	7.0	7.8

[a]From Catlin FI. Otolaryngolic disorders. In: Welch KJ, Randolph JG, Ravitch MM, O'Neill JA, Rowe MI, eds. Pediatric surgery, 4th ed. Chicago: Year Book Medical Publishers, 1986:484.

0 to 1 year of life	T3-T4
2 to 6 years of life	T4-T5
7 to 12 years of life	T5-T6
In adults	T4-T6

However, if the subject is erect, the tracheal bifurcation is in a lower position.

De Lorimier (43) presents a few practical points for determining the diameter of the trachea such as (*a*) the distal interphalangeal joint of the baby's index finger; (*b*) the size of the normal nostril; and (*c*) the formula for internal diameter in millimeters (age plus 18 divided by 4) (Table 13.12).

ASSOCIATED ANOMALIES

According to Ferguson and Ferguson (73), Ehlers-Gaylos syndrome and cutis laxa are associated with tracheobronchomegaly.

Bronchial dilation and male sterility were reported by Ben-Miled (126).

SYMPTOMS AND DIAGNOSIS

The only symptom is the early appearance of upper respiratory tract disease, which becomes chronic. The youngest patient in whom the disease has been recognized was 8 years of age. The diagnosis was by tracheography. Plain radiographs and bronchography established the diagnosis.

TREATMENT

Treatment appears to have been limited to prevention of respiratory tract infection, although surgical resection of the redundant mucosa should prove feasible.

Tracheal Diverticula and Tracheocele (Bronchial Diverticulum)

Diverticula of the trachea are rare. True diverticula—those that have all components of the tracheal wall—represent supernumerary bronchi arising from the trachea, most often on the right. Such bronchi usually serve part of the right upper lobe of the lung, but occasionally they may end blindly (127). These are discussed later in this chapter.

False pulsion diverticula (tracheocele) may be acquired from long exposure to high tracheal pressures, such as are found in some occupations. Similar diverticula may appear in patients with tracheobronchomegaly. Such diverticula develop as herniations of the mucosa through congenitally weakened musculus trachealis. They usually bulge to the right of the esophagus. They are asymptomatic unless they become large enough to retain their secretions and produce chronic respiratory disease (120).

As a general rule, congenital diverticula of the trachea are located at the right lateral wall. Diverticula found on the posterior wall are usually acquired.

Taybi (128) discussed congenital malformations of the larynx, trachea, bronchi, and lungs.

Fistula of the Trachea

TRACHEOESOPHAGEAL FISTULA

If the separation of the foregut into trachea and esophagus is incomplete, a communication between the two may persist into postnatal life. This common malformation is discussed in Chapter 3, "The Esophagus."

TRACHEOBILIARY FISTULA

Anatomy. Trifurcation of the trachea, with a median bronchus passing through the esophageal hiatus to connect with the biliary tract, has been reported three times (129–131). The findings were similar in two more recent cases. The anomalous duct resembles a bronchus in the thorax, having cartilage in the walls, and it resembles the biliary tract in the abdomen. In one case (130) (Fig. 13.11), there was an area of stratified squamous epithelium. Lindahl and Nyman (132) were able to collect only 12 cases from the literature.

Embryogenesis. Because the developing trachea is never close to the developing liver, this anomaly is difficult to explain. Bremer (133), commenting on Neuhauser's (130) case, could only suggest an anomalous, continued growth of the trachea beyond the bifurcation of the lung buds and its junction with an anomalous bud from the biliary tract. Although this explanation rings hollow, we can offer no better one.

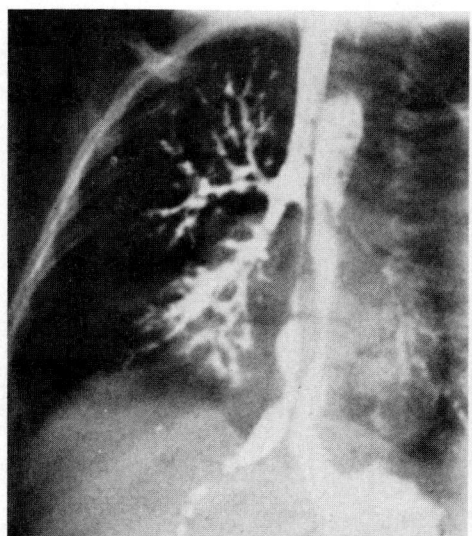
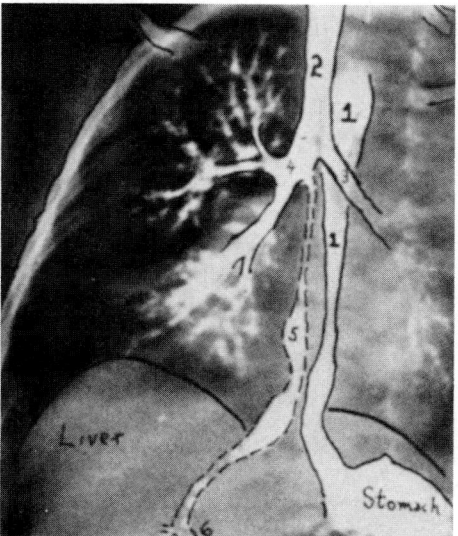
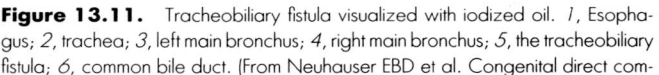

Figure 13.11.   Tracheobiliary fistula visualized with iodized oil. *1,* Esophagus; *2,* trachea; *3,* left main bronchus; *4,* right main bronchus; *5,* the tracheobiliary fistula; *6,* common bile duct. (From Neuhauser EBD et al. Congenital direct communication between biliary system and respiratory tract. Am J Dis Child 1952;83:654–659.)

Chittmittrapap et al. (134) reported 253 infants with esophageal atresia; 48% had 213 other anomalies. They further believe that esophageal atresia is associated with other congenital anomalies in 40 to 57% of affected individuals but lacks any link to the existence of fistula.

Perhaps genetics play a role in the genesis of esophageal atresia since familial cases have been reported (135). Essien and Maderious (136) believe that the morphogenesis of the laryngoesophageal complex in mice is perhaps controlled by a genetic factor. Zaw-Tun (38) questioned the presence of a tracheoesphageal septum in humans which might be responsible for the formation of the atresia; Kluth et al. (39) also denied its presence in the chick. Lister (137) blames the blood supply of the esophagus at the area of the level of the aortic arch; however, Skandalakis et al. (138) believe that the esophageal blood supply, segmental or not, is adequate especially for intramural anastomosis. As a matter of fact, Orringer (139) believes that poor technique, not poor blood supply, is responsible for leakage in end-to-end esophageal anastomosis.

Kirwan et al. (140) believe that abnormal budding from the early esophagus is responsible for the formation of duplications which perhaps are the results of a split notochord.

Symptoms and Diagnosis. In the cases of Neuhauser (130) and Bremer (133), bile-tinged sputum was observed. Enjoji's (131) patient had cough, fever, and cyanosis. Bronchography and cholangiography failed to demonstrate the communication, and no other anomalies were present.

Treatment. In other cases (130, 131) the infants survived untreated for several months. An unsuccessful attempt was made to locate the fistula in one case (131), and a cholecystojejunostomy was performed for a supposed atresia of the common duct. The patient died shortly after surgery. Once familiar with such a case, the physician will recognize the clear diagnostic signs. The apparently consistent path of the fistulous duct should result in early diagnosis and successful treatment. Several cases of successful surgical correction have been reported (132).

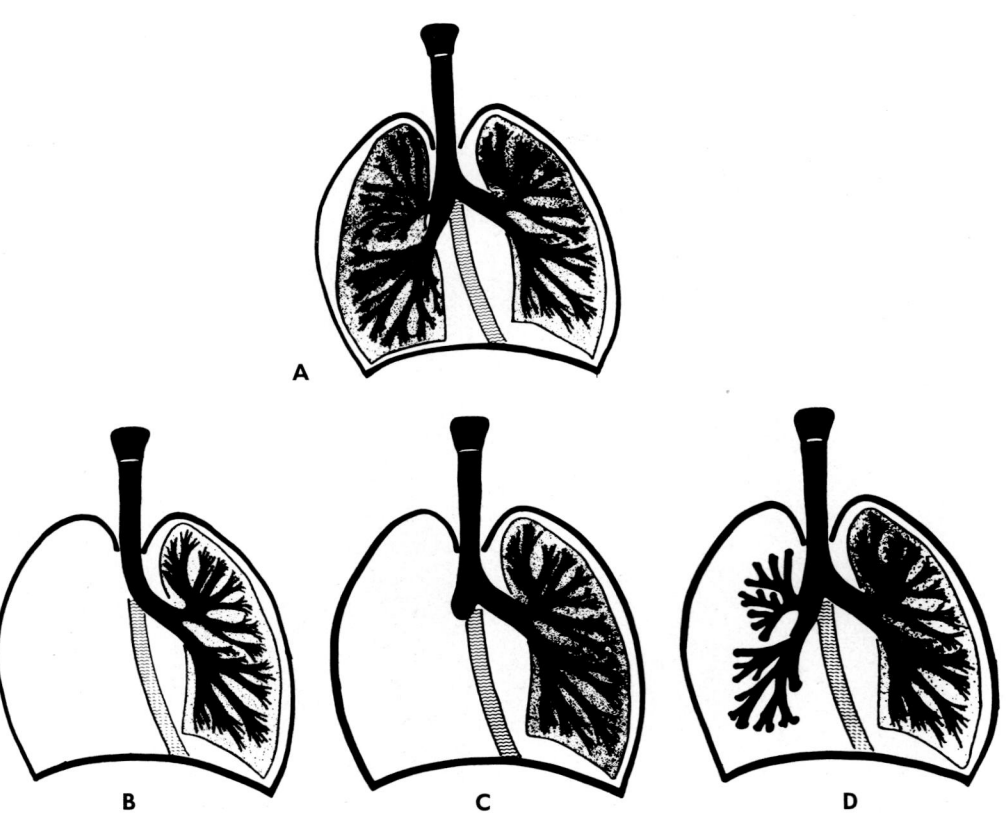

Figure 13.12. A, Normal lungs. **B**, Pulmonary aplasia, with complete absence of both bronchial and alveolar tissue. **C** and **D**, Pulmonary dysplasia. Some bronchial elements are present, but there are no alveoli. Enlargement of the sound lung and the resulting displacement of the heart and mediastinum are not shown. (From Schechter DC. Congenital absence or deficiency of lung tissue: the congenital subtractive bronchopneumonic malformations. Ann Thor Surg 1968;6:286–313.)

Unilateral Agenesis, Aplasia, and Hypoplasia of the Lung

DEFINITION

The definitions of pulmonary unilateral agenesis (complete absence of bronchus, parenchyma, and vessels) and hypoplasia (various degrees of underdevelopment) by Raffensperger (141) are pragmatic.

ANATOMY

Congenital deficiency of lung tissue was classified into four groups by Schechter (142) as follows:

Class I: bronchopneumonic aplasia (Fig. 13.12, *B*); unilateral (or bilateral) absence of the entire lung and bronchial tree. This was called "agenesis of the lung" in earlier classifications.

Class II: bronchopneumonic dysplasia (Fig. 13.12, *C* and *D*); interrupted formation of the bronchial tree, with absence of alveoli. This was "aplasia of the lung" in earlier classifications.

Class III: bronchopneumonic hypoplasia (Fig. 13.13, *A* to *C*). The entire lung is reduced in size or one lobe of the lung is absent.

Class IV. Bronchopneumonic ectoplasia (Fig. 13.13, *D* to *F*). Displacement of part or all of a lung, with bronchoesophageal fistula, has occurred.

Only the first three of Schechter's classes concern us here. Class IV, which is very rare, has a separate although perhaps not unrelated embryonic origin. It is one of the defects of tracheal and esophageal separation (see Chapter 3, "The Esophagus").

Defects of classes I and II occur in equal proportions, but the incidence of hypoplasia has been placed as low as 10% (143) and as high as 46% (142). The high frequency in the latter series is due in part to the inclusion of hypoplasia of the lung secondary to malformations of the diaphragm and of the great vessels. Bilateral congenital pulmonary agenesis is a rare lethal anomaly first described by Morgagni (144). Only 11 cases were reported in 1985 by Torriello and Bauserman (145).

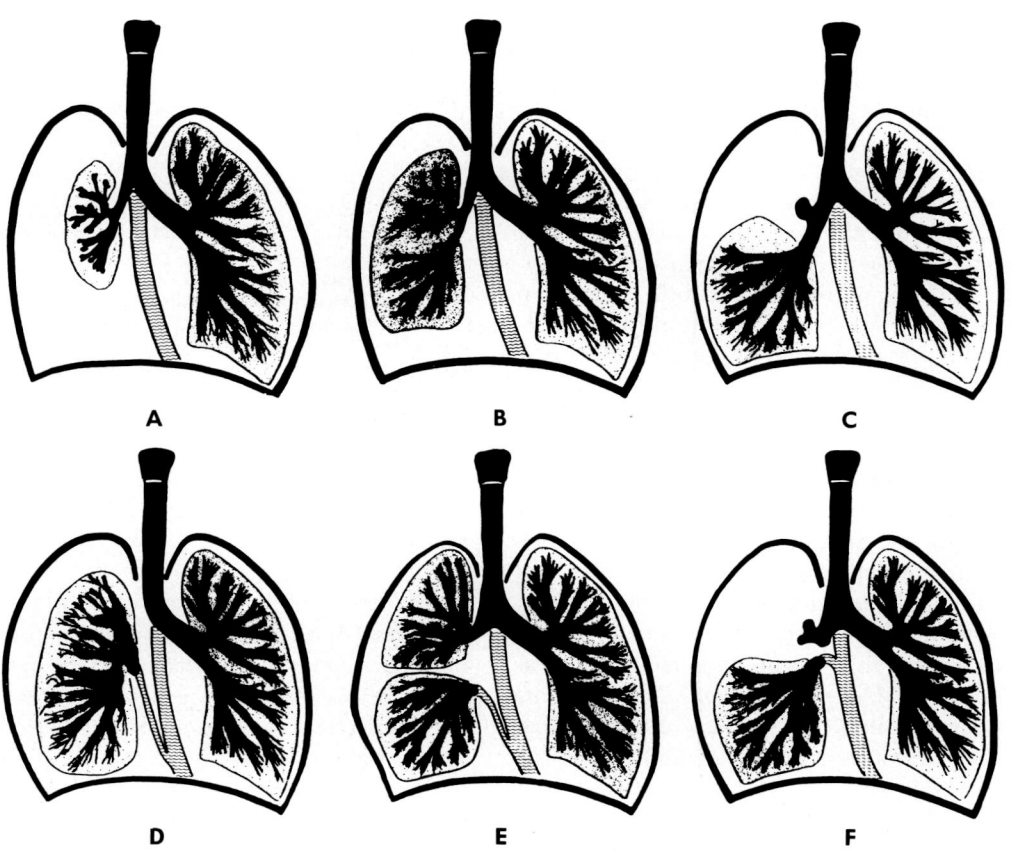

Figure 13.13. **A** to **C**, Pulmonary hypoplasia. Three conditions of different embryogenesis that all result in a smaller than normal lung. **A**, Alveolar tissue not functional. **B**, Reduced size of one lung. **C**, Hypoplasia resulting from lobar dysplasia. The accompanying mediastinal shift is not shown. **D** to **F**, Pulmonary ectoplasia. Part or all of one lung is attached to the esophagus and usually is supplied by a systemic artery. **D**, Bronchoesophageal fistula. **E**, Sequestration of right lower lobe. **F**, Sequestration of lower lobe and dysplasia of upper lobe. (From Schecter DC. Congenital absence or deficiency of lung tissue: the congenital subtractive bronchopneumonic malformations. Ann Thor Surg 1968;6:286–313.)

This classification is embryologically sound, and the type of any particular anomaly is easily determined at autopsy. With increasing radiologic diagnosis during life, however, it is easier to group classes I and II together and to modify class III:

Classes I and II: Aplasia: no lung tissue visible.
Class III: Hypoplasia (primary): lung greatly reduced in size; may or may not be contained within the mediastinum.

Oyamada and his colleagues (49) assigned 66% of cases to classes I and II and 33% to class III. Even this classification has pitfalls, however, because a segmental bronchus of the existing lung may supply lung tissue on the side of the absent lung (146).

In cases of complete unilateral agenesis no pleural cavity can be found on the affected side (147), but the heart and remaining lung occupy the whole of the thorax. The remaining lung is larger than normal even in the fetus. Smart (148) showed that, whereas emphysema may occur, most of the increase in size results from hyperplasia. The radiographic picture does not resemble that following pneumonectomy.

In primary hypoplasia the rudimentary lung is usually without air. It may be displaced by the heart and the other lung. In one case (149) the hypoplastic left bronchus turned to the right and lay posterior to the normal right lung.

This hypoplasia is very different from the hypoplasia found secondary to diaphragmatic hernia, in which the growth retardation of the affected lung results from lack of normal room to develop in the thorax. In such secondary hypoplasia, the lung is usually aerated, and often achieves its normal size following reduction of the herniated viscera and repair of the diaphragmatic defect (see Chapter 15 "The Diaphragm"). Stocker (150) reported etiologic factors and anomalies associated with pulmonary hypoplasia (Table 13.13 and Table 13.14).

Bilateral and often fatal pulmonary hypoplasia may be associated with severe chest wall growth abnormalities such as Jeune's syndrome or congenital asphyxiating thoracic dystrophy. It is not clear whether the hypoplasia is secondary to inadequate room within the thorax in this compromised chest wall deformity or whether the failure of the chest wall growth follows the anomalous bilateral hypoplasia of the lung. The parenchyma of the lung in such babies appears histologically normal; and therefore most clinicians believe this is primarily an abnormality in chest wall development with secondary hypoplasia of the lung rather than a primary pulmonary defect. Recent surgical attempts to expand the chest wall in the few babies who survive the first weeks of life have been encouraging, but there have been few long-term survivors.

Instances of agenesis of a specific secondary bronchus with otherwise normal lungs have been reported (151,

Table 13.13.
Etiologic Factors in Pulmonary Hypoplasia[a]

Intrathoracic mass with compression effect
Extrathoracic compression of thorax
Abnormal or absent fetal breathing movements
Decreased blood flow to the lung
Primary mesodermal defect
Unknown

[a]From Stocker JT. Congenital and development diseases. In: Dail DH et al., eds. Pulmonary pathology. New York: Springer-Verlag, 1988:41–71.

Table 13.14.
Anomalies Associated with Pulmonary Hypoplasia[a]

Frequent
   Diaphragmatic hernia
   Renal agenesis, bilateral
   Renal dysgenesis, bilateral
   Obstructive uropathy
   Renal polycystic disease
Unusual
   Diaphragmatic hypoplasia or eventration
   Extralobar pulmonary sequestration
   Hemolytic disease
   Musculoskeletal abnormalities such as thoracic dystrophies
   Oligohydramnios caused by prolonged amniotic fluid leakage
   Chromosomal including trisomy 13, 18, 21
   Anencephaly
   Scimitar syndrome
Rare
   Pleural effusion
   Ascites secondary to congenital infection
   Thoracic neuroblastoma
   Phrenic nerve agenesis
   Right-sided cardiovascular malformation as with hypoplastic right ventricle
   Gastroschisis
   Upper cervical spinal cord injury
   Laryngotracheoesophageal cleft

[a]From Stocker JT. Congenital and development diseases. In: Dail DH, Hammar SP, eds. Pulmonary pathology. New York: Springer-Verlag, 1988:41–71.

152). Such hypoplastic lobes may be cystic and infected. Mediastinal unilobar single lobe was reported by Markowitz et al. (153).

EMBRYOGENESIS

The rarity of bilateral agenesis of the lung (compared with unilateral agenesis) indicates that the latter is not a simple arrest of normal development. Rather, it is a failure to maintain the developmental balance between the two lung buds, perhaps due to failure of the primitive pulmonary buds. Normal development requires that the bronchial anlage be divided reasonably equally between the two buds. If this balance is not established, one side will develop normally while the other will fail completely (aplasia) or undergo only limited development (dysplasia or hypoplasia). We must not think that the normal balance depends on an exactly equal division of the bronchial primordium. The division need only leave an adequate cell population—not necessarily of the same size—on each side. What the minimum population needed for normal development is we do not know, but it is probably much less than one-half of the developing lung bud.

These defects, therefore, arise at the time the caudal tip of the tracheal primordium bifurcates. This occurs about the end of the fourth week after fertilization (stage 12), when the embryo is 4 mm long. Aplasia does not represent an error that occurred earlier than that causing hypoplasia; the difference is quantitative rather than temporal.

Therefore, when bronchial agenesis occurs, failure of pulmonary formation follows. In unilateral bronchial aplasia, the lung also is not formed. In unilateral or bilateral bronchial hypoplasia, one or both lungs are hypoplastic and not well developed.

ASSOCIATED ANOMALIES

Somewhat more than 50% of patients with pulmonary agenesis have other anomalies. If the left lung is the one present, it is frequently trilobed (147). Esophageal atresia (154) and tracheoesophageal fistula (147) have both been observed. Hemivertebra, spina bifida and fused ribs (155, 156), patent ductus arteriosus, cleft palate, ipsilateral deformed ear and ipsilateral absent hand (91), imperforate anus (143), and cardiac defects (147) have all been reported.

Stocker (150) made an excellent presentation of the anomalies associated with pulmonary hypoplasia (Table 13.14).

Oligohydramnios and prune belly syndrome were reported by Prouty and Myers (157). Sbokos and McMillan (158) stated that patients may have a normal life expectancy if other associated anomalies are not present. Mardini and Nyhan (159) stated that the life expectancy is 6 years for right pulmonary agenesis and 16 years for the left.

HISTORY

The earliest mentions of congenital absence of the lung were by de Pozzi (160) in 1674 and Riviere (161) in 1679. The descriptions are brief and leave some doubt about the exact findings. Riviere's patient had a diaphragmatic defect and the lung was probably secondarily hypoplastic (144). Haberlein (162) is usually credited with the first adequate description, which he published in 1787. Fewer than 36 cases were reported before 1900. Gilkey (163) in 1928 made the first diagnosis in a living patient, although in a few earlier cases the diagnosis had been suspected before death. The first adequate review of the subject in English was provided by Hurwitz and Stephens (164) in 1937, at which time they found 34 acceptable cases. Since then a number of reviews have appeared (49, 143, 148,

165). Oyamada and his colleagues (49) found 73 authentic cases of unilateral pulmonary agenesis, 38 cases of aplasia, and 21 other cases which they considered to be incompletely described. In 1968 Schechter (142) reviewed 414 cases from the world literature. His review may be consulted for details.

INCIDENCE

No statistics exist for the incidence of pulmonary aplasia but it appears to be of the order of 1:15,000 autopsies (142). There is a slight preponderance of females affected, but the difference is not significant. Both lungs are affected in equal proportions, although patients with aplasia of the left lung have a considerably better prognosis. Aplasia has been reported in both members of two sets of identical twins (166), but no familial tendency has been observed.

Maltz and Nadas (167) presented eight cases of agenesis of the lung and reviewed the literature. Half of the cases were associated with multiple anomalies such as cardiac defects, vascular anomalies, skeletal anomalies, and genitourinary anomalies.

In 1986 De Lorimier (43) stated that approximately 200 cases of unilateral pulmonary agenesis and aplasia had been reported. Pulmonary hypoplasia was reported by Wigglesworth et al. (168) and by Reale and Esterly (169).

When discussing this condition the water is muddy; perhaps in the future a better classification and associated anomalies will be described—for example, perhaps one of the features of scimitar syndrome is bilateral pulmonary hypoplasia.

SIGNS AND SYMPTOMS

Asymmetry of the thorax, with or without scoliosis, is a common but by no means universal finding. Chronic unproductive cough and signs of respiratory insufficiency, such as rapid breathing, dyspnea, harsh breath sounds, and cyanosis, are frequently encountered. Infants may fail to gain weight normally. Correct diagnosis is rarely made on the basis of history or physical findings alone.

DIAGNOSIS

Until recently, the diagnosis was usually made at autopsy. However, percussion and auscultation, radiography, bronchoscopy, and bronchography together will establish the diagnosis without doubt in most cases. Ferguson and Neuhauser (91) were able to recognize five cases in 6 years at the Boston Children's Hospital. While Smart (148) in 1946 could find only 17 cases diagnosed in life, Oyamada et al. (49) found 38 in 1953, and Bariety and Choubrac (170) found 50 by 1957.

The chest on the affected side is usually dull to percussion, and breath sounds are absent. On x-ray examination the heart and mediastinum are shifted toward the affected side, which appears opaque in contrast to the normal side. The diaphragm on the affected side is elevated but not immobilized. Some thoracic asymmetry, not visible on gross inspection, may be recognized.

Bronchoscopy will reveal the absence or underdevelopment of the main bronchus on the affected side, and bronchography with iodized oil will confirm the condition. Iodized oil should not be used, however, if tracheal or bronchial stenosis is present (84). The use of angiopneumography as a diagnostic aid is discussed by Bariety and Choubrac (170), who recommend that toleration to contrast media be tested beforehand.

Hypoplasia with a normal sized bronchus seen at bronchoscopy may be distinguished from atelectasis by radiographic films taken several months apart. The presence of any lateral aerated lung tissue should rule out aplasia. If a main bronchus tumor is suspected, bronchial washings should be examined cytologically.

TREATMENT

While the absent lung cannot now be restored, perhaps the future will include transplantation—thus every effort must be made to avoid infection of the remaining lung. All but the most essential surgery for associated abnormalities should be deferred until the single lung has attained its maximal size and development.

Resection of grossly hypoplastic lung tissue or functionless bronchial stubs, both of which may be sources of respiratory infection, has been suggested by Schechter (142).

However, the hypoplastic lung associated with congenital diaphragmatic hernia should not be resected at the time of the hernia repair since, with time, the hypoplastic lung will recover some respiratory function (171).

MORTALITY AND PROGNOSIS

Fifty percent of children born with pulmonary aplasia are stillborn or die within the first 5 years of life, and more than 20% die at birth or in the first month of life from concomitant anomalies. For the survivors, respiratory tract infections are the greatest danger. At least three children have died from inhaling foreign bodies which obstructed the single bronchus they possessed (147). In spite of this prognosis, some individuals have lived a normal life span with their deformity (142).

Shaffer (172) constructed survival curves from data of Oyamada and his colleagues (49) and showed that twice as many children with absence of the right lung have died by the age of 10 years as have those with absence of the left lung.

The incidence of respiratory infection is higher in patients with class II and III defects than in those with class I defects. Schechter (142) suggests that the bronchi on the affected side provide a constant source of infection for the normal lung. Similarly, there is a greater ventilation deficiency in aplasia than in dysplasia or hypoplasia, in which functionless bronchi contribute to the dead air space. In none of the classes, however, is there any evidence of an increased predisposition to lung cancer.

Anomalies of Lobulation

The grossly visible variations in the divisions of the lungs may be ranked into three groups:

Group 1: Variations of external fissures without alteration of the underlying bronchial pattern
Group 2: Superficial septation produced by an extrinsic blood vessel
Group 3: Variations of the bronchial pattern with or without external evidence

GROUP 1

Boyden (173) would prefer to consider these examples of supernumerary fissures rather than as supernumerary lobes. They are of no clinical significance and rarely come to the attention of their possessor or the patient's physician. A few are constant enough to be named (Fig. 13.14).

Some Bronchial Anomalies. Accessory cardiac bronchus (174) and segmental bronchial atresia (175) were reported in 1988. Jederlinic et al. (176) collected 82 cases with congenital bronchial atresia and reported four cases of their own. Aberrant bronchi and cardiovascular anomalies were reported by Evans (177) in 1990.

Cardiac Lobe. This condition, which occurs normally in some animals, is formed by a fissure separating the medial basal bronchopulmonary segment of the right lower lobe from the remainder. About 33% of affected individuals have at least traces of such a fissure (122), according to Dévé (178).

Dorsal Lobe. The superior bronchopulmonary segment of either lower lobe may be separated from the remainder by a fissure. This is present on the right in about 20% of the population, on the left in about 8%, and bilaterally in another 7%.

Absent Fissures. Normal fissures may be incomplete or absent. The fissure between upper and lower lobes on either side is absent in 30% of individuals, and the fissure between upper and middle right lobes is incomplete in 67% and absent in 21%, according to Kent and Blades (179) (Fig. 13.14). Absent fissures do not, however, indicate an alteration of the basic lobular pattern of the lungs.

GROUP 2

Azygous Lobe. The azygous lobe is not a true pulmonary lobe, but results from a septum impressed on the lung by an aberrant azygos vein (the embryonic postcar-

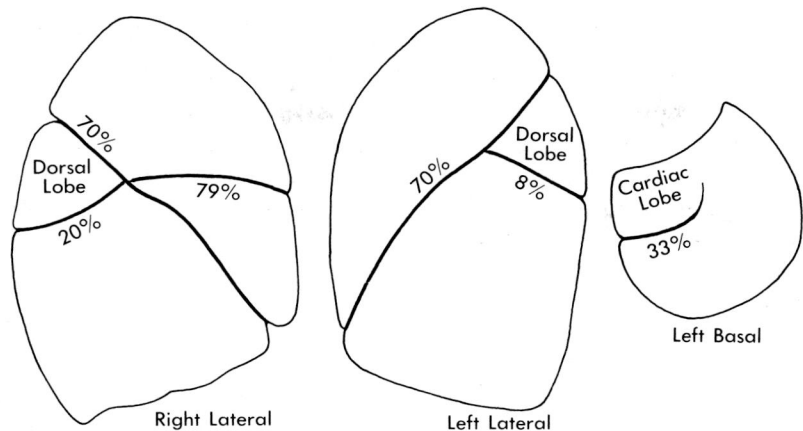

Figure 13.14. External fissures of the lungs, and the frequency of their occurrences. Absence of a fissure does not imply alteration in the underlying bronchial pattern. The less common fissures create dorsal and cardiac lobes.

dinal vein). The resulting fissure (unlike other fissures, which are composed of two infolded layers of visceral pleura) contains four layers because the parietal pleura enveloping the azygous vein as the mesazygos also is included. Bilateral cases are known (173). This anomalous lobe in the apical portion of the right upper lobe of the lung has been observed since 1777 (180). Stibbe (181) divided azygous fissures into three groups:

Group 1: Fissures that are more or less horizontal, cutting the lung below the apex.
Group 2: Fissures that are more nearly vertical, dividing the apex into two portions.
Group 3: Fissures that are vertical, cutting off a small, tongue-shaped lobe from the mediastinal surface.

Among roentgenograms from 30,000 male recruits at United States Armed Forces induction stations, Etter (182) found 130 cases of azygous lobes, of which 41% were group 1, 32% were group 2, and 27% were group 3. The overall incidence was 0.43%. In England, Clive (148) examined 30,000 female recruits and found only 32 azygous lobes, or 0.11%. This may indicate a gender difference. Krasovskii and his colleagues (184) found the defect in 0.6% of patients with chronic pulmonary infection.

GROUP 3

In these anomalies, alterations occur in the bronchial tree that may or may not be indicated by anomalous fissures.

Left Eparterial Bronchus. The existence of this structure as a suppressed homologue of the normal eparterial bronchus on the right has been postulated. Boyden (127) found five cases of such a bronchus, but he did not consider it to be identical to the normal right eparterial bronchus. It arises from two left upper lobe buds instead of from the normal single bud at the 7- to 8-mm stage of development. Its frequency is about 1%.

Tracheal Lobe. Very rarely a portion of the right upper lobe may be supplied by a bronchus arising directly from the trachea. Boyden (127) distinguishes between a displaced apical bronchus which, although arising abnormally, supplies a portion of the lung normally supplied by one of the three segmental bronchi of the upper lobe, and a true supernumerary bronchus that occurs in addition to the usual three upper lobe bronchi (Fig. 13.15, *B* and *C*).

True supernumerary bronchi may end blindly, in which case they are termed *tracheal diverticula* (Fig. 13.15, *E*), or they may lead to aerated or bronchiectatic lung tissue (Fig. 13.15, *D*). They may then be termed *tracheal lobes* or *apical accessory lungs* (185–187) (see Chapter 14, "Pulmonary Circulation").

A tracheal lobe represented by a cystic tumor connected to the trachea by a fibrous band, which showed no trace of bronchus or blood vessels, was reported as a mediastinal tumor (188). Gruenfeld and Gray (189) considered these tracheal lobes to be atavistic because they are normally present in some mammals.

Such lobes are usually asymptomatic, but in one patient a bronchiectatic tracheal lobe produced symptoms of chronic bronchitis and required surgical removal (187). The lobe was recognized by bronchoscopy and bronchography before surgery.

Tracheal buds are not rare in embryos (190) (Fig. 13.16), but they are less frequent in postnatal life. Le Roux (191) found right upper lobe anomalies in 3% of patients undergoing bronchography, but the incidence in the general population must be much less.

Duplication of the Lung. A single case has been described in which a left supernumerary bronchus served not an apical lobe but an entire duplicate right lung, complete with three lobes. Both right lungs were in separate pleural cavities. Repeated episodes of pneumonia in an 8-year-old boy led to bronchoscopy; the defect was revealed by

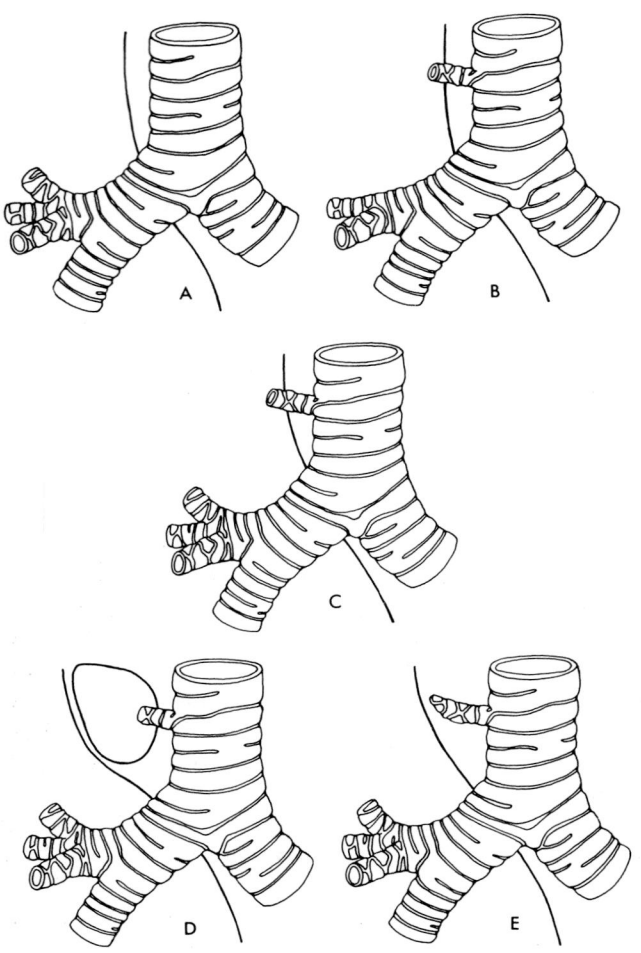

Figure 13.15. Forms of tracheal bronchi. **A**, Normal right bronchus. **B**, Apical bronchus displaced to trachea. **C**, Apical bronchus normal, supernumerary tracheal bronchus. **D**, Supernumerary tracheal bronchus ending in a tracheal accessory lung. **E**, Tracheal diverticulum with no surrounding lung tissue.

bronchoscopy and subsequently confirmed at an operation performed to remove a cystic lower lobe of the upper right lung (192) (Fig. 13.17). The authors suggested that the duplication was an extreme manifestation of a tracheal lobe, but it seems more probable that it represented an accidental splitting of a lung bud in the fifth week (stage 13). It is interesting to observe that, had there not been a cystic lobe of the upper lung, this remarkable anomaly might have gone undetected. No symptoms were present.

Pulmonary Isomerism. The lungs are slightly asymmetric and, therefore, may be found completely reversed along with the other viscera (situs inversus) or, in the absence of situs inversus, the left lung may have three lobes as does the normal right lung (left isomerism). Such anomalies are frequently associated with anomalies of the spleen and almost always with anomalous pulmonary venous drainage (Fig. 13.18).

Among 105 cases of absence of the spleen collected by Brandt and Liebow (193), the left lung was trilobed in 56 cases and had more than three lobes in 8 other cases. The pulmonary drainage was almost always abnormal, emptying into the superior vena cava or right atrium in about 50% of cases and into the portal, gastric, azygos, or innominate veins or the inferior vena cava in the remainder. The superior vena cava was bilateral in 40% of cases.

All of the 37 individuals with multiple spleens had eparterial bronchi and middle lobe bronchi on both sides, but the gross lobulation was more often normal in these patients than in patients with asplenia. (See Chapter 10, "The Spleen" for further discussion of the relationship between splenic and pulmonary anomalies.)

Anderson et al. (194) reported on 1042 autopsies on children which investigated the spleen, lung lobation,

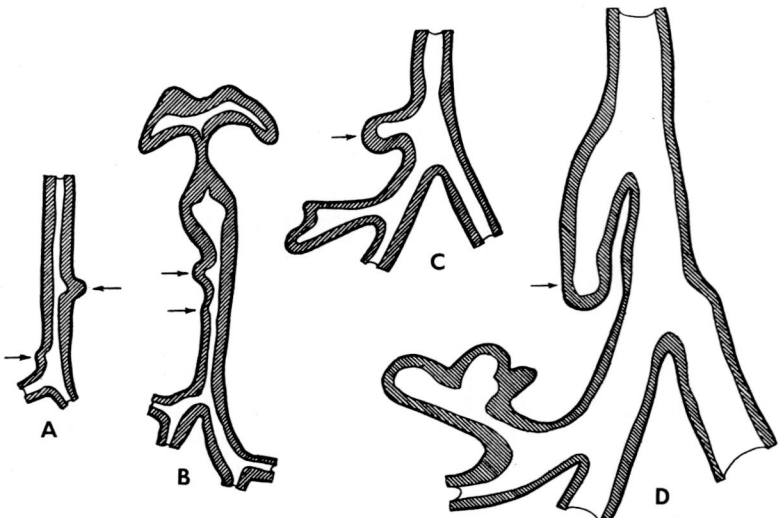

Figure 13.16. Trachea and tracheal bifurcation in human embryos of 6.25 mm (**A**), 8 mm (**B**), 10.6 mm (**C**), and 16.5 mm (**D**), in frontal view. In **B** are included the frontal section of the pharynx above the enlargement which is to form

the larynx. *Arrows* point to the tracheal bronchial outgrowths. Various magnifications. (From Bremer JL. Accessory bronchi in embryos: their occurrence and probable fate. Anat Rec 1932;34:361–364.)

bronchi arrangement, morphology of atrial appendage, cardiac anomalies, vascular anomalies, and malformations of abdominal organs. In this classic paper, the authors report: isomerism of left atrial appendages, 0.77%; isomerism of right atrial appendages, 1.25%; multiple spleens without isomerism of the atrial appendage,

0.67%; normal spleen with right and left atrial appendage isomerism, two patients.

The morphology of the atrial appendages and the arrangement of the atria is not accurately predicted by the type of the spleen, according to Anderson et al. (194). They advise the making of a detailed description for each patient of lung lobation, vessels, type of spleen, and any other malformation within the peritoneal cavity.

Sequestrations of the Lungs and Accessory Lungs

These anomalies are fundamentally vascular in nature and are considered in Chapter 14, "Pulmonary Circulation."

Cystic Duplications of the Trachea and Bronchi

Not all thoracic cysts lined with respiratory epithelium can be considered "duplications" of the trachea or bronchi. A distinction must be made between those duplications arising from the primitive foregut, the trachea, and the lungs (Fig. 13.19). Respiratory epithelium (pseudostratified ciliated) appears to be a potentiality of all primitive foregut epithelium. These thoracic cysts are classified by their anatomic characteristics and relationships in Table 13.15.

Evans (177) reported four autopsies in children with aberrant bronchi and cardiovascular anomalies. He stated that he had found 38 other cases of aberrant bronchi and several with some also exhibiting other defects. He reported that cardiac defects were more common with supernumerary bronchi.

ANATOMY

These congenital cysts were found in the mediastinum, associated with the lower part of the trachea or the bronchi. They are lined with ciliated, columnar, or pseudostratified columnar epithelium and have elastic tissue, smooth muscle, and sometimes cartilage in their walls. They may be attached to the trachea or bronchi. Some duplications may communicate with the trachea (195),

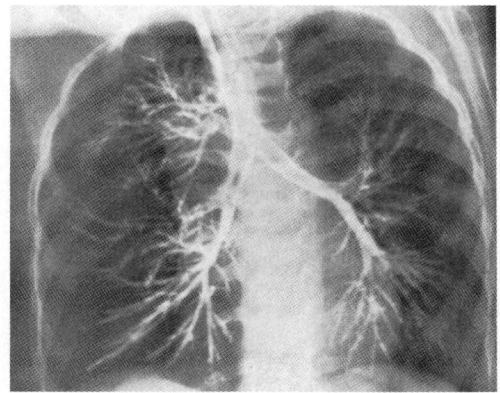
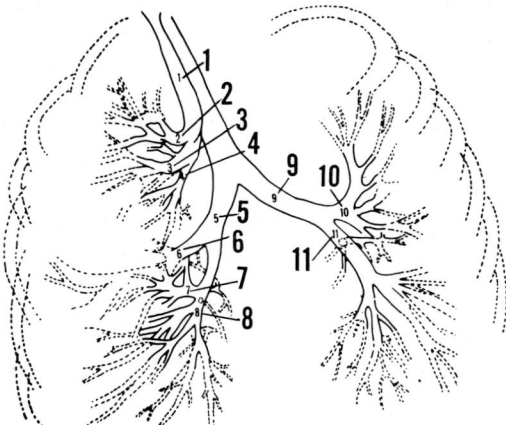

Figure 13.17. Duplication of the right lung, each lung having three lobes. Postoperative bronchogram, left anterior oblique view. *1*, Anomalous bronchus supplying right upper lung. *2* to *4*, Upper, middle, and lower lobe bronchi of right upper lung. *5*, Main-stem bronchus, right lower lung. *6* to *8*, Upper, middle, and lower lobes of right lower lung. *9* to *11*, Left mainstem, upper, and lower lobe bronchi. (From Brownlee RT, Dafoe CS. Complete reduplication of the right lung. J Thorac Cardiovasc Surg 1968;55:653–656.)

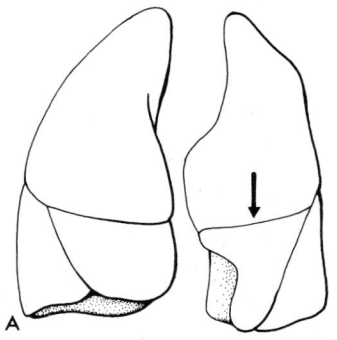
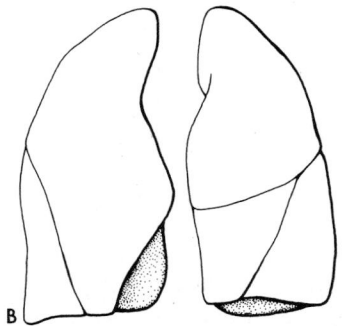

Figure 13.18. **A**, Pulmonary isomerism, which is associated with asplenia and anomalous pulmonary drainage. **B**, Situs inversus.

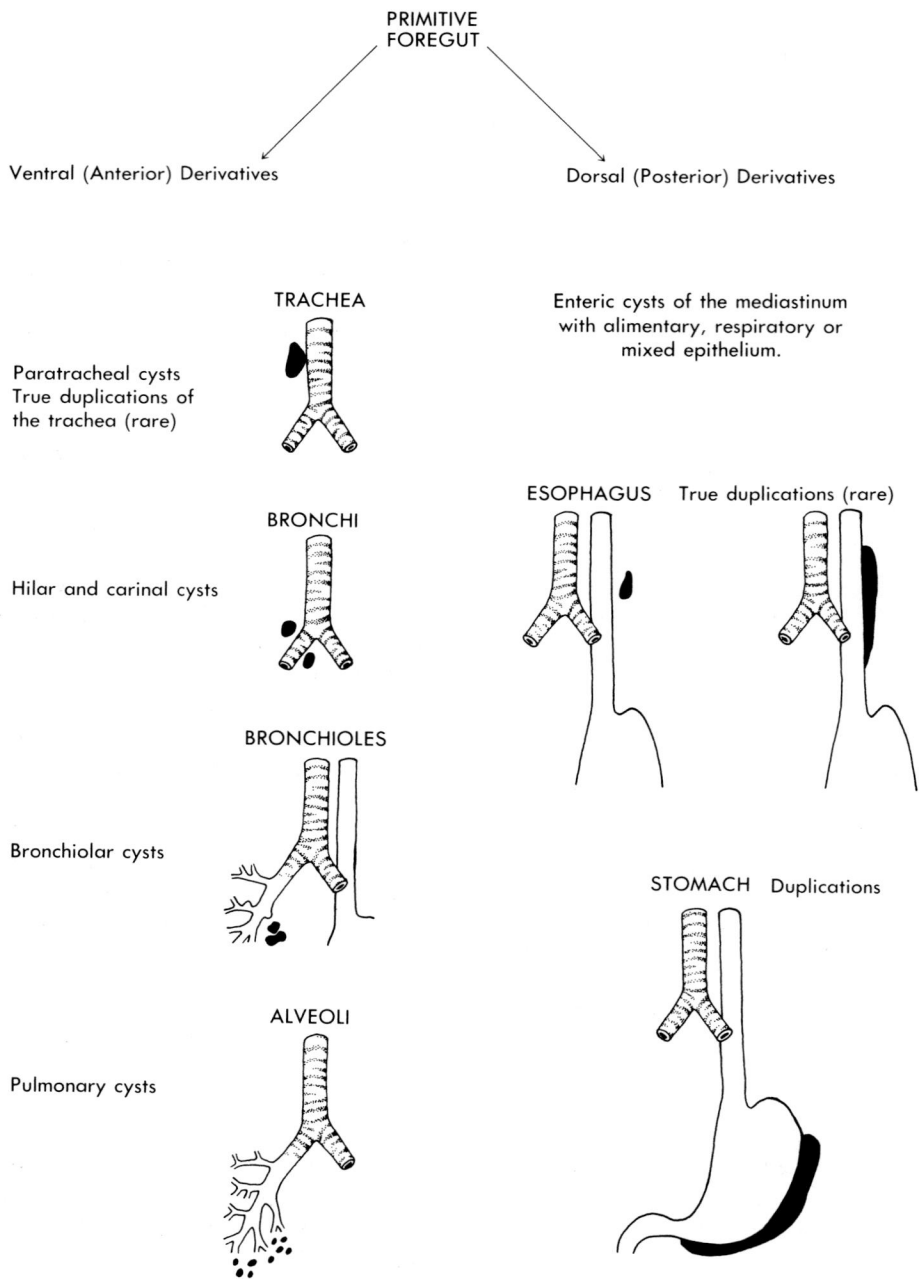

Figure 13.19. Duplications and cystic masses derived from the ventral (tracheopulmonary) and the dorsal (esophageal) portions of the embryonic foregut.

Origin of a duplication can rarely be determined from the type of epithelium lining its lumen.

but most tracheal diverticula are acquired through congenital weakness of the tracheal wall. Three groups of cystic duplications may be distinguished: paratracheal, hilar or carinal, and esophageal cysts.

Paratracheal Cysts (Duplication of the Trachea). These are attached to the right lateral tracheal wall, usually just above the bifurcation but sometimes more craniad. One cyst extended from the level of the glottis to the level of the sixth tracheal rib (196). Paratracheal cysts are rarely

found, perhaps because they are usually asymptomatic. At least one death from tracheal compression has been reported (197).

Hilar and Carinal Cysts (Duplications of the Bronchi). Most bronchogenic cysts are located at the hilus of the lung or around and beneath the bifurcation of the trachea. They are usually solitary, but there may be several in a row. They are usually attached to the trachea or a bronchus by a strand of tissue indicative of their embryonic origin.

Table 13.15.
Key to Thoracic Cysts Lined with Respiratory Epithelium

Cysts	Origin	Location	Communication	Blood Supply
Dorsal enteric cysts of the embryonic foregut ("duplications of the esophagus")	Week 2	Posterior mediastinum	None, or with esophagus	Esophageal arteries
Bronchogenic paratracheal cysts[a] ("duplications of the trachea")	Week 6	Right lateral tracheal wall	None, or with trachea or bronchus	Bronchial arteries or aorta
Intralobar sequestrations of the lung	Week 8 or later	Usually part of posterior basal segment of left lung	None, or with trachea or bronchus	Anomalous elastic artery from aorta; drainage through pulmonary veins
Extralobar sequestrations of the lung[b] (accessory lungs; Rokitansky lobes)	Week 6 or later	Separated from lung; posterior, usually on left; rarely subdiaphragmatic	None, or with bronchus, esophagus or stomach	Anomalous artery from aorta; drainage into azygos veins

[a]Hilar, carinal, and pulmonary cysts are not considered here.
[b]Apical accessory lungs are not considered here.

Hilar cysts frequently project into the pleural cavity as they enlarge. Their walls are bronchial in structure.

Esophageal Cysts with Respiratory Epithelium (Fig. 13.19). These are the paraesophageal cysts of Maier's classification (198). Although they are lined with ciliated epithelium, they are attached to, or embedded in, the wall of the esophagus rather than the trachea. (See Table 13.15 for the differential diagnosis of cysts lined with ciliated epithelium.)

Cysts of this type are derivatives of the primitive foregut prior to its differentiation into trachea and esophagus. They represent an earlier sequestration than do paratracheal, carinal, or hilar cysts. (For further discussion of these cysts, see Chapter 3, "The Esophagus.")

EMBRYOGENESIS

Hilar and carinal bronchogenic cysts represent groups of epithelial cells from the developing trachea and lung buds that have become separated from the tracheobronchial tree. Unlike the isolated bronchial buds around which sequestered lobes of the lung form, they were not distal enough to reach pulmonary mesenchyme, which might have stimulated them to further development. They form the middle group of a series of abnormal foregut derivatives (Fig. 13.19). Earlier separation results in the formation of enterogenous cysts or esophageal duplications, whereas later separation results in sequestration of the lung or accessory lungs. The earliest separation is usually dorsal—that is, from the presumptive esophageal portion of the foregut—whereas the later separations are from the ventral or tracheal portion of the foregut.

The rare paratracheal cysts have been considered to be derived from tracheal diverticula and subsequently cut off from the parent organ (198). Bremer (190) described tracheal diverticula in human and animal embryos.

Whether they would have formed supernumerary bronchi, become cysts, or been resorbed without a permanent trace cannot, of course, be determined.

HISTORY AND INCIDENCE

The earliest recognition of this malformation was by Hare (199) in 1899; well over 100 cases have since been reported. Lyons and his colleagues (200) examined 782 mediastinal masses, of which 22 were cystic. Of these 22, only 2 were of bronchogenic origin. Bronchogenic cysts rarely were found in children before 1945, but Opsahl and Berman (201) collected 31 cases in 1962.

SYMPTOMS

Compression of adjacent structures by the cyst produces the symptoms encountered. Respiratory difficulty with wheezing and cough may appear soon after birth or may follow an acute respiratory infection at an early age. Dyspnea and cyanosis may develop later, and death may ensue. Maier (198), who reviewed the cases in the literature, felt that the earlier the symptoms appeared, the more grave the prognosis.

When symptoms are not progressive, a dull chest pain and dry cough with frequent respiratory infections may become chronic. A few cases are asymptomatic and are discovered accidentally on routine chest x-ray examination or at autopsy.

DIAGNOSIS

Carinal cysts are not readily seen on x-ray examination. Hilar cysts, on the other hand, often suggest a diagnosis of mediastinal teratoma although the latter is usually in the anterior mediastinum, whereas bronchogenic cysts are more posterior.

Paratracheal cysts are more visible radiologically and

usually lie to the right of the trachea, in distinction to thyroid tumors (which surround the trachea) and to thymic tumors (which are bilaterally disposed around it). In Grafe's series (202) of 43 cysts, 12 were not seen directly on x-ray examination.

The usual radiographic findings of a bronchogenic cyst is that of homogenous radiodensity with sharply delineated borders unless obscured by other mediastinal structures. CT scan clearly delineates the main lesion and has become the diagnostic test of choice (203). MRI is of great value in distinguishing bronchogenic cysts from other intrathoracic congenital abnormalities (204).

TREATMENT

Excision of the cyst is the only effective treatment, and every effort must be made to destroy the epithelial lining to prevent recurrence. Maier (198) warns that the possible presence of anomalous pulmonary veins must be kept in mind. Injury to tracheal or bronchial walls must be avoided. Occasionally, the cyst and bronchus have a common wall between them rendering simple excision impossible. Grafe et al. (202) reported only one death in 31 operations for bronchogenic cysts.

Ectopic Bronchial Tissue

Bronchial or tracheal tissue may be found in the esophagus (see Chapter 3, ''The Esophagus''), in intestinal duplications, and in several locations not associated with the alimentary tract.

Bronchial tissue also has been reported within the pericardium (205, 206) and in the vicinity of pericardial defects (207). In the patient of Pierce and his colleagues (206), the tissue was found by angiocardiography and removed by surgery.

A unique case was reported by Seybold and Clagett (208) in which a subcutaneous tumor over the junction of the manubrium and body of the sternum was found to be a cyst lined with pseudostratified ciliated epithelium with cartilage in its wall. It appeared to be derived from a fragment of bronchial tissue pinched off from the developing lung by the closure of the sternal bars.

Park and Buford (209) described a large cyst lying behind the left sternocleidomastoid muscle in the lower neck of an 18-year-old boy. The cyst extended into the superior mediastinum and could be forced into the base of the neck by the Valsalva maneuver. It contained thick, yellowish, gelatinous material and was lined with ciliated epithelium, and its wall contained cartilage and glands. Cystic masses had been removed from the same region twice before.

Rubio et al. (210) reported ciliated gastric cells, and found that, in these cells, abnormal ciliogenesis resembles a possibly reversible altering of bronchial epithelium

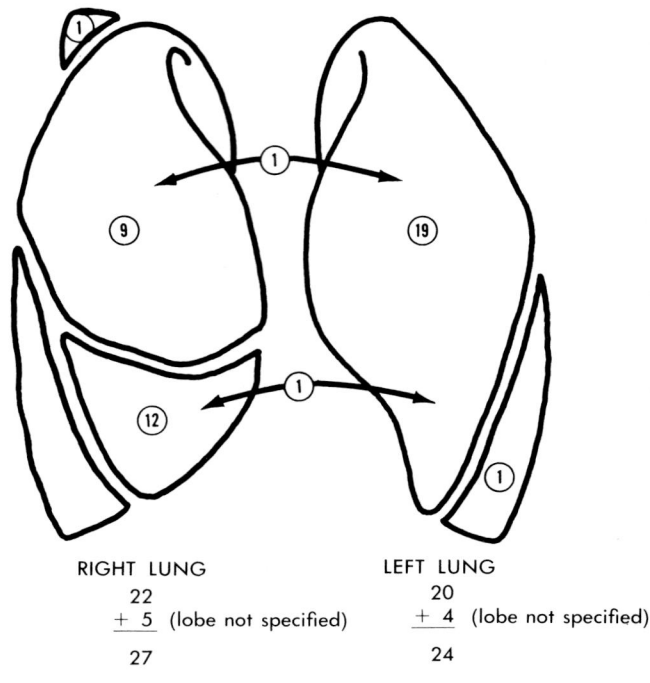

Figure 13.20. Sites of congenital lobar emphysema in 53 cases collected from the literature. In only two patients were both lungs involved. Involvement of an accessory apical lobe is indicated in the right lung.

which accompanies stasis of secretion and chronic inflammation.

Congenital Pulmonary Lobar Emphysema

ANATOMY

Emphysematous enlargement of a lobe or a segment of a lobe may appear early in postnatal life as a result of a valve-like congenital obstruction of a lobar or segmental bronchus.

Either of the upper lobes, or the right middle lobe, is usually affected. Two patients who had one affected lobe in each lung have been reported (211). In one patient an accessory apical lobe was affected (212). Figure 13.20 shows the locations of 53 cases from the literature.

The affected portion of the lung is dilated to many times its actual size. The normal lobes are compressed and the mediastinum is shifted toward the unaffected side.

Keith (213) reported congenital lobar emphysema. Miller et al. (214), in reporting bilateral involvement of lobar emphysema in infancy with congenital heart disease, were able to collect four cases in the American and British literature with proven bilateral involvement, and they also presented their own case (Table 13.16).

Table 13.16.
Summary of Data from Five Patients with Bilateral Lobar Emphysema of Infancy[a]

Authors	Sex	Birth Wt.	Age at Onset of Symptoms	Initial Symptoms	Lobes involved[b]	Treatment	Results
Floyd et al. (1963)	Male	8 lb 5 oz (3770 gm)	Birth	Tachypnea	L.U.L.	Lobectomy at 13 weeks	Alive Asymptomatic at 3½ yr
					R.M.L.	Lobectomy at 8 months	
May et al. (1964)	Male	7 lb 8 oz (3409 gm)	5 days	Cyanotic spell and "stiffening"	L.U.L.	Lobectomy at 17 days	Alive Asymptomatic at 21 mo
					R.M.L.	Lobectomy at 7 mo	
Leape and Longino (1964)	Male (case 2)	Not stated	Birth	Not stated	L.U.L.	Lobectomy at 3 mo	Alive Asymptomatic at 3 yr
					R.M.L.	Lobectomy at 6 mo	
	Not Stated (case 7)	Not stated	2 days	Not stated	L.U.L. R.M.L.	Medical	Died
Miller et al. (1968)	Male	7 lb 8 oz (3409 gm)	6 weeks	Dyspnoea and cyanosis	L.U.L.	Lobectomy at 2½ mo	Alive and well but signs of V.S.D. persist
					R.M.L.	Lobectomy at 4 mo	

[a]Modified from Miller CG, Woo-Ming MO, Carpenter RA. Lobar emphysema of infancy: case report of bilateral involvement with congenital heart disease. West Indian Med J 1968;17:35.
[b]*L.U.L.*, Left upper lobe; *R.M.L.*, right middle lobe.

Miller et al. (208) and Keith (207) reported left upper lobe involvement in 47% of cases; right middle lobe, 28%; right upper lobe, 20%; and lower lobe, 50%. Other reports (201, 215–217) gave lobe involvement as: left upper lobe, 42%; right upper lobe, 21%; right middle lobe, 35%; and lower lobe, 1% (Figure 13.21).

Warner et al. (218) discussed congenital lobar emphysema in a case with bronchial atresia and abnormal bronchial cartilages.

PATHOGENESIS

A variety of malformations may produce the obstruction that causes the emphysema. Stovin (212) divided such cases into three groups:

Group 1: Obstruction caused by collapse of bronchi on expiration, as a result of reduction in the number and size of cartilaginous plates in the bronchial wall. This appears to be a form of chondromalacia that is limited to one or a few bronchi.

Group 2: Obstruction caused by extrinsic pressure of an anomalous pulmonary artery or vein or by an abnormally large ductus arteriosus.

Group 3: Idiopathic obstruction, for which no cause can be recognized.

EDITORIAL COMMENT

In this group may fall the few dramatic clinical cases of bronchial atresia associated with overdistension of the pulmonary tissue, which should have been served by the absent bronchus. In such instances chronic symptoms of dyspnea on exertion may be reported. Such patients often have difficulty with competitive sports

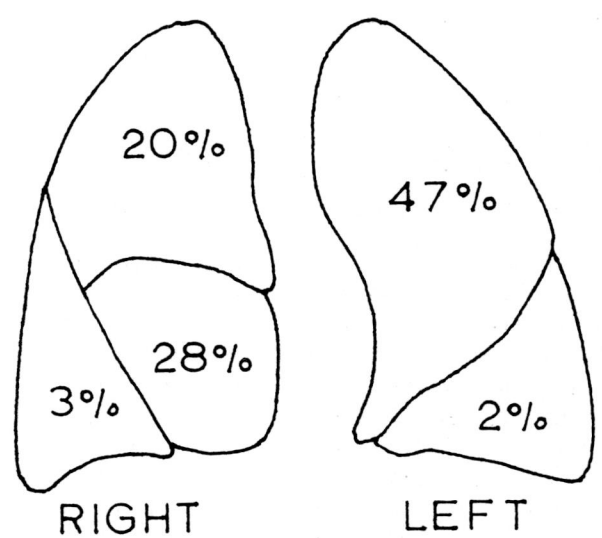

Figure 13.21. Distribution by percentage of lobar involvement in congenital lobar emphysema (205 cases). (From Keith HH. Congenital lobar emphysema. Pediatr Ann 1977;6(7):34, 452–458.)

and are found to have hyperinflated lobes which become overdistended with rapid breath and exertion. At surgery, they are found to have an absent bronchus and inflation of the emphysematous lobe by collateral ventilation through the pores of Kahn. Following resection of these abnormal lobes, the remainder of the pulmonary tissue expands normally and the children become asymptomatic (JAH/CNP).

About 33% of reported cases fall into each group. It is probable that some of the cases thought to be of extrinsic

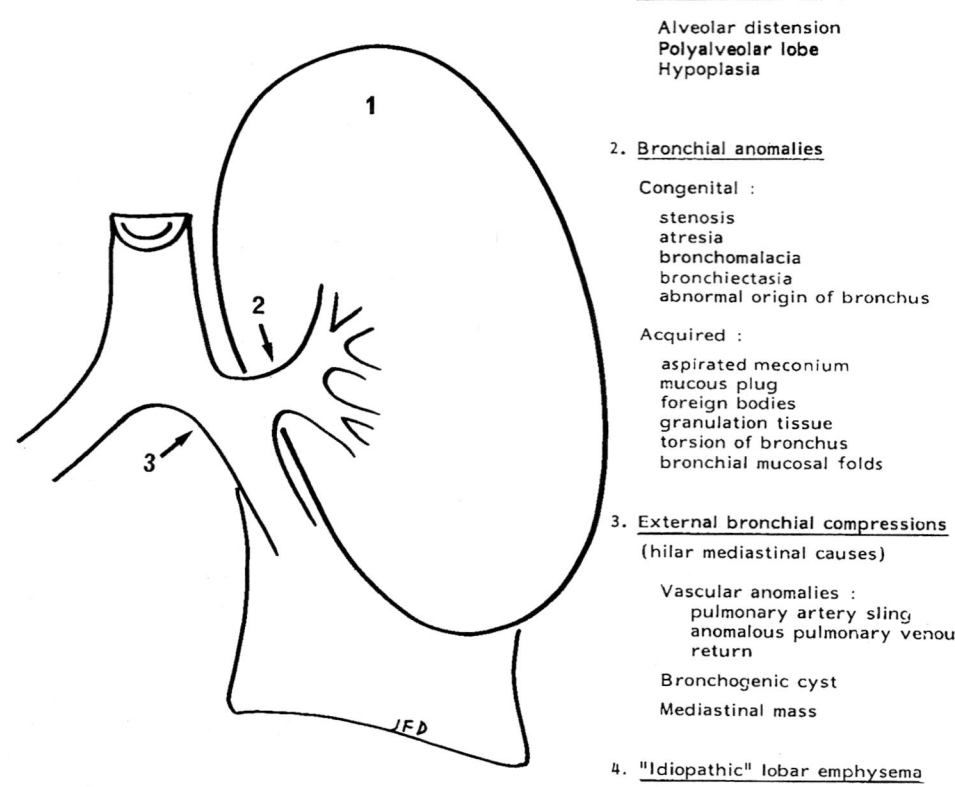

1. <u>Parenchymal anomalies</u>

   Alveolar distension
   Polyalveolar lobe
   Hypoplasia

2. <u>Bronchial anomalies</u>

   Congenital :

   stenosis
   atresia
   bronchomalacia
   bronchiectasia
   abnormal origin of bronchus

   Acquired :

   aspirated meconium
   mucous plug
   foreign bodies
   granulation tissue
   torsion of bronchus
   bronchial mucosal folds

3. <u>External bronchial compressions</u>
   (hilar mediastinal causes)

   Vascular anomalies :
       pulmonary artery sling
       anomalous pulmonary venous
       return

   Bronchogenic cyst

   Mediastinal mass

4. <u>"Idiopathic" lobar emphysema</u>

Figure 13.22. Causes of infantile lobar emphysema. (From Fallis JC, Filler RM, Lemoine G: Pediatric thoracic surgery. New York: Elsevier, 1991.)

origin are imaginary and belong to the idiopathic group. The problem awaits more careful study of specimens.

Dyon et al. (48) reported the causes of infantile lobar emphysema (Fig. 13.22). Ferguson and Ferguson (73) summarized the causes of bronchial obstruction (Table 13.17).

HISTORY AND INCIDENCE

The earliest identifiable case is that of Royes (219) in 1938. In 1939 Overstreet (220) drew attention to the defective bronchial cartilages. Fischer and his colleagues (221) performed the first successful lobar resection for the disease in 1943. Stovin (212) collected 51 cases in 1959, and at least 15 more have since been added to the English language literature (211, 222–224).

Although the cases are few, those in group 1 (cases caused by bronchial cartilage defects) appear to occur with equal frequency in males and females, whereas in the other two categories together, there were 24 males and 6 females.

SYMPTOMS AND DIAGNOSIS

Acute respiratory distress with dyspnea and cyanosis appear soon after birth (often within the first few days).

Radiography will demonstrate an expanded, radiolucent lobe, with a mediastinal shift to the opposite side. Angiography shows decrease in peripheral vascularization of the affected lobe, and displaced and compressed vessels in adjacent lobes. The lung tissue which surrounds the pathologic lobe is compressed.

In 1500 bronchograms in children and adults, Remy et al. (225) reported seven left tracheal bronchi, four of them associated with obstructive emphysema in the same area. They speculated that, for unknown reasons, the left tracheal bronchi is more often pathogenetic than the right.

TREATMENT

Conservative treatment is useless, and although patients have lived as long as 6½ years, they showed no improvement (212). Immediate excision of the distended lobe will permit the compressed normal lobes to expand to fill the thorax.

Pediatric surgeons disagree about the treatment of lobar emphysema. Some advocate conservative treatment, and others recommend surgery: segmental or lobar. Eigen et al. (226) stated that surgical or nonsurgical treatment has, for all practical purposes, the same

Table 13.17.
Causes of Bronchial Obstruction[a]

Intrinsic
    Hypoplastic, deficient, or dysplastic bronchial cartilages
    Redundant bronchial mucosal folds
    Inspissated mucous plugs or inflammatory exudates
    Bronchial atresia or stenosis
    Kinked bronchus
    Bronchial granulations
Extrinsic
    Cardiovascular
        Patent ductus arteriosus
        Pulmonary artery sling
        Hypertensive, dilated pulmonary arteries
        Pulmonic stenosis
        Tetralogy of Fallot with absent pulmonic valve
        Dilated superior vena cava in anomalous pulmonary venous
           return
    Others
        Bronchogenic cyst
        Esophageal duplication cyst
        Mediastinal adenopathy
        Mediastinal teratoma or neuroblastoma
        Accessory diaphragm

[a]From Ferguson TB Jr, Ferguson TB. Congenital lesions of the lung and emphysema. In: Sabiston DC Jr, Spencer FC, eds. Surgery of the chest, 5th ed. Philadelphia: WB Saunders 1990:778. Modified from Berlinger NT, Porto DP, Thompson TR: Infantile lobar emphysema. Ann Otol Rhinol Laryngol 1987;96:106.

results. In the majority of patients with infantile lobe emphysema, lobectomy has excellent results.

Congenital Cysts of the Lungs

Like cystic diseases elsewhere in the body, cystic lesions of the respiratory tract are obscure and confusing. No completely satisfactory arrangement of the widely varying pathologic pictures included under the heading "cysts of the lung" has been proposed. We suggest the following classification on an embryologic basis, while recognizing that the criteria are often difficult to apply.

    I. Multiple cysts of the pulmonary parenchyma
        A. Bronchiolar cysts: Cysts lined with ciliated respiratory epithelium, solitary or multiple, air or fluid filled. They may be diffuse or localized. The term *cystic bronchiectasis* has been applied to multiple cysts.
        B. Alveolar cysts: Air-filled cysts lined with epithelium ranging from cuboidal to simple squamous, without cilia. No cartilage or muscle is present, and no respiratory passages open distally from them. They may be solitary (pneumatocele) or multiple. If multiple, they may be localized or diffuse; the term *cystic emphysema* has been applied to them.
    II. Solitary cysts
    III. Miscellaneous cysts of endothelial or mesothelial origin: The confusion continues. We agree with Sieber (44) about the controversies over embryology, pathology, nomenclature, and etiology of these cysts. Therefore we do not plan to change our traditional classification.

According to Stovin (227), congenital pulmonary cysts are the end results of an abnormal growth of the bronchial epithelium or "the building process of the extracellular matrix." Chavrier (228) stated—rightly so—that the pathologic autonomy of the intrapulmonary lesions is still difficult to explain. DeLarue et al. (229) were perhaps the first to describe congenital bronchopulmonary lesions.

Subdiaphragmatic bronchogenic cyst with communication to the stomach was reported by Keohane et al. (230).

MULTIPLE CYSTS OF THE PULMONARY PARENCHYMA

    Anatomy.

    A. Bronchiolar cysts: Bronchiolar cysts are lined with ciliated pseudostratified epithelium and may have glands, smooth muscle, or even cartilage in their walls. Unlike bronchogenic cysts, they are always in communication with the bronchial tree although the communication may be small and tortuous. It is frequently possible to demonstrate alveoli and ducts distal to them. The cysts usually are multiple and generally restricted to a single lobe. They may be filled with air, fluid, or both (231). Various descriptions of the gross appearance of the cystic lung (e.g., resembling a sponge, berry, or honeycomb) have been used. Willis and Almeyda (232) reported an association between the size of the cysts and their origin from large, medium, or terminal bronchioles.

    B. Alveolar cysts: Alveolar cysts are lined with cuboidal or squamous epithelium without cilia. No muscle or cartilage appears in the walls, but there may be connective tissue hyperplasia. No passages distal to the cysts can be demonstrated.

Both types of cysts affect the right lung more frequently than the left, and lower lobes more frequently than upper lobes. Figure 13.23 shows the distribution of 85 cases reported at the Royal Chest Hospital, London, from 1928 to 1942 (232).

    Pathogenesis. Grawitz (233) suggested a congenital origin for cystic lung disease in 1880, but doubts have been maintained by many workers (234–236). Among those who believe that at least some cases are congenital, there is often the idea that a distinction cannot be drawn between these and acquired types (237). Koontz (238) considered that lack of pigment differentiates congenital from acquired cysts, but this criterion is inadequate for explaining cysts in infants and children. Absence of an epithelial lining suggests acquired disease, but secondary inflammation may destroy the epithelium. Franchel and his colleagues (239) set up a number of criteria which they felt would support the congenital origin of pulmonary cysts in particular cases. These criteria included:

    1. Presence of associated malformations
    2. Absence of a history of disease

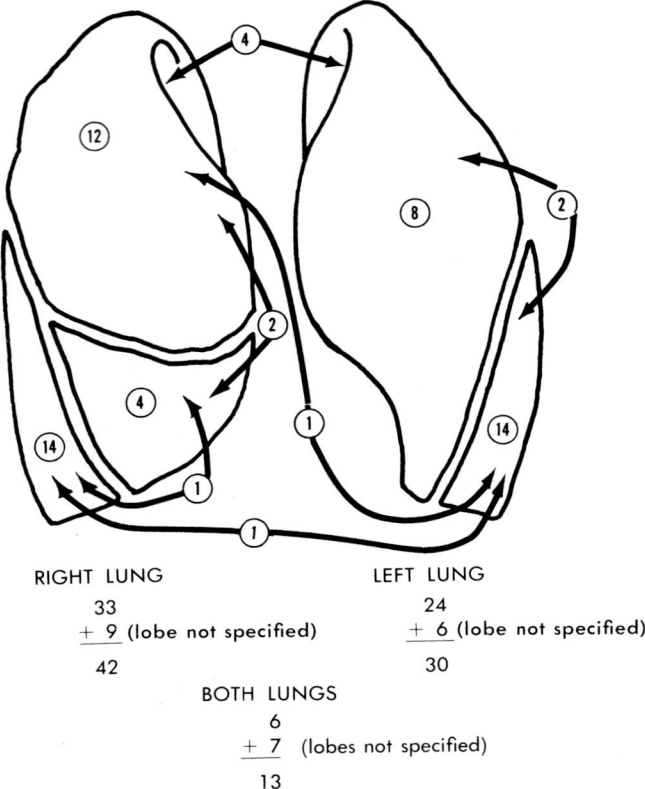

RIGHT LUNG
33
+ 9 (lobe not specified)
42

LEFT LUNG
24
+ 6 (lobe not specified)
30

BOTH LUNGS
6
+ 7 (lobes not specified)
13

Figure 13.23. Sites of alveolar cysts in 85 patients (Willis FES, Almeyda J. Cystic disease of the lung (broncho-alveolar cysts). Tubercle 1943;24:27–36, 43–58.) *Numbers with arrows* indicate the number of patients with more than one lobe affected.

3. Absence of primary communication with bronchi
4. Absence of a specific histologic lesion
5. Presence of a surgical plane of cleavage
6. Presence of at least two histologic bronchial elements

Using these criteria, Franchel et al. (239) found only two of 22 cases to be congenital. We can only say at present that cysts often are found in the lungs of stillborn infants and that similar cysts may be found in the lungs of older infants and children. While the actual process of cyst formation has not been observed, three unsupported hypotheses have been put forward by Willis and Almeyda (232).

1. The cysts are preformed but collapsed at birth, expanding at the first few breaths.
2. Bronchiectatic dilations exist at birth and enlarge rapidly as a result of obstruction of their orifices.
3. Fluid-filled cysts rupture into the bronchi and become secondarily filled with air.

If the cysts are preformed, they may represent peripheral respiratory tissue that has become separated from the respiratory tree, by partial pulmonary entrapment.

History. Recognition of pulmonary cysts has been attributed to Fontanus in 1638 and in 1687 to Bartholinus (240, 241), but no evidence exists concerning the nature of these cysts. Not until Koontz (238) reviewed 108 cases and reported the first U.S. case in 1925 did pulmonary cysts receive attention in the United States. Schenck (242) in 1936 collected 374 cases, of which 66% were non–American. Willis and Almeyda (232) reviewed 85 British cases in 1943. Conway (235), Cooke and Blades (243), and Moffat (244) contributed to efforts to find a satisfactory classification.

Incidence. The incidence of cystic pulmonary disease is not easy to judge in view of conflicting opinions over which forms should be included. Lenk (245) found six cases in 10,000 radiographs. Willis and Almeyda (232) found 11 among 27,255. Cooke and Blades (243) found 42 cases among 100,000 patients at Walter Reed Hospital, Washington, DC, over a period of 4 years. These give an incidence of 0.04 to 0.06% of patients. More males than females are affected (ratio of 1.5:1).

Only 10% of 362 cases collected by Schenck (242) were recognized at birth. Another 14% were discovered in the first year of life, and 57% were found in patients over the age of 15 years. Schenck found 42% on the right; 32% on the left; and 21% bilateral. Willis and Almeyda (236) agree with distribution.

Ramenofsky et al. (246) reported 12 intrapulmonary bronchogenic cysts and eight mediastinal. About three to one were located at the right side and were multiple or multilocular. However, other investigators, among them Raffensperger (141), maintain that lung cysts are different from bronchogenic cysts. According to Raffensperger, the location will give the diagnosis. Lung cysts are definitely within the pulmonary parenchyma, and bronchogenic cysts are either paratracheal or mediastinal. The confusion, therefore, continues.

EDITORIAL COMMENT

One additional reason for the confusion regarding the incidence of true congenital cystic disease of the lung was the earlier erroneous assumption that all such cystic changes represented "congenital bronchiectasis of the lung." Since many children in past decades (1930–1950) with congenital cystic disease of the lung presented clinically with recurrent infections and required resection because of septic complications, it was assumed by many thoracic surgeons that this represented end-stage bronchiectasis. It is now known that bronchiectasis is the end-stage of recurrent infection in terminal bronchi which may become dilated and saccular and thus simulate cystic disease. With the decrease in chronic pulmonary infections due to widespread use of antibiotics and better understanding of recurrent pulmonary infections, the incidence of late-stage bronchiectasis has diminished so much that now it is clear that many of the children with so-called congenital bronchiectasis truly had infected congenital cystic disease of the lung. To add to the confusion, however, congenital abnormalities of the lung, including congenital cystic disease and sequestration of the lung, may have secondary infection and thus appear to be histologically identical to late-stage bronchiectasis with infection (JAH/CNP).

Symptoms. **Many cysts seem to have check valves, which** lead to failure of air escape and thus to their progressive enlargement, producing symptoms of compression. Most, however, are asymptomatic until infection occurs.

Dyspnea and thoracic pain are common, together with a cough that becomes progressive with alveolar but not with bronchial cysts. Hemoptysis, clubbing of fingers, and tracheal displacement are all associated with the bronchial type, according to Willis and Almeyda (232).

Complications are spontaneous pneumothorax and chronic infection.

Diagnosis. Hyperresonance to percussion, with diminished breath sounds, is indicative of air-filled cysts. The heart may be shifted toward the unaffected side.

The diagnosis of congenital lung cysts is suggested from a chest x-ray examination. On x-ray films, multiple cysts are seen as circular, translucent areas. However, among 20 cases of such cysts in infants collected by Opsahl and Berman (201), the cysts could be visualized radiographically in only 14. CT scanning is of great benefit in diagnosing these lesions (247).

Treatment. The treatment of congenital lung cysts is resection of the cysts. Although lobectomy may be necessary in some cases, simple removal of the cyst should always be considered and performed, if possible, to conserve normal pulmonary tissue.

Read et al. (248) advised complete surgical excision of bronchogenic cysts, because of recurrence. Miller et al. (249) reported a similar case.

Spontaneous regression of untreated cysts has been reported by Caffey (236), who believes that most cysts in infants are not of congenital origin.

Prognosis. If respiratory symptoms are present in infancy, the outcome without surgery is uniformly fatal. Of 25 infantile cases collected by Opsahl and Berman (201), 11 unoperated patients died, whereas 12 of 14 patients who underwent surgery survived.

SOLITARY CYSTS

Mack and his colleagues (250) described a 9-year-old boy with an air-filled cyst that arose from a discrete left lingular lobe. It filled most of the hemithorax, compressing the upper and lower lobes (Fig. 13.24). The cyst was thin walled, with tortuous arteries and calcified plaques. Islands of lung parenchyma were present in the wall. The lining was of columnar and stratified squamous epithe-

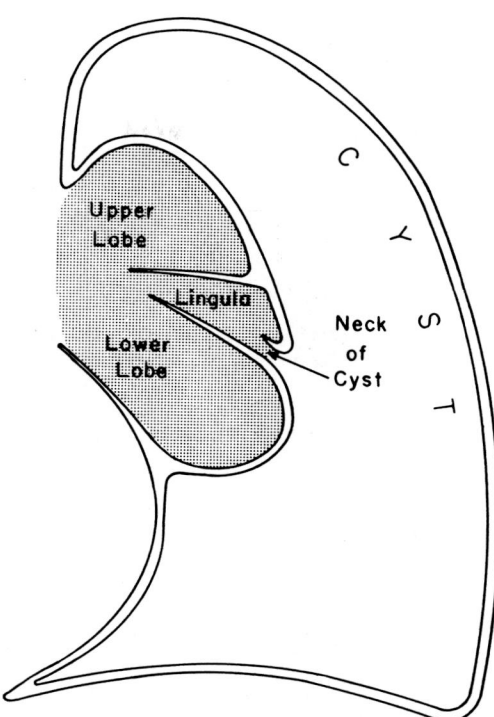

Figure 13.24. Solitary congenital cyst of the lung in a 9-year-old boy. The cyst, arising from a discrete lingular lobe of the left lung, filled the hemithorax, compressing the normal lobes of the lung. (From Mack RM et al. Gigantic solitary congenital cyst of the lung in a nine-year-old boy: case report. Am Surg 1966;32:549–556.)

lium. The lining suggests an origin from the foregut, whereas the position suggests a cystic bronchiole.

The patient showed dyspnea on exertion and at high altitude and growth was markedly retarded. There was minimal diaphragmatic movement, and no breath sounds were heard on the left side. Vital capacity was 70% of normal. Following excision of the cyst, the vital capacity, height, and weight all increased.

Boyden (251) described, in an embryo of 7 weeks gestation, what might later have become a similar cyst. The pathologist should remember that the histology of the cystic wall will give the answer as to the origin of the cyst.

MISCELLANEOUS CYSTS OF ENDOTHELIAL OR MESOTHELIAL ORIGIN

Congenital pulmonary cystic lymphangiectasis was described in 1856 by Virchow (252). About 23 cases were reported up to 1959 (253, 254); all were found at autopsy in stillborn or newborn infants.

The cysts are subpleural, septal, and peribronchial. They are lined with squamous epithelium and form a network of communicating channels. Laurence (253) suggests that the channels represent the proportion of lymphatic tissue existing during the 12th to 16th weeks of

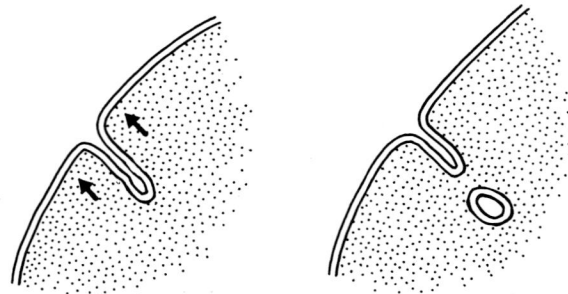

Figure 13.25. Mode of formation of mesothelial cysts of the lung. Sequestration of visceral pleural in fissures takes place with growth of the lung tissue.

development and that the anomaly represents a persistence of lymphatic growth in place of the cessation that normally takes place in the fifth month. Frank and Piper (254) consider the defect to be at least potentially a generalized rather than a specific disease of the lung.

Moffat (244) has called attention to cysts lined with squamous or fusiform cells, formed where the pleura dips into the septa of the lungs. Desquamated cells and giant cells are found in these cysts. They are interpreted by Moffat as a "nipping off" of the pleural surface by the final generation of lung buds (Fig. 13.25).

PULMONARY ADENOMATOID HAMARTOMA

In 1949 Chin and Tang (255) described a cystic disease of the lung, which they called "congenital adenomatoid malformation." Goodyear and Shillitoe (256) in 1959 discussed the same condition under the name "adenomatoid hamartoma."

Some 28 cases were reported as of 1959 (257) since Stoerk (258) described the first in 1897. A successful lobar resection for this lesion was performed by Graham and Singleton (259).

The essential feature of this disease is an overgrowth of bronchioles with almost complete suppression of alveolar development. Usually only a single lobe is affected. The overgrowth represents failure of the distal twigs of the bronchial tree to develop into alveoli. The defect may originate in the pulmonary mesenchyme. The majority of infants affected are stillborn; and anasarca, hydramnios, and prematurity are often seen concomitantly.

Congenital cystic adenomatoid malformation produces a multicystic rubbery malformation which becomes rapidly larger because of air trapped in the cystic structures.

The clinical picture is one of respiratory distress due to over distension of the involved lobe with resulting depression of the normal lung and shift of the mediastinal structures to the noninvolved side.

Diagnosis. The diagnosis can be made by roentgenographic examination, and should be distinguished from diaphragmatic hernia.

EDITORIAL COMMENT

More and more frequently, cystic adenomatoid malformations are being diagnosed prenatally by sonographic studies. This diagnosis can be made as early as the 12th to 14th week of intrauterine life, and with such consecutive studies, the pathogenesis of the anomaly is becoming better understood. There is a large cystic variety which has a better prognosis unless there is so much distension of the large cyst that compression of the remainder of the lung and shift of the mediastinum interferes with fetal viability. The other variety is microcystic which unfortunately often involves both lungs and, therefore, is a more diffuse parenchymal disease. It is this latter type which is most frequently associated with polyhydramnios and fetal hydrops—hence, the frequent impression that there is fetal death in utero. We now know that the large cystic variety does not have a high fetal death rate, and it is this group of children which is most likely to present with severe respiratory distress requiring an emergency operation in the first few hours of life (JAH/CNP).

Treatment. Resection of the involved lobe is the treatment of choice. This may be performed on an emergency basis if the patient is in respiratory distress, or electively in the asymptomatic patient (260). In a retrospective 10-year review of 23 cases, Neilson et al. (261) reported five deaths, including two therapeutic abortions and three postoperative fatalities. They emphasized the wide spectrum of severity of congenital cystic adenomatoid formation from an asymptomatic mass which may regress to one which can result in fetal death from hydrops and/or pulmonary hypoplasia.

Stocker et al. (260, 262) also described three types of cystic adenomatoid malformations:

I. Large cysts with thick walls
II. Multiple small cysts
III. Huge cysts that can occupy the whole lung or only one lobe

The following features, according to Bain (257), differentiate these cysts from other lung cysts:

1. Absence of bronchial cartilage
2. Absence of bronchial tubular glands
3. Presence of tall columnar mucinous epithelium
4. Overproduction of terminal bronchiolar structures without alveolar differentiation
5. Massive enlargement of the affected lobe

Congenital Alveolar Dysplasia

In 1948 MacMahon (263) described a pulmonary lesion found in infants who died shortly after birth. Their lungs were of normal size, but firm, rubbery, and red and weighed 10 to 15 gm more than average. He called this condition "congenital alveolar dysplasia."

Microscopically, there is an excess of connective tissue and a reduction in the number of alveoli, which are unevenly distributed and bordered by connective tissue and nests of flattened epithelial cells. After death, the pulmonary arteries and veins are filled with blood and the right atrium and ventricle are dilated. Cyanosis precedes death from asphyxia in many infants, but some may live a few weeks. Berba and Eitzen (264) believe there is a diffuse form of the disease which is fatal, and a localized form which is compatible with life.

In 1987 Miller et al. (265) postulated that tracheobronchial abnormalities should be considered in children with bronchopulmonary dysplasia.

Bailey et al. (266) provide a good review of the varieties of congenital bronchopulmonary malformations seen in 45 patients from birth to 13 years of age from 1977 to 1988. Thoracotomy with excision of the lesion by lobectomy or pneumarectomy resulted in survival of 42 (93%) patients.

Congenital Chylothorax

For the lymphatic aspects of congenital chylothorax, see Chapter 24, "The Lymphatic System."

DEFINITION

Accumulation of milky, clear, or straw-colored fluid in one or both pleural cavities.

ETIOLOGY

The etiologic factors are unknown. Andersen et al. (267) reported rupture of the thoracic duct.

HISTORY

Stewart and Linner (268) reported the first case, and Depp (269) collected 33 cases from the literature.

SYMPTOMS

Respiratory distress, cyanosis, dyspnea, and tachypnea are the symptoms, but the severity depends on the amount of accumulated fluid. Chylothorax is more common in the right than on the left thoracic cavities.

ASSOCIATED ANOMALIES

Polyhydramnios, Down's syndrome, Turner's syndrome, and others are the associated anomalies.

DIAGNOSIS

Prenatal diagnosis may be made by ultrasound examination, according to Defoort et al. (270) and Jaffa et al. (271). Chest x-ray examinations or thoracocentesis will confirm the diagnosis.

TREATMENT

Treatment consists of the following:
  Repeated thoracocentesis
  Respiratory support
  Tube thoracostomy
If fluid reaccumulates, thoracotomy for correction of the problem (e.g., with thoracic duct ligation) is necessary. Pleuroperitoneal shunting was reported as successful by Azizkhan (272).

Khoury et al. (273), Evans et al. (69), and Lubinsky (274) described multiple congenital anomalies including tracheal agenesis and the VACTERL association (vertebral defects, anorectal malformation, cardiac defects, tracheoesophageal fistula, renal anomaly and radial dysplasia, and limb defects).

REFERENCES

1. Aeby C. Der Bronchialbaum der Säugethiere und des Menschen nebst Bemerkugen über den Bronchialbaum der Vögel und Reptillien. Leipzig: Englemann 1880.
2. His W. Zur Bildungsgeschichte der Lungen beim menschlichen Embryo. Arch Anat Entw 1887;89–106.
3. Heiss R. Zur Entwicklung und Anatomie der menschlichen Lunge. Arch Anat Physiol (Anat Abt) 1919:1–129.
4. Ekehorn G. Ueber die Entwicklung der Lunge und insbesondere des Bronchialbaums beim Menschen. Z Anat Entw 1921;62:271–351.
5. Palmer DM. Early development stages of the human lung. Ohio J Sci 1936;36:69–79.
6. Wells LJ, Boyden EA. The development of the bronchopulmonary segments in human embryos of horizons XVII–XIX. Am J Anat 1954;95:163–202.
7. Smith EI. The early development of the trachea and esophagus in relation to atresia of the esophagus and tracheoesophageal fistula. Contrib Embryol Carnegie Inst Wash 1957;36:41–57.
8. Hjortsjö CH. Studies on the earliest pulmonary development in mammals. Lunds Univ Arsskrift NF AVD 1950;(2)46:4.
9. Bremer JL. Pleuroperitoneal membrane and bursa infracardiaca. Anat Rec 1943;87:311–318.
10. Rosenthal AH. Congenital atresia of the esophagus with tracheoesophageal fistula: report of eight cases. Arch Pathol 1931;12:756–772.
11. Rudnick D. Developmental capacities of the chick lung in chorioallantoic graft. J Exp Zool 1933;66:125–154.
12. Dameron F. Influence de diverse mésenchymes sur la différenciation de l'épithélium pulmonaire de l'embryon de poulet en culture in vitro. C R Acad Sci (Paris) 1961;252:3879–3881.
13. Dameron F. Influence de diverse mésenchymes sur la différenciation de l'épithélium pulmonaire de l'embryon de poulet en culture in vitro. J Embryol Exp Morphol 1961;9:628–633.
14. Alescio T, Cassini A. Introduction in vitro of tracheal buds by pulmonary mesenchyme grafts on tracheal epithelium. J Exp Zool 1962;150:83–94.
15. Alescio T, Cassini A. L'interazioni epiteliomesenchimale nell'organogenesi del polmone embrionale di topo coltivato in vitro. Z Anat Entw 1962;123:369–396.
16. Bucher U, Reid L. Development of the intrasegmental bronchial tree: the pattern of branching and development of cartilage at various stages of intrauterine life. Thorax 1961;16:207–218.
17. Bucher U, Reid L. Development of the mucus-secreting elements in human lung. Thorax 1961;16:219–225.

18. Dubreuil G, Lacoste A, Raymond R. Les étapes du développement du poumon humain et son appareil elastique. C R Soc Biol (Paris) 1963;121:244–246.

19. Dubreuil G, Lacoste A, Raymond R. Observations sur la développement du poumon humaine. Bull Hist Appl Physiol 1936;13:235.

20. Broman I. Zur Kenntnis der Lungenentwicklung. Verh Anat Ges 1923;23:83.

21. Emery JL, Mithal A. The number of alveoli in the terminal respiratory unit of man during late intrauterine life and childhood. Arch Dis Child 1960;35:544–547.

22. Cudmore RE, Emery JL, Mithal A. Postnatal growth of the bronchi and bronchioles. Arch Dis Child 1962;37:481–484.

23. Mithal A, Emery JL. The postnatal development of alveoli in premature infants. Arch Dis Child 1961;36:449–450.

24. Dunnill MS. Postnatal growth of the lung. Thorax 1962;17:329–333.

25. Ham AW, Baldwin KW. A histological study of the development of the lung with particular reference to the nature of alveoli. Anat Rec 1941;81:363.

26. Boyden EA. Differentiation of the lung between infancy and childhood. Anat Rec 1968:160:320.

27. Weibel ER, Gomez DM. Architecture of the human lung. Science 137;1962:577–585.

28. Emery JL. The postnatal development of the human lung and its implications for lung pathology. Respiration 1970;27(suppl):41–50.

29. Hogg JC, Williams J, Richardson JB, Macklem PT, Thurlbeck WM. Asge as a factor in the distribution of lower airway conductance and in the pathologic anatomy of obstructive lung disease. N Engl J Med 1970;282:23.

30. Snyder FF, Rosenfeld M. Intrauterine respiratory movements of the human fetus. JAMA 1937;108:1946.

31. Windle WF, Becker RF, Barth EE, Schulz MR. Aspiration of amniotic fluid by the fetus: an experimental roentgenological study in the guinea pig. Surg Gynecol Obstet 1939;69:705.

32. Potter EL, Bohlender GP. Intrauterine respiration in relation to development of the fetal lung, with report of two unusual anomalies of the respiratory system. Am J Obstet Gynecol 1941;42:14–22.

33. Carmel JA, Friedman F, Adams FH. Fetal tracheal ligation and lung development. Am J Dis Child 1965;109:452–456.

34. DeBlasio A, Ambrosio G, D'Amora G. Sui movimenti respiratori endouterini del feto umano a termine. Pediatria (Napoli); 1960;68:1124–1141.

35. Thurlbeck WM. Lung growth. In: Thurlbeck WM, ed. Pathology of the lung. New York: Thieme, 1988.

36. Tibboel D, Kluth D. Embryology of congenital lesions of the tracheobronchial tree. In: Lube TE, ed. Tracheal reconstruction in infancy. Philadelphia: WB Saunders, 1991.

37. O'Rahilly R, Muller F. Chevalier Jackson lecture: respiratory and alimentary relations in staged human embryos—new embryological data and congenital anomalies. Ann Otol Rhinol Laryngol 1948;93:421–429.

38. Zaw-Tun HA. The tracheo-esophageal septum: fact or fantasy?—origin and development of the respiratory primordium and esophagus. Acta Anat (Basel) 1982;114(1):1–21.

39. Kluth D, Steding G, Seidel W. The embryology of foregut malformations. J Pediatr Surg 1987;22(5):389–93.

40. Kluth D, Habenicht R. The embryology of usual and unusual types of esophageal atresia. Pediatr Surg Int 1987;2:223–227.

41. Kavlock RJ et al., eds. Abnormal functional development of the heart, lungs and kidney. Clin Biol Res 1983;140.

42. Sadler TW. Langman's medical embryology, 6th ed. Baltimore: Williams & Wilkins, 1990.

43. De Lorimier AA. Congenital malformations and neonatal problems of the respiratory tract. In: Welch KJ, Randolph JG, Ravitch MM, O'Neill JA, Rowe MI, eds. Pediatric surgery, 4th ed. Chicago: Year Book Medical Publishers, 1986:631–644.

44. Sieber WK. Lung cysts, sequestration, and bronchopulmony dysplasia. In: Welch KJ, Randolph JG, Ravitch MM, O'Neill JA, Rowe MI, eds. Pediatric surgery, 4th ed. Chicago: Year Book Medical Publishers 1986:645–654.

45. Goldstein JD, Reid LM. Pulmonary hypoplasia resulting from phrenic nerve agenesis and diaphragmatic amyoplasia. J Pediatr 1980;97:282.

46. Kitagawa M et al. Long hypoplasia in congenital diaphragmatic hernia: a quantitative study of airway artery, and alveolar development. Br J Surg 1971;58:342.

47. Ravitch MM, Matzen RN. Pulmonary insufficiency in pectus excavatum associated with left pulmonary agenesis, congenital clubbed feet and ectromelia: improvement following operation. Dis Chest 1968;54:58.

48. Dyon JF, Baudain P, Alibeu JP. Malformation of the lung mass. In: Fallis JC, Filler RM, Lemoine G, eds. Pediatric thoracic surgery. New York: Elsevier, 1991.

49. Oyamada A, Gasul BM, Holinger PH. Agenesis of the lung: report of a case, with a review of all previously reported cases. Am J Dis Child 1953;85:182–201.

50. Devi B, More JRS. Total tracheopulmonary agenesis: associated asplenia, agenesis of umbilical artery and other abnormalities. Acta Pediatr Scand 1966;55:107.

51. Claireaux AE, Ferriera HP. Bilateral pulmonary agenesis. Arch Dis Child 1958;33:364–366.

52. Kleinschmidt HJ. Beitrag zur kenntnis der bilaternalen Lungenagenesien. Zentralbl Allg Pathol 1962;104:34–39.

53. Von Schmit H. Ein Fall von vollständiger Agenesie beider Lungen. Virchow Arch Pathol Anat 1893;134:25–32.

54. Allen, Affelbach: Congenital absence of both lungs. Surg Gynecol Obstet 1925;41:375–376.

55. Tuynman PE, Gardner LW. Bilateral aplasia of the lung. Arch Pathol 1952;54:306–313.

56. Beneke R. Ueber Bauchlunge und Hernia diaphragmatico spuria. Verh Deutsch Ges Kreislaufforsch 1905;9:202.

57. Walcher K. Angeborener Mangel der Trachea. Deutsch Z Ges Gerichtl Med 1928;12:292.

58. Marek JJ. Congenital deformity of the trachea. Ohio State Med J 1940;36:1308.

59. Kessel I, Smith JN. Congenital absence of the trachea. Thorax 1953;8:266–268.

60. Sandison AT. Partial absence of the trachea with live birth. Arch Dis Child 1955;30:475–477.

61. Payne WA. Congenital absence of the trachea. Brooklyn Med J 1900;14:568.

62. Milles G, Dorsey DB. Intrauterine respiration-like movements in relation to development of the fetal vascular system: discussion of intrauterine physiology based upon cases of congenital absence of the trachea, abnormal vascular development and other anomalies. Am J Pathol 1950;26:411–425.

63. Hwang WS. Pulmonary agenesis and bronchial atresia. Singapore Med J 1968;9:48–51.

64. Buchino JJ, Meagher DP Jr, Cox JA. Tracheal agenesis: a clinical approach. J Pediatr Surg 1982;17:132.

65. Effman EL et al. Tracheal agenesis. AJR 1975;125:767.

66. Warfel KA, Schulz DM. Agenesis of the trachea: report of a case and review of the literature. Arch Pathol Lab Med 1976;100:357.

67. Koltai PJ, Quiney R. Tracheal agenesis. Ann Otol Rhinol Laryngol 1992;101:560–566.

68. Chiu T, Cuevas O, Cuevas L, Monteiro C. Tracheal agenesis. South Med J 1990;83:925–930.

69. Evans JA, Reggin J, Greenberg C. Tracheal agenesis and associated malformations: a comparison with tracheoesophageal fistula and the VACTERL association. Am J Med Genet 1985; 21:21.

70. Ashley DJB. A case of congenital tracheal obstruction with oesophageal atresia. J Pathol 1972;108:261.

71. Peison B, Levitzky E, Sprowls JJ. Tracheoesophageal fistula associated with tracheal atresia and malformation of the larynx. J Pediatr Surg 1970;5:464.

72. Chaurasia BD. Aplasia of the trachea in a malformed human foetus with single umbilical artery. Anatomischer Anzeiger 1976;139(5):480–485.

73. Ferguson TB Jr, Ferguson TB. Congenital lesions of the lung and emphysema. In: Sabiston DC Jr, Spencer FC, eds. Surgery of the chest, Vol 1, 5th ed. Philadelphia: WB Saunders, 1990.

74. Faro RS, Goodwin CD, Organ CH Jr. Tracheal agenesis. Ann Thorac Surg 1979;28(3):295–299.

75. Landing BH, Dixon LG. Congenital malformations and genetic disorders of the respiratory tract. Am Rev Respir Dis 1979;120:151–185.

76. Levin SJ, Adler P, Shere RA. Collapsible trachea (tracheomalacia): a nonallergic cause of wheezing in infancy. Ann Allergy 1964;22:20–25.

77. Davies MRO, Cywes S. The flaccid tracheal and tracheoesophageal congenital anomalies. J Pediatr Surg 1978;13:363–367.

78. Benjamin B, Cohen D, Glassom M. Tracheomalacia in association with congenital tracheoesophageal fistula. Surgery 1976;79:504–508.

79. Glason M. Tracheomalacia in association with tracheoesophageal fistula. Aust Paediatr J 1974;10:238.

80. Filler RM. Tracheomalacia. In: Fallis JC et al., eds. Pediatric thoracic surgery. New York: Elsevier, 1991.

81. Vallas J-S, de Beaujeu MJ. Discussion. In: Fallis JC et al., eds. Pediatric thoracic surgery. New York: Elsevier, 1991.

82. Fallis JC, Filler RM, Lemoine G. Pediatric thoracic surgery. New York: Elsevier, 1991.

83. Ruhrmann G. Stridor congenitus durch funktionelle stenose der trachea. Arch Kinderheilk 1963;169:170–177.

84. Wolman IJ. Congenital stenosis of the trachea. Am J Dis Child 1941;61:1263.

85. Hirsch W, Loewenthal M, Swirsky S. Congenital stridor and malformation of the trachea. Ann Paediatr 1954;182:1–9.

86. Gumbiner CH, Mullins CE, McNamara DG. Pulmonary artery sling. Am J Cardiol 1980;45:311–315.

87. Sade RM et al. Pulmonary artery sling. J Thorac Cardiovasc Surg 1975;69:333–346.

88. Backer CL, Idriss FS, Holinger LD, Mauroudis C. Pulmonary artery sling: results of surgical repair in infancy. J Thorac Cardiovasc Surg 1992:103(4):683–691.

89. Nakayama DK, Harrison MR, De Lorimier AA, Brasch RC, Fishman NH. Reconstructive surgery for obstructing lesions of the intrathoracic trachea in infants and small children. J Pediatr Surg 1982;17(6):854–868.

90. Putney FJ, Baltzell WH. Agenesis of the lung with tracheal stenosis. Ann Otol 1952;61:677.

91. Ferguson CF, Neuhauser EBD. Congenital absence of the lung (agenesis) and other anomalies of the tracheobronchial tree. AJR 1944;52:459–471.

92. Heikel PE. Congenital tracheal stenosis combined with truncus arteriosus cordis: a case diagnosed intravitam. Ann Paediatr Fenn 1957;3:22–26.

93. Lobe TE, Swischuk LE. Signs and symptoms of congenital tracheal stenosis: diagnostic considerations. In: Lobe TE, ed. Tracheal reconstruction in infancy. Philadelphia: WB Saunders, 1991.

94. Houston IB, Mackie DG. Congenital tracheal stenosis. Thorax 1961;16:94–96.

95. Stewart S, Pinkerton HH. Unusual stenosis of trachea in an adult. Br J Anaesth 1955;27:492–494.

96. Berdon WE et al. Complete cartilage-ring tracheal stenosis associated with anomalous left pulmonary artery: the ring-sling complex. Radiology 1984;152(1):57–64.

97. Cundy RL, Bergstrom LB. Congenital subglottic stenosis. J Pediatr 1973;82:282.

98. Devine P et al. Completely cartilaginous trachea in a child with Crouzon syndrome. Am J Dis Child 1984;138:40.

99. Paparo GP, Symchych PS. Postintubation subglottic stenosis and cor pulmonale. J Pediatr 1977;90:97.

100. Parkin JL, Stevens MH, Jung AL. Acquired and congenital subglottic stenosis in the infant. Ann Otol Rhinolaryngol 1976;85:573.

101. Ratner I, Whitefield J. Acquired subglottic stenosis in the very-low-birth-weight infant. Am J Dis Child 1983;137:40.

102. Hirschberg J, Lellei I. Stenose respectivement d'une obstruction de la trachea des nourrisons et des petits enfants. Therapeutische umbshaul revue therapeutique. Bund 39 Heft 12:997–1004, 1982.

103. Guisez J. Malformation congénitale de la trachée: trachéoscopie, trachéotomie. Bull d'oto Rhinolaryngol 1927;25:289–292.

104. Gebauer PW. Reconstructive tracheobronchial surgery. Surg Clin North Am 1956;36:893–911.

105. Tonkin ILD, Hollabaugh R, Hannissian A. Balloon dilatation of bronchial stenosis. In: Lobe TE, ed. Tracheal reconstruction in infancy. Philadelphia: WB Saunders, 1991.

106. Messineo A, Forte V, Joseph T, Silver MM, Filler RM. The balloon posterior tracheal split: a technique for managing tracheal stenosis in the premature infant. J Pediatr Surg 1992;27:1142–1144.

107. Bagwell CE, Talbert JL, Tepas JJ III. Balloon dilatation of long-segment tracheal stenoses. J Pediatr Surg 1991;26:153–159.

108. Campbell DN, Lilly JR. Surgery for total congenital tracheal stenosis. J Pediatr Surg 1986;21:934–935.

109. Mambrino LJ, Kenna MA, Seashore J. Surgical management of tracheal stenosis in an infant with multiple congenital anomalies: when is baby inoperable? Ann Otol Rhino Laryngol 1991;100:198–200.

110. Idriss FS et al. Tracheoplasty with pericardial patch for extensive trachea stenosis in infants and children. J Thorac Cardiovasc Surg 1984;88:527–536.

111. Grillo HC, Zannini P. Management of obstructive trachea disease in children. J Pediatr Surg 1984;19:414.

112. Maeda M, Grill HC. Effects of tension on tracheal growth after resection and anastomosis in puppies. J Thorac Cardiovasc Surg 1973;64:658–668.

113. Janik JS et al. Congenital funnel-shaped tracheal stenosis: an asymptomatic lethal anomaly of early infancy. J Thorac Cardiovasc Surg 1982;83:761–768.

114. Van Meter CH Jr, Lusk RM, Muntz H, Spray TL. Tracheoplasty for congenital long-segment intrathoracic tracheal stenosis. Am Surg 1991;57:157–190.

115. Branscheid D, Krysa S, Voigt-Moykopf I. Discussion: tracheal stenosis. In: Fallis JC, Filler RM, Lemoine G, eds. Pediatric thoracic surgery. New York: Elsevier, 1991.

116. de Lorimier AA, Harrison MR, Hardy K, Howell LJ, Adzick NS. Tracheobronchial obstructions in infants and children: experience with 45 cases. Ann Surg 1990;212:277–289.

117. Czyhlarz ER. Ueber ein pusionsdivertikel der trachea mit elastischen fasern an normalen tracheen und bronchien. Zentralbl Allg Pathol 1897;8:721–728.

118. Mounier-Kuhn P. Dilatation de la trachée; constattions radiographiques et bronchoscopiques. Lyon Méd 1932;150:106–109.

119. Katz I, LeVine M, Herman P. Tracheobronchiomegaly: the Moun-

ier-Kuhn syndrome. Am J Roentgenol Rad Therm Nucl Med 1962;88:1084–1094.

120. Surprenant EL, O'Loughlin BJ. Tracheal diverticula and tracheobronchomegaly. Dis Chest 1966;49:345–351.

121. Diaz CJ. Un caso de megatráquea idiopatica con traqueomalacia. Rev Clin Esp 1940;1:432–433.

122. Gay S, Dee P. Tracheobronchomegaly: the Mounier-Kuhn syndrome. Br J Radiol 1984;57(679):640–644.

123. Engle WA et al. Neonatal tracheobronchomegaly. Am J Perinatol 1987;4(2):81–85.

124. Butz RO Jr. Length and cross-section growth patterns in the human trachea. Pediatrics 1968;42:336–341.

125. Grant JCB, Basmajian JV. Grant's method of anatomy. Baltimore: Williams & Wilkins, 1965:496.

126. Ben-Miled MT. [Association between bronchial dilatation and male sterility]. Poumon Coeur 1983;39(1):17–24.

127. Boyden EA. The distribution of bronchi in gross anomalies of the right upper lobe, particularly lobes subdivided by the azygos vein and those containing pre-eparterial bronchi. Radiology 1952;58:797–807.

128. Taybi H. Congenital malformations of the larynx, trachea, bronchi and lungs. Prog Pediatr Radiol 1967;1:231–255.

129. Ballantyne JW. Manual of antenatal pathology and hygiene. Edinburgh: W Green & Sons, 1904.

130. Neuhauser EBD, Elkin M, Landing B. Congenital direct communication between biliary system and respiratory tract. Am J Dis Child 1952;85:654–659.

131. Enjoji M, Watanabe H, Nakamura Y. A case report: congenital biliotracheal fistula with trifurcation of bronchi. Ann Paediat (Basel) 1963:321–332.

132. Lindahl H, Nyman R: Congenital bronchobiliary fistula successfully treated at the age of three days. J Pediatr Surg 1986;21:734.

133. Bremer JL. Congenital anomalies of viscera. Cambridge: Harvard Univ Press, 1957.

134. Chittmittrapap S, Spitz L, Kiely EM, Brereton RJ. Oesophageal atresia and associated anomalies. Arch Dis Child 1989;64:364–368.

135. Jaubert F, Danel C. Discussion: intrathoracic malformations of foregut derivatives. In: Fallis JC, Filler RM, Lemoine G, eds. Pediatric thoracic surgery. New York: Elsevier, 1991.

136. Essien FB, Maderious A. A genetic factor controlling morphogenesis of the laryngo-esophageal complex in the mouse. Teratology 1981;24:235–239.

137. Lister J. The blood supply of the eosophagus in relation to oesophageal atresia. Arch Dis Child 1964;39:131–137.

138. Skandalakis JE, Gray SW, Skandalakis LJ. Surgical anatomy of the eosophagus. In: Surgery of the oesophagus. Edinburgh: Churchill Livingston, 1988.

139. Orringer MB. Complications of esophageal surgery and trauma. In: Greenfield LJ, ed. Complications in surgery and trauma. Philadelphia: JB Lippincott, 1984.

140. Kirwan WO, Walfaum PR, McCormack RJM. Cystic infrathoracic derivatives of the foregut and their complications. Thorax 1972;28:424–428.

141. Raffensperger JG. Congenital malformations of the lung. In: Raffensperger JG, ed. Swenson's pediatric surgery. Norwalk, CT: Appleton & Lang, 1990:743.

142. Schechter DC. Congenital absence of deficiency of lung tissue: the congenital subtractive broncho-pneumonic malformations. Ann Thorac Surg 1968;6:286–313.

143. Wexels P. Agenesis of the lung. Thorax 1951;6:171–192.

144. Morgani JB. The seats and causes of disease investigated by anatomy (transl). New York: Hafner, 1960.

145. Torriello HV, Bauserman SC. Bilateral pulmonary agenesis. Am J Med Genet 1985;21:93.

146. Huizinga E, van Weering IF. Bronchography in agenesis and hypoplasia of the lung. Ann Otol 1964;73:26–33.

147. Thomas LB, Boyden EA. Agenesis of the right lung: report of three cases. Surgery 1952;31:429–435.

148. Smart J. Complete congenital agenesis of a lung. Q J Med 1946;15:125–140.

149. Field CE. Pulmonary agenesis and hypoplasia. Arch Dis Child 1946;21:61–75.

150. Stocker JT. Congenital and developmental diseases. In: Dail DH, Hammer SP, eds. Pulmonary pathology. New York: Springer-Verlag, 1988.

151. Hepburn D. Note on a right lung which resembled a left lung in presenting only apical and basal lobes. J Anat 1925;59:326–327.

152. Feofilov GL. Hypoplasia of the lungs. Khirurgiia 1968;44:74–78.

153. Markowitz RI et al. Single, mediastinal, unilobar lung: a rare form of subtotal pulmonary agenesis. Pediatr Radiol 1987;17:2669.

154. Paul F. Fehlbildungen im bereiche der atmungsoragane. Virchow Arch [A] 1928;267:295–317.

155. Garside VOB. Agenesis of the lung. Br J Radiol 1943;16:69–71.

156. Fost WH, Lilien BB. Congenital aplasia of the lung: a report of two cases. J Newark Beth Israel Hosp 1950;1:272–277.

157. Prouty LA, Myers TL. Olighydramnios sequence (Potter's syndrome). South Med J 1987;80:585.

158. Sbokos CG, McMillan IKR. Agenesis of the lung. Br J Dis Chest 1977;71:183.

159. Mardini MC, Nyhan WL. Agenesis of the lung: report of four patients with unusual anomalies. Chest 1985;87:522.

160. de Pozzi A. Miscellaneous curiosa medico-physico, dec 1, an 14, obs 30. Frankfort-Leipzig, 1673–1674.

161. Rivière L. In: Benetus T: Sepulchretum, sive anatomia practica ex cadaveribus morbo denatis, hib III, Sect XVIII. Genevae, 1679.

162. Haberlein C. Case cited in: [Anon]. Abhandlungen von einigen widernatürlichen Bildungen des Herzens und seiner allernächsten Gefässe (Geschichte einer widernatürlichen Beschaffenheit und Lage der Brusteigneweide, und einer ganz eigenen Structur der Herzgefässe. "Unser erster fall." Abhandl römiach. KK josephlinischen medicine-chirug Academie zu Wien 1787? (1788).

163. Gilkey HM. Congenital absence of lung: report of a case. J Missouri Med Assoc 1928;25:296–297.

164. Hurwitz S, Stephens HB. Agenesis of the lung: a review of the literature and report of a case. Am J Med Sci 1937;193:81.

165. Valle AR. Agenesis of the lung. Am J Surg 1955;89:90–100.

166. Young F. Agenesis of the right lung in each of identical twins. Arizona Med 1948;5:48.

167. Maltz DL, Nadas AS. Agenesis of the lung: presentation of eight new cases and review of the literature. Pediatrics 1968;42:175.

168. Wigglesworth JS, Desai R, Guerrini P. Fetal lung hypoplasia: biochemical and structural variations and their possible significance. Arch Dis Child 1981;56:606.

169. Reale FR, Esterly JR. Pulmonary hypoplasia: a morphometric study of the lungs of infants with diaphragmatic hernia, anencephaly and renal malformations. Pediatrics 1973;51:91.

170. Bariéty M, Choubrac P. Intérêt et l'angio-pneumographie dans l'agénésie pulmonaire. Acta Chir Belg 1960;59:171–177.

171. Wohl ME et al. The lung following repair of congenital diaphragmatic hernia. J Pediatr 1977;90(3):405–414.

172. Schaffer AJ. Diseases of the newborn. Philadelphia: WB Saunders, 1960.

173. Boyden EA. Developmental anomalies of the lungs. Am J Surg 1955;89:79–89.

174. Sotile SC, Brady MB, Brogdon BG. Accessory cardiac bronchus: demonstration by computed tomography. J Comput Tomogr 1988;12(2):144–146.

175. Finck S, Milne EN. A case report of segmental bronchial atresia: radiologic evaluation including computed tomography and magnetic resonance imaging. J Thorac Imag 1988;3(1):53–57.

176. Jederlinic PJ, Sicilian LS, Baigelman W, Gaensler EA. Congenital bronchial atresia: a report of 4 cases and review of the literature. Medicine 1987;66(1):73–83.

177. Evans JA. Aberrant bronchi and cardiovascular anomalies. Am J Med Genet 1990;35(1):46–54.

178. Dévé MF. Les lobes surnuméraires du poumon: le lobe posterieur—le lobe cardiaque. Bull Mem Soc Anat (Paris) 1900;75:341.

179. Kent EM, Blades B. The surgical anatomy of the pulmonary lobes. J. Thorac Surg 1942;12:18–30.

180. Wrisberg HA. Observationes anatomicae de vena azyga duplici asiisque hujus venae varietatibus. Novis Comment Soc Reg Scient Gottingen 1777;8:14.

181. Stibbe EP. The accessory pulmonary lobe of vena azygo. J Anat 1919;53:305–314.

182. Etter LE. Variations in the position of the azygos septum and its incidence in fifty thousand roentgen examinations. AJR 1947;58:726–729.

183. Clive FT. Mass radiograph in women: review of 30,000 examinations in WAAF recruits. Tubercle 1943;24:63–67.

184. Krasovskii VV, Protopopov AN, Toropko IV. [Developmental anomalies of the lungs in children.] Vop Okhr Materin Dets 1967;12:11–14.

185. Herxheimer G. Ueber einen Fall von echter Neben lunge. Zentralbl Allg Pathol 1901;12:529–532.

186. Duval JM, Dubois de Montreynaud JM, Lefaucher C. A propos d'un cas de bronche trachéale documents bronchographiques et cliné-endoscopiques. C R Assoc Anat 1966;135:358–363.

187. Chofnas I. Tracheal lobe of the right lung. Am Rev Respir Dis 1963;87:280–283.

188. Kohlhardt M, Heinemann G, Friederiszick F. Nebenlungen als Mediastinal-zysten. Med Welt 1962;50:2688–2690.

189. Gruenfeld GE, Gray SH. Malformations of the lung. Arch Pathol 1941;31:392–397.

190. Bremer JL. Accessory bronchi in embryos: thier occurrence and probable fate. Anat Rec 1932;54:361–364.

191. Le Roux BT. Anatomical abnormalities of the right upper bronchus. J Thorac Cardiovasc Surg 1962;44:225.

192. Brownless RT, Dafoe CS. Complete reduplication of the right lung. J Thorac Cardiovasc Surg 1968;55:653–656.

193. Brandt HM, Liebow AA. Right pulmonary isomerism associated with venous, splenic, and other anomalies. Lab Invest 1958;7:469–504.

194. Anderson C, Devine WA, Anderson RH, Debich DE, Zuberbuhler JR. Abnormalities of the spleen in relation to congenital malformations of the heart: a survey of necropsy findings in children. Br Heart J 1990;63(2):122–128.

195. Stibbe EP. True congenital diverticulum of the trachea in a subject showing also right aortic arch. J Anat 1929;64:62–66.

196. Brosnan ML. Report of a case of double trachea. J Laryngol 1959;73:853–855.

197. Blackader AD, Evans DJ. A case of mediastinal cyst producing compression of the trachea ending fatally in an infant of nine months. Arch Pediatr 1911;28:194.

198. Maier HC. Bronchogenic cysts of the mediastinum. Ann Surg 1948;127:476–502.

199. Hare HA. The pathology, clinical history and diagnosis of affections of the mediastinum other than those of the heart and aorta. Philadelphia: P Bakiston's Son, 1899.

200. Lyons HA, Calvy GL, Sammona BP. The diagnosis and classification of mediastinal masses. I. A study of 782 cases. Ann Int Med 1959;51:897–932.

201. Opsahl T, Berman EJ. Bronchiogenic mediastinal cysts in infants: case report and review of the literature. Pediatrics 1962;30:372–377.

202. Grafe WR, Goldsmith EI, Redo SF. Bronchogenic cysts of the mediastinum in children. J Pediatr Surg 1966;1:384–393.

203. Rodgers BM, Moazam F, Talbert JL. Bronchopulmonary foregut malformations. Ann Surg 1986;203:517.

204. Brasch RC, Gooding CA, Lallemand DP, Wesbey GE. Magnetic resonance imaging of the thorax in childhood. Radiology 1984;150:463.

205. Nössen H. Tod unter dem Bilde, der Lungenembolie durch Zyste im Perikard. Deutsch Med Wschr 1925;51:1150.

206. Pierce EC II, Manion WC, Dabbs CH. Intrapericardial bronchiogenic cyst: embryological and gross anatomical aspects. Anat Rec 1957;127:347.

207. Rusby NL, Sellors TH. Congenital deficiency of the pericardium associated with a bronchogenic cyst. Br J Surg 1945;32:357.

208. Seybold WD, Clagett OT. Presternal cysts: report of a case. J Thorac Surg 1945;14:217–220.

209. Park OK, Buford CH. Bronchogenic cyst of neck and superior mediastinum. Ann Surg 1955;142:130–133.

210. Rubio C, Hayashi T, Stemmermann G. Ciliated gastric cells. A study of their phenotypic characteristics. Mod Pathol 1990;3(6):720–723.

211. May RK, Meese EH, Timmes JJ. Congenital lobar emphysema: case report of bilateral involvement. J Thorac Cardiovasc Surg 1964;48:850–854.

212. Stovin PGI. Congenital lobar emphysema. Thorax 1959;14:254–266.

213. Keith HH. Congenital lobar emphysema. Pediatr Ann 1977;6(7):34–41.

214. Miller CG, Woo-Ming MO, Carpenter RA. Lobar emphysema of infancy: case report of bilateral involvement with congenital heart disease. West Indian Med J 1968;17:35.

215. Carter D, Bibro MC, Touloukian RJ. Benign clinical behavior of immature mediastinal teratoma in infancy and childhood: report of two cases and review of the literature. Cancer 1982;49:398–402.

216. Sealy WC, Weaver WL, Young WG Jr. Severe airway obstruction in infancy due to the thymus gland. Ann Thorac Surg 1965;1:389–402.

217. Sieger L et al. Acute thymic hemorrhage. Am J Dis Child 1974;128:86–87.

218. Warner JO, Rubin S, Heard BE. Congenital lobar emphysema: a case with bronchial atresia and abnormal bronchial cartilages. Br J Dis Chest 1982;76(2):177–184.

219. Royes K. Localized hypertrophic emphysema. Br Med J 1938;2:659.

220. Overstreet RM. Emphysema in a portion of the lung in the early months of life. Am J Dis Child 1939;57:861.

221. Fischer CC, Tropea F, Bailey CP. Congenital pulmonary cysts: report of an infant treated by lobectomy with recover. J Pediatr 1943;23:219.

222. Reid JM, Barclay RS, Stevenson JG, Welsh TM. Congenital obstructive lobar emphysema. Dis Chest 1966;49:359–361.

223. Salomon JS, Levy MJ. Segmental emphysema of lung: congenital. Dis Chest 1966;49:214–216.

224. Staple TW, Hudson HH, Hartmann AT, McAlister WH. The angiographic findings in four cases of infantile lobar emphysema. AJR 1966;97:195–202.

225. Remy J, Smith M, Mararche P, Nuyts JP. La bronche "tracheale" gauche pathogene: revue de la litterature a propos de 4 observations. J Radiol Electrol Med Nucl 1977;58:621–630.

226. Eigen H, Lemen RJ, Waring WW. Congenital lobar emphysema: long-term evaluation of surgically and conservatively treated children. Am Rev Respir Dis 1976;113:823.

227. Stovin PGI. Early lung development. Thorax 1985;40:401–404.

228. Chavrier YPM. Intrapulmonary lesions. In: Fallis JC, Filler RM, Lemoine G, eds. Pediatric thoracic surgery. New York: Elsevier, 1991.

229. DeLarue J, Paillas J, Abelanet R, Chomette G: Les broncho-pneumopathies congénitales. Bronches 1959, 9:114–211.

230. Keohane ME, Schwartz I, Freed J, Dische R. Subdiaphragmatic bronchogenic cyst with communication to the stomach: a case report. Hum Pathol 1988;19(7):868–71.

231. Rogers LF, Osmer JC. Bronchogenic cyst: a review of 46 cases. AJR 1964;91:273–283.

232. Willis FES, Almeyda J. Cystic disease of the lung (bronchoalveolar cysts). Tubercle 1943;24:27–36, 43–58.

233. Grawitz P. Ueber Angeborne Bronchiectasie. Virchow Arch [A] 1880;82:217–237.

234. Pierce CB. Cystic disease of the lung. AJR 1940;44:848–852.

235. Conway DJ. The origin of lung cysts in childhood. Arch Dis Child 1951;26:504–529.

236. Caffey J. On the natural regression of pulmonary cysts during early infancy. Pediatrics 1953;11:48–64.

237. Guest JL Jr, Yeh TJ, Ellison LT, Ellison RG. Pulmonary parenchymal air space abnormalities. Am Thorac Surg 1965;1:102.

238. Koontz AR. Congenital cysts of the lung. Bull Johns Hopkins Hosp 1925;37:340–361.

239. Franchel F, Pesle G, Chevallier A, Rochainzamir A. Exist-t-il des kystesbronchogéniques congénitaux intrapulmonaires? Rev Tuberc (Paris) 1962;26:949–959.

240. Bartholinus T. Malpighii opera omnia, Vol 2. Leyden, 1687.

241. Meyer H. Ueber angeborene blasige Missbildung der Lungen, nebst einigen Bemerkungen über Cyanose aus Lungenleiden. Virchow Arch [A] 1859;16:78–94.

242. Schenck SG. Congenital cystic disease of the lungs. AJR 1936;35:604–629.

243. Cooke FN, Blades B. Cystic disease of the lungs. J Throac Surg 1952;23:546–569.

244. Moffat AD. Congenital cystic disease of the lungs and its classification. J Pathol Bact 1960;79:361–372.

245. Lenk R. Das charakteristische Röntgenbild der offenen Wabenlunge. Fortschr Geb Rontgenstrehlen 1933;48:418–426.

246. Ramenofsky ML, Leape LL, McCauley RGK. Bronchogenic cyst. J Pediatr Surg 1979;14:219.

247. Putnam CE, Goodwin JD, Silverman PM, Foster WL. CT of localized lucent lung lesions. Semin Roengenol 1984;19:173.

248. Read CA, Moront M, Carangelo R, Holt RW, Richardson M. Recurrent bronchogenic cyst: an argument for complete surgical excision. Arch Surg 1991;126:1306–1308.

249. Miller DC, Walter JP, Guthaner DF, Mark JBD: Recurrent mediastinal bronchogenic cyst: cause of bronchial obstruction and compression of superior vena cava and pulmonary artery. Chest 1978;74:218–220.

250. Mack RM, Stevenson JK, Graham CB. Gigantic solitary congenital cysts of the lung in a nine-year-old boy: case report. Am Surg 1966;32:549–556.

251. Boyden EA. Bronchogenic cysts and the theory of intralobar sequestration: new embryologic data. J Thorac Surg 1958;35:604.

252. Virchow R. Gesammelte Abhandlungen zur wissenschaftliche Medicin. Frankfort: Meidinges John, 1856.

253. Laurence KM. Congenital pulmonary lymphangiectasis. J Clin Pathol 1959;12:62–69.

254. Frank J, Piper PG. Congenital pulmonary cystic lymphangiectasis. JAMA 1959;171:1094–1098.

255. Chin KY, Tang MY. Congenital adenomatoid malformation of one lobe of a lung with general anasarca. Arch Pathol 1949;48:221–229.

256. Goodyear JE, Shillitoe AJ. Adenomatoid hamartoma of the lung in a newborn infant. J Clin Pathol 1959;12:172–174.

257. Bain GO. Congenital adenomatoid malformation of the lung. Dis Chest 1959;36:430–433.

258. Stoerk O. Ueber angeborene blasige Missbildungen der Lunge. Wien Klin Wschr 1897;10:25.

259. Graham GG, Singleton JW. Diffuse hamartoma of the upper lobe in an infant. Am J Dis Child 1955;89:609–611.

260. Stocker JT, Madewell JE, Drake RM. Congenital cystic adenomatoid malformation of the lung. Hum Pathol 1977;8:155.

261. Neilson IR et al. Congenital adenomatoid malformation of the lung: current management and prognosis. J Pediatr Surg 1991;26:975–981.

262. Rosado de Christenson ML, Stocker JT. Congenital cystic adenomatoid malformation. Radiographics 1991;11:865–886.

263. MacMahon HE. Congenital alveolar dysplasia. Pediatrics 1948;2:43–57.

264. Berba AM, Eitzen O. Congenital alveolar dysplasia. Ohio Med J 1961;57:792–793.

265. Miller RW, Woo P, Kellman RK, Slagle TS. Tracheobronchial abnormalities in infants with bronchopulmonary dysplasia. J Pediatr 1987;111:779.

266. Bailey PV et al. Congenital bronchopulmonary malformations: diagnostic and therapeutic considerations. J Thorac Cardiovasc Surg 1990;99:597–603.

267. Andersen EA, Hertel J, Petersen SA, Sorensen HR. Congenital chylothorax: management by ligature of the thoracic duct. Scand J Thorac Cardiovasc Surg 1984;18:193–194.

268. Stewart CA, Linner HP. Chylothorax in the newborn infant. Am J Dis Child 1926;31:654–656.

269. Depp DA, Atherton SO, McGough EC. Spontaneous neonatal pleural effusion. J Pediatr Surg 1974;9:809–812.

270. DeFoort P, Thiery M. Antenatal diagnosis of congenital chylothorax by gray scale sonography. J Clin Ultrasound 1978;6:47–48.

271. Jaffa AJ, Barak S, Kaysar N, Peyser MR. Antenatal diagnosis of bilateral congenital chylothorax with pericardial effusion. Acta Obstet Gynecol Scand 1985;64:455–456.

272. Azizkhan RG, Canfield J, Alford BA, Rodgers BM. Pleuroperitoneal shunts in the management of neonatal chylothorax. J Pediatr Surg 1983;18:842–850.

273. Khoury MJ et al. A population study of the VACTERL association: evidence for its etiologic heterogeneity. Pediatrics 1983;71:815–820.

274. Lubinsky M. Invited editorial comment: associations in clinical genetics with a comment on the paper by Evans JA et al. on tracheal agenesis. Am J Med Genet 1985;21:35–38.

CHAPTER 14

PULMONARY CIRCULATION

John Elias Skandalakis / Stephen Wood Gray / Panagiotis Symbas

*The neonatal pulmonary circulation is an ephemeral phase in the dramatic
metamorphosis of the pulmonary circulation that takes place during the passage
from fetal to adult life.*
—*WALKER A. LONG (1990)*
FETAL AND NEONATAL CARDIOLOGY, W. B. SAUNDERS

DEVELOPMENT

Development of the Pulmonary Arteries

Our understanding of the development of the pulmonary
arteries owes much to the work of Federow (1) and Bremer (2), who established the basic pattern from rabbit and
guinea pig embryos. Congdon (3) in 1922 confirmed their
work and elaborated the details in the human. A number
of more recent workers have refined the earlier studies
and added new information.

The earliest primordium of the pulmonary circulation
appears as a capillary net extending caudad from the aortic sac at the 4-mm stage (stage 13). The net grows
between the pharyngeal floor and the pericardium and
along the ventral and lateral surfaces of the tracheal outgrowth from the pharynx. From the dorsal aorta, a similar
capillary net develops over the future esophageal portion
of the foregut. These two nets fuse to form the vascular
plexus of the foregut and will eventually separate again
into pulmonary and esophageal portions.

The ventral plexus from the aortic sac develops two
main channels, which become the primitive pulmonary
arteries. By the 5.5-mm stage (stage 14), they are joined
by buds growing ventrad from the dorsal aorta (Fig.
14.1). These channels are the sixth pair of aortic arches.
Proximal to the junction with the sixth arch, the primitive
pulmonary artery is usually considered to be the proximal
(ventral) sixth arch although this terminology could be
questioned.

In the sixth week, symmetric sixth arches exist, which
are divided into proximal (ventral) and distal (dorsal) segments at the junction with the pulmonary arteries (Figure
14.2). The right distal segment disappears in the seventh
week (13 mm). If it persists (in anomalous cases), it is the
right ductus arteriosus when patent, or the right ligamentum arteriosum when fibrotic.

The proximal segments of the sixth arch arise as primitive pulmonary arteries from the aortic sac. At first as lateral branches from the sac, they subsequently migrate
over the dorsal surface of the sac until they fuse into a
single orifice arising from the upper portion of the truncus arteriosus (the aortic sac) on the left dorsolateral
aspect. This asymmetry results in the formation of the
definitive pulmonary arteries. The final result is that the
left proximal sixth arch becomes absorbed to form
the bifurcation of the pulmonary arteries, the left distal
portion becomes the ductus arteriosus, and the left pulmonary artery corresponds to the primitive pulmonary
artery distal to the arch. On the right the adult pulmonary
artery is composed of the right proximal sixth arch and
the primitive pulmonary arterial trunk (3). Anderson and
his colleagues (4) postulated that the asymmetry of the
blood flow in the fourth arch, which results in the formation of the normal definitive aorta on the left, causes
the regression of the right distal 6th arch and hence
determines the asymmetry of the pulmonary arteries. Figure 14.3 shows the derivation of the definitive pulmonary
arteries.

In summary: (a) The main pulmonary artery is formed
by fusion of the two sixth arches and by small participation of the aortic sac; (b) the left pulmonary artery is
developed from angioblasts which are not related to the
artery; (c) the right pulmonary artery is formed by the
proximal part of the right sixth arch; and (d) the left ductus arteriosus (the right disappears between the sixth and
seventh week together with the right aorta) is the product
of the left dorsal portion of persistent distal sixth arch.

Separation of the truncus arteriosus by the aorticopulmonary septum into pulmonary and arterial trunks
during the second month is discussed elsewhere in this
book.

Unlike most arteries of the body, which grow slowly in
size as functional demands on them increase, the pulmonary arteries receive a sudden increased load at birth. The
lumen of the artery is small compared with the thickness
of its wall at birth, but with age the relative size of the
lumen increases. Dammann et al. (5) plotted the change
from birth to maturity (Fig. 14.4). A number of studies of

these changes have been made (6–8), and the authors of the reports are in essential agreement. The arteries are thus constricted by their architecture and, according to Thomas (8), partly by chronic vasoconstriction. Persis-

tence of this fetal constriction can lead to primary pulmonary hypertension. Premature dilation can result in pulmonary edema and heart failure.

The interested reader will find useful information about developmental pulmonary circulatory physiology in Chapter 7 of *Fetal and Neonatal Cardiology* by Walker A. Long (9), who mentioned the following points:

1. The definite role of oxygen levels and pH in pulmonary vascular tone
2. The role of alveolar hypoxia as vasoconstrictor
3. The role of resistance of blood flow in a certain vessel in health and disease in association with pulmonary vasoconstriction, which may influence pulmonary vascular resistance, especially during the neonatal period when the pulmonary vessels are small
4. That the premature pulmonary circulation is unknown, a terra incognita
5. The need for more studies to understand pulmonary vasoconstriction and vasodilation

Campbell et al. (10) in 1980 reported aberrant left pulmonary artery (pulmonary sling) arising from the right and coursing behind the trachea and anterior to the esophagus. The origin of one pulmonary artery from the ascending aorta was documented by Fong et al. (11) in 1989. Unilateral absence of the pulmonary artery was reported by Werber et al. (12)

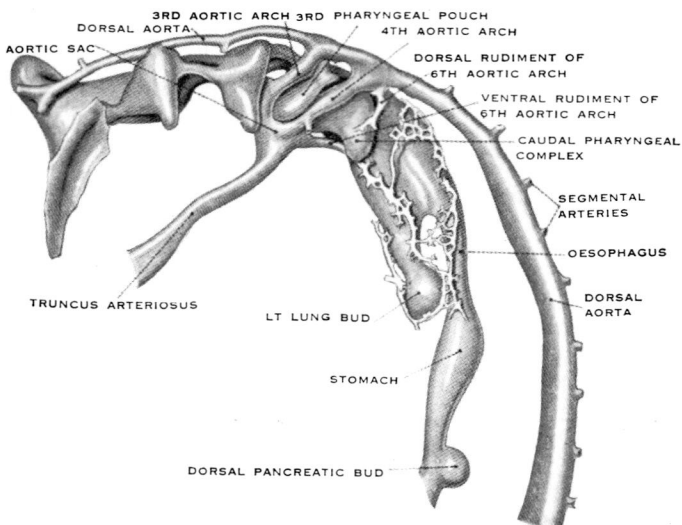

Figure 14.1. Reconstruction of the foregut and the bronchial arteries of a 5-mm human embryo. The sixth aortic arch is not yet complete and definitive pulmonary arteries are not yet established. (From Hamilton WJ, Mossman HW. Human embryology, 4th ed. Baltimore: Williams & Wilkins, 1972:265.)

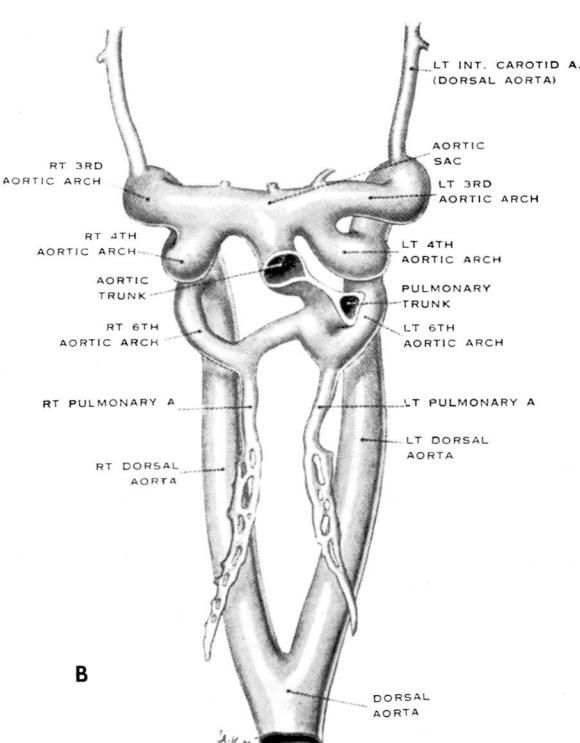

Figure 14.2. Reconstruction of the foregut and the bronchial arteries of an 11-mm human embryo. **A,** Lateral view. **B,** Ventral (anterior) view. The truncus arteriosus is divided into aortic and pulmonary trunks, the sixth arches are com- plete, and the pulmonary arteries are present. The tracheopulmonary and esoph- ageal vasculatures are separated. (From Hamilton WJ, Mossman HW. Human embryology, 4th ed. Baltimore: Williams & Wilkins, 1972:266–267.

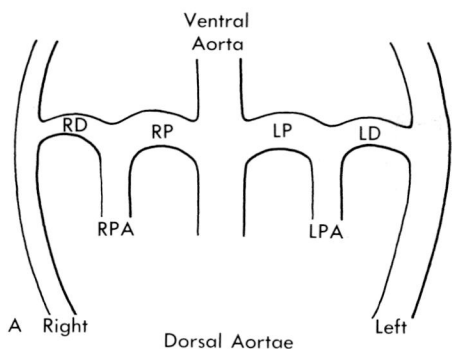

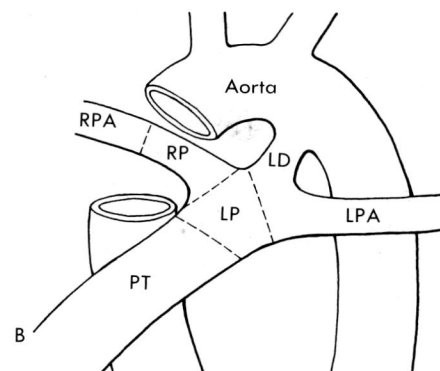

Figure 14.3. Diagram of the embryonic sixth arches (**A**) and schema showing their contribution to the adult pulmonary arteries (**B**). The right distal sixth arch (*RD*) and the right dorsal aorta completely disappear before birth. The left distal sixth arch (*LD*) is the ductus arteriosus, which will disappear after birth. *RD* and *LD*, Right and left distal sixth arch; *RP* and *LP*, right and left proximal sixth arch; *RPA* and *LPA*, right and left pulmonary arteries; *PT*, pulmonary trunk.

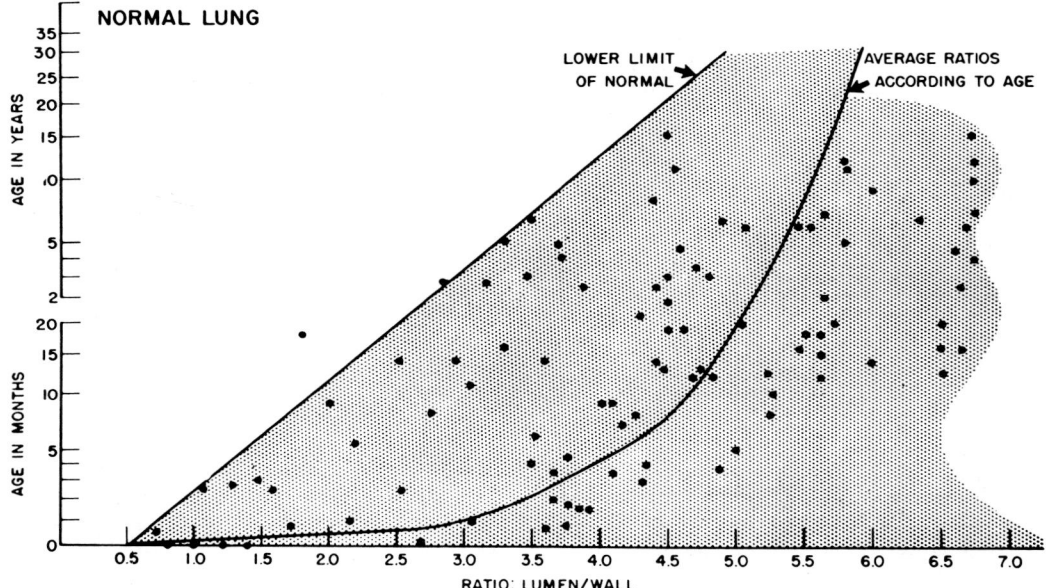

Figure 14.4. Graph of the ratio of lumen size and wall thickness in small muscular pulmonary arteries in normal patients of varying ages. Note the relative increase in lumen size and the decrease in wall thickness occurring with age. (From Dammann JF Jr, Thompson WM, Sosa O, Christlieb I. Anatomy, physiology and natural history of simple ventricular septal defects. Am J Cardiol 1960;5:136.)

Gikonyo et al. (13) in 1989 reported 130 cases (7 of their own) of pulmonary vascular sling (60% males; 40% females). Ninety percent of the cases were diagnosed during the first year of life. The diagnosis was done by esophagogram in most of the cases. Tracheobronchial anomalies were found in 40% of 68 autopsy cases.

Development of the Pulmonary Veins

In a classic paper Flint (14) described the development of the pulmonary veins in the embryo pig. However, he left a number of problems unsettled. Federow (1) described the outgrowth of vessels from the heart but believed they gave rise to the whole pulmonary venous system. Brown (15), taking a contrary view, thought the forward growth of the lungs brought the foregut venous plexus into contact with the heart. The subsequent work of Auër (16), Butler (17), and Neill (18) has shown that the growing pulmonary vein makes contact with the already established foregut plexus.

In the fourth week (2.5 to 3 mm), the primordium of the common pulmonary vein appears as a solid outgrowth from the sinoatrial region of the heart, projecting craniad into the dorsal mesocardium (17). At this stage two transitory, caudad evaginations appear, which Auër (16) suggested might in some cases form anomalous pulmonary

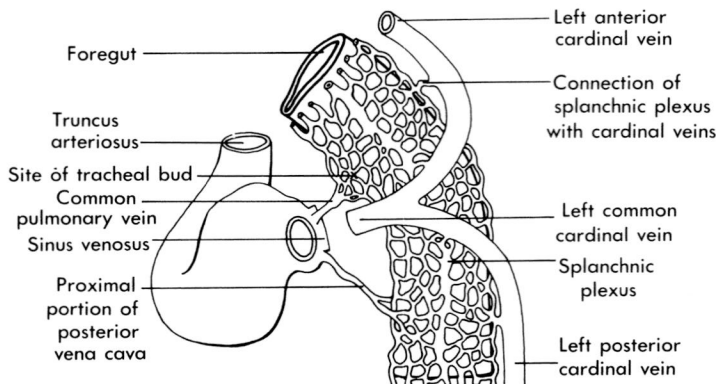

Figure 14.5. The foregut (splanchnic) plexus and its vascular connections in a 4.5-mm cat embryo. The tracheal bud is not evident on the ventral surface of the foregut, but the common pulmonary vein has grown out of the sinoatrial region of the heart and has tapped the vascular plexus, which was previously drained only by the cardinal veins. (After Brown AJ. The development of the pulmonary veins in the domestic cat. Anat Rec 1913;7:299–329.)

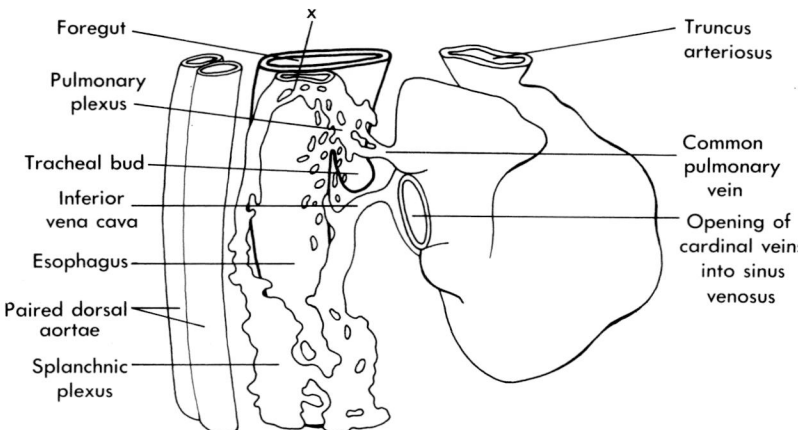

Figure 14.6. The foergut plexus and its vascular connections in a 5.18-mm cat embryo. The tracheal bud is present, and the foregut plexus is dividing into (a) a dorsal (splanchnic) plexus of the esophagus that drains into the cardinal veins (removed in this figure) and into the developing posterior vena cava, and (b) a ventral (pulmonary) plexus that is drained only by the pulmonary veins. The area in which the two plexuses are still joined is marked by X. (After Brown AJ. The development of the pulmonary veins in the domestic cat. Anat Rec 1913;7:299–329.)

veins if they persisted long enough to connect with the foregut plexus. By the 6- to 7-mm stage (stage 14), the cranial stem has become patent and has joined the plexus just caudal to the bifurcation of the lung buds. Its cardiac opening now lies on the atrium to the left of the septum primum (Figs. 14.5 and 14.6).

The foregut plexus at this stage drains into both anterior and posterior cardinal veins and is continuous with the gastric plexus, which drains into the portal vein (17). The venae comitantes of the vagus nerve are remnants of the connections between dorsal (esophageal) and ventral (pulmonary) portions of the primitive foregut plexus (19). These anastomotic connections are of little importance in the normal circulation, but they may become sites of anomalous pulmonary drainage.

The common pulmonary vein normally divides into left and right branches, which immediately divide again. The growing left atrium encroaches on the proximal end of the common pulmonary vein and eventually absorbs into the atrial wall not only the common vein but also the proximal portions of its branches, resulting in four pulmonary veins with separate atrial orifices. This is accomplished by the 25-mm stage (stage 20) (Fig. 14.7, B and C).

Remember that (a) angioblasts around the bronchi and lungs are responsible for the genesis of the pulmonary veins; (b) the common pulmonary vein is an outgrowth of the left atrium from its superior wall (18); and (c) later, the common pulmonary vein is absorbed and in the process produces the two pulmonary veins which enter the atrium by further subdivision.

Development of the Bronchial Arteries and Veins

Although the bronchial arteries and veins in the normal adult clearly belong to the systemic circulation, in many anomalies of the pulmonary circulation, they become

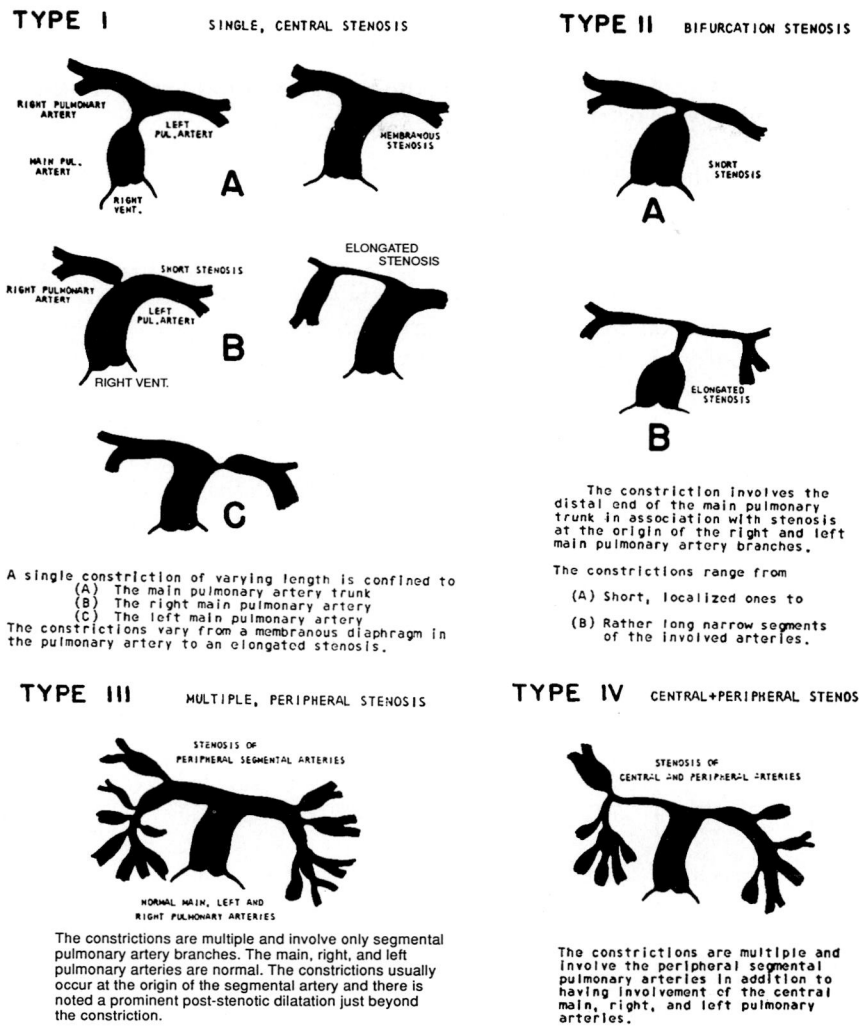

Figure 14.7. Varieties of coarctation of the pulmonary arteries and their branches. (From Gay BB, Franch RH, Shuford WH, Rogers JV. The roentgenologic features of single and multiple coarctations of the pulmonary artery and branches. AJR 1963;90:599–613.)

"pulmonized" and serve as the major vascular supply to the lungs.

This system develops very late, approximately between the 20 to 32 weeks, forming precapillary anastomoses with the arterioles of the pulmonary circulation. Most likely, however, these anastomoses do not survive too long. According to Wagenvoort et al. (7) they may be observed early in 2-year-old children.

The bronchial arteries, together with the esophageal arteries, are the remnants of the originally segmental arterial supply from the aorta to the foregut plexus, which includes vessels of the esophagus, trachea, and lung buds (15, 20). At the level of the main bronchi, they anastomose with each other across the midline. Bronchial arteries usually contribute branches to the esophagus, and these esophageal arteries send small branches into the pulmonary ligament. These vessels anastomose with

the pulmonary artery from the sixth arch during the fifth week.

Similarly, the even smaller bronchial veins represent the primitive drainage of the foregut plexus into the subcardinal veins (azygos or hemiazygos system), segmental intercostal veins, or (on the right) into the inferior or superior vena cava (21). Slavochinskaya (22) described the details of the fetal bronchial circulation.

Critical Events in the Development of the Pulmonary Vascular Supply

The separation of the embryonic foregut into a dorsal alimentary tube and a ventral respiratory tube is a hazardous step in organogenesis. Not only do the endodermal structures have to divide successfully (see Chapter 3, "The Esophagus," and Chapter 13, "The Trachea and

Lungs''), but the vascular plexus surrounding the foregut also must separate, and the two portions must acquire separate connections with the heart. Failure of correct closure of certain vascular channels and persistence of others produce anomalies that have small effect on the fetus but which may kill or handicap the newborn infant.

The fact that an infant may live with a normal blood supply to only one lung or with only half of the pulmonary drainage entering the right heart gives the vascular surgeon an especially good opportunity to correct the defects and restore the patient to a normal life.

The galaxy of symptoms and syndromes of pulmonary artery and vein anomalies are many. We present only a few of them as examples. The interested reader will find beautiful material in the work of Askin (23), Katzenstein and Askin (24), Dehner (25), and several others. Since we used their work extensively, we want not only to recommend their books but also to express appreciation to them for making our job less difficult.

ANOMALIES OF THE VASCULAR SUPPLY TO THE LUNGS (TABLE 14.1 AND FIG. 14.8)

Anomalous Arterial Supply to the Lungs

CLASSIFICATION

Two sets of arteries, the pulmonary arteries arising from the pulmonary trunk and the bronchial arteries arising from the descending aorta, normally supply the lungs with blood. Anomalies of this arterial pattern are uncommon, but they are unusually diverse. However bizarre the arrangement, an anomaly rarely affects the well-being of the fetus, which is not dependent on its lungs for oxygen.

Classification of these anomalies is difficult. The following groups are the most convenient to use:

A. *Aberrant Pulmonary Arteries* (Fig. 14.9). Tesler et al. (26) cited five cases of aberrant left pulmonary artery (vascular ring). Penkoske et al. (27) reported pulmonary artery branch originating from ascending aorta. These and

Table 14.1.
Anomalies of the Vascular Supply to the Lungs

Anomaly	Origin of Defect	First Appearance	Sex Chiefly Affected	Relative Frequency	Remarks
Aberrant pulmonary arteries					
I: Bilateral, persistent truncus arteriosus	Early week 5	At birth	Male	Rare	Usually fatal in infancy; ventricular septal defect common
II–IV: Unilateral, one artery with abnormal origin	Week 5	At birth	Equal	Rare	Affected lung is hypoplastic; tetralogy of Fallot and patent ductus arteriosus are usually associated
Absence of pulmonary artery					
Unilateral	Week 5	At birth	Equal	Rare	Affected lung is hypoplastic
Bilateral (pulmonized bronchial arteries)	Early week 5	At birth	Equal	Rare	Prognosis is better than in type I aberrant pulmonary arteries (persistent truncus arteriosus)
Intralobar sequestration of the lung	Unknown	At any period of life	Equal	Rare	Anomalous arterial supply usual
Extralobar sequestration of the lung (accessory lung)	Unknown	At any period of life	Equal	Rare	Predominantly left sided
Retrotracheal left pulmonary artery	Week 5	At birth	Male	Very rare	
Coarctation of the pulmonary artery	After mo 3	Childhood	Equal	Rare	Cardiac anomalies are common
Anomalous venous drainage of the lungs	Late week 5	Total anomalous drainage: at birth; 50% or more anomalous: in infancy; less than 50% anomalous: asymptomatic	Male	Uncommon	Cardiac anomalies are common
Right lung hypoplasia with anomalous vessels	Week 5	In childhood or never	Equal	Rare	Often asymptomatic
Pulmonary arteriovenous fistula	Pre- or postnatal	At any age	Equal	Rare	Familial

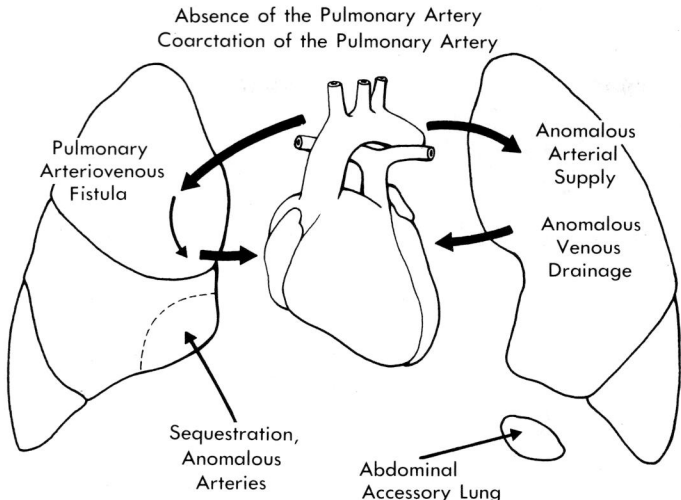

Absence of the Pulmonary Artery
Coarctation of the Pulmonary Artery

Pulmonary
Arteriovenous
Fistula

Anomalous
Arterial
Supply

Anomalous
Venous
Drainage

Sequestration,
Anomalous
Arteries

Abdominal
Accessory Lung

Figure 14.8. Anomalies of the vascular supply to the lungs.

other multiple vascular anomalies were noted by Berdon and Baker (28).

   I. No pulmonary trunk present; pulmonary arteries arise from the ascending aorta. This is one form of persistent truncus arteriosus (type I) (see Chapter 28, "The Thoracic and Abdominal Aorta").
   II. The pulmonary trunk leads to one pulmonary artery; the other arises from the ascending aorta.
   III. The pulmonary trunk leads to one pulmonary artery; the other arises from the innominate or subclavian artery.
   IV. The pulmonary trunk leads to one pulmonary artery; the other arises from a persistent ductus arteriosus.

B. *Absence of One or Both Pulmonary Arteries* (Figs. 14.9 and 14.10). Barbero-Marcial et al. (29) reported the absence of the pulmonary trunk and the central pulmonary artery. Presbitero et al. (30) reported absent or occult pulmonary artery. We agree with Askin (23) that this is an interruption of the proximal part of the pulmonary artery since the vascular tree of the parenchyma is intact.

   V. The pulmonary trunk leads to one pulmonary artery; the other lung is supplied by bronchial arteries from the descending aorta (unilateral absence of the pulmonary artery).
   VI. Neither pulmonary trunk nor pulmonary arteries are present; both lungs are supplied by bronchial arteries from the descending aorta (bilateral absence of the pulmonary arteries).

C. *Accessory Arteries to the Lungs* (Figs. 14.9 and 14.10).
   VII. Pulmonary trunk and arteries are normal or hypoplastic; accessory artery to one or both lungs arises from descending aorta. Accessory lobe or sequestered lung tissue may be present.

Loser et al. (31) and Kamio et al. (32) reported isolated stenosis of branches of the pulmonary artery. McCue et al. (33) found 20 cases of coarctation of the pulmonary artery and also reviewed 319 cases from the literature. Pernot et al. (34) noted stenosis of the pulmonary artery associated with skin discoloration.

Vascular resistance of the right lung secondary to anomalous origin of the right pulmonary artery from the ascending aorta was cited by Seki et al. (35). However, dysplasia of the ipsilateral lung was reported in three cases by Hislop et al. (36) in their paper on unilateral congenital dysplasia of the lung with vascular anomalies. Hypoplasia of the pulmonary arteries secondary to congenital rubella was reported by Taug et al. (37).

Goldstein et al. (38) noted a constellation of anomalies in an infant with hypoplastic pulmonary arterial branches, abnormal pulmonary venous connection, and both lungs receiving systemic arterial blood.

ANATOMY AND EMBRYOGENESIS

Type I. Both pulmonary arteries arise from the ascending aorta. The process of septation, which normally divides the truncus arteriosus into aortic and pulmonary channels, fails to take place. The pulmonary arteries may arise from the lateral walls of the aorta (persistent truncus arteriosus, type Ia; see Chapter 28, "The Thoracic and Abdominal Aorta"), or they may arise close together from the left dorsolateral side (persistent truncus arteriosus, type Ib). In both cases, developmental arrest occurred at the 4- to 6-mm stage (early fifth week) of development (3).

Type II. When only one pulmonary artery arises from the ascending aorta, it is on the right; the left artery is a continuation of the pulmonary trunk. The anomaly is reversed in the presence of a right aortic arch (39).

Normally, the right sixth arch "migrates" across the dorsal surface of the aorta to join the left sixth arch prior to septation of the pulmonoaortic truncus. Failure of this

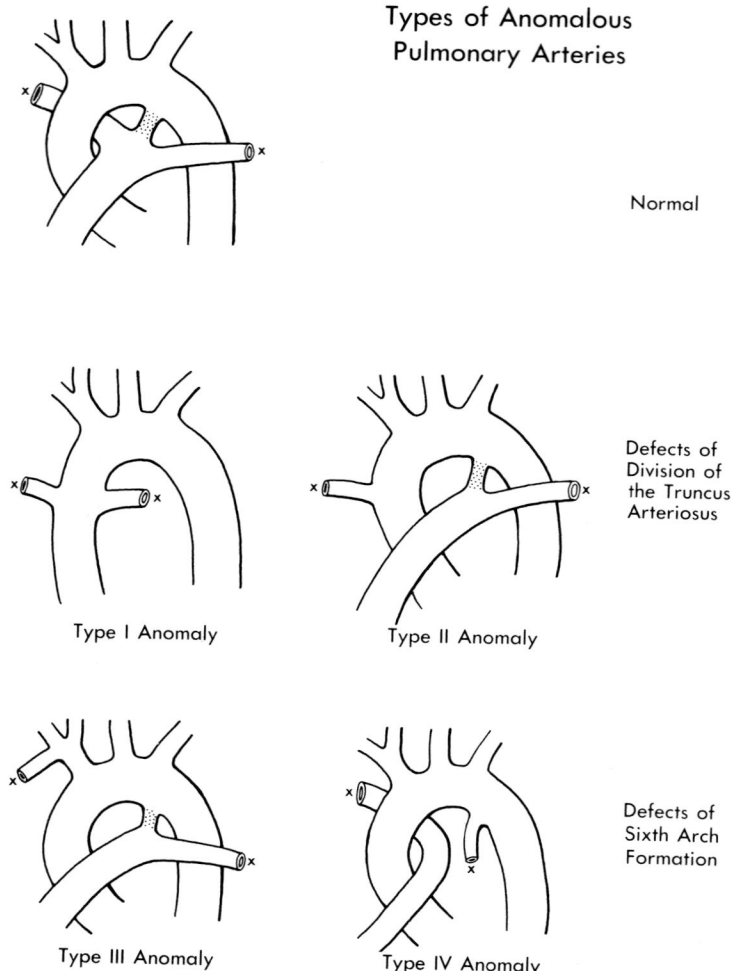

Figure 14.9.   Types of anomalous pulmonary arteries resulting from defective division of the primitive truncus arteriosus or from defects in formation of the sixth aortic arches. The pulmonary arteries are indicated by *x*.

migration to occur leaves the left arch on the pulmonary side of the septum and the right arch on the aortic side. This anomaly, like that of type I, arises early in the fifth week (40).

A single example of a left pulmonary artery arising from the ascending aorta and crossing in front of a normal right pulmonary artery has been reported (41). The aortic arch turned to the left (Fig. 14.11).

Anomalous origin of the right pulmonary artery from the ascending aorta was reported by Seki et al. (35).

Unilateral absence of the pulmonary artery in eight children was described by Werber et al. (12), seven in the right. In four of those patients, the anomaly was isolated without associated cardiac anomalies.

Anomalous origin of the pulmonary artery from the ascending aorta was reported by Fong et al. (11) in 1989.

Burrows et al. (42) wrote an illustrated, excellent article on the morphology and imaging of specific cardiovas-

cular anomalies that involve the pulmonary arteries. Anjos et al. (43) reported a case of tetralogy of Fallot with unusual blood supply to the left lung from the transverse aortic arch.

Type III. The right pulmonary artery arising from the innominate or right subclavian artery represents a persistent, distal, right sixth arch (right ductus arteriosus) with disappearance of the normally persistent proximal right sixth arch. This has been termed *proximal interruption of the pulmonary arch* by Anderson and his colleagues (4). This condition should be viewed in contradistinction to distal interruption, which normally takes place on the right early in fetal life and on the left after birth (obliteration of the ductus arteriosus).

A type III defect occurs on the left with a right aortic arch about as often as it occurs on the right (44, 45).

Type IV. In type III, the "absent" pulmonary artery is on the side opposite that of the descending aorta. In type

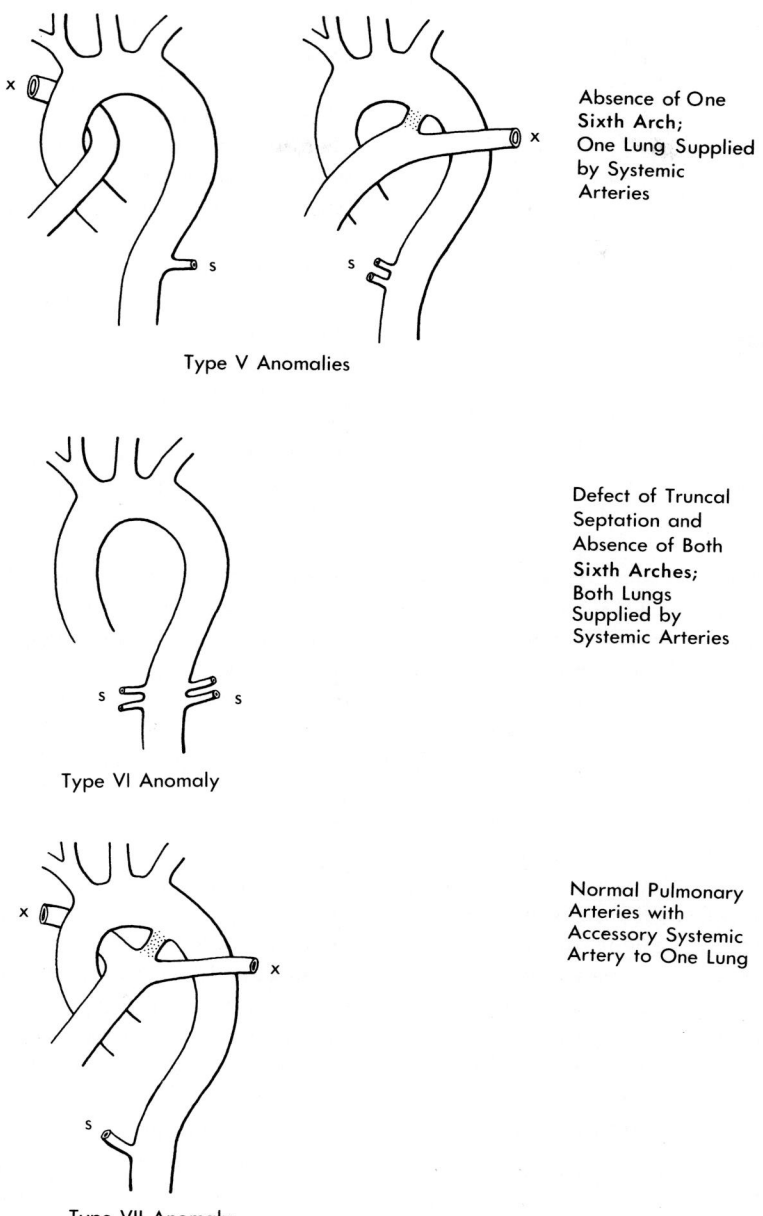

Type V Anomalies

Absence of One
Sixth Arch;
One Lung Supplied
by Systemic
Arteries

Type VI Anomaly

Defect of Truncal
Septation and
Absence of Both
Sixth Arches;
Both Lungs
Supplied by
Systemic Arteries

Type VII Anomaly

Normal Pulmonary
Arteries with
Accessory Systemic
Artery to One Lung

Figure 14.10. Types of anomalous pulmonary circulation with systemic arteries supplying one or both lungs. True pulmonary arteries are marked *x*, and systemic (bronchial) arteries, *s*.

IV, on the other hand, the left pulmonary artery arises from the left ductus arteriosus and a normal left aortic arch. Here, the proximal left sixth arch has disappeared, while the distal arch (ductus arteriosus) has persisted.

Type V. An absent right pulmonary artery implies absence of both proximal and distal portions of the sixth arch on the right. The lung receives blood from the enlarged bronchial arteries or from segmental arteries arising from the aorta above or below the diaphragm (46). The defect usually is associated with an otherwise normal

heart. A mirror image of this anomaly with a right aortic arch and an absent left pulmonary artery has been described (47). In this patient the left lung was hypoplastic.

An absent left pulmonary artery implies the absence of the left primitive pulmonary artery distal to the sixth arch as well as the distal portion of the arch itself. This is in contrast to type IV, in which the distal sixth arch (ductus arteriosus) persists. This defect almost always is associated with the tetralogy of Fallot and is rare.

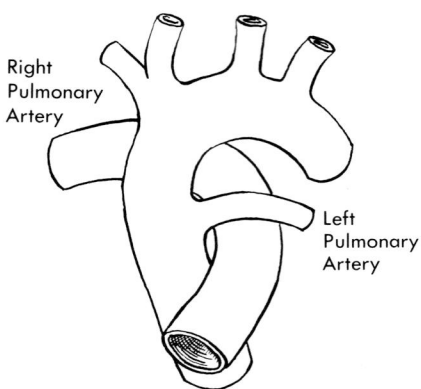

Figure 14.11. Type II anomaly in which the left, instead of the right, pulmonary artery arises from the ascending aorta. (From Stewart JR, Kincaid OW, Edwards JE. An atlas of vascular rings and related malformation of the aortic arch system. Springfield, IL: Charles C Thomas, 1964.)

Type VI. When both pulmonary arteries are absent and the lungs are served by bronchial arteries arising from the descending aorta, the truncus arteriosus remains undivided. Thus bilateral absence of the pulmonary arteries can be considered a form of persistent truncus arteriosus (48, 49) (see Chapter 28, "The Thoracic and Abdominal Aorta").

It is not apparent in the bilateral form whether the sixth arch failed to develop or whether secondary atresia occurred. The latter explanation seems far more probable. Regardless of the cause, the bronchial arteries become the only arterial supply to the primitive plexus of vessels around the developing foregut, the ventral portion of which will form the pulmonary vascular network. Enlarged bronchial arteries may be associated with an insufficient as well as an absent pulmonary artery (46, 50).

Type VII. Anomalous arteries to the lungs, arising from the aorta below the hila of the lungs or even below the diaphragm, will be discussed in the following section.

SUMMARY OF EMBRYOGENIC FACTORS (FIG. 14.12)

Aberrant pulmonary artery
   Truncus arteriosus defects
      Failure of truncus septum formation: type I
      Failure of migration of right pulmonary artery: type II
   Sixth arch defects
      Loss of proximal segments: type III
      Loss of proximal segments and persistence of distal segments: type IV
Absent pulmonary artery
   Sixth arch defects
      Early atresia of both proximal and distal segments: type V
      Enlarged bronchial arteries: type VI

ASSOCIATED ANOMALIES

Among the 46 cases collected by Pool et al. (44) in 1962, only seven appeared to have absent or aberrant pulmo-

nary arteries unaccompanied by other cardiovascular anomalies. Tetralogy of Fallot was present in 10 of 18 cases with anomalous left pulmonary artery. In eight cases, a right aortic arch occurred. A patent ductus arteriosus on the right or left was common. Among patients with anomalous right pulmonary arteries, both patent ductus arteriosus and patent foramen ovale were common.

Among patients with type I defects, the undivided truncus usually overrides a ventricular septal defect. The septum may be completely absent, resulting in a single ventricle. A right aortic arch frequently is present.

When the defect is unilateral (types II to V), the affected lung is usually smaller than the normal lung, but it is aerated, and cystic changes have been reported only rarely (51). In one case there was a hypoplastic lower lobe with venous drainage to the inferior vena cava (52).

In 1980, Campbell et al. (10) reviewed their successful repair of an aberrant left pulmonary artery (pulmonary artery sling), performed 24 years previously. The defect, which may arise from the right, was located between the trachea and the esophagus of their patient. This surgery took place only 2 years after Potts (53) performed his first successful operation.

Clements et al. (54) analyzed 25 cases with congenital bronchopulmonary vascular malformations. All 25 patients had abnormalities of the tracheobronchial tree; 9 patients lacked connection to the abnormal segment. The aberrant arterial blood supply was single in 16 cases and multiple in 9. Of those patients, 17 had anomalous venous drainage.

Barbero-Marcial et al. (29) reported a patient with pulmonary atresia, ventricular septal defect, and no extraparenchymal pulmonary arteries. All the bronchopulmonary arterial segments connected to systemic pulmonary collaterals.

Vigneswaran and Pollock (55) cited the case of a 41-year-old man with pulmonary atresia with ventricular septal defect and coronary artery fistula. A similar case was presented by Jowett et al. (56) in 1989. Fistulous connections between a solitary coronary artery and the pulmonary arteries were the primary source of pulmonary blood supply in tetralogy of Fallot with pulmonary valve atresia.

HISTORY

A pulmonary artery arising from the innominate artery was first described by Breschet in 1826, as noted by Poynter in 1916 (57). Aberrant pulmonary arteries from the ascending aorta were reported by Tiedemann (58) in 1831. An absent right pulmonary artery was described by Fraentzel (59) in 1868. However, an absent left pulmonary artery was not reported until 1941 (60), according to Emanuel and Pattison (61). In 1843 Calori (62) described a case with complete bilateral absence of the

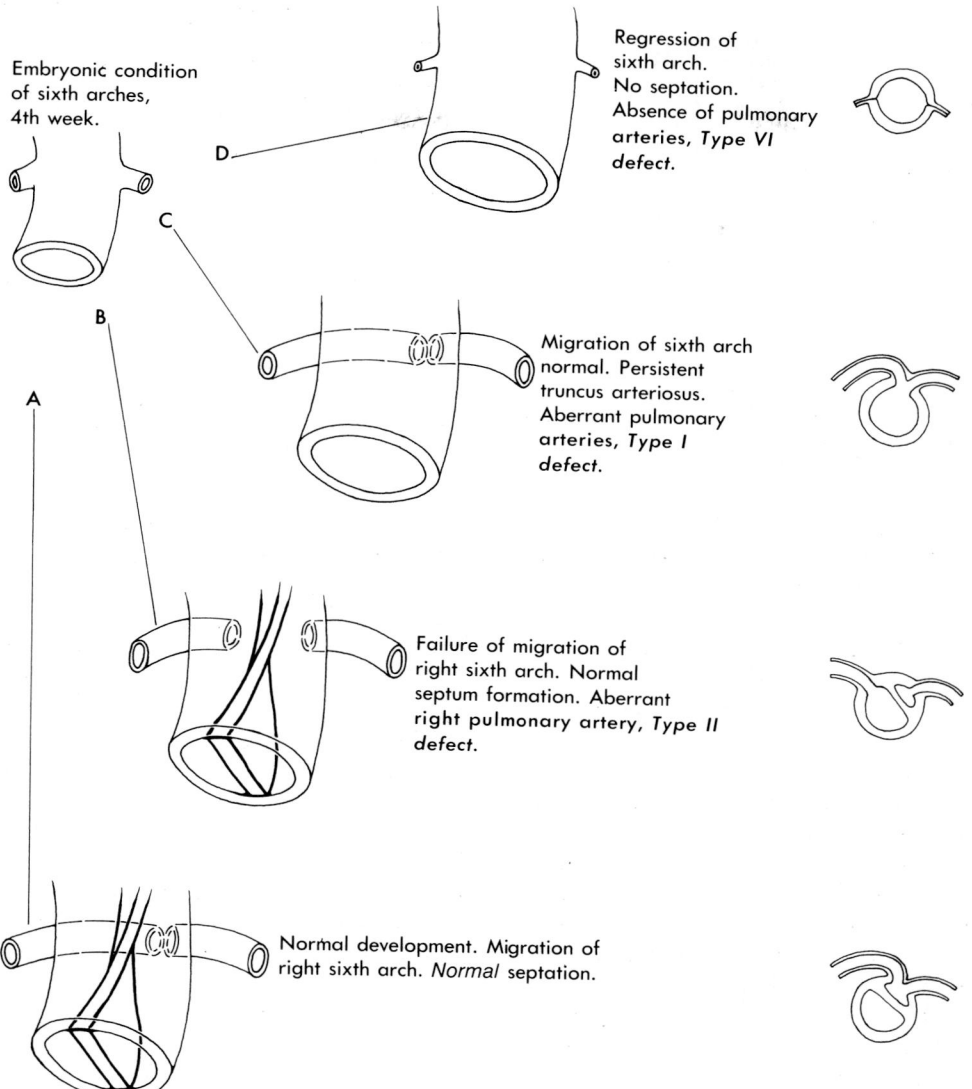

Embryonic condition of sixth arches, 4th week.

Regression of sixth arch. No septation. Absence of pulmonary arteries, *Type VI defect.*

Migration of sixth arch normal. Persistent truncus arteriosus. Aberrant pulmonary arteries, *Type I defect.*

Failure of migration of right sixth arch. Normal septum formation. Aberrant right pulmonary artery, *Type II defect.*

Normal development. Migration of right sixth arch. *Normal* septation.

Figure 14.12. Normal development of the truncus septum and migration of the orifices of the sixth arch (**A**). Defects resulting from failure of sixth arch migration (**B**), failure of septation (**C**), or both (**D**). Sketches on the right are cross-sections through the truncus at the level of pulmonary arteries.

pulmonary arteries. By 1952 Madoff et al. (63) were able to collect nine cases from the literature and add one of their own, which was the first to be diagnosed in a living patient before surgery. Schneiderman (40) collected 46 cases in 1958 but doubted the validity of many of those diagnosed by angiography only. Pool and his colleagues (44) made a thorough review in 1962, collecting 46 confirmed and 32 probable cases.

INCIDENCE

Type I appears to be the most prevalent of these anomalies; about 60 cases were collected by 1949 (48). Of types II to V, Pool et al. (44) were able to find 36 confirmed cases by 1962. Sixteen cases of type VI have been collected (64). Males are affected with type I defects twice as

frequently as are females. In the other types, both sexes are equally affected.

SYMPTOMS AND DIAGNOSIS

For clinical purposes, the types of anomalous pulmonary arteries may be reclassified as follows (Fig. 14.13):

1. Entire pulmonary circulation is from the aorta; pathophysiology is that of persistent truncus arteriosus (types I and VI).
2. Pulmonary supply to one lung is normal, supply to other lung is from systemic circulation (types II, III, IV, and V).
3. Pulmonary circulation to both lungs is normal or hypoplastic; an accessory artery serves a portion of one or both lungs; pathophysiology is that of sequestration of the lung (type VII).

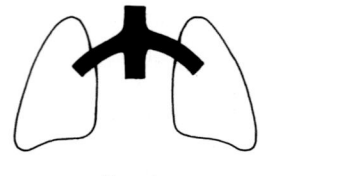

Type I

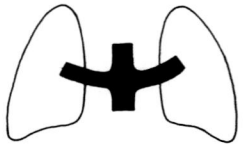

Type VI

Systemic pressure
in both lungs

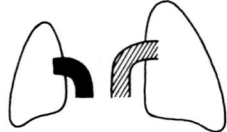

Types II & III

Systemic pressure and decreased
flow in right lung (often hypoplastic).
Increased pressure and flow in
left lung

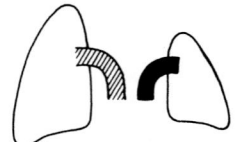

Type IV

Systemic pressure and decreased
flow in left lung (often hypoplastic).
Increased pressure and flow in
right lung

Type V   Either right or left lung may be affected as
          in Types II and III or Type IV

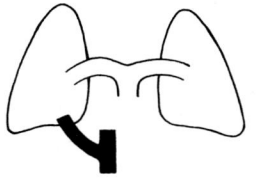

Type VII

Normal pulmonary pressure in both
lungs except for portion served
by anomalous systemic artery

Figure 14.13. Classification of anomalies according to hemodynamic factors.

Entire Pulmonary Circulation From the Aorta. In infancy and childhood, type I defects produce little or no cyanosis although there may be some depletion of the systemic circulation by excessive blood flow to the lungs at birth. Pulmonary vascular changes later in life eventually reduce the volume of blood reaching the lungs so that cyanosis, clubbing of the fingers, and polycythemia appear.

With type VI defects, cyanosis is present at birth. Polycythemia develops in infancy because the bronchial arteries are of inadequate caliber. Slight improvement of symptoms may occur with age. Exercise tolerance is impaired.

In both types, radiography will show an enlarged aorta and no pulmonary trunk. Selective angiography demonstrates filling of the truncus from either ventricle. Retrograde aortography outlines the arteries to the lungs.

Pulmonary Circulation to One Lung Normal. A unilateral aberrant pulmonary artery or a pulmonized bronchial artery does not usually carry the same amount of blood as does a normal pulmonary artery. Because of this, the affected lung is often smaller than the normal lung. Diagnosis may be suggested by an asymmetry of the thorax and a shift of the heart and mediastinum toward the affected side. A difference in the vascularity of the two lung fields may be apparent on radiography.

Although one lung receives blood through a normal pulmonary artery, both the flow and the pressure are increased since this artery receives the entire right ventricular output. The other lung receives a smaller than normal blood flow, but it is at systemic pressure. Pulmonary hypertension is thus present in both lungs (65).

As we have already mentioned, Schneiderman (40) questioned the accuracy of many diagnoses of absent pulmonary artery made by radiography during life. Failure to visualize a pulmonary artery must be accompanied by visualization of the anomalous artery to the affected lung before the diagnosis can be considered acceptable.

Radiographic evidence of absence of a pulmonary artery will not distinguish between a true congenital absence and an acquired attenuation of the artery. In true absence, the lung is normal and small, with slightly reduced ventilation. The collateral flow is good, and the radiopacity appears normal. In acquired attenuation of the artery, there is usually a mediastinal shift with impaired ventilation and abnormal breath sounds. The lung is often hyperlucent on the radiograph because collateral circulation is never as large as in the congenital form. Massumi and Donohoe (66) believe more than 50% of reported cases are not of congenital origin.

Accessory Pulmonary Arteries. Malformations in this group are discussed later.

TREATMENT

Pneumonectomy to relieve recurring hemorrhages in the affected lung was suggested in 1951 by Findlay and Maier (46). However, there is little evidence for its necessity in those patients who live long enough to be subjected to it since ligation of the artery to the affected lung has been found to be equally effective (67).

When one aberrant pulmonary artery arises from the ascending aorta, the logical treatment is to transplant it to the pulmonary trunk. This has been done successfully in some patients (39, 65, 68, 69) (Fig. 14.14).

Burrows et al. (42) in 1985 recommended thorough investigation of the pulmonary vascular bed by total evaluation of pulmonary arteries.

PROGNOSIS

When both pulmonary arteries arise from the ascending aorta (type I), death from heart failure usually occurs in less than a year although a few affected persons may live for as long as 10 years. When bronchial arteries from the descending aorta supply the lungs (type VI), 50% of patients may live 10 years or longer.

Patients who have only one anomalous pulmonary artery and a normal heart also have a better life expectancy. Seven of 37 patients with proven cases mentioned by Pool et al. (44) lived over 10 years. Among their "probable" cases, 16 were diagnosed in infancy or childhood, and 21 after the age of 10 years. Seven patients lived over 30 years.

Sequestration of the Lung and Accessory Lung

ANATOMY

The term *sequestration* is applied to a pulmonary lobe or portion of a lobe which is supplied separately by a large anomalous artery arising from the aorta or one of its

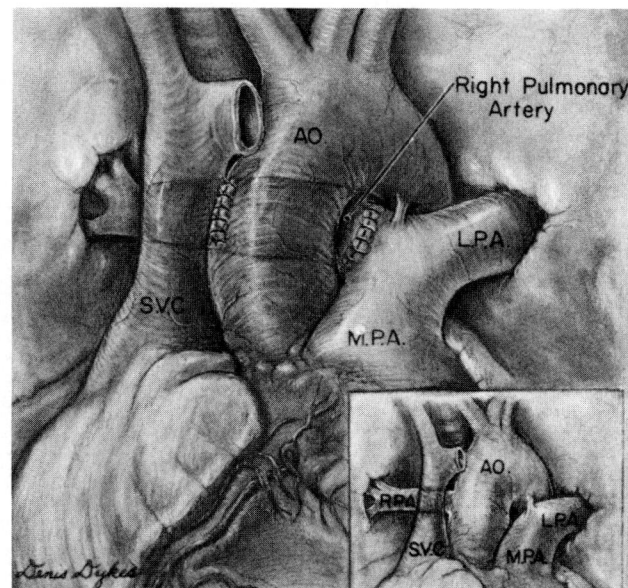

Figure 14.14. Transplantation of a right pulmonary artery (*RPA*) from the aorta (*AO*) to the pulmonary trunk (*MPA*). The *inset* shows the anomaly before operation. The left pulmonary artery (*LPA*) was located in its normal position. *SVC*, superior vena cava. (From Stanton RE, Durnin RE, Fyler DC, Lindesmith GG, Meyer BW. Right pulmonary artery originating from ascending aorta. Am J Dis Child 1968;115:403–413.)

branches and which is usually drained by anomalous veins. Such a lobe is usually composed of one or more cysts and may be physiologically or anatomically cut off from the remainder of the lung. There may be a fistulous connection between the sequestered lung tissue and the esophagus (70). It is convenient to divide the condition into intralobar sequestration, in which the isolated portion is anatomically part of a normal lobe of the lung within the visceral pleura, and extralobar sequestration or accessory lung outside the visceral pleura, in which the isolated tissue is separated from the normal lung. See Table 14.2 for a differential diagnosis of various thoracic cysts lined with respiratory epithelium.

Roe et al. (71) reported bilateral sequestration, and Savic and colleagues (72) documented intralobar and extralobar coexisting.

It is extremely difficult to classify all types of sequestration and their associated anomalies. However, the pathology may involve a pulmonary segment, a lobe, or even an entire lung. Landing and Dixon (73) reported such a pathology due to the main bronchus originating from the esophagus. Parts of both lungs may be involved. In addition, pulmonary tissue may be located under the diaphragm, where it is totally isolated or in communication with the lung through abnormal vessels.

Extrathoracic tissue within the pulmonary parenchyma has been reported. Corrin et al. (74) in 1985

Table 14.2.
Classification of Pulmonary Sequestration and Related Anomalies[a]

True sequestration
  Intralobar
  Extralobar
Bronchopulmonary-foregut malformation
  Intralobar or extralobar sequestration with communication to esophagus or stomach
Pseudosequestration
  Bronchial obstruction by foreign body and/or inflammatory mass; recurrent infection with enlargement of normal pulmonary ligament arteries
Vascular anomalies
  Systemic arterial supply to otherwise normal lung
  Venolobar syndromes; abnormal venous drainage of true sequestration, scimitar syndrome and its variants and some cases of horseshoe lung

[a]From Katzenstein ALA, Askin FB. Surgical pathology of non-neoplastic lung disease. Philadelphia: WB Saunders, 1990.

Table 14.3.
Contrasting Features of Intralobar and Extralobar Sequestrations[a]

	Intralobar	Extralobar
Age at diagnosis	50% > 20 yr	60% < 1 yr
Sex distribution	M:F–1:1	M:F–4:1
Relation to lung	Within	Separate (outside of visceral pleura)
Side affected	Left, 60%	Left, 90%
Venous drainage	Pulmonary	Systemic or portal
Associated anomalies	Rare	Pectus excavatum, diaphragmatic defects
Pathogenesis	Acquired or congenital	Congenital anomaly

[a]From Katzenstein ALA, Askin FB. Surgical pathology of non-neoplastic lung disease. Philadelphia: WB Saunders, 1990. Adapted from Askin FB. Pediatric lung disease. In: Thurlbeck WM, ed. Pathology of the lung. New York: Thieme Medical Publishers, 1988:115–146; Askin FB. Respiratory tract disorders in the fetus and neonate. In: Wigglesworth JS, Singer DB, eds. Pathology of the fetus and neonate. Oxford: Blackwell Scientific, 1989; Landing BH, Dixon LG. Congenital malformations and genetic disorders of the respiratory tract (larynx, trachea, bronchi and lungs). Am Rev Respir Dis 1979; 120:151; and Stocker JT. Sequestrations of the lung. Semin Diagn Pathol 1986; 3:106.

reported such a case with pancreatic tissue within the sequestration. Flye and Izant (75) reported extralobar sequestration with esophageal communication. Similar cases of foregut communication were reported by several investigators (76–78).

Horseshoe lung and sequestration was reported by Cipriano et al. (79), Frank et al. (80), and Freedom et al. (81). Katzenstein and Askin (24) tabulated several hundred cases of several authors and summarized the features of intralobar and extralobar sequestrations (Table 14.3).

According to Clements and Warner (82), the terms *intralobar* and *extralobar sequestration* provide no definite information on the morphology within these lesions. As a matter of fact, after objecting to the word "sequestration," Clements and Warner propose a new name, "malinosculation," (Latin: mal = abnormal; in = in; osculum = mouth), to describe the abnormal communications which are present in this pathological entity—that is, communication or anastomoses of vessels or other tubular structures.

We believe these authors are correct even though the medical profession, including authors and editors, still use the term *sequestration*. Clements and Warner tried to clear the muddy water surrounding pulmonary "sequestration" (malinosculation) by presenting a new, logical classification using the anatomic entities composing the lung (Table 14.4). Also, to explain the developmental pathology, they present an acceptable "wheel." We like it and present this "wheel" to our readers (Fig. 14.15).

Intralobar Sequestration. Pryce (83, 84) described three types of intralobar sequestration (Fig. 14.16):

1. The anomalous artery supplies normal lung tissue (type I).
2. The anomalous artery supplies normal lung and the sequestered lobe (type II).

3. The anomalous artery supplies the sequestered lobe only (type III).

The aberrant artery is large and of the elastic type thus resembling the normal pulmonary artery rather than a systemic branch of the aorta. There is no accompanying bronchial artery. Atherosclerotic changes are usual. Occasionally, the aberrant artery arises from the celiac axis or the intercostal arteries instead of from the aorta (85). In at least some cases branches of the anomalous artery anastomose with the normal pulmonary circulation. Cole and his colleagues (86) were able to demonstrate such connections in an artery and sequestered lobe removed surgically. In another similar case they found no such anastomosis. In intralobar sequestration, in contrast to extralobar sequestration, the venous drainage often is through the normal pulmonary veins only.

In 1986 Holder et al. (87) proposed that most intralobar sequestrations represent either systemic adenomatoid malformations that clinically are unrecognized until they become secondarily infected or developmentally normal lung supplied by a systemic artery. They reported 15 cases with an aberrant systemic artery to normal or abnormal lung.

In 1990 Katch et al. (88) reported a case of systemic origin of an aberrant artery to the basal segments of the left lung. By arteriography, the artery was large and originated from the descending aorta. It supplied the left posterior basal segment, which had no pulmonary arteries. The bronchial tree was normal, and a left lower lobectomy was performed with good results.

The sequestered area is usually, but not always, the posterior and basal segment of the lower lobe of the left

Table 14.4.
Classification of Pulmonary Malinosculation (First Step Defining Basic Abnormality of Tracheobronchopulmonary Airway Connection, Arterial Blood Supply, or Both, Followed by Description of Associated Anomalies of Venous Drainage and Lung Parenchyma)[a]

Abnormality of Tracheobronchopulmonary Airway and/or Arterial Blood Supply	Examples of Recognised Entities	Venous Drainage	Lung Parenchymal Abnormalities
Bronchopulmonary malinosculation (normal pulmonary artery blood supply)	Tracheal—tracheal stenosis Bronchial—bronchial stenosis or atresia, bronchogenic cyst Parenchymal—congenital lung cyst, cystic adenomatoid malformation, lobar emphysema	Normal Anomalous Multiple Mixed Mismatched	*Site of the lesion* Intrapulmonary, extrapulmonary
Arterial pulmonary malinosculation (normal bronchopulmonary airway)	Area of lung with systemic blood supply		*Within the lesion* Cystic, adenomatous, emphysematous, ectopic, foregut inclusions
Bronchoarterial pulmonary malinosculation (abnormal bronchopulmonary airway with systemic arterial blood supply)	Bronchopulmonary airway patent but abnormal—congenital cystic bronchiectasis, lobar emphysema with systemic arterial supply, scimitar syndrome Bronchopulmonary connection absent—classical sequestration, congenital lung cysts with systemic arterial blood supply		*Associated abnormalities of surrounding lung* Abnormal lobation, lobulation, hypoplasia

[a]From Clements BS, Warner J. Pulmonary sequestration and related congenital bronchopulmonary-vascular malformations: nomenclature and classification based on anatomical and embryological considerations. Thorax 1987;42:401–408.

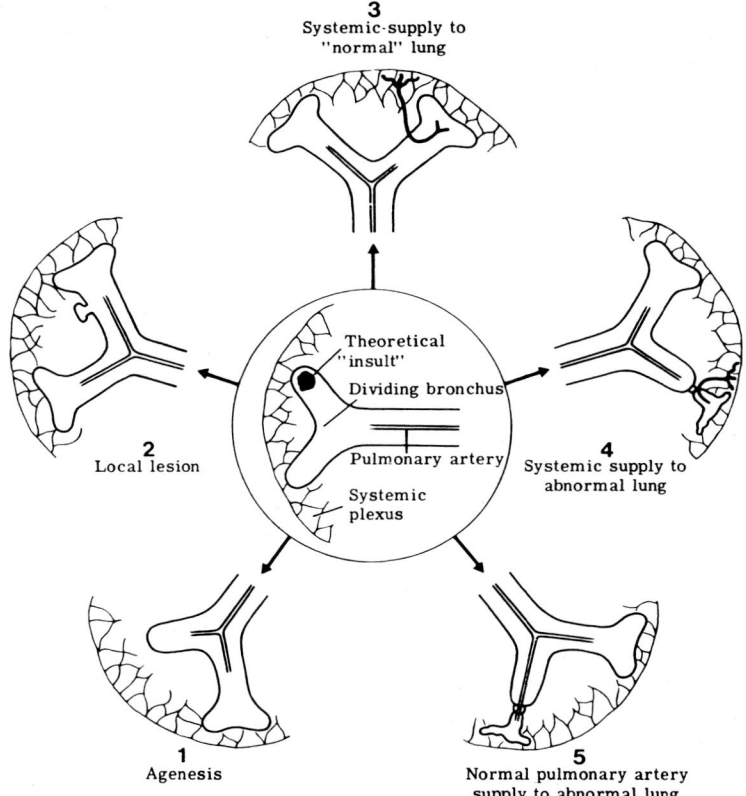

Figure 14.15. The "wheel" theory of abnormal lung development. After a theoretic "insult" to the tip of a dividing bronchus (shown in the center of the diagram), each satellite sketch represents a possible pathologic consequence at the next stage of development. This forms the basis of the eventual lesion. (From Clements BS, Warner JO. Pulmonary sequestration and related congenital bronchopulmonary-vascular malformations: nomenclature and classification based on anatomical and embryological considerations. Thorax 1987;42:401–408.)

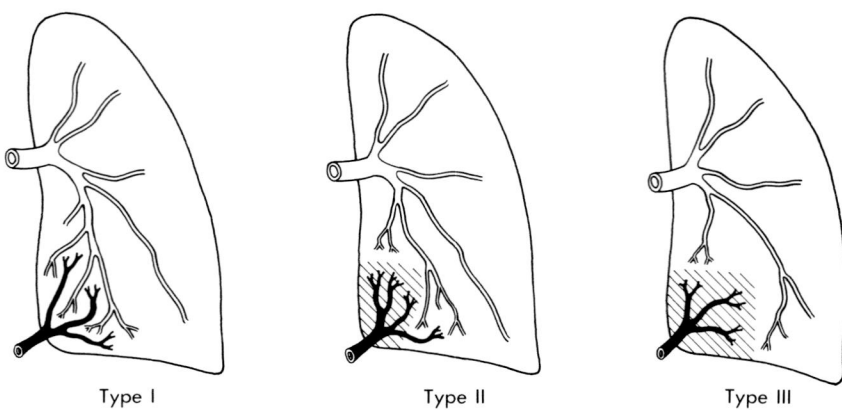

Figure 14.16. Pryce's types of intralobar sequestration. (See text for discussion.)

lung. Its size and extent are variable. It may form a single cyst or multiple cysts, or a mass of bronchi may occur parallel to the artery. The tissue is usually truly sequestered, but in about 20% of cases, there is communication with normal bronchi (89). Many such communications are probably secondary to the original pathologic condition. The cysts are usually lined with respiratory epithelium and are filled with thick mucoid material, blood, pus, or air. The walls contain all the elements of the normal bronchial wall. There is, therefore, a strong resemblance to a bronchogenic cyst. Some investigators (89, 90) believe that only the presence of the anomalous artery distinguishes an intralobar sequestration from a bronchogenic cyst. Others (91) have considered the presence or absence of bronchial communication to be the real criterion and have ignored the aberrant artery. We do not concur with this later view.

Three cases of intralobar sequestration having a fistulous tract connecting the esophagus with a bronchus or with a cystic space of the sequestration have been reported (92–94). In one case the muscular esophagus-like fistula arose subdiaphragmatically and was 10 cm long (92). In addition to these patent fistulae, Halasz and his colleagues (95) collected three cases and added one of their own, in which an esophageal connection existed but was not patent. In two cases (96, 97) the blind pulmonic end of the tube contained pancreatic tissue (Fig. 14.17). In the third case (98) the connection was fibrous and without a lumen.

Acker and his colleagues (99) reported a case of intralobar sequestration with partial anomalous pulmonary venous drainage from the opposite lung. The sequestered lobe was successfully removed.

Extralobar Sequestration (Accessory Lung). The sequestered tissue is separated from the normal lung, in contradistinction to intralobar sequestration (Fig. 14.18). It may occur in the upper portion of the thorax, the lower portion of the thorax, or the abdomen. It may have a

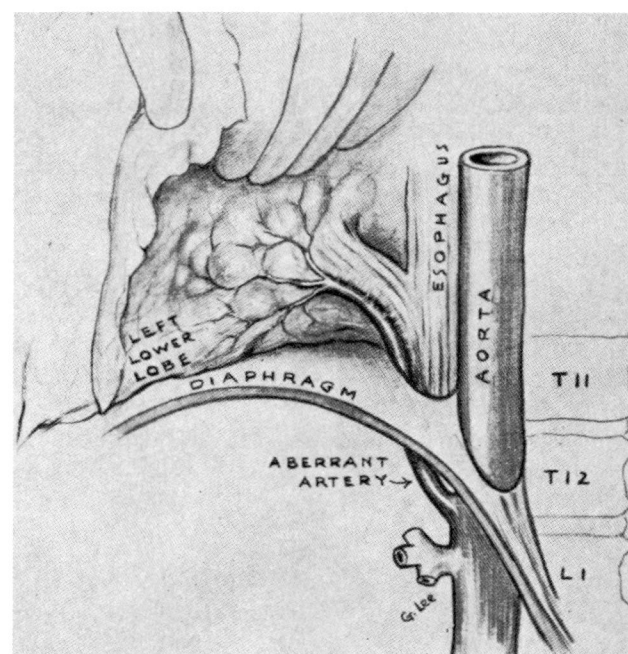

Figure 14.17. Intralobar sequestration with esophageal communication containing pancreas tissue. (From Beskin CA. Intralobar enteric sequestration of the lung containing aberrant pancreas. J Thorac Cardiovasc Surg 1961;41:314–317.)

bronchial connection with the normal respiratory tree, the trachea, or the digestive tract. As in the intralobar type, there is often an anomalous arterial supply from the thoracic or abdominal aorta. The venous drainage is into the azygos vein more frequently than is the case with intralobar sequestration.

Apical Accessory Lung (Tracheal Lobe).
This variety of accessory lung is rare. The blood supply is usually from the subclavian artery; there may be a connection with the trachea (100), in which case the term *tracheal lobe* is appropriate. An esophageal fistula that is

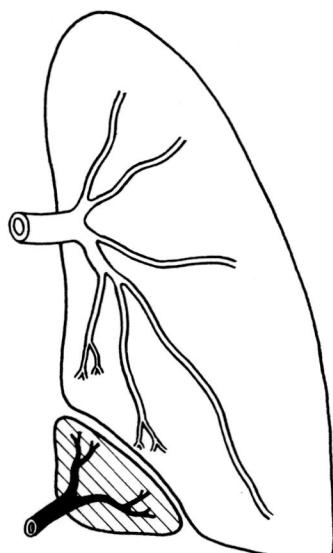

Figure 14.18.   Extralobar sequestration. The affected lobe is anatomically as well as physiologically sequestered.

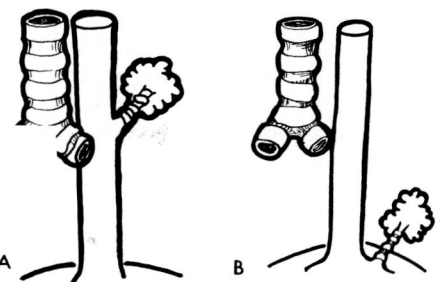

Figure 14.19.   Accessory lung. **A**, Thoracic accessory lung, with bronchus from the esophagus. **B**, Abdominal accessory lung, with bronchus arising from the stomach. Such lung tissue is supplied by systemic arteries from the aorta, if thoracic, or from the celiac artery, if abdominal. Both are very rare.

bronchial in structure may exist (101). It has been seen at least once in an embryo (102) (see Chapter 13, "The Trachea and Lungs"). The first case was reported in 1901 by Herxheimer (103). Cotton and his colleagues (100) successfully removed an apical accessory lung in an infant in 1952.

Lower Accessory Lung (Rokitansky Lobe).
In this type the arterial supply is from the aorta, arising either above or below the diaphragm, as in intralobar sequestration. The lower lobe is the most common site of extralobar sequestration. About 10 cases have been described (104). The chief distinction between intralobar sequestration and lower accessory lung is that the latter is anatomically separated from the remainder of the lung. A bronchial connection may be present and the tissue may contain air (105), but usually there is no connection (106, 107). Nearly all of these structures are on the left (Fig. 14.19, *A*).

In seven reported cases, the sequestered tissue had a fistulous connection with the stomach (108) (Fig. 14.19, *B*) or with the esophagus (70, 95, 109). In one case the tube was lined with gastric mucosa; in another (104), a bronchial structure lined with respiratory epithelium arose from the distal esophagus. In still another patient (110), there was intestinal mucosa. Pancreatic tissue has been found in similar fistulae associated with intralobar sequestration.

Most lower accessory lobes are on the left, but at least two have been found on the right (70, 109).

Abdominal Accessory Lung.
Lung tissue below the diaphragm is extremely rare. Two cases in adults were described by Vogel (111) in 1899. In

one, two arteries from the thoracic aorta passed through the aortic hiatus and supplied lung tissue medial to the left kidney. In the other the lung tissue was above the left kidney, was supplied from the celiac axis and the phrenic artery, and was drained by the suprarenal vein. Valle and White (112) found lung tissue below the left diaphragm in a 9-month-old infant.

EMBRYOGENESIS

There is little agreement about the embryologic origin of sequestration of the lung. A number of relatively unsatisfactory theories have been advanced. The fact that intra- and extralobar sequestration have been considered to have different origins (113) may have helped to confuse the picture. The chief theories proposed are as follows:

1. Supernumerary foregut lung bud formation caudal to the normal esophagotracheal groove (95, 114): Although this theory would seem to explain only those cases having a bronchoesophageal fistula, there is evidence that such anomalous connections may disappear before birth (95).
2. Adhesion of embryonic lung-forming cells to other organs, which, by traction of differential growth, separates them from the remainder of the lung tissue (107): This adhesion theory would seem to apply only to extralobar sequestration, especially to those few instances of pulmonary tissue below the diaphragm.
3. Capture of the developing bronchial buds by the anomalous artery, which, with growth of the lung, detaches the buds from their bronchial connections: The anomalous artery is the primary defect (83). This view is not in accord with our knowledge of vascularization. While large arteries in the adult may exert traction on an organ, the developing blood vessels of the embryo do not determine the location of an organ or its parts, but instead arise as preferred channels in a capillary plexus to supply blood where it is needed and in the quantity called for by the tissue.
4. Failure of the pulmonary artery to develop fast enough to supply the whole of the growing lung leads to formation (or persistence) of a collateral aortic supply, which is the

anomalous artery: An area so supplied undergoes cystic or fibrous degeneration after birth (113). This explanation appears to be inherently more reasonable than the others. The anomalous artery is one of the caudal vessels of the primitive vascular plexus around the foregut described by Bremer (115) which, having become established, enlarges at the same time as does the pulmonary trunk. Normally these vessels of the primitive plexus are represented by very small arteries of the pulmonary ligament (83). We suspect that the elastic wall of these abnormally persistent vessels may be induced by pulmonary mesenchyme rather than resulting from hemodynamic factors alone.

The absence of reports of the anomaly in newborn infants led Gebauer and Mason (116) to suggest an acquired rather than a congenital origin for sequestration in 1959, but Boyden (90) had described an anomalous artery arising from the aorta in a 41-mm embryo the year before. In the same paper Boyden also described symmetric upper lobe cysts in a 31-mm embryo that was without anomalous arteries.

No adequate explanation for the pronounced left-sided predominance of the anomaly is offered in any of the proposed theories.

Although we may in this manner account for the anomalous artery, the sequestration must result from a secondary pulmonary outgrowth of the foregut in those cases in which an esophageal or gastric fistula is present. There can be no doubt these represent development of cells from the ventral foregut that were not incorporated into the original tracheal formation.

When extralobar sequestration exists without a fistulous connection with either bronchial tree or esophagus, the explanation of Cockayne and Gladstone (107)—that it results from adhesions—is undoubtedly correct. The tissue culture experiments of Dameron (117) indicate that, if only a few isolated cells of the epithelial bronchial tree are present, they will continue to develop in the presence of lung mesenchyme. Hence, only a few cells need be "sequestered" during lung formation to produce a sequestered lobe.

In this sense the relationship to bronchogenic cysts pointed out by Gallagher and his colleagues (89) in 1957 is clear. Bronchogenic cysts derive from more proximal portions of the respiratory tree and occur earlier; sequestrations are more distal and occur later. Whether they are intralobar or extralobar depends upon their distance from the normal lung. Abdominal sequestrations represent the extreme separation which takes place before the formation of the diaphragm (see Table 13.15).

However, Pendse et al. (118) reported intralobar and extralobar sequestration in a child and raised the question of an anomaly of foregut budding. Iwai et al. (119) expressed the opinion that an accessory bronchopulmo-

nary bud from the foregut is responsible for the genesis of this malformation. Similar thoughts were expressed by Albrechtsen (120). Holder and Langston (87) believe intralobar sequestration results when an accessory lung bud is enveloped by normal lung.

Some authors, however, question the congenital origin of intralobar sequestration and support the view that the pathology is the result of chronic inflammation, since such cases have not been reported in newborn infants (87, 121, 122). These authors believe the systemic arterial supply present in intralobar communication is the result of inflammation. This is puzzling, since arterial branches from the aorta were reported in the pulmonary ligament by Stocker and Malczak (122) in 1984. Stocker (perhaps) changed his mind 2 years later (121).

ASSOCIATED ANOMALIES

Diaphragmatic hernia or eventration may be associated with Pryce's type I anomalies—that is, those in which the anomalous arteries supply normal lung tissue (86).

Diaphragmatic hernia is even more frequent with accessory lungs. Davies and Gunz (123) found it in about 20% of the cases they reviewed. The anomalous vessels pass through the diaphragmatic defect. The patient of St. Raymond and his colleagues (104) had a large hiatal hernia through which passed an artery from the aorta near the renal vessels to an accessory thoracic lung, connected by a fistula to the lower esophagus. Venous drainage was to the portal vein. The symptoms were chiefly those of hiatal hernia.

Alivizatos et al. (124) reported pulmonary sequestration complicated by anomalies of pulmonary venous return. Bell-Thomson et al. (125) noted carcinoma of the lung arising in sequestration. Clements and Warner (82) reported sequestration and bronchopulmonary vascular anomalies. Haworth et al. (126) reported scimitar syndrome associated with pulmonary hypertension and sequestration.

Table 14.2 (by Katzenstein and Askin [24]) gives a classification of pulmonary sequestration and associated anomalies.

John et al. (127) reported 41 children with associated disorders of the bronchopulmonary airway, the arterial supply to the lungs, and the lung parenchyma and its venous drainage.

In most cases intralobar sequestrations do not have other associated anomalies. However, Carter (128) stated that associated anomalies are common with extralobar sequestration (15 to 40%), with diaphragmatic hernia being the most common.

In 1983 Thilenius et al. (129) reported a spectrum of pulmonary sequestrations with several other anomalies such as bronchoesophageal communications and pulmonary hypoplasia.

In 1987 a new classification of sequestration, according to the four major components of the lung tissue, was presented by Clements and Warner (82):

1. Tracheobronchial airway
2. Lung parenchyma
3. Arterial supply
4. Venous drainage

Any combination may take place. A similar opinion was reported by John et al. (127) in 1989.

HISTORY

In 1777 Huber (130) first described an anomalous artery arising from the aorta at the level of the seventh thoracic vertebra and entering the right lower lobe of the lung in a 2-year-old girl. In 1802 Maugars (131) described a child in whom the anomalous artery arose from the abdominal aorta, passed through the esophageal hiatus of the diaphragm, and divided to reach the lower lobes of each lung.

Accessory lungs were seen independently by Rektorzik (132) and by Rokitansky (111) in 1861 (hence the name "Rokitansky lobe"). Cockayne and Gladstone (107) discussed the defect at length and collected 29 human and 3 animal cases in 1917.

Attention was called to the anomalous artery in 1940 when Harris and Lewis (133) reported the fatal outcome of severing such a vessel while performing a lobectomy.

In 1946 Pryce (83) was able to find only 12 cases of anomalous pulmonary arteries in the literature, none of which described the co-existing bronchial anomaly. He described the pulmonary sequestration, determined the elastic nature of the aberrant artery, and established the anatomy of the lesion. Pryce also performed the first successful resection of the sequestration. Since 1946 the literature has expanded considerably, and Eaker and his colleagues (134) collected a total of 106 cases in 1958.

The first diagnosis of an accessory lung in a living patient is credited to Valle and White (112) in 1947. In 1950 DeBakey and his colleagues (106) reported a successful resection which had been performed in 1946. Later in 1950, Leahy and MacCallum (105) reported a similar operation performed in 1948. Das and his associates (92) reviewed the cases of accessory lungs having foregut communications in 1959, and Halasz et al. (95) reexamined all reported pulmonary foregut fistulae.

Sequestration, the anomalous artery, and the esophageal fistulae still need thorough investigation; the nature of the defect or defects is still obscure.

INCIDENCE

Intralobar sequestration would seem to be more common than its early history suggests. Pryce et al. (84) found six cases among 336 pulmonary excisions.

Up to 1950 some 40 cases of extralobar sequestration were collected by DeBakey and co-workers (106). Twenty-two cases were found in animals (135) as of 1938. Extralobar sequestration may manifest itself at an earlier age than intralobar sequestration which is rarely recognized in infancy. In neither type is there a sex difference.

Sixty percent of intralobar and 90% of extralobar sequestrations occur on the left side. A few bilateral intralobar lesions have been reported (136). In 1979 Savic et al. (72) collected 540 cases.

SYMPTOMS

Sequestered lung tissue may give little evidence of its presence for years. When symptoms do occur, they are often nonspecific. Repeated acute episodes of pulmonary infection with cough, chills, fever, and hemoptysis lead to diagnoses of pneumonia, empyema, or bronchiectasis (137). Symptoms may be present from birth or be of only short duration in adulthood. One 36-year-old patient had chest pains for 2 weeks and cough for 6 months (104). In one case, in which an esophageal connection was present, the defect was discovered in an 18-year-old girl on a routine school physical examination (70).

For all practical purposes, in most cases extralobar sequestration is asymptomatic and discovered by accident. Recurring infection is the characteristic of intralobar sequestration.

DIAGNOSIS

Plain roentgenography may give a clue to the condition, but only when it already has been suspected. Absence of breath sounds in the lower left thorax, with increased radiopacity, may be indicative. The murmur from an anomalous artery may sometimes be detected on auscultation.

Thoracic aortography has been successfully used (137, 138) for demonstration of anomalous arteries, and tomography has been helpful in some cases (139). Where an esophageal fistula exists, it may be revealed by a barium swallow; in at least one case (104) it was not detected. Esophagoscopy demonstrated the fistulous opening in a patient of Gans and Potts (140).

Naidich et al. (141) recommend magnetic resonance imaging (MRI) for intralobar sequestration, and Ikezoe et al. (142) presented 24 cases diagnosed by computed tomographic (CT) scan to assess bronchopulmonary sequestration. Plain film and angiography were used by Riebel and von Windheim (138) for the diagnosis of pulmonary sequestration.

Thilenius et al. (129) stated that pulmonary sequestration is a spectrum of related lesions any of which may be absent or present; therefore diagnosis should be directed toward each component of the spectrum.

TREATMENT

The condition is not incompatible with life if associated congenital defects are not fatal, but recurrent respiratory infections are not without danger. The treatment of choice is resection of the sequestered lobe after ligation and section of the anomalous artery or esophageal fistula. No circulatory disturbance follows ligation of the artery, even in Pryce's type I anomaly in which the artery supplies normal lung (86).

The great surgical hazard attending the condition is that of accidentally cutting the anomalous artery during pulmonary resection (143, 144). Since the first report of such an accident (133) it has become mandatory to search for and ligate the artery before proceeding with the resection. The great size of the vessel, while aiding in its identification, makes its transection catastrophic.

In summary, surgery is the procedure of choice in symptomatic patients with extralobar or intralobar sequestration. The extralobar lesion is mobilized after ligating the vessels and then removed. The intralobar lesion requires lobectomy, isolating, and ligating all the abnormal vessels to prevent accidental bleeding (138).

Retrotracheal Left Pulmonary Artery

ANATOMY

In this rare anomaly the pulmonary trunk follows the course of the right pulmonary artery, giving off the left pulmonary artery to the right of the esophagus and trachea, outside the pericardium. The left pulmonary artery courses anteriorly and superiorly to the right primary bronchus and passes posteriorly to the trachea and left primary bronchus. The right bronchus and the esophagus may be compressed (Fig. 14.20). The ligamentum arteriosum arises from the pulmonary trunk and joins the aorta at its normal site (145–147).

Wells et al. (147) describe the anatomy of sling of left pulmonary arteries in association with other anomalies.

EMBRYOGENESIS

The developmental error occurs not in the left sixth arch itself, which forms normally, but in the embryonic left pulmonary artery, which extends caudad from the arch to join an arterial twig from the pulmonary plexus. This junction normally occurs at the cranial end of the plexus on the ventral surface of the lung bud during the fifth week (4 mm) (3). The anomaly arises when the junction forms with a median twig from the dorsal portion of the pulmonary plexus and the persistent channel passes to the right of the developing trachea (Fig. 14.21).

The anomalous left artery at term thus represents only the embryonic pulmonary artery; the elongated pulmo-

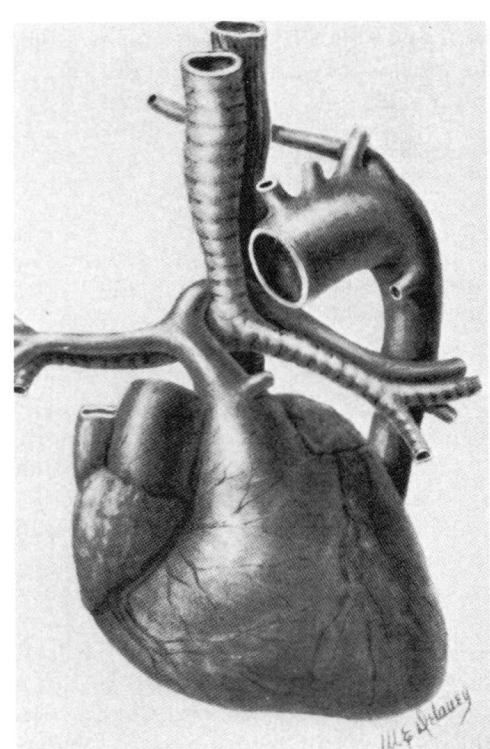

Figure 14.20. Retrotracheal left pulmonary artery. The distal trachea narrows, and a retroesophageal right subclavian artery is also present. (From Wittenborg MH, Tantiwongse T, Rosenberg BF. Anomalous course of left pulmonary artery with respiratory obstruction. Radiology 1956;67:339–345.)

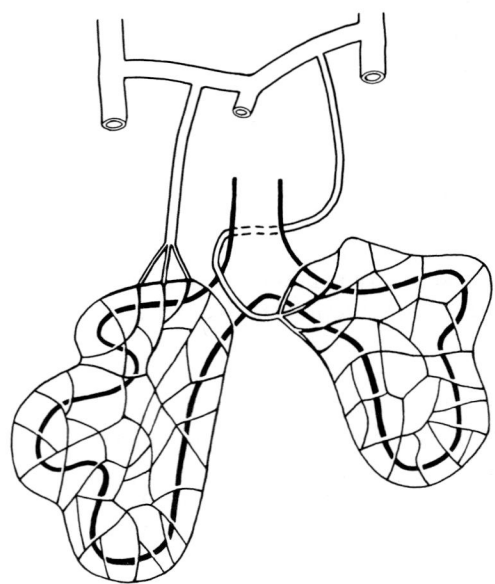

Figure 14.21. Course of primitive pulmonary arteries between the sixth aortic arch and the vascular plexus of the lung buds. The right artery has formed normally; the left artery has passed in front of the bronchus and behind the trachea, resulting in a retrotracheal artery.

nary trunk represents fusion of the proximal left sixth arch with the proximal right arch; and the ligamentum arteriosum represents the normally atrophied distal left sixth arch.

This explanation, first suggested by Contro and his colleagues (148) in 1958, is reasonable. It is curious, however, that among all the conceivable anomalous connections between the embryonic pulmonary artery and the pulmonary vascular plexus, only this specific one is known to occur—and this only on the left side. There is remarkably little variation in the few cases of this anomaly recorded (145).

The defect may be an isolated one (148), or there may be associated malformations (149). In one patient, who had a retrotracheal pulmonary artery, there was an aberrant right subclavian artery and a persistent left superior vena cava as well as absence of one kidney and malrotation of the gut. Persistent left superior vena cava and atrial septal defects are most frequently encountered.

INCIDENCE

The first case was described in 1897 by Glaevecke and Doehle (150). By 1965 there were 29 cases in the literature (146), 23 of which were confirmed at necropsy. Seventeen occurred in males, twelve in females.

SYMPTOMS

Respiratory distress, with prolonged, wheezing respiration, is present at birth. Emphysema on the right with mediastinal shift to the left may develop postnatally. There are often episodes of cyanosis. Dysphagia may occur, but it is not common (149). In three cases symptoms were mild or absent (146).

DIAGNOSIS AND DIFFERENTIAL DIAGNOSIS

A lateral esophagram will demonstrate an anterior constriction of the esophagus at the level of the carina. This is in contrast to a posterior constriction produced by a retroesophageal subclavian artery. Deviation of the trachea to the left and constriction of the right bronchus may be seen on a bronchogram (144).

TREATMENT

Untreated patients usually die within 6 months from generalized emphysema and pneumonia. One case has been reported in a 79-year-old man who suffered from dysphagia in the last few months of life only (151).

In 1954 Potts (53) performed the first successful repair by sectioning the left pulmonary artery at its origin and rejoining the ends at the same site anterior to the trachea. Fourteen such operations were performed, with four survivals, according to Jue et al. in 1965 (146). Mustard and his associates (152) obtained relief of symptoms

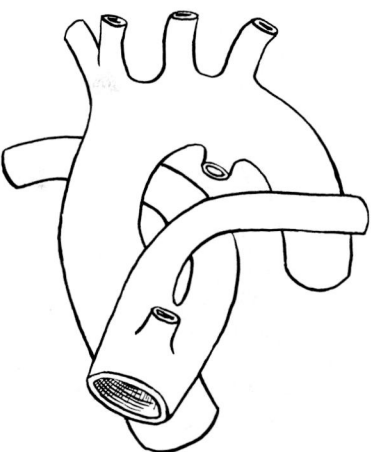

Figure 14.22. Crossed pulmonary arteries. The cut ends of the ductus arteriosus are shown. (After Jue KL, Lockman LA, Edwards JE. Anomalous origins of pulmonary arteries from pulmonary trunk ("crossed pulmonary arteries"): observation in a case with 18 trisomy syndrome. Am Heart J 1966;71:807–812.)

for patients by sectioning the ligamentum arteriosum, thus opening the vascular ring surrounding the trachea.

Crossed Pulmonary Arteries

In an apparently unique pulmonary arterial anomaly, the left pulmonary artery arose from the right side of the pulmonary trunk, crossing in front of the right pulmonary artery (146). The appearance was that of a normal pulmonary arterial bifurcation rotated 120 degrees counterclockwise. The pulmonary circulation was not altered by this arrangement (Fig. 14.22).

The patient was a newborn female with chromosome 18 trisomy. The usual stigmata of micrognathia, arched palate, low-set ears, limited adduction of hip joints, and overlapping of the third and fourth fingers by the index and little fingers, as well as an atrial septal defect, were present.

Coarctation of the Pulmonary Arteries

Although coarctation of the aorta has been known for centuries, only in the past few decades has it been appreciated that similar congenital narrowing can occur in the pulmonary trunk or in more distal branches of the pulmonary artery.

ANATOMY

The stenosis may affect the main pulmonary trunk, the right or left pulmonary artery, or segmental branches of the pulmonary arteries. Gay and his colleagues (154) classified the stenoses as follows (Fig. 14.7):

Type I: Single stenosis involving the pulmonary trunk or the right or left pulmonary artery

Type II: Stenosis of the pulmonary trunk at its bifurcation, extending into both pulmonary arteries

Type III: Multiple stenoses of the segmental arteries to one or both lungs

Type IV: Stenoses of type I or II, combined with those of type III

The stenoses may be very short, or they may form a long, narrowed segment of artery; often there is a distal, thin-walled enlargement. The narrowed segment shows fibrous proliferation of the intima, while the dilated segment shows a loss of elastic fibers in the tunica media.

Intimal hyperplasia with deficiency of the tunica media in even more distal pulmonary arteries has been described by Rubin and Strauss (155) and may be a variety of Gay and associates' (154) type III stenoses.

ASSOCIATED ANOMALIES

In 65 of 105 cases of pulmonary coarctation reviewed by Gay and his colleagues (154), associated cardiac anomalies were present. Pulmonary valvular stenosis occurred in 30%, and atrial septal defect, ventricular septal defect, and tetralogy of Fallot each were present in 15%.

EMBRYOGENESIS

No reasonable developmental explanation has been put forward to account for all the types of pulmonary coarctation. Types I and II have been related to the possible presence of ductus arteriosus tissue in the pulmonary artery (see the discussion on the "Skodiac" theory in Chapter 28, "The Thoracic and Abdominal Aorta") (156). This, however, will not explain type III stenoses. The association of pulmonary coarctation with valvular pulmonary stenosis suggests a widespread pulmonary vascular defect rather than a simple malformation of sixth arch development.

HISTORY AND INCIDENCE

In 1909 Schwalbe (157) mentioned pulmonary artery stenosis. Falkenbach et al. (158) could find only 23 cases by 1959. Gay and co-workers (154) at Emory University, who introduced the present classification, found 105 cases and added 15 of their own in 1963. By 1965 McCue and her colleagues (33) had found 319 cases in the literature, to which they added 20 others. Son et al. (159) added 10 cases in 1966. This great increase in reported cases is the result of increased use of angiocardiography; it suggests pulmonary coarctation is not a rare lesion.

Four families with two or more affected members each have been reported. No sex difference has been mentioned. The majority of cases were recognized in childhood, but several have been reported in adults, according to Franch and Gay (160).

SYMPTOMS

Symptoms are not specific and may be obscured by the presence of other cardiac defects. Dyspnea, reduced resistance to fatigue, growth retardation, and frequent respiratory infection are the most usual symptoms. Their severity depends on the degree of pulmonary resistance present.

DIAGNOSIS

The only basis for a firm diagnosis of pulmonary coarctation is angiocardiographic visualization of the pulmonary artery and its branches.

Catheterization of the pulmonary artery will show a pressure gradient across the constricted area. There will be a wide pulse pressure and a marked dicrotic notch in pulmonary artery pressure tracings. The electrocardiogram may show right ventricular strain, but otherwise it is unremarkable. Diminished pulmonary vascular markings may appear on a plain chest radiograph.

TREATMENT

Pulmonary coarctations of types I and II are amenable to surgery. A longitudinal incision, with a transverse closure, was performed by Thrower et al. (161). Baxter and his colleagues (162) relieved a right pulmonary artery stenosis with a Teflon graft. In at least one patient a tetralogy of Fallot was corrected with resection of a stenotic pulmonary bifurcation (33). Types III and IV must be considered inoperable at present.

PROGNOSIS

Coarctation affecting only one of the pulmonary arteries may produce few symptoms and may not adversely affect the life span of the patient. Bilateral narrowing of the arteries will produce elevation of right ventricular pressure. Intimal proliferation may be progressive, and the poststenotic dilations may become aneurysms, with eventual rupture and hemorrhage.

In a number of cases the prognosis is governed by the severity of the associated cardiac defect rather than by the pulmonary coarctation itself.

Variations of the Bronchial Arteries

The systemic arterial supply to the lungs, which are the nutrient arteries of the organ and also supply the bronchial glands and partially the esophagus and pericardium, normally consists of one right and two left bronchial arteries arising from the thoracic aorta or from an intercostal artery, but there are many variations. Cauldwell et al. (163) found the following combinations in 150 cadavers:

One right, two left: 40.7%
One right, one left: 21.3%

Two right, two left: 20.7%
Two right, one left: 9.3%
Other combinations: 8.0%

In nearly 90% of the population, the right bronchial arteries arise from the fifth or sixth right intercostal arteries, occasionally from as high as the third or from as low as the seventh intercostal arteries. The left bronchial arteries usually arise from the aorta, the upper one sometimes having a common stem with the right bronchial artery.

Enlarged bronchial arteries may be the chief or even the only supply of blood to the lungs in the absence of, or with hypoplasia of, the pulmonary arteries (Fig. 14.10, *type VI*). O'Rahilly et al. (164) reported subclavian origin of the bronchial arteries. Menke (165) noted right anomalous bronchial artery from the right subclavian artery.

Variations of the Pulmonary Veins

Two right and two left pulmonary veins emptying into the left atrium is the normal state. A common left or right pulmonary vein, representing incomplete absorption of the primitive common vein into the atrial wall, is present in nearly 25% of individuals (166). Almost all of these are on the left. In contrast, if the drainage is anomalous, a right common pulmonary vein is more frequent.

A third vein may be present on either side, more often on the right (1.6%, according to Healey [166]). Four, five, and even six pulmonary veins have been reported; all but the last configuration having been on the right side. One or more of these multiple veins usually open at an anomalous site. Multiple veins represent excessive resorption of the pulmonary veins into the atrial wall.

According to Lucas et al. (167) the pulmonary veins are thin walled and do not have any valves. The intima is one to two cell layers thick. The internal elastic lamina is present, but the external is rarely, if ever, present. There is no distinction between media and adventitia.

Nasrallah et al. (168) successfully treated a 16-month-old boy with a right pneumonectomy after the diagnosis of unilateral pulmonary vein atresia was made.

Niimi et al. (169) reported a patient with three pulmonary veins present on the right side which emptied into the left atrium, one of the veins arising from the upper lobe.

Stenosis of the Common Pulmonary Vein (Cor Triatriatum)

In this anomaly, the left atrium appears to be doubled; the pulmonary veins empty into the supernumerary chamber, and there is no alternative pulmonary drainage (Figs. 14.23, 14.24, and 14.25, *D*).

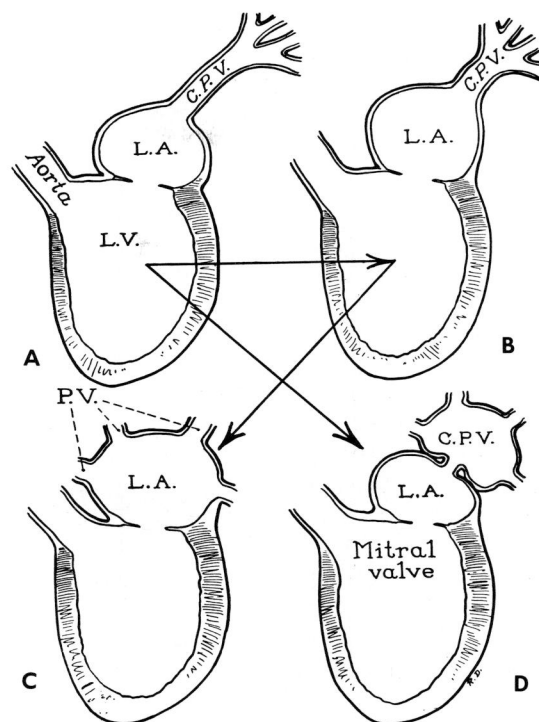

Figure 14.23. The developmental basis of cor triatriatum. In normal development (**A** to **C**), the pulmonary veins join to form the common pulmonary vein (*C.P.V.*), which subsequently becomes incorporated into the wall of the left atrium (*L.A.*). **D,** The anomaly occurs when the common pulmonary vein has not been absorbed into the atrium and becomes dilated until it resembles a third atrium. *P.V.,* Pulmonary veins; *L.V.,* left ventricle. (From Edwards JE, DuShane JW, Alcott DL, Burchell HB. Thoracic venous anomalies. Arch Pathol 1951;51:446–460.)

Loeffler (170) divided these defects into three groups, of increasing severity: (*a*) those with adequate atrial opening but with a large extra atrial sinus, (*b*) those in which the stenotic opening is small, and (*c*) those in which the communication is entirely obliterated and venous return from the lungs is impossible. Patients who fall into the first group may have a normal life span. However, those in the second group, which is the largest, die in infancy with right ventricular enlargement. Those in the third group have no pulmonary return and die at birth. One case of only partial pulmonary drainage into such an accessory chamber has been reported (171).

The accessory "atrium" represents the dilated embryonic common pulmonary vein. It fails to become absorbed into the atrial wall and dilates as a result of a stenotic opening into the true atrium (Fig. 14.23). The stenosis or atresia, which appears to be the primary defect, dates from before the eighth week. Edwards et al. (172) provided the true explanation of the anomaly. They proposed the term *congenital stenosis of the common pulmonary vein* to supersede the older *cor triatriatum.*

The first case was described as a double left atrium by Church (173) in 1868. Jimenez-Martinez et al. (174)

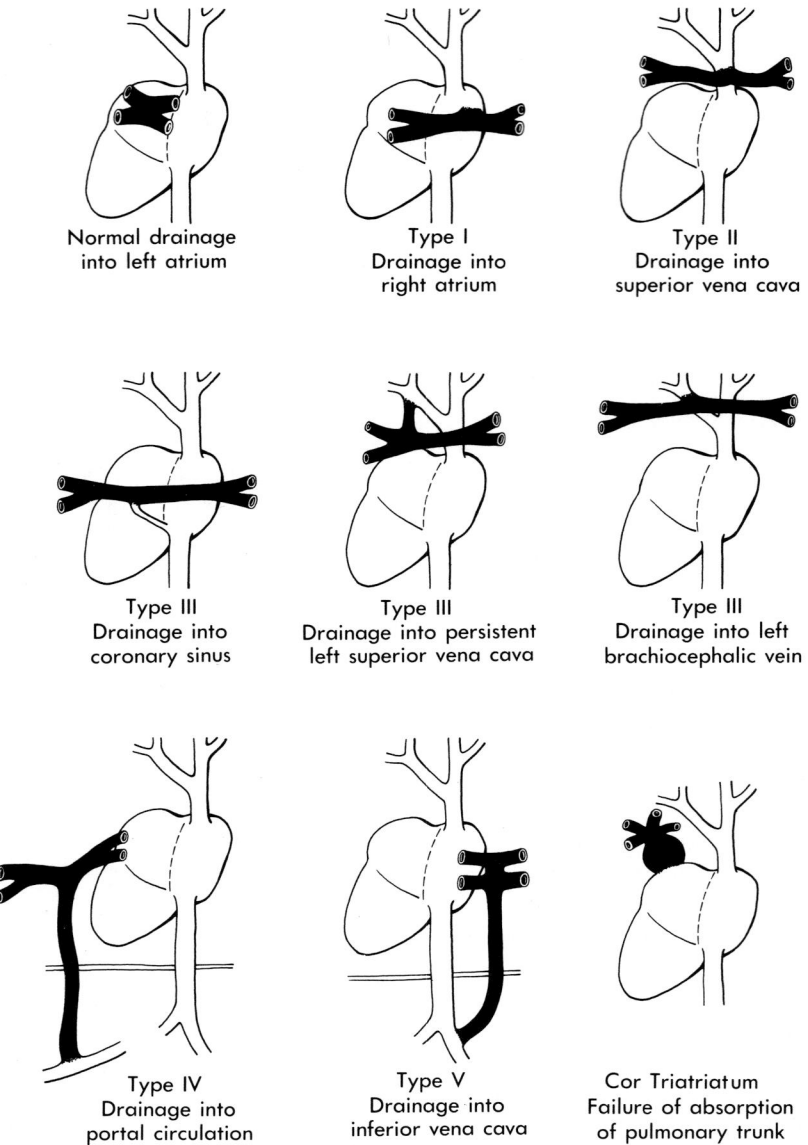

Figure 14.24.   Sites of anomalous drainage of the pulmonary veins. Drainage may be total (as shown in the diagrams), or it may
be only partial.

could find only 72 cases in 1969. They added a case of
their own, in which the defect was associated with agenesis of the pericardium. The first successful repair was by
Vineberg and Gialloretto (175) in 1956.

Hammon et al. (176) stated that the operative mortality is difficult to estimate due to the small number of
reported cases.

Stenosis of Branches of the Pulmonary Veins

Pulmonary stenosis also is unilateral or bilateral involving
right, left, or both pulmonary veins. Edwards (177) and
Lucas et al. (178) studied this anomaly well. In 1986 Reid
et al. (179) presented a fine paper covering this topic.

Reid et al. (179) noted a case of a 16-year-old girl with
right pulmonary vein stenosis. The laveophase test
showed no venous return on the right. They performed a
successful right pneuomonectomy.

Adey et al. (180) reported seven patients with congenital pulmonary vein stenosis. They stated that the left-
sided pulmonary veins are more involved. They emphasized that this anomaly may be suspected when asymmetry
of pulmonary vascularity appears in one lung with chest
film.

Pappas (181) noted two cases with left pulmonary vein
stenosis associated with dextrotransposition of the great
arteries and without ventricular septal defect. Dev and
Shrivastava (182) reported a 1½-year-old female with ste-

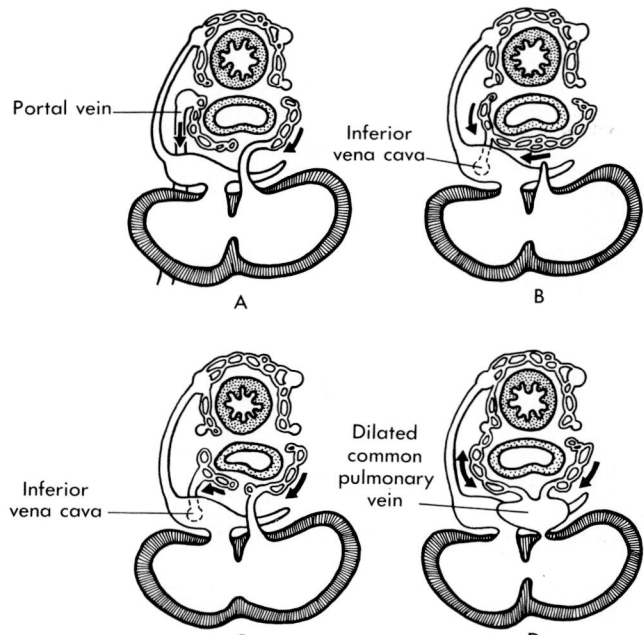

Figure 14.25. Abnormal development of the venous drainage of the foregut. **A**, Type IV. Partial anomalous pulmonary drainage into the umbilicovitelline system (portal vein or hepatic vein). **B**, Type V. Total anomalous pulmonary drainage into the posterior cardinal system (inferior vena cava). **C**, Type V. Partial anomalous pulmonary drainage into the inferior vena cava with right lung hypoplasia ("scimitar syndrome"). **D**, Cor triatriatum. Stenosis with proximal dilation of the common pulmonary vein and partial anomalous drainage into the superior vena cava (type II).

nosis of left upper and middle lobe pulmonary veins, arterial hypertension, and atrial and ventrical septal defects.

Muhler et al. (183) reported a case of stenosis of all pulmonary veins producing pulmonary hypertension which was diagnosed by cineangiography by selective injections into the right and left pulmonary artery branches. Surgery was not successful, and the authors feel congenital stenosis of all pulmonary veins is a rapidly progressive congenital anomaly.

Anomalous Venous Drainage of the Lungs

CLASSIFICATION

If one or more of the pulmonary veins empties into the systemic circulation instead of into the left atrium, respiratory efficiency is impaired.

A number of varieties of such anomalous pulmonary drainage are known. On an embryologic basis, they may be divided into five types as follows (Fig. 14.24):

  I. Drainage into the right atrium
  II. Drainage into the derivatives of the right cardinal system (superior vena cava, azygos vein)
  III. Drainage into the derivatives of the left cardinal system (persistent left superior vena cava, coronary sinus, left brachiocephalic vein)

  IV. Drainage into the umbilicovitelline system (hepatic portal vein, ductus venosus)
  V. Drainage into the inferior vena cava.

This classification is modified from that of Neill (18). Other classifications have been proposed by Darling and his colleagues (184) and by Edwards and Helmholz (185). Taussig (186) lumped together the first three groups and classified them according to whether the anomalous venous return was negligible, partial, or total.

From the viewpoint of physiologic function and clinical evaluation, the most useful division of these anomalies is that of Brody (187) and many subsequent writers (188, 189).

  1. Partial drainage into the right atrium
  2. Total drainage into the right atrium with no associated cardiac anomalies
  3. Total drainage into the right atrium with associated cardiac anomalies.

In the terms of these classifications, we may state:

  1. Most anomalous pulmonary drainage is partial rather than total.
  2. About 50% of patients with anomalous pulmonary drainage have associated cardiac anomalies.
  3. Most total anomalous pulmonary drainage is into the superior vena cava.
  4. Most partial anomalous pulmonary drainage is into the right atrium.

Lucas et al. (167) reported 49 cases of total anomalous pulmonary venous connection. They made an anatomical comparison of the frequency site of connection with the cases of Burrows and Edwards (190) and Delisle et al. (191).

According to Dehner (25), total anomalous pulmonary vein return with drainage into the superior vena cava or right atrium is one of the more frequent anomalies. Such cases were reported by Delisle et al. (191), Duff et al. (192), and Haworth and Reid (193).

Holder and Ashcroft (194) classified anomalous total pulmonary venous drainage according to the route that blood follows from the common pulmonary vein to the right atrium (Fig. 14.26). Of course, they recognized that the blood may follow different routes and pathways to reach the heart.

ANATOMY

Pulmonary Drainage into the Right Atrium. Partial drainage to the right atrium is found in about 25% of reported cases of anomalous pulmonary return. It is slightly less frequent in patients with complete anomalous drainage. The term *transposition of pulmonary veins* has been used by Nadas (195) for this defect.

Pulmonary Drainage into Derivatives of the Right Cardinal System. The superior vena cava is the most common site

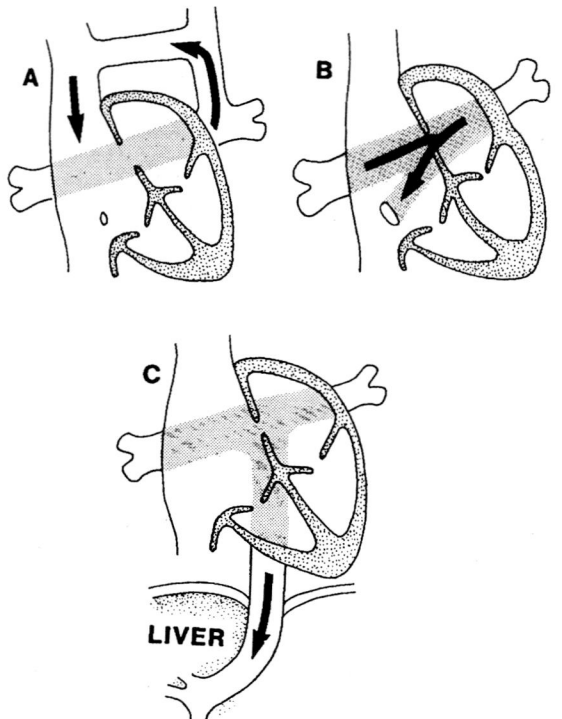

Figure 14.26. Total anomalous pulmonary venous drainage is classified according to the route by which blood from the common pulmonary vein drains to the right atrium. In addition to the three pictured here, there are varieties of mixed drainage, wherein pulmonary drainage may reach the heart by different routes. **A,** Supracardiac total anomalous pulmonary venous drainage is the most common type. The blood flow from the common pulmonary veins reaches the heart by way of an ascending vein, across the innominate vein, and down through the superior vena cava. Mixed caval blood is then distributed, partly to the right and partly to the left ventricle through the atrial septal defect, so that oxygen saturation in the aorta and pulmonary artery are very nearly equal. **B,** The cardiac level drainage from the confluent pulmonary veins is by way of the coronary sinus. **C,** The infracardiac type drains through the diaphragm and usually into the portal system below the liver. Because of the interposed hepatic vascular bed, the venous pressure is considerably increased, making this the most lethal of the types of total anomalous pulmonary venous drainage. Oxygenated blood in this instance reaches the right atrium by way of the inferior vena cava. (From Holder TM, Ashcraft KW. Cardiac surgery. In: Welch KJ, Randolph JG, Ravitch MM, O'Neill JA, Rowe MI, eds. Pediatric surgery. Chicago: Year Book Medical Publishers, 1986:1383.)

Table 14.5.
Sites of Total Anomalous Pulmonary Drainage[a]

Site	Associated Cardiac Defects		Total	Percentage
	Present	Absent		
Type I			30	18.1
Right atrium	13	17		
Type II			31	19.0
Right superior vena cava	14	12		
Right innominate vein	2	0		
Azygos vein	3	0		
Type III			74	45.4
Left innominate vein	10	41		
Coronary sinus	0	18		
Left superior vena cava	5	0		
Type IV			24	14.7
Portal vein	10	7		
Ductus venosus	2	4		
Hepatic vein	0	1		
Type V			4	2.5
Inferior vena cava	2	2		
	61	102	163	100.0

[a]Figures taken from Burroughs JT, Edwards JE. Total anomalous pulmonary venous connections. Am Heart J 1960;59:913–931.

the confluence of the pulmonary veins to join the brachiocephalic vein (197).

Drainage also may be into the proximal remnant of the left cardinal system—the left horn of the sinus venosus—which becomes the coronary sinus in the adult heart.

In 1988 Lucas et al. (167) reported 18 cases of total anomalous pulmonary vein connection to the left innominate vein. In their comments, the authors reported that the vertical vein, whether obstructed or not, was abnormal.

Pulmonary Drainage into the Umbilicovitelline System. Anomalous pulmonary veins occasionally penetrate the diaphragm to empty into the portal vein, the ductus venosus, or the hepatic veins. Although Brody found no such cases in 1942 (187), at least 37 cases were reported 20 years later (198). Butler (17) collected 13 cases, of which four had no other serious cardiac anomalies and in which the anomalous vein drained directly into the ductus venosus. In eight other cases, the pulmonary vein drained into a grossly dilated left gastric vein, which emptied into the portal vein. Cardiac anomalies were present in most of this second group of patients. In one case (199) the anomalous vein divided to enter the ductus venosus (obliterated), the portal vein, and intrahepatic veins of the quadrate lobe.

Lucas et al. (167) reported anomalous connection to the portal vein in 10 cases and to the ductus venosus in one. The same authors presented four cases of intrathoracic obstruction of the anomalous vein. The portal vein connection produced severe intrahepatic obstruction.

of partial anomalous drainage. Less often, it receives all the pulmonary veins (196). If the pulmonary veins enter the azygos vein, the superior vena cava may appear to enter the azygos or to receive the azygos, depending on its size.

Lucas et al. (167) reported six cases of pulmonary venous drainage by means of an anomalous vein to the right superior vena cava close to the right atrium.

Pulmonary Drainage into Derivates of the Left Cardinal System. The left brachiocephalic (innominate) vein is the most common site of total anomalous drainage (Table 14.5). A partially persistent left superior vena cava ascends from

Pulmonary Drainage into the Inferior Vena Cava. Total anomalous pulmonary drainage into the inferior vena cava below the diaphragm is rare (200, 201) (Fig. 14.25, *B*).

Kittle and Crockett (202) collected 13 cases in which blood from the right lung drained to the inferior vena cava. There were no cardiac anomalies other than atrial septal defects. When malformation is associated with right lung hypoplasia and systemic pulmonary arteries, it has been called the "scimitar syndrome" by Neill and her colleagues (203) and the "vena cava bronchovascular syndrome" by Kittle and Crockett (202). This complex is discussed separately later.

Vitarelli et al. (204) reported three patients with total anomalous pulmonary venous drainage, two supracardiac (left vertical vein or right superior vena cava) and one infracardiac to the inferior vena cava.

Miscellaneous Anomalous Drainage. Multiple sites of anomalous drainage of pulmonary veins have been reported frequently (205).

Five cases of total anomalous pulmonary venous connection to the coronary sinus was reported by Lucas et al. in 1988 (167). Of these, two cases exhibited draining in both coronary sinuses and the left innominate vein; in one of these cases the right pulmonary vein was trapped between the left pulmonary artery and the left main stem bronchus with severe narrowing in the point of entrapment. The third case included connection of the right upper pulmonary vein to the right superior vena cava and the remaining vein to the pulmonary vein. In the fourth case, the left pulmonary veins and the right middle pulmonary vein joined a stenotic vertical vein, which communicated with the left innominate vein. In the fifth case, the hypoplastic right pulmonary veins were connected to the ductus arteriosus through a hypoplastic anomalous vein.

Vogel et al. (206) studied four patients with transposition of the great arteries and unilateral pulmonary vein stenosis, all on the left side. The authors believe this type of congenital pathology becomes progressive as a result of postnatal preferential flow to the right lung.

According to Askin (23), lymphangiectasis may be prominent in the pulmonary parenchyma.

RELATIVE FREQUENCY

Occasionally, some or all of the pulmonary veins end blindly, without connecting with the heart or other vessels. What pulmonary return exists is usually anomalous (207, 208). A study of three patients with atresia of the common pulmonary vein is presented in Table 14.6.

Extent of the Anomalous Pulmonary Drainage. Of 86 cases of incomplete anomalous drainage of the lung collected by Healey (166), there were 22 cases in which blood from the

Table 14.6.
Clinical Findings in Three Patients with Atresia of the Common Pulmonary Vein[a]

Site of Connection	Burroughs & Edwards[b] 113 Cases (%)	Lucas et al. 49 Cases (%)	Delisle et al.[c] 93 Cases (%)
Left innominate vein	36	37	26
Coronary sinus	16	16	18
Right atrium	15	2	8
Right superior vena cava	11	12	15
Portal system	13	23	24
Multiple sites	7	10	5
Unknown or other	2	0	4

[a]From Lucas RV et al. Gross and histologic anatomy of total anomalous pulmonary venous connections. Am J Cardiol 1988;62(4):229–300.
[b]Burroughs JT, Edwards JE. Total anomalous pulmonary venous connection. Am Heart J 1960;59:913–931.
[c]Delisle G et al. Total anomalous pulmonary connection: report of 93 autopsied cases with emphasis on diagnostic and surgical considerations. Am Heart J 1976;91:99–122.

whole of the right lung drained abnormally and 11 in which blood from the whole of the left lung did so. When only a portion of one lung was involved, it was usually the upper lobe.

ASSOCIATED ANOMALIES

Cardiac anomalies are present concomitantly in about 50% of these patients. Cor biloculare, cor triloculare biatriatum, dextrocardia, transposition of great vessels, atrioventricularis communis, truncus arteriosus, coarctation of the aorta, and atrioventricular septal defects have all been reported (188). Among the various types of total anomalous drainage, only that into the coronary sinus is rarely accompanied by other cardiovascular defects. A patent foramen ovale is present in all cases of total anomalous drainage.

Total anomalous pulmonary venous connection with right isomerism was reported by DiDonaho et al. (209).

EMBRYOGENESIS

The common pulmonary vein forms as an endothelial outgrowth from the sinoatrial region of the developing heart, to the left of septum primum, and to the left of the left valve of the sinus venosus. The outgrowth makes contact with the pulmonary venous plexus surrounding the developing lung buds at the end of the fifth week (stage 14; 6 to 7 mm). Normally, the anterior (ventral) portion of the plexus of veins around the foregut becomes the pulmonary plexus of the lung buds and separates from the posterior (dorsal) portion, which is associated with the esophagus except for anastomoses with the bronchial circulation. When the common pulmonary vein reaches the

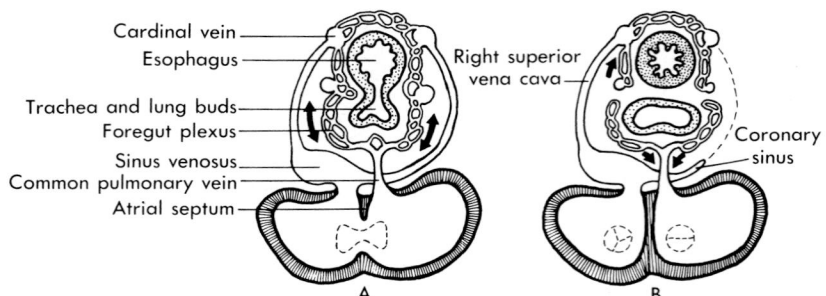

Figure 14.27. Schematic diagram of the normal development of venous drainage of the embryonic foregut. **A,** Tracheal bud and esophagus are not separated. Venous drainage is through the anterior cardinal system and through the common pulmonary vein. **B,** Separation of the trachea and lung buds from the esophagus. The venous plexus normally separates so that esophageal veins drain through the anterior cardinal system on the right side (superior vena cava) into the sinus venosus and the right atrium. Pulmonary veins drain entirely through the common pulmonary vein into the left atrium.

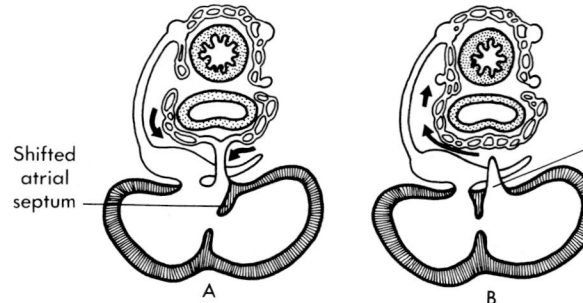

Figure 14.28. Abnormal development of the venous drainage of the foregut. **A,** Type I. Total anomalous pulmonary drainage into the right atrium. The atrial septum and the common pulmonary vein are transposed. **B,** Type II. Total anomalous pulmonary drainage through derivatives of the right cardinal system (usually superior vena cava). The common pulmonary vein is absent.

pulmonary plexus, connection with the cardinal system disappears (Fig. 14.27). The common pulmonary vein is later resorbed into the wall of the growing atrium so that four pulmonary veins enter the atrium separately (Fig. 14.23). The development of each of the anomalous types may now be considered.

Type I (Fig. 14.28, A). Neill (18) speculated that a type I anomaly would result from a slight shift of the location of the atrial septum to the left. The normal opening of the common pulmonary vein is very close to the septum. If this explanation is correct, the error occurs in the late fifth or early sixth week.

Type II (Fig. 14.28, B). Failure of the common pulmonary vein to form, or its subsequent resorption, results in persistence of a connection between the pulmonary venous plexus and the right cardinal vein (superior vena cava). Such a connection is ontogenetically a bronchial vein; when it assumes the role of a pulmonary vein, it is a "pulmonized bronchial vein" (21, 187).

Edwards and his colleagues (172) described a case in which atresia of the proximal portion of the common pulmonary vein had occurred, which might have produced dilation and the appearance of an accessory "atrium." However, because of a persistent connection with the superior vena cava, no dilation of the atretic vein occurred.

Type III (Fig. 14.29). In these cases the persistent pulmonary plexus connection is with the left horn of the sinus venosus, possibly after the common pulmonary vein has formed and subsequently separated from the atrium (18) (Fig. 14.29, A). This occurs in the fifth or sixth week. An alternate theory positing a connection between the foregut plexus and the normally transitory, paired caudal outpocketings from the sinus region in the fourth week, was proposed by Auër (16) to account for this anomaly.

If the left sinus horn then atrophies proximal to the entrance of the common pulmonary vein, a short persistent left superior vena cava will join the right superior vena cava by way of the innominate vein. The pulmonary return will be to the right atrium (Fig. 14.29, B).

If the left sinus horn atrophies distal to the entrance of the common pulmonary vein, the drainage is through the coronary sinus to the right atrium (Fig. 14.29, C).

Type IV (Fig. 14.25, A). Failure of the common pulmonary vein to tap the pulmonary venous plexus must be assumed, together with loss of connection with the cardinal system. Drainage is through the primitive connection, with the splanchnic plexus of the foregut following

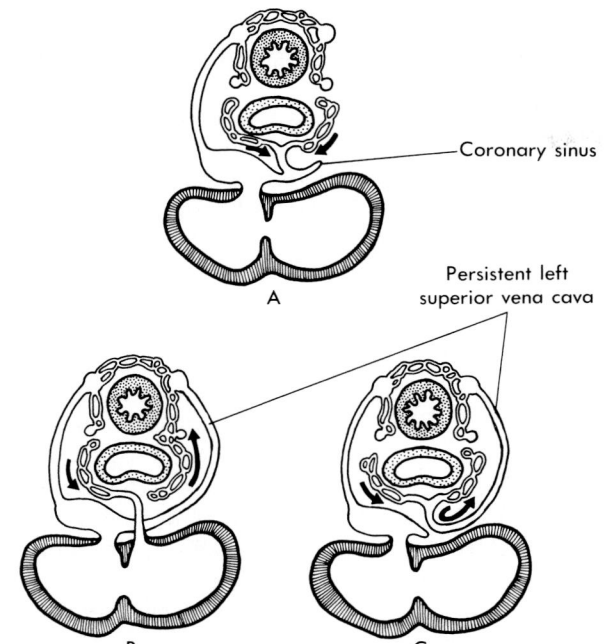

Figure 14.29. Type III abnormal development of the venous drainage of the foregut. **A,** Total anomalous pulmonary drainage into the coronary sinus and thence into the right atrium. **B,** Partial anomalous pulmonary drainage into a persistent left superior vena cava, which opens into the coronary sinus. **C,** Total anomalous pulmonary drainage through a persistent left superior vena cava into the right superior vena and thence to the right atrium.

the esophagus to the portal vein or the ductus venosus. This anomaly appears to date from the fifth week.

Type V (Fig. 14.25, B and C). This defect probably represents the absence of true pulmonary veins. The vessels that penetrate the diaphragm to reach the inferior vena cava represent persistent embryonic connections of the primitive foregut plexus with the posterior cardinal system secondarily absorbed by the inferior vena cava.

Total anomalous drainage at this site is known, but the usual form involves the right side only, with right lung hypoplasia. The "scimitar syndrome," as it has been called, is discussed separately in this text.

HISTORY

In 1739 Winslow first reported an anomalous pulmonary vein draining into the superior vena cava (187), and in 1798 Wilson (210) first described total anomalous pulmonary drainage. Not until 1942, when Brody (187) collected 106 cases, was an attempt made to analyze these anomalies. Smith (188), Healey (166), and Parsons et al. (189) brought the number to 155. Neill (18) in 1956 discussed the embryology of the various types of pulmonary vein anomalies. In 1960 she and her colleagues (203) added an analysis of patients with anomalous drainage into the inferior vena cava. Kittle and Crockett (202) col-

lected 180 cases of anomalous drainage of the right lung and 40 of the left lung.

INCIDENCE

The incidence of partial anomalous pulmonary veins in cadavers was found by Healey (166) to be 0.62%, or 1:160. Because many individuals with one anomalous vein (and a few with two) have no symptoms, the clinical incidence is less than the above figures would indicate.

Total anomalous drainage was found in 12 autopsies among 304 in which the cause of death was congenital cardiovascular disease (211).

Males are predominantly affected in types I to IV defects, whether the anomalous drainage is complete or incomplete. Smith (188) found 131 males and 57 females affected. Kittle and Crockett (202) found an equal distribution of sexes in patients with venous drainage to the inferior vena cava (type VI).

SYMPTOMS AND PROGNOSIS

The degree of functional impairment of the circulation resulting from anomalous pulmonary venous drainage depends upon the proportion of pulmonary blood shunted into the systemic circulation, rather than on the site of the anomalous drainage. A single pulmonary vein opening into the right side of the heart is usually asymptomatic and will be detected clinically only by accident. With the presence of a larger shunt, symptoms become increasingly marked. Brody (187) set the upper limit for continued survival: "When less than 50% of the pulmonary return is abnormally carried into the major venous circulation, there is little likelihood of decompensation, and such persons reach adult age."

Holder and Ashcraft (194) summarized the symptoms and prognosis as follows: Pulmonary venous hypertension with severe hypoxia is noted in the infracardiac type when the anomalous pulmonary venous drainage enters the portal system. When the coronary sinus is involved, the so-called cardiac type, again pulmonary venous hypertension is developed. The supracardiac type where the right and left pulmonary vein join behind the heart and drain into the SVC with the help of an ascending vein, is the least often associated with pulmonary venous hypertension.

The prognosis with the infracardiac type is not good. Bove et al. (212) reported a mortality of 25–30% due to acidosis in neonates.

Partial Anomalous Drainage. When the drainage is only partly anomalous, and an open foramen ovale exists, cardiac enlargement begins after birth but is not progressive, and a reasonably normal life span may be expected. If the foramen ovale closes, right heart enlargement is progressive until death, which occurs 4 to 6 months after birth.

Dyspnea, tachypnea, cyanosis on crying, and distension of neck veins are frequent symptoms. The patient may tire easily, gain weight slowly, and develop chest asymmetry. The liver is usually enlarged. Cardiac murmurs may or may not be present.

The smaller the amount of anomalous drainage and the larger the atrial septal defect, the better the prognosis. Among Brody's collected cases (187), all but two patients with only one anomalous vein (75% return to the left atrium) survived to adulthood. The presence and nature of other cardiac anomalies greatly influence the prognosis.

Total Anomalous Drainage. Unless a large compensatory shunt is present, total pulmonary return to the right heart is fatal at birth. Healey (166) found 11 of 61 patients who had survived for more than 1 year. One lived for 4 years (200). Two had patent ductus arteriosus, one had an atrial septal defect, two had a single atrium, and six had patent foramen ovale. Taussig (186) believed that although the increased pressure of the right atrium tends to keep the foramen open, there is a corresponding tendency for it to close with increasing age despite the pressure difference. Cyanosis may be absent at birth, but it becomes more marked as the heart increasingly enlarges. Death results from right heart failure.

Burroughs and Edwards (190) suggested that the shorter the route taken by the blood from the lungs and the wider the interatrial defect, the better the prognosis. Thus patients with total anomalous drainage to the superior vena cava, coronary sinus, or right atrium (types I to III) and those with an atrial septal defect have a longer life expectancy than do those with drainage to the portal vein or ductus venosus (type IV) and with a patent foramen ovale. This simply means that, the less the resistance in the venous return, the lower the pulmonary pressure and the longer right heart failure is postponed.

DIAGNOSIS

Increasing enlargement of the right side of the heart, beginning during the first month of life, is the most significant indication of abnormal pulmonary return. Increased vascularity of the lung fields and prominent pulmonary arteries also may appear radiographically (213). The electrocardiogram may show right axis deviation. Cyanosis appears only late in the course of the disease.

Cardiac catheterization and angiocardiography are necessary to confirm the diagnosis and to determine the site of anomalous return. Oxygen saturation is high in the right atrium; if the anomalous return is total, it is higher in the right than in the left atrium. These determinations will rule out coarctation or aortic atresia. The septal defect alone will not produce a decrease in arterial oxygen with exercise. If the catheter can be passed into an anomalous vein, the diagnosis is, of course, confirmed.

It should be kept in mind that atrial septal defects in these patients provide a life-saving right-to-left shunt to compensate for the left-to-right shunt formed by the anomalous pulmonary veins.

Long et al. (214) reported that helpful radiographic features include: small heart, congested lungs, perhaps plural effusion, and visualization of the anomalous trunk overlying the liver. Umbilical catheterization was pathognomic in three cases.

TREATMENT

Surgical repair for total anomalous venous return was not deemed feasible even as late as 1947 (215). The use of the heart-lung bypass methods introduced by Cooley and his associates (216, 217) has made successful correction easier.

Anastomosis of the pulmonary trunk to the left atrium with repair of the atrial septal defect is the operative procedure. The atrial septum may have to be shifted to provide a left atrium of adequate size. Because of inadequacy of the left atrium, it may be necessary to leave some of the septal defect unclosed to keep left atrial pressure within normal limits.

Both partial and total anomalous pulmonary return have been treated surgically with marked success. Zubiate et al. (218) reported 23 successful operations in 35 patients.

With total anomalous pulmonary venous drainage, the oxygenated venous blood is mixed in toto in the right atrium with systemic venous blood. Several procedures are used for the correction of this anomaly:

1. Enlargement of the atrial septal defect
2. Retrocardial open anastomosis, used by Breckenridge et al. (219)
3. Transantrial open anastomosis, used by Hawkins and associates (220)

Holder and Ashcraft (194) reported 12 cases with good results.

Podzolkov et al. (221) reported several cases of total drainage of pulmonary veins into the coronary sinus. The above authors advise widening the atrial septal defect in patients over 1 year of age, resecting the part of the interatrial septum between the defect and the coronary sinus, and closure by graft of the newly formed defect. The coronary sinus and the abnormal veins were transferred into the left atrium. Podzolkov and colleagues do not advise excision of the interatrial septum in patients under 1 year of age.

Right Lung Hypoplasia with Anomalous Arteries and Veins (Scimitar Syndrome)

ANATOMY

Sequestration of the lung with an anomalous artery occurs predominantly on the left side—to be more spe-

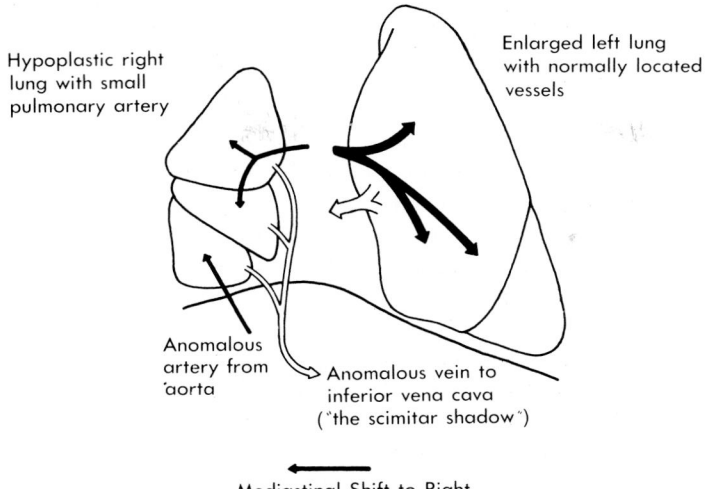

Figure 14.30. Characteristics of the "scimitar syndrome."

cific and topographicoanatomically correct, the usual location is close to the esophagus and the aorta at the left posterior costodiaphragmatic angle (postbasal segment). Characteristically, the sequestrated segment has no communication with the tracheobronchial tree, and its blood supply originates from the systemic circulation (thoracic or abdominal aorta or intercostal arteries). The above definition will clear any confusion and differentiate between scimitar syndrome and sequestration. A somewhat similar anomaly is restricted to the right. There is no sequestration of lung tissue, but the entire lung is hypoplastic without cystic changes. Only two lobes may be present; the lower lobe may be supplied by an anomalous artery from the aorta, with one or both lobes draining into the inferior vena cava, usually below the diaphragm because of anomalous pulmonary vein draining. The normal right pulmonary artery is reduced in size. The heart is usually shifted to the right because of the right lung hypoplasia (Fig. 14.30). The radiologic picture, in which the anomalous pulmonary vein crosses the right border of the heart, has led to the term *scimitar syndrome*. Raffensperger (222), quoting Kittle and Crockett (202) and Derksen (223), stated that scimitar syndrome is a right-sided lesion since sequestration occurs on either side.

EMBRYOGENESIS

The scimitar syndrome is limited to the right side because a left inferior vena cava is not normally present. Theoretically, a similar condition could be found on the left side if a left inferior vena cava persisted.

Neill and her colleagues (203) consider this defect to be primarily a malformation of the right lung bud rather than a specific anomaly of the pulmonary veins. They believe it to arise earlier than Streeter's horizon XIV (stage 14; early sixth week) at which time most other pul-

monary vein anomalies arise. The scimitar syndrome probably represents a unilateral agenesis of the true pulmonary veins, the functional drainage being a persistent part of the primitive venous plexus around the foregut.

Partridge et al. (224) group congenital pulmonary anomalies under the name "dysmorphic lung."

HISTORY AND INCIDENCE

The syndrome was first described by Park (225) in 1912; however, Jimenez et al. (226) stated that the scimitar syndrome was first described by Chassinet in 1836. Halasz et al. (227) were able to collect 21 cases by 1956. Dotter et al. (228) made the first clinical diagnosis by the use of angiography in 1949. Neill and her group (203) reviewed 14 cases in 1960 and found the anomaly present in a father and daughter. Kittle and Crockett (202) collected 43 cases and proposed the name "vena cava bronchovascular syndrome" in 1962. Apparently the sexes are equally affected.

ASSOCIATED ANOMALIES

Scimitar syndrome with horseshoe lung was reported by Beitzke et al. (229), and associated horseshoe lung also was presented by Frank et al. (80) in 1986 and Clements and Warner (82) in 1987.

Blaysat et al. (230) reported 12 cases of scimitar syndrome in children with anomalous pulmonary venous drainage, hypoplasia of right pulmonary artery and parenchyma, and several varieties of sequestrations above and below the diaphragm, forming a constellation of pathologic findings.

Khalife et al. (231) reported a young adult with a scimitar image related to a pure pulmonary vessel sequestration by a right subphrenic artery. They contend that, if there is no abnormality of pulmonary venous return, other anatomic entities and anomalies may produce the scimitar "sign."

SYMPTOMS

No specific symptoms are associated with this syndrome. Shortness of breath and repeated respiratory infections may be present. There may be no symptoms at all, or only a history of respiratory symptoms in childhood may be found (203). Foreman and Rosa (232) reported two cases of scimitar syndrome in two adults, one with a benign course who was practically asymptomatic and the other with severe symptomatology of recurrent upper respiratory tract infections. There may be a visible deformity of the chest. The degree of hypoplasia of the lung may account for the difference between symptomatic and asymptomatic cases.

DIAGNOSIS

An apparent dextrocardia is the most significant finding. On x-ray examination, a scimitar shaped density on the right cardiac border is considered diagnostic. The left-to-right shunt may amount to 50% of the pulmonary venous return; however, severe pulmonary hypertension is rare. An atrial septal defect may be present. Angiocardiography and bronchography will confirm the diagnosis and reveal the severity of the lesion. Cases of scimitar syndrome presented by Alfano et al. (233) were diagnosed by angiographic studies. Godwin and Tarver (234) diagnosed the defect by CT scan, and Gikonyo et al. (235) noted other cardiovascular anomalies which accompany the syndrome.

Jimenez et al. (226) reported the first inferior vena cava stenosis in scimitar syndrome; the diagnosis was made by two-dimensional echocardiographic Doppler color flow mapping.

TREATMENT

Patients without symptoms and cardiac enlargement and with normal pulmonary pressure require no treatment.

When the lung is hypoplastic with bronchiectasis, or when it shows other degenerative changes, pneumonectomy rather than vascular reconstruction is the operation of choice. However, right-sided pneumonectomy should be reserved for older symptomatic patients, according to Canter et al. (236). If anomalous drainage is limited to the lower lobe, lobectomy is indicated.

If the lung tissue is normal, surgical correction of the venous drainage will restore normal hemodynamic conditions without loss of pulmonary capacity.

Kirklin and his associates (237) transplanted an anomalous vein to the right atrium opposite an existing atrial septal defect to promote flow to the left atrium across the defect. When the anomalous vein is long enough to be transplanted to the left atrium, normal circulation can be

completely restored. In one patient encountered by Sanger et al. (238), the anomalous vein bifurcated to enter both the left atrium and the inferior vena cava. Ligation of the latter branch was all that was required.

Anomalous arteries from the aorta should be identified and occluded along with the normal pulmonary artery during surgery to avoid rupture of the lung from high arterial pressure. According to Honey (239), surgical treatment of scimitar syndrome in infancy is difficult and mortality is high.

Pulmonary Arteriovenous Fistula (Pulmonary Telangiectasia)

This lesion is one of the specific manifestations of hereditary hemorrhagic telangiectasia (Rendu-Osler-Weber syndrome). A number of tissues and organs besides the lungs may be affected: liver, retina, conjunctiva, thyroid, intestine, kidney, adrenal, and spinal meninges have all been mentioned. There may or may not be skin lesions (240).

According to Katzenstein and Askin (24), most arteriovenous fistulae are of congenital origin. They could be solitary or multiple, and the latter types are associated with Rendu-Osler-Weber syndrome, as reported by Trell et al. (241) and Utzon and Brandrup (242).

ANATOMY

The fistulae are formed by an afferent artery and distended efferent veins, connected by an aneurysmal sac or a labyrinth of distended vascular channels that are not recognizable as either veins or arteries. The extent of the dilation depends on the length of time it has existed. Rupture of the thin-walled vessels eventually takes place.

The lesion may lie deep in the lung or merely beneath the pleura. In about 66% of affected individuals, solitary lesions are found: as there is a tendency for new fistulae to form with age, earlier records, which are based on autopsy cases, showed a higher percentage of multiple lesions.

In about 20% of patients, both lungs are affected. When only one lung is involved, the right is implicated about twice as frequently as the left, and the right lower lobe is the most frequently affected site. Distribution of lesions in 129 cases were collected by Stringer et al. (243) (Fig. 14.31).

Pulmonary artery and systemic arteries are involved, but more responsibility for these malformations belong to the pulmonary artery. Brundage et al. (244) reported two cases of systemic artery to pulmonary vessel fistulae.

ASSOCIATED ANOMALIES

About 70% of patients also will have cutaneous telangiectases (245), and cardiac anomalies are not uncommon.

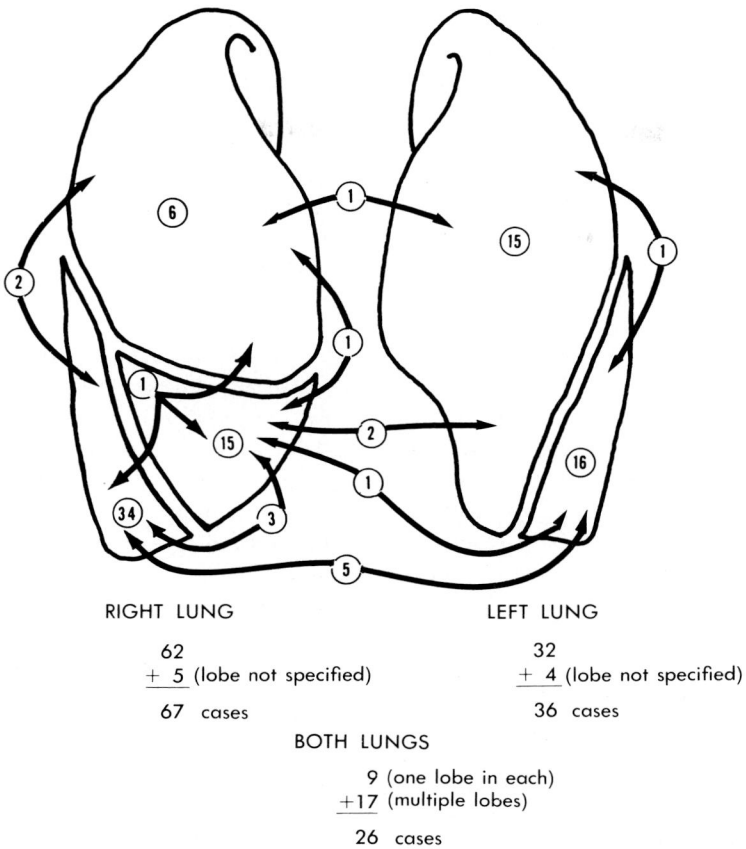

RIGHT LUNG

62
+ 5 (lobe not specified)

67 cases

LEFT LUNG

32
+ 4 (lobe not specified)

36 cases

BOTH LUNGS

9 (one lobe in each)
+17 (multiple lobes)

26 cases

Figure 14.31. Location of pulmonary arteriovenous fistulae (cavernous hemangiomas) in 129 patients reported by Stringer and his colleagues. The right lower lobe is most frequently affected. *Numbers* and *arrows* indicate the frequencies with which more than one lobe, or more than one lung, were involved. (Data from Stringer CJ et al. Pulmonary arteriovenous fistula. Am J Surg 1955;89:1054–1080.)

Gula et al. (246) reported four male patients with pulmonary arteriovenous fistula, with a familial occurrence in two brothers, and a 4-day-old baby with a large arteriovenous fistula affecting the whole upper right lobe and a ventricular septal defect. The other three patients had multiple fistulae in both lungs.

Masson et al. (247) reported isolated bronchial telangiectasia. Pulmonary hypertension with multiple fistulae and Rendu-Osler-Weber syndrome was reported by Trell et al. (241).

PATHOGENESIS

These vascular formations are essentially hamartomas or overgrowths of normal tissue. They are benign and nonneoplastic. Though genetically determined, they are not always present at birth.

HISTORY

Understanding of the disease developed gradually from a number of originally isolated observations. Babington (248) described hereditary epistaxis in 1865. Rendu (249) made the first detailed observations of telangiectasia in 1896. Osler (250) associated the epistaxis with the cutaneous lesions in 1901, and in 1924 Weber (251) completed the picture of the syndrome.

Churton (252) first reported the pulmonary manifestation of the disease in 1897, having found multiple arteriovenous fistulae in the lungs of a child at autopsy. His brief report was reprinted by Stringer et al. (243). The first radiologic observation of the disease was made in 1917 by Wilkins (253), although he recognized the nature of the radiologic picture only after autopsy of the patient. In 1939 Smith and Horton (254) made the first clinical diagnosis, for which they employed angiocardiography. Hepburn and Dauphinee (255) in 1942 reported the first surgical treatment. They performed a pneumonectomy on a 23-year-old woman whose right lung was affected.

Yater and his colleagues (256) reviewed the condition in 1949, finding 45 cases in the literature. Purriel and Muras (245) found 170 cases and added two of their own in 1957.

Przybojewski and Maritz (257) and Burke et al. (258) studied the subject extensively.

FAMILIAL INCIDENCE

Hemorrhagic telangiectasia is a familial disease; up to 1959 some 264 family lines containing the gene were reported (253). Among 1622 individuals composing 112 families who were examined in detail, 56% were affected.

Hodgson et al. (253) studied six generations and 231 members of an affected family. Ninety-one had telangiectasia, and 14 (15.4%) of these had pulmonary arteriovenous shunts. Males and females were equally affected with the primary disease and its pulmonary manifestation. Although the disease may be present at birth, there is a tendency for the telangiectases to appear or increase in number with age, eventually affecting 90% of the family members by the sixth decade of life.

The gene behaves as dominantly, and there is no sex linkage. Both white and black races are known to be affected. One example of a homozygous individual is known: In this person, telangiectases were present at birth and multiplied rapidly, becoming fatal in 11 weeks (259). This suggests that complete dominance is lethal and that the heterozygous condition is merely "semidominant."

Not all patients with pulmonary arteriovenous fistulae have a positive family history. Purriel and Muras (245) found a negative history in 42% of cases collected from the literature. This low correlation may reflect inadequate search, spontaneous mutation, or a nonfamilial type of the disease. Gula et al. (246) reported two brothers with obvious familial occurrence.

SYMPTOMS

Cyanosis, clubbing of the fingers, dyspnea, and epistaxis are the chief complaints; the severity of all but the last depend on the extent of the arteriovenous shunt. About 50% of patients are asymptomatic, presumably because their fistulae are small or because they are in the bronchial rather than the pulmonary circulation. Burke et al. (258) stated that 13 to 56% of patients are asymptomatic. In later stages of the disease, central nervous system symptoms may be manifested. Several patients have had brain abscesses, presumably resulting from emboli that passed through the pulmonary shunt to enter the cerebral circulation.

Dines et al. (260) reported a female preponderance. Kintzer et al. (261) reported hemothorax as a complication of an arteriovenous fistula. The mediastinum and chest wall may be involved.

DIAGNOSIS

All patients with mucocutaneous telangiectases and all patients from families showing the disease should be suspected of having pulmonary arteriovenous fistulae.

Large fistulae produce polycythemia, with increases in blood volume, red blood cell count, and hematocrit values. These increases may be marked if there is chronic bleeding from telangiectases, especially in the intestine. Blood pressure is normal, as are cardiac output and electrocardiogram recordings. The oxygen saturation is low. An extracardiac bruit is usually audible over the site of the lesion. Right-to-left shunt with cyanosis is present.

On radiography, one or more lobulated opacities with band-like densities connected with the hilum may be seen. On fluoroscopy, these may be seen to pulsate. The opacities may be observed to decrease on expiration against the closed glottis. Angiocardiography will confirm the suspected diagnosis of cardiac malformation as a possible cause of the cyanosis and clubbing.

According to Perloff (262) in 1989, detection of hereditary hemorrhagic telangiectasia may be the first clue to the diagnosis of an associated pulmonary arteriovenous fistula. Angiography of both lungs is the diagnostic procedure of choice.

PROGNOSIS

The prognosis in untreated cases is poor. Pulmonary thrombosis from the polycythemia, fatal hemorrhage from the rupture of the thin, distended vessels of the lesion, and intracranial thrombosis from emboli passing through the open shunt all present dangers to the patient.

TREATMENT

Complete cure following resection of the affected area was claimed for 17 of 26 patients, whose cases were collected from the literature by Yater and his colleagues (256). Burke et al. (258) reported a 5% surgical mortality with minimal morbidity and recurrence. Reidy et al. (263) showed that the treatment of choice for multiple fistulae is balloon embolotherapy after selective angiography. The current philosophy calls for embolotherapy even in single lesions.

REFERENCES

1. Federow V. Ueber die Entwicklung der Lungenvene. Arb Anat Inst Wiesbaden 1910;40:529–603.
2. Bremer JL. The development of the aorta and aortic arch in rabbits. Am J Anat 1912;13:126–128.
3. Congdon ED. Transformation of the aortic-arch system during the development of the human embryo. Contrib Embryol Carnegie Inst Wash 1922;14:47.
4. Anderson RC, Char F, Adams P. Proximal interruption of a pulmonary arch (absence of one pulmonary artery): case report and a new embryologic inerpretation. Dis Chest 1958;34:73–86.
5. Dammann JF Jr, Thompson WM, Sosa O, Christlieb I. Anatomy, physiology and natural history of simple ventricular septal defects. Am J Cardiol 1960;5:136.
6. Civin WH, Edwards JE. Postnatal structural changes in intrapulmonary arteries and arterioles. Arch Pathol 1951;51:192–200.

7. Wagenvoort CA, Neufield HN, Edwards JE. The structure of the pulmonary arterial tree in fetal and early postnatal life. Lab Invest 1961;10:751–762.

8. Thomas MA. Adult pattern of pulmonary vessels in newborn infants. Arch Dis Child 1964;39:232–235.

9. Long WA. Developmental pulmonary circulatory physiology. In: Fetal and neonatal cardiology. New York: WB Saunders, 1990:76.

10. Campbell CD, Wernly JA, Koltip PC, Vitullo D, Replogle RL. Aberrant left pulmonary artery (pulmonary artery sling): successful repair and 24 year follow-up report. Am J Cardiol 1980;45(2):316–320.

11. Fong LV, Anderson RH, Siewers RD, Trento A, Park SC. Anomalous origin of one pulmonary artery from the ascending aorta: review of echocardiographic, catheter, and morphological features. Br Heart J 1989;62(5):389–395.

12. Werber J, Ramilo JL, London R, Harris VJ. Unilateral absence of a pulmonary artery. Chest 1983;84(6):729–732.

13. Gikonyo BM, Jue KL, Edwards JE. Pulmonary vascular sling: report of seven cases and review of the literature. Pediatr Cardiol 1989;10(2):81–89.

14. Flint JM. The development of the lungs. Am J Anat 1907;6:1–137.

15. Brown AJ. The development of the pulmonary veins in the domestic cat. Anat Rec 1913;7:299–329.

16. Auër J. The development of the human pulmonary vein and its major variations. Anat Rec 1948;101:581–594.

17. Butler H. An abnormal disposition of the pulmonary venous drainage. Thorax 1952;7:249–254.

18. Neill CA. Development of the pulmonary vein: with reference to the embryology of anomalies of pulmonary venous return. Pediatrics 1956;18:880–887.

19. Konaschko PI. Ueber das system der anastomesen die lungenvenen und den linken vorhof mit den venen des grossen kreislaufes verbinden. Z Anat Entw 1929;89:672–695.

20. Huntington GS. The morphology of the pulmonary artery in the mammalia. Anat Rec 1919;17:165.

21. Geddes AC. Abnormal superior vena cava. Anat Anz 1912;41:449–453.

22. Slavochinskayà LB. Some developmental aspects of the blood supply of the bronchial tree [Russian]. Trudy Tadzhinsk Med Inst 1964;63:131–134.

23. Askin FB. Pulmonary disorders in the neonate infant and child. In: Thurlbeck WM, ed. Pathology of the lung. New York: Thieme Medical Publishers, 1988:116–146.

24. Katzenstein ALA, Askin FB. Surgical pathology of nonneoplastic lung disease. Philadelphia: WB Saunders, 1990.

25. Dehner LP. Pediatric surgical pathology, 2nd ed. Baltimore: Williams & Wilkins, 1987.

26. Tesler UF, Balsara RH, Niguidula FN. Aberant left pulmonary artery (vascular sling): report of five cases. Chest 1974;66:402–407.

27. Penkoske PA, Castaneda AR, Fyler DC, Van Praagh R. Origin of pulmonary artery branch from ascending aorta: primary surgical repair in infancy. J Thorac Cardiovasc Surg 1983;85:537–545.

28. Berdon WE, Baker DH. Vascular anomalies and the infant lung: rings, slings and other things. Semin Roentgenol 1972;7:39–64.

29. Barbero-Marcial M et al. Correction of pulmonary atresia with ventricular septal defect in the absence of the pulmonary trunk and the central pulmonary arteries (so-called truncus type IV). J Thorac Cardiovasc Surg 1987;94(6):911–914.

30. Presbitero P, Bull C, Haworth SG, deLaval MR. Absent or occult pulmonary artery. Br Heart J 1984;52:178–185.

31. Loser H, Osswald P, Apitz J, Schmalta AA. Periphere pulmonalstenosen: mogliche ursachen und syndromale zusammenhange. Klin Padiatr 1977;189:137–145.

32. Kamio A, Fukushima K. Takebayashi S, Toshima H. Isolated stenosis of the pulmonary artery branches: an autopsy case with review of the literature. Jpn Circ J 1978;42:1289–1296.

33. McCue CM, Robertson LW, Lester RG, Mauck HP. Pulmonary artery coarctations: a report of 20 cases with review of 319 cases from the literature. J Pediatr 1965;67:222–238.

34. Pernot C, Deschamps J-P, Didier F. Stenose de l'artere pulmonaire, taches cutanees pigmentaires et anomalies du squelette: quatre observations. Arch Franc Pediatr 1979;28:593–603.

35. Seki S et al. [Vascular resistance of the right lung in the anomalous origin of the right pulmonary artery from the ascending aorta: right pulmonary arterial vascular resistance as a key point for operative indication (author's transl)]. Kyobu Geka 1980;33(9):681–685.

36. Hislop A, Sanderson M, Reid L. Unilateral congenital dysplasia of lung associated with vascular anomalies. Thorax 1973;28:435–441.

37. Taug JS, Kauffman SL, Lynfield J. Hypoplasia of the pulmonary arteries in infants with congenital rubella. Am J Cardiol 1971;27:491–496.

38. Goldstein JD, Rabinovitch M, Van Praagh R, Reid L. Unusual vascular anomalies causing persistent pulmonary hypertension in a newborn. Am J Cardiol 1979;43(5):962–968.

39. Weintraub RA, Fabian CE, Adams DF. Ectopic origin of one pulmonary artery from the ascending aorta. Radiology 1966;86:666–676.

40. Schneiderman LJ. Isolated congenital absence of the right pulmonary artery: a caution as to its diagnosis and a proposal for its embryogenesis—report of a case with review. Am Heart J 1958;55:772–780.

41. Stewart JR, Kincaid OW, Edwards JE. An atlas of vascular rings and related malformation of the aortic arch system. Springfield, IL: Charles C Thomas, 1964.

42. Burrows PE, Freedom RM, Rabinovitch M, Moes CA. The investigation of abnormal pulmonary arteries in congenital heart disease. Radiol Clin North Am 1985;23(4):689–717.

43. Anjos RT, Suzuki A, Ho SY. A rare case of tetralogy of Fallot with unusual blood supply to the left lung. Int J Cardiol 1989;24(3):303–306.

44. Pool PE, Vogel JHK, Blount SG Jr. Congenital unilateral absence of a pulmonary artery. Am J Cardiol 1962;10:706–732.

45. McKim JS, Wiglesworth FW. Absence of the left pulmonary artery. Am Heart J 1954:47:845–859.

46. Findlay CW Jr, Maier HC. Anomalies of the pulmonary vessels and their surgical significance: with a review of literature. Surgery 1951;29:604–641.

47. Steinberg I, Miscall L, Goldberg HP. Congenital absence of left pulmonary artery with patent ductus arteriosus. JAMA 1964;190:394–396.

48. Collett RW, Edwards JE. Persistent truncus arteriosus: a classification according to anatomic types. Surg Clin North Am 1949;29:1245–1270.

49. Manhoff LJ, Howe JS. Absence of the pulmonary artery: a new classification for pulmonary arteries of anomalous origin. Arch Pathol 1949;48:155–170.

50. Ferencz C. Congenital abnormalities of pulmonary vessels and their relation to malformations of the lung. Pediatrics 1961;28:993–1010.

51. Ambrus G. Congenital absence of right pulmonary artery with bleeding into right lung. J Tech Methods 1936;15:103–109.

52. Maier HC. [Discussion.] Of: Read CT. Absence of hypoplasia of a pulmonary artery with anomalous systemic arteries to the lung. J Thorac Surg 1954;28:161.

53. Potts WJ, Holinger PH, Rosenblum AH. Anomalous left pulmo-

nary artery causing obstruction to right main bronchus: report of a case. JAMA 1954;155:1409–1411.

54. Clements BS, Warner JO, Shinebourne EA. Congenital broncho-pulmonary vascular malformations: clinical application of a simple anatomical approach in 25 cases. Thorax 1987;42(6):409–416.

55. Vigneswaran WT, Pollock JC. Pulmonary atresia with ventricular septal defect and coronary artery fistula: a late presentation. Br Heart J 1988;59:387–388.

56. Jowett NI, Thompson DR, Pohl JE. Temporary transvenous cardiac pacing: 6 years experience in one coronary care unit. Postgrad Med J 1989;65(762):211–215.

57. Poynter CWM. Arterial anomalies pertaining to the aortic arches and the branches arising from them. Stud Zool Lab Univ Nebraska 1916;16:229.

58. Tiedemann F. Abweichende Anordnung des Pulsaderstämme des Herzens. Z Physiol 1831;4:287.

59. Fraentzel O. Ein Fall von abnormer Communication der Aorta mit der Arteria pulmonalis. Virchow Arch [A] 1968;43:420–426.

60. Thomas HW. Cardiovascular anomalies: congenital cardiac malformations. J Tech Meth 1941;21:58.

61. Emanuel RW, Pattison JN. Absence of the left pulmonary artery in Fallot's tetralogy. Br Heart J 1956;18:289–295.

62. Calori L. Iperencefalo umano. Mem Soc Med Chir Bologna 1843;3:417.

63. Madoff IM, Gaensler EA, Strieder JW. Congenital absence of the right pulmonary artery. N Engl J Med 1952;247:149.

64. Fontana RS, Edwards JE. Congenital cardiac disease: a review of 357 cases studied pathologically. Philadelphia: WB Saunders, 1962.

65. Rosenberg HS, Hallman GL, Wolfe RR, Latson JR. Origin of the right pulmonary artery from the aorta. Am Heart J 1966;72:106–115.

66. Massumi RA, Donohoe RF. Congenital versus acquired attenuation of one pulmonary artery. Circulation 1965;31:436–447.

67. Hopkins WA. Personal communication, 1968.

68. Wilcox BR, Croom RD. Aortic origin of the right pulmonary artery. Ann Thorac Surg 1968;5:165–170.

69. Stanton RE, Durnin RE, Fyler DC, Lindesmith GG, Meyer BW. Right pulmonary artery originating from ascending aorta. Am J Dis Child 1968;115:403–413.

70. Moscarella AA, Wylie RH. Congenital communication between the esophagus and isolated ectopic pulmonary tissue. J Thorac Cardiovasc Surg 1968;55:672–676.

71. Roe JP, Mack JW, Shirley JH. Bilateral pulmonary sequestrations. J Thorac Cardiovasc Surg 1980;80:8.

72. Savic B et al. Pulmonary sequestration. Ergebn Kinderheilk 1979;43:57.

73. Landing BH, Dixon LG. Congenital malformations and genetic disorders of the respiratory tract (larynx, trachea, bronchi and lungs). Am Rev Respir Dis 1979;120:151–185.

74. Corrin B et al. Intralobar pulmonary sequestration of ectopic pancreatic tissue with gastropancreatic duplications. Thorax 1985;40:637–638.

75. Flye MW, Izant RJ. Extralobar pulmonary sequestration with esophageal communication and complete duplication of the colon. Surgery 1972;71:744–752.

76. Heithoff KB et al. Bronchopulmonary foregut malformations: a unifying etiological concept. AJR 1976;126:46–55.

77. Leithiser RE Jr, Capitanio MA, Macpherson RI, Wood BP. "Communicating" bronchopulmonary foregut malformations. AJR 1986;146:227–231.

78. Lewis JE, Murray RE. Pulmonary sequestration with broncho-esophageal fistula. J Pediatr Surg 1968;3:575–579.

79. Cipriano P, Sweeney LJ, Hutchins GM, Rosenquist GC. Horse-shoe lung in an infant with recurrent pulmonary infections. Am J Dis Child 1975;129:1343–1345.

80. Frank JL, Poole CA, Rasas G. Horseshoe lung: clinical, pathologic and radiologic features and a new plain film finding. AJR 1986;146:217–226.

81. Freedom RM, Burrows PE, Moes CAG. "Horseshoe" lung: report of five new cases. AJR 1986;146:211–215.

82. Clements BS, Warner JO. Pulmonary sequestration and related congenital bronchopulmonary-vascular malformations: nomenclature and classification based on anatomical and embryological considerations. Thorax 1987;42:401–408.

83. Pryce DM. Lower accessory pulmonary artery with intralobar sequestration of the lung: a report of seven cases. J Pathol Bact 1946;58:457–467.

84. Pryce DM, Sellors TH, Blair LG. Intralobar sequestration of lung associated with an abnormal pulmonary artery. Br J Surg 1947;35:18–29.

85. Batts M Jr. A pulmonary artery arising from the abdominal aorta. J Thorac Surg 1939;8:565–569.

86. Cole FH, Alley FH, Jones RS. Aberrant systemic arteries to the lower lung. Surg Gynecol Obstet 1951;93:589–596.

87. Holder PD, Langston C. Intralobar pulmonary sequestration (a nonentity?). Pediatr Pulmonol 1986;2(3):147–153.

88. Katch S et al. [A case of systemic origin of an aberrant artery to the basal segments of the left lung]. Nippon Kyobu Geka Gakkai Zasshi 1990;38(1):154–159.

89. Gallagher PG, Lynch JP, Christian HJ. Intralobar bronchopul-monary sequestration of the lung: report of two cases and review of the literature. N Engl J Med 1957;257:643–650.

90. Boyden EA. Bronchiogenic cysts and the theory of intralobar sequestration: new embryologic data. J Thorac Surg 1958;35:604.

91. Tosatti E, Gravel JA. Two cases of bronchiogenic cyst associated with anomalous arteries arising from the thoracic aorta. Thorax 1951;6:82–88.

92. Das JB, Dodge OG, Fawcett AW. Intralobar sequestration of lung, associated with foregut diverticulum (oesophagobronchial fistula) and an aberrant artery. Br J Surg 1959;46:582–586.

93. Berman JK, Test PS, McArt BL. Congenital esophago-bronchial fistula in an adult. J Thorac Surg 1953;24:493.

94. Polák E, Levinský L, Jedlička J, Jedlička V, Žák F. Operativer verschluss eines angeborenen ductus esophagobronchialis. Schweiz Z Tuberk 1958;15:92.

95. Halasz NA, Lindskog GE, Liebow AA. Esophagobronchial fistula and bronchopulmonary sequestration. Ann Surg 1962;155:215–220.

96. Baar HS, d'Abreau AL. Duplications of the foregut: superior accessory lung (2 cases); epiphrenic oesophageal diverticulum; intrapericardial teratoid tumour; and oesophageal cyst. Br J Surg 1949;37:220–230.

97. Beskin CA. Intralobar enteric sequestration of the lung containing aberrant pancreas. J Thorac Cardiovasc Surg 1961;41:314–317.

98. Wechsberg F. Ueber eine seltene form von angborener missbildung der lunge. Zentralbl Allg Pathol 1900;11:593.

99. Acker JJ, Brawer JN, Rawls WJ, Shuford WH, Schlant RC. Pulmonary sequestration associated with partial anomalous pulmonary venous return from the opposite lung. Am J Med 1966;40:470–476.

100. Cotton BH, Spaulding K, Penido JRF. An accessory lung. J Thorac Surg 1952;23:508–512.

101. Gans SL, Potts WJ. Anomalous lobe of lung arising from the esophagus. J Thorac Surg 1950;21:313–318.

102. Hammar JA. Ein Fall von Nebenlunge bei einem Menschenfötus von 11.7 mm Nackenlänge. Beitr Pathol Anat 1904;36:518–527.

103. Herxheimer G. Ueber einen Fall von echter Nebenlunge. Zentralbl Allg Pathol 1901;12:529–532.

104. St. Raymond AH Jr, Hardy JD, Robbins SG. Lower accessory lung communicating with esophagus and associated with congenital diaphragmatic hernia. J Thorac Surg 1956;31:354–358.

105. Leahy LJ, MacCallum JD. Cystic accessory lobe: report of a case. J Thorac Surg 1950;20:72–76.

106. DeBakey M, Arey JB, Brunazzi R. Successful removal of lower accessory lung. J Thorac Surg 1950;19:304–311.

107. Cockayne EA, Gladstone RJ. A case of accessory lungs associated with hernia through a congenital defect of the diaphragm. J Anat 1917;52:64–96.

108. Scheidegger S. Lungenmissbildungen (Beitrag zur Entstehung der Nebenlunge). Frankfurt Z Pathol 1936;49:362.

109. Warner FS, McGraw CT, Peterson HG Jr, Cleland RS, Meyer BW. Lung ectopia and agenesis with heart dextrorotation. Am J Dis Child 1961;101:514–518.

110. Morton DR, Klassen KP, Baxter EH. Lobar agenesis of the lung. J Thorac Surg 1950;20:665–670.

111. Vogel R. Zwei Fälle von abdominalen Lungengewebe. Virchow Arch [A] 1899;155:235.

112. Valle AR, White ML Jr. Subdiaphragmatic aberrant pulmonary tissue. Dis Chest 1947;13:63–68.

113. Smith RA. A theory of the origin of intralobar sequestration of the lung. Thorax 1956;11:10–24.

114. Eppinger H, Schauenstein W. Krankheiten der Lungen. A. Angeborene Krankheiten Ergebn. Allg Pathol 1902;8:267–275.

115. Bremer JL. Congenital anomalies of viscera. Cambridge, MA: Harvard University Press, 1957.

116. Gebauer PW, Mason CB. Intralobular pulmonary sequestration associated with anomalous pulmonary vessels: A nonentity. Dis Chest 1959;35:282–288.

117. Dameron F. Influence de divers mésenchymes sur la différenciation de l'épithélium pulmonaire de l'embryon de poulet en culture in vitro. C R Acad Sci (Paris) 1961;252:3879–3881.

118. Pendse P, Alexander J, Khademi M, Gross DB. Pulmonary sequestration: coexisting classic intralobar and extralobar types in a child. J Thorac Cardiovasc Surg 1972;64:127.

119. Iwai K et al. Intralobar pulmonary sequestration, with special reference to developmental pathology. Am Rev Respir Res 1973;167:911–920.

120. Albrechtsen D. Pulmonary sequestration. Scand J Thorac Cardiovasc Surg 1974;8:64.

121. Stocker JT. Sequestrations of the lung. Semin Diagn Pathol 1986;3:106.

122. Stocker JT, Malczak HT. A study of pulmonary ligament arteries: relationship to intralobar pulmonary sequestration. Chest 1984;86:611–615.

123. Davies DV, Gunz FW. Two cases of lower accessory lung in the human subject. J Pathol Bact 1944;56:417–427.

124. Alivizatos P, Cheatle T, de Laval M, Stark J. Pulmonary sequestration complicated by anomalies of pulmonary venous return. J Pediatr Surg 1986;20:76.

125. Bell-Thomson J, Misser T, Sommers S. Lung carcinoma arising in bronchopulmonary sequestration. Cancer 1979;44:334.

126. Haworth SG, Sauer U, Buhlmeyer K. Pulmonary hypertension in scimitar syndrome in infancy. Br Heart J 1983;50(2):182–189.

127. John PR, Beasley SW, Mayne V. Pulmonary sequestration and related congenital disorders: a clinico-radiological review of 41 cases. Pediatr Radiol 1989;20(1–2):4–9.

128. Carter R. Pulmonary sequestration: collective review. Ann Thorac Surg 1969;7:68.

129. Thilenius OG et al. Spectrum of pulmonary sequestration: association with anomalous pulmonary venous drainage in infants. Pediatr Cardiol 1983;4(2):97–103.

130. Huber JJ. Observationes aliquot de arteria singulari pulmoni concessa. Act Heln 1777;8:85.

131. Maugars A. Descriptions d'une artère pulmonaire considérable, naissant de l'aorte abdominale. J Med Paris 1802;3:453.

132. Rektorzik E. Ueber akzessorische Lungenlappen. Wchnbl KK Gesellsch Aerzte Wien 1861;12:4–6.

133. Harris HA, Lewis L. Anomalies of the lungs with special reference to the danger of abnormal vessels in lobectomy. J Thorac Surg 1940;9:666–671.

134. Eaker AB, Hannon JL, French SW III. Pulmonary sequestration: a review of the English literature with a report of 4 cases. Am J Surg 1958;95:31–39.

135. Sjolte IP, Christiansen MJ. Zehn Fälle von Nebenlungen bei Tieren. Virchow Arch [A] 1938;302:93–117.

136. Natucci G. Sopra un caso raro di anomalia delle arterie bronchiali. Pathologica 1939;31:514–519.

137. Simopoulous AP, Rosenblum DJ, Mazumdar H, Kiely B. Intralobar bronchopulmonary sequestration in children. Am J Dis Child 1959;97:796–804.

138. Riebel T, von Windheim K. [Pulmonary sequestration (author's transl)]. Monatsschr Kinderheilkd 1982;130(4):233–238.

139. Buchanan MC. Sequestration of the lung. Arch Dis Child 1959;34:137–139.

140. Gans SL, Potts WJ. Anomalous lobe of lung arising from the esophagus. J Thorac Surg 1950;21:313–318.

141. Naidich DP, Rumancik WM, Lefleur RS, Estioko MR, Brown SM. Intralobar pulmonary sequestration: MR evaluation. J Comput Assist Tomogr 1987;11(3):531–533.

142. Ikezoe J, Murayama S, Godwin JD, Done SL, Verschakelen JA. Bronchopulmonary sequestration: CT assessment. Radiology 1990;176(2):375–379.

143. Lintermans JP, Guntheroth WG, Figley MM. Extensive accessory pulmonary arteries in the presence of relatively normal primary pulmonary arteries. Am Heart J 1966;71:527–532.

144. Sherman FE. Anomalous course of left pulmonary artery: a cause of obstructive emphysema in infants. J Pediatr 1959;54:93–98.

145. Wittenborg MH, Tantiwongse T, Rosenberg BF. Anomalous course of left pulmonary artery with respiratory obstruction. Radiology 1956;67:339–345.

146. Jue KL, Rahbig G, Amplatz K, Adams P, Edwards JE. Anomalous origin of the left pulmonary artery from the right pulmonary artery. AJR 1965;95:598–610.

147. Wells TR, Gwinn JL, Landing BH, Stanley P. Reconsideration of the anatomy of sling left pulmonary artery: the association of one form with bridging bronchus and imperforate anus—anatomic and diagnostic aspects. J Pediatr Surg 1988;23(10):892–898.

148. Contro S, Miller RA, White H, Potts WJ. Bronchial obstruction due to pulmonary artery anomalies. I. Vascular sling. Circulation 1958;17:418–423.

149. Fontan A, Verger P, Bricaud H. Anomalie de division de l'artère pulmonaire avec trajet récurrent de la branche gauche et obstruction respiratoire chronique. Ann Pediatr (Paris) 1964;11:333–340.

150. Glaevecke and Doehle. Ueber eine seltene angeborene Anomalie der Pulmonalarterie. Munchen Med Wschr 1897;44:950–951.

151. Dumler MP. A rare cause of dysphagia. JAMA 1966;197:513–514.

152. Mustard WT, Trimble AW, Trusler GA. Mediastinal vascular anomalies causing tracheal and esophageal compression and obstruction in childhood. Can Med Assoc J 1962;87:1301–1305.

153. Jue KL, Lockman LA, Edwards JE. Anomalous origins of pulmonary arteries from pulmonary trunk ("crossed pulmonary arter-

ies"): observation in a case with 18 trisomy syndrome. Am Heart J 1966;71:807–812.

154. Gay BB, Franch RH, Shuford WH, Rogers JV. The roentgenologic features of single and multiple coarctations of the pulmonary artery and branches. AJR 1963;90:599–613.

155. Rubin E, Strauss L. Occlusive intrapulmonary vascular anomaly in the newborn. Am J Pathol 1961;39:145.

156. Søndergaard T. Coarctation of the pulmonary artery. Danish Med Bull 1954;1:46–48.

157. Schwalbe E. Morphologie der Missbildunger. Jena: Gustav Fischer, 1909.

158. Falkenbach KH, Zheutlin N, Dowdy AH, O'Loughlin BJ. Pulmonary hypertension due to pulmonary arterial coarctation. Radiology 1959;73:575.

159. Son RS, Maranhao V, Ablaza SG, Goldberg H. Coarctation of the pulmonary artery. Dis Chest 1966;49:289–297.

160. Franch RH, Gay BB. Congenital stenosis of the pulmonary artery branches: a classification with postmortem findings in two cases. Am J Med 1963;35:512–529.

161. Thrower WB, Abelmann WH, Harken DE. Surgical correction of coarctation of the main pulmonary artery. Circulation 1960;21:672.

162. Baxter CF, Booth RW, Sirak HD. Surgical correction of congenital stenosis of the right pulmonary artery accompanied by agenesis of the left pulmonary artery. J Thorac Cardiovasc Surg 1961;41:796.

163. Cauldwell EW, Siekert RG, Lininger RE, Anson BJ. The bronchial arteries: an anatomic study of 150 human cadavers. Surg Gynecol Obstet 1948;86:395.

164. O'Rahilly R, Debson H, King TS. Subclavian origin of bronchial arteries. Anat Rec 1950;108:227–238.

165. Menke JF. An anomalous a. bronchialis dextra from the a. subclavia dextra, secondarily connected to the aorta thoracalis. Anat Rec 1936;65:55–58.

166. Healey JE. Anatomical survey of anomalous pulmonary veins: their clinical significance. J Thorac Surg 1952;23:433–444.

167. Lucas RV Jr, Lock JE, Tandon R, Edwards JE. Gross and histologic anatomy of total anomalous pulmonary venous connections. Am J Cardiol 1988;62(4):292–300.

168. Nasrallah AT, Mullins CE, Singer D, Harrison G, McNamara DG. Unilateral pulmonary vein atresia: diagnosis and treatment. Am J Cardiol 1975;36(7):969–973.

169. Niimi T, Kajita M, Matsuyama T. A case of unusual branching and aberrant course of segemental vein (V2) in the upper lobe of the right lung. J Jpn Assoc Thorac Surg 1991;39:935–937.

170. Loeffler E. Unusual malformation of the left atrium: pulmonary sinus. Arch Pathol 1949;48:371–376.

171. Kalmansohn RB, Maloney JV, Kalmansohn RW. Partial anomalous venous connection with unusual variations. N Engl J Med 1961;264:1233–1235.

172. Edwards JE, DuShane JW, Alcott DL, Burchell HB. Thoracic venous anomalies. Arch Path 1951;51:446–460.

173. Church WS. Congenital malformation of the heart: abnormal septum in left auricle. Trans Pathol Soc Lond 1868;19:188.

174. Jiménez-Martínez M, Franco-Vázquez JS, Guitiérrez-Bosque R, Pérez-Alverez JJ, Agüero-Sánchez R. Cor triatriatum with pericardial agenesis. Thorax 1969;24:667–672.

175. Vineberg A, Gialloretto O. Report of a successful operation for stenosis of common pulmonary vein (cor triatriatum). Can Med Assoc J 1956;74:719.

176. Hammon JW et al. Total anomalous pulmonary venous connection in infancy. J Thorac Cardiovasc Surg 1980;80:544.

177. Edwards JE. Congenital stenosis of pulmonary veins: pathogenic and developmental considerations. Lab Invest 1960;9:46–66.

178. Lucas RV Jr et al. Congenital causes of pulmonary venous obstruction. Pediatr Clin North Am 1963;10:781–836.

179. Reid JM, Jamieson MPG, Cowan MD. Case reports: unilateral pulmonary vein stenosis. Br Heart J 1986;55:599–601.

180. Adey CK, Soto B, Shin MS. Congenital pulmonary vein stenosis: a radiographic study. Radiology 1986;161:113–117.

181. Pappas G. Left pulmonary vein stenosis associated with transposition of the great arteries. Ann Thorac Surg 1986;161:113–117.

182. Dev V, Shrivastava S. Diagnosis of pulmonary venous obstruction by Doppler echocardiography. Int J Cardiol 1989;22:129–133.

183. Muhler E et al. Congenital pulmonary vein stenosis as a rare cause of pulmonary hypertension. Klin Padiatr 1991;203:137–140.

184. Darling RC, Rothney WB, Craig JM. Total pulmonary drainage into the right side of the heart. Lab Invest 1957;6:44–64.

185. Edwards JE, Helmholz HF Jr. A classification of total anomalous pulmonary venous connection based on developmental consideration. Proc Mayo Clin 1956;31:151–160.

186. Taussig HB. Congenital malformations of the heart, Vol 2. Cambridge, MA: Harvard University Press, 1960.

187. Brody H. Drainage of the pulmonary veins into the right side of the heart. Arch Pathol 1942;33:221.

188. Smith JC. Anomalous pulmonary veins. Am Heart J 1951;41:561–568.

189. Parsons HG, Purdy A, Jessup B. Anomalies of the pulmonary veins and their surgical significance. Pediatrics 1952;9:152–166.

190. Burrows JT, Edwards JE. Total anomalous pulmonary venous connections. Am Heart J 1960;59:913–931.

191. Delisle G et al. Total anomalous pulmonary venous connection: report of 93 autopsied cases with emphasis on diagnostic and surgical considerations. Am Heart J 1976;91(1):99–122.

192. Duff DF, Nihill MR, McNamara DG. Infradiaphragmatic total anomalous pulmonary venous return: review of clinical and pathological findings and results of operation in 28 cases. Br Heart J 1977;39:619–626.

193. Haworth SG, Reid L. A morphometric study of regional variation in lung structure in infants with pulmonary hypertension and congenital cardiac defect: a justification of lung biopsy. Br Heart J 1978;40:825.

194. Holder TM, Ashcraft KW. Cardiac surgery. In: Welch KJ, Randolph JG, Ravitch MM, O'Neill JA, Rowe MI, eds. Pediatric surgery. Chicago: Year Book Medical Publishers, 1986:1385.

195. Nadas AS. Pediatric cardiology. Philadelphia: WB Saunders, 1957.

196. Anderson HN, Guntheroth WG, Winterscheid LC, Merendino KA. Congenital communications of the right pulmonary veins with the azygous vein: report of a case with surgical correction. Circulation 1964;30:439–443.

197. Winter FS. Persistent left superior vena cava: summary of world literature and reports of 30 additional cases. Angiology 1954;5:90–132.

198. Leal del Rosal P, Márquez Monter H, Avila L, Arce Gómez F. Anomalous entry of the pulmonary veins into the umbilical vein and the vena portae: presentation of a case and of the autopsy findings. Rev Med Hosp Gen (Mex) 1962;25:535–541.

199. Arnold J. Ein Fall von Cor Triloculare biatriatum: communication der Lungenvenen mit der Pfortader und Mangel der Milz. Virchow Arch Pathol Anat 1868;42:449–477.

200. Ainger LE. Infradiaphragmatic anomalous pulmonary venous connection: report of an unusual case. Am J Dis Child 1962;104:662–668.

201. Trinkle JK, Danielson GK, Noonan JA, Stephens C. Infradiaphragmatic total anomalous pulmonary venous return: report of a new and correctable variant. Ann Thorac Surg 1968;5:55–60.

202. Kittle CF, Crockett JE. Vena cava bronchovascular syndrome: a

triad of anomalies involving the right lung. Ann Surg 1962;156:222–233.

203. Neill CA, Ferencz C, Sabiston DC, Sheldon H. The familial occurrence of hypoplastic right lung with systemic arterial supply and venous drainage "scimitar syndrome." Bull Johns Hopkins Hosp 1960;107:1–21.

204. Vitarelli A, Scapato A, Sanguigni V, Caminiti MC. Evaluation of total anomalous pulmonary venous drainage with cross-sectional colour-flow Doppler echocardiography. Eur Heart J 1986;7(3):190–195.

205. Gott VL, Lester RG, Lillehei CW, Varco RL. Total anomalous pulmonary return: analysis of 70 cases. Circulation 1956;13:543–552.

206. Vogel M et al. Congenital unilateral pulmonary vein stenosis complicating transposition of greater arteries. Am J Cardiol 1984;54:166–71.

207. Lucas RV, Woolfrey BF, Anderson RC, Lester RG, Edwards JE. Atresia of the common pulmonary vein. Pediatrics 1962;29:729.

208. Hastreiter AR, Paul MH, Molthan ME, Miller RA. Total anomalous pulmonary venous connection with severe pulmonary venous obstruction. Circulation 1960;25:916.

209. DiDonaho R et al. Palliation of cardiac malformations associated with right isomerism (asplenia syndrome) in infancy. Ann Thorac Surg 1987;44:35.

210. Wilson J. On a very unusual formation of the human heart. Phil Trans R Soc London 1798;18:332–337.

211. Sherman FE, Bauersfeld SR. Total, uncomplicated, anomalous pulmonary venous connection; morphologic observations on 13 necropsy specimens from infants. Pediatrics 1960;25:656–668.

212. Bove EL et al. Infradiaphragmatic total anomalous pulmonary venous drainage: surgical treatment and long-term results. Ann Thorac Surg 1981;31:544–550.

213. Lester RG, Mauck HP, Grubb WL. Anomalous pulmonary venous return to the right side of the heart. Semin Roentgenol 1966;1:102–119.

214. Long WA, Lawson EE, Harned HS Jr, Henry GW. Infradiaphragmatic total anomalous pulmonary venous drainage: new diagnostic, physiologic, and surgical considerations. Am J Perinatol 1984;1:227–235.

215. Brantigen OC. Anomalies of the pulmonary veins: their surgical significance. Surg Gynecol Obstet 1947;184:653–658.

216. Cooley DA, Collins HA. Anomalous drainage of entire pulmonary venous system into the left innominate vein. Circulation 1959;19:486.

217. Cooley DA, Balas PE. Total anomalous pulmonary venous drainage into the inferior vena cava: report of a successful surgical correction. Surgery 1962;51:798.

218. Zubiate P, Magidson O, Kay JH. Surgical correction of total and partial anomalous pulmonary venous connections. Dis Chest 1962;41:518–523.

219. Breckenridge IM et al. Correction of total anomalous pulmonary venous drainage in infancy. J Thorac Cardiovasc Surg 1973;66:447–453.

220. Hawkins JA, Clark EB, Doty DB. Total anomalous pulmonary venous connection. Ann Thorac Surg 1983;36:548–560.

221. Podzolkov KP et al. Total anomalous drainage of pulmonary veins into the coronary sinus (clinical aspects, diagnosis and surgical treatment). Grud Serdechnosudistaia Khir 1991;5:15–18.

222. Raffensperger JG. Swenson's pediatric surgery. Norwalk, CT: Appleton-Lange, 1990:743–753, 755–762.

223. Derksen OS. Scimitar syndrome and pulmonary sequestration. Radiol Clin 1977;46:81.

224. Partridge JB, Osborne JM, Slaughter RE. Scimitar etcetera: the dysmorphic right lung. Clin Radiol 1988;39:11–19.

225. Park EA. Defective development of the right lung, due to anomalous development of the right pulmonary artery and vein, accompanied by dislocation of the heart simulating dextrocardia. Proc NY Pathol Soc 1912;12:88–93.

226. Jimenez M, Hery E, van Doesburg NH, Guerin R, Spier S. Inferior vena cava stenosis in scimitar syndrome: a case report. J Am Soc Echocardiogr 1988;1(2):152–154.

227. Halasz NA, Halloran KH, Liebow AA. Bronchial and arterial anomalies with drainage of the right lung into the inferior vena cava. Circulation 1956;14:826.

228. Dotter CT, Hardisty NM, Steinberg I. Anomalous right pulmonary vein entering the inferior cava: two cases diagnosed during life by angiocardiography and cardiac catheterization. Am J Med Sci 1949;218:31.

229. Beitzke A, Gypser G, Sager WD. [Scimitar syndrome with horse-shoe lung (author's transl)]. Rofo Fortschr Geb Rontgenstr Nuklearmed 1982;136:265–269.

230. Blaysat G et al. [Scimitar syndrome in infants. Physiotherapy and therapeutic implications in 12 cases.] Arch Franc Pediatr 1987;44:245–251.

231. Khalife K et al. The scimitar sign: a pulmonary vein or systemic artery?—apropos of a case of pure vascular sequestration. Rev Pneumol Clin 1985;41:410–412.

232. Foreman MG, Rosa U. The scimitar syndrome. South Med J 1991;84:489–494.

233. Alfano R et al. [Scimitar syndrome with or without the "scimitar sign"]. Pediatr Med Chir 1982;4(3):291–296.

234. Godwin JD, Tarver RD. Scimitar syndrome: four new cases examined with CT. Radiology 1986;159(1):15–20.

235. Gikonyo DK, Tandon R, Lucas RV Jr, Edwards JE. Scimitar syndrome in neonates: report of four cases and review of the literature. Pediatr Cardiol 1986;6(4):193–197.

236. Canter CE et al. Scimitar syndrome in childhood. Am J Cardiol 1986;56:652.

237. Kirklin JW, Ellis FH Jr, Wood EH. Treatment of anomalous pulmonary venous connections in association with interatrial communication. Surgery 1956;39:389.

238. Sanger PW, Taylor FH, Robicsek F. The "scimitar syndrome." Arch Surg 1963;86:580–587.

239. Honey M. Anomalous pulmonary venous drainage of right lung to inferior vena cava (scimitar syndrome): clinical spectrum in older patients and role of surgery. Q J Med 1977;46:463.

240. Willis RA. The borderland of embryology and pathology. London: Butterworth, 1958.

241. Trell E et al. Familial pulmonary hypertension and multiple abnormalities of large systemic arteries in Osler's disease. Am J Med 1972;53:50.

242. Utzon F, Brandrup F. Pulmonary arteriovenous fistulas in children: a review with special reference to the disperse telangiectatic type illustrated by report of a case. Acta Paediatr Scand 1973;62:422–432.

243. Stringer CJ, Stanley AL, Bates RC, Summers JE. Pulmonary arteriovenous fistula. Am J Surg 1955;89:1054–1080.

244. Brundage BH et al. Systemic artery to pulmonary vessel fistulas: report of two cases and a review of the literature. Chest 1972;62:19.

245. Purriel P, Muras O. Aneurismas arteriovenosos de pulmón. Thorax 1957;6:101–158.

246. Gula G, Nakvi A, Radley-Smith R, Yacoub M. The spectrum of pulmonary arteriovenous fistulae: clinico-pathological correlations. Thorac Cardiovasc Surg 1981;29:51–54.

247. Masson RG, Altose MD, Mayock RL. Isolated bronchial telangiectasia. Chest 1974;63:450.

248. Babington BG. Hereditary epistaxis. Lancet 1865;2:362.

249. Rendu. Epistaxis repetée chez un sujet porteur de petits angiomes cutanés et mugueaux. Bull Mém Soc Méd Hôp Paris 1896;13:731.

250. Osler W. A family form of recurring epistaxis associated with multiple telangiectases of the skin and mucous membrane. Bull Johns Hopkins Hosp 1901;11:333.

251. Weber FP. Developmental telangiectatic hemorrhages and so-called "telangiectasia," familial and non-familial. Br J Child Dis 1924;21:198.

252. Churton T. Multiple aneurysm of pulmonary artery. Br Med J 1897;1:1223.

253. Hodgson CH, Burchell HB, Good CA, Clagett OT. Hereditary hemorrhagic telangiectasia and pulmonary arteriovenous fistula. N Engl J Med 1959;261:625–636.

254. Smith HL, Horton BT. Arteriovenous fistula of the lung associated with polycythemia vera: report of a case in which the diagnosis was made clinically. Am Heart J 1939;18:589.

255. Hepburn J, Dauphinee JA. Successful removal of hemanangioma of the lung followed by disappearance of polycythemia. Am J Med Sci 1942;204:681.

256. Yater WM, Finnegan J, Giffin HM. Pulmonary arteriovenous fistula (varix): review of the literature and report of two cases. JAMA 1949;141:581–589.

257. Przybojewski JZ, Maritz F. Pulmonary arteriovenous fistulas: a case presentation and review of the literature. S Afr Med J 1975;57:355.

258. Burke CM, Safai C, Nelson DP, Raffin TA. Pulmonary arteriovenous malformation: a critical update. Am Rev Respir Dis 1986;134:334.

259. Snyder LH, Doan CA. Studies in human inheritance: is homozygous form of multiple telangiectasia lethal? J Lab Clin Med 1944;29:1211–1216.

260. Dines DE, Seward JB, Bernatz PC. Pulmonary arteriovenous fistulas. Mayo Clin Proc 1983;58:176.

261. Kintzer JS Jr, Jones FL Jr, Phatt WF. Intrapleural haemorrhage complicating pulmonary arteriovenous fistula. Br J Dis Chest 1978;72:155.

262. Perloff JK. Congenital heart disease in adults. In: Kelley WN, ed. Textbook of internal medicine. New York: JB Lippincott, 1989:229.

263. Reidy JF et al. Embolisation procedures in congenital heart disease. Br Heart J 1985;54:184.

CHAPTER 15

THE DIAPHRAGM

John Elias Skandalakis / Stephen Wood Gray / Richard R. Ricketts

There is a certain large, circular muscle rightly called the diaphragm
[διάφραγμα, barrier] since it separates the instruments of respiration from the
receptacles of the nutriment; for it lies above all the latter and beneath the former.
—*GALEN, ON THE USEFULNESS OF THE PARTS OF THE BODY*

DEVELOPMENT

The mammalian diaphragm is of complex origin, and not all the details of its development are known. The classic picture of the embryonic components of the diaphragm is that of Broman (1), who showed that the developing diaphragm receives contributions from the transverse septum, the mediastinum, and the musculature of the body wall. Final closure of central areas on each side by the pleuroperitoneal membranes completes the diaphragm. There are, therefore, two paired and two unpaired components of the diaphragm in the adult (Fig. 15.1 and Table 15.1).

During the fourth week, progressively caudal splitting of the lateral mesenchyme forms the beginning of the embryonic celom. The lateral cavities thus formed communicate cranially with the unpaired pericardial cavity and laterally with the extraembryonic celom (see Fig. 25.1). At the same time the advancing head fold brings the heart and pericardial cavity upward and under the embryonic body. These movements create the transverse septum, the first of the diaphragmatic components to appear (Fig. 15.2, A).

The septum formed in this manner is an incomplete mesenchymal partition, bound cranially by the pericardial cavity and caudally by the open midgut in the midline. From the gut, on the caudal side of the septum, the liver cords invade the mesenchyme of the septum (Fig. 15.3, A and B). Dorsally, the transverse septum joins the mediastinum, containing the foregut. Dorsal to the septum, on either side of the mediastinum, are the pleural canals connecting the pericardial and peritoneal cavities (Fig. 15.2, B). The subsequent history of the diaphragm is concerned with the closure of these dorsal pleural canals and the formation of the pleural cavities.

The lung buds, developing within the mediastinum during the fourth week, bulge into the pleural canals, which are the future pleural cavities. Partitions forming at both ends will separate these pleural cavities from the pericardium cranially and from the peritoneal cavity cau-

dally. The relationships between these cavities can be understood only if one remembers that, in the embryo at 4 weeks, the pericardial cavity is very large and the pleural canals are quite small.

The cranial partition—the pleuropericardial membrane—will separate the pleural cavity from the pericardial cavity. Two lateral ridges of mesenchyme, containing the common cardinal veins on their way to the heart, bulge into the pleural canal and fuse with the mediastinum on the opposite side during the fifth and sixth weeks. While they help define the pleural cavity, they contribute to the diaphragm only by providing the path for the phrenic nerves from the third and fourth cervical somites. Whether or not myoblasts follow the nerves to the diaphragm is not a settled question (Fig. 15.4).

The formation of the pleuroperitoneal membranes results from the progressive narrowing of the opening between the growing pleural cavities and the pericardium (see Fig. 25.4). Bremer (2) believes the suprarenal glands are a major factor in the closure of the canal. In cases of congenital absence of the suprarenal gland, however, the diaphragm is not usually defective. Both Bremer (2) and Wells (3) have shown that the narrowing of the pleuroperitoneal canal leaves only a very small aperture to be covered by the membrane (Fig. 15.5) proposed by Broman (1). The actual closure takes place during the eighth week (20-mm stage) (2).

Two small celomic spaces (pneumatoenteric recesses), one on either side of the mediastinum, are isolated during the fusion of the sides of the pleuroperitoneal canal. The recess on the left is transitory; the one on the right becomes the infracardiac bursa. It is a flattened, elongated, mesothelial-lined space lying in the esophageal hiatus (4). The space is about 1 cm long at birth and may become obliterated in the adult (5) (see Fig. 25.9). It is larger in some animals than in humans and has been called by Mall the "third pleural space" (6).

Following closure of the pleuroperitoneal canals, the pleural cavities enlarge as the lungs grow. Cranially, they

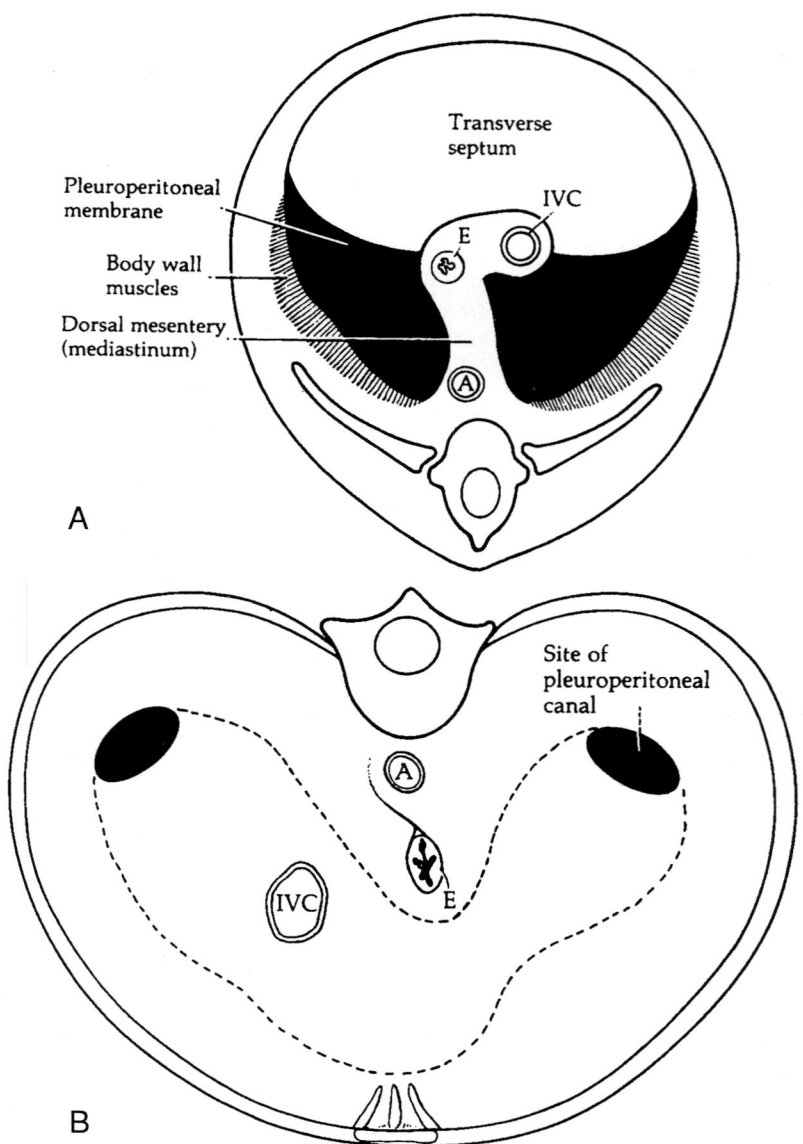

Figure 15.1. **A,** The four embryonic components of the diaphragm. **B,** The adult diaphragm. The sites or the closed pleuroperitoneal canals occupy a relatively small area in the adult diaphragm. **E,** esophagus; **IVC,** inferior vena cava; **A,** aorta. (From Skandalakis JE, Gray SW, Rowe JS Jr, Skandalakis LJ. Surgical anatomy of the diaphragm. In: Nyhus LM, Baker RJ, eds. Mastery of surgery. Boston: Little, Brown, 1992).

expand past the end of the pericardial space; caudally, they extend into the body wall by a process described by Bremer (2) as "burrowing." It is this process during the third month that forms the costal component of the diaphragm. This expansion on the dorsal side transfers the suprarenal gland and the innermost thoracic muscles to the diaphragm (the "glandular" component), from which the crura of the diaphragm are formed (Fig. 15.6). Laterally and anteriorly, a second group of thoracic muscles from the innermost layer is stripped from the thoracic wall and added to the diaphragm by a similar process. The

triangular space at which these two muscle groups join is the lumbocostal trigone, which may remain unfused and become the site of diaphragmatic hernia through the foramen of Bochdalek. The transfer of inner thoracic musculature to the diaphragm explains the presence of three muscle layers in the thoracic wall, with the intimal intercostal forming the deepest, third layer.

Against this explanation of the origin of diaphragmatic muscles is the fact that the diaphragm is innervated by the phrenic nerve from the third and fourth cervical segments. Lewis (7) believed that premuscle masses derived

Table 15.1.
Embryology Part Formation and Congenital Defects of the Diaphragm

Embryologic Entities	Definition/Origin	Time	Fusion	Parts Formed	Herniation
Septum transversum	A single mesodermal entity partially separating the pericardial and peritoneal cavities because it is located between the thoracic cavity and the stalk of the yolk sac	Weeks 3 and 4	With the pleuroperitoneal membranes and the ventral esophageal mesenchyme	Central tendon of diaphram	Pericardial, ventral diaphragmatic defect
Pleuroperitoneal membranes	Bilateral, located to start with at C2 and later at L2-L3	Weeks 7 and 8	With the septum transversum and dorsal esophageal mesentery	Primitive diaphragm	Bochdalek, posterolateral defect
Esophageal mesenteries	Bilateral dorsal		With the septum transversum and the pleuroperitoneal membranes	Median portion of diaphragm	
			Later on, myoblasts invade the dorsal mesentery	Diaphragmatic crura	
Body wall	Lungs and pleural cavities "burrow" and "excavate," as Moore stated, into the mesoderm of the lateral body wall, which is split in two layers—outer abdominal and inner diaphragmatic	Weeks 9–12	With the peripheral portion of the diaphragm from the dorsal and lateral body wall	Peripheral muscular diaphragmatic parts (ventrolateral and dorsal)	Morgagni Eventration

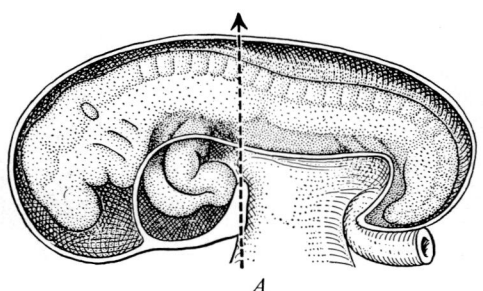
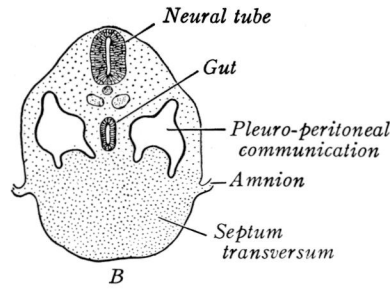

Figure 15.2. Relationship of the transverse septum to the pericardial and abdominal cavities in a human embryo of 4 weeks. **A,** Opened celom, viewed from the left. **B,** Cross-section through the embryo at the *dashed line* in **A,** showing the earliest formed elements of the future diaphragm. (From Arey LB. Developmental anatomy, 7th ed. Philadelphia: WB Saunders, 1965.)

from the caudal end of the infrahyoid mesoderm migrate with the phrenic nerve. Because the phrenic nerve originates from the third and fourth cervical segments, most authors have assigned the diaphragmatic musculature to these segments. This is in accordance with the principle that muscles, however modified, retain their original segmental innervation. It may be that myoblasts from upper cervical myotomes accompany the phrenic nerve, but some of the innervation must be subsequently transferred to muscle masses derived from the thoracic wall. That the central tendon is primarily fibrous and is never provided with muscle fibers (3) provides further evidence against the theory of migration of myoblasts.

It is interesting to note that, while Broman (8) presented a schematic diagram of the adult diaphragm, indicating the areas derived from the various embryonic components, no subsequent workers have revised this diagram. Indeed, Wells (3) stated that boundaries (on the adult diaphragm) could not be drawn from the knowledge available to him.

While the additions to the primitive transverse septum occur as described above, the position of the diaphragm

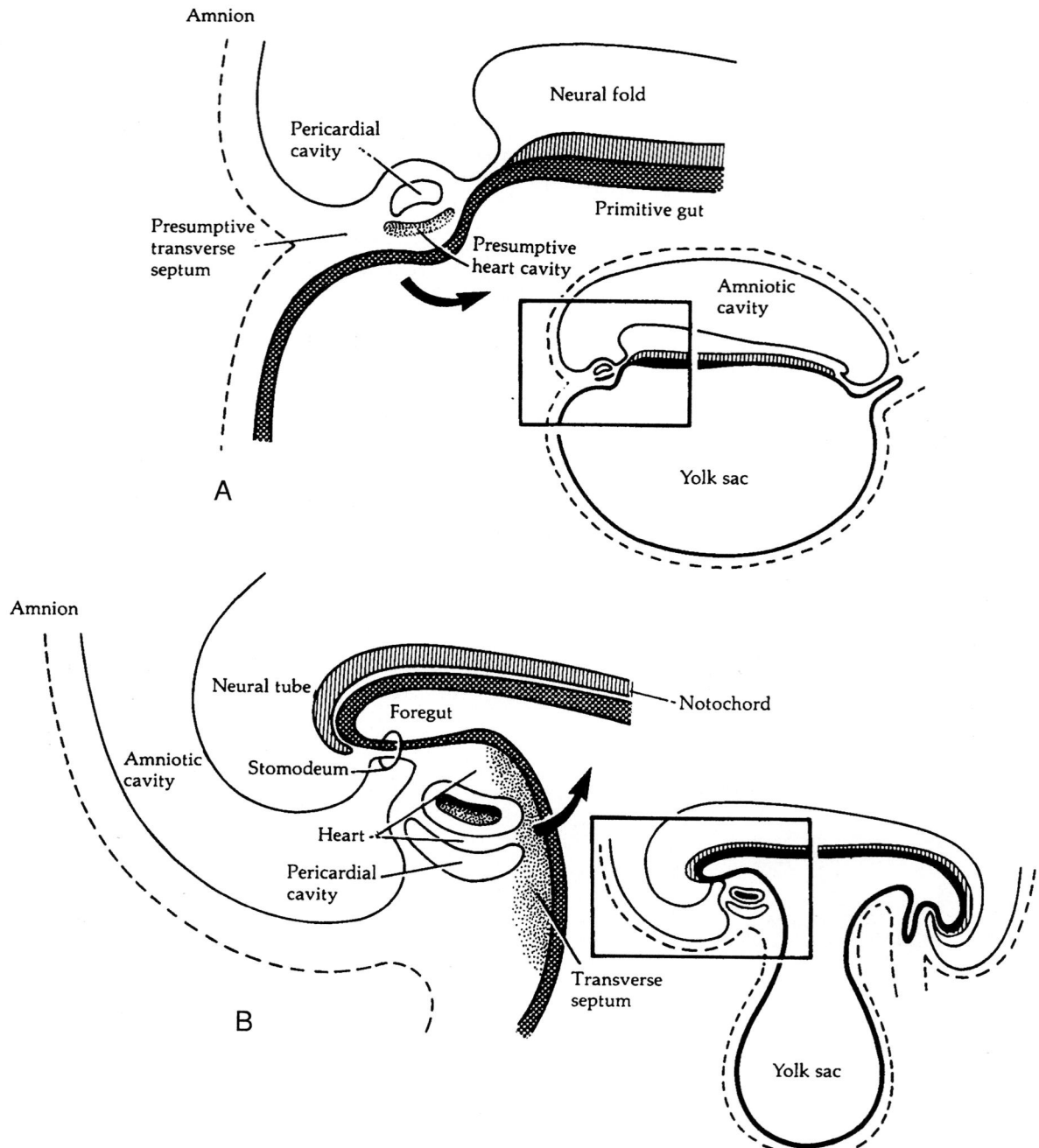

Figure 15.3. Formation of the transverse septum. **A,** The heart and pericardium form anterior to the head of the embryo in the third week. **B,** Rapid growth of the head rotates the heart and the mesoderm, which will become the transverse septum, in the direction indicated by the *arrows* by the fourth week. (From Skan-dalakis JE, Gray SW. Rowe JS Jr, Skandalakis LJ. Surgical anatomy of the diaphragm. In: Nyhus LM, Baker RJ, eds. Mastery of surgery. Boston: Little, Brown, 1992).

in the body shifts. At its first formation, the plane of the transverse septum would, if extended, intercept the dorsal axis of the body at the first cervical segment. By the end of the second month, it has "descended" to the definitive level of the first lumbar segment (Figs. 15.7 and 15.8).

This descent of 19 somites represents anterior growth of the more dorsal structures and the great increase in relative size of the cervical and thoracic body.

A second change, which occurs in the primitive septum, is the emergence of the liver from the substance of the septum beginning in the fourth week. This emergence causes the septum to remain a thin membrane rather than the thick wall it was at its formation.

Carmi et al. (9) added evidence supporting the possible existence of an X-linked midline mutant gene. They reported familial congenital diaphragmatic defects associated with other midline anomalies such as cleft palate and omphalocele in brothers.

Czeizel and Kovacs (10) and Cunniff et al. (11) also reported genetic studies of diaphragmatic defects for determination of chromosomal, genetic, and nongenetic patterns.

Carmi et al. (12) suggested an X-linked dominant inheritance in a family with thoracoabdominal syndrome (diaphragmatic and ventral herniae plus hypoplastic lung and cardiac anomalies).

Similar cases of a condition referred to as Fryns syndrome were reported by Ayme et al. (13), who stated that

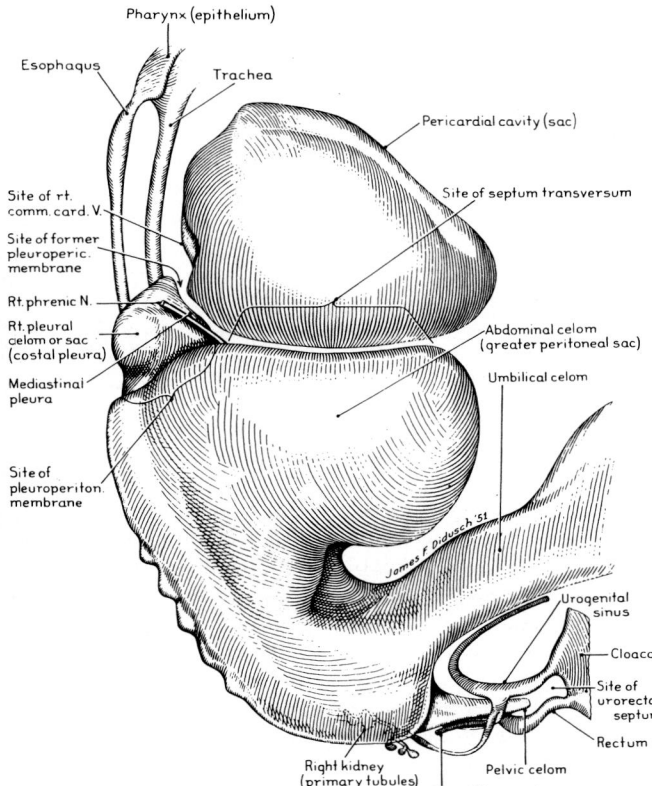

Figure 15.4. Relationships of pericardium, right pleura, and peritoneum, with all other structures removed, in a 12.6-mm human embryo (6 weeks), in which the pleuroperitoneal canals have closed. Note that the pleural sac is still very small in comparison with the pericardial sac. (From Wells LJ. Development of the human diaphragm and pleural sacs. Contrib Embryol Carnegie Inst Wash 35:109, 1954.)

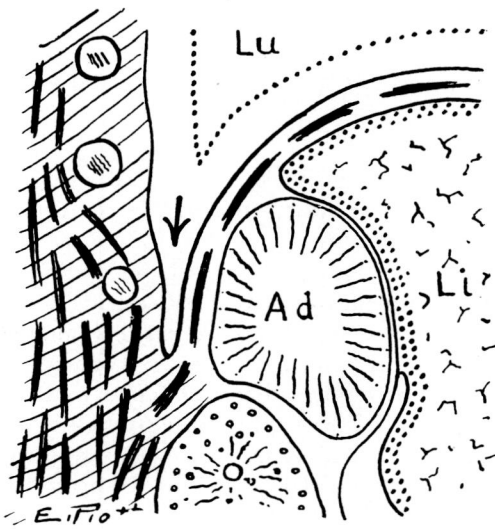

Figure 15.6. Section of the right side of a 30-mm embryo, showing the splitting off of muscle fibers from the lower ribs and their transfer to the developing diaphragm by a process of "burrowing" (indicated by *arrow*). *Lu*, lung; *Ad*, suprarenal gland; *Li*, liver. (From Bremer JL. The diaphragm and diaphragmatic hernia. Arch Pathol 1943; 36:539–549. Copyright 1943, the American Medical Association.)

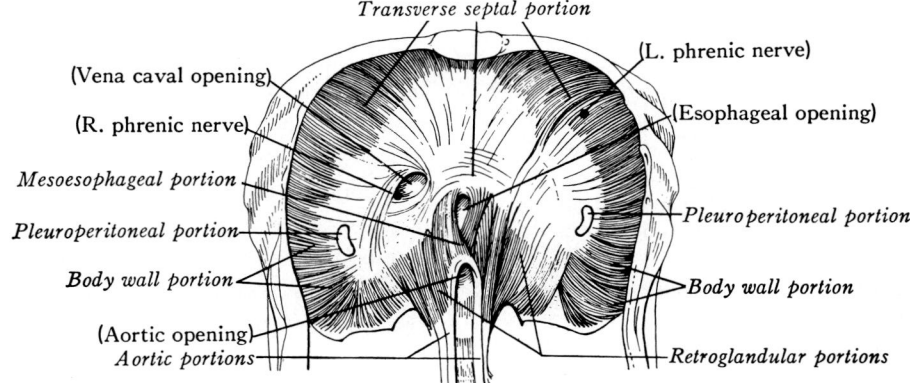

Figure 15.5. The components of the definitive diaphragm. No distinct boundaries can be drawn and the extent of the portions contributed by the pleuroperitoneal membranes can only be estimated. (From Arey LB. Developmental anatomy, 7th ed. Philadelphia: WB Saunders, 1965. After Wells.)

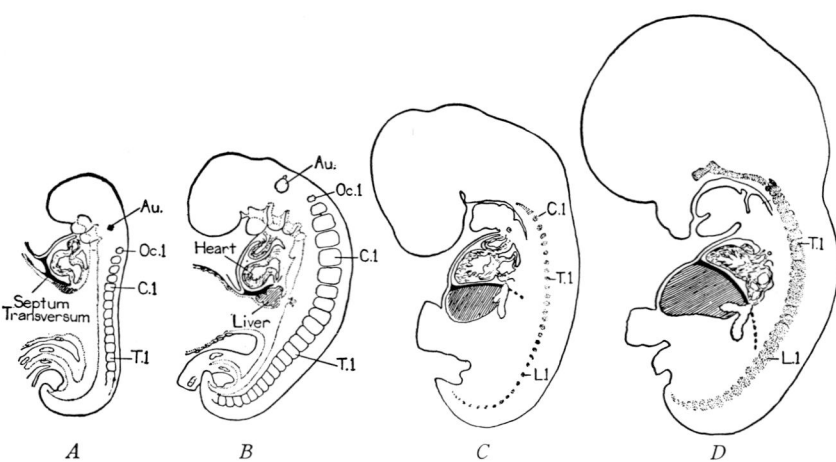

Figure 15.7. "Descent" of the transverse septum from its site of origin to its final position. **A,** At 2 mm. **B,** At 3.6 mm. **C,** At 11 mm. **D,** At 25 mm (8 weeks). *Au.,* Auditory vesicle; *Oc. 1,* first occipital vertebra; *C. 1,* first cervical vertebra; *T. 1,* first thoracic vertebra; *L. 1,* first lumbar vertebra. Drawn at varying magnifications. (From Arey LB. Developmental anatomy, 7th ed. Philadelphia: WB Saunders, 1965. After Patten.)

this is autosomal recessive, and by Cunniff et al. (14), who stated that there are approximately 25 cases of Fryns syndrome in the literature.

Cullen et al. (15) reported that diaphragmatic hernia is as much an enigma today as it was during the time of Bochdalek. There is both parenchymal and vascular hypoplasia and, despite tremendous progress in understanding the pathophysiology, effective treatment has eluded physicians. Survival rates are still poor.

Anomalies of the diaphragm are associated with multiple other congenital malformations. To present them in toto is not possible, and to name all syndromes is not practical for a book such as this. The authors hope the reader or the investigator will forgive this.

Remember the diaphragmatic decalogue:

1. The pericardioperitoneal canal is a large opening located at the septum transversum on either side of the foregut because of the inability of the septum transversum to perform a complete separation between thoracic and abdominal cavities.
2. The formation of the lung buds is within the pericardioperitoneal canal.
3. The thin pleuropericardial fold is a single embryologic entity between the septum transversum and the sternal xiphoid process, owing its genesis to the ventrally and laterally growing pulmonary expansions.
4. The pleuropericardial fold envelops the phrenic nerves and the short common cardinal veins before they enter the sinus horn.
5. The pleuropericardial folds fuse together forming the pericardium and the pleural cavities.
6. The final step of the genesis of the diaphragm is the penetration by myoblasts from the body wall into the membranes of the general peripheral part.
7. The adult diaphragm now is formed.
8. The etiology and mechanism of genesis of a diaphra-

matic hernia are not known. The most logical explanation is failure to fuse rather than failure to form. In other words, all the responsible embryologic entities are present but not fused. Therefore, around the 10th to 12th weeks of gestation, the returning intestinal loops find the diaphragm formed, and they remain within the abdominal cavity. If for some reason, there is nonfusion or delayed closure, some abdominal viscera will enter the thorax producing a hernia and preventing union of the embryologic parts of the diaphragm. Therefore early upward migration of the abdominal viscera into the thorax is perhaps an acceptable speculation. Large amounts of abdominal viscera in the thorax and a small-sized diaphragmatic defect supports early migration and a secondary effect of the embryologic entities to close the defect. The hernia of Bochdalek results from this etiologic mechanism, probably as a maldevelopment of the pleuroperitoneal membrane caused by the inability to close the pericardioperitoneal canal around the sixth week. Both Moore (16) and Sadler (17) agree.

EDITORIAL COMMENT

While it is reasonable that abdominal viscera herniated through the pleuroperitoneal canal would prevent fusion of the pleuroperitoneal canal and the result would be a patent canal or hernia, the real question is why the pleuroperitoneal canal is still open at the time the abdominal *viscera* return from their umbilical herniation site. Is it not just as reasonable to assume that the closure of the pleuroperitoneal canal results from the failure of development of the tracheobronchial tree and, specifically, the lung buds, which should at this time be filling the developing pleural space? If there is an abnormality in this development with marked hypoplasia of these tissues, this could itself have an effect on the normal closure of the pleuroperitoneal canal, and the subsequent vasculature and parenchymal abnormalities associated with diaphragmatic hernia

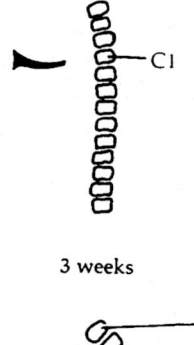

3 weeks

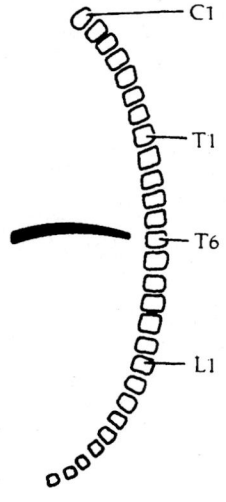

6 weeks

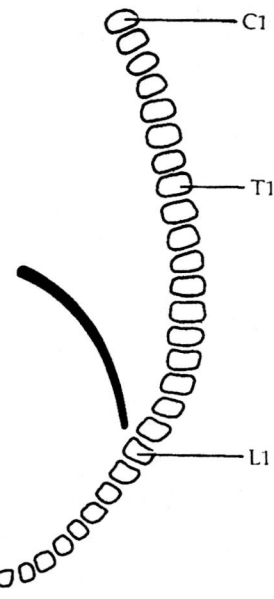

8 weeks

Figure 15.8. The descent of the diaphragm during development. The phrenic nerve arises from the third to the fifth cervical segments and follows the diaphragm down to its final position. (From Skandalakis JE, Gray SW, Rowe JS Jr, Skandalakis LJ. Surgical anatomy of the diaphragm. In: Nyhus LM, Baker RJ, eds. Mastery of surgery. Boston: Little, Brown, 1992.)

may actually be primarily rather than secondarily due to compression of the lungs by the herniated viscera! This embryologic process has not been carefully studied, but it is just as viable (and perhaps somewhat more logical) an explanation for the failure of closure since the former explanation does not give any etiologic factors for the patency of the pleuroperitoneal canal through which the abdominal viscera herniates.

In summary, there is no good embryologic basis for the current, most popular theory of diaphragmatic hernia formation—namely, that the returning intestine slips up through the pleuroperitoneal canal and thus blocks its closure. In view of the commonly altered development of the lung associated with diaphragmatic hernia, it is just as reasonable that the primary defect is a lung bud anomaly with underdevelopment and abnormal vascular parenchymal relationship which does not contribute to the normal closure of a pleuroperitoneal canal. Thus it is patent when the intestine comes back, but it is not the intestine going through it which keeps it from closing. The best evidence for this position is the recent documentation of more than 25% of sonographically studied human embryos who eventually show herniated intestine into the pleural cavity as late as 20 weeks, although prior to that no evidence of any herniation of abdominal viscera through the defect into the chest was present.

It should also be pointed out that the foramen of Bochdalek hernia does not actually go through the pleuroperitoneal canal but is medial to this in the developing muscular part of the diaphragm. Thus the original description by Bochdalek may very well have been a rare type of diaphragmatic hernia, not the common one which goes through the pleuroperitoneal canal (JAH/CNP).

9. Occasionally, however, a part of the muscular diaphragm does not develop. Perhaps the myoblastic invasion is not complete, permitting the formation of gaps, and the presence of a hernia. The so-called parasternal hernia of Morgagni belongs to this group, as perhaps does eventration.

10. Concerning the pulmonary hypoplasia which develops from pressure of the abdominal viscera in the thorax (and which is a possible cause of death from respiratory failure), the reader should remember the steps of development of the bronchial tree. This development starts around the fifth week of gestation and continues until birth (and for at least 7 years thereafter). Reid (18) and Dibbins (19) studied damage of the respiratory epithelium as well as the vasoconstriction of the lungs. Early insult stops the embryologically normal process which can start again after repair by production of small numbers of alveoli and pathologic changes in the vessels that may be responsible for pnemoneal hypertension.

EDITORIAL COMMENT

As noted above, there is no good evidence that pulmonary hypoplasia associated with diaphragmatic hernia is *caused* by pressure of the abdominal viscera in the thorax. Experimental animal prep- arations using silastic balloons have demonstrated that displace- ment of the lung during early development can cause hypoplasia, but none of these animal models develops the abnormal pulmo- nary vasculature that results in pulmonary hypertension, which is the hallmark of the baby with diaphragmatic hernia. Thus the pul- monary hypoplasia may be a primary defect associated with fail- ure of closure of the diaphragmatic tissue (JAH/CNP).

Critical Events in Development

Failure of closure of the pleuroperitoneal canal by the pleuroperitoneal membranes in the eighth week is the source of several diaphragmatic defects. An especially serious one occurs with the return of the intestines before complete separation of pleural and peritoneal cavities.

Delay in elongation of the esophagus during the sev- enth and eighth weeks may be responsible for the enlarged esophageal hiatus of the diaphragm, which later produces hiatal hernia. This, however, has not been unequivocally established.

Congenital short esophagus—myth or not—should be considered as an explanation of esophageal hernia.

ANOMALIES OF THE DIAPHRAGM (TABLES 15.2 AND 15.3 AND FIG. 15.9)

Fusion Defects of the Diaphragm

The diaphragm, being constructed from several fused embryonic components, is subject to a number of defects.

From the developmental point of view, three fundamen- tal types of defects occur.

COMPLETE OR PARTIAL ABSENCE OF THE DIAPHRAGM

This results from failure of one or more of the compo- nents to form or from failure of the components to join properly. In such cases, if the diaphragm is present, there is a large or small perforation providing open communi- cation between the thorax and abdomen. Regardless of the size of the opening, no hernial sac is present. Defects of this type have been termed *embryonic*, in contradistinc- tion to *congenital* defects belonging to the second group. To this group belong absence of the diaphragm, herniae into the pericardium, and many posterolateral (foramen of Bochdalek) herniae (Figs. 15.10 and 15.11).

FAILURE OF COMPLETE MUSCULARIZATION

In this group of defects normal fusion of the embryonic components of the diaphragm occurs, but there is a sub- sequent failure of the muscular tissue to spread over the entire area. In such cases the portion unprotected by muscle will bulge into the thoracic cavity, forming a her- nial sac. This thin, bulging membrane may or may not rupture. If it ruptures in prenatal life or early in infancy, no trace of it may appear at operation. When the sac is present, the hernia is often called "true," and when it is absent, "false." The distinction is of surgical but not developmental significance. To this group of defects belong eventration, many posterolateral (foramen of Bochdalek) herniae, all retrosternal (foramen of Morga-

Table 15.2.
Anomalies of the Diaphragm

Anomaly	Origin of Defect	First Appearance	Sex Chiefly Affected	Relative Frequency	Remarks
Absence of the diaphragm	Week 8 onward	At birth	?	Rare (unilateral): very rare (bilateral)	
Posterolateral defects of the diaphragm (Bochdalek)	Weeks 8–10	At birth or later	Equal	Common	
Parasternal defects of the diaphragm (Morgagni)	Week 7	At any age, usually in adulthood	Equal	Uncommon	
Eventration of the diaphragm	Week 10	At any age	Male	Uncommon	
Defect of the septum transversum	Unknown	At any age	?	Very rare	Often with ectopia cordis
Defects of the esophageal hiatus					
Hiatal hernia	Weeks 7–8	At middle age or later	Female	Common	Distinguishable only at operation
Congenital short esophagus	Week 7	In childhood	Male	Uncommon	
Accessory diaphragm	Week 8	At any age, or not at all	?	Very rare	

Table 15.3.
Congenital Hernias of the Diaphragm[a]

Congenital Hernias	Anatomy	Sac and Herniated Organs	Remarks
Eventration of the diaphragm	Congenital hernia. Diaphragm is thin with sparsely distributed, but normal muscle fibers. Either or both sides may be affected. Phrenic nerve appears normal.	"Sac" is formed by the attenuated diaphragm. Contents: Normal abdominal organs under elevated dome of hemidiaphragm.	Heart and mediastinum shifted to contralateral side. Ipsilateral lung collapsed, but normal. Malrotation and inversion of abdominal viscera are common.
Hernia through the foramen of Bochdalek; posterolateral hernia of the diaphragm	Congenital hernia through the lumbocostal trigone. May expand to include almost whole hemidiaphragm. More common on left.	Sac present in 10–15%. Contents: Small intestine, usual; stomach, colon, spleen, frequent. Pancreas and liver, rare. Liver only in right-sided hernia.	Heart and mediastinum shifted to contralateral side. Ipsilateral lung hypoplastic. Contralateral lung also hypoplastic to variable degrees. Secondary malrotation is common. Craniorrhachischisis, tracheoesophageal fistula and heart defects occasionally associated.
Hernia through the foramen of Morgagni; retrosternal hernia; parasternal hernia; anterior diaphagramatic hernia	Congenital potential hernia through muscular hiatus on either side of the xiphoid process. Usually on the right; bilateral cases are known. Actual herniation usually the result of postnatal trauma.	Sac present at first. May rupture later, leaving no trace. Contents: Infants: Liver. Adults: Omentum May be followed by colon and stomach later.	Rare in infants and children.
Peritoneopericardial hernia; defect of the central tendon; defect of the transverse septum	Congenital hernia through central tendon and pericardium.	Sac rarely present. Contents: Stomach, colon.	Has been seen in newborns and in adults. Perhaps traumatic in adults. Very rare.

[a]From Gray SW, Skandalakis JE: Atlas of surgical anatomy for general surgeons, Philadelphia: WB Saunders, 1985: 62, Plate 3-4; 63, Plate 3-4.

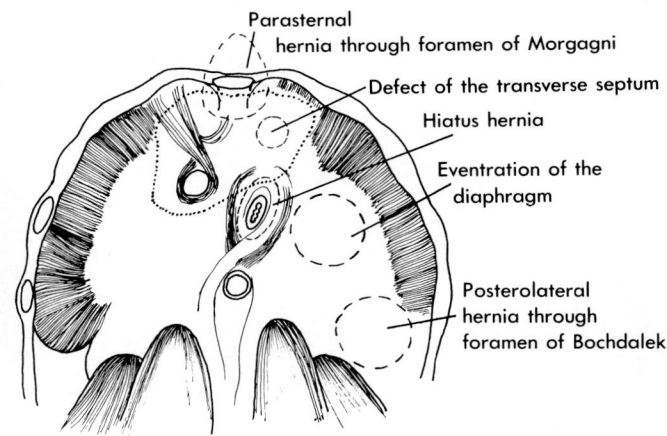

Figure 15.9. Sites of diaphragmatic anomalies.

gni) herniae, and herniae through the dome of the diaphragm.

CONGENITALLY ENLARGED ESOPHAGEAL HIATUS

The diaphragm forms completely and normally, but as a result of delay in descent of the stomach, the esophageal hiatus is slightly larger than necessary. This leaves a space between the diaphragm and the esophagus. Hiatal herniae of various types, with or without a hernial sac, belong to this group. The hiatal defect is the congenital malformation; the herniation of the stomach is an acquired lesion.

Because the presence or absence of a hernial sac is not usually recognized on radiography and often is not determined even at operation, the embryologic classification is not convenient clinically. A more practical classification of congenital diaphragmatic defects must rest largely on morphology and anatomic location:

1. Partial or complete absence of the diaphragm
2. Posterolateral defects of the pleuroperitoneal membrane (foramen of Bochdalek)
3. Parasternal defects (foramen of Morgagni)
4. Eventration of the diaphragm
5. Defects of the septum transversum
6. Defects of the esophageal hiatus

In the infant herniation through the foramen of Bochdalek is the most frequently encountered. With increasing age, other forms of herniation, especially those through the esophageal hiatus, become more common. When all ages are considered, hiatus hernia accounts for about 50% of diaphragmatic herniae. Figure 15.12 shows the percentage of developmental defects of the dia-

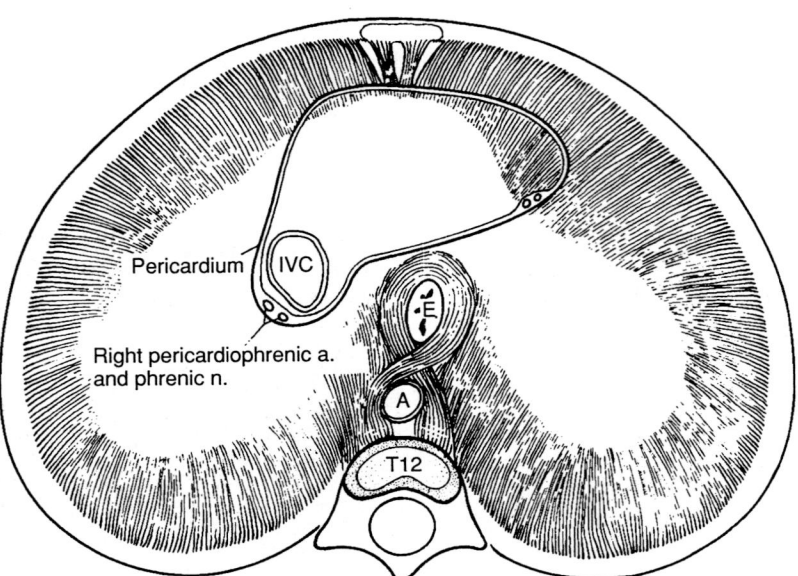

Figure 15.10. The diaphragm viewed from below. The area in contact with the pericardium is indicated. The pericardial fibrous tissue is continuous with that of the diaphragm. (From Skandalakis JE, Gray SW, Rowe JS Jr, Skandalakis LJ. Surgical anatomy of the diaphragm. In: Nyhus LM, Baker RJ, eds. Mastery of surgery. Boston: Little, Brown, 1992.)

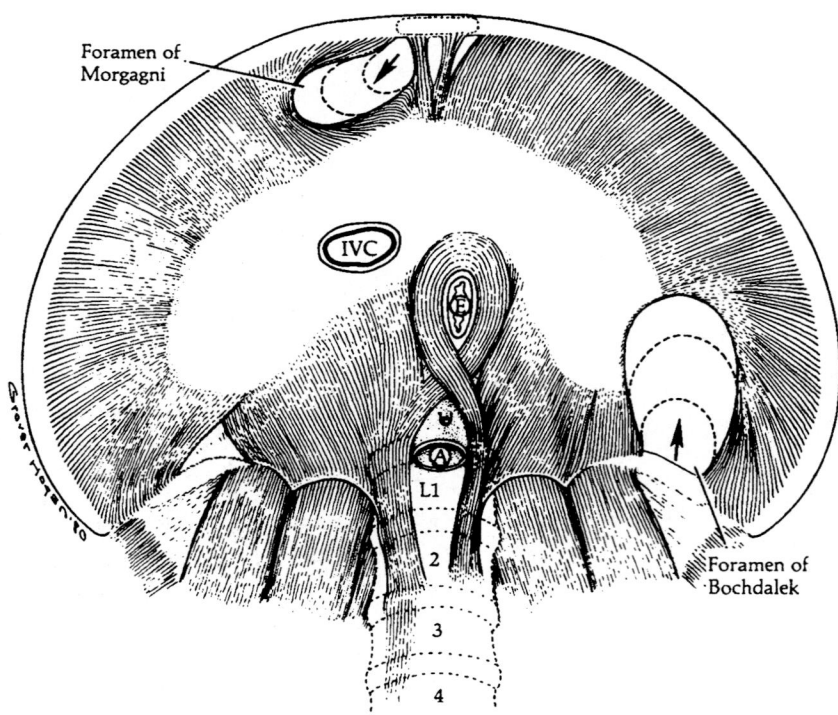

Figure 15.11. The diaphragm from below, showing the foramen of Bochdalek and the foramen of Morgagni. Both are weak areas of potential herniation. *Arrows* indicate the direction of enlargement after herniation has begun. (From Skandalakis JE, Gray SW, Rowe JS Jr, Skandalakis LJ. Surgical anatomy of the diaphragm. In: Nyhus LM, Baker RJ, eds. Mastery of surgery. Boston: Little, Brown, 1992.)

phragm by location. The relative incidence of various types of congenital herniae of the diaphragm also was presented by Kiesewetter (20) (Fig. 15.13).

OVERALL ASSOCIATED ANOMALIES

Malrotation of the gut is the most common associated congenital anomaly, according to Irving and Booker (21). The same authors present their experience with 153 cases of congenital diaphragmatic herniae (Table 15.4).

EDITORIAL COMMENT

Malrotation of the gut is a very serious complication of posterolateral diaphragmatic hernia because, when the bowel is replaced in the abdomen, midgut volvulus may occur as a result of the failure of fixation of the mesentery. In various series, 5 to 10% of patients with diaphragmatic herniae will have partial to complete intestinal obstruction and occasionally full necrosis of the midgut following successful repair of the diaphragmatic hernia. For this reason, most pediatric surgeons believe that the best approach to closure of the diaphragmatic defect is transabdominal, rather than transthoracic, so that the intestine can be brought back under direct vision and replaced in the abdomen in an untwisted fashion. If this is carried out from the transthoracic route, the intestine is pushed blindly through the defect into the abdomen and may become twisted.

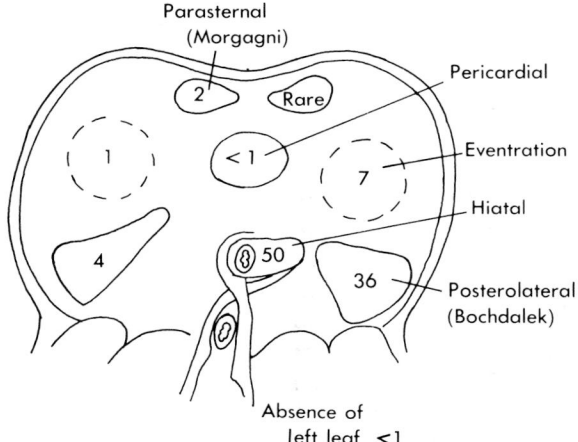

Figure 15.12. Percentage of developmental defects of the diaphragm at various locations for persons of all ages. Posterolateral (Bochdalek) defects are by far the most frequently found in infants; esophageal hiatus defects rarely manifest themselves before adulthood.

Table 15.4.
Congenital Diaphragmatic Hernia: Associated Anomalies in 153 Cases (Excluding Pulmonary Hypoplasia)[a]

Malrotation		63
Congenital heart lesions		
Patent ductus arteriosus	3	
Hypoplastic left heart	2	
VSD	1	8
ASD + coarctation of aorta	1	
Pulmonary stenosis	1	
Undescended testes		8
Meckel's diverticulum		7
Skeletal anomalies		
Minor deformities of hands	3	
Talipes	2	7
Multiple hemivertebrae	1	
Craniostenosis	1	
Myelomeningocele		3
Renal anomalies		
Ectopic (thoracic) kidney	1	
Ectopic (pelvic) kidney	1	3
PUJ obstruction	1	
Inguinal hernia		2
Extralobar pulmonary sequestration		2
Cystic adenomatoid malformation of lung		1
Duodenal atresia		1
Hirschsprung's disease		1
Esophageal atresia		1
Choanal atresia		1

[a]From Irving IM, Booker PD. Congenital diaphragmatic hernia and eventration of the diaphragm. In: Lister J, Irving IM: Neonatal surgery, 3rd ed. London: Butterworth, 1990.

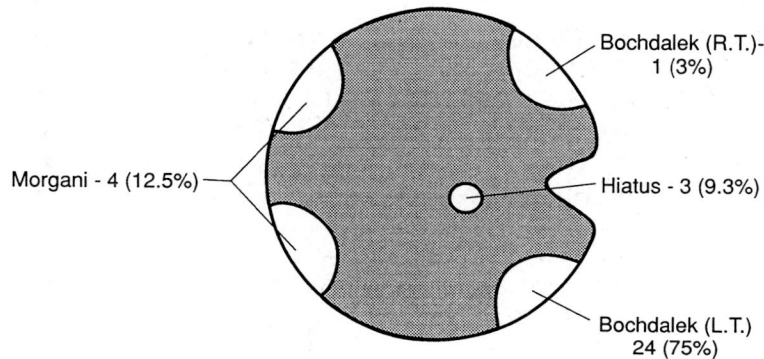

Figure 15.13. The relative incidence of various types of congenital herniae of the diaphragm. (From Kiesewetter WB, Gutierrez IZ, Sieber WK. Diaphragmatic hernia in infants under one year of age. Arch Surg 1961; 83:561–572.)

ABSENCE OF THE DIAPHRAGM

Complete Absence of the Diaphragm. Absence of both leaves of the diaphragm is occasionally seen in monstrous fetuses; rarely have such individuals survived. Coca and Landin (22) described the findings at surgery in a 19-year-old male who complained only of gastric pain. The patient had an infantile, hypoplastic pituitary habitus, cranial osteoporosis, and sacral spina bifida. The entire right diaphragm was absent, and the left diaphragm was represented by a 2-cm semilunar fold covering the spleen. The hepatic flexure of the colon was in the right thorax, and most of the stomach was in the left thorax. No diaphragmatic repair was attempted, and the patient survived.

Absence of the Hemidiaphragm. Absence of one leaf of the diaphragm, usually the left one, is more frequently encountered, although it is still rare. Sagal (23) was able to find only 13 cases up to 1933 although he overlooked some. All but one were on the left side. While some cases are detected in infancy (24, 25), many patients are of advanced age at the time of discovery (26). One example of this anomaly, associated with phocomelia and other defects, was reported in a suspected but unconfirmed case of 17–18 trisomy (27).

Hatzitheofilou et al. (28) presented a case of agenesis of the right hemidiaphragm.

The first successful repairs were made in 1954 by Neville and Clowes (24) and by Cornet et al. (29).

Slim et al. (30) reviewed 52 cases of congenital diaphragmatic defects: 36 of Bochdalek hernia, 13 of eventration, and 3 of agenesis. The operative mortality of diaphragmatic agenesis was 100%.

POSTEROLATERAL DEFECTS OF THE DIAPHRAGM: HERNIA THROUGH THE FORAMEN OF BOCHDALEK (FIG. 15.14)

The foramen of Bochdalek includes the site of the pleuroperitoneal membrane; hence, the resulting hernia is often called "hernia through the pleuroperitoneal canal" (Fig. 15.15). However, because the pleuroperitoneal membrane forms only a small portion of the area of the defect, we prefer not to use this term. It is through this type of defect that most diaphragmatic herniae—other than esophageal hiatus herniae—occur (Fig. 15.16).

According to Reynolds (31), in 20% of left Bochdalek herniae, there is a sac.

Anatomy. The defect, when small, consists of an opening in the posterolateral portion of the diaphragm. When large, it may extend almost to the midline and beyond the dome, leaving only an anterolateral shelf of diaphragmatic muscle. There appears to be a gradation from defects of 1 cm or less to almost complete absence of one-half of the diaphragm.

Most of the herniae through the foramen of Bochdalek are "false"—that is, without a membrane. The pleura

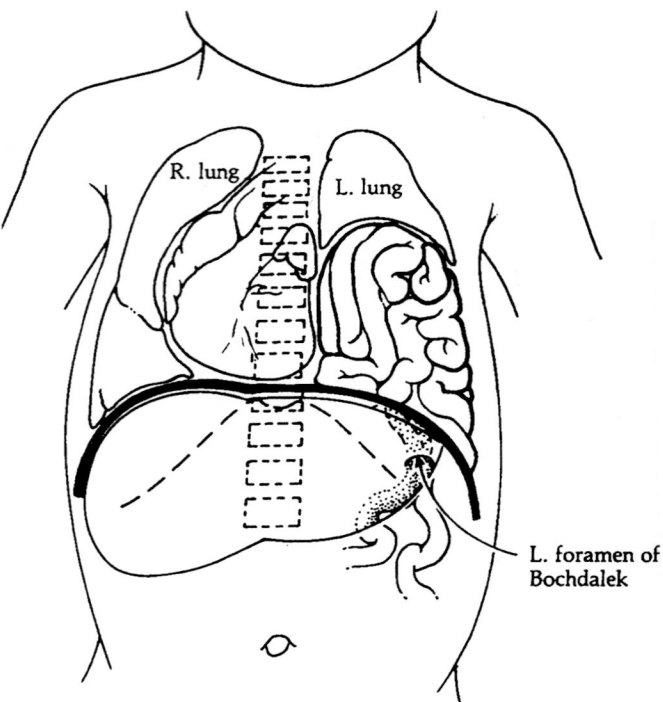

Figure 15.14. Herniation of intestines through the foramen of Bochdalek compressing the left lung. The mediastinum is shifted to the right, reducing the volume of the right lung also. (From Skandalakis JE, Gray SW, Rowe JS Jr, Skandalakis LJ. Surgical anatomy of the diaphragm. In: Nyhus LM, Baker RJ, eds. Mastery of surgery. Boston: Little, Brown, 1992.)

and peritoneum are continuous over the edge of the aperture.

In from 10 to 15% of patients, the presence of a sac can be demonstrated. The left side is affected in 85 to 90% of patients. Blank and Campbell (32) reported right-sided congenital posterolateral defects. Butler and Claireaux (33) found, among 60 infants, 55 with defects on the left, 4 with defects on the right, and 1 with defects on both sides (Fig. 15.17).

The rarity of bilaterality was emphasized by Nicolisi et al. (34) and Zamir (35).

The small intestine is involved in about 90% of diaphragmatic herniae; the stomach, colon, and spleen in more than 50%. The pancreas and liver are occasionally involved. In the rare right-sided herniae, the liver is usually the only organ to enter the thorax.

Incomplete rotation of the intestine, with anomalous mesenteric attachments, is usual. The heart and mediastinum usually are displaced markedly to the right by the abdominal organs in the left thorax.

No relationship is seen between the size of the diaphragmatic defect and the mass of the herniated organs (Fig. 15.16).

Pathophysiology. The infant with a congenital diaphragmatic hernia faces two distinct but interrelated patho-

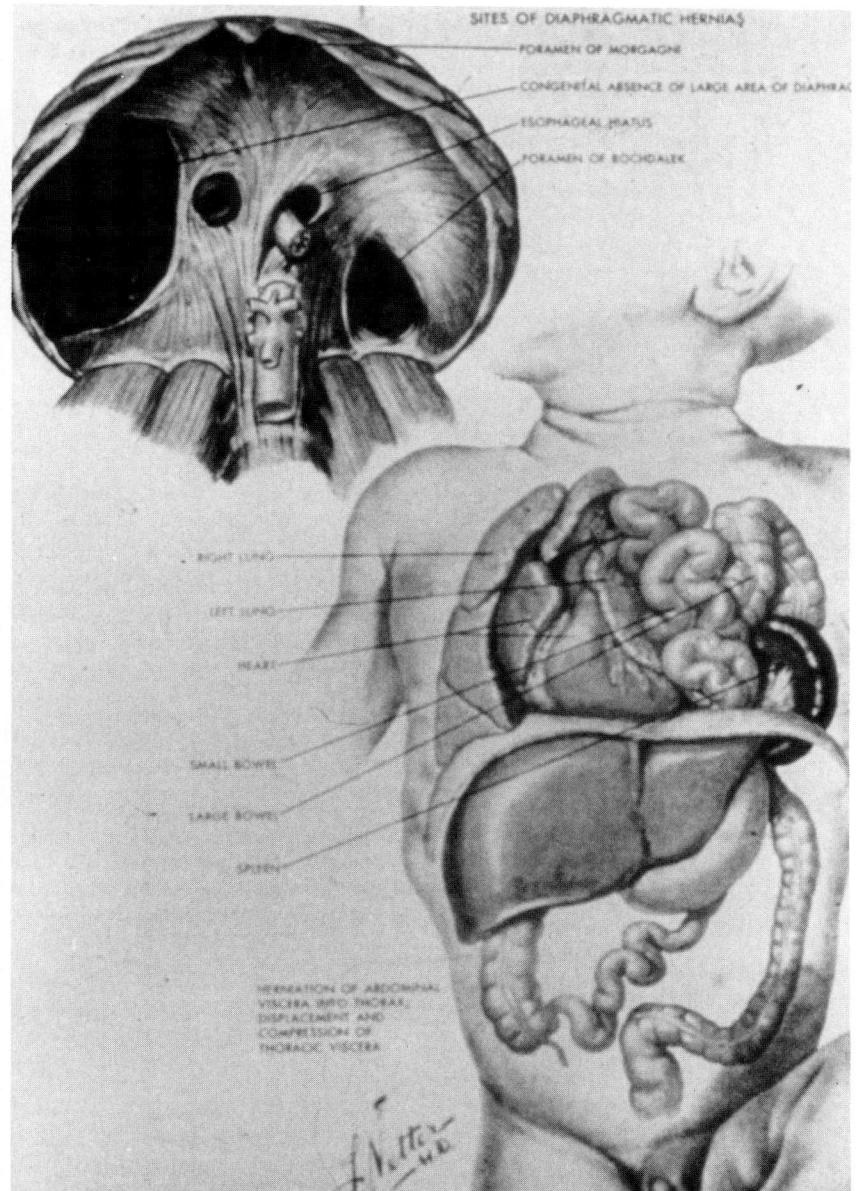

SITES OF DIAPHRAGMATIC HERNIAS

FORAMEN OF MORGAGNI
CONGENITAL ABSENCE OF LARGE AREA OF DIAPHRAGM
ESOPHAGEAL HIATUS
FORAMEN OF BOCHDALEK

RIGHT LUNG
LEFT LUNG
HEART
SMALL BOWEL
LARGE BOWEL
SPLEEN

HERNIATION OF ABDOMINAL
VISCERA INTO THORAX,
DISPLACEMENT AND
COMPRESSION OF
THORACIC VISCERA

Figure 15.15. Schematic illustration of a left-sided congenital diaphragmatic hernia through the foramen of Bochdalek. (From Netter FH. The CIBA collection of medical illustrations. Vol 3, Digestive system. Part II, Lower digestive tract. Summit NJ: CIBA Pharmaceutical Co., 1979.)

physiologic abnormalities, either one of which can result in death.

First, there is a variable degree of pulmonary hypoplasia affecting the ipsilateral lung and, to a lesser degree, the contralateral lung. Postmortem examination of the lungs of infants who have died from congenital diaphragmatic hernia showed decreased lung volume and lung weight compared to normal controls (36–38). Simson (37) found that lung weights in patients dying from congenital diaphragmatic hernia were consistently less than one-half the normal lung weights of controls. There is significant hypoplasia of both lungs: The ipsilateral lung weight was 31% and the contralateral lung weight 60% of that of controls. Bohn (36) also found a severe reduction in total alveolar number when compared to normal newborn control values. Thus pulmonary hypoplasia is present to a certain degree in all infants with congenital diaphragmatic hernia; there is a degree of pulmonary hypoplasia which is incompatible with life regardless of the therapeutic modalities used. However, at the present time, and utilizing all the clinical and laboratory data available, it is impossible to determine which infant has

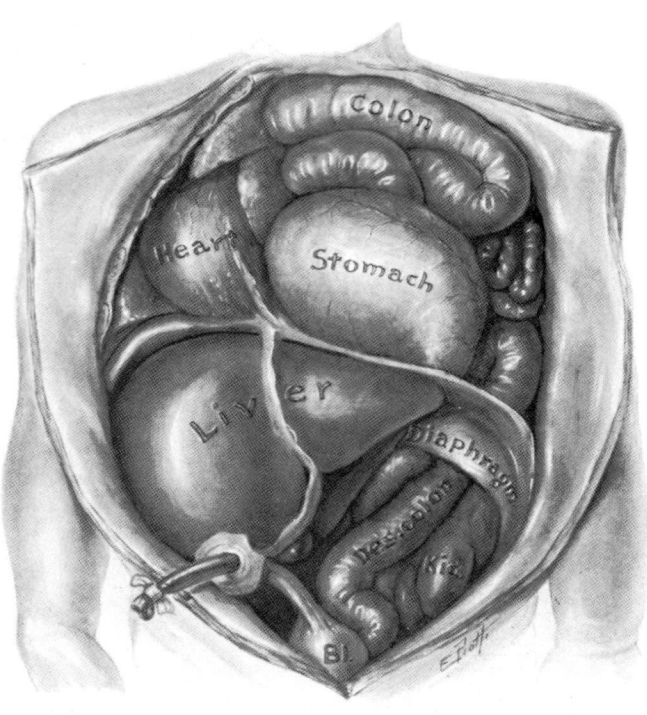

Figure 15.16. Diaphragmatic hernia through the posterolateral foramen of Bochdalek in an infant. The infant died 4 hours after birth, after exhibiting severe cyanosis and respiratory distress. There is no sac surrounding the viscera in the thorax. (From Gross RE. The surgery of infancy and childhood. Philadelphia: WB Saunders, 1953.)

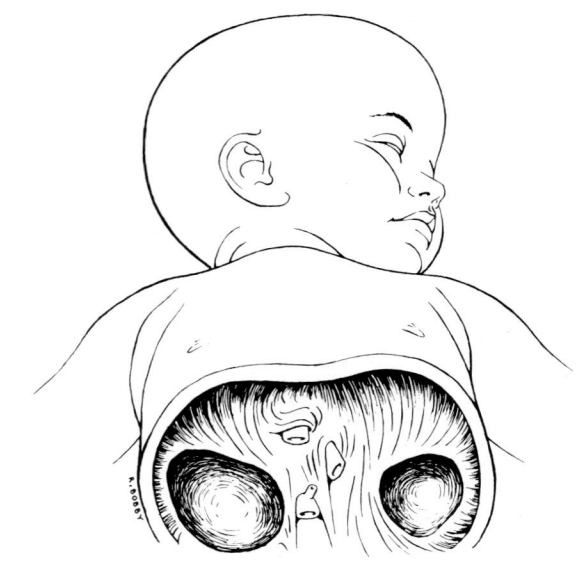

Figure 15.17. An unusual example of bilateral posterolateral diaphragmatic (Bochdalek) defect in an infant. (From Fitchett CW, Tavarez V. Bilateral congenital diaphragmatic herniation: case report. Surgery 1965; 57:305–308.)

that degree of pulmonary hypoplasia that precludes survival.

A distinct but related pathophysiologic abnormality is persistence of pulmonary vascular hypertension which these infants manifest. There are abnormalities not only in the pulmonary parenchymal architecture but also in the pulmonary vascular architecture (36, 38, 39). There is a significant increase in muscle mass in the small pulmonary arteries in infants with congenital diaphragmatic herniae when compared to age-matched controls (39) (Fig. 15.18).

EDITORIAL COMMENT

While it is true there are two distinct pathophysiologic additions—namely, hypoplasia of the lung and persistent pulmonary artery hypertension with congenital diaphragmatic hernia—the one which is by far the most lethal is the persistent pulmonary artery hypertension. Hypoplasia of the lung alone, if the lung tissue is normal, does not result in obstruction to pulmonary blood flow, and thus there is no pulmonary artery hypertension. There is good clinical and experimental evidence to indicate that a pneumonectomy in a newborn baby is well-tolerated without the development of pulmonary vascular hypertension. It is the rare baby with dia-

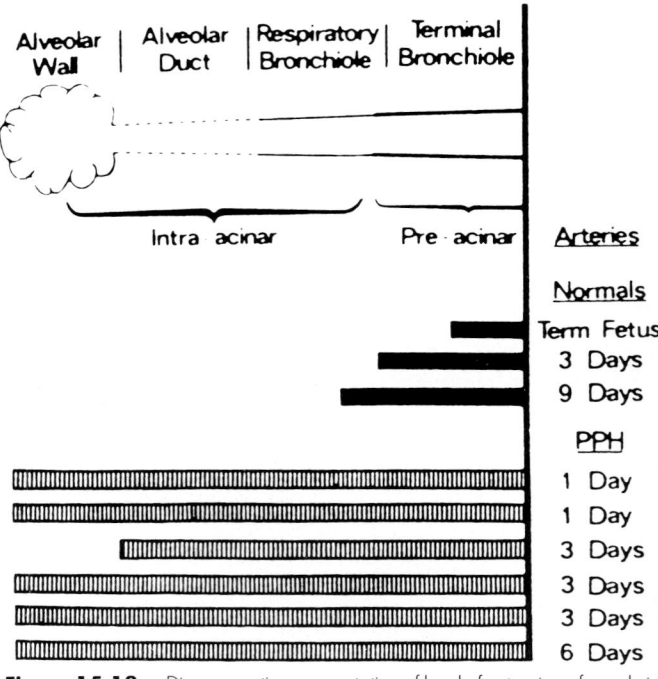

Figure 15.18. Diagrammatic representation of level of extension of muscle in the walls of the intraacinar arteries of normal infants and those with persistent pulmonary hypertension (PPH). (From Shochat SJ: Pulmonary vascular pathology in congenital diaphragmatic hernia. Pediatr Surg Int 1987; 2:331–335; reproduced from Reid LM: Pathological changes in humans. In: Sandor GGS, Macnab AJ, Rastogi RB, eds. Persistent fetal circulation. Mount Kisco, NY: Futura Media Services, 1982:37.)

phragmatic hernia which does not have more than one-half of normal pulmonary tissue. Therefore it is the pulmonary vascular abnormality which is lethal, not the lack of pulmonary tissue (JAH/CNP).

In addition, there is a decrease in the total size of the pulmonary vascular bed, a decrease in the number of vessels per unit of lung, and an elevated pulmonary vascular resistance resulting in right-to-left shunting through the fetal channels (patent ductus arteriosus and patent foramen ovale) (38). This abnormal pulmonary vascular bed demonstrates an exaggerated response to normal physiologic stimuli, such as hypoxia, acidosis, and hypercarbia, that produce pulmonary vasoconstriction in the newborn (39).

Whereas pulmonary hypoplasia cannot be altered in the newborn, pulmonary vascular hypertension can. Thus therapeutic interventions in infants with congenital diaphragmatic hernia are now directed toward treating or preventing pulmonary vasospasm utilizing hyperventilation with oxygen, medication (Fig. 15.19), and (recently) extracorporeal membrane oxygenation (ECMO) (40).

Associated Anomalies. In approximately 60% of patients, congenital diaphragmatic hernia is the only severe malformation, apart from those normally associated with the presence of abdominal viscera in the thorax, such as malrotation. These patients have a favorable outcome with a 55% survival rate. Forty percent of patients have one or more severe extra diaphragmatic malformations; these patients have a dismal outcome, with only 14% surviving (41). Most of the associated abnormalities involve the heart, brain, genitourinary system, craniofacial region, or limbs.

Of those patients diagnosed in utero with prenatal ultrasound, 40% have other severe congenital malformations (42). Furthermore, 16% of these fetuses have chromosomal abnormalities (43). Only 24% of patients diagnosed prenatally will be expected to survive even with the most sophisticated medical and surgical therapy, including ECMO (43).

Embryogenesis. The studies of Broman (1) assigned a large area of the diaphragm to the pleuroperitoneal membrane, and explanations of posterolateral diaphragmatic defects usually are based on his concept. Bremer (2) and Wells (3) showed that the membrane accounts for a very small area of the adult diaphragm and that the foramen of Bochdalek is not coincident with the site of the pleuroperitoneal canal (see Fig. 15.5).

Failure of the pleuroperitoneal canal to be reduced to a small slit early in the eighth week will not prevent the opening from becoming covered by a membrane but will

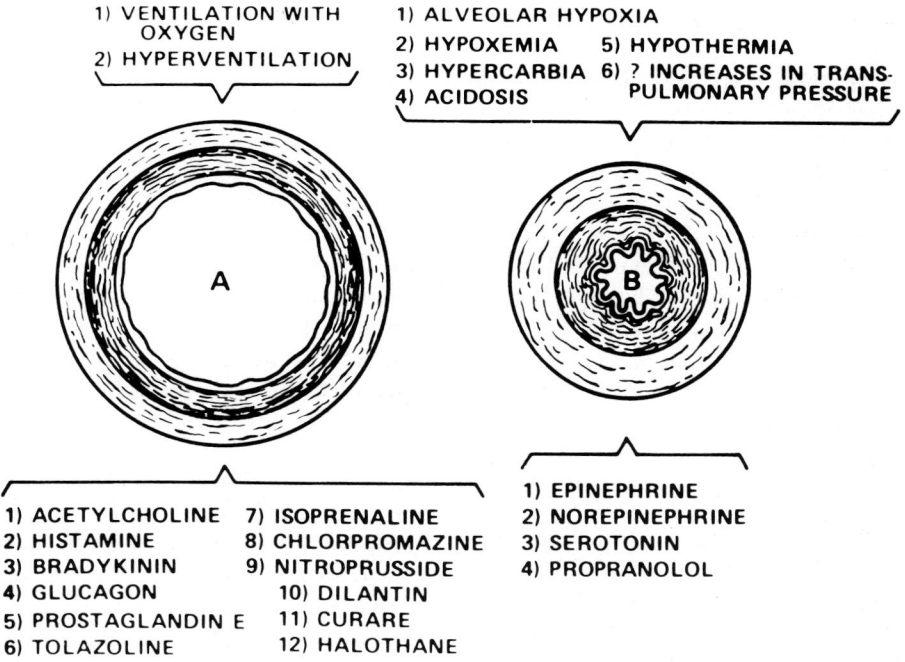

VENTILATORY AND METABOLIC FACTORS

1) VENTILATION WITH OXYGEN
2) HYPERVENTILATION

1) ALVEOLAR HYPOXIA
2) HYPOXEMIA   5) HYPOTHERMIA
3) HYPERCARBIA   6) ? INCREASES IN TRANS-
4) ACIDOSIS   PULMONARY PRESSURE

1) ACETYLCHOLINE   7) ISOPRENALINE
2) HISTAMINE   8) CHLORPROMAZINE
3) BRADYKININ   9) NITROPRUSSIDE
4) GLUCAGON   10) DILANTIN
5) PROSTAGLANDIN E   11) CURARE
6) TOLAZOLINE   12) HALOTHANE

1) EPINEPHRINE
2) NOREPINEPHRINE
3) SEROTONIN
4) PROPRANOLOL

Figure 15.19. Factors that affect pulmonary vascular tone. **A,** Vasodilation, decreased pulmonary artery resistance, and increased pulmonary blood flow. **B,** Vasoconstriction, increased pulmonary artery resistance, and decreased pulmonary blood flow. (From Shochat SJ. Pulmonary vascular pathology in congenital diaphragmatic hernia. Pediatr Surg Int 1987; 2:331–335.)

leave the dorsal and lateral costal contributions less closely approximated than usual. Thus the lumbocostal trigone, with its apex at the site of the pleuroperitoneal membrane, is without muscle fibers. This triangle, plus the pleuroperitoneal orifice, forms the foramen of Bochdalek (see Fig. 15.12).

Normally, firm closure of the canal and the trigone must occur before the return of the intestines from the umbilical cord to the abdominal cavity during the 10th week. Should the pleuroperitoneal membrane be incomplete when the intestines return, they will pass into the thorax. The membrane will be unable to close the defect; the result will be a herniation without a sac.

If the closure of the pleuroperitoneal canal and the lumbocostal trigone is membranous only—that is, if the muscular component is lacking—and the edges of the muscle are widely separated, the pressure of the returning viscera will push up the unreinforced portion and form a "true" diaphragmatic hernia, with a sac that may subsequently rupture.

Whether there is a delay in the closure of the pleuroperitoneal canal and lumbosacral trigone, an actual arrest in their development, or a premature return of the intestines, the results will be the same. The rarity of the defect on the right side supports the view that closure is usually only delayed and not arrested. The liver usually protects the right leaf from pressure from the returning intestine until closure is complete. In a few instances a portion of the liver itself is found above the diaphragm, with an aperture sufficient only for the passage of its vessels (see Chapter 8, "The Liver").

Almost nothing is known about the etiology of the defect. Warkany and his colleagues (44) were able to produce diaphragmatic herniae in rats from vitamin A–deficient mothers. Andersen (45) reported differences in the frequency of hernia among the offspring of different genetic strains of rats fed the same vitamin A–deficient diet. Kluth et al (46) developed an animal model for the study of diaphragmatic herniae in rats, utilizing Nitrofen to induce hernia formation in the developing diaphragm. With this model, he hopes to study which parts of the diaphragm are affected during the early stages of the malformation. Questions to be explored include when signs of pulmonary hypoplasia become visible, and whether pulmonary hypoplasia occurs as a primary event or the result of displaced intrathoracic viscera.

Since the defect is more common on the left side, Moore (16) emphasized that this may be explained due to an earlier closure of the right pleuroperitoneal opening. Does the developing liver participate in this phenomenon? Perhaps.

History. Parè described two cases of traumatic diaphragmatic hernia in 1610 (47). The first congenital case described appears to be that of Riverius early in the 17th

century; it is included in Bonetus's *Sepulchretum* of 1679 (48). Morgagni (49) reviewed the cases up to 1761 and credited Stehelinus with observing hypoplasia of the lung in a fetus with diaphragmatic hernia. In the same discussion Morgagni mentioned a patient with a substernal diaphragmatic hernia (hernia of Morgagni). The pulmonary hypoplasia was described again in 1819 by Zwanziger, whose description is quoted at length by Korns (50). Bochdalek (51) described the hernia with and without a hernial sac. The name "foramen of Bochdalek" antedates the understanding of the development of the pleuroperitoneal canals.

Irving and Booker (21) carefully studied the original paper of Bochdalek (51) and raised several embryologic and topographicoanatomic questions. They concluded that the term *Bochdalek's hernia* is inaccurate—a misnomer, an inaccuracy also mentioned by White and Suzuki (52).

Keith (53) in 1910 reviewed 34 examples of congenital diaphragmatic defects with anatomic specimens and attempted an embryologic explanation. Hedblom (47) reviewed 378 cases of diaphragmatic hernia in 1925, of which 37 were congenital, and advocated early surgery. However, although Aue (54) performed the first successful repair in 1902 (the report of which was published only in 1920), there was little cause for optimism in 1925. By 1929 Greenwald and Steiner (55) found only 25 cases diagnosed during life among 81 cases in infants and children reported between 1912 and 1929. By 1935 Truesdale (56) had found 44 reports of operations, of which 24 were successful. A number of these cases were his own.

Ladd and Gross (57) reviewed the world literature up to 1940 and found 31 cases treated by surgery in the first year of life, with 17 (55%) of these patients surviving. Gross's results of surgically treating infants and young children for left posterolateral diaphragmatic herniae at Boston Children's Hospital from 1940 to 1951 revealed only 7 deaths in 53 cases (85% survival) (58).

None of the historic data takes into consideration the "hidden mortality" of congenital diaphragmatic hernia (59). Many fetuses with diaphragmatic hernia are aborted or die shortly after birth from the hernia or other coexisting lethal anomalies and therefore do not reach neonatal treatment centers. Currently, the mortality of all babies born with congenital diaphragmatic hernia is well over 50% (37, 40, 43, 60).

Incidence. Congenital diaphragmatic hernia occurs in approximately 1:4000 live births. Since about one-half of infants with diaphragmatic hernia are stillborn or die immediately, the true incidence is about 1:2000 (61, 62). The incidence at Los Angeles County–University of Southern California Women's Hospital from June 1972 to June 1977 was one case in every 2644 births (60). Puri and Gorman (63) reported an incidence of 1:2097 births.

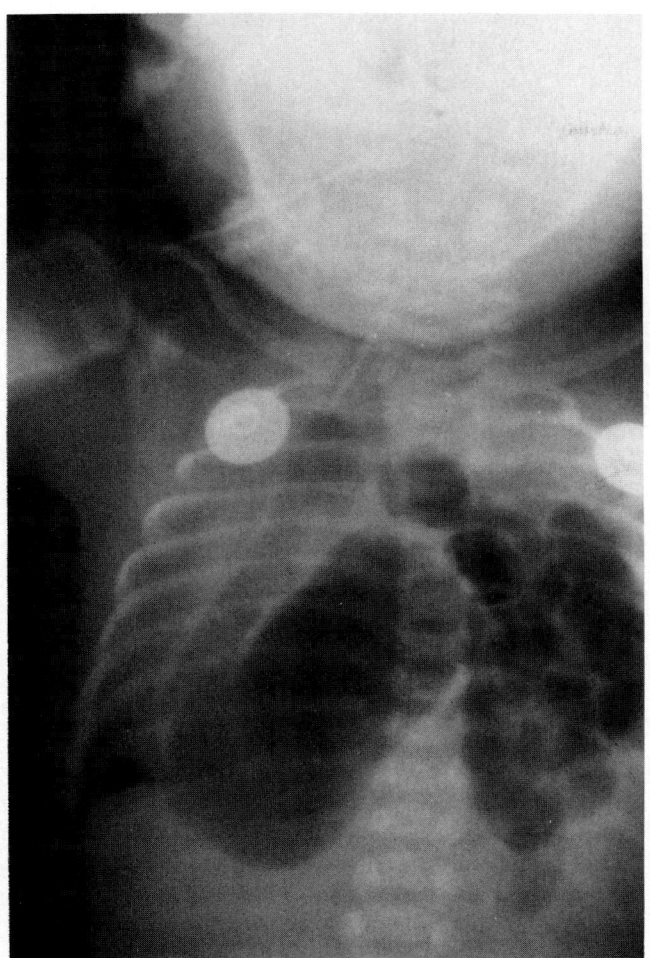

Figure 15.20. Chest radiograph of an infant with a left-sided congenital diaphragmatic hernia. Note the gas-filled intestinal loops in the left hemithorax displacing the mediastinal structures to the right.

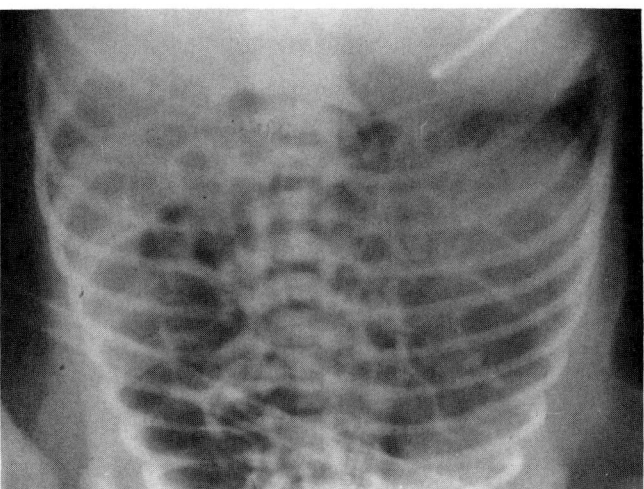

Figure 15.21. Chest radiograph of the same infant as in Figure 15.20.

Both sexes have an equal incidence. Most cases are sporadic, although rare familial cases have been reported.

Symptoms and Diagnosis.

Infants.

Dyspnea and cyanosis are the usual symptoms in the newborn infant with diaphragmatic hernia. They may become progressive as inspiratory movements suck more intestines into the thorax. The abdomen may be scaphoid, and the chest movements may be asymmetric. The heart is displaced, usually to the right, and breath sounds are absent on the affected side. Intestinal sounds auscultated in the chest are considered diagnostic. Riker (64), however, believes they are usually not recognized or interpreted correctly.

Radiographic examination will reveal gas-filled loops of intestine in the thorax (Figs. 15.20 and 15.21). If a hernial sac is present and intact, the intestines will not extend to the top of the thorax. There is general agreement that barium-enhanced radiographic studies should not be done in infants. Indeed, the additional information obtained will rarely influence the subsequent surgical procedure unless there is a question about congenital cystic lung disease such as congenital cystic adenomatoid malformation, which could be approached surgically via a thoracotomy (whereas a diaphragmatic hernia is repaired transabdominally) (Fig. 15.22).

The radiographic picture of diaphragmatic hernia may be simulated by large intrathoracic duplications of the intestine, but these latter are not usually accompanied by respiratory distress. They are rare and are often correctly diagnosed only at operation (page 89).

Young et al. (65) used computed tomography (CT) to diagnose diaphragmatic hernia. Today, prenatal ultrasonography is the procedure of choice for diagnosis, according to Bell and Ternberg (66). With ultrasonography, Adzick et al. (67) were able to diagnose 88 of 94 infants with congenital diaphragmatic herniae.

Adults.

Untreated congenital diaphragmatic hernia is not necessarily fatal. Kirkland (68) reviewed 25 cases, including one of his own, of individuals over age 12 years who had such herniae. Six of the patients, whose average age was 39 years, had no symptoms. Another 14, whose average age was 47 years, had a long history of vague or minor symptoms before acute attacks occurred. Five patients, with an average age of 19 years, had definite, long-standing clinical symptoms.

Gastrointestinal, rather than respiratory symptoms predominate in adults and older children (69). Abdominal pain is present in 50% of the patients. In addition, vomiting, dyspnea, chest pain, and cardiovascular symp-

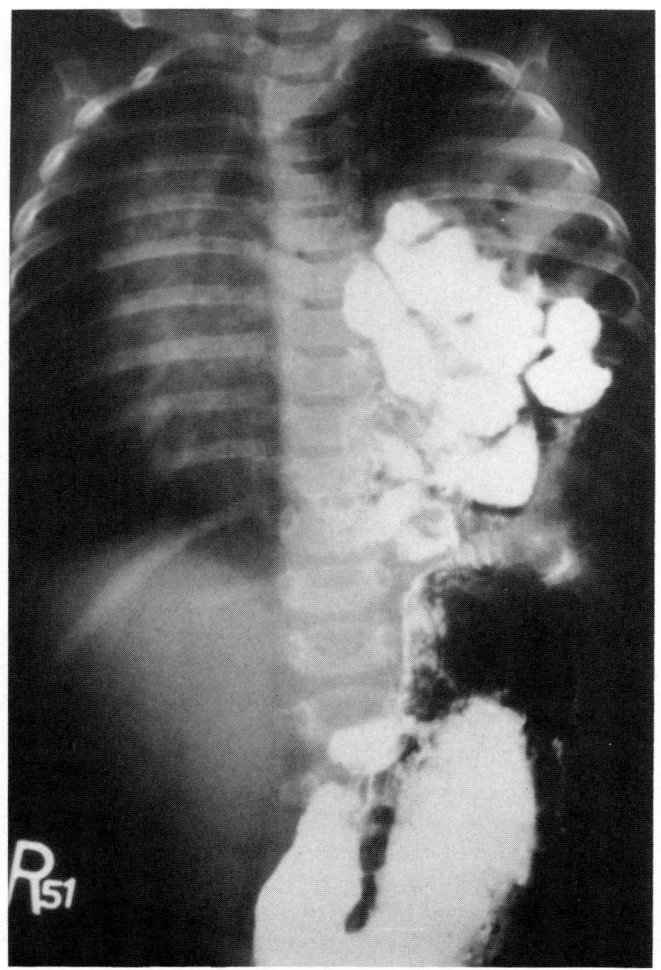

Figure 15.22. Upper gastrointestinal contrast-enhanced radiographic study in an infant with a left-sided congenital diaphragmatic hernia in which the differential diagnosis included congenital cystic lung disease.

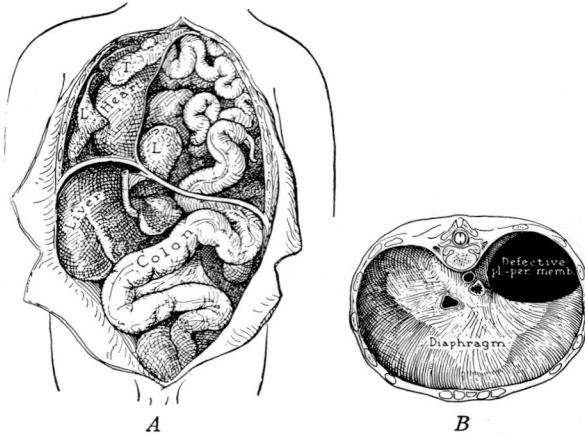

Figure 15.23. Herniation of the intestines through the posterolateral triangle (foramen of Bochdalek) in an adult. **A,** Loops of intestines in the thorax compressing the left lung and shifting the heart to the left. **B,** View of the defective diaphragm seen from below. In spite of the compression of the lungs, such patients may show more gastrointestinal than respiratory symptoms. (From Arey LB. Developmental anatomy, 7th ed. Philadelphia: WB Saunders, 1965.)

that pulmonary growth and development are normal and there is no pulmonary artery hypertension. Otherwise, these patients would have the usual symptoms which result in poor operative correction (JAH/CNP).

Treatment. Preoperative preparation of the infant includes several measures designed to improve the mechanics of ventilation and to prevent pulmonary vasospasm. These measures include:

1. Administration of 100% oxygen prevents alveolar hypoxia, which is a potent stimulus to pulmonary vasospasm.
2. Endotracheal intubation is used if assisted ventilation is required. Bag and mask ventilation is contraindicated since increasing gaseous distension of the stomach and small bowel will worsen the ventilatory abilities of the infant because of further compression of the contralateral lung.
3. Insertion of an oral gastric tube connected to suction prevents further distension of the gastrointestinal tract with air.
4. Hyperventilation to lower the Pco_2 to less than 40 mm Hg prevents hypercarbia, which is another potent stimulus to pulmonary vasospasm.
5. Acidosis is corrected with sodium bicarbonate or tris (hydroxymethyl) aminomethane (THAM); acidosis is another potent stimulus for pulmonary vasospasm.

EDITORIAL COMMENT

It is important to recall that sodium bicarbonate is actually an *acidic* solution. It only corrects acidosis if CO_2 can be blown off. Therefore, it is critically important that good ventilation and adequate pul-

toms are present in about 25% of patients. Obstruction is rare (Fig. 15.23).

EDITORIAL COMMENT

Clearly, patients outside the newborn period who have no symptoms and who, indeed, are only found to have diaphragmatic herniae on incidental physical or chest x-ray examination must have no pulmonary component to their diaphragmatic hernia. It would be most interesting to know if these are patients with a congenital diaphragmatic hernia without herniation of the intestine in utero. If so, there has been no interference with normal pulmonary growth and development. The other possibility is that there is a defective diaphragmatic closure; however, for some reason, the pressure relationships between the pleural space and the abdominal cavity do not result in herniation. For whatever reason, we must assume

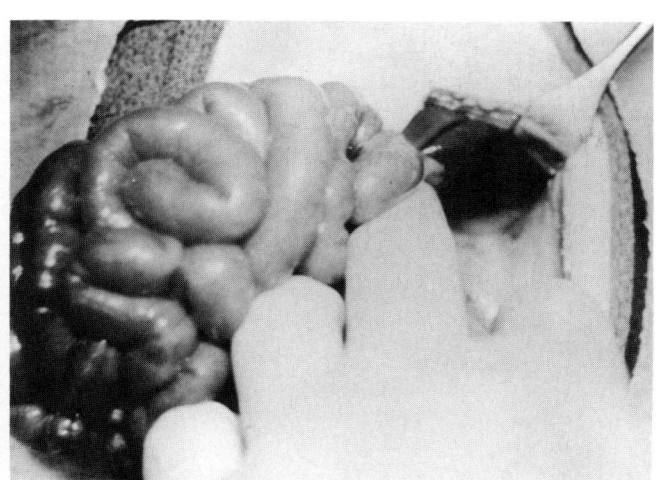

Figure 15.24. Transabdominal repair of a left-sided congenital diaphragmatic hernia. The retractor is elevating the anterior rim of the diaphragm; note the remnant of the posterior rim. The bowel has been reduced from the chest; there is no hernia sac.

monary tissue be present *before* the sodium bicarbonate is given; otherwise, there will simply be an increase in acidosis (JAH/CNP).

6. The systemic vascular volume and blood pressure is supported with intravenous fluids and cardiotonic agents, such as dopamine, as required.
7. Normal body temperature is maintained.
8. Prophylactic antibiotics are administered anticipating the need for early surgical intervention.
9. Placement of preductal and postductal arterial lines quantitates the amount of right-to-left shunting through fetal channels.
10. Pulmonary vasodilators such as tolazine are used, if necessary.

The preferred approach for left-sided diaphragmatic herniae is transabdominal through a left subcostal incision. The bowel may be more easily reduced from the abdominal approach, and the defect can more easily be repaired under direct vision (Fig. 15.24).

EDITORIAL COMMENT

In addition, the small intestine can be so placed within the abdomen that there is minimal danger of midgut volvulus since such intestine does not have normal mesentery fixation. Finally, if the intestine is tremendously distended with gas and fluid, it may not be possible to close the abdomen without compromising diaphragmatic function. A temporary fascial defect may thus be necessary to prevent such intraabdominal pressure which would alter diaphragmatic motion (JAH/CNP).

In some cases a prosthetic patch may be required. If necessary, the abdominal wall can be stretched to allow for accommodation of the replaced bowel. Exploration for associated anomalies and surgical correction of these may be accomplished if the patient's condition allows. Right-sided diaphragmatic herniae are generally approached transabdominally as well. However, if only the liver has herniated through the defect, a right thoracotomy may be employed with satisfactory results. The surgical anatomy and technique of repair have been described recently by Skandalakis et al. (70).

The prior dictum of immediate surgical repair of all congenital diaphragmatic herniae is currently in dispute (71). There is an increasing trend to delay repair until the patient's cardiopulmonary status can be maximized, utilizing jet ventilation if necessary. If this fails to stabilize the patient, ECMO may be utilized preoperatively (40). This approach avoids perioperative barotrauma and protects the infant from the pulmonary function deterioration and worsening pulmonary hypertension that often accompany operative repair. This technique probably saves some patients who otherwise would not survive the standard preoperative preparation and operative procedure. On the other hand, this approach may sustain patients with profound pulmonary hypoplasia through the operative procedure and initial postoperative course, only to have them succumb later from a lack of sufficient pulmonary tissue to sustain life.

West et al. (72) studied the cases of 111 newborns with congenital diaphragmatic herniae who were treated before and after the advent of extracorporeal membrane oxygenation. They reported 43% survival with emergency surgery and 67% with surgery delayed and use of extracorporeal membrane oxygenation. West and her colleagues emphasized that survival was best in newborns in whom prosthetic material was used to correct large defects.

Falterman and Adolph (73) stated that neonatal extracorporeal membrane oxygenation is a new tool in the armaments of pediatric surgeons and neonatologists. They emphasized that it is no longer an experimental technique; rather, it is now a standard for certain respiratory problems.

Since pulmonary hypoplasia is a major factor in the mortality of patients with congenital diaphragmatic hernia, Harrison and his colleagues have been working for over a decade in utero (74–77). This research culminated in 1990 in an initial clinical trial in which six highly selected fetuses with severe congenital diaphragmatic hernia were treated by open fetal surgery (78). Although all of these fetuses expired, subsequent efforts have resulted in survival. By correcting the defect in the fetus in utero, it is anticipated that the affected lung will be able to continue to grow throughout the remainder of gestation to a degree which will support the infant's existence after delivery. This is an exciting and monumental contribution to the field of pediatric surgery.

EDITORIAL COMMENT

One word of caution is in order: We do not know for sure that the herniated intestine causes the pulmonary hypoplasia. Therefore, we may find that operating in utero corrects the diaphragmatic defect but does not cure the underlying pathophysiologic condition. Furthermore, cautious clinical studies are clearly indicated and are awaited with great interest (JAH/CNP).

Prognosis. The overall mortality for infants with diaphragmatic hernia remains approximately 50%. According to Adolph et al. (79) postoperative general postsurgical diaphragmatic hernia of congenital origin still is a fatal disease and a difficult problem for the pediatric surgeon. Neonates presenting in the delivery room or within the first few hours of life have a higher mortality when compared to those who present clinically after 12 hours of life. Of those diagnosed in utero, the mortality is 80%. Many of these fetuses are aborted or stillborn or have lethal associated malformations (77). Even when prenatally diagnosed infants are treated postnatally with the most aggressive therapy available, including preoperative and postoperative ECMO, the mortality is still 76% (43). Prenatal predictors of poor clinical outcome include: (*a*) polyhydramnios, which is present in 69% of patients and which is associated with only an 18% survival rate; (*b*) chromosomal abnormalities; and (*c*) diagnosis prior to 25 weeks gestation (77). Postnatal predictors of a poor clinical outcome include: (*a*) an intrathoracic stomach, which occurs in approximately one-third of such patients and carries a 75% mortality (80) and (*b*) the inability to achieve a Pco_2 less than 40 mm Hg and a ventilatory index (respiratory rate $\times$ mean airway pressure) of less than 1000 (36).

PARASTERNAL DEFECTS OF THE DIAPHRAGM: HERNIA THROUGH THE FORAMEN OF MORGAGNI

Anatomy. The foramina of Morgagni (spaces of Larrey, parasternal spaces) are small triangular areas of the diaphragm on either side of the inferior end of the sternum. They are bound medially by muscle fibers from the xiphoid process and laterally by those from the costal cartilages. These small gaps in the diaphragmatic musculature permit the passage of the superior epigastric vessels; they may also be the site of herniation of abdominal contents (retrosternal or parasternal hernia) (Fig. 15.25).

If herniation takes place, it is almost always on the right side, but bilateral cases have been reported (81) (Fig. 15.26).

A hernial sac always is formed although it may have ruptured and left no subsequent trace (82). If the sac is

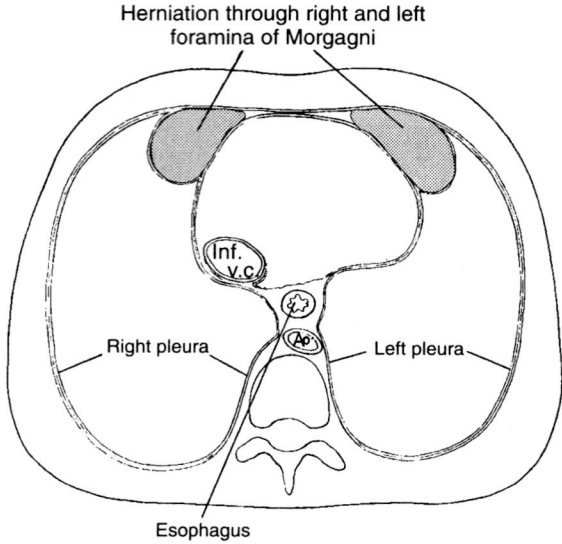

Figure 15.25. Location of herniation through the foramen of Morgagni; The left side rarely is affected. (From Boyd DP, Wooldridge BF. Diaphragmatic hernia through the foramen of Morgagni. Surg Gynec Obstet. 1957; 104:727–732.)

present and intact, the superior epigastric artery is located lateral to it. In infants and children the hernial sac often contains the liver; in adults the inclusion of the omentum is usual. Colon may be present in young and old alike, and the stomach may follow the colon after several years.

Embryogenesis. Embryologically, the foramen of Morgagni represents the junction of the septum transversum, the lateral component of the diaphragm, and the anterior thoracic wall. The area is congenitally weak, but to what extent its weakness varies from individual to individual is unknown. An enlarged space between muscles has been attributed to retardation of the fusion of the lower ribs with the xiphisternum during the seventh week (83). The interposition of fat between the muscles has been said also to predispose the patient to herniation.

Actual herniation through the foramen is almost always the result of trauma and usually occurs in adults.

History and Incidence. The first case was reported in an elderly man by Morgagni (49) in 1761. Subsequently, little interest was manifested and few cases were reported. Neither Keith (53) in 1910 nor Hume (84) in 1922 included retrosternal hernia in their classifications of herniae. Only eight cases were reported in children from 1921 to 1951, and none was proven to be congenital (85). Four of these children had Down's syndrome. In 1977 Thomas and Clitherow (86) cited four cases only.

The incidence is low. In most series, hernia through the foramen of Morgagni occurs once in every 20 herniae through the foramen of Bochdalek (82, 87). The sexes are equally affected, on the whole, but there are more males

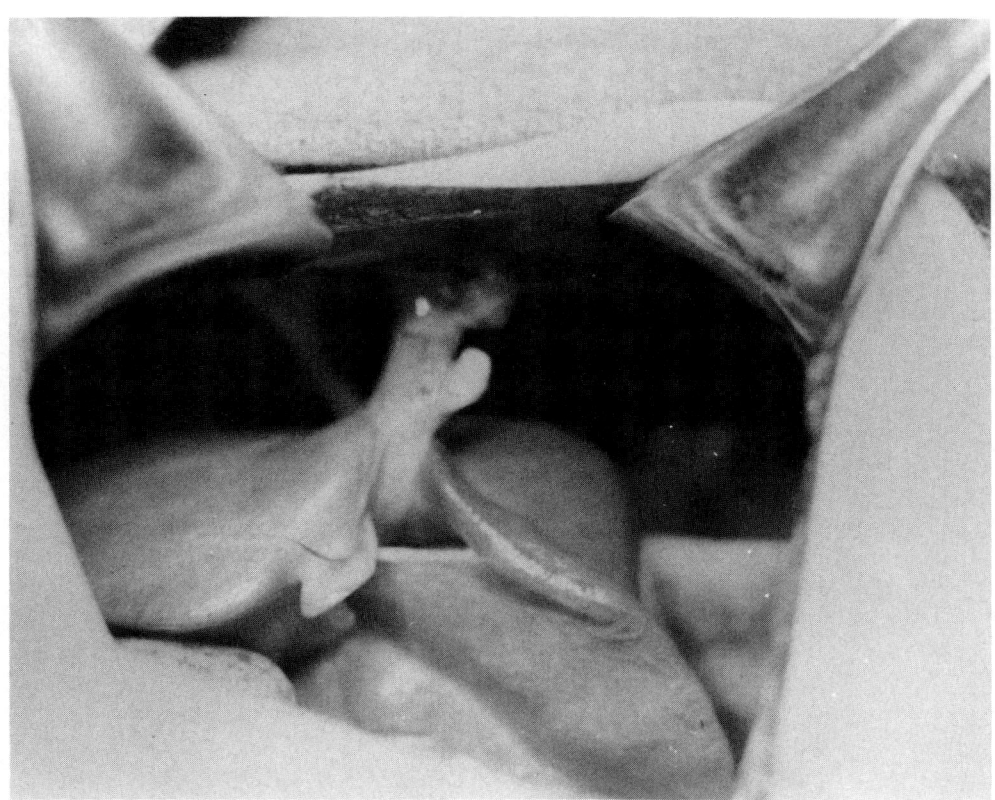

Figure 15.26. Bilateral foramen of Morgagni hernia; note the falciform ligament and the remaining central attachment of the diaphragm.

among the older adults (85). The hernia is rare in infants and children (88).

Symptoms. Symptoms of retrosternal hernia are less marked than those of pleuroperitoneal hernia, or they may be absent. Indigestion, abdominal pain, and occasionally cough and dyspnea may be present. Obstruction is rare although sometimes it follows incarceration of the stomach (85).

Diagnosis. The symptoms may mimic those of gallbladder disease, or those of diseases of stomach, pancreas, or colon. Because of the presence of the heart shadow, radiographic diagnosis is difficult; lateral x-ray films may be more helpful than anteroposterior films (89). A barium meal will help if stomach or intestine is herniated but not if the omentum is involved. A barium enema will help if the colon has herniated through the defect (Figs. 15.27 and 15.28). Pneumoperitoneal studies have been suggested (83). Often a diagnosis of low anterior thoracic mass is the best that can be made.

Pokorny et al. (90) stated that, occasionally, respiratory distress will be present if loops of small bowel enter the chest. Herniation of intestine into the pericardium was observed by Ravitch (91).

Treatment. Surgical repair of the foramen after reduction of the hernia may be achieved through either a trans-

thoracic or a transabdominal route. The authors prefer the latter. As congenital absence of musculature is not involved, no prosthesis to span the gap is required. The diaphragm and the posterior sheath of the rectus muscle usually may be sutured directly.

EVENTRATION OF THE DIAPHRAGM

Anatomy. "Eventration" refers to the abnormal elevation of one leaf of the diaphragm. It differs from true diaphragmatic hernia with a sac in that, in eventration, the entire leaf bulges upward from the pressure of the abdominal viscera (Figs. 15.29 and 15.30). Whereas in hernia, the diaphragm retains its normal position and the viscera bulge through a localized defect in its surface. Considerable dissatisfaction with the name has been expressed (92, 93), but no better one has been proposed. Eventration may be congenital, arising from aplasia of the diaphragm, or it may develop in later life, resulting from paralysis. Only the congenital type is considered here.

In congenital eventration, the phrenic nerve is normal, and the muscle fibers present are not atrophic. The whole or only a part of the hemidiaphragm may be involved. The entire leaf may be thinner than usual, or no muscle fibers may be present at all, the leaf being represented by a translucent membrane. Scattered muscle fibers may be

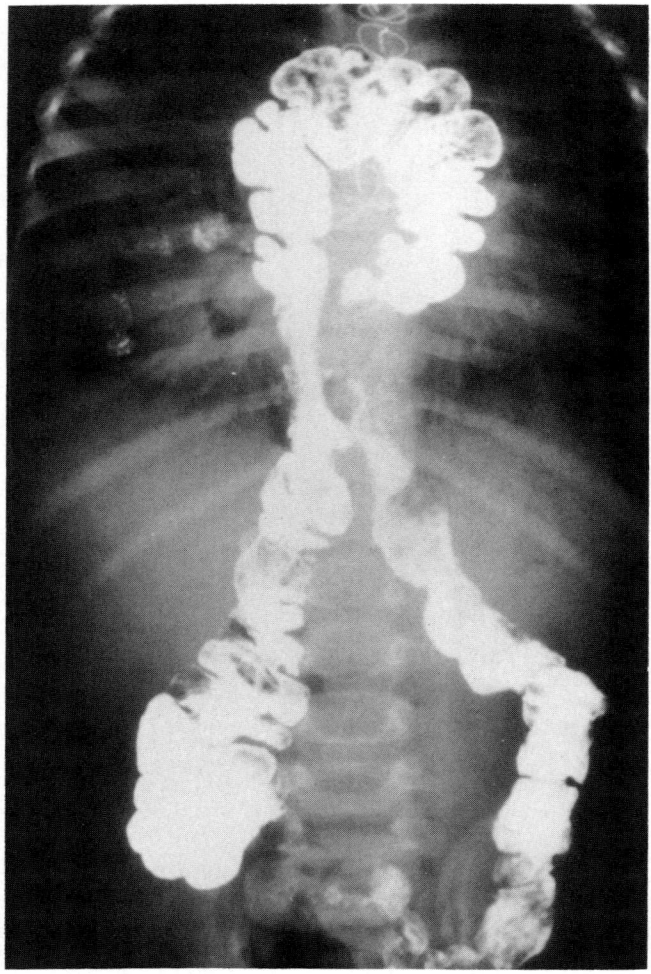

Figure 15.27. Anteroposterior view of a barium enema in a child with a congenital diaphragmatic hernia through the foramen of Morgagni.

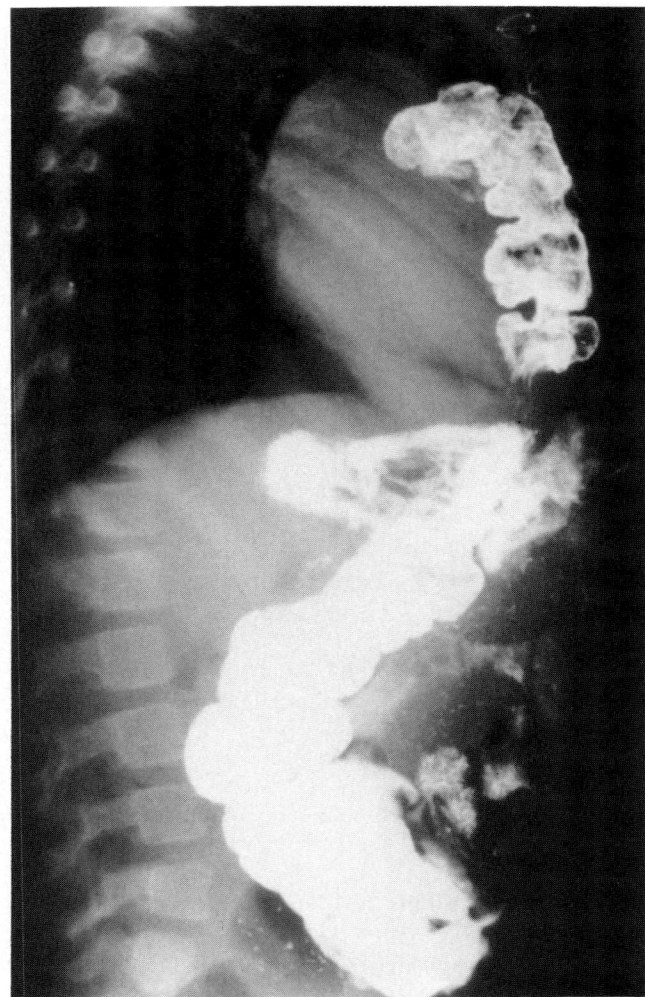

Figure 15.28. Lateral view of patient in Figure 15.27.

present, or some areas may be muscular and others not. Usually the eventrated leaf consists of peritoneum, a fascial layer, and pleura.

However, injury of the phrenic nerve during delivery may produce eventration which may be diagnosed as congenital, as reported by McNamara et al. (94) and Haller et al. (95).

In some cases only a portion of the leaf of the diaphragm shows thinning. The eventration is said to be partial. The defect is usually in the diaphragmatic dome, which is not a point of junction of the embryonic components. Either side may be involved, and at least three patients with bilateral eventration have been reported (94).

Ravitch and Hendelsman (95) described such defects surrounded by a ring of muscle in the right diaphragm. In one patient there were two such areas. When the areas are small, the effect is that of a diaphragmatic hernia with a sac rather than that of a typical eventration.

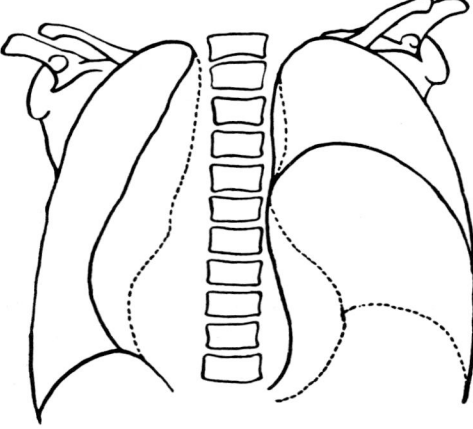

Figure 15.29. Eventration of the left leaf of the diaphragm. *Solid line* indicates original position of the diaphragm and the mediastinum. *Broken line* indicates position following repair of the eventration. (From Beck WC. Etiologic significance of eventration of the diaphragm. Arch Surg 1950; 60:1154–1160.)

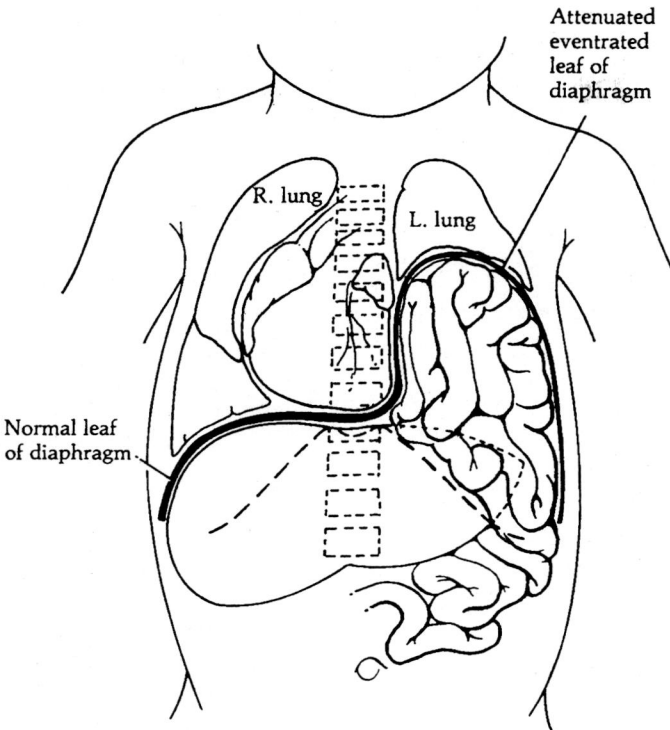

Table 15.5.
Eventration of Diaphragm: Associated Anomalies in Nine Cases (Excluding Pulmonary Hypoplasia)[a]

Malrotation		4
Cardiac anomalies		
Coarctation of aorta	1	
Ventral septal defect	1	3
Partial anomalous pulmonary venous drainage	1	
Renal anomalies		
Thoracic kidney	1	
Pelvic kidney	1	3
Solitary dysplastic pelvic kidney	1	
Deformities of pinna		2
Meckel's diverticulum		1
Perineal anus		1
Single umbilical artery		1
Undescended testis		1
Vertebral anomalies		1
Down's syndrome		1

[a]From Irving IM, Booker PD. Congenital diaphragmatic hernia and eventration of the diaphragm. In: Lister J, Irving IM, eds. Neonatal surgery, 3rd ed. London: Butterworth, 1990.

Figure 15.30. Eventration of the (left) diaphragm. The herniated abdominal organs remain beneath the attenuated by intact leaf of the diaphragm. Both lungs are compressed and the mediastinum is shifted to the right. Compare with Figure 15.14. (From Skandalakis JE, Gray SW, Rowe JS Jr, Skandalakis LJ. Surgical anatomy of the diaphragm. In: Nyhus LM, Baker RJ, eds. Mastery of surgery. Boston: Little, Brown, 1992.)

Briggs et al. (98) reported fetal rubella; Becroft (99) and Wayne et al. (100), cytomegalovirus; Wexler and Poole (101), trisomic chromosomal anomalies; and Stauffer and Rickham (102), familial incidence.

Associated Anomalies. Partial or complete inversion of the stomach and malrotation of the intestines usually accompany congenital eventration. Transposition of abdominal organs, megacolon, hypospadias, and other defects have been encountered (92, 93). Roberts (103) reported an association between eventration and arthrogryposis in sheep. The possibility these represent a common neuromuscular disturbance has been suggested (104). Hypoplasia of the ipsilateral lung was first reported by Korns (50) in a patient with eventration; this is a common finding at autopsy or during surgery on neonatal infants. In spite of this appearance of the lung in neonates, it seems to attain nearly normal size within several weeks after surgery, as does the hypoplastic lung in diaphragmatic hernia (page 502).

Irving and Booker (21) presented the associated anomalies (Table 15.5).

Embryogenesis. Phrenic nerve paralysis is the most common cause of acquired diaphragmatic eventration.

Among 1235 patients with paralytic poliomyelitis in Copenhagen, Christensen (105) found permanent eventration in seven patients and temporary eventration in 333 patients. Greenebaum and Harper (106), as well as others, have suggested that injury to the phrenic nerve during delivery may account for some congenital examples.

That diaphragmatic eventration might be an embryonic malformation appears to have been suggested in 1882 (50) and was emphasized in 1916 by Bayne-Jones (107). The frequent disruption of the normal pattern of gut rotation and abnormal mesenteric attachments are the strongest arguments that the defect exists in fetal life. The presence of a normal phrenic nerve, shown by histologic section at autopsy in some cases and implied by synchronous motion of the halves of the diaphragm in many others, is evidence that phrenic nerve injury is not responsible for most eventrations.

Congenital eventration is a failure of muscularization of the diaphragm, not a failure of fusion of its parts. Whether the defect is primarily muscular or is secondary to a defective distribution of phrenic nerve fibers is not known. It is more readily explained as failure of the migration of myoblasts along the phrenic nerve than by Bremer's theory of muscle formation from the thoracic wall (2).

History. The first recognizable description of the condition should be credited to Petit in 1774 (108). Cruveilhier (109) first used the term *eventration*, which he ascribed to Béchard. In the *Anatomie Pathologique* of 1829, he made the distinction between eventration and diaphragmatic hernia. The first clinical case was that of Marsh (110) in 1867.

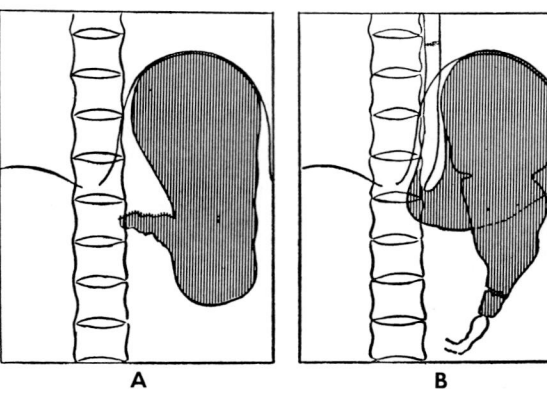
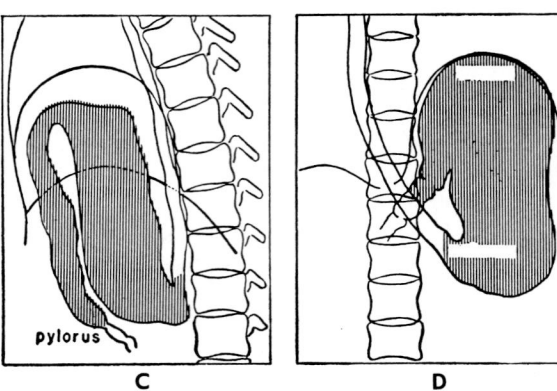
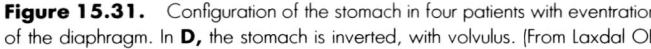

Figure 15.31. Configuration of the stomach in four patients with eventration of the diaphragm. In **D,** the stomach is inverted, with volvulus. (From Laxdal OE McDougall H, Mellin G et al. Congential eventration of the diaphragm. New Eng J Med 1954; 250:401–408.)

Preoperative diagnosis was not readily made even after the advent of radiography. Korns (50) recounts the case of one patient, Frederich Schneider, who was seen in numerous hospitals and described by various authors in 1890, 1900, 1904, 1905, and twice in 1906; finally, autopsy findings were published in 1912. The conflicting diagnoses were dextrocardia, diaphragmatic hernia, and eventration of the diaphragm.

Morrison (111) performed the first repair of an eventration in 1923, but in 1935 Reed and Borden (92) were pessimistic about the value of surgical intervention.

Korns (50) reviewed 22 proven and 43 probable cases in 1921. Reed and Borden (92) increased these to 47 and 136, respectively, in 1935. Laxdal and his colleagues (93) found over 300 cases in the literature by 1954. Bisgard (112) performed the first succesful operation on an infant. Bingham (113) surgically treated a case with phrenic nerve paralysis.

Incidence. From a survey of reported cases, the incidence among adults has been placed at about 1:10,000 (93, 114). From 412,000 mass radiographs in England, Chin and Lynn (115) detected 32 cases (1:13,000), but among 107,778 similar radiographs in Denmark, Christensen (105) found 38 (1:2800). Not all of these were of congenital origin. Among infants, the frequency may be higher because eventration is often fatal in the perinatal period.

Males are more frequently afflicted than are females; the ratio has been placed as high as 2:1 (93) and as low as 4:3 (92). The left side is involved eight times as often as the right.

Eventration corresponds to 5% of all diaphragmatic defects, according to David and Illingworth (116).

Symptoms. The symptoms of eventration are those resulting from inadequate ventilation and displacement of the mediastinum. Respiratory distress, cyanosis, and tachycardia are usual, and the stomach may undergo volvulus or may be inverted, with consequent abdominal pain (Fig. 15.31). The symptoms of eventration are less severe than those of diaphragmatic hernia; in many cases no symptoms are present and the condition is recognized only on routine chest x-ray films (64). In such cases symptoms may first appear late in life.

Diagnosis. Radiography is necessary for diagnosis. Ideally, the elevated diaphragm will be visualized high in the thorax. This is in distinction to the picture seen in diaphragmatic hernia, in which the diaphragm is located normally, with intestine above. Lateral and oblique x-ray films may be helpful.

Ultrasound or fluoroscopy can be used to watch diaphragmatic excursion during breathing. The side with the eventration will not move, whereas the other side will move normally. In phrenic nerve paralysis, on the other hand, there will be paradoxic movement of the diaphragm (elevation with inspiration on the affected side).

Observation of respiratory movements of the infant in the supine position shows a characteristic pattern in eventration (117), but few surgeons see enough cases to become sufficiently familiar with it to make a firm diagnosis.

Treatment. Treatment is required only when respiratory, cardiac, or gastrointestinal symptoms are present. Stabilization of the mediastinum, restoration of pulmonary capacity, and replacement of abdominal organs are the aims of surgical repair. Excision, overlapping, or plication of the weakened area of the diaphragm through a transthoracic approach will restore the diaphragm to its normal level. Because of the risk of injury to the phrenic nerve, excision is the least desirable operative procedure (Fig. 15.32). Reynolds (31) advises surgery through the chest for right eventration and through the abdomen for left eventration.

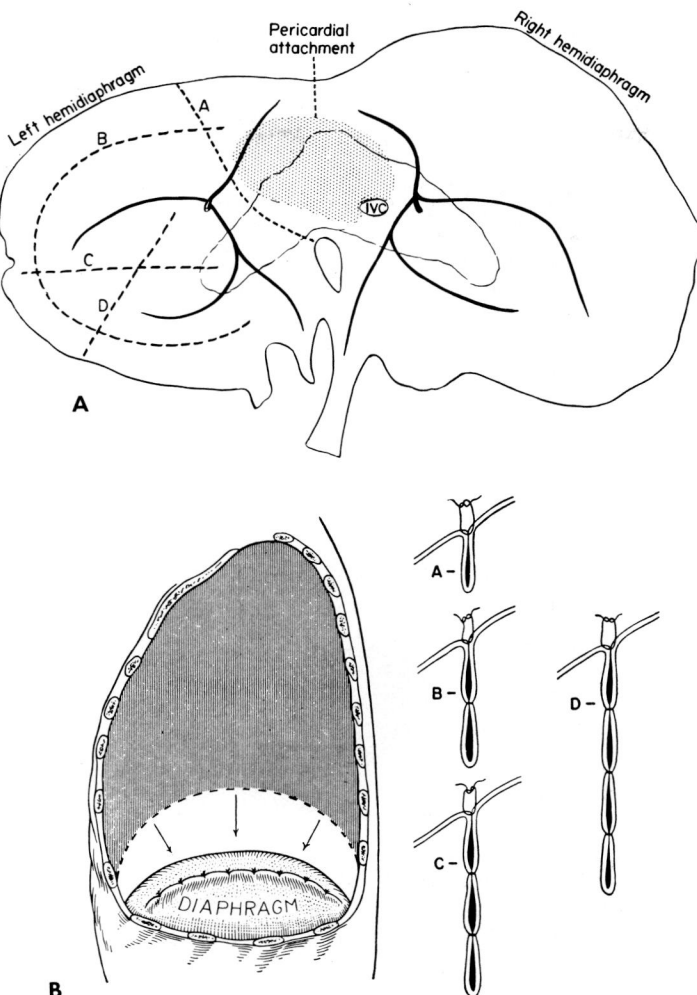

Figure 15.32. Considerations in diaphragmatic repair. **A,** *Solid lines* show the distribution of branches of the phrenic nerve; *broken lines* show the locations at which incisions may be made without significant effect on diaphragmatic function. (From Merendino KA. The intradiaphragmatic distribution of the phrenic nerve. Surg Clin NA 1964; 44:1217–1226. **B,** Imbrication procedure for repair of eventration. (From Laxdal OE. McDougall H, Mellin G. Congenital eventration of the diaphragm. N Engl J Med 1954; 250:401–408.)

The results of early surgical intervention were reported to be good by Stone et al. (118). Conservative treatment is contraindicated, as advised by Stauffer (119).

DEFECT OF THE SEPTUM TRANSVERSUM (DEFECT OF THE CENTRAL TENDON)

Anatomy. This anomaly, which results in a communication between the peritoneal and pericardial cavities, is the rarest and least understood of the diaphragmatic defects that result in herniation (Fig. 15.33). Its congenital nature seems unassailable since, in at least five cases, it was reported in newborn infants (120). The remainder of the 12 cases reported up to 1958 were in adults between 47 and 70 years of age. In several of the adult

cases traumatic rupture of the diaphragm cannot be excluded (121, 122).

Anatomic findings are confusing. No hernial sac has been reported among adult patients, but Keith (53) found a sac in a newborn infant, and Wilson et al. (120) reported traces of a sac found at surgery on an infant. In still another case (123) no membranes could be found, even though none of the abdominal organs actually had herniated through the opening into the pericardial cavity.

The earliest reported case is that of Grenier de Cardenal and Bourderou (124) in 1903. Keith (53) in 1910 found three specimens in pathology collections. By 1947 Wilson and his colleagues (120) could find only eight cases, to which they added one of their own. O'Brien

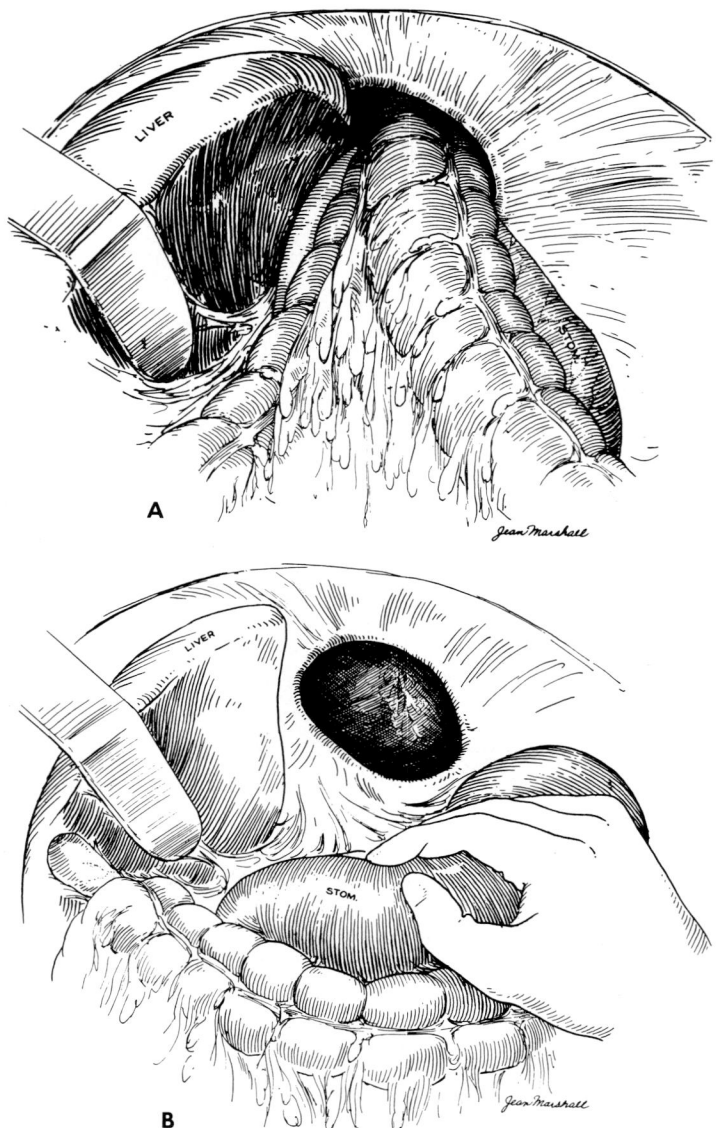

Figure 15.33.   Herniation into the pericardium. **A,** Diaphragmatic defect containing herniated stomach and colon. **B,** Diaphragmatic defect after reduction of the hernia; the heart is visible through the defect. (From Rogers JF, Lane WL, Gibbs R. Herniation through the diaphragm into the pericardium. Conn Med J 1958; 22:653–656.)

(125) mentions the occurrence of this defect in four dogs and a donkey.

Embryogenesis. The defect involves the transverse septum, the earliest of the diaphragmatic components to be formed. Complete failure of the septum to appear would be incompatible with subsequent viable development since this septum is the site of formation of the liver as well as of the ducts of Cuvier, which receive the embryonic venous return to the heart. Since the septum is not paired, there is no fusion defect; a secondary rupture of the septum in embryonic life must therefore be postulated. We suggest that the most probable time for such a rupture is during the fourth week, when the rapidly growing liver is expanding out of the septum and the septum itself is decreasing in relative thickness.

Defects of the Esophageal Hiatus: Hiatal Hernia

Hiatus hernia may be defined as the protrusion of a portion of the stomach into the thoracic mediastinum through the esophageal hiatus of the diaphragm. A hernial sac is present. Åkerlund (126) was one of the first to classify hernia in this area, and he may have been first to use the term *hiatus hernia.* He recognized three types of

Table 15.6.
Hernia Through the Esophageal Hiatus[a]

Hernia	Anatomy	Sac and Contents	Remarks
Hiatus hernia: Sliding hiatus hernia Fixed hiatus hernia	Congenital potential hernia. G-O junction and cardia are displaced upwards to enter the mediastinum above diaphragm. The phrenoesophageal membrane is attenuated. The herniated stomach may move freely or become fixed in the thorax	Sac lies anterior and to the left of herniated stomach. Contents: cardia, stomach	A large hiatus (admitting three fingers) may be a predisposing factor. Actual herniation usually occurs in middle life but has been seen in newborn.
'Pure' paraesophageal hernia	Congenital potential hernia. G-O junction and the cardia are in normal position. The fundus has herniated through the hiatus into the thorax beside the esophagus	Sac lies anterior to esophagus and posterior to pericardium. Contents: cardia and fundus of stomach	An enlarged hiatus may be a predisposing factor. Actual herniation occurs in adult life.
Combined sliding and paraesophageal hernia	Congenital potential hernia. G-O junction, cardia and much of greater curvature of stomach has herniated into the thorax	Sac lies anterior to esophagus and posterior to pericardium in right posterinferior mediastinum. Sac may contain fundus and body of stomach, omentum, transverse colon, spleen	A hiatus already enlarged by a hiatus hernia. Progresses to complete thoracic stomach with volvulus
Short esophagus	Congenital hernia. G-O junction and cardia are displaced upwards and fixed in the thorax	No sac present	This lesion is rare. It appears to result from failure of the embryonic esophagus to elongate enough to bring the G-O junction into the abdomen.

[a]From Jamieson GG. Surgery of the oesophagus. Edinburgh: Churchill Livingstone, 1988.
[b]G-O, Gastroesophageal.

hernia: sliding, paraesophageal, and congenital short esophagus. Today, however, a fourth category has been added (Table 15.6).

Sliding Hiatus Hernia. The esophagus moves freely through the hiatus with the gastroesophageal junction being in the thorax or in the normal position at different times. It is found usually in the normal position at autopsy. Sliding herniae make up 90% of all hiatus hernia (Fig. 15.34). Although these herniae do slide back and forth through the hiatus, they are called sliding herniae because the stomach makes up part of the wall of the hernial sac. Thus, they are analogous with sliding inguinal herniae.

A sliding hernia may become secondarily fixed in the thorax by adhesions. The esophagus in these patients appears to be too short to reach the diaphragm because of contraction of the longitudinal muscle coat. This type is uncommon.

Paraesophageal Hiatus Hernia. The gastroesophageal junction remains in its normal location. The gastric fundus and greater curvature bulges through the hiatus anterior to the esophagus. Volvulus of the herniated stomach is a major complication (Fig. 15.34, *C*).

Combination Hiatus Hernia. Combination hiatus hernia was described by Payne and Ellis (127) and several other surgeons. The gastroesophageal junction is displaced upwards, such as in a sliding hernia, and the fundus and

greater curvature are herniated, such as in a paraesophageal hernia. They believe that most paraesophageal herniae are of the combined type (Fig. 15.34, *D*). Further weight to this view has been provided by Walther et al. (128), who found that over half of their patients with paraesophageal herniae had abnormal gastroesophageal reflux.

Congenital Short Esophagus. This defect has long been the subject of debate. Three conditions must be considered under this general term.

Grossly Normal Esophagus.
In this condition, the lower portion of the esophagus is lined with gastric mucosa (Barrett's esophagus) (129). This may be described also as heterotopic gastric mucosa. Far from being a benign anomaly, as we believed in 1979 (130), it may be a precursor of adenocarcinoma (131, 132). This metaplasia often is associated with gastro-esophageal reflux (133, 134).

Irreducible Partially Supradiaphragmatic True Stomach.
In this condition, the stomach has herniated into the thorax through an enlarged diaphragmatic esophageal hiatus and become fixed. This is true fixed hiatus hernia.

Partially Supradiaphragmatic True Stomach Existing from Birth and Not Reducible.
This is true "congenital short esophagus" (Fig. 15.34, *E*) and is very rare.

Barrett (135) believed congenital short esophagus

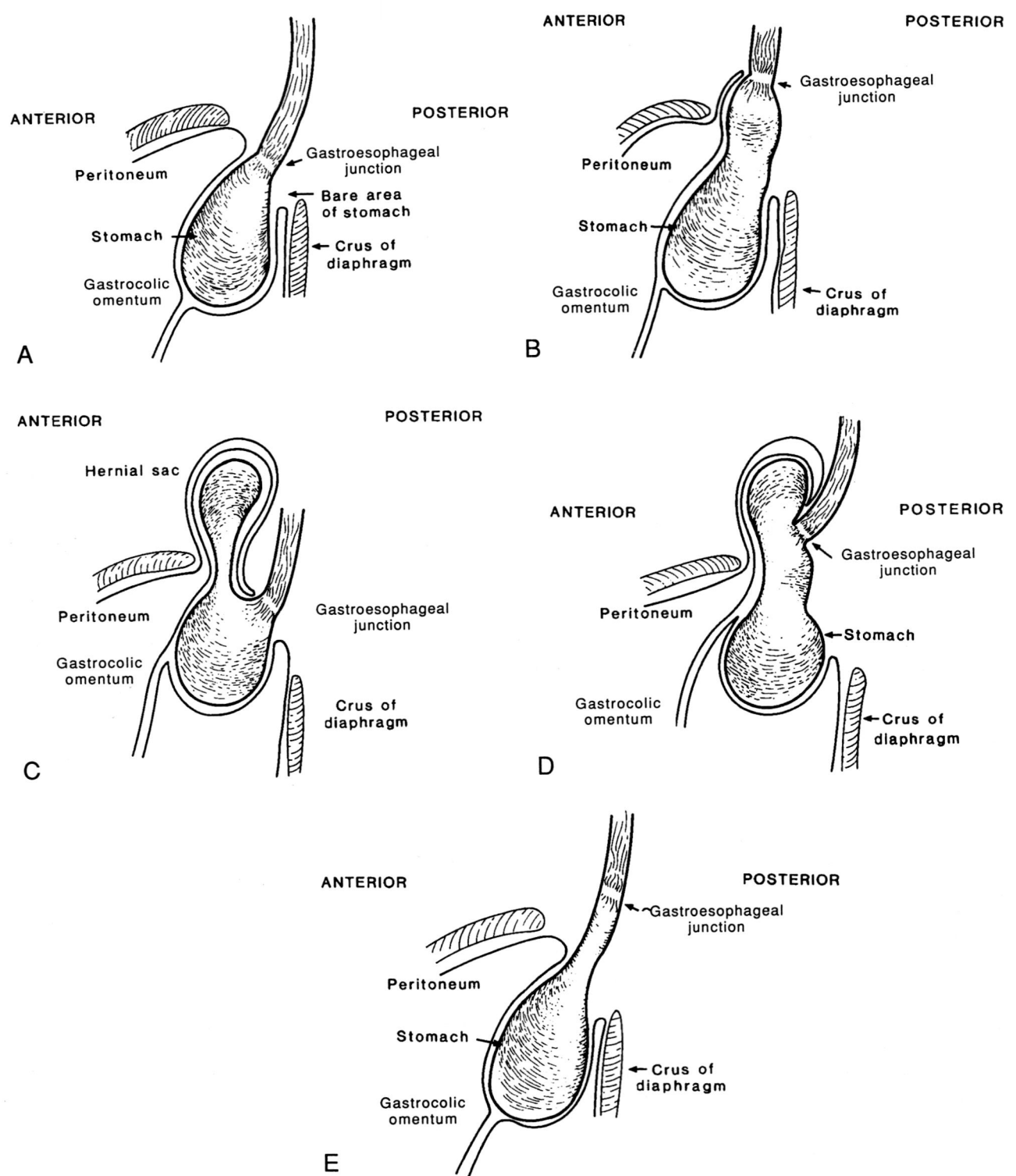

Figure 15.34. The diagram shows the esophageal hiatus in sagittal section with the (a) normal anatomy and the various abnormalities described in the text, (b) sliding hiatus hernia, (c) paraesophageal hiatus hernia, (d) combined or mixed hiatus hernia, (e) congenital short esophagus. (From Gray SW, Skandalakis LJ, Skandalakis JE. Classification of hernias through the oesophageal hiatus. In: Jamieson GG, ed. Surgery of the oesophagus. Edinburgh: Churchill Livingstone, 1988.)

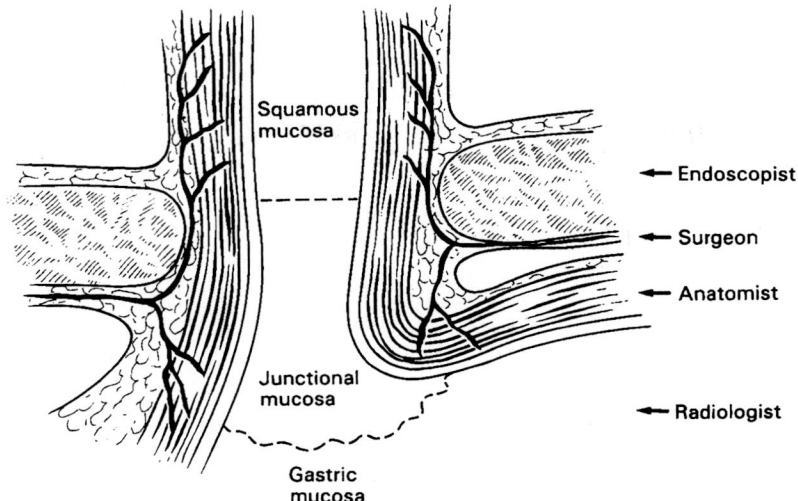

Figure 15.35. The concept of the ''gastroesophageal junction'' by four specialties. Each must be considered to be correct. (From Skandalakis JE, Gray SW, Rowe RS Jr, Skandalakis LJ. Surgical anatomy of the diaphragm. In: Nyhus LM, Baker RJ, eds. Mastery of surgery. Boston: Little, Brown, 1984.)

could be recognized by the absence of a hernial sac. Branches of the left gastric artery do not pass upwards through the hiatus. Only a small percentage of hiatal hernias belong to this group.

ABDOMINAL ESOPHAGUS AND GASTROESOPHAGEAL JUNCTION

External Junction. The gastroesophageal junction lies in the abdomen just below the diaphragm. It has been defined succinctly by Gahagan (136) as ''the termination of the tube, the oesophagus and the beginning of a pouch, the stomach.''

The abdominal esophagus is said to be from 0.5 to 2.5 cm in length, although Pearl (137) states that it may be as long as 7 cm. Allison (138) has pointed out that, by taking the level of the lowest connective tissue fibers attaching the esophagus to the diaphragm as the inferior limit of the mediastinum, there is technically no abdominal esophagus. In spite of this view, the surgeon has access to an appreciable length of esophagus below the diaphragm (139).

The abdominal esophagus lies at the level of the 11th or 12th thoracic vertebra. Relations with surrounding structures are as follow. Anteriorly lies the posterior surface of the left lobe of the liver, the left vagal trunk, and the esophageal plexus. Posteriorly are one or both crura of the diaphragm (140), the left inferior phrenic artery, and the aorta. The caudate lobe of the liver lies to the right, and the fundus of the stomach lies to the left of the esophagus. The abdominal esophagus partially is covered by peritoneum in front and on its left lateral wall.

Internal Junction. The histologic junction between esophagus and stomach is marked by an irregular boundary between stratified squamous epithelium and simple columnar epithelium. In the cadaver this epithelial boundary lies about 1 cm above the external gross junction (141). Above the boundary, islands of columnar gastric epithelium may be present at all levels of the esophagus (142). Allison (143) found the lower esophagus lined by gastric mucosa in 9.3% of the subjects he examined. The origin of such mucosa has provoked much discussion. A biopsy specimen to identify histologic changes in the mucosa should be taken more than 2 cm above the epithelial junction to avoid most of these patches (144).

Part of the problem of defining the gastroesophageal junction is the fact that this mucosal boundary does not coincide with the external junction described above. In the living patient the situation is even less simple. The submucosal connective tissue is so loose that the mucosa moves freely over the underlying muscularis, bulging in folds into the stomach at each swallow (145). Even at rest, the junctional level may change. Palmer (146), using silver markers on the epithelial boundary, found that the junction was lower in the full stomach than in the empty one. Figure 15.35 shows the internal gastroesophageal junction from the point of view of four specialties.

The columnar epithelium at the internal junction forms a mucosa unlike that of the remainder of the stomach. Its glands contain no chief or parietal cells. There are the cardiac glands of the histologist. Hayward (147) opposes the use of the word *cardia* and terms derived from it as insufferably vague. He has proposed the term *junctional epithelium* for this region between typical esophageal and typical gastric mucosae.

''Cardiac Sphincter.'' As one may stand on one's head without losing the contents of one's stomach, it follows that there is a sphincter at the cardiac orifice of the stomach that normally permits swallowing but not reflux. No

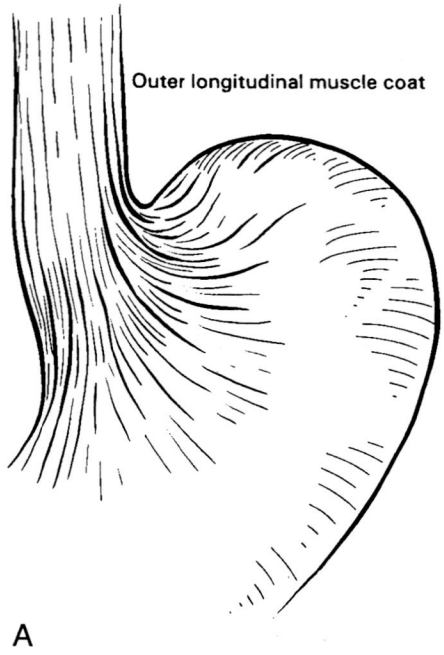

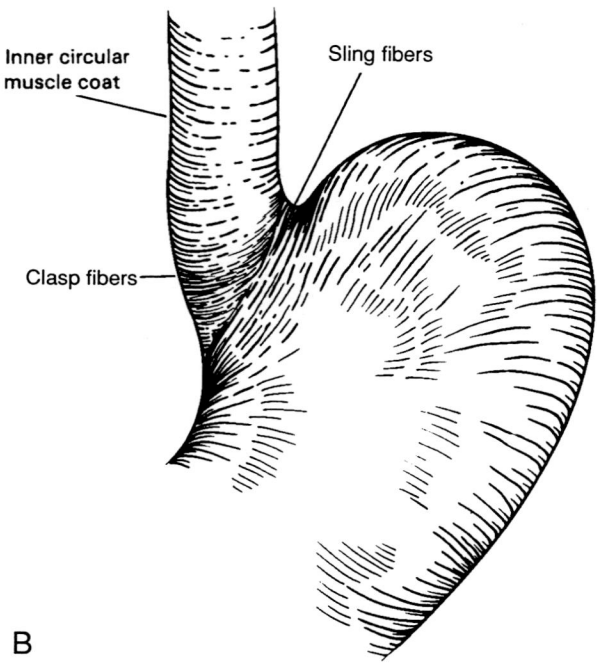

Figure 15.36. The gastroesophageal junction. **A,** Longitudinal muscle fibers. **B,** "Clasp fibers," gastric sling, and circular muscle coat. (From Skandalakis JE,

Gray SW, Rowe RS Jr, Skandalakis LJ. Surgical anatomy of the diaphragm. In: Nyhus LM, Baker RJ, eds. Mastery of Surgery. Boston: Little Brown, 1984.)

specialized muscular ring, such as is found at the pylorus, guards this orifice. A slight thickening of the circular musculature of the distal esophagus has been described (148–150). Such a thickening was grossly visible in only 21 of 33 cadavers (64%) examined by Bombeck and colleagues (141).

Several other structures have been held responsible for closing the cardia: the angle (of His) at which the esophagus enters the stomach, the pinchcock action of the diaphragm, a plug of loose esophageal mucosa (mucosal rosette), the phrenoesophageal membrane, and the sling of oblique fibers of the gastric musculature. These have been evaluated by Mann et al. (151); some or all may play a part in closure of the cardia.

The theory of the sling of oblique gastric muscle has received the greatest support (151–153). In a thorough study of the gastroesophageal musculature, Liebermann-Meffert and associates (151) described a sphincter-like thickening of the circular muscle coat which they call the oblique gastroesophageal ring. Muscle bundles of the external layer of the muscularis run parallel to the long axis of the esophagus and continue longitudinally along the greater and lesser curvatures. On the anterior and posterior gastric walls below the ring, the fibers turn upwards towards the fundus, interlacing with fibers of the internal muscle layer (Fig. 15.36, A).

The internal muscle layer of the lower esophagus is arranged in semicircular bundles designated "clasps." They continue down the lesser curvature of the stomach about 2.5 cm and insert into the submucosal connective tissue at the margin of the long oblique fibers which form the gastric sling (Fig. 15.36, B).

Regardless of the mechanisms, there is normally an area—the "lower esophageal high pressure zone" (154)—with a resting pressure of more than 15 cm of water. This pressure resists esophageal reflux. By no means will all patients with hiatal hernia demonstrate reflux; the sphincter may function satisfactorily in the thorax. Conversely, in a few patients esophageal reflux may exist without evidence of hiatal hernia (155) (Fig. 15.37). Fisher (153) believes pressure of the lower esophageal sphincter is the most important factor in preventing reflux in the unoperated patient.

EDITORIAL COMMENT

Practically all newborn infants demonstrate gastroesophageal reflux. However, it is extremely rare to have a hiatal hernia in an otherwise healthy infant. Therefore, gastroesophageal reflux in the infant and young child is not the result of a hiatal hernia. With normal maturation of the lower esophageal sphincter, gastroesophageal reflux becomes less common by the time a child reaches 1 year of age and is normally absent thereafter. Thus, unless there is significant aspiration of gastric contents or interfer-

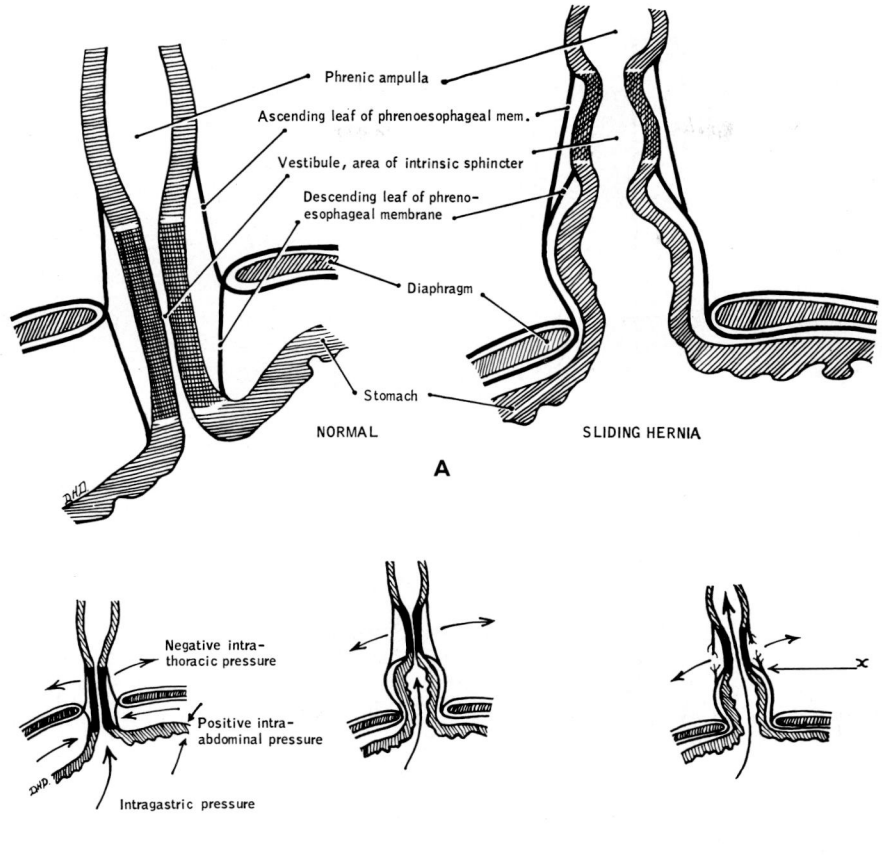

Phrenic ampulla
Ascending leaf of phrenoesophageal mem.
Vestibule, area of intrinsic sphincter
Descending leaf of phreno-esophageal membrane
Diaphragm
Stomach
NORMAL
SLIDING HERNIA
A

Negative intra-thoracic pressure
Positive intra-abdominal pressure
Intragastric pressure

B NORMAL   **C** HERNIA WITHOUT REFLUX   **D** HERNIA WITH REFLUX

Figure 15.37. Diagrammatic representations of the esophageal hiatus. **A,** In the normal hiatus (at left), the intrinsic sphincter (*cross-hatched*) is protected from distracting mechanical influences by the phrenoesophageal membrane. In sliding hernia (at right) the change of relationships of the normal structures is shown. **B** to **D,** Mechanical and hydrodynamic factors affecting function of the intrinsic sphincter are depicted. The sphincteric area is shown in *solid black*. In **B,** the normal, the sphincter combats only that intragastric pressure which is greater than intraabdominal pressure since the intraabdominal pressure imparted to the lumen of the stomach and lower esophagus is canceled out by an equal pressure against the outside of the abdominal esophagus. In **C,** a sliding hiatal hernia is shown. The sphincter has lost the benefit of reinforcement of intraabdominal pressure, but there is no interference from the phrenoesophageal membrane. In **D,** stretching of the membrane has resulted in an abnormal pull which opposes the action of the intrinsic sphincter and results in reflux. (From Dillard DH. Esophageal sphincter and reflux. Surg Clin North Am. 1964; 44:1201–1209.)

ence with swallowing to result in failure to thrive, the simple presence of gastroesophageal reflux in a small infant is not an indication for an antireflux procedure (JAH).

ESOPHAGEAL HIATUS AND THE CRURA

The esophageal hiatus is an elliptic opening in the muscular part of the diaphragm through which the esophagus passes. It lies to the left of the midline, about 1 cm from the posterior border of the central tendon at the level of the 10th thoracic vertebra. The margins of the hiatus are formed by the arms of the diaphragmatic crura and the median arcuate ligament when it is present.

The diaphragmatic crura arise from the anterior surface of the first three or four lumbar vertebrae on the right, or the first two or three lumbar vertebrae on the left, as well as from the intervertebral discs and the anterior longitudinal ligament (Fig. 15.38). The crural fibers pass upward and forward to give rise to the arms of muscle that form the hiatal ring (156). Anteriorly, the fibers of the arms insert in the transverse ligament of the central tendon of the diaphragm. The origins of the right and left arms from the crura are variable. The most frequent configurations are those in which both right and left arms arise from the right crus or the left arises from the right crus and the right arm rises from both crura (140) (Fig. 15.39).

The descending diaphragmatic crura are thick, musculotendinous bundles becoming more tendinous and less muscular near their vertebral origin. In nine of the

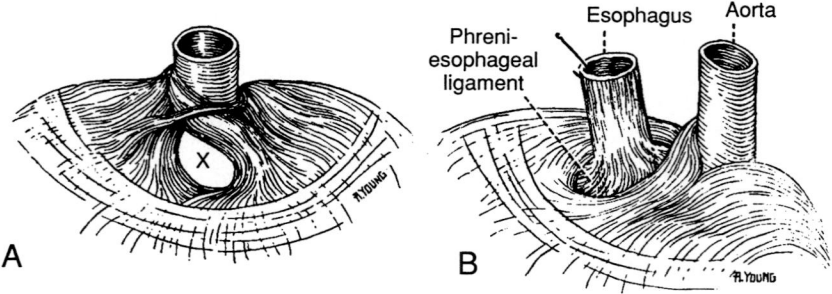

Figure 15.38. Sketches of the diaphragm from above. **A,** Aorta and (*X*) esophageal hiatus, showing accessory bundle of muscle fibers from left crus passing to the right, posterior to the hiatus. **B,** Esophagus and phrenoesophageal ligament viewed from the left. (From Carey JM, Hollinshead WH. Anatomy of the esophageal hiatus related to repair of hiatal hernia. Proc Staff Meet Mayo Clin 1955; 30:223–226.)

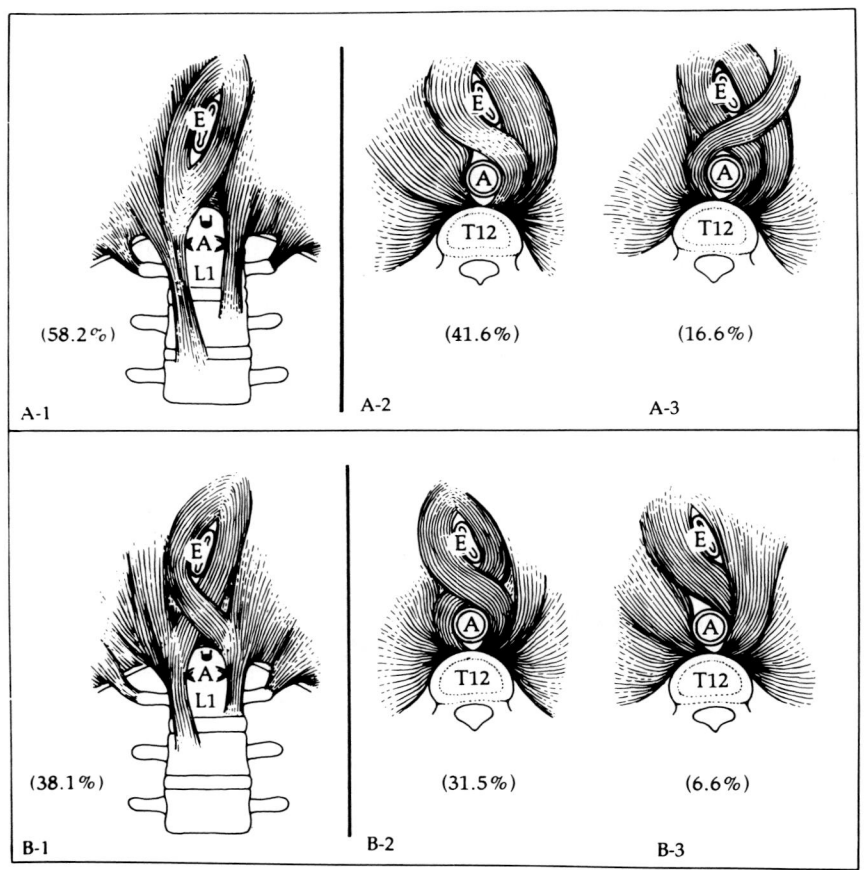

Figure 15.39. The most common patterns of the diaphragmatic crura. **A-1** and **B-1** seen from below. **A-2, A-3, B-2,** and **B-3** seen from above. (Data from Pataro VA et al. Anatomic aspects of the esophageal hiatus: distribution of the crura in its formation. J Int Coll Surg 1961; 35:154.)

ten cadavers with hiatal hernia we examined, the crura between the 10th thoracic and the first lumbar vertebrae were tendinous posteriorly and medially. In one specimen, the posterior tendinous portion did not extend to the medial aspect (130, 157) (Fig. 15.40). From the surgeon's view (anterior), there was no medial tendinous portion in this specimen through which sutures could have been placed. This variation in the extent of tendi-

nous and muscular portions of the crura may explain the recurrence rate in hiatal hernia repair. In our specimens the crural ring was friable and fibrotic for about 2 cm from the margin, except anteriorly, where the stretched opening extended to the central tendon of the diaphragm.

Where the esophagus passes from the thorax into the abdomen through the diaphragmatic hiatus, a strong, flexible, airtight seal is necessary. The seal must be strong enough to resist the abdominal pressure that tends to push the stomach into the thorax and flexible enough to give with the pressure changes incidental to breathing and the movement incidental to swallowing. The structure forming this seal is known as the phrenoesophageal ligament or membrane (Fig. 15.41).

The ligament should consist, in principle, of the following (147): pleura; subpleural (endothoracic) fascia; phrenoesophageal fascia (of Laimer); transversalis (endoabdominal subdiaphragmatic) fascia; and peritoneum (158).

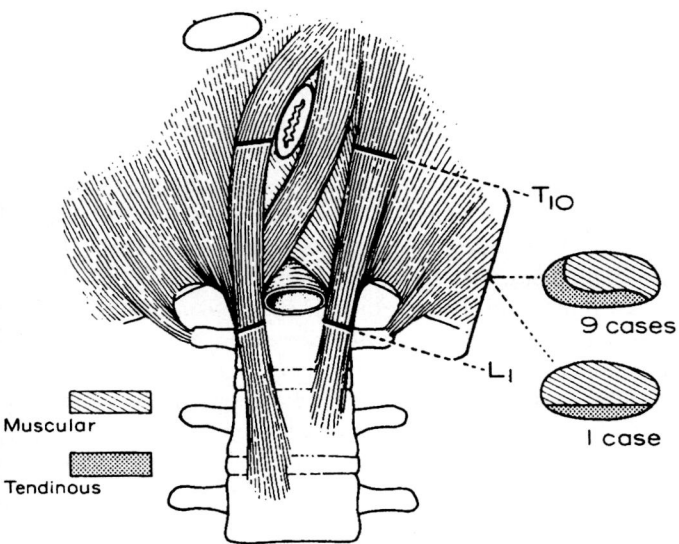

Figure 15.40. The crura consist of both tendinous and muscular tissue; only the tendinous portion holds sutures. In nine out of ten cadavers examined, the medial edge of the crura is tendinous. (Gray SW, Rowe JS Jr, Skandalakis JE. Surgical anatomy of the gastro-esophageal junction. Am Surg 1979; 45:575–587.)

The first and last of these elements provide the requirement for airtightness, and the middle three provide flexibility and strength. Most anatomists do not recognize the phrenoesophageal fascia as a separate entity.

The chief sources of disagreement are over the relative importance of the endothoracic and endoabdominal components and the extent of their esophageal attachment. In some published descriptions, the ligament is shown arising largely from the endoabdominal (subdiaphragmatic) fascia (141, 147). In others, the ligament is shown arising from both sub- and supradiaphragmatic fasciae (159, 160). Attachments to the esophagus are drawn as single (above the hiatus), double (above and below the hiatus), and multiple. Hill (161) considers the strongest attachment of the ligament to be the posterior fibers that insert in the preaortic fascia and the median arcuate ligament.

Peters' description (162) of the ligament remains the best. In all subjects, collagen and elastic fibers from the abdominal aspect of the hiatal margin insert into the circumference of the esophagus with extensions both above and below, blending into the adventitia over about 2 cm of esophagus. They may be traced into the intermuscular connective tissue of the muscularis externa. The insertion is usually proximal to the epithelial junction. In some subjects there is a comparable but more diffuse sheet of fibers arising from the thoracic surface of the hiatal margin and passing downwards to attach to the esophagus below the hiatus (Fig. 15.42).

We compared the ligament in fresh cadavers of 10 stillborn infants and 10 middle-aged subjects having no pathology of the hiatus or gastroesophageal junction with its appearance in cadavers of 10 adult subjects having clinical, radiologic, and anatomic evidence of sliding hiatal hernia. The ligament is best seen in infants. With age,

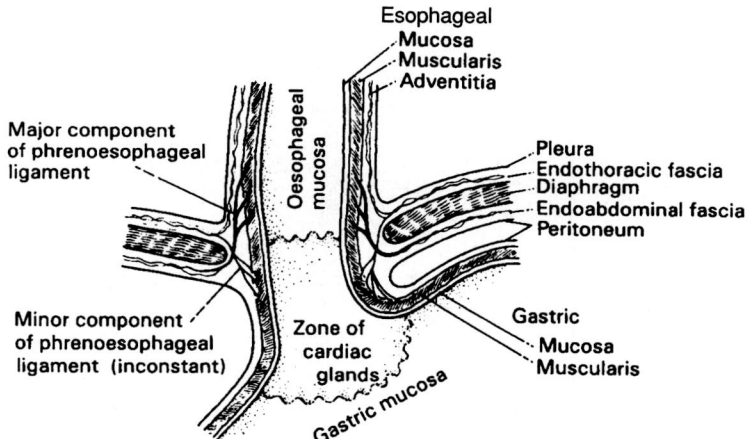

Figure 15.41. Diagrammatic section through the gastroesophageal junction showing the elements of the phrenoesophageal membrane. It is rarely so well defined in adults. (From Gray SW, Rowe JS Jr, Skandalakis JE. Surgical anatomy of the gastro-esophageal junction. Am Surg 1979; 45:575–587.)

the esophagus becomes less firmly fixed in the hiatus; the ligament becomes less definite; and fat appears between the attenuated fibers. In our specimens the ligament had lost much of its identity by middle age. For all practical purposes the ligament does not exist in adult patients with long-standing hiatal hernia (157) (Figs. 15.43 and 15.44).

MEDIAN ARCUATE LIGAMENT

The esophageal hiatus is separated from the aortic hiatus by fusion of the arms of the left and right crura. If the tendinous portions of the crura are fused, the median arcuate ligament is present as a fibrous arch passing over the aorta, connecting the right and left crura. If the fusion is muscular only, the ligament is ill-defined or absent.

The median arcuate ligament passes in front of the aorta at the level of the first lumbar vertebra just above the origin of the celiac trunk (Figs. 15.14 and 15.45). The celiac ganglia lie just below and anterior to the celiac trunk. The ligament and the origin of the celiac artery become slightly lower with increasing age. In 16% of patients, a low median arcuate ligament covers the celiac artery and may compress it. At angiography, such compression may simulate atherosclerotic plaques. Adequate collateral circulation exists since such patients usually do not have symptoms.

If there is no true ligament, and the muscular arms of the crura are thinned by posterior extension of the esophageal hiatus, the aortic and esophageal openings may become practically confluent, although there is always some connective tissue between them.

COMPLICATIONS OF HIATAL HERNIA

Obstruction and sometimes strangulation may occur with paraesophageal hernia. Ulcerative erosion, with hemor-

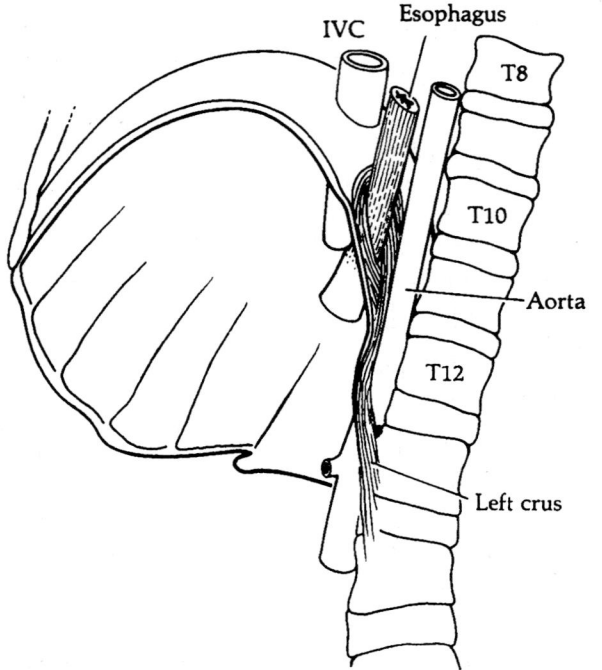

Figure 15.42. The diaphragmatic openings for the inferior vena cava, the esophagus, and the aorta as seen from the left. (From Skandalakis JE, Gray SW, Rowe JS Jr, Skandalakis LJ. In: Nyhus LM, Baker RJ, eds. Mastery of surgery. Boston: Little, Brown, 1992.)

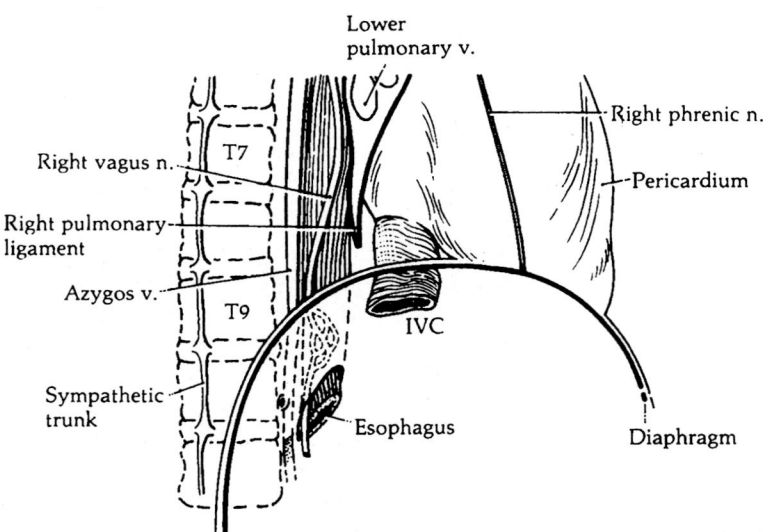

Figure 15.43. Structures in the inferior portion of the right mediastinum. (From Skandalakis JE, Gray SW, Rowe JS Jr, Skandalakis LJ. In: Nyhus LM, Baker RJ, eds. Mastery of surgery. Boston: Little, Brown, 1992.)

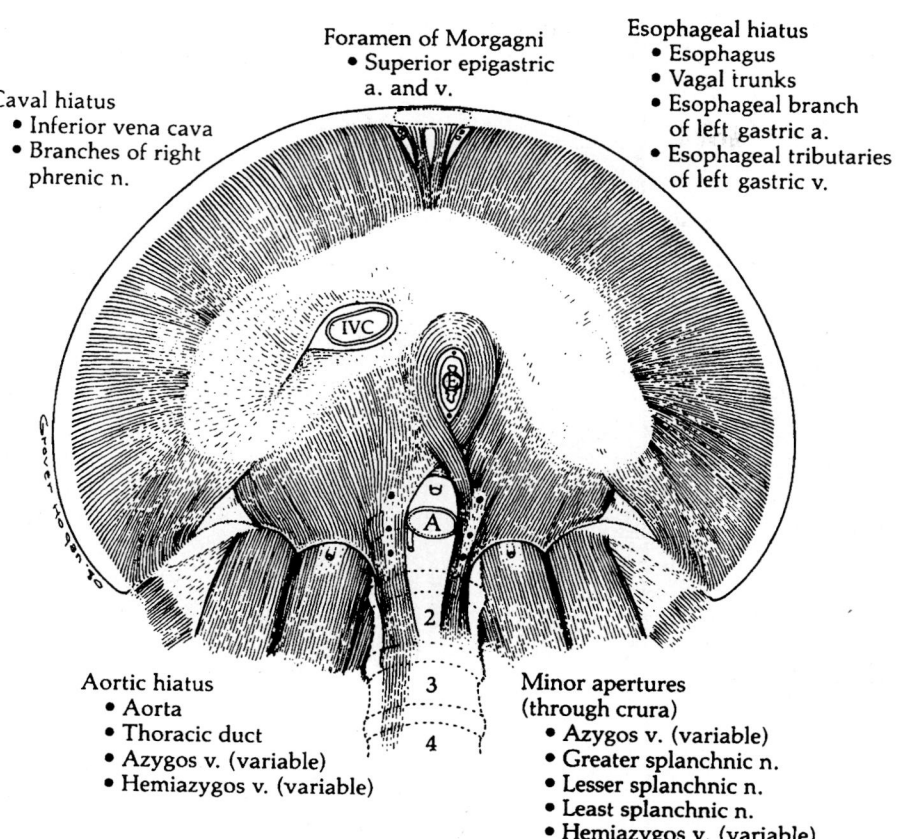

Caval hiatus
- Inferior vena cava
- Branches of right phrenic n.

Foramen of Morgagni
- Superior epigastric a. and v.

Esophageal hiatus
- Esophagus
- Vagal trunks
- Esophageal branch of left gastric a.
- Esophageal tributaries of left gastric v.

Aortic hiatus
- Aorta
- Thoracic duct
- Azygos v. (variable)
- Hemiazygos v. (variable)

Minor apertures (through crura)
- Azygos v. (variable)
- Greater splanchnic n.
- Lesser splanchnic n.
- Least splanchnic n.
- Hemiazygos v. (variable)

Figure 15.44. The apertures of the diaphragm seen from below and the structures transversing them. (From Skandalakis JE, Gray SW, Rowe JS Jr, Skandalakis LJ. In: Nyhus LM, Baker RJ, eds. Mastery of surgery. Boston: Little, Brown, 1992.)

rhage from either stomach or esophagus, often appears in cases of long standing, and esophageal stricture with achalasia is not rare.

There is reason to believe that an enlarged esophageal hiatus permits the cardia of the stomach to enter the mediastinum during forceful vomiting. In this location, the esophagus is susceptible to mucosal tearing (Mallory-Weiss syndrome) because the rise in intragastric pressure of vomiting is not balanced by the rise in intraabdominal pressure (163).

Adler and Rodriguez (164) called attention to the association of malignancy with hiatal hernia; they found 21 cases among 814 herniae. More than 5% of males with hiatal hernia developed gastric malignancy, whereas less than 1% of females did so. Our own experience with small muscle tumors of the esophagus (165) indicates a relatively high incidence (4.2%) of associated hiatal hernia. That reflux esophagitis may predispose the individual to carcinoma is possible, but that it can influence the muscle coats of the esophagus is doubtful. Some of the incidence of associated lesions probably results from concentrated attention on the esophagus in studying one condition, during which the other—either hernia or tumor—is detected more often than would otherwise be the case.

EMBRYOGENESIS

The congenital nature of an enlarged esophageal hiatus is by no means well established. A reasonable but unconfirmed explanation is that there is a delay in the elongation of the esophagus and hence in the descent of the stomach during the seventh to eighth weeks while the diaphragmatic muscle fibers are forming. The hiatus thus forms around the upper portion of the gastric dilation rather than around the esophagus itself, and subsequent further descent of the stomach results in an esophagus lying in a hiatus that is too large for it (Figs. 15.46 and 15.47). This condition predisposes the individual to a hiatal hernia later in life (Fig. 15.48). As under similar conditions elsewhere in the body, such a potential hernia may never become actual. Other causes, such as tight corseting, obesity, or chronic esophagitis, are undoubtedly contributory. Nevertheless, hiatal hernia has been found in stillborn infants (166).

When esophageal elongation is permanently arrested

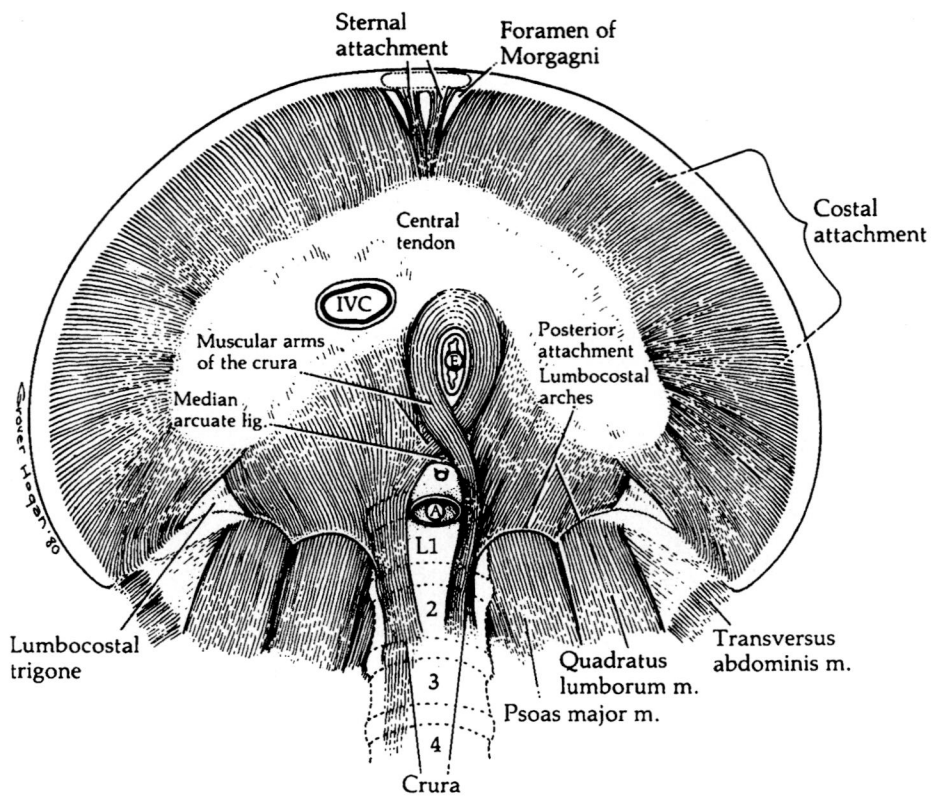

Figure 15.45. The attachments of the muscles of the diaphragm seen from below. (From Skandalakis JE, Gray SW, Rowe JS Jr, Skandalakis LJ. In: Nyhus LM, Baker RJ, eds. Mastery of surgery. Boston: Little, Brown, 1992.)

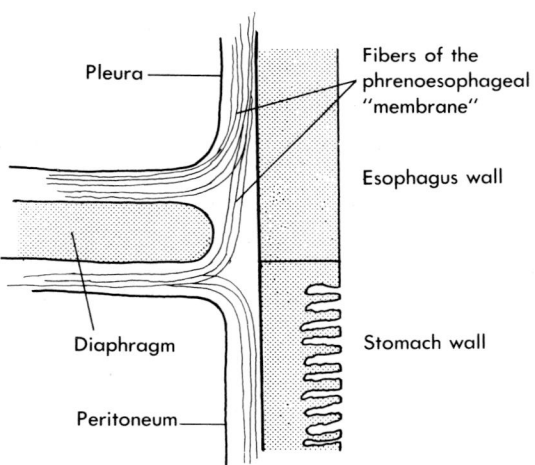

Figure 15.46. Diagram showing arrangement of the fibers of the phreno-esophageal membrane in the newborn. (Drawn from the description by Botha GSM. Organogenesis and growth of the gastroesophageal region in man. Anat Rec. 1959; 133:219–239.)

(congenital short esophagus), the stomach is never fully descended. Although the clinical condition is similar to that of enlarged esophageal hiatus, the embryogenesis and local anatomy are different (see page 98).

Moore (16) discusses predisposing factors concerning the enlarged esophageal hiatus, while Sadler (17) speculates about congenital short esophagus.

HISTORY

The earliest clear description of hiatal hernia was written in 1761 by Morgagni (De Sedibus LIV:11, 12), who collected and discussed a number of earlier observations. In 1836, Bright (167) described a massive hiatal hernia in the autopsy of a 19-year-old girl who had suffered from gastric distress from infancy. As the thoracic stomach was enveloped in a peritoneal sac, the lesion must be considered a hiatal hernia; however, its probable congenital nature led to confusion between hiatal hernia and congenital short esophagus. Subsequent workers were not always able to distinguish between acquired and congenital thoracic stomach. Although hiatal hernia was mentioned among diaphragmatic herniae in general, it received little attention and was considered rare until the 1920s.

In 1923 Richards (168) collected nontraumatic cases of diaphragmatic hernia and was able to find only 22 cases of hiatal hernia over a period of 23 years. In 1924 Abbott (169) called attention to paraesophageal herniae. Healey in 1925 (170) reported 53 cases, and Morrison (111) described the radiologic picture. In 1926 Åkerlund (124) presented a classification of esophageal hiatal herniae. With these studies, it became apparent that hiatal hernia is a relatively common lesion. It has not lacked attention since then.

INCIDENCE

Fewer than 5% of hiatal herniae are paraesophageal; the remainder are esophageal. About 80% of the latter are of the sliding type.

Mobley and Christensen (171) found 153 cases of hiatal hernia in 13 years in Rochester, Minnesota, a city of 30,000. They considered the incidence to be between 0.5 and 0.8 per 1000 per year, and the prevalence to be 5:1000. From this data, they concluded that about 800,000 cases exist in the United States. Unlike most congenital anomalies, hiatal hernia is better diagnosed on radiography than at autopsy because the esophagus relaxes after death, and in the sliding type of hernia, the stomach returns to the abdomen.

In most series, from 60 to 70% of the patients are females (164, 171, 172), but a few investigators have reported a preponderance of males (173, 174).

Hiatal hernia is rare before the age of 30 years, and over half of those affected will be between the ages of 50

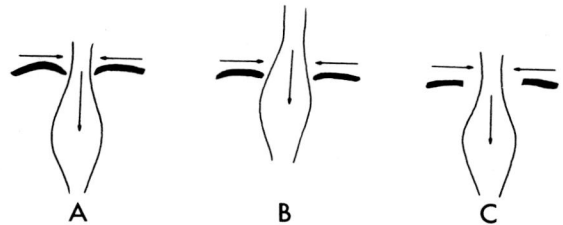

Figure 15.47. Possible embryogenesis of hiatal hernia, showing descent of the embryonic stomach and closure of the hiatus. **A,** Normally descended stomach and normally closed hiatus. **B,** Delayed descent of the stomach and closure of the hiatus. **C,** Eventual normal descent of the stomach with abnormally large hiatus.

and 70 years. The occurrence of hernia in later life was attributed by Harrington (175) to progressive elastic atrophy of the phrenoesophageal membrane. Obesity, along with a rise in intraabdominal pressure and decreased muscle tone, further encourages herniation. Trauma, on the other hand, is not an important factor.

Symptoms in infants are usually, if not always, those of short esophagus rather than of hiatal hernia (176).

SYMPTOMS

Hiatal Hernia. Symptoms range from mild epigastric discomfort to substernal pain and frank bleeding from the esophagus. Anemia may be present without evidence of hemorrhage. An intrinsic factor defect in the anemia of hiatal hernia has been suggested (177).

The pain may simulate that caused by peptic ulcer, cholelithiasis, or coronary artery disease (178). Nuzum (179) found 25 cases of hiatal hernia among 100 patients diagnosed as having angina pectoris. In a similar series, Gilbert (180) found 17% with hiatal hernia.

Esophagitis, with dysphagia and regurgitation, is present in about 25% of patients. Back pain is frequently associated (181), and obesity is a common physical finding.

Some 21% of patients in the series of Mobley and Christensen (171) had no symptoms. This is higher than that usually reported, but it reminds one that the condition may remain silent for years before the patient is motivated to seek medical advice. Diagnosis is made more difficult by the fact that peptic ulceration or biliary disease also may be present. Rex and his colleagues (182) at the Mayo Clinic found duodenal ulcers in 8% of patients with hiatal hernia, and gallbladder disease in 19%.

Congenital Short Esophagus. Dysphagia from birth is the most common symptom of congenital short esophagus. It is associated with reflux vomiting and eventually results in esophagitis and stricture. Barrett (129) noted that the higher the gastric mucosa extends up into the thoracic portion, the less severe will be the reflux esophagitis.

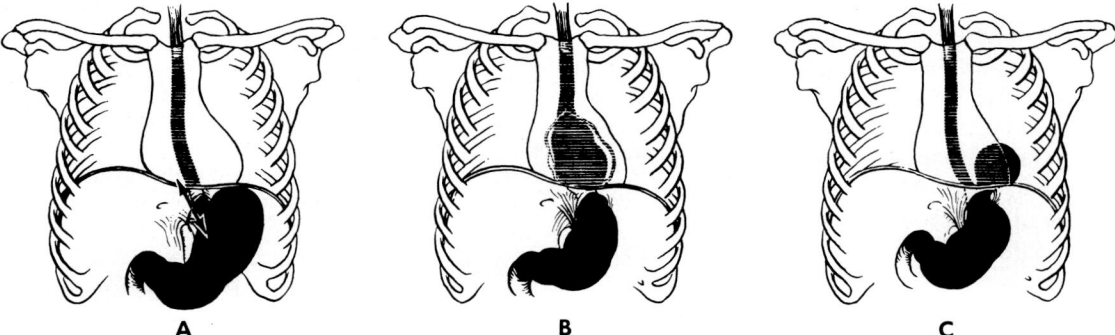

Figure 15.48. Types of hiatal hernia. **A,** Sliding hiatal hernia. **B,** Fixed hiatal hernia. This type appears identical radiographically to the rare congenital short esophagus; the two can be distinguished only at surgery or at necropsy. **C,** Para- esophageal hernia. (From Rex JC et al. Esophageal hiatal hernia: a 10-year study of medically treated cases. JAMA 1961; 178:271–274.)

Vomiting appears early and may become severe when transition to solid food is begun; malnutrition is common (particularly in babies and children); and death from starvation is possible. Blood often appears in the vomitus, and frank or occult blood may be found in stools. Anemia and failure to gain weight are common findings. As a result of frequent vomiting, aspiration pneumonia is an ever present danger. Bleeding and pain are less common in infants and children than in adults. Males are more frequently and more severely affected than are females (183) (see the discussion on gastroesophageal retlux).

DIAGNOSIS

Radiologic examination is the primary means of diagnosis. It serves to distinguish the condition from achalasia, esophageal diverticulum, and defects elsewhere in the diaphragm. Negative radiologic findings in a patient should not be trusted since a sliding esophageal hernia may be temporarily reduced; several pictures taken at different times may be required. Endoscopic examination should always accompany radiographic study to determine the condition of the lower esophagus or to detect ulceration, diverticula, or carcinoma. The presence of these complications may materially affect the choice of treatment.

Shackelford (184) observed that the gastroesophageal junction is a complex of structures which may be defined differently by the anatomist, the surgeon, the radiologist, and the endoscopist (Fig. 15.49).

Gross Anatomic: "the termination of the tube, the esophagus and the beginning of a pouch, the stomach" (136)
Microscopic: the squamocolumnar junction
Surgical: just below the diaphragm at the upper border of the reflection of the peritoneum from the stomach on to the distal esophagus
Radiologic: an imaginary line from the angle of His to the middle of the junctional mucosa at the lesser curvature; longitudinal mucosal folds of esophagus change to transverse folds of stomach
Endoscopic: the junction of the pale pink esophageal mucosa with the bright red gastric mucosa (Z line)

Since precise definition of the gastroesophageal junction is practically impossible in living patients with or without sliding hiatus hernia, it is difficult to relate specific symptoms to specific anatomic structures and their function. Only the squamocolumnar Z line can be located precisely by direct vision (185). Even this line is highly mobile over the other tissues.

Radiology. Anatomic entities not always demonstrated radiographically are:

1. The squamocolumnar epithelial junction (Z line) (This may show as a B or Schatzki ring.)
2. The lower esophageal sphincter (LOS) (The upper limit may correspond with the A ring.)
3. The gastric sling (rare exceptions)

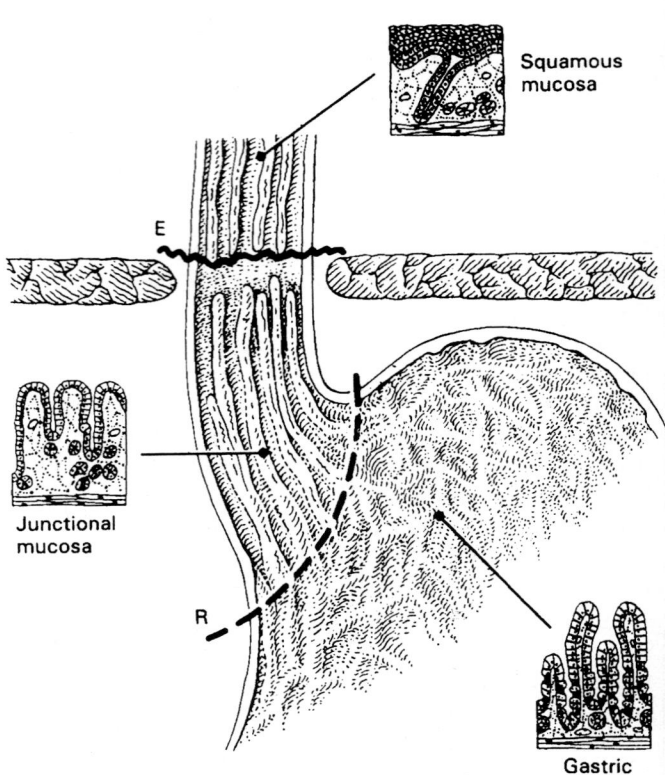

Figure 15.49. The gastroesophageal junction. *E*, Endoscopic gastroesophageal junction; *R*, anatomic gastroesophageal junction. (From Gray SW, Skandalakis LJ, Skandalakis JE. Classification of hernias through the oesophageal hiatus. In: Jamieson GG, ed. Surgery of the oesophagus. Edinburgh: Churchill Livingstone, 1988.)

Anatomic entities usually demonstrable by radiography are:

1. The angle of His
2. The phrenic ampulla, that part of the distal esophagus which balloons slightly when it is in the intrathoracic position. (It is probably that part of the esophagus encompassed by the phrenoesophageal ligament. Peristaltic waves cease at the proximal ampullary region.)
3. The "submerged segment" which is the abdominal esophagus
4. Under fluoroscopy, concentric contractions which are observed in the ampulla and submerged segment of the distal esophagus
5. Due to the oblique gastric sling, the cardia, which shows flaccidity or nonconcentric contractions

The gastroesophageal function of the radiologist is the imaginary line of the gastric sling from the angle of His to the lesser curvature. The diagnosis of hiatus hernia can be made if a supradiaphragmatic gastric pouch, contracting nonconcentrically, can be identified.

Paraesophageal herniae are recognized readily on plain x-ray films with the stomach partly above the level

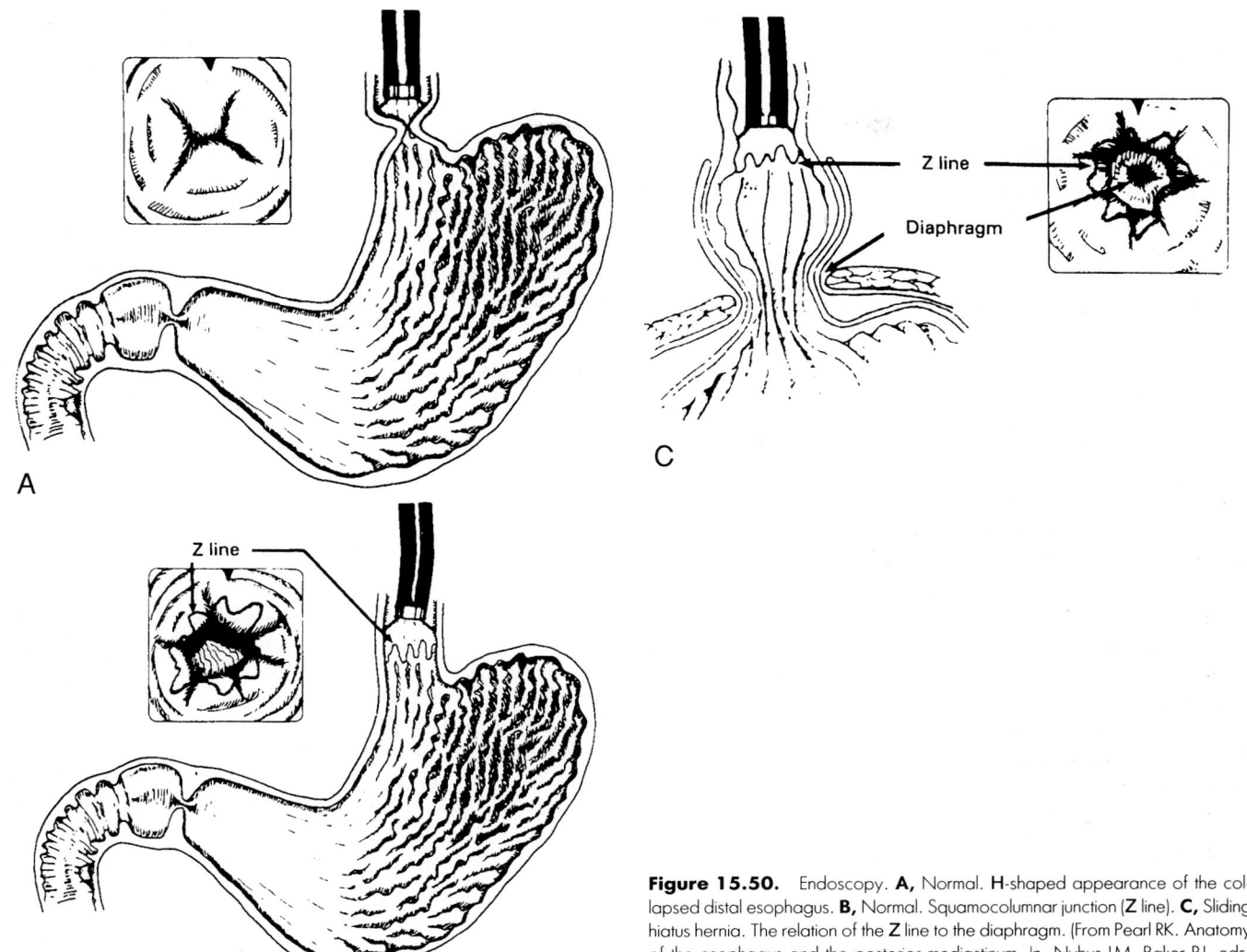

Figure 15.50. Endoscopy. **A,** Normal. **H**-shaped appearance of the collapsed distal esophagus. **B,** Normal. Squamocolumnar junction (**Z** line). **C,** Sliding hiatus hernia. The relation of the **Z** line to the diaphragm. (From Pearl RK. Anatomy of the esophagus and the posterior mediastinum. In: Nyhus LM, Baker RJ, eds. Mastery of surgery. Boston: Little, Brown, 1984.)

of the diaphragm. The gastroesophageal junction is at or below the diaphragm.

Endoscopy. The normal cardiac opening appears as a contracted rosette of pale esophageal mucosa, descending during inspiration and ascending during expiration. In hiatus hernia the cardiac opening does not descend during inspiration but opens widely, displaying pink gastric mucosa in longitudinal folds (Fig. 15.50, *A* and *B*).

Normally, with the **Z** line under direct vision, when the patient is asked to sniff two or three times, the esophageal orifice contracts or is obliterated, probably by contraction of the diaphragm. If there is a hiatal hernia, endoscopy will reveal the **Z** line above the level of luminal obliteration when the patient sniffs (Fig. 15.50, *C*). The endoscopist can quantitate the hiatus hernia by measuring the distance between the **Z** line and the area of contracted lumen during the sniff.

The epithelial junction (**Z** line) can be readily visualized endoscopically and is thus the most precisely defined of the elements of the gastroesophageal junction. These observations apply to sliding hiatus herniae. Endoscopic findings in patients with paraesophageal hiatus herniae are usually negative.

TREATMENT

Hiatal Hernia. In the absence of symptoms from a radiographically demonstrable hernia, surgery need not be undertaken. Weight reduction and the avoidance of tightly fitting garments should be encouraged. When mild symptoms exist, the surgeon must use his or her own judgment. Hernial repair during surgery for other upper abdominal lesions may be desirable when equivocal symptoms are present.

The objectives of surgical treatment are reduction of

the hernia, obliteration of the sac, contraction of the hiatus, and fixation of the esophagus (Fig. 15.51).

The surgical approach may be transthoracic or transabdominal. Allison (186), Sweet (187), and others advocate the transthoracic approach, while Harrington (150) prefers the transabdominal route. A number of pertinent papers may be found in the book edited by Mulholland and his colleagues (188). Handelsman (181) advocates the transthoracic approach under the following conditions:

1. When there are concurrent thoracic lesions
2. When the hernia has recurred
3. When more than half the stomach is in the thorax
4. When the stomach is fixed above the diaphragm

Harrington (150) observed that it is more difficult to reduce the size of a diaphragmatic opening than it is to close it completely. In the light of this, Meredino and his colleagues (189) designed a method of making a new diaphragmatic orifice, completely closing the old one. In contrast, Nissen (190) made no effort to close the hiatus, preferring to fix the stomach to the anterior abdominal wall.

Temporary and occasionally permanent interruption of the left phrenic nerve often has been employed to relax the diaphragm and allow complete healing before diaphragmatic function returns (3 to 5 months). Many surgeons, however, doubt the usefulness of this (191).

The authors believe that all of these procedures have their merits and that evaluation of each individual patient is necessary. Those who advocate a particular procedure exclusively, and support their choice dogmatically, are perhaps as correct as those who insist on an ideal anatomic repair. Why demand the perfect repair of a hiatal hernia in an elderly person, who already has several other medical problems when one can help the patient with simpler measures? In many instances gastropexy is not a mark of inferior surgical skill, but rather a sign of mature surgical judgment.

Congenital Short Esophagus

The problem of the congenital short esophagus differs from that of ordinary hiatal hernia in that the stomach cannot be returned to the normal position, never having been there. Mobilization of the esophagus up to the aortic stricture may be safely performed without damage to the circulation, and this may provide sufficient length. Otherwise, the problem is to elevate the diaphragm to a position above the stomach.

Effler and Groves (192) advocate advancement of the hiatus to the highest point available on the diaphragm, which is immobilized by phrenic interruption. This method appears to share the advantages of the Merendino operation for forming a new esophageal hiatus in

the case of ordinary hiatus hernia. Finney pyloroplasty was used by Burford and Lischer (193) in 16 patients with short esophagus. Interposition of a jejunal segment, accompanied by bilateral vagotomy, was performed by Merendino and Dillard (194) in 12 cases with achalasia, esophageal varices, and congenital short esophagus. When stricture is present, Ellis and his colleagues (195) advocated esophagogastrectomy for treatment of short esophagus. Sweet (187) criticized this procedure, questioning the adequacy of the blood supply to the gastric remnant.

Accessory Septum Transversum: Accessory Diaphragm

Duplication of the septum transversum occurred in a newborn with respiratory distress thought clinically to be due to diaphragmatic paralysis. Surgical plication of the "floppy" diaphragm was attempted via a transabdominal approach. The anomalous septum transversum was perceived to be the diaphragm and was plicated. The central tendon of the diaphragm was redundant and surgical plication may have improved respiratory function. In this first case report, embryology of the diaphragm is reviewed and correlated with autopsy findings. A surgical approach to possible correction is proposed.

Accessory diaphragm is a rare congenital anomaly that consists of a fibromuscular membrane separating the affected hemithorax into two cavities. In three of the 21 reported cases, the accessory diaphragm was innervated by the phrenic nerve. It may interfere with respiration causing respiratory distress in the neonatal period, recurrent respiratory infection during infancy and childhood, and chronic pulmonary inflammation in adult life (196).

We report a unique and previously unreported developmental anomaly that embryologically represents an accessory septum transversum. This structure produces similar clinical symptoms and possibly has similar embryologic roots as the entity known as accessory diaphragm. However, marked differences exist in the anatomic structure, location, and extent of these two anomalies—and consequently in the surgical approach to their corrections.

CASE REPORT

A 2180 gm, 34½-week-gestation, black female was born to a 21-year-old, para 1-0-0-1 mother after a pregnancy that was uneventful until the onset of premature labor on the day of delivery. A cesarean section was performed without complications. The infant had Apgar scores of 1 at 1 minute and 2 at 5 minutes and required mechnical ventilation as well as intravenous sodium bicarbonate and calcium gluconate. The infant was also transfused with 10

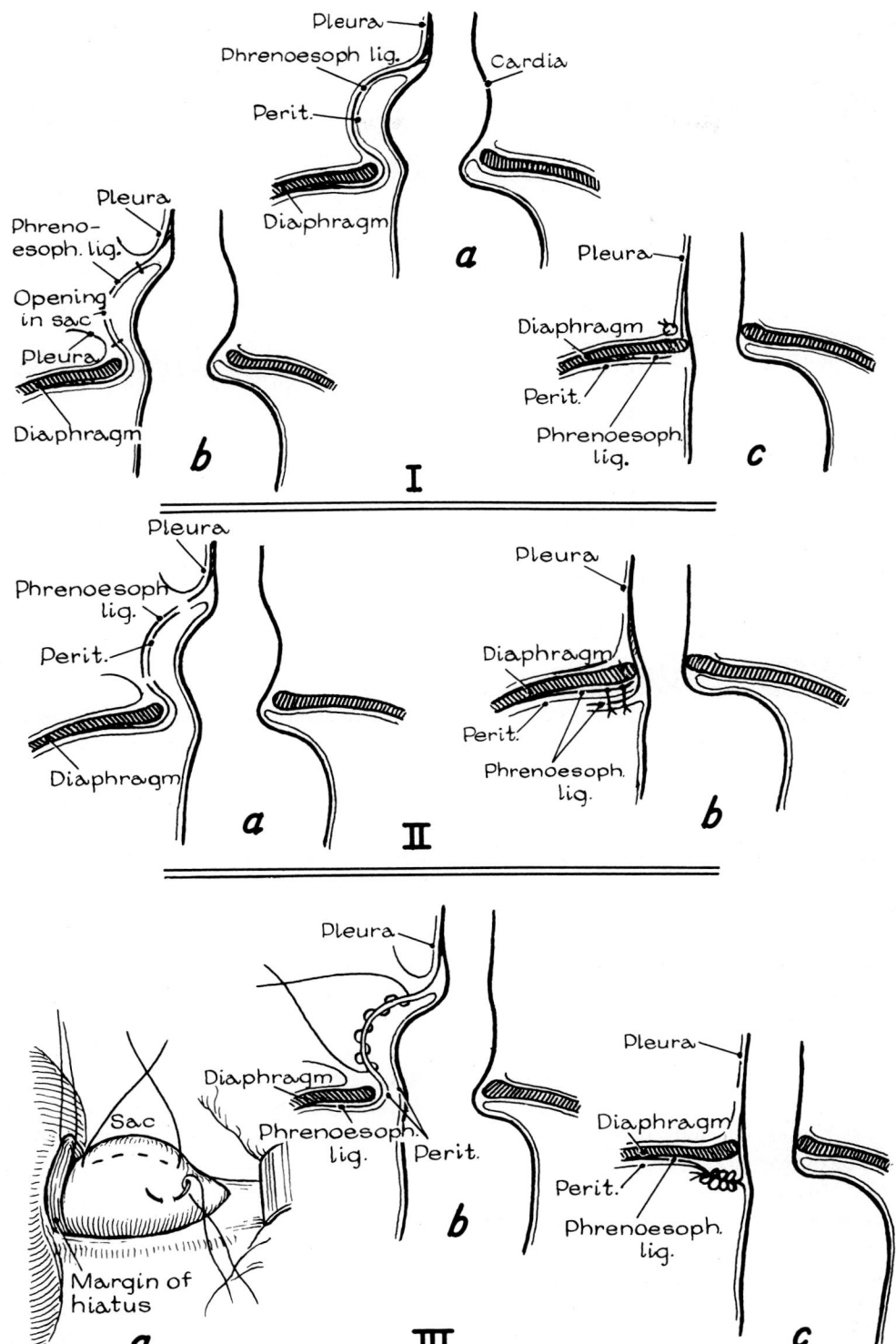

Figure 15.51. Procedures for repair of hiatal hernia. **Ia,** The pathologic relationships of sliding hiatal hernia. **Ib,** Pleural incision, with removal of the sac. **Ic,** Reduction of the hernia and repair of the pleural incision. **IIa,** Removal of the sac. **IIb,** Suturing of the ligament and peritoneum to abdominal side of the diaphragm; closure of the pleural incision (Allison). **IIIa** to **c,** Plication sutures to obliterate the hernial sac (Sweet). In each procedure, closure of the muscular ring of the hiatus completes the repair of the hernia. (From Madden JL. Atlas of technics in surgery, ed 2. vol 2. New York: Appleton-Century-Crofts, 1958.)

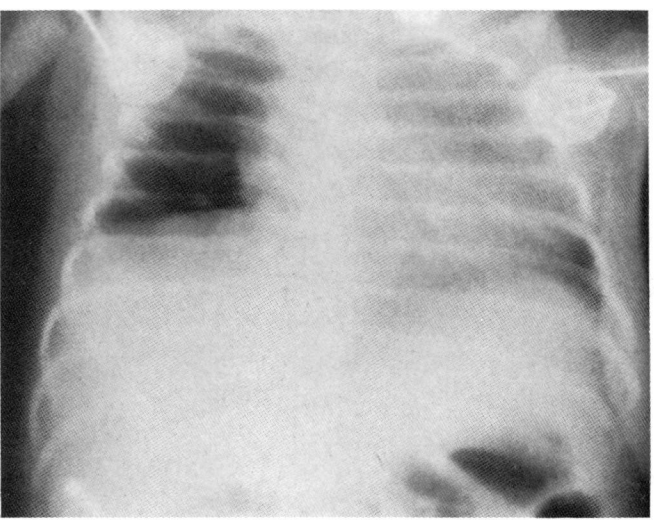

Figure 15.52. Chest x-ray film in the third day of life at maximum excursion on inspiration. (From Krzyzaniak R, Gray SW. Accessory septum transversum. The first case report. Am Surg 1986; 52(5):278–281.)

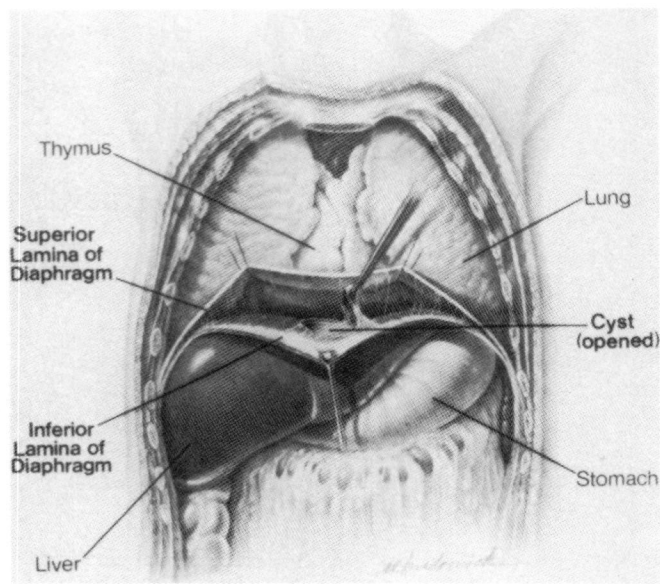

Figure 15.53. Drawing of the relationships of the superior and inferior laminae of the diaphragm in a patient. (From Krzyzaniak R, Gray SW. Accessory septum transversum. The first case report. Am Surg 1986; 52(5):278–281.)

cc/kg packed red blood cells for hypotension, decreased perfusion, and a hematacrit of 35%.

Physical examination revealed growth parameters at the 25th percentile for gestational age, epicanthal folds, oblique palpebral fissures, a sloping forehead, and a prominent occiput. There were no adventitious breath sounds, but a grade II/IV systolic ejection murmur was heard at the left upper sternal border radiating to the left lower sternal border. Also noted were hypoplastic fingernails, bilateral talipes equinovarus, bilateral overlapping of the thumb and index finger over the third finger, and marked abduction of the hips.

Chest x-ray films showed hypoexpansion of the lungs (Fig. 15.52) with the maximal excursion to the T6 level. Fluoroscopy on the third day of life revealed elevated diaphragms, which, without mechanical ventilation, ascended poorly. Multiple attempts to discontinue mechanical ventilation were unsuccessful, as was a trial of negative pressure mechanical ventilation. Findings from muscle biopsy, electromyography, nerve conduction studies, and a cranial ultrasound study were normal.

On the 29th day of life, a transabdominal, bilateral diaphragmatic plication was performed. Right upper lobe atelectasis developed and apneic episodes occurred. One week postoperatively, bilateral rales and increased tracheal secretions were noted. The Gram stain showed negative rods and Gram-positive cocci. Intravenous ampicillin and gentamycin were begun, but there was no clinical improvement. On the 44th day of life the patient died.

Pertinent Autopsy Findings. External examination confirmed the dysmorphic features. A 12.5-cm suture, midline abdominal incision and a 2-cm scar on the right ante-

rior thigh were present from the previous diaphragmatic plication and muscle biopsy, respectively.

Internal examination disclosed a duplicated right ureter. The diaphragm was elevated resulting in decreased pleural volume and lung size. Diaphragmatic duplication was present and consisted of a normal diaphragm which had moderate redundancy of its central tendon (Fig. 15.53), normal composition of muscle, and normal pericardial and body wall attachments. A substantial musculofibrous septum completely separated the abdominal cavity from the diaphragm. The central fibrous area was surgically plicated from an inferior approach. This accessory septum attached to the anterior, lateral, and dorsal thoracic body wall. The inferior surface of the diaphragm partially served as a dorsal attachment site, being formed by a diffuse network of membranes and filaments. Anterior to the inferior vena cava, in the midline and extending 15 cm to the left, was a prominent, pneumoenteric recess measuring 1.5 cm in diameter. The superior and lateral surfaces of the pneumoenteric recess were the major membranous structure, uniting the accessory septum transversum to the dorsal inferior diaphragm. The dorsal body wall, however, was its primary dorsal attachment. The accessory septum transversum was composed of approximately 50% muscle, primarily located posterolaterally. The anterocentral portion was a thick musculofibrous septum that was adherent to the superior surface and formed hepatic attachments normally made with the peritoneal surface of the diaphragm.

Microscopic examination revealed that both the diaphragm and the accessory septum transversum were composed of striated muscle, fibrous tissue, and nerve. The diaphragm, however, contained more muscle. The lungs showed changes of mild interstitial pneumonitis, alveolar spaces that were frequently lined by thin layers of fibroblasts, and areas of distended alveolar spaces adjacent to atelectatic areas.

The authors feel the appellation of accessory diaphragm would be an appropriately descriptive name for the anatomic anomaly described in this case. Since this name has been used already to describe a dissimilar entity, the term accessory septum transversum is chosen to refer to this anomaly.

The observed anomaly is embryologically explained by duplication of the septum transversum with persistence of the left pneumoenteric recess between the leaves of the accessory septum transversum and the diaphragm. That both the diaphragm and the accessory septum transversum were innervated by the phrenic nerve suggests that formation of the accessory septum transversum occurred at approximately 4 weeks of gestation. At this time the septum transversum normally develops at the level of the third and fourth cervical somites and is invaded by the phrenic nerve. Additional evidence supporting this hypothesis is that the diaphragm was totally separated from the liver. The accessory septum transversum assumed the intimate developmental association and attachments that normally occur between the liver and the mesenchyme of the septum transversum, a process also initiated during the fourth gestational week.

Accessory diaphragm, a dissimilar anomaly, may have similar embryologic roots, as reported by Minnis and Reingold (197), Patten (198), Nayarion et al. (199), Ikeda et al. (200), Karkola et al. (201), Wedel et al. (202), Hart et al. (203), and Merten et al. (204).

The findings presented in the case report of Krzyzaniak and Gray (205) are evidence for the potential for duplication or splitting of the septum transversum early in embryogenesis. Accessory diaphragm may represent a similar early splitting of the septum transversum. However, in this anomaly, the superior leaf (or leaves) of the bifid septum transverum plays the accessory role. Premature arrest in the descent of the superior accessory leaf (leaves) usually results in a fibromuscular band across one hemithorax, which may compromise pulmonary function and manifest clinical symptoms. Fusion of such anomalous schisms may be a frequent, undetected event.

Although CT was not performed in this case, it might have elucidated or suggested the anomaly. Contrast material injected into the pleural and abdominal cavities should make the anatomy apparent. If simple CT scanning suggests the anomaly, contrast injected into the "diaphragmatic space" should visualize the abnormality.

Hopkins and Davis (206) reported a case of a neonate with accessory right diaphragm. They emphasized the need for lateral chest x-ray films for the diagnosis.

Correction of the anomaly should attempt to unite the two diaphragms. Injection of a sclerosing agent such as tetracycline in conjunction with initial surgical plication and union of the leaves may offer an approach to correction. The effectiveness of the floppy diaphragm would be increased by eliminating redundancy of the central tendon. Uniting the accessory septum transversum to the true diaphragm early in infancy should allow appositional defects to be grown over and improve inspiratory performance with union of the muscle masses. Fusing the diaphragm with the accessory septum transversum would also unite the liver to the diaphragm. Thus many important hepatodiaphragmatic ligamentous attachments would be achieved. This would result in effective muscular contraction and production of negative intrapleural pressure.

This report is the first recorded case of such an extensive duplication of diaphragmatic structures. The finding of such an anomaly has both clinical and morphogenetic ramifications. Clinically, it indicates the potential for similar or identical anomalies which may be amenable to correction. Morphogenetically, it suggests that the origin of diaphragmatic musculature may primarily be derived from elements intrinsic within the septum transversum and/or from myoblasts which migrate with the phrenic nerve. The process of "burrowing" suggested by Bremer (2) is less tenable in light of these findings. Using this hypothesis to explain this anomaly becomes extremely difficult. Discovery and documentation of additional similar anomalies may contribute to a better understanding of the morphogenesis of the diaphragm.

ANATOMY

Complete or partial duplication of the diaphragm is very rare. Only 21 cases have been encountered in the literature, and most involved the right diaphragm, according to Krzyzaniak and Gray (205). A complete duplication was reported by Sullivan (207) in a 4-year-old male patient. The upper part of the right thorax was partitioned off by a muscular wall. This wall arose from the normal diaphragm anteriorly and passed over the bronchus and vessels of the middle and lower lobes to attach to the posterior thoracic wall. The upper lobe was represented by a bronchial stub.

An almost complete duplication, which lay in the oblique fissure of the right lung, was found incidentally at autopsy in a 57-year-old woman. A small aperture near the mediastinum admitted the normal bronchovascular elements to the lower lobe. The accessory diaphragm was largely membranous, while the normal diaphragm was muscular (208).

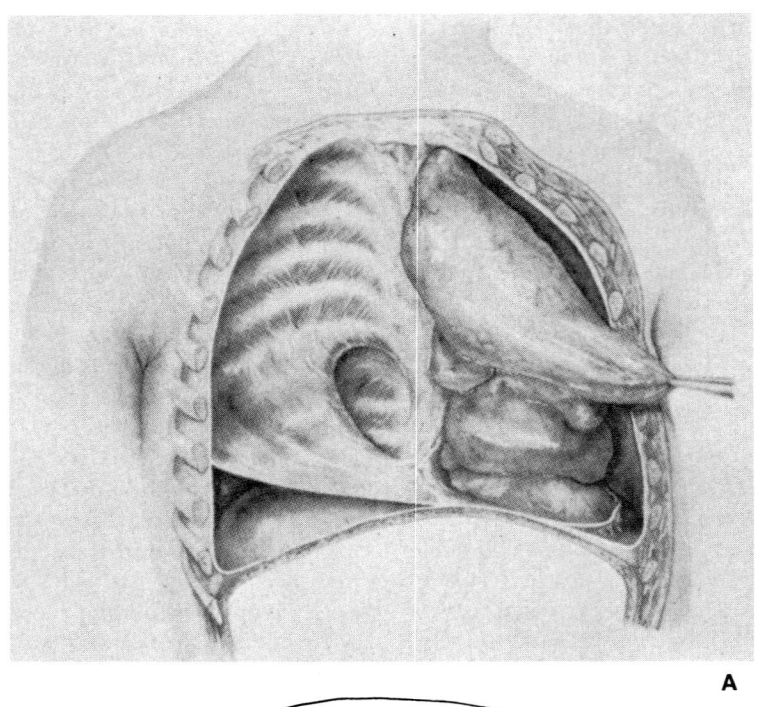

A

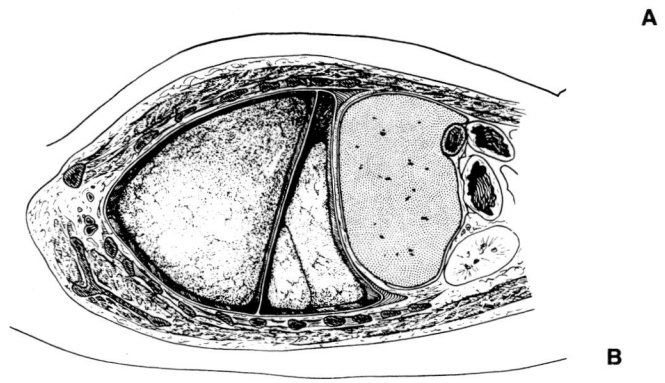

B

Figure 15.54. Accessory diaphragm. **A,** The middle and lower lobes of the right lung have been delivered through the hiatus in the accessory diaphragm, and the entire right lung has been retracted medially to show the position of the acces-sory diaphragm. **B,** Paramedian section, showing the contents of the two right thoracic cavities. (From Hashida Y, Sherman FE. Accessory diaphragm associated with neonatal respiratory distress. J Pediatr 1961; 59:529–532.)

In three cases the accessory diaphragm was incom-plete, and all lobes of the lung were present. In one 24-year-old patient (209), the accessory organ arose from the dome of the diaphragm and divided the lower lobe to attach posteriorly 2 inches above the normal diaphragm. An anomalous pulmonary vein passed through the nor-mal diaphragm to enter the vena cava. In two other cases the partial accessory diaphragm arose at the pericardial junction with the diaphragm. In one patient (210) the accessory diaphragm was muscular, while the normally placed diaphragm was fibrous. In the other case (211) the diaphragm was muscular, while the accessory membrane contained only a few muscle fibers (Fig. 15.54).

An even more rudimentary duplication was described in an adult cadaver, an individual with no known medical history, by Allen (212). A pair of muscles arose from the central tendon of the right diaphragm and passed through an oblique fissure in the lung to attach to the sixth rib (Fig. 15.55).

EMBRYOGENESIS

These rare anomalies represent duplications of the pleu-roperitoneal membrane, with the more cranial portion acquiring some—or in the patient of Sappington and Daniel (210), almost all—of the lateral muscle mass derived from the fourth and fifth cervical myotomes. In Sullivan's patient (207) it is possible that premature for-mation of the membrane occurred since no lung tissue lay

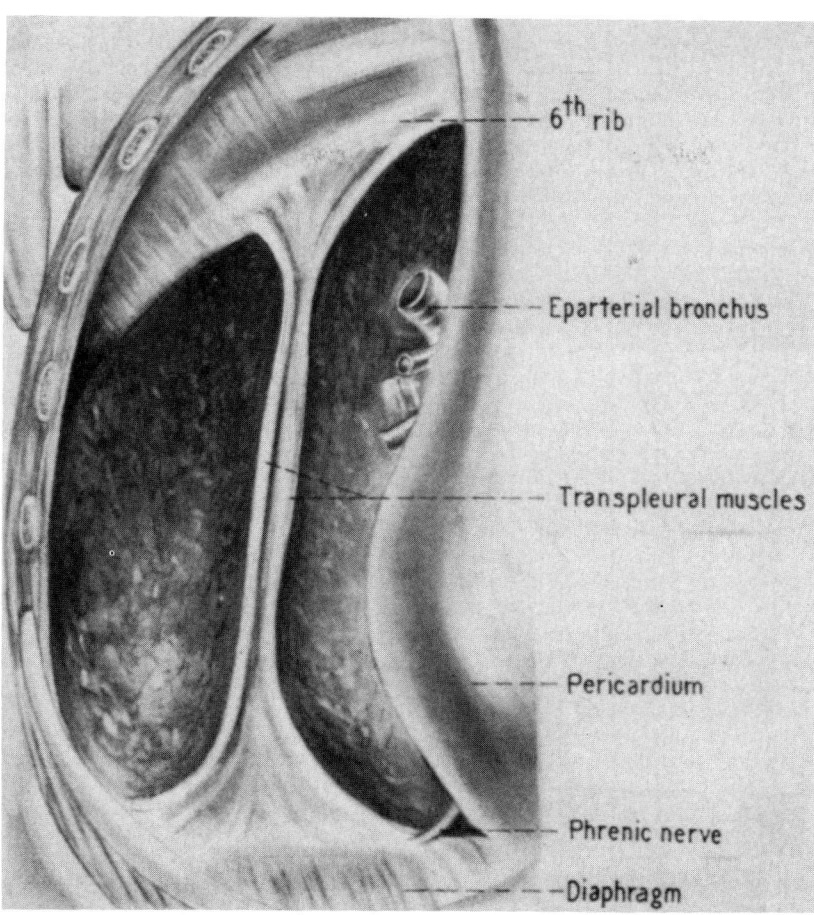

Figure 15.55. Accessory diaphragm represented by a transpleural muscular band. The upper and middle lobes of the right lung have been removed to show the anomalous band in the oblique fissure. (From Allen L. Transpleural muscles. J Thor Surg 1950; 19:290–291.)

above it. In the other cases development of the lungs preceded the formation of the accessory membrane.

A few cases are known in which lung tissue lies beneath the normal diaphragm. These result from abnormal formation of bronchial buds from the foregut, rather than resulting from an abnormal position of the diaphragm (page 469).

SYMPTOMS AND DIAGNOSIS

Symptoms are not diagnostic. Persistent cough and frequent upper respiratory tract infections were present in three cases. One patient died immediately after birth because of pneumothorax of the left (normal) lung (211). Allen's patient (212) had died of other causes and may have had no symptoms from his anomaly.

TREATMENT

In the three surgically treated cases, the accessory diaphragm was resected, with reduction of respiratory distress.

REFERENCES

1. Broman I. Ueber die Entwicklung und Bedeutung der Mesenterien und der Körperhöhlen bei den Wirbeltieren. Ergeb Anat Entw 1905;15:332–409.
2. Bremer JL. The diaphragm and diaphragmatic hernia. Arch Pathol 1943;36:539–549.
3. Wells LJ. Development of the human diaphragm and pleural sacs. Contrib Embryol Carnegie Inst Wash 1954;35:109.
4. González de Santander R. Contribucion al estudio de la morfologia y desarrollo de la bursa omentalis en embriones humanos. An Desarrollo 1962;10:269–298.
5. Botha GSM. The gastro-oesophageal region in infants. Arch Dis Child 1958;33:78–94.
6. Mall FP. Determination of the age of human embryos and fetuses. In: Keibel F, Mall FP, eds. Manual of human embryology. Philadelphia: JB Lippincott, 1910.
7. Lewis WH. The development of the muscular system. In: Keibel F, Mall FP, eds. Manual of human embryology. Philadelphia: JB Lippincott, 1910.
8. Broman I. Ueber die entwicklung der Zwerchfells beim Menschen. Verh Anat Ges 1902;21:9–17.
9. Carmi R, Meizner I, Katz M. Familial congenital diaphragmatic defect and associated midline anomalies: further evidence for an X-linked midline gene? Am J Med Genet 1990;36(3):313–315.

10. Czeizel E, Kovacs M. Genetic study of diaphragmatic defects. Orv Hetil 1990;131(22):1193–1195.

11. Cunniff C, Jones KL, Jones MC. Patterns of malformation in children with congenital diaphragmatic defects. J Pediatr 1990;116(2):258–261.

12. Carmi R, Barbash A, Mares AJ. The thoracoabdominal syndrome (TAS): a new X-linked dominant disorder. Am J Med Genet 1990;36(1):109–114.

13. Ayme S et al. Fryns syndrome: report on 8 new cases. Clin Genet 1989;35(3):191–201.

14. Cunniff C et al. Fryns syndrome: an autosomal recessive disorder associated with craniofacial anomalies, diaphragmatic hernia, and distal digital hypoplasia. Pediatrics 1990;85(4):499–504.

15. Cullen ML, Klein MD, Philippart AI. Congenital diaphragmatic hernia. Surg Clin North Am 1985;65:1115–1138.

16. Moore KL. The developing human, 4th ed. Philadelphia: WB Saunders, 1988.

17. Sadler TW. Langman's medical embryology, 6th ed. Baltimore: Williams & Wilkins, 1990.

18. Reid L. The lung: its growth and remodeling in health and disease. AJR 1977;129:777.

19. Dibbins AW. Congenital diaphragmatic hernia, hypoplastic lung, and pulmonary vasoconstriction. Clin Perinatol 1978;5:93.

20. Kiesewetter, WB, Gutierrez, IZ, Sieber WK. Diaphragmatic hernia in infants under one year of age. Arch Surg 1961;83:561–572.

21. Irving IM, Booker PD. Congenital diaphragmatic hernia and evantration of the diaphragm. In: Lister J, Irving IM, eds. Neonatal surgery, 3rd ed. London: Butterworths 1990:199–220.

22. Coca MA, Landin F. Malformations congénitales multiples avec absence presque complète de diaphragme. Semin Hop Paris 1957;33:3839.

23. Sagal Z. Absence of left diaphragm associated with inverted thoracic stomach. AJR 1933;30:206–214.

24. Neville WE, Clowes GHA Jr. Congenital absence of hemidiaphragm and use of a lobe of liver in its surgical correction. Arch Surg 1954;69:282–290.

25. Shaffer JO. Prosthesis for agenesis of the diaphragm. JAMA 1964;188, 1000–1002.

26. Jenkinson EL. Absence of half of the diaphragm (thoracic stomach; diaphragmatic hernia). AJR 1931;26:899–903.

27. Kajii T, Oikawa K, Itakura K, Ohsawa T. A probable 17-18 trisomy syndrome with phocomelia, exomphalos, and agenesis of hemidiaphragm. Arch Dis Child 1964;39:519–522.

28. Hatzitheofilou C, Conlan AA, Nicolaou N. Agenesis of the diaphragm: a case report. S Afr Med J 1982;62(26):999–1001.

29. Cornet E, Dupon H, Fertil P. Six cas de malformation congénitale du diaphragme (hernies et eventrations) chez le nouveau-né et le jeune enfant. Mem Acad Chir (Paris) 1954;85:165–167.

30. Slim MS, Akel S, Baraka A, Mounla N. Congenital diaphragmatic hernia and eventration. Middle East J Anesthesiol 1987;9(1):55–69.

31. Reynolds M. Diaphragmatic anomalies. In: Raffensperger JG, ed. Swenson's pediatric surgery, Norwalk, CT: Appleton & Lange, 1990:721.

32. Blank E, Campbell JR. Congenital posterolateral defect in the right side of the diaphragm. Pediatrics 1976;57:807.

33. Butler N, Claireaux AE. Congenital diaphragmatic hernia as a cause of perinatal mortality. Lancet 1962;1:659–663.

34. Nicolisi CR, Leaf D, Schulenberg R. Bilateral congenital posterolateral diaphragmatic hernia. Minn Med 1977;60:791.

35. Zamir O, Eyal F, Lernau OZ, Nissan S. Bilateral congenital posterolateral diaphragmatic hernia. Am J Perinatol 1986;3(1):56–57.

36. Bohn D et al. Ventilatory predictors of pulmonary hypoplasia in congenital diaphragmatic hernia, confirmed by morphologic assessment. J Pediatr 1987;111:423–431.

37. Simson JNL, Eckstein HB. Congenital diaphragmatic hernia: a 20 year experience. Br J Surg 1985;72:733–736.

38. Levin DL. Congenital diaphragmatic hernia: a persistent problem. J Pediatr 1987;111:390–392.

39. Shochat SJ. Pulmonary vascular pathology in congenital diaphragmatic hernias. Pediatr Surg Int 1987;2:331–335.

40. Connors RH et al. Congenital diaphragmatic hernia repair on ECMO. J Pediatr Surg 1990;25:1043–1047.

41. Benjamin DR, Juul S, Siebert JR. Congenital posterolateral diaphragmatic hernia: associated malformations. J Pediatr Surg 1988;23:899–903.

42. Nakayama DK et al. Prenatal diagnosis and natural history of the fetus with a congenital diaphragmatic hernia: initial clinical experience. J Pediatr Surg 1985;20:118.

43. Adzick NS et al. Fetal diaphragmatic hernia: ultrasound diagnosis and clinical outcome in 38 cases. J Pediatr Surg 1989;24:654–658.

44. Warkany J, Roth CB, Wilson JG. Multiple congenital malformations: a consideration of etiologic factors. Pediatrics 1948;1:462.

45. Anderson DH. Effect of diet during pregnancy upon the incidence of congenital diaphragmatic hernia in the rat. Am J Pathol 1949;25:163–185.

46. Kluth D et al. Nitrofen-induced diaphragmatic hernias in rats: an animal model. J Pediatr Surg 1990;25:850–854.

47. Hedblom CA. Diaphragmatic hernia: a study of three hundred and seventy-eight cases in which operation was performed. JAMA 1925;85:947–953.

48. Bonetus T. Sepulchretum sive anatomia practica et cadareribus morbo denatus. Geneva [Genevae], 1679.

49. Morgagni JB. The seats and causes of disease investigated by anatomy. Alexander B (transl). New York: Hafner, 1960.

50. Korns HM. The diagnosis of "eventration" of the diaphragm. Arch Intern Med 1921;28:192–212.

51. Bochdalek V. Einige Betrachtungen ueber die Einstellung des angeborenen Zwerchfellbruches als Beitrag zut pathologischen Anatomie des Herniun. Viertelijahrs Prakt Heilk 1848;19:89.

52. White JJ, Suzuki H. Hernia through the foramen of Bochdalek: a misnomer. J Pediatr Surg 1972;7:60–61.

53. Keith A. Diaphragmatic herniae. Br Med J 1910;2:1297.

54. Aue O. Congenital dipahragmatic hernia. Deutsch Z Chir 1920;160:14.

55. Greenwald HM, Steiner M. Diaphragmatic hernia in infancy and childhood. Am J Dis Child 1929;38:361–392.

56. Truesdale PE. Diaphragmatic hernia in children with a report of thirteen operative cases. N Engl J Med 1935;213:1159.

57. Ladd WE, Gross RE. Congenital diaphragmatic hernia. N Engl J Med 1940;223:917.

58. Gross RE. The surgery of infancy and childhood: its principles and techniques. Philadelphia: WB Saunders, 1953:441.

59. Harrison MR, Bjordal RI, Langmark E. Congenital diaphragmatic hernia: the hidden mortality. J Pediatr Surg 1978;13:227.

60. Harrison MR, deLorimier AA. Congenital diaphragmatic hernia. Surg Clin North Am 1981;61:1023–1035.

61. Anderson KD. Congenital diaphragmatic hernia. In: Welch KJ, Randolph JG, Ravitch MM, O'Neill JA, Rowe MI, eds. Pediatric surgery, 4th ed. Chicago: Yearbook Medical Publishers, 1986:590.

62. Collins DL. Diaphragmatic hernia. In: Holder TM, Ashcraft KW, eds. Pediatric surgery. Philadelphia: WB Saunders, 1980:229.

63. Puri P, Gorman F. Lethal nonpulmonary anomalies associated

with congenital diaphragmatic hernia: implications for early intra-uterine surgery. J Pediatr Surg 1984;19:29–32.

64. Riker WL. Congenital diaphragmatic hernia. Arch Surg 1954;69:291–308.

65. Young WC, Haines JE, Larson SM. Diagnosis of posterolateral congenital diaphragmatic (Bochdalek) hernia by liver scintigram: case report. J Nucl Med 1976;17:110.

66. Bell MJ, Ternberg JL. Antenatal diagnosis of diaphragmatic hernia. Pediatrics 1977;60:738.

67. Adzick NS et al. Diaphragmatic hernia in the fetus: prenatal diagnosis and outcome in 94 cases. J Pediatr Surg 1985;20:357–361.

68. Kirkland JA. Congenital posterolateral diaphragmatic hernia in the adult. Br J Surg 1959;47:16–22.

69. Hermann RE, Barber DH. Congenital diaphragmatic hernia in the child beyond infancy. Cleveland Clin Q 1963;30:73–80.

70. Skandalakis JE, Gray SW, Mansberger AR Jr, Colborn GL, Skandalakis LJ. Hernia: surgical anatomy and technique. New York: McGraw Hill Information Services, 1989:305–378.

71. Langer JC et al. Timing of surgery for congenital diaphragmatic hernia: is emergency operation necessary? J Pediatr Surg 1988;23:731–734.

72. West KW, Bengston K, Rescorla FJ, Engle WA, Grosfeld JL. Delayed surgical repair and ECMO improves survival in congenital diaphragmatic hernia. Ann Surg 1992;216:454–462.

73. Falterman KW, Adolph VR. Uses of extracorporeal membrane oxygenation in non-neonatal respiratory patients: an update. Surg Clin North Am 1992;72:1341.

74. Harrison MR, Jester JA, Ross NA. Correction of congenital diaphragmatic hernia in utero. I. The model: intrathoracic balloon produces fatal pulmonary hypoplasia. Surgery 1980;88:174.

75. Harrison MR et al. Correction of congenital diaphragmatic hernia in utero. II. Simulated correction permits fetal lung growth with survival at birth. Surgery 1980;88:260.

76. Harrison MR, Ross NA, deLorimier AA. Correction of congenital diaphragmatic hernia in utero. III. Development of a successful surgical technique using abdominoplasty to avoid compromise of umbilical blood flow. J Pediatr Surg 1981;16:934.

77. Adzick NS et al. Correction of congenital diaphragmatic hernia in utero. IV. An early gestational fetal lamb model for pulmonary vascular morphometric analysis. J Pediatr Surg 1985;20:673.

78. Harrison MR et al. Correction of congenital diaphragmatic in utero. V. Initial clinical experience. J Pediatr Surg 1990;25:47–57.

79. Adolph V, Arensman RM, Falterman KW, Goldsmith JP. Ventilatory management casebook: congenital diaphragmatic hernia meeting criteria for extracorporeal membrane oxygenation. J Perinatol 1990;10:202–205.

80. Burge DM, Atwell JD, Freeman NV. Could the stomach site help predict outcome in babies with left-sided congenital diaphragmatic hernia diagnosed antenatally? J Pediatr Surg 1989;24:567–569.

81. Fitchett CW, Tavarez V. Bilateral congenital diaphragmatic herniation: case report. Surgery 1965;57:305–308.

82. Carter REB, Waterston DJ, Aberdeen E. Hernia and eventration of the diaphragm in childhood. Lancet 1962;1:656–659.

83. Craighead CC, Strug LH. Diaphragmatic deficiency in the retrocostoxiphoid area. Surgery 1958;44:1062–1069.

84. Hume JB. Congenital diaphragmatic hernia. Br J Surg 1922;10:207–215.

85. Saltzstein HC, Linkner LM, Scheinberg SR. Subcostosternal (Morgagni) diaphragmatic hernia. Arch Surg 1951;63:750–765.

86. Thomas GG, Clitherow NR. Herniation through the foramen of Morgagni in children. Br J Surg 1977;64:215–217.

87. Baffes TG. Diaphragmatic hernia. In: Benson CD, Mustard WT, Ravitch MM, Snyder WH Jr, Welch KJ, eds. Periatric surgery, Vol 1. Chicago: Year Book Medical Publishers, 1962.

88. Bentley G, Lister J. Retrosternal hernia. Surgery 1965;57:567–575.

89. Hunter WR. Herniation through the foramen of Morgagni. Br J Surg 1959;47:22–27.

90. Pokorny WJ, McGill CW, Harberg FJ. Morgagni hernias during infancy: presentation and associated anomalies. J Pediatr Surg 1984;19:394.

91. Ravitch MM. Congenital deformities of the chest wall and their operative correction. Philadelphia: WB Saunders, 1977:1–306.

92. Reed JA, Borden DL. Eventration of the diaphragm. Arch Surg 1935;31:30–64.

93. Laxdal OE, McDougal H, Mellin GW. Congenital eventration of the diaphragm. N Engl J Med 1954;205:401–408.

94. McNamara JJ, Eraklis AJ, Gross RE. Congenital posterolateral diaphragmatic hernia in the newborn. J Thorac Cardiovasc Surg 1968;55:55.

95. Haller JA Jr et al. Management of diaphragmatic paralysis in infants with special emphasis on selection of patients for operative plication. J Perinat Surg 1979;14:779–785.

96. Lundstrom CH, Allen RP. Bilateral congenital eventration of the diaphragm: case report with roentgen manifestation. Maer J Roentgenol 1966;97:216–217.

97. Ravitch MM, Handelsman JC. Defects in right diaphragm of infants and children with herniation of liver. Arch Surg 1952;64:794–802.

98. Briggs VA, Reilly BJ, Loewig K. Lung hypoplasia and membranous diaphragm in the congenital rubella syndrome: a rare case. J Can Assoc Radiol 1973;24:126–127.

99. Becroft DMO. Prenatal cytomegalovirus infection and muscular deficiency (eventration) of the diaphragm. J Pediatr 1979;94:74–75.

100. Wayne ER, Burrington JD, Myers DN, Cotton EN, Block W. Bilateral eventration of the diaphragm in a neonate with congenital cytomegalic inclusion disease. J Pediatr 1973;83:164–165.

101. Wexler HA, Poole CA. Neonatal diaphragmatic dysfunction. AJR 1976;127:617–622.

102. Stauffer UG, Rickham PP. Acquired eventration of the diaphragm in the newborn. J Pediatr Surg 1972;7:635–643.

103. Roberts JAF. The inheritance of a lethal muscle contracture in sheep. J Genet 1929;21:57–69.

104. Beck WC. Etiologic significance of eventration of the diaphragm. Arch Surg 1950;60:1154–1160.

105. Christensen P. Eventration of the diaphragm. Thorax 1959;14:311–319.

106. Greenebaum JV, Harper FG. Right-sided transient paralysis of the diaphragm in a newborn infant. J Pediatr 1946;28:483–487.

107. Bayne-Jones S. Eventration of diaphragm: with report of a case of right-sided eventration. Arch Intern Med 1916;17:221–237.

108. Petit JL. Traites des maladies chirurgicales et des operations qui leus conviennent. Paris: TF Didot, 1774.

109. Cruveilhier J. Anatomie pathologique du corps humaine, VI, Book 17. Paris, 1829.

110. Marsh FH. On abnormal conditions of the diaphragm. Lancet 1867;1:298.

111. Morrison JMW. Eventration of the diaphragm due to unilateral phrenic paralysis: radiological study, with special reference to differential diagnosis. Arch Radiol Electrother 1923;28:111–123.

112. Bisgard JD. Congenital eventration of the diaphragm. J Thorac Surg 1947;16:484–491.

113. Bingham JAW. Two cases of unilateral paralysis of the diaphragm in the newborn treated surgically. Thorax 1954;9:248–252.

114. Newcomet WS, Spackman EW. Eventration and hernia of the diaphragm as incidental finding. Radiology 1936;27:36–43.

115. Chin EF, Lynn RB. Surgery of eventration of the diaphragm. J Thorac Surg 1956;32:6–14.

116. David TJ, Illingworth CA. Diaphragmatic hernia in the south-west of England. J Med Genet 1976;13:253.

117. Michelson E. Eventration of the diaphragm. Surgery 1961;49:410–422.

118. Stone KS et al. Long-term fate of the diaphragm surgically plicated during infancy and early childhood. Ann Thorac Surg 1987;44:62.

119. Stauffer UG. Diaphragmatic paralysis due to birth trauma. Helv Paediatr Acta 1972;27:253.

120. Wilson AK, Rumel WR, Ross OL. Peritoneopericardial diaphragmatic hernia: report of a case in a newborn infant, successfully corrected by surgical operation with recovery of patient. AJR 1947;57:42–49.

121. Rogers JF, Lane WZ, Gibbs R. Herniation through the diaphragm into the pericardium. Conn Med J 1958;22:653–656.

122. Wetzel H. Parasternale Zwerchfellhernie mit Verlagerung des Colon in den Herzbeutel. Fortschr Rontgenstr 1963;98:501–503.

123. Casey AE, Hidden EH. Nondevelopment of septum transversum, with congenital absence of anterocentral portion of the diaphragm and the suspensory ligament of the liver and presence of an elongated ductus venosus and a pericardioperitoneal foramen. Arch Pathol 1944;38;370–374.

124. Grenier de Cardenal, Bourderou. Hernie diaphragmatique du grand épiploon et d'une anse du côlon transverse dans le péricarde chez un adulte. J Med Bordeaux 1903;33:222–224.

125. O'Brien HD. Pericardio-peritoneal communication: description of a rare type of diaphragmatic hernia. J Anat 1939;74:131–134.

126. Åkerlund Å. Hernia diaphragmatica hiatus oesophagi. Vom anatomischen und röntgenologischen Gesichtspunkt. Acta Radiol 1926;6:3–24.

127. Payne WS, Ellis WS, Ellis FH Jr. Esophagus and diaphragmatic hernias. In: Schwartz SI, ed. Principles of surgery. New York: McGraw-Hill, 1984.

128. Walther B et al. Effects of para-esophageal hernia on sphincter function and its implications on surgical therapy. Am J Surg 1984;147:111–116.

129. Barrett NR. Chronic peptic ulcer of the oesophagus and oesophagitis. Br J Surg 1950;38:175–182.

130. Gray SW, Rowe JS Jr, Skandalakis JE. Surgical anatomy of the gastro-esophageal junction. Am Surg 1979;45:578–587.

131. Starnes VA, Adkins RB, Ballinger JF, Sawyers J. Barrett's esophagus: a surgical entity. Arch Surg 1984;119:563–567.

132. Saubier EC, Gouillat C, Samaniego C, Guillaud M, Moulinier B. Adenocarcinoma in columnar-lined Barrett's esophagus: analysis of 13 esophagectomies. Am J Surg 1985;150:365–372.

133. Skinner DB, Belsey RHR, Hendrix TR, Zuidema GD. Gastroesophageal reflux and hiatal hernia. Boston: Little, Brown, 1972.

134. Sanfey H, Hamilton SR, Smith RL, Cameron JL. Carcinoma arising in Barrett's esophagus. Surg Gynecol Obstet 1985;161:570–574.

135. Barrett NR. Hiatus hernia: a review of some controversial points. Br J Surg 1954;42:231–243.

136. Gahagan T. The function of the musculature of the esophagus and stomach in the esophagogastric sphincter mechanism. Surg Gynecol Obstet 1962;114:293–303.

137. Pearl RK. Anatomy of the esophagus and the posterior mediastinum. In: Nyhus LM, Baker RJ, eds. Mastery of surgery. Boston: Little, Brown, 1984.

138. Allison PR. Peptic ulcer of the oesophagus. Thorax 1948;3:20–42.

139. Skandalakis JE, Gray SW, Rowe JS Jr. Anatomical complications in general surgery. New York: McGraw Hill, 1983.

140. Listerud MB, Harkins HN. Anatomy of the esophageal hiatus: anatomic studies on two hundred and four fresh cadavers. Arch Surg 1958;76:835–842.

141. Bombeck CT, Dillard DH, Nyhus LM. Muscular anatomy of the gastro-esophageal junction and role of phrenoesophageal ligament: autopsy study of sphincter mechanism. Ann Surg 1966;164:643–652.

142. Rector LE, Connerley ML. Aberrant mucosa in the oesophagus in infants and in children. Arch Pathol 1941;285–294.

143. Allison PR. Hiatus hernia: a 20-year retrospective survey. Ann Surg 1973;178:273–277.

144. Bynum TE. Histopathologic alterations in oesophageal mucosa secondary to gastro-esophageal reflux. South Med J 1978;71:53–55.

145. Botha GSM. Mucosal folds at the cardia as a component of the gastro-oesophageal closing mechanism. Br J Surg 1958;45:569–580.

146. Palmer ED. An attempt to localize the normal esophagogastric junction. Radiology 1953;60:825–831.

147. Hayward J. The lower end of the oesophagus. Thorax 1961;16:36–41.

148. Lerche W. The oesophagus and pharynx in action: a study of structure in relation to function. Springfield, IL: Charles C Thomas, 1950.

149. Pisko-Dubienski ZA. Anatomy of sliding hiatal hernia. In: Nyhus LM, Harkins HN, eds. Hernia. Philadelphia: JB Lippincott, 1964.

150. Liebermann-Meffert D, Allgower M, Schmid P, Math D, Blum AL. Muscular equivalent of the lower oesophageal sphincter. Gastroenterology 1979;76:31–38.

151. Mann DV, Greenwood RK, Ellis FH. The oesophageal junction. Surg Gynecol Obstet 1964;118:853–862.

152. Didio LJA, Anderson MC. The "sphincters" of the digestive system. Baltimore: Williams & Wilkins, 1968.

153. Fisher RS. Lower esophageal sphincter as a barrier to gastroesophageal reflux before and after anti-reflux surgery. South Med J 1978;71:22–25.

154. Liebermann-Meffert D, Schwizer W, Vosmeer S, Allgower M. Myogenic activity relationship between the lower esophageal sphincter and pylorus of the cat in normal peristalsis and provoked retroperistalsis. Scand J Gastroenterol 1983;19:17–20.

155. Woodward ER. Surgical accomplishments in enhancing lower esophageal sphincteric competency. South Med J 1978;71:38–40.

156. Hayward J. Sliding oesophageal hiatus hernia. In: Nyhus LM, Harkins HN, eds. Hernia. Philadelphia: JB Lippincott, 1964.

157. Androulakis JA, Skandalakis JE, Gray SW. Contributions to the pathological anatomy of hiatal hernia. J Med Assoc Ga 1966;55:295–296.

158. Gray SW, Skandalakis JE. Embryology for surgeons. Philadelphia: WB Saunders, 1972.

159. Dillard DH. Esophageal sphincter and reflux. Surg Clin North Am 1964;44:1201–1209.

160. Listerud MB. Details of interest and controversy in the anatomy of the esophageal hiatus and hiatal hernia. Surg Clin North Am 1964;44:1211–1216.

161. Hill LD. An effective operation for hiatal hernia: an eight year appraisal. Ann Surg 1967;166:681–690.

162. Peters PM. Closure mechanisms at the cardia with special reference to diaphragmatic oesophageal elastic ligament. Thorax 1955;10:27–36.

163. Young H, Gray SW, Skandalakis JE. Traumatic vomiting: the Mallory-Weiss syndrome. J Med Assoc Ga 1967;56:362–364.

164. Adler RH, Rodriguez J. The association of hiatus hernia and gastroesophageal malignancy. J Thorac Surg 1959;37:553–569.

165. Gray SW, Skandalakis FE, Shepard D. Smooth muscle tumors of the esophagus. Surg Gynecol Obstet 1961;113:205–220.

166. Tarnay TJ. Diaphragmatic hernia. Ann Thorac Surg 1968;5:66–92.

167. Bright R. Account of a remarkable misplacement of the stomach. Guy Hosp Rep 1936;1:598–603.

168. Richards LG. Nontraumatic hernia of the diaphragm. Ann Ital Rhinol Laryngol 1923;32:1145–1196.

169. Abbott DP. The early diagnosis of true hernia of the diaphragm. JAMA 1924;83:1898.

170. Healey TR. Symptoms observed in fifty-three cases of non-traumatic diaphragmatic hernia. AJR 1925;13:266–271.

171. Mobley JE, Christensen NA. Esophageal hiatal hernia: prevalency diagnosis and treatment in an American city of 30,000. Gastroenterology 1956;30:1–11.

172. Kaiser E. Die operativ behandlung der hiatushernien. Schweiz Med Wschr 1959;89:526.

173. Harrington SW. Various types of diaphragmatic hernia treated surgically: report of 430 cases. Surg Gynecol Obstet 1948;86:735–755.

174. Master AM, Dack S, Stone J, Grishman A. Differential diagnosis of hiatus hernia and coronary artery disease. Arch Surg 1949;58:428–449.

175. Harrington SW. Esophageal hiatal diaphragmatic hernia. Surg Gynecol Obstet 1955;100:227–292.

176. Harp RA, Gonzalez, JL, Graham J. Total gastric hiatal herniation in an infant. Surgery 1965;57:302–304.

177. Michaelides GJ, Philis HC. Pathogenesis and treatment of the anaemia associated with hiatus hernia. Lancet 1959;1:552.

178. Posey EL, Stephenson SL Jr, Fyke FE Jr. Sliding esophageal hiatus hernia: manifestations, pathophysiology, and management—findings in 100 consecutive cases. South Med J 1958;51:809–819.

179. Nuzum FR. Hernia of esophageal hiatus: its relationship to angina pectoris. Am Heart J 1947;33:724.

180. Gilbert NC. Recurrent esophageal hiatus hernia. Med Clin North Am 1948;32:213.

181. Handelsman JC. Esophageal hiatal hernia. Surgery 1962;52:803–809.

182. Rex JC, Andersen HA, Bartholomew LG, Cain JC. Esophageal hiatal hernia: a 10-year study of medically treated cases. JAMA 1961;178:271–274.

183. Burke JB. Partial thoracic stomach in childhood. Br Med J 1959;2:787–792.

184. Shackelford RT. Surgery of the alimentary tract. Philadelphia: WB Saunders, 1978.

185. Skinner DB, Belsey RHR, Hendrix TR, Zuidema GD. Gastroesophageal reflux and hiatal hernia. Boston: Little, Brown, 1972.

186. Allison PR. Reflux esophagitis, sliding hiatal hernia and the anatomy of repair. Surg Gynecol Obstet 1951;92:419–431.

187. Sweet RH. Esophageal hiatus hernia of the diaphragm: the anatomical characteristics, technic of repair, and results of treatment in 111 consecutive cases. Ann Surg 1952;135:1.

188. Mulholland JH, Ellison, EH, Friesen SR, eds. Current surgical management. Philadelphia: WB Saunders, 1957.

189. Merendino KA, Varco RL, Wangensteen OH. Displacement of the esophagus into a new diaphragmatic orifice in the repair of para-esophageal and esophageal hiatus hernia. Ann Surg 1949;129:185–197.

190. Nissen R. Repair of esophageal hiatal hernia by fixation to the abdominal wall. In: Mulholland JH, Ellison EH, Friesen SR, eds. Current surgical management, Vol 2. Philadelphia: WB Saunders, 1960.

191. Hill LD, Tobias J, Morgan EH. Newer concepts of the pathophysiology of hiatal hernia and esophagitis. Am J Surg 1966;111:70–79.

192. Effler DB, Groves LK. Short esophagus, mechanism of pain, and surgical therapy. Arch Surg 1957;75:639.

193. Burford TH, Lischer CE. Treatment of short esophageal hernia with esophagitis by Finney pyloroplasty. Ann Surg 1956;144:647.

194. Merendino KA, Dillard DH. The concept of sphincter substitution by an interposed jejunal segment for anatomic and physiologic abnormalities at the esophagogastric junction: with special reference to reflux esophagitis, cardiospasm and esophageal varices. Ann Surg 1955;142:486.

195. Ellis FH Jr, Andersen HA, Clagett OT. Treatment of short esophagus with stricture by esophagogastrectomy and antral excision. Ann Surg 1958;148:526.

196. Willie L, Holthusen W, Willich E. Accessory diaphragm: report of 6 cases and a review of the literature. Pediatr Radiol 1975;4:14–20.

197. Minnis JF, Reingold M. Accessory diaphragm: report of a case. Dis Chest 1963;44:554–557.

198. Patten BM. Human embryology, 3rd ed. New York: McGraw-Hill, 1968:246, 407.

199. Nayarion M et al. Accessory diaphragm: report of a case with complete physiological evaluation and surgical correction. J Thorac Cardiovasc Surg 1971;61:293–299.

200. Ikeda T et al. Accessory diaphragm associated with congenital posterolateral diaphragmatic hernia, aberrant systemic artery to the right lower lobe, and anomalous pulmonary vein: review and report of a case. J Thorac Cardiovasc Surg 1972;64:18–25.

201. Karkola P, Kairaluoma MI, Larmi TKF. Accessory diaphragm with total anomalous right pulmonary venous drainage and aplasia of the middle lobe. Scand J Thorac Cardiovasc Surg 1977;11:133–136.

202. Wedel MK, Dickman RW, Land GW. Accessory diaphragm. Minn Med 1981;64:21–23.

203. Hart JC, Cohen I, Ballantine VN, Varrano LF. Accessory diaphragm in an infant. J Pediatr Surg 1981;16:947–949.

204. Merten DF, Bowie JD, Kirks DR, Grossman H. Anteromedial diaphragmatic defects in infancy: current approaches to diagnostic imaging. Radiology 1982;142:361–365.

205. Krzyzaniak R, Gray SW. Accessory septum transversum. Am Surg 1986;52:278–281.

206. Hopkins RL, Davis SH. Haziness of the right hemithorax in a newborn. Chest 1988;94(3):662–663.

207. Sullivan HJ. Supernumerary diaphragm with agenesis of upper lobe. J Thorac Surg 1957;34:544–547.

208. Nigogosyan G, Ozarda H. Accessory diaphragm: a case report. AJR 1961;83:309–311.

209. Drake EH, Lynch JP. Bronchiectasis associated with anomaly of the right pulmonary vein and right diaphragm: report of a case. J Thorac Surg 1950;19:433.

210. Sappington TB Jr, Daniel RA Jr. Accessory diaphragm: a case report. J Thorac Surg 1951;21:212–216.

211. Hashida Y, Sherman FE. Accessory diaphragm associated with neonatal respiratory distress. J Pediatr 1961;59:529–532.

212. Allen L. Transpleural muscles. J Thorac Surg 1950;19:290–291.

CHAPTER 16

THE ANTERIOR BODY WALL

John Elias Skandalakis / Stephen Wood Gray / Richard Ricketts / Lee John Skandalakis

*Best known are man's external parts, but it is just the opposite as far as the
internal parts are concerned. For least known of all things is the structure of
men's bodies, so that it is necessary to consider the individual parts, comparing
them to the parts of other animals which they by nature resemble.*
—ARISTOTLE

DEVELOPMENT

The development of the human embryo may be said to begin with the establishment of the posterior body wall and end with the formation of the anterior body wall.

The anterior wall is at first represented only by the somatopleure of the overhanging hand and tail folds of the embryo, the middle portion being occupied by the body stalk and the open midgut (Fig. 16.1). Closure proceeds simultaneously from cranial, caudal, and lateral directions, centering on the site of the future umbilical ring (1, 2) (Fig. 16.2). The reduction in size of the body stalk, relative to that of the umbilical cord, and the final separation of the cord at birth completes the development of the anterior body wall.

Anterior Thoracic Wall

The thoracic wall and epigastric portion of the abdominal wall are first represented by the ventral portion of the head fold of the embryo. The caudal limit of the thorax is established by the early formation of the transverse septum cranial to the midgut. The cranial limit is as yet unmarked. Most of the primitive wall consists of somatopleure covering the ventral wall of the pericardial cavity (Fig. 16.1, C).

The somatopleure comprises a layer of ectoderm and mesoderm; it is almost transparent and is without muscles, blood vessels, or nerves. Skin will form from its ectodermal layer, but the other components of the definitive body wall will derive from invading dorsal mesoderm.

During the sixth week, the dorsolateral mesoderm begins to expand into the lateral body wall, forming a sheet in which the segmental character of the somites becomes obliterated. Extensions of the lateral vertebral processes, the future ribs, accompany the mesodermal extension. By the end of the sixth week (9 mm), however, they lag behind the invading mesoderm from the myotomes. The most cranial elements reach the midline

first, and the heart moves caudally to this area of fusion to assume its normal thoracic position (3).

The advancing edge of the mesoderm forms a longitudinal rectus thoracis, which corresponds to the rectus abdominis of the lower body wall. It is usually transitory, but occasionally remains on one or both sides as the sternalis muscle (Fig. 16.3). The greater part of the mesodermal sheet splits to form three layers: the external intercostal muscles, the internal intercostal muscles, and an inner layer represented by the transverse thoracic muscle. Other portions of this innermost layer probably contribute to the diaphragm (4). All of these layers are differentiated by the middle of the seventh week.

The sternum appears during the sixth week as a pair of parallel mesenchymal bands of condensed mesenchyme. They begin to chondrify almost at once. At about the same time a median cranial rudiment, the presternum, appears, associated with the developing shoulder girdle (Fig. 16.4, A). Much later (the sixth month), the paired suprasternal cartilages appear cranially and laterally to the presternum. These usually fuse with the presternum to form part of the manubrial articulation with the clavicle.

Ruge (5), who first described the development of the sternum in 1880, thought that the lateral sternal bands were derived from the distal ends of the ribs. Paterson (6, 7) considered the median cranial primordium to be part of the anterior limb girdle and the sternal bands to be caudal outgrowths from it. The suggestion proposed by Whitehead and Waddell (8) and by Hanson (9) that the sternal elements arise in situ has been confirmed by Chen (3). He observed the formation of the sternum in isolated tissue culture explants from the anterior thoracic wall of embryonic mice.

Following the appearance of the presternum and the lateral sternal bands, the lateral bands fuse with the presternum cranially and with the tips of the ribs laterally. During the seventh week, the sternal bands join at their

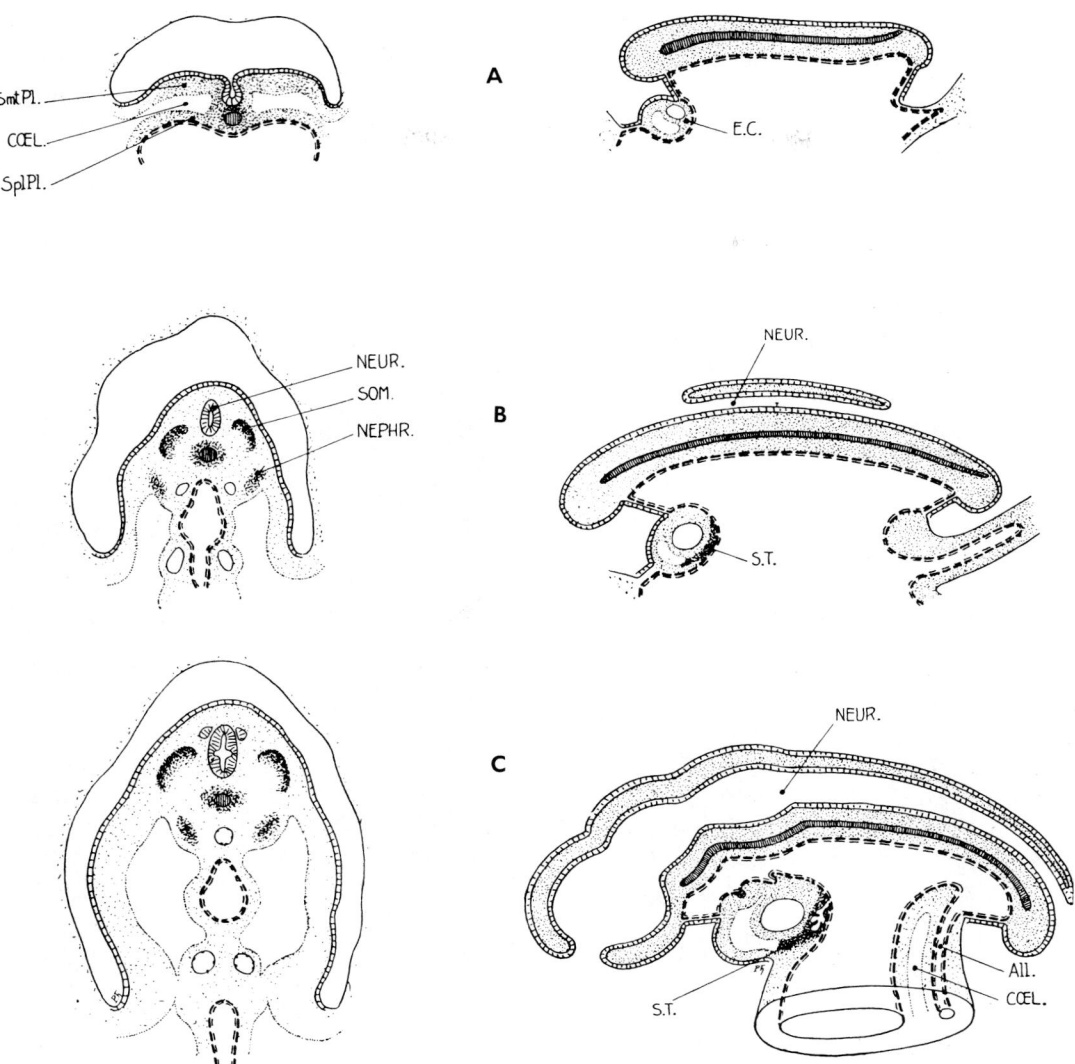

Figure 16.1. Schematic transverse and longitudinal sections through human embryos. **A,** 2 mm. **B,** 2 mm. **C,** 3 mm. In **C** the elements of the anterior body wall are present, but in very different proportions from those of the adult. *SmtPl.,* Somatopleure; *COEL,* celom; *SplPl.,* splanchnopleure; *NEUR.,* neural tube; *SOM.,* somite; *NEPHR.,* nephrotome; *E.C.,* endocardium; *S.T.,* septum transversum; *All.,* allantois. (From Duhamel B. Embryology of exomphalos and allied malformations. Arch Dis Child 1963;38:142.)

cephalic ends and gradually fuse in the midline, throughout their length. The fusion progresses with decreasing rapidity and ceases during the ninth or tenth weeks, by which time it is usually complete. The most caudal portion—the xiphoid process—however, often remains bifid or with a median aperture (Fig. 16.4, *B*).

At first, the approximation of the lateral halves of the sternum was considered to be the result of rib elongation. In tissue culture, however, the medial movement is inherent in the sternal rudiment and occurs in the absence of ribs. The normal sequence of chondrification is maintained [3].

Division of the sternum into segmental sternebrae is not apparent in the chondrification process. This segmentation appears later, with the dividing lines forming opposite the ends of the ribs. In primates, subsequent refusion of the middle sternebral segments results in formation of three sections: a body, a cranial manubrium, and a caudal xiphoid process. Unlike chondrification, later ossification is not band-like, but originates from a number of isolated centers. Ossification starts in the manubrium and upper part of the sternal body at the sixth month, in the middle of the sternal body at the seventh month, in the lower part of the body during the first postnatal year, and in the xiphoid process between the years 5 and 18. The number of centers varies (Fig. 16.4, *C*). Coalescence of the ossification centers in the sternal body does not take place until after puberty. In old age there may be bony fusion between the manubrium and the body, and between the body and the xiphoid process, but these are exceptions rather than the rule. Trotter (10) found synostosis between manubrium and body in about 10% of 877 adults, without respect to age. The greatest incidence was found among white females.

Suprasternal elements are variable. They usually coalesce with the manubrium but may form separate ossicles at the upper border of the manubrium, near the clavicular articulation. When present, they may articulate with the manubrium by a diarthrodial joint or a synchondrosis (Fig. 16.5). If not indistinguishably fused with the manubrium, they ossify between 17 and 23 years of age. Cobb (11) has discussed them in great detail. Their presence is

not associated with sternal defects or with cervical ribs. They appear to be highly variable vestiges of the epicoracoid element of the primitive vertebrate shoulder girdle. Cobb found them in 6.8% of white and 2.2% of black cadavers.

Late in the sixth week, before the embryonic wall is completely invaded by the dorsolateral mesoderm, two lateral ridges of thickened ectoderm appear between the bases of the anterior and posterior limb buds (Fig. 16.6, A). In human embryos, the caudal two-thirds and the most cranial portion of this embryonic milk line are tran-

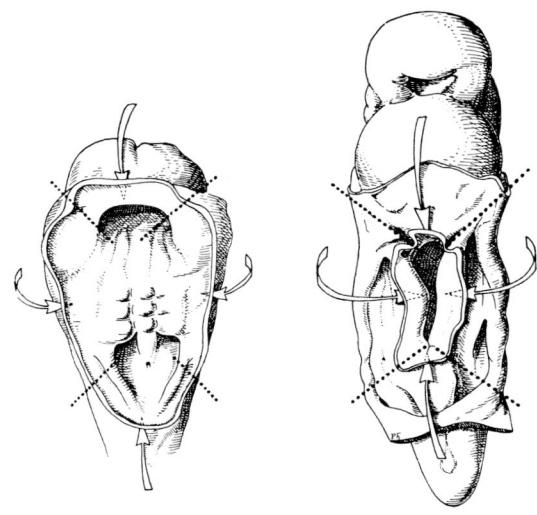

Figure 16.2. Ventral views of human embryos of 2 and 3 mm. The body stalk has been cut distal to the site of the future umbilical ring. *Arrows* show the direction of infolding; *dotted* lines indicate the arbitrary boundaries of the four inholdings. (From Duhamel B. Embryology of exomphalos and allied malformations. Arch Dis Child. 1963;38:142–147.)

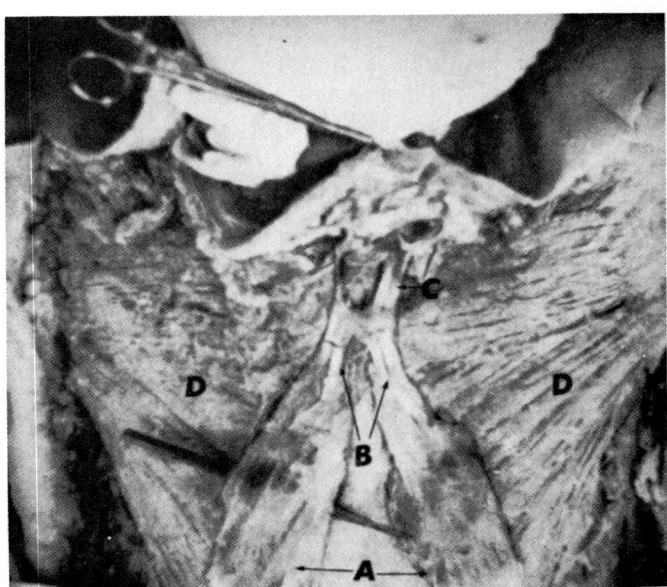

Figure 16.3. Well-developed, bilateral sternalis muscle in an adult male cadaver. Traces are said to be present in about 4% of the population and in about 50% of anencephalic infants. *A,* Belly of sternalis muscle. B, Tendon of sternalis muscle inserting on tendon of sternocleidomastoid muscle (C). D, Pectoralis major. (Courtesy of Charles B. Blair, Jr., College of Veterinary Medicine, University of Georgia.)

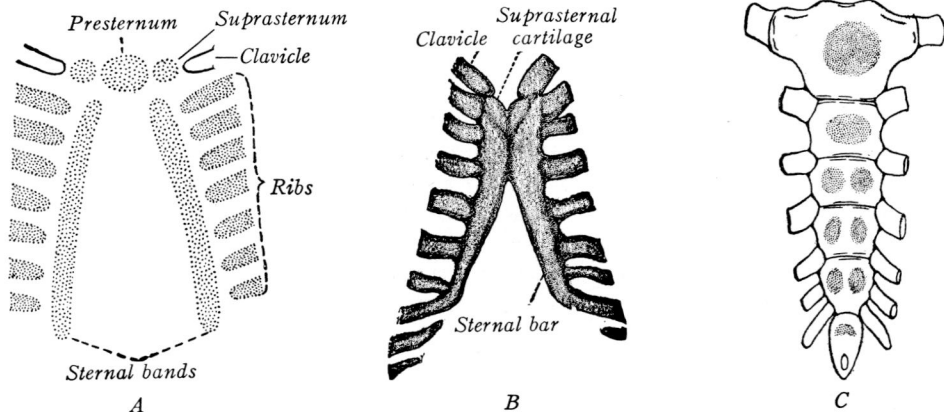

Figure 16.4. Development of the sternum. **A,** Mesenchymal stage (sixth week). **B,** Cartilaginous stage (ninth week). **C,** Ossification centers appearing after birth. (From Arey LB. Developmental Anatomy, 7th ed. Philadelphia: WB Saunders, 1965.)

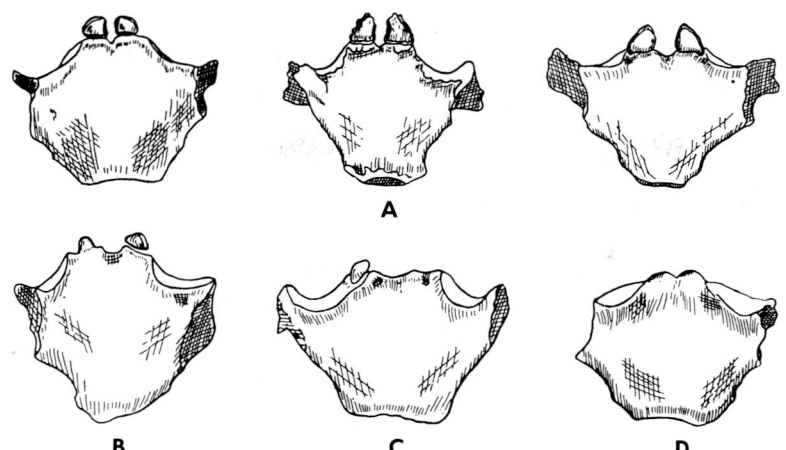

Figure 16.5. Variations of the suprasternal ossicles. **A,** Paired and separate ossicles. **B,** One ossicle separate, one fused. **C,** One ossicle separate, one absent. **D,** Paired and fused ossicles. (From Cobb WM. The ossa suprasternalia in whites and American negroes and the form of the superior border of the manubrium sterni. J Anat 1937;71:245–291.)

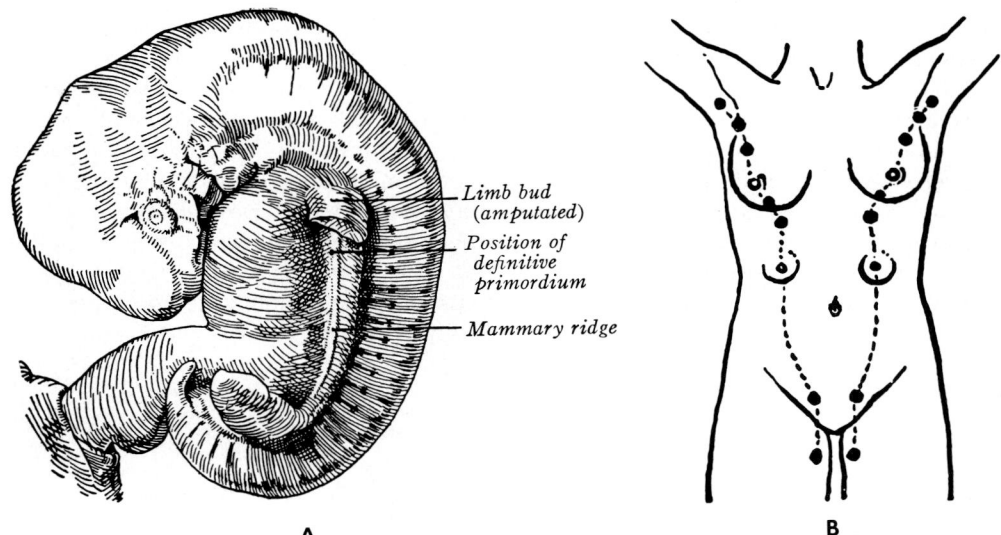

Limb bud (amputated)

Position of definitive primordium

Mammary ridge

Figure 16.6. The milk line. **A,** Unusually prominent mammary ridge in a 13-mm human embryo. **B,** Position and extent of the lines along which supernumerary mammary structures may appear in women. (From Arey LB. Developmental Anatomy, 7th ed. Philadelphia: WB Saunders, 1965.)

sitory (Fig. 16.6, *B*). From the remainder will form the mammary glands. By the sixth week, glandular cells can be found in the basal epithelial layer of the ectoderm. By the twelfth week, 16 to 24 buds of glandular cells grow down into the underlying corium of the developing skin. These buds become canalized during the eighth or ninth month, the canals being the lactiferous ducts. The region from the junction of the ducts to the surface is at first an epidermis-lined pit, which at term or shortly afterward becomes everted by mesenchymal growth to form the nipple. The areola is said to be visible from the fifth month onward.

With a few exceptions, embryonic organs tend to develop in the same sequence in which they appeared in vertebrate evolution. Since mammary glands are mammalian structures without precursors among their reptilian predecessors, it is surprising to find them originating as early as the sixth week of embryonic life. The presence of circulating maternal hormones must be considered to be responsible for the precocious differentiation of the embryonic mammary glands as well as for their better known, transient functional activity at birth.

Remember the following:

1. The paraxial mesoderm is responsible for the genesis of the ribs. The ribs are formed from the mesenchymal costal processes of the thoracic vertebrae. They are at first cartilaginous, but later ossify.

2. The vertical sternal bars, right and left, of mesenchymal origin (somatic mesoderm) are responsible for the formation of the sternum by a ventrolateral and craniocaudal union of the two bars. To start with, the sternal elements are cartilaginous, and later on ossification takes place.

Anterior Abdominal Wall

Most of the abdominal wall of the embryo forms during closure of the midgut and reduction in the relative size of the body stalk. As in the thorax, the primitive wall is somatopleure, composed of ectoderm and mesoderm without muscle, vessels, or nerves. The somatopleure of the abdomen and the thorax is secondarily invaded during the sixth week by mesoderm from the myotomes lying on either side of the vertebral column. The segmental pattern of the mesodermal mass is lost, and it migrates laterally and ventrally as a sheet. The leading edges of the advancing sheets differentiate while still widely separated to form the right and left musculi rectus abdominis, whose final approximation in the midline will close the body wall (Fig. 16.7, A).

While the primordia of the recti are still separated, the main body of the mesodermal sheet splits into three layers: the external layer differentiates into the external oblique muscle ventrally and the serratus muscle group dorsally; the middle layer forms the internal oblique muscle; and the inner layer forms the musculus transversus abdominis. All of these muscles can be recognized by the middle of the seventh week (Fig. 16.7, B).

In the infraumbilical region, the invasion of the somatopleure by the somatic mesoderm is preceded by a layer of mesoderm that arises from the primitive streak just behind the cloaca. This "secondary mesoderm" surrounds the margin of the cloaca and invades the abdominal wall caudal to the body stalk, separating the layers of ectoderm and endoderm of the cranial end of the cloacal plate (12). It provides primary closure of the body wall between the phallus and the body stalk and forms part of the musculature of the bladder (13). The secondary mesoderm is in position by the seventh week (Fig. 16.8); it will be followed by the somatic mesoderm which fuses externally to it by the 12th week.

Approximation of the two recti proceeds from both cranial and caudal ends, becoming essentially closed by the 12th week, except for the umbilical ring itself. At the ring, the body wall with its developing muscles gives way to undifferentiated somatopleure over the surface of the umbilical cord. Although true skin may grow a short distance beyond the body, the cord remains embryonic in its structure.

Klippel (14) suggested a new theory about the development of the anterior abdominal wall. He considers the embryo as a vector field and uses the modern mathematic science of vector analysis. He reported that the development of the embryo progresses not by lateral infolding of the embryologic entities closing at the future umbilicus, but by an outward process from a fixed midpoint, perhaps from the middle to the periphery.

This concept is very interesting but revolutionary

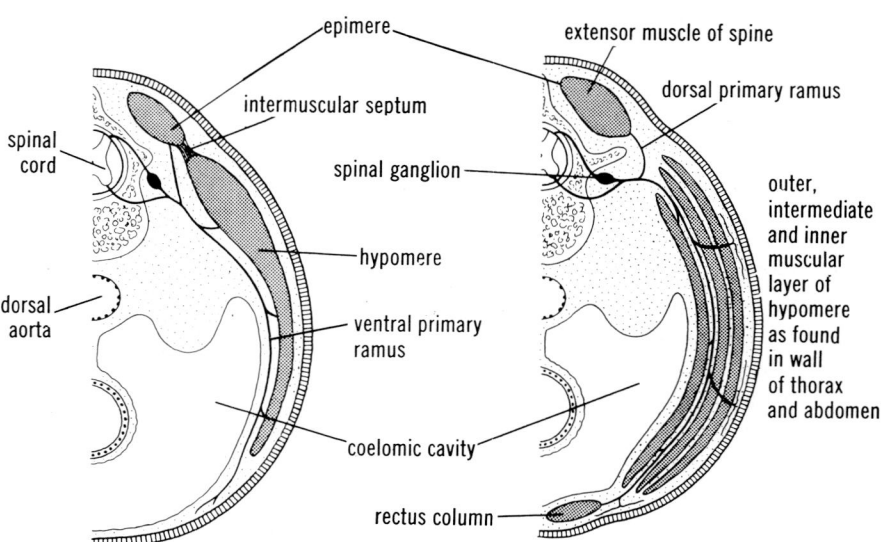

Figure 16.7. Schematic diagram showing the differentiation of myotomes and the establishment of the primordia of the chief muscle groups of the abdomen. A, Transverse section through the thoracic region of a 5-week embryo. The dorsal portion of the body wall musculature (epimere) and the ventral portion (hypomere) are innervated by a dorsal primary ramus and a ventral primary ramus, respec- tively. B, Similar section as in A, at a later stage of development. The hypomere has formed three separate muscle layers and a ventral longitudinal muscle. (From Sadler TW. Langman's Medical Embryology, 6th ed. Baltimore: Williams & Wilkins, 1990.)

enough to demand further practical and theoretic investigations.

Remember the following:

1. Somites of parietal mesodermal origin are responsible for the formation of the anterior abdominal wall by permitting myoblasting invasion into the somatopleurae (approximately the sixth week) and splitting and elongating of the future muscles.
2. Failure of closure may be difficult to discern from rupture of a weak anterior wall. Such is the case in exstrophy of the bladder, where nonunion and rupture after weak wall development are nearly impossible to differentiate.

Critical Events in Body Wall Closure

Duhamel (2) has described failure of closure of the four "folds" of the anterior body wall as celosomia. Failure of closure of individual components of the wall results in a variety of mild to severe embryonic defects.

1. Failure of the cephalic fold to close (upper celosomia): sternal defects
2. Failure of the caudal fold to close (lower celosomia): exstrophy of the bladder and, in the extreme case, exstrophy of the cloaca
3. Failure of lateral folds to close: umbilical hernia and, in the extreme cases, omphalocele

Most frequently, ectopia cordis is primarily the result of malposition of the heart, and the body wall defect is secondary. Most omphaloceles are the result of failure of intestinal return in the 10th week, and here, too, the body

wall defect is secondary. In a few cases in which a large abdominal wall hiatus was present, the abdomen may have failed to retain the normally returned intestines.

Wolff (1) related absence of the limbs (ectromelia) to defects of the body wall. While both body wall and limbs arise from somatic mesoderm, their defects are rarely related. When Wolff studied it, ectromelia was exceedingly rare. Those cases resulting from thalidomide poisoning are rarely accompanied by body wall defects.

The defects of primary closure of the body wall were well reviewed by Hutchin (15).

ANOMALIES OF THE ANTERIOR BODY WALL (FIG. 16.9 and TABLE 16.1)

Anomalies of the Thorax

CONGENITAL CHEST DEFORMITIES

Anatomy.

Sternum Deformities.

Depression deformities. Pectus excavatum—also called funnel chest, trichterbrust, and chonechondrosternon—is a striking deformity in which the normal shape of the thorax is altered by a depression of the sternum. This causes a conical depression of the chest in which the apex is at the lower end of the body of the sternum just above the xiphoid process (Fig. 16.10). The depression may or may not be symmetric. In some severe cases the xiphoid process almost touches the vertebral column (Figs. 16.11 and 16.12, *A* and *B*). In other cases it bends outward at the tip. The third to eighth ribs are angulated, protruding laterally and depressed medially. The result is an individual with a chest hollowed in front, a potbelly, a rounded back, and a head thrust forward.

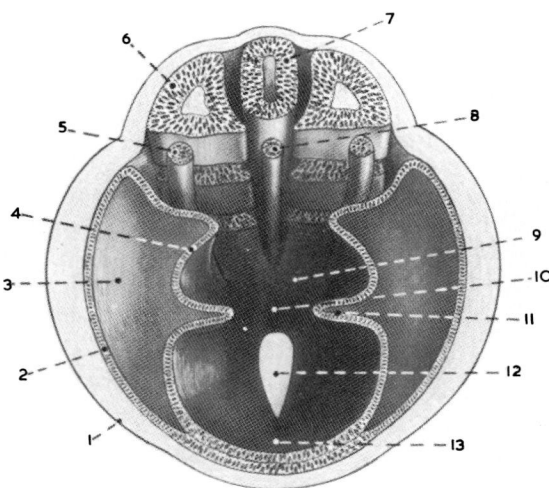

Figure 16.8. Diagram of the disposition of the mesoderm in the embryo below the body stalk. *1,* External cleft and midline fusion defect in a newborn infant. *2,* Same patient as in *1* after removing the attenuated skin overlying the heart and middle portion of the diaphragm. *3,* Same patient as in *1* after having the sternal halves approximated with interrupted wire sutures. (From Glenister TW. A correlation of the normal and abnormal development of the penile urethra and of the infraumbilical abdominal wall. Brit J Urol 1958;30:117–126.)

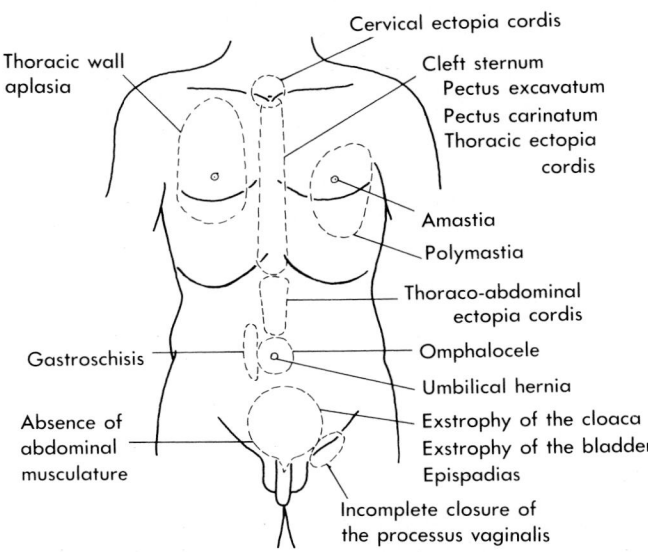

Figure 16.9. Sites of abnormal development of the anterior body wall.

Table 16.1.
Anomalies of the Anterior Body Wall

Anomaly	Origin of Defect	First Appearance	Sex Chiefly Affected	Relative Frequency	Remarks
Deformities of the thorax	Late in fetal life	At birth or in infancy	Male	Common	Familial tendency
Unilateral thoracic wall aplasia	Weeks 6–7	At birth	Male	Very rare	
Sternal defects:					
Simple defects	Week 7	At any age	Male	Rare	
Ectopia cordis	Week 3	At birth	Male	Rare	Few affected persons reach maturity; common in nonviable monsters
Amastia	Week 6	At birth	Female	Very rare	Familial tendency
Polymastia	Week 6	At any age	Equal?	Common	Familial tendency
Umbilical hernia	Week 10	At birth	Equal	Common	Usually disappears spontaneously
Omphalocele	Week 10	At birth	Equal	Uncommon	Failure of normal intestinal return
Gastroschisis	Weeks 6–7	At birth	Male	Uncommon	Herniation through defect in abdominal wall
Incomplete closure of the processus vaginalis	Around birth	In infancy	Male	Common	Results in inguinal hernia or hydrocele
Epispadias[a]	Week 4	At birth	Male	Uncommon	
Exstrophy of the bladder[b]	Week 6	At birth	Male	Uncommon	Untreated patients die eventually from pyelonephritis
Exstrophy of the cloaca[b]	Week 5	At birth	Equal	Very rare	All should be reared as females.
Absence of abdominal musculature with urinary tract defects	Week 7	In infancy	Male	Rare	
Aplasia of abdominal musculature without urinary tract defects	Week 7	In infancy	Male?	Very rare	

[a]See Chapter 21.
[b]See Chapter 18.

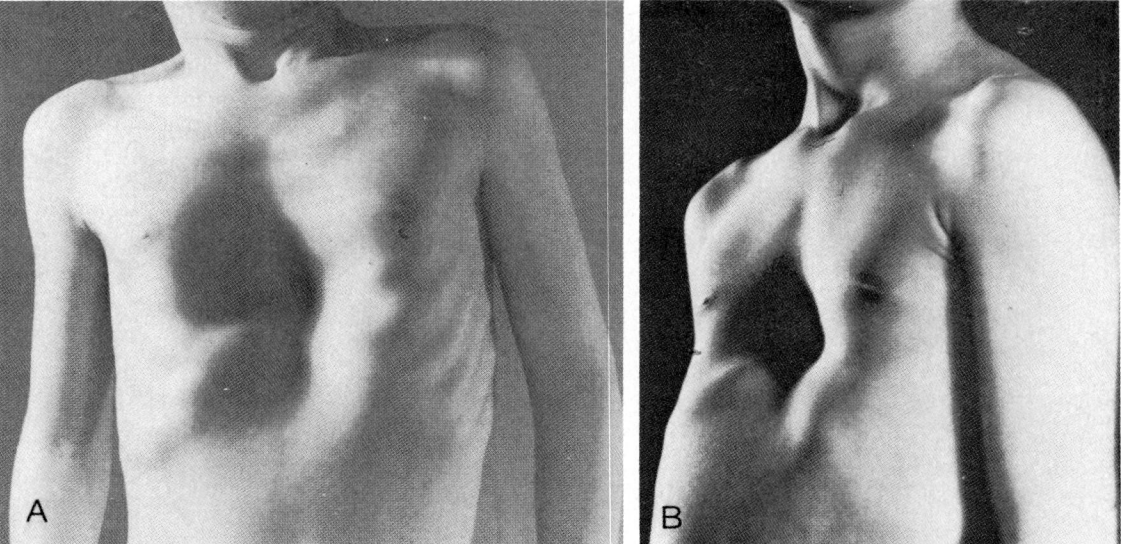

Figure 16.10. Anterior and oblique views of a 7-year-old boy with depression deformity of the chest (pectus excavatum). (From Ravitch MM. The operative treatment of pectus excavatum. Ann Surg 1949;129:429–444.)

While the deformity may be recognizable at birth, especially during crying spells, it progressively worsens during childhood, sometimes producing cardiac and respiratory impairment.

Protrusion deformities. Pectus carinatum, or pigeon breast, is an abnormal protrusion of the anterior chest wall (Fig. 16.13). Strictly speaking, the term *pectus carinatum* should be applied only when the sternum protrudes in the midline, but asymmetric protrusions of the costochondral junction or even of the costal arch are usu-

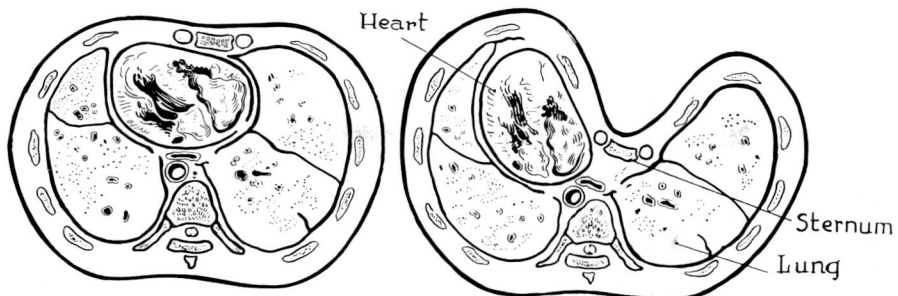

Figure 16.11. Diagrammatic cross-sections through the thorax at the level of the fourth costal cartilage. **A,** Normal thorax. **B,** Thorax with depression deformity. The deformity is asymmetric, the sternum is deviated to the right, and the heart is displaced into the left hemithorax. The transverse diameter of the thorax is increased. (From Ochsner A and DeBakey M. Chone-chondrosternon: report of a case and review of the literature. J Thor Surg 1939;8:469–511.)

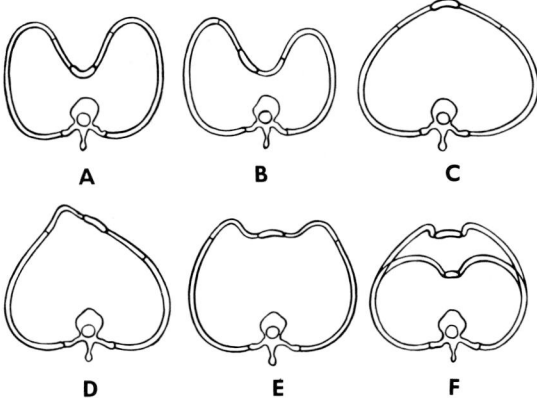

Figure 16.12. Varieties of chest deformities diagrammed in cross-section. **A** and **B,** Depression deformities. **C** and **D,** Protrusion deformities. **E,** Bilateral protrusion. **F,** Chondromanubrial protrusion with gladiolar depression. (From Sanger PW et al. Deformities of the anterior wall of the chest. Surg Gynec Obstet 1953;116:515–522.)

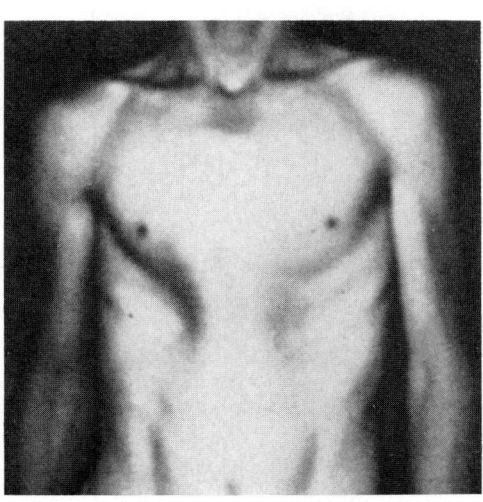

Figure 16.13. Anterior view of an 18-year-old boy with protrusion deformity of the chest (pectus carinatum). (From Ravitch MM. The operative correction of pectus carinatum (pigeon breast). Ann Surg 1960;151:705–714.)

ally also included in this category (Fig. 16.12, *C* and *D*). Typically, the sternum curves forward, but sometimes the greatest protrusion is at the xiphoid process.

Mixed deformities. In addition to those cases in which protrusion extends the length of the thorax, there are examples, not readily classified, in which the lower sternum is retracted, while the upper sternum protrudes (Figs. 16.12, *F,* and 16.14, *E*). This has been called "pouter pigeon breast" by Ravitch (16).

Fusion deformities. This is a nonunion of the right and left sternal halves.

Rib Deformities. Rib and cartilage may be deformed, absent, or separated and associated or not associated with other soft tissue or skeletal anomalies (Poland's anomaly).

Remember that incomplete fusion of the cartilaginous sternal elements may produce cleft sternum.

Combined Deformities. Combined deformities of sternum and ribs occur with or without other associated skeletal anomalies.

Complications of Chest Deformities. Lester (17) emphasized the psychologic distress of patients with chest deformities. Affected children shun all activities in which their deformity might be revealed, with the result that they become physically underdeveloped and socially withdrawn. With this connection, Lynn (18) observed that more cases come to medical attention in regions in which swimming is a leading pastime among children because exposure of the defect is less avoidable than it is in regions in which disrobing is uncommon.

The physiologic effects of chest deformities are respiratory and cardiac complications. Respiratory problems result from decreased lung capacity and restricted movement of the diaphragm. These complications are absent usually in childhood but become increasingly severe after adolescence. However, Polgar and Koop (19) failed to find a correlation between respiratory impairment and severity of the chest defect.

Cardiac symptoms also increase with age. In funnel chest, the heart may be displaced to the left or may actu-

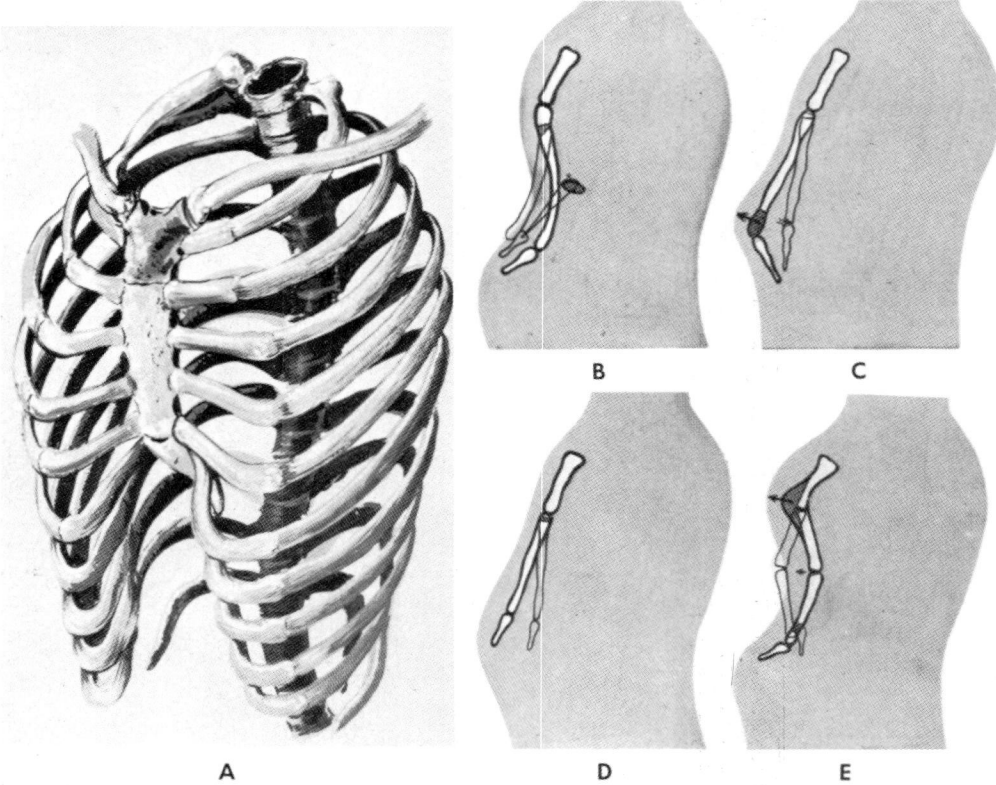

Figure 16.14. **A,** The bony thorax of pectus excavatum. **B** to **E,** Lateral diagrams of various chest deformities, with technique of surgical correction indicated in each. (From Sanger et al. Deformities of the anterior wall of the chest. Surg Gynec Obstet 1963;116:515–522.)

ally be compressed by the sternum. Although severe cardiac distress rarely occurs, a large number of young adults have some degree of intolerance to exercise and frequent minor cardiac symptoms. Ravitch (20) reviewed the cardiac symptoms of a number of patients and reported a case in which chronic heart failure resulted from cardiac displacement.

Bevegard (21) reported that, because of the impaired ventricular filling, the working capacity and stroke volume were less than in normal subjects. Beiser et al. (22) agree with Bevegard. These authors also showed, using cardiac catheterization, that pectus excavatum can reduce the pumping capacity of the heart during exercise in the upright position and that hemodynamic improvement occurs after surgical correction. Cahill (23) studied preoperative and postoperative pulmonary function tests in patients with pectus excavatum. They demonstrated that, postoperative, patients demonstrated a small improvement in total lung capacity and a significant improvement in maximal voluntary ventilation. In addition, exercise performances were improved following correction of the pectus excavatum as quantified both by the total exercise time and maximal oxygen consumption.

Ravitch (24) operated on many pairs of siblings with pectus excavatum. He also operated on a father and a daughter, but he thinks most of his patients represented isolated or sporadic instances. Concerning the cause, he thinks, most likely, a disproportionate growth of the osteocartilaginous structures of the chest wall is perhaps responsible for the genesis of these deformities.

Smith (25) reported that thoracic deformities may occur concomitantly with abdominal muscle weakness, with a number of neurologic disorders, with some genetic connective tissue disorders, and with a number of recognized syndromes.

Embryogenesis. Because funnel chest usually is not apparent at birth and because the deformity increases with age, it is not surprising that 19th century physicians such as Woillez (26) considered chest deformities to be the result of malnutrition. As the congenital nature of the deformities became clear, attention was directed first to the sternum itself and then to the ribs and diaphragm.

Two mechanical factors, overgrowth of the ribs and pull of the diaphragm, are usually involved. Bauhinus (27) in 1600 suggested that diaphragmatic pull might cause funnel chest. This view was revived by Brown (28), who believed that the abnormality lay in a short central tendon

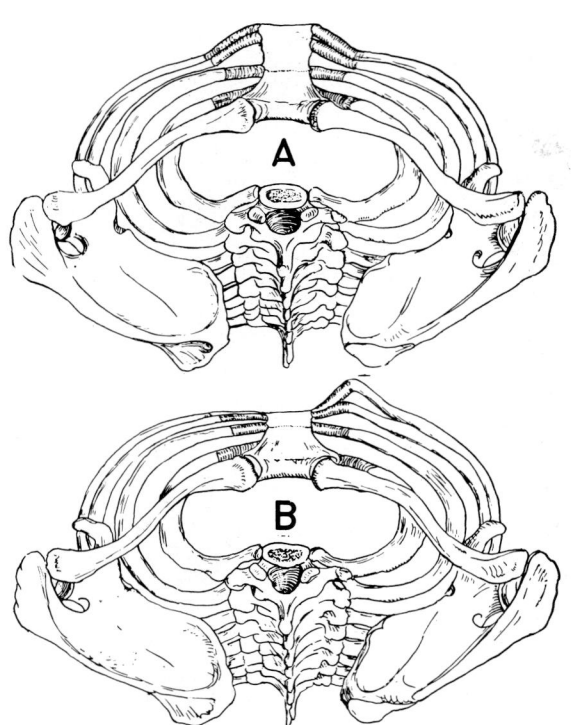

Figure 16.15. The genesis of protrusion deformities proposed by Lester. *A*, Mechanism of middle protrusion deformities. Proportionate overgrowth of the third, fourth, and fifth pairs of ribs causes them to buckle at the costochondral junctions and push the midportion of the sternum forward. *B*, Mechanism of lateral protrusion deformities. Proportionate overgrowth of the ribs on one side of the anterior chest wall produces forward angulation at the costochondral junctions. (Lester CW. Pigeon breast, funnel chest, and other congenital deformities of chest. JAMA 1954;156:1063–1067.)

of the diaphragm. Lester (29, 30) explained protrusion defects as resulting from disproportional growth of the ribs on one or both sides (Fig. 16.15). There is no stage in human development during which protrusion of the thorax is normal (31). Other explanations put forward to explain protrusion and depression deformities are summarized by Ochsner and De Bakey (32).

That the mechanical action of the ribs and diaphragm is capable of producing forces that can distort the thorax is unquestionable. Indeed, one may wonder why chest deformity is so rare. On the other hand, very little is known of those forces that oppose deformation in normal development. Whether the defects are in morphology or in the timing of the pertinent developmental processes is entirely speculative at present.

Despite that depression deformities of the chest develop late and that no sound embryonic basis can be found, there is a familial tendency for them to recur. Nowak (33) found 12 cases among school children in Vienna. In families of these children, 41 of 106 relatives were similarly affected. Lester (30) believes the hereditary factor to be a nonsex-linked, recessive gene.

History. The earliest description of funnel chest is that of Bauhinus (27) in 1600. The first great display of interest in the deformity, however, did not come until the middle of the 19th century when a medical student with a funnel chest was seen by Rokitansky (34) in 1857. During the next 10 years, half a dozen papers, including a classic description of the deformity by Woillez (26) in 1860, appeared describing this patient.

Brown (28) considers that modern interest in chest deformities dates from the work of W. Ebstein (35) in 1882. The condition was reviewed in 1909 by E. Ebstein (36).

The operative history began in 1913 when Sauerbruch (37) operated successfully on a young man with severe respiratory and cardiac symptoms. Brown (28) in 1939 and Lester (17) since 1946 have made the most significant contributions to the treatment of these deformities. Ravitch (24) reviewed the surgical history up to 1951 and summarized the current state of knowledge of the deformities.

Incidence. From a number of series the incidence of funnel chest has been put at about 0.06% (32). Boys are affected much more frequently (78% of patients) than are girls. The estimate of total cases is probably low because mild cases often do not receive medical attention (38).

Although Lester (17) found a ratio of only 28 cases of protrusion deformities out of 122 cases of depression deformities, he believes that protrusion defects are nearly as common as are depression defects.

Welch and Vos (39) reported that pectus excavatum comprised 95% of cases and pectus carinatum 5% at the Boston Children's Hospital. According to Ravitch (24), the ratio of pectus carinatum in most series is 1:6 to 1:10.

Symptoms. Both depression deformities and protrusion deformities may be recognized on inspection. In funnel chest, respiration may be paradoxic, with the lower sternum being pulled inward on inspiration. Dorsal kyphosis is usual. In severe cases respiratory insufficiency, frequent and prolonged respiratory infections, and even cardiac irregularities as a result of displacement of thoracic viscera may appear later in life. The patient often is introverted and withdrawn. Physical underdevelopment in older children is related to their avoidance of athletic activities because of self-consciousness.

Diagnosis and Differential Diagnosis. A history of thoracic trauma or rickets should be excluded; visible enlargement of the costochondral junctions and a groove extending laterally from the xiphoid cartilage above the costal margin (Harrison's groove) are the recognizable stigmata of childhood rickets.

Among infants suspected of developing pectus excavatum, paradoxic respiration resulting from respiratory disease may appear to represent the onset of the deformity (17). This acquired "pseudo–pectus excavatum" is never present at birth and always follows the onset of respiratory distress. Spontaneous recovery of the chest wall follows cure of the respiratory distress. Clemmens and Reyes (40) described nine cases, of which seven had hyaline membrane disease.

Treatment. The overall treatment of congenital deformities of the chest wall may be studied in the classic work by Ravitch (41). The reconstruction of pectus deformities and Poland's syndrome was discussed recently by Garcia et al. (42), who presented their own approach to the operative management. In summary, the treatment is as follows:

1. Fusion Defects of Sternum: Correction in newborn period when ribs are soft, by approximation of the right and left parts of the sternum.

2. Pectus Excavatum: Operation is indicated in: *(a)* symptomatic cases; *(b)* asymptomatic cases with severe deformity, which may be expected to produce symptoms later; and, *(c)* asymptomatic cases for cosmetic or psychologic reasons. The procedure involves subperichondrial resection of the costal cartilages and elevation of the depressed sternum, with internal or external fixation of the sternum (Fig. 16.14). Ravitch, one of the pioneers of such operations, prefers internal fixation (43). There has been one death among 135 patients treated.

3. Pectus Carinatum: If surgery is indicated, elevation of the lateral gutters parallel to the protrusion by subperichondrial resection is the procedure of choice.

RIB ANOMALIES

Unilateral Thoracic Wall Aplasia. In a study of 6 million chest x-ray films reviewed for costal anomalies, the incidence was 0.31%, as reported by Bergman et al. (44), who also stated that cervical ribs occur in about 0.5 to 1% of cadavers and that lumbar ribs occur in 8%.

Absence of costal cartilages and musculi pectoralis on one side of the thorax is a rare condition, limited to males. First reported in 1826 by Lallemond (45), only 12 cases could be found up to 1934 by Colman and Bisgard (46).

In all cases cartilages of the third and fourth ribs were absent on one side. In four patients, three cartilages were affected: in two, four cartilages were absent; and in one, the first five cartilages were missing. In eight cases the defect was on the right; in four it was on the left. The pectoralis major and pectoralis minor were absent or greatly reduced in all cases, and the nipple was absent or small in six patients (Fig. 16.16). The axillary hair on the affected side was displaced down the arm. In all of the left-sided cases, the heart was displaced to the right.

The initial embryonic defect appears to reside in the failure of the ribs to fuse with the sternum. The musculi pectoralis arise from the medial side of the limb bud late in the sixth week. Their fibers, however, do not attach to

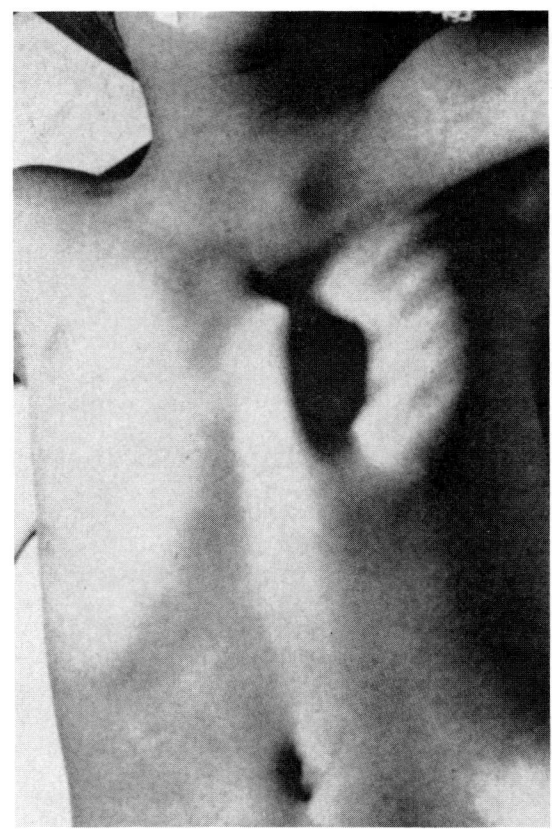

Figure 16.16. Unilateral absence of pectoralis major and minor muscles in a 10-year-old girl. The left breast is absent and there is an asymmetric depression deformity of the chest. (From Martin LW, Helmsworth JA. The management of congenital deformities of the sternum. JAMA 1962;179:82–84. Copyright 1962, American Medical Association.)

the sternum and ribs until the end of the seventh week (47). Failure of full development of the ribs results in failure of the musculi pectoralis mass to migrate to its normal position.

Placement of nonabsorbable synthetic prostheses to bridge the defect is the recommended procedure for absence of costal cartilage (48).

Rib deformities may or may not be associated with other skeletal or soft tissue abnormalities. Absent ribs, fused ribs, or supernumerary ribs are well known to the radiologist. Absence of costal cartilages accompanies the absence of the ribs. Ravitch, of course, is right to use the words "atypical" and "bizarre."

Some deformities are totally asymptomatic and represent an incidental finding on routine chest x-ray films. Some of them, however, are identified as a result of associated paradoxic movements, arrhythmias, and respiratory problems.

According to Bergman et al. (44), there is an asymmetry of the costal cartilages, which may articulate in an

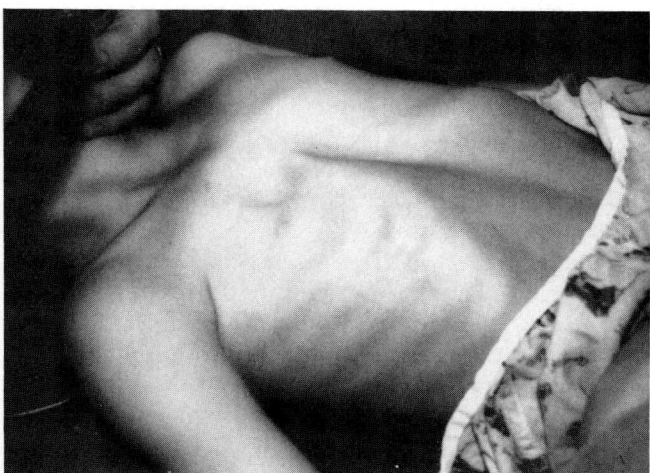

Figure 16.17. Poland's anomaly. Note the pectus excavatum, the absence of the ribs in the region of the right nipple, and the absence of the pectoralis minor and a large portion of the pectoralis major muscle.

alternating pattern. The same authors report absence of the xiphoid, an abnormally long xiphoid extending to the umbilicus, or a perforated one.

We tentatively theorize that: the costal cartilage agenesis and pectoralis agenesis are related. They may share a common cause rather than having the causal relationship stated. The authors think the defect is in the local mesoderm destined to become connective tissue (nonmyotome). If supporting connective tissues of the musculi pectoralis do not develop (deep muscle fascia, tendinous fibers), then the pectoralis muscles are absent or reduced. There is considerable evidence of a separate development for muscle (invasive myotome) and its connective tissue components (tendons, deep fascia).

Poland's Syndrome (Fig. 16.17). According to Ravitch (24), the father of this syndrome is Alfred Poland of Guy's Hospital, who in 1841 reported the first case, and the godfather is Patrick Clarkson, who in 1962 described Poland's syndactyly. Poland's syndrome consists of the following:

1. Absence of costal cartilages and portions of the second to fourth ribs
2. Hypoplasia or absence of nipple and breast
3. Minimal subcutaneous fat, if any
4. Absence of axillary hair
5. Absence of musculus pectoralis minor
6. Absence of costosternal portion of musculus pectoralis major

Diagnosis.

The diagnosis is made by observation of obvious paradoxic motion of the chest wall due to the absence of cartilage and muscles.

Associated Anomalies.

Associated anomalies such as syndactylism, missing phalanges with short fingers and forearm, and spinal anomalies may be present.

Treatment.

Correction of the sternal depression follows those principles outlined for correction of pectus excavatum deformities. Bilateral subperichondrial cartilage resection and sternal osteotomy allow for anterior displacement of the sternum and correction of any rotational anomalies of the sternum. In patients lacking ribs on one side, a rib graft is obtained from the contralateral side to fill in the defect. Placement of a synthetic mesh across the defect may be required to reconstitute the integrity of the chest wall. It is necessary to correct the chest wall deformity, particularly in females, to allow for reconstruction of the ipsilateral breast at the time of full development. If the underlying chest wall deformity is not corrected, ideal breast reconstruction is difficult (24, 49).

THORACIC DYSTROPHY

Thoracic dystrophy is associated with a small thoracic cage (microthorax?) and pulmonary hypoplasia with asphyxiating symptoms.

Jeune et al. (50) described this anomaly for the first time, and later, several papers appeared in the literature such as that of Finegold et al. (51), Hull and Barnes (52), and Karjoo et al. (53) who treated the problem by splitting the sternum, holding the halves with steel struts.

DEFECTS OF THE ANTERIOR THORACIC WALL AND ECTOPIA CORDIS

Ravitch (24), a true scholar of the subject, classifies the sternal clefts in three major groups:

1. Cleft sternum without associated anomalies.
   a. V- or U-shaped clefts of the upper sternum, involving manubrium and one or two sternebrae
   b. Lower sternum cleft with the xiphoid process united
   c. Entire sternum is a cleft
2. True ectopia cordis with varying degrees of cleft sternum with the heart outside the chest wall, usually internally malformed and with other malformations
3. Cantrell's (54) pentalogy (syndrome), which is composed of the following anomalies:
   a. Cleft or absence of the distal sternum
   b. Crescenting ventral diaphragmatic defect
   c. Midline ventral abdominal defect or omphalocele
   d. Defect at the apical pericardium with communication with the peritoneal cavity
   e. Cardiac defects

Thoracic wall defects arise from the absence of part or all of the sternum; from the failure of sternal elements to fuse in the midline; or from fusion and subsequent rupture. The defects may involve the sternum only, or there may be accompanying defects of the abdominal wall and the diaphragm. Associated with the more severe defects is a condition of displacement or eventration of the heart, *ectopia cordis.*

Ravitch (24) divides ectopia cordis into three groups: cervicothoracic; thoracoabdominal; and an uncommon one associated with complete sternal cleft. He stated that, for all practical purposes, the thoracoabdominal ectopia cordis, which is presented by a distal sternal defect, is most likely part of the Cantrell's (54) pentalogy (syndrome). He advises surgery during early infancy with an attempt to correct all the anomalies, if possible—something that was accomplished by Mulder et al. (55), Murphy et al. (56), and Symbas and Ware (57).

We would love to abstract in extensa Ravitch's (24) excellent and classic work, *Congenital Deformities of the Chest Wall and Their Operative Correction,* but obviously this is not possible.

Anatomy.

Sternal Defects without Displacement of the Heart.

Absence of sternal elements. The xiphoid process is the element most frequently absent; in extreme cases, the manubrium alone remains (58). A patient has been reported in whom the clavicles and upper ribs were attached to a reduced manubrium, while the lower ribs were attached to a sternum separated by some distance from the manubrium. (59) (Fig. 16.18).

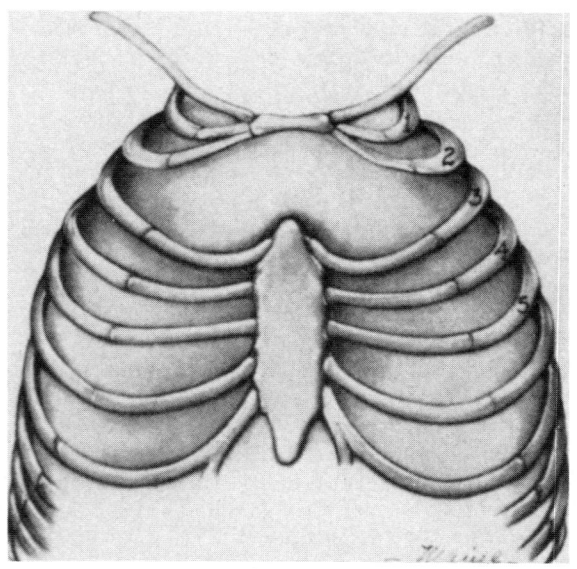

Figure 16.18.   Absence of sternal elements with separation of the manubrium from the remainder of the sternum. (From Martin LW, Helsworth JA. The management of congenital deformities of the sternum. JAMA 1962;179:82–84. Copyright 1962, American Medical Association.)

Complete absence of all elements is rare, but successful repair was reported by Asp and Sulamaa (60). Ravitch (61) also described successful repair in an infant who lacked sternal elements and had pericardial and diaphragmatic defects as well as a gross abdominal wall defect. Skin covered the abdominal and thoracic defects and the heart was not ectopic. Except for the presence of the heart in the thorax, all of the characteristics of thoracoabdominal ectopia (see discussion later in this chapter) appear to have been present (Fig. 16.19).

Failure of sternal fusion.   Although complete failure of fusion usually is associated with eventration of the heart, one case was reported in which the skin was intact over the defect and the thoracic viscera had not herniated. Repair was successful (62) (Fig. 16.20). Greenberg et al (63) recommended repair in early infancy when the bony thorax is most compliant. The authors also successfully treated such a case, as is shown in Figures 16.21 to 16.23.

Failure of superior sternal fusion.   In this anomaly, there may be a V-shaped cleft in the upper sternum, or as in the patient of Longino and Jewett (64), the separation may extend down to the xiphoid process. Nine cases have been reported (65). In three of the nine patients, there were hemangiomas of the head and neck, and in three, there was a midline abdominal raphe, indicating an incipient midline fusion defect. True ectopia cordis was not present, although the heart pulsated visibly under the skin of the unprotected area. Crying may accentuate the rather alarming appearance, even though the heart is normal and in its proper location.

Sternal Defects with Ectopia Cordis.

The presence of the living, beating heart outside the thorax is perhaps the most alarming and distressing of all congenital anomalies. The severity of the defect, its rarity, and the frequent existence of internal cardiac malformation combine to make the outlook for the affected infant very poor.

Depending on the location of the protruding heart and on the extent of the body wall defect, ectopias may be grouped into cervical, thoracic, thoracoabdominal, or abdominal types.

Among 224 cases of ectopia in the literature, 197 are described well enough to be classified as follows:

Cervical ectopia	6
Thoracic ectopia	126
Thoracoabdominal ectopia	36
Abdominal ectopia	29

The heart was uncovered in 41%, covered with a serous membrane in 31%, and covered with skin in 27% (66).

It is important to distinguish between thoracic or cervical cardiac ectopia and failure of sternal fusion in which the heart, though protruding ventrally through the sternal gap, is not otherwise dislocated (Fig. 16.19). Such

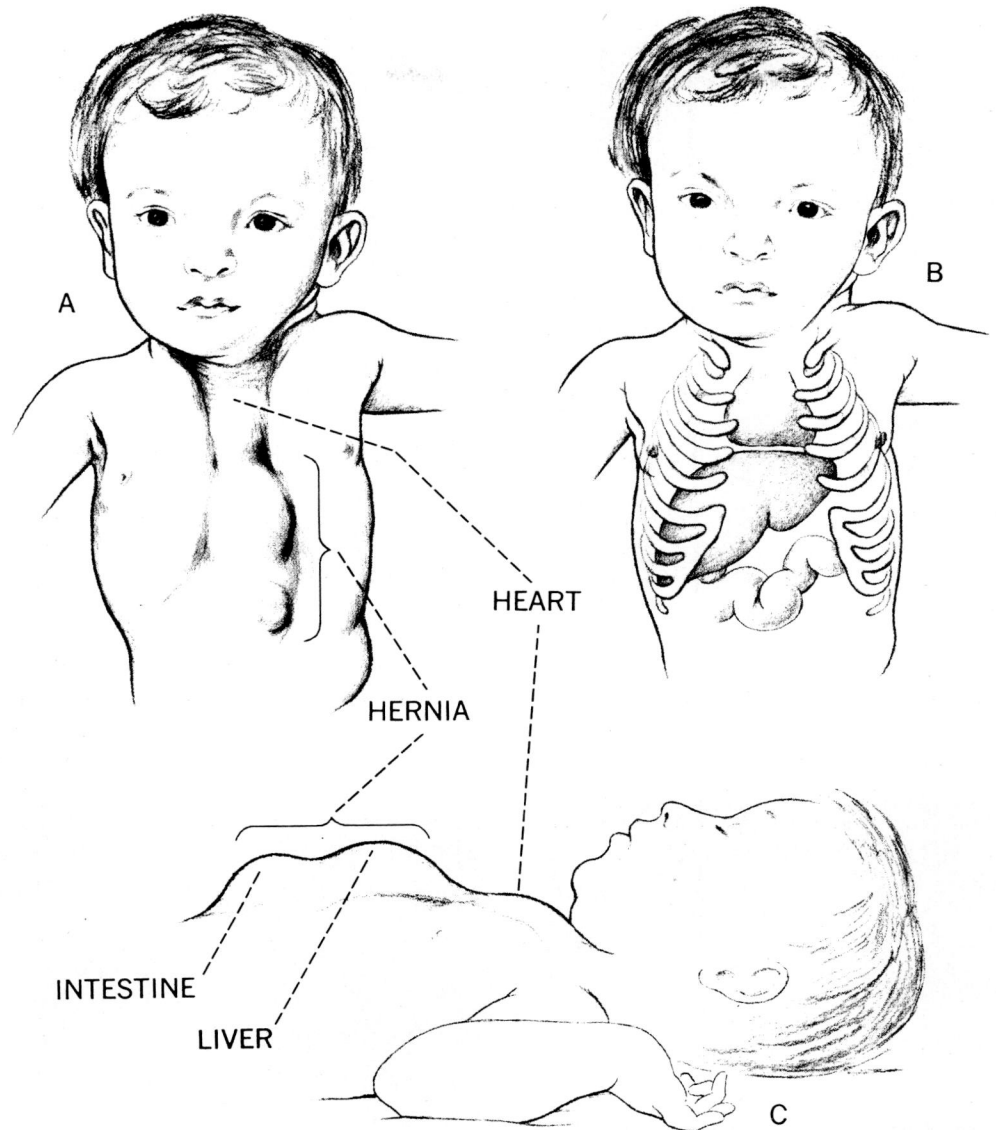

Figure 16.19. *Absence of the entire sternum. The defect was covered by skin, fat, and serosa. A ventral diaphragmatic hernia opened into the pericardial cavity, so that the pericardial diaphragmatic and sternal defects required repair, which was successfully completed in two stages. (From Ravitch MM. Congenital absence of sternum. In: American College of Surgeons, Clinical Congress. Advancing with surgery: spectacular problems in surgery. Sommerville, NJ: Ethicon, 1963.)*

hearts are usually without internal malformations. Most of the cases reported as thoracic ectopia with intact skin are probably examples of failure of sternal fusion.

In thoracoabdominal ectopia, the body wall usually remains unclosed as far as the umbilicus. The diaphragm has a V-shaped hiatus. The anterior and inferior portion of the pericardium may be absent. The heart itself may be congenitally abnormal as well as displaced (Figs. 16.24 and 16.25). Due to the diaphragmatic defect, the cardiac ectopia is usually downward; the surface of the liver may be hollowed out to receive it (67).

Both cervical and abdominal ectopia may occur without cleft sternum. Abdominal ectopia cordis strictly does not belong to this group of anomalies because the defect is diaphragmatic and does not involve the anterior body wall. The known cases include that of a veteran soldier of the Napoleonic wars whose heart was situated at the level of the left kidney. The left kidney itself was absent and the man died of nephritis of the remaining kidney (68). A few other cases have been reported (69, 70).

Associated Cardiovascular Anomalies.

Where cardiac ectopia is complete, internal cardiac anomalies generally occur (71). Interventricular septal defects usually are present and interatrial septal defects

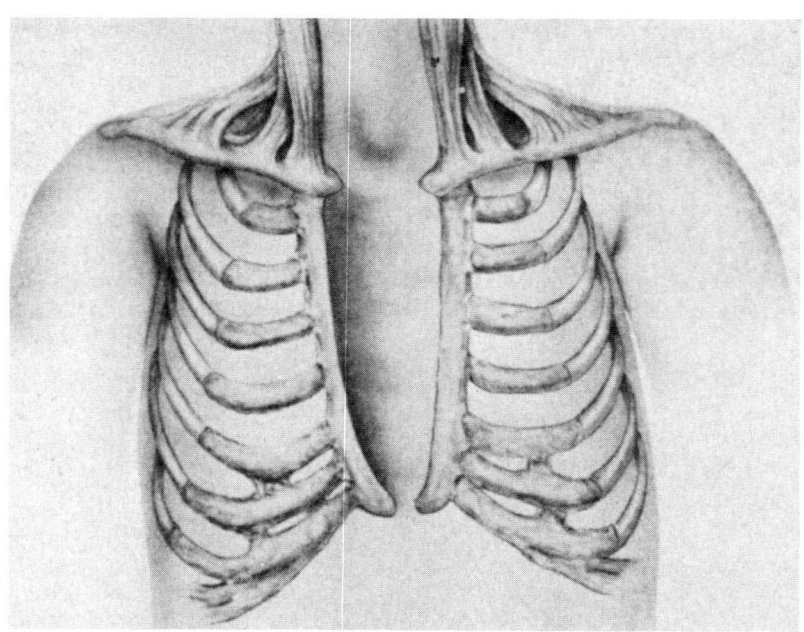

Figure 16.20. Failure of sternal fusion. In this patient the sternum and ribs appear to have ceased their normal medial migration at about the sixth week of development and to have ossified in that position. The skin was intact over the bony defect. Compare with Figure 16.4, **A.** (From Maier HC, Bortone F. Complete failure of sternal fusion with herniation of pericardium. J Thor Surg 1949;18:851–859.)

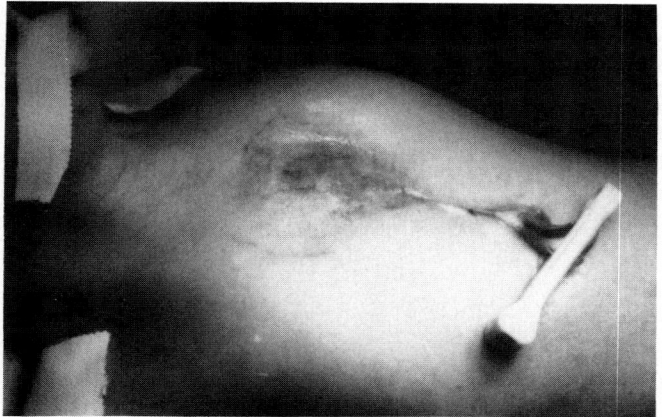

Figure 16.21. External cleft and midline fusion defect in a newborn infant.

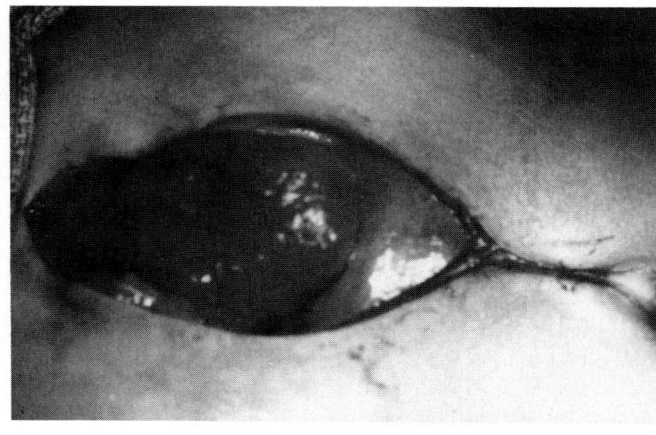

Figure 16.22. Same patient as in Figure 16.21 after removing the tenuated skin overlying the heart and middle portion of the diaphragm.

are common. The tetralogy of Fallot has been found frequently. Cantrell and his colleagues (54) suggested that five conditions constitute a syndrome among the cases of thoracoabdominal cardiac ectopia: (1) cleft of lower sternum, (2) supraumbilical abdominal wall defect, (3) deficiency of the anterior diaphragm, (4) defect of the pericardium, and (5) intracardiac defects. Twenty-three examples have been reported (54, 55). In at least four patients, a left ventricular diverticulum was observed (Fig. 16.25) (see also "Diverticula of the Heart"). In one case there were no intracardiac defects (72).

Jewett and his colleagues (65) noted that, in at least four cases of cleft sternum among 10 reported between 1947 and 1962 hemangiomas of the face and neck were present (Fig. 16.24, *A*). No explanation has been suggested.

Embryogenesis. Failure of inferior sternal fusion after the seventh week appears to represent a simple arrest in

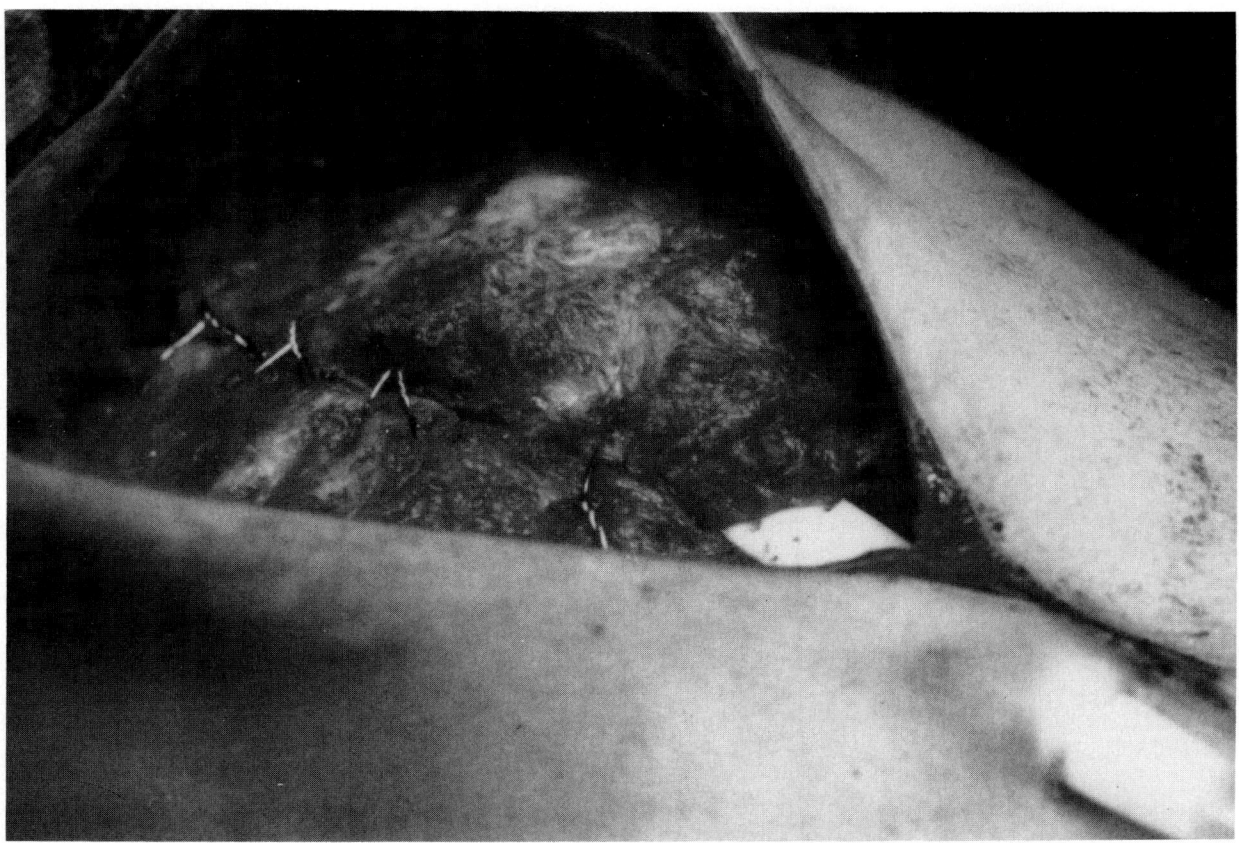

Figure 16.23. Same patient as in Figure 16.21 after the sternal halves were approximated with interrupted wire sutures.

development. Failure of superior sternal fusion is paradoxic since fusion normally proceeds from the cephalic end. The only explanation lies in primary absence of the cephalic unpaired element or a secondary splitting of the developing sternum.

Where true ectopia cordis is present, the failure of sternal fusion appears to be secondary to a primary malposition of the heart itself. Failure of the heart to descend into the thorax during the third week may leave it trapped above the closing upper portion of the sternum, creating a cervical ectopia.

More difficult to explain are the thoracic and abdominothoracic ectopias. The diaphragmatic defect associated with the latter suggests a defect of the transverse septum. Such a defect can hardly be primary because the septum is not a paired structure. Kanagasuntheram and Verzin (73) suggest that excessive pericardial celom formation may perforate the transverse septum and allow the heart to emerge ventrally (Fig. 16.26, *B*). It is tempting to apply this explanation to defects of the central tendon of the diaphragm that result in a communication between the pericardial and peritoneal cavities (page 515)

and to consider them to be a mild form of a condition which, when severe, produces thoracoabdominal ectopia cordis. Whether or not this speculation is true, both anomalies result from defects of the transverse septum.

History. The early reports all concern ectopia cordis. Stenson in 1671 described a child born with a divided sternum and upper abdomen and who had almost complete visceral ectopia (74).

Several similar reports appeared during the 18th century (75). In a thesis at Berlin in 1818, Weese (76) endeavored to classify the types of the condition and proposed the terms ectopia cordis *cum sterni fissura, suprathoracica,* and *subthoracica.* In 1939, Roth (77) and Blatt and Zeldes (78) in 1942 together reported 142 cases from the literature. Schao-tsu (66) in 1957 collected 210 cases. About 16 more cases were described up to 1961 (73). A dog embryo with ectopia cordis was reported by Kanagasuntheram and Perumal Pillai (79).

It should be noted that some of these patients had sternal defects without ectopia cordis since the heart, though visible, did not protrude. Among older case histories the distinction is not always clear.

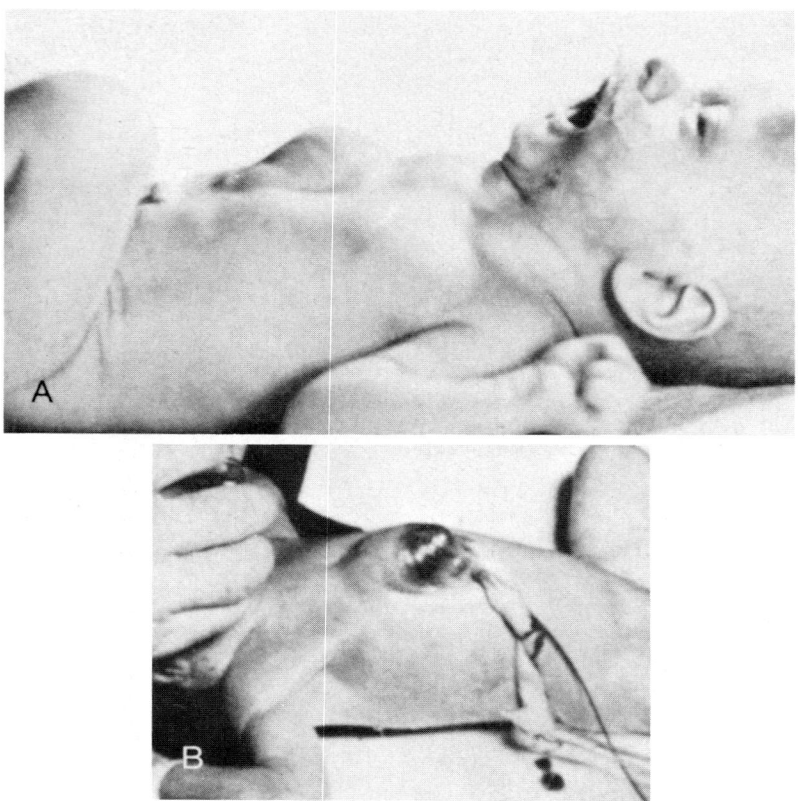

Figure 16.24. Ectopia cordis. **A,** Thoracic ectopia with absence of the sternum. The defect was covered with membranous skin. (From Asp K, Sulamaa M. Ectopia cordis. Acta Chir Scand 1961;123(suppl):52–56.) **B,** Thoracoabdominal ectopia. The base of the heart was covered by skin and the greater portion of the ventricles by pericardium, but the apex was completely uncovered. (From Brown JJM. Ectopia cordis. J R Coll Surg Edin 1960;5:231–232.)

Greig (75) collected 39 cases of cleft sternum up to 1926. Of these, he considered 19 to be true ectopia cordis, while 20 had no cardiac displacement.

Incidence. Schao-tsu (66) cited German figures for cardiac ectopia as high as 5.5:1000 births at Tubingen and 0.4:1000 at Munich. Abbott (80) included eight cases in her series of 1000 congenital heart defects. The great majority of these cases were lethally deformed monsters, either stillborn or with no prospect of survival.

More males than females are affected. Blatt and Zeldes (78) found 25 males and 14 females in their series.

Symptoms and Diagnosis. The diagnosis of simple cleft sternum is by palpation. In severe cases, without ectopia cordis, there may be a history of dyspnea and repeated respiratory tract infection. The dyspnea is the result of an unstable chest wall, which causes the skin over the defect to alternately balloon out and suck in with each breath.

Diagnosis of complete cervical, thoracic, or thoraco-abdominal ectopia is usually made at birth. At least one case was diagnosed in utero during labor by location of the fetal heart beat (81).

The problem is in determining whether the heart, unprotected by the sternal covering, is ectopic or in its normal location. Because the unrestrained heart may bulge into the defect on exertion, the diagnosis may be difficult. A correct diagnosis must be made to evaluate the possibility of corrective surgery.

Treatment. Surgical repair of ectopia cordis has been attempted in 27 recorded cases since 1888, when Lannelongue (82) successfully covered the heart of a 12-day-old girl with a skin flap and followed up on her for 20 years. Subsequently, at least nine successful operations have been performed (60). Five were performed on patients with thoracic ectopia, three on thoracoabdominal ectopia patients, and one on a cervical ectopia patient. In no cases were other cardiac anomalies present.

The greatest problem in replacing the heart in the thorax lies with the inadequate size of the thorax itself. Cardiac or respiratory embarrassment is the frequent result of replacement.

Our experience with ectopia cordis associated with Cantrell's (54) pentalogy involves five patients (Figs. 16.27 to 16.29), two of whom had true ectopia cordis and three of whom had the heart covered by skin. One of the patients with true ectopia cordis was treated utilizing the silo technique (as described under the section "Gastros-

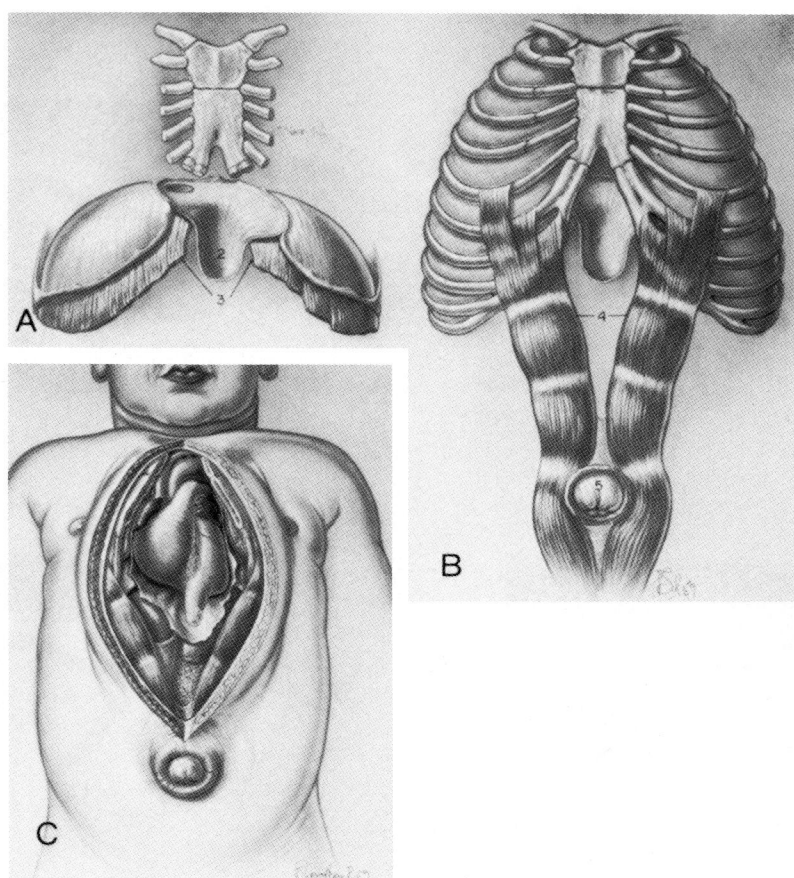

Figure 16.25. Thoracoabdominal ectopia cordis. **A,** *1,* Sternal defect; *2,* pericardial defect; *3,* diaphragmatic defect. **B,** *4,* Diastasis recti; *5,* umbilical hernia. **C,** Left ventricular diverticulum that passed through the pericardial and diaphragmatic defects. (From Mulder DG et al. Complete repair of a syndrome of congenital defects involving the abdominal wall, sternum, diaphragm, pericardium and heart; excision of left ventricular diverticulum. Ann Surg 1960;151:113–122.)

chisis"). The other patient had the heart covered with skin flaps. Both of these patients died from intracardiac defects. Two of the patients with Cantrell's (54) pentalogy and ectopia cordis (covered with skin) had the associated omphalocele treated conservatively with topical antiseptics. One died from severe intracardiac anomalies and the other is still alive awaiting repair of his congenital heart defects. The third patient with a skin-covered ectopia cordis associated with Cantrell's (54) pentalogy is alive 6 years following treatment. In that patient, a diaphragm was constructed using the left rectus muscle to separate the thoracic from the abdominal cavities. This patient has undergone normal growth and development.

The authors recommend strongly that the interested reader consult the classic work of Ravitch and Streichen (41), *Atlas of General Thoracic Surgery.*

Prognosis. The prognosis in cases of simple cleft sternum is good. The sight of the heart visibly pulsating beneath the skin is alarming, and the organ undoubtedly is more exposed to trauma by the absence of the sternal covering, but when no intrinsic cardiac defects are present, there is no danger to life. In some cases the body defect may be great enough to embarrass respiration on exertion (60).

The prognosis in cases of ectopia cordis is far poorer. Of 138 patients for whom there are follow-up or survival records, 23 were stillborn and 42 more died on the first day. Only 32 patients have survived for more than 1 month after birth. Seven are known to have reached maturity, and 19 others survived infancy and were alive at the time their cases were reported. The oldest patient was 75 years old (58).

Among patients with thoracic ectopia, over 50% died within 1 day. Only seven have lived to maturity or, from prognosis after surgery, have hopes of doing so. Most of the survivors originally suffered only from partial ectopia.

Cervical ectopia also carries with it a poor prognosis, with only two patients having survived to adulthood (83, 60).

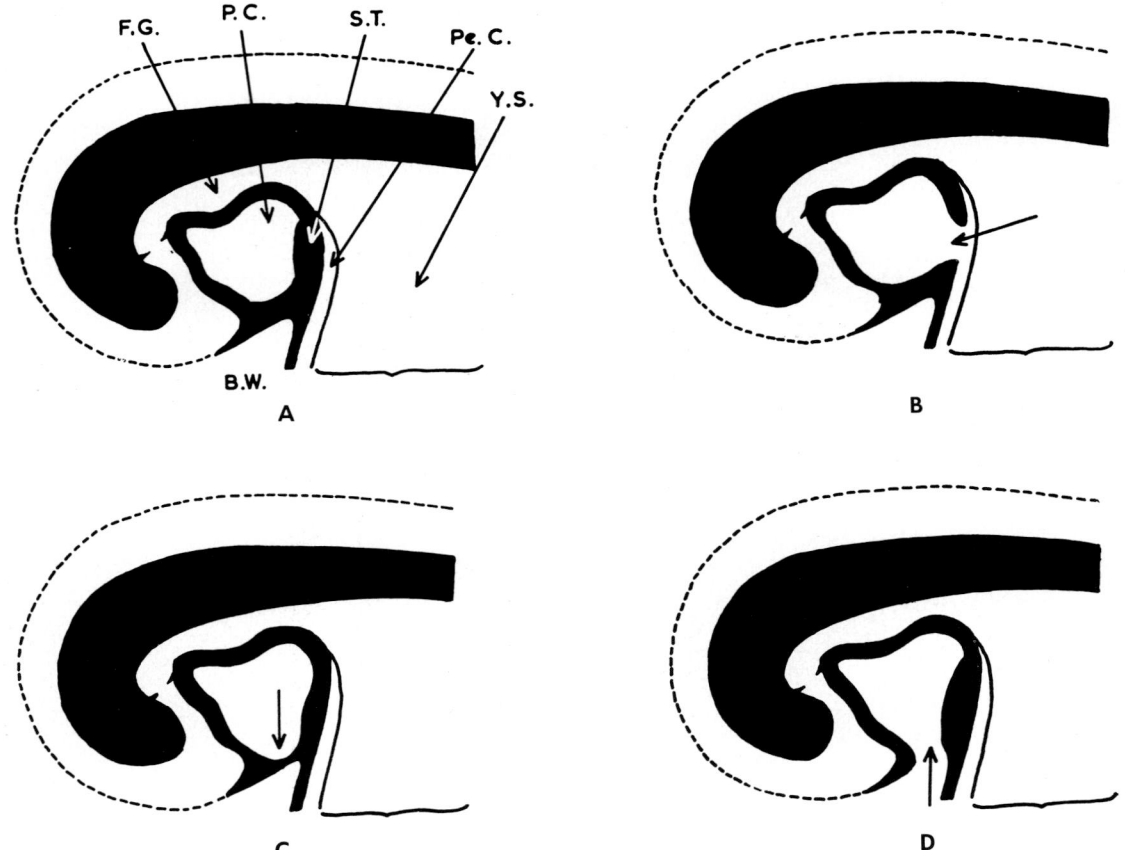

Figure 16.26. Hypothetical stages in the formation of ectopia cordis. **A,** Normal development of the transverse septum and the pericardium in the fourth week. **B,** Abdominal and thoracoabdominal ectopia. *Arrow* indicates the site of destruction of the transverse septum by excessive pericardial coelom formation. **C** and **D,** Cervical and thoracic ectopia. *Arrows* indicate anterior body wall rupture. *F.g.,* Foregut; *P.C.,* pericardial cavity; *S.T.,* transverse septum; *Pe.C.,* peritoneal cavity; *Y.S.,* yolk stalk (midgut); *B.W.,* body wall. (From Kanagasuntheram R, Verzin JA. Ectopia cordis in man. Thorax 1962;17:159–167.)

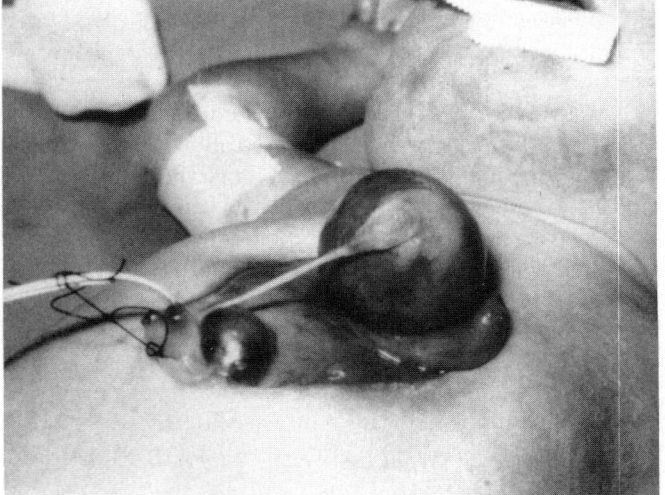

Figure 16.27. Ectopia cordis with a left ventricular diverticulum.

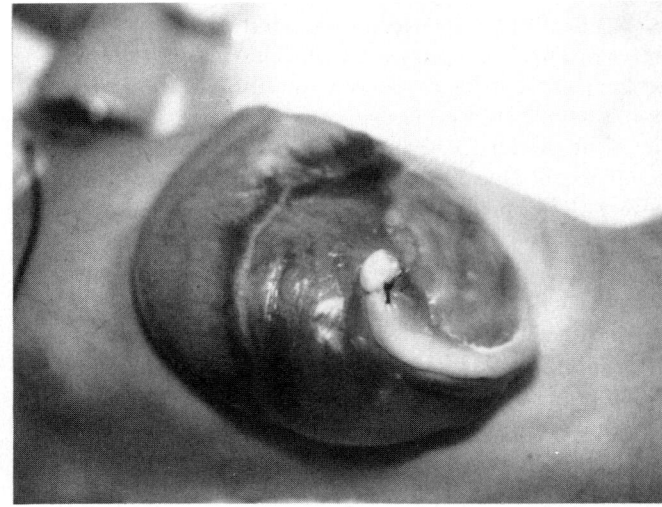

Figure 16.28. Pentalogy of Cantrell with a large omphalocele, cleft distal sternum, and skin-covered heart.

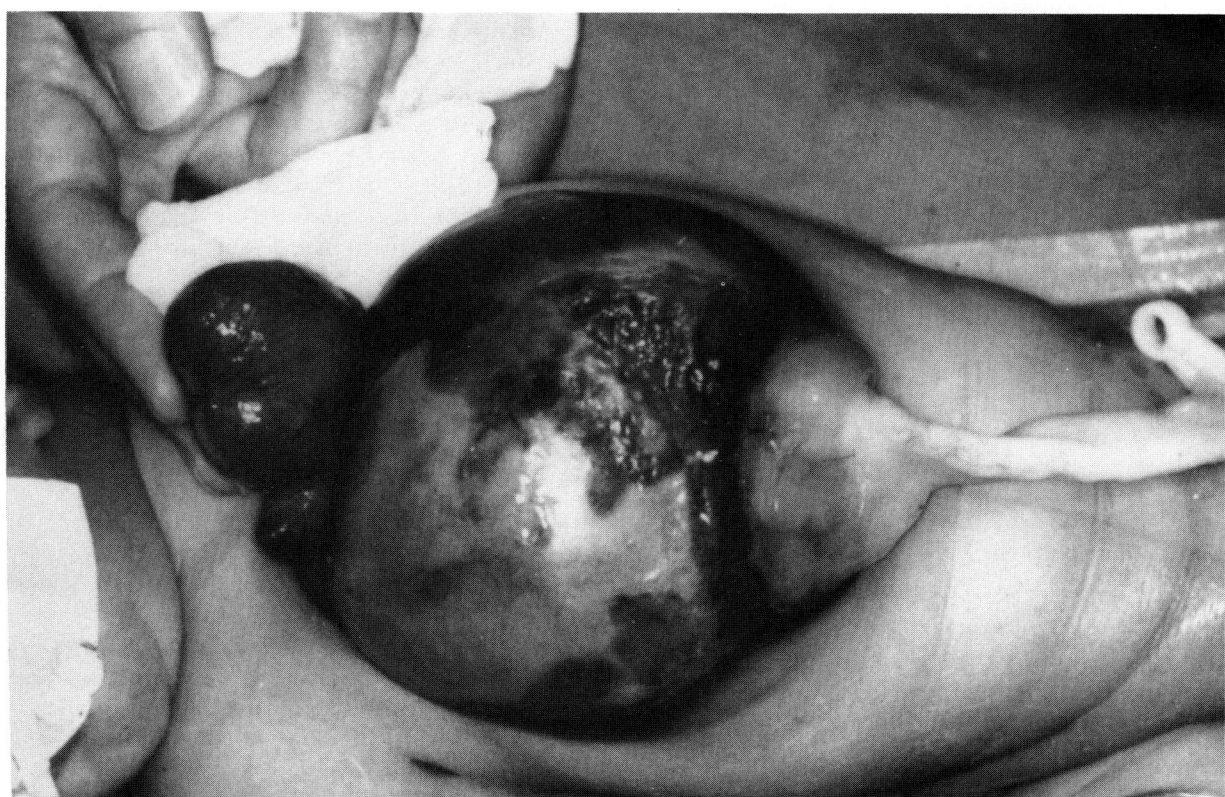

Figure 16.29. Pentalogy of Cantrell with a true ectopia cordis.

The prognosis in cases of thoracoabdominal ectopia is slightly better; six of 36 patients have survived.

Abdominal cardiac ectopia does not appear to be incompatible with life. Five patients were stillborn or died on the first day after birth, but at least 10 of 17 patients who were followed up have survived. In general, the survivors are those without associated congenital cardiac defect.

Congenital Anomalies of the Breast

DEVELOPMENT

In early embryonic development (at 35 days approximately), an ectodermal, thick band (milk line or milk ridge) develops in the ventral area of the body, starting from the yet unformed axilla to the inguinal area on each side, sometimes extending into the triangle of Scarpa. The pectoral part of the ridge will produce the mammary primordium on each side, and the proximal and distal extrapectoral ridge disappears.

The ectodermal thickening of the mammary primordium grows into the dermis producing 16 to 24 solid cords of cells within the mesenchymal tissue, which later will proliferate and produce the lactiferous ducts as well as the alveoli. Around the eighth to ninth month of intrauterine life, the nipple appears first as a depression and later as an elevation when ready to accept the lactiferous ducts.

We agree with Langebartel (84) that the female breast is mostly a mound of fat, with fasciae and fibrous strands and the mammary gland. This harmonious cooperation of ectoderm (epithelial ductal lining and acini) and mesenchyme (supporting elements such as the skin) occasionally is interrupted, and the congenital anomalies of the breast are produced.

CONGENITAL ANOMALIES

Congenital anomalies of the breast can be categorized as follows:

1. Amastia: bilateral or unilateral
2. Athelia: bilateral or unilateral
3. Polymastia
4. Polythelia
5. Mammary asymmetry
   a. Megalomastia: bilateral or unilateral
   b. Micromastia: bilateral or unilateral

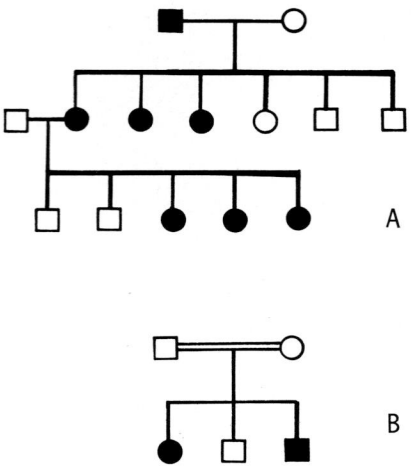

A. FRASER (1956)

B. KOWLESSAR AND ORTI (1968)

Figure 16.30. Two lineages with congenital absence of the breast. **A,** Three generations, with seven affected members. (From Fraser FC, Dominant inheritance of absent nipples and breast. Novant anni delle leggi mendeliane. Roma. Instituto Gregorio Mendel, 1956, pp. 360–362.) **B,** First cousin marriage with two affected offspring. (From Kowlessar M, Orti E. Complete breast absence in siblings. Amer J Dis Child 1968;115:91–93.)

Amastia and Athelia

Absence of the breast is rare. Deaver and McFarland (85) collected only 20 instances up to 1918, and Trier (86) in 1965 was able to collect only 43 cases from the literature since 1839.

In seven cases, all in males, the absence of breasts was associated with a thin, dry skin, absence of hair and sweat glands, saddle nose, atrophic nasal mucosa, and underdeveloped or missing teeth. These patients seem to have a generalized defect of ectodermal tissues rather than simple amastia. In contrast to this group, most examples of amastia show otherwise normal ectodermal structures but do have local mesodermal defects, such as absence of musculus pectoralis major and occasionally of one or more ribs or costal cartilages.

Unilateral absence of the breast was reported in 20 cases, four of which occurred in males. Right and left sides were equally affected, and the pectoral muscles were absent on the affected side in all but two individuals (see the section on "Unilateral Thoracic Wall Aplasia," Fig. 16.16).

Bilateral absence has been described in 16 patients of whom two were male.

A familial tendency has been observed by several investigators (87, 89). Two of the pedigrees are shown in Figure 16.30.

Amastia may result from the absence of the milk lines or from their excessive obliteration later. The presence of areolae without nipples or glandular tissue in one case (90) implies that a fragment, insufficient to induce an entire breast, might have been the only portion to persist. Where breast tissue is present but without a nipple, the condition is termed *athelia*. This is rare at the normal site but is not infrequent in accessory mammary structures at other locations.

Treatment may occasionally be required for cosmetic or psychologic reasons. Trier (86) suggests skin grafts from the labia minora to form a nipple and silastic gel implants in subcutaneous pockets to form a breast. Currently, however, there are concerns about the use of breast implants.

SUPERNUMERARY BREASTS: POLYMASTIA AND POLYTHELIA

Anatomy. Breasts are said to be *accessory* if they lie on the embryonic milk line, which at its greatest development runs on the ventrolateral body wall from the axilla to the groin, with extensions on the inner surfaces of the upper arm and the inner side of the thigh. Breast tissue found outside of this milk line is said to be *ectopic* (Fig. 16.6).

Accessory Breasts.

The great majority of supernumerary breasts are accessory and are nearly always axillary or thoracic. Among Caucasians it usually is considered an accepted fact that about 95% of examples are found just below the normal breast, of which fewer than 5% are abdominal. The remaining 4 to 5% are axillary (Fig. 16.31).

The figures of Iwai (91), however, seem to show that accessory breasts among the Japanese are found above the normal breast in 95% of female cases and in 60% of the male cases.

Accessory breasts below the thorax are rare. Breast tissue in the vulva was first reported by Crumpe (92) in 1854, and a total of 17 cases were reviewed by Tow and Shanmuharatnam (93) in 1962. Of these four were bilateral, and three were sites of malignant tumors. Curiously, in five patients the supernumerary organ was discovered only during the third or a later pregnancy. In only two cases was there an actual discharge of milk.

Examples of normal mammary glands at any location along the milk line may be found among one or another of mammalian species. Deaver and McFarland (85) provide a discussion of the comparative anatomy.

Ectopic Breasts.

Breast tissue, occasionally even functional breasts, have been reported from a variety of locations outside the embryonic milk line (Fig. 16.32). De Cholnoky (94) collected cases in the following locations:

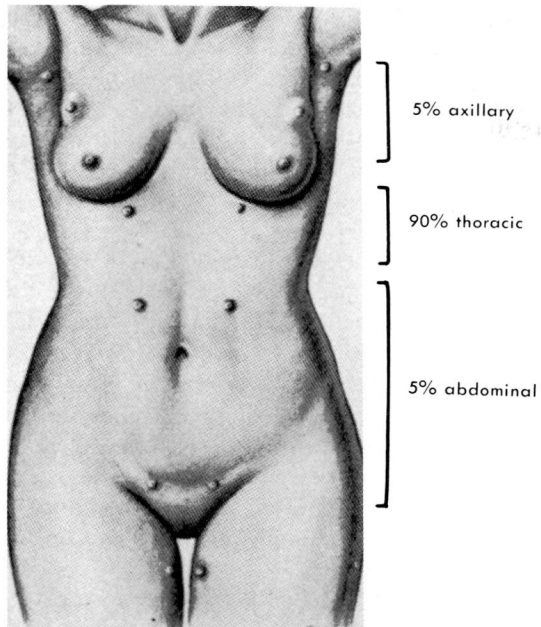

Figure 16.31. The sites of accessory breast tissue along the embryonic milk line and the relative frequencies of their occurrence in Caucasians. (From De Cholnoky T. Supernumerary breasts. Arch Surg 1939;39:926–941. Copyright 1939. American Medical Association.)

Cheek	2	Shoulder	3
Ear	2	Back	9
Neck	1	Flank and hip	4
Buttock	1	Dorsolateral thigh[a]	7

In addition to these, a few cases of midline thoracic or abdominal breast tissue have been described. These may represent displacement of the milk line anlage, or they may be true ectopia. The only naturally occurring mammae in the midline are found in opossums.

Structure of Supernumerary Mammary Organs.
Not all supernumerary mammary structures deserve to be called breasts. Any combination of one, two, or all three of the elements of the normal breast glandular tissue, areola, and nipple may be present. The presence of entire extra breasts is referred to as *polymastia*, whereas the presence of extra nipples only is called *polythelia*. While these terms are useful, the division by Kajava and his associates (95) into eight types, although cumbersome, gives a greater understanding of the actual clinical findings. We have modified the headings:

---

[a]In one South American rodent, *Lagastomus*, the dorsolateral thigh is the normal location.

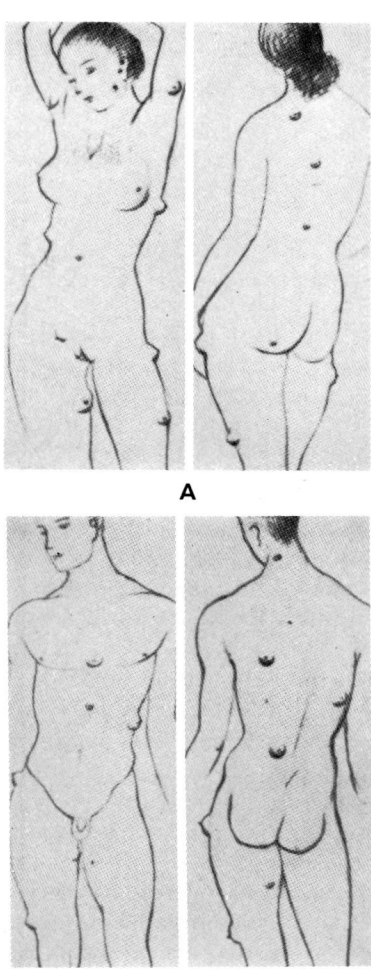

B

Figure 16.32. Ectopic breast tissue. **A,** Reported sites in women. **B,** Reported sites in men. (From De Cholnoky T. Supernumerary breasts. Arch Surg 1939;39:926–941. Copyright 1939. American Medical Association.)

1. *Polymastia*
   a. Complete breast with glandular tissue, areola, and nipple
   b. Glandular tissue with nipple only
   c. Glandular tissue with areola only
   d. Glandular tissue without nipple or areola
2. *Pseudomammae*
   a. Nipple and areola, deeper swelling of fat only, and no glandular tissue
3. *Polythelia*
   a. Nipple only
   b. Areola only
   c. Patch of hair only (*polythelia pilosa*)

The polythelias are the most common. They occasionally may be found on a normal breast, and an accessory nipple may even lie within the areola of a normal breast, although this is rare.

Pseudomammae may be indistinguishable from lipomas, and even after removal and sectioning their exact nature may be in doubt (96).

Number of Supernumerary Mammary Organs.
About 60 to 65% of affected individuals have a single supernumerary organ; 30 to 35% have two; 3.5 to 4% have three; and 1.5 to 2% have four. Reports have included a male and a female with eight, a female with nine (94), and two females with ten supernumerary structures (97).

Associated Anomalies. Polymastia and polythelia are not usually accompanied by other congenital defects. Curiously left-handedness appears to be more frequent among individuals with supernumerary breasts (98).

The association between the number of nipples and litter size in mammals has inevitably led to an investigation of the frequency of multiple births among women with supernumerary breasts. Leichtenstern (99) and Iwai (100) concluded that the incidence of twin births in polymastic women was higher than normal, but later investigators have been less convinced (101). There is no physiologic reason why there should be a connection. Bell's multinippled sheep bred for twinning have been cited, but it has been shown that there is no genetic linkage between twinning and the number of nipples (102). Haagensen (103) stated that these anomalies occur in about 1% of all females, and inheritance is responsible.

Embryogenesis. The location of mammary tissue in mammals is determined by continued development of specific portions of the embryonic milk line and suppression of other portions. What controls which part of the milk line will persist is unknown, but the site or sites are relatively constant for each mammalian species. In the 19th century, under the influence of Darwinism, supernumerary breasts were considered atavistic, implying a "throwback" to the condition found in an evolutionary ancestral form. True atavism, representing a rarely expressed but still present gene, is not common, but examples—such as the occasional appearance of lateral toes in horses—are known. There is little reason to believe that multiple breasts fall into this category. No immediate human ancestor possessed them.

As with some other structures in the body, the definite appearance of the normal breasts suppresses the development of the remainder of the potential breast-forming tissue. Failure of this suppression mechanism permits the development of breast tissue in other parts of the line. This presumably occurs during the sixth week of development. That the suppression mechanism is only weakened, not entirely abolished, is evident from the fact that accessory breasts are frequently very small and are always smaller than the normal breasts. Usually only the epidermal structures are formed (polythelia), and little or no secretory parenchyma appears.

While accessory breasts may be explained in the context of developmental patterns, ectopic breasts on the neck, the ear, the back, and the buttock are not so easily accounted for. Efforts have been made to deny the existence of such structures, especially those described in the 18th and 19th centuries. While some cases may be apocryphal, there are enough well-documented cases that they cannot be disregarded.

Excellent descriptions of these cases may be found in Deaver and McFarland's text (85). These rare but striking cases are explicable only on the basis that mammary glands are related to sweat glands and apocrine glands. Von Saar (104) long ago showed that a complete series of epidermal glands exists, starting from small, coiled sweat glands and passing through apocrine sweat glands and glands of Montgomery to culminate in mammary glands. With this view, the skin everywhere on the body has the necessary tissues for mammary gland formation and lacks only the local organizer. Champneys (105), in fact, put forward the theory that these ectopic breasts are actually enlarged sweat glands and not true breasts. It is interesting to note that the patient of Fraser (87), who had no breasts, also had no axillary apocrine glands. How the stimulus for mammary gland formation can act in ectopic locations, even though the potentiality for glandular development may be present in the skin, remains as great a mystery as it ever was.

Moore (106) believes that supernumerary breasts and nipples most likely develop from displaced segments of the mammary zygotes.

History. Although known since antiquity, supernumerary breasts were long considered to be a freak of nature, more comic than tragic. Geoffroy St. Hilaire (107) in 1836 first suggested a phylogenetic explanation for accessory breasts. Leichtenstern (99) in 1878 collected 105 cases, and the following year Bruce (108) in England collected 61 cases among 3956 hospital patients. Von Bardeleben (109) studied polymastia in males. Among German military conscripts, he found more than 8500, which he tabulated anatomically and geographically in 1893. Williams (110) in 1891 reviewed the subject in English. In 1907 Iwai (91, 100) published two papers in *Lancet*, describing 1680 cases of supernumerary breasts in Japanese men and women. Deaver and McFarland (85) thoroughly reviewed the entire literature up to 1918, noting 10,895 cases. No comparable effort has been made since that time.

Incidence. As our previous statements have implied, supernumerary breasts are not uncommon. Kajava and his associates (95) found an incidence of 2.8% in Finland. Iwai (91) estimates a 4% incidence among Japanese. Speert (101) concluded that the actual incidence was closer to 1%. However, because of its known familial tendency, it may be higher in some geographic areas than in others. Cellini and Offidani (111) reported three cases of supernumerary breasts in the same family.

Iwai (91) found a predominance of females in his series and stated that the incidence was 1.68% for males and 5.19% for females. Kajava (95) believed from his survey of Finns that more males than females were affected. The fact that, in males, supernumerary breasts are asymptomatic and are usually mistaken for moles makes their detection difficult. Conversely, the relative ease with which large numbers of unclothed males may be examined at recruiting centers provides a larger sampling of males. The true sex ratio is at present unknown.

Most writers agree that, when they are unilateral, supernumerary breasts are more frequently found on the left than on the right. Among von Bardeleben's (109) male recruits, 31% had bilateral accessory breasts; in 30%, the right side only was affected; and in 39%, the left side only was affected. Among Japanese males, 53% were found on the left side, and among females, 51.5% were on the left.

Subhuman primates are equally subject to polymastia. Speert (101) found a 1.4% incidence among 1000 Rhesus monkeys examined. Old and New World monkeys, as well as gibbons, orangutans, and chimpanzees, have been reported with supernumerary breasts (112).

Symptoms. Unless glandular tissue is present, there are no symptoms. Where glandular tissue exists, enlargement may lead to discovery in the female at puberty. More often, swelling in late pregnancy is the presenting complaint. If a nipple is present, milk is secreted; if not (polymastia type 3 or 4), the accessory breast may become painful until involution takes place. In nonpregnant women, there may be a tender mass, which becomes more painful before each menstrual period.

In men, no symptoms are present, and accessory breasts may be considered to be moles. In a few cases, pseudomammae may cause embarrassment and require removal for cosmetic reasons (96).

Diagnosis. The diagnosis is not always easy. An axillary tail of a normal breast may appear to be an axillary accessory breast. Elsewhere in the body, a lipoma or even a fibroma may simulate a breast. The situation is further confused by the fact that the lipoma may actually have a core of breast tissue. In other cases an areola and a nipple may be associated with a lipoma containing no glandular tissue. Such pseudomammae may be quite equivocal (96). Especially in the male, one might have great difficulty in deciding the nature of pigmented areas in the thorax along the embryonic milk line. Fortunately, recognition is usually of little clinical importance.

We do not know how to explain embryologically or endocrinologically the peculiar phenomenon of asymmetry.

Several combinations can take place, such as small breast occurs with large breast; both breasts are very large; both breasts are atrophic but not absent; very small atrophic breasts occur with an underdeveloped breast.

This type of classification is done with one purpose only: not to confuse but to remind the reader about these possible anomalies with their possible combinations.

Differential Diagnosis. Rule out giant fibroadenoma.

Treatment. Accessory or ectopic breast tissues should be removed because of the discomfort of periodic swelling (in females) and because of the frequency with which such structures undergo neoplastic changes, as well as for cosmetic reasons.

Augmentation mammoplasty or reduction mammoplasty are employed for psychologic and cosmetic reasons.

Abdominal Defects

CLASSIFICATION

The terminology of the abnormal conditions in which some portion of the viscera of the newborn infant lies outside the abdominal cavity is by no means agreed upon. Some who have complained most about the ambiguities of nomenclature have themselves further confused the picture.

A convenient and embryologically sound terminology is that originally proposed by Moore and Stokes (113):

1. Umbilical Hernia. This is essentially an enlarged umbilical ring. The slightly protruding viscera are covered with normal skin.

2. Omphalocele (Exomphalos, Amniocele). The opening is bound by the umbilical ring, which may be very large. Herniation is into the umbilical cord. The covering of the viscera is a thin avascular membrane derived from the covering of the cord. The cord inserts onto the apex of the hernial sac or onto its remnants.

3. Gastroschisis. The defect is not continuous with the umbilical ring, the cord being inserted normally. No hernial sac is present, and the intestines usually are imbedded in a gelatinous mass.

4. Intussusception at the Umbilicus. The umbilical ring may be normal, but Meckel's diverticulum is patent. The intestinal mass consists of ileum, which has prolapsed through the patent diverticulum. The extraabdominal intestine is everted, with the mucosal surface to the outside. No sac is present.

SURGICAL ANATOMY OF THE UMBILICAL REGION

In a study of the umbilical region, Orda and Nathan (114) found that in most individuals (74%), the round ligament of the liver passed over the superior margin of the umbilical ring and crossed the ring to attach to the inferior margin (Fig. 16.33, *A*). In about one-fourth of subjects, the round ligament bifurcated and attached to the superior

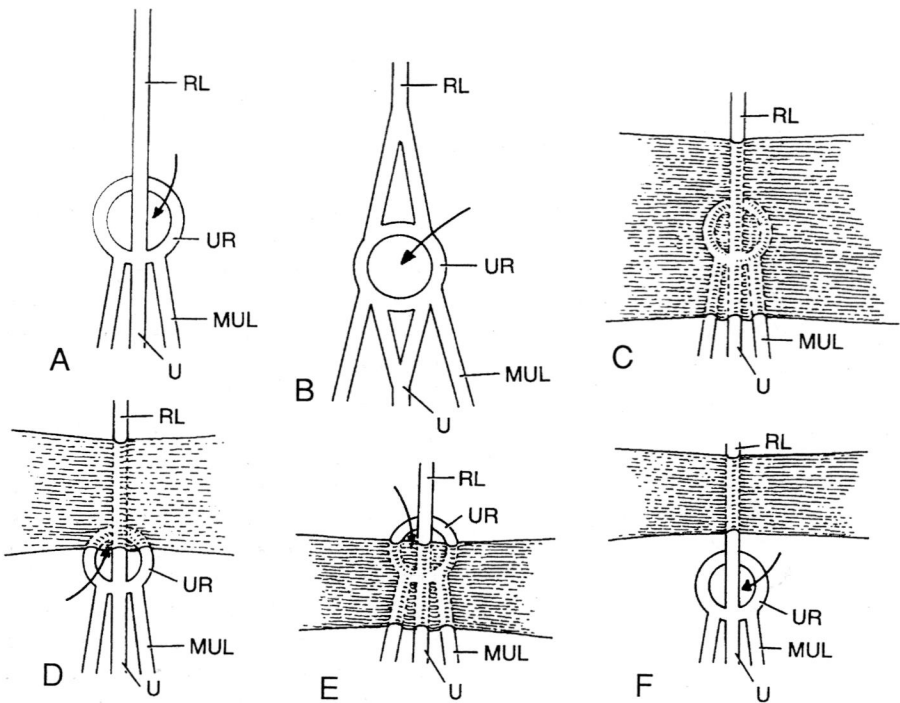

Figure 16.33. Variations in the umbilical ring and the umbilical fascia as seen from the posterior (peritoneal) surface of the body wall. *Arrows* indicate:

A. Usual relations (74%) of the umbilical ring (*UR*), the round ligament (*RL*), the urachus (U), and the medial umbilical ligaments (*MUL*). The round ligament crosses the umbilical ring to insert on its inferior margin.

B. Less-common configuration (24%). The round ligament splits and is attached to the superior margin of the umbilical ring.

C. The thickened transversalis fascia which forms the umbilical fascia covers the umbilical ring (36%).

D. The umbilical fascia covers only the superior portion of the umbilical ring (38%).

E. The umbilical fascia covers only the inferior portion of the umbilical ring (6%).

F. Though present, the umbilical fascia does not underlie the umbilical ring (4%). The fascia is entirely absent in 16%.

(From Orda R, Nathan H. Surgical anatomy of the umbilical structures. Int Surg 1973;58(7):454–464.)

margin of the ring (Fig. 16.33, *B*). In such cases the floor of the ring was formed by transversalis fascia and peritoneum only.

The floor of the umbilical ring may be further strengthened by a thickening of the transversalis fascia in this area, the fascia umbilicalis. This thickened fascia may cover the umbilical ring entirely (Fig. 16.33, *C*) or partially (Fig. 16.33, *D* and *E*). It may fail to cover the ring (Fig. 16.33, *F*). It was completely absent in 16% of specimens.

There are thus two structures, the round ligament and the fascia umbilicalis, that protect the umbilical area. If both are absent (Fig. 16.33, *B* and *F*), the floor of the umbilical ring is relatively unsupported. Herniation through such a ring has been called "direct" umbilical hernia by Orda and Nathan (114).

Where the umbilical fascia partly covers the ring (Fig. 16.33, *D* and *E*), the superior or inferior edge may form a fold or recess through which a hernia may occur. Such an "indirect" umbilical hernia descends into the umbili-

cal ring from a superior fascial fold or ascends into the ring from an inferior fold. A combination of the variations shown in Figures 16.33, *B, D,* and *E* would appear to predispose the individual to herniation through the umbilical ring. Far from supporting the ring in such cases the umbilical fascia may predispose the individual to hernia.

ANATOMY OF THE UMBILICAL CORD

The covering of the umbilical cord at its junction with the body is a simple epithelium continuous distally with the amnion and proximally with the skin. At term the cord contains the stroma of the embryonic connective tissue (Wharton's jelly) as well as the following structures: *(a)* two umbilical arteries; *(b)* one left umbilical vein; and *(c)* vestige of the allantoic duct (urachus) (Fig. 16.34 and Table 16.2).

These structures pass through the abdominal wall at the umbilical ring, an opening in the linea alba about 1 cm in diameter (Figs. 16.35 to 16.37).

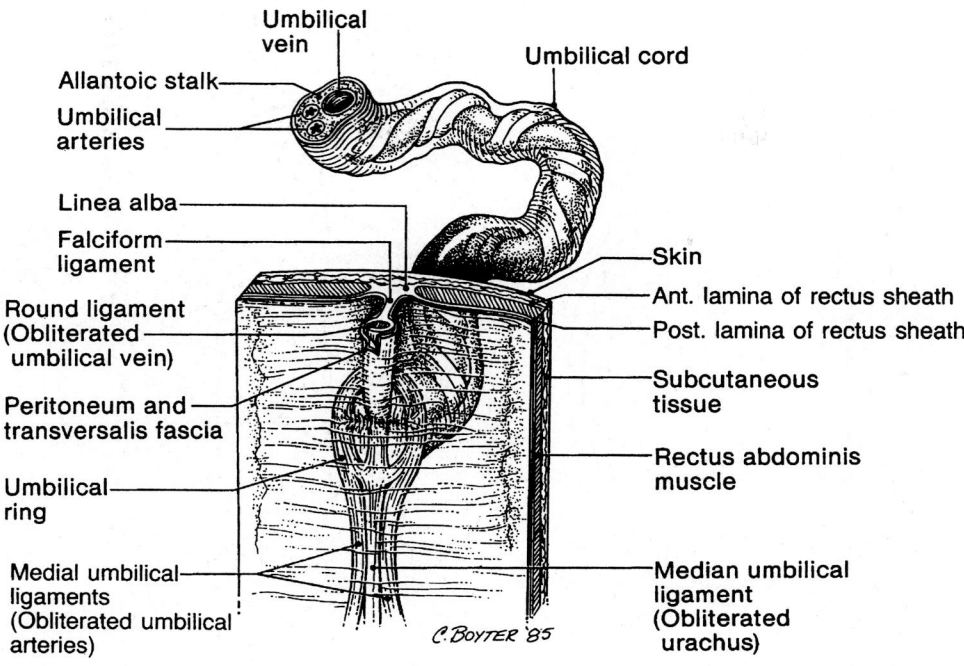

Figure 16.34. Surgical anatomy of the umbilical region. The posterior surface of the anterior abdominal wall of a newborn infant is seen from inside the abdomen. The umbilical cord is still attached. The medial umbilical ligaments (obliterated umbilical arteries) and the urachus (obliterated allantoic duct) participate in the formation of the fibrous umbilical ring. The round ligament (obliterated umbilical vein) arises from the inferior margin of the ring and passes superiorly in the falciform ligament. (From Skandalakis JE, Gray SW, Mansberger AR Jr, Colborn GL, Skandalakis LJ. Hernia: surgical anatomy and technique. New York: McGraw-Hill, 1989.)

Table 16.2.
Structures Associated with the Umbilical Cord and Umbilicus

In the Primitive Body Stalk	At the Umbilicus at Term	In the Neonatal Abdomen	Pathology
Yolk stalk (vitelline duct)	Absent or vestigial	Absent	Meckel's diverticulum or umbilical sinus or fistula
Extraembryonic celom	Absent	None	
Herniated intestine	Returned to abdomen	Returned to abdomen	Failure of return: omphalocele
Vitelline arteries	Absent	Celiac, superior, and inferior mesenteric arteries	
Vitelline veins	Absent	Part of portal vein	
Allantois	Absent or vestigial	Urachus (median umbilical ligament)	Patent urachus; undescended bladder
Umbilical arteries	Both present	Medial umbilical ligaments	Single umbilical artery (1%)
Umbilical veins	Only left vein present	Round ligament in falciform ligament	
Undifferentiated mesenchyme	Embryonic connective tissue at cord	None	

From Skandalakis JE, Gray SW, Mansberger AR Jr, Colborn GL, Skandalakis LJ. Hernia. New York: McGraw-Hill 1989.

UMBILICAL HERNIA

Anatomy. The most minor of the congenital defects at the umbilicus is umbilical hernia. The umbilical ring is slightly enlarged, but the protruding abdominal contents are covered with normal skin (Fig. 16.38). Rarely is there obstruction of a trapped intestinal loop, even though the ring may be as much as 4 cm in diameter.

The anatomic entities associated with the umbilical area are as follows:

1. Median umbilical ligament (obliterated urachus)
2. Medial umbilical ligaments (obliterated umbilical arteries)
3. Lateral umbilical folds containing inferior (deep) epigastric vessels

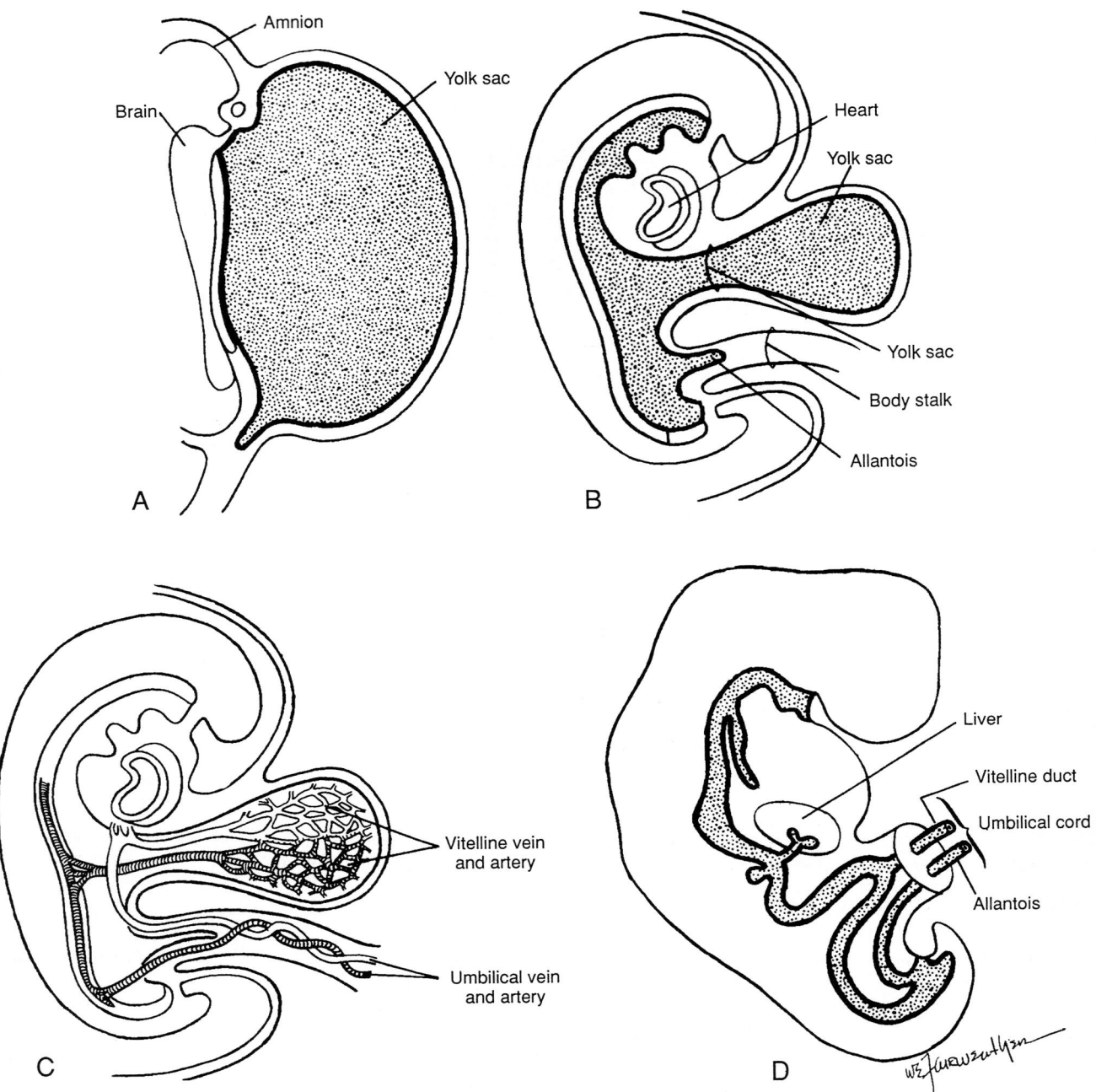

Figure 16.35. Development of umbilical cord. **A,** Embryonic disk. Yolk sac in contact with entire ventral surface. **B,** Ventral attachment of yolk sac narrowed and lengthened as a result of folding of embryo. Intracelomic portion of yolk sac forms gut. Allantois buds from hindgut into body stalk. **C,** Vitelline and umbilical vessels develop in yolk and body stalks, respectively. **D,** Yolk and body stalks fused into umbilical cord. Development of abdominal wall narrows umbilical ring. (From Shaw A. Disorders of the umbilicus. In: Welch KJ, Randolph JG, Ravitch MM, O'Neill JA Jr, Rowe MI, eds. Pediatric surgery, 4th ed. Chicago: Year Book Medical Publishers, 1986.)

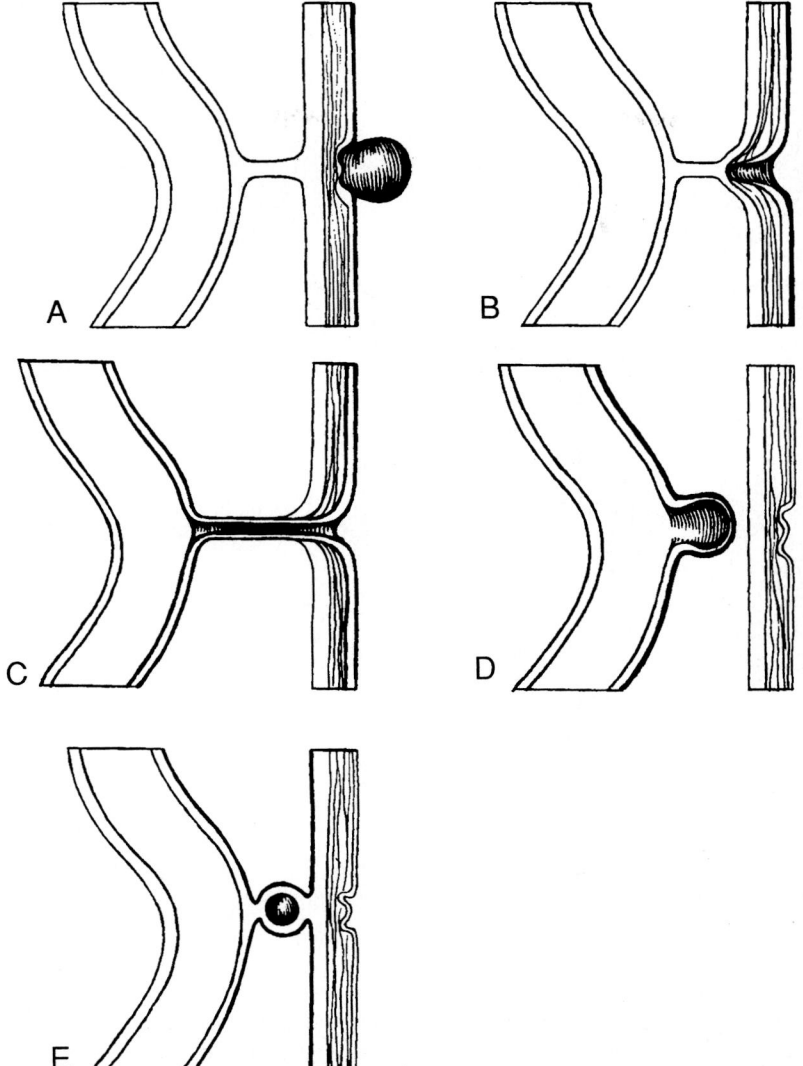

Figure 16.36. Vestiges of vitelline (omphalomesenteric) duct. **A,** mucosal polyp (with band from bowel to umbilicus). **B,** Sincus. **C,** Fistula. **D,** Meckel's diverticulum. **E,** Cyst. (From Shaw A. Disorders of the umbilicus. In: Welch KJ, Randolph JG, Ravitch MM, O'Neill JA Jr, Rowe MI, eds. Pediatric surgery, 4th ed. Chicago: Year Book Medical Publishers 1986.)

4. Falciform ligament
5. Round ligament (left umbilical vein) at the free edge of the falciform ligament
6. Umbilical fascia (thickening of the transversalis fascia)

The etiology of the umbilical hernia is embryologic as well as anatomic, with anomalies and variations of the anatomic entities "guarding" the umbilicus.

Embryogenesis. The defect is in the failure of the recti to approximate in the midline after the return of the intestines to the abdomen. Small umbilical herniae usually spontaneously regress as the infant grows. Halpern (115) reported that 81% of herniae under 1 cm in diameter, and 56% of larger herniae, disappear spontaneously in untreated patients.

Remember that umbilical hernia is a secondary umbilical herniation, whereas omphalocele is retention of the primary herniation of the midgut.

Incidence. Umbilical hernia has been estimated to be present in 18.5% of white infants (116) and in 42.3% of black infants (117).

However, Blumberg (118) stated that the difference in occurrence between black and white babies is very small. The condition is more frequent in premature infants, twins, and those with long umbilical cords (116). Although the sex ratio varies in different series, the sexes are probably equally affected (119).

Symptoms. A painless swelling at the umbilicus, noticed by the mother, is the chief complaint.

Treatment. Spontaneous regression of small umbilical

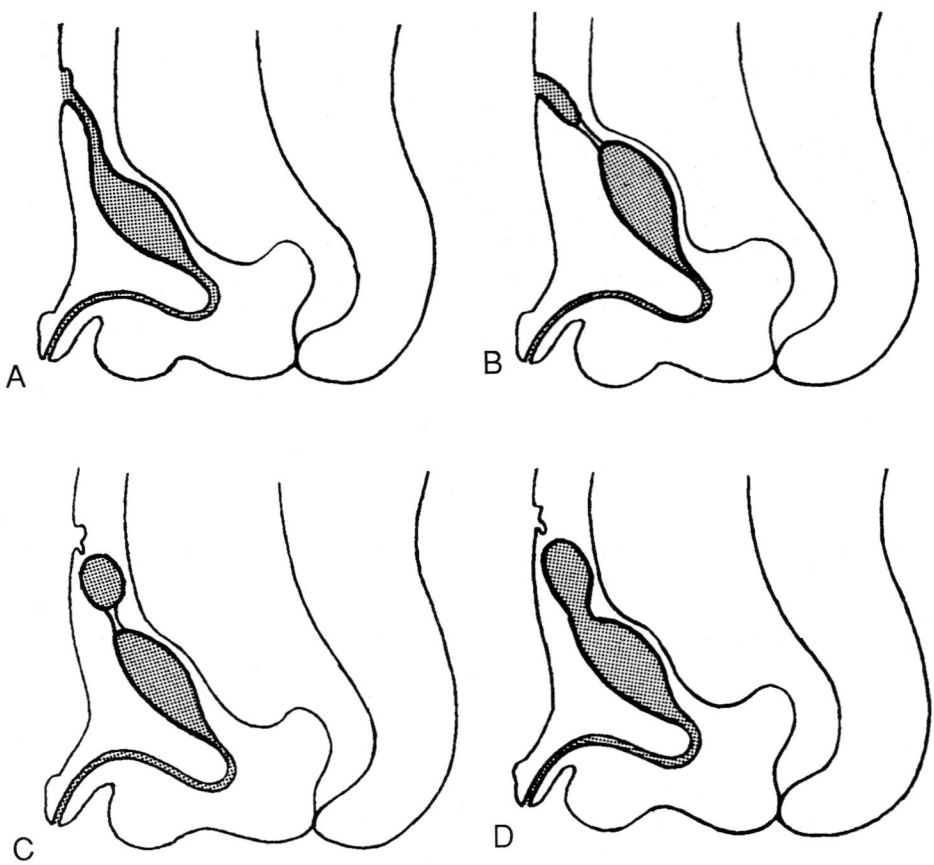

Figure 16.37. Vestiges of urachus. **A,** Fistula. **B,** Sinus. **C,** Cyst. **D,** Bladder diverticulum. (From Shaw A. Disorders of the umbilicus. In: Welch KJ, Randolph JG, Ravitch MM, O'Neil JA Jr, Rowe MI, eds. Pediatric surgery, 4th ed. Chicago: Year Book Medical Publishers, 1986.)

herniae usually occurs by the age of 5 to 6 years. Elective surgical repair is indicated if the hernia has not closed by that time. The rate of spontaneous closure decreases greatly after the fifth or sixth year of life.

OMPHALOCELE (EXOMPHALOS)

Definition. Benson et al. (120) defined omphalocele as herniation through a 4 cm in diameter umbilical and supraumbilical portion of the abdominal wall into a sac formed by peritoneum and amniotic membrane; hernia of the umbilical cord is the same as omphalocele but has a diameter of less than 4 cm and a sac containing intestinal loops.

Etiology. Most researchers ascribe to the original theory of Duhemel (2) which holds omphalocele results from failure of the lateral body wall folds to close. Whether the primary event is failure of body wall closure or failure of the midgut to return to the abdominal cavity is, we think, speculation.

Gross and Blodgett (121) and Ladd and Gross (122) posited an arrest of the development of the abdominal

cavity in the third month of fetal life. Through some mechanism, the midgut is not allowed to return to the abdominal cavity at 10 weeks.

Margulies (123) theorized that abnormal development of the parietes in early embryonal life (3 weeks ?) will not permit the return of the midgut into the peritoneal cavity.

Anatomy. In omphalocele, most or all of the intestine and frequently other abdominal organs lie outside the body in a thin, transparent, avascular sac on the apex of which the umbilical cord inserts. The enlarged umbilical ring, through which the intestines pass, is usually less than 5 cm in diameter but may be as large as 15 cm (Fig. 16.39).

The sac may be small, with only a single loop of intestine, or large, enclosing the stomach, heart, and liver as well as the intestines (124). There is no relationship between the size of the sac and the diameter of the umbilical ring (Fig. 16.40).

Although a sac always is present in omphalocele, it may rupture before or during delivery or postnatally. If no trace of a sac can be found, the defect in the abdominal wall probably was located not at the umbilicus but at the

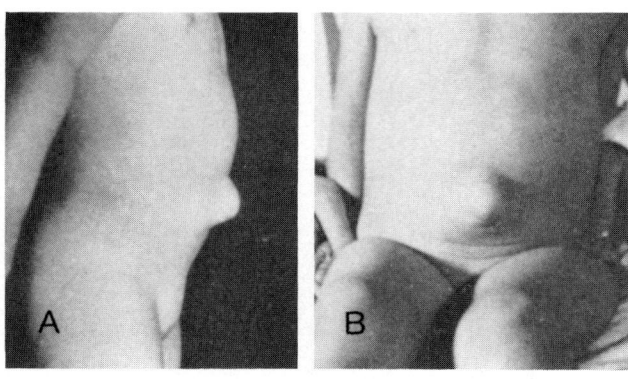

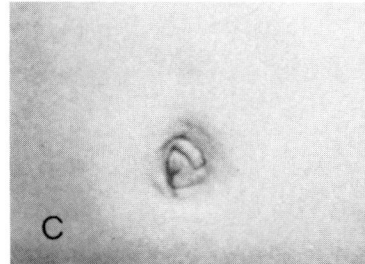

Figure 16.38. **A** and **B,** Umbilical hernia in a 3-year-old boy. Photograph taken after surgical repair. (From Gross RE. The surgery of infancy and childhood. Philadelphia: WB Saunders, 1953.)

congenitally weakened spot in the abdominal musculature (see the section on "Gastroschisis.") Because the sac is thin and without a blood supply, it dries out on exposure to air and is easily ruptured (Fig. 16.41).

In omphalocele, the abdominal cavity is almost always too small to accommodate the mass of eventrated viscera when an attempt is made to replace it, and the lower thorax is less flared than normal.

Associated Anomalies. About 50% or more of infants with omphalocele have other congenital anomalies (121, 125, 126). Anencephaly is present in about 20%. Congenital heart disease, spina bifida, diaphragmatic hernia, and hydrocephalus are not uncommon. Malrotation of the intestines is usual (Table 16.3.)

Greenwald et al. (127) reported that 19.5% of such patients had congenital heart disease, the most common being tetralogy of Fallot, followed by atrial septal defect of the secundum type and other anomalies.

Raffensperger (128), however, reported cardiac anomalies occurred in up to 35% of patients with omphalocele, as did several other defects including the Beckwith-Wiedemann syndrome (umbilical defects, macroglossia, and hypoglycemia).

Abnormal karyotypes are also frequently present

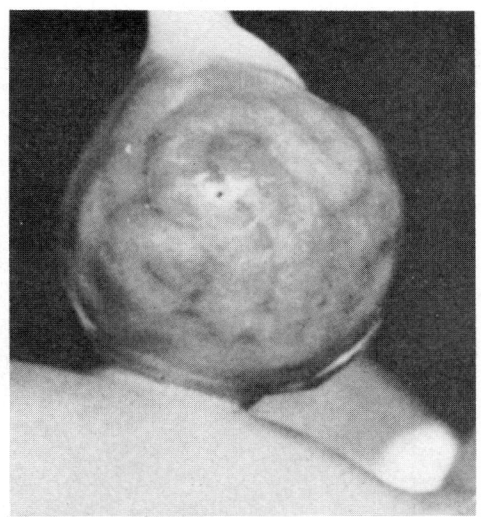

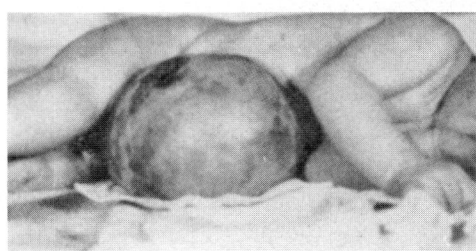

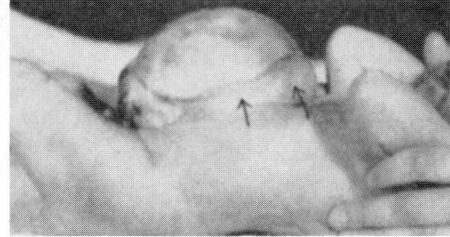

Figure 16.39. Omphalocele. **A,** Newborn infant with an omphalocele in large, transparent sac and a 3-cm defect in the abdominal wall. **B,** Two views of a large omphalocele containing colon, intestines, and a part of the liver. *Arrows* indicate the narrow rim of skin at the base. A two-stage repair was required. (From Gross RE. The surgery of infancy and childhood. Philadelphia: WB Saunders, 1953.)

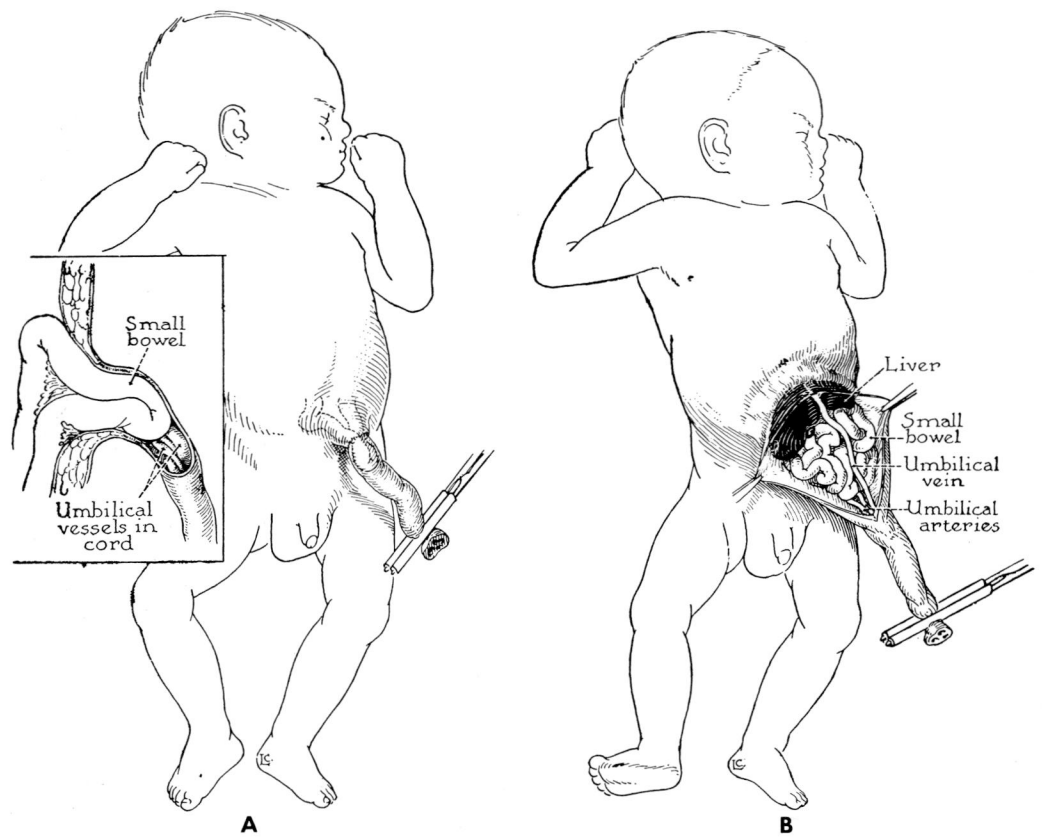

Figure 16.40. Omphalocele. **A,** Small omphalocele, with a single loop of small intestine protruding. **B,** Large omphalocele, containing most of the abdominal viscera. (From Zimmerman LM, Anson BJ. Anatomy and surgery of hernia. Baltimore: Williams & Wilkins, 1967.)

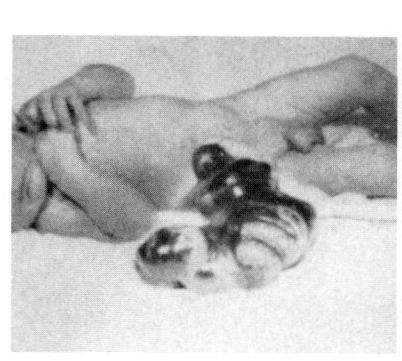
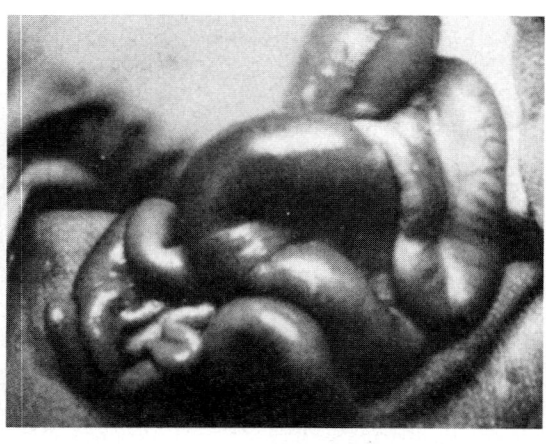

Figure 16.41. Two infants with rupture of the omphalocele sac. **A,** Rupture before birth. Intestines are thickened, edematous, and adherent. **B,** Rupture after delivery. Intestines are smooth, moist, and not adherent. Condition **B** has a better prognosis than that of **A.** (From Gross RE. The surgery of infancy and childhood. Philadelphia: WB Saunders, 1953.)

(129). One of the most severe associated anomalies is the OEIS complex, consisting of an **O**mphalocele, **E**xtrophy of the cloaca, **I**mperforate anus, and **S**pinal defects (130).

The associated anomalies are well recorded by Martin and Torres (131). It is the associated anomalies which determine the prognosis for patients with omphalocele (132).

Embryogenesis. Omphalocele represents developmental arrest at the stage in which the growing intestines are normally herniated into the umbilical cord (page 184).

Table 16.3.
Malformation Associated with Omphaloceles

Type	Number
Gastrointestinal	18
Cardiovascular	15
Genitourinary	15
Central nervous system	9
Diaphragmatic	6
Extremity deformities	5
Ear, nose, and throat	5
Absent sternum	2
Pulmonary	1
Eye	1
Pancreas	1
Imperforate anus	6
Exstrophy of bladder and myelomeningocele	5
Ileal atresia	4
Ileal stenosis	1
Colon atresia	2
Incomplete jejunal wall	1
Partial absence of segment of colon	2
Persistent omphalomesenteric duct	2

From Smith WR, Leix F. Omphalocele. Am J Surg 1966;111:450–456.

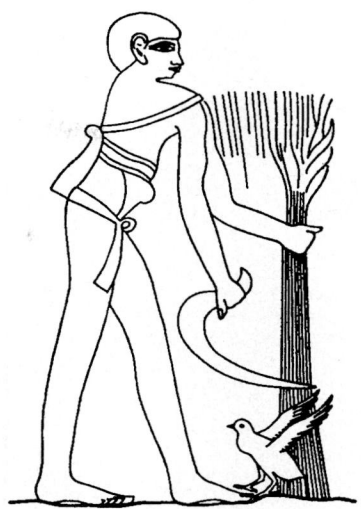

Figure 16.42. Diseased harvester. After a Fifth Dynasty relief from Saqqara. A man suffering from an umbilical hernia and abdominal distension is shown harvesting grain with a long sickle. Bandages are tied around him from the shoulders down around the abdomen and the waist (Courtesy Dr. Ragab, Papyrus Institute, Giza, Egypt).

Return to the abdomen normally occurs in the 10th week. It is this return which has failed to take place or is incomplete in omphalocele. The space in which the eventrated viscera lie is the extraembryonic celom and the sac is the covering of the umbilical cord itself. This covering, three to five cells thick, is similar to and continuous with the upper surface of the placenta, with the amnion distally, and with the skin of the abdomen proximally. The transition to skin is abrupt, and may be part way up the base of the sac. Because the sac is derived from amnion, not from abdominal wall, the term *amniocele* may be applied.

The inadequacy of the abdominal cavity to contain the intestines has been considered to be the cause of their failure to return by Bergglas (133). Most embryologists, however, believe the absence of the visceral mass removes the necessary stimulus for normal growth of the abdominal wall. The fact that about 25% of omphaloceles contain liver, heart, and stomach, which normally are not outside the abdomen during development, has been taken to indicate that the abdominal wall is at fault. On the other hand, there is no pressure on the wall from developing organs as long as the cavity is open anteriorly, so that other viscera may eventually protrude from the defect as they grow in size. We believe the fault lies with failure of the intestines to return to the abdomen, which then would have enlarged sufficiently to contain the intestines had they been present.

Papez (134) described a 61-year-old male cadaver in whom the entire small intestine was contained in a separate sac within the abdominal cavity. He interpreted this to represent the extraembryonic celom surrounded by the covering of the umbilical cord. The entire proximal cord containing the intestines was assumed to have intussuscepted into the abdomen to form an "internal omphalocele" at the time of normal intestinal return. There was no evidence of pathology resulting from the presence of the sac (see Figs. 6.12 and 6.13).

History. Omphalocele and umbilical hernia were familiar to the ancient Egyptians, as indicated by tomb drawings (Figs. 16.42 and 16.43). Reference to omphalocele may be found in Celsus and in Paulus Aegineta (135). Jarcho (136) credits Scarpa (137) with separation of congenital from acquired forms in 1809. Aribat (138) in 1901 collected 160 cases, of which only nine were reported before 1800. Approximately 350 published cases appeared in the literature by 1937 (136). However, because of the high incidence of neonatal mortality in infants with omphalocele, many cases are neither treated nor recorded.

Incidence. Jarcho (136) estimated the incidence of omphalocele at 1:6600 births, but other authors have placed it higher. McKeown and his colleagues (139) placed the incidence at 1:3200 in Birmingham, England, between 1941 and 1951. In the United States, Hebert (140) placed it at 1:1860. Ivy (141) found it to rank 14th among congenital anomalies recognized at birth in Pennsylvania. Several large series have been reported (123, 136). (142, 126) Mahour (143) stated that the incidence is 1:3200 total births or 1:10,000 live births.

When omphalocele is associated with anencephaly, there is a predominance of males, but otherwise the sexes are equally affected. If anencephalic infants are excluded,

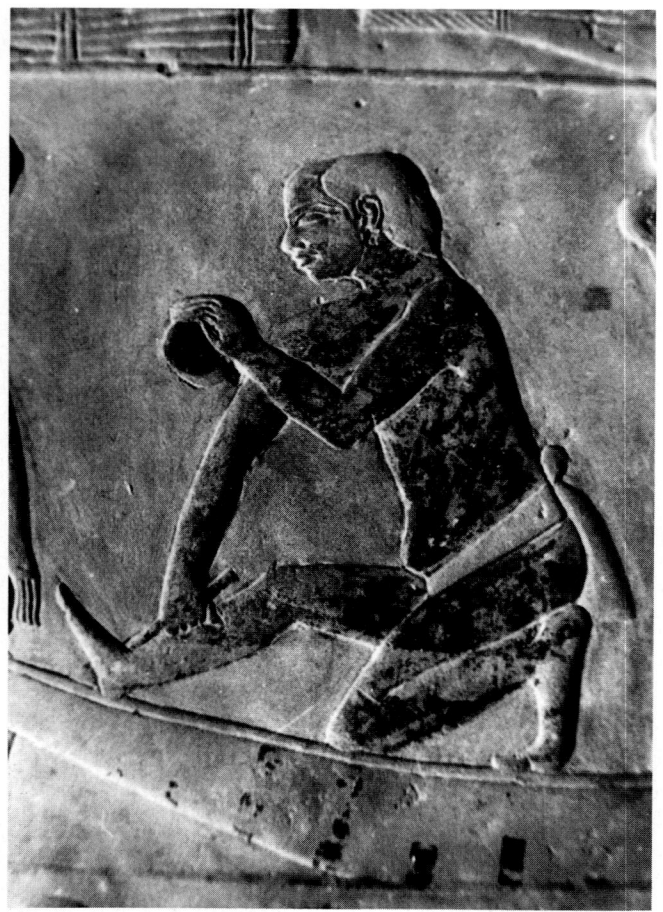

Figure 16.43. Stone cutter with umbilical hernia (Courtesy Omar Askar).

there is a higher incidence among infants of older mothers (139). No familial tendency has been confirmed.

Symptoms. Except for the visible herniation, the infant usually appears normal. There is no evidence of pain or discomfort.

Diagnosis. Omphalocele differs from umbilical hernia in that the intestines are not covered by skin. The condition may be distinguished from gastroschisis because the latter is not exactly in the midline and there is no trace of a sac. In umbilical intussusception, the intestines are turned inside out, while in omphalocele, the serosal surfaces are visible and normal.

Small omphaloceles must be diagnosed before the cord is tied at birth. Cases have been reported in which a portion of protruding intestine has been tied with the cord, with fatal results (144).

Treatment. Omphaloceles may be divided into three groups according to the size of the herniated mass (gastrointestinal tract, liver) and by the treatment required (145).

Small Omphalocele, 2 to 4 cm in Diameter.
This requires reduction and one-stage repair of the fascia and skin.

Medium Omphalocele, 4 to 6 cm in Diameter.
This requires skin closure only, forming a ventral hernia to be closed later.

Gross (146), who first performed this operation in 1948, achieved primary closure of the defect by wide lateral mobilization of the skin, with closure over the unopened sac. This procedure avoids forcing the intestines back into the abdominal cavity. At the second operation, several months or even years later, the redundant peritoneum and skin may be excised, and the rectus fascia may be brought together (Fig. 16.44).

Wide mobilization of skin flaps is no longer recommended since the ventral hernia thus formed grows as the infant grows, making secondary fascial closure difficult. Rather, manual stretching of the abdominal wall, mobilization of a 2-cm skin flap circumferentially, and placement of the viscera into the (stretched out) abdominal cavity with subsequent skin closure, leaving the fascia open, is successful in most cases (147). Closure of the small resultant ventral hernia later is readily accomplished.

Holcomb (148) advocates removal of the sac to free adhesions and to search for anomalies before primary closure. Others advocate leaving the amniotic sac intact and inverting it during repair of the defect (149, 150).

Massive Omphalocele, 7 to 10 cm in Diameter.
In this defect, the abdominal cavity is inadequate. A prosthetic "chimney" or "silo" may need to be constructed if the method described above is not possible.

A massive omphalocele can contain parts of the liver, stomach, pancreas, spleen, transverse colon, or urinary bladder, in addition to the small intestine. These organs cannot be placed into the inadequate abdominal cavity. A prosthetic "chimney" or "silo" must be constructed to contain them. Gentle, continuing pressure must be applied to stimulate enlargement of the space within the abdominal cavity (Figs. 16.45 and 16.46).

Remember that the abdominal cavity is usually too small to receive the herniated mass all at once. Forcible attempts to reduce the hernia may result in fatal respiratory embarrassment from pressure on the diaphragm or reduced venous return to the heart due to compression of the inferior vena cava (Fig. 16.47).

Conservative Treatment.
In Italy, conservative treatment for large, unruptured omphaloceles has been advocated by Soave (151). Under sterile dressings, the sac hardens and then epithelializes over the course of 2 to 3 months, by which time the abdomen has enlarged sufficiently to contain the intestines. Among the 25 cases reported, 5 died without treatment;

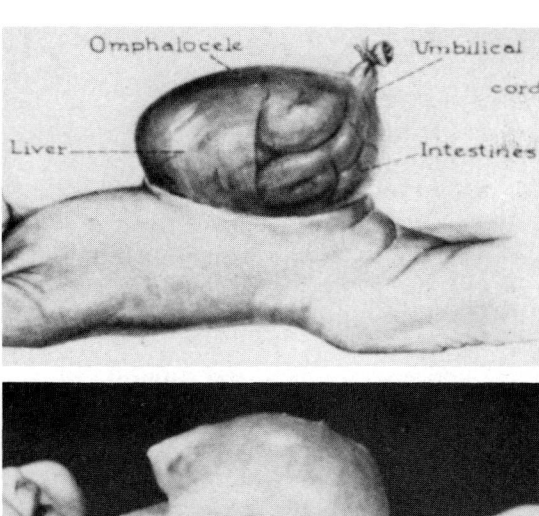
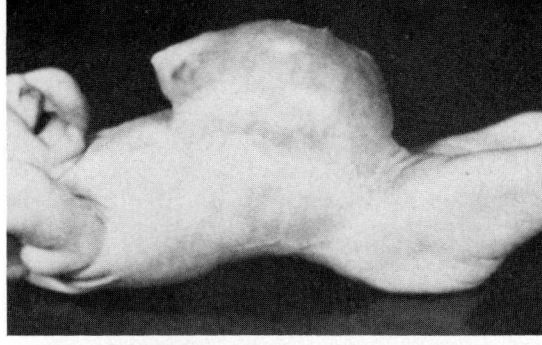
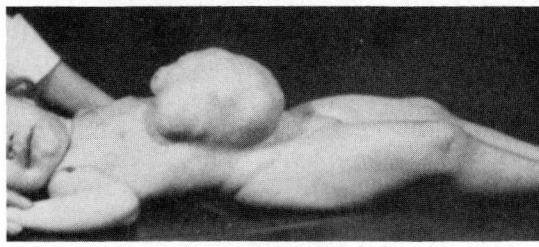
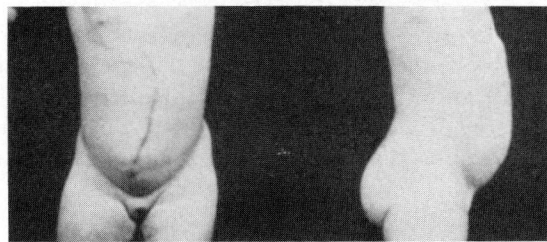

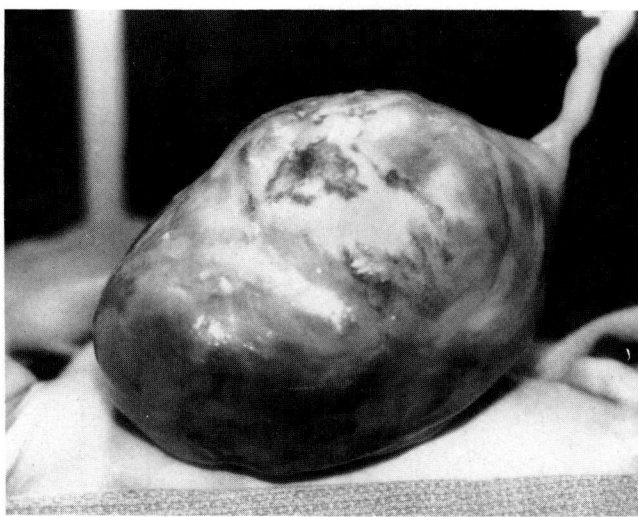

Figure 16.45. Giant omphalocele demonstrating the herniated viscera including liver and intestines within a sac with the umbilical cord coming of the apex of the sac.

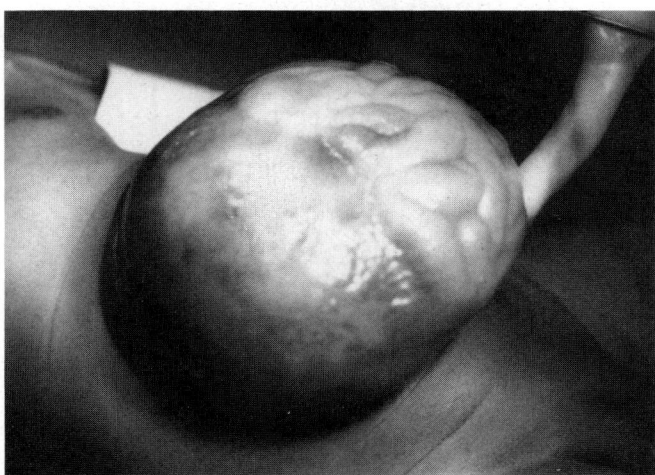

Figure 16.46. Giant omphalocele demonstrating the herniated viscera including liver and intestines within a sac with the umbilical cord coming of the apex of the sac.

Figure 16.44. Repair of omphalocele in two stages. **A,** Original lesion at birth. The presenting visceral mass is about the same size or a little larger than the abdominal cavity of the infant. **B,** The condition 2 weeks after closure of skin at the first operation. **C,** The condition 9 months after the first operation and just prior to the second operation. **D,** The condition 2 months after the second operation. (From Gross RE. The surgery of infancy and childhood. Philadelphia: WB Saunders, 1953.)

14 were treated surgically, with 7 deaths; and 6 were treated conservatively, with no deaths. This is the treatment of choice for infants with huge omphaloceles or for those who have other life-threatening or chromosomal defects.

Mortality and Prognosis. The earliest successful repair has been credited to Visick (152). Prior to 1900 there were 47 recoveries (69%) among 68 cases treated with radical surgery. From 1900 to 1930, 69 patients (76%) among 91 surgical cases recovered (136). Gross (146) reported a 66% survival rate among his cases between 1940 and 1950. These figures, however, represent selected cases and cannot be taken as the general prognosis. Fully 50% of affected infants are stillborn (139), and of those born living, more than 54% have other serious congenital defects.

Omphalocele is a real emergency. Mortality rises sharply with delay. Among cases collected by O'Leary and

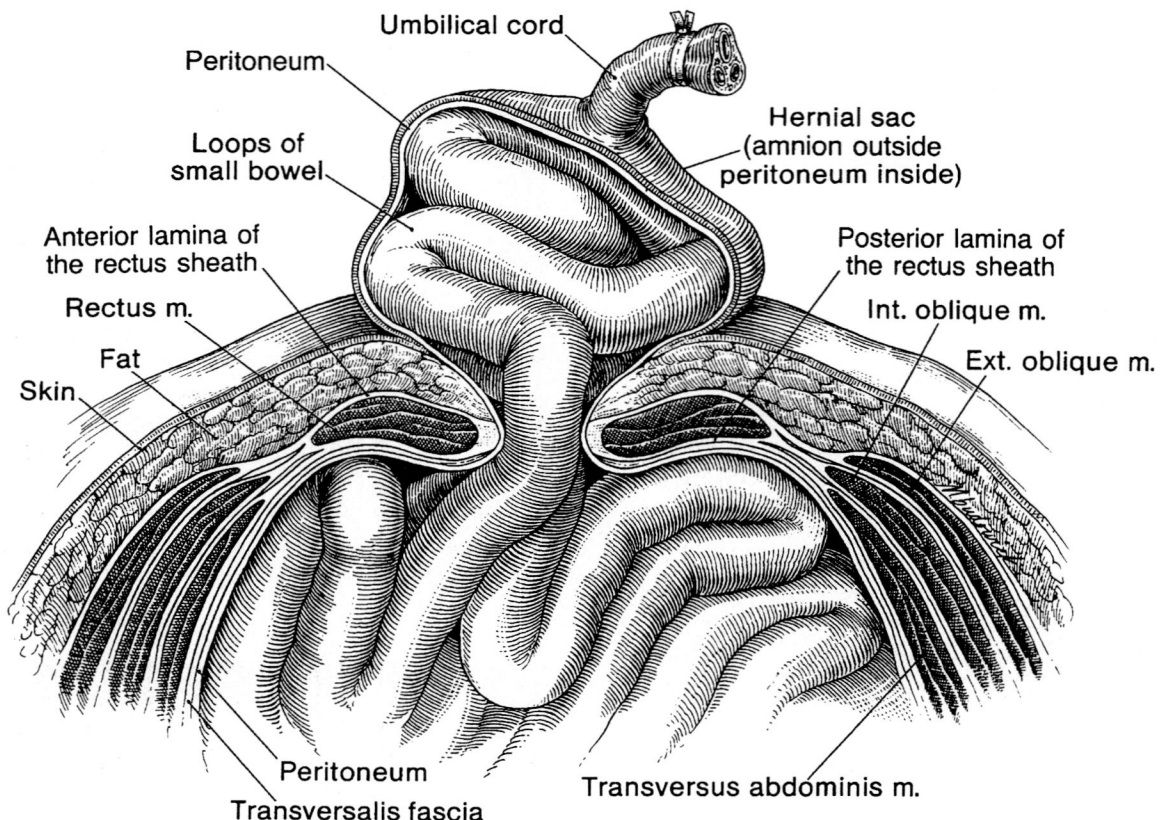

Figure 16.47. Diagram of a sagittal section through a small omphalocele. The herniated viscera are covered with a vascular amnion continuous with the skin of the abdominal wall. Care must be taken to avoid rupture of the sac. . (From Skandalakis JE, Gray SW, Mansberger AR Jr, Colborn CL, Skandalakis LJ. New York: McGraw-Hill, 1989.)

Clymer (153), the mortality was 21.4% in infants operated on within 12 hours after birth, 44% in those operated on between 12 and 24 hours after birth, and 61.6% in those operated on after 36 hours.

Mortality increases also as birth weight decreases (154) and as the size of the defect increases. Similar reports were presented by Moore and Nur (155), Stringel and Filler (156), Mayer et al. (157) and Schwartzberg et al. (158).

Rupture of the sac was once considered to be fatal, but since 1949 some patients have been saved. Smith and Leix (126) reported survival in eight of 32 patients. Similar survival has been reported in England in patients with postnatal rupture of the sac (142). Prenatal rupture carries a much poorer prognosis.

Raffensperger (128) found a 35% mortality with massive omphaloceles and a 17% mortality in small omphaloceles.

GASTROSCHISIS

Anatomy. Gastroschisis resembles omphalocele, but there is neither a sac nor a trace of one. The defect is not at the umbilicus and usually is found to the right of the midline. The margins of the defect are smooth and it may be several centimeters in diameter. In one patient (159) there was more than one defect. The herniated intestinal loops are cyanosed, leathery, and embedded in a gelatinous material. The intestine is grossly shortened, without normal rotation (Fig. 16.48). Gastroschisis may be associated with other severe defects in stillborn monsters, but it is usually the only anomaly in live affected infants (Fig. 16.49).

Embryogenesis. "And now at the beginning of the 20th century, there are so many cases of gastroschisis on record that the mere task of collecting all of the references is arduous," wrote Ballantyne (160) in 1904.

Fifty years later Moore and Stokes (113) reported that the defect is extraumbilical and without a sac. In 1963 Moore (161) collected 31 cases from the literature.

We agree with Schuster (162) that the developmental anatomy of gastroschisis is based on speculation.

In the first edition of this book, we stated that "the defect lies in the failure of the musculature migrating from the dorsal myotomes completely to invade the splanchnopleure of the embryonic abdominal wall." We accept the criticism of Schuster (162), who showed that the rectus muscle should present more diastasis and per-haps a defect.

As a matter of fact, we had the opportunity to dissect a stillborn baby with Dr. Gray. The umbilicus was found

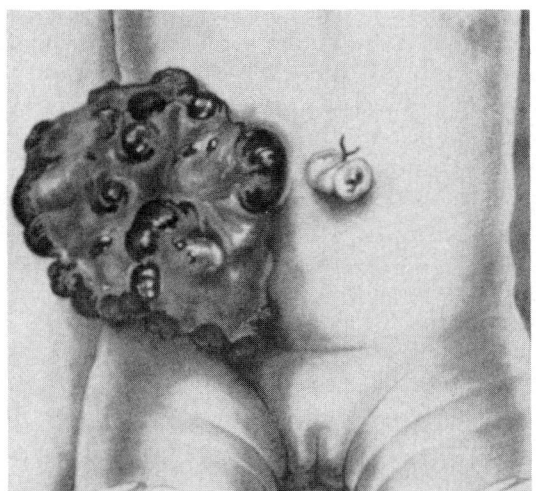

Figure 16.48. Gastroschisis. The intestinal loops are leathery and embed-ded in gelatinous material. In this patient, there were multiple intestinal atresias. Observe that the lesion is not in the midline. (From Moore TC, Stokes GE. Gas-troschisis; report of two cases treated by modification of Gross operation for omphalocele. Surgery 1953;33:112–120.)

intact. There was a small hole in the skin close to the umbilicus on the left, from which loops of small bowel protruded without sac.

The abdominal wall beneath the recti was normal, but the defect was close to the midline and therefore close to the umbilicus in the aponeurosis approaching the midline. A strip of normal skin was noticed, forming a bridge-like formation between the umbilicus and the "hole."

"The abdominal wall muscles are normally formed in a newborn with omphalocele or gastroschisis," according to Schuster (162).

Still there are many questions to be answered about the embryology and the topographic anatomy of the defect. How does the defect develop and why? Is the bowel eviscerated and never returned to the peritoneal cavity, as in intrauterine catastrophe? How does the par-aumbilical defect develop? Is there any way to reconstruct the crime? The authors are afraid not.

Is Shaw (163) correct with his "myth of gastroschisis," Duhamel (2) with his teratogenic actions, or perhaps Noordijk and Bloemsma-Jonkman (164) with "gastros-chisis: no myth"? There are several postulations but none satisfy the author. Gastroschisis is an enigmatic clinical entity. Various environmental teratogens, risk factors, and maternal demographic and reproductive factors have

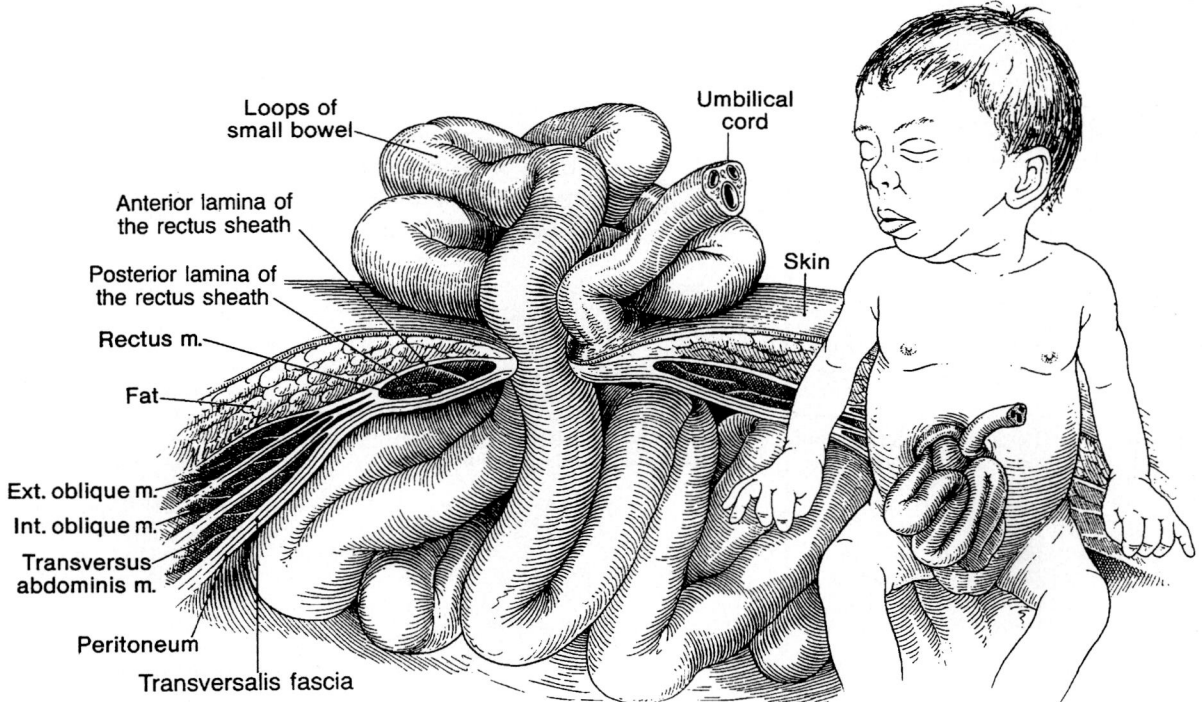

Figure 16.49. Diagram of gastroschisis—parasagittal section. Diagram of a parasagittal section through a patient with gastroschisis. The defect lies to the right of the insertion of the umbilical cord. The herniated mass is usually composed of small intestine only. There is no sac. (From Skandalakis JE. et al. Hernia. New York: McGraw-Hill, 1989.)

been implicated in the etiology of gastroschisis (165–167), but none is conclusive.

History and Incidence. Gastroschisis is rare. Moore and Stokes (113) found only five cases, while Simpson and

Caylor (168) were able to collect 16. Rickham (169) added 13 cases in 1963. The earliest identifiable case is that of Calder (170), who in 1733 described herniated intestines in an infant with the "navel entire, and a perforation half an inch above it, through which the guts had fallen out. . . ." Bernstein (171) considered that five cases had been reported before Calder's, the earliest being that in Lycosthenes in 1557. While it is possible these were cases of gastroschisis, their descriptions leave much doubt.

This defect is more frequent in male infants. It is also known to occur in domestic animals (172).

Having in mind the works of Randolph (173), Moore and Khalid (174), Noordijk and Bloemsma-Jonkman (164), Shaw (163), and Raffensperger (128), we were able to formulate Table 16.4.

The destiny of the abdominal wall depends on the harmonious cooperation of the three embryologic folds—namely, the cephalic, caudal, and lateral folds, which are formed by somatic and splanchnic layers.

The splanchnic layer, by definition, is involved in gut, not body wall, development. Table 16.5 lists splanchnic tissue involved in visceral, not body wall, morphogenesis.

Treatment. The problem is essentially the same as that encountered in omphalocele, and the treatment is the same as for an omphalocele with prenatal rupture of the sac. Watkins (175) has been credited with the first successful repair.

If the fascia and/or skin cannot be primarily closed the treatment is the same procedure used for massive omphalocele with silo or chimney prosthesis (147, 176–179).

Hebra and Ross (180) reported prolonged intestinal dysfunction in children after repair of gastroschisis and advise a waiting period of 3 to 4 months. They stated it would be unwise to be heroic initially with these patients, trying to dissect conglomerate masses of intestinal loops.

Mortality. Of the 16 cases collected from the literature

Table 16.4.
Differences Betweeen Omphalocele and Gastroschisis[a]

Omphalocele	Gastroschisis
Uncommon	Rare
Possible genetic origin	Possible environmental origin
Incomplete fusion of the four somatic plates	Rupture of the cord membrane where attached to the umbilical skin
Avascular sac formed by the peritoneum and amniotic membrane	No hernial sac; bowel is exposed to amniotic fluid
Intestinal rotation with small omphalocele but no rotation with large omphalocele	No intestinal rotation
Most likely none	Inflammatory areas on the loops with severe adhesions
Few associated gastrointestinal malformations	Gastrointestinal malformations present in 14–16%
Liver is attached to the upper surface of the sac and not to the diaphragm	Liver does not participate in the evisceration
74% with severe cardiac or neuromuscular defects	Associated birth defects (except gastrointestinal) rare
Both rectus abdominis muscles are intact	If the defect is on the right side of the abdominal wall, the right rectus abdominis muscle is partially defective; if on the left, the left rectus abdominis muscle is partially defective; left gastroschisis is very rare

[a]NOTE: For all practical purposes, the abdominal wall muscles in both omphalocele and gastrochisis have a normal development since the mesoderm develops normally.

Table 16.5.
Splanchnic Tissue Involved in Visceral Morphogenesis

Folds	Somatic	Splanchnic	Observation
Cephalic (the folds of the foregut)	Thoracic and epigastric wall and septum transversum	Surrounds heart, great vessels, and participates in closure of the foregut	Early failure of somatic layer will produce an upper midline epigastric hernia
			Associated anomalies: diaphragmatic hernia, cardiac anomalies, etc.
Lateral	Surrounds the embryo, forms the wall and the umbilical ring		Failure of fusion = large umbilical ring
	Hypogastric abdominal wall	Closes the hindgut in front	Failure of somatic-hypogastric wall absent; if both layers fail to form, then hypogastric hernia, extrophy of bladder
Caudal (the fold of the hindgut)			

by Simpson and Caylor (168), repair was attempted in 14 and was successful in eight. There were about a dozen survivals reported up to 1963. Two recent series, with over 100 infants each, report an identical survival rate of 88% (147, 176).

Although omphalocele and gastroschisis are frequently discussed together when considering abdominal wall defects in newborns, they are really quite different embryologically and their management and prognosis differs as well (as can be gleaned from reading the previous section. Several reviews compare and contrast the management of these anomalies, to which the reader is referred (181-185).

INTUSSUSCEPTION AT THE UMBILICUS

Prolapse of the ileum through a patent vitelline duct may occasionally resemble other umbilical defects. However, the exteriorized intestine is always everted, with its mucosal side out. If it is large, it is often T-shaped, with two stomata leading to the proximal and the distal intestine, respectively.

Such intussusception through a congenital umbilical fistula also may occur through a fistula produced by clamping a small omphalocele containing an ileal loop or a patent Meckel's diverticulum. It is not always possible to tell whether the prolapse is through a natural, congenital fistula or through a rent in the intestine caused by injury to the umbilical cord (186).

Further discussion of the defect causing intussusception at the umbilicus may be found in Chapter 6, pages 215–216.

Variations in the Muscles of the Lower Abdominal Wall

Because of their relationship to the problem of inguinal hernia, the muscles of the lower abdominal wall have been studied intensively and their variations have been described in detail. The interested reader should consult the papers of Chandler and Schadewald (187) and Kreig (188) and Anson and his colleagues (189). Only brief observations on the more important variations are presented here.

APONEUROTIC CLEFTS OF THE EXTERNAL OBLIQUE LAYER

The lenticular cleft, through which the spermatic cord of the male and the round ligament of the female emerge, varies from little more than a ring at the lowest portion near the body of the pubic bone to a fusiform hiatus extending to the anterosuperior iliac spine itself. The gap was limited to the medial half of Hesselbach's triangle in only 11% of the specimens examined by Anson and his

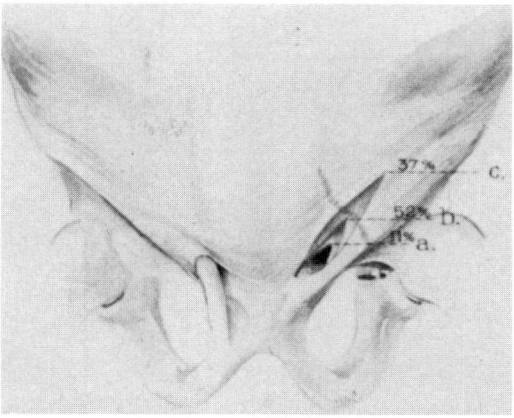
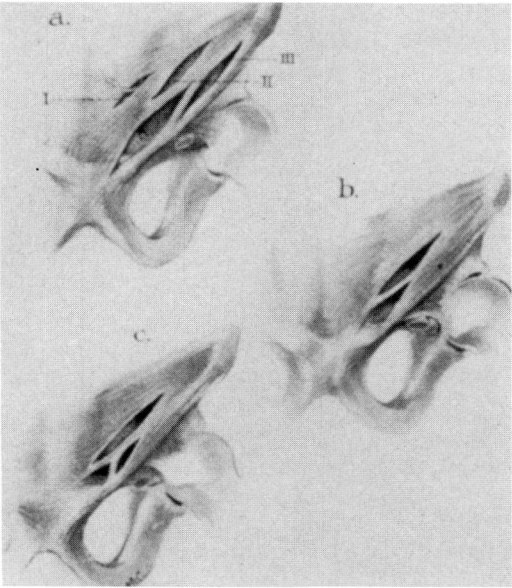

Figure 16.50. Variations in the aponeurotic cleft of the external oblique muscle. **A,** The triangular fault shown in relation to the epigastric vessels at the lateral boundary of Hesselbach's triangle. In 37% of 66 body halves examined, the cleft extended beyond the epigastric fold. **B,** Examples of accessory clefts in the aponeurosis of the external oblique muscle. (From Anson BJ et al. Surgical anatomy of the inguinal region based upon a study of 500 body halves. Surg Gynecol Obstet 1960;111:707–725.)

colleagues. (189) In a few cases accessory aponeurotic clefts were observed (Fig. 16.50).

INTERNAL OBLIQUE MUSCLE

The inferior extent of the muscular portion of the internal oblique layer is extremely variable. Rarely does it extend to the level of the inguinal canal (189). Among Chandler and Schadewald's (187) specimens, it covered the whole of Hesselbach's triangle in 21% and none of the triangle in 33%. Musculoaponeurotic defects were present in about 50% of the 500 body halves examined by

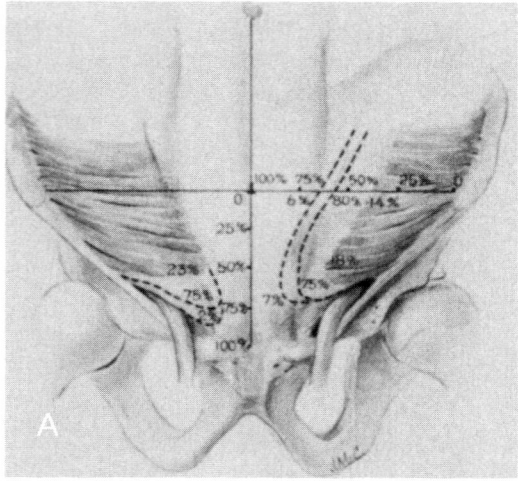

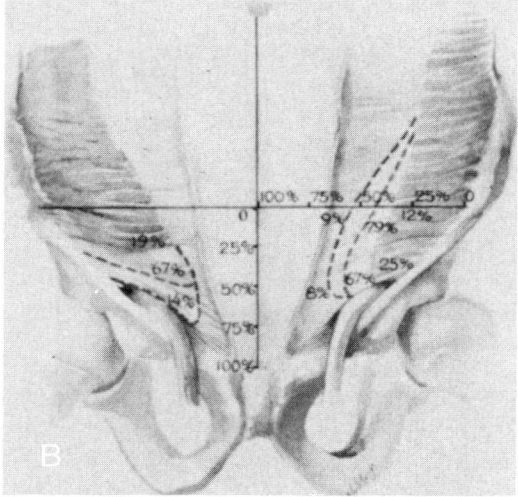

Figure 16.51. **A,** Variations of the internal oblique muscle. Inferior extent *(left)* and medial extent *(right)*. Percentages encountered in a study of 425 inguinal regions. **B,** Variations of the transverse abdominal muscle. (From Anson BJ et al. Surgical anatomy of the inguinal region based upon a study of 500 body halves. Surg Gynec Obstet 1960;111:707–725.)

Anson and his colleagues (189) (Fig. 16.51, *A*). Macalister (190) reported a highly developed internal oblique muscle that was traversed by the spermatic cord.

TRANSVERSUS ABDOMINIS LAYER

The most variable of the layers of the body wall in the inguinal region is the transversus abdominis. In only 4.2% of specimens examined did transversus muscle fibers cover Hesselbach's triangle (187). In 50% of cases the triangle was less than half covered. Musculoaponeurotic defects were present in 13% of the cadavers examined by Anson and his colleagues (189). Great variation in the attachment of the aponeurotic portion of the transversus abdominis layer may be found (Fig. 16.51, *B*).

According to Bergman et al. (44), the muscle has been found fused with the internal oblique or perhaps was absent.

Incomplete Closure of the Processus Vaginalis: Inguinal Hernia and Hydrocele

DEFINITION

The groin has been succinctly defined by Condon (191) as "that portion of the anterior abdominal wall below the level of the anterior superior iliac spines." In this area a viscus may protrude, forming a visible and usually palpable swelling. Three types of herniae—direct inguinal, indirect inguinal, and external supravesical—may emerge through the abdominal wall by way of the external ring above the inguinal ligament. A fourth type, femoral hernia, emerges beneath the inguinal ligament by way of the femoral canal. These four types make up 90% of all herniae.

Other inguinal herniae, although not common, are important to the surgeon. In this chapter we also discuss female and male pediatric inguinal herniae and hydrocele.

ANATOMY

Following the descent of the testes into the scrotum during the seventh to ninth month of fetal life, the internal inguinal ring becomes closed and the lumen of the *processus vaginalis testis* above the testis is obliterated. In the adult male, the neck, or funicular process, is represented by a fibrous band, while the scrotal portion remains as a peritoneum-lined cavity (Fig. 16.52), the tunica vaginalis, around the anterior surface of the testis. In the female, the canal of Nuck corresponds to the processus vaginalis testis and opens into the labium majus, the homologue of the scrotum. The canal of Nuck usually becomes obliterated in the seventh month, earlier than does the processus vaginalis of the male, and it never becomes large.

Failure of prompt and complete closure of the processus vaginalis or of the canal of Nuck soon after birth may leave a peritoneal diverticulum into which abdominal viscera may herniate, or it may result in a fluid-filled, cystic cavity (a *hydrocele*). These defects of closure may be classified as follows:

1. Diverticular defects
   a. Processus vaginalis, open throughout its length; herniation of abdominal organs may take place at birth or shortly afterward. This is "congenital indirect hernia."
   b. Upper portion of processus (funicular process), opens into the peritoneal cavity; lower portion is closed. Herniation of abdominal organs may occur later in life. This is "acquired indirect hernia."
2. Cystic defects
   a. Processus is closed, or nearly closed, only at the

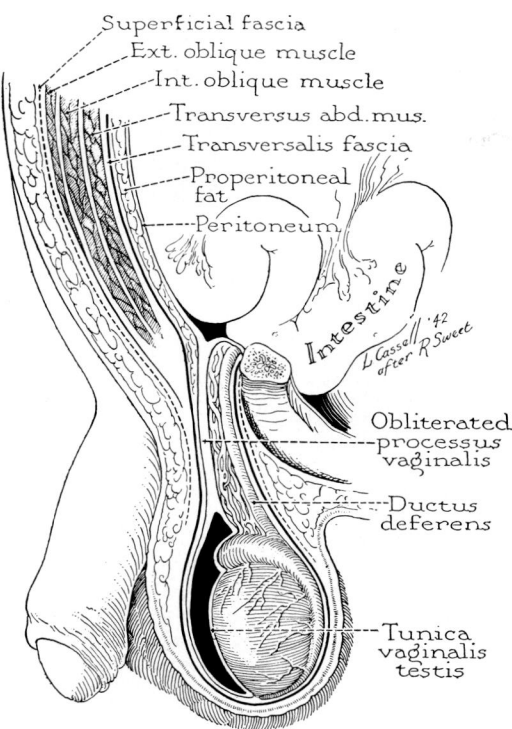

Figure 16.52. Diagramatic section showing the normal, complete obliteration of the processus vaginalis after normal testicular descent. (From Zimmerman LM, Anson BJ. Anatomy and surgery of hernia, 2nd ed. Baltimore: Williams & Wilkins, 1967.)

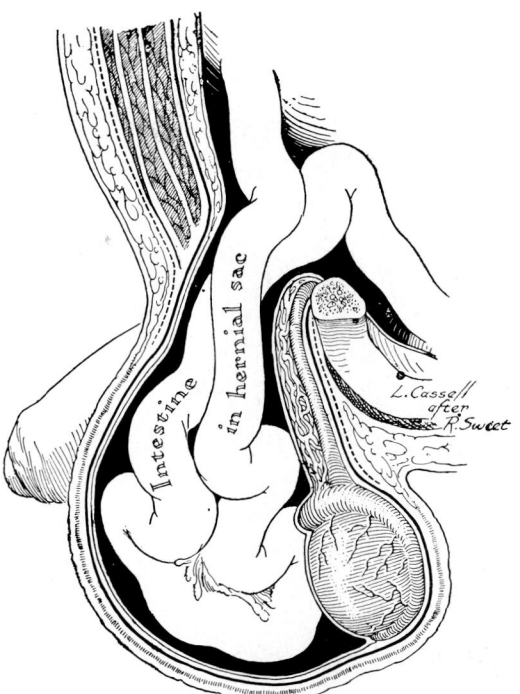

Figure 16.53. Failure of normal closure of the processus vaginalis. Congenital indirect inguinal hernia. The testis may or may not have descended. (From Zimmerman LM, Anson BJ. Anatomy and surgery of hernia, 2nd ed. Baltimore: Williams & Wilkins, 1967.)

abdominal orifice; the remainder is fluid filled. This is called "infantile hydrocele."

b. Processus is closed above and below a fluid-filled cystic remnant. This is called "cystic hydrocele," "funicular hydrocele," or "hydrocele of the spermatic cord."

These hydroceles are not to be confused with adult vaginal hydroceles, in which the fluid collects in the normally formed tunica vaginalis and no defect of the processus vaginalis exists.

Open Processus Vaginalis. When the processus vaginalis is open throughout its length, abdominal viscera are free to enter it, forming an indirect inguinal hernia. Because the open canal is present before birth, herniation into it is called congenital even though actual herniation may not occur until after birth. In males, herniation may precede testicular descent or follow it (Fig. 16.53).

Failure of the testis to enter the internal inguinal ring at or near birth leaves the processus vaginalis with nothing to prevent other abdominal contents from moving into it under the increased abdominal pressure produced by the crying and coughing of postnatal life. Thus indirect inguinal hernia and cryptorchidism are frequently associated with the condition. This type of hernia is more frequent in premature than in full-term infants.

In most cases of congenital indirect hernia, the herniating organs follow the testis through the internal inguinal ring and enter the scrotum through the yet unclosed processus. Although such herniae usually are easily reduced, they occasionally become incarcerated. Six percent of herniae treated at the Children's Hospital in Boston before 1938 were incarcerated (192); in subsequent years, the percentage fell to below 2% (146). Most incarcerations are on the right side, presumably related to the fact that testicular descent and closure occur later here than on the left.

Occasionally the cecum descends through the inguinal canal in back of the processus vaginalis, following the actual course of the descending testis and hence remaining retroperitoneal. Such a hernia is known as a sliding hernia, and the cecum lies beside the empty processus rather than within it.

In women, the canal of Nuck rarely is patent into the labium. Indirect herniae are usually bubonic or pubic rather than labial.

In the inguinal region with indirect hernia, the layers of the abdominal wall are:

1. Skin
2. Subcutaneous fascia (Camper's and Scarpa's fasciae)
3. External oblique aponeurosis
4. Cremasteric fascia (internal oblique muscle)

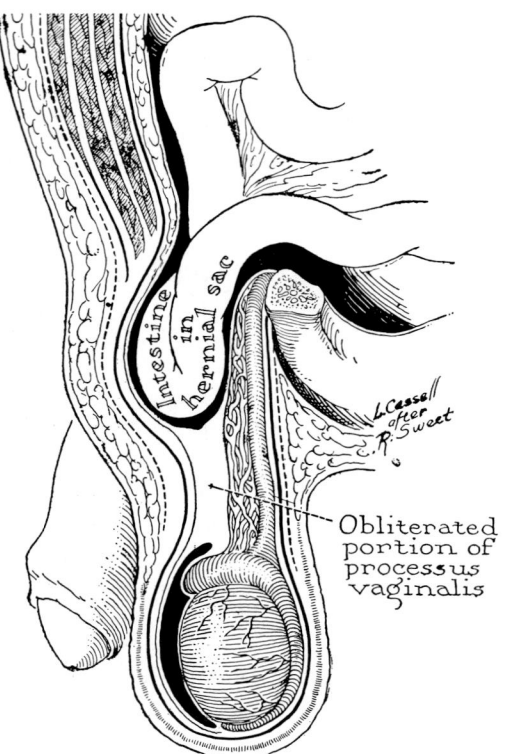

Figure 16.54. Normal closure of the distal portion only of the processus vaginalis, with a proximal, blind peritoneal sac where an acquired, indirect inguinal hernia may occur in postnatal life. The hernial sac will lie beside the tunica vaginalis instead of within it. Compare with Figure 16.53. (From Zimmerman LM, Anson BJ. Anatomy and surgery of hernia, 2nd ed. Baltimore: Williams & Wilkins, 1967.)

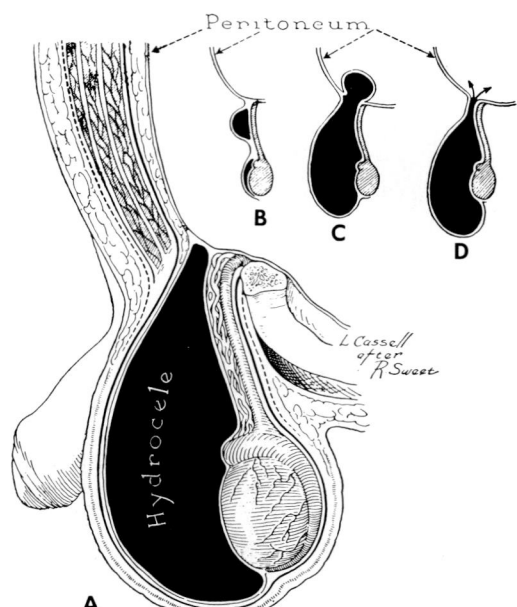

Figure 16.55. Hydrocele. **A,** Closure of the internal inguinal ring only. Fluid accumulation in the distal processus and tunica vaginalis. **B,** Open midportion of the processus vaginalis. The hydrocele does not communicate with the tunica vaginalis or the peritoneal cavity. **C,** Infantile type of hydrocele, which bulges into the abdominal cavity. **D,** Communicating hydrocele. A small aperture at the internal inguinal ring allows some escape of fluid. Hydrocele may be reduced by gentle pressure, but soon returns. (From Zimmerman LM, Anson BJ. Anatomy and surgery of hernia, 2nd ed. Baltimore: Williams & Wilkins, 1967.)

5. Internal spermatic sheath (transversalis fascia)
6. Preperitoneal fat
7. Hernial sac

In the scrotal region, the layers are (see Fig. 20.10):

1. Skin
2. Dartos tunica, dartos scroti (Scarpa's fascia)
3. External spermatic fascia (external oblique fascia)
4. Cremasteric fascia (internal oblique aponeurosis)
5. Internal spermatic fascia (transversalis fascia)
6. Preperitoneal fat
7. Peritoneum (tunica vaginalis)

Closure of the Lower Processus Vaginalis Only. If the lower portion of the neck of the processus vaginalis closes normally but leaves a blind peritoneal sac (funicular process) opening from the abdominal cavity, an acquired indirect inguinal hernia may occur in later life. In such a condition the hernial sac will extend into the scrotum to lie beside the tunica vaginalis instead of opening into it, as in the congenital type of hernia (Fig. 16.54).

The female normally has no persisting tunica vaginalis, and the distinction between congenital and acquired herniae therefore does not apply.

Burton (193) studied the possible pathology of the processus vaginalis. Rowe et al. (194) reported the patency of the processus vaginalis: 60% during the first year of life are open; in the second year, 40% will continue to be open.

The authors observed cases of "hydrocele" secondary to ascites due to cirrhosis and pancreatitis.

Closure of the Internal Inguinal Ring Only. If only the abdominal orifice of the processus vaginalis is closed, fluid may accumulate in the cavity to form a hydrocele around the testis and spermatic cord (Fig. 15.55, *A*). If the upper end of the hydrocele bulges into the peritoneal cavity, it may be described as an *abdominoscrotal hydrocele* (Fig. 16.55, *C*). Although it is frequently termed *infantile*, the condition is not limited to infants.

Occasionally the internal orifice of the processus vaginalis is too small to permit herniation, yet fluid may enter, forming a hydrocele. The fluid may be forced out of the scrotum by gentle pressure, but it will return later. This condition has been designated *congenital* or *communicating hydrocele* (Fig. 16.55, *D*).

Open Midportion of the Processus Vaginalis. A hydrocele that communicates neither with the abdominal cavity above nor with the tunica vaginalis below is called a *cystic* or *funicular hydrocele*. It is a fluid-filled, isolated portion of the funicular process lying next to the spermatic cord (Fig. 16.55, *B*).

CONTENTS OF THE HERNIAL SAC

Serous fluid is always present and may compose the contents of the hernial sac. In male infants and children an ileal loop is usually the structure involved. Because of its position on the ileum, Meckel's diverticulum may also enter the sac (Littrè's hernia). In female infants and children the ovary and uterine tube are most often present.

The omentum is too short in children to reach the internal inguinal ring, but in adults it is the most frequently encountered structure. Occasionally, the uterus is herniated in women (195), and sometimes, even in unsuspected male pseudohermaphrodites.

EMBRYOGENESIS

That indirect inguinal hernia can occur results from two evolutionary changes widely separated in time, coupled with a minor developmental anomaly. The mechanism of testicular migration from the abdomen to the scrotum became established early in the development of the mammals, while the assumption of an erect posture appeared much later with the rise of the higher primates. The first change caused weakening of the abdominal wall; the second change moved the weakened area from a region of relatively minor stress in a quadruped mammal to a region of major stress in a biped mammal.

The extraabdominal positioning of the testis may be described as occurring in three steps: A passage is made through the abdominal wall, which seriously weakens the wall; the testis passes quickly through the opening into the scrotum; and the passage is reclosed to restore the integrity of the wall. The first step in the process rarely causes trouble because the intraabdominal pressure in the fetus is low when the processus vaginalis is formed. The second step is a major source of trouble. The testis may be slow in entering the scrotum, or it may fail to descend at all. In the first instance the testis may be followed closely by an intestinal loop, before closure can be accomplished (Fig. 16.53); in the second instance the loop may enter the canal, which is left open for the descent of a testis that fails to appear on schedule.

Even if the testis passes through the inguinal canal with dispatch, the third step of closure of the internal inguinal ring and obliteration of the funicular process of the processus vaginalis may be inadequate to restore the abdominal wall to the strength required for the stresses of later life in an erect posture.

The order of events during closure has been described by Frazer (196):

Step 1: Closure of the processus vaginalis at the internal inguinal ring

Step 2: Closure of the processus just above the testis

Step 3: Atresia of the processus between the two constrictions

Although this is the order in which the canal normally closes, obviously it does not always take place in that way (197). The defects that result from failure during individual steps of the closure may be tabulated as follows:

1. Congenital indirect hernia: Failure of closure of the internal ring and of all subsequent steps (Fig. 16.53). Later constriction of the internal ring may produce strangulation.
2. Acquired indirect hernia: Failure of closure of the internal ring, with successful completion of the second and third steps (see Fig. 20.10).
3. Infantile hydrocele: Inguinal ring closed; the second and third steps are not completed (Fig. 16.54, *A* and *C*).
4. Cystic hydrocele: Only the third step is not completed (Fig. 16.54, *B*).

The governing mechanism of closure of the processus is unknown. Although gonadotropins will induce testicular descent (see Chapter 20, "The Ovary and Testis"), obliteration of the processus vaginalis does not automatically follow. This failure of the inguinal canal to close behind a testis induced to descend means that surgery for removal of the hernial sac cannot be avoided.

PREDISPOSING CONDITIONS

A number of factors have been said to be responsible for the actual herniation of viscera into an open funicular process (acquired hernia). A few of these are worth mentioning.

Body Build. Moskalenko (198) suggested that husky men with narrow hips are more immune than are others to acquired inguinal hernia.

Inguinal Ligament. Harris and White (199) measured the inguinal ligament in 500 men and concluded that those with ligaments less than 11 cm long had little tendency toward inguinal hernia; ligaments from 11 to 15 cm long were associated with indirect inguinal hernia; and longer ligaments were associated with direct inguinal hernia.

Nutrition. Watson (200) and Maitland (201) emphasized the role of poor diet, hard work, and loss of fat in producing herniae.

Familial Tendency. It has long been known that predisposition to inguinal hernia runs in certain families. As early as 1864 Kingdon (202) stated that 34% of herniae occurred in families having other members similarly afflicted. Iason (203) estimated that 25% of herniae were familial. Fathers seem to transmit the predisposition to sons, while mothers transmit to daughters.

Trauma. Despite the readiness of the public to believe in the traumatic origin of inguinal hernia, most studies show that few patients are able to identify a specific traumatic event as a cause of their hernia.

In those cases in which a definite strain can be shown, the position of the body at the time is important. Stephens (204) considers that strenuous effort, with the legs widely separated on the ground or with one foot on the ground and the other braced higher on a step or against a wall, is likely to be the most dangerous. The more sudden the strain, the greater the risk, as the internal ring is less well-guarded when the strain catches the abdominal musculature at a time when it is relaxed. There is no doubt that a single trauma or strain may be the precipitating cause of an inguinal hernia, but only in unusual circumstances.

Harper et al. (205) reported that the incidence of inguinal hernia in premature infants with a weight of less than 1000 gm is 30%.

Weiner (206) reported congenital inheritance, and Bakmin (207) reported congenital hernia in twins.

That potential herniae tend to wait until middle life to manifest is due largely to the factor of absolute size. The strength of growing tissues increases as the square of their dimensions increases, but their weight—and hence the mechanical stresses they bear—increases as the cube of the same dimension. The active adult works much closer to the point of mechanical failure than does the active child. An adult lifting 300 lbs at maximum effort is far more likely to force the internal inguinal rings than is a youngster who proudly demonstrates a barely developed ability to raise 100 lbs from the ground.

In infancy, whooping cough, chronic constipation, and lengthy crying spells may be considered precipitating causes. The common factor is the accompanying rise in intraabdominal pressure. All such causes become effective only when an unclosed processus vaginalis is already present.

The failure of the patient to identify the precipitating cause probably results from the gradual forcing of the internal ring under strain. Once past the ring, the hernia may proceed rapidly downward under conditions of less than maximal exertion. Recognition by the patient often occurs during the latter phase, and hence he or she searches in vain for an immediate strain of unusual violence to account for the injury.

Since this means that the processus vaginalis is not closed, the question arises of whether to employ bilateral repair in a child with obvious unilateral hernia. Raffensperger (128) advised bilateral repair for girls under 1 year of age and in boys if there is any suggestion of thickness of the cord or of the so-called silk sign.

HISTORY

Although inguinal hernia has been recognized since time immemorial, the first mention of the processus vaginalis appears to be that of Celsus in the second century after Christ. Based on Alexandrian surgery, the writings of Celsus were essentially unknown until they were printed in 1478 in Florence.

The earliest reference to inguinal hernia in women appears in the work of Soranus of Ephesus who confirmed the existence of the suspensory ligament of the ovary by stating that he had seen it in an operation for hernia. The canal of Nuck was specifically described in 1672.

The intraabdominal origin of the testis was first observed by Haller (208) in 1755, and testicular descent was described in detail by Hunter in 1762 (209). Cloquet (210) observed an open processus vaginalis in an adult and emphasized the absence of evidence for violent rupture of tissues at the hernial site.

Although the view that acquired indirect inguinal hernia takes place through an unclosed funicular process was suggested several times earlier in the 19th century, Russell (211) in 1899 brought the "saccular theory" to the attention of surgeons. For many years Keith (212) opposed Russell's views of the essentially embryonic nature of acquired indirect inguinal hernia. At present, however, there is little reason to doubt that all indirect inguinal herniae are the result of defective closure of the processus vaginalis. When the testis is ectopic rather than undescended, the processus vaginalis usually is closed.

Incidence of Hernia. An undescended testis is an indication of an open processus vaginalis. Unless the testis is arrested in the inguinal canal, the open processus is the site of a potential congenital indirect inguinal hernia. The incidence of nondescent is high among premature infants (213) and decreases with age (214, 215) (see Fig. 20.31 and Table 16.6).

The incidence of a partially closed processus vaginalis with an open funicular process and a normally descended testis is harder to estimate. Anson and his colleagues (189) found at least one processus open and empty in 13 of 254 consecutive cadavers (5.1%). Watson's (200) older figures of 33% for males and 20% for females cannot be taken to represent an unselected adult series.

Actual inguinal herniae may be expected to appear in about 5% of males and 1% of females. The findings of Anson and his colleagues (189) suggest that about as

Table 16.6.
Incidence of Undescended Testis

Age Group	Study	Percentage
Premature infants	Scorer, 1955 (213)	30.30
Full-term infants	Scorer, 1955	3.40
5-year-old children	East Anglian Survey, 1959 (214)	4.30
8-year-old children	East Anglian Survey, 1959	4.50
11-year-old children	East Anglian Survey, 1959	3.50
14- to 17-year-old children	East Anglian Survey, 1959	0.60
Military recruits (Europe and the United States)	Campbell 1963 (215)	0.28

many herniae remain potential as become actual. Thus an individual with an unclosed funicular processus has about a 50% chance of developing an actual acquired indirect inguinal hernia in his or her lifetime.

A high incidence of herniae among large groups of soldiers has often been reported (201). These results must be interpreted with care because they depend on the effectiveness of the screening of draftees, the extent to which repair while in the service is contemplated, and the actual occurrence of new cases of hernia after acceptance into the service.

Specific Incidence.

Age.

There is an increased incidence of inguinal hernia during the first year of life (216).

The congenital type of hernia may be present at birth, but more frequently, it occurs in the first few months of life in both girls and boys. The acquired type of indirect inguinal hernia is most frequently found between the ages of 30 and 50 years, during which period about 60% occur.

Sex.

The incidence of inguinal hernia is greater in males, according to Holder and Ashcraft (217).

Location.

```
Males:    60% right
          30% left
          10% bilateral
Females:  60% right
          32% left
          8% bilateral (218)
```

The preponderance of right-sided herniae is said to reflect the later descent of the right testis and hence a processus vaginalis that is open for a longer period of time than that on the left.

Among the acquired indirect inguinal herniae of later life, there is also a right-sided preponderance, suggesting that closure of the right processus not only occurs later, but also tends to be less complete. In female infants, herniation into the canal of Nuck shows only a slight right-sided preponderance (195).

Family History.

There is an increased incidence in twins and in parents with inguinal hernia, according to Bronsther et al. (216) and Czeizel and Gardonyi (219).

Other Populations.

Rowe and Lloyd (220) reported an incidence of herniae in 37% of general surgical operations in a pediatric hospital. According to Bronsther and colleagues (216) the incidence of inguinal hernia in children is from 0.8% to 4.4%. Harper et al. (205) reported the incidence of inguinal hernia as up to 30% in premature children.

INCIDENCE OF HYDROCELE

Among 3509 male infants operated on for inguinal hernia by Gross (146), 586 (16.6%) were found to have an associated hydrocele.

SYMPTOMS AND DIAGNOSIS

The diagnosis of an unclosed processus vaginalis may be made in the following ways:

1. By presumption, if the testis cannot be palpated in the scrotum or in the inguinal canal.
2. By the "silk sign," if the sac is empty. The two sides of the sac rubbing on each other produce the sensation of silk surfaces rubbing together. Presence of this sign is a positive indication of an unclosed sac, but absence of the sign is meaningless.
3. By observation of a bulge or by palpation of a swelling in the inguinal region or the scrotum, if the processus contains abdominal organs or fluid. The presence of an inguinal or scrotal mass requires further diagnostic procedures:
   a. The mass, although reported by parents, is not always visible on examination. Crying in the infant or coughing and straining in the older child may serve to bring the mass down. In other patients the mass may be apparent at examination and be easily reduced in the recumbent position. In either case diagnosis of indirect inguinal hernia can be made.
   b. The mass may be reported by the parents to change size and to be smaller in the morning after sleep than in the afternoon after play. If reducible, reduction is slow and gradual. These indications point to an infantile hydrocele, with a very small abdominal opening, through which fluid passes slowly into the lower, unclosed portion of the processus (Fig. 16.37, *D*).
   c. If the inguinal or scrotal mass fails to reduce, incarcerated hernia, torsion of the testis, torsion of the appendix testis, or hydrocele must be considered.

With incarceration or torsion, the mass is painful; symptoms of intestinal obstruction will appear within a few hours when incarceration is present.

Cystic hydrocele of the cord is painless and mobile; it can be transilluminated. Frequently the upper, closed portion of the inguinal canal can be palpated above the swelling.

TREATMENT

The repair of inguinal hernia is thoroughly described in most standard textbooks of surgery and need not be repeated here. However, the following principles should be kept in mind:

1. All inguinal herniae should be repaired as soon as they are diagnosed, regardless of age, unless a concomitant illness precludes surgery. A truss should not be employed.
2. Operate only on the side with the hernia, unless a contra-

lateral hernia is suspected by the presence of cord thickening or by a good history from a reliable observer.

3. When only a hydrocele exists in a newborn infant, allow 6 to 12 months for possible absorption of the fluid before operating.

Remember that the vas deferens as well as the testicular vessels should be protected by very careful technique. According to Janik and Shandling (221) pressure may produce damage to the ductus.

According to Wiklander (222) and Sloman (223), long-standing incarceration will produce testicular atrophy in 12 to 15% of testes.

Moss and Hatch (224) reported their experience with 384 infants less than 2 months of age who were operated for inguinal herniorrhaphies and presented the following informative statistic analysis:

1. Incarcerated hernias found in 24% of patients and with preoperative reduction in 96%
2. Contralateral surgery was performed in 96%, and herniae found in 85%
3. Recurrence rate: 1%
4. Complication rate: 2.3%

The authors recommend repair in the first 2 months of life.

Varicocele

DEFINITION

Varicosities of the pampiniform plexus when present, usually occur in the left scrotum (90%), rarely bilateral (9%), and very rarely (only 1%) in the right scrotum according to Wilms et al. (225). As a matter of fact, Wilms et al. reported two cases of varicocele with situs inversus. Yarborough et al. (226) stated that varicocele is present in 15% of the general adult population. According to Belker (227), it is present in up to 35% of men with infertility problems.

ANATOMY OF THE SCROTUM

One cannot fully describe the inguinal area and completely omit the scrotum, testicles, and epididymis. It is outside the scope of this chapter to describe the morphology of these organs, but we think certain features should be mentioned. (Table 16.7).

The **scrotal skin** is elastic and corrugated, thinner and more pigmented than the inguinal skin. After puberty, this skin has less hair than inguinal skin, but possibly it has more sebaceous glands and sweat glands. The raphe between the right and left halves of the scrotum is a median ridge continuous with the raphe of the penis and perineum.

The **dartos** is the superficial fascia of the scrotum. The superficial portion is contributed by Camper's fascia which covers the abdominal wall, penis, perineum, thigh,

Table 16.7.
The Corresponding Layers of the Abdominal Wall, Scrotum and Thigh

Abdominal Wall	Scrotum	Thigh
Skin	Skin	Skin
Superficial fascia	Dartos	Fat and cribriform fascia
Innominate fascia	External spermatic fascia	Fascia latae
Internal oblique muscle and aponeurosis	Cremasteric fascia and muscle	
Transversus abdominis muscle and aponeurosis	Cremasteric fascia and muscle	None
Transversalis fascia	Internal spermatic fascia	Femoral sheath
Preperitoneal fat	Preperitoneal fat	None
Peritoneum	Tunica vaginalis	None

From Skandalakis JE et al. Surgical anatomy of the inguinal area. I and II. Contemp Surg 1991; 38(2):34.

and buttocks. The deep portion derives from Scarpa's fascia and is continuous over the abdominal wall to the penis and to the perineum (Colles' fascia).

Connective tissue and smooth muscle fibers compose the dartos. It is attached to the skin. Colles' fascia is attached laterally to the periosteum of the pubic arch of the lower abdominal wall. The space deep to the dartos may allow extravasated urine to collect.

The **external spermatic fascia** is the scrotal continuation of the fascia of the external oblique muscle (innominate or Galluadet's fascia).

The **cremaster muscle** is derived from the internal oblique aponeurosis, muscle and fascia, and perhaps the transverse muscle of the abdomen. The fibers are not under voluntary control although they are composed of striated muscle.

The **internal spermatic fascia** is a prolongation of the transversalis fascia. The covering of the spermatic cord is formed from layers three, four, five, and six.

Preperitoneal Fat. The **tunica vaginalis** is a serous membrane of peritoneum.

Within these eight layers (layers seven and eight are part of the cord) of the scrotum, the testes move freely. Only the skin and the dartos are fixed.

Blood is supplied to the scrotum primarily by the external (superficial and deep) and internal pudendal arteries as well as by twigs from the testicular and cremasteric arteries. Remember that the terminal branches of vessels to the skin of the scrotum lie transversely; therefore, scrotal exploration should be done through a transverse incision to minimize bleeding.

Approximately 12 scrotal veins from the posterior testicular surface and epididymis form the pampiniform plexus. This plexus travels upward into the spermatic cord by three routes: (*a*) around the testicular artery; (*b*) around the vas deferens; and (*c*) alone. These veins gradually join together to form four, three, two, and finally one vein—the testicular vein. The left testicular vein drains into the left renal and the right into the inferior vena cava.

Lymphatic drainage from the scrotum and the skin of the inguinal area is to the superficial lymph nodes.

EMBRYOGENESIS OF THE SCROTUM

Stages of Development. Remember that the *embryo* is the stage of development taking place with the womb at the first 8 weeks of conception. From week 9 until birth it is called a *fetus*.

Stage I: The genesis and opening of the genital tubule takes place during later embryonic or early fetal development, together with the solid urethra, which becomes longer.

Stage II: The sandwich becomes present:
Upper outer layer—skin
lower middle layer—deep body wall
innermost layer—peritoneum

Stage III: The formation of the right and left labioscrotal folds takes place. The acceptance of the deep body wall (fasciae superficial and deep) within the sacs and finally the movement within the sac of the peritoneum (processus vaginalis) and the formation of the scrotum by fusion of the scrotal folds takes place.

ETIOLOGY

Etiologically, the explanation of varicocele is enigmatic, and embryologically and anatomically perhaps without explanation. There are several speculations:

1. Ahlberg et al. (228) reported the absence of valves in the left testicular vein, an observation reinforced by Kuypers et al. (229). Kuypers et al. (229) reported, as a possible etiologic factor in varicocele, the absence of valves in 25 subjects on the left and 8 subjects on the right testicular vein with a significant statistical difference $P<.001$.
2. Shafik et al. (230) thought that this was a mechanical phenomenon resulting from disruption of the venous pump, which is enveloped by the fasciomuscular covering of the spermatic cord.
3. Compression of the left renal vein occurs between the abdominal aorta and the superior mesonephric aortas.
4. Saypol et al. (231) said the right-angle insertion of the long left testicular vein, in comparison with the right into the left renal vein, produces a higher hydrostatic pressure in the standing position.
5. Williams et al. (232) support the opinion that there is extrinsic pressure to the left renal vein by the sigmoid colon.
6. Epinephrine (adrenalin) from the left suprarenal (adrenal) vein draining into the renal vein could cause contraction of the orifice of the left testicular vein, resulting in a variocele. We agree with Basmajian (233) that this spec-

ulation is ingenious. By the way, we could not discover the author of this explanation.

SYMPTOMS, DIAGNOSIS, DIFFERENTIAL DIAGNOSIS

Symptoms include testicular discomfort or pain and perhaps infertility. The "bag of worms" sign at the left scrotum from the varicose veins is more than obvious when patient is standing and disappears in the supine position.

A low sperm count and reduced spermatic motility are perhaps attributable to varicocele. However, it would be good practice to rule out any possible renal mass or thrombosis of the left renal vein or inferior vena cava.

TREATMENT

With concrete indications, varicosclerostomy is the procedure of choice; however, it has a failure rate of 5 to 15%, according to Belker (227).

Congenital Aplasia of the Abdominal Muscles Without Urinary Tract Defects

PRUNE BELLY SYNDROME

According to Bergman (44) the muscles of the anterior abdominal wall may be absent in toto, attenuated, or partially absent or may have innumerable variations in origin or attachment. Some muscles may be well developed or normal on one side, and highly abnormal or absent on the other side.

It is not the purpose of this chapter to present the multiple variations of these muscles but to deal only with their complete absence and the sequelae.

In a few cases muscular aplasia of the abdominal wall is not accompanied by a urinary bladder defect. The body wall aplasia is more limited and does not produce the flaccid, "prune belly" appearance seen in the more widespread hypoplasia discussed previously. The abdomen presents a lateral bulge in the lower quadrant on one or both sides, without a neck or a hernial ring. The internal and external oblique muscles are attenuated or reduced to a fibrous lamella; the rectus also may be involved. Sheldon and Heller (234) described a unilateral defect of this type in a 24-year-old man, with accompanying cryptorchidism. Stoica and his colleagues (235) described a similar bilateral defect in a child; they used the term *eventration* for the defect.

A few other similar but poorly described cases may be found in the literature cited by Stoica and his colleagues (235).

Chronic urinary retention may result from the absence of abdominal muscles to assist in voiding, and urinary infection may follow. Jona (236) stated that he observed three children with the prune belly syndrome who urinated through the urachus and not from the urethra. Hydronephrosis with renal dysplasia and dilated tortuous ureter was reported also by Raffensperger (128).

Several urogenital anomalies were reported by Nunn and Stephens (237), who believe that failure of the musculature of the abdominal wall and urinary system to develop is the cause of this syndrome.

Repair is effected by overlapping the hypoplastic layer and fixing it to the linea alba, the crest of the ileum, and the ribs. Excess skin was removed and used to reinforce the defect in Stoica's (235) patient.

Duckett (238) doubts the good result of plication of the abdominal wall and the results of reconstruction of the urinary tract. However, Randolph (239) proposes more radical procedures, such as resection of the lower abdominal wall and resection, tapering, and reimplantation of ureter.

Congenital Absence of the Abdominal Muscles Associated with Urinary Tract Defects

ANATOMY

The syndrome consists of absence or hypoplasia of the abdominal musculature, hypertrophy of the bladder, cryptorchidism, hydroureter, and hydronephrosis. Other malformations are frequently present.

Abdominal Muscular Defects. In extreme cases the musculi rectus abdominis, obliquus externus abdominis, obliguus internus abdominis, transversus abdominis, and quadratus lumborum are absent or rudimentary on both sides. More commonly, the lower halves of the recti are absent, and the external and internal oblique muscles and the transversus abdominis are deficient. The muscles may be entirely absent, represented by a few fibers, or only thinned. The defect is usually bilateral though the deficiency may be greater on one side than on the other. The umbilicus is often slit-like.

Urinary Tract Defects. The bladder is dilated and hypertrophied in almost all cases. It is often fixed at the umbilicus, and a patent urachus or umbilicovesical fistula may be present (240). The bladder musculature is thinned or patchy (237).

Hydroureter and hydronephrosis on one or both sides are nearly always present. The kidneys may be palpable, and the enlarged ureters may be visible beneath the thin, flaccid abdominal wall. In addition, the ureteral muscularis may be deficient.

While the clinical picture is one of lower urinary tract obstruction, an anatomic cause for obstruction is not easily demonstrated. In a few cases urethral atresia, stenosis, or urethral valves have been observed, and hypertrophy of the colliculus seminalis has been mentioned. In general, earlier workers (241) found no obstruction, while other reports (242) mentioned a wide variety of obstructing causes. It is probable that not all megaloureters result from lower urinary tract obstruction.

Genital Defects. In only three cases have the testes been normally descended; they are usually abdominal. Prostatic maldevelopment also has been reported (237).

Other Associated Anomalies. Pigeon breast and flaring of the costal margins, with Harrison's groove marking the diaphragmatic attachment, are usually present (Fig. 16.56). The diaphragm is flattened and vital capacity is markedly reduced. Intestinal anomalies, usually of rotation and fixation, are present in about 20% of patients. About 25% have clubfoot or other deformities of the lower extremities, including congenital dislocation of the hip.

Cardiac malformations appeared five times in Lattimer's (243) series of 22 patients.

EMBRYOGENESIS

As might be expected, this extensive anomaly has been given many explanations.

The wrinkled, sac-like abdomen has suggested to some that pressure in the obstructed urinary tract produces bladder distension in utero and that this distension is responsible for dysgenesis of the abdominal musculature. The presence of the defect without urinary obstruction in some cases, and the absence of muscular defects in many other instances of urinary obstruction, greatly weaken this argument.

Embryologically, the lower abdominal wall receives "secondary" mesoderm from the primitive streak posterior to the cloaca (13). This provides the primary closure of the infraumbilical body wall and also contributes to the bladder musculature. There appears to be no failure of this component to form.

The somatic mesoderm invades the ventral body wall and is complete by the 12th week (70 mm). The individual muscles, however, are differentiated as early as the seventh week (14 to 16 mm) although they lie far lateral to their final positions. The defect under consideration goes back to this earlier period, for it is not a failure of myogenesis in the normal mesoderm. Those rudimentary portions of the muscles that exist are in their normal location. The center of the hypoplasia appears to lie in the first lumbar segment, from which the greater part of the transverse and oblique muscles develop, and the hypoplasia decreases in severity both craniad and caudad. The occasional lower limb defects indicate that the dysgenesis may involve the lower lumbar and upper sacral myotomes, and the frequent absence of the upper part of the rectus indicates an extension of the dysgenesis to the lower thoracic segments (Fig. 16.57).

Another theory suggests the urinary malformation is the result of the muscular defect, implying that emptying of the bladder may be inhibited by the flaccid abdomen. Lattimer (243) pointed out that bladder dilation does not accompany omphalocele and that in a few cases the bladder is not distended. Unquestionably, the bladder is

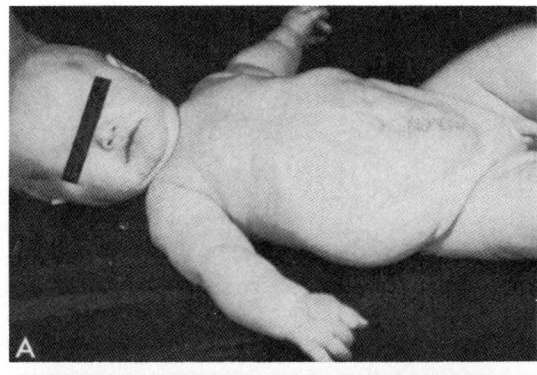
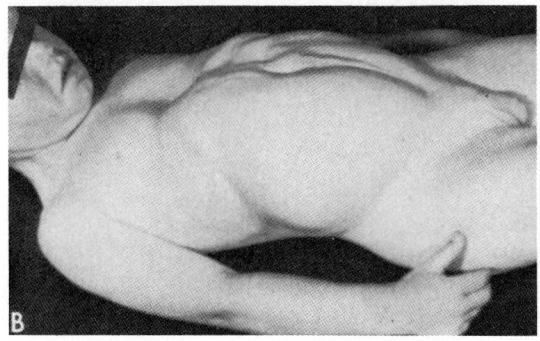
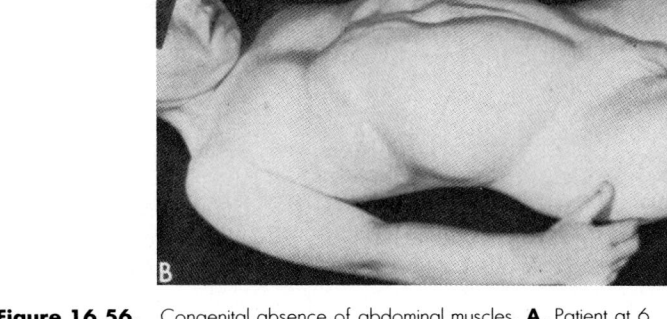
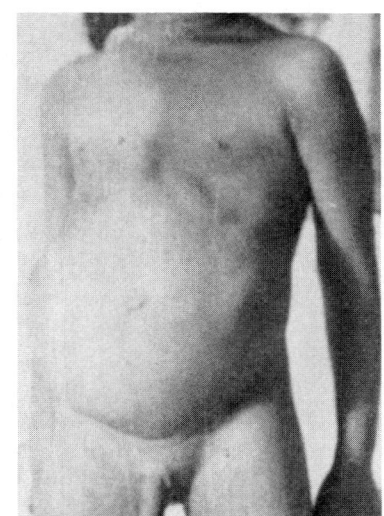

Figure 16.56. Congenital absence of abdominal muscles. **A,** Patient at 6 months. **B,** Same patient at 6 years. On effort of raising the head, the upper recti draw the umbilicus craniad and the weaker lower abdomen bulges. **C,** Four-year-old boy. Note the distended abdomen and the characteristic flaring of the lower ribs. (**A** and **B,** From Nunn IN, Stephens FD. The triad syndrome: a composite anomaly of the abdominal wall urinary system and testes. J Urol 1961;86:782–794; **C,** from Metrick S et al. Congenital absence of the abdominal musculature and associated anomalies. Pediatrics 1957;19:1043–1052.)

enlarged and often is high in the abdomen and fixed at the umbilicus; often the urachus is patent. These result from much later defective developmental processes than do the muscular defects. Normally, the urachus closes in the fourth or fifth month, whereas the bladder "descends" near birth, carrying the urachal remnant with it. Presumably, descent fails because the urachus is still patent and the bladder is not free from the abdominal wall. In this sense, bladder deformation is probably secondary to the muscular dysgenesis. The distension of the bladder accounts for the frequent patent urachus and perhaps for the failure of testicular descent as well. It is also responsible for megaloureter and hydronephrosis, although defects in the musculature are equally to blame. Aganglionosis has been suggested (241), but it has not been confirmed (237).

No familial tendency has been found, nor is there any explanation for the preponderance of males. Prematurity and oligohydramnios are no more frequent than would be expected, and no correlation of the defect with parity of the mother has been noted.

HISTORY

Parker (244) in 1895 described a male infant with a thin, flaccid abdomen, who lacked both external and internal oblique abdominal muscles. Hypertrophied bladder, enlarged kidneys, and undescended testes were present. At least three earlier cases had been reported briefly: Frölich (245) and von Ammon (246) in infants, and Henderson (247) in an adult. Urinary tract defects were not mentioned in the first two and seem not to have been present in Henderson's 60-year-old patient.

By 1950 Silverman and Huang (241) were able to collect 45 cases (one of which they questioned) and added three of their own. In 1957 Metrick (242) and his colleagues collected 38 more cases and added four of their own. By 1961 at least 47 more cases had been reported, bringing the total to about 140.

INCIDENCE

In the first 100 years since the initial report, only 38 cases were recorded. In the following 30 years, 81 cases appeared, and in 1958 Lattimer (243) stated that one to three new cases were recognized at a single New York hospital each year between 1947 and 1958. Of 137 patients, only six were females.

SYMPTOMS

Urinary obstruction or respiratory embarrassment is often the presenting complaint.

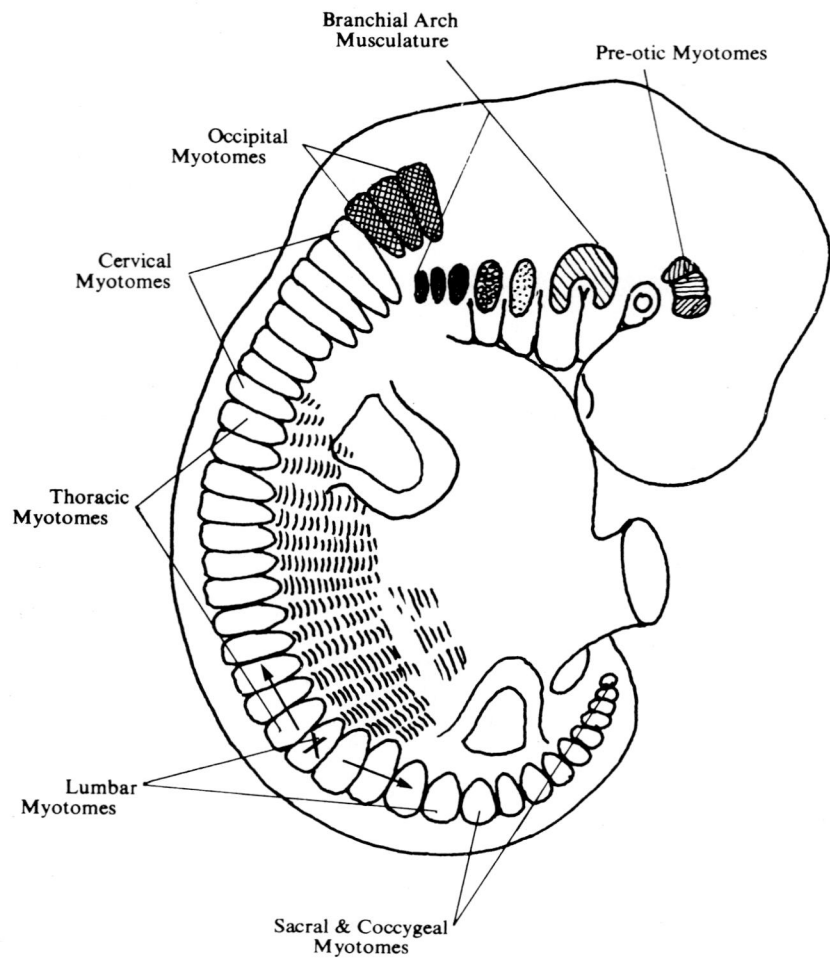

Figure 16.57. Absence or hypoplasia of the abdominal musculature centers on derivatives of the first lumbar myotome (indicated by X), but other myotomes above and below (indicated by *diverging arrows*) may be involved in severe hypoplasia. (From Allan FD. Essentials of human embryology. New York: Oxford University Press, 1960.)

DIAGNOSIS

The diagnosis is made by inspection. The thin, lax, wrinkled abdomen ("prune belly") is pathognomonic. If the blood urea nitrogen (BUN) level is not markedly elevated, excretory urography should be used to outline the urinary tract. Cystoscopy may be necessary to evaluate obstruction at the bladder neck. Cystograms are useful also in confirming the presence of vesicoureteral reflux. Retrograde pyelography may be required to rule out renal agenesis or hypoplasia.

TREATMENT

The abdominal wall can be managed conservatively with an elastic bandage which will support and protect the viscera and make breathing easier. It can also be reconstructed as advocated by Randolph et al (239, 248) and more recently by Monfort et al (249).

The primary concern is the protection of renal function. Cutaneous ureterostomy may be necessary to afford good drainage and provide time for evaluation of the lower urinary tract. Relief of bladder neck obstruction and partial resection and reimplantation of redundant or incompetent ureters may be required. If proper drainage cannot be established, permanent cutaneous ureterostomy, ileal loop diversion, or ureterosigmoidostomy should be considered.

PROGNOSIS

Among 108 patients, 44 died in early infancy, most of them from uremia, pneumonia, or other infection.

If the patient survives infancy, the outlook is reasonably good. One patient was reported well at age 20 years (250), and at least three other patients have reached puberty. Two other patients were reported alive at age 60 and 70 years and another at age 60 years (241).

REFERENCES

1. Wolff E. La Science des monstres. Paris: Gallimard, 1948.
2. Duhamel B. Embryology of exomphalos and allied malformations. Arch Dis Child 1963;38:142–147.
3. Chen JM. Studies on the morphogenesis of the mouse sternum. I. Normal embryonic development. II. Experiments on the origin of the sternum and its capacity for self-differentiation in vitro. J Anat 1952;86:373–386,387–401.
4. Bremer JL. Pleuro-peritoneal membrane and bursa infracardia. Anat Rec 1943;87:311–319.
5. Ruge G. Untersuchungen über Entwicklungsvorgänge am Brustbein und der Sternoclavicularverbindung der Menschen. Morphol Jahrb 1880;6:362–414.
6. Paterson AM. The sternum: its early development and ossification in man and mammals. J Anat Physiol 1900;35:21–32.
7. Paterson AM. Development of the sternum and shoulder girdle in mammals. Br Med 1902;2:777.
8. Whitehead RH, Waddell JA. Development of the human sternum. Am J Anat 1911;12:89–106.
9. Hanson FB. The ontogeny of phylogeny of the sternum. Am J Anat 1919;26:41–115.
10. Trotter M. Synostosis between manubrium and body of the sternum in whites and Negroes. Am J Phys Anthropol 1934;18:439–442.
11. Cobb WM. The ossa suprasternalia in whites and American Negroes and the form of the superior border of the manubrium sterni. J Anat 1937;71:245–291.
12. Wyburn GM. The development of the infra-umbilical portion of the abdominal wall with remarks on the aetiology of ectopia vesicae. J Anat 1937;71:201–231.
13. Glenister TW. A correlation of the normal and abnormal development of the penile urethra and of the infraumbilical abdominal wall. Br J Urol 1958;30:117–126.
14. Klippel CH Jr. The embryo considered as a vector field. In: El Shafie M, Klipper CH Jr, eds. Associated congenital anomalies. Baltimore: Williams & Wilkins, 1981:157–163.
15. Hutchin P. Somatic anomalies of the umbilicus and anterior abdominal wall. Surg Gynecal Obstet 1965;120:1075–1090.
16. Ravitch MM. The operative correction of pectus carinatum (pigeon breast). Ann Surg 1960;151:705–714.
17. Lester CW. The etiology and pathogenesis of funnel chest, pigeon breast and related deformities of the anterior chest wall. J Thorac Surg 1957;34:1–10.
18. Lynn HB. Pectus excavatum. J Lancet 1963;83:106–110.
19. Polgar G, Koop CE. Pulmonary function in pectus excavatum. Pediatrics 1963;32:209–215.
20. Ravitch MM. Pectus excavatum and heart failure. Surgery 1951;30:178–194.
21. Bevegard S. Postural circulatory changes after and during exercise in patients with a funnel chest, with special reference to factors affecting stroke volume. Acta Med Scand 1962;171:695.
22. Beiser GC et al. Impairment of cardiac function in patients with pectus excavatum, with improvement after operative correction. N Engl J Med 1972;287:267.
23. Cahill JL, Lees GM, Robertson HT. A summary of preoperative and postoperative cardiorespiratory performance in patients undergoing pectus excavatum and carinatum repair. J Pediatr Surg 1984;19:430–433.
24. Ravitch MM. Congenital deformities of the chest wall and their operative correction. Philadelphia: WB Saunders, 1977:81.
25. Graham JM Jr. Smith's recognizable patterns of human deformation, 2nd ed. Philadelphia: WB Saunders, 1988:35.
26. Woillez E. Sur un cas de difformité thoracique considérable , avec déplacement inoffensif de plusieurs organes et signes stéthoscopiques particuliers. Union Med J Interets Corps Med 1860;6:515.
27. Bauhinus J. Observationum medicarim. Francfurti, 1600₁:264.
28. Brown AI. Pectus excavatum (funnel chest). J Thorac Surg 1939;9:164–184.
29. Lester CW. Pigeon breast, funnel chest, and other congenital deformities of chest. JAMA 1954;156:1063–1067.
30. Lester CW. Pectus carinatum, pigeon breast and related deformities of the sternum and costal cartilages. Arch Pediatr 1960;77:399–405.
31. Popva-Latkins NV. On the development of the shape of the human thorax during the embryonic period. Med Inst Astrakhan Dokl Biol 1961;135:886–889.
32. Ochsner A, DeBakey M. Chone-chondrosternon: report of a case and review of the literature. J Thorac Surg 1939;8:469–511.
33. Nowak H. Die erbliche Trichterbrust. Deutsch Med Wschr 1936;62:2003–2004.
34. Rokitansky C. Lehrbuch der pathologischen Anatomie. Vienna [Wien]: W Braumüller, 1855-1861.
35. Ebstein W. Ueber die Trickterbrust. Deutsch Arch Klin Med 1882;30:411–428.
36. Ebstein E. Ueber die angeborene und erworbene Trichterbrust. Samml Klin Vertr Leipzig 1909;541.
37. Sauerbruch EF. Die Chirurgie der Brustorgane, 3rd ed. Berlin; J Springer, 1928.
38. Lindskog GE, Felton WL. Pectus excavatum: a report of eight cases with surgical correction. Surg Gynecol Obstet 1952;95:615–622.
39. Welch K, Vos A. Surgical correction of pectus carinatum (pigeon breast). J Pediatr Surg 1973;8:659–667.
40. Clemmens RL, Reyes AG. Pseudo pectus excavatum in the newborn due to lower respiratory tract disease. Am J Dis Child 1959;97:864–867.
41. Ravitch MM, Steichen FM. Atlas of general thoracic surgery. Philadelphia: WB Saunders, 1988:10–49.
42. Garcia VF, Seyfer AE, Graeber GM. Reconstruction of congenital chest-wall deformities. Surg Clin North Am 1989;69(5):1103–1118.
43. Ravitch MM. The chest wall. In: Benson CD et al. eds. Pediatric surgery, vol 1. Chicago: Year Book Medical Publishers, 1962:227–250.
44. Bergman RA, Thompson SA, Afifi AK, Saadeh FA. Compendium of human anatomic variation. Baltimore: Urgan & Schwarzenberg, 1988:204.
45. Lallemond: Absence de trois côtes simulant un enfoncement accidental. Ephém Med Montpel 1826;1:144.
46. Colman JK, Bisgard JD. Congenital aplasia of costal cartilages. Am J Surg 1934;25:539–542.
47. Lewis FT. The early development of the entodermal tract and the formation of its subdivisions. In: Keibel F, Mall FP, eds. Manual of human embryology, Vol 2. Philadelphia: JB Lippincott, 1912.
48. Ravitch MM. The operative treatment of congenital deformities of the chest. Am J Surg 1961;101:588–597.
49. Shamberger RC, Welch KJ, Upton III J. Surgical treatment of thoracic deformity in Poland's syndrome. J Pediatr Surg 1989;24:760–766.
50. Jeune M, Beraud C, Carron R. Dystrophic thoracique asphysiante de caractere familial. Arch Franc Pediatr 1955;12:886–891.
51. Finegold MJ, Katzew H, Genieser NB, Becker MH. Lung structure in thoracic dystrophy: case reports. Am J Dis Child 1971;122:153.
52. Hull D, Barnes ND. Children with small chests. Arch Dis Child 1972;47:12–19.

53. Karjoo M, Koop CE, Cornfeld D, Holtzapple PG. Pancreatic exocrine enzyme deficiency associated with asphyxiating thoracic dystrophy. Arch Dis Child 1973;48:143–46.

54. Cantrell JR, Haller JA, Ravitch MM. A syndrome of congenital defects involving the abdominal wall, sternum, diaphragm, pericardium and heart. Surg Gynecol Obstet 1958;197:602–614.

55. Mulder DG, Crittenden IH, Adams FH. Complete repair of a syndrome of congenital defects involving the abdominal wall, sternum, diaphragm, pericardium, and heart: excision of left ventricular diverticulum. Ann Surg 1960;151:113–122.

56. Murphy DA, Aberdeen E, Dobbs RH, Waterston DJ. The surgical treatment of a syndrome consisting of thoracoabdominal wall, diaphragmatic, pericardial, and ventricular septal defects, and a left ventricular diverticulum. Ann Thorac Surg 1969;6:528.

57. Symbas PN and Ware RE. A syndrome of defects of the thoracoabdominal wall, diaphragm, pericardium, and heart. J Thorac Cardiovasc Surg 1973;65–914.

58. Byron F. Ectopia cordis: report of a case with attempted operative correction. J Thorac Surg 1948;17:717–722.

59. Martin LW, Helmsworth JA. The management of congenital deformities of the sternum. JAMA 1962;179:82–84.

60. Asp K, Sulamaa M. Ectopia cordis. Acta Chir Scand 1961;123(Suppl):52–56.

61. Ravitch MM. Congenital absence of sternum. In: American College of Surgeons, Clinical Congress. Advancing with surgery: spectacular problems in surgery. Somerville, NJ: Ethicon, 1962.

62. Maier HC, Bortone F. Complete failure of sternal fusion with herniation of pericardium. J Thorac Surg 1949;18:851–859.

63. Greenberg BM, Becker JM, Pletcher BA. Congenital bifid sternum: repair in early infancy and literature review. Plast Reconstr Surg 1991;88:886–889.

64. Longino LA, Jewett TC Jr. Congenital bifid sternum. Surgery 1955;38:610–614.

65. Jewett TC Jr, Butsch WL, Hug HR. Congenital bifid sternum. Surgery 1962;52:932–936.

66. Schao-tsu VL. Ectopia cordis congenita. Thorax 1957;5:197–212.

67. Major JW. Thoraco-abdominal ectopia cordis: report of a case successfully treated by surgery. J Thorac Surg 1953;26:309–317.

68. Breschet G. Mémoir sur l'ectopie de l'appareil de la circulation et particulièrement sur celle du coeur. Rep Gen Anat Physiol Pathol Clin Chir (Paris) 1826;2:1.

69. Ramel MFB. Sur un coeur situé au-dessous du diaphragme. J Chir Pharm 1778;64:423–428.

70. Huchard H. Un cas d'ectrocardie épigastrique. Bull Mem Soc Med Hôp Paris 1888;5:300.

71. Medina-Escobedo G, Reyes-Mugica M, Arteaga-Martinez M. Ectopia cordis: autopsy findings in four cases. Pediatr Pathol 1991;11:85–95.

72. Reese HE, Stracener CE. Congenital defects involving the abdominal wall, sternum, diaphragm and pericardium. Ann Surg 1966;163:391–394.

73. Kanagasuntheram R, Verzin JA. Ectopia cordis in man. Thorax 1962;17:159–167.

74. Willius FA. An unusually early description of the so-called tetralogy of Fallot. Proc May Clin 1948;23:316–320.

75. Greig DM. Cleft-sternum and ectopia cordis. Edinb Med J 1926;33:480–511.

76. Weese C. De cordis ectopia [Inaug Dissert]. Berlin: JF Starck, 1818.

77. Roth F. Morphologie und Pathogenese der ectopia cordis congenita. Frankfurt Z Pathol 1939;53:60–100.

78. Blatt ML, Zeldes M. Ectopia cordis: report of a case and a review of the literature. Am J Dis Child 1942;63:515–529.

79. Kanagasuntheram R, Perumal Pillai C. Ectopia cordis and other anomalies in a dog embryo. Res Vet Sci 1960;1:172.

80. Abbott ME. Atlas of congenital cardiac disease. New York: American Heart Association, 1936.

81. Lumsden JFW. A case of ectopia cordis diagnosed clinically in utero. J Obstet Gynaecol Br Commw 1960;67:299–300.

82. Lannelongue O. De l'ectocardie et de sa cure par l'autoplastie. Acad Sci Paris 1888;106:1336–1339.

83. Laliberté JH. Ectopia cordis. Bull Med Quebec 1918;20:241.

84. Langebartel D. The anatomical primer. Baltimore: University Park Press. 1977.

85. Deaver JB, McFarland J. The breast: its anomalies, its diseases and their treatment. London: William Hunman, 1918.

86. Trier WC. Complete breast absence: case report and review of the literature. Plast Reconstr Surg 1965;36:430–439.

87. Fraser FC. Dominant inheritance of absent nipples and breast. Novant' anni delle leggi mendeliane. Rome: Instituto Gregorio Mendel, 1956:360–362.

88. Goldenring H, Crelin ES. Mother and daughter with bilateral congenital amastia. Yale J Biol Med 1961;33:466–467.

89. Kowlessar M, Orti E. Complete breast absence in siblings. Am J Dis Child 1968;115:91–93.

90. Batchelor HT. Absence of mammae in a woman. Br Med J 1888;2:876.

91. Iwai T. A statistical study of polymastia of the Japanese. Lancet 1907a;2:753–759.

92. Crumpe F. Dublin Q J Med Sci 1854;17:466.

93. Tow SH, Shanmuharatnam K. Supernumerary mammary gland in the vulva. Br Med J 1962;2:1234–1236.

94. de Cholnoky T. Supernumerary breast. Arch Surg 1939;39:926–941.

95. Kajava Y, Schroderus M, Wallenius M, Wichmann SE. Das Vorkommen überzähliger Milchdrüsen bei der Bevölkerung in Finland. Act Soc Med Fenn Duodecim 1921;2:1–163.

96. Weinshel LR, Demakopoulos N. Supernumerary breasts. Am J Surg 1943;60:76–80.

97. Graham-Campbell R. Polythelia. Br Med J 1936;1:471.

98. Landauer W. Supernumerary nipples, congenital hemihypertrophy and congenital hemi-atrophy. Hum Biol 1930;2:447–472.

99. Leichtenstern O. Über das Vorkommen und die Bedeutung supernumerärer (accessoricher) Bruste und Brustwarzen auf Grund 13 eigener und 92 aus der Literatur gesammelter Beobachtungen. Virchow Arch [A] 1878;72:222–256.

100. Iwai T. The relation of polymastia to multiparous birth. Lancet 1907b;2:818–820.

101. Speert H. Supernumerary mammae, with special reference to the Rhesus monkey. Q Rev Biol 1942;17:59–68.

102. Castle WE. The genetics of multi-nippled sheep. J Hered 1924;15:75–85.

103. Haagensen CD. Diseases of the breast, 3rd ed. Philadelphia: WB Saunders, 1986.

104. von Saar G. Die gutartigen Geschwülste der Brustdrüse im Lichte neuer Forschungen. Ergebn Chir Orthop 1910;1:413–450.

105. Champneys FH. On the development of mammary functions by the skin of lying-in women. Med Chir Trans (London) 1886;69:419–442.

106. Moore KL. The developing human: clinically oriented embryology, 4th ed. Philadelphia: WB Saunders, 1988.

107. Geoffroy St. Hilaire I. Histoire générale et particulière des anomalies de l'organization chez l'homme et les animaux. Paris: JB Baillière, 1832–1836.

108. Bruce JM. On supernumerary nipples and mammae. J Anat Physiol 1879;13:425.

109. Von Bardeleben K. Massenuntersuchungen über Hyperthelie beim Mann. Verh Anat Ges 1893;7:171–185.

110. Williams WR. Polymastism, with special reference to mammae erraticae and the development of neoplasms from supernumerary structures. J Anat Physiol 1891;25:225–255.

111. Cellini A, Offidani A. Familial supernumerary nipples and breasts. Dermatology 1992;185:56–58.

112. Elder JH. Report of a case of inherited polymastia in chimpanzee. Anat Rec 1936;65:83–98.

113. Moore TC, Stokes GE. Gastroschisis: report of two cases treated by modification of gross operation for omphalocele. Surgery 1953;33:112–120.

114. Orda R, Nathan N. Surgical anatomy of the umbilical structures. In: Skandalakis JE et al, eds. Hernia: surgical anatomy and technique. Int Surg 1973;58(7):454–456.

115. Halpern LJ. Spontaneous healing of umbilical hernias. JAMA 1962;182:851–852.

116. Woods GE. Some observations on umbilical hernia in infants. Arch Dis Child 1953;28:450–462.

117. Crump EP. Umbilical hernia. I. Occurrence of the infantile type in Negro infants and children. J Pediatr 1952;40:214–223.

118. Blumberg NA. Infantile umbilical hernia. Surg Gynecol Obstet 1980;150:187.

119. Sibley WL III, Lynn HB, Harris LE. A twenty-five year study of infantile umbilical hernia. Surgery 1964;55:462–468.

120. Benson CD, Penherthy GC, Hill EJ. Hernia into the umbilical cord and omphalocele (amniocele) in the newborn. Arch Surg 1949;58:833.

121. Gross RE, Blodgett JB. Omphalocele (umbilical eventration) in the newly born. Surg Gynecol Obstet 1940;71:520–527.

122. Ladd WE, Gross RE. Abdominal surgery of infancy and childhood. Philadelphia: WB Saunders, 1941.

123. Margulies L. Omphalocele (amniocele). Am J Obstet Gynecol 1945;49:695.

124. Buchanan RW, Cain WL. A case of a complete omphalocele. Ann Surg 1956;143:552–556.

125. Soper RT, Green EW. Omphalocele. Surg Gynecol Obstet 1961;113:501–508.

126. Smith WR, Leix F. Omphalocele. Am J Surg 1966;3:450–456.

127. Greenwald RD, Rosenthal A, Nada AS. Cardiovascular malfunctions associated with omphalocele. J Pediatr Surg 1974;85:181.

128. Raffensperger JG, ed. Swenson's pediatric surgery. Norwalk, CT: Appleton & Lange, 1990.

129. Benacerraf BR, Saltzman DH, Estroff JM, Frigoletto FD Jr. Abnormal karyotype of fetuses with omphalocele: prediction based on omphalocele contents. Obstet Gynecol 1990;75:317–319.

130. Smith NM, Chambers HM, Furness ME, Haan EA. The OEIS complex (omphalocele-exstrophy-imperforate anus-spinal defects): recurrence in sibs. J Med Genet 1992;29:730–732.

131. Martin LW, Torres AM. Omphalocele and gastroschisis. Surg Clinic North Am 1985;65(5):1238.

132. Tucci M, Bard H. The associated anomalies that determine prognosis in congenital omphaloceles. Am J Obstet Gynecol 1990;163:1646–1649.

133. Bergglas B. Zur Genese und Therapie der Nabelschnurbrueche. Arch Gynaek 1933;152:214.

134. Papez JW. A rare intestinal anomaly of embryonic origin. Anat Rec 1932;54:195–215.

135. Paul of Aegina: The seven books of Paulus Aegineta. Francis Adam (transl.). London: Sydenham Society, 1846.

136. Jarcho J. Congenital umbilical hernia. Surg Gynecol Obstet 1937;65:593–600.

137. Scarpa A. Traité pratique des hernies. Baylor (transl.). Paris: Gabon, 1812.

138. Aribat P. Contribution à l'eétude des herniaes ombilicales congénitales [Thesis]. Paris, 1901.

139. McKeown T, MacMahon B, Record RG. An investigation of 69 cases of exomphalos. Am J Hum Genet 1953;5:168–175.

140. Herbert AF. Hernia funiculi umbilicalis, with report of three cases. Am J Obstet Gynecol 1928;15:86–88.

141. Ivy RH. Congenital anomalies, as recorded on birth certificates in the Division of Vital Statistics of the Pennsylvania Department of Health, for the period 1951–1955, inclusive. Plast Reconstr Surg 1957;20:400–411.

142. Eckstein HB. Exomphalos: a review of 100 cases. Br J Surg 1963a;50:405–410.

143. Mahour GH. Omphalocele. Surg Gynecol Obstet 1976;143:821.

144. Landor JH, Armstrong JH, Dickerson OB, Westerfeld RA. Neonatal obstruction of bowel caused by accidental clamping of small omphalocele: report of two cases. South Med J 1963;56:1236–1238.

145. Skandalakis JE, Gray SW, Mansberger AR Jr, Colborn GL, Skandalakis LJ: Hernia: surgical anatomy and technique. New York: McGraw-Hill, 1989.

146. Gross RE. The surgery of infancy and childhood. Philadelphia: WB Saunders, 1953.

147. Luck SR, Sherman JO, Raffensperger JG, Goldstein IR. Gastroschisis in 106 consecutive newborn infants. Surgery 1985;98:677–683.

148. Holcomb GW Jr. Omphalocele. Am J Surg 1961;101:598–604.

149. de Lorimier AA, Adzick NS, Harrison MR. Amnion inversion in the treatment of giant omphalocele. J Pediatr Surg 1991;26:804–807.

150. Yokomori K, Ohkura M, Kitano Y, Hori T, Nakajo T. Advantages and pitfalls of amnion in version repair for the treatment of large unruptured omphalocele: results of 22 cases. J Pediatr Surg 1992;27:882–884.

151. Soave F. Conservative treatment of infant omphalocele. Arch Dis Child 1963;38:130–134.

152. Visick C. An umbilical hernia in a newly-born child. Lancet 1873;1:829.

153. O'Leary CM, Clymer CE. Umbilical hernia. Am J Surg 1941;52:38–43.

154. Eckstein HB. Weights of children with major congenital abnormalities of the intestinal tract. Arch Dis Child 1963b;38:173–175.

155. Moore TC, Nur K. An international survey of gastroschisis and omphalocele (490 cases). I. Nature and distribution of additional malformations. Pediatr Surg Int 1986;1:46–50.

156. Stringel G, Filler R. Prognostic factors in omphalocele and gastroschisis. J Pediatr Surg 1979;14:515.

157. Mayer T, Black R, Matlak M, Johnson D. Gastroschisis and omphalocele. Ann Surg 1980;192:783.

158. Schwartzberg S, Pokorny W, McGill C, Hasbeg F. Gastroschisis and omphalocele. Am J Surg 1982;144:650.

159. Berman EJ. Gastroschisis, with comments on embryological development and surgical treatment. Arch Surg 1957;75:788–792.

160. Ballantyne JW. Manual of antenatal pathology and hygiene. Edinburgh: William Green & Sons, 1904.

161. Moore TC. Gastroschisis with antenatal evisceration of intestines and urinary bladder. Ann Surg 1953;158:263.

162. Schuster SR. Omphalocele and gastroschisis. In: Welch KJ, et al., eds. Pediatric surgery. Chicago: Year Book Medical Publishers, 1986:740–763.

163. Shaw A. The myth of gastroschisis. J Pediatr Surg 1975;10:235.

164. Noordijk JA, Bloemsma-Jonkman F. Gastroschisis: no myth. J Pediatr Surg 1978;13:47.

165. Werler MM, Mitchell AA, Shapiro S. Demographic, reproductive, medical and environmental factors in relation to gastrochisis. Teratology 1992;45:353–360.

166. Orongowski RA, Smith RK Jr, Coran AG, Klein MD. Contribution of demographic and environmental factors to the etiology of gastrochisis: a hypothesis. Fetal Diagn Ther 1991;6:14–27.

167. Goldbaum G, Daling J, Milham S. Risk factors for gastroschisis. Teratology 1990;42:397–403.

168. Simpson RL, Caylor HD. Gastroschisis. Am J Surg 1958;96:675–678.

169. Rickham PP. The incidence and treatment of etopia vesicae. Proc Roy Soc Med 1961;54:389–392.

170. Calder J. Medical essays and observations. Edinburgh, 1733.203.

171. Bernstein P. Gastroschisis, a rare teratological condition in the newborn. Arch Pediatr 1940;57:505–513.

172. Kiesewetter WB. Gastroschisis: report of a case. Arch Surg 1957;75:28–30.

173. Randolph J. Omphalocele and gastrochisis: different entities, similar therapeutic goals. South Med J 1982;75(12):1517–1519.

174. Moore T, Khalid N. An international survey of gastroschisis and omphalocele (490 cases). I. Nature and distribution of additional malformations. II. Relative incidence, pregnancy and environmental factors. Pediatr Surg Int 1986;1:46,109.

175. Watkins DE. Gastroschisis, with case report. Va Med Month 1943;70:42–44.

176. Swartz KR, Harrison MW, Campbell TJ, Campbell JR. Selective management of gastroschisis. Ann Surg 1986;203:214–218.

177. Swift RI, Singh MP, Ziderman DA, Silverman M, Elder MA, Elder MG. A new regime in the management of gastrochisis. J Pediatr Surg 1992;27:61–63.

178. Stringer MD, Brereton RJ, Wright VM. Controversies in the management of gastroschisis: a study of 40 patients. Arch Dis Child 1991;66:34–36.

179. Shah R, Woolley. Gastroschisis and intestinal atresia. J Pediatr Surg 1991;26:788–790.

180. Hebra A, Ross AJ. Abdominal wall defects: omphalocele and gastroschisis. Post Grad Surg 1992;4:32–37.

181. Yang P, Beaty TH, Khoury MJ, Chee E, Stewart W, Gordis L. Genetic-epidemiologic study of omphalocele and gastroschisis: evidence for heterogeneity. Am J Med Genet 1992;44:668–675.

182. Chang PY, Yeh ML, Sheu JC, Chen CC. Experience with treatment of gastroschisis and omphalocele. J Formos Med Assoc 1992;91:447–451.

183. Sauter ER, Falterman KW, Arensman RM. Is primary repair of gastroschisis and omphalocele always the best operation? Am Surg 1991;57:142–144.

184. Sipes SL, Weiner CP, Sipes DR II, Grant SS, Williamson RA. Gastroschisis and omphalocele: does either antenatal diagnosis or route of delivery make a difference in perinatal outcome? Obstet Gynecol 1990;76:195–199.

185. Kohn MR, Shi EC. Gastroschisis and exomphalos: recent trends and factors influencing survival. Aust NZ J Surg 1990;60:199–202.

186. Anthony JE Jr., Brawley WG. An unusual complication associated with omphalocele. J Med Assoc Ga 1963;52:363–364.

187. Chandler SB, Schadewald M. Studies on the inguinal region. I. The conjoined aponeurosis versus the conjoined tendon. Anat Rec 1944;80:339–343.

188. Krieg EGM. Anatomy and physiology of the inguinal region in the presence of hernia. Ann Surg 1953;137:41–56.

189. Anson BJ, Morgan EH, McVay CB. Surgical anatomy of the inguinal region based upon a study of 500 body-halves. Surg Gynecol Obstet 1960;111:707–725.

190. Macalister A. Observations on muscular anomalies in the human anatomy. Trans R Irish Acad Sci 1875;25:1–130.

191. Condon RE. The anatomy of the inguinal region and its relationship to groin hernia. Nyhus LM, Condon RE, eds. Hernia, 2nd ed. Philadelphia: JB Lippincott, 1978:14.

192. Thorndike A Jr., Ferguson CF. Incarcerated inguinal hernia in infancy and childhood. New Engl J Med 1938;218:205–211.

193. Burton CC. The embryologic development and descent of the testis in relation to congenital hernia. Surg Gynecol Obstet 1958;107:294.

194. Rowe MI, Copelson LW, Clatsworthy HW. The patent processus vaginalis and the inguinal hernia. J Pediatr Surg 1969;4:102.

195. Arnheim EE, Linder JM. Inguinal hernia of the pelvic viscera in female infants. Am J Surg 1956;92:436–440.

196. Frazer JE. In: Buchanan's manual of anatomy, 6th ed. London: Bailliere, Tindall & Cox, 1937.

197. Mitchell GAG. The condition of the peritoneal vaginal processes at birth. J Anat 1939;73:658–661.

198. Moskalenko V. Konstitutionelle veranlagung zu inguinal hernia. Arch Orthop Unfallchir 1928;26:503–519.

199. Harris FI, White AS. The length of the inguinal ligament. JAMA 1937;109:1900–1903.

200. Watson LF. Hernia: anatomy, etiology, symptoms, diagnosis, differential diagnosis, prognosis, and the operative and injective treatment, 2nd ed. St. Louis: CV Mosby, 1938.

201. Maitland AIL. A survey of incidence of inguinal hernia in different racial groups. Br J Surg 1948;34:408–410.

202. Kingdon JA. On the causes of hernia. Roy Med Chir Trans London 1864;47:295–321.

203. Iason AH. Hernia in infancy and childhood. Am J Surg 1945;68:287–296.

204. Stephens P. Etiology of inguinal hernia. Surg Clin North Am 1942;22:1107–1113.

205. Harper RC, Carcia A, Sia C. Inguinal hernia: a common problem of premature infants weighing 1000 grams or less at birth. Pediatrics 1975;56:112.

206. Weiner BR. Congenital inheritance of inguinal hernia. J Hered 1949;40:219.

207. Bakmin H. Inguinal hernia in twins. J Pediatr Surg 1971;6:165.

208. Haller A. Opusculla pathologica. (Lausanne): Bousquet et Soc. 1755.

209. Hunter J. Observation on certain parts of the animal oeconomy. London, 1786.

210. Cloquet J. Recherches anatomiques sur les hernies de l'abdomen [Thesis]. Paris, 1817.

211. Russell RH. The etiology and treatment of inguinal hernia in the young. Lancet 1899;2:1353–1358.

212. Keith A. On the origin and nature of hernia. Br J Surg 1924;11:455–475.

213. Scorer CG. Descent of the testicle in the first year of life. Br J Urol 1955;27:374–378.

214. Society of Medical Officers of Health, East Anglian Branch Survey. Med Offr 1958;100:379.

215. Campbell M. Urology. Philadelphia: WB Saunders, 1963.

216. Bronsther B, Abrams M, Elboim C. Inguinal hernia in children: a study of 1,000 cases and a review of the literature. J Am Med Women Assoc 1972;22:522.

217. Holder TM, Ashcraft KW. Groin hernias and hydroceles. In: Textbook of pediatric surgery. Philadelphia: WB Saunders, 1980:594.

218. Rowe MI, Clatworthy HW. The other side of the pediatric inguinal hernia. Surg Clinic North Am 1971;51;1371.

219. Czeizel and Gardonyi J. A family study of congenital inguinal hernia. Am J Med Genet 1979;4:247.

220. Rowe MI, Lloyd OA. Inguinal hernia. In: Welch KJ et al., eds. Pediatric surgery. Chicago: Year Book Medical Publishers, 1986:779–93.

221. Janik and Shandling B. The vulnerability of the vas deferens. II. The case against routine bilateral inguinal exploration. J Pediatr Surg 1982;17:585.

222. Wilkander O. Incarcerated inguinal hernia in childhood. Acta Chir Scand 1951;101:303.

223. Sloman JG. Testicular infarction in infancy: in association with irreducible inguinal hernia. Med J Aust 1958;45:242.

224. Moss RL, Hatch EI Jr. Inguinal hernia repair in early infancy. Am J Surg 1991;161:596–599.

225. Wilms G et al. Solitary or predominantly right-sided varicocele, a possible sign for situs inversus. Urol Radiol 1988;9:243–246.

226. Yarborough MA, Burns JR, Keller FS. Incidence and clinical significance of subclinical varicoceles. J Urol 1989;141:1372–1374.

227. Belker AM. Surgery for male infertility. In: Glenn JE, ed. Urologic surgery, 4th ed. Philadelphia: JB Lippincott, 1991.

228. Ahlberg NE, Bartley O, Chidekel N. Right and left gonadal veins: an anatomical and statistical study. Acta Radiol 1966;4:593–601.

229. Kuypers P, Kang N, Ellis N. Valveless testicular veins: a possible etiological factor in varicocele. Clin Anat 1992;5:113–118.

230. Shafik A, Khalil AM, Saleh M. The fascio-muscular tube of the spermatic cord. J Urol 1972;44:147–151.

231. Saypol DC, Howards SS, Turner TT, Miller ED. Influence of surgically induced varicocele on testicular blood flow, temperature and histology in adult rats and dogs. J Clin Invest 1981;68:39–45.

232. Williams PL, Warwick R, Dyson M, Bannister L. Gray's anatomy, 37th ed. Edinburg: Churchill Livingston, 1989.

233. Basmajian JV. Grant's method of anatomy, 8th ed. Baltimore: Williams & Wilkins, 1971.

234. Sheldon JG, Heller EP. Congenital defect of the anterior abdominal wall and cryptorchism. J Miss Med Assoc 1922;19:493–495.

235. Stoica T, Andor G, Ganea Z. Angeoborene Eventration infolge Aplasie der schrägen Bauchdeckenmuskulatur. Zentralbl Chir 1959;84:325–329.

236. Jona JZ. Umbilical anomalies. In: Raffensperger JG, ed. Swenson's pediatric surgery. Norwalk, CT: Appleton & Lange, 1990:194.

237. Nunn IN, Stephens FD. The triad syndrome: a complete anomaly of the abdominal wall, urinary system and testes. J Urol 1961;86:782.

238. Duckett J. Prune belly syndrome. In: Welch K et al., eds. Pediatric surgery. Chicago: Year Book Medical Publishers, 1986:1195.

239. Randolph JG. Total surgical reconstruction for patients with abdominal muscular deficiency (prune belly syndrome). J Pediatr Surg 1977;12:1033–1043.

240. Greene LF, Emmett JL, Culp OS. Urologic abnormalities associated with congenital absence or deficiency of abdominal musculature. J Urol 1952;68:217–229.

241. Silverman FN, Huang N. Congenital absence of abdominal muscles: report of cases and review of literature. Am J Dis Child 1950;80:91–124.

242. Metrick S, Brown RH, Rosenblum A. Congenital absence of the abdominal musculature and associated anomalies. Pediatrics 1957;19:1043–1052.

243. Lattimer JK. Congenital deficiency of the abdominal musculature and associated genitourinary anomalies: a report of 22 cases. J Urol 1958;79:343–352.

244. Parker RW. Absence of abdominal muscles in an infant. Lancet 1895;1:1252.

245. Fröhlich F. Der mangel der muskeln, insbesondere der seitenbauch-muskein. Würzburg: Zürn, 1839.

246. von Ammon FA. Die angebornen chirurgischen krankheiten des menschen in abbildungen dargestellt und durch erläuternden tex erklärt. Berlin: FA Herbig, 1842.

247. Henderson B. Congenital absence of abdominal muscles. Glasgow Med J 1890;33:63.

248. Randolph JG, Cavett C, Eng G. Abdominal wall reconstruction in the prune belly syndrome. J Pediatr Surg 1981;16:960–964.

249. Monfort G, Guys JM, Bocciardi A, Coquet M, Chevallier D. A novel technique for reconstruction of the abdominal wall in the prune belly syndrome. J Urol 1991;146:639–640.

250. Riparetti PP, Charnock DA. Urological problems in agenesis of abdominal wall musculature. Trans West Sect Am Urol Assoc 1953;20:57–66.

CHAPTER 17

THE KIDNEY AND URETER

Thomas S. Parrott / John Elias Skandalakis / Stephen Wood Gray

Did Nature really need two instruments to remove the serous liquid? I ask because
if it was better to have two, she would seem to have been negligent when she made
only one spleen and one gall bladder, and again, if one is sufficient, she would
seem to have made a superfluous left kidney in addition to the right. Or must we
even in this admire her skill?
—*GALEN, ON THE USEFULNESS OF THE PARTS THE INSTRUMENTS OF NUTRITION*

DEVELOPMENT

Human nephric organs arise from a portion of the paraxial mesoderm which becomes demarcated with formation of somites during the fourth week of gestation. The particular region, the nephrotome, lies lateral to the somite and medial to the lateral plate from which the body musculature arises (Fig. 17.1). Because of this position, it is called the *intermediate mesoderm;* in view of its fate, that part of the intermediate mesoderm from the level of the seventh somite caudad may be called the *nephrogenic mesoderm.*

During the fourth and fifth weeks of development a wave of differentiation starts at the cranial end of this nephrogenic mesoderm and proceeds caudally, culminating in the formation of the true kidney (metanephros), and leaving various modified and vestigial structures in its wake (Fig. 17.2).

Although the essential facts remain the same, the path of development may be viewed in two ways. The classic interpretation, which Felix (1) elucidated in a magnificent chapter in Keibel and Mall's *Manual of Human Embryology,* emphasized ontogenetic recapitulation of phylogeny, which for many years had been the most important guiding principle in embryology. In the jawless fishes *(Cyclostomes),* an excretory organ, the pronephros, forms from the more cranial somites; in the true fishes and amphibians, more caudal segments form the permanent kidney, the mesonephros; whereas in birds and mammals a still more caudal region forms the definitive metanephric kidney.

With this comparative background it was easy to convince oneself, in studying mammalian embryology, that one observed the early appearance of a vestigial pronephros, the later appearance of a mesonephros and the ultimate development of the badge of the higher vertebrates, the metanephros.

Although this sequence has been widely accepted, as early as 1879 Balfour and Segwick (2)—and later embryologists—thought that the division of nephrogenic activity into three stages was arbitrary and misleading. They constitute the "holonephric" school, whose chief defenders have been Fraser (3) and Torrey (3). To proponents of this school of thought, kidney development occurs in a continuous wave of formation of glomeruli and tubules, which proceeds caudally in the nephrogenic mesoderm. It is followed by a similar wave of degeneration and reabsorption that leaves only the most caudal and the last formed units as the definitive kidney of the adult (Fig. 17.2).

This holonephric concept has much to recommend it to the embryologist. It is hard to justify a distinction between pronephros and mesonephros among the anterior tubules. The metanephros, whose units arise from a common branch of the wolffian duct, should perhaps be considered a single compound nephric unit comparable with one of the mesonephric units, each of which arises independently from the wolffian duct. This is in accord with the shift from large glomeruli with short tubules at the cranial end to small glomeruli with long tubules at the caudal end of the series (5).

Whether or not the kidney is considered to form as three discrete organs or as a continuum, it is necessary for our purposes to discuss separately the cranial portion that degenerates before birth and the caudal portion that forms the adult kidney.

Embryonic Kidney (Pronephros and Mesonephros)

In the latter half of the fourth week, tubules appear in the intermediate mesoderm. They form successively, starting occasionally as high as the second somite, but usually extending from the seventh somite onward. They are not

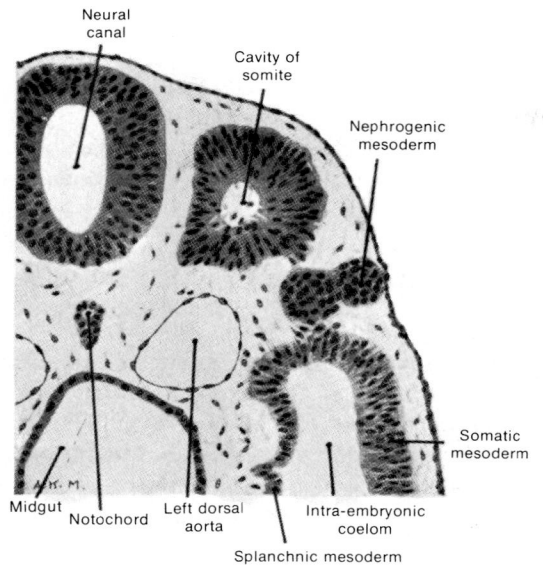

Figure 17.1. A section through a 14-mm human embryo at the level of the tenth somite. The lateral mesoderm appears dorsally as the somite and ventrally as splanchnic and somatic mesoderm, separated by the celom. Between these, a solid mesodermal region, the future mesonephric capsule and tubular area lie medially and the future wolffian duct, laterally. (From Hamilton WJ, Boyd JD, Mossman HW. Human embryology, 3rd ed. Baltimore: Williams & Wilkins, 1962.)

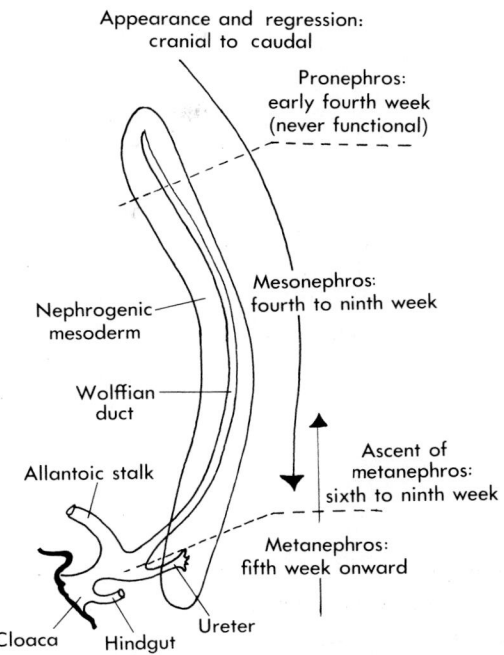

Figure 17.2. Diagram of the development of nephric structures of the human embryo. Development, maturation, and regression proceed caudad. Only the most caudal portion of the nephrogenic mesoderm persists to become the adult kidney. This organ then moves cranially to reach its normal position in the abdomen.

metameric; eventually there are many more tubules than there are somites. The most cranial tubules disappear before the caudal ones are formed.

The first seven tubules to appear are those considered by Felix (1) to be pronephric. Only occasionally has a glomerulus been described (6), and Torrey (4, 7) doubts true glomeruli are formed in these cranial tubules. The chief distinction between those tubules called pronephric and the later, more caudal tubules is their contribution to the formation of the wolffian duct. Felix (1) described the beginning of the duct as springing from the coalescence of pronephric tubules, starting at the ninth somite. Heuser (6) and later Torrey (4) consider the duct to arise *in situ* just as the first tubules become delimited from the nephrogenic mass.

After initial appearance, the duct grows caudally toward the cloaca in the mesenchyme just beneath the celomic epithelium. It is at first solid in its elongating portion, and its tip reaches the cloaca at the 26 to 28 somite stage. It is completely hollow by the time 36 somites are present, near the end of the fifth week.

Tubules appearing below the level of somite 14 join the already formed duct. A total of 83 tubules may be formed, although only about half are present at any one time (Fig. 17.3). Felix (1) considered that the caudal proliferation and cranial degeneration of tubules shifted the entire mesonephros backward; but Davies and Davies (5), using landmarks peculiar to sheep mesonephros, believe

that elongation of the embryo rather than cranial degeneration is responsible for most of the caudal shift. They observed degeneration of only the cranial six to twelve tubules and felt that union with the gonad (vasa efferentia) involved the succeeding six tubules. Felix placed genital union at the level of tubules 58 to 69. There may, of course, be species differences.

Simultaneous movements of the digestive organs change the abdominal relations rapidly. At 4 mm, the head of the mesonephros is at the level of the liver bud and the tubules extend almost to the junction of the intestine and cloaca. Beyond the last tubules, the nephrogenic mesoderm is undifferentiated. By 5.5 mm, the cranial end of the wolffian duct reaches the level of the lower part of the stomach, and the nephrogenic mesoderm at the caudal end is being invaded by the ureteric bud. At 8 mm (sixth week), elongation of the stomach and esophagus has brought the head of the mesonephros to the level of the lower part of the esophagus. By 14.5 mm (seventh week), only degenerating tubules lie above the cardia of the stomach, and the last tubules are at the level of the body stalk; the metanephros has begun its ascent. By 23 mm (end of the eighth week), the metanephric hilus lies at the head of the mesonephros, all of which now lies at the level of the greatly expanded stomach (Fig. 17.4, *E*). These relationships have been described by Shikinami (8).

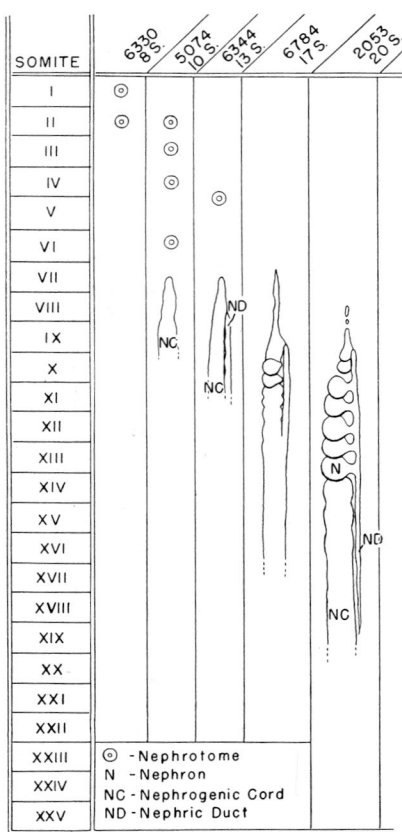

Figure 17.3. Formation of the earliest tubules of the embryonic kidney. The wolffian duct first appears at the level of somite 8 in embryos of 13 somites. *Column heading* gives specimen identification and number of somites present. (From Torrey TW. The early development of the mesonephros. Contrib Embryol Carnegie Inst Wash 1954;35:175–197.)

At its greatest development, each mesonephric tubule consists of a glomerulus surrounded by a Bowman's capsule, which is drained by a tubule that passes laterally, dorsally, and medially to form a loop, which again turns laterally to join the wolffian duct. There are no secondary or tertiary divisions of the tubules in mammals, such as there are in the chick. Mesonephric arteries supplying the glomeruli arise as parallel, right-angled branches from the aorta; vessels form and degenerate with the glomeruli they supply. Drainage occurs into the postcardinal veins. A mesonephric portal system does not seem to become established in the human embryo.

From about the 13-mm stage (beginning of the seventh week), there is an absolute decrease in the number of mesonephric units, and by 40 mm (10th week), no intact units are left (9). In the degenerating tubules, the capsular epithelium thickens and the capillary tufts of the glomerulus withdraw. The capsular epithelium thickens and the capillary tufts of the glomerulus withdraw. The capsule becomes a blind end of the tubule, with an epithe-

lium indistinguishable from that of the remainder of the tube.

Vestigial remains of the mesonephric tubules occur regularly in both sexes, and some may undergo pathologic changes. These remnants usually are associated with the reproductive tract of the adult and are discussed in Chapters 21 and 22.

Functional State of the Mesonephros

Altschule (9) concluded that the mesonephros was anatomically capable of functioning, but he was unable to demonstrate that it did. Gersh (10) showed that mesonephric glomeruli can excrete ferrocyanide and mesonephric tubules excrete phenol red in fetal rabbits, cats, and pigs. In the rabbit the mesonephros produces glomerular filtrate, but its ability to concentrate the filtrate appears to be very poor (11–13). There is no similar proof of mesonephric function in humans, but from the morphologic appearance, it is reasonable to believe that there is some excretion.

Functional or not, the mesonephros inexorably degenerates even when no metanephros develops to supersede it: Renal agenesis does not result in mesonephric persistence. A single case (14) has been reported in which the mesonephroi and their ducts persisted and may even have functioned in an otherwise normal adult (Fig. 17.5).

The Adult Kidney (Metanephros)

The formation of the adult kidney depends on the existence of the embryonic kidney, or at least on the presence of a mesonephric duct from which the ureter will arise. The interdependence of the metanephros, the genital ducts, and the suprarenal cortex, as well as the consequences of arrest at various developmental states, are illustrated in Table 17.1.

By the 4-mm stage, the wolffian duct has reached the cloaca, bending at the level of the first sacral vertebra to join the cloaca at almost a right angle. At this point, the ureter appears as a dorsal bud, growing from the wolffian duct, and turns cephaladly into the undifferentiated nephrogenic mesenchyme (nephric blastema) lying caudal to the mesonephros. By the 9- or 10-mm stage, the tip of the ureteric bud has elongated craniodorsally and produced several secondary buds, which will form the primitive pelvis and calyces (Fig. 17.6, A). The mesenchyme is condensed visibly about this expanded tip. Grobstein (15, 16) has shown that formation of secondary and subsequent generations of buds from the ureteric tip is the result of induction by nephrogenic mesoderm acting on the ureteric epithelium.

The secondary buds of the primitive pelvis mark the beginning of rapid dichotomous branching and reab-

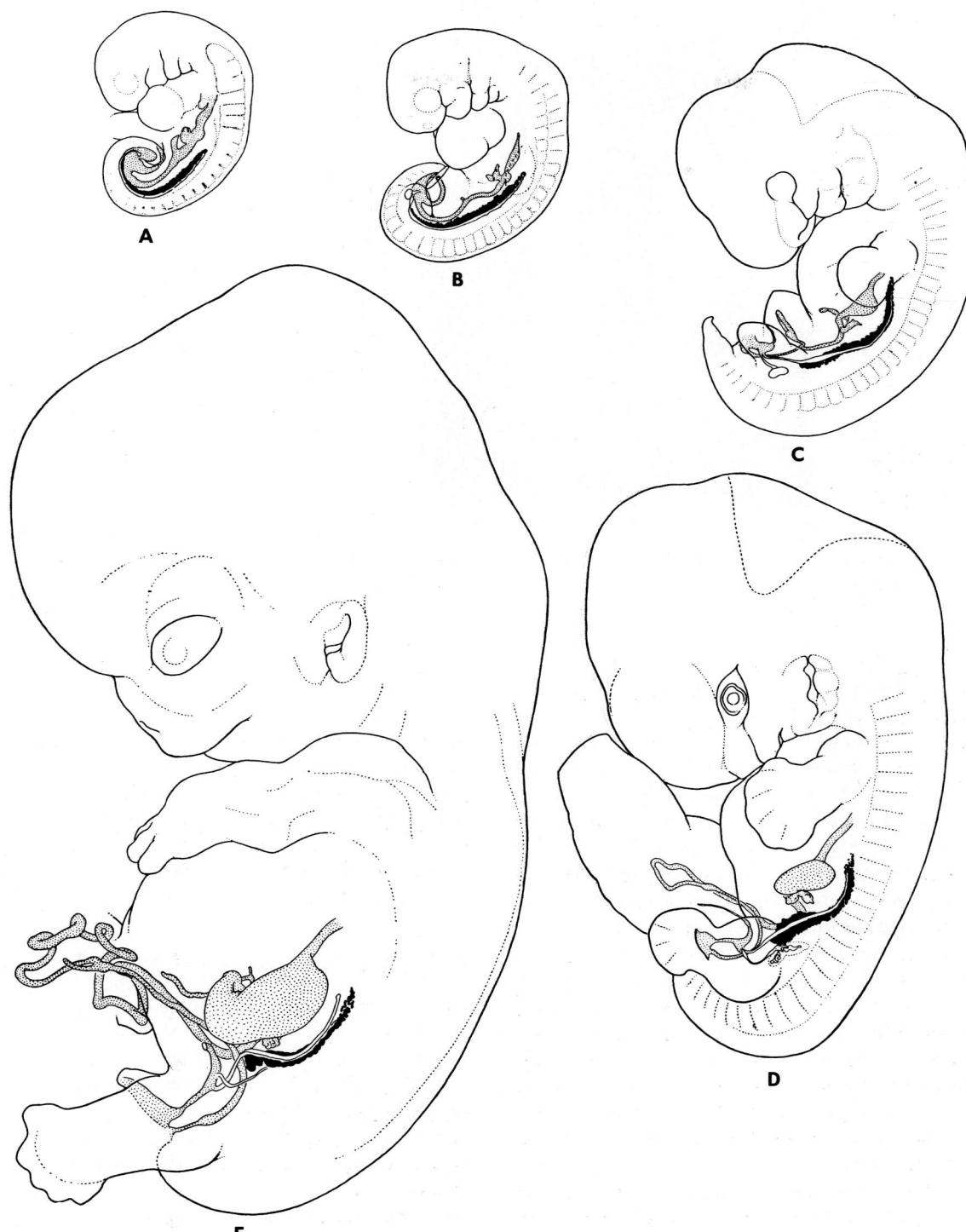

Figure 17.4. Drawings based on projection of human embryos to show the relationships of the mesonephros *(solid black)* and alimentary tract. **A,** 4 mm (fifth week). **B,** 5.5 mm (early sixth week). **C,** 8 mm (sixth week). **D,** 14.6 mm (seventh week). **E,** 23 mm (eighth week). (From Shikinami J. Detailed form of the wolffian body in human embryos. Contrib Embryol Carnegie Inst Wash 1926;18:49–61.)

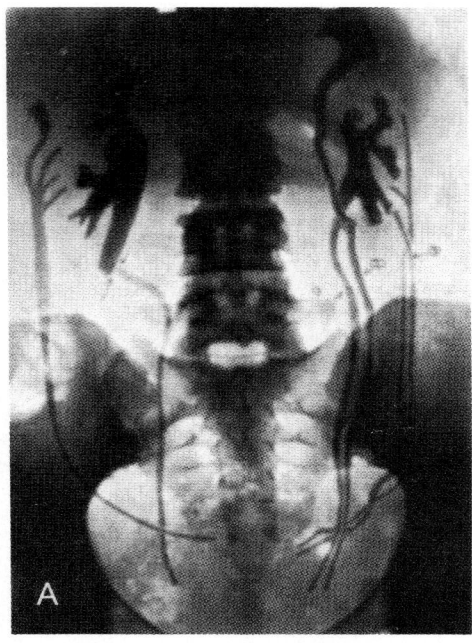
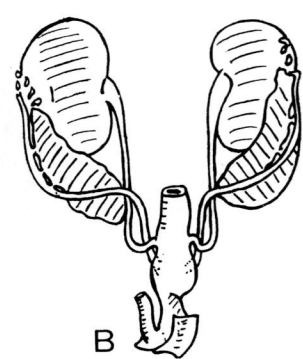

Figure 17.5 **A,** Unique example of probable persistence of the mesonephros. Both mesonephric duct and ureter are seen on the right and left, and on the left, both structures are duplicated. It was not possible to tell which structures were anterior at the crossing in the pelvis. **B,** Drawing of the urinary tract relationships in a 23-mm fetus. The mesonephric duct passes anterior to the ureter (From Begg RC. Sextuplicitas renum: a case of six functioning kidneys and ureters in an adult female. J Urol 1953;70:686–693.)

sorption of septa between branches. By the count of Osathanondh and Potter (17), the renal pelvis and major calyces arise from generations three to five, and the minor calyces arise from generations three to six. The renal papilla, on the other hand, is composed of generations four to six in the middle, and of generations nine to ten in the polar regions (Fig. 17.6, *B*). The papillary ducts are six to eleven generations removed from the ureter and are removed by six to nine more generations of branches from the collecting tubules of each papillary duct.

The ureteral bud and the nephrogenic blastema having joined, the future kidney begins its ascent and rotation. At 7 mm, the kidney is at the level of the second and third sacral vertebrae. At 9 mm, the kidney lies just caudal to the umbilical arteries. The upper pole turns ventrally, with rapid lengthening of the kidney and pelvis, and by 12 mm, the kidney passes the level of the umbilical arteries (18). By the 18-mm stage, the kidney has come into contact with the descending suprarenal body and has become wider and shorter. By 25 mm, the caudal pole has passed the artery and the kidney has reached its final position (Fig. 17.7).

There has been considerable debate about the mechanical factors involved in this "ascent." Felix (1) argued that elongation of the ureter was responsible, but this possibility seems remote. The renal blastema moves upward even when the ureter is absent (19). Brockmann

(20) and Gruenwald (18) believe that the migration is effected by the straightening of the embryo, which occurs at this time. No other external force acting on the kidney has ever been seriously proposed.

The kidneys face ventrally at first, then undergo a rotation of 90 degrees during the seventh and eighth weeks (Fig. 17.8). The alteration in position results from differential growth, with more tubules being formed on the ventrolateral side than on the dorsomedial side (21).

Glomerulus Formation

The ureteric bud and its subsequent branches form the renal pelvis, the calyces, and the collecting tubules. The nephrons themselves arise from the nephrogenic mesenchyme by induction. The earliest recognizable response to the induction is an increase in the rate of synthesis of RNA (22). At first a solid mass, the primordium of the nephron acquires a lumen that eventually connects with that of the collecting tubule. The distal end forms the capsule, while the remainder elongates to form proximal and distal convoluted segments and the loop of Henle (Fig. 17.9).

As with other organs, neither the pelvis nor the blastema can develop when cultured by itself. Only kidney mesoderm can induce calyceal development of the ureteric tip, but submaxillary gland epithelium can induce

Table 17.1.
Developmental Relations of Some of the Urogenital Organs

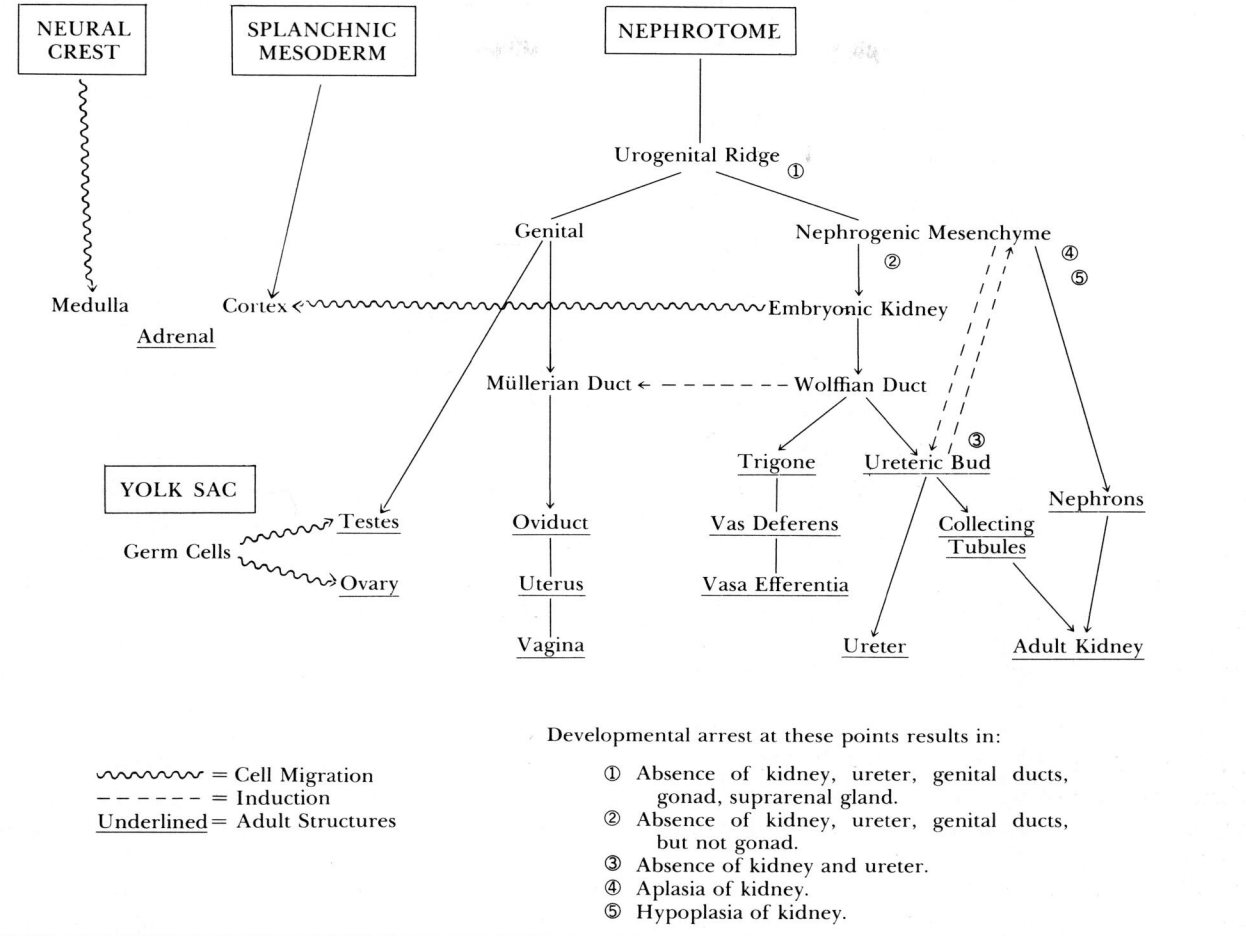

Developmental arrest at these points results in:

① Absence of kidney, ureter, genital ducts, gonad, suprarenal gland.
② Absence of kidney, ureter, genital ducts, but not gonad.
③ Absence of kidney and ureter.
④ Aplasia of kidney.
⑤ Hypoplasia of kidney.

〰〰〰〰〰 = Cell Migration
– – – – – = Induction
Underlined = Adult Structures

tubule formation in the nephrogenic blastema (15, 23).

Remak (24) in 1855 described the formation of the malpighian corpuscle as an invagination of the blind end of the tubule by glomerular vessels. This view was challenged in 1900 by Herring (25), who observed glomerular capillaries forming *in situ*. This mode of formation has been confirmed by Lewis (26), Kurtz (27), Vernier and Birch-Anderson (28), and Jokelainen (29).

Kurtz (27), using the electron microscope, concluded that the glomerular space develops as a cleft in the epithelial cells of the developing nephron. The cleft is not created by invagination but by separation of already differentiated glomerular and tubular epithelial cells. The capillary tuft forms within the mass, leaving a single capsular layer inside. The cells of this layer, the visceral epithelium, develop foot processes and invade the glomulerulus as the capillary loops develop. Figure 17.9 shows the stages of development as described by Jokelainen (29).

The presence of these capillaries is an exception to the rule that only axial vessels develop in situ, whereas lateral vessels arise as buds from existing vessels. Not only do capillaries develop locally, but there is also a suggestion that erythrocytes may be formed from nephrogenic mesenchyme (29). Hemopoiesis has been observed in the nephric blastema, which was not stimulated to develop by a ureteric bud (30).

Gruenwald and Popper (31) put forth the concept that the visceral epithelium of Bowman's capsule ruptures at birth, when the capillary tuft expands. This has not been confirmed by electron microscopic studies (28), and there is no evidence of an abrupt change in glomerular permeability at or near birth (32).

Foot processes of the visceral epithelium of the capsule appear late, and the epithelial cells are at first closely applied to the capillary. The basement membrane of the glomerular capillaries is thinner than that of the adult and lacks the perforations found at maturity (33).

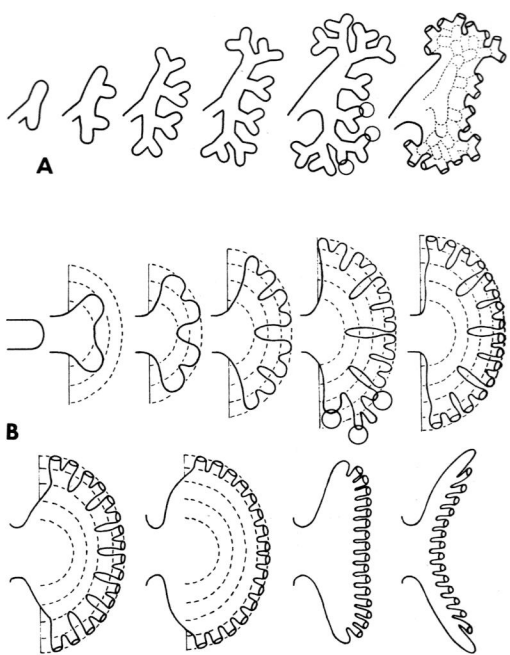

Figure 17.6 **A,** Development of renal pelvis, showing branches of ureteral bud. Circles indicate possible locations of minor calyces at level of third, fourth, or fifth generation branches. Figure at right shows ureteral bud branches that may dilate to form renal pelvis. **B,** Development of minor calyx and papilla, showing formation of multiple short branches. The proximal portions expand gradually and become confluent, forming a single cavity. Urinary secretion and continued growth of tubules is responsible for the compression and lateral expansion of the minor calyx. *Circles* indicate attachment of collecting tubules at level of third, fourth, or fifth generation branches distal to the generation initiating calyceal formation. (From Osathanondh V, Potter EL. Development of human kidney as shown by microdissection. Arch Pathol 1963;76:271–302.)

Pattern of Nephron Formation

Nephron formation has been divided into four stages by Osathanondh and Potter (17) (Figs. 17.10 and 17.11). During the first stage, from week 5 to 14 or 15, nephrons appear at the ends of the branches of the actively growing collecting tubules. The first nephrons appear at the ends of the third generation branches in the middle of the kidney and on fifth generation branches at the poles. Contrary to the views of Kampmeier (34), most of the nephrons thus formed are carried forward with the branching; only an occasional nephron is left behind to lose its attachment and degenerate. At the end of the first stage, few nephrons are attached to any but the last generation of collecting tubules.

At term, glomeruli occasionally may be found in the connective tissue around interlobar vessels. Efferent vessels to these ectopic glomeruli serve the pelvic mucosal plexus. These vessels remain, but the glomeruli have vanished in the adult (35).

During the second stage, from week 14 or 15 to week 20 or 22, the collecting tubules no longer divide. New nephrons are induced at the ends of the branches, even though a nephron already is present. New nephrons displace older nephrons and form "arcades," in which the most distal units are the oldest (Fig. 17.10, *B*). Peter (36), who first described the arcades, believed the stem of the arcade to be of collecting tubule origin, but Osathanondh and Potter (17) believe it to be of nephric origin. Arcades usually contain four nephrons but may have as many as eight. While a few nephrons not carried forward subsequently degenerate, there appear to be no clear-cut "vestigial" and "provisional" zones, such as were described by Kampmeier (34).

During the third stage of development, lasting from week 20 or 22 until week 32 to 36, the tips of the collecting tubules elongate without branching and without carrying the older nephrons forward (Fig. 17.11, *A*). They induce from four to seven new nephrons, after which the developing tips of the tubules disappear.

In the final stage, from 32 to 36 weeks onward, the collecting tubules drain 10 to 14 nephrons, of which the proximal four to seven are in an arcade and the distal five to seven arise from a single stem. These constitute the definitive renal cortex.

The time at which new glomerulus formation ceases has been the subject of a surprising amount of debate. Felix (1) believed that new units were formed even a few days after birth, but subsequent writers (37) placed cessation of activity much earlier. MacDonald and Emery (38) divided glomerulogenesis into (a) a nephrogenic phase, during which new glomeruli are formed, which occurs up to week 36; (b) a stage at which all glomeruli are present but most are immature lasting from 36 weeks' gestational age to 3 to 5 years of age; and (c) a stage of maturation of glomeruli, ending by 12 years of age. Potter and Thierstein (39) found immature glomeruli in most kidneys of infants born before week 35 and concluded that glomerular development depended on fetal size rather than on gestational age. Rożynek (40) concluded that the converse was true, but agreed that glomerular formation was complete in fetuses of 2300 to 2500 gm, regardless of age.

Although glomeruli are probably mature at birth, their size continues to increase with age (28). Fetterman and his colleagues (41) measured glomeruli, with the following results:

Glomerular size at term	0.08 to 0.150 mm (average, 0.120 mm)
Glomerular size at 3½ years:	0.160 to 0.240 mm (average, 0.200 mm)
Glomerular size in adult	0.220 to 0.360 mm (average, 0.290 mm)

The proximal convoluted segment is small relative to the glomerulus at birth, but it grows rapidly in the first few postnatal months.

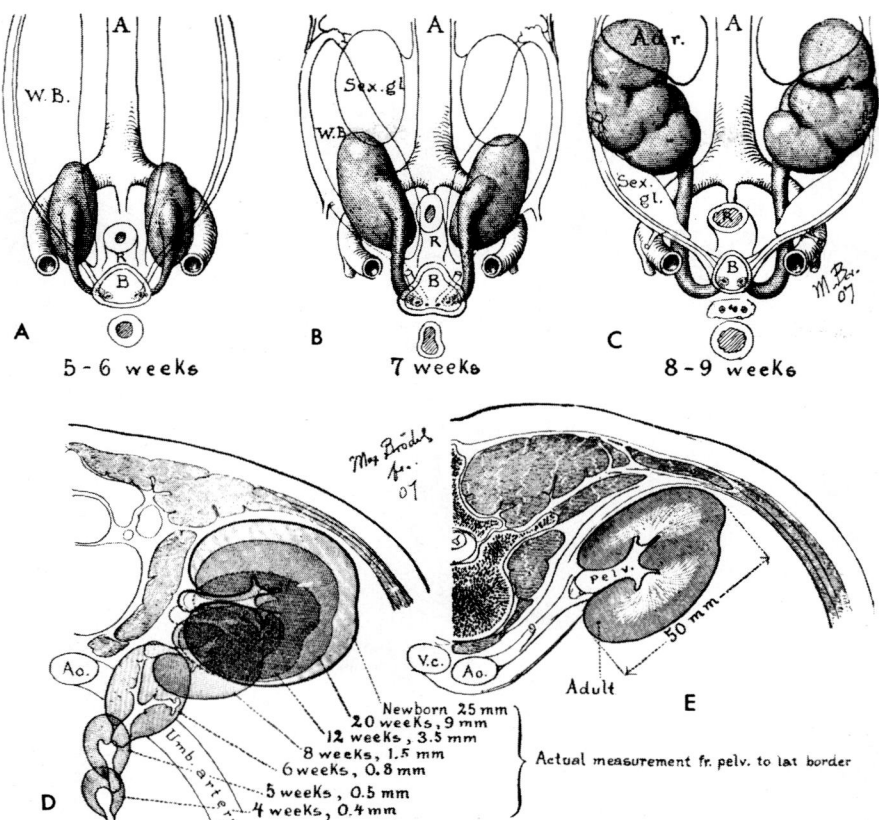

Figure 17.7 Changes in the position of the developing kidney. **A** to **C,** Ventral view, showing ascent of the kidneys from the pelvis to the abdomen and their medial rotation as they cross the iliac arteries. **D,** Composite diagram illustrating rotation and increase in size. **E,** Cross-section of adult body, showing final position with pelvis facing medially. *A,* Aorta; *Ao.,* aorta; *Adr.,* suprarenal gland; *B,* bladder; *R,* rectum; *Sex. gl.,* gonad; *V.c.,* inferior vena cava; *W. B.,* mesonephros (From Kelly HA, Burnam CF. Disease of the kidneys, ureters and bladder, Vol 1. New York: Appleton, 1914.)

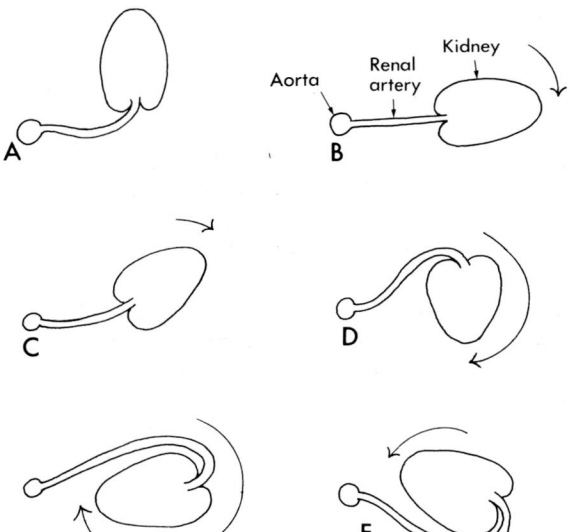

Figure 17.8. Rotation of the kidney during its ascent from the pelvis. The left kidney with its renal artery and the aorta are viewed in transverse section to show normal and abnormal rotation during its ascent to the adult site. **A,** Primitive embryonic position, hilus faces ventrad (anterior). **B,** Normal adult position, hilus faces mediad. **C,** Incomplete rotation. **D,** Hyperrotation, hilus faces dorsad (posterior). **E,** Hyperrotation, hilus faces laterad. **F,** Reverse rotation, hilus faces laterad.

Critical Events in Development

Three events appear to be critical in the development of the normal kidney:

1. Appearance of the ureteric bud from the mesonephric duct at the end of the fifth week.
2. Junction of the growing ureter with the nephrogenic blastoma in the sixth week. Failure of development at either stage 1 or 2 results in absence, aplasia, or hypoplasia of the kidney. Splitting of the ureteric bud as it grows into the blastoma results in various duplications of the kidney and ureter.
3. The ascent of the kidneys during the sixth and seventh weeks; involves possible fusion of the two kidneys with one another (horseshoe kidney). Failure or arrest of ascent at this time may leave the kidney in the pelvis.

ANOMALIES OF THE UPPER URINARY TRACT (TABLE 17.2 AND FIG. 17.12)

Congenital Anomalies of the Kidneys

Congenital anomalies of the kidneys are fairly common, but not always clinically significant. Although various classifications of renal congenital malformations exist,

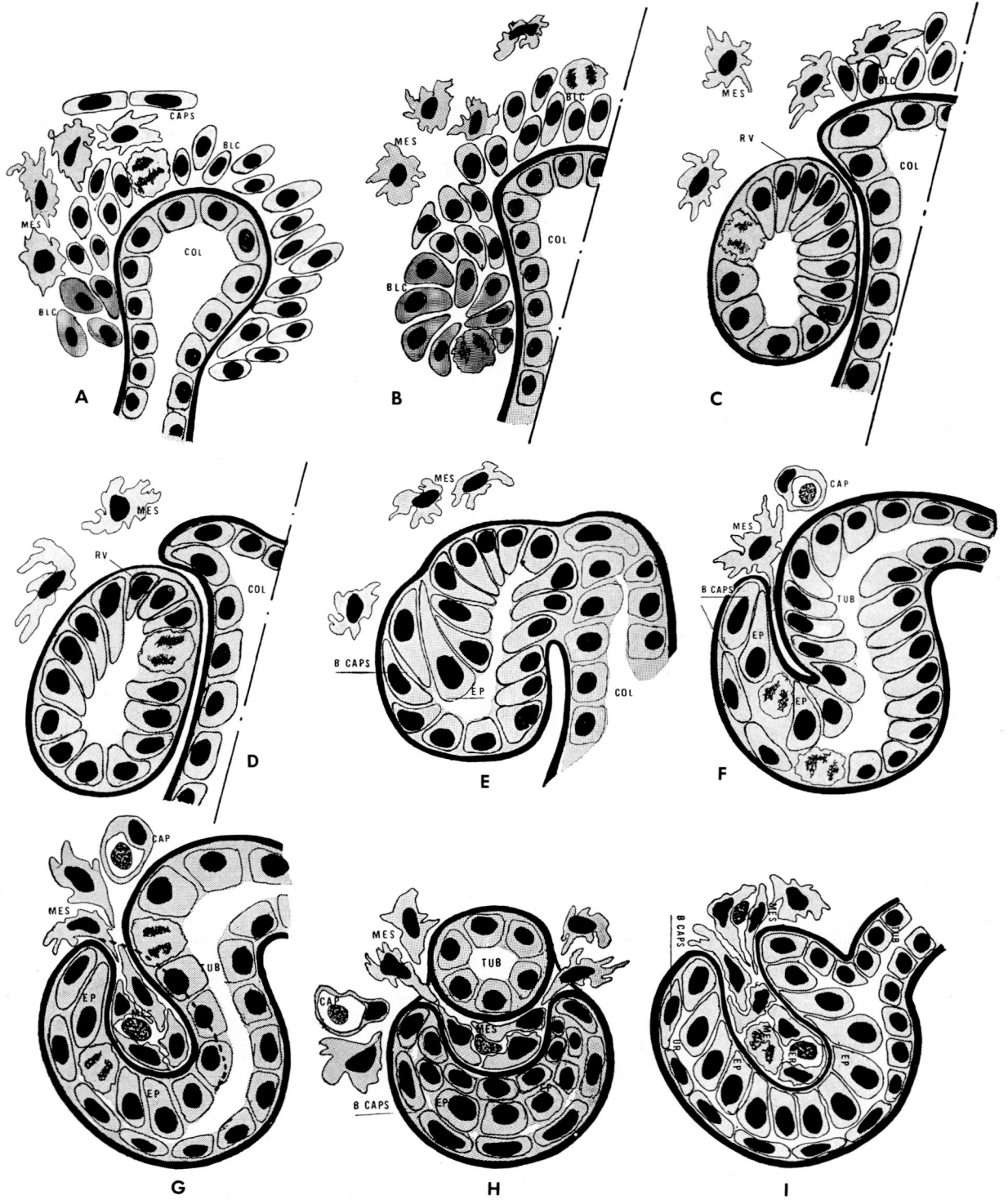

Figure 17.9. Development of the nephron in the rat. Drawings based on electron micrographs. **A,** Nephrogenic mesenchymal cells *(B1.C)* surrounding the end of the collecting tubule *(COL)* derived from the ureteral bud. The *heavy line* is the basal lamina of the tubule epithelium. **B,** Differentiation of blastemal cap cells *(BLC)* from stromal mesenchyme cells *(MES)*. **C,** Formation of the renal vesicle *(RV)* by the glastema cells. **D,** Multiplication of the vesicular cells. **E,** Disappearance of the basal laminae between the collecting tubule and the vesicle: differentiation of presumptive parietal layer of Bowman's capsule *(B CAPS)* and visceral layer *(EP)*. **F,** Proliferation of capsular cells and appearance of the glomerular space. **G,** The S-shaped stage; mesenchymal cells occupy the enlarging glomerular space; a capillary *(CAP)* is nearby. **H,** Section at right angles to that in **G. I,** Two layers of capsular epithelium are evident and the urinary space *(UR)* is indicated. The glomular space is filled with presumptive glomerular endothelium and an erythrocyte *(ER)*. (From Jokelainen P. An electron microscope study of the early development of the rat metanephric nephron. Acta Anat (Basel) 1963;52(Suppl):47.)

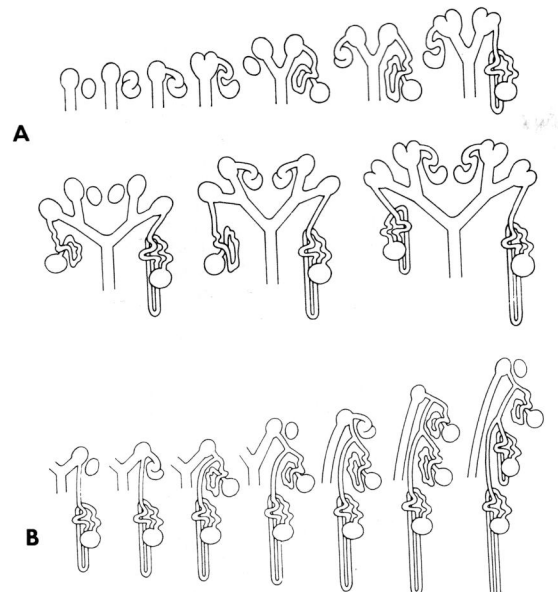

Figure 17.10. Kidney development. **A,** First stage. Development of nephrons on growing collective tubules. The first four drawings correspond to the stages shown in Figure 17.9. **B,** Second stage. Arcade formation. (From Osathanondh V, Potter EL. Development of the human kidney as shown by microdissection. Arch Pathol 1963;76:271–302.)

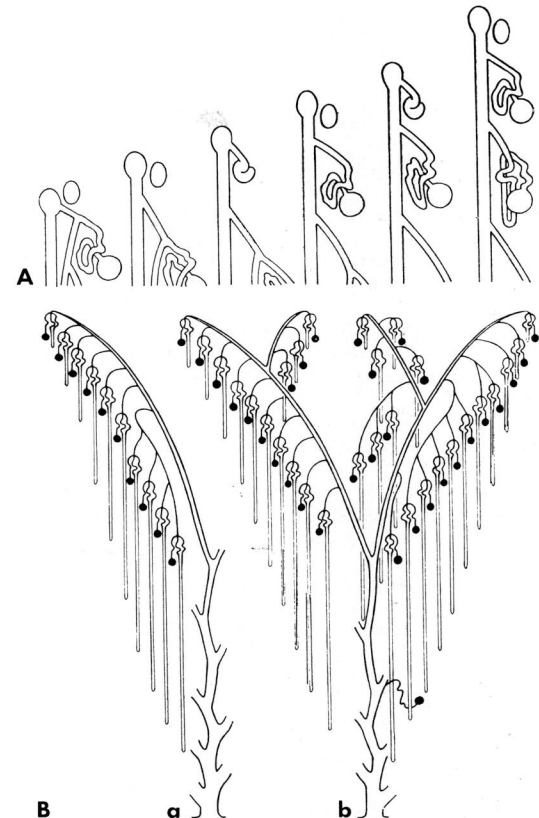

Figure 17.11. Kidney development. **,** Third stage. Direct attachment of distal nephrons. **B,** Arrangement of nephrons at birth. a, Usual patter; b, possible variations. (From Osathanondh V, Potter EL. Development of the human kidney as shown by microdissection. Arch Pathol 1963;76:271–302.)

they most commonly are grouped into four general categories: abnormalities in the amount of renal tissue; abnormalities in orientation; placement, and form; abnormalities of histologic differentiation (dysplasia); and abnormalities secondary to heritable disorders, which include genetic forms of renal cystic disease (42, 43).

Complete Absence of the Urinary Tract

At least one infant has been born alive with complete absence of kidneys, ureters, bladder, urethra, external genitalia, and anus. The legs were fused, the testes and vasa deferentia were present, and there was a single umbilical artery (44). The chain of events that resulted in this malformation illustrates the interdependence of developmental processes.

The initial defect occurred before the end of the second week of development. A few cells of the inner cell mass at the future caudal end of the embryonic disc failed to delaminate to form endodermal cells; hence, with the formation of the tail fold, the hindgut was abnormally short. This shortened hindgut failed to extend far enough caudally to form an allantoic diverticulum or a cloacal plate. All allantoic and cloacal derivatives thus failed to form. Absence of the cloacal plate in turn withheld the necessary stimulus for the formation of the genital folds by the ectoderm. The hind limb buds were permitted to touch and fuse with one another because of the absence

of the midline cloaca. Although the wolffian duct formed, its failure to join the absent cloaca inhibited the formation of the midline cloaca, the ureteral bud, and hence, the kidneys.

Survival of this deformed fetus in utero depended on the presence of the single umbilical artery. In most such cases the absence of an allantois would produce early death through failure of placental vascularization by allantoic vessels. In this case a single vessel reached the placenta and permitted continued intrauterine development.

Persistent Mesonephric Remnants

The normal regression of the mesonephros leaves a number of vestigial structures associated with the reproductive tract of both the male (see Chapter 21) and the female (see Chapter 22). In addition to these, more extensive remnants of the mesonephros have occasionally been found associated with the upper urinary tract.

The presence of persistent wolffian ducts in females has been claimed in three instances (45–47). In each case

Table 17.2.
Anomalies of the Upper Urinary Tract[a]

Anomaly	Origin of Defect	First Appearance		Sex Chiefly Affected	Relative Frequency	Remarks	
		Unilateral	Bilateral			Unilateral	Bilateral
Renal Agenesis	Late week 4	At any age; usually adulthood	At birth	Male	Common (unilateral)	May remain asymptomatic	Fatal within a few days
Aplasia	Week 5	At any age; usually adulthood	At birth	Equal	Rare	May remain asymptomatic	Fatal within a few days
Hypoplasia	Week 6 or later	At any age; usually adulthood	In childhood	Equal	Common (unilateral)	May remain asymptomatic	Renal parathyroid dwarfism
Abortive double ureter (ureteric diverticulum)	Week 5	In early adulthood		Female	Common	Usually asymptomatic enlargement occurs	
Uteropelvic junction obstruction	?	At any age		Male	Common	May remain asymptomatic	
Double pelvis and ureter	Week 5	At any age, usually in early adulthood		Female	Common	Asymptomatic complications of infection only	
Supernumerary kidney	Week 5	In adulthood		Equal	Rare	Complications of infection only	
Pelvic kidney	Week 6	In adulthood		Male	Uncommon	May associate with genital anomalies in female	
Thoracic kidney	Week 9	In early adulthood		Male	Very rare	Usually discovered in routine chest x-ray	
Crossed ectopia	Late week 6	In early adulthood		Male	Uncommon	Asymptomatic	
Malrotation	Weeks 7–8	Rarely symptomatic		Male	Uncommon	Usually asymptomatic	
Horseshoe kidney	Late week 6	In early adulthood		Male	Common	May produce symptoms in absence of other pathology	
Retrocaval ureter	Week 7	In adulthood		Male	Uncommon	Right side only: hydronephrosis	
Retroiliac ureter	?	?		?	?	?	
Ureteral valves	Late in development?	At any age		Equal	Rare	Produce symptoms of obstruction	
Mega	?	In childhood		Equal	Rare	Reflux may or may not be present	

[a]Cystic diseases of the kidney, see Table 17.6.

a tube extended from above the normal kidney to become continuous with Gartner's duct in the broad ligament. The presumption is strong that these tubes were persistent mesonephric ducts, but the possibility that they were blind ureteral duplications with ectopic openings cannot be excluded.

An even more striking case has been reported by Begg (14). The findings were from pyelograms of a 42-year-old woman who understandably opposed confirmatory laparotomy in the absence of disease. In addition to a normal right ureter and complete duplication of the left ureter, the patient had three widely separated lateral ureters, one on the right and two on the left. These lateral ureters received multiple horizontal calyces without the appearance of pelves (Fig. 17.5). We agree with Begg that these lateral ureters can be explained only as persistent mesonephric (wolffian) ducts, serving still functioning mesonephroi. No similar case is known.

Abnormalities of the Amount of Renal Tissue: Renal Agenesis, Aplasia, and Hypoplasia

DEFINITIONS

Degrees of defective renal development range from complete failure of the kidney to form to the occurrence of varying quatities of kidney tissue of less than normal size. This failure may be arbitrarily divided into the following:

1. Agenesis: Complete failure of the kidney to form—no trace of nephrogenic tissue exists at the normal site of the kidney (Fig. 17.13, A). This condition must be distinguished from crossed ectopia, in which a kidney has migrated and fused with the kidney on the other side of the body.
2. Aplasia (dysplastic hypoplasia): Only a small mass of undifferentiated or very poorly differentiated tissue is present at the normal site of the kidney. The ureter, if present, does not reach the organ, and there is no evidence of kidney function (Fig. 17.13, B).

3. Hypoplasia (simple hypoplasia): The organ is present and recognizable, but it is small and often infantile. Excretory functioning occurs, but usually much below normal (Fig. 17.12, *C*).

Some authors would abolish the category termed *aplasia* on the grounds that it is merely extreme hypoplasia (48). Others would classify aplastic kidneys under the term *dysplastic hypoplasia* and would reserve the term *simple hypoplasia* for small kidneys of normal structure (49). Embryologically, there is a continuous series of forms from complete absence to a fully normal kidney. The division of these gradations depends on whether structure,

function, or symptomatology is emphasized. We believe the terms *agenesis, aplasia,* and *hypoplasia* are the most accurate and the least confusing.

BILATERAL RENAL AGENESIS

Anatomy. A common defect in embryogenesis is probably responsible for both unilateral and bilateral renal agenesis. Normal kidney development depends on a satisfactory union of the metanephric blastema with the ureteral bud. Absence or interruption of ureteral bud development from the mesonephric duct prevents maturation of the metanephric blastema into adult kidney tissue. Whatever causes the insult at the origin of the ureteric bud occurs during early gestation, probably at 4 to 6 weeks of embryogenesis. The close embryologic proximity of the müllerian duct, mesonephric duct (i.e., wolffian), and ureteral bud may explain the high incidence of malformed or absent müllerian duct structure in females, and similarly abnormal wolffian structures in males with renal agenesis.

Bilateral renal agenesis fortunately is rare, incompatible with life, and of little consequence to the clinician. The condition was found once in every 2721 pediatric autopsies in Campbell's series (50), and Potter (51) estimated its occurrence once in every 4800 births. Males with the condition outnumber females by three to one. There appears to be no predisposing condition, as neither advanced maternal age, maternal illness, nor specific complications of pregnancy seem to influence its development (52). Although a familial tendency has been recorded (53), it seems that, if there is a genetic predisposition to the syndrome, it must have a low level of penetration (54).

Bilateral renal agenesis may be detected prenatally by

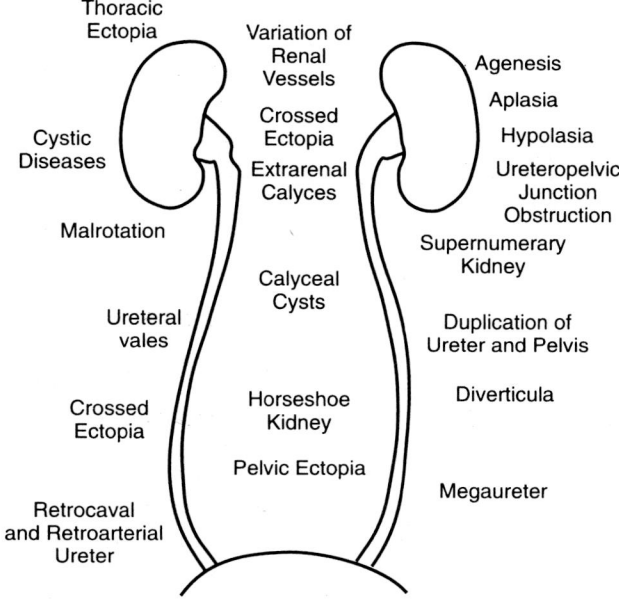

Figure 17.12. Sites of anomalies of the kidney and ureter.

Thoracic Ectopia

Variation of Renal Vessels

Agenesis

Aplasia

Hypolasia

Cystic Diseases

Crossed Ectopia

Extrarenal Calyces

Ureteropelvic Junction Obstruction

Malrotation

Calyceal Cysts

Supernumerary Kidney

Ureteral vales

Duplication of Ureter and Pelvis

Crossed Ectopia

Horseshoe Kidney

Diverticula

Pelvic Ectopia

Megaureter

Retrocaval and Retroarterial Ureter

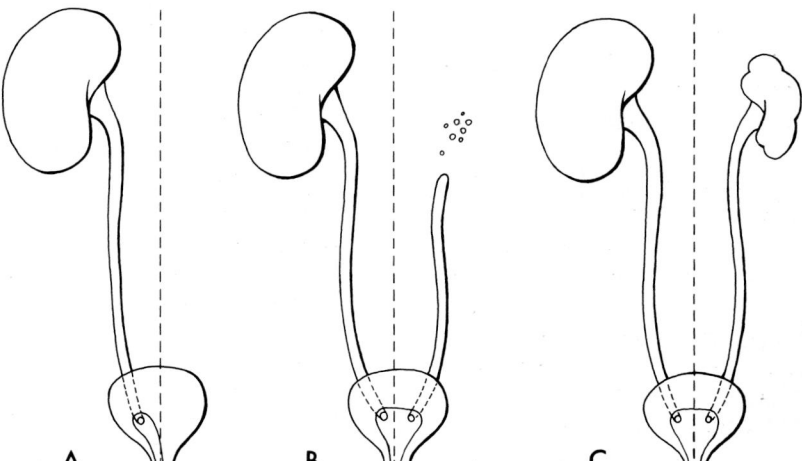

A   B   C

Figure 17.13. Unilateral kidney insufficiency. **A,** Agenesis. Complete absence of left kidney and ureter; left half of trigone is absent. **B,** Aplasia of the left kidney. The kidney is represented by a few cystic remnants, and the ureter ends blindly. **C,** Hypoplasia of the left kidney, which remains fetal external lobulation.

a maternal fetal ultrasound examination. Normal kidneys can be detected sonographically by week 20 of gestation. When the kidneys are not visualized by that time, failure to demonstrate the bladder within 1 to 2 hours after intravenous administration of Lasix to the mother is considered confirmatory (55). A pregnancy complicated by significant oligohydramnios should alert the clinician to the probability of a defect in fetal urine production, the most severe cause of which is bilateral renal agenesis. Other severe abnormalities often occur in association with oligohydramnios, where the uterine wall presses on the fetus, restricting fetal chest movements, bending the extremities, and wrinkling and distorting fetal facies (Fig. 17.14). The recognition of the association of pulmonary hypoplasia, bowel abnormalities, clubbed lower extremities, typical facial features, and bilateral renal agenesis led Potter (51) to her classic description in 1965 of the syndrome which bears her name. Pulmonary hypoplasia, presumably caused by restricted chest movement in utero is usually the cause of death soon after birth in these infants. In addition to the absence of functioning kidneys, each ureter is either wholly or partially absent. Interestingly, the lower urinary tract is often absent or at most minute, usually with urethral atresia. As one might expect, the gonads are usually present in this condition; however, it has been reported that 10% of boys with absent kidneys also have absent testicles, indicating a more severe embryologic defect. The vas deferens is absent in most cases, and uterine abnormalities are common in females (56).

Associated Anomalies. About 25% of infants with bilateral renal agenesis have no other anomalies (52). Among the remainder, hypoplasia of the lungs, malformations of

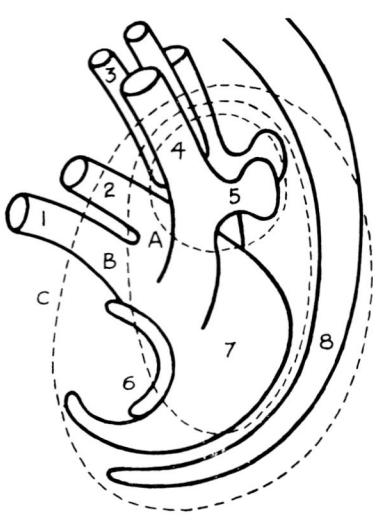

Figure 17.15. Diagram of early stage in embryonic development of lower end of body, showing possible variation in extent of the disturbance responsible for renal agenesis. *1,* Allantois; *2,* hindgut; *3,* paramesonephric (müllerian) duct; *4,* mesonephric duct; *5,* ureteral bud; *6,* cloacal membrane; *7,* cloaca; *8,* spinal cord. *Zone A:* Area of abnormality limited to lower proportion of mesonephric and paramesonephric ducts. *Zone B:* Area of abnormality also includes hindgut and cloacal membrane. *Zone C:* Area of involvement includes entire caudal end of embryo. (From Potter EL. Bilateral absence of ureters and kidneys: a report of 50 cases. Obstet Gynecol 1965;25:3–12.)

the external genitalia, imperforate anus, and malformations of the lower extremities account for 90% of the defects (51, 52). Spina bifida, hydrocephalus, congenital heart defects, esophageal and intestinal atresias and fistulae account for less than 10%. This is a complete reversal of the normal distribution of congenital anomalies found in the general population (57), in which the first group makes up only 5% and the second makes up 90% of all defects. Neural, cardiac, and gastrointestinal defects may be considered entirely incidental findings.

Embryogenesis. Agenesis of the kidney itself is discussed under unilateral renal agenesis (page 608). Briefly, Dubois (58), Moore (59), Sadler (60), and Datta (61) speculate that failure of development of the ureteric bud (metamorphic diverticulum), early degeneration of the ureteric bud, failure of penetration of the metanephric mesoderm by the ureteric bud, and failure to proliferate the metanephric elements due to the lack of induction are responsible for such a phenomenon.

Potter (51) discussed variation in the morphogenetic disturbance, which may include the entire posterior portion of the developing embryo. Figure 17.15 illustrates the relationships and extent of such defective development.

History and Incidence. Excluding formless and parasitic monsters, the earliest report of bilateral renal agenesis was by Wolfstrigel (62) in 1671. Coen (63) collected 32 cases in 1884. In 1954 Davidson and Ross (52), in an

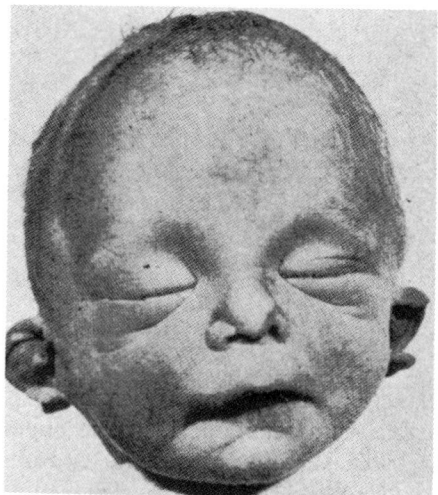

Figure 17.14. Characteristic appearance of infants with bilateral renal agenesis (the Potter facies). (From Potter EL. Facial characteristics of infants with bilateral renal agenesis. Am J Obstet Gynecol 1946;51:885–888.)

Table 17.3.
Diagnosis of the Absent or Hypoplastic Kidney

	Symptoms		Cystoscopy	Pyelogram		Differential Diagnosis From:	Treatment
	Bilateral	Unilateral		Retrograde	Excretory		
Agenesis	Anuria and death	None	Hemilateral absence of trigone and ureteral orifice	No kidney mass visible; no ureteral orifice	No visualization	Aplasia, hypoplasia	None
Aplasia	Anuria and death	Rarely, pain (late)	Hemilateral absence of trigone or normal trigone	No kidney mass visible; ureter rarely patent; orifice small	No visualization	Agenesis, hypoplasia, secondary atrophy	Occasionally, ureterectomy
Hypoplasia	Renal hyperparathyroidism in childhood	Rarely, pain (late)	Trigone and orifices (normal)	Ureter may be normal; pelvis small with few calyces	Visualization poor to absent	Aplasia, crossed ectopia, secondary atrophy	None or renal transplant

excellent review, found 232 authentic cases in the literature.

The incidence among autopsies of infants and children ranges from 0.028% (the average of six series compiled by Davidson and Ross [52] in 1954) to 0.37% (among 19,046 in Campbell's [64] 1963 series). Sylvester and Hughes (65) in England found an incidence of 0.042% among 9940 deliveries. More than twice as many males as females are affected. In a number of cases gender is doubtful because of malformations of the genitalia, both external and internal (66).

Gestational History. There is no significant relationship between bilateral renal agenesis and maternal age or parity (52), and no hereditary tendency is known. In some sets of twins, only one of the pair has been affected (67). Some genetic strains of rats also are known to be subject to the anomaly (68–70). No chromosomal aberration has been identified (71).

Sixty-six percent or more of these infants are reported as premature (under 2500 gm), but Bain and Scott (72) suggest that this reflects a failure to gain weight after the 34th week, rather than a shortened gestation time. Oligohydramnios may be present in as many as 70% of the cases, in contrast to polyhydramnios which is usually encountered when other developmental anomalies occur. Oligohydramnios is found in about 3% of normal births (72).

Breech presentation of infants with bilateral renal agenesis is usual. Bain and Scott (72) found 30 examples in their series of 50 cases of bilateral and unilateral renal agenesis.

Symptoms and Diagnosis. The "Potter facies," fused lower extremities (sirenomelia), and oligohydramnios are all pathognomonic of severe kidney malformation, but are not specific to bilateral agenesis. Amnion nodosum—a condition in which small, white, keratinized nodules of 1 to 3 mm in diameter stud the surface of the amnion—is associated with oligohydramnios and, hence, with severe kidney defects (73–75). The presence of any of these signs warrants immediate pyelography (Table 17.3).

Renal agenesis will produce anuria without the distension associated with lower urinary tract obstruction. Pulmonary hypoplasia will produce signs of respiratory insufficiency. The diagnosis, however, is usually confirmed only at autopsy.

Mortality. All infants with bilateral renal agenesis will soon die. About 33% will be stillborn, and most of the others will die in less than 24 hours. Respiratory insufficiency is the usual cause of death, but about six patients have survived long enough to die of uremia. The longest survival has been 39 days (76).

UNILATERAL RENAL AGENESIS

Absence of one kidney may go undetected throughout a lifetime because, it is thought, in most instances the contralateral kidney enlarges and assumes a greater workload to keep renal function normal.

Incidence. Since it is often silent, the incidence of unilateral renal agenesis is not reliably known, although estimates derived from autopsy studies suggest it occurs once in every 1100 births (79).

Unilateral renal agenesis is encountered about five times as frequently as bilateral agenesis. Campbell (64) found unilateral absence in 1:552 autopsies and bilateral absence in 1:2721 autopsies, while Ashley and Mostofi (56) found 47 bilateral and 232 unilateral cases in their series. The incidence of unilateral agenesis is probably much greater than this because the condition may be asymptomatic throughout life. Older estimates are more conservative than that of Campbell: Fortune (78), compiling records from 21 series, found 1:1290 autopsies, and Collins (79) computed a ratio of 1:920. Longo and Thompson (80) estimated the incidence to be 1:1000 autopsies. Unilateral renal agenesis, according to Sadler (60), occurs in 1:1500 individuals.

The incidence of aplasia is more difficult to estimate. Nation (81) found 16 cases of aplasia and 17 of agenesis among 27,000 autopsies. Two of his examples of aplasia seem at least questionable, so that true aplasia is perhaps slightly less common than is agenesis. Strict discrimination between the two conditions requires histologic evidence of the absence of renal tissue. Gutierrez (82) found an incidence in 92,690 autopsies of 1:400 for renal aplasia and considered it to be four times as frequent as agenesis.

The left kidney is more frequently absent than is the right. Fortune (78) found over twice as many cases with absence on the left, while Collins (79) and others found the proportions to be about 1.3:1. The earlier writers (77, 83, 84) found that the two sides were nearly equally affected in women and that a left-sided preponderance occurred among males. Recent studies have not been broken down in this manner.

Males are more commonly affected than are females; however, as we have already stated, accompanying genital defects are more frequent among females. Collins (79) found a sex ratio of 1.22:1, while the older series of Ballowitz (83) had a ratio of 1.46:1. Campbell (64) found more than twice as many males among his cases (2.26:1).

Unilateral agenesis may be discovered at any age, and unquestionably many cases are never discovered. It has been recognized in embryos (85), but the majority of patients are adults.

Both agenesis and aplasia occur spontaneously in animals other than humans. In addition to Morgagni's (86) dog and rabbit (see the section on "History"), the anomalies have been described in rats (87) and at least eight times in cats (88, 89). In Reis's (88) specimen, the left kidney had a total of 125 glomeruli, and its ureter entered the urethra. In addition, the left half of the trigone was undeveloped. This may have been a case of hypoplasia rather than of true aplasia. In lower vertebrates (anuran amphibia) having a mesonephric kidney, experimental destruction of the pronephros, along with failure to develop a wolffian duct, results in aplasia, not agenesis, of the mesonephros (90).

No evidence exists for a hereditary basis for renal agenesis or aplasia in humans, but the defect has been found to be hereditary in a strain of rats (87). The agenesis is always on the left and always associated with genital anomalies, indicating a failure of wolffian duct formation rather than failure of the ureteric bud to form.

As in bilateral agenesis, there is a male preponderance for this condition, although the incidence is less. The left kidney is more often absent. Like the bilateral condition, there seems to be a familial tendency without a definite inheritance pattern. The diagnosis is often made from pyelograms or ultrasound examinations performed for evaluation of urinary tract infection or hematuria, as there are no obvious pathognomonic clinical signs of the condition.

The Solitary Kidney. Clinical interest in unilateral renal agenesis arises from the possibility that the solitary kidney may be prone to congenital abnormalities or more liable to disease. Certainly, varying degrees of malrotation and ectopia are frequently seen, and ureteral widening is often encountered. Dees (91) suggested that congenitally single kidneys are twice as prone to disease as those left behind following contralateral nephrectomy. The series of Emanuel et al. (92) indicated a significant morbidity and mortality for the congenital solitary kidney. Forty-two percent of their patients were diagnosed as having unilateral agenesis in the first year of life, most of them associated with imperforate anus, whereas 75% were diagnosed in the first 5 years, often during the workup for cardiac anomalies or urinary tract infection. Hydronephrosis owing to vesicoureteral reflux was commonly found; these authors, as have others (93), stress the association of unilateral agenesis with multiple organ system involvement.

Associated Anomalies. Associated abnormalities in systems other than the genitourinary tract occur frequently. Syndromes such as Turner's, Poland's and Klippel-Feil have been shown to involve absence of a kidney (94, 95). Contrasted to these reports is the work of Longo and Thompson (80) in which anomalies of the contralateral kidney other than ectopia and malrotation were infrequently encountered, suggesting that unilateral agenesis with an otherwise normal contralateral kidney is not incompatible with normal longevity. In addition to the kidney, any or all of the urinary or reproductive structures associated with the fetal urogenital ridge may be absent.

The ureter as well as the kidney was absent in 60% of Ashley and Mostofi's cases (56) of unilateral renal agenesis. The lower end of the ureter was present in about 8%, but in no case was there a fully developed ureter extending to the site of the absent kidney (Table 17.1, *site 3*). The ureteral orifice was missing, and the trigone was hemiatrophied in 53% (Fig. 17.13, *A*).

In about 10% of patients with unilateral renal agenesis, the homolateral suprarenal gland also is absent (56, 78). This frequency is greater than that observed in bilateral renal agenesis (Table 17.1, *site 1*).

Nearly all affected females have associated anomalies of the reproductive tract either on the side of the absent kidney or on both sides (Table 17.1, *site 2*). Burwell and Kent (96) found the vagina absent in 51.3%, the uterus absent in 40.1%, one or both tubes absent in 25.6%, and one or both ovaries absent in 23.1%. Absence of one-half of the uterus or a bifid uterus is common (97). So closely associated are renal and genital defects in females that discovery of a renal anomaly should lead to a search for genital anomalies, and vice versa.

Fewer males show concomitant reproductive defects. About 33% of male patients will have atrophic ductus deferens and seminal vesicle on the affected side, with or without involvement of the testis or epididymis (Table 17.1, *site 2*).

As in bilateral renal agenesis, deformed ears (98, 99) and pulmonary hypoplasia are often present but unilateral. The pulmonary pathologic condition is less severe and does not usually cause death. Prematurity is common, but less so than when bilateral agenesis occurs.

Among Collin's (79) 581 collected cases of unilateral renal agenesis, 89% of females and 41% of males had other anomalies. The distribution of these anomalies lies between that found in bilateral agenesis and that in the general population (Table 17.4).

Embryogenesis. Agenesis and aplasia result from failure of the ureteric bud from the wolffian duct to make contact with the nephrogenic blastema at the proper time. This mishap may spring from the absence of the wolffian duct, the failure of the ureteric bud to form, the failure of the bud to reach the blastema before its upward migration, or the absence of the metanephrogenic mesenchyme itself (Table 17.1).

A genetic basis for renal aplasia or hypoplasia has been found in a mutant mouse. The mutation is complete and lethal in homozygotes, while heterozygotes have unilateral aplasia or bilateral hypoplasia of the kidney. Both ureteric induction of mesoderm and the response of the

Table 17.4.
Anomalies Associated with Kidney Agenesis[a]

Defects	Bilateral Agenesis (%)	Unilateral Agenesis (%)	Anomalies in General Population (%)[b]
Extremities Anorectal Genital Pulmonary Single umbilical artery	89.5	60.5	5.0
Spina bifida Esophageal and intestinal stenoses and atresias Hydrocephalus Anencephalus Cardiac	7.25	32.5	90.0

[a]Percentages in bilateral and unilateral agenesis were calculated from data of Davidson WM, Ross GIM. Bilateral absence of the kidneys and related congenital anomalies. J Pathol Bact 1954;68:459–474.
[b]From Murphy DP. Congenital malformations: a study of parental characteristics with special reference to the reproductive process, 2nd ed. Philadelphia: JB Lippincott, 1947.

mesoderm itself appear to be affected (100). This suggests that failure of induction may be more than an accidentally missed appointment between two tissues.

A 9-mm human embryo without ureteric buds but with apparently normal wolffian ducts and metanephrogenic blastema present has been described (19). Absence of one ureteric bud and the fusion of metanephric blastemas have been seen in a 10-mm embryo (85).

The extent of the defect in the adult depends on the portion of the developmental sequence affected. This sequence is shown in Table 17.1, together with its relationships to the reproductive tract and the suprarenal gland.

The most severe condition results from failure of the urogenital ridge to form. All internal genital and upper urinary tract structures, including the trigone on the affected side, will fail to form. The mildest form appears when the ureteric bud fails to reach or penetrate the nephrogenic mesoderm at the right time to induce kidney formation. The mesodermal blastema may completely disappear (agenesis), or it may form a few abortive cysts and tubules (aplasia). Occasionally, the unstimulated blastema may form large cystic structures (see the section on "Congenital Multicystic Kidney," page 629).

In a few remarkable cases, a kidney is present in the absence of the homolateral ureter. This occurs when the solitary ureter bifurcates and one branch crosses the midline to stimulate the contralateral nephrogenic blastema to form a kidney (101) (Fig. 17.16, *E*).

History. Unilateral absence of the kidney has been known since antiquity. Aristotle (102) mentions its occurrence in animals in *Generatione Animalium* (IV:iv:771a).

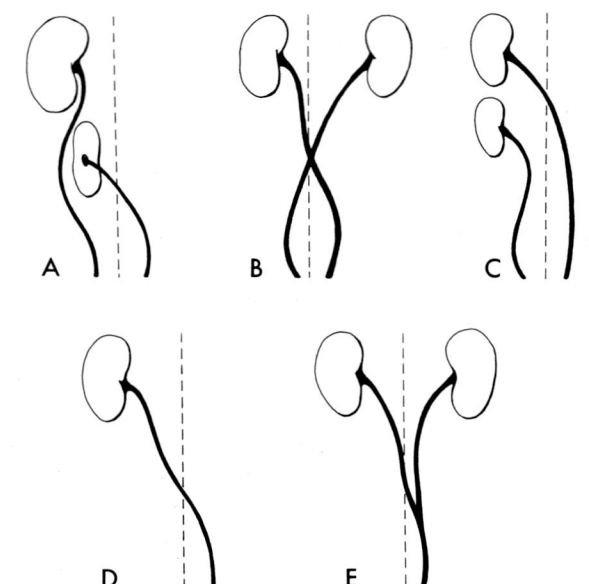

Figure 17.16. Crossed ectopia. **A** and **C,** Crossing without fusion. **B,** Double crossed ectopia. **D,** Solitary crossed ectopia. **E,** Crossed ectopia from solitary bifurcated ureter.

Riolan in 1610 observed the compensatory hypertrophy of the solitary kidney: "If one solitary kidney be found, it generally equals the magnitude of both" (Morgagni XLVIII:16). Morgagni (86) in 1761 collected 26 cases in humans and mentions the condition in a rabbit and a dog. He distinguished between solitary double kidney and crossed, fused ectopia. At least one of the collected cases, that of Poupart (103) in 1700, appears to have been renal aplasia.

Mosler (104) collected a number of cases in 1863. The first thorough review was made in 1895 by Ballowitz (83), who assembled records of 213 cases from the literature. By 1932 Collins (79) was able to list 581 cases and mentioned 49 others he was unable to consult. Radasch (97) in 1908 evaluated the associated genital defects in 255 cases. In 1925 Bagg (105) was able to produce both agenesis and aplasia of the kidney in the offspring of irradiated mice.

Symptoms. While an adequately functioning solitary kidney is asymptomatic, Longo and Thompson (80) have catalogued the circumstances that brought the patients to seek medical advice in 94 cases. In 11, the discovery was incidental; 23 had pain, usually on the side of the existing kidney; 12 exhibited a genital anomaly; and in 10, the complaint was urinary frequency and burning. Nine patients had hematuria, five had hypertension, and the remainder had miscellaneous urinary complaints.

Diagnosis. The diagnosis of unilateral agenesis usually is entertained when there is failure of visualization of contrast medium in one kidney on intravenous pyelography

(IVP), although left-sided agenesis may be suggested on the plain abdominal x-ray film by the presence of a splenic flexure gas pattern in the renal fossa (106). Absence of observed contrast medium due to agenesis must be distinguished from failure of function. Renal ultrasonography identifies most cases of nonopacified kidney, although it occasionally misses a very small organ or one ectopically located. Dimercaptosuccinic acid (DMSA) radionuclide scanning is indicated when only one kidney has been identified and doubt exists about the presence of a second kidney (107). Cystoscopy and retrograde pyelography generally require anesthesia but occasionally are useful investigations—if there is no ureter, there is no kidney. Nevertheless, the cystoscopist must be aware that the ureteric orifice can sometimes be missed; even when a clearcut hemitrigone is seen, a ureter may be present but ectopic (108).

The diagnosis may be suspected during physical examination when the vas deferens is missing or when a septate or absent vagina is seen. Genital anomalies are found in 25 to 50% of females and 10 to 15% of males with unilateral renal agenesis, and these also include unicornuate ureter with absence of a horn and fallopian tube or a bicornuate uterus. Complete or incomplete midline fusion of the müllerian ducts leading to a septate uterus, cervix, or vagina may occur and may be associated with stenosis of one vagina leading to hematocolpos or hydrocolpos (53, 109).

Treatment. There is no therapy for the absence of a kidney, but the few aplastic kidneys that produce symptoms must be removed.

All efforts must be aimed at supporting the solitary functional kidney; any evidence of disease in it must be taken very seriously. A patient with congenital absence of a kidney should be watched as carefully as one who has had a kidney removed surgically.

RENAL HYPOPLASIA (SIMPLE HYPOPLASIA)

Anatomy. The term *renal hypoplasia* has been misused frequently and often alludes to all forms of small kidneys. True renal hypoplasia can be taken to describe only the miniature kidney with normal-appearing calices (although often with a smaller number), essentially normal parenchyma, and a normal ureter. This limited description is necessary to distinguish truly hypoplastic kidneys from similarly small kidneys that are dysplastic (a primary phenomenon, a histologic diagnosis) or atrophic (originally normal kidneys "damaged" by vascular insufficiency, infection, radiation, etc.). To meet the criteria for diagnosis of true hypoplasia, no dysplastic or embryologic elements should be present. True hypoplasia occasionally is seen as a unilateral condition. However, it may be extremely difficult to distinguish from the small kidney resulting from renal arterial stenosis or renal venous thrombosis. In such cases, renal arteriography may demonstrate a narrow renal artery that is wide and funnel-shaped at its origin, suggesting that the renal artery was once wider but contracted. This angiographic finding may indicate that the kidney was originally larger and therefore not hypoplastic by definition (110). Kidneys associated with vesicoureteral reflux also may be small. Controversy exists regarding the exact nature of small kidneys associated with vesicoureteral reflux—whether they are dysplastic and therefore small because of a congenital predisposition or whether they are contracted and/or atrophic as a result of damage associated with urinary tract infection. Ambrose and co-workers (111) defined a population of patients with small kidneys and vesicoureteral reflux, from whom renal tissue was available for histologic evaluation either by biopsy, partial nephrectomy, or nephrectomy. Normal renal tissue was not found in the specimens, indicating that true hypoplasia is rarely if ever encountered in patients with small kidneys and vesicoureteral reflux.

Embryogenesis. While agenesis represents failure of kidney development, hypoplasia represents an insufficient response of the metanephrogenic mesoderm to the stimulus of the ureteric bud. Why the response is insufficient is difficult to determine. Three possibilities exist: The ureteric bud may not have been capable of organizing all of the available mesenchyme (Fig. 17.17, *B*); the mesenchyme may have been incapable of a full response (Fig. 17.17, *C*); or the ureter may have reached the mesenchyme after the optimum response period had passed (Fig. 17.17, *D*).

We lean toward the first possibility, largely because the pelvis of the hypoplastic kidney is reduced in size. Had the deficiency been wholly in the mesenchyme, one might expect the pelvis and calyces to be of normal size and the kidney substance itself to be thinner. The mesenchyme normally proliferates around the branches of the embryonic pelvis as they appear; hence, the hypoplasia would seem to be the result of inadequate growth potential of the ureteric primordium itself (Fig. 17.17, *B*).

Incidence. Campbell (64) found unilateral hypoplasia in 1:577 autopsies of children and in 1:462 autopsies of adults. Dees (112) estimated that hypoplasia constituted 6% of upper urinary tract anomalies. Smith and Orkin (113) found it in 7.4% of a similar series. Bilateral hypoplasia is rare. Campbell mentioned two cases, and Kruglich and Minnick (114) described one. The fact that acquired atrophy is not easily distinguishable from congenital hypoplasia makes any estimate of incidence unreliable. A case of renal hypoplasia with hydroureter was reported in an adult marmoset (Mico) by Hill (115).

Symptoms and Diagnosis. If hypoplasia is bilateral with an overall shortage of nephrons, there may be hypertrophy of the elements that are present and therefore distortion of the normal microscopic appearance. "Oligomeganephronia" is a distinct clinical entity and probably represents the most common form of true renal hypoplasia (116, 117). This is a nonfamilial condition presenting early in childhood, usually with vomiting and dehydration. Investigation usually reveals poor renal concentration, slight proteinuria, and progressive uremia. Small kidneys with insufficient numbers of calices may be found on IVP. The diagnosis, often made in infancy, usually is followed by a period of stable azotemia lasting many years. Growth retardation may be marked. Hypertension is not usually a part of the picture. Shortly after the onset of puberty, there is a rapidly progressive worsening of the condition and dialysis becomes necessary. In differential diagnosis, one should keep in mind the similarity of this condition with medullary cystic disease of nephronophthisis complex. The latter entity, however, has a later age of onset and a familial incidence (50 to 80%), and the defects of tubular function precede those of glomerular insufficiency (118).

Differential Diagnosis. So difficult is it in practice to distinguish congenital hypoplastic kidneys from those which have become atrophic from disease that some writers have avoided the use of the term *renal hypoplasia*, preferring instead *small kidney*, which has no etiologic implications. Emmet and his colleagues (119) analyzed 400 cases

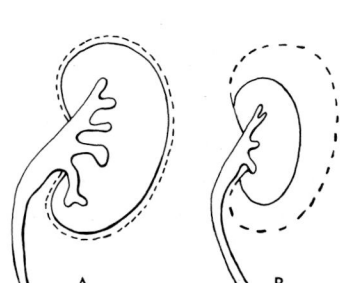
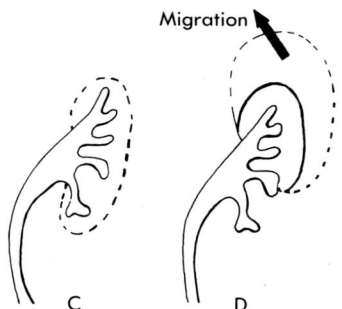

Figure 17.17. Development of hypoplastic kidney. **A,** Normal ureteric bud including normal sized kidney. **B,** Inadequate ureteral bud inducing small kidney; *dashed line* indicates normal area of potential kidney mesoderm. **C,** Normal ureteric bud inducing small kidney from insufficient potential mesoderm. **D,** Delayed arrival of a normal ureter reaching only the posterior portion of the potential kidney mesoderm, which has already started to ascend.

of kidneys that were two-thirds of normal size or smaller and selected 183 without obvious disease. They divide these into two groups; those with evidence of past or present infection and those without such evidence. However, they were unable to find symptoms, pyelographic characteristics, or other qualities that would separate the two groups. They concluded that, while there is a difference in the genesis of the two types, it is impossible to distinguish chronic atrophic pyelonephritis from congenital hypoplastic kidney. Simple hypoplasia is an embryonic lesion; perhaps demonstrated unequivocally only during infancy or childhood.

Renal hyperparathyroidism accompanying bilateral hypoplasia is not pathognomonic. It may be produced by renal insufficiency from any cause, and the renal disease may be the result of a primary hyperparathyroidism rather than the cause of it, although primary parathyroid disease is rare in infants and children.

Treatment. Renal transplantation should be considered in bilateral renal hypoplasia with severe impairment of function.

Abnormalities in Placement, Form, and Orientation

SIMPLE RENAL ECTOPIA

Anatomy. The kidney that is not ptotic and does not occupy its normal position in the lumbar fossa is classified as ectopic. Failure of the kidney to pass from its embryonic position (at the level of the second and third sacral segments) to its adult position (at the level of the first four lumbar vertebrae) results in simple ectopia, without crossing or fusion. Simple ectopia of one kidney is common; rarely are both affected.

Ectopic kidneys frequently are classified by the position in which they lie, and as a consequence, it is not always easy to translate one author's terminology into that of another. "Pelvic," "iliac," "iliolumbar," "lumbar," and "abdominal" all express varying degrees of ascent. About 60% of ectopic kidneys are pelvic in location (Fig. 17.18).

The lower the kidney, the nearer to the midline it will be, the less it will have rotated from the primitive ventral facing position, and the more numerous will be its blood vessels. Perirenal fat is absent. Multiple arteries arise from the inferior mesenteric artery, the common or the external iliac artery, or the middle sacral arteries. Anson and Riba (120) described the anatomic details of an ectopic kidney.

Failure of ascent of the kidneys may occur in combination with other renal anomalies. About 10% of unascended kidneys are solitary (121).

Embryogenesis. Just as the mechanics of the ascent of the kidneys are unknown, so the causes of failure to complete the ascent are unknown. From the distribution of ectopic kidneys, it appears that, in most cases, the process

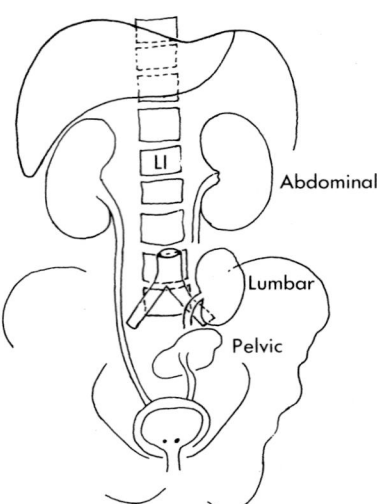

Figure 17.18. Incomplete ascent of kidney. The kidney may halt at any level of the ascent from the pelvis.

of ascent never takes place at all. In other cases ascent starts and is interrupted before completion. Although the umbilical vessels form a slight barrier in the path of ascent, it is not clear how they can block the upward passage of kidneys in some embryos and not in others, or how one kidney passes the vessels to reach the adult position, whereas the other does not (Fig. 17.7). Moore (59) believes that the cause of renal ectopia is failure of the kidney to "ascend." Sadler (60) proceeds further, stating that diminution of the body curvature and the growth of lumbar and sacral regions are the causes of malascent.

The vascularization of the ectopic kidney is the normal embryonic vascularization of the level at which the kidney has remained. With ascent, caudal vessels drop out and cranial vessels appear. In ectopia, the vascularization pattern remains "frozen" at whatever developmental stage the ascent ceased. The picture therefore is one of arrest, not malformation.

Incidence.

Bilateral Simple Ectopia.
Strube (122) in 1894 was able to find only four cases in which both kidneys were ectopic. Fowler (123) in 1941 collected 40 cases, of which 22 were clinical and 18 were from autopsy. Among the clinical cases, which were diagnosed by pyelography, there were twice as many males as females.

Unilateral Simple Ectopia.
Estimates of frequency range from 1:800 (64) to 1:1220 (121). Clinically, Culp (124) found three cases in 747 routine pyelograms. Here, too, more males than females are affected; the left kidney is involved about 1.3 times as often as the right (125).

Symptoms. Ectopia, whether bilateral or unilateral, produces no symptoms by itself. Pain, which is reported in about 33% of affected patients, results from the usual complications of hydronephrosis, pyelonephritis, or lithiasis, but the atypical position of the kidney makes the location and nature of the pain misleading. The pain is in the lower abdomen and is usually thought to involve the appendix or the male pelvic organs. It is possible that ectopic kidneys are no more subject to disease than are normally placed kidneys, the apparent frequency reflecting the more common discovery of ectopia in diseased kidneys.

Complications of Pregnancy. Cragin (126) in 1898 mentioned the obstruction to normal delivery produced by a pelvic kidney. Anderson and his colleagues (127) assembled 98 cases from 1828 to 1948 in which ectopic kidney was a complication of pregnancy. Of these cases 85 were simple unilateral ectopia, 5 were solitary, and 3 were bilateral simple ectopia. The remaining five cases were fused ectopia.

In 86% of cases in which the affected side was reported, the offending kidney was on the left. Because simple ectopia occurs on the left in only 56% of all cases of ectopia, it would appear that left-sided ectopia predisposes the individual to dystocia much more often than does right-sided ectopia.

Cesarean section should be performed at once if there appears to be dystocia caused by a pelvic kidney. Dyspareunia reported before pregnancy should lead the physician to anticipate dystocia during delivery, and pelvic kidney should be kept in mind while seeking the cause of the dyspareunia.

Diagnosis. The condition is diagnosed by IVP and nuclear scanning technique. Particularly helpful is 99^m-Tc dimercaptosuccinic acid (DMSA) or 99^m-Tc diaminotetraethylpentacetic acid (DPTA) scanning when renal function is poor and when the collecting system is difficult to visualize because of overlying bowel gas or superimposed bony structure (Fig. 17.19). The presence of a pelvic mass may occasionally suggest the diagnosis, but pyelograms are necessary for confirmation. In the absence of a pyelogram, the pelvic mass may be mistaken for a uterine or ovarian tumor. Nephroptosis is the only condition requiring differentiation. In this acquired dislocation, the ureter is of normal length since the kidney originally had ascended completely. In ectopia, on the other hand, the ureter is short because ascent has never taken place.

Treatment. Treatment of the diseased ectopic kidney is similar to that of the diseased kidney in the normal location.

THORACIC RENAL ECTOPIA

Anatomy and Embryogenesis. Renal ectopia usually implies failure of ascent of the kidney, but occasionally ascent continues beyond the normal location, and in extreme cases the kidney lies above the diaphragm.

Congenital thoracic kidney may occur through a diaphragm intact but for a "ureteral foramen" (128), through a congenitally open foramen of Bochdalek (129),

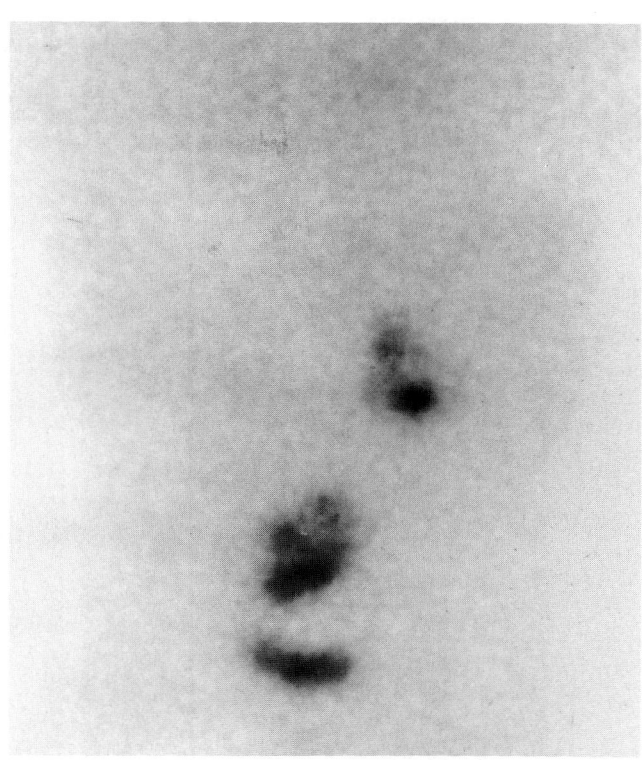

Figure 17.19. Pelvic kidney. DTPA renal scan showing pelvic left kidney above normal bladder and normal right kidney.

or through a large diaphragmatic defect. In the last instance the thoracic location of the kidney is probably secondary to the diaphragmatic defect. In a number of cases location has been determined radiographically only (Fig. 17.20). In these, the possibility of traumatic diaphragmatic hernia cannot be eliminated completely.

The condition occurs with equal frequency on the right or left side, but we have not encountered a bilateral case. About 30 cases have been diagnosed clinically (130, 131). All but three have been in males. Campbell (64) found two cases among 15,919 autopsies in children.

One patient had a wide variety of pulmonary, cardiac, and pericardial anomalies in addition to a thoracic kidney (131). Another had 16 to 18 trisomy and a translocated chromosome (130). In most cases there are no other anomalies.

Symptoms. Urologic symptoms are sometimes present and may be chronic, such as in the patient of Spillane and Prather (132), who had suffered from urinary frequency and nocturia for most of his 71 years. For the most part, the symptoms have been thought to come from a chest condition (133, 134), or discovery has been accidental. Routine chest x-ray films have been the means of discovery in several cases (129, 133). Other cases have been found incidentally at surgery or autopsy.

Diagnosis. A chest x-ray film with a suspicious supradiaphragmatic shadow may be rechecked with retrograde pyelograms or excretory urograms. The possibility of

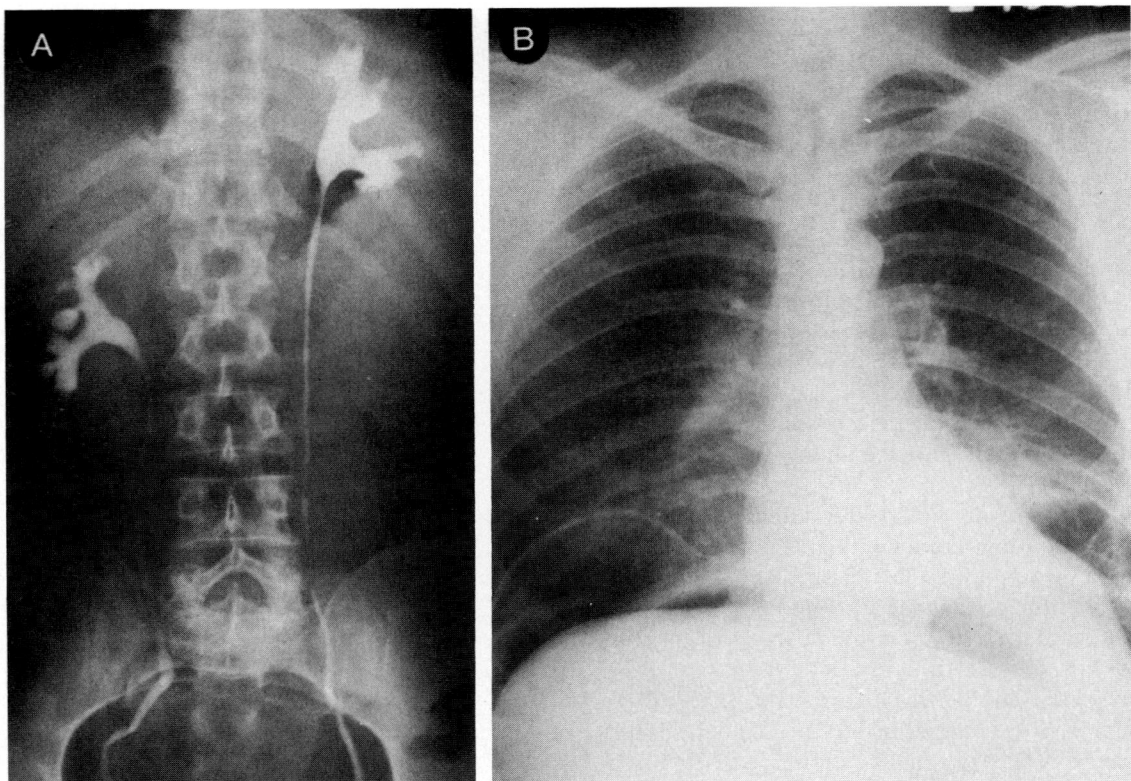

Figure 17.20.   Radiograph of a thoracic kidney. The left kidney lies above the diaphragm. **A,** Diagnostic urogram. **B,** Diagnostic pneumoperitoneum. (From Hill JE, Bunts RC. Thoracic Kidney: case report. J Urol 1960;84:460–462.)

supradiaphragmatic liver tissue (pages 286–288) may thus be excluded. Hiatal hernia may likewise be excluded by visualization of the stomach and esophagus with barium.

Treatment. No treatment is required if the thoracic kidney is not diseased. Replacement of the kidney in the abdomen, with repair of the herniated diaphragm, may be undertaken if blood vessels permit enough movement.

PELVIC KIDNEY

Etiology. Sadler (60) believes that the arterial fork of the umbilical arteries and the failure of one or both kidneys to pass cause pelvic kidney.

Pelvic kidney perhaps deserves special recognition because of the apparently higher incidence of pathologic conditions involving both the ectopic kidney and its contralateral mate. Some 50% of pelvic kidneys are involved in a disease process that causes poor function (135). Especially common is vesicoureteral reflux and high ureteral insertion into the pelvis leading to hydronephrosis. The opposite kidney is likewise often abnormal and may be absent in 10% of affected patients.

Skeletal abnormalities should be expected in more than half of the patients with pelvic kidney. Vertebral anomalies are common as are those of ribs and skull. Car-

diovascular and gastrointestinal anomalies also are seen with increased frequency and include valvular septal defects, imperforate anus, and malrotation of the gut. Low set or absent ears are likewise seen with increased frequency in this condition (136).

CROSSED RENAL ECTOPIA

Anatomy. In crossed ectopia, the kidney from one side of the body lies on the opposite side; its ureter crosses the midline and opens normally into the bladder. Several varieties may be distinguished.

Crossed Ectopia with Fusion.
This is the most common type of crossed ectopia; the ectopic and the normal kidney are fused with one another in various positions. In the great majority of cases the ectopic kidney is smaller and lies inferior to or at the same level as the normal kidney. Six different arrangements of the two kidneys have been described.

1. End-to-end fusion with the crossed kidney inferior; both pelves face the same way, usually anteriorly (Fig. 17.21, *A*).
2. S-shaped, end-to-end fusion; the upper pelvis faces medially, and the lower pelvis faces laterally. Both kidneys have rotated normally (Fig. 17.21, *B*).
3. Lump kidney, resulting from fusion without retaining the

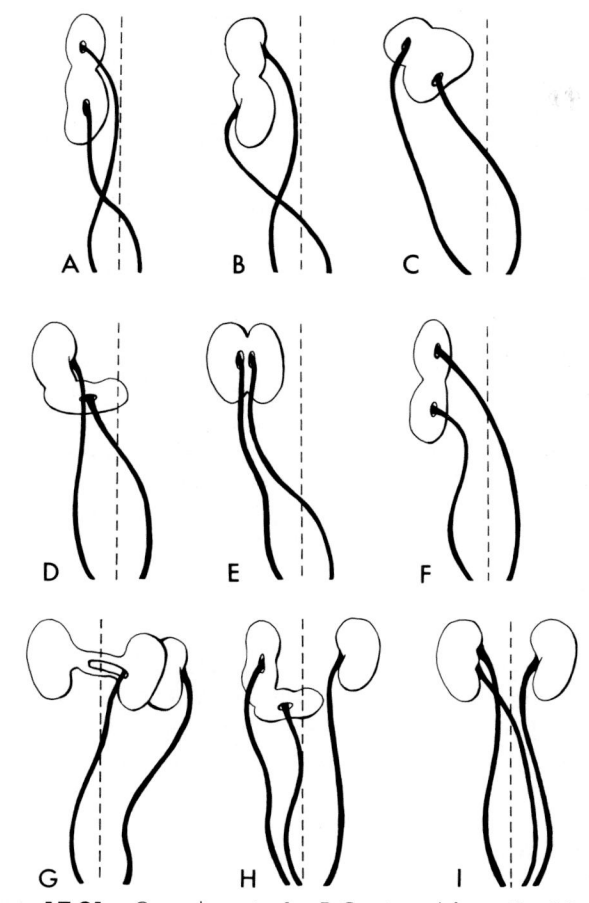

Figure 17.21. Crossed ectopia. **A** to **F,** Crossing with fusion. **G** to **I,** Bizarre forms of crossed ectopia.

shapes of the two kidneys; both pelves usually face anteriorly (Fig. 17.21, C). This is generally associated with failure of ascent as well as of rotation.

4. L-shaped, right-angle fusion, with the ectopic kidney lying transversely. The normal pelvis faces medially, or both face anteriorly (Fig. 17.21, D).
5. Medial border fusion; pelves face each other, or nearly so (Fig. 17.21, E).
6. As in type 1, but the crossed kidney is superior (Fig. 17.21, F).

In addition to these classifiable anomalies, there are a number of bizarre arrangements known. Potampa and his colleagues (137) reported a patient who had fused crossed ectopia, as well as a third kidney connected across the midline with the ectopic kidney by a broad common pelvis (Fig. 17.21, G). On the basis of this latter finding, they classified it as a combined tandem and horseshoe kidney. Paoletti (138) described a patient with an L-shaped fusion on the right, in which the ureter of the transverse kidney crossed back to its proper side. There was a normal kidney on the left, although there was an anatomically crossed ureter; in this case, embryologically, it was a uni-

lateral duplication of the kidney (Fig. 17.21, H). A case of doubling, with fusion and crossed ectopia, was reported by Pia (139). A lump kidney was composed of a crossed left kidney and a double right kidney. Two ureters opened into the bladder, and one opened into the urethra.

Still another combination of anomalies was present in a patient described by Sebening (140). In addition to crossed fused ectopia, there was an uncrossed supernumerary kidney occupying the site left vacant by the crossed kidney (Fig. 17.21, I).

A case of pseudo–crossed ectopia in a patient with a large retroperitoneal cyst was found by Konrad and his colleagues (141) in 1949. The cyst displaced a double right kidney across the midline, simulating a congenital crossed ectopia.

Crossed Ectopia without Fusion.
In 10 or 15% of crossed ectopias, the two kidneys remain unfused. As with fused ectopia, the crossed kidney is generally the lower of the two (Fig. 17.16, A). In a single instance (142) the crossed kidney lay above the kidney (Fig. 17.16, C).

Double Crossed Ectopia.
A unique case in which each kidney had crossed to the opposite side was described by Bugbee and Losee (143) in 1919 (Fig. 17.16, B). It was the first case of crossed ectopia to be diagnosed by pyelogram, according to Diaz (144), and no similar case has been described.

Solitary Crossed Ectopia.
A few cases of crossed ectopia of a kidney in the absence of a contralateral kidney have been reported (145–147) (Fig. 17.16, D).

Three cases are mentioned by Braasch (101) in which a solitary ureter was divided; one limb crossed the midline to serve a contralateral kidney, while the other served the ipsilateral kidney (Fig. 17.16, E). This may represent crossed ectopia of a supernumerary kidney with contralateral agenesis, or a simple crossing of a ureteral branch to induce a normal kidney *in situ*.

Embryogenesis. Crossed renal ectopia remains something of a mystery. Two general hypotheses present themselves immediately: *(a)* The developing ureter wanders across the midline and induces formation of a kidney from the contralateral nephrogenic mesoderm, and the true ipsilateral kidney never forms (Fig. 17.22, A); or *(b)* the developing ureter induces normal kidney formation from the nephrogenic mesoderm on its own side, and during ascent to the adult level, the trailing kidney becomes attached to the leading kidney and is dragged by it across the midline (Fig. 17.22, B). Neither hypothesis will account for all the variations that have been encountered.

Against the first hypothesis are the following:

1. The crossed kidney frequently receives its blood supply from vessels that have crossed with it.

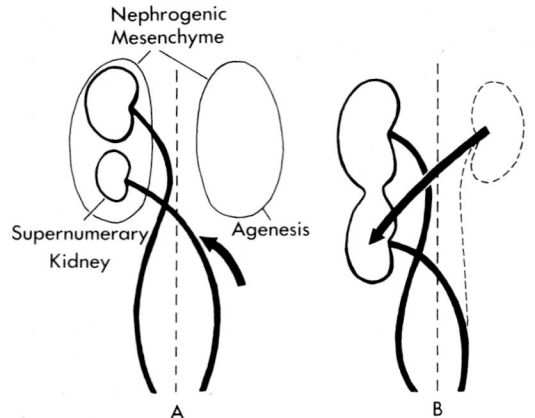

Figure 17.22. Two ways in which crossed ectopia may occur. **A,** The left ureter has grown across the midline and induced a supernumerary kidney on the right; there is complete agenesis of the left kidney. **B,** The left kidney has crossed the midline carrying its ureter with it. This may have resulted from fusion of the two kidneys during ascent.

2. The extent of fusion is less than is found in true double pelvis kidney, in which two ureters on the same side have reached the same nephrogenic mesenchyme; the total kidney mass is also larger than that of the double pelvis kidney.

Against the second hypothesis are the following:

1. Crossed ectopia without fusion, and especially crossed ectopia of a solitary kidney, cannot be explained by adherence.
2. Ectopia with a superior crossed kidney cannot be explained by adherence.

At the time the ureters bud from the mesonephric duct (5-mm stage), their course from origin to contact with the nephrogenic mesenchyme is too short to permit deviation by bending. To reach the contralateral mesenchymal mass, the bud would have to arise from the dorsomedial aspect of the mesonephric duct, rather than from the dorsal aspect. If, on the other hand, the growing ureter encountered no competent mesenchyme on its own side, it might deviate medially during elongation. In either case there would be no midline structures to prevent such crossing.

No direct evidence exists for such crossing of the ureters, but it seems to be the only way to account for crossed ectopia in a solitary kidney and for the unique double crossed ectopia (Fig. 17.16, *B*). This hypothesis also would explain the existence of crossed ectopia without fusion.

The second hypothesis, suggested by Felix (1), and enlarged upon by Joly (148), explains crossed fused ectopia by assuming that one kidney is slightly in advance of the other during its ascent out of the pelvis. The kidney tilts while passing the umbilical arteries (at the 10- to 11-mm stage), bringing its inferior (caudal) pole upward and

inward, where it makes contact and fuses with the superior pole of the trailing kidney. The leading kidney continues its ascent, carrying its attached mate across the midline and upward behind it.

This series of events is compatible with the anatomic arrangement in the adult. The inferior kidney usually receives its blood supply from the aorta (or iliac artery) at a level lower than normal. Joly (148) points out that the vessels are similar to those "supplying a simple ectopic kidney placed at the brim of the true pelvis." As might be expected, the superior kidney, having completed its ascent, often completes its rotation as well. The inferior kidney is more likely to retain the primitive position, with its pelvis in the anterior position.

With these hypotheses, most observed anomalies can be explained, but neither hypothesis alone will suffice. Because of this, still a third hypothesis—postulating some unknown force that pushes one kidney across the midline—is sometimes wistfully suggested by those who prefer a single, all-embracing explanation, regardless of its improbability.

History. The finding of the first case of crossed ectopia has been credited to Panaroli (149) in 1654 by Wilmer (150). Numerous other cases were subsequently found at autopsy and sometimes at surgery. The introduction of pyelography in 1906 by Voelker and von Lichtenberg (150, 151) greatly increased the number of cases recognized. Wilmer collected 192 cases from the literature and added 94 of his own. Abeshouse (152) added 51 cases, making the total 337. Ten years later, McDonald and McClellan (153) added 39 more cases.

The first case of unfused crossed ectopia was seen in 1861 by Rokitansky (154). By 1949 Lee (155) was able to collect 29 cases. Since then, at least 15 more have been added by Caine (156), McDonald and McClellan (153), Ma and his colleagues (157), Shih and co-workers (158), Winram and Ward-McQuaid (159), Burford and Burford (160), and Diaz (144).

Incidence. The incidence has been placed as low as 1:7600 autopsies (150) and as high as 1:1300 (64). Among Abeshouse's (152) 3684 urologic admissions at Mt. Sinai Hospital, the relative proportions of simple ectopia, crossed ectopia with fusion, and crossed ectopia without fusion were 6:2:1.

Among cases reported up to 1957, there were 220 males to 152 females. The left kidney crossed to the right side 222 times, compared to 139 times for the converse situation (153).

Clinical discovery is most frequent in the third decade of life, although the condition has been found at any time, from prematurity to senescence. Cases found at autopsy tend to occur in a younger group than might be expected; hence, it is possible that crossed ectopia may reduce life expectancy. Thompson and Allen (161) consider that there is an increased likelihood of affected individuals developing hydronephrosis.

Symptoms. Pain is present in from 65 to 80% of symptomatic patients with fused crossed ectopia; dysuria and frequency of urination are present in about 20% of patients. A palpable mass is mentioned in about 60% of patients, and pyuria is present in about 50%. No other symptoms are usual.

A wide variety of pathologic conditions have been found in patients with crossed ectopia. In 17 of 57 patients there was no associated pathologic condition (153).

Symptoms in unfused crossed ectopia do not differ from those in fused ectopia. Of 34 cases, 15 had no symptoms.

Diagnosis. Intravenous or retrograde pyelograms will demonstrate the ectopia clearly in most cases. Tracing the course of the ureters is important to distinguish the condition from unilateral duplication accompanied by contralateral agenesis. It may be necessary to rule out horseshoe kidney.

Forty-nine of 57 cases collected by McDonald and McClellan (153) were diagnosed clinically and only four confirmed at operation; the remainder required no surgery. In addition to cystoscopy and pyelography, Hillenbrand (162) induced retropneumoperitoneum to demonstrate fusion of the kidneys.

The greatest care must be taken to demonstrate the presence of a functional contralateral kidney before starting any surgical procedure. Five of twelve operative deaths up to 1947 were the result of unwitting total nephrectomy (152).

Treatment. With unfused crossed ectopia, it is theoretically possible to restore the ectopic organ to its proper location. Diaz (144) performed this operation successfully. However, anomalous vascularization of the ectopic kidney frequently makes such repair impossible. Vessels are usually more numerous and have varied origins. In many cases such vessels cannot be spared.

MALROTATION OF THE KIDNEYS

Anatomy. The pelvis of the normal kidney faces the midline as a result of developmental movements at the end of the second month. Deviation from this position is called malrotation; it results from defects in the normal pattern of development and may need to be distinguished from acquired malposition or torsion.

The malrotated kidney may become fixed in a number of positions, which have been grouped by Weyrauch (163) into the following locations.

Ventrally (Anteriorly) Facing Kidney.
This is the primitive position and represents complete failure of rotation to take place (Fig. 17.8, *A*). It is the most common malrotation. Weyrauch (163) illustrated a

remarkable case in which the ventral position of the hilus resulted from a 360-degree malrotation rather than from nonrotation. The artery and vein passed posterior to the kidney and around the lateral side, to enter the anteriorly facing hilus. Accessory vessels were present at both poles.

Ventromedially Facing Kidney.
This position represents incomplete rotation, which stopped during the seventh week, leaving the kidney rotated 45 degrees instead of 90 degrees (Fig. 17.8, *C*).

Laterally Facing Kidney.
This position may result from excessive rotation through 270 degrees, in which case the blood vessels pass posterior to the kidney to reach the hilus (Fig. 17.8, *E*), or from reverse rotation of 90 degrees, in which case the renal vessels pass anterior to the kidney to reach the lateral hilus (Fig. 17.8, *F*). Weyrauch (163) found both conditions among five laterally facing kidneys in his series of 23 malrotations.

Dorsally (Posteriorly) Facing Kidney.
The reverse of the primitive condition results from excessive rotation of 180 degrees; the renal vessels pass posteriorly to reach the hilus (Fig. 17.8, *D*). This is the rarest form of malrotation.

Embryogenesis. At the end of the sixth week, the process of cranial elongation of the ureter slows, and the renal pelvis lies at the level of the second lumbar vertebra. At this stage the developing kidney faces ventrally (Fig. 17.8, *A*). During the next 2 weeks of embryonic development (20 to 30 mm), the kidney will rotate outwardly through 90 degrees to face medially (Fig. 17.8, *B*). Failure of this process to proceed normally results in a kidney facing ventrally (anteriorly), dorsally (posteriorly), or laterally.

Two theories to account for malrotation were put forward by Weyrauch (163). One suggests that a slightly delayed ureteric bud might make a more lateral contact with the renal blastema; hence, the kidney would develop in an abnormal plane of rotation. Although this explanation would account for an anomalous initial position of the kidney, it fails to account for the rotation from the initial to the final position.

The second theory, elaborated by Priman (21), is based on the observation of Felix (11) that the progressive branching of the ureteral tree into what will become collecting tubules proceeds by the sending out of two ventral branches for one dorsal branch, with the appropriate multiplication of cells of the nephrogenic blastema. So-called rotation therefore may be the result of asymmetric growth in a lateroventral direction, with consequent turning of the pelvis in a medial and dorsal direction. This theory will not account for extremes of hyperrotation.

Both of these "intrarenal" theories obviate the need for normal external rotational forces. The chief extrarenal force that has been suggested is the pull of blood vessels on the enlarging kidney. It is argued that, if the renal artery and vein do not elongate, and the dorsomedial mesenchyme prevents expansion in that direction, the expanding kidney will be forced to turn laterally and ventrally. Against this argument is the principle that developing blood vessels are as long and as large as the demands on them require: They rarely govern and nearly always follow. Against it also is the fact that vessels do elongate in the cases of reverse rotation and laterally facing kidney.

Incidence. Campbell (64) found 17 cases of renal malrotation among 32,834 autopsies on adults (1:1939). In only one case were both kidneys involved, although both right and left were about equally affected. More males than females exhibited malrotation. Smith and Orkin (105) consider the incidence to be much higher (1:390) and state that malrotation accounts for 10% of upper urinary tract anomalies. Such wide differences in reported incidence depend on the degree of malrotation considered to be anomalous by the particular writers.

Malrotation of the kidney has been reported in from 33 to 50% of patients with gonadal dysgenesis (Turner's syndrome) (164, 165).

Symptoms. Malrotation produces no specific symptoms, although many cases are revealed by the concomitant presence of kidney disease. Infection and hydrone-

phrosis are found in some cases of malrotation. Connective tissue bands fixing the pelvis and upper ureter, as well as vascular compression and angulation of the ureter, all predispose such individuals to stasis and infection.

Diagnosis. Laterally facing kidneys are easily visualized by pyelography, but lateral or stereoscopic films may be necessary to differentiate dorsally and ventrally facing kidneys. The narrow anteriorly facing pelvis may suggest compression from a neoplasm unless the possibility of nonrotation is considered.

The pelves of horseshoe kidneys are usually abnormally rotated, and this malformation should always be suspected in the presence of malrotation.

Treatment. No treatment is required for malrotation of the kidney, but disease of such a kidney should be treated as one would treat a similar condition in a normal kidney.

HORSESHOE KIDNEY

As we have already stated, in the last several stages in their development, the kidneys may fuse with one another. Early fusion of bilateral masses of nephric tissue results in an amorphous renal mass lying in the pelvis. This is the rare discoid or lump kidney (page 622).

A possible occurence at the other end of the time scale is fused crossed ectopia, in which two relatively normal

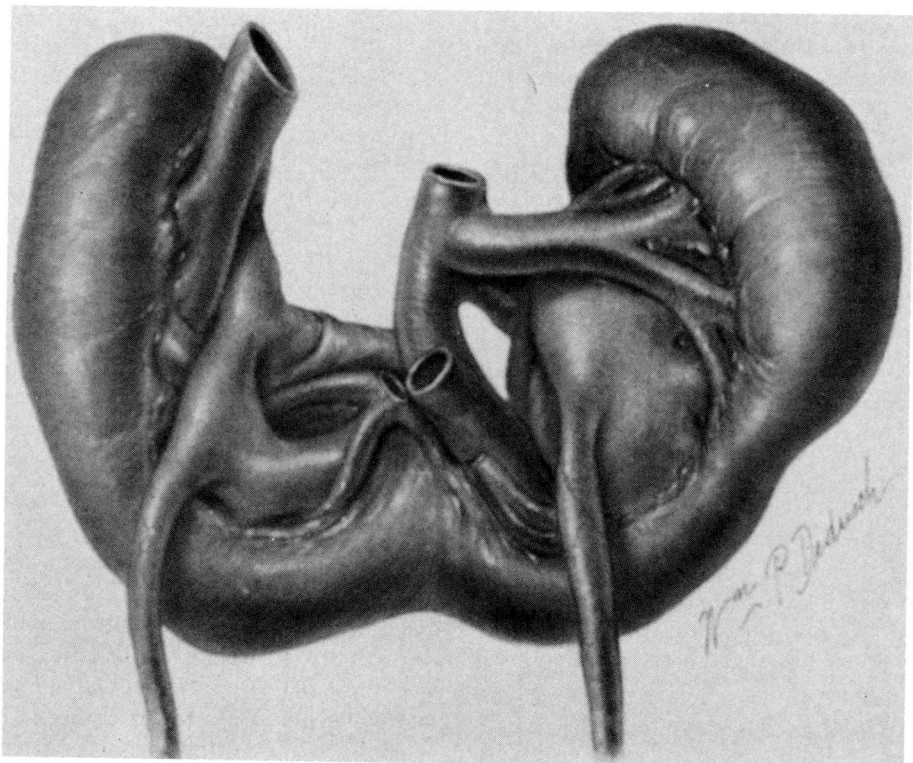

Figure 17.23. A typical horseshoe kidney. (From Didusch WP. A collection of urogenital drawings. New York: American Cystoscope Makers, 1952.)

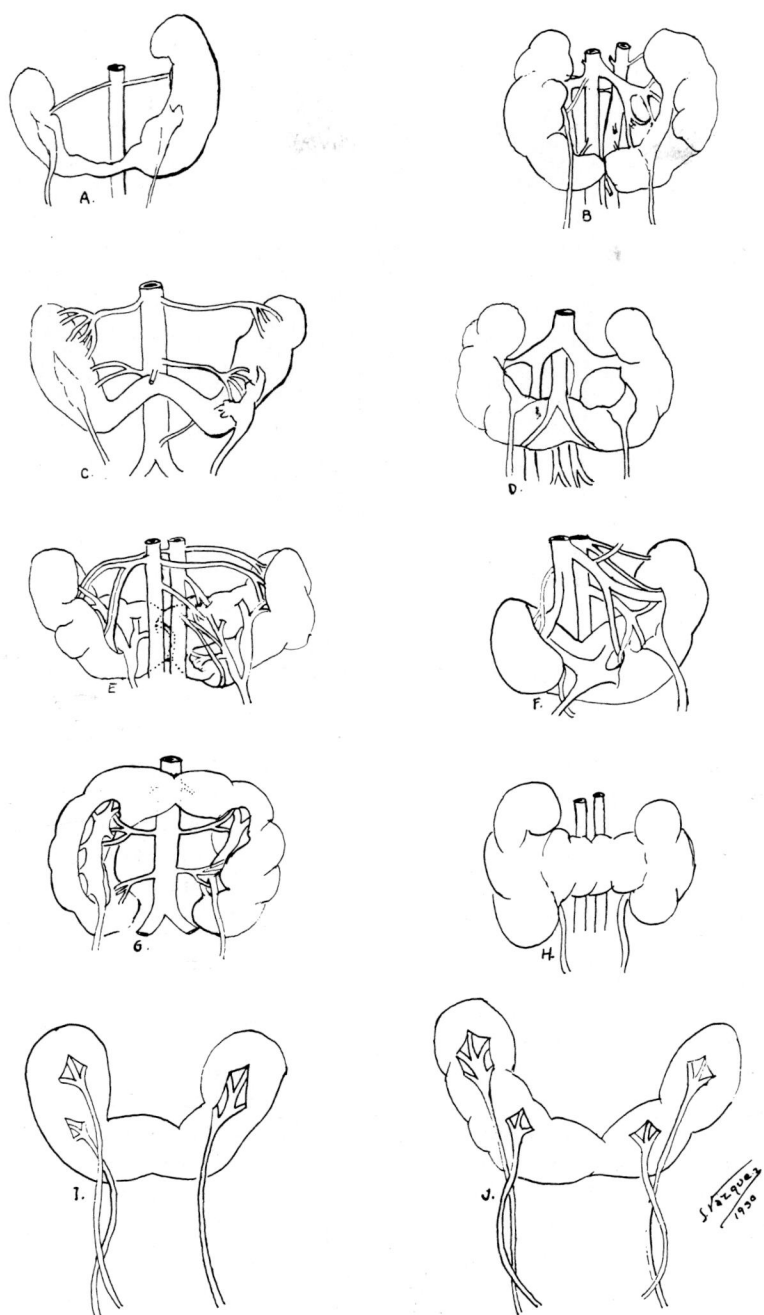

Figure 17.24. Variations in the shape of horseshoe kidneys and the number of their ureters. (From Gutierrez R. The clinical management of horseshoe kidney. Am J Surg 1931;14:657–688.)

kidneys become attached and lie one above the other, on the same side of the body (page 614).

Between these extremes, and much more common than either, is the condition called "horseshoe kidney" (Fig. 17.23).

Anatomy. There are many variations of horseshoe kidney, some of which are shown in Figure 17.24. In 95% of horseshoe kidneys, the lower poles of the two kidneys are joined. A simple fusion of two otherwise normally shaped kidneys may result in a V-shaped kidney. More often, a band of tissue, the isthmus, connects the lower poles. This isthmus is from 5 to 6 cm long, strap shaped, and usually of normal kidney tissue, but occasionally it is of fibrous tissue derived from the capsule only. The isthmus lies at the level of the fourth lumbar vertebra, just beneath the origin of the inferior mesenteric artery, in about 40% of

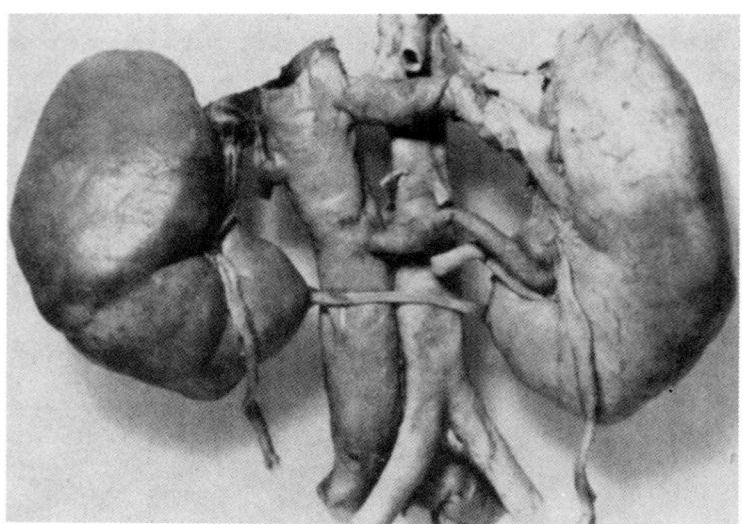

Figure 17.25. Aberrant arterial communication between kidneys. The single right renal artery is posterior to the inferior vena cava; there are three renal arteries on the left. (From Guggemos E, Nystrom BA, Peppy SJ, Sinatra C, Brody H. A rare case of arterial connection between the left and right kidneys. Ann Surg 1962;156:940–943.)

cases (Fig. 17.24). The artery may pass through a notch in the isthmus. In another 20% of cases, the isthmus is in the pelvis; in the remainder, it lies at the level of the lower poles of normal kidneys. In general, the more complete the fusion, the lower the kidneys lie.

An isthmus of capsular connective tissue may be transitory, its existence marked by only an aberrant artery. In one case a branch of a polar renal artery crossed the midline to serve the pole of the contralateral kidney. No parenchyma was present (166) (Fig. 17.25).

The isthmus of the usual horseshoe kidney lies anterior to the aorta and the vena cava. A few cases have been reported in which the isthmus was posterior to the vena cava (167) or to the aorta and vena cava (168) (Fig. 17.24, E) (see the discussion of postcaval and postarterial ureters, pages 656–658.) A single case in which the ureters lay beneath the isthmus was reported over a century ago (169), and another case is known in which one ureter passed beneath the isthmus (170).

The blood supply to a horseshoe kidney is usually anomalous. Papin (171) studied 127 cases and found more than two arteries present in 100. Even when only two arteries are present, they arise from the aorta below the normal level. When three arteries are present, one supplies the isthmus. The greater the number of arteries, the more frequent is their extraaortic origin. As many as 10 arteries were present in two of Papin's cases.

Fusion of the upper poles instead of the lower poles results in an "inverted horseshoe kidney." About 5 to 10% of horseshoe kidneys are of this type (Fig. 17.24, G). Even more rare is the "doughnut kidney" in which both upper and lower poles are fused to form a ring-shaped structure with medial ureters.

In addition to fusion, there is usually failure of rota-

tion of the kidneys; hence, the pelves are usually anterior. They are often extrarenal. Duplication of the ureters is not rare, and therefore three or four pelves and ureters may be associated with the renal mass (172) (Fig. 17.24, I and J).

Associated Anomalies. Nonurinary tract defects often accompany horseshoe kidneys. Cardiovascular and gastrointestinal anomalies are present in more than the expected number and anorectal defects are especially common.

Embryogenesis. During the passage of the kidneys out of the pelvis during the sixth week, they cross the umbilical arteries, which constrict the passage into the abdomen. Contact between the two kidneys at this time may result in fusion. If the caudal pole of the leading kidney fuses with the cranial pole of the trailing kidney, the trailing kidney will follow the leading kidney to the same side of the body and the result will be crossed ectopia with fusion (page 614).

It has been assumed that horseshoe kidney occurs when both kidneys lie at the same level and their caudal poles come into contact. Subsequent divergence produces the isthmus connecting them. The joined kidneys continue to ascend until the inferior mesenteric artery, branching from the aorta, halts them. Not only is ascent halted, but rotation of the kidneys also is prevented, so that the pelves usually remain facing anteriorly (Fig. 17.26).

In some cases one or both members of the fused pair rotate normally, so that the pelvis is medial. Campbell (64) has suggested that this indicates later fusion than in cases in which the pelves retain their primitive anterior position.

A number of embryos showing the development of this

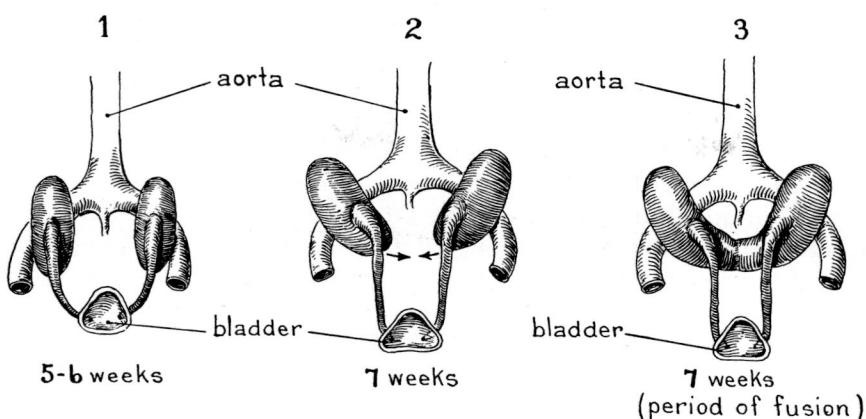

Figure 17.26. Embryogenesis of horseshoe kidney. The lower poles of the two kidneys touch and fuse as they cross the iliac arteries. Ascent is stopped when the fused kidneys reach the junction of the aorta and inferior mesenteric artery. (From Gutierrez R. The clinical management of horseshoe kidney. Am J Surg 1931;14:657–688.)

anomaly have been found (173), the youngest dating from the sixth week (10 mm) (174).

History. The earliest observation of a horseshoe kidney was by daCarpi (175) in 1521 at Bologna. In 1564 Botallo (176) illustrated such a kidney and showed the separate artery to the isthmus. His dissection appears to have been excellent and his figure shows an additional anomaly of a renal vein draining into the left common iliac vein as well as into the inferior vena cava. The descriptions of both daCarpi and Botallo, together with the figure of the latter, may be found in a paper by Benjamin and Schullian (177).

Horseshoe kidneys are present in other animals than humans. The earliest reference is in a 17th century work on Talmudic Law quoted by Boyden (174).

Incidence and Associated Conditions. Horseshoe kidney, the most common fusion anomaly, has been said to occur once in every 400 births (178). It is more common in males and is found with even greater frequency in infants and children who come to autopsy, suggesting a higher risk of mortality in these children, not so much because of renal disease but rather because of the severity of associated anomalies. Zondek and Zondek (179) found that only 5% of infants with horseshoe kidney found at autopsy died of disease in the horseshoe kidney. In addition to lethal conditions involving other organ systems, there is an increased incidence of genitourinary abnormalities in patients with horseshoe kidney. Most common are ureteral duplication anomalies, vesicoureteral reflux, undescended testis, and hypospadias (180). Nonlethal extragenitourinary anomalies are found with increased incidence but are less common than those associated with renal ectopy and are generally milder. Boatman (181) documented the increased incidence of this entity with chromosomal abnormalities such as Turner's syndrome and trisomy 18.

Of interest is the reported increased incidence of Wilms' tumor and other renal malignancies associated

with horseshoe kidney. Dische and Johnston (182) reported a significant increase over the expected normal incidence of tumors in horseshoe kidney.

Hydronephrosis is the most common complication of horseshoe kidney as well as of other forms of malrotated kidney. It was formerly customary to identify the point where the ureter crosses the isthmus as the site of obstruction. However, this is, in fact, very infrequently observed (183). Rather, a true obstruction at the ureteropelvic junction may occur, requiring surgical intervention with dismembered pyeloplasty, particularly if infection or calculus formation occurs.

Symptoms. The division of patients with horseshoe kidney into three groups by symptoms, suggested by Gutierrez (184), can hardly be improved on:

1. The anomaly is present but asymptomatic.
2. Horseshoe kidney disease is present, but there is no demonstrable pathologic condition.
3. The kidneys are diseased.

About 66% of patients fall into group 3, and most of the remainder belong in group 1.

Horseshoe kidney disease (Rovsing syndrome) consists of nausea, abdominal discomfort, and pain on hyperextension. No renal pathologic condition can be shown. The pain has been related to compression of the ureters over the isthmus, although this has not been proved. More often, obstruction and infection complicate the condition as a result of the abnormal course of the ureters and the anomalous blood supply, both of which may interfere with normal drainage. About 30% of patients have calculi (178).

Complications of Pregnancy. Horseshoe kidney is less likely to complicate pregnancy than is simple pelvic renal ectopia, but it cannot be entirely ignored. About 33% of women with horseshoe kidneys have had mild complications of pregnancy, while 5% have had severe difficulties in labor. Division of the isthmus in some cases has been followed by uneventful pregnancies (185).

Diagnosis. Pain, localized at the umbilicus, and Rovsing's sign are suggestive but not diagnostic.

The relatively low kidneys can often be palpated, and sometimes the isthmus itself can be distinguished. In the pyelogram, the long axes of the kidney are inclined inward and downward with the ureters crossing the lower calyces. A calyx draining the isthmus is sometimes present. Both pelves and their calyces lie below the last rib. The pelves usually are anterior because of rotational failure, but this is not invariably the case. The shadow of the psoas muscle is interrupted by the isthmus.

In the absence of symptoms, many cases remain undiagnosed until discovered at autopsy.

Treatment. Surgical intervention is required in about 25% of horseshoe kidney cases.

Division of the isthmus and nephropexy often will straighten the course of the ureters and provide better drainage. Division was first performed by Martinow (186) in 1910, and the procedure was discussed in detail by Rovsing (187) the following year. These early symphysiotomies were approached transperitoneally. Papin (171) first successfully divided the isthmus by an extraperitoneal approach. Donohue (188) reported the first U.S. operation. Technical details for surgery in horseshoe kidney, whether pyeloplasty or ureterocalicostomy, with emphasis on aberrant blood supply, is readily available (189).

It has been suggested that horseshoe kidneys are almost always associated with disease (105). However, others have found this in error. In Glenn's (178) study, 60% remained symptom free over a 10-year followup. Only 13% had persistent urinary tract infection; 17% developed recurrent calculi; and surgery to remove stones or obstruction was necessary in only 25%. Division of the isthmus for relief of pain is no longer tenable (190).

Prognosis. In their study of renal anomalies, Smith and Orkin (105) considered horseshoe kidneys the anomaly most susceptible to kidney disease. In their series, less than 5% could be considered asymptomatic. While one must keep in mind the fact that the frequency of the asymptomatic anomaly is as hard to estimate as that of the undetected murder, there is a general agreement that, while it was not incompatible with long life, horseshoe kidneys are a real handicap to their possessors. Campbell (64) pointed out that the incidence of horseshoe kidney among autopsies of children was 1:312, while among autopsies of adults, it was 1:538.

Shoup and his colleagues (191) collected 47 cases of renal neoplasms occuring in horseshoe kidneys, and added one case of their own. Beck and Hlivko (192) collected seven cases of Wilm's tumor and reported the first preoperative diagnosis.

FUSED PELVIC KIDNEY (LUMP, DISCOID, OR CAKE KIDNEY)

Anatomy. Fused pelvic kidneys have been variously described as "lump," "cake," or "discoid," according to their gross form. Since few cases are alike, these descriptive terms are not helpful. The most that can be said of these structures is that there is an irregular mass of renal tissue, usually in the midline, with two or more pelves and a weight approximately equal to that of two normal kidneys. Although most are pelvic, cases are known of irregular kidney masses found at the normal location of one kidney. These might be considered as crossed ectopia with fusion, except for their irregular shape (139, 193).

Careful dissection may reveal a line of fusion, but this line is usually not apparent externally. The pelves face anteriorly and are separate as a rule, although in the case described by Kron and Meranze (194), they communicated with one another (Fig. 17.27). Most patients are male.

Embryogenesis. This extreme type of fusion occurs earlier than that which produces horseshoe kidney or fused crossed ectopia. The primary defect is probably the failure of the kidneys to ascend, with fusion resulting from their enlargement at their primitive pelvic location. The

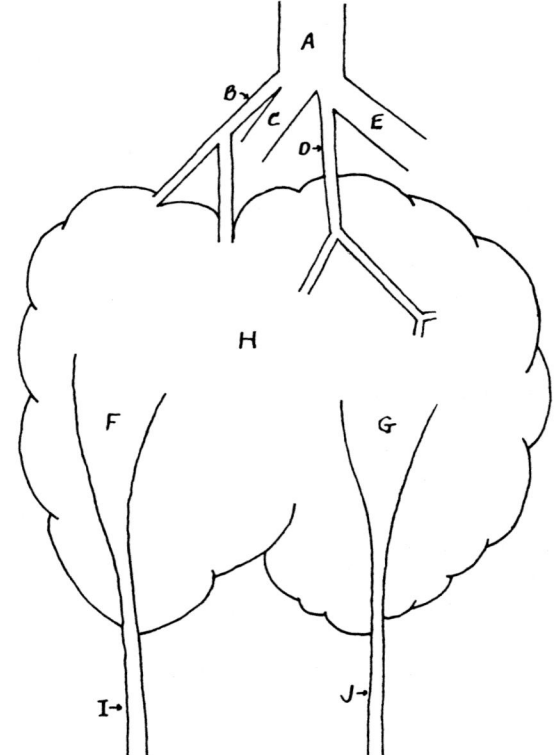

Figure 17.27. Fused pelvic kidney. *A,* Aorta; *B and D,* renal arteries; *C and E,* iliac arteries; *F and G,* visible pelves; *H,* intercommunication of pelves within kidney; *I and J,* ureters. No two such kidneys are exactly alike. (From Kron SD, Meranze DR. Completely fused pelvic kidney. J Urol 1949;62:278–285.)

existence of patients with unfused bilateral pelvic ectopia indicates that these factors do not always produce a fused kidney.

History. Morgagni (86) cites several cases of what may have been lump kidneys, including a case from Vesalius (De Sedibus XLVIII:16). He emphasized the midline position but did not discuss their pelvic location. Morris (193) lists six or seven 19th century cases. We have not seen an adequate review of the cases in the literature.

Incidence. Campbell (64) found three examples among 51,880 autopsies.

Symptoms and Diagnosis. Symptoms are only those of obstruction and infection. An uncomplicated fused pelvic kidney is not incompatible with longevity: A case was reported in a 70-year-old man (195).

Pyelograms showing both renal pelves close together below the pelvic brim indicate bilateral pelvic ectopia and suggest fusion of the kidneys. Retrograde pyelograms may be required in the presence of calculi or other obstruction. The pelves are frequently bizarre.

The kidney mass, abnormal in shape and location, is often palpable, but this may lead to an incorrect diagnosis of neoplasm.

Treatment. The primitive, multiple arterial supply to these renal masses makes surgical resection impossible in some cases. Their lack of similarity to one another in shape and the arrangement of pelves, ureters, and blood vessels reduces the value of even the most carefully described examples.

Severe obstruction, calculi, infections, or tumors may dictate surgical intervention. Although mortality in the past was high, currently available techniques of renal parenchymal suturing and vascular repair have greatly decreased the danger of surgery.

Variations of the Renal Arteries

ANATOMY

The vascular anatomy of the kidney is important to renal surgery, and lends itself well to study because of the ease with which the variations may be tabulated in large series.

Our knowledge of the arterial supply to the kidney rests largely on the work of Graves (196, 197). Five arterial branches supply each kidney. As these are end arteries, without collateral connections between them, the kidney is thus divided into five segments: posterior, upper anterior, middle anterior, and two polar. The arrangement of these segments is shown in Figure 17.28.

NUMBER OF RENAL ARTERIES

Although these five arterial segments appear to be fundamental, the pattern of arterial branching to supply them is subject to great variation. The number of renal arteries entering the kidney has been studied so often that

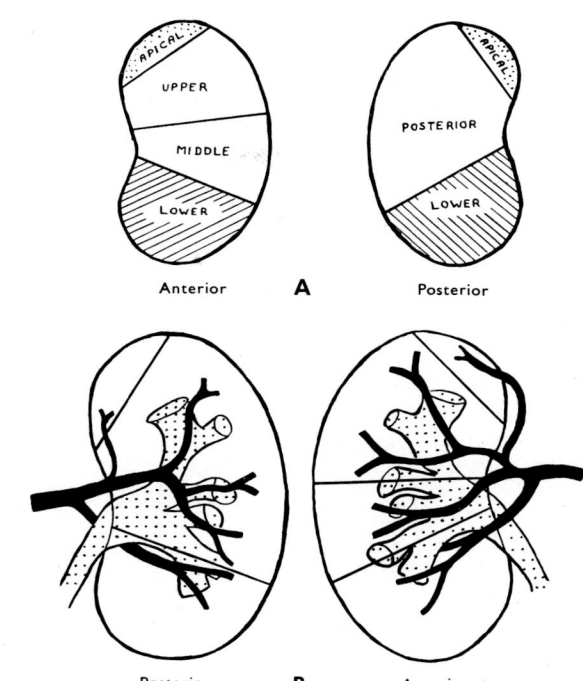

Figure 17.28. *Usual pattern of arteries to the kidney.* **A,** *The five vascular lobes of Graves.* **B,** *Relationships of renal artery branches and renal pelvis to the five lobes. (From Graves FT. The anatomy of the intrarenal arteries and their application to segmental resection of the kidneys. Br J Surg 1954;42:132–139.)*

in 1958 Merklin and Michels (198) were able to collect the experience of 45 authors who had examined 10,987 kidneys. Their findings are summarized in Table 17.5.

Because of differences in the manner of computation by different authors, the total adds up to more than 100%. The frequency of the less common varieties in particular may be overestimated. It is interesting to note that there are fewer variations in the cat and dog than there are in humans (199).

In any of these varieties, true aberrant small arteries may occasionally enter the kidney from the suprarenal, ovarian, or internal spermatic arteries. A unique case, in which a branch of a left inferior polar artery emerged from the left kidney to cross to the inferior pole of the right kidney, appears to represent a transient fusion of the kidneys, with subsequent separation (Fig. 17.25) (166).

The terminology of multiple renal arteries presents some difficulties. The vessels represent variable extrarenal branching to form the five normal segmental arteries; hence, they are not "accessory" in any sense. We agree with Geyer and Poutasse (200) that the term *aberrant* should be reserved for arteries that originate from vessels other than the aorta, even though urologists use the term for arteries that compress the pelvis or ureter. This use is justified on a functional, but not on an anatomic, basis. When a separate extrarenal artery supplies one of the

Table 17.5.
Variations in the Arterial Supply to the Kidney

	Condition	Percentage
	1 Hilar artery	71.1
	1 Hilar artery and 1 upper pole branch	12.6
	2 Hilar arteries	10.8
	1 Hilar artery and 1 upper pole aortic artery	6.2
	1 Hilar artery and 1 lower pole aortic artery	6.9
	1 Hilar artery and 1 lower pole branch	3.1
	3 Hilar arteries	1.7
	2 Hilar arteries, one with upper polar branch	2.7
	Other variations	—

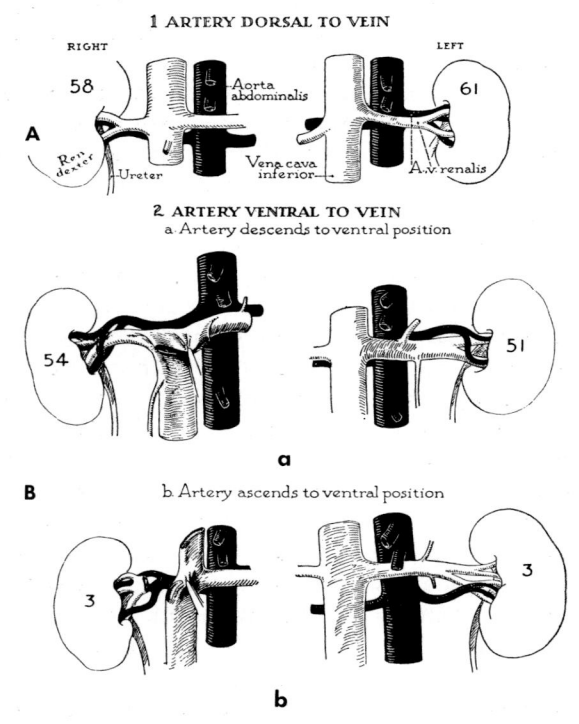

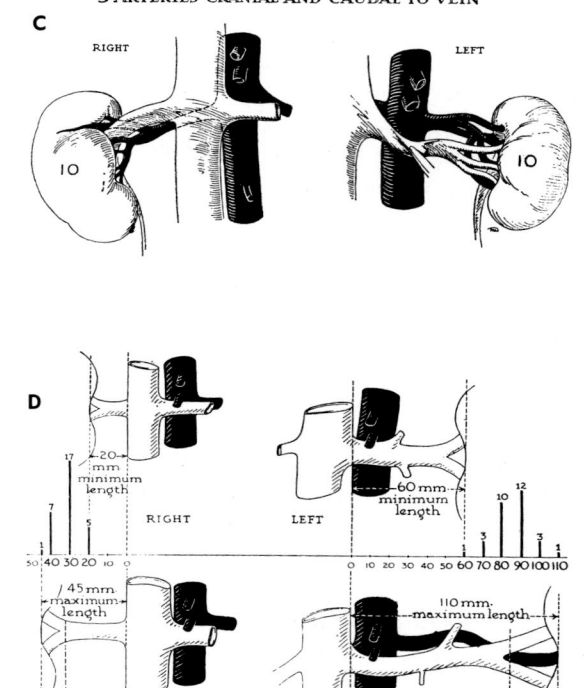

Figure 17.29. Relationships of renal arteries and veins. **A,** Artery dorsal to vein (47.6%). **B,** Artery ventral to vein (**Ba,** 42%; **Bb,** 2.4%). **C,** Artery cranial and caudal to vein (8.0%). **D,** Maximum, minimum, and average lengths of the renal pedicle in 30 successive specimens. (From Anson BJ, Daseler EH. Common variation in renal anatomy affecting blood supply, form, and topography. Surg Gynecol Obstet 1961;112:439–449.)

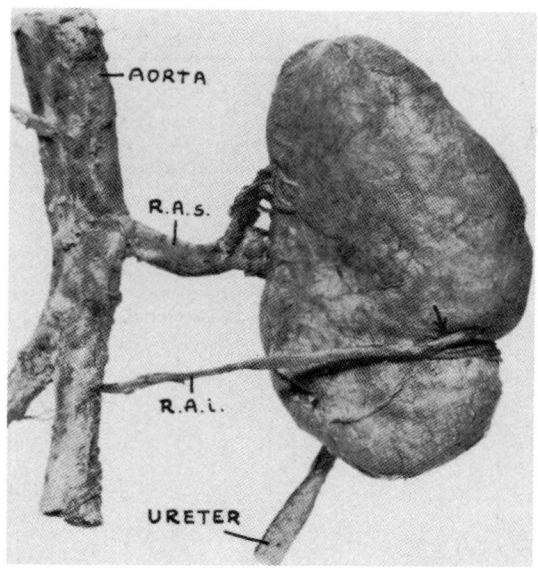

Figure 17.30. Kidney with its vascular connections seen from behind. A right inferior renal artery *(R.A.i.)* runs over the posterior surface to reach the hilus, which faces anterolaterally. This appears to be an example of reversed rotation of the kidney (see Fig. 17.8, **F**). *R.A.s.,* Right superior renal artery. (From Nathan H. Aberrant renal artery producing developmental anomaly of kidney associated with unusual course of gonadal ovarian vessels. J Urol 1963;89:570–572.)

polar segments of a normally placed kidney, it should be termed a superior or inferior *polar artery.* When more than one artery supplies the hilus, it is a superior or inferior *renal artery* or a superior, inferior, anterior, or posterior *branch of the renal artery.*

POSITIONS OF RENAL ARTERIES

In addition to variations in number of renal arteries, there are variations in their position with respect to the renal veins. The artery lay posterior (dorsal) to the vein in 47.6% of 250 kidneys examined by Anson and Daseler (201). The artery became anterior to the vein at the hilus by curving over the vein in 42% or by curving under the vein in 2.4%. In the remaining cases the artery emerged from the aorta cranial or caudal to the vein (Fig. 17.29). A case in which an inferior renal artery crossed the kidney anteriorly and passed around the lateral border to reach the hilus from behind has been reported (202) (Fig. 17.30).

EMBRYOGENESIS

The renal arteries represent a reduction of a series of segmental arteries from the aorta which originally supplied the mesonephric kidney in the embryo. Which arteries persist and which drop out depend on the final position of the kidney. Complete reduction of the primitive arterial supply results in a single renal artery, branching at the hilus to supply the five arterial segments of the kidney.

Less complete reduction results in extrarenal branching or in multiple arteries arising independently from the aorta. Small vessels from spermatic, ovarian, or suprarenal arteries are vestiges of segmental mesonephric arteries that have persisted.

The ectopic kidney frequently is supplied by arteries that represent lower segmental arteries, which would normally have atrophied had the kidney reached its normal location (203). They may be considered to be the normal embryonic arterial supply for the stage of ascent at which arrest took place.

SYMPTOMS

A lower polar artery may sometimes produce constriction where it crosses the ureter. The constriction may be primary (congenital), or it may occur only after renal ptosis has changed the original relationships. This constriction produces ureteral obstruction and hydronephrosis. Even the most severe hydronephrosis may be asymptomatic, but symptoms of flank or abdominal pain may occur, with acute distension of the renal pelvis, resulting from diuresis or a sudden increase in the degree of obstruction. Secondary infection of the kidney is not uncommon and may result in pain and fever. The hydronephrotic kidney is more easily injured; pain and hematuria may be the first indication of the lesion. It has been suggested that hypertension of renal origin might be related to the presence of multiple renal arteries. However, aortography in 381 patients with hypertension has shown that there is no higher incidence of multiple renal arteries among these patients than in non-affected patients, nor is there a higher incidence of occlusive renal artery disease in patients with multiple arteries (200).

DIAGNOSIS

Urography will demonstrate the hydronephrosis and may show a line of demarcation between the distended upper ureter and the normal or only partially filled lower ureter. Aortography may be useful in delineating the artery.

Frequently a primary stricture of the ureteropelvic junction is found on exploration to be the cause of the hydronephrosis. The apparent obstruction by the artery is caused by bulging of the distended renal pelvis between the vascular structures. This may mislead the surgeon into thinking that the artery is the sole cause of obstruction. In these cases correction of the hydronephrosis will eliminate the arterial pressure on the ureter.

TREATMENT

When the primary obstruction is caused by the artery, the vessel must be sectioned or the position of the ureter changed by ureteroneopyelostomy or pyelopyelostomy. The latter is preferable if there is demonstrable ischemia when the artery is temporarily occluded.

Table 17.6.
Comparison of Cystic Diseases of the Kidney

Defect	Origin of Defect	Age at Onset	Preferred Location	Sex Chiefly Affected	Remarks
Simple cyst	Unknown	Adults	Unilateral, lower pole	Female	Considered by many to be acquired
Multicystic disease	5th week	Infancy	Unilateral, whole kidney	Equal	A form of renal dysplasia; pelvis, and ureter absent or rudimentary
Sponge kidney	Unknown	Most ages 30 to 50	Bilateral, pyramids of medulla	Male	
Calyceal diverticula	6th week?	Adulthood	Unilateral, medullary	Equal	Usually located at poles
Polycystic disease	Unknown	I Recessive at birth	Bilateral	Equal	Fatal
		II Dominant ages 30–60	Bilateral (unilateral form exists)	Equal	Progressively severe; eventually fatal; an inherited disease
Cystadenoma	Unknown	Middle age	Unilateral, cortical	Equal	Benign neoplasm

Abnormalities of Histologic Differentiation: Cystic Diseases of the Kidney

More than other organs of the body, the kidney is subject to cyst formation. Cysts may be found in all sizes and may be solitary or multiple. They may affect one or both kidneys and may manifest themselves at any age from birth to senescence.

All agree that cystic disease comprises several disease entities, but the number of these entities and their precise definition is subject to debate. Most are considered to be of congenital origin, but their embryogenesis is no more certain than is their classification. Included are those cystic kidneys whose origin is hereditary, developmental but not hereditary, and acquired (Table 17.6).

Cystic diseases of the kidney are heterogenous and not easy to classify. The most widely utilized schemes in the past have been based on morphologic and radiographic observations, modified by clinical findings (204, 205). The original scheme of Osathanondh and Potter (206) is based on microdissection studies and has little direct application to the clinical setting. Most recently, attempts have been made to link the observed clinical entities with a genetic predisposition (118, 207).

Cystic diseases that appear to be of embryonic origin may be divided into nine groups and can be distinguished from cystic disease of nonembryonic origin. We are concerned here with the embryonic group only:

A. Renal cysts of probable embryonic origin
   1. Simple cysts (including "solitary" and "multilocular" cysts)
   2. Congenital multicystic kidney ("multicystic dysplastic kidney")

3. Calyceal or pelvic diverticula
4. Cystic adenoma of the kidney
5. Glomerulocystic disease
6. Cystic dilation of renal pyramids ("sponge kidney")
7. Medullary cystic disease—familial juvenile nephrophthisis complex
8. Polycystic kidney disease
9. Renal cysts associated with multiple malformation syndrome
  B. Renal cysts of nonembryonic origin
1. Retention and inflammatory cysts
2. Cysts associated with neoplastic disease (excluding cystadenoma)
3. Cysts associated with calculi or infection
4. Parasitic cysts

EMBRYOGENESIS OF RENAL CYSTS

As early as 1855 Virchow (208) suggested that intrinsic tubular obstruction was responsible for cyst formation in the kidney. By 1892 he inclined to the view that fibrous occlusion from prenatal inflammation was responsible. Hanau (209) in 1890 suggested that a primary aplasia of the tubules was responsible, thus anticipating the "failure of union" theory of Hildebrand (210). Brigidi and Severi (211) suggested the neoplastic theory of origin of the cysts, and McKinlay (212) suggested epithelial hyperplasia. A thorough review of the history of speculations of the pathogenesis of cystic kidneys is to be found in the paper of Osathanondh and Potter (206).

Among the many theories of developmental origin of renal cysts, three are the most likely as well as the most widely held. No one view, however, is expected to fit all the cystic conditions of congenital origin. The specific applicability of these views will be considered under the discussion of each lesion.

Developmental Insufficiency. Two explanations of cyst formation have been based on the idea that one of the two embryonic components of the kidney might be inadequate. We have discussed the origin of the multicystic or aplastic kidney from nephrogenic mesenchyme in the absence of the normal ureteric component. Beeson (213) suggested the opposite explanation for the infantile form of polycystic disease. Observing the small number of glomeruli present in such kidneys, Beeson proposed that the nephrogenic mesenchyme was unable to induce enough nephrons to cap the developing ends of the ureteric tree. The small number of glomeruli represents not destruction by pressure, but failure of glomerular formation. Cysts arise from the tips of the fruitlessly branching tubules of the ureteric bud.

Failure of the Primordia to Unite. Hildebrand (210) in 1894 and von Mutach (214) in 1895 suggested that failure of the developing nephrons to unite with the collecting tubules from the ureteric bud during development would produce cystic enlargement of the isolated nephrons.

Felix (1) agreed with this view, which is perhaps the most widely accepted one. Lambert's (215) reconstructions of nephrons of polycystic kidneys in 1947, however, have shown that cyst formation in the adult form of the diseases can occur even when there is demonstrable continuity of the tubules (Fig. 17.31). Norris and Herman (216) suggest that there is no failure of union of the two nephric components, but subsequent abnormal degeneration of tubules already united. In terms of Kampmeier's hypothesis (discussed in the next section, "Persistence of Vestigial Nephrons"), an excessive number of metanephrons are "provisional."

Persistence of Vestigial Nephrons. Kampmeier (34) described the development of the kidney in three concentric zones, of which only the outermost forms the definitive cortex. The earliest formed nephrons in the hilar region are vestigial. The next three sets of nephrons differentiate and join the second to fourth orders of collecting tubule branches, but degenerate before birth. From these vestigial and provisional tubules cystic disease may develop. Rall and Odel (217) and Spence (218) have accepted this explanation for polycystic kidney disease, but not for other cystic conditions.

A second source of cysts is from persistence of mesonephric structures incorporated in the adult kidney. Interestingly, cystic disease of the mesonephros of lower vertebrates is known to occur.

Rożynek (40) reported the presence of deformed glomeruli in the subcapsular zone, which represents the most recently formed nephrons rather than the oldest. He felt that glomerular and tubular cysts may be seen in practically every fetal kidney. If this is true, such cysts must normally be reabsorbed rather than persisting to cause cystic disease.

Microdissection Studies. Osathanondh and Potter (206, 219–222) repudiated all the above explanations on the basis of microdissection studies of diseased kidneys. They proposed the following list for classification and pathogenesis of cystic disease. (As noted previously, this classification scheme has little clinical usefulness, but we decided to keep it for historical reasons.)

1. Cysts resulting from hyperplasia of interstitial portions of collecting tubules: There is no change in number or pattern of nephrons, and cysts may also be present in the liver. The condition is familial, probably produced by a homozygous recessive gene. The clinical synonyms consist of polycystic kidney of the newborn, sponge kidney, and hamartomatous kidney (Fig. 17.32, *A to C*).
2. Cysts resulting from the inhibition of collecting tubule development: Nephrons are reduced in number and poorly developed; convoluted tubules are short. The kidney may be larger or smaller than normal; the ureter is irregularly dilated or atretic. Developing tubules failed to branch normally and induced few nephrons. The cyst

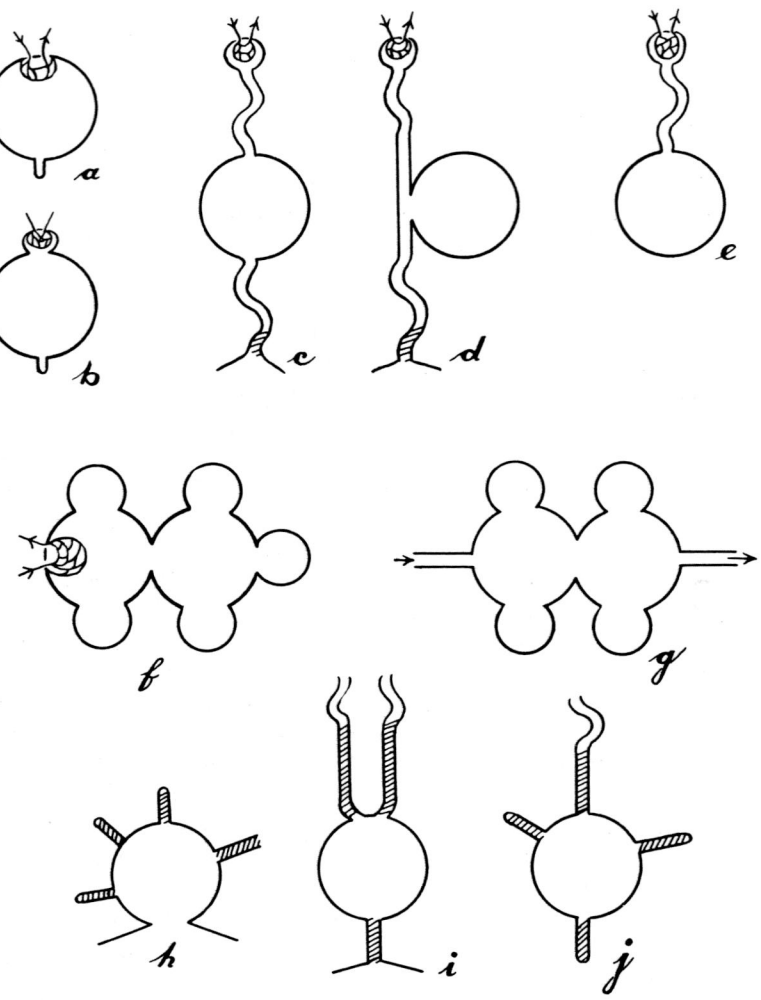

Figure 17.31. Various types of cysts seen in adult polycystic kidneys. **A,** Glomerular cyst with blind tubule. **B,** Subglomerular cyst. **C,** Bipolar cyst in an open nephron. **D,** Unipolar cyst in an open nephron. **E,** Terminal cyst in a closed nephron. **F,** Multilocular glomerular cyst. **G,** Multilocular tubular cyst. **H,** Cyst of the calyx. **I,** Tripolar excretory cyst. **J,** Excretory cyst unconnected with the pelvis. Types **C, D, H,** and **I** do not block urinary channels and are not found in the infantile forms of the disease. Collecting tubules are *shaded*. (From Lambert PP. Polycystic disease of the kidney: a review. Arch Pathol 1947;44:34–58.)

fluid is not glomerular filtrate. Clinical synonyms consist of polycystic kidney of the adult (enlarged kidney) and multicystic kidney (partial involvement) (Fig. 17.32, *D* and *E*).

3. Cysts resulting from multiple abnormalities: Normal nephrons and collecting tubules are mixed with abnormal forms. Cysts form in any part of the abnormal tubule or nephron. Developing tubules divided irregularly with independent rates, producing irregular architecture of the kidney. The kidney is enlarged, both sides are usually affected. The lesion is progressive and is often associated with other malformations (Fig. 17.32, *F* to *H*).

4. Cysts resulting from congenital urethral obstruction: The bladder and ureters are distended. Cysts are subcapsular and at the ends of collecting tubules, in Bowman's capsule, or in the loop of Henle of the last one or two generations of nephrons. Damage is from pressure in fetal life while the final few orders of nephrons are developing (Fig. 17.33).

SIMPLE CYSTS OF THE KIDNEY

Anatomy. DeWeerd and Simon (223) set seven criteria for simple renal cysts. These are: *(a)* the cysts must be unilocular; *(b)* they must have no communication with the pelvis; *(c)* they must be lined with epithelium; *(d)* they can have no renal elements within; *(e)* they must be localized in the kidney; *(f)* the uninvolved kidney tissue should be normal; and *(g)* the ureter and pelvis should be present and patent.

The disease is usually unilateral, more often on the right (224). Hepler (225) found cysts on both kidneys in only 3.5% of his series. About 80 to 90% of simple cysts are found at the poles of the kidney. While cysts are usually single ("solitary cysts"), more than one cyst may be present (Fig. 17.34).

The lining is usually flattened epithelium; in spite of the above criteria, in most large cysts epithelium is for the most part absent. The cysts may become very large, not uncommonly with a diameter of 12 to 15 cm. Carson (224) cites a cyst with a capacity of 13 liters. The contents are usually serous, but blood or traces of blood may be found in some. A few are calcified, and cartilage and bone sometimes form.

Pathogenesis. Nothing is known for certain of the development of solitary renal cysts. Kampmeier (226) observed cystic degeneration of nephrons near the hilus in the normal fetal kidney and concluded that one of these nephrons might form a solitary cyst instead of being reabsorbed. The fact that such cysts have been associated with solitary cysts of the liver and spleen suggests a less localized explanation.

Some authors consider these cysts to be acquired rather than congenital. Hepler (225) produced cysts experimentally in rabbit kidneys by fulguration of the papilla and ligation of a branch of the renal artery. He concluded that simple cysts were the result of tubular obstruction along with circulatory disturbance, but there is no evidence that spontaneous simple cysts form in this manner.

History and Incidence. Although Hildanus (227) saw renal cysts early in the 17th century, and Morgagni (86) in 1761 described what were probably simple cysts (DeSedibus XXXVIII:39–41), it is difficult to be sure of the nature of cystic diseases mentioned in the early literature. Rayer (228) classified cysts by their contents, but Laveren (229) distinguished between simple cysts and polycystic disease of the kidney. Harpster and his colleagues (230) collected 95 cases from the literature in 1922, and Hepler (225) in 1930 collected 256 serous and hemorrhagic "solitary cysts." He considered them all to be acquired. By 1956 the varieties of cystic disease in the literature had so multiplied that DeWeerd and Simon (223) felt it necessary to redefine simple cysts.

Simple renal cysts are twice as frequent in females as in males and are only rarely diagnosed in infancy or childhood. Carson (224) found only four children among the 145 cases he collected. Campbell (64) found 11 among 19,046 autopsies of infants and children. Solitary cysts also have been seen in two varieties of lemurs: *Microcebus* (231) and *Cheirogaleus* (115).

Symptoms. The symptoms are those produced by compression of the kidney parenchyma and of the surrounding organs. Pain, hematuria, and hypertension are unusual but have been reported. A palpable abdominal mass is almost always present.

Diagnosis. Diagnosis is by renal ultrasound, urography,

and rarely aortography, with the cyst appearing as a mass with a filling defect of pelvis and calyces. The kidney axis, and even the kidney itself, may be displaced by a large cyst (232).

Treatment. Since exploration is occasionally necessary to differentiate the cyst from a tumor, partial excision of the cyst wall is generally performed, usually with excellent results. Rarely is nephrectomy indicated or performed.

MULTILOCULAR CYSTS

Multilocular cysts have been reported in infants and adults. It is a rare condition closely simulating a tumor, and its pathologic differentiation from cystic and relatively benign forms of nephroblastoma (Wilms' tumor) is difficult. It is bulky, well encapsulated, and noninfiltrating (Fig. 17.35). It rarely, if ever, metastasizes (233) although Beckwith and Palmer (234) report metastases from cystic Wilms' tumor, with which multilocular cysts may be confused or which is possibly a part of a spectrum.

Radiologically and on ultrasonography, multilocular cysts cannot be readily distinguished from nephroblastoma. Computed tomography (CT) scan likewise is not reliable enough to specifically differentiate among cystic Wilms' tumor, benign multilocular renal cyst, or multilocular cyst with foci of Wilms' tumor or adenocarcinoma (118). Neither arteriography, radionuclide studies, nor cyst puncture seem to add to diagnostic capability, and they have little place in the evaluation of these lesions.

Treatment for this condition is nephrectomy or partial nephrectomy removing only the cystic lesion. The surgeon who performs the more limited procedure should be prepared to return and remove the residual kidney tissue should histologic examination confirm malignancy in the removed specimen. Essential in the discussion of treatment of the affected kidney is absolute knowledge of the status of its mate.

CONGENITAL MULTICYSTIC KIDNEY (MULTICYSTIC DYSPLASTIC KIDNEY)

Renal Dysplasia. A great deal of confusion exists regarding the definition and meaning of various terms used to describe maldevelopment or abnormal appearance of the kidney. We previously defined *hypoplasia* of the kidney as the miniature kidney with normal appearing calices which may be reduced in number, essentially normal parenchyma and a normal ureter. Small kidneys displaying other than normal histologic renal tissue may be *dysplastic* or *atrophic,* and when associated with vesicoureteral reflux, they should be described as manifesting *reflux nephropathy.* Further descriptive terms possibly adding to the confusion are *aplasia,* which is an extreme form of dysplasia in which a "nubbin" of nonfunctioning dysplastic tissue is identified in the renal fossa, and *agenesis,*

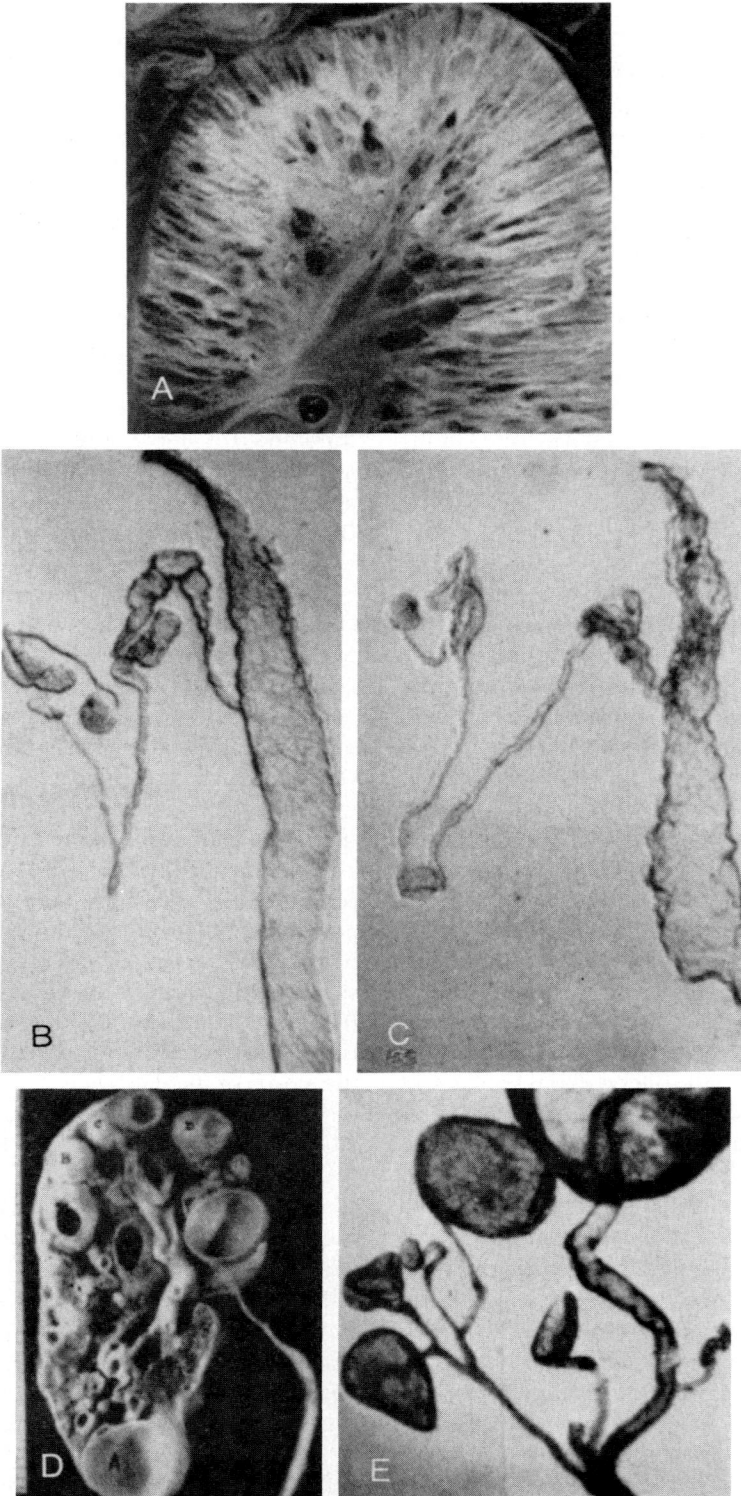

Figure 17.32.   Cystic kidney disease. Potter's classification. *(See text.)* **A,** Gross appearance of kidney, showing uniformly enlarged collecting tubules. **B** and **C,** Microdissection, showing nephrons attached to dilated collecting tubules. **B,** Dilation of proximal convoluted segment. **C,** Small cyst in loop of Henle. **D,** Innumerable cysts are visible in the partially dissected kidney. Calyces, pyramids, and pelvis are absent, the upper end of the ureter is atretic, and the bladder is not expanded. **E,** Collecting tubules end in cysts, no nephrons are present.

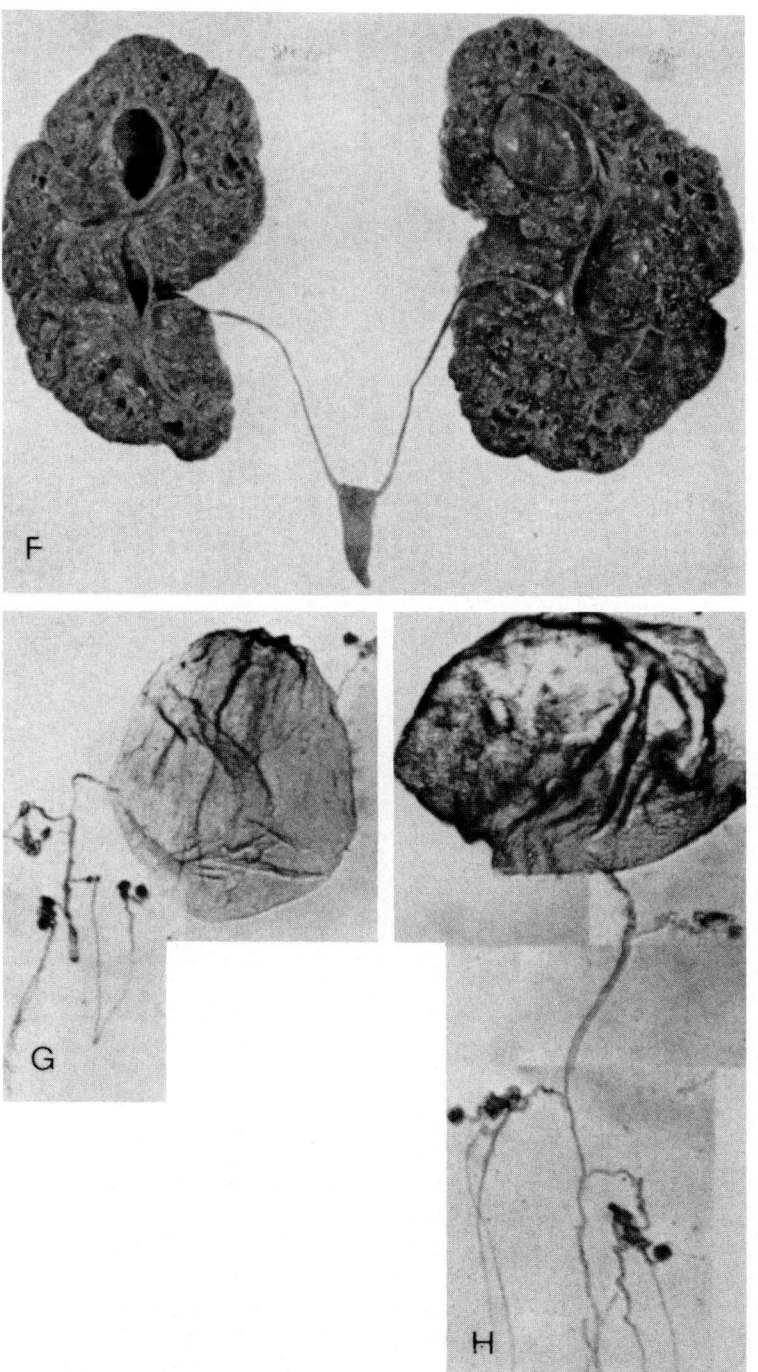

Figure 17.32.—*continued*
F, Sagittal section of kidneys showing tubular pelvis and calyces; no demarcation of cortex and medulla; and large cysts and innumerable small cysts. The large cysts are not dilated portions of the pelvis. **G,** A large cyst of Henle's loop in the youngest of four nephrons of an arcade. **H,** Large cyst at the end of a collecting tubule. Three nephrons are attached to the normal, proximal portion of the tubule. (From Osathanondh V, Potter EL. Pathogenesis of polycystic kidneys type 1–3. Arch Pathol 1964;77:466–501.)

which essentially describes congenital absence of the kidney. The term *dysmorphic* describes the gross shape of the kidney and its caliceal system. It is a term that is best used to describe the radiologic appearance of a misshapen kidney or a kidney with an abnormal or unusual caliceal configuration—it should not have any histologic implications.

Renal dysplasia is a histologic diagnosis and should not be regarded as a specific malformation, but rather as a group of malformations characterized by abnormal

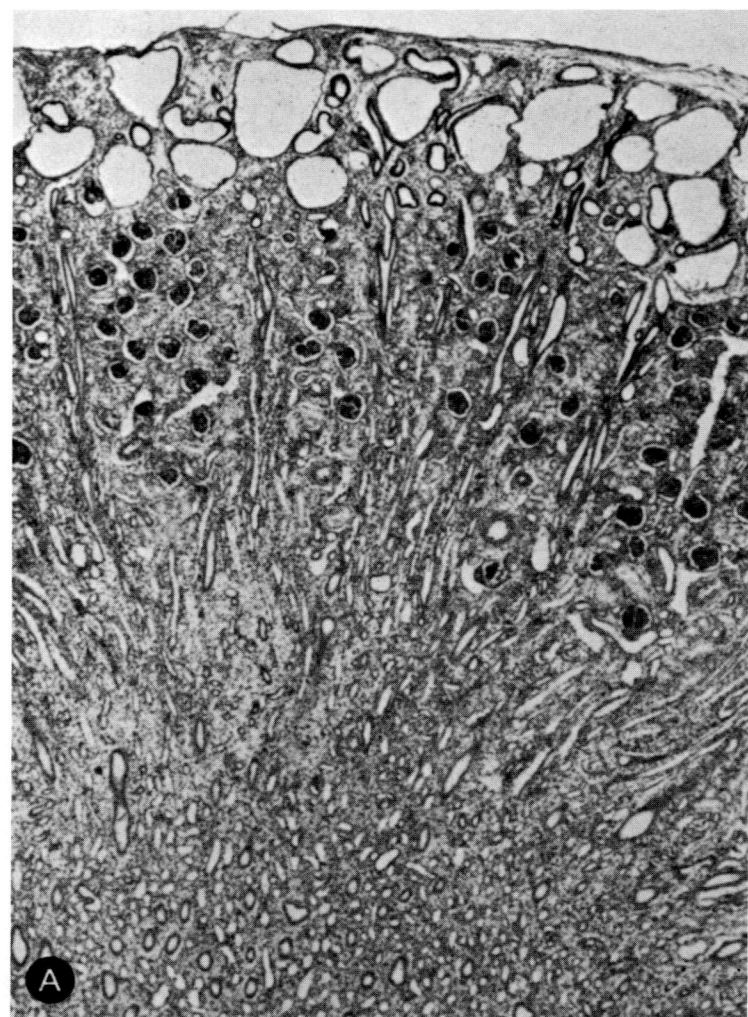

Figure 17.33. Cystic kidneys resulting from congenital ureteral or ureteral obstruction. **A,** Slightly dilated collecting tubules, subcapsular cysts, and absence of the nephrogenic zone.

parenchymal development. It may be diffuse, segmental, or focal. Cysts may or may not be present. The abnormalities that constitute dysplasia do not correspond to normal stages of fetal development, and dysplasia is not simply a retention of fetal renal structures (235, 236). The irrefutable feature by which renal dysplasia may be recognized on histologic examination is the finding of primitive ducts, structures found in the renal medulla that are lined by cuboidal or tall columnar epithelium which are often ciliated (237, 238). Supportive evidence for the diagnosis of dysplasia includes the presence of cartilage, primitive tubules, primitive ductules, primitive glomeruli, and loose mesenchymal and fibrous tissue. Some of the findings lending supportive evidence have been demonstrated in acquired conditions or have been experimentally induced and, therefore, are not included as

irrefutable evidence. When dysplasia occurs in an otherwise small kidney, the term *hypodysplasia* is appropriate.

Ask-Upmark kidney refers to a specific form of segmental renal hypodysplasia first described in 1929, well before the significance of vesicoureteral reflux was recognized (239). In the original description, the hypodysplastic segment is characterized by one or more deep grooves on the lateral convexity of the kidney. Beneath the grooves, the parenchyma is composed mostly of "thyroid-like" cubules, without the presence of inflammatory cells or glomeruli. It is a condition that probably should not be identified as a separate category but rather should be included within the spectrum of reflux nephropathy—it is now recognized to be associated almost universally with reflux or with a strong suggestion of a previous history of reflux (240, 241). It is not clear whether the seg-

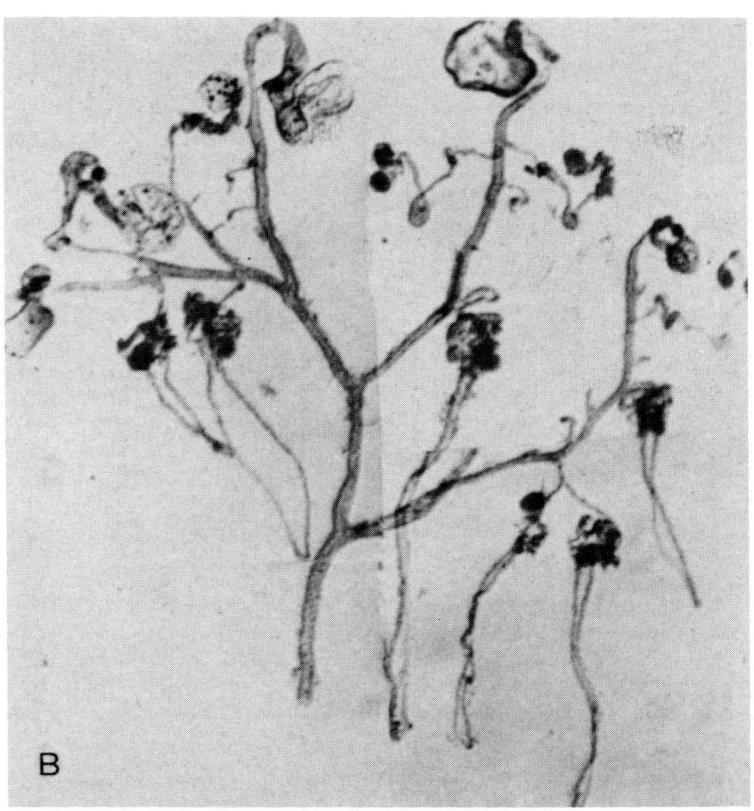

B

Figure 17.33.—*continued*
B, Microdissection of collecting tubule with 15 nephrons attached; the tubules show abnormal cortical branching. Most nephrons are directly attached to the tubule; only one arcade of two nephrons is visible *(lower right)*. Three young nephrons have small cysts in Henle's loop and the terminal branches of the tubules end in cysts where glomeruli would normally form. (From Osathanondh V, Potter EL. Pathogenesis of polycystic kidneys type 4 due to urethral obstruction. Arch Pathol 1964;77:502–509.)

mental hypoplasia characteristic of an Ask-Upmark kidney is the end stage of pyelonephritis, represents segmental hypodysplasia, or is a combination of both.

Multicystic Kidney. An easily recognizable clinical entity, multicystic kidney (MCK) is pathologically an extreme form of dysplasia associated with an atretic ureter. Characteristically, there is a lack of the normal reniform shape; when the cysts are larger, there is very little stroma between them, giving the appearance of a "bunch of grapes" (Fig. 17.36). There seem to be two distinct forms of the disease based on size of the cysts and the amount of dysplastic stroma. The kidneys range from being extremely large, crossing the midline with very large cysts and little stroma, to small kidneys having microscopic cysts and a greater amount of stroma. Some have used the term *solid cystic dysplasia* to define the latter condition. Both are currently thought to represent the same entity and are only variations of multicystic dysplasia.

Classically, the condition is unilateral. However, bilateral multicystic kidneys have been reported in stillborns with oligohydramnios and Potter's facies. In the much more common unilateral condition, the opposite kidney is noncystic but at high risk for another abnormality (242, 243). This contralateral disease process is most often ureteropelvic junction (UPJ) obstruction but also may be due to vesicoureteral reflux or obstructive megaureter. There seems to be no gender predilection; however, the left side is favored.

Characteristically, the MCK presents as a mass in the abdomen of the newborn infant. In most studies it has been reported as the most common entity leading to an abdominal mass in neonates (244). The increasing use of prenatal ultrasonography accounts for the current increased number of diagnoses of the condition made prior to birth (245).

Often no mass is palpable, and the infant is otherwise asymptomatic, a situation which creates some controversy regarding management. Approximately 30% of the neonatal cases have been discovered due to symptoms of associated congenital anomalies (246). Gastrointestinal (esophageal atresia) and cardiac anomalies are frequently encountered. In adults with a retained MCK, abdominal mass (tumor), urinary infection, hematuria, and abdominal pain have led to investigations which revealed the presence of the abnormal kidney (247). There are other reports of malignancy developing in an MCK (246).

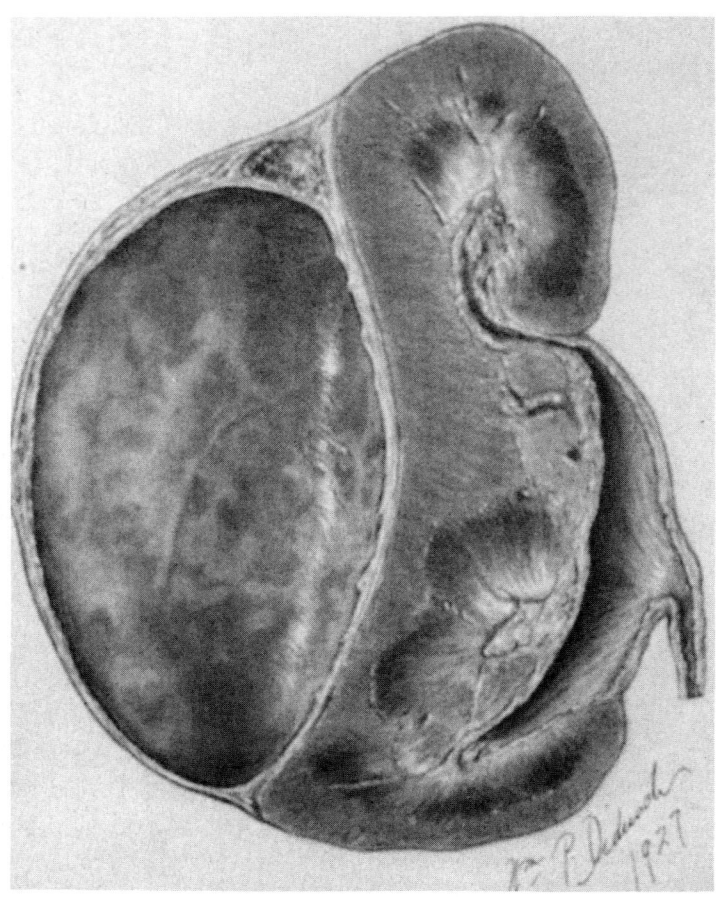

Figure 17.34.   A simple calcified renal cyst. The cyst has severely compressed the otherwise normal pelvis. (From Didusch WP. A collection of urogenital drawings. New York: American Cystoscope Makers, 1952.)

In the past the neonatal diagnosis of MCK was suspected on physical examination and the finding of nonfunction on IVP. Retrograde pyelography often demonstrated atresia of the ipsilateral ureter, most commonly at the junction of the upper ureter with the multicystic kidney. However, variations do exist (243). Surgery was generally thought necessary to confirm the clinical impression. Advances in the past decade in ultrasonography and renal nuclear imaging have, however, produced diagnostic accuracy rates exceeding 90% (248).

The greatest problem comes from distinguishing MCK from a poorly functioning UPJ obstruction. Complete reliance on current imaging techniques may be misleading. However, a 1978 survey of urologists treating children revealed a number of diagnostic inaccuracies, usually when MCK and UPJ obstruction were confused (249). Nuclear medicine studies are of help in differentiating a poorly functioning hydronephrotic kidney from an MCK. In most cases of hydronephrotic kidneys that do not visualize on IVP, some evidence of renal tissue is found on DMSA scan, whereas renal concentration rarely is demonstrated in the MCK (118). Likewise, the uptake

curve on DTPA renal imaging is flat, indicative of a paucity of blood flow to the cystic kidney. In an otherwise fit child, the above features alone may be sufficient for diagnosis. Nevertheless, there is always concern about the possibility of confusion with hydronephrosis, and additional procedures may be warranted. Percutaneous cyst puncture is readily performed; injection of opaque medium does not produce an antegrade pyelogram in the MCK since it outlines one or a few of the cysts only, and ureteral atresia prevents descent of the contrast medium down the ureter. Confusion may still exist between classic MCK and the "hydronephrotic form" (250) in which all of the cysts appear to communicate (Fig. 17.36). However, most often, in this condition the cysts are not of similar size and lack the radial configuration around a large central pelvis which is seen with hydronephrosis. In some cases a voiding cystourethrogram (VCUG) will demonstrate reflux into the ipsilateral atretic ureter. However, the inclusion of cystography in the diagnostic armamentarium of this condition is, more importantly, to evaluate the opposite ureter and bladder outlet.

Traditionally, most kidneys thought to be multicystic

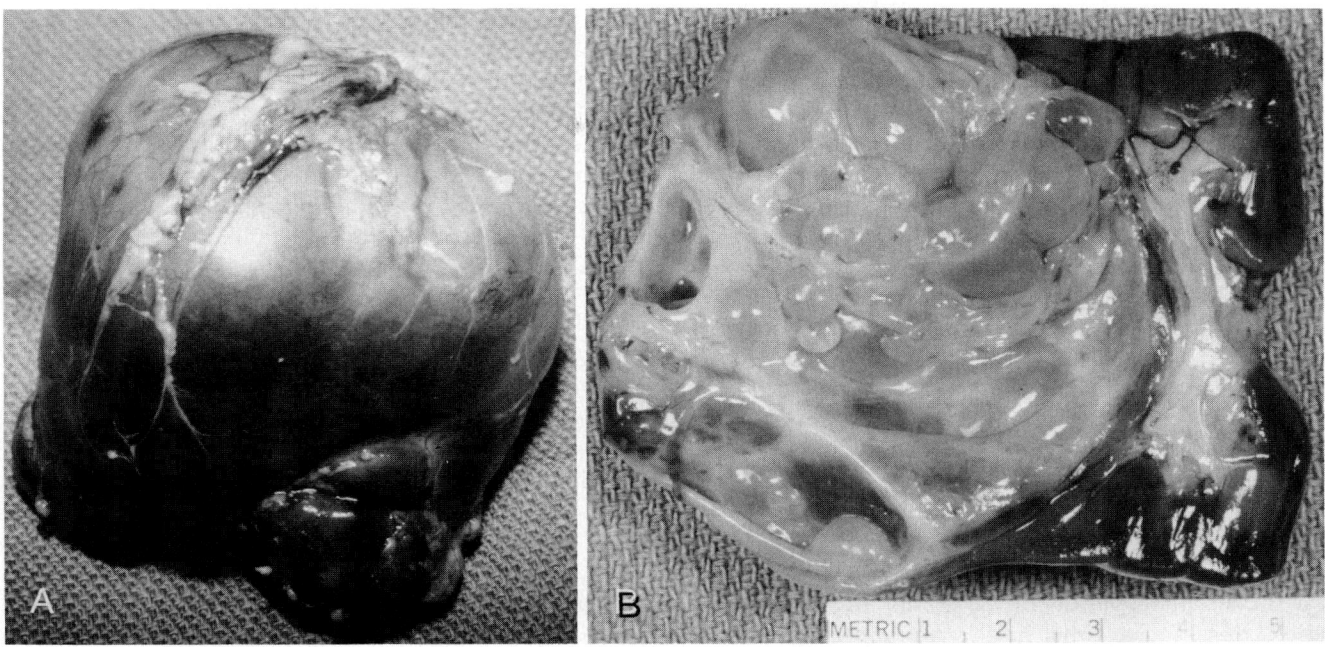

Figure 17.35. Multilocular cyst. **A,** Total nephrectomy specimen. **B,** Cut surface with normal kidney on the left.

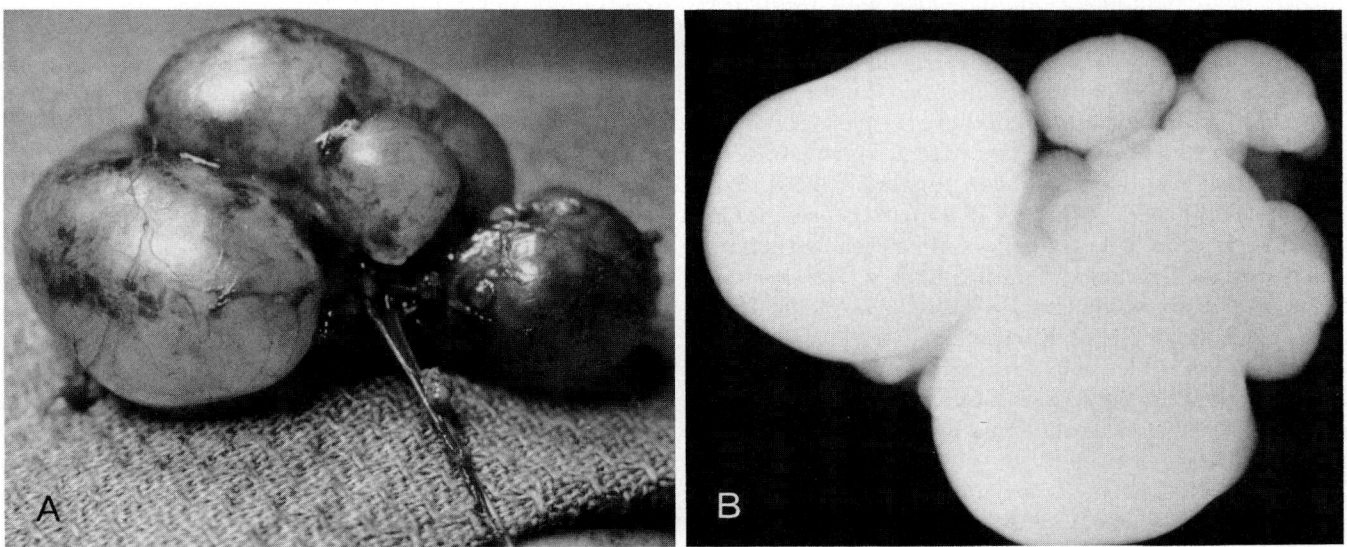

Figure 17.36. Multicystic kidney. **A,** Gross specimen showing typical upper ureteral atresia. **B,** Injection of contrast with x-ray may reveal hydronephrotic variety.

have been explored and removed because of the concern for misdiagnosing the condition and leaving instead an unrelieved obstructive uropathy. Williams and Risdon (108) suggested that a large MCK forming an easily palpable and visible swelling is best removed surgically, whereas smaller ones are thought harmless and may be left *in situ.* Hartman et al. (246), who do not include the small nonpalpable variety of MCK in their discussion, would remove all palpable kidneys presenting in the new-

born period. Germane to any discussion of whether MCKs can be left *in situ* is a knowledge of the natural history of the condition. Stanisic (251) reminds us that many of these larger lesions presenting at birth shrink to minimal proportions when observed for several months. Furthermore, it is suggested that many such lesions must have been left in place over the years for lack of detection; and yet, given such a large historic population at risk for morbidity associated with retention of such kidneys, only a small number of reports of problems with retained multicystic kidneys have emerged (246).

An individualized approach would seem appropriate when a physician is confronted with what seems to be multicystic kidney after appropriate diagnostic modalities have been employed. The parents of an affected child should be told that the natural history of the retained MCK is not actually known, but that both surgical removal under expert pediatric anesthesia and sonographic follow-up offer the patient low-risk options. Certainly, in kidneys that remain large or when the diagnosis of MCK is not entirely clear, the kidney should be removed. When the diagnosis is clear, postponing elective extirpation to 6 months of age to avoid even the slightest increase in anesthesia-related morbidity or mortality seems the proper course of action (252).

CALYCEAL CYSTS AND DIVERTICULA

Anatomy. By definition, a calyceal diverticulum is lined with transitional epithelium. It lies in the kidney substance, distal to a calyx and communicating with it through a narrow channel. It is filled with urine and frequently contains calculi. The upper calyx is most frequently involved and the middle calyx least frequently (253). Similar diverticula outside the substance of the kidney are discussed with ureteric diverticula (page 650).

Embryogenesis. Theories of both an acquired and congenital origin of these diverticula have been proposed. An achalasia, or functional muscular defect, which interferes with calyceal emptying has been suggested (254). Yow and Bunts (253) believe that the diverticula represent failure of regression of lower orders of calyceal branching, which normally disappear during kidney development. These diverticula would be the ureteric equivalents of the provisional nephrons of Kampmeier, which may themselves be responsible for cyst formation. This explanation fails to account for the solitary nature of these diverticula; one might well expect several provisional calyces to fail to regress in the same kidney.

History and Incidence. Rayer (228) first described this condition in 1841, but because of confusion in terminology, it is difficult to determine how often the disease has been encountered since then. Yow and Bunts (253) collected 82 cases from the literature and added 19 cases of their own in 1955. The majority are reported in adults, and the sexes are equally affected.

Symptoms. Pain, varying from chronic to severely acute, is usually present. Other symptoms are those secondary to infection. In addition, pyuria is common.

Diagnosis. Excretory pyelograms may outline the diverticulum, and retrograde pyelograms will almost certainly do so. Calculi are present in about 50% of affected patients. Diverticula range from 1 to 5 cm in diameter. Simple cysts do not communicate with the pelvis and

thus appear as filling defects, in contrast to the situation with calyceal diverticula. Pyelonephritis of a calyx may be difficult to distinguish from a diverticulum.

Treatment. Surgery is rarely necessary and should be restricted to those patients with recurrent or persistent urinary tract infection or those with obstructing or infected stones (118). Complete excision of the diverticulum wall, with obliteration of its neck, is the procedure of choice.

CYSTIC ADENOMA

Cystic adenoma is a rare, benign neoplasm that has been related to functionally isolated renal or mesonephric elements (255). Usually found accidentally, it may consist of single or multiple cysts in the cortex or at the surface of the kidney; rarely, it is bilateral. Cystic adenoma may be diagnosed at any age. If not found in infancy, its discovery often is delayed until middle age, when the onset of other diseases begins to focus attention on the kidney. No gender difference has been observed.

The cysts are thick walled, with a connective tissue capsule derived from the renal capsule itself. The epithelium stains more deeply than does that of normal kidney. Glomeruli are never present. The cyst cavity may be filled with papillary projections of epithelium.

Symptoms usually are absent, but hematuria is occasionally reported. The diagnosis is usually that of malignant neoplasm. Nephrectomy is recommended for all cases because recurrence is possible.

GLOMERULOCYSTIC DISEASE

This is a rare form of cystic disease that is confined to the renal cortex. The cysts are smaller and more uniform than those seen in dominant polycystic kidney and are characterized predominantly as dilations of Bowman's capsule, the cysts involving primarily the glomeruli. There is no suggestion that this is a familial disorder. The prognosis is variable in the few cases that have been reported (118). Most of the cases have reported some element of renal failure although in some, renal function was normal (256).

CYSTIC DILATION OF THE RENAL PYRAMIDS (SPONGE KIDNEY DISEASE)

Sponge kidney disease, also known as medullary sponge kidney, has been confused with the medullary cystic disease (juvenile nephronophthasis complex). For this reason alone perhaps, "medullary" should be dropped and the entity should be known simply as sponge kidney disease (SKD). It is similar to the above-named complex in one aspect only: In both entities the cysts are located in the renal medulla although the exact location with the medulla is different (Fig. 17.37).

Anatomy. Numerous small cysts, 5 mm or less in size,

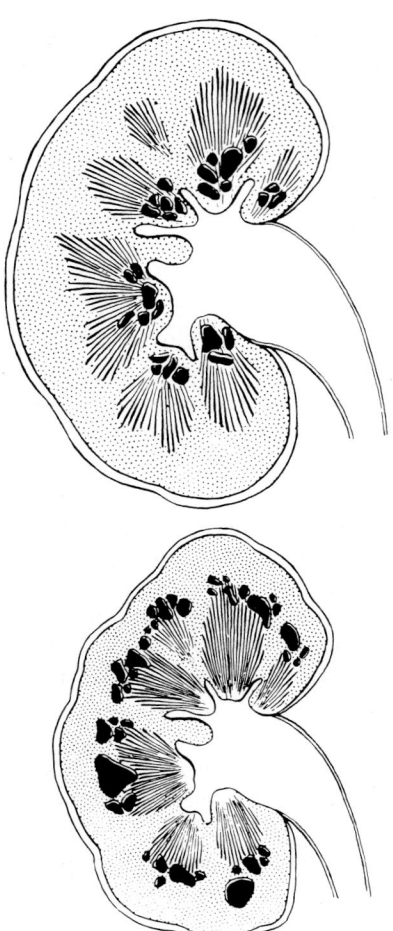

Figure 17.37. **A,** Sponge kidney disease (cysts near tips of papillae). **B,** Medullary cystic disease—familial juvenile nephronophthesis (cysts at corticomedullary junction) (From Spence HM, Singleton R. What is sponge kidney disease and where does it fit in the spectrum of cystic disorders? J Urol 1972;107:176.)

are found in the renal pyramids and papillae only. The gross appearance of porosity of the pyramids on sectioning of the kidney gives rise to the term *sponge kidney.* All pyramids and usually both kidneys are affected.

The cysts are elongated in the axis of the pyramid and are lined with cuboidal or flattened epithelium. About 50% of patients have small calculi in some of the cysts.

Cacchi and Ricci (257) described the cysts as chains of dilations along the collecting tubules, associated with other closed spheric cysts. The latter contain calculi, and whether they are in collecting tubules or separate, the cysts do not communicate with the calyces. An increase in pyramidal connective tissue has been described. There is usually evidence of obstruction of the collecting tubules and the nephrons proximal to the cystic region.

Embryogenesis. The condition is known in the newborn, and most authorities believe it to be congenital. While a number of theories have been proposed for the development of these cysts (64), all are completely speculative.

History and Incidence. This disease was first described in 1939 by Lenarduzzi (258). In 1960 Abeshouse and Abeshouse (259) collected 131 cases and added five to the literature. They mentioned 23 other cases not available to them for study. Ekström (260) and his colleagues reviewed 44 cases in 1959. Felts (262) and his co-workers estimated that over 175 cases had been found by 1964. The majority of cases have been reported in the Italian, Swedish, and French literature; up to 1962 only 25 were from the United States (262). Whether this represents a real geographic difference or a reluctance to accept the disease as an entity is not yet clear.

Although the disease has been reported in the newborn, about 60% of the cases are diagnosed between the ages of 30 and 50 years. Nearly 75% have been found in males.

Symptoms. Clinically, the condition may exist in an asymptomatic state indefinitely and become apparent only when IVPs are done for some unrelated purpose. Even more likely, it may be uncovered when hematuria, urinary tract infection, nephrocalcinosis, or frank stones come under investigation (205). It usually presents after 20 years of age but, on occasion, is seen in children. One-third of patients are found to have hypercalceuria (260).

Diagnosis. The classical finding on IVP is radial streaking in the papillae, which correspond to the enlarged collecting tubules filled with contrast medium. Because the cysts are so small, sonography is rarely helpful. The cysts seldom fill on retrograde studies.

Treatment. Obviously, no measures can correct the underlying structural defects; treatment is limited to the management of the complications, especially urinary tract infection and calculi.

Prognosis. Murphy and his colleagues (263) concluded that the condition is compatible with a normal life and that the symptoms result from complications, which may frequently be avoided until the seventh decade of life (262).

MEDULLARY CYSTIC DISEASE (JUVENILE NEPHRONOPHTHISIS COMPLEX)

Most authorities regard these entities as a single disease with different modes of inheritance. Medullary cystic disease seems to be inherited as a dominant disorder, whereas juvenile nephronophthisis demonstrates a recessive mode of inheritance (264). The vast majority of patients with recessively inherited disease present in the first two decades of life, while those with dominantly inherited disease often present in the third decade of life or later. The major manifestations of the complex are small kidneys and progressive renal failure although initially polyuria, polydipsia, and enuresis may be seen because of the severe concentrating defect. Proteinuria is usually mild or absent and hematuria does not occur.

Hypertension is seen only as an end-stage event. Other names which this condition has gone by or with which it has been confused include uremic sponge kidney, uremic medullary cystic disease, and sponge kidney (Fig. 17.37). From a terminologic standpoint, the condition must be distinguished from the nongenetic forms of medullary cystic disease where the prognosis is much more favorable and the clinical presentation is considerably different (see the discussion on sponge kidney).

POLYCYSTIC KIDNEY DISEASE

Anatomy. Because polycystic kidney disease can sometimes be recognized before the cysts have become so large that all traces of their origin are obliterated, the anatomy of the lesion is better understood than is that of other cystic lesions of the kidney.

In 1947 Lambert (215), by reconstruction from serial sections, demonstrated five types of cystic structures:

1. Cysts of Bowman's capsule, containing glomeruli and always ending blindly (Fig. 17.31, *A* and *B*)
2. Cysts of convoluted tubules, either ending blindly or opening into collecting tubules (Fig. 17.31, *C* to *E*)
3. Cysts of collecting tubules (Fig. 17.31, *F* and *G*)
4. Cystic vesicles without communication with other elements (Fig. 17.31, *I* and *J*)
5. Cysts communicating only with the calyces (Fig. 17.31, *H*)

In the disease in the newborn, glomerular and closed tubular cysts are the only ones present. In adults, all types are present, but the tubular cysts of the open type permit excretion to continue. Lambert (215), and subsequently Bricker and Patten (265), demonstrated inulin excretion through cystic tubules.

This anatomic study, together with the peculiar age distribution of the disease, confirmed the belief of many that the infantile and adult forms of the disease were different.

AUTOSOMAL RECESSIVE (INFANTILE) POLYCYSTIC KIDNEYS [ARPK]

The often used terms *infantile polycystic kidney disease* and *adult polycystic kidney disease* can be misleading, particularly when it is realized that the latter condition often manifests during infancy and childhood. For this reason, it would seem advisable to refer to the former condition as autosomal recessive polycystic kidney disease (ARPK) and to polycystic kidneys appearing primarily in adulthood as dominant polycystic kidneys (ADPK), as their known mode of genetic inheritance indicates.

ARPK is a congenital renal abnormality affecting both kidneys and having no gender predilection. Blyth and Ockenden (266) described four types corresponding to pathologic and genetic differences as well as clinical features. The most severely involved group exhibited massive renal enlargement; the child was often stillborn or died soon after birth, and at least 90% of the renal tubules were affected by cystic dilation.

Occasionally, this condition has been diagnosed prenatally on ultrasonography and usually is associated with oligohydramnios (245). In the second group, approximately 60% of the tubules were involved, and the neonates presented with bilaterally enlarged kidneys associated with renal failure and salt-wasting. Death usually occurred within 6 weeks. In the third group, infants were found to have enlarged kidneys and a palpable liver. Some degree of renal failure was present, but hepatic involvement with portal hypertension was the prominent factor. These children often survived a number of years and at postmortem were found to have 25% of tubules involved. The fourth group presented later in childhood, often with hepatomegaly; a diagnosis of congenital hepatic fibrosis was often made, and subsequent renal evaluation revealed some 10% of tubules to be affected by cystic change. Genetic studies seemed to indicate that the four groups were separate and that a different gene mutation was responsible in each case. Other workers have not found so clear-cut a distinction (108).

Liver involvement seems to be a universal finding in all patients with the recessive form of polycystic kidneys. This may vary histologically from biliary ectasia to severe degrees of portal hepatic fibrosis. While the literature is confusing about what percentage of patients with congenital hepatic fibrosis manifest ARPK, it can at least be said that the vast majority of patients with congenital hepatic fibrosis will be found to have renal changes compatible with ARPK.

As outlined by Blyth and Ockenden (266), the mode of presentation of ARPK depends on the amount of renal tubules involved. This seems to correlate with the age of the patient at presentation—the older patients have less renal involvement, and tend to suffer liver disturbances predominantly.

The diagnosis of ARPK often is made on clinical grounds, particularly when a second sibling is involved. High-dose IVP with delayed radiographic films often shows the characteristic radial streaking of contrast medium–filled dilated collecting tubules (Fig. 17.38). Ultrasound examination is essential to rule out hydronephrosis as a cause of bilaterally enlarged kidneys in the neonate. Bilateral mesoblastic nephroma or bilateral Wilms' tumor may be more difficult to differentiate from ARPK by ultrasound alone. However, the combination of high-dose IVP with ultrasonography should leave few diagnostic dilemmas.

Treatment is essentially the management of renal failure or hepatic insufficiency. Venous shunting to correct portal hypertension may be necessary. In some surviving

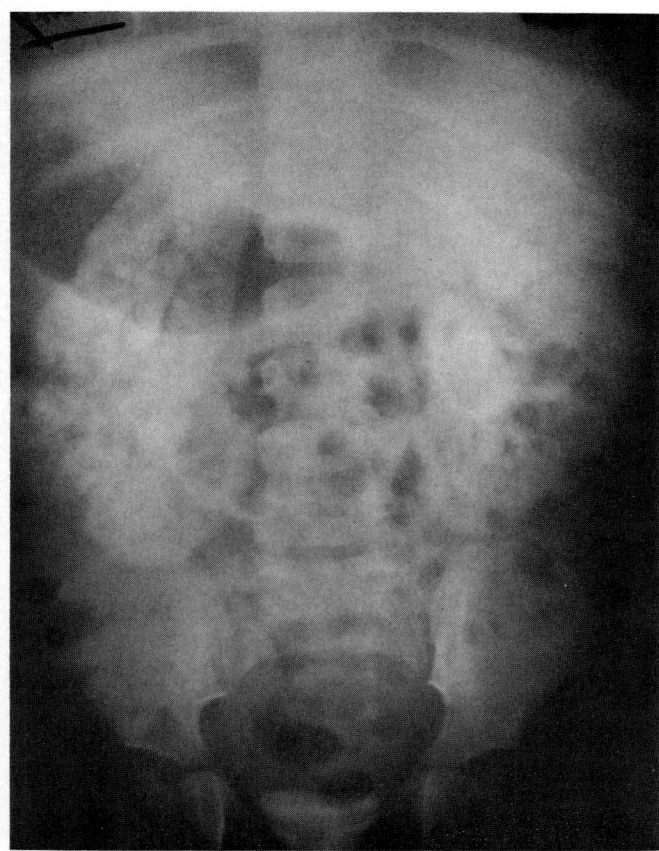

Figure 17.38. Autosomal recessive polycystic kidney. IVP in a neonate.

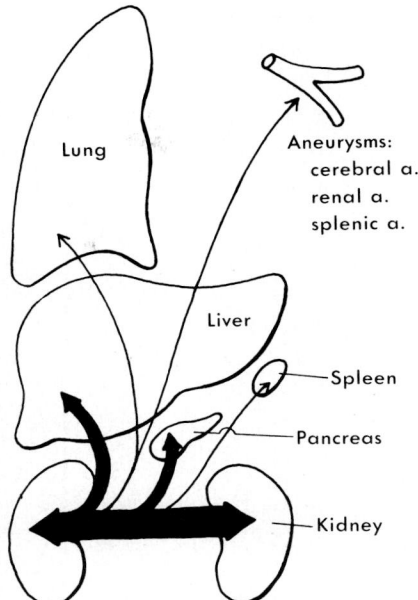

Figure 17.39. Autosomal dominant polycystic kidney disease is usually bilateral and is frequently associated with cysts elsewhere in the body. The width of the *arrows* indicates relative frequencies of association. Aneurysms of certain arteries are often found.

patients with predominantly renal involvement, dialysis and transplantation must be considered.

AUTOSOMAL DOMINANT (ADULT) POLYCYSTIC KIDNEYS (ADPK)

ADPK is the most common form of cystic kidney disease in humans, ranking third among causes of end-stage renal disease (267). It is inherited as an autosomal dominant trait and appears in several generations of affected families. The age of onset was thought by Dalgaard (268) to be similar within any family; however, that impression has not held up. It is likely that the disease will be diagnosed at a much earlier age in the future, as affected family members choose to have other family members screened with ultrasound.

The disease can present at any time during life, but classically presents after the age of 30 years. Reports of 29 cases of ADPK appearing in infants under 6 months of age have been summarized by Glassberg and Filmer (118) and reveal a relatively poor prognosis for those who survive the initial diagnostic period. Adults with ADPK may present with hematuria, flank pain or mass, or symptoms related to progressive azotemia. One-third of patients

with ADPK are found to have cysts of the liver and less frequently of other organs (e.g., pancreas, spleen, and lungs) (Fig. 17.39). Unlike the recessive form, no hepatic dysfunction is seen in those with liver involvement. Berry aneurysms of the brain are not uncommon in ADPK, and approximately 9% of adult patients die of subarachnoid hemorrhage (269).

Associated Disease. Autopsy often reveals cysts of other organs accompanying polycystic kidney disease (64, 217, 268). The liver has cysts in about 33% of patients (Fig. 17.40); pancreas, lung, spleen, or other organs have cysts in about 11%. Aneurysm of cerebral, renal, or splenic arteries is not unusual (Fig. 17.40).

The cystic kidneys of von Hippel-Lindau disease (270)—associated with liver or pancreatic cysts, cysts of the cerebellum, and angiomas of the retina or brain—do not resemble those associated with polycystic disease, nor do they produce abdominal symptoms.

In 1953 Bigelow (271) collected 32 cases of patients with polycystic kidney and aneurysm of basal cranial arteries. Dalgaard (268) questioned whether more careful autopsy of individuals who died of polycystic kidneys has produced misleading figures, and he also queried whether the aneurysms are secondary to the hypertension. He concluded that polycystic kidney, polycystic liver, and congenital aneurysm of the basal cranial arteries can be tentatively considered to be a syndrome produced by a single gene.

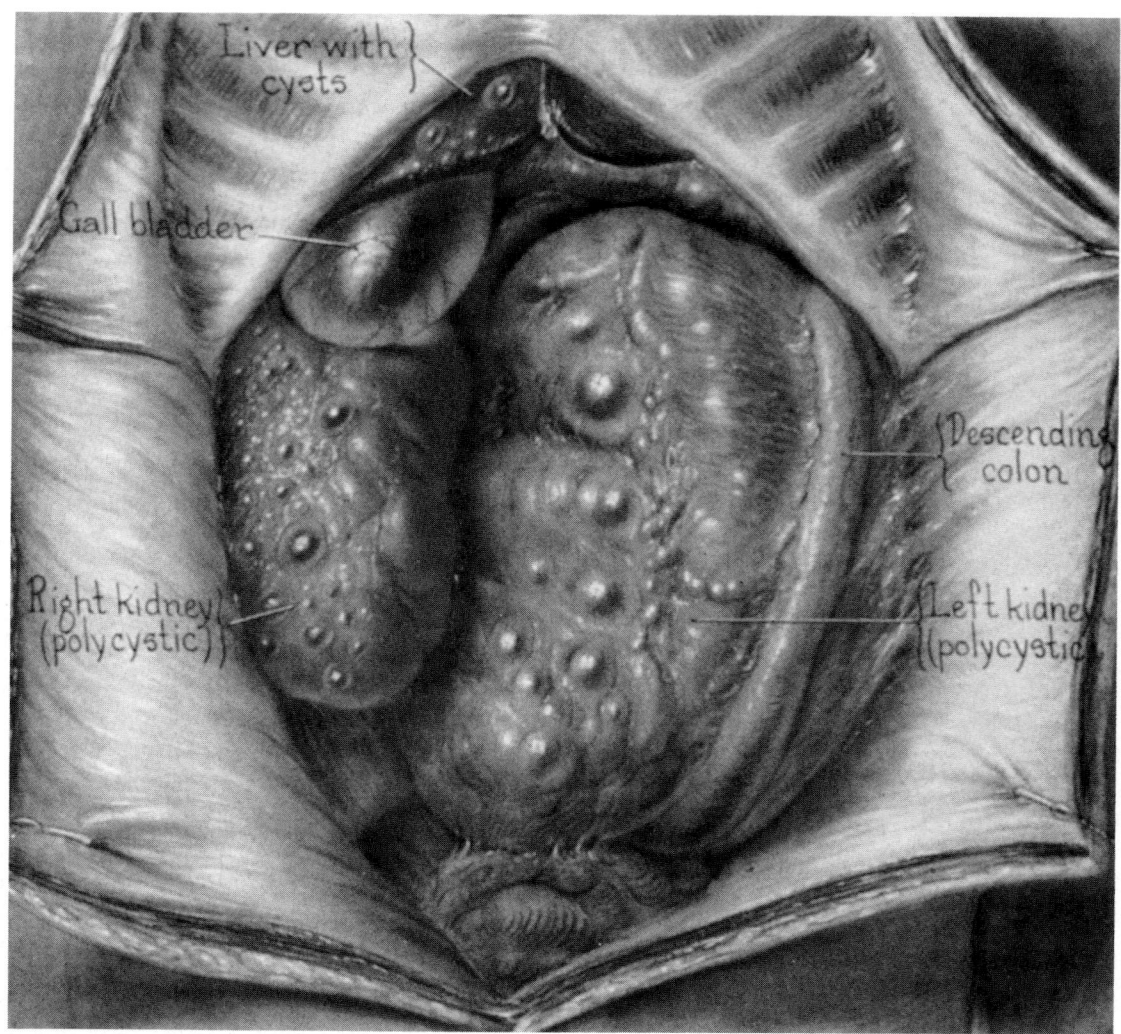

Figure 17.40.   Polycystic disease of the kidney. Both kidneys are affected. The left kidney forms a mass reaching from diaphragm to pelvis. The colon is adherent to the kidney. The liver is cystic and the gallbladder is enlarged. (From Didusch WP. A collection of urogenital drawings. New York: American Cystoscope Makers, 1952.)

Familial Tendency. Polycystic kidney disease in the adult is inherited. A number of reports of the occurrence of the disease in members of the same family appeared during the 19th century, and in 1899 Steiner (272) postulated a hereditary tendency. Cairns (273) collected 23 families with more than one case of polycystic disease, with 11 of them having affected members in two or more generations. Rall and Odel (217) found positive family histories in 34% and questionable histories in another 27% of their 207 cases. Goldstein (274) found 27 definite and 9 doubtful histories among the parents of 36 patients.

Two detailed genetic analyses of the disease have been made by Arrigoni and his colleagues (275) and by Dalgaard (268). Arrigoni and co-workers found 45 affected individuals in 15 pedigrees and concluded that the disease resulted from an autosomal dominant gene with varying expressivity.

Dalgaard (268) confirmed the autosomal location of the gene and showed there was no sex linkage and no linkage with blood groups involved. He believed the disease to be recessive rather than dominant, but considered complete proof lacking. Penetrance approaches 100% by age 80 years. If we estimate the frequency for polycystic kidney disease at 0.001, and the number of children born to women with polycystic disease as from 60 to 80% of the number born to normal women, the mutation rate (in Denmark) appears to be between $6.5 \times 10^{\cdot}ms^5$ and $12 \times 10^{\cdot}ms^5$ mutations per gene per generation. This rate is high compared with calculated rates for other human genes.

History. Laveren (229) first distinguished polycystic kidney disease from other renal cystic disease, although Meckel (276) and Virchow (208) were acquainted with it. Steiner (272) established the hereditary nature of the disease. Braasch (277) in 1916 made one of the first large clinical studies and emphasized the progressive nature of the disease. Dalgaard (268) thoroughly reviewed the state of our knowledge of the disease up to 1957.

Incidence. In adults, the clinical incidence has been reported to be from 1:2438 to 1:5000. The largest series collected, that of Braasch and Schacht (278), places it at 1:3523. The autopsy incidence varies from 1:222 to 1:1019, the most frequent values reported being between 1:260 and 1:780.

Most series show a slight preponderance of women over men, but at least one (279) shows the opposite. The sexes are probably equally affected.

The autosomal dominant type of polycystic disease is rare in children; about 3% of all cases are reported in the first decade. Between 70 and 80% of adult cases are found between the ages of 30 and 60 years (217, 268, 279, 280). The distribution is remarkably constant over time and place.

Symptoms. The symptoms of polycystic kidney disease are insidious and progressive. In adults, the progress is slow. Although the time of onset is not easily determined, usually three phases of the disease are recognizable:

Early Stage.
Pain, which may be aroused by walking or vigorous movement, may be persistent and radiating or intermittent and severe. Lumbar tenderness is often present. Pain is present at some time in about 60% of patients, more frequently in women.

Proteinuria, in slight to large amounts, is present in 75 to 95% of patients.

Middle Stage.
In 60 to 80% of patients, one or both kidneys become palpable as they enlarge.

Although it is not among the earliest symptoms, hematuria is often the symptom that leads the patient to seek medical advice. About 50% of patients will have hematuria, either gross or microscopic.

Inflammation, with its usual symptoms, may be expected in about 50% of patients. It is more frequent in women than in men.

Last Stage.
Cardiac pain, edema, dyspnea, and hypertension eventually appear in about 50% of patients.

Weakness and weight loss are common symptoms in the terminal stage of the disease; about 75% of patients with the disease can be expected to show these symptoms.

Uremia is of slow onset, and while it is frequent, it appears in only 50 to 60% of patients. Women are affected more commonly.

Diagnosis. Renal ultrasonography is now the major imaging modality in the diagnosis of the dominant form of polycystic kidney. Confirmation of the suspicion of polycystic kidney disease requires excretory urography with nephrotomography. CT scanning is also helpful in confirming the presence of this disease.

Elongation and irregular enlargement of the calyces occur, sometimes with evidence of cysts that impinge on the calyceal outline (Figs. 17.41 and 17.42). The enlargement must be distinguished from that of hydronephrosis or compensatory hypertrophy. Billing (281) suggested that a kidney length of more than 14 cm and a parenchyma thickness of more than 3 cm indicate a polycystic kidney. The nephrographic phase of aortography (the moment when the renal capillaries are filled) will show a characteristic worm-eaten appearance.

The literature on radiographic diagnosis is too large to conveniently discuss here. A good summary may be found in Dalgaard's (268) monograph of the disease.

In actual practice, Simon and Thompson (279) found that the diagnosis was made radiologically in 79% of 366 patients at the Mayo Clinic. Among Dalgaard's (268) 56 patients seen between 1950 and 1953 in Copenhagen, 9% were diagnosed clinically, 41% by radiography, 20% at surgery, and 30% at autopsy.

In children suspected of having ADPK, the major investigation centers around a good family history of at least three generations. The renal ultrasound is the most sensitive imaging technique of the diagnosis. However, it should be emphasized that a negative finding in a study performed for screening purposes in early childhood does not necessarily rule out presentation of the disease in later life. The most common finding on IVP has been enlargement of the kidneys, at times asymmetrically, with distortion of the calices by enlarged cysts (Fig. 17.42).

Treatment. Nonsurgical procedures include avoidance of, or relief of, kidney infection and relief of anemia and hypertension. A high fluid and low protein diet, rest, control of acidosis, and transfusions may be helpful.

Surgically, pelvilithotomy may be required for the removal of stones, nephrostomy for renal infection, and cystotomy for severe, persistent hematuria or for a renal neoplasm. Nephrectomy for polycystic disease alone is not indicated. Every effort should be made to avoid exploratory operations without having already ruled out polycystic disease.

In 1911 Rovsing (282) described and advocated multiple puncture of the cysts of polycystic kidneys. In spite of a number of studies of the effect of cyst puncture on prognosis (268, 274, 279, 283, 284), there is no incontrovertible evidence that multiple puncture of cysts increases the life expectancy of the patient. Temporary relief of pain, however, often results.

Transplantation is a very viable option in the adult with

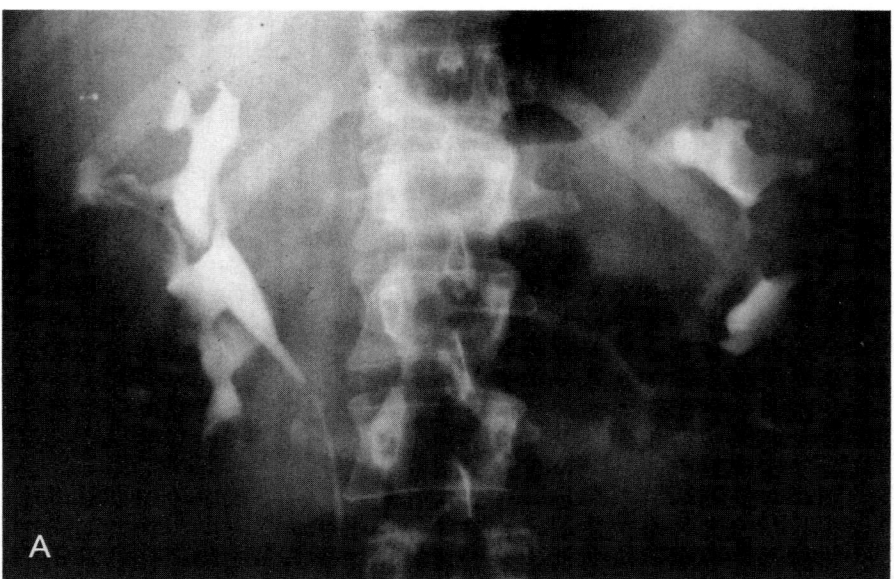

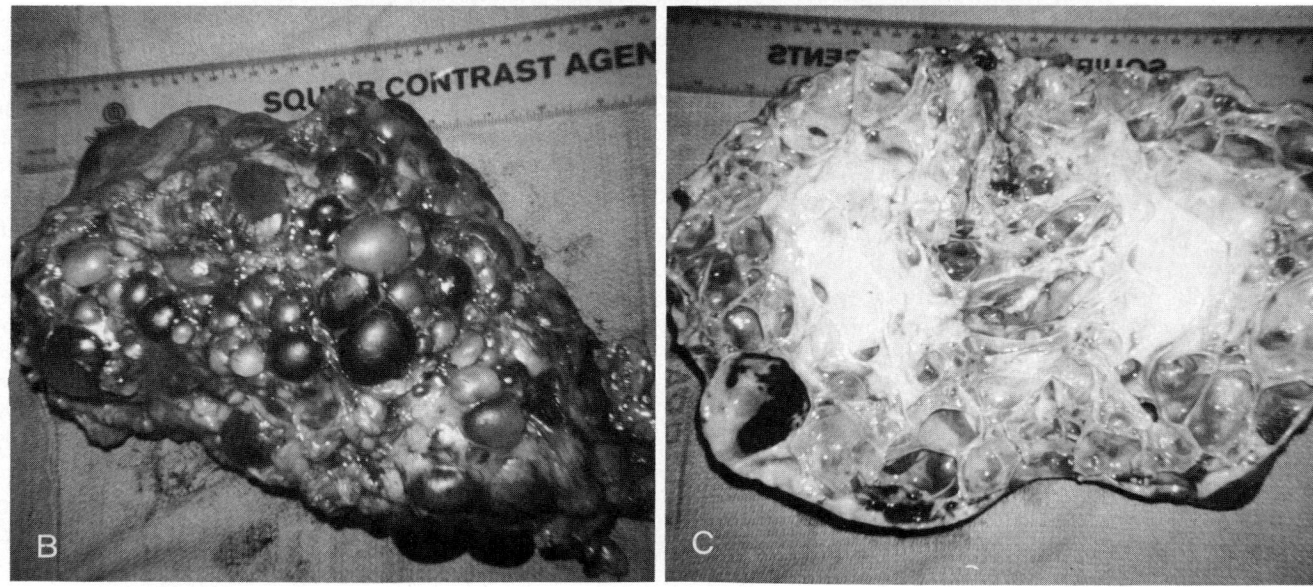

Figure 17.41.   Autosomal dominant polycystic kidney. **A,** IVP in adult showing classically splayed calyces. **B,** Gross specimen.
C, Cut surface.

renal failure due to ADPK because this condition as well as other forms of hereditary disease, such as nephron-ophthisis or medullary cystic disease, should not recur in transplant recipients if the donor kidney is free of disease (285).

Prognosis. Among adults, 5- and 10-year survival rates have been computed (Table 17.7) (279).

The longest survival time was 26 years. When patients are divided according to sex and into groups of those over and under the age of 50 years, it has been found that women survived longer than men at any age.

The majority of children with symptomatic ADPK present in the terminal stages of their disease, whereas

others may be candidates for dialysis and transplantation. Some older children and young adults may survive with suitable management of the complications of the disease, such as hypertension, infection, and renal failure. Palpable kidneys, hematuria, hypertension, and uremia, in that order, give an increasingly poor prognosis. Patients with normal renal function have an 85% 5-year survival rate, whereas those with impaired function have only a 21% 5-year survival rate (268).

Among Dalgaard's cases, the mean age at onset was 40.7 years, the mean age at diagnosis was 47.2 years, and the mean age at death was 51.5 years.

Genetic prognosis. Use of contraceptive methods (278)

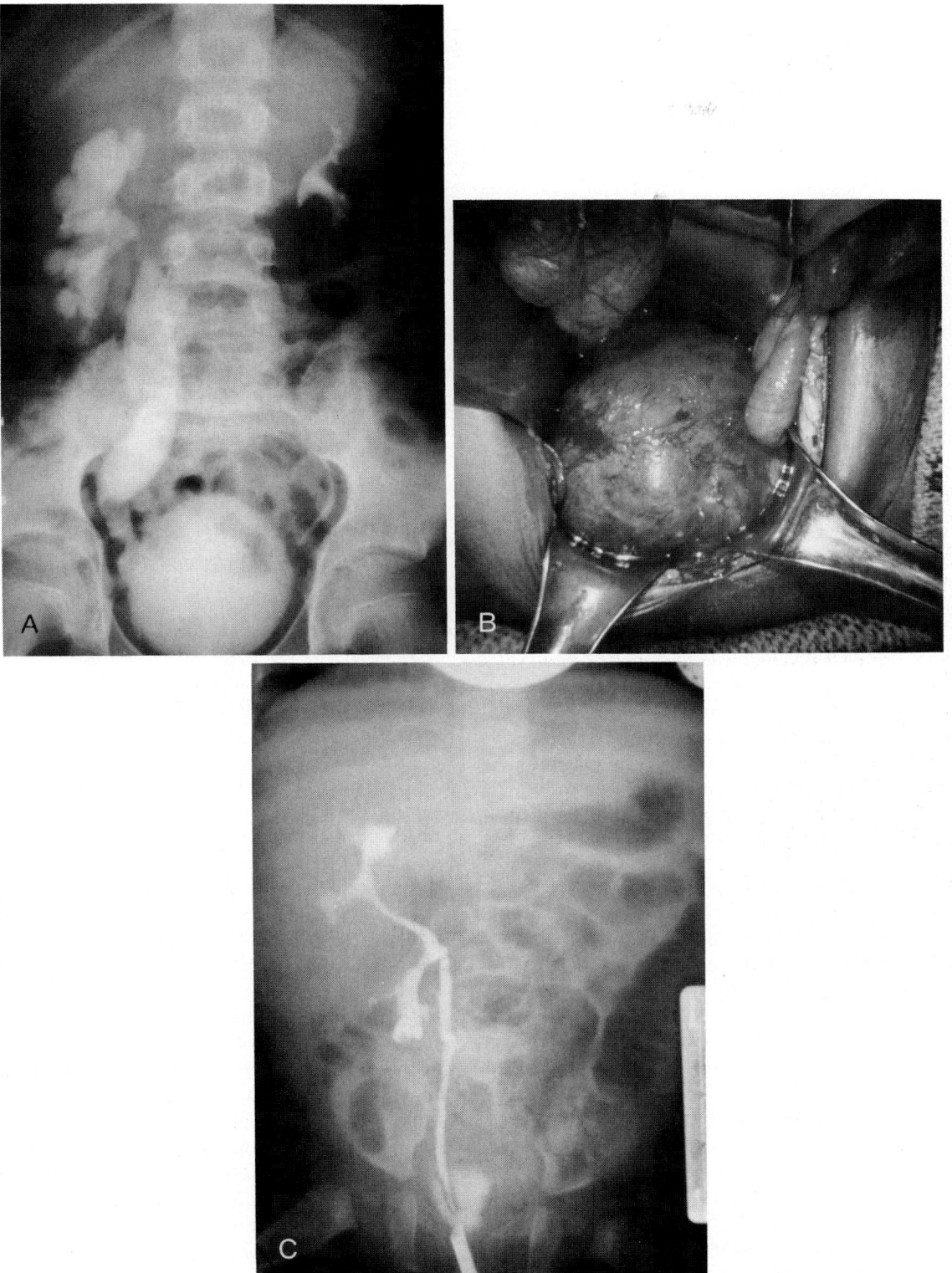

Figure 17.42. Autosomal recessive polycystic kidney. **A,** IVP in infant showing splayed calyces. **B,** Typical findings on retrograde
pyelogram (RPG). **C,** Exposure of infantile kidney prior to biopsy showing macroscopic cysts of varying size.

Table 17.7.
Survival Rates for Polycystic Kidney Disorder[a]

Survival Time from Diagnosis	Normal Expected Survival (%)	Patients with Polycystic Kidney Disease (%)
5 years	96	56 (of 288 patients)
10 years	90.5	38 (of 248 patients)

[a]Data from Simon HB, Thompson GJ. Congenital renal polycystic disease. JAMA 1955; 159:657–662.

and even compulsory sterilization of individuals with polycystic kidney disease has been advocated (286), although the diagnosis often is not made until late in the childbearing period. This disease satisfies the requirements of the Danish Abortion Act, which permits termination of pregnancy if there is danger of the child having an incurable inherited disease (268).

RENAL CYSTS ASSOCIATED WITH MULTIPLE MALFORMATION SYNDROME

A number of inherited malformation syndromes have been associated with renal findings which usually involve large cystic dilations within the renal parenchyma, subcapsular cortical "microcysts," or even severe renal dysplasia. The various syndromes associated with renal cysts are listed in Table 17.8. The most common of these relatively rare inherited disorders is tuberous sclerosis, which is characterized by adenoma sebaceum, mental retardation, epilepsy, and renal masses which (in addition to cysts) may be histologically classified as hamartomas (204). The cysts rarely exceed 3 cm and may be present at birth. These cysts can impair renal function by diffuse involvement or by compression of normal tissue (287).

Congenital Anomalies: Renal, Pelvic, and Ureteral

EXTRARENAL CALYCES

Occasionally, a kidney is encountered in which major calyces as well as the pelvis occur outside the mass of the kidney. The earliest report we have found, by Richmond (288) in 1884–1885, described a case in which the pelvis was 4 inches away from the kidney. Connection was by four elongated calyces. A case with more moderate separation is discussed by Malament and his colleagues (289) (Fig. 17.43). They reported eight cases, but were able to collect only six earlier references to malformation.

Malament (289) and his co-workers suggested that these cases reflect branching of the ureteric bud prior to its junction with the metanephric blastema. If this interpretation is true, extrarenal calyces represent a stage between agenesis or aplasia and the normal kidney. A slightly longer delay in ureteric growth would have ended with a blind, unbranched ureter and no kidney. The condition represents normal but delayed ureteric growth,

Table 17.8.
Renal Cysts Associated with Multiple Malformation Syndromes[a]

Mendalian (Single-Gene) Disorders
  I. Autosomal dominant cystic disease
     Tuberous sclerosis
     Von Hippel-Lindau disease
  II. Autosomal recessive
     Meckel's syndrome
     Jeune's asphyxiating thoracic dystrophy
     Zellweger's cerebrohepatorenal syndrome
  III. X-linked dominant
     Orofaciodigital syndrome, type I
Chromosome Disorders
  Trisomy D (Patau's syndrome)
  Trisomy E (Edwards' syndrome)
  Down's syndrome
  Turner's XO syndrome

[a]Glassberg KI, Filmer RB: Renal dysplasia, renal hypoplasia and cystic diseases of the kidney. In: Kelalis PP, King LR, Belman AB, eds. *Clinical pediatric urology*, 2nd ed, Vol 2. Philadelphia, WB Saunders, 1985:946.

rather than the insufficient growth that produces aplasia.

Extrarenal calyces are usually asymptomatic, although they may fail to drain normally and, hence, become a site of disease. They may be recognized in retrograde pyelography by their location outside the kidney shadow.

URETEROPELVIC JUNCTION OBSTRUCTION

The most common site of obstruction of the upper urinary tract is the uteropelvic junction. Whether from intrinsic, extrinsic, or a combination of causes, the ultimate result is hydronephrosis to some degree.

Hydronephrosis secondary to UPJ obstruction is one of the most common anomalies. By definition, a UPJ obstruction is impedance to flow between the renal pelvis and the upper ureteral system. This results in decreased drainage with progressive dilation of the collecting system which causes further delay in pelvic emptying. Initially, there is hypertrophy of the renal pelvic musculature with a concomitant decrease in glomerual infiltration rate. Eventually, the renal parenchyma atrophies with permanent loss of renal function.

UPJ obstruction occurs in utero and presents clinically in childhood and infancy. Although the incidence of this entity was thought to be on the rise, it would appear that this is artifactual and really only reflects the increased use of prenatal ultrasound examinations.

UPJ obstruction is found in all age groups. The highest incidence appears to be in the group under 1 year of age and particularly in the group less than 6 months of age. Williams and Kenawi (290) quote a 25% incidence in the group less than 1 year of age. With increased use of prenatal ultrasound one can expect that this condition will be diagnosed even more frequently in the early stages (245, 291, 292). Male predominance by a 2:1 ratio is well documented (293). In unilateral cases the left side is far more

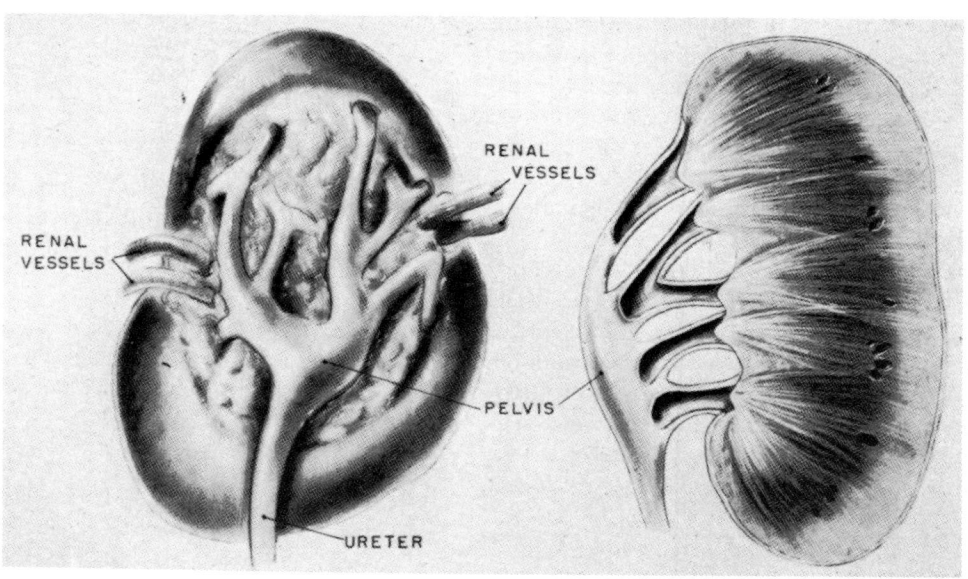

Figure 17.43. Extrarenal calyces. These represent delayed rather than insufficient ureteral growth. (From Malament M, Schwartz B, Nagamatsu GR. Extrarenal calyces: their relationship to renal disease. AJR 1961;86:823–829.)

common than the right. The study of Johnston and colleagues (293) in 1977 cited 139 left-sided lesions and 61 right-sided lesions for a total of 200 cases sampled with known UPJ obstruction. Others have confirmed the almost 2:1 predominance of the left side over the right side (290).

In males, particularly newborns, the condition is frequently bilateral (10 to 40%) (293, 294). With increased age, unilaterality is more common and the side predominance disappears. Beyond puberty and into adulthood, UPJ obstruction (congenital) is rare.

Pathogenesis. The predominance of obstructions at the UPJ are congenital in nature. They are caused by an anatomic narrowing secondary to intrinsic stenosis or extrinsic compression by a fibrous band of tissue or aberrant blood vessel. Other obstructions may be classified as functional and are due to incoordinate contraction of the renal pelvis secondary to abnormal development, injury, or neurologic disease (295).

UPJ obstruction can be broken down into three major categories of etiology: intrinsic, extrinsic, and secondary.

Intrinsic abnormalities are the most predominant cause of obstruction. The abnormal muscle bundle (either by congenital defect or acquired defect) causes impaired passage of urine in the renal pelvis to the ureter. Hanna et al. (295) define the problem as a narrow, aperistaltic segment, secondary to replacement of the normal muscle spiral by longitudinal fibers. Continued distension leads to further elongation of the fibers without a concomitant increase in girth. The pelvis thus elongates and narrows instead of widening and becoming conical, as is seen in normal circular fibers. Whatever the etiology,

muscle fibers are replaced by fibrous tissue causing obstruction. Ruano-Gil et al. (296) point out that the ureter goes through an embryologic solid phase. This solid phase, in normal development, recanalizes. UPJ obstruction may represent failure in part or in toto to recanalize.

The abnormal UPJ, as well as the more "normal" pelvis and ureter adjacent to it, have been examined under the electron microscope. Hanna et al. (295) noted an improved quality of the muscle cells the more cephalad one got from the UPJ (Figs. 17.44 and 17.45). With severe hydronephrosis, when muscle damage has occurred, increases in collagen and ground substance were found diffusely throughout the pelvis, but were most abundant around the junction of the pelvis with the ureter.

Whitaker (297) in 1975 and later Hanna (295) reported that it was the lack of the funnel shape of the pelvis which causes ineffective propulsion of the fluid bolus with diuresis, particularly of a rapid nature. The pelvis distends and this further retards emptying.

Regardless of the cause, physiologically, the end result is the failure of the peristaltic wave to propagate from the pelvis to the ureter. Ineffective pelvic peristaltic waves eventually cause hydronephrosis by incompletely emptying the pelvic contents.

Kinking, abnormal bands, and angulation of the UPJ can be seen even in the absence of inflammation (298). The angulation produced may cause obstruction. The pelvis dilates and the ureter is pulled proximally so the dependent portions of the pelvis fail to drain. Particularly prone to this displacement are high insertion pelves. The anterior and medially inserted pelvis starts off in a non-dependent position. With diuresis, spheric distension occurs. The UPJ is raised higher and the ureter becomes compressed against the pelvicoureteric fascia. This leads to a functional obstruction early on. As the diuresis abates, the obstruction is relieved. However, with persistent intermittent elevation, adhesions form between the ureter and the fascia, which may lead to permanent obstruction (299).

Valvular **mucosal folds** were described by Maizels and Stevens (300) in 1980. The explanation offered was that persistent fetal convolutions gave rise to these folds. These are exceedingly rare. Congenital folds, a variant of valves, are first seen in the upper ureter at the fourth month in utero. They often persist into the newborn period. These mucosal infoldings may fail to flatten when the ureter distends, causing a functional and (with time) an anatomic obstruction.

Polyps of the upper ureter as the cause of UPJ obstruction are rare but they do occur. This makes it most important to explore the upper ureter even when release of adhesions seems to relieve the "kink" in the upper ureter (298). Polyps are narrow, finger-like fronds with a connective tissue core lined with transitional cell epithelium (290). On IVP, they are seen as a filling defect. More commonly, they are not appreciated preoperatively and are found at the time of laparotomy. Pathologically, they are hamartomas (i.e., not neoplastic) and require only local excision.

Multiple ureteral polyps have been reported with Peutz-Jegher's syndrome.

Extrinsic compression is most commonly caused by aberrant or accessory vessels to the lower poles of the kidney. Nixon (301) reported that 25 out of 78 cases of UPJ obstruction were caused by aberrant vessels. Aberrant vessels are probably present in at least one-third of patients with UPJ obstruction, an incidence that is much higher than found in the general population (298).

Early branching of the renal vessels (accessory arteries) and anteriorly located arteries to the lower pole of the kidney (aberrant arteries) are the main vascular variance which cause UPJ obstruction. As the pelvis fills with urine, its anterior expansion is prevented by the offending vessel. The pelvis becomes draped over the vessel and angulated and thus leads to obstruction. Rarely, the pelvis distends to such a degree as to encircle the vessel. The vasculature is compressed and the renal tissue becomes ischemic.

Particularly prone to obstruction by aberrant vessels are duplicated ureteral systems and pelves with a high insertion.

In most of the ureters compressed by aberrant vessels and accessory vessels, there is also an associated intrinsic defect. It has been speculated that abnormal vessels

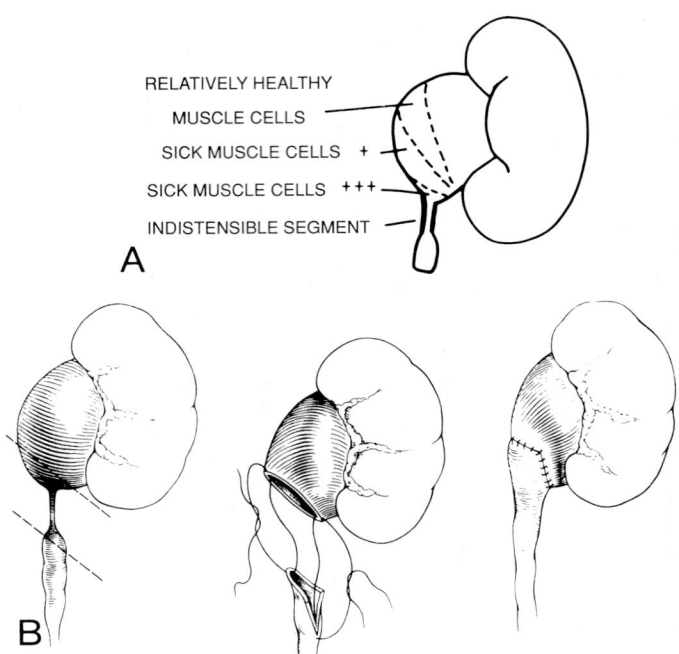

Figure 17.44. Ureteropelvic junction obstruction. **A,** Typical histologic findings. **B,** Dismembered pyeloplasty, the operation of choice for most cases of UPJ obstruction. (**A,** From Hanna MK, Jeffs RD, Sturgess JM, Barklin M. Congenital ureteropelvic junction obstruction and primary obstructive megaureter. J Urol 1976;116:725; **B,** from Kelalis PP. Renal pelvis and ureter. In: Kelais KK, King LW, Belman AB, eds. Clinical pediatric urology. Philadelphia: WB Saunders, 1985.)

merely exacerbate an existing problem rather than act as the primary cause of the obstruction. Some authors have actually speculated that the vessels cause pressure on the ureter which induced the primary intrinsic abnormality. The hard correlation between aberrant vessels and intrinsic disease is not coincidental. Further work will be needed to delineate whether one effect causes the other or if they co-exist and create the pathology, in combination and simultaneously.

Secondary Etiology. UPJ obstruction can be imitated by vesicoureteral reflux (302). Urine refluxes causes overload of the pelvis. It is unable to handle the excess load of urine and thus dilates. As the ureters dilate, they elongate. More distal obstructions, such as with urethral valves, also may cause a secondary UPJ obstruction. The hallmark of true secondary UPJ obstruction caused by reflux is a voiding cystourethrogram showing reflux to the pelvis in the face of an IVP which demonstrates hydronephrosis. On IVP, the ureters appear tortuous and kinked at the UPJ. If reflux remains uncorrected, inflammation between the ureter and pelvis can occur. This can cause stenosis and adhesions of adjacent ureteral segments.

Associated Anomalies. Up to 50% of the patients with a

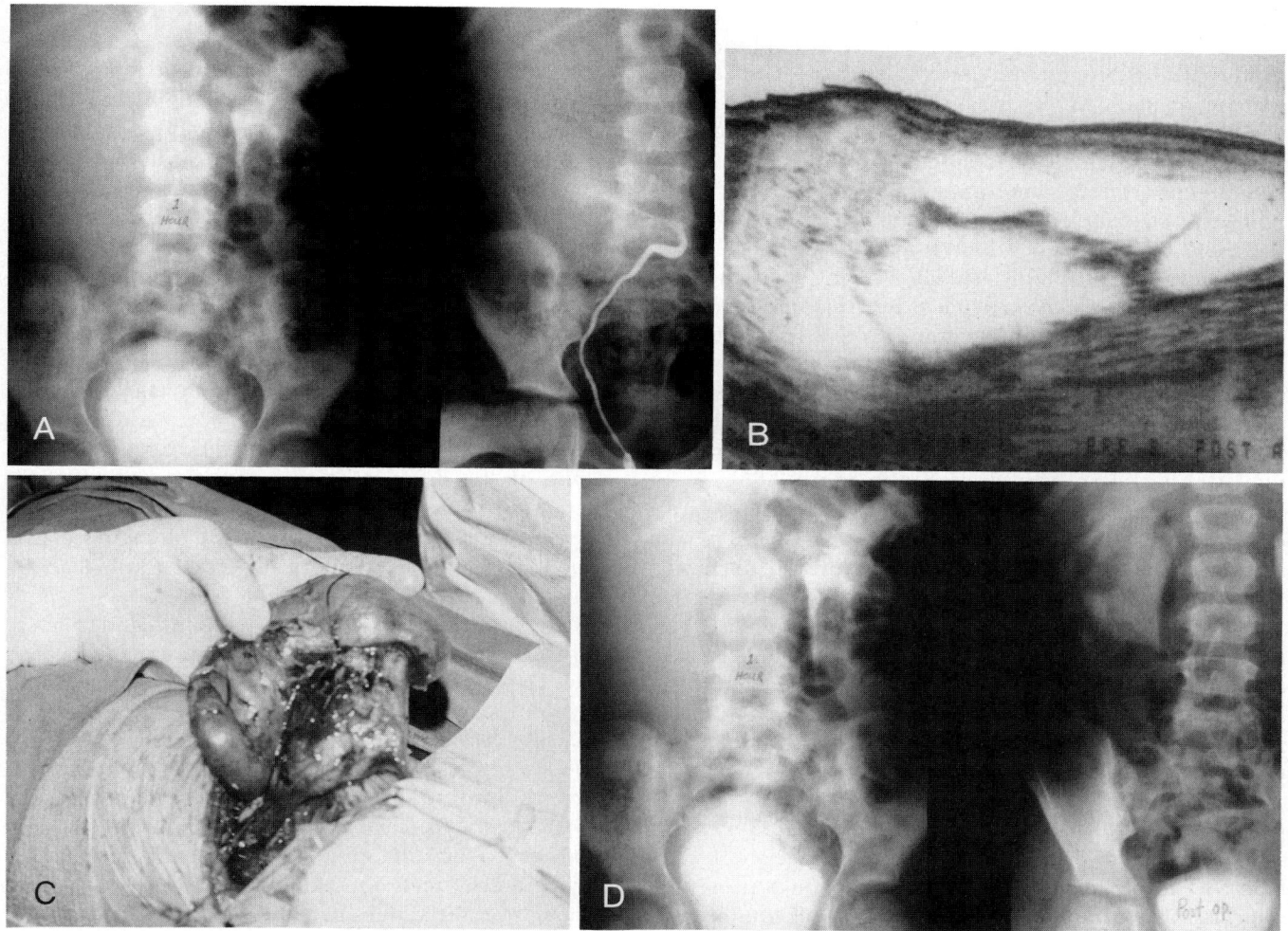

Figure 17.45. Ureteropelvic Junction Obstruction. **A,** *Left,* IVP showing poor visualization; *right,* RPG showing displacement of ureter across midline with typical jet of contrast medium past the obstruction. **B,** Renal ultrasound. **C,** Kidney mobi-lized at time of pyeloplasty with tape around proximal ureter. **D,** Comparison of pre- and postoperative IVP results.

UPJ obstruction may have a second renal and/or urinary anomaly (294). UPJ obstruction also is associated with vertebral anomalies, imperforate anus, congestive heart disease, diaphragmatic herniae, and esophageal anomalies. Although the pattern and frequency are not constant, it is well documented that they are associated.

The most common associated anomaly (10 to 40%) is a contralateral UPJ obstruction (293, 303). Bilaterality is relatively common in children, particularly in the group under 6 months of age.

Other associations include unilateral agenesis of the kidney (293, 304), horseshoe kidneys, ectopic ureters, and malrotation of the kidneys.

Vesicoureteral reflux has been reported in 40% of children with UPJ obstruction (290) although this is not often thought to contribute to the obstruction.

Clinical Features. The presenting symptoms of UPJ obstruction are variable. An asymptomatic palpable mass is the most common presentation in the newborn, found in 50% of patients in that age group (293, 304). This is particularly true if the obstruction is bilateral. Other presenting symptoms include failure to thrive, decreased tolerance for feedings, and sepsis. Colicky pain, anemia, and polycythemia are less common presentations. To a large extent, the presenting symptomatology is changing, owing to the increased use of prenatal ultrasound. Currently, many asymptomatic but surgically important obstructions are initially diagnosed on prenatal ultrasound screening (245). Older children with UPJ obstruction are often erroneously diagnosed initially as having gastrointestinal diseases (298). From 33 to 50% of the patients present with vague periumbilical abdominal pain, nausea, and vomiting (290, 298). These children are frequently worked up for appendicitis, spastic colon, herniae, and other gastrointestinal disorders, including gastroenteritis.

Colicky flank pain, particularly after large fluid intake and particularly in older adolescents, is the second most common presenting symptom.

Twenty-five percent of patients present with hematuria, even in the absence of trauma or associated with minor trauma (290, 303). This is thought to be due to rupture of a distended renal pelvic mucosal vessel. Infections with frank pyelonephritis are rare. If found, these should arouse suspicion of reflux before suspicion of a UPJ obstruction. Hypertension secondary to transient ischemia of the renal parenchyma and vessels by a dilated pelvis is caused by activation of the renin angiotensin system. This is a common presentation in adults (305).

Extravasation and frank rupture of the pelvis are extremely rare causes of pain and ascites. Stone disease is seen in a small percentage of the cases of UPJ obstruction. Greater than 90% of these are in adolescents and in adults. In addition, the asymptomatic obstruction may be found when urologic x-ray or ultrasound examinations are performed for an unrelated problem (e.g., hypospadias, Hirschsprung's disease, cardiac catheterizations). Azotemia in a patient with bilateral disease or solitary kidney occasionally is seen as well.

Diagnosis. Currently, most investigations for abdominal mass, pain, urinary tract infection and (often) hematuria commence with an ultrasound examination of the kidneys and bladder. When UPJ obstruction is present, the classical sonographic findings of multiple symmetric sonoluscent filling defects capping a distended pelvis will be found (Fig. 17.45). Ultrasound is useful in showing the absence of a distended ureter, so that retrograde pyelography to confirm the anatomic site of obstruction is rarely necessary.

Classically, the IVP seen with UPJ obstruction reveals a dilated renal pelvis with nonvisualization of the ureter below the renal pelvis. Delayed films are helpful in confirming the level of obstruction and thus the diagnosis. To maximize the diagnostic capabilities of the IVP in diagnosing UPJ obstruction, the patient must be well hydrated. A small dose of diuretic may help in accentuating the IVP findings.

In mild or partial obstruction, the IVP may show a very dilated pelvis with normal caliceal configurations. The more severe degrees of obstruction lead to caliceal clubbing. Infants present with a higher degree of hydronephrosis. With high-grade obstruction and severe hydronephrosis, caliceal crescents may be seen. These are collections of contrast medium lying in transversely oriented calices. The transverse orientation is due to extrinsic compression of the calices by dilated collecting ducts

(crescent sign). These "crescents" are seen early in the IVP and disappear with time. The appearance and disappearance of the crescents imply functioning renal parenchyma. Consequently, the crescent sign is a fairly reliable indicator of recoverable renal function (298).

An IVP should be done on a patient with intermittent pain during an attack, with the hope of documenting the obstruction. Judicious administration of a diuretic may again help to augment the findings.

As mentioned above, vesicoureteral reflux may masquerade as UPJ obstruction because reflux of a bolus of urine into the kidney, and the inability of the pelvis to handle this, may lead to hydronephrosis. Because reflux has been shown to occur fairly commonly as an associated condition in cases of UPJ obstruction, a **voiding cystourethrogram** should be obtained in all cases.

One of the differentiating points between the UPJ obstruction and reflux is that, with reflux, the ureters are well seen. Reflux can cause kinking and ultimate scarring of the UPJ, so that both reflux and true UPJ obstruction can co-exist.

With the improvement of ultrasound and nuclear imaging, **retrograde pyelogram** studies are rarely used today. They do have a place in patients with a radiographically nonfunctioning kidney or when the ureter cannot be clearly delineated on IVP or ultrasound. The retrograde studies are predominantly done with the patient asleep just prior to surgical exploration so he or she need not be exposed to more than one anesthetic. **Percutaneous access** to the kidney is a safe and effective method for studying a nonfunctioning kidney, and has replaced the use of retrograde studies in many instances. The ureteral orifices are not traumatized as in retrograde studies. An accurate diagnosis can be made readily.

Lack of ureteral edema is key if the surgeon plans a tubeless pyeloplasty (298). **Arteriography** is indicated in patients with renovascular hypertension when the diagnosis cannot be made by less invasive techniques. It is useful to delineate the anatomy of the collecting system and the renal vessels, particularly with the UPJ obstruction, which is secondary to aberrant or accessory vessels.

Radioisotopes have developed to the point that **nuclear imaging** is an excellent technique for defining the function and anatomy of the kidneys. Assessing the preoperative renal function in a hydronephrotic kidney can be done readily. The degree of the obstruction can be well demonstrated. In addition, surgical repair can be followed serially with minimal radiation exposure to the patient. The DMSA scan is an excellent method of quantitating the percentage of renal function in each kidney. Radionuclide renography is a valuable tool for assessing renal blood flow and the degree of obstruction (306, 307). The DTPA scan coupled with the use of intravenously administered furosimide can be helpful in delineating true UPJ obstruction from the distended nonobstructed renal pelvis. Analysis of the excretory phase of the renogram curve can provide useful information about possible obstruction, as the nonobstructed dilated system will return to baseline levels when challenged by the diuretic. However, caution must be exercised in interpreting the response to furosimide if there is poor urinary function or gross dilation of the collecting system.

Truly equivocal obstructions not really clarified by radiographic or nuclear studies are rare. **Perfusion studies** may provide the only accurate way to assess the problem. A major drawback is the invasiveness of the technique. The percutaneous catheter is introduced into the collecting system above the possible site of obstruction by ultrasound under fluoroscopic control. A Foley catheter is inserted into the bladder. Constant infusion through the nephrostomy catheter is started and pressure readings of the pelvic and bladder pressures are made at set intervals. A difference of 10 to 14 cm of water with an empty bladder or 10 cm with a full bladder is thought to be the upper limits of normal (308). Equivocal studies after surgical repair can be delineated by this method.

Treatment. Two basic issues must be resolved once the UPJ obstruction has been documented. First, one must decide whether surgical intervention is required. Second, if surgery is indicated, one must decide whether removal of the kidney or pyeloplasty is indicated.

In the case of an IVP demonstrating minimal caliectasis and well-cupped calices over a period of years in an asymptomatic patient, no intervention should be undertaken. Progressive caliectasis, symptomatic disease, loss of renal function, and infection all mandate surgical repair.

The goal of all upper tract urologic management is maximizing the amount of functional renal tissue left after the intervention. Children particularly have amazing recuperative potential. Conservatism is further warranted if one considers that bilaterality may appear over a period of years. Nephrectomy may lead to overload of the remaining kidney, thus precipitating obstruction in the heretofore unobstructed kidney.

Total absence of demonstrable function, cystic/dysplastic changes, and severe parenchymal infection are indications for nephrectomy. Fortunately, if treated early and effectively, less than 5% of UPJ obstructions require nephrectomy. The DMSA scan has provided urologists with an excellent method of assessing renal function where standard urologic studies often were equivocal. Obstructed kidneys showing 10 to 15% of total renal function on DMSA scanning should certainly be salvaged, as the potential for even greater return of function is possible after relief of the obstruction. This is particularly true in the infant and young child (291, 309). The technique is rapid, effective, accurate, and noninvasive.

Temporary Diversion.
A medically unstable patient, particularly a newborn, may well benefit from temporary diversion of urine before definitive repair is undertaken. A percutaneous nephrostomy tube is easy to insert into a dilated pelvis. This can be directed with ultrasound under local anesthesia with minimal complications (310). The major disadvantage to this is that perirenal scarring may make the definitive repair more difficult at a later date.

Definitive Repair.
Multiple methods for performing pyeloplasty have been reported. Any method used should by necessity create a dependent funnel-shaped UPJ of good caliber. The most common method of repair in use today is the dismembered pyeloplasty, first described in 1949 and updated 14 years later (311) (Fig. 17.44).

Renal function generally improves following pyeloplasty, particularly in cases of bilateral obstruction when initially compromised renal function was documented. Surgery is beneficial for infants and young children (290, 212); the operation is easily tolerated by neonates and small infants (309) with minimal complications. Success is equal to that obtained in older infants and children.

Even if improvement in renal function following pyeloplasty is difficult to prove, diminished caliectasis or relief of symptoms should be demonstrable in 90% of the cases. Where caliectasis is worse or symptoms persist, diuresis renography, percutaneous pressure/perfusion studies, or both should clarify the picture.

Duplications of the Upper Urinary Tract

Upper urinary tract duplications are always the result of a doubling of the ureteric primordium. The extent of the ureteral duplication depends on the time at which the initial separation of the primordia occurred, whereas the extent of the kidney duplication depends on the distance to which the two primordia diverge from one another before reaching the nephrogenic blastema. These relationships are diagrammed in Table 17.9.

Embryologically, there is a complete gradation of forms from occult to complete. For diagnostic purposes and for surgical considerations, this sequence is best divided into (a) double ureter, in which there is no gross renal parenchymal separation, and (b) supernumerary kidney, in which parenchymal separation is complete.

DOUBLE PELVIS AND URETER

Anatomy. A so-called double kidney is provided with two pelves, each with a ureter draining it, but it is a single kidney. The lower pelvis is usually larger and appears less deformed than the upper. The ureter draining it is also larger in diameter. The pelves are usually in tandem, but occasionally they may lie side by side. They rarely com-

Table 17.9.
Gradations in Ureteral and Kidney Duplications

Temporal Relationships	Spatial Relationships

Abortive duplication of ureter (early)

Incomplete duplication of ureter (late)

Complete duplication of ureter (early)

Inverted Y ureter ← Rejoined tips of ureteric buds

Ureteral diverticulum ← Blindly ending branch

Bifid pelvis ← Narrow divergence of ureteric buds

Double pelvis ← Medium divergence of ureteric buds

Supernumerary kidney ← Wide divergence of ureteric buds

municate, but their calyces may interdigitate, making surgical separation of the two portions impossible.

Most such kidneys have two distinct sets of blood vessels, as well as two pelves, but in some cases they are served by branches from common renal vessels. The latter arrangement makes surgery more difficult.

Level of Ureteral Bifurcation.
The extent of the ureteral duplication is variable. It may be complete, the two ureters having independent orifices in the bladder (Fig. 17.46, *D*), or incomplete, with bifurcation occurring at any level (Figs. 17.46, *C*, and 17.47). Roughly 25% divide in the distal third, 50% in the middle third, and 25% in the proximal third. At the lower end, bifurcation may be within the bladder wall. At the upper end, doubling may be indicated merely by a bifid pelvis,

the mildest form of duplication (Fig. 17.46, *A* and *B*). The division is usually unequal, and it is the superior calyx that tends to separate from the remainder of the pelvis.

A few cases are known in which the ureters are fused above and enter a single pelvis, but later divide to form two orifices in the bladder (Fig. 17.46, *L*). Campbell (313) illustrates an example.

Abortive Duplication (Ureteral Diverticula).
Not all ureteral duplications generate double pelves; so-called ureteral diverticula represent duplicate ureters not associated with nephric tissue. In most cases they terminate before reaching the kidney (314) (Fig. 17.46, *G*), and occasionally they reach the kidney only to end blindly. In one case a duplication with a separate orifice was confined to the bladder wall (315).

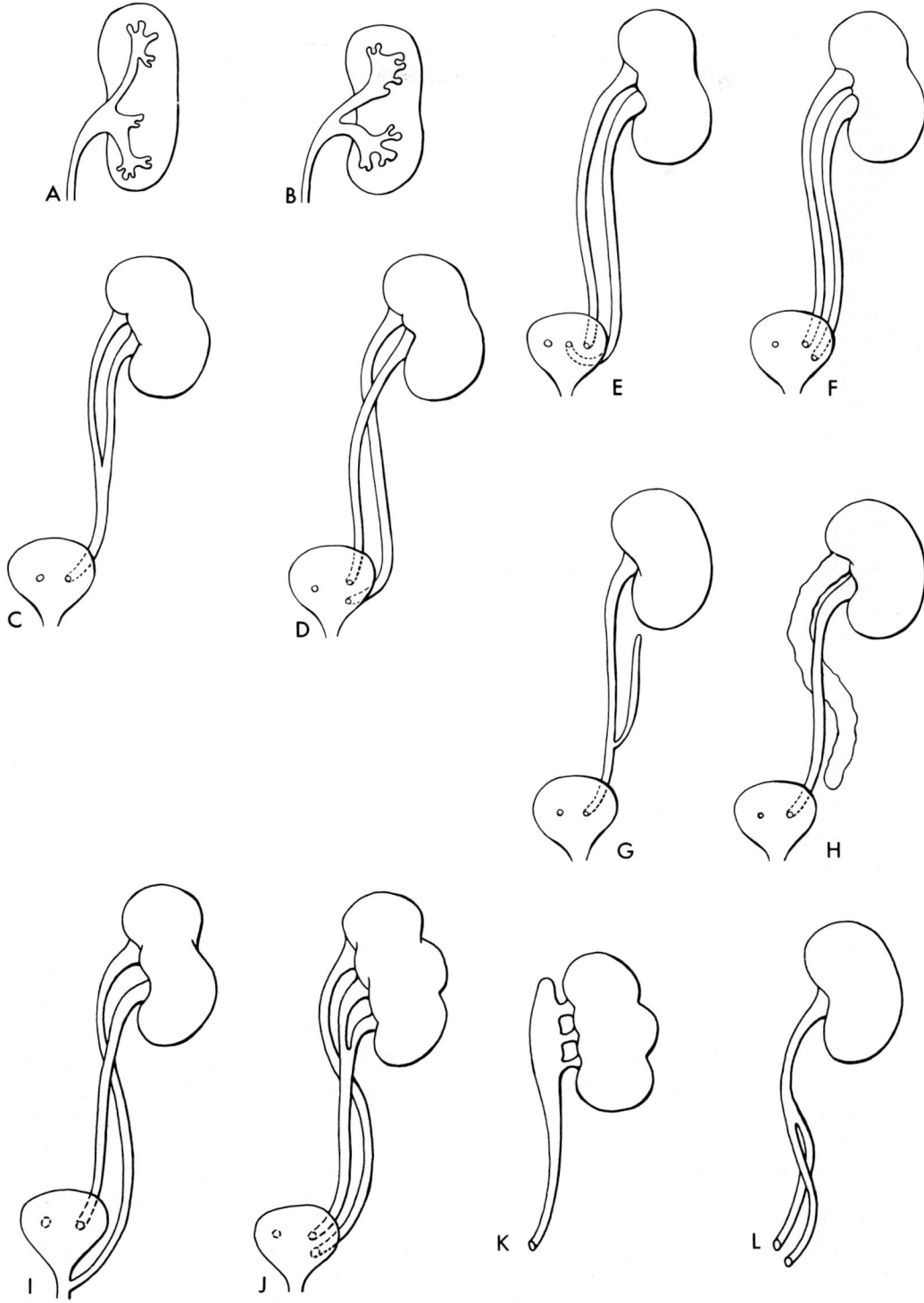

Figure 17.46. Doubling of the pelvis and ureter. **A** and **B,** Bifid pelvis, the mildest form of duplication. **C,** Bifurcation of the ureter. **D,** Complete duplication of the ureter with separate orifices in the bladder; upper pelvis drains to lower orifice in bladder. **E,** Unusual form of double ureter without crossing. **F,** Rare form of parallel ureters without crossing (compare with **D** and **E**). **G,** Doubling of the ureter with one aborted limb; normal kidney. **H,** Blind-ending ureter from upper pelvis. Such a ureter will be greatly enlarged and its renal tissue will be atrophic. **I,** Ectopic opening of one ureter into the urethra. **J,** Triple ureters becoming double; complete triple ureters are also known. **K,** Trifid pelvis with single ureter. **L,** Inverted **Y** duplication with a single ureter becoming doubled before reaching the bladder.

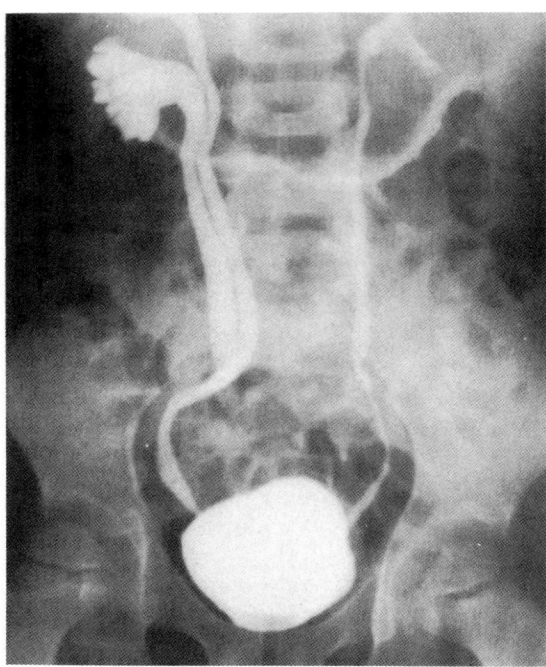

Figure 17.47. Radiologic appearance of a kidney with two pelves and bifurcated ureter.

Ectopic Ureteral Openings.
Low implantation into the urethra is not uncommon (Fig. 17.46, *I*). A supernumerary ureter may end blindly, usually in the region of the urethra. It will be enlarged, and its kidney tissue atrophic (316) (Fig. 17.46, *H*). The ureter from the superior pelvis most often ends ectopically. Ectopic ureteral orifices are discussed in detail on page 695.

Triplication of the Ureter.
In addition to duplication, triplication and even higher orders of replication have been found. In 1946 Smith (317) collected 11 cases of triplicate ureters, and about nine have been added since. The earliest case is that of Wrany (318), which was found at autopsy. The next case (319) was identified on pyelography and at surgery. The kidney with triple ureters was ectopic, hypoplastic, and hydronephrotic.

Triple ureters may be classified into four groups:

1. Complete triple ureters with separate orifices, of which about nine cases are known (320, 321)
2. Complete double ureter, one bifid (Fig. 17.46, *J*), of which about four cases have been reported (318, 322)
3. Single trifid ureter, of which about seven cases are known (317, 323)
4. Trifid pelvis (Fig. 17.18, *K*)

Quadruple ureters also have been reported (324). At autopsy of a 65-year-old man, Fürstner (325) found five

ureters to one kidney and a sixth to a supernumerary kidney on the same side. All six joined to form a common ureter. Campbell (64) mentions an adult with six-branched ureters on each side. In another case (288) what appeared to be an example of quadruple ureter was a completely extrarenal pelvis, with four elongated calyces (page 644).

Embryogenesis. Duplications of the upper urinary tract may arise from two separate deviations from normal development: splitting of the tip of the growing ureteric bud and formation of an accessory ureteric outgrowth of the wolffian duct.

Splitting of the Ureteric Bud.
Late in the fourth week the ureteric bud branches off the posterior portion of the wolffian duct and, within a short distance, makes contact with the nephrogenic mesoderm. Throughout the following week, the ureter elongates and forms the primary calyces at its cranial end. If division occurs at the very beginning of its growth, two complete ureters and pelves will be formed. Bifurcation will later produce incomplete ureteral duplication. Finally, if division occurs at the end of the growing period (fifth week), only a bifid pelvis will result (Table 17.8). The distance separating the ureteral tips when they reach the nephrogenic mesoderm determines whether a double pelvis or a free supernumerary kidney will be formed (Fig. 17.48). Complete duplication is therefore seen when two buds arise from one wolffian duct. Clinically, at cystoscopy, the ureteral orifice serving the upper pole is inferior and medial to the lower pole orifice. The lower pole ureter separates early from the wolffian duct and takes a supero-lateral position relative to the upper pole (Meyer-Weigert law). The clinical implications of the embryology are that, as a rule, the upper ureter is more likely to be ectopic in location and/or obstructive, whereas the lower pole ureter more frequently refluxes. Orifices at the extreme of placement, either laterally or caudally (into the urethra), are often associated with renal abnormalities. Mackie and Stephens (326) believe that the greater the distance of the ureteral bud from the middle of the wolffian duct, the greater the renal anomaly is likely to be, with renal dysplasia being the most significant abnormality encountered. Vesicoureteral reflux is seen with increased frequency in duplication anomalies. One or both of the orifices may reflux; however, more severe degrees of reflux usually occur in the lower pole ureter.

Accessory Ureteric Bud.
When two ureteric buds arise from the wolffian duct at a short distance from each other, this occasionally leads to complete duplication of the upper urinary tract. Wharton (327) described a 9.6-mm human embryo of 30 to 32 days of age with double ureters and two kidneys on the left side. The ureters arose separately at about the same time,

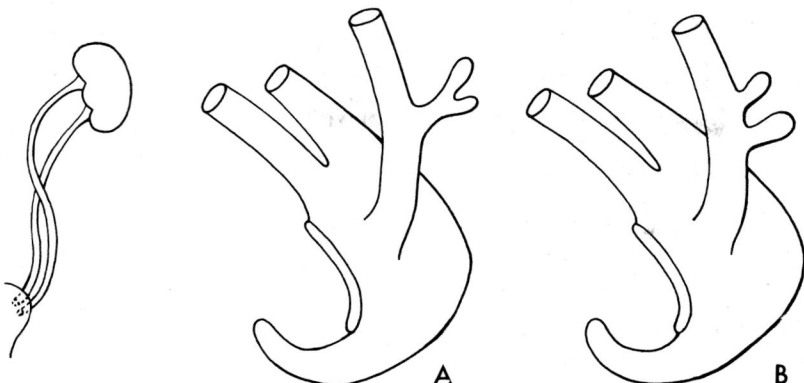

Figure 17.48. Embryogenesis of ureteral duplication. **A,** Splitting of the ureteric bud. The point of division will determine whether partial or complete duplication will result. **B,** Accessory ureteric bud from wolffian duct. Complete duplication usually results.

and the nephrogenic tissue was divided between them to form masses of potential kidney. Whether the two masses would have fused to form a double kidney or whether a supernumerary kidney would have resulted could not be determined. In another, slightly smaller embryo, a rudimentary ureteric bud was present in addition to a normal ureter, with its developing kidney. This bud, if not absorbed, would have formed a blind ending ureter or a ureteral diverticulum (Fig. 17.46, *G*) (314). Occasionally, instead of the two buds diverging, their tips come into contact and they coalesce to form the rare, "inverted Y" type of duplication (Fig. 17.46, *L*).

Triplications and other multiple formations are likewise the result of accessory ureteric buds and of the splitting of their tips in various combinations.

Crossing of the Double Ureters.
In most cases of double ureter the two ureters cross so that the one from the upper pelvis enters the bladder below the one from the lower pelvis (Fig. 17.46, *D*). The usual type of crossed ureteral duplication is the result of formation of two separate ureteric buds. The lower (caudal) bud is, with the caudal portion of the wolffian duct, absorbed by the expanding bladder first and carried upward with it. The accessory (cranial) bud is incorporated into the bladder wall at the same level as was the upper bud, but it is carried upward for a shorter distance and at a later time. Frazer (328) described this development during the 18- to 28-mm stages and later.

The crossing of the ureter is usually at the brim of the bony pelvis. More rarely, the lower ureter swings around the end of the upper ureter and thus avoids crossing (Fig. 17.46, *E*). Dougherty (329) described a case in which the two ureters were parallel and the upper ureter inserted in the bladder above the lower one. He mentioned only three other cases with this arrangement (Fig. 17.46, *F*).

The greater the distance between the normal and the accessory ureteric buds, the lower the latter will be implanted. At the extreme is the urethral implantation found in females (Fig. 17.46, *I*) and the seminal vesical implantation in males. Single as well as duplicate ureters may be found to open at these sites (Fig. 18.29).

When the ureters run parallel without crossing (Fig. 17.46, *F*), the condition has resulted from an originally bifid ureter, in which the bifurcation was so near its origin from the wolffian duct that incorporation into the bladder wall barely absorbed the common ureteric stem. Had bifurcation occurred at a lower level, the ureters would have crossed; had it occurred at a higher level, only a bifid ureter would have been produced.

Incidence. Bifid pelvis is at once the mildest and the most frequent form of upper urinary tract duplication. Campbell (64) stated that 10% of pelves show incipient doubling. Others, who include only more marked cases of doubling, place the frequency at 2 to 4% (330).

Duplication of the ureter is found in about 0.7 to 0.9% of all autopsies. Nation (331) found a frequency of 1:143 among 16,000 autopsies and Campbell (313) found a frequency of 1:117 among 32,834 adult autopsies.

These duplications may be complete (separate ureteric orifices) or incomplete (single ureteric orifice), and they may be bilateral or unilateral (Table 17.10).

Table 17.10.
Incidence of Urinary Tract Duplication

	Complete (%)[a]	Incomplete (%)	Total (%)
Bilateral	9	6	15
Unilateral	41	44	85
TOTAL	50	50	100

[a]Taken from data of Braasch WF, Scholl AJ Jr. Primary tumors of urethra. Ann Surg 1922; 76:246–259 and from Harpster CM, Brown TH, Delcher A. Solitary unilateral large serous cysts of the kidney with report of two cases and review of the literature. J Urol 1924; 11:157–175.

In some series (202, 334), bilateral duplication has been found more frequently.

A preponderance of duplications on one side or the other has been reported in various series, but the differences are probably not significant.

About three times as many females as males appear to have renal duplication. However, since ureteral ectopia is commonly found along with duplication and since ectopic ureters cause incontinence in females and not in males, the difference may be more apparent than real. The sex ratio found at autopsy is more nearly equal than is the sex ratio at pyelography (331).

Pathology. Hydronephrosis, infection, and lithiasis commonly affect kidneys with double pelves and ureters. The summation of Nation's (331) findings is represented in Table 17.11.

In bilateral clinical cases, 77% had disease in one or both kidneys.

Other renal anomalies are associated with duplication of the ureter and pelves. In order of frequency, ectopia, ureteral stenosis, hypoplasia, ectopic orifice, agenesis, polycystic disease, and aplasia have been found (331). Ureterocele also is associated frequently with ureteral duplication and usually involves the orifice draining the superior renal unit (See Fig. 18.37).

Among patients in whom renal and ureteral duplication is discovered in life, about 66% have symptoms that lead to the discovery of the anomaly, whereas in the other 33% discovery is incidental to examination for other unrelated diseases (335).

Infection is the most common cause of symptoms arising from ureteral duplication. These symptoms may be general, such as fever, malaise, fatigability, and weight loss, or they may be local, such as flank or bladder pain, dysuria, and frequency of urination. Signs such as flank tenderness, mass, hematuria, and pyuria also occur.

Obstruction without infection may result in pain, palpable mass, or tenderness.

A classical persistent, constant *incontinence* is usually associated with urethral or vaginal ureteral ectopia in the female; a normal voiding pattern usually is also present.

Diagnosis. IVP will detect those anomalies in which functioning of both portions of the kidney is good. Retrograde pyelograms may be necessary when functioning is impaired. Where double ureteric orifices are present and visible, ureteral catheterization is most effective; however, the possibility of ectopic orifices must be kept in mind.

It has been recognized that complete ureteral duplication is a predisposing factor to vesicoureteral reflux (336). The two ureters usually enter the bladder through the same muscular hiatus—with the ureter from the lower pole almost always entering at a point closer to the

Table 17.11.
Kidneys with Double Pelves and Ureters Affected by Hydronephrosis, Infection, and Lithiasis[a]

	Percentage of Patients with Disease	
	On Affected Side	On Normal Side
Autopsy cases	16	12
Clinical cases	50	30

[a]Data from Nation EF. Duplication of the kidney and ureter: a statistical study of 230 new cases. J Urol 1944; 51:456–465.

hiatus than the ureter from the upper pole. The resulting short intravesical segment of the ureter from the lower pole is incompetent and permits reflux. Changes consistent with pyelonephritis in the lower division of the kidney should always suggest reflux. Cystoscopy will reveal the anatomic defect of the vesicoureteral junction, and cystograms will confirm it. Rarely, the ureter from the superior portion of the kidney will enter the bladder ectopically, and the muscular hiatus also will be ectopic. The resulting short intravesical segment will allow reflux into this ureter.

Incompletely duplicated ureters may become dilated above the point of junction. Asynchronous peristalsis in the two limbs often results in a peristaltic wave descending one limb and passing up the other, rather than continuing down the common stem (337). This is known as ureteroureteral reflux or the "yo-yo" phenomenon. If the lesion is severe, ureteropyelostomy with excision of one of the dilated ureters will correct the dysfunction.

Treatment. Functional defects resulting from ureteral duplication—and the complications such as pyelonephritis, hydronephrosis, calculi, and incontinence arising from these defects—will dictate a variety of surgical procedures designed to correct the functional deficiency or to remove the diseased portion of the tract. The necessary surgical procedures are widely documented in the urologic literature and should be studied if operative intervention is contemplated. A synopsis of symptoms, diagnosis, and treatment of ureteral and renal duplication is presented in Table 17.12.

SUPERNUMERARY KIDNEY

Anatomy. This is the most extreme form of upper urinary tract duplication, as well as the rarest. Two completely separate—but usually unequal—kidneys are formed, with no parenchymatous connection between them. They are separately encapsulated and have independent pelves. The smaller, or supernumerary, kidney usually is below the larger, although it may be above. It is often hypoplastic and histologically less organized than the normal. Function is proportional to the extent of nor-

Table 17.12.
Synopsis of Symptoms, Diagnosis, and Treatment of Ureteral and Renal Duplication

Condition	Symptoms	Cystoscopy	Cystography	Pyelography		Treatment
				Retrograde	Excretory	
Ureteral diverticulum (abortive duplication)	Usually none; occasionally obstructive	Usually no extra orifice	May reveal ureteral reflux	Incomplete ureteral duplication readily visualized. Complete duplication demonstrable only if extra orifice is found and catheterized	Diverticulum readily visualized	Diverticulectomy
Double ureter	None; concomitant disease only	Extra orifice on affected side present in complete ureteral duplication; absent in incomplete duplication	May reveal ureteral reflux	Incomplete ureteral duplication readily visualized. Complete duplication demonstrable only if extra orifice is found and catheterized	Doubled structures visualized if both portions of kidney are functional	Uretero-ureterostomy, uretero-pyelostomy, pyelo-pyelostomy, partial nephrectomy and ureterectomy, revision of ureterovesical junction
Supernumerary kidney	None; concomitant disease only	Extra orifice on affected side present in complete ureteral duplication; absent in incomplete duplication	May reveal ureteral reflux	Incomplete ureteral duplication readily visualized. Complete duplication demonstrable only if extra orifice is found and catheterized	Both sets of structures usually visualized	Removal of supernumerary structure

mal development. Vascularization is usually separate, but anastomoses are common and must be sought in each case to be treated surgically.

The ureters from the supernumerary kidneys join the normal ureters (Fig. 17.49, *B* and *C*) about as commonly as they enter the bladder separately (Fig. 17.49, *A*). In the latter cases three orifices are present in the trigone. In one patient the extra ureter entered the upper vagina (338) and was at first considered to be a vesicovaginal fistula. In two patients the ectopic ureter opened into the vestibule (339, 340).

In the gradations of duplication, a distinction is sometimes made between "free" and "fused" supernumerary kidneys. In the fused type, there is a common connective tissue bond between the two organs, without the parenchymatous fusion found in the double kidney. Embryologically, the difference is one of degree, not of kind.

Usually excluded from the category of supernumerary kidney are small detached masses of metanephrogenic tissue which, although without ureteral connection, often undergo some differentiation. These were designated "beinieren" in 1914 by Neckarsulmer (341).

Embryogenesis. The origin of the supernumerary kidney is similar to that of the double pelvis described previously (page 649). If the duplicated ureteric buds reach the nephrogenic mesenchyme near one another, the kidney substance induced by the two will fuse into a typical double pelvis kidney. If the ends of the two buds diverge sufficiently, the two kidney masses will be far enough apart to remain separate and to form both a normal and a supernumerary kidney (Table 17.9).

History and Incidence. A supernumerary kidney was first mentioned in 1656 by Blasius (342) in reporting a case found by Martisu several years earlier, and only 30 satis-

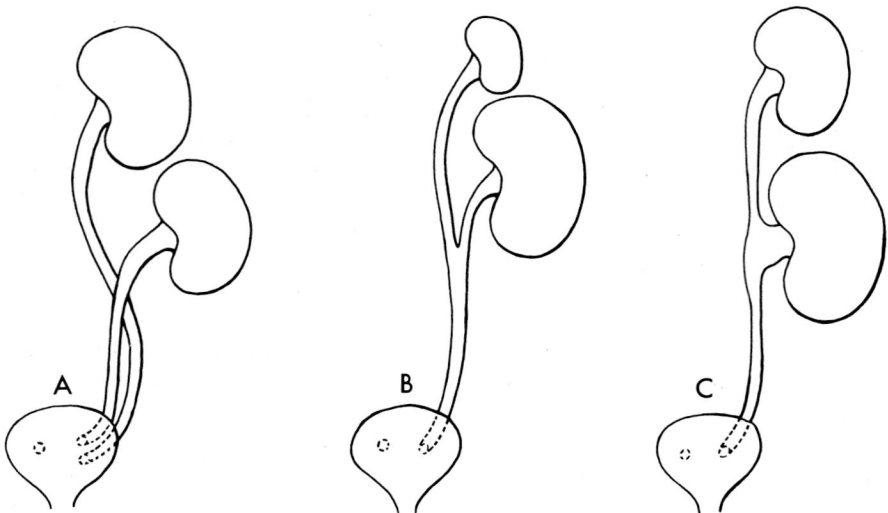

Figure 17.49. Duplication of the ureter and supernumerary kidney. **A,** Divergent ureters induce two separate kidneys. **B** and **C,**
Separate kidneys formed by bifurcated ureters.

factory cases could be assembled by Kretschmer (343) by 1929. Geisinger (344) added 10 more by 1937; Exley and Hotchkiss (345) six more by 1944; and Carlson (346), discarding one of Kretschmer's cases, collected 51 in 1950. Three more were added by Campbell in 1954 (313). The condition has been reported in the cow and pig (344).

The sexes seem to be about equally affected; there have been 21 males and 25 females described. There is no preponderance of either side; 25 supernumerary kidneys have been found on the left and 22 on the right. Only one bilateral case seems to be recorded (313).

Pathology. The supernumerary kidney is pathologically affected slightly more frequently than is the normal kidney. Occasionally, both kidneys may be affected. Lithiasis, ptosis, pyonephrosis, hydronephrosis, and infection have been reported. Hypoplasia of the supernumerary organ is usual. Exley and Hotchkiss (345) reported a case of carcinoma in a supernumerary kidney.

Symptoms. There are no specific symptoms: Pain and palpable mass are often but not invariably present. Instead, presenting symptoms usually are related to the specific pathologic condition. A number of cases are not pathologic, give no symptoms, and are found only incidentally or at autopsy.

Diagnosis. Diagnosis is rare before the age of 20 years. Kretschmer (343) mentioned a case in an infant, but Geisinger (344) excluded it, considering the organ too poorly developed to be more than a metanephrogenic fragment (beineiren). Excluding this case, over 25% of those reported were diagnosed in the third decade of life and the rest in later decades.

Only six cases were diagnosed preoperatively by 1954, although retrograde pyelography should uncover many more. In a few cases this procedure will not reveal the defect because the extra ureter ends blindly (347, 348). Excretory urography often is useless, as the supernumerary kidney may not excrete the dye. Aortography and a renal scintiscan may be of value in delineating the suspected lesion.

Treatment. Nephrectomy and ureterectomy of the supernumerary kidney may be required. It is essential that a supernumerary kidney be differentiated from crossed ectopia, in which the apparently extra organ is the normal kidney from the other side of the body. Because renal surgery should never be undertaken without proof of the presence of a healthy contralateral kidney, the existence of crossed ectopia should always be recognized in time to preserve the kidney.

Preureteral Vena Cava (Retrocaval Ureter)

ANATOMY

The anomaly in which the right ureter lies behind the inferior vena cava instead of in front of it is usually designated "retrocaval ureter." Because the resulting dysfunction is ureteral and not caval, it is treated by the urologist. Embryologically, however, the ureter is in its normal position and the vena cava is displaced anteriorly.

In most reported cases the anomaly is on the right. When the vena cava is double, the ureter lies behind the right limb only. Left retrocaval ureter associated with left inferior vena cava was reported by Pierro et al. (349). The association of horseshoe kidney with retrocaval ureter has been reported in six instances (350). One bilateral case in an acardiac monster has been observed (351).

EMBRYOGENESIS

The posterior vena cava forms during the seventh week from a system of three pairs of veins running roughly parallel to one another in the posterior part of the body. Two pairs, the posterior cardinals and the supracardinals, lie dorsally (posteriorly). Normally, the postrenal vena cava is formed from the right supracardinal vein. The left supracardinal vein and both postcardinal veins vanish, and the two subcardinal veins become the internal spermatic veins.

In patients with preureteral vena cava, it is the right subcardinal vein that has become the definitive postrenal segment of the vena cava, which, therefore, lies anterior to the ureter. There seems to be no reason why the left subcardinal might not persist, producing a left postcaval ureter, but the only such case reported was Gladstone's monster (351). Where double venae cavae are found, the right supracardinal vein and right subcardinal vein both persist, with the ureter passing under the latter and over the former (352). In other cases the right subcardinal vein and left supracardinal vein make up the double vena cava, and again the ureteral anomaly is only on the right (353). Figure 29.5 illustrates these relationships.

In 1925, the development of the abdominal veins was first clarified by McClure and Butler (354), who believed that the preureteric vein was the right cardinal vein. Gruenwald and Surks (352) showed that it was actually a persistent right subcardinal vein, and that the subcardinal-supracardinal anastomosis is lower than normal when the right subcardinal vein forms the vena cava. Huntington (355) analyzed all the possible variations that might account for his unique case of fused crossed ectopia, in which the crossed ureter was anterior to the vein, while the uncrossed ureter was posterior to it.

HISTORY

Hochstetter (356) reported the first case. In 1935 Kimbrough (357) performed the first operation for relief of hydronephrosis, sectioning the ureter below the UPJ and reanastomosing it anterior to the vena cava. In 1952 Cathro (358) ligated and sectioned the vena cava to preserve a postcaval ureter. Pick and Anson (353) collected 26 cases in 1940 and added one. By 1960 there were 90 published cases (359), and in 1964 Spaziante (360) published a report on a case, which he considered to bring the total of cases to 144. In 1989 Varma (361) reported on the association of retrocaval ureter with transitional cell carcinoma and suggested that slightly fewer than 200 cases of retrocaval ureter had been reported.

INCIDENCE

Heslin and Mamonas (362), assembling the experiences of four authors, reported five cases encountered among 7410 cadavers (1:1500).

From three to four times as many males as females have been reported; however, this ratio is probably too high because of the predominance of males in dissecting rooms. Although (obviously) the condition is congenital, rarely is a clinical diagnosis made in children (363). Most operative cases have been in adults. One case of solitary kidney has been reported (364). Retrocaval ureters are associated not infrequently with gonadal dysgenesis and Turner's syndrome.

The condition has been seen in rabbits, sheep, cats, and hedgehogs. In cats it occurs on the right in 4.3%, on the left in 1.5%, and on both sides in 3.3% (353). It does not seem to produce hydronephrosis in quadrupeds.

SYMPTOMS

The symptoms of retrocaval ureter are those of chronic partial ureteral obstruction with hydronephrosis and, frequently, infection.

The condition is clinically important if hydronephrosis secondary to obstruction is present. Dilation of the proximal one-third of the ureter associated with pyelectasis and choliectasis should raise a high index of suspicion for retrocaval ureter.

DIAGNOSIS

In the presence of a retrocaval ureter, anterior pyelography shows hydronephrosis on the right, with a long ureteral segment involved. The right ureter makes a characteristic S curve to, or beyond, the midline at the level of the third to fifth lumbar vertebrae. In an oblique pyelogram, the postcaval ureter remains against the vertebral column, instead of falling away from it. Confirmation by use of radiopaque medium in the vena cava (365, 366) has been obtained. Such venography is unnecessary for diagnosis but may be useful when planning operative procedures in difficult cases.

TREATMENT

The extent to which hydronephrosis has injured the kidney must be carefully estimated. In about 66% of patients, the kidney will be worth saving; in the rest, nephrectomy is indicated.

To bring the ureter to its normal position, anterior to the vena cava, one of the two structures must be cut and rejoined. Kimbrough (357) divided the ureter in 1935, but because of stricture formation at the site of anastomosis, Harrill (367) divided the pelvis above the UPJ. Harrill's operation is considered to be the most promising (64, 368–370). Common points of technique for a superior operation in this condition should include the following: (a) resection of that portion of the ureter lying beneath the vena cava; (b) transposition of the two ureteral or pelvis "halves" anterior to the vena cava; and (c) wide spatulated anastomosis, preferably using adjunctive

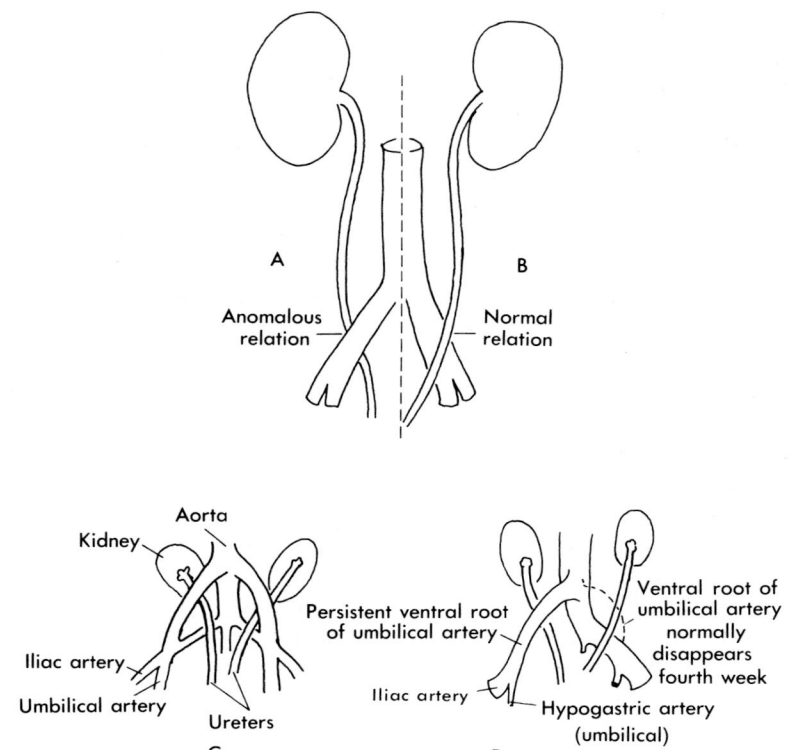

Figure 17.50. Retroiliac ureter. **A,** Anomalous relationship of ureter and artery. **B,** Normal relationship of ureter and artery. **C,** Relationships of ureter and iliac and umbilical arteries in the embryo. **D,** Development of normal iliac channel on the right, anomalous iliac channel (persistence of proximal umbilical artery) on the left.

nephrostomy and ureteral stent. Section of the distal ureter with reimplantation into the bladder has not been successful (371).

The second alternative, section of the vena cava, was first performed in 1952 by Cathro. Goodwin and his colleagues (368) later reported section and reanastomosis of the vena cava behind the ureter. This procedure must be considered seriously if the affected kidney is the only functioning one.

Retroiliac Ureter (Preureteral Iliac Artery)

In three instances (372–374) the ureter has been observed to pass behind the iliac artery—in one case on the left and in one on the right side. In one patient the ureteral opening was ectopic, and in another it was suspected to be so. Hanna (375) reported one case of bilateral retroiliac ureters associated with vesicoureteral reflux and horseshoe kidney. Nguyen et al. (376) reported a male newborn with left retroiliac ureter, ectopic left vas deferens, ectopic ureter, and imperforate anus.

This anomaly is a vascular malformation, like the retrocaval ureter previously described. At the end of the fourth week the primitive ventral root of the umbilical artery normally is replaced by a more dorsal intersegmental aortic branch, which forms a shunt between the aorta and distal umbilical artery. This new dorsal root becomes the iliac trunk, and the primitive ventral root disappears. Failure of the dorsal root to form, along with persistence of the ventral root, would place the iliac artery ventral to the ureter (Fig. 17.50).

An alternate explanation offered by Dees (372) is based on the redundancy of the overlying iliac artery in his patient. He suggests that the kidney has passed dorsal to the iliac artery during migration; furthermore, he suggests that, when this happens bilaterally, horseshoe fusion results, with a postaortal and postcaval isthmus. He cites three cases of this latter anomaly (see page 620).

Ureteral Diverticula

ANATOMY

Diverticula of the ureter may be divided into three groups:

1. Abortive duplications of the ureter (bifid ureter), which have been considered on page 650 (Fig. 17.46, *G*)
2. True congenital diverticula, in which all layers are present

3. Acquired diverticula, which are true herniations without muscularis

None of these is common. Culp (124), reviewing the literature in 1947, found 14 bifid ureters, 10 congenital diverticula, and 5 acquired diverticula. Since then, Williams and Goodwin (377) have reported a 17th congenital case. Pratt and his colleagues (378) reported 36 cases, but they did not distinguish between congenital and acquired deviations.

Congenital diverticula have been found just above the ureterovesical junction (379), in the midportion of the ureter (380), and at the UPJ (377, 381). At least three have been very large: Richardson's (380) diverticulum was 18 cm in diameter and contained 3600 cc of fluid; Culp's (124) patient had a diverticulum containing 1600 cc (Fig. 17.51); and McGraw and Culp's patient (381) had an even larger diverticulum that extended from the costal margin to the pelvic brim. Its volume was not determined.

EMBRYOGENESIS

We agree with Rank and his colleagues (382) that all congenital diverticula of the midportion and of the vesiculoureteral region represent abortive ureteral buds. Rathbun's patient (379) with bilateral diverticula can have no other explanation.

Although the distinction between a bifid ureter and a congenital diverticulum has no embryonic basis, the clinical distinction between a long duplication parallel to the ureter and a balloon-shaped diverticulum of the ureteric wall is sound. Once such a diverticulum has begun to expand under pressure, it seems to continue to do so until repaired. If such expansion never starts, the true bifid ureter rarely causes symptoms.

Ureteropelvic diverticula appear to be primitive calyces that failed to encounter nephrogenic mesenchyme and hence remained extrarenal. They do not differ from intrarenal diverticula (page 636); their enlargement from calculi or infection is secondary.

SYMPTOMS

Pain is present in most cases, yet those patients with the largest diverticula (those of Richardson (380), Culp (124), and McGraw and Culp (381)) complained only of abdominal distension.

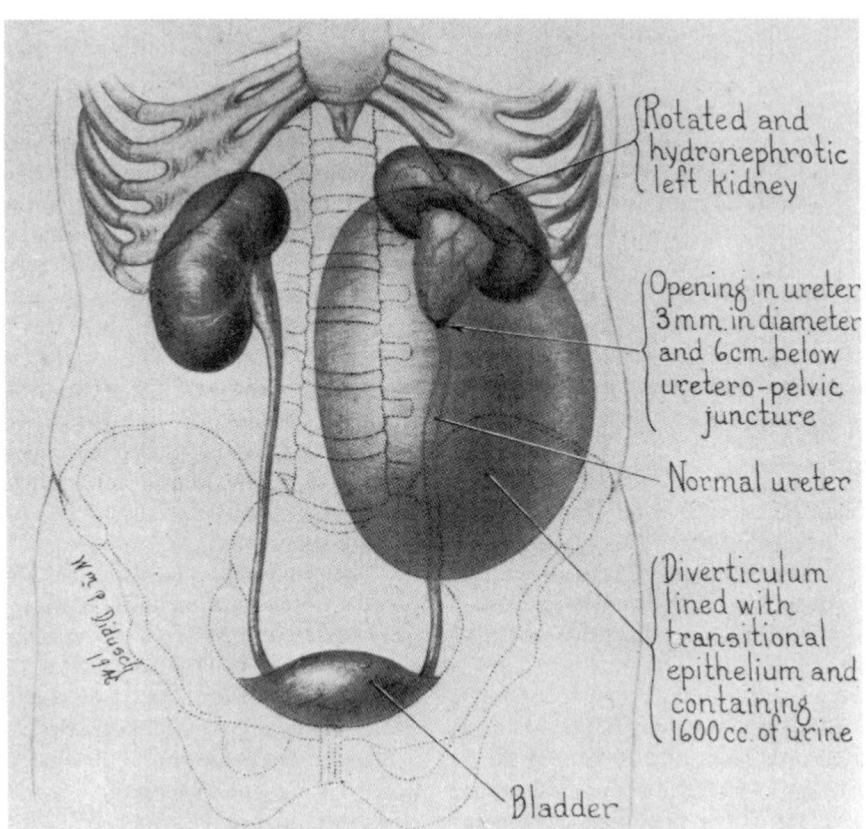

Figure 17.51. Congenital diverticulum of left ureter containing 1600 cc of urine. The kidney was hydronephrotic. (From Culp OS. Ureteral diverticulum: classification of literature and report of authentic case. J Urol 1947;58:309–321.)

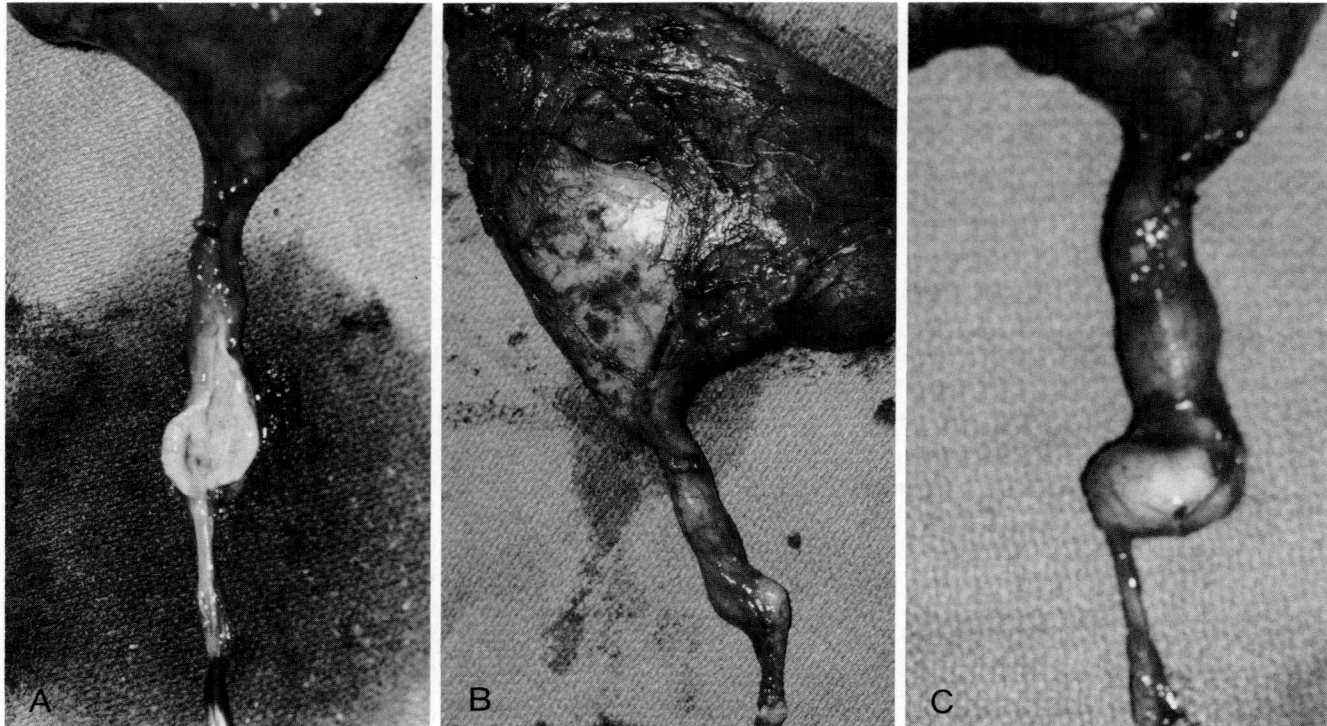

Figure 17.52. Ureteral valve. **A** to **C,** Operative specimen.

DIAGNOSIS

Visualization of the ureter will usually reveal ureteral diverticula if they are present. Large ones have been recognized by the coiling of a ureteral catheter within them.

TREATMENT

Removal of the diverticulum, with repair of the ureteral wall, is the preferred operation if the kidney can be saved. In the case of huge diverticula, resection with end-to-end anastomosis may be necessary (380).

Ureteral Valves and Strictures

Transverse folds of redundant ureteral mucosa are not uncommon in the newborn. Wölfler (383), who first described them in 1887, found them present in about 5% of autopsies, and Campbell (313) estimated them to be present in 10%. Such mucosal folds produce no obstruction and usually disappear.

In a few cases the structures persist and cause obstruction. Wall and Wachter (384) reviewed a number of such case reports and accepted only four, adding one of their own. Pasaro and Smith (385) in 1960 reported what seems to be the 10th case. The valves have been found in patients of either sex and on either or both sides and may be located in any part of the ureter. They have been found in both children (385) and adults (386, 387). They may be

cusplike, or more commonly, they may be diaphragms with or without a central orifice (Fig. 17.51). In 1927 Chwalle (388) demonstrated the closure of the embryonic ureteral lumen by an epithelial membrane during the separation of the ureter and wolffian duct at the 10- to 12-mm stage (sixth week). This membrane normally breaks down during the eighth week, but it may persist even longer. Vermooten (389) believed he could demonstrate radiographically the occasional persistence of this membrane as a valve-like structure at the ureteral orifice of infants. Hydroureter and hydronephrosis due to the persistence of Chwalle's membrane has been reported in rat fetuses with pantothenic acid deficiency (390). The membrane also is considered to play a part in ureterocele formation (page 700).

Pain, nocturia, incontinence, and other symptoms of obstruction are present. The ureter may be dilated and mild hydronephrosis may occur; in one case, hypertension resulted (391). Intravenous pyelography usually indicates ureteral obstruction, but this may be extrinsic rather than valvular. The obstruction may not appear on a retrograde pyelogram because the valve encourages flow in only one direction. Campbell (64) illustrated a visualized ureter with three valves, later confirmed at autopsy. The occurrence of symptoms late in life casts doubt on the congenital origin of some of these valves. Foroughi and Turner's (392) 68-year-old patient had had symptoms for only 3 weeks. Docimo et al. (393) reported from Boston Children's Hospital on seven cases of midureteral obstruction due to ureteral valve or stricture occurring over a 17 year period. Owing to the fact that three of their cases had contralateral renal dysgenesis, they felt that an underlying ureteral bud abnormality might play a major role in embryogenesis.

Allen (394), in analyzing 95 cases of ureteral strictures, found only three occurring in the midureter. The remainder were located at the UPJ or ureterovesical junction. Each of these, however, occurred where the ureter passed over the pelvic brim. Unlike ureteral valves, strictures present histologically as a localized segment of decreased diameter and reduced muscle bulk.

Megaureters (Wide Ureters)

Megaureters should be approached as a radiographic diagnosis necessitating further evaluation to rule out reflux or other etiologies as a cause of ureterovesical junction obstruction. Multiple systems of classification of megaureters are in existence, and all attempt to differentiate between obstructed and nonobstructed conditions. Whitaker (297, 308) has given us a rational classification scheme which sorts out wide ureters into groups of refluxing or nonrefluxing, primary or secondary, and obstructed or nonobstructed. **Primary refluxing megaureter** is due to a foreshortened or absent intravesical ureteral segment, periureteral diverticulum, or other abnormalities of the ureterovesical junction, whereas **secondary refluxing megaureters** are due to reflux and associated neurogenic bladder or intravesical obstruction. **Primary nonobstructing nonrefluxing megaureters** (congenital megaureters) are without obstruction at the ureterovesical junction, without reflux or bladder abnormalities or bladder outlet obstruction.

The lesion, which has been called "megaloureter" by Lewis and Kimbrough (395) and "ureteral achalasia" by Creevy (396), is known as *congenital megaureter* since the publications of Hendren (397, 398) popularized this nomenclature. Its mildest nonrefluxing form consists of a localized, fusiform dilation of the distal ureter just above its entrance to the bladder. The intravesical segment is normal, and there is no evidence of obstruction and no vesicoureteral reflux. Active peristalsis is visible except at the distal end of the dilated segment. There is no evidence of nervous system disease (Fig. 17.52).

The undilated intramural segment, distal to the dilation, has suggested a similarity with congenital megacolon (399), and resection of the normal appearing distal segment and reimplantation of the ureter (ureteroneocystostomy) has been performed successfully (395). A study of vesical ganglion cells in children with megaloureter, megacystis, and megacolon has shown no absence or unusual distribution of neural elements (400). Success of the surgical procedure was probably due to the reimplantation rather than to the segmental resection. Although the condition is often found incidentally in adults, it is more often a cause of significant morbidity in children. In one surgical series, congenital megaureter accounted for over one-half of wide ureters undergoing operative intervention (401).

The major cause of a **primary obstructed megaureter** is a narrow ureterovesical junction which impedes peristalsis and the passage of urine. By definition, one should be unable to pass a ureteral catheter past the narrow area cystoscopically. Physiologic studies to rule out the nonobstructive condition, such as antegrade perfusion or Lasix renogram, should be performed in making this diagnosis. However, many of the clinical studies in the past which tried to look at the primary etiology of wide ureters thought to be of obstructive etiology often did not employ these physiologic parameters and may have included both the obstructive and nonobstructive varieties (402, 403). Differentiation from the nonrefluxing nonobstructed megaureter usually is based on the presence of the distal adynamic segment found in congenital megaureter and the ability to pass a ureteral catheter in the nonobstructed condition.

Fetal screening during maternal ultrasonography has changed the mode of presentation of patients with megaureter. In a recent series from Children's Hospital of Philadelphia (404) over a 6-year period one-half of the megaureters presenting in neonates and infants were detected antenatally. Others (405, 406) report a similar high incidence of prenatal detection. Symptomatic megaureter with or without caliectasis usually presents with infection. This may be due to cystitis and may have no relation to the upper urinary tract lesion. Hematuria and abdominal pain are also presenting complaints. Ureterectasis may be found during an abdominal operation such as appendectomy. Uremia, anemia, renal rickets, and failure to thrive are rarely found as presenting complaints, but most commonly are found in infants. Bilaterality occurs in less than 25% of the patients, but is more common in children diagnosed at less than 1 year of age. Males are affected two to five times as often as females, and the left ureter is affected more frequently than the right side.

Most patients with congenital megaureter, particularly older children and adults, have nonobstructive megaureters which require no specific surgical therapy. Pediatric patients with nonobstructing megaureter often show progressively less dilated ureters as growth occurs (407). In the Children's Hospital of Philadelphia series, 87% of the patients were managed without surgical intervention despite the fact that 16 of 44 renal units were graded as moderate to severe hydronephrosis. The authors of this

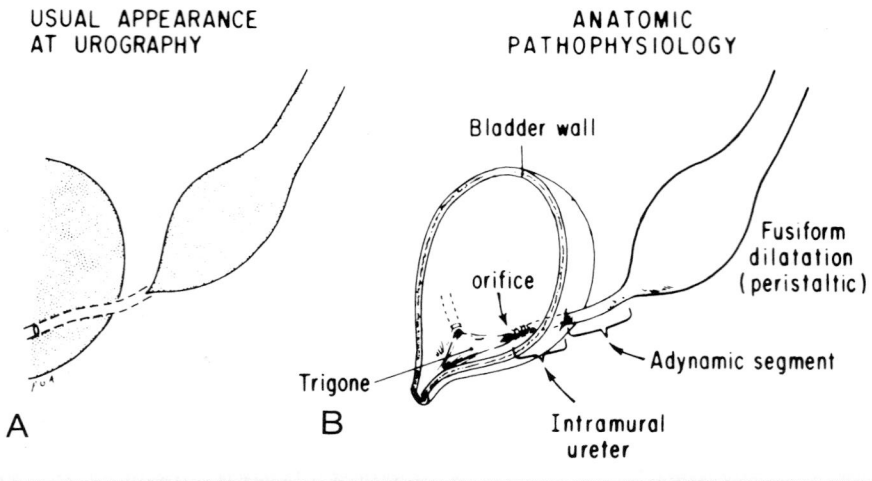

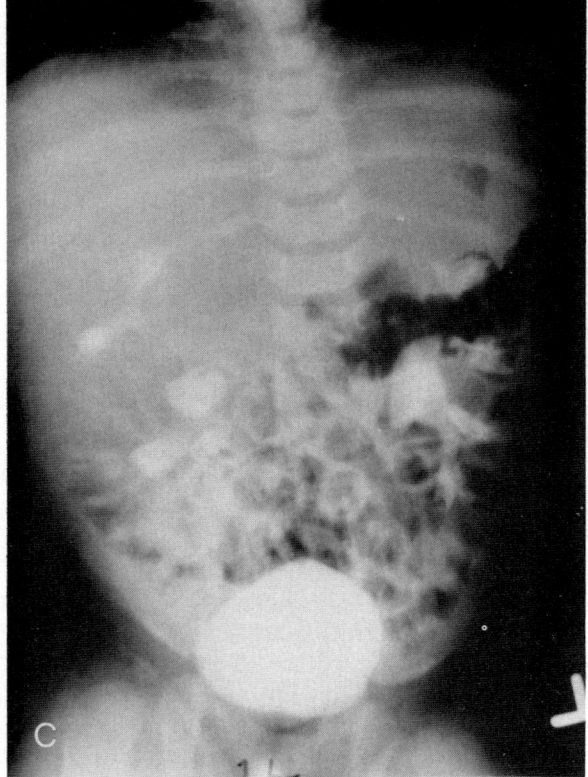

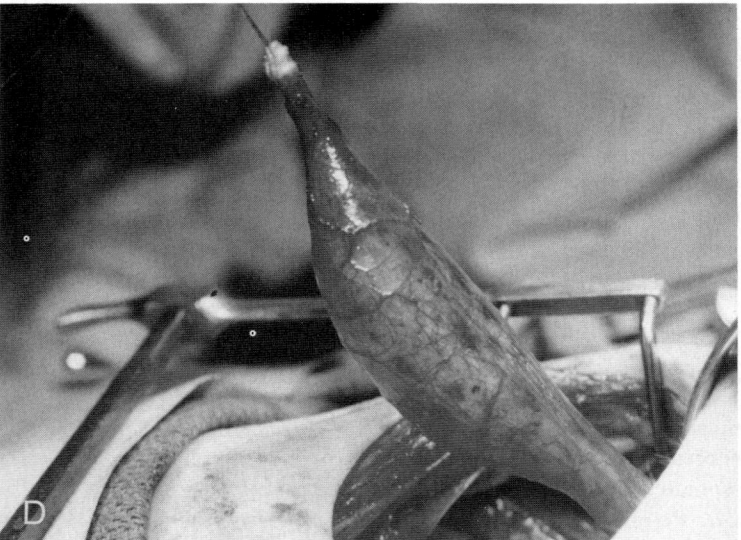

Figure 17.53. Megaureter. **A,** Usual appearance at urography. **B,** Anatomic pathophysiology. **C,** IVP appearance of congenital magaureter with significant associated caliectasis. **D,** Operative appearance of small distal segment with proximal hydroureter.

series believed that their data supported a contention that the neonatal congenital megaureter in many cases represents a different entity than those that commonly presented before the advent of prenatal diagnosis.

Indications for surgery include progressive ureteral dilation with severe hydronephrosis and/or parenchymal loss and radiologic evidence (DTPA with Lasix, Whitaker test) which unequivocally demonstrates obstruction. Persistent infections in children may indicate the need for surgical intervention. Ureteral tapering with excision or infolding remains the surgical technique most used today (401).

EDITORIAL COMMENTS

The decade of the 1980s witnessed the maturation of technology which allowed for the routine antenatal diagnosis of hydronephrosis and other abnormalities of the urinary system. In addition, this technology has made it possible to define further our concept of "obstructive uropathy," because many conditions which previously were thought to be obviously "obstructive" are now considered to be merely dilated but without harmful elevated pressure effects. Real-time ultrasonography of the fetal urinary tract may show dilated kidneys or extrarenal collecting systems, such as is seen with UPJ obstruction and megaureter. Such scanning may reveal unilateral renal agenesis, cystic kidneys, ectopic kidneys, and the unfortunate bilateral renal agenesis associated with deficient amniotic fluid volume. Prenatally diagnosed ureteropelvic junction "obstruction" is a common entity in pediatric urologic practice. Without prenatal ultrasonography, the newborn infant with this condition may escape diagnosis unless a mass is felt. Currently, diligent effort is focused on accurate diagnosis of true (i.e., harmful) obstruction rather than dilation without obstruction. Nuclear imaging techniques are at the forefront in this endeavor, as DTPA and DMSA renal scans are used much more commonly in practice than IVPs and retrograde pyelograms. Ideally, the future will enhance our understanding of the natural history of these asymptomatic renal and ureteral dilations.

Evidence is mounting to suggest that children who are born with only one kidney, or those who undergo unilateral nephrectomy at an early age, are at risk for developing proteinuria and possibly renal insufficiency later in life (408). Whether this is due to the so-called Brenner hypothesis of nephron hyperperfusion with resultant glomerulosclerosis is difficult to prove, as rarely is adequate biopsy material available (409). It is uncertain whether efforts at early restriction of protein intake will influence the eventual outcome, if indeed hyperperfusion is a real entity. Further research is necessary to determine if patients with a solitary kidney will benefit from such efforts.

Classification of cystic renal disease has always been a challenge. Anyone interested in urinary embryology should be familiar with the early microdissection studies of Osathanondh and Potter, which laid the foundation for our understanding of renal cystic disease based on microhistology. Of more clinical interest (and germane to the focus of this book) is the effort to divide cystic lesions into those that are of embryonic origin from those of non-embryonic basis. Further subdivision can be made on the basis of heredity (e.g., polycystic kidneys). No longer is it suitable to use the terms *adult polycystic* and *infantile polycystic,* as the former have been regularly diagnosed during infancy, and some patients with the latter have lived into young adulthood. Recessive and dominant modes of transmission are responsible for the clinical presentation of "infantile" and "adult" forms of polycystic kidneys, and it is now preferable to refer to these entities according to the mode of genetic transmission. The discussion of multicystic kidney in this chapter includes our effort to put forth our current understanding of the pathophysiology of this entity. We try to show the similarity between multicystic kidney and UPJ obstruction. It appears that the timing during embryogenesis of the ureteral obstruction and the severity of the obstruction are responsible for whether cystic pathology or hydronephrosis results. Furthermore, nonsurgical management of multicystic kidney is routinely considered at most pediatric centers, especially when the kidney is not palpable (TSP).

REFERENCES

1. Felix W. The development of the urinogenital organs. In: Keibel F, Mall FP, eds. Manual of human embryology, Vol 2. Philadelphia: JB Lippincott, 1912.
2. Balfour FM, Segwick A. On the existence of rudimentary head-kidney in the embryo chick. Q J Micr Sci Lond 1879;19:1–20.
3. Fraser EA. The pronephros and early development of the mesonephros in the cat. J Anat 1920;54:287–304.
4. Torrey TW. The early development of the human nephros. Contrib Embryol Carnegie Inst Wash 1954;35:175–197.
5. Davies J, Davies DV. The development of the mesonephros of the sheep. Proc Zool Soc Lond 1950;120:73–93.
6. Heuser CH. A human embryo with 14 pairs of somites. Contrib Embryol Carnegie Inst Wash 1930;22:135–153.
7. Torrey TW. Morphogenesis of the vertebrate kidney. In: DeHaan RL, Ursprung H, eds. Organogenesis. New York: Holt, Rinehart & Winston, 1965.
8. Shikinami J. Detailed form of the wolffian body in human embryos. Contrib Embryol Carnegie Inst Wash 1926;18:49–61.
9. Altschule MD. The changes in the mesonephric tubules of human embryos ten to twelve weeks old. Anat Rec 1930;46:81–91.
10. Gersh I. The correlation of structure and function in the developing mesonephros and metanephros. Contrib Embrol Carnegie Inst Wash 1937;26:35–38.
11. Davies J, Routh JI. Composition of the foetal fluids of the rabbit. J Embryol Exp Morphol 1957;5:32–39.
12. Stanier MW. The function of the mammalian mesonephros. J Physiol 1960;151:472–478.
13. McCance RA, Stainer MW. The function of the metanephron in fetal rabbits and pigs. J Physiol 1960;151:479–483.
14. Begg RC. Sextuplicitas renum: a case of six functioning kidneys and ureters in an adult female. J Urol 1953;70:686–693.
15. Grobstein C. Inductive interaction in the development of the mouse metanephros. J Exp Zool 1955;130:319–340.
16. Grobstein C. Some transmission characteristics of the tubule inducing influence on mouse metanephrogenic mesenchyme. Exp Cell Res 1957;13:575–587.
17. Osathanondh V, Potter EL. Development of human kidney as shown by microdissection. Arch Pathol 1963;76:271–302.
18. Gruenwald P. The normal changes in the position of the embryonic kidney. Anat Rec 1943;85:163–176.
19. Gruenwald P. The mechanism of kidney development in human embryos as revealed by an early stage of agenesis of the ureteric buds. Anat Rec 1939;75:237–247.
20. Brockmann AW. Bemerkungen zu einer Arbeit Sarkenstein: "Ueber die Anlage und Wanderung der Nachniere beim Menschen." Morphol Jahrb 1938;81:21–23.
21. Priman J. A consideration of normal and abnormal positions of the hilum of the kidney. Anat Rec 1929;42:355–364.
22. Miettinen H, Ellem KAO, Saxen L. Studies of kidney tubulogenesis. VII. The response of RNA synthesis of mouse metanephrogenic mesenchyme to an inductive stimulus. Ann Med Exp Fenn 1966;44:109–116.
23. Grobstein C. Inductive epithelio-mesenchymal interaction in cultured organ rudiments of the mouse. Science 1953;118:52–55.
24. Remak R. Untersuch: Ueber d. Entwicklung. d. Wirbeltheir, Berlin, 1855.

25. Herring PT. The development of the malpighian bodies of the kidney and its relation to the pathological changes which occur in them. J Pathol Bact 1900;6:459–496.

26. Lewis OJ. The vascular arrangement of the mammalian renal glomerulus as revealed by a study of its development. J Anat 1958;92:433–440.

27. Kuntz SM. The electron microscopy of the developing human renal glomerulus. Exp Cell Res 1958;14:355–367.

28. Vernier RL, Birch-Anderson A. Studies of the human fetal kidney. I. Development of the glomerulus. J Pediatr 1962;60:754–768.

29. Jokelainen P. An electron microscope study of the early development of the rat metanephric nephron. Acta Anat (Basel) 1963;52(Suppl):47.

30. Hickey MF. Extra-medullary haematopoiesis in the solitary hypoplastic kidney of a malformed full-term foetus. Proc Anat Soc Great Br Ireland 1964;26:34.

31. Gruenwald P, Popper H. The histogenesis and physiology of the renal glomerulus in early postnatal life: histological examinations. J Urol 1940;43:452–458.

32. Alexander DP, Nixon DA. The foetal kidney. Br Med Bull 1961;17:112–117.

33. Kuntz SM, Feldman JD. Experimental studies on the formation of the glomerular basement membrane. J Ultrastruct Res 1962;6:19–27.

34. Kampmeier OF. The metanephros or so-called permanent kidney in part provisional and vestigal. Anat Rec 1926;33:115–120.

35. Moffat DB, Fourman J. Ectopic glomeruli in the human and animal kidney. Anat Rec 1964;149:1–11.

36. Peter K. Untersuchungen über Bau und Entwicklung der Niere. Jena (Germany): Fischer-Verlag, 1927.

37. Tsuda K. Histologic investigation of the foetal kidney. Jpn J Obstet Gynecol 1943;17:227–341.

38. Macdonald MS, Emery JL. The late intrauterine and postnatal development of human renal glomeruli. J Anat 1959;93:331–340.

39. Potter EL, Thierstein ST. Glomerular development in the kidney as an index of fetal maturity. J Pediatr 1943;22:695–706.

40. Rożynek M. Badania histopatologiczne nerek plodnow i noworodkow. Poznan Towarzy Przyjac Nauk Wydz Led 1962;22:235–270.

41. Fetterman GH, Shuplock NA, Phillipp F, Gregg HS. The growth and maturation of human glomeruli and proximal convolutions from term to adulthood: studies by microdissection. Pediatrics 1965;35:601–619.

42. Kissane JM, Smith MG. Pathology of infancy and childhood. St. Louis: CV Mosby, 1967:521.

43. Someren A (Ed.). Urologic pathology with clinical and radiologic correlations. New York: MacMillan Publishing, 1989:18.

44. Boulgakow B. The effect of non-development of the allantois as illustrated by a case of sympodia. J Anat 1929;63:253–258.

45. Greig DM, Herzfeld G. On the persistence of complete wolffian ducts in females. Endinb Med J 1927;34:701–724.

46. Spitzer WM, Wallin IE. Supernumery ectopic ureters. Ann Surg 1928;88:1053–1062.

47. Troup J. Persistence of the complete wolffian duct. Br Med J 1931;1:707–708.

48. Arnold JH. A clinico-histologic consideration of renal malformations. J Urol 1960;84:510–516.

49. Rubenstein M, Meyer R, Berstein J. Congenital abnormalities of the urinary system. I. A postmortem survey of developmental anomalies and acquired congenital lesions in a children's hospital J Pediatr 1961;58:356–366.

50. Campbell MF. Embryology and anomalies of the urogenital tract. In: Clinical pediatric urology. Philadelphia: WB Saunders, 1951.

51. Potter EL. Bilateral absence of ureters and kidneys: a report of 50 cases. Obstet Gynecol 1965;25:3–12.

52. Davidson WM, Ross GIM. Bilateral absence of the kidneys and related congenital anomalies. J Pathol Bact 1954;68:459–474.

53. Rizza JM, Downing SEP. Bilateral renal agenesis in the female siblings. Am J Dis Child 1971;121:60.

54. Perlmutter AD, Retik AB, Bauer SB. Anomalies of the upper urinary tract. In: Harrison JH, Gittes RF, Perlmutter AD, Stamey TA, Walsh PC, eds. Campbell's urology. Philadelphia: WB Saunders, 1979:1310.

55. Wladimiroff JW. Effect of furosemide on fetal urine production. Br J Obstet Gynecol 1975;82:221.

56. Ashley DJB, Mostofi FK. Renal agenesis and dysgenesis. J Urol 1960;83:211–230.

57. Murphy DP. Congenital malformations: a study of parental characteristics with special reference to the reproductive process, 2nd ed. Philadelphia: JB Lippincott, 1947.

58. DuBois AM. The embryonic kidney. In: Muller AF, ed. The kidney: morphology, biochemistry, physiology. New York: Academic Press, 1969.

59. Moore KL. The developing human: clinically oriented embryology, 4th ed. Philadelphia: WB Saunders, 1988.

60. Sadler TW. Langman's medical embryology, 6th ed. Baltimore: Williams & Wilkins, 1990.

61. Datta AK. Essentials of human embryology, 2nd ed. Calcutta: Current Books International, 1991.

62. Wolfstrigel L. Miscellanea curiosa medico-physica academiae naturae curiosorum. Jena, 1671;2:36.

63. Coen E. Descrizione anatomica di un feto senza reni e senza utero, con altre anomalie. Ann Univ Med Chir 1884;267:52.

64. Campbell MF. Urology, 3 vols. Philadelphia: WB Saunders, 1963.

65. Sylvester PE, Hughes DR. Congenital absence of both kidneys: a report of four cases. Br Med J 1954;1:77–79.

66. Carpentier PJ, Potter EL. Nuclear sex and genital malformation in 48 cases of renal agenesis, with especial reference to nonspecific female pseudohermaphroditism. Am J Obstet Gynecol 1959;78:235–258.

67. Levin H. Bilateral renal agenesia. J Urol 1952;67:86–91.

68. Ratcliffe HL, King HD. Developmental abnormalities and spontaneous diseases found in rats of the mutant strain, stub. Anat Rec 1941;81:283–305.

69. Bagg HJ. Hereditary abnormalities of the limbs: their origin and transmission. Am J Anat 1929;43:167–220.

70. Danforth CH. Developmental anomalies in a special strain of mice. Am J Anat 1930;45:275–287.

71. Passarge E, Sutherland JM. Potter's syndrome: chromosome analysis of three cases with Potter's syndrome or related syndromes. Am J Dis Child 1965;109:80–84.

72. Bain AD, Scott JS. Renal agenesis and severe urinary tract dysplasia: a review of 50 cases, with particular reference to associated anomalies. Br Med J 1960;1:841–846.

73. Thompson VM. Amnion nodosum. J Obstet Gynaecol Br Commw 1960;67:611–614.

74. Bain AD, Beath MM, Flint WF. Sirenomelia and monomelia with renal agenesis and amnion nodosum. Arch Dis Child 1960;35:250–253.

75. Bryans AM, Balis JU, Haust MD. Amnion nodosum: report of a case. Am J Obstet Gynecol 1962;84:582–585.

76. Woolf RB, Allen WM. The frequent simultaneous occurrence of congenital malformations of the reproductive and urinary tracts. Obstet Gynecol 1953;2:236–265.

77. Doroshow LW, Abeshouse BS. Congenital unilateral solitary kidney: report of 37 cases and a review of the literature. Urol Surv 1961;11:219.

78. Fortune CH. The pathological and clinical significance of congenital one-sided kidney defect, with the presentation of three new cases of agenesia and one of aplasia. Ann Intern Med 1927;1:377–399.

79. Collins DC. Congenital unilateral renal agenesia. Ann Surg 1932;95:715–726.

80. Longo VJ, Thompson GJ. Congenital solitary kidney. J Urol 1952;68:63–68.

81. Nation EF. Renal aplasia: a study of sixteen cases. J Urol 1944;51:579–586.

82. Gutierrez R. Surgical aspects of renal agenesis with special reference to hypoplastic kidney, renal aplasia and congenital absence of one kidney. Arch Surg 1933;27:686–735.

83. Ballowitz E. Ueber angebornen, einseitigen, vollkommenen Neirenmangel. Virchow Arch Path Anat 1895;141:309–390.

84. Gérard G. Les anomalies congénitales du rein chez l'homme: essai de classification d'après 527 cas. J Anat Physiol 1905;41:241, 411.

85. Boyden EA. Congenital absence of the kidney: an interpretation based on a 10-mm human embryo exhibiting unilateral renal agenesis. Anat Rec 1932;52:325–349.

86. Morgagni JB. The seats and causes of disease investigated by anatomy. B. Alexander (transl). New York: Hafner Publishing, 1960.

87. Hain AM, Robertson EM. Congenital urogenital anomalies in rats including unilateral renal agenesis. J Anat 1936;70:566–576.

88. Reis RH. Renal aplasia, ectopic ureter and vascular anomalies in a domestic cat *(Felis domestica)*. Anat Rec 1959;135:105–107.

89. Pierson DL, Grollman SS. Absence of one kidney and abnormal development of the uterus in the domestic cat. Acta Anat (Basel) 1960;40:385–390.

90. Manelli H. Richerche sperimentali sulla morfogenesi dell'apparato renale degli Anfibi Anuri: bufo bufo e rana esculenta. Arch Ital Anat Embriol 1962;66:364–382.

91. Dees JE. Prognosis of the solitary kidney. J Urol 1960;83:550–552.

92. Emanuel B, Nachwan R, Avonson N, Weiss H. Congenital solitary kidney: a review of 74 cases. J Urol 1974;111:394.

93. Parrott TS. Urologic implications of imperforate anus. Urol 1977;10:407.

94. Marc JW, Kaplan JM, Schauberger JE. Poland's syndrome: report of seven cases and a review of the literature. Clin Pediatr 1972;11:98.

95. Moore WB, Matthews TJ, Rabinowitz R. Genitourinary anomalies associated with Klippel-Feil syndrome. J Bone Joint Surg 1975;57:355.

96. Burwell RG, Kent SG. The solitary ectopic pelvic kidney: case report with a review. Br J Urol 1959;31:254–264.

97. Radasch HE. Congenital unilateral absence of the urogenital system and its relation to the development of the wolffian and müllerian ducts. Am J Med Sci 1908;136:111–118.

98. Hilson D. Malformation of ears as sign of malformation of genitourinary tract. Br Med J 1957;2:785–788.

99. Vincent RW, Fyan RF, Longenecker CG. Malformations of the ear associated with urogenital anomalies. Plast Reconstruct Surg 1961;28:214–220.

100. Waelsch SG, Rota TR. Development on organ tissue culture of kidney rudiments from mutant mouse embryos. Develop Biol 1963;7:432–444.

101. Braasch WF. The clinical diagnosis of congenital anomaly in the kidney and ureter. Ann Surg 1912;56:726–737.

102. Aristotle. Generation of animals. Peck AL (transl). Cambridge, MA: Harvard University Press (The Loeb Classical Library), 1943.

103. Poupart E. Diverse observations anatomiques. Paris: Historical Acadamy of Royal Science, 1700:35.

104. Mosler F. Beiträge zur Pathologie und Therapie der Krankheiten der Harnivege. Arch Heilk 1863;4:289.

105. Bagg HJ. Hereditary abnormalities of the viscera. I. A morphological study with special reference to abnormalities of the kidneys in the descendants of x-rayed mice. Am J Anat 1925;36:275–311.

106. Mascatello V, Liebowitz R. Malposition of the colon in left renal agenesis and ectopia. Radiology 1976;120:371.

107. Britton KE, Maisey MN. Renal radiouclide studies. In: Maisey MN, Britton KE, Gilday DL, eds. Clinical nuclear medicine. London: Chapman & Hall, 1983.

108. Williams DI, Risdon RA. Hypoplastic, dysplastic and cystic kidneys. In: Williams DI, Johnston JH, eds. Pediatric urology. London: Butterworths, 1982.

109. Thompson DP, Lynn HB. Genital anomalies associated with solitary kidney. Mayo Clin Proc 1966;41:538.

110. Portsman W. Renal angiography in children. Prog Pediatr Radiol 1970;3:51.

111. Ambrose SS, Parrott TS, Woodard JR, Campbell WG. Observations on the small kidney associated with vasicoureteral reflux. J Urol 1980;123:349.

112. Dees JE. The clinical importance of congenital anomalies of the upper urinary tract. J Urol 1941;46:659–666.

113. Smith EC, Orkin LA. A clinical and statistical study of 471 congenital anomalies of the kidney and ureter. J Urol 1945;53:11–26.

114. Kruglich T, Minnick S. Bilateral hypoplasia of the kidneys with report of case. Arizona Med 1947;4:34–36.

115. Hill WCO. Congenital abnormalities of the urinary tract in primates. Folia Primat 1964;2:111–118.

116. Scheinman JI, Abelson HT. Bilateral renal hypoplasia with oligonephonia. J Pediatr 1970;76:369.

117. Carter JE, Lireuman DS. Bilateral renal hypoplasia with oligomeganephoma: Oligomeganephonic renal hypoplasia. Am J Dis Child 1970;120:537.

118. Glassberg KI, Filmer RB. Renal dysplasia, renal hypoplasia and cystic disease of the kidney. In: Kelalis KK, King LW, Belman AB, eds. Clinical pediatric urology. Philadelphia: WB Saunders, 1985.

119. Emmett JL, Alverez-Ierena JJ, MacDonald JR. Atrophic pyelonephritis versus congenital renal hypoplasia. JAMA 1952;148:1470–1477.

120. Anson BJ, Riba LW. The anatomical and surgical features of ectopic kidney. Surg Gynecol Obstet 1939;68:37–44.

121. Thompson GJ, Pace JM. Ectopic kidney: a review of 97 cases. Surg Gynecol Obstet 1937;64:935–943.

122. Strube G. Ueber congenitale Lage und bildungsanomalien der Nieren. Virchow Arch [A] 1894;137:227–264.

123. Fowler HA. Bilateral renal ectopia: report of 4 cases. J Urol 1941;45:795–812.

124. Culp OS. Treatment of horseshoe kidneys. Ann Surg 1944;119:777–787.

125. Anderson GW, Rice GG, Harris BA Jr. Pregnancy and labor complicated by pelvic ectopic kidney anomalies. Obstet Gynecol Surv 1949;4:737–769.

126. Cragin EB. Congenital pelvic kidneys obstructing the parturient canal. Am J Obstet 1898;38:36–41.

127. Anderson GW, Rice GG, Harris BA Jr. Pregnancy and labor complicated by pelvic ectopic kidney. J Urol 1951;65:760–776.

128. Frančisković V, Martinčić N. Intrathoracic kidney. Br J Urol 1959;31:156–158.

129. Barloon JW, Goodwin WE, Vermooten V. Thoracic kidney: case reports. J Urol 1957;78:356–358.

130. Shapira E, Fishel E, Levin S. Intrathoracic kidney in a premature infant. Arch Dis Child 1965;40:86–88.

131. Fusonie D, Molnar W. Anomalous pulmonary venous return, pulmonary sequestration, bronchial atresia, aplastic right upper lobe,

pericardial defect and intrathoracic kidney: an unusual complex of congenital anomalies in one patient. AJR 1966;97:350–353.

132. Spillane RJ, Prather GC. High renal ectopy: a case report. J Urol 1949;62:441–445.

133. Hill JE, Bunts RC. Thoracic kidney: case report. J Urol 1960;84:460–462.

134. Paul ATS, Uragoda CG, Jayewardene FLW. Thoracic kidney with a report of a case. Br J Surg 1960;47:395–397.

135. Kelalis PP. Anomalies of the urinary tract. In: Kelalis KK, King LW, Belman AB, eds. Clinical pediatric urology. Philadelphia: WB Saunders, 1985.

136. Malek RS, Kelalis PP, Burke EC. Ectopic kidney in children and frequency of association of other malformations. Mayo Clin Proc 1971;46:461.

137. Potampa PB, Hyman MD, Catlow CA. An unusual renal anomaly: combined tandem and horseshoe kidney. J Urol 1949;61:340–343.

138. Paoletti M. Crossed dystopia. Ann Radiol Diagn (Bologna) 1950;22:276–298.

139. Pia R. Crossed ectopy of the left kidney: supernumerary right kidney. Urologia 1951;19:284–286.

140. Sebening W. In welchen Darmabschnitt wird das Avertin wirksam resorbeirt? Erwiderung auf die Mitteilung von L Treplin Zentralbl Chir 1930;57:1539–1540.

141. Konrad J, Kubik M, Pour S. Voluminous retroperitioneal cyst associated with double homolateral kidney. Cas Lek Cesk 1949;88:16–20.

142. Ghoshal L. A case of both kidneys on the right side with total absence of kidney on the left side. Indian Med Gaz Calcutta 1905;40:58.

143. Bugbee HG, Losee JR. The clinical significance of congenital anomalies of the kidney and ureter with notes on the embryology and foetal development of the kidney. Surg Gynecol Obstet 1919;28:97–116.

144. Diaz G. Renal ectopy: report of a case of crossed ectopy without fusion with fixation of kidney in normal position by the extraperitoneal route. J Int Coll Surg 1953;19:158–169.

145. Alexander JC, King KB, Fromm CS. Congenital solitary kidney with crossed ureter. J Urol 1950;64:230–234.

146. Magri J. Solitary crossed ectopic kidney. Br J Urol 1961;33:152–156.

147. Purpon I. Crossed renal ectopy with solitary kidney: a review of the literature. J Urol 1963;90:13–15.

148. Joly JS. Fusion of the kidneys. Proc Roy Soc Med 1940;33:697–706.

149. Panaroli D. Iatrologismorum seu medicinalium observationum pentecostae quinque, utilibus praeceptis, singularibut medelis, reconditis, speculationibus, portentosis casibus refertae, quibus diversa, eaque curisa (prout adversa pagina indicabit) in calce adduntur opuscula. Hanover [Hanoviae]: J Bayer, 1654.

150. Wilmer HA. Unilateral fused kidney: a report of five cases and a review of the literature. J Urol 1938;40:551–571.

151. Voelker F, von Lichtenberg A. Pyelographie. München Med Wschr 1906;53:105.

152. Abeshouse BS. Crossed ectopia with fusion. Am J Surg 1947;73:658–683.

153. McDonald JH, McClellen DS. Crossed renal ectopia. Am J Surg 1957;93:995–1002.

154. Rokitansky C. Lehrbuch der pathologische Anatomie, Vol 3. Vienna [Wein]: W Brumüller, 1861.

155. Lee HP. Crossed unfused renal ectopia with tumor. J Urol 1949;61:333–339.

156. Caine M. Crossed renal ectopia without fusion. Br J Urol 1956;28:257–258.

157. Ma YC, Li CA, Wu CW. Congenital crossed ectopia of left kidney without fusion: a case report. J Chin Surg 1955;3:615–619.

158. Shih HE, Sun WH, Chén HK. Crossed unfused renal ectopia. Chin Med J (Peking) 1957;75:841–848.

159. Winram RG, Ward-McQuaid JN. Crossed renal ectopia without fusion. Can Med Assoc J 1959;81:481–483.

160. Burford EH, Burford CE. Crossed renal ectopia: report of 9 cases and review of the literature. Missouri Med 1957;54:237–240.

161. Thompson GJ, Allen RB. Unilateral fused kidney. Surg Clin North Am 1934;14:729–742.

162. Hillenbrand HJ. Retropneumoperitoneum in crossed renal dystopia. Z Urol 1953;46:485–486.

163. Weyrauch HM Jr. Anomalies of renal rotation. Surg Gynecol Obstet 1939;69:183–199.

164. Jeune M, Bertrand J, Deffrenne P, Forget H. Fréquence des malformation de l'arbre urinaire au cours du syndrome de Turner. Pediatrie 1962;17:897–907.

165. Hung W, LoPresti JM. Urinary tract anomalies in gonadal dysgenesis. AJR 1965;95:439–441.

166. Guggemos E, Nystrom BA, Peppy SJ, Sinatra C, Brody H. A rare case of arterial connection between the left and right kidneys. Ann Surg 1962;156:940–943.

167. Meek JR, Wadsworth GH. A case of horseshoe kidney lying between the great vessels. J Urol 1940;43:448–451.

168. Jarman WD. Surgery of the horseshoe kidney with a postaortic isthmus: report of two cases of horseshoe kidney. J Urol 1938;40:1–9.

169. Durham AE. Misplacement and mobility of the kidneys in reference to the diagnosis of abdominal tumors. Guy Hosp Rep 1860;6:404–420.

170. Perruchot EV, Courbin. Rein unique en fer à cheval avec deux hiles. J Med Bordeaux 1913;43:420.

171. Papin E. Valeur de la phénolphtaleine comme moyen d'exploration de la fonction rénale. J Urol Med Chir 1922;13:33–37.

172. Beer E, Mencher WH. Heminephrectomy in disease of the double kidney: report of fourteen cases. Ann Surg 1938;108:705–729.

173. Zondek T. Notes on the topography of the fetal horseshoe kidney. Br J Urol 1952;24:201–206.

174. Boyden EA. Description of a horseshoe kidney associated with left inferior vena cava and disc-shaped suprarenal glands, together with a note on the occurance of horseshoe kidneys in human embryos. Anat Rec 1931;51:187–211.

175. daCarpi JB. Isagogae breves Balogna 1522 [A short introduction to anatomy]. Lind LR (transl). Chicago: University of Chicago Press, 1959.

176. Botallo L. De catarrho commentarius: addita est in fine monstrorum renum figura, nuper in cadauere repertorum. Paris, 1564.

177. Benjamin JA, Schullian DM. Observations on fused kidneys with horseshoe configuration: the contribution of Leonardo Botallo (1564). J Hist Med 1950;5:315–326.

178. Glenn JF. Analysis of 51 patients with horseshoe kidneys. N Engl J Med 1959;261:684–687.

179. Zondek LH, Zondek T. Horseshoe kidney and associated congenital malformations. Urol Int 1964;18:347.

180. Segura JW, Kelalis PP, Burke EC. Horseshoe kidney in children. J Urol 1972;108:333.

181. Boatman DL, Kolln CP, Flocks RH. Congenital anomalies associated with horseshoe kidney. J Urol 1972;107:205.

182. Dische MR, Johnston R. Teratoma in horseshoe kidneys. Urology 1979;13:435.

183. Williams DI. Anomalies of the kidney. In: Pediatric urology. London: Butterworth, 1982.

184. Gutierrez R. The clinical management of horseshoe kidney. New York: Paul B Hoeber, 1934.

185. Bell ET. Renal diseases, 2nd ed. Philadelphia: Lea & Febiger, 1950.

186. Martinow A. Operatiner Eingriff bei Hufeisenmiere. Z Chir Leipz 1910;39:134–136.

187. Rovsing T. Beiträge zur Symptomatologie, Diagnose und Behandlung der Hufeisenniere. Zentralbl Chir 1911;38:407.

188. Donahue PF. Division of horseshoe kidney for relief of ureteropelvic obstruction. J Urol 1932;27:59–72.

189. Woodard JW. Renal ectopia and fusion anomalies. In: Glenn JR, ed. Urologic surgery. Hagerstown, MD: Harper & Row, 1975:143.

190. Pitts WR, Mueka EC. Horseshoe kidneys: a 40-year experience. J Urol 1975;113:743.

191. Shoup GD, Pollack HM, Dou JH. Adenocarcinoma occurring in a horseshoe kidney. Arch Surg 1962;84:413–420.

192. Beck WC, Hilvko AE. Wilms' tumor in the isthmus of a horseshoe kidney. Arch Surg 1960;81:803–806.

193. Morris H. Surgical diseases of the kidney and ureter, Vol 1. London: Cassel, 1901.

194. Kron SD, Meranze DR. Completely fused pelvic kidney. J Urol 1949;62:278–285.

195. Looney WW, Dodd, DL. An ectopic (pelvic) completely fused (cake) kidney associated with various anomalies of the abdominal viscera. Ann Surg 1926;84:522–524.

196. Graves FT. The anatomy of the intrarenal arteries and their application to segmental resection of the kidneys. Br J Surg 1954;42:132–139.

197. Graves FT. The aberrant renal artery. J Anat 1956;90:553–558.

198. Merklin RJ, Michels NA. The variant renal and suprarenal blood supply with data on inferior phrenic, ureteral and gonadal arteries. J Int Coll Surg 1958;29:41–76.

199. Reis RH, Essenther G. Variation in the pattern of renal vessels and their relation to the type of posterior vena cava in man. Am J Anat 1959;104:295–318.

200. Geyer JR, Poutasse EF. Incidence of multiple renal arteries on aortography. JAMA 1962;182:120–125.

201. Anson BJ, Daseler EH. Common variation in renal anatomy affecting blood supply, form, and topography. Surg Gynecol Obstet 1961;112:439–449.

202. Nathan H. Aberrant renal artery producing developmental anomaly of kidney associated with unusual course of gonadal (ovarian) vessels. J Urol 1963;89:570–572.

203. Neidhardt JH, Bouchet A, Morin A, Guelpa G, Giraud R. A génésies rénales et malformations associeés. Bull Assoc Anat 1967;136:718–728.

204. Bernstein J, Gardner KD Jr. Cystic disease of the kidney and renal dysplasia. In: Harrison JH, ed. Campbell's urology, Vol 2, 4th 3d. Philadelphia: WB Saunders, 1979:1399.

205. Spence HM, Singleton R. What is sponge kidney disease and where does it fit in the spectrum of cystic disorders? J Urol 1972;107:176.

206. Osathanondh V, Potter EL. Pathogenesis of polycystic kidneys: historical survey. Arch Pathol 1964;77:459–465.

207. Stephens FD. Congenital malformations of the rectum, anus, and genito-urinary tracts. Edinburgh: E & S Livingstone, 1963.

208. Virchow R. Discussion über den vortrag des Herrn A. Ewald: Zur totalen cysteschen Degeneration der Nieren. Lin Wschr 1892;29:104.

209. Hanau L. Ueber congenitale Cystennieren [Inaug Dissert]. Munich: C Geissen, 1890.

210. Hildebrand A. Weiterer Beitrag zur pathologischen Anatomie der Nierengeschwülste. Arch Klin Chir 1894;48:343–371.

211. Brigdi V, Severi A. Contributo alla patogenesi delle cisti renale. Le Sperimentale 1880;46:1.

212. McKinlay CA. Epithelial hyperplasia in congenital cystic kidneys. J Urol 1920;4:195–207.

213. Beeson HG. Polycystic disease in a premature infant. J Urol 1933;30:285–298.

214. von Mutach A. Beitrag zur Genese der congenitalen Cystennieren. Virchow Arch [A] 1895;142:46–86.

215. Lambert PP. Polycystic disease of the kidney: a review. Arch Pathol 1947;44:34–58.

216. Norris RF, Herman L. The pathogenesis of polycystic kidneys: reconstruction of cystic elements in four cases. J Urol 1941;46:147–176.

217. Rall JE, Odel HM. Congenital polycystic disease of the kidney: review of the literature and data on 207 cases. Am J Med Sci 1949;218, 399–407.

218. Spence HM. Congenital unilateral multicystic kidney: an entity to be distinguished from polycystic kidney disease and other cystic disorders. J Urol 1955;74:693–706.

219. Osathanondh V, Potter EL. Pathogenesis of polycystic kidneys type 1 due to hyperplasia of interstitial portions of collecting tubules. Arch Pathol 1964;77:466–473.

220. Osathanondh V, Potter EL. Pathogenesis of polycystic kidneys type 2 due to inhibition of ampullary activity. Arch Pathol 1964;77:474–484.

221. Osathanoondh V, Potter EL. Pathogenesis of polycystic kidneys type 3 due to multiple abnormalities of development. Arch Pathol 1964;77:485–501.

222. Osathanondh V, Potter EL. Pathogenesis of polycystic kidneys type 4 due to urethral obstruction. Arch Pathol 1964;77:502–509.

223. DeWeerd JH, Simon HB. Simple renal cysts in children. J Urol 1956;75:912–921.

224. Carson WJ. Solitary cysts of the kidney. Ann Surg 1928;87:250–256.

225. Hepler AB. Solitary cysts of the kidney: report of 7 cases and observations on pathogenesis of these cysts. Surg Gynecol Obstet 1930;50:668–687.

226. Kampmeier OF. A hitherto unrecognized mode of origin of congenital renal cyst. Surg Gynecol Obstet 1923;36:208–216.

227. Hildanus F. Opera omnia. Frankfurt: J Bejerus, 1646.

228. Rayer PFC. Traité des maladies des reins et des altérations de la sécrétion urinaire, 3 Vols. Paris: 1837–1841.

229. Laveren A. De la degenerescence kystique des reins chez l'adulte. Gaz Hedb Med Chir 1876;63:756–776.

230. Harpster CM, Brown TH, Delcher HA. Abnormalities of the kidney and ureter: a case of double kidney and double ureter with a review of the literature. J Urol 1922;8:459–490.

231. Scott HH. Congenital malformations of the kidney in reptiles, birds, and mammals. Proc Zool Soc Lond 1925;95:1259–1270.

232. Bartholomew TH, Slovis TL, Kroovand RL. The sonographic evaluation and management of simple renal cysts in children. J Urol 1980;123:732.

233. Joshi VV. Cystic, partially differentiated nephroblastomas: an entity in the spectrum of infantile renal neoplasia. Perspect Pediatr Pathol 1980;5:217.

234. Beckwith JB, Palmer NF. Histopathology and prognosis of Wilms' tumor: results from First National Wilms' Tumor Study. Cancer 1978;41:1937.

235. Bernstein J. Developmental abnormalities of the renal parenchyma: renal hypoplasia and dysplasia. In: Sommies SC, ed. Pathology annual. New York: Appleton-Century-Crafts, 1968.

236. Risdon RA. Renal dysplasia. I. A clinicopathological study of 76 cases. J Clin Pathol 1971;24:57.

237. Ericcson NO, Ivemark BI. Renal dysplasia and pyelonephritis in infants and children. Arch Pathol 1958;66:255.

238. Berstein J. The morphogenesis of renal parenchymal maldevelopment (renal dysplasia). Pediatr Clin North Am 1971;18:395.

239. Ask-Upmark E. Uber juvinile molgne Nephrosklerose und ihr Verhaltuis 3u storangen in der nierenentwicklung. Acta Pathol Microbiol Scand 1929;6:383.

240. Habid R, Courtecuisse V, Ehrenspeager J. Hypoplasie segmentaire du rein aver hypertension arterielle chez l'enfant. Am Pediatr (Paris) 1965;12:262.

241. Arant BS, Sotelo-Anile C, Bernstein J. Segmental hypoplasia of the kidney (Ask-Upmark). J Pediatr 1979;95:931.

242. Green LF, Feinzaig W, Dahlin DC. Multicystic dysplasia of the kidney with special reference to the contralateral kidney. J Urol 1971;105:482.

243. DeKlerk D, Marshall FF, Jeffs RD. Multicystic dysplastic kidney. J Urol 1977;118:306.

244. Longino LA, Martin LW. Abdominal masses in the newborn infant. Pediatr 1958;21:596.

245. Parrott TS, Woodard JR, Hawkins B, Mendleson M. Spot uropathy earlier with ultrasound. Contemp Obstet Gynecol 1985;27(6):101.

246. Hartman GE, Swalik LM, Shochat SJ. The dilemma of the multicystic dysplastic kidney. Am J Dis Child 1986;140:925.

247. Ambrose SS, Gould RA, Trulock TS, Parrott TS. Unilateral multicystic renal disease in adults. J Urol 1982;128:366.

248. Stuck KJ, Koff SA, Silver TM. Ultrasonic features of multicystic dysplastic kidney: expanded diagnostic criteria. Radiology 1982;143:217.

249. Bloom DA, Brosman S. The multicystic kidney. J Urol 1978;120:211.

250. Felson B, Cussen LJ. The hydronephrotic type of congenital multicystic disease of the kidney. Semin Roentenol 1975;10:113.

251. Stanisic TH. Review of "the dilemma of the multicystic dysplastic kidney" [Editorial]. Am J Dis Child 1986;140:865.

252. Betts EK. Anesthesia in the neonate and young infant. Dialog Pediatr Urol 1981;4(12):3–8.

253. Yow RM, Bunts RC. Calyceal diverticulum. J Urol 1955;73:663–670.

254. Moore T. Hydrocalicosis. Br J Urol 1950;22:304–319.

255. Kretschmer HL, Doehring C. Adenoma of the kidney. Surg Gynecol Obstet 1929;48:629–634.

256. Taxy VJ, Filmer RB. Glomerulo-cystic kidney. Arch Pathol Lab Med 1976;100:186.

257. Cacchi R, Ricci V. Sur une rare maladie kystique multiple des pyramides rénales le "rein en éponge." J Urol (Paris) 1949;55:497–519.

258. Lenarduzzi G. Reperto pielografico poco comune (dilatozione delta vie urinaire intrarenali). Radiol Med Torino 1939;26:346–347.

259. Abeshouse BS, Abeshouse GA. Sponge kidney: a review of the literature and report of five cases. J Urol 1960;84:252–267.

260. Ekström T, Engfeldt B. Lagergren C, Lindvall N. Medullary sponge kidney. Stockholm: Almgrist & Wiksell, 1959.

261. Felts JH, Headley RN, Whitley JE, Yount EH. Medullary sponge kidneys: clinical appraisal. JAMA 1964;188:233–236.

262. Miller F. Sponge kidney: report of a case in a 70-year-old man. J Urol 1962;87:770–773.

263. Murphy WK, Palubinskas AJ, Smith DR. Sponge kidney: report of 7 cases. J Urol 1961;85:866–874.

264. Chamberlain BC, Hagge WW, Stickler GK. Juvenile nephronophthisis and medullary cystic disease. Mayo Clin Proc 1977;52:485.

265. Bricker NS, Patton JF. Cystic disease: dynamics and chemical composition of cyst fluid. Am J Med 1955;18:207–219.

266. Blyth H, Ockenden BG. Polycystic disease of kidneys and liver presenting in childhood. J Med Genet 1971;8:257.

267. Advisory Committee to the Renal Transplant Registry. The 11th report of the Human Transplant Registry. JAMA 1973;226:1197.

268. Dalgaard OZ. Bilateral polycystic disease of the kidneys. Acta Med Scand 1957;32(Suppl):13–155.

269. Grantham JJ. Polycystic renal disease. In: Earley LE, Gottschalk CW, eds. Strauss and Welt's diseases of the kidney. Boston: Little, Brown, 1979.

270. Lindau A. Aortitis gonorrhoica ulcerosa (gonococcal endaortitis with the formation of an aneurism). Acta Pathol Microbiol Scand 1924;1:263–275.

271. Bigelow NH. The association of polycystic kidneys with intracranial aneurysms and other related disorders. Am J Med Sci 1953;225:485–494.

272. Steiner. Ueber grosscystiche Degeneration der Nieren und der Leber. Deutsch Med Wschr 1899;25:677–678.

273. Cairns HWB. Heredity in polycystic disease of the kidneys. Q J Med 1925;18:359–393.

274. Goldstein AE. Polycystic renal disease with particular reference to author's surgical procedure. J Urol 1951;66:163–172.

275. Arrigoni G, Cresseri A, Lovati G. Richerche genetiche sul rene policistico. Ium Sumposium Internationale Geneticae Medicae, 1954.

276. Meckel JF. Beschreibung Zweier, durch sehr ähnliche Bildungs-Ab-weichungen entstellter Geschwister. Deutsch Arch Physiol 1822;7:99–172.

277. Braasch WF. Clinical data of polycystic kidney. Surg Gynecol Obstet 1916;23:697–702.

278. Braasch WF, Schacht FW. Pathological and clinical data concerning polycystic kidney. Surg Gynecol Obstet 1933;57:467–475.

279. Simon HB, Thompson GJ. Congenital renal polycystic disease. JAMA 1955;159:657–662.

280. Küster E. Die chirurgische Frankheiten der Nieren. Stuttgart: A Bonz, 1902.

281. Billing L. The roentgen diagnosis of polycystic kidneys. Acta Radiol 1954;41:305–315.

282. Rovsing T. The treatment of multilocular kidney cystoma (congenital cystic kidney) by means of multiple punctures. Am J Urol 1912;8:120–124.

283. Meltzer M. Echinococcus cysts of the kidney. Am J Surg 1929;7:418–423.

284. Walters W, Braasch WF. Surgical aspects of polycystic kidney. Surg Gynecol Obstet 1934;58:647–650.

285. Steinmuller DR. Evaluation and selection of candidates for renal transplantation. Urol Clin North Am 1983;10:217.

286. Weidner O. Die polycystiche Degeneration der Nieren, ihre Klinishen Symptome und ihre Bedeutung als Erbkrankheit. Z Urol 1938;32:339–344.

287. Okada RD, Platt MA, Fleishman J. Chronic renal failure in patients with tuberous sclerosis association with renal cysts. Nephron 1982;30:85–88.

288. Richmond WS. Abnormal ureters. J Anat Physiol 1885;19:120.

289. Malament M, Schwartz B, Nagamatsu GR. Extrarenal calyces: their relationship to renal disease. AJR 1961;86:823–829.

290. Williams DI, Kenawi JM. The prognosis of pelviureteric obstruction in childhood: a review of 190 cases. Eur Urol 1976;2:57.

291. King LR, Coughlin PW, Bloch EC. The case for immediate pyeloplasty in the neonate with ureteropelvic junction obstruction. J Urol 1984;132:725.

292. Roth DR, Gonzales ET. Management of ureteropelvic junction obstruction in infants. J Urol 1983;129:108.

293. Johnston JH, Evans JP, Glassberg KO, Shapiro SR. Pelvic hydroephrosis in children: a review of 219 personal cases. J Urol 1977;117:97.

294. Lebowitz RL, Griscom NT. Neonatal hydronephrosis: 146 cases. Radiol Clin North Am 1977;15:49.

295. Hanna MK, Jeffs RD, Sturgess JM, Barkin M. Congenital ureteropelvic junction obstruction and primary obstructive megaureter. J Urol 1976;116:725.

296. Ruano-Gil D, Coca-Payeros A, Tejedo-Maten A. Obstruction and recanalization of the ureter in the human embryo: its relation to congenital ureteric obstruction. Eur Urol 1975;1:287.

297. Whitaker RH. Some observations and theories on the wide ureter and hydronephrosis. Br J Urol 1975;47:377.

298. Kelalis PP. Renal pelvis and ureter. In: Kelalis KK, King LW, Belman AB, eds. Clinical pediatric urology. Philadelphia: WB Saunders, 1985.

299. Johnston JH. The pathogenesis of hydronephrosis in children. Br J Urol 1969;41:724.

300. Maizels M, Stephens FD. Valves of the ureter as a cause of primary obstruction of the ureter. J Urol 1980;123:742.

301. Nixon HH. Hydronephrosis in children: a clinical study of 78 cases with special reference to the role of aberrant renal vessels and the results of conservative operations. Br J Surg 1953;40:601.

302. Hutch JA, Hinman F Jr., Miller ER. Reflux as a cause of hydronephrosis and chronic pyelonephritis. J Urol 1962;88:169.

303. Kelalis PP, Culp OS, Stickler GB, Burke EG. Ureteropelvic obstruction in children: experiences with 109 cases. J Urol 1971;106:98.

304. Williams DI, Karloftis CM. Hydronephrosis due to pelviureteric obstruction in the newborn. Br J Urol 1966;38:138.

305. Grossman IC, Cromie WJ, Wein AJ. Renal hypertension secondary to uretero-pelvic junction obstruction. Urology 1981;17:69.

306. Lupton EW, Testa HJ, O'Reilly PH. Diuresis renography and morphology in upper urinary tract obstruction. Br J Urol 1979;51:10.

307. Koff SA, Thrall JH, Keyes JW Jr. Diuretic radionuclide urography: a non-invasive method for evaluating nephroureteral dilatation. J Urol 1979;121:153.

308. Whitaker RH. Methods of assessing obstruction in dilated ureters. Br J Urol 1973;45:15.

309. Wolpert JJ, Woodard JR, Parrott TS. Pyeloplasty in the young infant. J Urol 1989;142:573–575.

310. Saxton HM. Percutaneous nephrostomy: technique. Urol Radiol 1981;2:131.

311. Anderson JC. Hydronephrosis: a 14 years' survey of results. Proc Roy Soc Med 1962;55:93.

312. Mayor G, Genton N, Torrado A. Renal function in obstructive nephropathy: long-term effect of reconstructive surgery. Pediatriatrics 1975;56:740.

313. Campbell MF. Urology. Philadelphia: WB Saunders, 1954.

314. Harris A. Ureteral anomalies with special reference to partial duplication with one branch ending blindly. J Urol 1937;38:442–454.

315. Hanlon FR. A rare anomaly of the ureter. J Urol 1929;21:123–127.

316. Kreutzmann HA. Unusual ureteral anomaly. J Urol 1937;38:67–73.

317. Smith I. Triplicate ureter. Br J Surg 1946;34:182–185.

318. Wrany H. Verdoppelung eines Ureters. Ost Jh Peadiat 1870;1:105–110.

319. Perrin WS. Ectopic kidney with triple ureter removed from a man, aged 41. Proc Roy Soc Med 1927;20:1806–1807.

320. Spangler EB. Complete triplication of the ureter. Radiology 1963;80:795–979.

321. Ringer MG Jr, MacFarlan SM. Complete triplication of the ureter: a case report. J Urol 1964;92:429–430.

322. MacKelvie AA. Triplicate ureter: case report. Br J Urol 1955;27:124.

323. Gill RD. Triplication of the ureter and renal pelvis. J Urol 1952;68:140–147.

324. Neimeyer CE. Singularis in foetu puellari recens edito abnormitatis exemplum descriptum et illustratum [Inaug Dissert]. Halle, 1814.

325. Fürstner C. Zwei seltene Fälle von Concrementbildung in den Harnorganen. Virchow Arch [A] 1874;59:401–406.

326. Mackie GG, Stephens FD. Duplex kidneys: a correlation of renal dysplasia with position of the ureteral orifice. J Urol 1975;114:274.

327. Wharton LR. Double ureter and associated renal anomalies in early human embryos. Contrib Embryol Carnegie Inst Wash 1949;33:103–112.

328. Frazer JE. The terminal part of the wolffian duct. J Anat 1935;69:455–468.

329. Dougherty J. Duplication of the upper part of the urinary tract. J Int Coll Surg 1954;21:160–166.

330. Nordmark B. Double formations of the pelves of the kidneys and the ureters: embryology, occurrence and clinical significance. Acta Radiol 1948;30:267–278.

331. Nation EF. Duplication of the kidney and ureter: a statistical study of 230 new cases. J Urol 1944;51:456–465.

332. Braasch WF, Scholl AJ Jr. Primary tumors of urethra. Ann Surg 1922;76:246–259.

333. Harpster CM, Brown TH, Delcher A. Solitary unilateral large serous cysts of the kidney with report of two cases and review of the literature. J Urol 1924;11:157–175.

334. Johnston JH. Urinary tract duplication in childhood. Arch Dis Child 1961;36:180–189.

335. Payne RA. Clinical significance of reduplicated kidneys. Br J Urol 1959;31:141–149.

336. Ambrose SS, Nicholson WP III. The causes of vesicoureteral reflux in children. J Urol 1962;87:688–694.

337. Lenaghan D. Bifid ureters in children: an anatomical, physiological and clinical study. J Urol 1962;87:808–817.

338. Samuuels A. Kern H, Sachs L. Supernumerary kidney with ureter opening into vagina. Surg Gynecol Obstet 1922;35:599–603.

339. Camina R. La concentración maxima en casos de riñónes suplementarios. Med Ibera Madrid 1920;12:216–219.

340. Rubin JS. Supernumerary kidney with aberrant ureter terminating externally. J Urol 1948;60:405–408.

341. Neckarsulmer K. Ueber Beinieren. Klin Wschr (Berlin) 1914;51:1641–1643.

342. Blasius G. Observations medicae rariores: accedit monstri triplicis historia. Amsterdam [Amstelodami]: Abraham Wolfgang, 1656.

343. Krestschmer HL. Supernumerary kidney: report of case with review of literature. Surg Gynecol Obstet 1929;49:818–831.

344. Geisinger JF. Supernumerary kidney. J Urol 1937;38:331–356.

345. Exley M, Hotchkiss WS. Supernumerary kidney with clear-cell carcinoma. J Urol 1944;51:569–578.

346. Carlson HE. Supernumerary kidney: a summary of 51 reported cases. J Urol 1950;64:224–229.

347. Clifford AB. Two cases of abnormal kidney. US Navy Med Bull 1908;2:37–39.

348. Alvarez L. Doble ureter con agenesia parcial renal. An Desarrollo 1962;10:325–330.

349. Pierro JA, Soleimanpour M, Bory JL. Left retrocaval ureter associated with left inferior vena cava. AJR 1990;155:545–546.

350. Fernandez M, Scheuch J, Seebode JJ. Horseshoe kidney with retrocaval ureter: a case report. J Urol 1988;140:362–364.

351. Gladstone J. Acardiac fetus (acephalus omphalositicus). J Anat Physiol 1905;40:71–80.

352. Gruenwald P, Surks SN. Preureteric vena cava and its embryological explanation. J Urol 1943;49:195–201.

353. Pick JW, Anson BJ. Retrocaval ureter: report of a case with a discussion of its clinical significance. J Urol 1940;43:672–685.

354. McClure CFW, Butler EG. The development of the vena cava inferior in man. Am J Anat 1925;35:331–383.

355. Huntington GS. Harvey lectures. Philadelphia: JB Lippincott, 1906–1907.

356. Hochstetter F. Entwicklungeschichte des Venensystems der Amnioten. Morphol Jahrb 1893;20:543.

357. Kimbrough JC. Surgical treatment of hydronephrosis. J Urol 1935;33:97–107.

358. Cathro AJMcG. Section of inferior vena cava for retrocaval ureter. J Urol 1952;67:464–475.

359. Rowland HS Jr, Bunts RC, Iwana JH. Operative correction of retrocaval ureter: a report of four cases and review of the literature. J Urol 1960;83:820–833.

360. Spaziante G. Uretere retrocavale. Urolgia 1964;31(Suppl):88–99.

361. Varma KT. Transitional carcinoma associated with retrocaval ureter. J Okla State Med Assoc 1989;82:463–645.

362. Heslin JE, Mamonas C. Retrocaval ureter: report of four cases and review of literature. J Urol 1951;65:212–222.

363. Hradcová L, Kafka V. Retrocaval ureter in childhood. Urol Int 1963;16:103–116.

364. Laughlin V. Retrocaval (circumcaval) ureter associated with solitary kidney. J Urol 1954;71:195–199.

365. Duff PA. Retrocaval ureter: case report. J Urol 1950;63:496–499.

366. Presman D, Firfer R. A diagnostic method for retrocaval ureter. Am J Surg 1956;92:628–631.

367. Harrill HC. Retrocaval ureter: report of a case with operative correction of the defect. J Urol 1940;44:450–457.

368. Goodwin WE, Burke DE, Muller WH. Retrocaval ureter. Surg Gynecol Obstet 1957;104:337–345.

369. Mayer RF, Mathes GL. Retrocaval ureter. South Med J 1958;51:945–950.

370. Voekel HH. Retrocaval course of the right ureter. Z Urol 1963;56:49–60.

371. Lowsley OS. Postcaval ureter with description of a new operation for its correction. Surg Gynecol Obstet 1946;82:549–556.

372. Dees JE. Anomalous relationship between ureter and external iliac artery. J Urol 1940;44:207–215.

373. Seitzman DM, Patton JF. Ureteral ectopia: combined ureteral and vas deferens anomaly. J Urol 1960;84:604–608.

374. Corbus BC, Estrem RD, Hunt W. Retro-iliac ureter. J Urol 1960;84:67–68.

375. Hanna MK. Bilateral retroiliac artery ureters. Br J Urol 1972;44:335.

376. Nguyen DH, Koleilat N, Gonzalez R. Retroiliac ureter in a male newborn with multiple genitourinary anomalies: case report and review of the literature. J Urol 1989;141:1400–1403.

377. Williams JL, Goodwin WE. Congenital multiple diverticula of the ureter. Br J Urol 1965;37:299–301.

378. Pratt JG, Gahagan HQ, Fichman JL. Diverticulum of the ureter: a review of the literature and a report of two additional cases. J Urol 1947;58:322–326.

379. Rathbun NP. Bilateral diverticula of the ureter. J Urol 1927;18:347–362.

380. Richardson EH. Diverticulum of the ureter: a collective review with report of a unique example. J Urol 1942;47:535–570.

381. McGraw AB, Culp OS. Diverticulum of the ureter: report of another authentic case. J Urol 1952;67:262–265.

382. Rank WB, Mellinger GT, Spiro E. Ureteral diverticula: etiologic consideration. J Urol 1960;83:566–569.

383. Wölfler A. Neue Beiträge zur chirurgischen Pathologie der Nieren. Arch Klin Chir 1887;21:694–725.

384. Wall B, Wachter E. Congenital ureteral valve: its role as a primary obstructive lesion, classification of the literature and report of an authentic case. J Urol 1952;68:684–690.

385. Passaro E Jr, Smith JP. Congenital ureteral valve in children: a case report. J Urol 1960;84:290–292.

386. Finby N, Begg CF. Congenital ureteral valves. NY J Med 1963;63:1827–1830.

387. Simon HB, Culp OS, Parkhill EM. Congenital ureteral valves: report of two cases. J Urol 1955;74:336–341.

388. Chwalle R. The process of formation of cystic dilatations of the vesical end of the ureter and of diverticula at the ureteral ostium. Urol Cutan Rev 1927;31:499–504.

389. Vermooten V. A new etiology for certain types of the dilated ureters in children. J Urol 1939;41:455–463.

390. Roux C, Dupuis R. Anomalies urogénitales par carence pantothénique. C R Soc Biol (Paris) 1961;155:2105–2106.

391. Ostry H. Hypertension associated with congenital ureteral valve. J Urol 1948;60:738–742.

392. Foroughi E, Turner JA. Congenital ureteral valve. J Urol 1959;81:272–274.

393. Docimo SG, Lebowitz RL, Coldny AH. Congenital midureteral obstruction. Urol Radiol 1989;11:156–160.

394. Allen TD. Congenital ureteral strictures. J Urol 1970;104:196.

395. Lewis EL, Kimbrough JC. Megaloureter: new concept in treatment. South Med J 1952;45:171–177.

396. Creevy CD. The atonic distal ureteral segment (ureteral achalasia). J Urol 1967;97:457–463.

397. Hendren WH. Functional restoration of decompensated ureters in children. Am J Surg 1970;119:477–482.

398. Hendren WH. Recent advances in the management of low urinary obstruction in the newborn. Prog Pediatr Surg 1971;2:115–145.

399. Caulk JR. Megalo-ureter: the importance of ureterovesical valve. J Urol 1923;9:315–330.

400. Leibowitz S, Bodian M. A study of the vesical ganglia in children and the relationship of the megaureter megacystic syndrome and Hirschsprung's disease. J Clin Pathol 1963;16:342–350.

401. Parrott TS, Woodard JR, Wolpert JJ. Ureteral tailoring: a comparison of wedge resection with infolding. J Urol 1990;144:328–329.

402. MacKinnon KJ, Foote JW, Wiglesworth FW. The pathology of the adynamic distal ureteral segment. Trans Am Assoc GU Surg 1969;61:63.

403. McLaughlin AP III, Leadbetter WF, Pfister RC. Reconstructive surgery of primary megaloureter. J Urol 1972;106:186.

404. Keating MA, Escala J, Snyder HM, Heyman S. Changing concepts in management of primary obstructive megaureter. J Urol 1989;142:636–640.

405. Peters CA, Mandell J, Lebowitz RL, Colodny AH. Congenital obstructed megaureters in early infance: diagnosis and treatment. J Urol 1989;142:641–645.

406. Dejter SW, Eggli DF, Gibbons MD. Delayed management of neonatal hydronephrosis. J Urol 1988;140:1305–1309.

407. Williams DI, Hulme-Moir I. Primary obstructive megaureter. Br J Urol 1970;42:140.

408. Argueso LR, et al. Prognosis of children with solitary kidney after unilateral nephrectomy. J Urol 1992;148:747–751.

409. Hakim RM, Goldszer RC, Brenner BM. Hypertension and protainuria: long-term sequelae of uninephrectomy in humans. Kidney Int 1984;25:930.

CHAPTER 18

THE BLADDER AND URETHRA

Thomas S. Parrott / Stephen Wood Gray / John Elias Skandalakis

*[They] are nothing at all ashamed, by the urine alone to deliver their
Delphian oracles concerning all diseases.*
—*THE DELPHIC ORACLE:*
ITS EARLY HISTORY, INFLUENCE AND FALL
T. DEMPSEY, OXFORD, ENGLAND, BH BLACKWELL, 1918

DEVELOPMENT

In contrast to the kidneys and ureter, which are of mesodermal origin, the structures of the lower urinary tract are formed from endoderm. Their development is intimately related to that of the anus and rectum (page 242) and to that of the lower reproductive tract (Chapters 21 and 22).

Formation of the Cloaca

At about the 13th day of development, the allantois, a ventral outgrowth from the hindgut, marks the site of the future bladder (Fig. 18.1). Soon after its appearance, the allantois reaches the chorion through the extraembryonic mesoderm of the body stalk. Its blood vessels—the umbilical arteries and vein—persist and enlarge to supply the placental area of the chorion, while the allantois itself fails to develop with the growing embryo. The part remaining within the umbilical cord becomes atretic, being barely identifiable at term.

With the appearance of the allantois, the hindgut may be considered to be the *cloaca,* and its closing plate (proctodeum) may be termed the *cloacal membrane* (Fig. 18.1, C).

At the end of the fourth week (4.9 mm), the cloacal membrane bounds the whole of the medioventral wall of the cloaca, from the allantoic stalk to the tailgut. The mesonephric (wolffian) ducts have reached the cloaca and enter it laterally, just caudal to the allantoic stalk. The formation of these ducts is described in Chapter 17.

Division of the Cloaca

During the fifth week, the division between the dorsal (rectal) and ventral (urogenital) cloaca begins to appear. Viewed from the side, the cloaca is a long triangle with the tailgut at the acute downward-pointing apex; at the top, the hindgut and the base of the allantois with the wolffian ducts make up the short side of the triangle; while the clo-acal membrane bounds most of the long ventral side (Fig. 18.2).

The division at the upper part of the cloaca becomes the urorectal septum, which grows caudad in a frontal plane by progressive fusion of lateral ridges to reach the cloacal membrane during the seventh week (Figs. 18.3 and 18.4).

The septum unites with the cloacal plate to form the perineal body. At about the same time, the cloacal plate ruptures, forming anal and urogenital orifices separated by the perineum. The subsequent history of the dorsal cloaca is discussed in Chapter 7.

Formation of the Bladder

During the sixth week, the ventral cloaca elongates and forms four segments: an expanded distal portion, the urogenital sinus; a tubular portion, the primitive urethra; an upper dilation, the future bladder; and a tubular portion, the urachus, which is continuous with the extraembryonic allantoic stalk.

Almost as soon as the wolffian duct reaches the cloaca, it gives rise to the ureteric bud (page 596). The exact means by which the ureters and wolffian ducts are altered to enter the urinary tract separately—the former laterally and high in the posterior bladder wall and the latter (in the male) medially and into the urethra—has been the subject of much debate. Several views have been put forward. Frazer (1) contended that the wolffian duct up to its junction with the ureter was obliterated by intussusception into the bladder, with subsequent resorption of the intussusceptum. Wesson (2) believed that the wolffian duct was simply resorbed by the growing bladder. Gyllensten (3) argued that the wolffian duct caudal to the ureteric junction becomes expanded and is eventually incorporated into the bladder wall, with subsequent replacement of ductal epithelium by bladder epithelium by the beginning of the seventh week.

By the end of the sixth week, the ureter opens into the

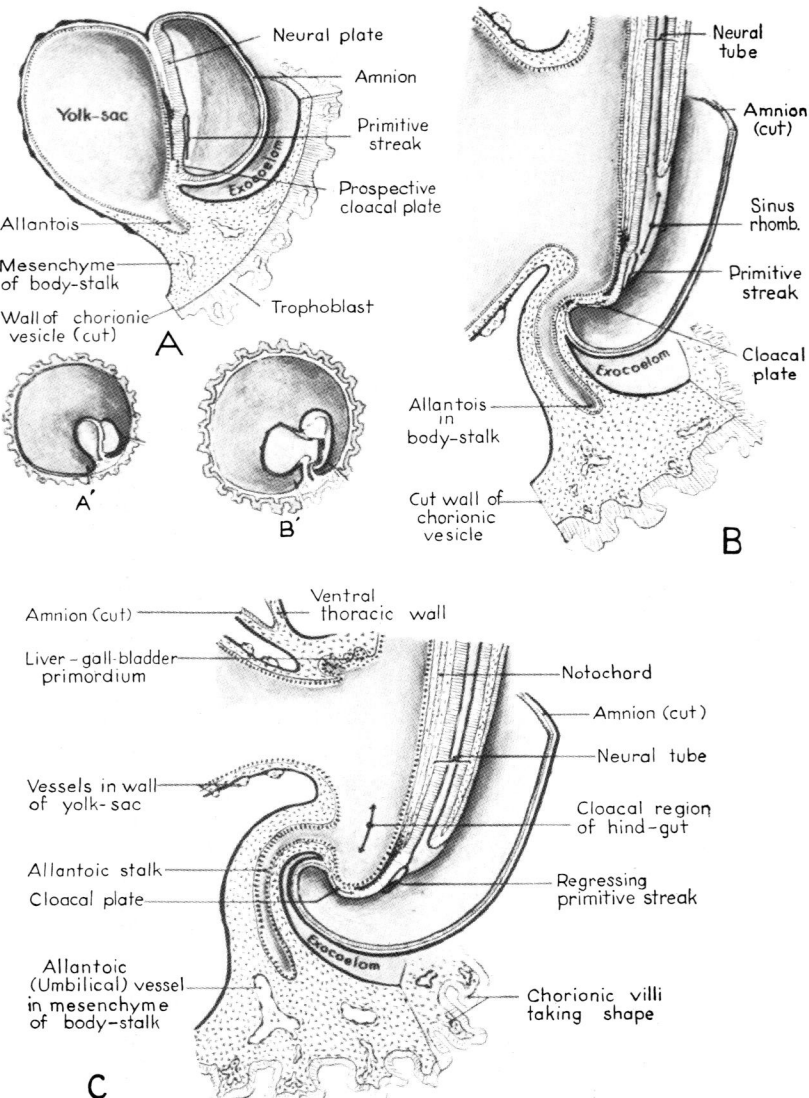

Figure 18-1. Early development of the cloacal region. **A,** Appearance of the allantois at 2 weeks. **B,** At 2½ weeks. **C,** At 3 weeks. The cloaca may now be said to be present. (A' and B' show orientation of **A** and **B.**) (From Patten BM, Berry A. The genesis of exstrophy of the bladder and epispadias. Am J Anat 1952;90:35–57.)

bladder, and the wolffian duct descends past this orifice and loops back up in the bladder wall to reach it (Fig. 18.5). The ureteric opening is temporarily obliterated by bladder epithelium forming Chwalle's membrane, which normally perforates at the beginning of the third month (3).

Resorption of the bladder wall separating the ascending loop of the wolffian duct brings the opening of this tube to its definitive location in the ureter, at the site of the entrance of the müllerian ducts (Fig. 18.5). Thus Müller's tubercle is established even before the müllerian ducts reach the site (see Chapter 22).

The path of the caudal migration of the wolffian duct is marked by the location of the orifices of duplicated ure-

ters. Such ectopic ureters drain the cranial portions of double kidneys and arise from secondary ureteral buds, which leave the wolffian duct cranial to the normal ureters. Because the wolffian duct forms a loop and reverses the direction of its course as it enters the bladder, these accessory ureters are absorbed into the bladder wall along a particular pathway extending from the normal ureteral orifice to the site of Müller's tubercle. The pattern of these ectopic ureteral orifices was originally described by Weigert (4) in 1877 and the description was expanded by Meyer (5) and Stephens (6). Its peculiar shape indicates that either there is torsion in the proximal part of the wolffian duct as it is resorbed or that accessory ureters, when located close to the normal ureter, arise

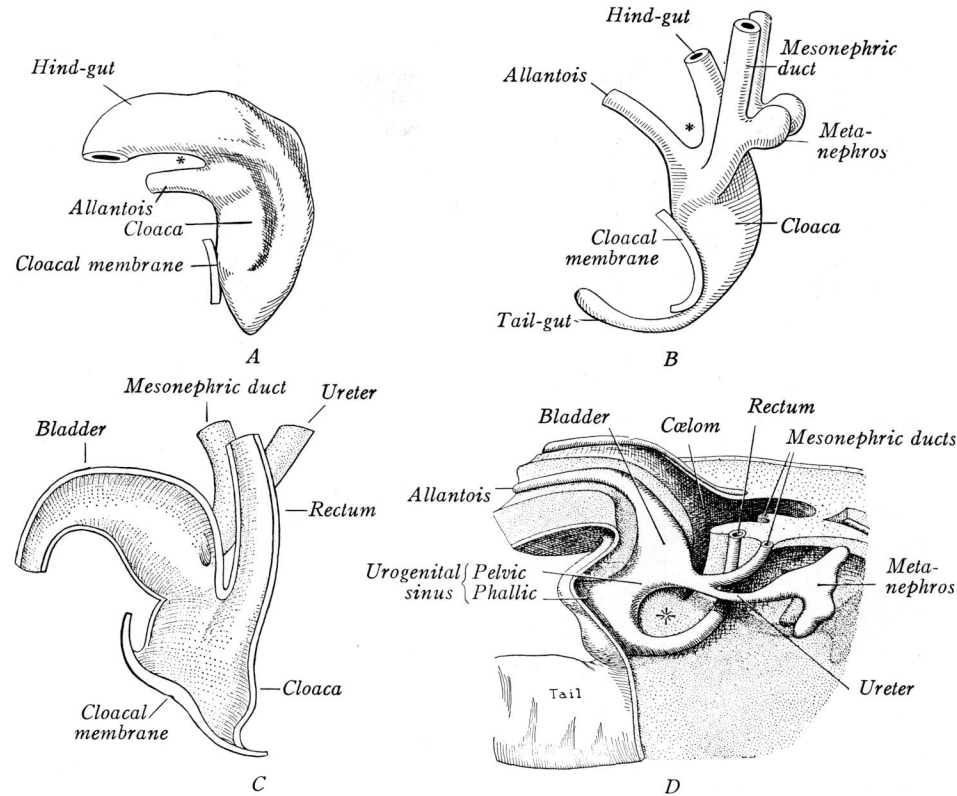

Figure 18.2. Stages in the division of the cloaca into dorsal and ventral positions. **A,** Cloaca at 3.5 mm. **B,** At 4 mm. The mesonephric (wolffian) ducts have joined the ventral cloaca. **C,** The ventral cloaca enlarges to form the bladder at the 8-mm stage, and division of the cloaca has started. **D,** At 11 mm. The allantois has stopped growing and the cloaca is almost divided. An *asterisk* indicates the site of the caudad growing cloacal septum. (From Arey LB. Developmental anatomy, 7th ed. Philadelphia: WB Saunders, 1965.)

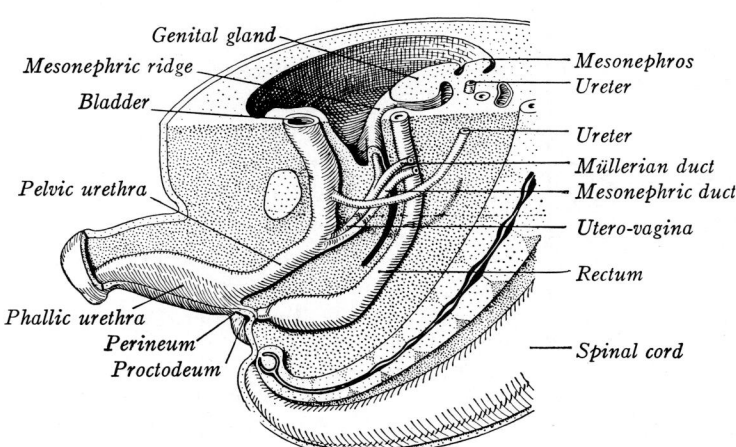

Figure 18.3. Final stage in the division of the cloaca at 9 weeks. The ventral portion has differentiated into phallic urethra, pelvic urethra, bladder, and the disappearing allantois (not shown). The site of the müllerian tubercle is indicated by the junction of the müllerian ducts with the pelvic urethra. (From Arey LB. Developmental anatomy, 7th ed. Philadelphia: WB Saunders, 1965.)

from the duct more medially than do those located farther away (Fig. 18.6).

The bladder epithelium originating from the endoderm of the urogenital sinus remains a single layer of epithelium up to the seventh week, then gradually assumes the appearance of transitional epithelium in the third month. The musculature appears as a longitudinal layer, chiefly on the dorsal surface, from the apex to the urethra during the eighth week; circular muscle appears slightly later, beginning at the apex. A third longitudinal layer

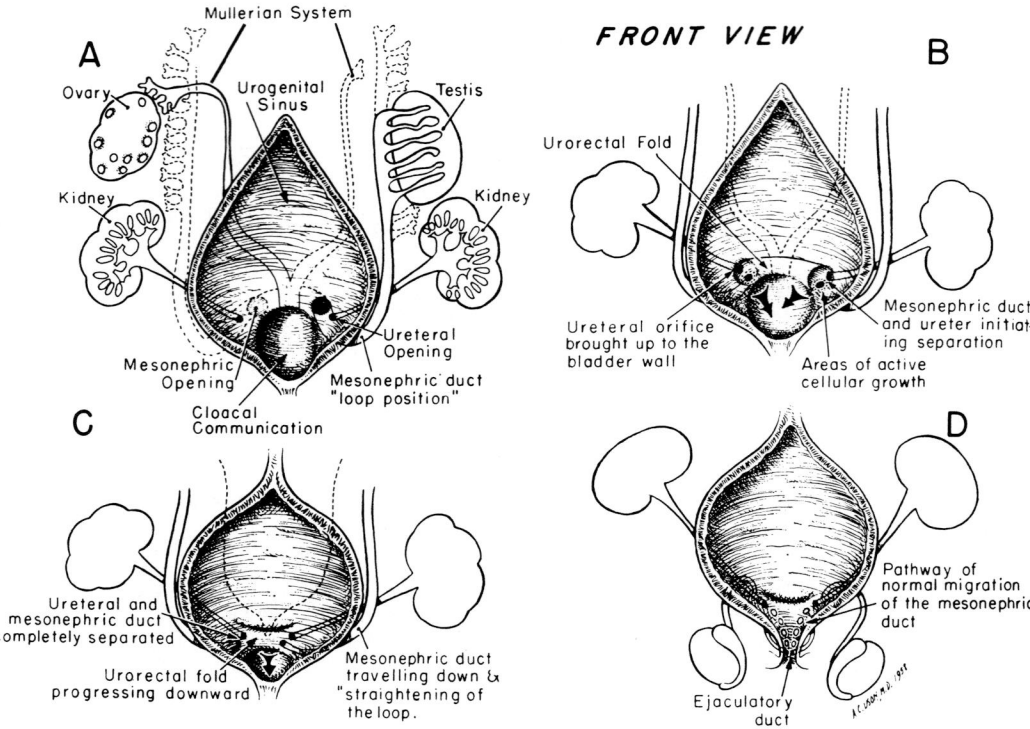

Figure 18.4. Schematic views of the division of the cloaca, viewed anteriorly with the anterior wall of the bladder removed. The migration of the associated ducts and their orifices is shown. **A,** The primitive stage for both sexes. **B** to **D,**

Development in the male. (From Uson AC, Donovan JT. Ectopic ureteral orifice. Am J Dis Child 1959;98:152–161.)

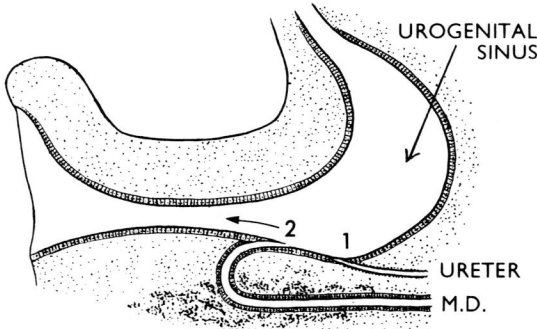

Figure 18.5. Diagrammatic parasagittal section showing the entrance of the ureter into the bladder at the site of Chwalle's membrane *(1)* and the loop of the mesonephric duct *(M.D.),* which will straighten out as the lower orifice *(2)* is carried downward to the site of the müllerian tubercle in the urethra. (From Williams DI. The development of the trigone of the bladder. Br J Urol 1951;23:123–128.)

appears still later, and the adult condition is essentially present during the fourth month.

The earliest muscle arises on the dorsal wall of the bladder from local mesenchyme, but the ventral wall receives a secondary reinforcement from mesenchyme, which has migrated from the primitive streak caudal to the cloaca. This "secondary" mesoderm also occupies the body wall between the allantoic stalk and the cranial end of the cloaca as the body elongates (7, 8) (see Chapter 16). The ureteral circular muscle first appears during the

eighth week, and the internal sphincter is visible in the fourth month (9).

LATER DEVELOPMENT OF THE URETHRA

The urogenital sinus, the most distal portion of the ventral cloaca, develops differently in the two sexes and will be discussed with the development of the male and the female reproductive systems (Chapters 21 and 22, respectively). However, remember that the epithelium in both sexes is of endodermal origin and that the connective tissue and smooth muscle are formed from the splanchnic mesenchyme.

Remember the following:

1. The urinary bladder is formed by the upper part of the urogenital sinus, and its epithelium in toto is of endodermal origin from the urogenital sinus.
2. The mucosa of the trigone of the bladder to start with is of mesodermal origin because of the incorporation of the caudal part of both mesonephric ducts and ureters, and later is replaced by epithelium of endodermal origin.
3. In the male the prostatic and membrane parts of the urethra are formed by the pelvic or tubular part of the urogenital sinus. In the female the entire urethra and the paraurethral glands are formed by the cranial part (vesicourethral part) of the endodermal cloaca. In both males and females the epithelium is of endodermal origin. However, in the female the caudal ends of the mesonephric

ducts disappear; whereas, in the male each seminal vesicle is formed from a lateral outgrowth of the caudal end of the mesonephric duct. Each ejaculatory duct is also of mesonephric origin and is formed by the part which is located between the urethra and the duct.

Critical Events in Development

"Capture" of the ureter by the developing urinary bladder occurs in the sixth week. If the ureteric bud, or a redundant ureteric bud, arises from the mesonephric (wolffian) duct higher than is usual, it may fail to become incorporated into the bladder wall and may open into the urethra or even into the vestibule in the female.

A patent urachus draining at the umbilicus may result from a failure of the upper portion of the ventral cloaca to regress in the third month or even later, or it may be secondary to urethral obstruction from urethral valves or stenoses.

ANOMALIES OF THE BLADDER AND URETHRA (FIG. 18.6 and TABLE 18.1)

Agenesis of the Bladder

Agenesis of the bladder is not uncommon in nonviable monsters with multiple anomalies (10); however, it is extremely rare in viable infants. Only 37 cases are reported in the world literature; 29 of those were in stillborn, and 7 of the 8 who survived were female (11).

Glenn (12) described a $3\frac{1}{2}$-year-old girl whose ureters opened with double orifices in the vestibule. There was a short, blind urethra but no bladder; the left kidney was double, and the uterus was bicornuate. Because of incontinence and hydronephrosis, the ureters were implanted into an ileal loop, which was brought to the outside in the right lower quadrant (Fig. 18.7).

The oldest patient to have been reported was a 27-year-old woman in whom the ureters opened into the vaginal wall (13). Incontinence and pain from chronic infection were the complaints. A sacral meningocele and bilateral clubbed feet were present at birth. No operation was attempted.

Embryogenesis

The defect lies in the cranial portion of the ventral cloaca, from which the bladder and urachus are derived. The presence of a urethral meatus as well as a normal vestibule in Glenn's patient (12) implies that the caudal end of the ventral cloaca was not affected. Absence of the allantoic diverticulum would account for the anomaly but for the presence of umbilical vessels. It is usually assumed that at least the temporary presence of the allantois is necessary for the formation of these vessels. However, in one fetus there were functional, although abnormal, umbilical vessels in the absence of any postvitelline endodermal derivatives (14). In general, allantoic defects must be lethal, and the few examples of survival are rare exceptions.

In most of the cases in which the bladder is absent, the ureters take the same course as do ureters with ectopic vestibular openings. From an anatomic and diagnostic standpoint, the presence of the urinary bladder may be appreciated between weeks 10 and 11 of gestation. Around the 13th week it may be demonstrated by imaging methods as reported by Campbell (15) and Wladimiroff and Campbell (15).

For a good image, the bladder should contain enough urine. Since a normal fetus voids approximately every hour, serial examination should reveal the presence or absence of the urinary bladder and thus the presence of unilateral or bilateral kidneys with good function.

The Urachus and Its Remnants

At the umbilicus of the fetus are two endodermal structures of considerable importance in the beginning of development, which must be severed at birth and their internal connections obliterated. One is the connection of the yolk sac to the midgut, and the other is the connection of the allantoic stalk to the cloaca. Neither extraembryonic structure has any function after the first few weeks of development, and both normally have almost disappeared by birth. In both structures, however, regression may remain incomplete and portions may persist into later life. The yolk sac remnants have already been considered (page 213), and our present concern is with the connection of the anterior cloaca with the allantois. This connection, normally a mere fibrous remnant from the apex of the bladder to the anterior body wall, is the urachus.

Despite the fact that the ventral cloaca is responsible for the genesis of the urachus which joins the allantois, the contributions of these two embryologic entities in the formation of the urachus is unclear, according to Arey (17). The allantois degenerates into a fibrous cord-like formation (third gestational month), while the urachal growth and elongation continues to become the bridge between the umbilicus and the urinary bladder (fifth gestational month).

Anatomy

THE NORMAL URACHUS IN THE ADULT

The adult urachus is between 3 and 5 cm long; the proximal portion is in the bladder wall, while the remainder lies in loose areolar tissue between the transversalis fascia and the peritoneum. In the fetus and occasionally in the newborn, the urachus is attached to the abdominal wall by a remnant of the primary ventral mesentery, the mesourachis (18); it has also been reported free in the

Table 18.1.
Anomalies of the Bladder and Urethra

Anomaly	Origin of Defect	First Appearance	Sex Most Affected	Relative Frequency	Remarks
Agenesis of the bladder	3rd week?	At birth	Female?	Very rare	Other genitourinary tract anomalies usually present
Urachal anomalies:					
Patent urachus	9th week or later	In infancy	Male	Very rare	
Umbilical sinus	9th week or later	At any age	?	Rare	Usually found only if infected
Vesical sinus	9th week or later	None	Equal	Common	
Urachal cyst	9th week or later	At maturity	Equal	Common	Small cysts may exist without symptoms
Duplication of the bladder:					
Bilateral	3rd week	At birth	Equal	Very rare	Usually with duplication of all hindgut derivatives
Frontal	?	In childhood	Female	Very rare	Redundancy of mucosa only
Hourglass	?	At any age	?	Very rare	Questionably congenital
Diverticula of the bladder	7th week	In infancy and childhood	?	Rare	Not to be confused with acquired diverticula in adult males
Exstrophy of the bladder	5th week	Birth	Male	Very rare	Associated with epispadias
Ectopic ureter	6th week	In childhood	Female	Common	Urinary incontinence in females; usually asymptomatic in males; often associated with double ureter
Ureterocele	8th week	1st year of life	Female	Common	Often associated with double ureter
Vesicoureteral reflux	?	Males - at birth; females - at age 4 yr	Probably female	Common	Associated with urinary tract infection
Posterior urethral valves	?	In childhood	Male	Common	
Aganglionic bladder	9th week	In childhood	?	Rare	With or without associated megacolon
Duplication of the urethra:					
Female	?	At birth	Female	Very rare	
Male	10–14 weeks	At birth	Male	Rare	Accessory urethra often hypospadiac

abdominal cavity, surrounded by a serosa of peritoneum (19).

The distal end may terminate as a cord, independent of the similar cord-like remnants of the umbilical vessels, or it may merge with either or both. It may be visibly tubular for a portion of its length, to become lost in the fascia as a fibrous prolongation (Fig. 18.8).

Commonly, the proximal (vesicular) end contains a tube of irregular transitional epithelium, about 1 mm in diameter and surrounded by smooth muscle. In about 50% of cases examined, the lumen is continuous with that of the bladder; in the remainder, it is closed by bladder mucosa (Fig. 18.9). The presence of valves at the orifice, described by Wutz (20), has not been confirmed by later visualization (18). The urachal arteries arise from the superior vesical arteries.

According to Noe (21) the urachus consists of three layers: outer muscular, medial vascular, and an innermost layer lined by epithelium of transitional or cuboidal type while the urachal lumen is in existence. The urachus is

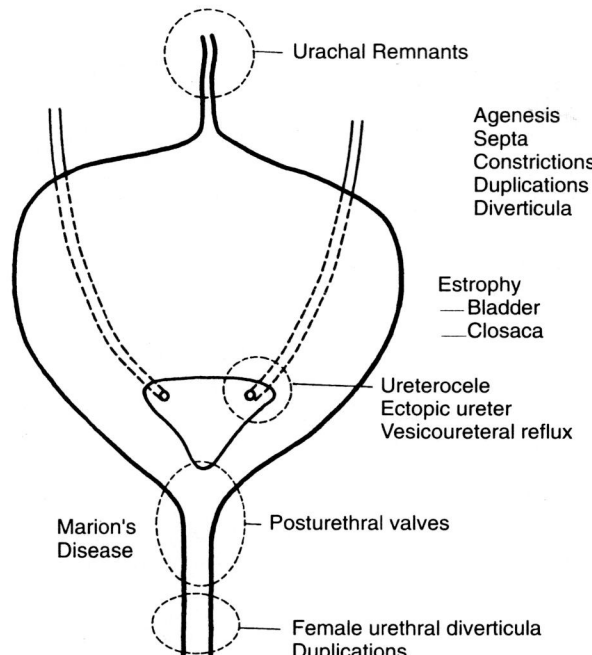

Figure 18.6. Sites of congenital anomalies in the bladder and urethra.

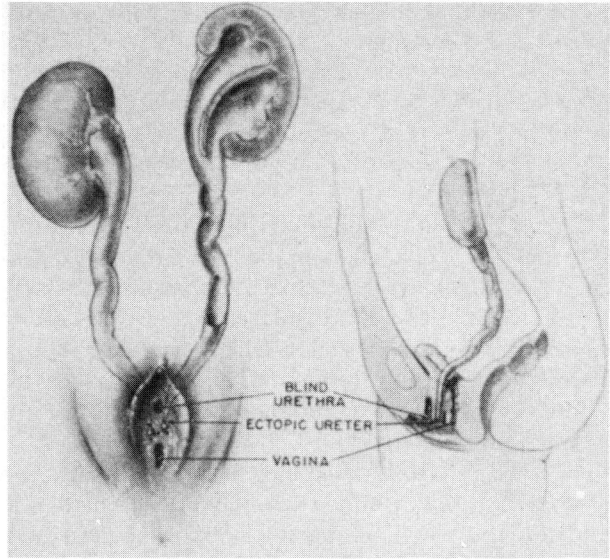

Figure 18.7. Agenesis of the bladder in a 3½-year-old girl. There was a short, blind urethra, no bladder, and stenosed vulvar openings of both ureters. Hydronephrosis, a bicornuate uterus, and an interventricular septal defect were present. The ureters were anastomosed to an isolated ileal loop brought out in the right lower quadrant. (From Glenn JF. Agenesis of the bladder. JAMA 1959;169:2016–2018.)

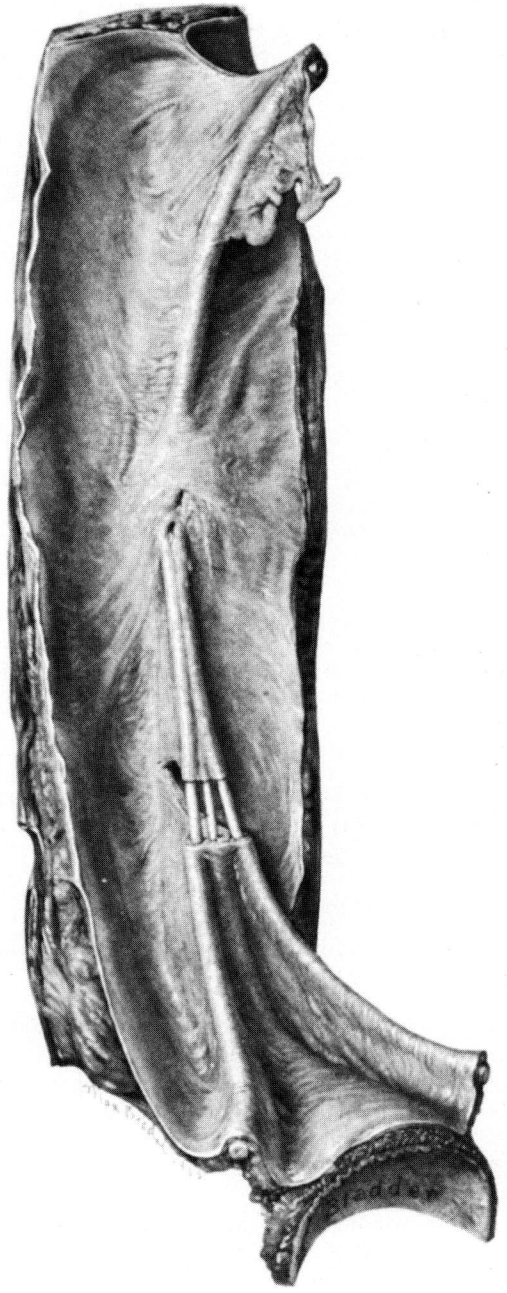

Figure 18.8. Posterior view of the umbilical region of the abdominal wall. The two obliterated umbilical (hypogastric) arteries are visible, together with the urachus, which arises from the dome of the bladder and extends partway toward the umbilicus. (From Cullen TS. Embryology: anatomy and diseases of the umbilicus together with diseases of the urachus. Philadelphia: WB Saunders, 1916.)

located in an isolated space which is formed, again according to Noe, as follows:

Anteriorly: Umbilicovesical fascia
Posteriorly: Umbilicovesical fascia
Laterally: Obliterated umbilical artery
Inferiorly: Home of bladder with extension over the

hypogastric vessels posteriorly and to the pelvic diaphragm anteriorly.

This space is completely separated from the peritoneum. Noe stated that infection or malignancy may be confined within this space.

Hammond et al. (18) studied the anatomy of the ura-

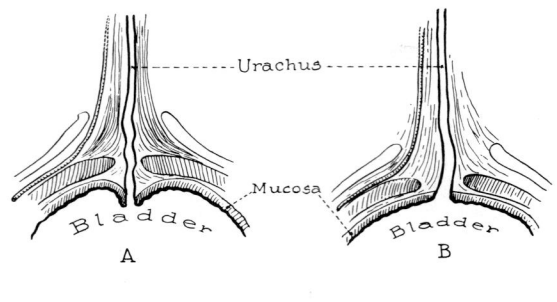

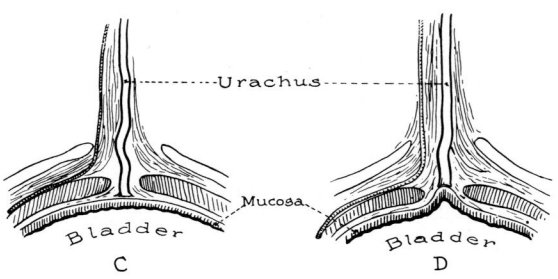

Figure 18.9. Four examples of the termination of the urachus at the dome of the bladder. **A** and **B,** A small communication exists between bladder and urachus. **C** and **D,** The urachus reaches the mucosa of the bladder and ends blindly. (From Begg RC. The urachus and umbilical fistulae. Surg Gynecol Obstet 1927;45:165–178.)

chus and its fasciae. Hinman (22), Blichert-Toft et al. (23), Bauer and Retik (24) presented several anatomic variants and umbilical disorders of urachal origin.

URACHAL ANOMALIES

Failure of the urachus to regress completely results in anomalies that may be classified as follows:

A. Bladder is located below the level of the umbilicus, and the urachus is a tube:
  1. Urachus is patent throughout (Fig. 18.10, A)
  2. Proximal portion is patent, opening into bladder (urachal diverticulum) (Fig. 18.10, B)
  3. Distal portion is patent, opening at umbilicus (urachal sinus) (Fig. 18.10, C)
  4. Midportion only is open, both ends are closed (urachal cyst) (Fig. 18.10, D)
B. Bladder is located at the level of the umbilicus, and a widely open umbilicovesical fistula is present (Fig. 18.10, E).

Although the urachus and the vitelline duct are in close approximation at the umbilicus, no unusual coincidence of patent urachus and patent vitelline duct has been noted. Nix and his colleagues (25) recorded only five cases.

Most large urachal cysts are mucinous. Ripmann (26) described one containing 52 liters, and Begg (27) described one nearly as large. As the transitional epithelium of the normal urachus is nonsecretory, these large

cysts apparently form only if epithelial metaplasia occurs. Jonathan (28) described a mucinous cyst lined with tall columnar epithelium, which had papillae resembling intestinal villi, and Trimingham and McDonald (29) found similar intestine-like epithelium in a patent urachus.

Infection, lithiasis, and malignant tumors have all been reported in urachal remnants. In one patient an abscessed cyst ruptured into the peritoneum (30). Seventy cases of carcinoma have been found, with all but three being in the intravesical portion of the urachus (31). Eight cases of sarcoma have been collected (32, 33); one occurred in a 4-month-old infant and three others were in children. The urachal origin of some of these cases has been questioned (34).

EMBRYOGENESIS

Two separate processes may produce a urinary opening at the umbilicus. In the usual case the bladder forms normally from the cloaca and the intraembryonic connection with the allantoic stalk remains as the urachus. It may fail to narrow before birth, leaving a connecting tube from the bladder to the umbilicus (median umbilical ligament). The top of the bladder lies below the level of the umbilicus, but it is higher than that of a normally descended bladder (Fig. 18.10, A).

In other cases no urachus is formed, and the entire ventral cloaca becomes the bladder. The top of the bladder lies at the level of the umbilicus, and the opening is an umbilicovesical fistula rather than a patent urachus (Fig. 18.10, E).

Begg (35) explored the embryology of the urachus and confirmed the conclusion of Felix (9) that it is wholly derived from the ventral cloaca rather than from the allantoic stalk. Only the transitory extraembryonic prolongation of the urachus should be considered allantoic. The urachus may be considered to represent presumptive bladder, which normally is not used to form the definitive organ in humans.

The urachus is thus created by failure of the distal ventral cloaca to enlarge and is subsequently attenuated and withdrawn from its attachment at the umbilicus by the descent of the bladder (Fig. 18.8). When the bladder is continuously distended from urethral obstruction, this descent does not take place and the urachus remains open (Fig. 18.10, E). Spontaneous closure after relief of the lower urinary obstruction sometimes occurs. Whether or not the bladder belatedly descends has not been reported.

Tsuchida and Ishida (36) associated urachal patency at birth with enlargement of the umbilical cord, perhaps secondary to urine extravasation into the cord.

Unlike patent vitelline duct and Meckel's diverticulum, patent urachus is not usually associated with other mal-

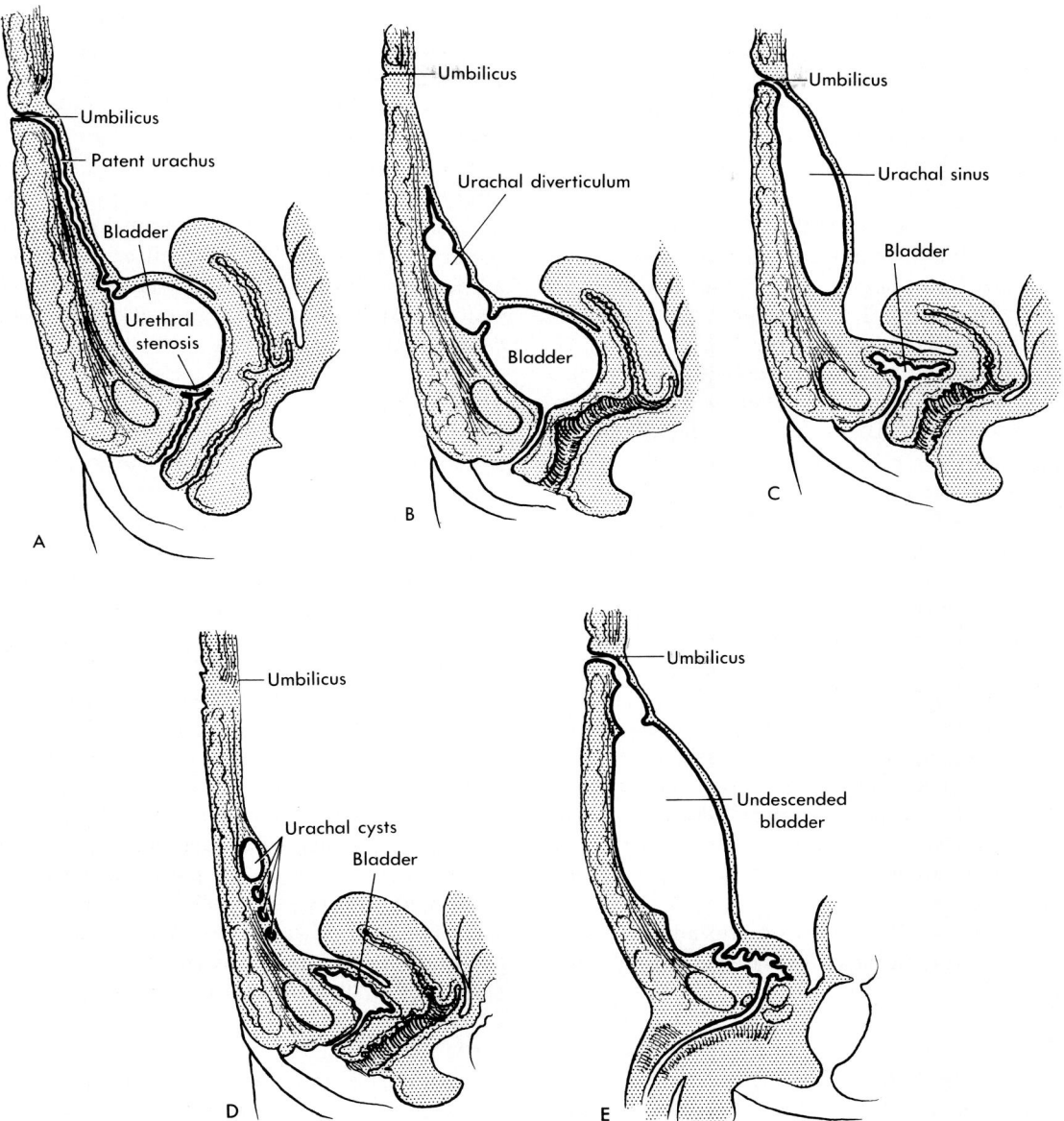

Figure 18.10. Urachal anomalies. **A,** Normally descended bladder with narrow, completely patent urachus and urethral stenosis. **B,** Proximal portion of urachus open; urachal diverticulum present. **C,** Distal portion of urachus patent; infected sinus opening at the umbilicus. **D,** Midportion of urachus open; urachal cyst present. **E,** Undescended bladder; widely open omphalovesical fistula. (Redrawn from Cullen TS. Embryology: anatomy and diseases of the umbilicus together with diseases of the urachus. Philadelphia: WB Saunders, 1916.)

formations. Renal and anorectal anomalies may sometimes be associated with urachal cysts.

Acquired Umbilical Fistula. In infants, the appearance of urine at the umbilicus implies a patent urachus, but occasionally urine appears in adults with no history of similar leakage. Phimosis, prostatic hypertrophy, and carcinoma are frequent findings.

Begg (35) denied that the urachus, once normally closed, can become patent in later life. However, a previously patent urachus may reopen if obstruction occurs at the urethra (37). However, if the urachus has never

been patent, the leakage in later life passes into the space of Retzius, between the peritoneum and the fascia transversalis, and then to the umbilicus. Herbst (38), who collected 155 cases of patent urachus in 1937, found at least 50% in adults, but he did not distinguish congenital from acquired cases, implying merely that a large number were acquired. Sterling and Goldsmith (39) collected 28 cases in patients "who had presented no observable signs or symptoms during infancy." Their patients ranged in age from 5 to 72 years.

A curious case of ectopic, patent urachus in a 30-year-old male patient was described by Vilanova and Raventós (40). The urachus ended in a papillary elevation just above the root of the penis. There was no urethral obstruction. No other example of such an extraumbilical urachal termination has been reported.

HISTORY

Cabrol (as reported by Herbst [38]) in 1550 described a young woman who had urinated from a protrusion at her navel all of her life. Cabrol opened the urethra, which had been congenitally occluded, and ligated the umbilical protrusion, effecting a complete cure.

During the 18th century, controversy arose over the anatomy of the urachus. Littré (41) believed that it contained a lumen, and von Haller (42) contended that it did not. The latter defended his position by stating that there is no allantois in humans, thus weakening the value of his observations. Peyer considered that there was a lumen until term, at which time it was obliterated (20). Wutz examined 74 cadavers and described the variations of the urachus, finding in most a channel that was patent for only a short distance from the bladder.

Paget and Bowman (43) in 1861 seem to have performed the first repair since Cabrol's time. They denuded and approximated the lips of the opening. Two years later Smith (44) ligated an umbilical protrusion in the same way as had Cabrol. A large number of papers and monographs on the urachus appeared toward the end of the 19th century. They were reviewed by Vaughan (45) in 1905 and by Cullen (46), who collected 60 cases of patent urachus up to 1916.

The 1927 studies of Begg (35) on the anatomy and embryology of the urachus have been the basis for all subsequent work.

INCIDENCE

Patent urachus is very rare. Nix and his colleagues (25) found only three cases in 200,000 hospital admissions in Boston and three in 1,168,760 admissions in New Orleans. McCauley and Lichtenheld (47) found two cases in 108,000 admissions. The incidence in pediatric autopsy series is 1:7610 for patent urachus and 1:5000 for urachal cysts (48). Males are affected twice as often as are females.

Over a period of 33 years Irving (49) observed six cases in newborns (four patent urachus and two urachal cysts; four males and two females).

Among domestic animals, patent urachus has been observed in horses, cows and pigs. It seems to be relatively common in horses, and as in humans, it affects more males than females (46).

Urachal diverticula opening into the bladder are usually asymptomatic and are detected only on autopsy. A small lumen in the proximal urachus is not rare.

Urachal sinuses opening at the umbilicus are much less common (29). Unless they become infected, they rarely come to the attention of the physician or patient (50). Careful probing or injection of radiopaque material is necessary to distinguish them from similar blind vitelline duct remnants.

Small urachal cysts are not rare, nor do they produce symptoms. Wutz (20) found them present in about 33% of cadavers. Larger cysts of clinical importance are less common. Yeorg (51) found three in 12,500 urologic admissions. Trimingham and McDonald (29) found eight over the same period of time in which they found only two cases of patent urachus.

SYMPTOMS

The obvious sign of a patent urachus is urine appearing at the umbilicus, either as a stream or, more usually, as drops. There may be a protruding structure, the remnant of the umbilical cord, or even a mucosal prolapse. Pain is often present, indicating infection.

A large urachal cyst usually presents as a tender midline mass beneath the umbilicus; intestinal disturbances or urinary frequency from pressure are chief complaints. Such cysts may reach great size even before birth. At least two cases of obstruction to delivery from distended urachal cysts have been reported (52, 53). In one infant the abdomen was distended to three times the diameter of the mother's pelvic outlet.

Not all urachal anomalies are discovered early in life. Thomford and his colleagues (54) reported three examples found in adults. In one patient a nearly complete patent urachus was revealed following infection in the umbilical portion. In two others, aged 63 and 76 years, the presence of carcinoma revealed the existence of a urachal diverticulum of the bladder. All three patients were men.

DIAGNOSIS

An umbilical tumor or a cystic dilation of the umbilical cord before separation may give warning of a patent urachus. The discharge should be tested for urine to be sure of its nature. In at least one case (55) what appeared to be urine from a patent urachus proved to be gastric juice from ectopic gastric mucosa in a patent vitelline duct.

Urachal sinuses must be distinguished from similar vitelline duct remnants. Careful probing or injection of radiopaque material is necessary. If doubt still remains, a mucosal biopsy will show the transitional epithelium of the urachus or the simple columnar epithelium of the vitelline duct.

Urachal cysts may be suspected from the presence of inflammation observed at cystoscopy at the apex of the bladder. Cystography may reveal a convex filling defect caused by the weight of the overlying cyst. Such cysts are difficult to distinguish from bladder diverticula.

If the cyst lies nearer to the umbilicus than to the bladder, there may be a visible protrusion, and pressure may expel pus at the umbilicus. In other cases the cyst has no communication in either direction. In Jonathan's patient (28) the cyst was calcified and, therefore, visible on radiography.

According to Persutte et al. (56) a urachal cyst is located in the distal or proximal one-third of the urachal remnant and may be diagnosed by CT scan or ultrasound plus cystogram.

TREATMENT

Excision of the patent urachus or urachal sinus is the proper treatment. A small portion of the apex of the bladder also may be removed. In addition, umbilical herniorrhaphy may be necessary (57).

Cysts require laparotomy and must be handled carefully, if they are infected, to avoid leakage of the contents into the peritoneal cavity.

Bilateral Duplication of the Bladder and Urethra

Bilateral duplication of the bladder and urethra is part of a rare and striking anomaly that involves the entire caudal end of the body. In its extreme form, there is symmetric doubling of the lower vertebral column, the colon, the rectum and anus, the uterus and vagina in females, and the external genitalia as well as the lower urinary tract in both sexes.

ANATOMY

Two bladders lie on either side of the midline. Each is supplied by a single normal ureter and each is drained by a separate urethra opening independently to the outside. Strictly speaking, the bladder is not doubled but is merely separated into lateral halves (Fig. 18.11, A and B).

If duplication of the bladder and urethra is complete, some other midline structures also are doubled (Fig. 18.12). The findings in 21 reported cases of duplication of the bladder and urethra are as follows:

Duplication of lumbar vertebrae	2
Duplication of anus and rectum	9
Duplication of rectum, with anus single	2
Rectum single with persistent cloaca	1
Anus single; rectum not explored	3
Anus and rectum single	4
Males with double penis	7
Males with single penis and two urethrae	1
Females with double uterus and vagina	8
Females with bicornuate uterus only	1
Females with partially doubled vagina only	2
Female with single uterus and vagina	1

In addition to these 21 cases, there are two in which only the urethra was doubled (58, 59). In two others the clitoris was bifid (58, 60).

Partial bladder duplications are known in which only the neck and the urethra are undivided (61).

The bladder may be divided into two portions by a sagittal septum only; an external groove may or may not indicate its presence. Such a septum may be complete (Fig. 18.11, C) or incomplete (Fig. 18.11, D); it may be composed of two layers of mucosa, or there may be a muscular core. Juetting (62) described the first case in 1838. In his patient both kidneys were double. Two ureters opened into the right side, which communicated with the urethra; one opened into the closed left side, and one ureter ended in the septum. When one ureter opens into the closed portion, the corresponding kidney is destroyed by the back pressure. Aplasia or hypoplasia may also exist. In one case (63) a triplicated colon accompanied the bladder deformity. In another example a rectourethral fistula existed on one side (64).

Incomplete sagittal septa have been reported eight times since Blasius (65) saw the first one in 1656. The septa ended with a crescentic opening at the bladder neck. Unlike a complete septum, an incomplete septum produces no symptoms. In one patient (66) the appendix and colon were duplicated.

EMBRYOGENESIS

These duplications are manifestations of a developmental disturbance of the caudal end of the body. In its extreme form, the disturbance seems to start with a divided notochord, which fuses again cranially to the separation. Beneath this paired notochord, the endoderm forms two hindguts, each of which gives rise to an allantoic stalk and a cloaca. When vertebral splitting does not occur, one must assume that the endoderm originated the duplication, in some cases bifurcating from the level of the midgut and in others dividing only at its caudal end. The existence of two allantoic stalks is supported by the presence of four umbilical arteries in a puppy having double bladder, urachus, urethra, and colon (67). That the allantoic duplication can occur without doubling of other hindgut derivatives is indicated by the occasional presence of a single bladder with doubling of the urachus (68) (see the section on "Colonic Duplications," in Chapter 7).

HISTORY AND INCIDENCE

The first adequate description of duplication of the lower urinary tract was by Schatz (69) in 1871. Three other cases were reported before 1900. Burns et al. (61) reviewed a number of cases up to 1947. Several cases of this defect have been reported in articles concerned with colonic and anal duplication, which are usually also present. Nineteen clear-cut cases have been described. Burns was able to find five cases of incomplete duplication of the bladder, the first of which was reported in 1670 by Cattirri (70). Sagittal septa are equally rare.

Complete Reduplication of Bladder

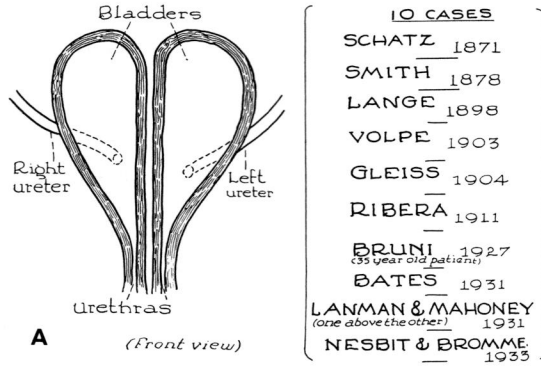

Incomplete Reduplication of Bladder

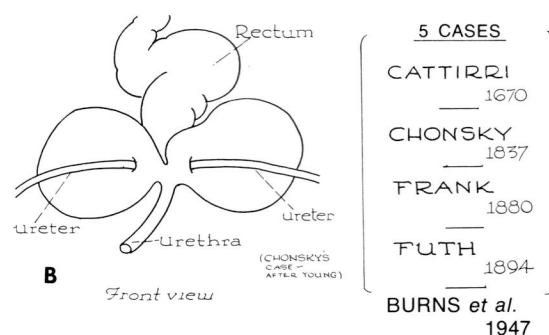

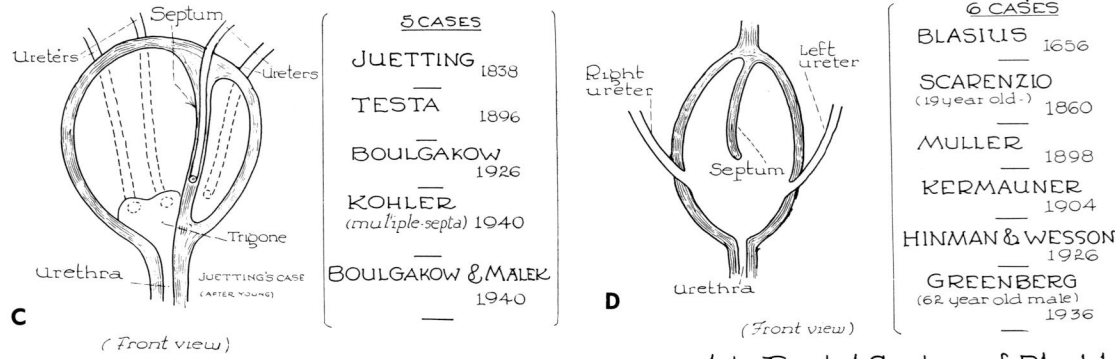

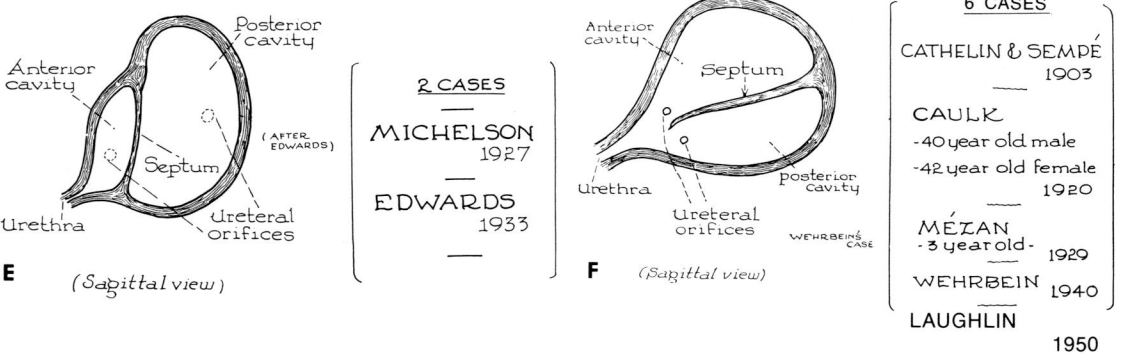

Figure 18.11.   Classification of reported cases of duplication of the urinary bladder. (From Burns E, Cummins H, Hyman I. Incomplete reduplication of the bladder with congenital solitary kidney. J Urol 1947;57:257–269.)

SYMPTOMS AND DIAGNOSIS

The condition is diagnosed usually by inspection at birth. Symptoms may arise from the presence of rectal fistulae (71), bladder exstrophy (72), rectal atresia (73), or ectopic ureter (74). While recognition of the anomaly is not difficult, a complete diagnosis demands exploration of all orifices to determine the anatomic relationships and the functional possibilities. Barium enema and cystourethography should be employed.

TREATMENT

Treatment is limited usually to procedures for maintaining normal function. No detailed recommendations are possible because of the variations among the individual

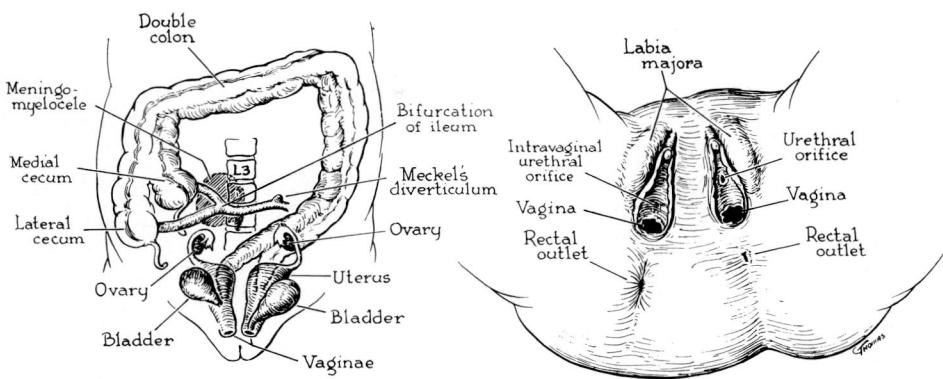

Figure 18.12. Bilateral duplication of the urethra, bladder, external genitalia, colon, and terminal ileum. One urethral orifice was ectopic, and there was a rectovaginal fistula on the right. (From Beach PD, Brascho DJ, Hein WR, Nichol WW, Geppert LJ. Duplication of the primitive hindgut of the human body. Surgery 1961;49:779–793.)

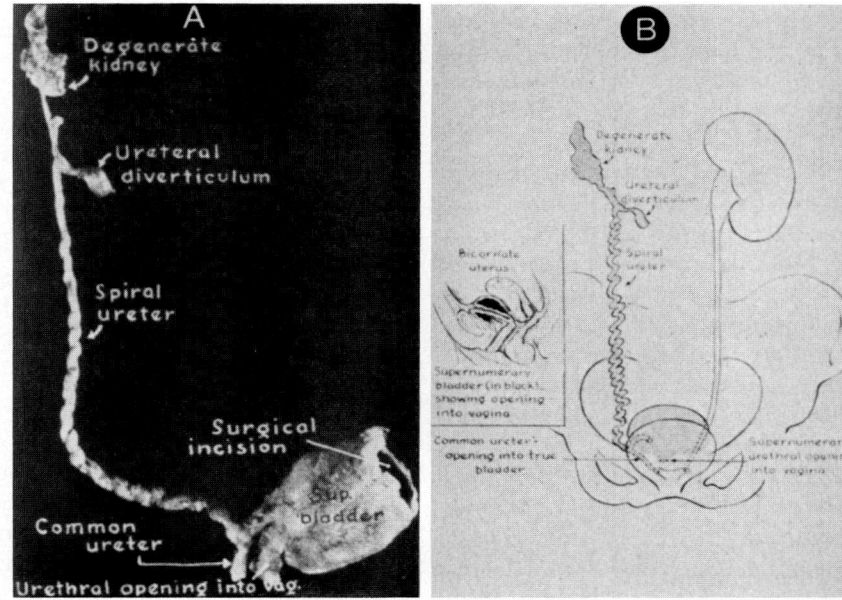

Figure 18.13. **A,** Supernumerary urinary bladder and associated structures removed at operation. **B,** Anatomic relationship of supernumerary bladder to remainder of urinary system. *Shaded* structures were removed at operation. *Insert* shows median sagital section of pelvis to illustrate complete separation of walls of two bladders. The supernumerary urethra opens into the vagina. (From Bowie CW, Garvey FK, Boyce WH, Pautler EE. Supernumerary urinary bladder and ureter, spiral deformity of the ureter, ureteral diverticulum, hypoplasia of the kidney and bicornate uterus: a case report. J Urol 1954;71:293–298.)

affected patients. Exstrophy of the bladder and rectal fistulae must be repaired. Blind colonic duplications must be anastomosed to provide for emptying. Also, plastic reconstructive procedures may be attempted on the genitalia.

Frontal Duplications, Septa, and Constriction of the Bladder

ANATOMY

Frontal Duplications. Two bladders, the anterior drained by a normal urethra and the posterior opening into the upper vagina, have been reported in a 17-year-old girl (75) (Fig. 18.13). The normal bladder received ureters from both kidneys. The posterior bladder received a ureter that branched from the normal right ureter; the right kidney was aplastic. The right kidney and ureter, together with the posterior bladder, were removed.

Frontal Septa. Only slightly more frequent than complete frontal duplication is the presence of a frontal mucosal septum. The condition has been termed *duplication,* but it is actually a single bladder divided by an anomalous septum, (Fig. 18.11, *E*) and is not accompanied by genital or rectal doubling. Complete partitioning is rare; a possible case is that of Senger and Santare (76). Abrahamson (77) considered most of the reported cases to be ureteroceles. Burns and his colleagues (61) accepted two cases (78, 79); in both of these a ureter opened into each cavity. Only one cavity was drained by the urethra, and in Edward's (79) patient the urethra was stenosed.

Incomplete frontal partitions have been described eight times. Meyer (80) found one in an 85-mm fetus. In two cases a ureter opened into each chamber (Fig. 18.11, *F*), and in one case the ureters opened on the septum (81). In Mézan's patient (82) both a complete and an incomplete septum were present; one ureter opened into the closed chamber.

Although the septum may be incomplete, it may be long enough to obstruct the ureteral opening. Under the term *redundant mucosa*, Campbell (83) described six examples found in a series of autopsies of more than 19,000 infants and children; he also treated four cases in living children. The mucosal flap may hang as a curtain from the posterior wall, or it may form an upwardly opening cup at the base of the trigone (trigonal curtain), such as that described by Harris (84).

A number of cases of prolapse of redundant bladder mucosa through the urethra in female infants have been discussed by Bernardo and Roth (85). They did not make clear whether or not the redundancy in these cases was in the form of a septum.

Multiple Septa. A single example of a bladder that was normal in shape but with numerous blind and communicating locules was reported by Kohler (86). Other genitourinary disturbances were present, and the infant died 10 days after birth.

Hourglass Bladder. Twenty-three cases of bladders with ring-like constrictions were reported up to 1944. One was in a 360-mm fetus (80); one was in a child; and the remainder were in adults. These have been reviewed by Zellermayer and Carlson (87) (Fig. 18.14). In three cases the ureters opened into the inferior chamber. The upper chamber was usually the larger, and the opening between upper and lower chambers was from 1 to 6 cm in diameter. Excepting the fetal specimen, there is no evidence the condition is a congenital anomaly. Megaureter and hydronephrosis were found in the case reported by Berariu and his colleagues (88).

EMBRYOGENESIS

There is no adequate explanation for the existence of mucosal bladder partitions. Watson (89) studied the bladder during late intrauterine life and suggested that undistended folds of mucosa or rugae might come into contact with one another and fuse to form a partition.

Mucosal redundancy has been considered to be secondary to chronic irritation of the bladder (90). The extreme youth of many of the patients reported makes

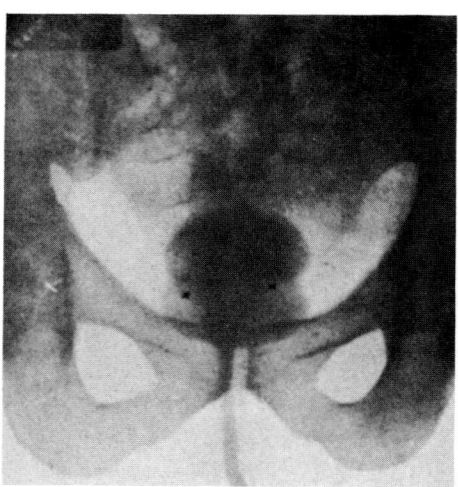

Figure 18.14. Example of an hourglass deformity of the bladder, probably of congenital origin. The sites of the ureteric orifices are indicated by X. (From Zellermayer J, Carlson HE. Congenital hourglass bladder. J Urol 1944;51:24–30.)

this explanation unsatisfactory for most cases. Bernardo and Roth (85) support the view that a congenital defect of the connective tissue attaching the mucosa to the muscularis is the cause.

If hourglass bladder is indeed of embryonic origin, the superior chamber may represent a dilated urachus, while the inferior chamber represents the bladder itself. When the superior chamber receives the ureters, however, this explanation cannot be correct.

HISTORY AND INCIDENCE

All of these bladder defects are rare. Cathelin and Sempé (91) list 17 reports published prior to 1900 as "doubtful but probable" cases of double bladder. Burns and his colleagues (61), in their excellent review, list all the cases in each category up to 1945. Abrahamson (77) studied these defects in 1961.

SYMPTOMS AND DIAGNOSIS

Incomplete septa produce no symptoms unless they are long enough to obstruct the bladder neck, in which case distension of the bladder, hydroureter, and hydronephrosis result. Unlike other such obstructions of the outlet, no resistance is made to passage of a retrograde catheter or cystoscope. The mucosal septum may be difficult to see if it is folded back against the bladder wall. Complete septa produce kidney destruction if a ureter opens into the loculus not drained by the urethra.

These septa frequently are difficult or impossible to distinguish from large ureteroceles prior to surgery.

Hourglass bladder usually is associated with a long history of cystitis and frequent, painful micturition. Diagnosis by cystography and cystoscopy is not difficult.

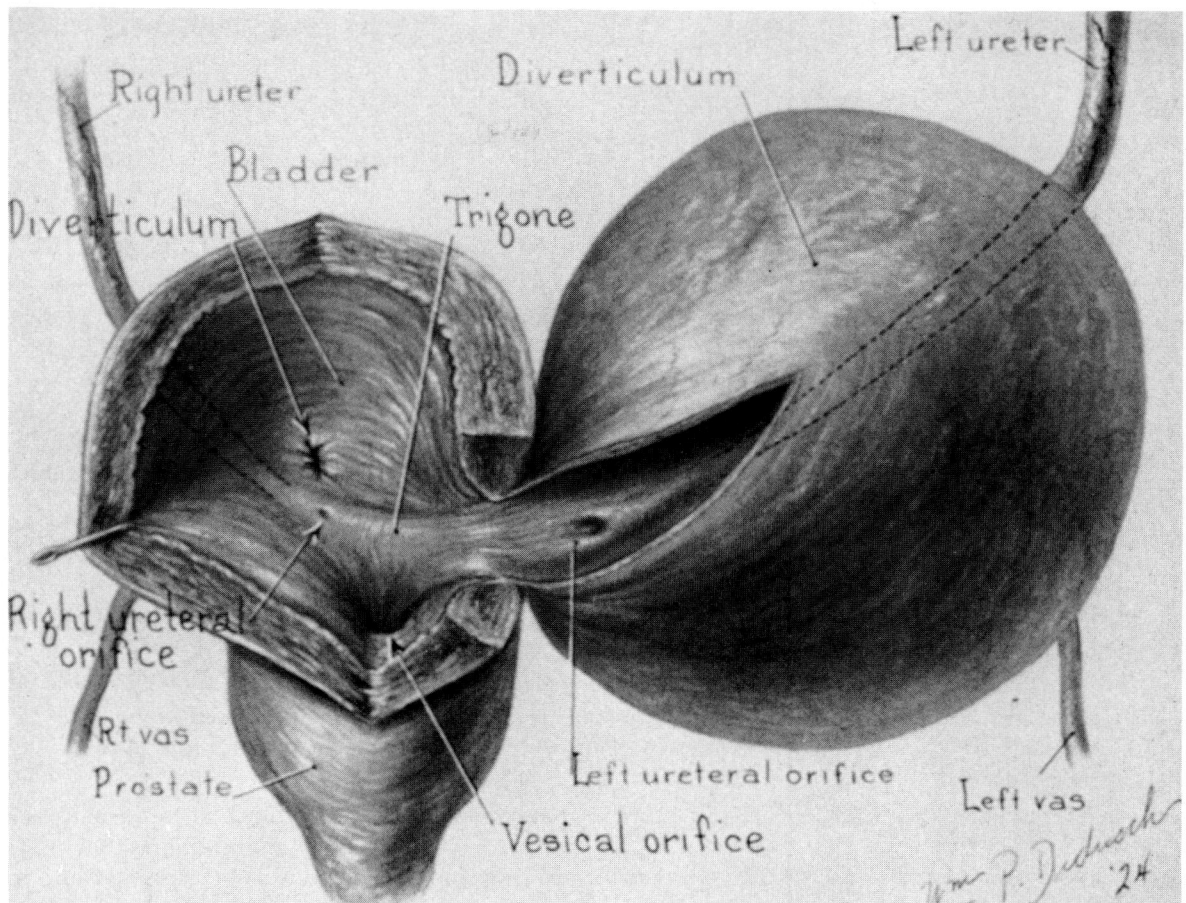

Figure 18.15. Diverticulum of the bladder found at autopsy. The bladder has been opened in front, exposing the trigone. The bladder wall was so incised down to the orifice of the diverticulum on left. The diverticulum was partially opened, exposing the left ureteral orifice within it. (From Didusch WP. A collection of urogenital drawings. New York: American Cystoscope Makers, Inc., 1952.)

TREATMENT

Resection of the redundant mucosal septum by cystotomy is the usual corrective procedure. Ureteronephrectomy may be necessary when obstruction to drainage of the bladder has been chronic.

Surgical removal of the constricting ring is the treatment of choice for hourglass bladder, if symptoms warrant surgical intervention.

Diverticula of the Bladder

Vesicular diverticula may be acquired or congenital. Most are acquired and are the late sequelae of mild urethral obstruction, which causes (in this order) chronic distension, trabeculation, cellule formation, and eventually diverticula. About 95% occur in men past the age of 50 years. They are associated with benign prostatic hypertrophy.

Diverticula of the bladder in infants and children are of different origin. The etiology of such congenital diverticula appears to be a weakness of the bladder muscle, often in the region of the ureterovesical hiatus. Normal voiding pressures are capable of causing diverticula to occur through these weakened muscular fibers. Unlike a saccule, which may not be evident at all except during voiding, a diverticulum forms a permanent protrusion.

The majority of these diverticula arise on the posterior wall of the bladder near the ureteric orifices. They have been related to the presence of abortive ureteric duplications, which become enlarged by pressures. These, as well as diverticula elsewhere in the bladder wall, are usually hernial sacs without a muscular coat. They may be the result of congenital deficiencies of the bladder muscularis, the actual diverticulum being formed later by intravesicular pressure (92) (Fig. 18.15). Diverticula may be formed in association with posterior urethral valves, neurogenic bladder, and vesicoureteral reflux, with which it is frequently termed a *Hutch diverticulum.*

Between 1859 and 1934 Kretschmer (93) collected 25 cases of hernia in infants and children, of which eight

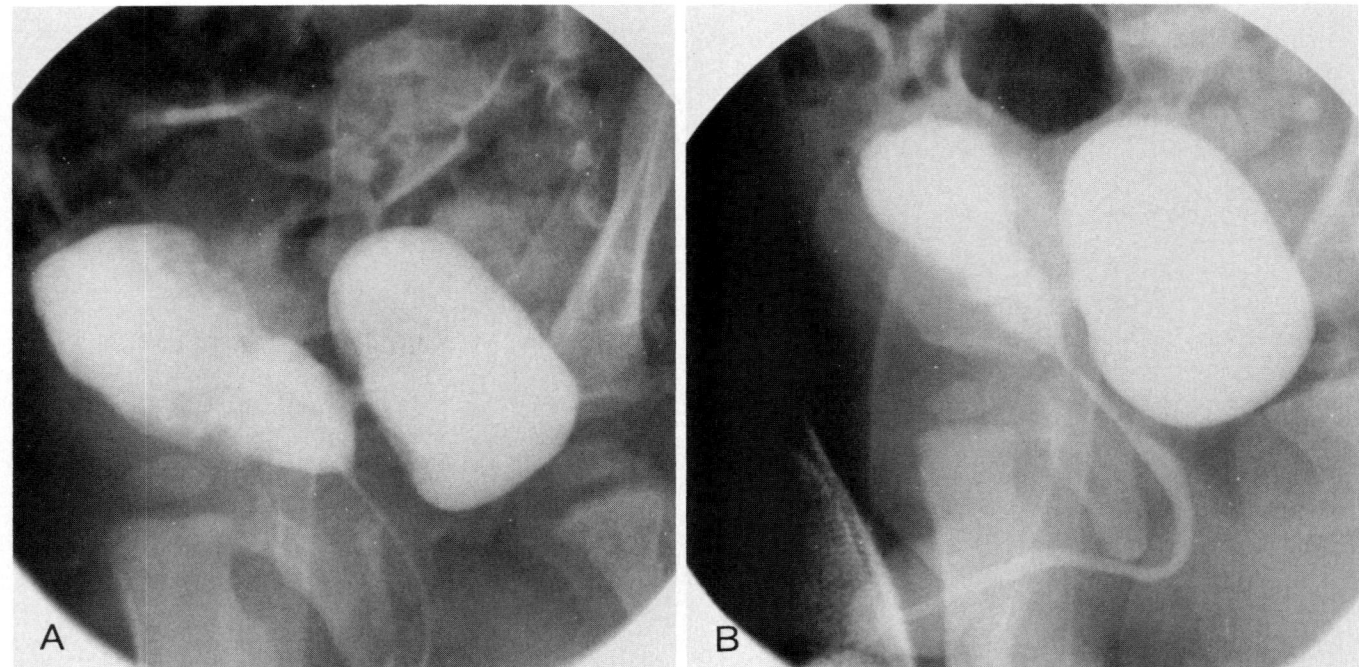

Figure 18.16.   Large bladder diverticulum causing bladder outlet obstruction and urinary retention in a male infant. Some dribbling urination occurred outlining normal urethra.

were 1 year old or younger. The muscular defect was first described by Anschütz (94) in 1922.

There are no constant symptoms except pain. Urinary retention in an infant from bladder outlet obstruction due to a large bladder diverticulum has been reported (95) (Fig. 18.16). The presence of other urinary defects often results in the discovery of the diverticulum. Cystoscopy and cystography are the means of confirming its suspected presence. Diverticulectomy is the treatment.

Exstrophy of the Bladder

ANATOMY

Incomplete exstrophy, or vesical fissure, is a suprapubic opening in the abdominal wall between the bladder and the outside. The pubic bones are united, and epispadias is not present. The condition is rare and is easily cured by simple closure of the defect.

Complete exstrophy is the most common type of the anomaly. Complete epispadias, wide separation of the pubic symphysis, and exposure and protrusion of the entire posterior bladder wall characterize the defect. The exposed bladder mucosa is bright red and sensitive at first, becoming pearl gray and less sensitive in later life as stratified squamous epithelium gradually replaces the normal transitional epithelium. The ureteral orifices are visible (Figs. 18.17 and 18.18).

The upper end of the defect may extend into the umbilical ring or end below it. If the defect reaches the ring, it is usually shorter than if it does not. If the umbilical ring is involved, the umbilicus is lower and the infraumbilical abdominal wall is reduced. Occasionally, the defect extends into the supraumbilical wall; the vitelline duct prolapses, and there is an amnion-covered sac above.

The lateral margins of the defect are formed by the medial borders of the rectus abdominis muscles above the symphyseal surfaces of the pubic bones below. Paul (96) demonstrated that no abdominal wall tissue is absent; instead, the failure is one of midline fusion.

The lower end of the defect is at the tip of the urethral gutter of the penis in the male or at the urethral orifice in the vestibule in the female. The penis and scrotum of the male are usually smaller than normal, and the scrotum is often bifid.

ASSOCIATED ANOMALIES

Undescended testes and bilateral inguinal herniae are common in males; duplication of the uterus and vagina may occur in females. Also, ureteral duplication is not unusual. The anus may be imperforate or stenosed, or there may be a rectovaginal fistula. Associated skeletal anomalies include cleft palate, vertebral malformation, spina bifida, congenital dislocation of the hip, and clubfoot.

Sixty percent of patients have renal anomalies and 72%

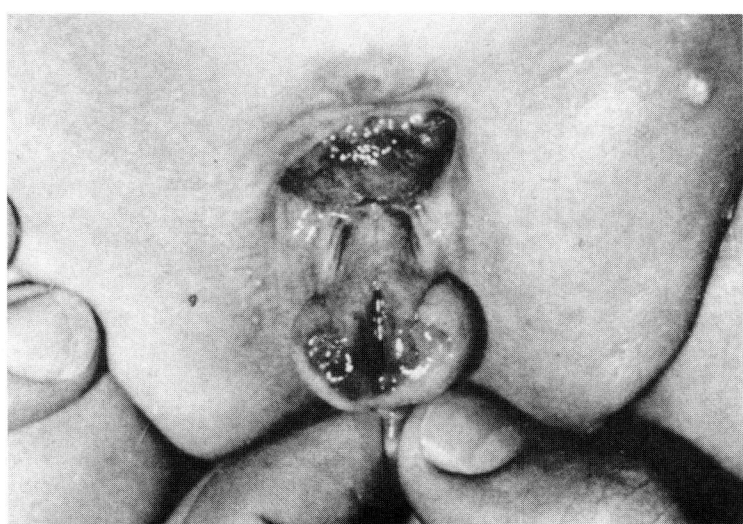

Figure 18.17.   Epispadias and exstrophy in male infant. (From Patten BM,   Berry A. The genesis of exstrophy of the bladder and epispadias. Am J Anat 1952;90:35–57.)

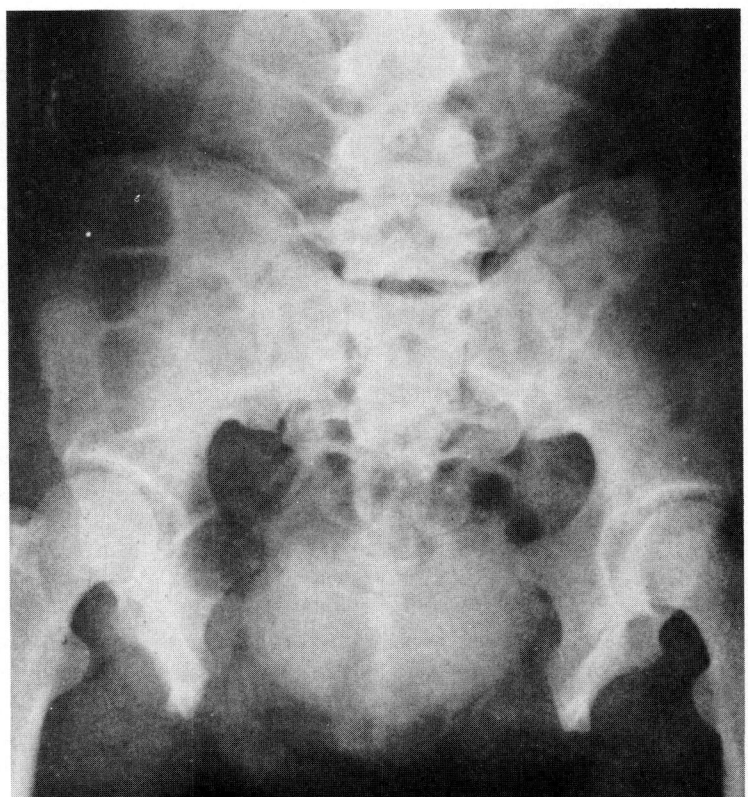

Figure 18.18.   Roentgenogram showing the widely separated pubic bones in exstrophy of the bladder. From Patten BM, Berry A. The genesis of exstrophy of the bladder and epispadias. Am J Anat 1952;90:35–57.)

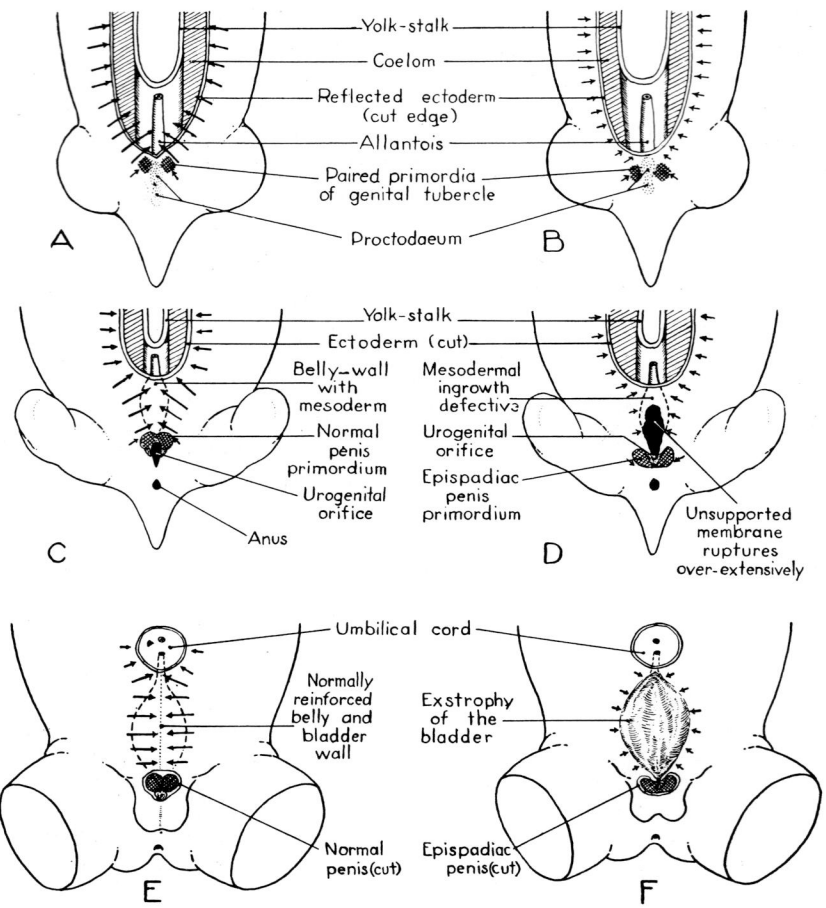

Figure 18.19. Schematic diagrams contrasting normal with hypothetical abnormal changes in the relationships of the primordium of the genital tubercle to the cloacal membrane and the urogenital orifice. **A, C,** and **E,** Normal stages. **B,**

D, and **F,** Stages in the genesis of exstrophy and epispadias. (From Patten BM, Berry A. The genesis of exstrophy of the bladder and epispadias. Am J Anat 1952;90:35–57.)

have skeletal anomalies, according to Soper and Kilger (97). Double inferior vena cava was reported by Muecke (98) in 1986.

EMBRYOGENESIS

Whereas epispadias is the result of an unusual ventral prolongation of the cloacal membrane beyond the phallic primordium, exstrophy results from a continuation of the cloacal cleft into the infraumbilical body wall. The rupture of the membrane, which consists of only two layers, has been attributed to the failure of the phallic primordium to form a mesodermal bar across the midline at the end of the cloacal groove. However, complete absence of the penis may occur without exstrophy.

More probably, the fault lies in the cloaca itself. At the end of the fourth week, the cloacal plate bounds the whole ventromedial portion of the cloaca from the allantoic stalk to the tail gut (1). No infraumbilical wall can be said to exist. Subsequent growth of the ventral cloaca (urogenital sinus) normally carries the insertion of the

allantois away from the anterior end of the cloacal plate at about the time the phallus forms (5 mm). If the anterior tip of the cloacal plate is carried upward by the elongation of the upper part of the urogenital sinus, instead of being left behind, the resulting extension of the cloacal plate and its eventual rupture would account for the open infraumbilical abdominal wall (Fig. 18.19).

Wyburn (99) recognized these defects as failure of the mesodermal components of the ventral abdominal wall to develop normally. He argued that the infraumbilical wall was supported by mesoderm arising from the primitive streak, surrounding the margin of the cloacal membrane, and invading the inferior side of the body stalk. If the "secondary mesoderm" fails to form, the endoderm of the urogenital sinus remains in contact with the skin ectoderm and eventually ruptures. Paul and Kanagasuntheram (100) argue that the mesoderm is not absent, but that its lateral halves have failed to fuse. Glenister (7) reconciled these views by observing that the single layered "secondary" mesodermal sheet that forms the musculature of the ventral bladder wall is eventually reinforced by extension of the primary somatic mesoderm, which forms the voluntary musculature of the remainder of the body wall. If the secondary mesoderm fails to unite at the midline, the somatic mesoderm also will be unable to unite, and the midline will remain a thin, double layer of ectoderm and endoderm. Thus, there is no absence of the

infraumbilical wall or of the anterior bladder wall in exstrophy, but a failure of midline fusion only.

One case appears to represent a borderline stage in the development of exstrophy (101). The patient had no external defect, but the bladder wall lay just beneath the skin, and the bladder musculature was in the fascia of the abdominal wall. In this patient, the secondary mesoderm had fused across the midline, and exstrophy was prevented, but little subsequent development of the somatic mesoderm had occurred. The chief clue to the existence of the defect was the wide separation of the pubic bones, which occurs only in the presence of urinary tract defects and which is rarely absent in complete epispadias or exstrophy (102) (Fig. 18.18).

In summary, the anatomy of the normal consists of following steps that take place for the production of exstrophy (Fig. 18.20 to Fig. 18.25).

1. Fusion of the two mesodermal ridges for the formation of the genital tubercle
2. Downward retraction of the cloacal membrane toward the perineum
3. Elements from mesodermal ridges reinforcing the lower anterior abdominal wall

The anatomy of the abnormal and the genesis of exstrophy consists of the following:

1. Abnormal retraction of the cloacal membrane, resulting in an inferior fusion of the two mesodermal ridges
2. Formation of the anterior wall of the urinary bladder by the cloacal membrane
3. Disappearance of the cloacal membrane (therefore the anterior wall of the urinary bladder does not exist anymore, resulting in expostion of the posterior wall of the

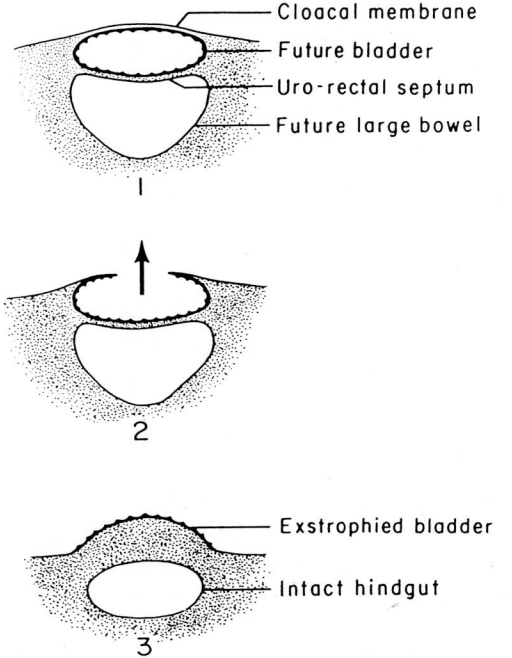

Figure 18.20. Diagram of events leading to classic exstrophy. (From Meucke EC. Exstrophy, epispadias and other anomalies of the bladder. In: Walsh PC, ed. Campbell's urology, 5th ed. Philadelphia: WB Saunders, 1986.)

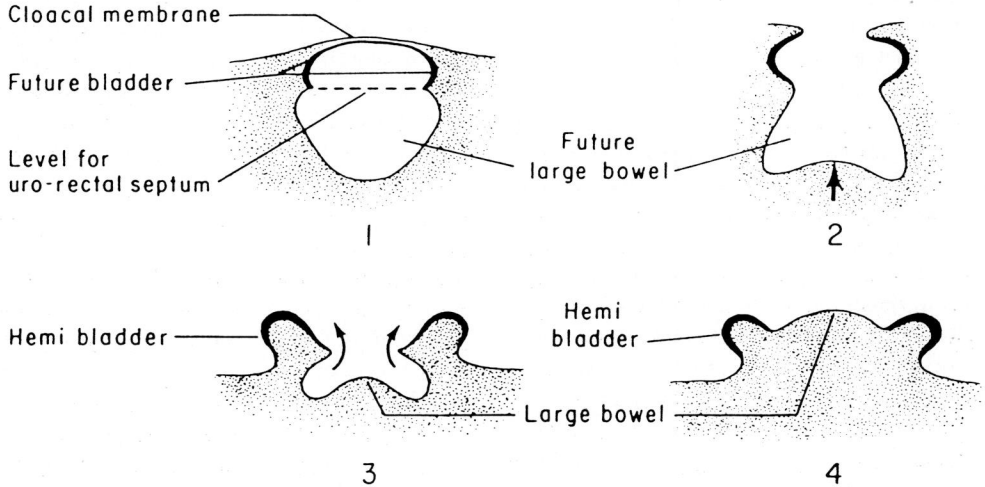

Figure 18.21. Diagram of eventration of cloaca to form cloacal exstrophy. (From Meucke EC. Exstrophy, epispadias and other anomalies of the bladder. In: Walsh PC, ed. Campbell's urology, 5th ed. Philadelphia: WB Saunders, 1986.)

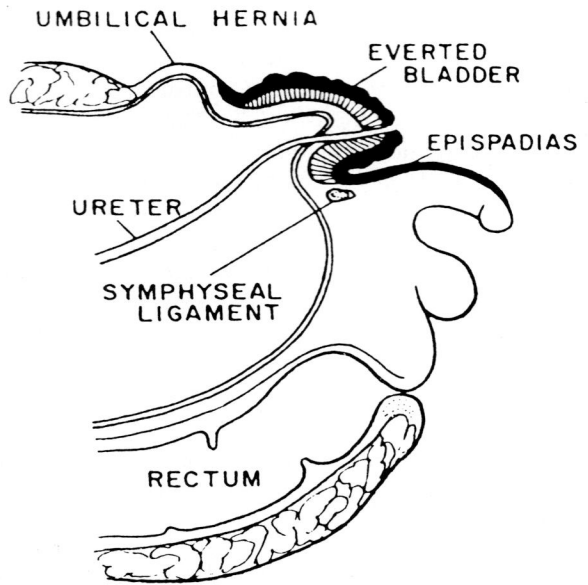

Figure 18.22. Descriptive drawing of classic exstrophy of the bladder in a male child. (From Meucke EC. Exstrophy, epispadias and other anomalies of the bladder. In: Walsh PC, ed. Campbell's urology, 5th ed. Philadelphia: WB Saunders, 1986.)

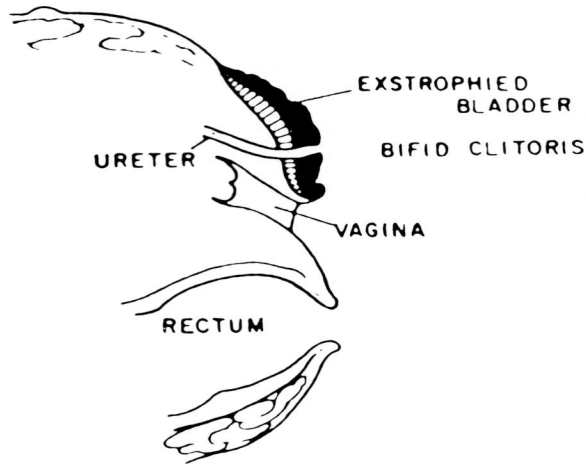

Figure 18.23. Female child with exstrophy of the bladder. A patulous anus was also present. (From Meucke EC. Exstrophy, epispadias and other anomalies of the bladder. In: Walsh PC, ed. Campbell's urology, 5th ed. Philadelphia: WB Saunders, 1986.)

urinary bladder, including ureters and urethra at the lower abdominal wall)

4. Division of the primitive cloaca by the anorectal septum before the disappearance of the membranes, resulting in cloacal exstrophy

HISTORY

Although exstrophy of the bladder must have occurred since antiquity, no record of it has survived. Von Grafenburg (102) described a case in 1598, and there is a reference to it in the *Historia Monstrosum* of Aldrovandus in 1646. The first adequate anatomic description was by Mowat, whose report is quoted in full by Connell (103).

The earliest effort at treatment was palliative. A silver bowl was placed over the exstrophy to protect it and to collect the urine. The device is first mentioned toward the end of the 18th century and ascribed to Jurine of Geneva (103). One feels it could well have been invented by the unhappy patient. Similar devices with a collecting reservoir are still in use today.

Sometime before 1811, Chaussier, who contributed to the reform of the curriculum of the medical schools of France after the Revolution, applied the term *exstrophic* to the malformation (103). By 1805 Duncan (104) collected 50 cases, and by 1833 Velpeau (105) was able to assemble 100. Hamilton (106) in 1835 reported the first U.S. case—that of a woman with exstrophy of the bladder who had been delivered of a child by cesarean section in 1787 by "Dr. Mather of the city of Hartford." The patient died in 1827 at the age of 80 years.

Lloyd (107) in 1851 and Simon (108) in the following year made the first attempts to transplant ureters into the colon of exstrophic patients, but neither patient survived.

During the latter half of the 19th century, skin flap operations to cover the defect were widely used. Pancoast in Philadelphia and Ayres in Brooklyn (109) achieved the first successful results in 1858. Pancoast's patient died from typhoid fever 2½ months after the operation. Ayres's patient, who had already borne a child, underwent two operations and was subsequently well and apparently continent.

According to Caldamone (110) the first successful operation for bladder coverage was performed in 1871 by Maury.

After the early failures of ureteral transplantation, this method was abandoned until Maydl (111) in 1894 presented two successful transplantations of the entire trigone into the sigmoid colon. He believed that the normal ureteral orifices would prevent reflux infection from the colon. Connell (103) has thoroughly reviewed the various operative procedures, both successful and unsuccessful, up the end of the 19th century.

INCIDENCE

Exstrophy of the bladder has been said to occur once in 30,000 to 40,000 births (112). Rickham (113) reported an incidence in Liverpool of 1:40,000 births before 1953 and 1:10,000 births between 1953 and 1960. Although a familial tendency has not been demonstrated, Lattimer and Smith (114) believe the risk of having a second exstrophic child in the same family is increased. Affected twins are known. In series of Harvard and Thompson (115), Uson and his colleagues (116), and Higgins (112), there were twice as many males as females; in those of

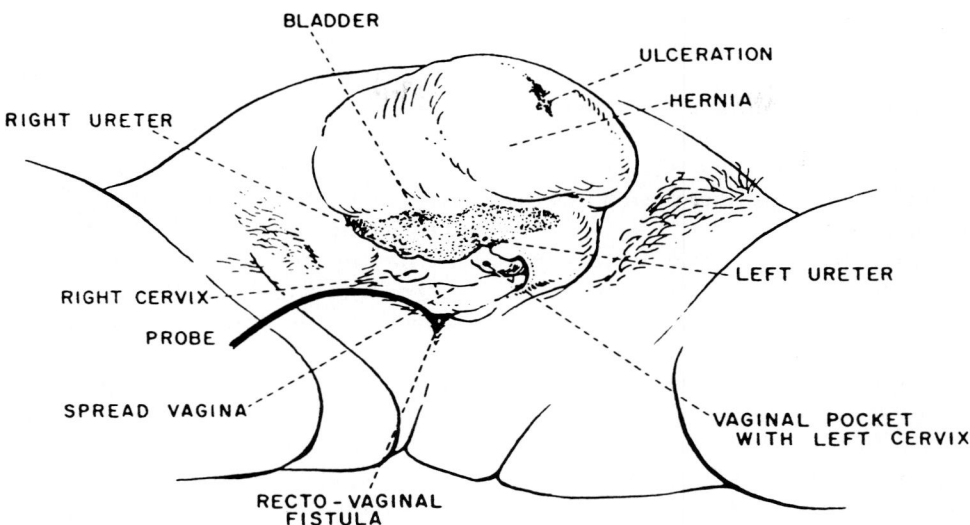

Figure 18.24. An extreme form of classic exstrophy in a young woman. The pubic bones were separated by 17 cm; two cervices and uteri were present, and the vagina communicated with the rectum (marked by probe). (From Meucke EC. Exstrophy, epispadias and other anomalies of the bladder. In: Walsh PC, ed. Campbell's urology, 5th ed. Philadelphia: WB Saunders, 1986.)

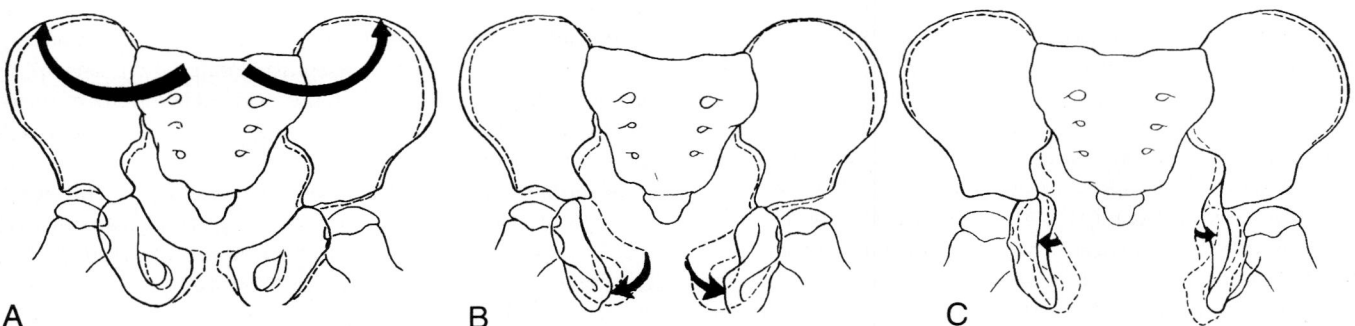

Figure 18.25. Sequential presentation of rotational and lateral deformities of the pelvic girdle in cases of exstrophy. **A,** Widening of the symphysis caused by outward rotation of the innominate bones, usually the only skeletal abnormality present in epispadias. **B,** An additional external (outward) rotation of the pubic bones: the characteristic skeletal changes in classic forms of exstrophy. **C,** The final addition of lateral inferior separation of the innominate bones present in the extreme manifestation of the complex, namely, cloacal exstrophy. (From Meucke EC. Exstrophy, epispadias and other anomalies of the bladder. In: Walsh PC, ed. Campbell's urology, 5th ed. Philadelphia: WB Saunders, 1986.)

Gross (117) and Lattimer and Smith (114), there were three times as many males. The ratio of male to female is 2.3:1, according to Jeffs and Lepor (118).

SYMPTOMS

The patient is odoriferous and as a consequence, is often socially withdrawn. In the young there is a characteristic waddling gait, which has been ascribed to the open pubic symphysis, but which Uson and his colleagues impute to the sensitivity of the bladder mucosa to the touch of the diaper (116).

DIAGNOSIS

Diagnosis is made by inspection. Excretory pyelograms should be made to reveal possible upper urinary tract anomalies.

TREATMENT

We agree with Raffensperger (119) that a successful repair of bladder exstrophy ought to meet the following postoperative results: restoration of the abdominal wall, prevention of rectal prolapse, dryness with good social life, and sexual functioning.

Ureterointestinal Transplantation. In 1911 Coffey (120) proposed a transplantation technique providing oblique entrance of the ureter into the intestine, and for many years this method, with several modifications (121), was the treatment of choice. During this period, efforts were made to design operations to avoid three chief problems: leakage, obstruction, and ascending infection.

Mucosa-to-mucosa anastomosis of ureter to bowel has prevented leakage and obstruction (122, 123). Leadbetter and Clarke (124) combined this procedure with tunneling of the ureter through the bowel wall for a short distance to prevent reflux. This is the method of choice today.

Following a successful implantation of the ureter into the colonic wall, the bladder mucosa must be removed, the abdominal wall defect closed, and the epispadias repaired. These operations are usually done a few months after the transplantation.

Another approach has been the revival of Gersuny's operation, common in the last century. In this operation, the ureters are transplanted to the excluded rectum, and the sigmoid colon is brought down, anterior to the rectum, through the anal sphincter, producing a double-barreled anus controlled by the sphincter. The advantages accruing from establishment of continence and the separation of urinary streams are obvious. However, this procedure must be delayed until one is certain that the child has a good anal sphincter.

Plastic Reconstruction. The goal of complete repair of the defect with a functioning, continent lower urinary tract has been sought for over 100 years. A successful operation by Young (125) was reported in 1942. He closed the bladder, reconstructed the body wall and created a continent urethra in a series of operations. Unfortunately, widespread success did not follow at once.

In 1966 Lattimer and Smith (114) reported 70 cases of primary repair of the bladder, and Williams and Savage (126) reported 51 cases. In both series very few patients were continent and most had ureteral reflux with infection. A number of them required subsequent urinary diversion. Williams and Savage concluded that primary closure should be attempted only in patients whose exstrophy borders on epispadias. Lattimer and Smith observed that, in the absence of detrusor function, free incontinence that avoids back pressure on the kidney is safer than continence with ureteral reflux.

Palliative Therapy. Campbell (127) advocated the use of antibiotic ointment, petrolatum, and electric light therapy for the macerated skin and bleeding mucosa of children for whom surgery must be delayed. He suggested the use of a sheet of plasticene over the mucosa and skin to reduce friction.

Ansel (128) advised closure within the first 48 hours after birth because of the elasticity of the tissues and the easiness of molding the bones of the pelvis.

Jeffs and Lepor (118) recommended primary neonatal bladder closure, interval treatment, vesical neck reconstruction, reimplantation of both ureters at age 3 or 4 years, and penile elongation and urethroplasty (one- or two-stage procedure) at age 4 to 5 years.

Kramer (129) stated that approximately 95% of all children with bladder exstrophy are amenable to closure early after birth. Mobility of the pelvic bones, preservation of the detrusor function, and avoidance of mucosal

metaplasia are the cardinal points of justification of early intervention. Bladder augmentation has been reported by Ritchey et al. (130) and Goldwasswer et al. (131).

MORTALITY AND PROGNOSIS

Most untreated patients with exstrophy of the bladder eventually will die of ascending pyelonephritis. Fifty percent will not survive early childhood, and only 33% will live past the age of 10 years. Campbell (127) found one patient who lived to age 30 years, and Connell (103) mentions three who lived over 70 years. Higgins (112) was able to report only seven hospital deaths among 132 patients with ureterointestinal anastomoses. Of those surviving for 5 years or more, 60% had mild to severe hydronephrosis. Gross (117) had no operative deaths among 54 operations.

In 1966 Spence (132) evaluated 31 patients with ureterosigmoid diversion. Six patients were followed for 5 years and 16 for 10 years. There were no operative deaths; three patients died subsequent to surgery. On the basis of urograms, degree of infection, blood chemistry, and clinical status of the patients, Spence concluded that acceptable results were attained in 24 of the 31 patients.

The life expectancy of patients treated for exstrophy of the bladder is still less than the desired level, but a number of patients are alive and well 30 or more years after their operations.

Malignant potentialities of the exstrophic bladder seem to be greater than those of the normal bladder. By 1956, 39 cases of carcinoma had been reported (133). The incidence of carcinoma was 4% among the 170 cases observed at the Mayo Clinic (133). McCown (134) considered carcinomas of the exstrophic bladder to be more frequent but less liable to metastasize than equivalent lesions of the normal bladder.

Mesrobian et al. (135) reported the rates of 55% satisfactory cosmetic appearance of the external genitalia

Table 18.2.
Urinary Continence After Exstrophy[a]

Reference	Patients	Continent (%)
Chisholm (1979)	95	45
Jeffs et al. (1982)	55	60
Mollard (1980)	16	69
Ansell (1983)	23	43
Jeffs & Lepor (1986)	22	86
Rickham & Stauffer (1984)	—	31
Duckett & Caldemone (1984)	—	60
Diamond & Ransley (1986)		
Augmented	14	85
Unaugmented	9	15
Mayo Clinic (1988)	18	76

[a]From Kramer SA. Exstrophy and epispadias. In: Glenn, JF, ed. Urologic surgery, 4th ed. Philadelphia: Lippincott, 1991:531.

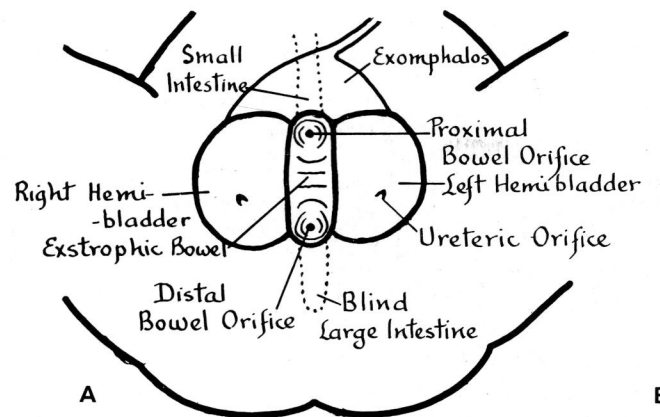

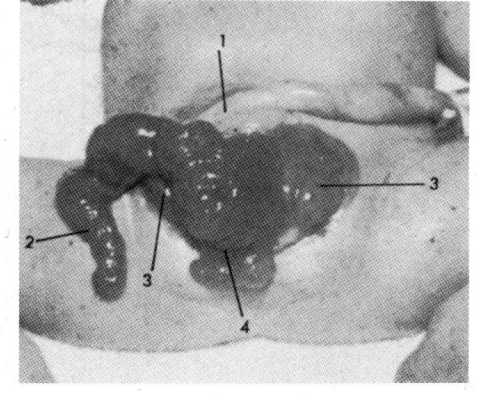

Figure 18.26. Exstrophy of the cloaca. **A,** Diagram of the external anatomy. **B,** Photograph of a patient showing exomphalos *(1)*, prolapsed ileum *(2)*, hemibladders lying on either side of exstrophic bowel *(3)*, distal bowel orifice *(4)*, and absence of anus and external genitalia. (From Johnston JH, and Penn IA. Exstrophy of the cloaca. Br J Urol 1966;38:302–307.)

and 100% erection with 61% ability for intercourse. Urinary continence after exstrophy was reported by Kramer (129) (Table 18.2).

Prognosis for Pregnancy. A number of women with exstrophy of the bladder have borne children. Randall and Hardwick (136) collected cases of 33 children who were born to 26 such women and of whom 25 were live and 8 stillborn. There was one set of twins (115). Eleven of the women had repaired exstrophy, and three more underwent repair after delivery. Six of the deliveries were by cesarean section; 27 were vaginal. Coulter and Sabbagh (137) described a patient who became pregnant 2 years after ureteral transplantation, excision of the bladder, and reconstruction of the abdominal wall, with vulval and vaginal plastic repair. Uterine prolapse almost always follows vaginal delivery in these patients and also may occur in the absence of pregnancy. Krisilof et al. (138) advised cesarean section for women who have undergone repair of bladder exstrophy.

Exstrophy of the Cloaca

ANATOMY

This is the most severe of the ventral wall defects as well as the most rare. It has been called "ileovesical fistula," which is a correct but misleading term.

Superficially, the anomaly resembles exstrophy of the bladder, but the defect is larger (Fig. 18.26). The lateral portion of the exposed mucosa represents the posterior wall of the bladder, but the central portion is intestinal epithelium. Superiorly, just below the umbilicus, the ileum opens to the surface and usually is prolapsed. On the exposed intestinal mucosa, one or occasionally two vermiform appendices open. At the inferior end of the mucosal surface, a segment of colon, which usually ends

blindly, opens. The ureters open low on the lateral bladder mucosa, and in males there may be two penes or hemipenes. Females may have müllerian duct orifices on the bladder mucosa, or two vaginae may end blindly. Exomphalos may extend the defect cranially, and the pubic bones are separated, as in exstrophy of the bladder (Fig. 18.18). Spina bifida, myelomeningocele, and a single umbilical artery are common. The best description of the defect is that of Johnson and Penn (139).

EMBRYOGENESIS

Exstrophy of the cloaca arises from the failure of secondary mesoderm from the primitive streak to cover the infraumbilical wall. It differs from exstrophy of the bladder in that midline rupture has occurred earlier (about the fifth week) before the fusion of the genital tubercles (hence, the double penis) and before the descent of the urorectal septum, which separates the cloaca into bladder and rectum. As the individual cloaca is exposed, its central portion is the posterior wall of the gut, while its lateral portions receive the ureters and differentiate into bladder mucosa (Fig. 18.27).

In some cases the exstrophic gut lies caudal to the bladder. In these cases the cloacal rupture took place after the urorectal septum began to descend, but before its descent was complete. These cases represent a stage between exstrophy of the bladder and typical exstrophy of the cloaca (Fig. 18.28). Thus cloacal rupture early in the fifth week results in cloacal exstrophy, while the same mishap in the seventh week results in vesicular exstrophy only.

The origin of the blind caudal intestinal segment is not entirely clear. Johnston (140) believed that the entire hindgut is shortened and exstrophic, while the blind caudal segment represents the persistent tailgut. This is reasonable, although it has not been proved.

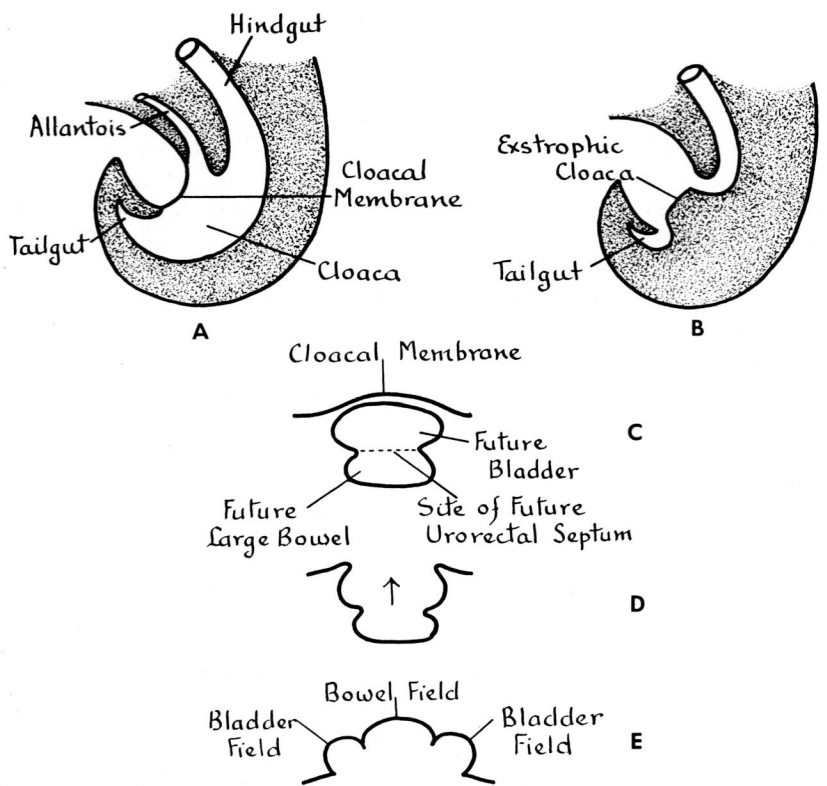

Figure 18.27. Presumed genesis of cloacal exstrophy. **A,** Normal condition of the embryo at 4 mm stage. **B,** Rupture of the cloacal membrane, perhaps from failure of local mesodermal development, leads to exstrophy. **C,** Transverse section through normal cloaca. **D, E,** Rupture of the cloacal membrane and resulting exstrophy. (From Johnston JH, Penn IA. Exstrophy of the cloaca. Br J Urol 1966;38:302–307.)

HISTORY AND INCIDENCE

Exstrophy of the cloaca was first described by Meckel (141) in 1812, and by 1909, 25 cases had been reported (142). Soper and Kilger (97) collected 57 cases in 1964. Males and females were equally represented; according to Kramer (129), its incidence is 1:200,000 births.

TREATMENT

While most of these malformed infants survive only a few hours, a few live long enough to be treated. Rickham (113) reported the first successful repair of exstrophy of the cloaca. Three stages were required: *(a)* repair of the intestinal defect and correction of the imperforate anus; *(b)* transplantation of the solitary ureter to an ileal loop brought to the outside; and *(c)* excision of the bladder fields. Eight months were required to complete all three stages, and the child was alive and well 22 months later.

In 1964 a second successful operation was performed by Zwiren and Patterson (143). The imperforate anus was corrected and intestinal continuity was restored in two stages. Reconstruction of the genitalia (male) was postponed.

In another patient, Ambrose (144) successfully closed

the bladder with a suprapubic cystostomy for drainage. The child is now over 20 years old.

Raffensperger (119) reported on his experience with 11 cases of cloacal exstrophy. He advised complete repair of bladder and bowel in one stage—recommending, however, the Howell procedure as safer. Howell et al. (145) reported a 85% long-term survival rate in 15 cases, advising repair of omphalocele, closure of the bladder, colostomy, and assignment of the female gender.

In summary, Howell et al. (145) and Ricketts et al (146) advise:

1. Preservation of the entire hindgut, including the terminal colon
2. End colostomy using the tailgut
3. Primary closure of omphalocele, if possible at once or in stages
4. Reapproximation of the bladder halves
5. Closure of the exstrophic bladder
6. Bladder augmentation at a later stage, using either bowel or stomach
7. Conversion to female gender
8. Staged abdominoperineal pull-through of the fecal stoma, or conversion to a continent ileostomy, depending on the anatomy and available bowel

Ectopic Ureter

ANATOMY

A ureter that opens anywhere but into the trigone of the bladder is considered ectopic. In males, ectopic ureters usually open into the prostatic urethra, the prostatic utricle or the seminal vesicle. In females, they usually open into the urethra, the vestibule, or the vagina. In a few cases in both sexes, other openings occur. Figure 18.29 shows the relative frequency of such ectopic ureteral openings at various locations (147).

Uterine or cervical openings are rare, and the uterus in such cases is often bicornuate (148, 149). In one patient a vesicovaginal fistula was present (150). In males the vas deferens is an uncommon site (151). Rectal ureteric openings have been found in at least four instances (152), and in a fifth case the opening was into a rectovaginal fistula (153). A bifurcated ureter with two vaginal openings 2 cm apart has been reported (154).

In addition to ectopic ureters that actively drain kidneys at some unusual location, ureters occasionally end blindly. These are almost always greatly dilated, and the kidney drained by them is atrophied. In one patient with unilateral agenesis of the kidney, the abortive ureteric bud remained as a diverticulum from the ejaculatory duct (155). In another patient the ureter opened into the closed half of a double vagina (156).

About 20% of ectopic orifices are associated with single ureters draining normal kidneys. The majority, however, are associated with the ureter draining the upper portion of a double kidney, with complete ureteral duplication. Figure 18.30 shows the distribution of ureteral and renal anomalies with which ectopic ureters are associated.

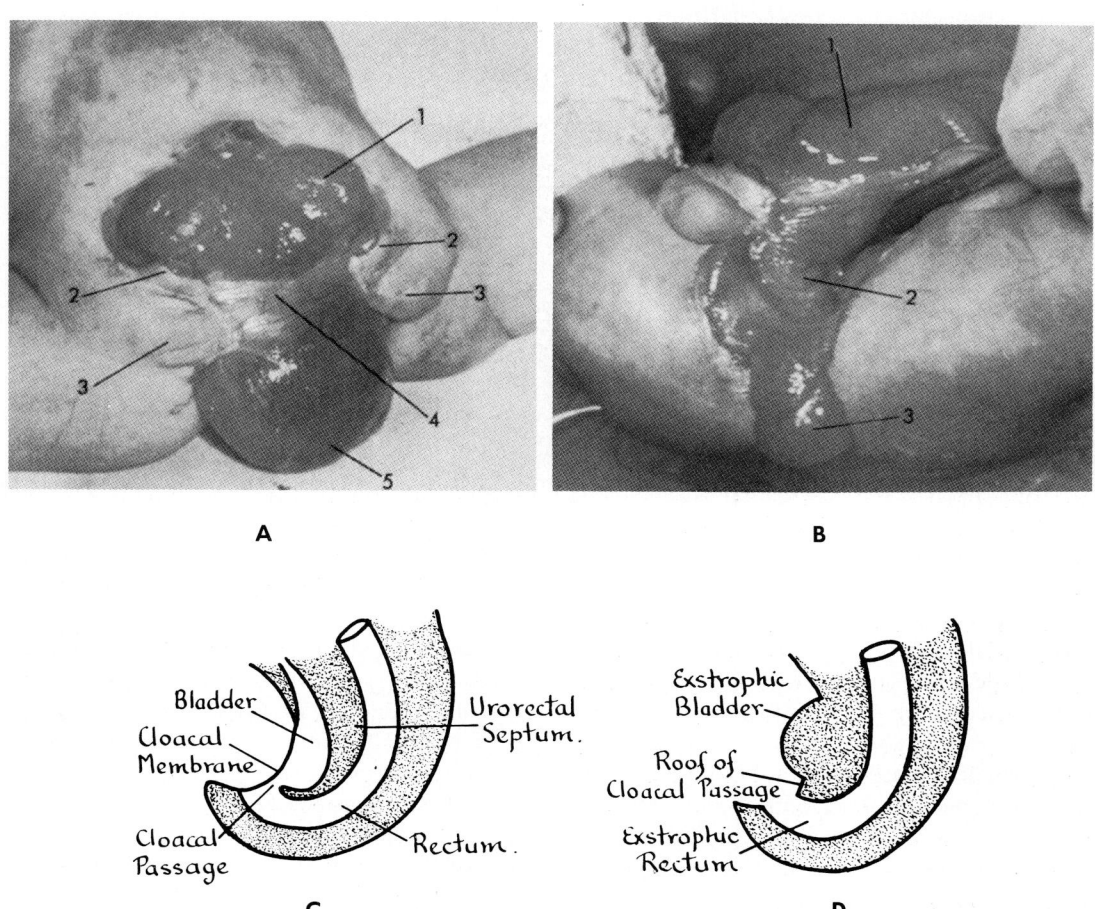

Figure 18.28. A type of cloacal exstrophy in which there is a single exstrophic bladder superior to the exstrophic bowel. **A,** Exstrophic bladder *(1),* paired epispadic phalli *(2),* hemiscrota *(3),* zone representing the roof of the cloaca *(4),* and prolapsed exstrophic rectum *(5).* **B,** Perineal view of same patient. Exstrophic bladder *(1),* exstrophic rectum reduced, showing wide orifice extending from the interpubic area to the coccyx and from one ischium to the other *(2);* coccygeal cyst *(3).* **C,** Normal development of the cloaca (slightly later than Fig. 18.27, *A).* **D,** Rupture of the cloacal membrane, resulting in exstrophy of the bladder craniad, the rectum caudad, and in between, the roof of the cloaca. (From Johnston JH, Penn IA. Exstrophy of the cloaca. Br J Urol 1966;38:302–307.)

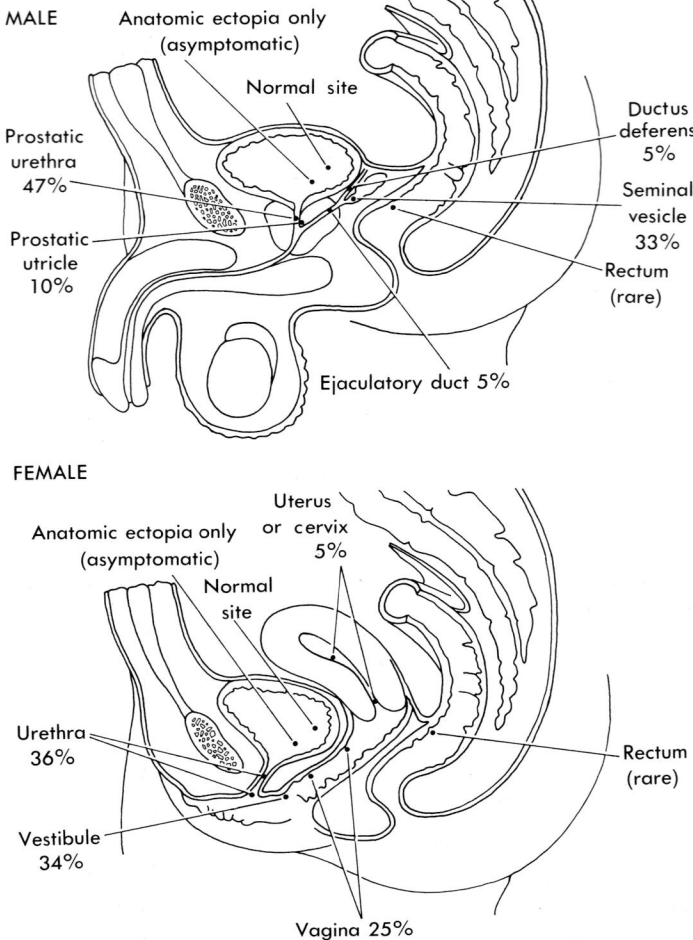

Figure 18.29.   Sites of ectopic ureteral orifices and their relative frequencies of occurrence in men and women.

EMBRYOGENESIS

Ectopic ureteral orifices result when a ureteric bud arises from the mesonephric (wolffian) duct more craniad than is usual. It may be the only bud, but more often it is a second outgrowth, with the first in the normal location. Because of this cranial location, the supernumerary bud is taken into the bladder wall during the seventh week at a lower level than is usual, or if it is sufficiently cranial in origin, it may not join the bladder at all.

Although abnormally located ureteral orifices within the bladder are not clinically "ectopic ureters," they are anatomically ectopic. They lie along a specific path, which starts at the site of the normal opening and ends at the neck of the bladder (Fig. 18.31). They may be recognized on cystoscopy, but they produce no symptoms.

If the orifice opens below the internal sphincter into the urethra, the ectopia becomes clinical as well as anatomic.

Should the ureter arise from the mesonephric duct at a still higher level, it will fail completely to become incorporated into the lower urinary tract and will remain confluent with the mesonephric duct in the male or with its vestiges in the female.

In the male, opening of a ureter into the ductus deferens or the seminal vesicle represents the primitive condition (Fig. 18.32). Subsequent resorption of the distal mesonephric duct may bring the junction medially until it lies at the prostatic utricle or is absorbed into the urethra itself (Fig. 18.33, *B*). Kidneys drained by such ectopic ureters usually function poorly or not at all and are often severely dysplastic.

In the female the distal portion of the mesonephric duct normally becomes vestigial and may remain in the wall of the cervix and vagina as the duct of the epoophoron, or Gartner's duct. It is into this channel that an ectopic ureter will drain (Fig. 18.33, *A*).

As the vestibule represents the termination of Gartner's duct, ectopic ureters would be expected to open there. Vaginal, cervical, and uteric orifices result from rupture of the thin partition between the vaginal or uterine cavity and Gartner's duct, which may have become distended by urine as a result of the anomalous connec-

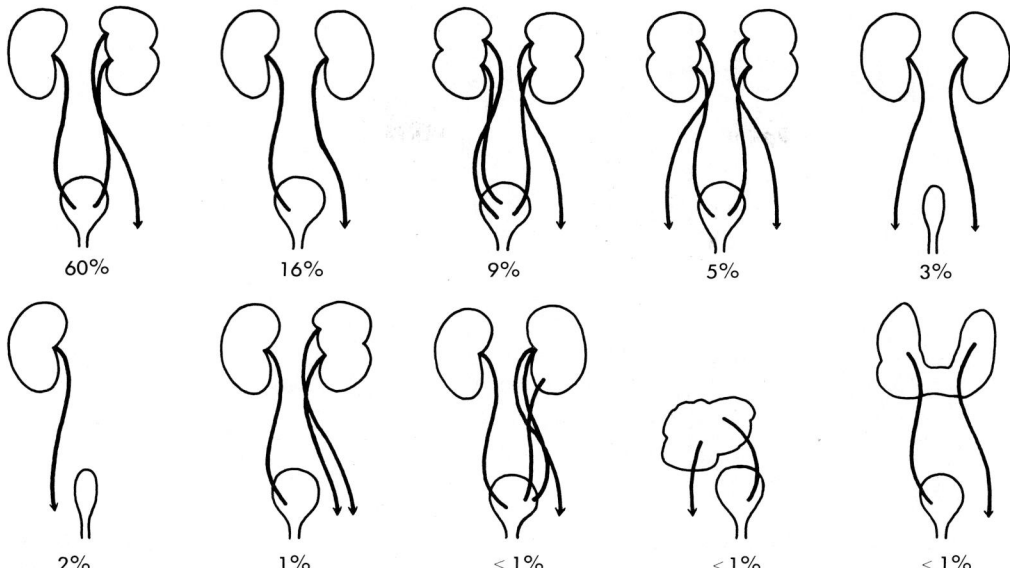

Figure 18.30. Frequencies of normal and anomalous kidneys and ureters associated with ectopic ureteral orifices (ending in *arrows*). (Percentages from Burford CE, Glenn JE, Burford EH. Ureteral ectopia: a review of the literature and 2 case reports. J Urol 1949;62:211.)

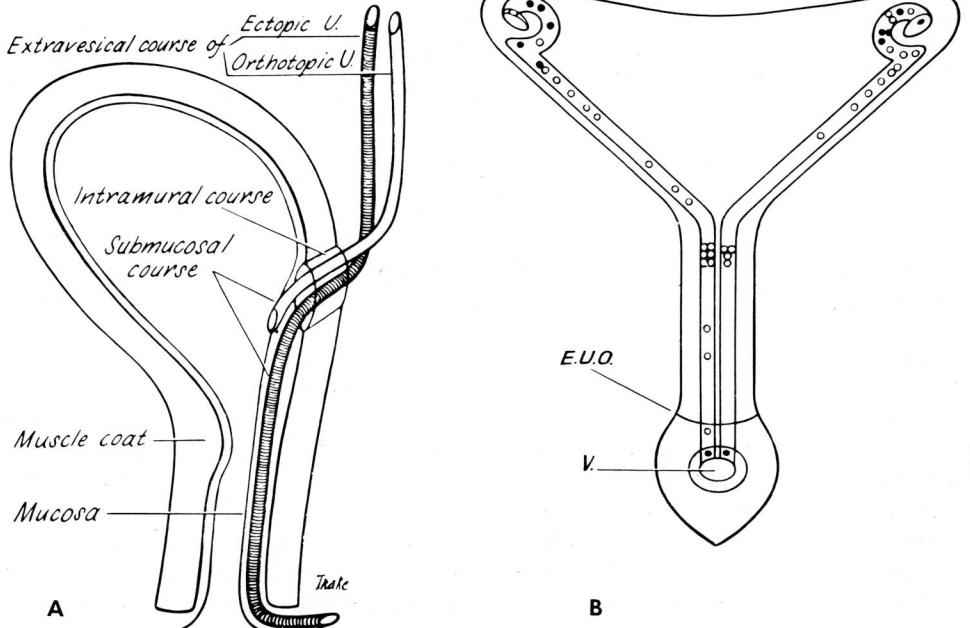

Figure 18.31. Ectopic ureter in the female. **A,** Diagram of the intramural course of an ectopic ureter. **B,** Positions of ectopic ureteral orifices along the "ectopic pathway" from the normal site to the vestibule. *EUO,* External urethral orifice; *V,* vagina. (From Stephens FD. Congenital malformation of the rectum, anus, and genitourinary tracts. Edinburgh: E&S Livingstone, 1963.)

tion (5). Rupture of a Gartner's duct cyst of the vagina during parturition has been observed (157).

Thus we may divide ectopic openings into two groups:

A. Anatomic but not clinical ureteral ectopia
1. Ureteral openings into the bladder medial to and below the normal site
B. Anatomic and clinical ureteral ectopia

1. Ureteral openings into some part of the urethra
   a. Openings into the prostatic urethra of the male
   b. Openings into the urethra of the female (incontinence)
2. Ureteral openings into the distal mesonephric duct in the male or into its vestiges in the female
   a. Openings into the seminal vesicle, ductus deferens, ejaculatory duct or prostatic utricle of the male

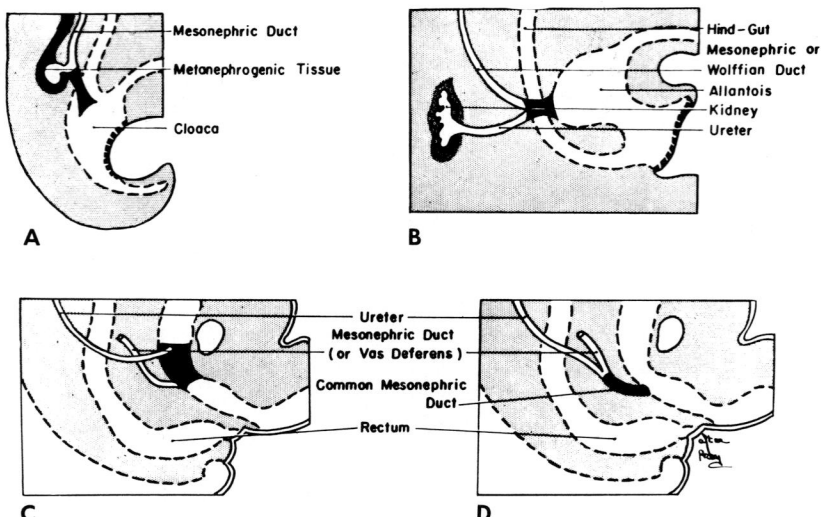

Figure 18.32. Ectopic ureter in the male. **A** to **C,** Stages in normal development in which a portion of the mesonephric duct (in *black*) is absorbed into the posterior bladder wall. (Compare with Fig. 18.5.) **D,** Failure of absorption of the mesonephric loop. The ureter thus opens ectopically into the ductus deferens or the seminal vesicle. (From Seitzman DM, Patton JF. Ureteral ectopia: combined ureteral and vas deferens anomaly. J Urol 1960;84:604–608.)

    b. Openings by way of Gartner's duct into the uterus, cervix, or vagina of the female (incontinence)
    c. Paravaginal openings by way of Gartner's duct into the female vestibule (incontinence)

Greig and Herzfeld (158) suggested that not all ectopic tubes associated with the ureters are of ureteric origin. They cite a number of cases in males in which the duct might be of müllerian origin and other cases in females in which the ducts might be persistent cranial portions of wolffian ducts. Two such cases which they describe seem to be acceptable. In both, the cranial end of the duct ended blindly near the kidney but had no renal tissue of its own.

HISTORY

The earliest description of an ectopic ureter appears to be that of Columbus (158, 159). The ureters were bilateral and opened near the urethral meatus. Columbus considered them to be duplications of the uterine tubes. Schrader (160) in 1674 described an extravesicular ureteral orifice (151), but the first adequately described case was probably that of Civiale in 1843 (161). The first important review was by Thom, who was able to find 185 cases in 1928. Eisendrath (162) found 255 cases by 1934, and Burford and his colleagues (161) found 525 by 1948. Ellerker (147) tabulated 494 ectopic orifices in 459 patients in 1958.

The importance of prenatal detection of hydronephrosis in duplications with ectopic ureters and ureteroceles was elucidated by Winters and Lebowitz (163). A sixfold increase in the diagnosis of these conditions was reported from 1982 to 1989 when prenatal detection was common, contrasted with the pre–ultrasound era.

INCIDENCE

Crenshaw (164) found one case among 81,150 patients in the records of the Mayo Clinic, but this is perhaps too low. Mills (165) found 112 ectopic orifices in 850 cases with ureteral duplications.

Females are more frequently afflicted than males, although series from the 1930's to the 1950's showed increasing numbers of cases detected in males. Mills (165) found 87 females and only 7 males; Burford and his colleagues (161) found 124 females and 25 males. Lowsley and Kerwin (166) estimated the ratio to be only 2:1, suggesting that even this may be too high. Because ureteral ectopia usually produces incontinence in females but not in males, discovery is far more likely to be made in females and to be made much earlier in life.

SYMPTOMS

Female. Incontinence is the constant symptom in cases of clinical ureteral ectopia, when the related kidney is functional (Fig. 18.34). Normal bladder emptying also is present when normal as well as ectopic ureters are found. When a ureter is from an aplastic or atrophic kidney, infection may be the only complaint. Patients may present with dribbling urination despite normal voiding at normal intervals. Frequently, the dribbling occurs only during the day because, at night, the supine patient's ureter has a large reservoir capacity. Stasis within the dilated segment may lead to infection and subsequent "vaginal" discharge in infants. In fact, young infants with a vaginal discharge in the face of no other pathology should be evaluated for the presence of ectopic ureter.

Male. Incontinence is not present. Epididymitis, pyuria, or pain may occur, and sterility was the complaint

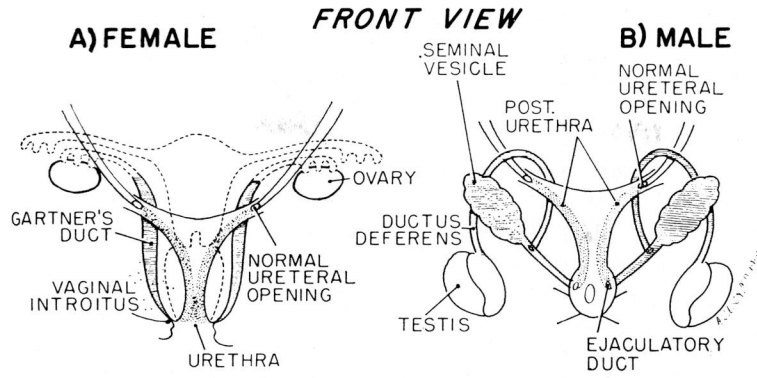

Figure 18.33. Ectopic ureteral orifices in female **(A)** and male **(B)**. *Stippled* and *shaded* areas indicate sites at which such openings may occur. (From Uson AC, Donovan JT. Ectopic ureteral orifice. Am J Dis Child 1959;98:152–161.)

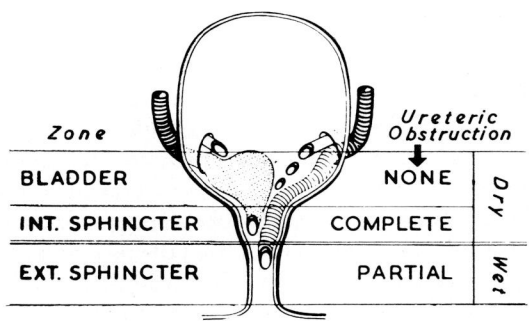

Figure 18.34. Ectopic ureteral orifices in the female. When the orifice is in the zone of the internal sphincter, the ureter is obstructed, but the patient is continent. When the orifice lies below the sphincter, the ureter is only partially obstructed, and the patient is incontinent. (From Stephens FD. Congenital malformation of the rectum, anus, and genitourinary tracts. Edinburgh: E&S Livingstone, 1963.)

in one patient (167). The epididymis may be grossly enlarged, and testicular pain has been reported (168).

DIAGNOSIS

Female. A carefully taken history of the incontinence is important.

The following distinctions can be made:

1. Complete incontinence: all functional ureters are ectopic
2. Incontinence along with normal voiding: normal as well as ectopic ureters are present
3. Incontinence varying with posture: ectopic orifice is located in neck of bladder

Excretory urography often will demonstrate the presence of an ectopic ureter, although the orifice may still be difficult to locate. Duplication, unless clearly of the complete type (bifid ureter), should reinforce a suspicion of ectopic ureteral orifice (Fig. 18.30). Presumptive evidence of an ectopic ureter on upper urinary tract studies may be shown by (a) abnormal number of calices and position of the calices; (b) rotation of the kidney down and out—"drooping lily"; and (c) malrotation of the calices and pelvis. A voiding cystogram may help to clarify the

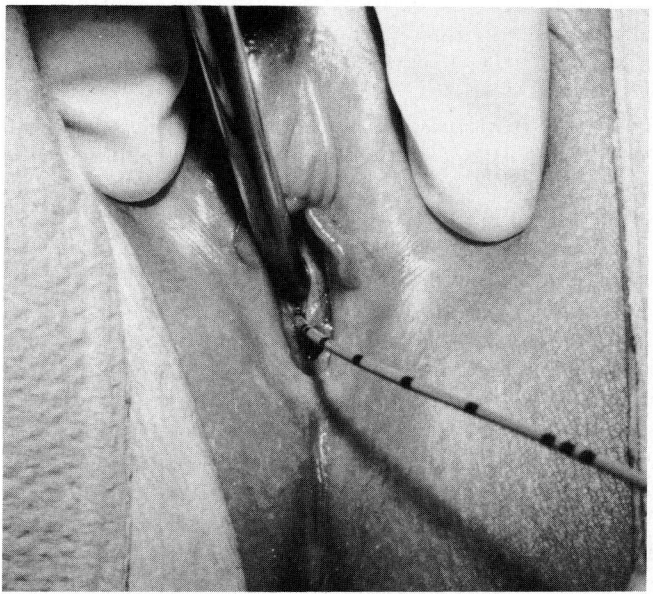

Figure 18.35. Ectopic ureteral opening in a female child with urinary incontinence. The child was said to be "always wet."

issue because often the ectopic ureter refluxes on voiding.

Intravenous indigo carmine injection usually will reveal the actual orifice in the vestibule, vagina, or urethra. For urethral search, normal ureters emptying into the bladder should be catheterized. When identified, ectopic ureters should be catheterized and retrograde pyelograms made (Fig. 18.35). The finding of one ectopic ureteral orifice by no means excludes the possibility of the existence of another. In about 5% of cases bilateral ectopic orifices are present. Multiple orifices also may be found on the same side. Ectopic orifices are frequently smaller than normal orifices.

Stress incontinence from the bladder may be distinguished from the incontinence of ectopic ureters by injecting methylene blue into the bladder and observing the leakage.

The greatest difficulty is in recognizing ureteral ectopia in childhood. It is rarely recognized before toilet training has been attempted and may be mistakenly treated as enuresis for many years.

Male. Seminal vesicular openings of ectopic ureters may often be detected by cystoscopic observation of bulging of the base of the lateral wall of the bladder, together with the absence of a normal orifice. Intravenous pyelograms are usually not helpful because of absence of secretion from the kidney involved, although renal ultrasound scanning will often show a hydronephrotic system. Vesiculography has been employed. Extension upward of the opaque medium is diagnostic of a ureteral connection (167).

In general, ectopic ureter in the male will only be suspected from intravenous pyelograms or renal/bladder ultrasound and must be confirmed at surgery.

TREATMENT

If the kidney drained by the ectopic ureter is single and healthy, transplantation of the ureter to the bladder is the operation of choice. A variety of ureteroneocystostomy procedures have been performed.

When the upper portion of a double kidney is involved, heminephrectomy and ureterectomy may be indicated if function of the upper pole is very poor. DMSA renal scanning, with split function between upper and lower poles, will reveal those upper poles that are worthy of salvage. In such instances anastomosis of the upper pole ureter to the lower pole renal pelvis is the procedure of choice (169). Occasionally, the condition of the kidney requires complete ureteronephrectomy.

Excision of the distal ureteral segment in the male may be extremely difficult. The posterior urethra and vas deferens should be tied off to prevent future epididymitis. Bilateral single ectopic ureters are a special challenge. Failure of both ureters to separate from the wolffian ducts results in failure of the bladder neck mechanism to form. Incontinence may be due to ureteral orifice ectopia and lack of a bladder neck mechanism. Total rehabilitation may require ureteral reimplantation and vesicourethroplasty. Females with this condition often wind up with small bladders due to lack of urine flow through the bladder. Ultimate rehabilitation in this situation may require enlargement of the bladder capacity with colocystoplasty or cecocystoplasty.

Ureterocele

ANATOMY

A ureterocele is a ballooning of the lower end of the ureter into the cavity of the bladder. Only the initial obstruction of the meatus can be considered to be the congenital defect; the ureterocele itself is a hyperplastic response that continues to produce an ever-increasing dilation until it fills the bladder. The thin, translucent wall is composed of bladder epithelium on the outside and ureteral epithelium within, with connective tissue and muscle fibers between. The orifice, which is often very small, is usually at the apex of the swelling; occasionally, it is on the underside, near the junction of the ureterocele with the normal bladder wall. The ureterocele may be as small as 1 cm, or it may fill the entire bladder and prolapse through the urethra (Fig. 18.36).

Ureteral duplication is present in about 75% of patients with ureterocele (170, 171) (Fig. 18.37). Renal agenesis, aplasia, pelvic ectopia, cystic disease, and other renal anomalies are common. Anomalies of other organ systems have been reported, but their frequencies are no higher than would be expected in a series of otherwise normal children.

EMBRYOGENESIS

It is generally agreed that ureterocele is the result of obstruction of the ureteral orifice. Persistence of Chwalle's membrane closing the ureteral lumen during the sixth embryonic week has been suggested as a cause of both ureterocele and congenital ureteric valves (172).

A more complete explanation may be found in the pattern of development of the intramural portion of the wolffian duct and the ureter, as described by Frazer (1). The growth of the bladder, which has absorbed the distal portion of the wolffian duct up to the junction with the ureter by the end of the sixth week, now carries the internal opening of the ureter upward, leaving the external ureterovesical connection at its earlier location. Thus the ureter enters the bladder wall at the region of the trigone, is fixed by the surrounding mesenchyme, and traverses the wall just beneath the epithelium to its internal orifice, which is carried upward by the growth of the bladder. Eventual destruction of the epithelial separation during the eighth week restores the internal opening to the level of the trigone. This septum dividing the ureter and bladder is probably the membrane described by Chwalle (172). Failure of this membrane to resorb provides the initial material for a ureterocele. The meatus of the ureterocele may be the embryonic internal orifice, whose diameter has not kept pace with the growing embryo, or it may represent a secondary rupture at a point at which resorption began but failed to continue (Fig. 18.38).

HISTORY

A case of ureterocele was first mentioned by Nöel in 1753 (170), and the first description of the condition was provided by Lechler (173) in 1834 under the name of "double bladder." Patron (174) in 1857 recognized the first case in which the ureterocele prolapsed through the urethra. Bostroem (175) in 1884 collected 26 cases of bilat-

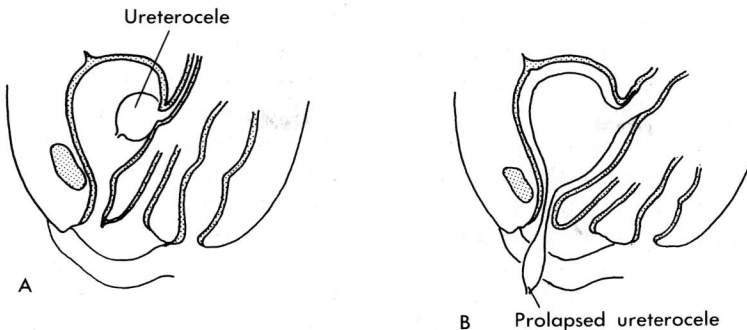

Figure 18.36. Ureterocele. **A,** Confined to the bladder. **B,** Enlarged and prolapsed through the urethra.

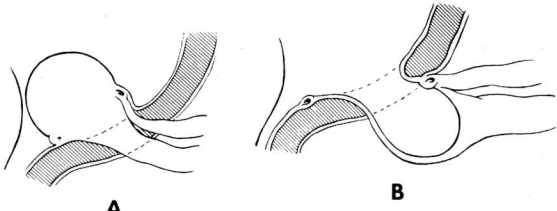

Figure 18.37. Ureterocele with double ureter. **A,** Ureterocele of lower orifice. **B,** Everted ureterocele of lower orifice carrying normal upper orifice with it. (From Ambrose SS, Nicholson WP. Ureteral reflux in duplicated ureters. J Urol 1964;92:439–444.)

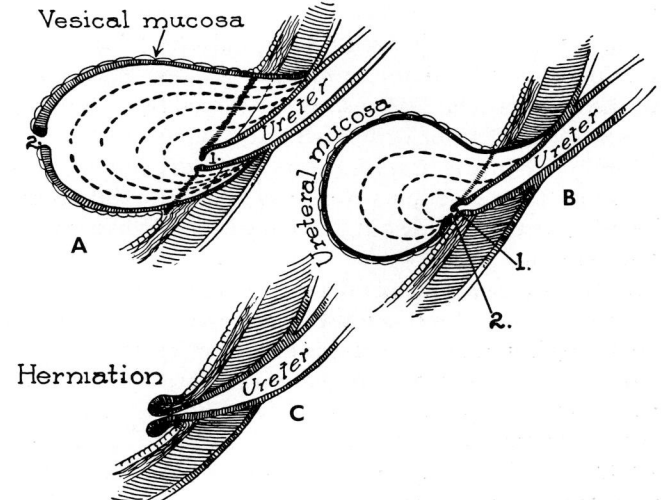

Figure 18.38. Development of ureterocele. **A,** Successive stages in the ballooning of the mucosa. **B,** Asymmetric ballooning, with the orifice on the under side of the ureterocele. **C,** Uretrovesical herniation, without ureterocele formation. *1,* Normal orifice; *2,* orifice of the cyst. (From Campbell M. Urology, 2nd ed. Philadelphia: WB Saunders, 1963.)

eral and 9 cases of unilateral ureterocele. The term *ureterocele,* however, was not applied to the condition until 1907 by Stoeckel (176). Although observed cystoscopically as early as 1899 (177), the first preoperative diagnosis was not made until 1904.

INCIDENCE

Gross and Clatworthy (178) estimated the frequency to be 1:12,000 general pediatric hospital admissions. Campbell (127) found one in 4000 autopsies and four in 100 children examined for pyuria. Campbell felt that the autopsy incidence was too low; because the ureterocele may collapse after death, some were doubtlessly overlooked. Uson and his colleagues (170) found 38 cases among 3800 new urologic pediatric hospital admissions and 6 in 3200 consecutive autopsies (1:533) of infants and children. There is a general agreement that ureterocele will be found in from 1 to 3% of all patients examined cystoscopically.

In Campbell's series (127), the two sides were equally affected. However, in two smaller series (170, 179), twice as many occurred on the left as on the right. About 15% are bilateral. Over twice as many are found in females as in males.

Most ureteroceles are discovered in the first year of life; one has been seen in a 7-month gestational age premature infant (170). Only three of Campbell's (127) series of 100 were over 11 years of age.

CLASSIFICATION

By definition, a ureterocele is a congenital cystic dilation of the terminal ureter. These may be divided into *simple* and *ectopic* varieties. The simple form is manifest by an outpouching of a normally positioned ureteral orifice. It bulges intraluminally into the bladder, its size and appearance varying with the ejection of urine through a stenotic meatus. With ectopic ureteroceles, the orifice is ectopically placed, usually into the urethra or bladder neck. The most accepted differentiation between a simple and an ectopic ureterocele deals with the location of the ureteral orifice; those of the simple variety are located within the bladder, whereas those classified as ectopic ureteroceles have their ureteric opening in a location other than normal, such as in the bladder neck or urethra (180).

Simple ureteroceles rarely occur in pediatric patients,

suggesting an acquired rather than a congenital etiology. The defect leading to this anomaly is thought to be a persistence of Chwalle's membrane with a consequent obstruction at the fusion point between the mesonephric duct and urogenital channel. Most commonly, patients with simple ureteroceles present with recurrent urinary tract infections. Pediatric patients often have solitary ureters, usually with ureterectasis and hyronephrosis, to a lesser degree than that found in adults (181).

Radiographic findings are pathognomic, and the diagnosis is often relatively straightforward. The classic excretory cystogram reveals a "cobra head" or "spring onion" deformity. Children tend to fill their ureteroceles less well, and thus the usual picture is one of a nanopacified filling defect in the bladder. Care must be taken not to confuse this with tumor, stone, blood clots, or feces/air in the rectum. The diagnosis is confirmed by cystoscopy. Cystic swelling at the orifice which changes with reflux of urine is diagnostic. Care must be taken to avoid overdistension of the bladder, which may obliterate the ureterocele or turn it "inside out," causing it to look like a diverticulum (Fig. 18.37).

Ectopic ureteroceles are currently diagnosed more commonly. Antenatal ultrasound often reveals fetal obstruction uropathy of which ectopic ureteroceles are often the cause (182). This condition is found more commonly in females, except when associated with a single ureter. Neither side predominates, and the bilateral condition is found in less than 10% of cases.

Cecoureteroceles are an uncommon form of ectopic ureterocele in which the intravesical portion dissects submucosally below the trigone and urethra. A dome-like protrusion into the bladder and urethra is seen. The lumen extends beyond the orifice like a tongue or "cecum." The orifice is often patulous and incontinent (Fig. 18.39). This condition is of particular interest to the surgeon because total excision is often quite difficult and risks damage to the bladder sphincter mechanism.

The orifice of the contralateral ureter may be obstructed by the ureterocele. Most commonly, the ipsilateral lower pole ureteral orifice likewise may be distorted, causing vesicoureteral reflux.

Ectopic ureteroceles and ectopic ureters are differentiated by their course. Ectopic ureteroceles run intravesically, whereas simple ectopic ureters run extravesically. In ectopic ureteroceles, the ureters enter the bladder in a common sheath and, by the nature of their submucosal course, provide distinctive cystoscopic and cystographic appearances.

Upper urinary tract anomalies with ureteroceles are common. Renal function in the affected segment is often decreased due to back pressure atrophy and/or pyelo-

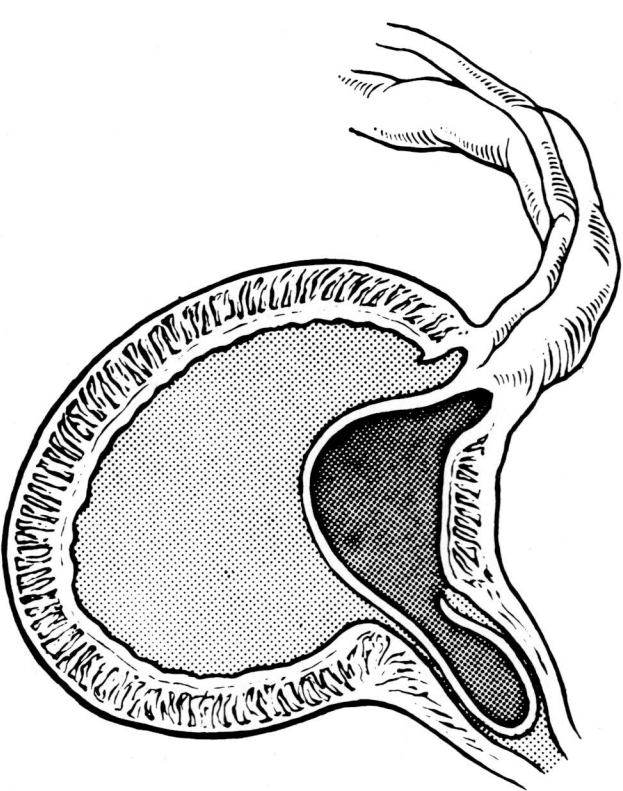

Figure 18.39. Cecoureterocele.

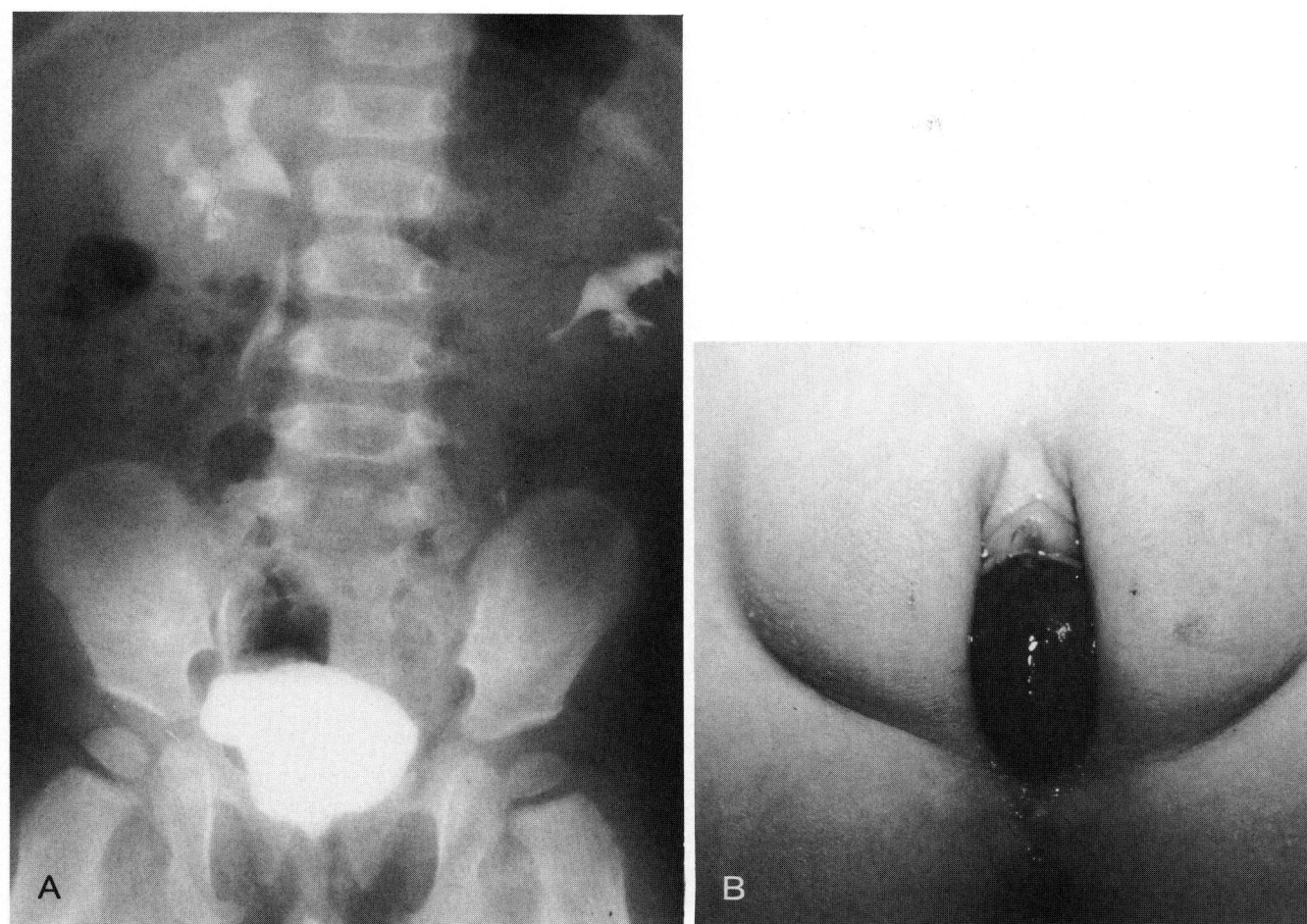

Figure 18.40. Prolapsed ectopic ureterocele. **A,** Typical IVP appearance showing "drooping lily" deformity of lower pole moiety. **B,** Clinical appearance of the prolapse in an infant.

nephritis. One-third of the patients in Williams and Woodard's study (180) showed renal dysplasia associated with the ectopic ureterocele. Renal anomalies, including ectopy and fusion, are not uncommon. Share and Lebowitz (183) coined the term *ureterocele disproportion* to describe that special clinical entity in which there is a striking dissimilarity in size between a large ureterocele and its diminutive ureter and calyces. The upper moiety did not function in their reported eight cases, and except for the ureterocele, the indirect urographic and direct sonographic signs of duplication were absent or subtle.

SYMPTOMS

Clinically, the patients with ureteroceles present with a mixture of obstruction and urinary infection. Infantile urinary infections may be severe and may lead to life-threatening urosepsis. Often, infants may present with severe renal failure, nausea and vomiting, and failure to thrive. Older children often present with pain, stranguria, and hematuria. The most common cause of urinary

retention in female infants is a ureterocele. Urinary incontinence results more from cystitis and severe urinary infection rather than from orifice ectopia, although true incontinence due to an incompetent urinary sphincter can be seen. Prolapse of the ureterocele in females may present as a cystic perimeatal swelling during voiding or the Valsalva maneuver (Figs. 18.36 and 18.40).

DIAGNOSIS

Ninety percent of ureteroceles can be diagnosed on the cystogram phase of the IVP or on low-dose voiding cystography. Stenosis of the orifice with severe obstruction causing nonfunction of the upper pole moiety has been found in up to 50% of the patients in some studies (184). Classically, the voiding cystogram will show a nanopacified filling defect (secondary to low concentration of the contrast medium in the ureterocele). Size may vary from 2 to 3 cm to a defect encompassing the whole bladder. The lesion is off-center and lies flush with the bladder floor. The size of the ureterocele may vary with the status

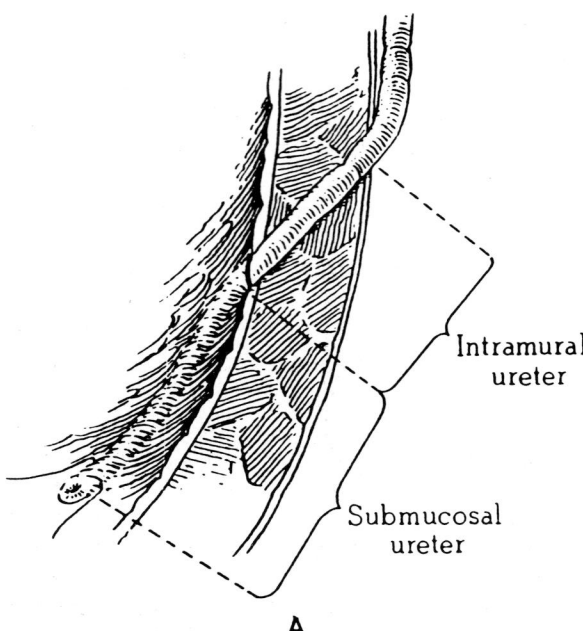
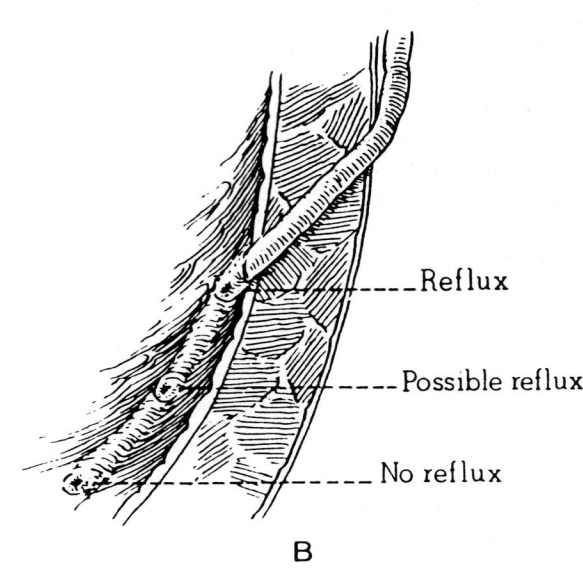

Figure 18.41. Mechanism of competence of ureterovesical junction. **A,** Normal. **B,** Refluxing. Same anatomic features as nonrefluxing orifice, except for inadequate length of intravesical submucosal ureter, are shown. Some orifices reflux intermittently with borderline submuscosal tunnels. (From Glenn JF, ed. Urologic surgery, 2nd ed. New York: Harper & Row, 1975.)

of bladder filling. Collapsed or contracted bladders may mask the ureterocele and cause a misdiagnosis. Small ureteroceles at the bladder neck are often not seen initially. Reflux is often found; in one series 50% of the patients with ectopic ureteroceles had ipsilateral lower pole reflux, whereas a lesser number had contralateral reflux (185).

Nuclear scans and ultrasound gives valuable preoperative information for ectopic ureters; evaluation of renal function by DMSA scanning may clarify the salvageability of the upper pole. Ultrasound may reveal a dilated upper pole ureter in addition to the ureterocele.

TREATMENT

Treatment usually involves excision of the upper pole segment and as much of the upper pole ureter as possible through a flank incision. Occasionally, renal function in the upper pole may be salvageable and proximal ureteroureterostomy is preferred. Approximately one-quarter to one-half of the patients treated in this fashion will require a subsequent operation to remove the ureterocele, to correct persisting reflux, or both (186). Some authors (187) have advocated marsupialization of the ureterocele, rather than total removal.

Delayed surgery for removal of the ureteral stump may be necessary because of persistent vaginal drainage, but reflux into the ipsilateral lower pole orifice seems to be less frequently encountered when ectopic ureter rather than ectopic ureterocele is found.

Monfort et al. (188) described a plan in which the ureterocele is incised endoscopically. This approach involves a small puncture rather than unroofing and offers a better chance of avoiding reflux. Tank (189) also enthusiastically adopted this approach. It is particularly attractive in managing the asymptomatic neonate with prenatally detected hydronephrosis.

Vesicoureteral Reflux

A normally functioning ureteral vesical junction (UVJ) allows for the smooth expulsion of urine from the ureter into the bladder without regurgitation of urine back up the ureter, either during bladder filling or upon voiding. If this valvular mechanism fails, from whatever etiology, urine flowing backward from the bladder into the ureter and/or the kidney is known as *vesicoureteral reflux*. The competence of the UVJ valvular mechanism depends on the length of the submucosal tunnel, which tends to increase with age and is the basis for expectant management of reflux (Fig. 18.41). Any factor which disturbs or distorts the normal anatomy of the UVJ, such as bladder outlet obstruction with secondary detrusor hypertrophy, can cause secondary reflux.

CLASSIFICATION OF REFLUX

Primary reflux results when there is congenital failure of the UVJ valvular mechanism. The reflux begins at the fifth month of life in utero when urine production starts.

This category includes all cases of reflux where no other documentable urologic pathology is seen, and it is due to a congenitally short submucosal tunnel.

Secondary reflux is caused by distortion of the UVJ by bladder outlet obstruction, such as occurs with posterior urethral valves or in neuropathic bladder. Reflux, secondary to detrusor instability, may be transient and resolve spontaneously. In the interim, upper urinary tract dilation can be severe. Allen (190) has shown that patients with unstable bladders and high voiding pressures are actually voiding against a closed external sphincter. The bladder assumes neuropathic changes in the absence of definite neurologic disease. Severe parenchymal disease can occur in a very short period of time. The most severe parenchymal damage actually may be seen in these secondary forms of reflux caused by high bladder pressures.

Rarely does recurrent urinary tract infection lead to reflux by causing UVJ edema and thereby disturbing the muscular sphincter mechanism. Although, strictly speaking, this is secondary reflux, it is highly probable in such cases that the UVJ was not entirely normal in the beginning.

The most commonly accepted scheme of classification of vesicoureteral reflux is the international classification (Fig. 18.42).

DIAGNOSIS OF REFLUX

Voiding cystourethrograms and nuclear cystograms are used to demonstrate vesicoureteral reflux because they may show reflux of urine from the bladder into the ureters and kidneys either upon filling or voiding. They also assist in assessing the bladder outlet for the possibility of intravesical obstruction. DMSA renal scans provide useful information regarding the degree of scarring, whereas

DTPA scans assess upper urinary tract drainage and hydronephrosis and assist in ruling out a concomitant ureteropelvic junction obstruction (Fig. 18.43).

Reflux may be suspected if the IVP shows parenchymal scarring, ureteral dilation, and tortuosity (without ureteral obstruction) which is increased with increases in bladder filling. Striations of the renal pelvis or ureters may suggest increased distensibility and supply indirect evidence for the presence of reflux. Ultrasound evaluations have been of little use in the evaluation of patients for reflux because significant reflux can be missed if the bladder is empty and the upper urinary tract is nondistended. Small scars may also be missed (191).

The complexity of radiographic findings in patients with reflux has been previously illustrated (192).

Most frequently, reported reflux is detected during the evaluation of recurrent urinary tract infections. Fully 30 to 50% of females with recurrent urinary infections have vesicoureteral reflux (193). A similar percentage of females with asymptomatic bacteriuria have reflux. Any male with a noniatrogenic urinary tract infection should be investigated for reflux. While formerly it was believed that females should be evaluated on the second or third

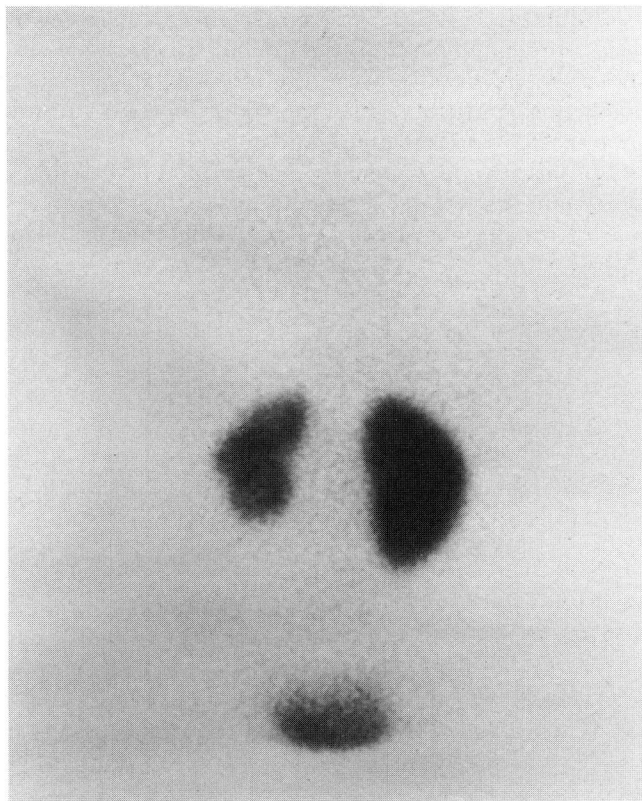

Figure 18.43. DSMA renal scan showing severe scarring of the left kidney, associated with vesicoureteral reflux. The left kidney contributes 28% of the total renal function.

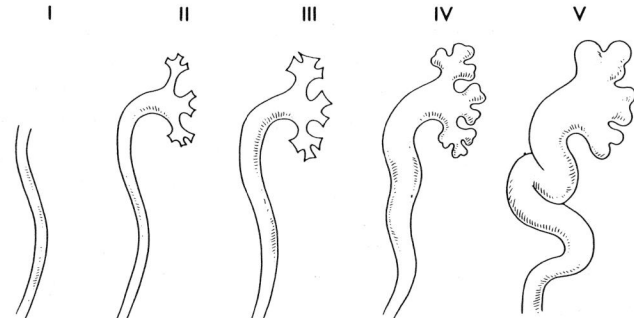

Figure 18.42. International classification of vesicoureteral reflux. Radiographic grades of reflux. *I*, Ureter only. *II*, Ureter and upper collecting system without dilation. *III*, Mild or moderate dilation of the ureter and mild or moderate dilation of the renal pelvis, but no or slight blunting of the fornices. *IV*, Moderate dilation and/or tortuosity of the ureter with moderate dilation of the renal pelvis and calyces and complete obliteration of the sharp angles of the fornices, but maintenance of papillary impressions in the majority of calyces. *V*, Gross dilation and tortuosity of ureters, renal pelves, and calyces. Papillary impressions are not visible in the majority of calyces.

urinary infection, it is now felt that all female children with a urinary tract infection should be evaluated after the first infection, except for those over age 5 years, whose initial infection is not associated with fever (194).

Infants with severe reflux may have small, scarred, dysplastic kidneys and present with overwhelming sepsis and/or renal failure. Males and females are equally affected during this period, in contradistinction to later life, when females predominate. Most authors postulate that severity is a combination of abnormal urinary defense mechanisms and predisposition to infection secondary to elevated residual urine. Males predominate during the neonatal period, probably because of the high incidence of vesicoureteral reflux associated with posterior urethral valves.

TREATMENT

In general, the majority of cases of reflux will resolve spontaneously with growth and maturation of the trigone and intramural ureter. The key to management is to prevent permanent injury while reflux is still present. Seventy-nine percent of ureters in 71% of children studied by Smellie and Normand (195) showed spontaneous resolution of reflux. Gross reflux (higher grades) are less likely to result. Forty-one percent of ectatic ureters and 85% of normal caliber ureters in Smellie and Normand's series spontaneously resolved. Renal scarring does not affect resolution of reflux, but it must be borne in mind that higher grades of reflux most often cause scarring and are less likely to resolve spontaneously.

Conservative management is advocated if the child is less than 6 years of age, is asymptomatic, has no progression of the degree of reflux or scarring, and has urine which remains sterile. If the patient is receiving antibiotic prophylaxis, parental compliance with giving the medicine may affect the management plan. Surgical repair is generally advocated in patients in whom the degree of reflux is severe or for whom compliance is a problem, for older children where reflux has persisted in the face of scarring, and in the presence of infection despite antibiotic therapy.

When surgery is indicated, the common goal of all operative techniques is to lengthen the submucosal portion of the ureter (Fig. 18.44). Reduction of ureteral diameter by tapering is occasionally necessary to achieve a 5-to-1 ratio of ureteral width to submucosal length (196).

Posterior Urethral Valves

Posterior urethral valves are by far the most common congenital obstructive lesion in the whole urethra.

ANATOMY

Three types of valvular structures in the male urethra have been described by Young and his colleagues (197) and Young (198) (Fig. 18.45).

Type 1 arises as a ridge from the colliculus seminalis and passes distally to divide into two membranes, which attach to the lateral walls of the urethra. This is the most common type.

Type 2 arises similarly, but from the proximal portion of the colliculus. It passes upward to divide into membranes, which attach laterally just below the sphincter. This type probably does not exist clinically.

Type 3 are diaphragms, usually with a central perfo-

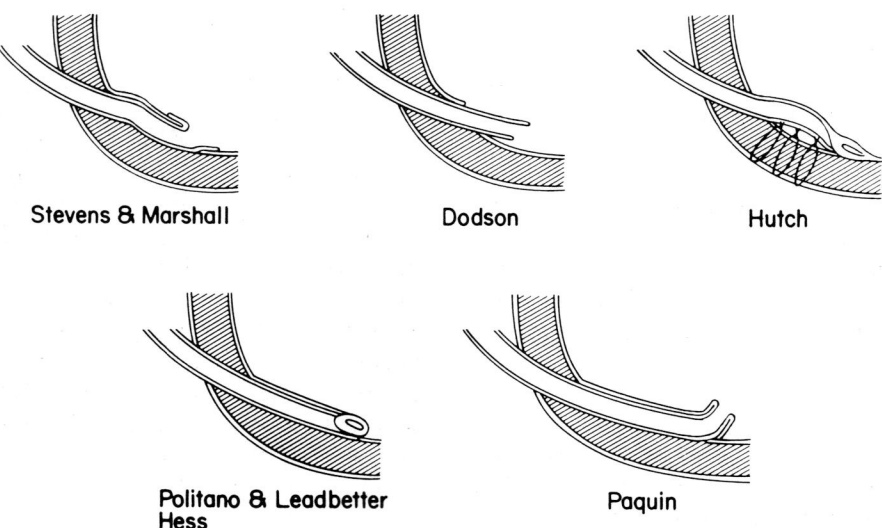

Figure 18.44. Five reported procedures for ureterovesical anastomosis using the "oblique valve" principle. (From Paquin AJ Jr. Ureterovesical anastomosis: a comparison of two principles. J Urol 1962;87:818–822.)

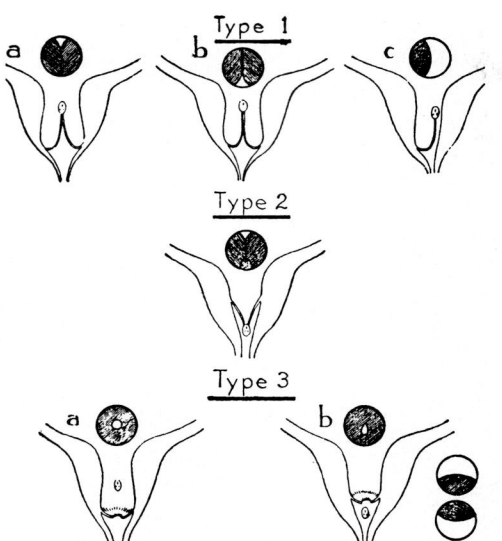

Figure 18.45. Valves of the posterior urethra. The *circles* above each sketch represent the cystoscopic view of the valves. *Type 1,* Valves distal to the colliculus seminalis (verumontanum). *Type 2,* Valves proximal to the colliculus. *Type 3,* Perforated diaphragms proximal or distal to the colliculus. (From Campbell M. Urology, 2nd ed. Philadelphia: WB Saunders, 1963.)

ration. They are not related to the colliculus and may be above or below it.

EMBRYOGENESIS

Urethral valves have been considered to be extreme developments of normally occurring folds and ridges of the urethral wall (199), the remnants of the urogenital membrane (200), the product of an anomalous junction of the ejaculatory duct and the prostatic utricle (201), the fusion of the epithelium of the colliculus with the roof of the urethra (202) and persistent distal extremities of the wolffian ducts (203).

None of these views is completely satisfactory, and none will explain the diaphragmatic type 3 obstruction. From an embryologist's standpoint, the theory of Lowsley (200) is the most attractive, but proof for any of the five theories is lacking.

Several authors, such as Grajewski and Glassberg (204), Kjellberg et al. (205), and Krueger and Churchill (206), reported posterior urethral valves in twins and siblings. Livne et al. (207) discussed the possible genetic etiology. Kelalis et al. (208) discussed heterogenous embryologic development.

HISTORY

Congenital valves of the posterior male urethra were first described by Morgagni (De Sedibus XL:29) in 1769. Some would reject this case because the patient was 50 years of age and showed signs of syphilitic infection, but the description is clearly that of Young's type 2 valves.

These valves were mentioned again in 1802 by Langenbeck (209, 210), but Tolmatschew (199) in 1870 was the first to study them seriously. Eigenbrodt (211) diagnosed them in a living patient in 1938, and Young (197) and his colleagues demonstrated them cystoscopically in 1919 and performed the first vulvectomy. Landes and Rall (212) reviewed 125 cases in 1935, and McCrea (213) collected 207 cases up to 1949. Pagano (214) presented 11 cases in 1965. Long-term follow-up of a large series of valve patients has been presented by Churchill et al. (215) and Parkhouse and Woodhouse (216).

INCIDENCE

Most cases are detected before the patient reaches the age of 10 years, but Landes and Rall (212) found 20% of their cases in patients over 20 years of age. Their oldest patient was 89 years of age. Opsomer et al. (217) reviewed the findings of adult males with posterior urethral valves, as did Heaton et al. (218). On the other hand, in some cases the obstruction has already produced dilation or ureters and pelves in intrauterine life (213). Valves may be suspected prenatally on maternal/fetal ultrasound examination and may be diagnosed prenatally by intrauterine cystography (220).

With a few exceptions, urethral valves are limited to males. Matheson and Ward (221) described valves in a female infant who was masculinized because of hypertrophic adrenal glands. The incidence has been calculated at one in 5000 to 8000 boys. Although some studies report that over 50% of patients are diagnosed before 1 year of age, others have reported that 20% were over age 20 years at the time of presentation (222). The spectrum varies from children with evidence of only mild obstruction to those with severe renal compromise.

DIAGNOSIS

Posterior urethral valves may be diagnosed prenatally, neonatally, and even into adulthood. The earliest diagnoses are made on maternal/fetal ultrasound screening; however, their presence should be suspected in the male neonate who cannot void at all. Urinary ascites may be suspected in an otherwise healthy neonate who becomes either obtunded or distended. Since the urinary ascites decompresses the kidneys, the degree of renal damage due to obstruction is often less than when ascites is absent. A similar renal-protective mechanism has been postulated for urinoma formations and the large bladder diverticula often seen in valve patients (223). Other presentations include fever of unknown origin, anemia, failure to thrive, weight loss, and seizures. One-third of male infants who present with azotemia have valves. Hematuria is also a frequent sign, more so in the older age groups with hypertrophied bladders. A distended bladder is the most common presenting sign in both the neonatal group as well as in toddlers. Laboratory studies will reflect deranged renal function, acidosis, anemia, and infection. Hypercloremic acidosis is associated with urinary ascites.

The hallmark radiographic study is the VCUG. The classical findings are a heavily trabeculated bladder, a hypertrophied bladder neck, and dilation of the prostatic urethra. A filling defect may or may not be seen at the site of the valves (Fig. 18.46). Vesicoureteral reflux occurs in 50% of patients.

TREATMENT

The management of posterior valves, after initial diagnosis and placement of a catheter for bladder drainage, can be divided into three categories: *(a)* transurethral resection of valves (224); *(b)* vesicotomy (225); and *(c)* a more proximal diversion for patients who present with severe hydronephrosis and azotemia that is unrelieved by distal drainage. Children who present with either severe infection or sepsis usually are candidates for proximal diversion, such as cutaneous pyelostomy or ureterostomy (226). Approximately 15 to 25% of patients diagnosed in infancy will require eventual renal transplantation before adulthood (227).

The nadir serum creatinine, within the first year of life, must fall below 1 mg% for the patient to avoid chronic renal insufficiency in later life.

Aganglionic Bladder

In about 4% of patients with congenital megacolon, the bladder also is involved. Swenson (228) considered the megabladder to represent a more extensive aganglionosis than that of uncomplicated Hirschsprung's disease. In addition to patients with megacolon, there is a large group of patients in whom Swenson (228) found aganglionosis of the bladder without aganglionosis of the colon. Bladder function in these patients is similar to that in dogs with parasympathetic enervation. There is an absence of bladder sensation with increased bladder pressure, and a large residual urine volume from deficient detrusor contraction. Among Emmett and Simon's cases (229), 90% had more than 30 cc of residual urine.

Harris and his colleagues (230) consider that the incontinence of neuromuscular dysfunction is an overflow incontinence, with physiologic obstruction at the outset, whereas that resulting from spinal cord defects is a true incontinence, with obstruction appearing later in life.

Infrequent urination with abdominal distension is the usual sign of an aganglionic bladder. Urinary tract infection eventually appears. Cystoscopic examination to rule out the presence of an anatomic obstruction is necessary to confirm the diagnosis.

Treatment is usually conservative. Swenson (228) rec-

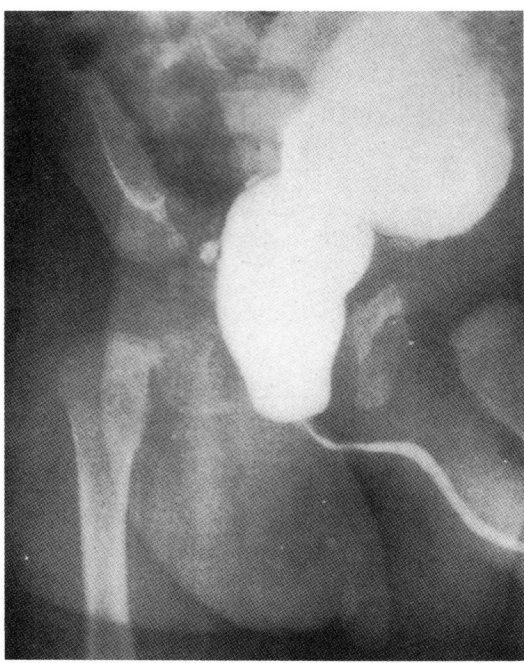

Figure 18.46. Radiographic diagnosis of urethral valve. The urethra above the valve is greatly distended, although a thin stream passes through the valve to the distal urethra.

ommended surgery to widen the bladder neck in some cases.

Marion's Disease

This is an extremely rare condition in infants, which simulates urethral stenosis; there is failure of the internal sphincter to dilate normally at urination.

The lesion occurs in infants and may prove to be fatal. Some light has been shed on it by Bodian (231), who dissected and histologically studied specimens from five infants who had died of the disease.

The prostate was elongated and extended from the bladder neck to the beginning of the corpus spongiosum. An increase in both fibrous and elastic elements of the gland was seen. The colliculus seminalis was hypertrophied in all cases. There was no aganglionosis of the bladder, and no evidence was found of a necrogenic basis for the obstruction. No etiology has been suggested for the prostatic changes; their embryonic origin remains doubtful.

Bladder distension, hydroureter, and hydronephrosis follow from this, as from urethral obstruction from other causes.

Duplication of the Urethra

Urethral duplication is not a single anomaly. It may arise as part of a general doubling of postvitelline structures,

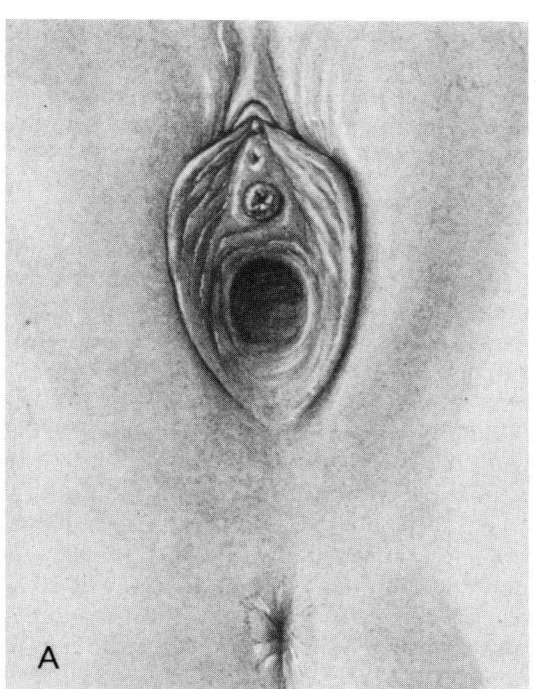

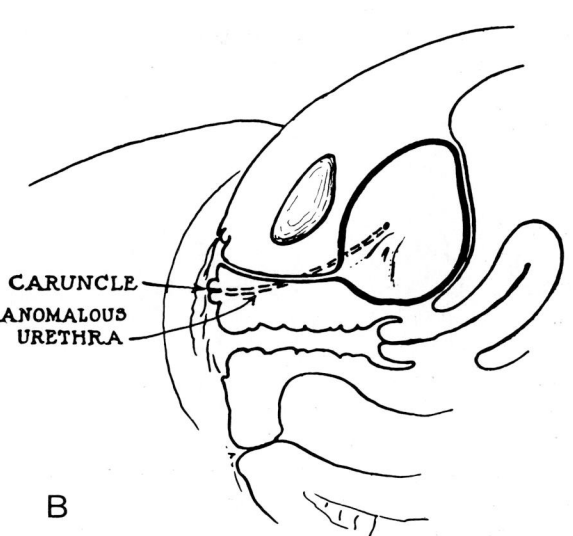

Figure 18.47. *Complete duplication of the female urethra.* **A,** *Caruncle at orifice of anomalous urethra is seen in the vestibule below the normal urinary* meatus. **B,** *Sketch of the course of the normal and anomalous urethrae. (From Dannreuther WT. Complete double urethra in a female. JAMA 1923;81:1016.)*

from a defect of urogenital sinus formation or in the male, from defective closure of the penile raphe.

ANATOMY

Bilateral Duplication of the Lower Urinary Tract. Two urethrae may drain separate hemibladders in those patients who also may have doubled genitalia and doubled rectum and anus. These have been discussed with the bladder (page 681) and with the anus and rectum (page 248). One patient was described (58) in whom only the urethra was doubled, but the presence of a bifid clitoris and widely separated pubic bones suggested this was a minimal expression of bilateral duplication of the lower urinary tract. This appears to be the only way in which true duplication of the female urethra can arise.

Persistence of Postvesicular Wolffian Ducts. Two male patients have been described who had two lateral accessory canals that opened from the bladder on either side of the normal urethra and joined it below the level of the prostate. In one case both lateral canals were complete (232), and in the other one of the canals ended blindly (233). These accessory canals are not of urethral origin, but represent persistence of the wolffian (mesonephric) ducts below the site of the ureteral branch. Such persistence in the absence of a connection with the bladder is ureteral ectopia (page 695). In these cases persistence of the distal duct has occurred even though the ureter opened normally into the bladder.

In two female patients, similar accessory urinary ducts have been reported (234, 235). In both cases an accessory urethra arose from above the bladder neck on one side and crossed the normal urethra to open near the midline, posterior to the normal urethral meatus (Fig. 18.47). These anomalous ducts are unilateral wolffian duct remnants comparable to those described previously in males. Functionally, they are accessory urethrae; embryologically, they are persistent wolffian ducts.

Midline Duplication of the Proximal Urethra in the Male. Duplications in which the two channels are both situated in the midline, one anterior to the other, are more frequently encountered than are bilateral duplications. They may be divided as follows:

1. Functional, complete duplication extending from the bladder to the skin: The external opening of the accessory urethra may be on the glans or on the dorsum or ventrum of the penis (Fig. 18.48, *A* to *D*)
2. Functional, incomplete duplication: Separate channels from the bladder unite to open at a single, normal meatus (Fig. 18.48, *E* and *F*)
3. Bifurcation of the distal urethra
4. Blind canal from the bladder or urethra
5. Blind canal from the surface of the penis

Only the first two categories shall be considered here. The remaining three are limited to the penile urethra and are discussed with anomalies of the male genitalia (see Chapter 21).

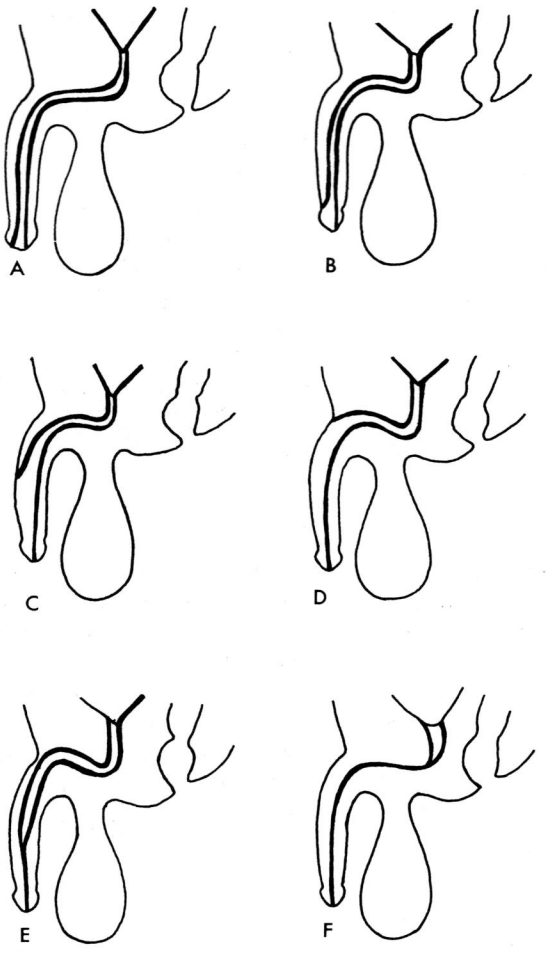

Figure 18.48. Duplications of the posterior urethra arising independently from the bladder. **A** to **D,** Complete separation of the urethrae. **E** and **F,** Separate urethrae becoming confluent distally.

Taruffi's classification (236) included an anomaly in which ejaculation proceeded from one channel, while urination proceeded from the other. Vesalius mentioned such a case, as did a few subsequent writers, but no case has been described in modern times. It seems probable that ejaculation in such patients occurred through the normal urethra, while urine passed incontinently through the accessory channel, which was not equipped with a sphincter. Bladder pressure may never have risen sufficiently high to produce relaxation of the sphincter guarding the normal urethra.

Woodhouse and Williams (237) have added to the classification the **Y** or **H** duplication which ends in the perineum, usually within the anal verge. Clinically, these patients present with two urinary streams or with infection. The patient with the **Y** duplication passes most or all of the urine from the rectum. Treatment consists of either surgically joining the duplication to the normal urethra or excising the extra channel. Management of the

rare **Y** duplication is more complex, because the penile urethra is usually rather stenotic. Most authors favor a staged approach in which the rectal urethra is mobilized to the perineum and then subsequently advanced using various graft and flap techniques (238).

EMBRYOGENESIS

Duplications of the urethra having separate vesicular orifices arise from abnormal relationships between the lateral anlagen of the genital tubercle and the ventral end of the cloacal membrane. Normally, the fusion of these anlagen in front of the urogenital portion of the cloacal membrane forms a bar to the ventral extent of the membrane. Should the tubercles unite slightly more posteriorly than usual, or should the membrane extend farther ventrally than usual, a portion of the membrane will remain in front of the tubercle. In its most extreme form, such ventral and cranial extension of the cloacal membrane produces exstrophy of the bladder (page 686). Less extreme deviation from the normal results in an epispadiac urethra only. The mildest result of such alteration of relationships is the urethral duplication with separate openings from the bladder (Fig. 18.48, *A* to *E*). The smallest deviation is represented by Figure 18.48, *A,* and the greatest by Figure 18.48, *D.* Certain types of defects are rare, and at least one, the hypospadiac accessory urethra, appears to be unique (58).

HISTORY AND INCIDENCE

These factors will be discussed with anomalies of the penis (see Chapter 21).

SYMPTOMS

Complete duplications may produce incontinence. Gross and Moore (239) found partial incontinence in three, and total incontinence in four of the 19 cases they reviewed. Even when incontinence is absent, an ectopic opening may be a nuisance to the patient.

Incomplete duplications of the proximal urethra are rare and asymptomatic, although incontinence might conceivably occur.

DIAGNOSIS

When the channels are of normal diameter, catheterization will provide the necessary information about the relationship of the accessory urethra to the normal urethra. Voiding cystourethrograms have been used (240).

TREATMENT

Complete duplication of the urethra requires treatment only if there is incontinence or if the accessory meatus is hypospadiac. Excision of the accessory urethra, with later repair of chordee, if necessary, is the only effective treatment. Such excision usually is not difficult; however, in

Rinker's case, in which a blind passage started at the glans and passed between the bladder and rectum to end at the level of the top of the bladder, three operations—penile, perineal, and abdominal—were required (241).

Diverticula of the Female Urethra

ANATOMY

The nature of these diverticula is obscure, partly because the anatomy of the female urethra has never been studied in detail. Most of the diverticula are infected when discovered. Their epithelial lining may be cuboidal or squamous, or there may be no epithelium. They lie posteriorly in the urethrovaginal septum. Among 21 diverticula, Wharton and Kearns (242) found eight in the posterior third, nine in the middle third, and four in the anterior third of the urethra. Some diverticula have been reported to have more than one opening into the urethra.

EMBRYOGENESIS

There is no agreement about the nature of these diverticula. They have been considered orifices of ectopic ureters or portions of Gartner's duct. Many appear to be infected paraurethral glands or mucosal crypts. Traumatic origin following parturition has been suggested, but about 33% occur in nulliparous women. They are rare in infants and children.

HISTORY AND INCIDENCE

Only recently have these diverticula received attention. Nine cases appeared in the literature prior to 1954, but four years later, Davis and TeLinde (243) were able to catalog 121.

In 1950 Wharton and Kearns (242) estimated their frequency as 1:2300 gynecologic admissions to hospitals. With the recent interest in the subject, the incidence will probably be found to be higher. Wishard and his colleagues (244) in 1960 estimated the incidence as 1:282 new gynecologic patients.

Few urethral diverticula have been found in infants or children. In Davis and TeLinde's (243) series, only 6.5% were under 20 years of age, while 65% were between 20 and 40 years of age.

SYMPTOMS

Frequency of urination is the presenting symptom in about 75% of patients. Dysuria and burning are present in more than 50%. Hematuria, stress incontinence, and dyspareunia are mentioned in about 25% of patients. In a very few the diverticula are asymptomatic.

DIAGNOSIS

Vaginal palpation of the vaginourethral septum usually reveals a mass from which pus may be expressed. Urethrography may yield further information. Calculi are not infrequent.

TREATMENT

Excision of the diverticulum or incision and drainage are the procedures which have been employed. In at least two cases, a postoperative urethrovaginal fistula has developed following excision (245). McLoughlin (246) reported carcinoma in a urethral diverticulum, and advised total inspection of the entire urethra during reconstructive surgery. Sheldon and Gilbert (247) use the appendix for urethral reconstruction in children with congenital anomalies of the urinary bladder. They advised against performing incidental appendectomies in the presence of bladder anomalies.

Pheochromocytoma of the Bladder

Sweetser et al. (248) presented a case of pheochromocytoma of the urinary bladder. They stated fewer than 200 cases have been reported since 1953 when Zimmerman et al. (249) reported the first case. They advised that the incidence is approximately 0.1% of all bladder tumors in males and females, with an equal gender ratio, and age variance from 11 to 78 years. The same authors estimated that 17% are nonfunctional and about 15% have malignant changes. The cardinal symptom is hypertension in most cases.

Surgical excision is the treatment of choice.

EDITORIAL COMMENTS

Prenatal diagnosis and subsequent management of conditions of the bladder and urethra is a major topic, just as are anomalies of the kidney and ureter. Ectopic ureters and ureteroceles, vesicoureteral reflux, and posterior urethral valves are now diagnosed prenatally, probably more often than when the diagnosis is made following the onset of symptoms such as infection, hematuria, or failure to thrive. Hydronephrosis due to obstructed upper poles is frequently encountered with both ectopic ureters and ureteroceles, as both conditions are most commonly associated with ureteral duplication anomalies. This hydronephrosis is easily detected on prenatal ultrasound screening. Usually the pregnancy is allowed to proceed to term, and the baby has a normal newborn examination. Under such circumstances, ectopic ureters and ureteroceles are treated similarly and involve management of the hydronephrosis via partial nephrectomy or ureteropyelostomy. Transurethral incision of some newborn ureteroceles seems appropriate, as it can reliably relieve hydronephrosis and is minimally invasive. Whether return of function in the hydronephrotic upper pole can be expected has yet to be definitely proven.

An interesting although unproven hypothesis of the embryogenesis of renal dysplasia associated with ectopic ureteroceles has been made by Machie and Stephens (250). Abnormal induction of the metanephric blastema by an anomalous ureteral bud is proposed, resulting in renal dysplasia in that portion of the kidney drained by the ureterocele. A correlation is made between the ectopic position of the ureteral orifice of upper pole segment with the degree of dysplasia. The hypothesis seems to fit fairly well when describing ureteroceles and ectopic ureters, as a fairly high percentage of upper pole segments drained by these ectopic systems are associated with dysplastic renal histology. However, caution must be observed when attempts are made to correlate this observation with primary vesicoureteral reflux. Patients with vesicoureteral reflux (and therefore laterally placed ureteral orifices [e.g., lateral ectopia]) have been shown to have a higher percentage of renal tissue showing histologic changes of chronic pyelonephritis rather than dysplasia (251).

Vesicoureteral reflux, like UPJ obstruction, megaureter, ureterocele, and urethral valves, is being diagnosed frequently prenatally through the increasing use of maternal/fetal ultrasonography. To be detectable on ultrasound, the reflux must necessarily be of a more severe degree and is found much more commonly in males. From an embryologic point of view, the most interesting aspect of this is that DMSA scanning has shown "damaged" kidneys associated with prenatally diagnosed reflux, even in the proven absence of urinary tract infection (252). Both global and focal parenchymal changes were found. This raises the question of the importance of the so-called water-hammer effect associated with severe reflux on the developing renal parenchyma. Could the intermittent bombardment of increased pressure from fetal bladder emptying in the presence of severe reflux lead to fibrosis in the embryonic kidney and present as disordered DMSA imaging? Ideally, animal models will be developed that will answer this intriguing question.

Proper management of patients presenting with urinary tract infection who are found to have vesicoureteral reflux of a degree slightly less than that commonly found on prenatal imaging has been controversial. To find out whether surgical or prolonged medical management was best for the treatment of international grades 3 and 4 reflux, a cooperative effort involving some of the leading medical institutions of Europe and the United States was devised. In 1991 the 5-year follow-up of these patients was completed. The results were summarized in a recent supplement to the *Journal of Urology* (253). Definition of the natural history of this degree of reflux (as gleaned from the medical arm of the study) was a goal, as was determination of surgical cure rates and the risk of surgical complications. Although some differences in results were found between the U.S. and European arms of the study, it seems safe to say that bilateral grade 3 or 4 reflux has significantly less chance of subsiding spontaneously after a 5-year follow-up than does its unilateral counterpart. Although progressive renal scarring can occur after successful surgical correction of reflux, its

occurrence is unlikely, whereas medical treatment is associated with a significantly increased risk. The complication rate from surgery is quite acceptable.

With the development of prenatal ultrasonography and the diagnosis of fetal hydronephrosis came the opportunity for treatment of the obstruction in the unborn child. An initial enthusiasm for intrauterine urinary drainage procedures in cases of suspected posterior urethral valves has been tempered most recently by the knowledge that prenatal relief of unilateral hydronephrosis does not improve renal function and that the number of cases of bilateral obstruction that will benefit from internalized drainage (e.g., pigtail shunts of fetal urine from bladder to amniotic space) is extremely small. By the time in gestation that most cases of bilateral hydronephrosis are diagnosed, there is a marked deficiency of amniotic fluid indicating that renal function is severely impaired. Renal dysplasia and cystic disease are commonly present and easily diagnosed on ultrasonography. If oligohydramnios is present, relief of the fetal obstructive uropathy by pigtail shunt will not influence the ultimately fatal outcome. The very few cases that might benefit from prenatal intervention are those in which oligohydramnios developed later in gestation. Analysis of fetal urine via bladder aspiration must reveal sodium of less than 100 mEq per liter, with a similarly low chloride level. Osmolality measurements must show ability of the fetal kidney to concentrate. Only in such circumstances is fetal intervention for relief of obstruction from posterior urethral valves warranted. Renal dysplasia and cystic disease, themselves closely related embryologically to obstructive uropathy, become the major determinants of survivability.

The long-term outlook for patients born with exstrophy of the urinary bladder is now much better from the quality of life standpoint than it was only a few years ago. Nevertheless, ultimate reconstruction requires multiple operations, many for management of significant complications. The basic philosophy for initial surgical management of males and females is to convert the open exstrophy to epispadias with incontinence by mobilizing and turning-in the bladder, bringing the pubic symphyses together, and leaving construction of the bladder neck antiincontinence mechanism for another day. In all but a few instances, this initial closure should be performed as early after birth as possible, preferably in the first few days of life. Creation of a sphincter mechanism is delayed until after the time of attainment of normal potty training. Reconstruction of the epispadias deformity may be accomplished at almost any time after the first 6 months. Extremely small bladders are closed similarly with the knowledge that ultimate reconstruction will involve augmentation using a suitable intestinal or stomach segment. Using this staged approach, encouraging results with respect to attainment of urinary continence were reported by Jeffs and the Hopkins group (254). Most successful surgeons dealing with this potentially devastating anomaly have adopted this approach, and reserve primary diversion for a very small number of cases (TSP).

REFERENCES

1. Frazer JE. The terminal part of the wolffian duct. J Anat 1935;69:455–468.
2. Wesson MB. Anatomical embryological and physiological studies of trigone and neck of bladder. J Urol 1920;4:279.
3. Gyllensten L. Contributions to the embryology of the urinary bladder. Acta Anat 1949;7:305–344.
4. Weigert C. Ueber einige Bildungsfehler der Ureteren. Virchow Arch [A] 1877;70:490.
5. Meyer R. Normal and abnormal development of the ureter in the human embryo: a mechanistic consideration. Anat Rec 1946;96:355–372.
6. Stephens FD. Anatomical vagaries of double ureters. Aust N Z J Surg 1958;28:27–33.
7. Glenister TW. A correlation of the normal and abnormal development of the penile urethra and of the infraabdominal wall. Br J Urol 1958;30:117–126.
8. Wyburn GM. The development of the infra-umbilical portion of the abdominal wall, with remarks on the aetiology of ectopia vesicae. J Anat 1937;71:201–231.
9. Felix W. The development of the urinogenital organs. In: Keibel F, Mall FP, eds. Manual of Human Embryology, Vol 2. Philadelphia: JB Lippincott, 1912.
10. Potter EL. Pathology of the fetus and the newborn. Chicago: Year Book Medical Publishers, 1952.
11. Bauer SB, Retik AB. Bladder diverticula in infant children. Urology 1974;3:712–715.
12. Glenn JF. Agenesis of the bladder. JAMA 1959;169:2016–2018.
13. Miller A. The aetiology and treatment of diverticulum of the bladder. Br J Urol 1958;30:43–56.
14. Boulgakow B. The effect of nondevelopment of the allantois as illustrated by a case of sympodia. J Anat 1929;63:253–258.
15. Campbell S. The antenatal detection of fetal abnormality by ultrasonic diagnosis. Proceedings of the Fourth International Conference on Birth defects. Vienna, 1973.
16. Wladimiroff JW, Campbell S. Fetal urine-production rates in normal and complicated pregnancy. Lancet 1974;1:151.
17. Arey LB. Developmental anatomy, 7th ed. Philadelphia: WB Saunders, 1965.
18. Hammond G, Yglesias L, Davis JE. The urachus, its anatomy and associated fasciae. Anat Rec 1941;80:271–287.
19. Haupt GJ, Keitel HK. Intestinal obstruction in a child with a peritonealized urachal remnant. J Pediatr 1960;57:741–743.
20. Wutz JB. Ueber urachus und urachuscysten. Virchow Arch [A] 1883;92:387.
21. Noe HN. Urachal anomalies and related umbilical disorders. In: Glenn JF, ed. Urologic surgery, 4th ed. Philadelphia: JB Lippincott, 1991.
22. Hinman F Jr. Surgical disorder of the bladder and umbilicus of urachal origin. Surg Gynecol Obstet 1961;113:605–614.
23. Blichert-Toft M, Koch F, Neilson OV. Anatomic variants of the urachus related to clinical appearance and surgical treatment of urachal lesions. Surg Gynecol Obstet 1973;137:51–54.
24. Bauer SB, Retik AB. Urachal anomalies and related umbilical disorders. Urol Clin North Am 1978;5:195–203.
25. Nix JT, Menville JG, Albert M, Wendt D. Congenital patent urachus. J Urol 1958;79:264–273.
26. Ripmann G. Eine seröse Cyste in der Bauchhöhle, mit einem Inhall von 50 Liter Flüssigkeit. Deutsch Klin 1870;22:267.
27. Begg RC. Enormous mucoid cyst of the urachus. J Urol 1947;57:870–873.
28. Jonathan OM. Mucinous urachal cyst: report of a case and review of the subject. Br J Urol 1956;28:253–256.
29. Trimingham HL, McDonald JR. Congenital anomalies in the region of the umbilicus. Surg Gynecol Obstet 1945;80:152–163.
30. Edeikin S, Hutchinson H, Grimm G. Ruptured urachal cyst abscess complicating pregnancy. Obstet Gynecol 1966;27:338–340.
31. Fisher ER. Transitional-cell carcinoma of the urachal apex. Cancer 1958;11:245–249.
32. Butler DB, Rosenberg HS. Sarcoma of the urachus. Arch Surg 1959;79:724–728.
33. Whittle CH, Coryllos E, Simpson JS Jr. Sarcoma of the urachus. Arch Surg 1961;82:443–444.
34. Shaw RE. Sarcoma of the urachus: report of a case and brief review of the subject. Br J Surg 1949;37:95–98.
35. Begg RC. The urachus and umbilical fistulae. Surg Gynecol Obstet 1927;45:165–178.
36. Tsuchida Y, Ishida M. Osmolar relationships between enlarged umbilical cord and patent urachus. J Pediatr Surg 1969;4:465–467.
37. Steck WD, Helwig EB. Umbilical granulomas, pilonidal disease, and the urachus. Surg Gynecol Obstet 1965;120:1043–1057.
38. Herbst WP. Patent urachus. South Med J 1937;30:711–719.
39. Sterling JA, Goldsmith R. Lesions of the urachus which appear in the adult. Ann Surg 1953;137:120–128.
40. Vilanova X, Raventós A. Pseudodiphallia, a rare anomaly. J Urol 1954;71:338–346.
41. Littré A. Histoire de l'Académie Royale des Sciences de Paris. Amsterdam, 1701.
42. von Haller A. De uracho pervio et allantoide humana. Gottingen, 1739.
43. Paget T, Bowman W. On an operation for previous urachus. Med Chir Trans Lond 1861;44:13.
44. Smith T. An open urachus. Med Times (London) 1863;1:320.
45. Vaughan GT. Patent urachus, review of cases reported. Trans Am Surg Assoc (Philadelphia) 1905;23:273–294.
46. Cullen TS. Embryology: anatomy and diseases of the umbilicus together with diseases of the urachus. Philadelphia: WB Saunders, 1916.
47. McCauley RT, Lichtenheld FR. Congenital patent urachaus. South Med J 1960;53:1138–1141.
48. Rubin A. Handbook of congenital malformations. Philadelphia: WB Saunders, 1967:334.
49. Irving IM. Umbilical abnormalities. In: Lister J, Irving IM, eds. Neonatal surgery. Boston: Butterworths, 1990:376.
50. Hinman FH Jr. Urologic aspects of the alternating urachal sinus. Am J Surg 1961;102:339–343.
51. Yeorg OW. Cysts of the urachus. Minn Med 1942;25:496.
52. Strickland CE, Bowes JE. Dystocia caused by anomalies of the fetal urogenital tract. Obstet Gynecol 1957;9:571–574.
53. Easton L. Obstructed labour due to foetal abdominal distention. J Obstet Gynaecol Br Commw 1960;67:128–130.
54. Thomford NR, Knight PR, Nusbaum JW. Urachal abnormalities in the adult. Am Surg 1971;37:405–407.
55. Newman SR, Landes RR, Eggleston RB. Dribbling from an umbilical fistula. JAMA 1960;172:448–449.
56. Persutte WH, Lenke RR, Kropp KA, Ghareeh C. Antenatal diagnosis of fetal patent urachus. J Ultrasound Med 1988;7:399–403.
57. McGowan AJ Jr, Willmarth CL. Patent urachus. Am J Dis Child 1965;109:255–258.
58. Boissonnat P. Two cases of complete double functional urethra with a single bladder. Br J Urol 1961;33:453–462.
59. Schinagel G. Bifurcated female urethra. Urol Cutan Rev 1936;40:398–399.
60. Swenson O, Oeconomopoulos L. Double lower genitourinary systems in a child. J Urol 1961;85:540–542.

61. Burns E, Cummins H, Hyman J. Incomplete reduplication of the bladder with congenital solitary kidney. J Urol 1947;57:257–269.

62. Juetting G. De ventriculi et vesicae urinariae duplicatae [Dissertation]. Berlin: Neitackianis, 1838.

63. Ravitch MM. Hind gut duplication: doubling of colon and genital urinary tract. Ann Surg 1951;137:588–601.

64. Cohen SJ. Diphallus with duplication of colon and bladder. Proc R Soc Med 1968;61:305.

65. Blasius G. Observationes medicae rariores: accedit monstri triplici historia. Amersterdam [Amstelodami]: A Wolfgang, 1656.

66. Menton ML, Denny HE. Duplication of the vermiform appendix, the large intestine and the urinary bladder. Arch Pathol 1945;40:345–350.

67. Mainland D. Posterior duplicity in a dog with reference to mammalian teratology in general. J Anat 1929;63:473.

68. Lang J. Ein seltener fall von gespaltenem urachus persistens. Act Chir Acad Sci Lung 1960;1:285–289.

69. Schatz F. Ein besonderer Fall von Missbildung des weiblichen Urogenitalsystems. Arch Gynaecol 1871;3:304.

70. Cattirri I. Obs Med Pietro Borello. Communicatae Francfort Obs 1670;20:85.

71. Volpé M. Dell'asta doppia. Policlinico [Chir] 1903;10:46–52.

72. Lanman TH, Mahoney PJ. Intravenous urography in infants and children. Am J Dis Child 1931;42:611.

73. Lange M. Ueber complete Verdoppelund des Penis, combinirt mit rudimentärer Verdoppelund der Harnblase und atresia ani. Beitr Z Pathol Anat, 1898;24:223–230.

74. Beach PD, Brascho DJ, Hein WR, Nichol WW, Geppert LJ. Duplication of the primitive hindgut of the human body. Surgery 1961;49:779–793.

75. Bowie CW, Garvey FK, Boyce WH, Pautler EE. Supernumerary urinary bladder and ureter, spiral deformity of the ureter, ureteral diverticulum, hypoplasia of the kidney and bicornate uterus: a case report. J Urol 1954;71:293–298.

76. Senger TL, Santare VJ. Congenital multilocular bladder. Trans Am Assoc Genitourin Surg 1951;43:114–119.

77. Abrahamson J. Double bladder and related anomalies: clinical and embryological aspects and a case report. Br J Urol 1961;33:195–214.

78. Michelson D. Ein seltener Fall von Doppelniere, kombiniert mit doppelter Harnblase und Divertikel der letzteren. Z Urol Chir 1927;23:15.

79. Edwards C. Congenital multilocular bladder. Med J Aust 1933;2:443.

80. Meyer R. Zwei Fälle von Missbildung der Harnblase bis Feten. Zentralbl Gynak 1932;56:1090–1105.

81. Roche AE. The late results of ureterocolis anastomosis. Br Med J 1952;1259–1316.

82. Mézan S. Contribution à l'etude clinique de la vessie multilocular. J Urol (Paris) 1929;27:31.

83. Campbell M. Urology, 1st ed. Philadelphia: WB Saunders, 1954.

84. Harris A. Congenital vesical neck obstruction in a female child due to cup-valve formation: open operation—complete recovery. Am J Surg 1933;20:64–69.

85. Bernardo P, Roth AA. Massive prolapse of redundant bladder mucosa. JAMA 1963;185:321–323.

86. Kohler HH. Septal bladder. J Urol 1940;44:63–66.

87. Zellermayer J, Carlson HE. Congenital hourglass bladder. J Urol 1944;51:24–30.

88. Berariu T, Scheau M, Popse E. Eine seltene Anomalie der Harnblase: Die Blase in Sanduhrform [hourglass bladder]. Z Urol Nephrol 1965;58:35–37.

89. Watson E. Developmental basis for certain vesical diverticula. JAMA 1920;75:1473–1474.

90. Mostofi FK. Potentialities of bladder epithelium. J Urol 1954;71:705–714.

91. Cathelin F, Sempé C. La vessie double. Ann Mal Org Gen Urin 1903;21:339–358.

92. MacKellar A, Stephens FD. Vesical diverticula in children. In: Stephens FD, ed. Congenital malformations of the rectum, anus and genito-urinary tracts. Edinburgh: EDS Livingstone, 1963.

93. Kretschmer HL. Diverticulum of the bladder in infancy and childhood. Am J Dis Child 1934;48:842–857.

94. Anschütz W. Congenital diverticulum of bladder. Z Urol Chir 1922;10:103–112.

95. Parrott TS, Bastuba M. Giant bladder diverticulum causing urethral obstruction in an infant. Br J Urol 1992;69(5):545–546.

96. Paul MA. The surgery of the congenital anomalies of the midline ventral abdominal wall. Ann Roy Coll Surg Eng 1953;13:313–355.

97. Soper RT, Kilger K. Vesico-intestinal fissure. J Urol 1964;92:490–511.

98. Muecke EC. Exstrophy, epispadias and other anomalies of the bladder. In: Campbell's urology, 5th ed. Walsh PC (ed.). Philadelphia: WB Saunders, 1986.

99. Wyburn GM. The development of the infra-umbilical portion of the abdominal wall with remarks on the aetiology of ectopia vesicae. J Anat 1937;71:201–231.

100. Paul M, Kanagasuntheram R. The congenital anomalies of the lower urinary tract. Brit J Urol 1956;28:64–74.

101. Mackenzie LL. Split pelvis in pregnancy. Am J Obstet Gyned 1935;29:255–257.

102. van Geddern CD. The etiology of exstrophy of the bladder. Arch Surg 1924;8:61–99.

103. Connell FG. Extrophy of the bladder. JAMA 1901;36:637–668.

104. Duncan A Jr. Systematic account of hernia of the inverted bladder. Edinburgh Med Surg J 1805;43:132.

105. Velpeau AAIM. Rapport sur un cas d'exstrophie congénitale de vessie. Mem Acad Med 1833;3:90–100.

106. Hamilton HA. Singular malformation. Boston Med Surg J 1835;11:93–96.

107. Lloyd. Ectrophia vesicae (absence of the anterior walls of the bladder): operation, subsequent death. Lancet 1851;2:370.

108. Simon J. Ectropia vesicae (absence of the anterior walls of the bladder and pubic abdominal parieties): operation for directing the orifices of the ureters into the rectum; temporary success; subsequent death; autopsy. Lancet 1852;2:568–570.

109. Gross SW. Congenital exstrophy of the urinary bladder and its complications, successfully treated by a new plastic operation by Daniel Ayres. North Am Med Clin Rev 1859;3:709–711.

110. Caldamone AA. Anomalies of the bladder and cloaca. In: Gillenwater JY, Grayhack JT, Howards SS, Duckett JW, eds. Adult and pediatric urology, Vol 2. Chicago: Year Book Medical Publishers, 1987.

111. Maydl K. Urber die Radikaltherapie der Blasenektopie. Med Wschr 1894;44:1113, 1169, 1209, 1256, and 1297.

112. Higgins CC. Exstrophy of the bladder: report of 158 cases. Am Surg 1962;28:99–102.

113. Rickham PP. Vesico-intestinal fissure. Arch Dis Child 1960;35:97–102.

114. Lattimer JK, Smith MJV. Exstrophy closure: a follow-up on 70 cases. J Urol 1966;95:356–359.

115. Harvard BM, Thompson GJ. Congenital exstrophy of the urinary bladder: late results of treatment by the Coffey-Mayo method of uretero-intestinal anastomosis. J Urol 1951;65:223–234.

116. Uson AC, Lattimer JK, Melicow MM. Types of exstrophy of urinary bladder and concomitant malformations: a report based on 82 cases. Pediatrics 1959;23:927–933.

117. Gross RE. The surgery of infancy and childhood. Philadelphia: WB Saunders, 1953.

118. Jeffs RD, Lepor H. Management of the exstrophy epispadias complex and urachal anomalies. In: Walsh PC, Cambpell's urology, 5th ed. Philadelphia: WB Saunders, 1986.

119. Raffensperger JG. Exstrophy. In Raffensperger JG, ed. Swenson's pediatric surgery, 5th ed. Norwalk, CT: Appleton & Lange, 1990.

120. Coffey RC. Physiologic implantation of the severed ureter or common bile-duct into the intestine. JAMA 1911;56:397–403.

121. Coffey RC. Further studies and experiences with the transfixion suture technic (Technic 3) for transplantation of the ureters into the large intestine. Northwest Med 1933;32:31–34.

122. Cordonnier JJ. Ureterosigmoid anastomosis. Surg Gynecol Obstet 1949;88:441–446.

123. Nesbit RM. Ureterosigmoid anastomosis by direct elliptical connection: a preliminary report. J Urol 1949;61:728–734.

124. Leadbetter WF, Clarke BG. Five years' experience with ureteroenterostomy by the "combined" technique. J Urol 1954;73:67–82.

125. Young HH. Exstrophy of the bladder: first case in which a normal bladder and urinary control have been obtained by plastic operation. Surg Gynecol Obstet 1942;74:729–737.

126. Williams DI, Savage J. Reconstruction of the exstrophied bladder. Br J Surg 1966;53:168–173.

127. Campbell M. Urology, 2nd ed. Philadelphia: WB Saunders, 1963.

128. Ansel JS. Exstrophy and epispadias. In: Clay JF, Urologic surgery, 3rd ed. Philadelphia: JB Lippincott, 1983:647–663.

129. Kramer SA. Exstrophy and epispadias. In: Glenn JF, ed. Urologic surgery, 4th ed. Philadelphia: JB Lippincott, 1991:523–537.

130. Ritchey ML, Kramer SA, Kelalis PP. Vesical neck reconstruction in patients with epispadias-exstrophy. J Urol 1988;139:1278–1281.

131. Goldwasser B, Barrett JM, Webster GD, Kramer SA. Cystometric properties of ileum and right colon after bladder augmentation, substitution, or replacement. J Urol 1987;138:1007–1008.

132. Spence HM. Ureterosigmoidostomy for exstrophy of the bladder: results in a personal series of 31 cases. Br J Urol 1966;38:36–43.

133. Wattenberg CA, Beare JB, Tormey AR Jr. Exstrophy of the urinary bladder complicated by adenocarcinoma. J Urol 1956;76:583–594.

134. McCown PE. Carcinoma in exstrophy of the bladder. J Urol 1940;43:533–542.

135. Mesrobian HG, Kelalis PP, Kramer SA. Long-term follow-up of cosmetic appearance and genital function in boys with exstrophy: review of 53 patients. J Urol 1986;136:256–258.

136. Randall LM, Hardwick RS. Pregnancy and parturition following bilateral ureteral transplantation for congenital exstrophy of bladder. Surg Gynecol Obstet 1934;58:1018–1020.

137. Coulter WJ, Sabbagh MI. Bladder exstrophy and pregnancy: report of a case. Obstet Gynecol 1958;11:104–107.

138. Krisilof M, Puchner P, Tretter W. Pregnancy in women with bladder exstrophy. J Urol 1978;119:478.

139. Johnston JH, Penn IA. Exstrophy of the cloaca. Br J Urol 1966;38:302–307.

140. Johnston TB. Extroversion of the bladder, complicated by the presence of intestinal openings on the surface of the extroverted area. J Anat Physiol 1913;48:89–106.

141. Meckel JF. Handbuch der pathologischen Anatomie. Leipzig, 1812.

142. Schwalbe E. Die Morphologie der Missbildungen der Menschen und Tiere. Jena: Fisher, 1909.

143. Zwiren GT, Patterson JH. Extrophy of the cloaca: report of a case treated surgically. Pediatrics 1965;35:687–691.

144. Ambrose SS. Personal Communication, 1969.

145. Howell G, Caldamone A, Snyder H, Ziegler M, Ducket J. Optimal management of cloacal exstrophy. J Pediatr Surg 1983;18:365–369.

146. Ricketts RR, Woodard JR, Zwiren GT, Andrews HG, Broecker BH. Modern treatment of cloacal exstrophy. J Pediatr Surg 1991;26:444–450.

147. Ellerker AG. The extravesical ectopic ureter. Br J Surg 1958;45:344–353.

148. Thom B. Harnleiter—und Nierenverdopplung mit besonder Berücksichtigung der extravesikalen Harnleitermundungen. Z Urol 1928;22:417–468.

149. Helper AB. Bilateral pelvic and ureteral duplication with uterine ectopic ureter. J Urol 1947;57:94.

150. Abeshouse BS. Rare case of ectopic ureter opening in uterus: review of literature. Urol Cutan Rev 1943;47:447.

151. Seitzman DM, Patton JF. Ureteral ectopia: combined ureteral and vas deferens anomaly. J Urol 1960;84:604–608.

152. Leef GS, Leader S. Ectopic ureter opening into the rectum: a case report. J Urol 1962;87:338–342.

153. Williams JI, Carson RB, Wells WD. Renal aplasia: a report of two cases. J Urol 1958;79:6.

154. Honke EM. Ectopic ureter. J Urol 1946;55:460.

155. Varney DC, Ford MD. Ectopic ureteral remnant persisting as cystic diverticulum of the ejaculatory duct: case report. J Urol 1954;72:802–807.

156. Constantian HM. Ureteral ectopia, hydrocolpos and uterus didelphs. JAMA 1966;197:54–57.

157. Fromme A. Über die operation grosser Bauchnarbenbrüche in der Mittellinie, besonders oberhalb des Nabels. Beitr Z Klin Chir 1926;137:690–700.

158. Greig DM, Herzfeld G. On the persistence of complete wolffian ducts in females. Edinb Med J 1927;34:701–724.

159. Columbus R. De re anatomica. Venetiis, 1559.

160. Schrader J. Observationes et historiae omnes et singulae e Guiljelmi Harvei libello de generatione animalium excerptae, et in accuratissimum ordinem redactae. Amsterdam [Amstedlodami]: A Wolfgang, 1674.

161. Burford CE, Glenn JE, Burford EH. Ureteral ectopia: a review of the literature and 2 case reports. J Urol 1949;62:211.

162. Eisendrath DN. Ectopic ureteral ending. Urol Cutan Rev 1938;42:404–411.

163. Winters WD, Lebowitz RL. Importance of prenatal detection of hydronephrosis of the upper pole. AJR 1990;155:125–129.

164. Crenshaw JL. Ureter with extravesical orifice; supernumerary ureter ending blindly; crossed ureteral ectopia; stones in extrapelvic cystocele: report of 11 cases. J Urol 1940;43:82–101.

165. Mills JC. Complete unilateral duplication of ureter with analysis of the literature. Urol Cutan Rev 1939;43:444–447.

166. Lowsley OS, Kerwin TJ. Clinical urology, 3rd ed., Vol 1. Baltimore: Williams & Wilkins, 1956.

167. Young JN. Ureter opening into the seminal vesicle: report on a case. Br J Urol 1955;27:57–60.

168. Szkodny A, Zielinski J. Abouchement de l'uretère dans la vésicule séminale. J Urol Nephrol (Paris) 1964;70:259–261.

169. Smith FL, Ritchie EL, Maizels M, Zaontz MR. Surgery for duplex kidneys with ectopic ureters: interlateral ureteroureterostomy vs. polar nephrectomy. J Urol 1989;142:532–534.

170. Uson AC, Lattimer JK, Melicow MM. Ureteroceles in infants and children. Pediatrics 1961;27:971–983.

171. Gummess GH, Charnock DA, Riddell HI, Stewart CM. Ureteroceles in children. J Urol 1955;74:331–335.

172. Chwalle R. Eine bemerkenswerte Anomalie der Harnblase bei enem menschlichen embryo von 32,5 mm. Virchow Arch [A] 1927;263:632.

173. Lechler. Fall einer doppelten Harnblase. Med Cor Bl Württemb Ärztl Ver 1834;4:23.

174. Patron J. Du renversement de la muqueuse de l'aréthre et de la muqueuse vesicale. Arch Gen Med 1857;10:689–709.

175. Bostroem E. Beiträge zur pathologischen Anatomie der Nieren. heft I. Freiburg and Tubingen: JCB Mohr, 1884.

176. Stoeckel W. Handbuch der Gynäkologie. Vol 1. Munich [Munchen]: JF Bergman, 1938.

177. Wershub LP, Kirwin TJ. Ureterocele, its etiology, pathogenesis and diagnosis. Am J Surg 1956;88:317–327.

178. Gross RE, Clatworthy HW Jr. Ureterocele in infancy and childhood. Pediatrics 1950;5:68.

179. Gross RE. The surgery of infancy and childhood. Philadelphia: WB Saunders, 1953.

180. Williams DI, Woodard JR. Problems in the management of ectopic ureteroceles. J Urol 1964;92:635.

181. Rabinowitz R, et al. Bilateral orthotopic ureteroceles causing massive ureteral dilatation in children. J Urol 1978;119:839.

182. Parrott TS. Urologic implications of anorectal malformations. Urol Clin North Am 1985;12:13–21.

183. Share JC, Lebowitz RL. Ectopic ureterocele without ureteral and calyceal dilatation (ureterocele disproportion): findings on urography and sonography. AJR 1989;152:567–571.

184. Williams DI. Male urethral anomalies. In: Williams DI, Johnston JH, eds. Pediatric urology, 2nd ed. London: Butterworths, 1982.

185. Brock WA, Kaplan WG. Ectopic ureteroceles in children. J Urol 1978;119:800.

186. Caldamone AA, Snyder HMcC, Duckett JW. Ureteroceles in children: follow-up of management with upper tract approach. J Urol 1984;131:1130.

187. Scherz HC, Kaplan GW, Packer MG. Ectopic ureteroceles: surgical management with preservation of continence—review of 60 cases. J Urol 1989;142:438–441.

188. Montfort G, Morrison-LaCombe G, Coqueet M. Endoscopic treatment of ureteroceles revisited. J Urol 1985;133:1031.

189. Tank ES. Management of ureterocele in the newborn. In: Gonzales ET, Roth D, eds. Common problems in pediatric urology. St. Louis: Mosby–Year Book, 1991.

190. Allen T. The non-neurogenic neurogenic bladder. J Urol 1977;117:232.

191. Whitaker RH, Sherwood T. Another look at diagnostic pathways in children with UTI. Br Med J 1984;288:839.

192. Someren A. Urologic pathology with clinical and radiologic correlations. New York: Macmillan, 1989.

193. Smellie JM, Normand C. The clinical features and significance of UTI in childhood. Proc R Soc Med 1966;59:415.

194. Smellie JM, Normand C. Bacteriuria, reflux and renal scarring. Arch Dis Child 1975;50:581.

195. Smellie JM, Normand C. Urinary tract infection: clinical aspects. In: Williams DI, Johnston JH, eds. Pediatric urology. London: Butterworths, 1982.

196. Parrott TS, Woodard JR, Wolpert JJ. Ureteral tailoring: a comparison of wedge resection with infolding. J Urol 1990;144:328–329.

197. Young HH, Frontz WA, Baldwin JC. Congenital obstruction of the posterior urethra. J Urol 1919;3:289–365.

198. Young HH. Genital abnormalities: hermaphroditism and related adrenal diseases. Baltimore: Williams & Wilkins, 1937.

199. Tolmatschew N. Ein Fall von semilunaren Klappen der Harnröhre und von vergrösserter Vesicula prostatica. Virchow Arch [A] 1870;49:348–365.

200. Bazy P. Rétricissement congenital de l' urètre chez l'homme. Presse Med 1903;1:215–217.

201. Lowsley OS. The development of the human prostate gland with reference to the development of other structures at the neck of the urinary bladder. Am J Anat 1912;13:299.

202. Watson E. Structural basis for congenital valve formation in posterior urethra. Trans Sect Urol AMA 1921;162.

203. Stephens FD. Congenital malformation of the rectum, anus and genitourinary tracts. Edinburgh: E & S Livingstone, 1963.

204. Grajewski RS, Glassberg KI. The variable effect of posterior urethral valves as illustrated in identical twins. J Urol 1983;130:1188.

205. Kjellberg SR, Ericsson NO, Rudhe U. Urethral valves. In: The lower urinary tract in childhood: some correlated clinical and roentgenologic observations. Stockholm: Almquisst & Wiksell, 1957:203–254.

206. Krueger RP, Churchill BM. Megalourethra with posterior urethral valves. Urology 1981;18:279.

207. Livne PM, Delaune J, Gonzales ET Jr. Genetic etiology of posterior urethral valves. J Urol 1983;130:781.

208. Kelalis PP, King LR, Belman AB. Posterior urethra. In: Kelalis PP, King LR, Belman AB eds. Clinical pediatric urology, 2nd ed. Philadelphia: WB Saunders, 1985:527.

209. Langenbeck CJM. Ueber eine einfache und sichere Methode des Steinschnittes, mit einer Vorrede von Dr. Johann Barthel Siebold. Wurzburg: G Stahel, 1802.

210. Counseller VS, Menville JG. Congenital valves of posterior urethra. J Urol 1935;34:268–277.

211. Eigenbrodt K. Ein Fall von Blasenhalsklappe. Beitr Z Klin Chir 1891;8:171–178.

212. Landes HE, Rall R. Congenital valvular obstruction of the posterior urethra. J Urol 1935;34:254–267.

213. McCrea LE. Congenital valves of the posterior urethra. J Int Coll Surg 1949;12:342.

214. Pagano F. Congenital valves of the urethra. Urologia 1965;32(Supp)16:64–109.

215. Churchill BM, McLorie GA, Khoury AE, Merguerian PA, Houle AM. Emergency treatment and long-term follow-up of posterior urethral valves. Urol Clin North Am 1990;17:343–360.

216. Parkhouse HF, Woodhouse CR. Long-term status of patients with posterior urethral valves. Urol Clin North Am 1990;17:373–378.

217. Opsomer RJ, Wese FX, Dardenne AN, Van Cangh PJ. Posterior urethral valves in adult males. Urology 1990;36:35–37.

218. Heaton ND, Kadow C, Yates-Bell AJ. Late presentation of congenital posterior urethral valves. Br J Urol 1989;64:98.

219. Connor JP, Burbige KA. Long-term urinary continence and renal function in neonates with posterior urethral valves. J Urol 1990;144:1209–1211.

220. Stoutenbeek P, de Jong TP, van Gool JD, Drogtrop AP. Intrauterine cystography for evaluation of prenatal obstructive uropathy. Pediatr Radiol 1989;19:247–249.

221. Matheson WJ, Ward EM. Hormonal sex reversal in a female. Arch Dis Child 1954;29:22.

222. Williams DI, Eckstein HB. Obstructive valves in the posterior urethra. J Urol 1965;93:236.

223. Fernbach SK, Feinstein KA, Zaontz MR. Urinoma formation in posterior urethral valves: relationship to later renal function. Pediatr Radiol 1990;20:543–545.

224. Gonzales ET Jr. Alternatives in the management of posterior urethral valves. Urol Clin North Am 1990;17:335–342.

225. Walker RD, Padron M. The management of posterior urethral valves by initial vesicostomy and delayed valve ablation. J Urol 1990;144:1212–1214.

226. Parrott TS. Pediatric urinary diversion. In: Glenn JF. ed. Urologic surgery. Philadelphia: JB Lippincott, 1991:1050.

227. Warshaw BL, Hymes LC, Trulock TS. Prognostic features in infants with obstructive uroprothy. J Urol 1985;133:240.

228. Swenson O. Pediatric surgery. New York: Appleton-Century-Crofts, 1958.
229. Emmett JL, Logan GB. Ureterocele with prolapse through the urethra. J Urol 1944;51:19–24.
230. Harris AP, Porch PP, Haines CE. Neuromuscular dysfunction of the lower urinary tract. J Urol 1962;87:742–746.
231. Bodian M. Some observations on pathology of congenital "idiopathic bladder neck obstruction." Br J Urol 1957;29:393–398.
232. Chauvin E. A propos des urètres doubles, en particulier de leurs variétés postérieures. J Urol (Paris) 1927;23:289–310.
233. Purcell HM. Another cause of urinary obstruction. J Urol 1949;62:748.
234. Dannreuther WT. Complete double urethra in a female. JAMA 1923;81:1016.
235. DeNicola RR, McCartney RC. Urethral duplication in a female child. J Urol 1949;61:1065–1067.
236. Taruffi A. Sui canali anomali del pene. Bull Sci Med (Bologna) 1891;2:275–301.
237. Woodhouse CR, Williams DI. Duplications of the lower urinary tract in children. Br J Urol 1979;51:481.
238. Belman AB. The repair of a congenital H-type urethrorectal fistula using a scrotal flap urethroplasty. J Urol 1977;118:659.
239. Gross RE, Moore TC. Duplication of the urethra. Arch Surg 1950;60:749–761.
240. Arnold MW, Kaylor WM. Double urethra: case report. J Urol 1953;70:746–748.
241. Rinker JR. Accessory urethra in a boy. J Urol 1943;50:331.
242. Wharton LR, Kearns W. Diverticula of the female urethra. J Urol 1950;63:1063–1076.
243. Davis HJ, TeLinde RW. Urethral diverticula: an assay of 121 cases. J Urol 1958;80:34–39.
244. Wishard WN, Nourse MH, Mertz JHO. Carcinoma in diverticulum of female urethra. J Urol 1960;83:409.
245. Parmenter FJ: Diverticulum of the female urethra. J Urol 1941;45:479–496.
246. McLoughlin MG. Carcinoma in situ in urethral diverticulum: pitfalls of marsupialization alone. Urology 1975;6:343.
247. Sheldon CA, Gilbert MD. Use of the appendix for urethral reconstruction in children with congenital anomalies of the bladder. Surgery 1992;112:805–812.
248. Sweetser PM, Dana AO, Thompson NW. Pheochromocytoma of the urinary bladder. Surgery 1991;5:677–681.
249. Zimmerman IJ, Biron RE, MacMahan HE. Pheochromocytoma of the urinary bladder. N Engl J Med 1953;249:25–26.
250. Machie GG, Stephens FD: Duplex kidneys: a correlation of renal dysplasia with position of the urethral orifice. J Urol 1975;114:274–280.
251. Ambrose SS, Parrott TS, Woodward JR et al. Observations on the small kidney associated with vesicoureteral reflux. J Urol 1980;123:349–351.
252. Burge DM, Griffiths MD, Malone PS, Atwell JD. Fetal vesicoureteral reflux: outcome following conservative postnatal management. J Urol 1992;148:1743–1745.
253. Olbing H et al. International reflux study in children. J Urol 1992;148(suppl):1643–1682.
254. Jeffs RD, Charrios R, Many M, Juransz AR. Primary closure of the exstrophied bladder. In: Scott R, ed. Current controversies in urologic management. Philadelphia: WB Saunders, 1972.

CHAPTER 19

THE SUPRARENAL GLANDS

John Elias Skandalakis / Stephen Wood Gray / William M. Scaljon /
Thomas Stephen Parrott / Richard R. Ricketts

*"Consentaneum esse duxi de quibusdam Renum glandulis ab aliis Anatomicis
negligenter praetermissis hoc loco scribere. Nam utrique Reni, in eminentiori
ipsorum regione (quae venam spectat) glandula adhaeret. Ejus substantia
quemadmodum et figura Renibus fere respondet: licet saepe depressa quoque
ad latera accurat, ut potius placentae quam Renis formam referre videatur . . .
Evenit tamen frequentius ut dextra, sicut etiam Reni, sinistram superet."*
—Description of the Discovery of the Adrenal Glands
by Bartholomeus Eustachius (1563).
From The Mammalian Adrenal Gland *by Geoffrey H. Bourne.*

DEVELOPMENT

The classic descriptions of suprarenal development are those of Wiesel (1) in 1902 and Zuckerkandl (2) in Keibel and Mall's 1912 *Manual of Human Embryology.* Kern (3) in 1911 and Lewis and Pappenheimer (4) in 1916 described the postnatal involution of the cortex, and Keene and Hewer (5) in 1927 supplied the name "fetal cortex." Other descriptions of the development of the organ include those of Uotila (6), Crowder (7), and Sucheston and Cannon (8).

The primordium of the suprarenal cortex becomes visible as early as the fourth week. The celomic epithelium of the posterior abdominal wall, in the angle between the mesentery and the head of the mesonephros, becomes more columnar and begins to divide, so that cords of epithelial cells invade the mesenchyme beneath the epithelial surface. These cells will form the primordium of the fetal suprarenal cortex. They are clearly visible early in the sixth week (Fig. 19.1, *A* to *C*). A secondary proliferation of celomic epithelial cells form a cap over the primitive cortical cells. This cap will form the zona glomerulosa of the definitive cortex (Fig. 19.1, *D*).

A contribution of elements from the cranial mesonephros was described by Uotila (6) but was not confirmed by Sucheston and Cannon (8). Mesenchymal cells included among the migrating epithelial cells (9) probably form the stroma of the definitive gland.

Barbet et al. (10) studied histologic assessments of gestational age in human embryos and fetuses. They reported that neuroblastic nests are normally found between 7 and 26 weeks of gestation. They advised that, for a definition of the profile of maturation, it is important to compare the degree of histologic maturation with clinical macroscopic and radiologic data. Hata et al. (11) used ultrasonography to identify and measure the human fetal adrenal gland in utero. They reported that, in 12 abnormal fetuses, the fetal adrenal gland measurements were always lower than the normal calculation. Fetal adrenal gland circumference was 75% of normal, and the length was 33.3% less than expected. Hata et al. (11) also advise that the circumference, length, and especially the area should be a pertinent diagnostic tool for the management and control of high-risk pregnancies.

The development of the adrenal arteries and veins was described very well by Davies (12) in the excellent book, *Surgery of the Adrenal Glands,* by Scott, a true scholar of the adrenal glands (Figs. 19.2 and 19.3). The aorta, vessels of the septum transversum, and mesonephric arteries are responsible for the rich blood supply of the adrenal glands from an embryologic standpoint (Fig. 19.4). The adrenal veins are developed from the inferior vena cava (IVC).

As always, there are several variations of the adrenal venous system. Monkhouse and Khalique (13) studied the formation, dimensions, and terminations of the central and superficial adrenal veins, reporting routes for venous adrenal blood to the heart via the azygos system and the superior vena cava (SVC) rather than via the IVC.

It is not within the scope of this book to represent details of the anatomy, physiology, and pathology of the adrenal gland because of the complexity. However, Figure 19.5 can help the student to summarize these organs. The mnemonic device of "*Good For Reason Mother*" (GFRM) can serve to remind students of the zones of the adrenal gland.

The cells that will give rise to the chromaffin tissue of the medulla have been identified in the neural crest by Crowder (7) as early as the 7-mm stage (stage 14). During the subsequent week, they accompany neural tissue, chiefly from the ganglia of the sixth to twelfth thoracic

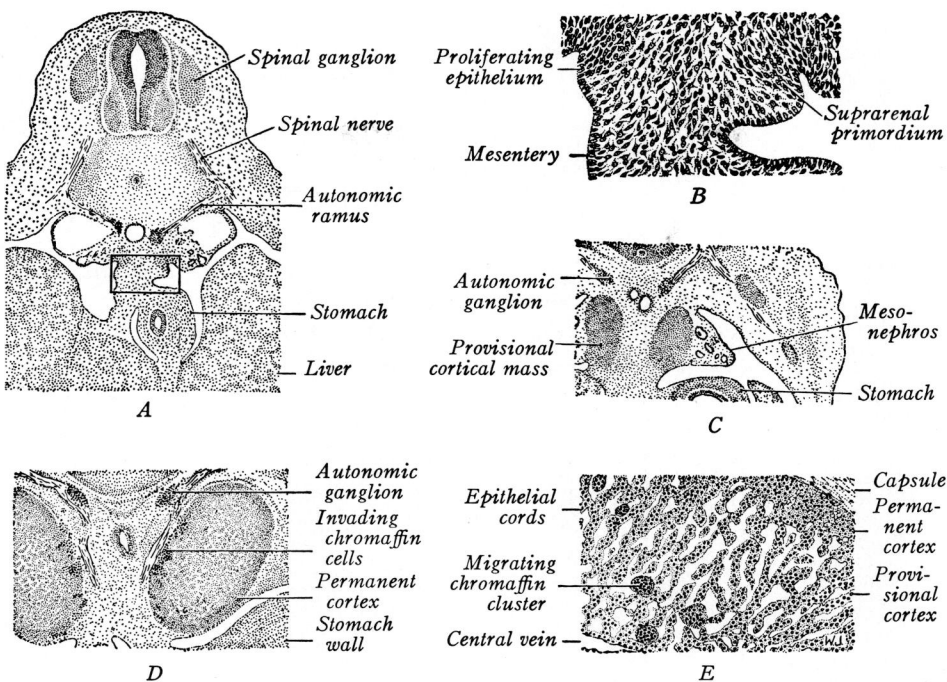

Figure 19.1. Development of the human suprarenal gland. **A,** Site of primordium of gland early in the sixth week (8 mm). **B,** Higher power view of area marked by the rectangle in **A. C,** Relationship of the provisional (fetal) cortex to the mesonephros late in the sixth week (12 mm). **D,** Invading chromaffin cells at the end of the seventh week (16 mm). **E,** The start of demarcation between permanent and provisional cortex. (From Arey LB. Developmental anatomy. Philadelphia: WB Saunders, 1965.)

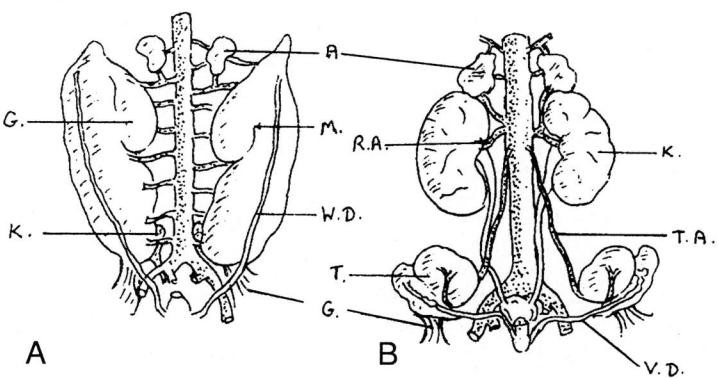

Figure 19.2. The development of the adrenal arteries. **A,** The large mesonephros, comprising about 40 nephric units, is supplied by multiple arteries from the dorsal aortae. The adrenal primordium receives arteries directly from the aorta and from an adjacent mesonephric artery. **B,** The mesonephros has regressed, become transposed into the pelvis, and transformed into the epididymis and associated structures (epoophoron and paraoophoron in female). The wolffian duct becomes the vas deferens and duct of the epididymis in the male and the vestigial duct of Gartner in the female. The metanephros or adult kidney is large and lies in a true retroperitoneal position and in contact with the adrenals, which are molded by it. The definitive adrenal arteries are derived from adjacent mesonephric arteries, one of which is selected from the renal artery, from the aorta, and from the phrenic arteries. A, Adrenal; G, glomeruli; K, kidney; M, mesonephron; R.A., renal artery; T, testis; T.A., testicular artery; V.D., vas deferens; W.D., wolffian duct. (From Davies J. Anatomy, microscopic structure, and development of the human adrenal gland. In: Scott HW, ed. Surgery of the adrenal glands. Philadelphia: JB Lippincott, 1990.)

segments, into the developing gland. These cells proliferate within the suprarenal gland. Differentiation into chromaffin cells begins about the beginning of the third month, continuing until 12 to 18 months after birth. The presence of adrenalin can be detected before the chromaffin reaction is present (Figs. 19.1, *E,* and 19.6).

Crowder (7) supports the idea that the formation of the fetal adrenal cortex as well as the formation of the final cortex with its zonations are phenomena resulting from a continuous and homogeneous development—a development which continues after birth. Differentiation of cortical zones begins in the eighth month by prolifer-

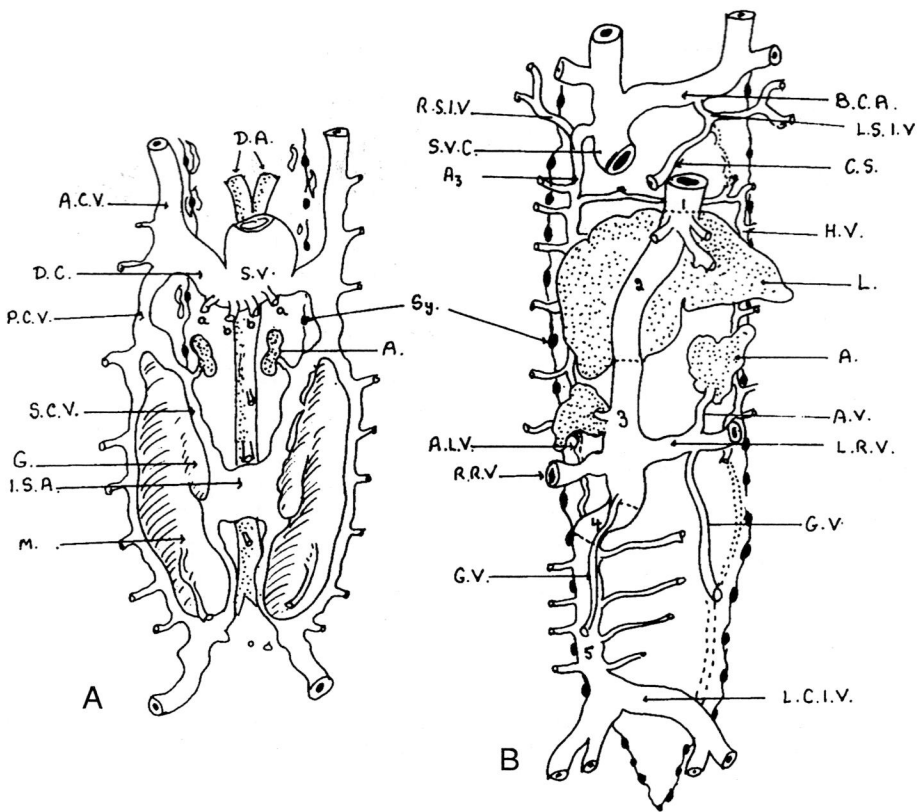

Figure 19.3. Development of the adrenal veins and inferior vena cava. **A,** The primitive system of veins in an early embryo of 5 weeks (cardinal, subcardinal, vitelline, and umbilical). The subcardinals on either side are developed specifically in relation to the urogenital structures. A large intersubcardinal anastomosis links them across the midline distal to the superior mesenteric (vitelline) artery. The earliest adrenal veins probably drain into the subcardinal veins cranially. **B,** The final modification of this system, accomplished in embryos of 15 to 20 mm. The segments of the inferior vena cava are 1, suprahepatic segment (terminal part of right vitelline vein); 2, a hepatosubcardinal anastomosis between the right subcardinal and the hepatic veins; 3, the right subcardinal above the intersubcardinal anastomosis; 4, a subcardinal-supracardinal anastomosis at the level of the intersubcardinal anastomosis; and 5, a right supracardinal segment that takes over the lumbar veins and the venous drainage of both legs via a right common iliac and a new anastomosis between the left and the right common iliac veins. The supracardinal veins are new veins developed after the degeneration of the posterior cardinal veins and lie near and around the sympathetic chain. They are sometimes called the perisympathetic system. The intersubcardinal anastomosis becomes the left renal vein. The right adrenal vein drains into the subcardinal segment of the inferior vena cava. The left adrenal vein is sometimes considered a remnant of the left subcardinal veins, as is the gonadal vein (testicular or ovarian). A, Adrenal; Az, azygous vein; aa, umbilical veins; A.C.V., anterior cardinal vein; A.V., adrenal vein; A.L.V., ascending lumbar vein; A3, part three of IVC; bb, vitelline veins; B.C.A., brachiocephalic (left innominate) anastomosis; C.S., coronary sinus; D.A., dorsal aortae; D.C., duct of Cuvier; G, gonad; G.V., gonadal vein; H.V., hemiazygos vein; I.S.A., intersubcardinal anastomosis; l, liver; L.C.I.V., left common iliac vein; L.R.V., left renal vein; L.S.I.V., left superior intercostal vein; M, mesonephros; P.C.V., posterior cardinal vein; R.R.V., right renal vein; R.S.I.V., right superior intercostal vein; S.C.V., subcardinal vein; S.V., sinus venosus; S.V.C., superior vena cava; Sy sympathetic chain. (From Davies J. Anatomy, microscopic structure, and development of the human adrenal gland. In: Scott HW, ed. Surgery of the adrenal glands. Philadelphia: JB Lippincott, 1990.)

ation of cells of the definitive cortex. The fetal cortex begins to decrease in size within a few hours after birth and has nearly vanished by the end of the first year of life. The zona glomerulosa remains unaltered and produces the greatly shortened zona reticularis and zona fasciculata of the adult cortex (Fig. 19.7). The zona reticularis does not attain the adult appearance until the age of 11 or 12 years (8).

According to Hubbard et al. (14), a definitive medulla is not present until after birth.

There is an absolute loss of weight of the suprarenal glands from birth to the fourth month of postnatal life, after which the gland again begins to grow (15). The stroma of the degenerating fetal cortex constitutes a large proportion of the gland of the infant; it has disappeared by the end of the second year (16).

The suprarenal gland is at first elongated, lying parallel to the mesonephros. By the eighth week (16 to 18 mm; stage 19), the ascending kidney meets the lower pole. The gland assumes first a conical shape and later becomes pyramidal, with a concave base fitted over the upper pole of the kidney. As Davies (12) stated, the fetal adrenal dwarfs the kidney in size. The huge enigmatic size of the fetal adrenal takes place around the eighth week; the fetal cortex (whose function is not known), possibly under pituitary control, bears the responsibility for it. At the fourth month of gestation, the adrenal is four times the size of the kidney, whereas at birth it is one-third of the

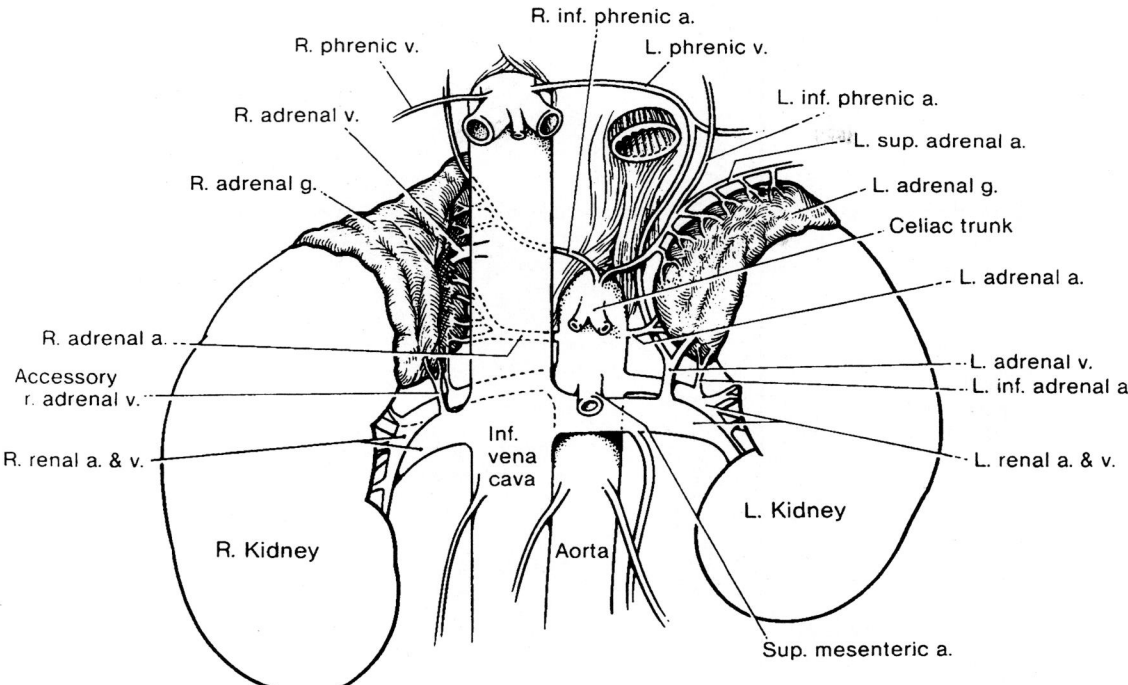

Figure 19.4. The arterial supply and venous drainage of the adrenal glands. As many as 60 arterial twigs may enter the adrenal gland. One or, occasionally, two veins drain the adrenal gland. (From Scaljon WM. Adrenal glands. In: Skandalakis JE, Gray SW, Rowe JS Jr. Anatomical complications in general surgery. New York: McGraw-Hill, 1983.)

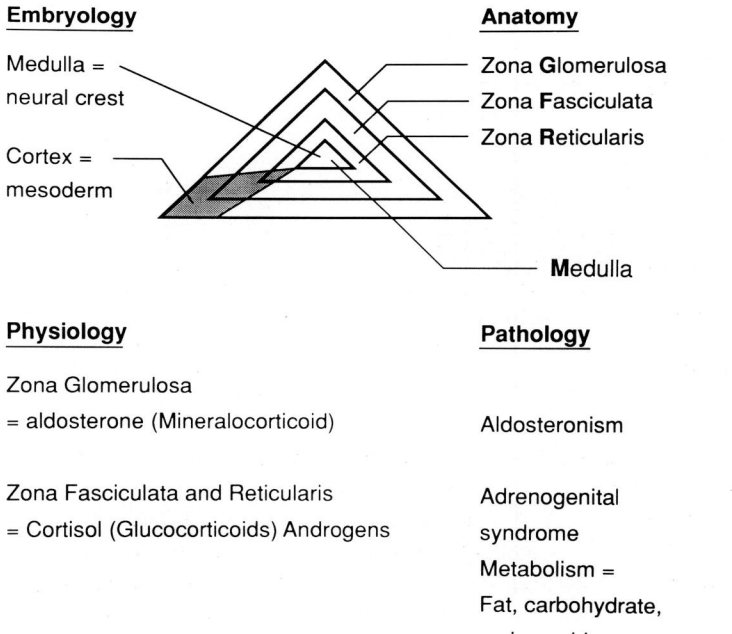

Figure 19.5. Condensation of embryology, anatomy, physiology, and pathology of the adrenal gland.

kidney size. At the end of the first year, the adrenal weighs about 1 gm and finally will reach the weight of 4 to 5 gm (12).

Kangarloo et al. (17) reported that after 1 year of age, the gland is similar to that of an adult. Unlike the kidney and the testis, the suprarenal gland undergoes no marked shift craniad or caudad during development (Fig. 19.8).

Remember the following:

I. The dual genesis of the adrenal gland (Figs. 19.9 and 19.10)

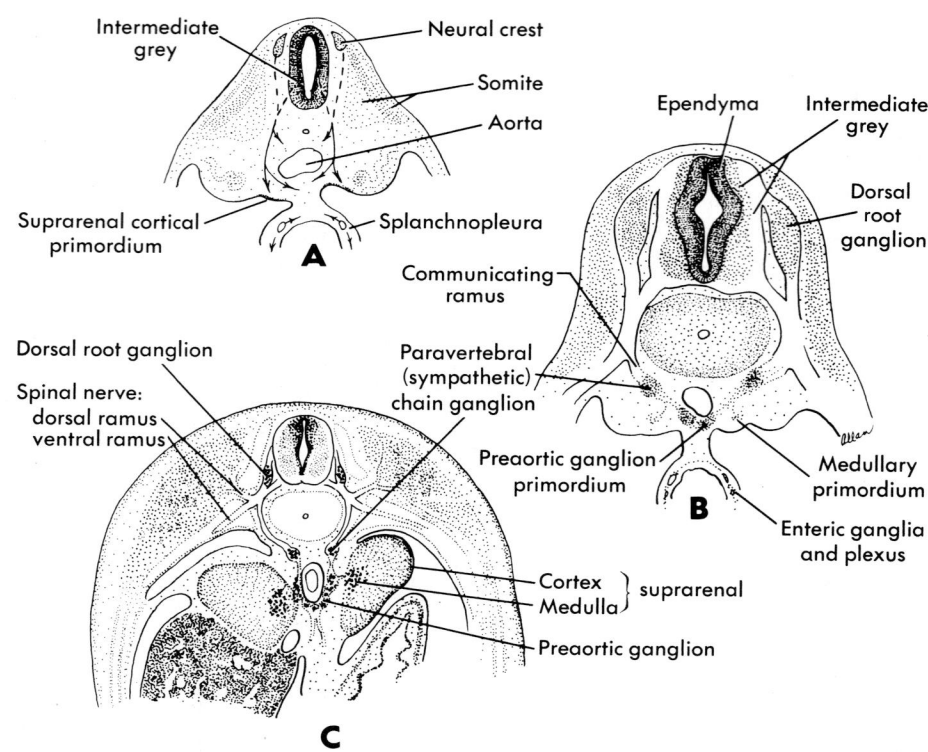

Figure 19.6. Development of the human suprarenal gland. **A,** Migration of sympathetic ganglion and chromaffin cells from the neural crest and neural tube. *Arrows* in the gut wall indicate enteric ganglion cells migrating from the vagus nerve. **B,** The formation of the sympathetic ganglia. **C,** The chromaffin cells of the future suprarenal medulla reaching the provisional cortex (compare with Figure 19.1, *D* and *E*.) (From Allan FD. Essentials of human embryology, 2nd ed. Toronto: Oxford University Press, 1969.)

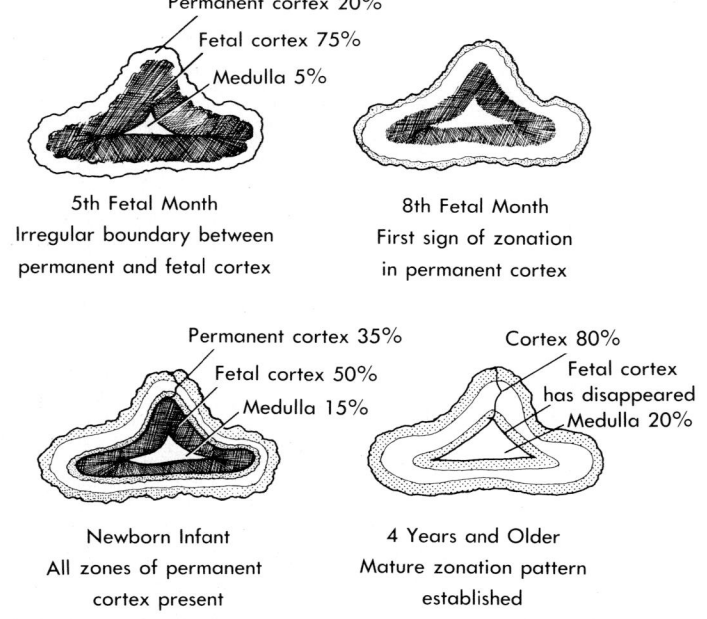

Figure 19.7. Internal development of the human suprarenal gland. The fetal cortex *(cross-hatched)* decreases in volume from the fifth fetal month to its complete disappearance in the first year of postnatal life. Zonation of the permanent cortex begins with the zona glomerulosa, indicated in the eighth fetal month; complete zonation is established by the fourth year of life. (Data from Sucheston ME, Cannon MS. Development of zonular patterns in the human adrenal gland. J Morphol 1968;126:477–492.)

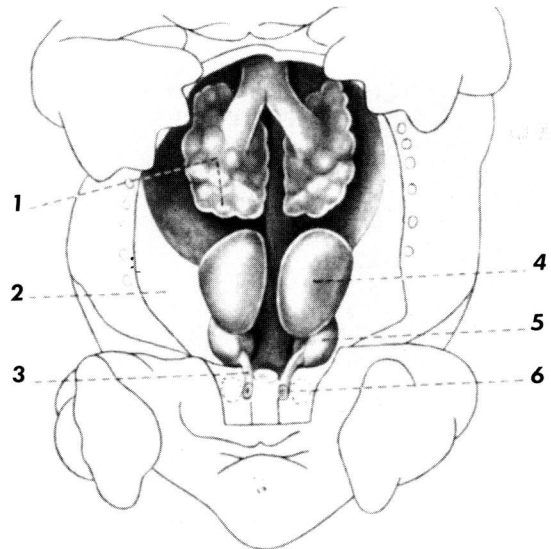

Figure 19.8. Relative sizes and positions of the suprarenal gland and the kidney in the eighth week (20 mm). The heart, diaphragm, liver, gut, and gonads have been removed. *1*, Lung; *2*, site of right lobe of liver; *3*, ureter; *4*, suprarenal gland; *5*, kidney; *6*, left umbilical artery. (From Blechschmidt E. The stages of human development before birth. Philadelphia: WB Saunders, 1961.)

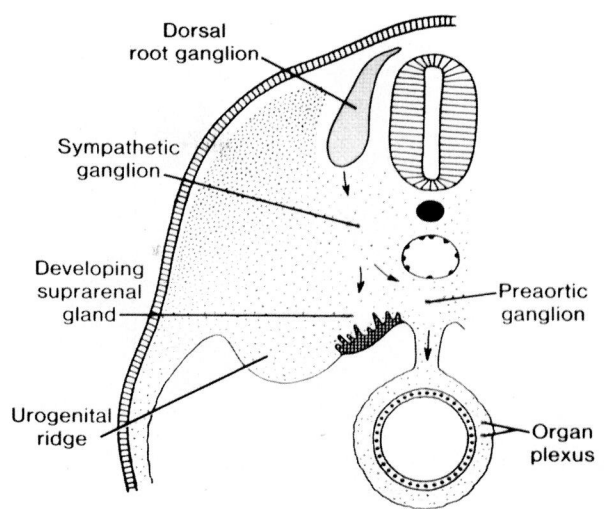

Figure 19.9. Mesothelial cells from mesenteric root differentiate to form the cortex. (From Sadler TW. Langman's medical embryology, 6th ed. Baltimore: Williams & Wilkins, 1990.)

1. Mesodermal from celomic epithelium (cortex)
2. Ectodermal from the neural crest (medulla)
   a. Formation of neural crest (Fig. 19.11)
   b. Migration of its cells and its derivatives (Figs. 19.12 and 19.13)
II. The possible sites of cortical and chromaffin tissue (Fig. 19.14)

Critical Events in Development

Agenesis of the suprarenal gland is bound up with the failure of the entire nephrogenic ridge to form early in the fourth week. Little else in the morphologic development of the organ can be called critical. Chemical differentiation, which is outside the scope of this book, has its own timetable.

ANOMALIES OF THE SUPRARENAL GLANDS (TABLE 19.1 AND FIG. 19.15)

Agenesis of the Suprarenal Gland

Unilateral agenesis of the suprarenal gland is almost always associated with agenesis of the kidney on the same side. The suprarenal gland is absent in about 10% of such cases (18, 19). It seems probable that the renal agenesis results from the absence of the whole nephrogenic ridge. Failure of the mesonephros to form causes absence of one of the two components of the suprarenal anlage. When the suprarenal gland is present but the kidney is absent, failure of the ureteric bud is the probable cause

of the renal agenesis. The mesonephros was probably formed normally. In the absence of the kidney, such suprarenal glands are usually flat discs of tissue rather than the usual pyramidal shape (20).

Adrenal Gland Hemorrhage

The adrenal gland is the second most common source of hemoperitoneum in the newborn (21). It may present as free hemoperitoneum or as an abdominal mass noted on physical examination and confirmed by ultrasound examination or computed tomographic (CT) scanning. Adrenal gland hemorrhage occurs on the right side in 70% of patients, on the left side in 25% of patients, and bilaterally in 5% of patients. Since the right gland drains directly into the inferior vena cava, it is more vulnerable to damage by increased caval pressure than is the left gland, which drains into the left renal vein (22). The neonatal adrenal gland is also susceptible to traumatic injury because of its relatively large size. Alternatively, hemorrhage may occur because of the physiologic involution of the inner fetal zone of the adrenal cortex, with resultant tearing of the unsupported central adrenal gland vessels (22). About 75% of babies who develop adrenal hemorrhage have had a breech or traumatic delivery (23).

A hematoma resulting from adrenal hemorrhage must be differentiated from a neonatal neuroblastoma of the adrenal gland (24). Both can present as abdominal masses in the newborn. Both can have flecks of calcification seen on abdominal radiographs. Adrenal gland hemorrhage is usually manifested by hypovolemic shock or corticosteroid deficiency, whereas neonatal adrenal neuroblastoma is not. An adrenal gland hematoma should regress in size

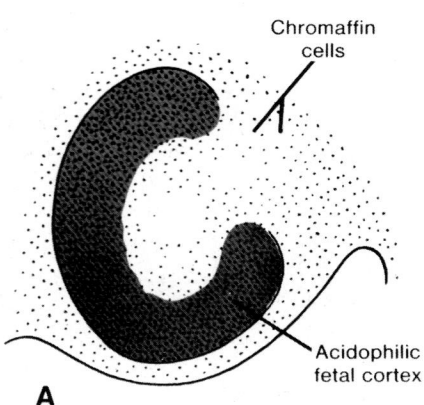

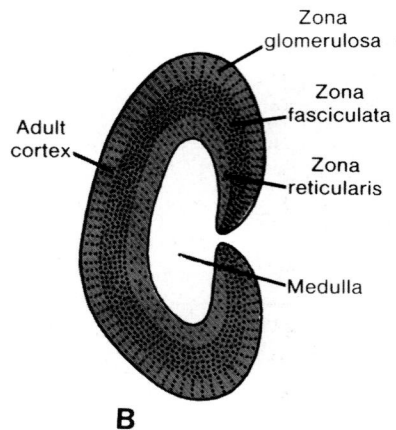

Figure 19.10. **A,** Drawing showing the chromaffin (sympathetic) cells penetrating the fetal cortex of the suprarenal gland. **B,** At a later stage of development, the definitive cortex surrounds the medulla almost completely. (From Sadler TW. Langman's medical embryology, 6th ed. Baltimore: Williams & Wilkins, 1990.)

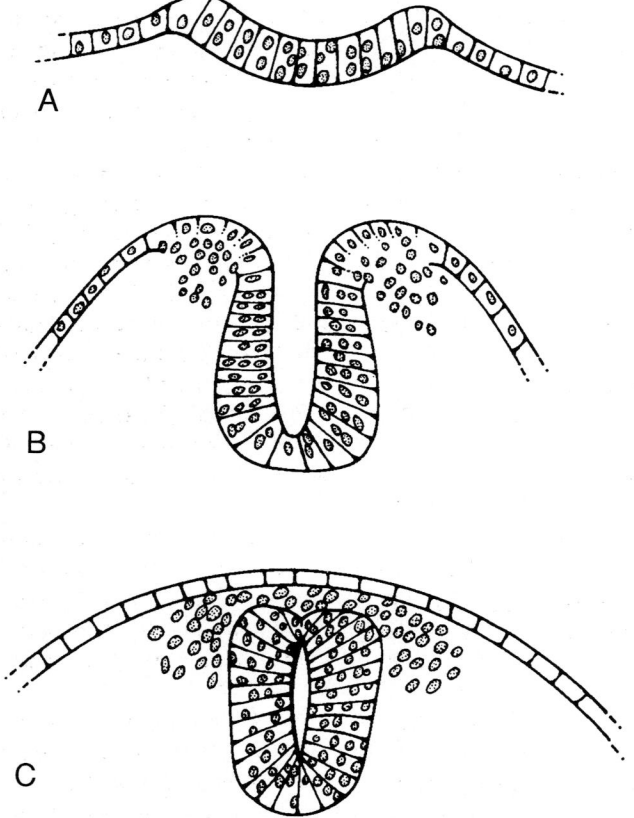

Figure 19.11. The formation of the neural tube and the origin of cells of the neural crest from the neurectoderm. (From Scaljon WM. Adrenal glands. In: Skandalakis JE, Gray SW, Rowe JS Jr. Anatomical complications in general surgery. New York: McGraw-Hill, 1983.)

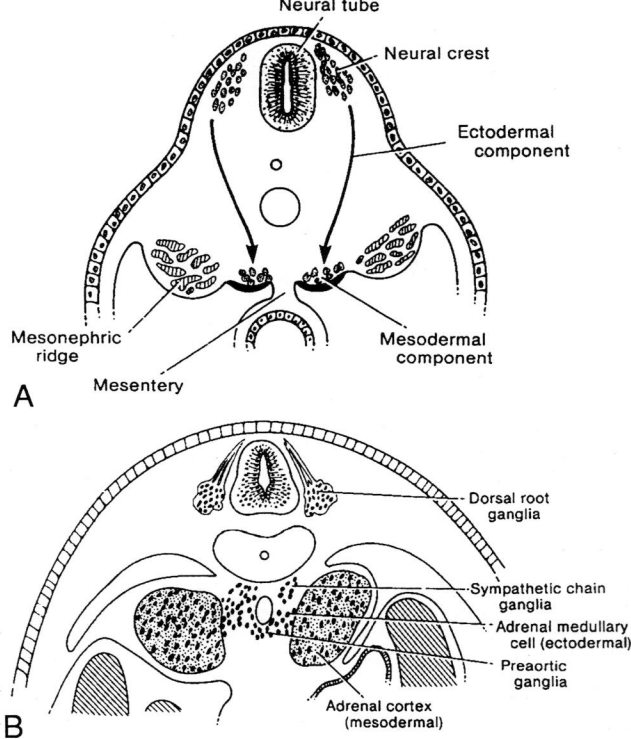

Figure 19.12. Migration of neural crest cells into the mesodermal components of the adrenal gland during **(A)** the sixth week and **(B)** the seventh week. (From Scaljon WM. Adrenal glands. In: Skandalakis JE, Gray SW, Rowe JS Jr. Anatomical complications in general surgery. New York: McGraw-Hill, 1983.)

on follow-up abdominal ultrasounds over a 4-week period, whereas a neonatal neuroblastoma will not. Neuroblastomas can be associated with elevated serum and urine catecholamines, whereas an adrenal hematoma is not. It is rare for a neonatal adrenal neuroblastoma to be associated with hemoperitoneum, according to Brock and Ricketts (24).

Neuroblastoma is the second most common tumor of infancy, second only to teratoma (excluding hemangiomas and lymphangiomas). Neuroblastoma is the most common neonatal abdominal tumor; approximately half of these arise in the adrenal, while the remaining tumors arise in the sympathetic chain (25).

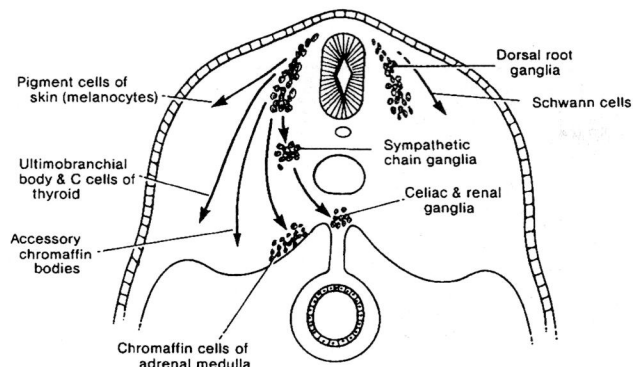

Figure 19.13. Derivatives of the neural crest. This is the origin of the chromaffin cells of the adrenal medulla and the aortic bodies. (From Scaljon WM. Adrenal glands. In: Skandalakis JE, Gray SW, Rowe JS Jr. Anatomical complications in general surgery. New York: McGraw-Hill, 1983.)

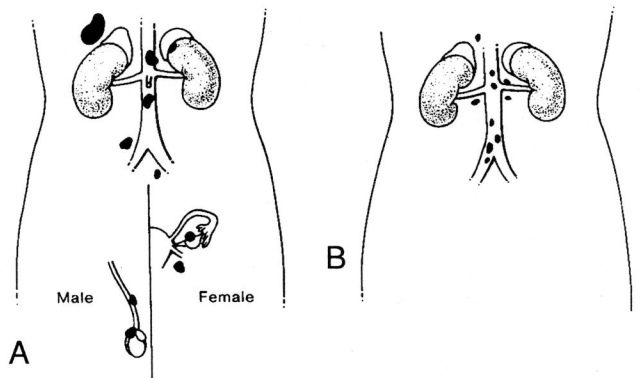

Figure 19.14. Sites of **(A)** heterotopic adrenal glands and nodules of cortical tissue and **(B)** chromaffin tissue. Masses on and near the aorta are the retroperitoneal extraadrenal paraganglia. (From Scaljon WM. Adrenal glands. In: Skandalakis JE, Gray SW, Rowe JS Jr. Anatomical complications in general surgery. New York: McGraw-Hill, 1983.)

Neuroblastoma

Because of the congenital nature of this neuroblastoma, it is appropriate to include a section on this tumor. It is the most frequent solid tumor in children, and represents one-half of all malignancies in neonates and one-third of those in infants in the first year (26–27). Neuroblastoma is found in approximately one in 10,000 children per year (26, 28–30). An even higher rate, 1:40 to 1:250, has been reported in infants less than 3 months old who die of other causes (26, 28).

Up to 1:7000 children will be affected by age 5 years (30) with a mean age at diagnosis of 2 years (26).

Males are affected slightly more often than females, and there is an equal racial distribution. Some cases appear to be familial, with an increased association of mother-daughter and father-son cases and autosomal dominant and autosomal recessive inheritance patterns. Familial cases tend to be diagnosed at a younger age and have multiple primary tumors (26).

In addition, neuroblastoma has been noted to occur in association with other congenital syndromes such as Hirschsprung's disease, fetal hydantoin syndrome, Beckwith-Wiedemann syndrome, and fetal alcohol syndrome (26, 28). Because of their origin in the neural crest, neuroblastomas can arise in any site of neural crest-derived tissue, including the ganglia in the neck, the posterior mediastinum, the retroperitoneum, and the pelvic organ of Zuckerkandl. The majority of these tumors (75%) are found in the abdomen or retroperitoneum, with 40% arising from the adrenal and 35% from the paraspinal ganglia. Of the remainder, 20% are found in the mediastinum, 3% in the pelvis, and 2% in the neck (26, 28).

Neuroblastoma is part of a spectrum of neural tumors. Ganglioneuroma (a truly benign tumor) is at one end; neuroblastoma (a tumor with malignant behavior) is at the other end; ganglioneuroblastoma can be placed in between. The latter can "mature" into a ganglioneuroma. This can occur spontaneously or in response to chemotherapy; and in the primary tumor or in metastases (26). These tumors also have been shown to regress spontaneously. This maturation and regression is thought to be influenced by the immune system.

Because of their neural crest origin, 80 to 95% of these tumors are capable of synthesizing and secreting catecholamines (26, 28–30). Since the cells are not fully differentiated, however, they tend to secrete compounds such as homovanillic acid (HVA) and vanillylmandelic acid (VMA) and, less frequently, cystathionine and homoserine. These are derivatives of the catecholamine precursors. The more immature the tumor cells, the earlier the precursor derivative they secrete. Thus immature tumors tend to secrete HVA, a dopamine derivative, while more mature tumors secrete VMA, a derivative of norepinephrine (26, 28).

Up to 80% of neuroblastoma cells contain chromosomal abnormalities. Hyperdiploidy, double minutes, homogenous staining regions, and deletions or rearrangements of the short arm of chromosome 1 (so-called marker chromosome 1) and of chromosome 17 have been found in advanced stage tumors (31, 32).

Neuroblastoma may be found incidentally (i.e., when calcifications are noted on a chest x-ray film, abdominal film, or ultrasonogram done for other reasons). In 50 to 75% of cases, children with abdominal neuroblastoma present with an abdominal mass or pain (28).

The mass may compress lymphatics, leading to lower extremity edema; or the spinal cord, causing pain or neurological deficits; or the renal artery, causing hypertension. Hypertension, which is found in 25% of cases, is less frequently a result of the catecholamines secreted by the tumor (33).

Less commonly, these children initially have only nonspecific signs and symptoms, such as fever, flushing, irritability, failure to thrive, myalgias, anemia, or thrombo-

Table 19.1.
Anomalies of the Suprarenal Glands

Anomaly	Origin of Defect	First Appearance (or Other Diagnostic Clues)	Sex Chiefly Affected	Relative Frequency	Remarks
Agenesis of the suprarenals	4th week	None, when unilateral	?	Uncommon	Associated with absence of kidney on the same side
Fusion of the suprarenals	6th week	None	Male	Rare	Associated with fused kidneys
Hypoplasia of the suprarenals	Probably late in gestation	At birth	Male	Very rare except in anencephalic infants	Usually lethal in infancy
Heterotopia of the suprarenals	8th week	None	?	Uncommon	Usually found within capsule of liver or kidney
Accessory suprarenal glands	4th-6th weeks	None	Probably equal	Common	Rarely contain medullary tissue

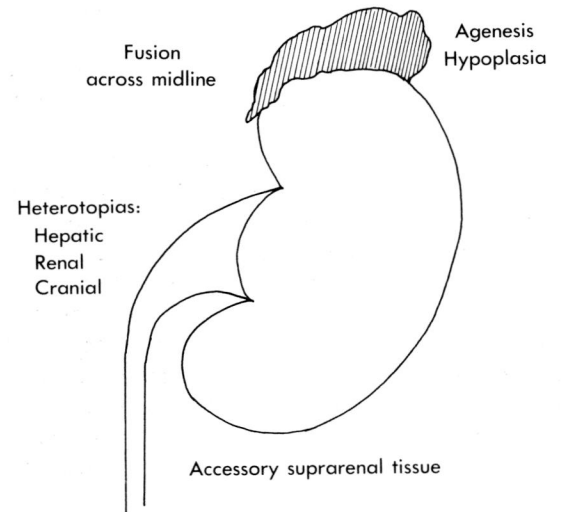

Figure 19.15. The chief congenital anomalies of the suprarenal glands.

cytopenia (34). The production of vasoactive intestinal peptides by the tumor may result in profuse diarrhea. Because the catecholamines can cross the placenta in congenital cases, the mother may report hypertension or episodes of flushing during the pregnancy (26).

Neuroblastoma can also produce a type of cerebellar ataxia. This syndrome—also called "dancing eyes, dancing feet" because of the nystagmus and myoclonic movements which characterize it—has been attributed to an autoimmune phenomenon and may not resolve with treatment of the tumor. This syndrome is more frequent in children under 1 year of age with a more mature, localized tumor (29). Finally, children may present with manifestations of metastases, such as bone pain or bilateral orbital ecchymoses.

Pertinent laboratory tests include: complete blood count with platelets; prothrombin time/partial thromboplastin time (PT/PTT) test; sequential multiple analysis

of 20 chemical constituents (SMA 20); and urine VMA, HVA and creatinine values. In 85 to 90% of cases, urinary VMA and HVA levels will be above the normal values. A kidney, ureters, and bladder (KUB) radiographic series and ultrasound should be done to determine the size and location of the tumor, to delineate whether it is solid or cystic, and to rule out adrenal hemorrhage as the cause of the mass (see the previous section on "Adrenal Hemorrhage").

A CT scan with or without contrast media or magnetic resonance imaging (MRI) may be necessary to confirm that the mass is separate from the kidney. Neuroblastoma, ganglioneuroblastoma, and ganglioneuroma cannot be differentiated radiologically although cystic masses are more often benign. If a mass with characteristics of neuroblastoma is found, a metastatic workup—including bone marrow aspiration and biopsy, chest x-ray examination, and skeletal survey—must be done.

As in other malignancies, staging of neuroblastoma is important for dictating treatment and predicting prognosis. A large number of staging systems have been proposed. The most commonly used is that of Evans et al. (35):

Stage I:	Tumor confined to organ or structure of origin
Stage II:	Tumor extending in continuity beyond the organ or structure or origin but not crossing the midline (Regional lymph nodes on the homolateral side may be involved.)
Stage III:	Tumor extending in continuity beyond the midline (Regional nodes bilaterally may be involved.)
Stage IV:	Remote disease involving skeleton, organs, soft tissues, or distant lymph node groups
Stage IV-S:	Patients less than 1 year of age who would otherwise be classified as stage I or II but who have remote disease confined only to one or more of the following: liver, skin, or bone marrow (without radiographic evidence of bone metastases on complete skeletal survey)

Standard treatment for neuroblastoma can be most clearly described on a stage-by-stage basis using the Evans system.

For stage I tumors, complete excision is curative (28, 36).

For stage II, complete resection is attempted. If this is not possible, a partial resection is performed, and radiation treatment or chemotherapy is given. Chemotherapy, particularly vincristine and cyclophosphamide, has also been used successfully for stage I and II tumors, in addition to surgery (36), although no increase in survival has been demonstrated by the addition of chemotherapy (28).

For stage III tumors, chemotherapy may be given prior to surgery to decrease tumor size and vascularity, thus making a more complete resection possible. Excision is followed by chemotherapy and radiation. Attempts at initial partial excision of stage IV tumors has not been shown to increase survival, so surgery is preceded by chemotherapy. In all cases where tumor resection is incomplete, a second-look operation is required after a period of treatment with radiation and/or chemotherapy (26, 28).

Treatment of stage IV-S tumors is controversial. Although some studies suggest that resection of the localized primary tumor should be attempted, others indicate that only chemotherapy—or no therapy—should be given (26, 28, 36). The role of autologous bone marrow transplantation for patients with stage IV neuroblastoma is under investigation by the Pediatric Oncology Group.

The prognosis for patients with neuroblastoma is dictated by the stage of the tumor and the age of the child at diagnosis. The rate of survival for 2 years or more for all patients with abdominal tumors in all age groups is 26.3%. Survival in children with mediastinal or pelvic tumors is higher. Based on age, the rates of survival for 2 years or greater for all stages and locations of neuroblastoma are: 75% for ages less than 1 year; 52% for ages 1 to 2 years; 16% for ages over 3 years (28).

Using the Evans system, survival is: 100% for stage I; 80 to 100% for stage II; 37% for stage III; 7 to 20% for stage IV (50% for children less than 1 year of age; 10% for those older than 1 year of age); and 79% for stage IV-S (28, 30).

The two-year survival rate for children with disseminated disease treated with bone marrow transplantation is 25 to 60% (28, 37). Hayes has found that, of patients with Evans stage II disease, 100% with negative nodes and 54% with positive nodes survive, and of those with either stage II or III disease, 83% with negative nodes and 31% with positive nodes survive (38). These results indicate that both surgical resectability of the primary tumor and the presence of lymph node involvement affect prognosis.

Recent research has detected other parameters which affect survival. First of all, the number of copies of the N-myc oncogene in the tumor cells correlates with the stage of disease (39–41). All tumors with 3 to 300 copies of this gene were Evans stage III or IV, and all stage I and II tumors contained only one copy (40). The number of copies varies with and may dictate aggressive behavior of the tumor, and the relationship between the number of copies and survival is independent of the age of the patient at diagnosis. Survival rates at 18 months for children with tumors with 1, 3 to 10, or greater than 10 copies of the N-myc gene per cell were 70, 30, and 5% for all tumors, respectively, and 61, 47, and 0% for stage IV tumors, respectively (40).

N-myc is a member of the c-myc oncogene family and is produced almost exclusively by neuroblastomas. N-myc encodes a protein similar in size to that encoded by c-myc. The c-myc protein, and thus probably the N-myc protein, has a high binding affinity for DNA. There may be a correlation between expression of the gene and prognosis (41).

Secondly, determination of DNA ploidy by flow cytometry (42) has also been used to determine prognosis. Look et al. (32) have shown that hyperdiploidy (1.07 to 2.42 times the normal diploid amount of DNA) has been associated with a decreased frequency of stage III and IV disease, an increased frequency of stage IV-S disease, an increased survival at 18 months, and a better response to chemotherapy in infants with unresectable tumors. Children with hyperdiploid or triploid tumor cells have a better prognosis than those with cells with diploid amounts, marker chromosome 1, double minutes, or homogenous staining regions (31).

A recent step toward improving the prognosis for children with neuroblastoma entails screening for this tumor in young infants. Preliminary studies in Japan (43) and Canada (36) have shown that screening for neuroblastoma is feasible, cost effective, and sufficiently accurate. In comparison with the other diseases for which neonates are screened, neuroblastoma is twice as frequent as phenylketonuria (PKU), ten times as frequent as galactosemia, and only slightly less frequent than hypothyroidism. In the Canadian study, urine VMA and HMA levels were measured in newborns. The test was found to be 86% sensitive and 99% specific for neuroblastoma. Proponents of initiating screening for neuroblastoma in the United States (30) have determined that it would cost $3.50 per infant screening and would save 260 lives per year.

Fusion of the Suprarenal Glands

In cases in which the two kidneys are fused, the suprarenal glands also may be joined across the midline, behind the aorta (20) (Fig. 19.16).

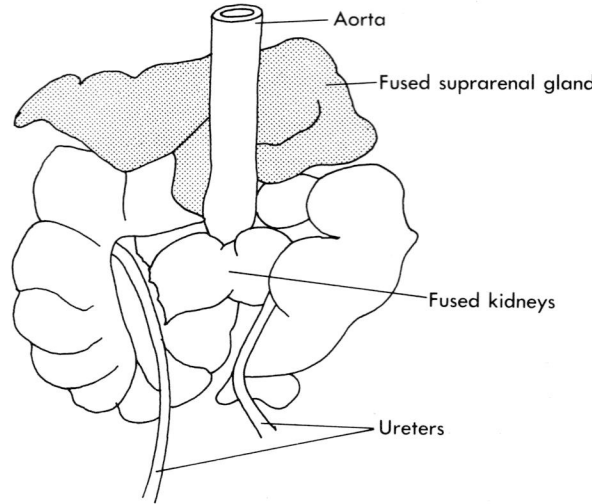

Figure 19.16. Fusion of the suprarenal glands posterior to the aorta. The kidneys are fused anterior to the aorta. These two defects often occur together. (Drawn from a photograph by Potter EL. Pathology of the fetus and the newborn. Chicago: Year Book Medical Publishers, 1952.)

Suprarenal Hypoplasia

Two types of suprarenal hypoplasia have been described by Kerenyi (44). One may be called the "anencephalic type," in which the suprarenal glands are greatly reduced in size, the fetal cortex is usually absent or hypoplastic, and the medullary tissue appears poorly developed (45). There is no evidence of premature atrophy of a normally formed fetal cortex. Four examples of nonanencephalic infants with this type of hypoplasia have been collected by Kerenyi (44), and a fifth has been reported by Winquist (46). None of these infants lived for more than a few days. In four of the cases there was an absence or a reduction of acidophils and an increase in basophils of the anterior pituitary. Hypoplasia of thyroid and gonads was usually but not always present. In Winquist's patient, pituitary acidophils amounted to 20%, about half the normal number, but symptoms of suprarenal insufficiency were present; the author considered the placenta or the maternal pituitary to be deficient. Others (47, 48) believe that there is a specific corticotropin for the fetal suprarenal cortex from the fetal pituitary. Because the hypothalamus and posterior lobe of the pituitary are absent or defective in anencephalic fetuses, deficiency of neurosecretory material has been suggested as a cause of early involution of the fetal cortex in these infants (49). Although there are known relationships between the pituitary and the suprarenal cortex, the coincidence of defects is not sufficient proof of a functional connection.

A second type of suprarenal hypoplasia has been found in which the fetal cortex is composed of very large, irregularly placed cells. No marginal, permanent cortex is present, and the medulla occurs in eccentric islets. The anterior pituitary appears normal, as do the other endocrine glands. All cases have been in males, and all patients have survived for a few months (44). This second type of hypoplasia appears to be an intrinsic defect, whereas the first type appears to be of pituitary origin.

Left vascular shrinking of adrenal gland was reported by Schonenberg (50) in association with other congenital anomalies in a 10-year-old girl. Turner and O'Herlihy (51) reported three cases of trisomy 18 with hypoplasia of fetal adrenal cortical zone.

Newman et al. (52) described a case of adrenal hypoplasia with pituitary agenesis in a normocephalic infant female and were able to collect 28 additional cases from the literature for review. In the 29 cases, 18 females and 11 males were affected with the abnormality. Five families were involved, and Newman and colleagues suggested an autosomal recessive inheritance.

Anomalous Location of Suprarenal Tissue

ANATOMY

Suprarenal Heterotopia. In this condition, the suprarenal gland is in its normal location, but it lies under the capsule of the kidney (suprarenal-renal heterotopia) or under the capsule of the liver (suprarenal-hepatic heterotopia).

Because of the dual genesis of the adrenal glands, mesodermal (celomic epithelium) and ectodermal (neural crest), extraadrenal tissue may be found anywhere in the peritoneal cavity in abundance, but it usually follows its embryologic destiny. In other words, cortical islands may be found anywhere in the peritoneal cavity, but characteristically they are located in the vicinity of or even within anatomic entities derived from the urogenital ridge (testicle, epididymis, vas, ovary, broad ligament, persistent mesonephric duct alongside uterus and vagina, and the so-called duct of Gartner) (Fig. 19.17.).

According to Fonkalsrud (53), adrenocortical rests, which may be found in 50% of newborns, disappear within a few weeks after birth. The same author reports that, in males with adrenogenital syndrome, one can often find ectopic adrenal tissue within an atrophic testicle.

Cortical and medullary tissue, adrenal in toto, also may be found together everywhere. However, medullary tissue usually rests alone along the dorsal root ganglia, the sympathetic chain. Coupland (54) reported, after histochemical and electron microscopic studies, that these tissues are part of the catecholamine-secreting organs.

Suprarenal-renal heterotopia was first described by Klebs (55) in 1876. By 1925 Weller (56) could find only 13 cases. By 1942 there were 26 cases in the literature

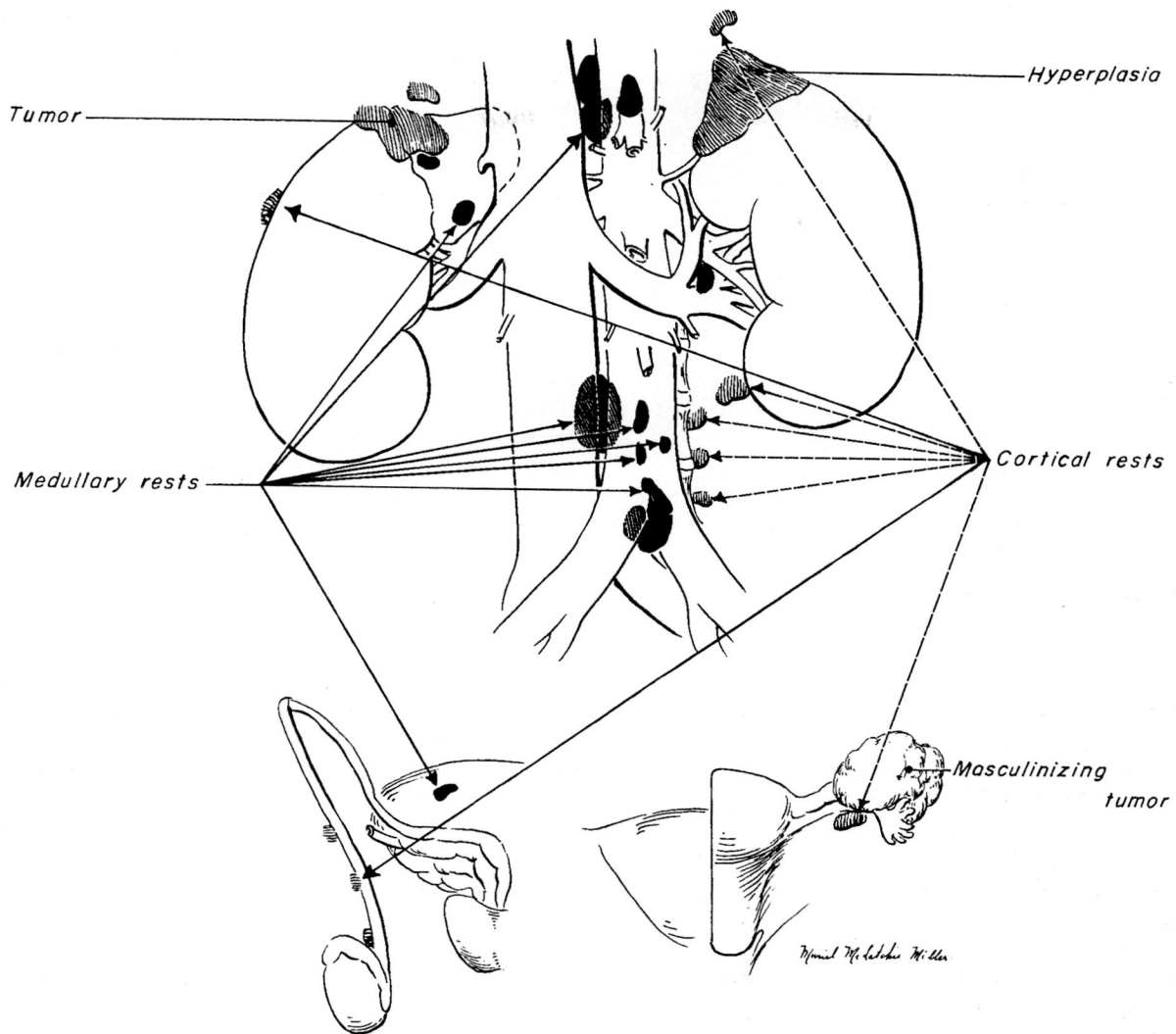

Figure 19.17. Composite drawing showing reported locations of rest of adrenal cortical and medullary tissues. These sites have surgical significance when the suspected lesion is not found within the substance of the normally situated adre- nal glands. (From Fonkalsrud EW. The adrenal glands. In: Welch KJ, Randolph JG, Ravitch MM, O'Neill JA, Rowe MI, eds. Pediatric surgery. Chicago: Year Book Medical Publishers, 1986:1115.)

(57). Either side may be affected, but the heterotopia is bilateral in most cases. Occasionally, there may be a normal suprarenal in addition to the subcapsular one.

Suprarenal-hepatic heterotopia has been reported less often, although Weller (56) found three cases in 800 autopsies. Only the right suprarenal was affected.

In these heterotopias, there is a thin connective tissue layer between the suprarenal parenchyma and the adjacent tissue, but this layer is almost always incomplete. Kidney tubules or bile ducts may be found among the suprarenal cells at the junction. The medullary component often is reduced, and is usually absent in that portion of the suprarenal closest to the kidney or liver tissue.

By far the most remarkable of the heterotopic supra-

renal glands are those that occur in the cranium. At least three cases have been reported (58–60). One patient lived to age 73 years and died of unrelated causes (59). Another patient (60) died of unrelated cerebral hemorrhage and was found at autopsy to have a suprarenal tumor $5.2 \times 3 \times 1.8$ cm, attached to the inferior surface of the left frontal lobe. Both cortex and medulla were present, and no suprarenals were found in the normal location (Fig. 19.18). There were no symptoms.

Accessory Suprarenal Glands. While most accessory suprarenal tissue is without a medullary component, in a few cases the structures are complete. Graham (61), investigating accessory structures near the aorta between the celiac axis and the superior mesenteric artery, found

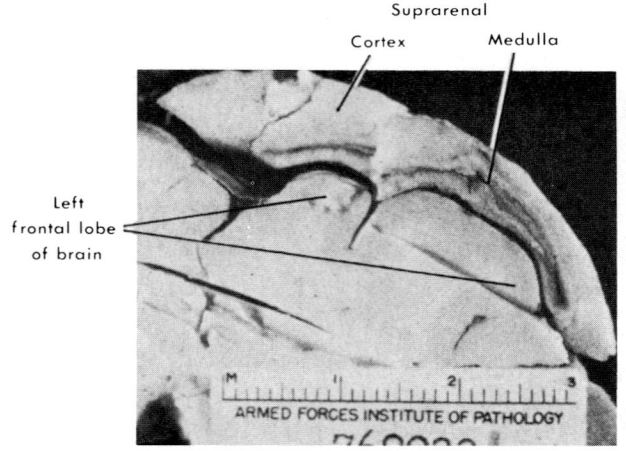

Figure 19.18. *Cranial suprarenal heterotopia. The suprarenal tissue, containing both cortex and medulla, was attached to the leptomeninges of the left frontal lobe in the anterior cranial fossa of a 49-year-old man. No suprarenal glands were present at the normal location. At least three such cases have been reported. (From Wiener MF, Dallgaard SA. Intracranial adrenal gland: a case report. Arch Pathol 1959;67:228–233.)*

among 100 consecutive autopsies 16 cadavers with complete accessory glands and another 16 with cortical rests only (Fig. 19.19). Histologic examination for all but the smallest nodules is necessary to prove the presence or absence of medullary elements.

Skandalakis et al. (62) reported a case of extraadrenal retroperitoneal "nonfunctioning" paraganglioma. Similar cases were reported by Olson and Abell (63) and Glenner and Grimley (64). Skandalakis and his colleagues stated that extraadrenal retroperitoneal paraganglioma is a rare tumor that may occur at any place along the sympathetic ganglionated chain. The most common location of the tumor is near the organs of Zuckerkandl, which are located at the origin of the inferior mesenteric artery on either side of the aorta. However, cases have been reported with the tumor located around and near the adrenals or kidneys, below the pancreas, around the abdominal aorta, etc. According to Pack and Tabah (65), the incidence of these tumors, in comparison with the pheochromocytomas (similar tumors arising from the paraganglionic cells of the adrenal medulla), is about one in 12 cases. Cases of intrathoracic paragangliomas have been reported (66).

The paraganglioma can be active or inactive. When active, according to Stout (67), it should be called "pheochromocytoma." We believe that the term *paraganglioma* should always apply to these extraadrenal, retroperitoneal, functioning (or nonfunctioning), chromaffin (or nonchromaffin) tumors. When functional, they act as a pure pheochromocytoma, presenting symptoms and signs of paroxysmal or sustained hypertension.

According to Kohn and Ganem and Cahill (58, 68),

chromaffin cells (cells which show chromaffin granules when brought into contact with potassium bichromate) can be found along the entire length of the autonomic nervous system. Such cells also can be found in the ganglia of the same system. However, it now is accepted that small islands of chromaffin and nonchromaffin tissue (both histologically similar) may be found in the retroperitoneal space and other spaces or organs of the human body (e.g., carotid body, vagus and glossopharyngeal nerves) (69).

There is confusion in the literature concerning these chromaffin and nonchromaffin tumors. The name "paraganglioma" is freely applied to both tumors. We agree with Scott and his associates (70) who stated in 1990 that the term *pheochromocytoma* cannot be discarded since it is so "deeply ingrained in medical literature" and that the functional neoplasm of the paraganglia should be classified according to anatomic location, hormonal secretion, and histopathology.

Table 19.2 indicates the differences between these two types of tumors, which are both termed *paraganglioma*.

Accessory Cortical Tissue. Accessory suprarenal cortical tissue nodules, or islands, may occur almost anywhere in the abdomen (Fig. 19.20). They were first described by Marchand (71) in 1883 although Morgagni (72) is said to have recognized them in 1740 (73). We have been unable to locate Morgagni's reference to them although he does speak of fat in the mediastinum testis (XLII:41) and of fat between the testis and epididymis (XLIII:37) and suggests that such bodies may be the source of tumors. These were almost certainly suprarenal cortical rests.

The most frequent sites of accessory suprarenal tissue are under the renal capsule (74), in the broad ligament in

Table 19.2.
Differences Between Chromaffin and Nonchromaffin "Paragangliomas" Extraadrenal Retroperitoneal Paraganglioma[a]

Chromaffin reaction	Chromaffin (Positive)		Chromaffin (Negative)	
Innervation	Efferent preganglionic sympathetic fibers (motor)		Sensory or afferent	
Secretion	Adrenalin Sympathin (?)		Acetylcholine (?)	
Origin	Related to certain tissues of the sympathetic nervous system		From parasympathetic neuroblasts (?)	
Clinical	*Active:* Paroxysmal or sustained hypertension	*Inactive:* Pressure signs only, if any	*Active:* Questionable	*Inactive:* Presure signs only, if any

[a]From Skandelakis JE et al. Extra-adrenal retroperitoneal "nonfunctioning" paraganglioma: report of a case and review of the literature. South Med J 1959;52(11):1368–1370.

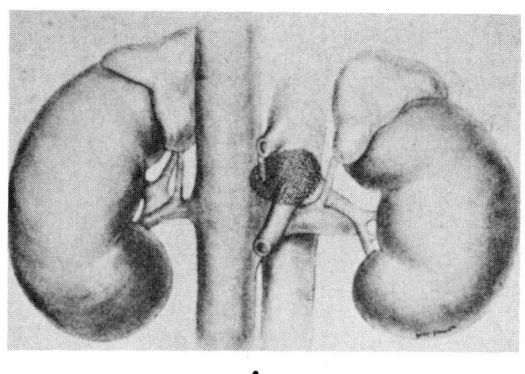

A

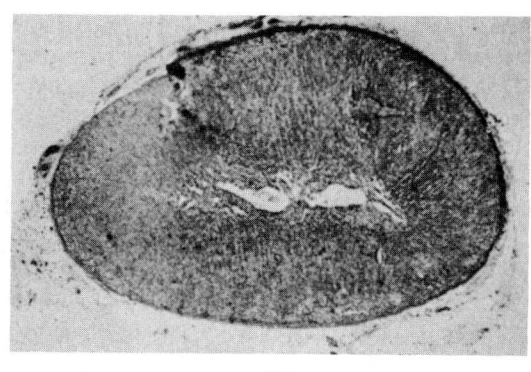

B

Figure 19.19.　Accessory suprarenal gland. **A,** Most frequent location of an accessory gland *(shaded area)* on the aorta between the celiac and superior mesenteric arteries. **B,** Section of the accessory gland showing the presence of both cortical and medullary tissue. (From Graham LS. Celiac accessory adrenal glands. Cancer 1953;6:149–152.)

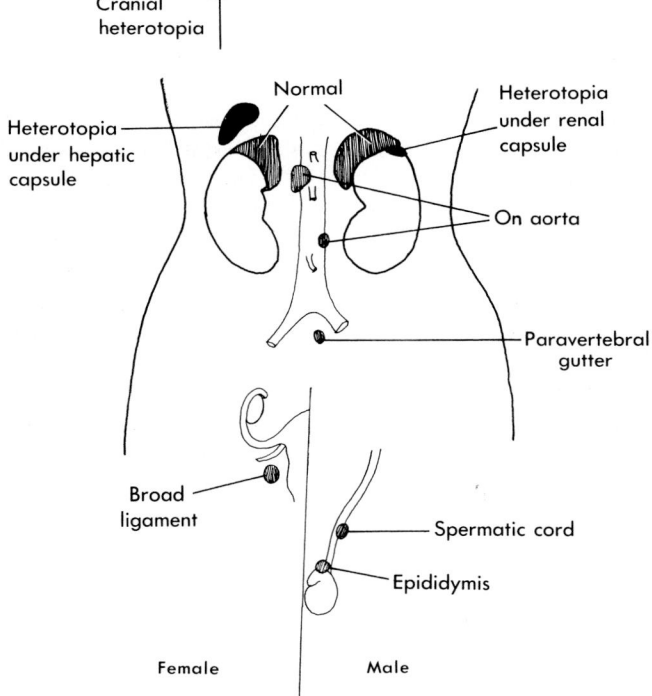

Figure 19.20.　Suprarenal heterotopia. The chief sites at which heterotopic and accessory suprarenal glands have been reported.

the female, and in the spermatic cord in the male. Falls (75) was able to find nine examples in 30 consecutive gynecologic laparotomies. This is in striking contrast to the fact that he was able to find only nine cases in adults in the literature since Marchand's original report. Bret and Brodi (76) added six more published cases.

The accessory nodules are beneath the peritoneum of the broad ligament, usually close to the ovarian vein or even within the ovary. They may or may not be embedded in fat. They have been found more frequently in children than in adults (77), but there is little reason to believe that they are not equally common in adults.

Dahl (78) examined testes from 100 male infants who died at the Mayo Clinic and found 15 suprarenal cortical nodules in 11 individuals. This incidence is in agreement with results from other, smaller series cited by Dahl. Six were in the connective tissue at the posterior margin of the epididymis, four were in or near the mediastinum testis, and five were in the connective tissue of the distal 1 cm of the spermatic cord. They have been found as well in hydroceles and in hernial sacs.

Finkbeiner et al. (79) described a patient with bilateral cryptorchism, ectopic splenic nodules on the left testicle, and adrenal cortical rest on the right testicle.

Hamazaki and Saito (80) reported a 3-month-old male infant with adrenal cytomegaly and adrenal rest tissue in the right testis and Beckwith-Wiedemann's syndrome. Accessory adrenal during orchiopexy was reported by Wolloch et al. (81).

Myelolipoma arising from an accessory adrenal gland, most likely anatomically located in the periadrenal fatty tissue, was reported by Kageyama et al. (82).

In 1985 Kenney et al. (83) found that, in 83% of congenital renal anomalies, the ipsilateral adrenal was identified as a disc-shaped paraspinal organ on CT scan. However, the adrenals retained their normal shape with acquired renal atrophy. Similar cases were discovered by Hadar et al. (84), who stated that the shape and position of the adrenal in patients with renal agenesis and ectopy was abnormal by CT.

In both males and females, the cortical tissue of adrenal nodules was normal. In young infants, the fetal cortex was present and underwent involution, as did that of the normal gland.

There is no doubt that accessory suprarenal structures are of wide occurrence in the human body, despite the paucity of reports. In rats, as many as 50% may be so affected, and in rabbits the frequency approaches 100% (73, 75). In 1926 Jaffe (85) found that, among suprarenalectomized rats, 35% died within 30 days, 46% lived 6 to 7 months, and 19% thrived indefinitely. All in the last group showed hypertrophic accessory suprarenal cortical tissue. Cases of compensatory hypertrophy of accessory cortical tissue following destructive lesions of the normal suprarenal glands in humans are cited by Falls (75).

It must be kept in mind that suprarenal cortical adenomas may occur in ectopic and heterotopic suprarenal tissues as well as in the normal gland.

Accessory Chromaffin Tissue. Extramedullary chromaffin tissue is distributed diffusely along the abdominal aorta and in discrete structures (organs of Zuckerkandl) around the origin of the inferior mesenteric artery. As these structures occur normally and are composed of chromaffin cells that were not incorporated into the suprarenal medulla, they cannot be considered to be anomalous accessory tissue although undoubtedly variations occur in the amount present in different individuals (Fig. 19.21).

Glowniak et al. (86) reported familial extraadrenal pheochromocytoma in the right renal hilum in a family over three successive generations.

EMBRYOGENESIS

Inclusion of the suprarenal gland under the capsule of the kidney or liver takes place during the eighth week of fetal development when the ascending kidney comes into contact with the lower pole of the developing suprarenal gland. The kidney, liver, and suprarenal are all enveloped in peritoneum and have the beginnings of their connective tissue capsules. It must be assumed that fusion between the organs takes place with subsequent destruction of the intervening layers of celomic epithelium. The process is analogous to the fusion that may occur between the two kidneys themselves in the formation of horseshoe kidney. What factors permit this fusion are unknown, but from the relative rarity of its occurrence and from the fact that there are no associated anomalies of connective tissue formation, one must conclude that the defect is a local one and perhaps reflects a transient pathologic condition.

The presence of suprarenal rests throughout the abdomen, and especially in association with the gonads, is not surprising when one remembers that the zone of development of the celomic portion of the primordium is almost contiguous with the genital portion of the nephrogenic ridge. As the suprarenal cortical cells migrate from the site of their formation, some must fail to reach their normal location. They are already in a position to be included in the descending gonad and its adnexa.

A second possibility is that the degenerating mesonephros, already being converted to the service of the

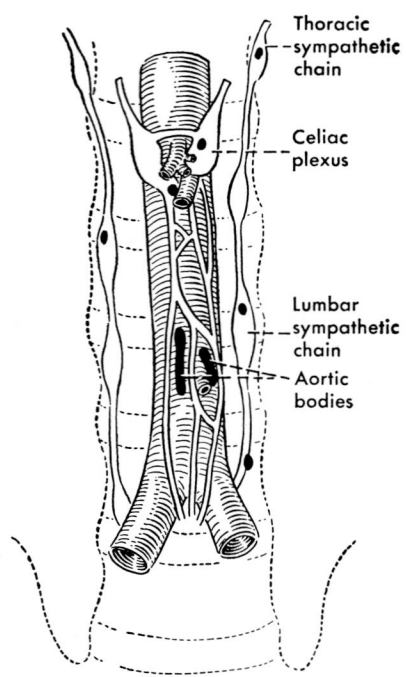

Figure 19.21. Common locations of ectopic chromaffin bodies: along the lower thoracic and lumbar parts of the sympathetic chain, in the prevertebral plexuses, and on the aorta close to the origin of the inferior mesenteric artery. (From Hollinshead WH. Anatomy for surgeons. New York: Hoeber Medical Division, Harper & Row, 1956.)

gonad, retains cells of cortical potentiality which may differentiate in their definitive location sometime later. That these cortical nodules have no medullary tissue is reasonable in view of the migration of the latter from a very different location to a rendezvous with the cortical migratory stream at the normal site of the suprarenal gland. In a few locations, such as the aorta, there are extrasuprarenal chromaffin cells, which would presumably be attracted by the presence of cortical cells in their vicinity and, hence, would form the complete suprarenal accessory found by Graham (61) (Fig. 19.19).

There remain the three reported cases of intracranial suprarenal glands to explain. Wiener and Dallgaard (60), who reported the most recent example, made a gallant attempt, suggesting a displaced blastomere or a cephalic pronephric segment as the source of the cortical tissue. It seems incredible that either of these circumstances could have occurred without producing other gross malformations. We are forced to admit that the embryogenesis of these three cases remains a mystery.

SYMPTOMS AND DIAGNOSIS

Neither heterotopic or accessory suprarenal tissue produces symptoms; hence, few cases are recognized clinically. However, Gualtieri and Segal (87) removed a $4 \times 3 \times 3$-cm accessory suprarenal from the scrotum, where it produced a visible and palpable tumor. With a few exceptions, there are no indications of the existence of abnormally situated suprarenal structures. The ectopic structures function entirely normally, wherever in the body they may be placed.

SURGICAL IMPLICATIONS

Accessory suprarenal tissue presents no direct surgical problem because its removal often is not necessary. Accidental removal at nephrectomy of a suprarenal gland beneath the capsule of the kidney is a possible danger (88). More important is the ineffectiveness of suprarenalectomy for advanced carcinoma of the breast or prostate in the presence of adequate accessory cortical nodules. If functional suprarenalectomy is desired, a search for accessory structures must be undertaken.

Congenital Adrenal Hyperplasia (Adrenogenital Syndrome)

It is not within the scope of this book to present this galaxy of diseases. Because we mention hyperplasia briefly, we want to emphasize that the congenital adrenogenital syndrome is not a morphologic phenomenon but an endocrinologic one. According to McDougal et al. (89), it results from a deficiency of 21-hydroxylase in 90% of the cases.

Congenital adrenal hyperplasia as a cause of female pseudohermaphrodism was reported by Larrea et al. (90). Heyns et al. (91) reported a 60-year-old female with pseudohermaphroditism and congenital adrenal hyperplasia with acute urinary retention secondary to benign "prostatic" hyperplasia and uterine leiomyomas.

RARE CASES

Bilateral adrenal lipoma associated with renal abnormalities and Laurence-Moon-Biedl syndrome was reported by Oochi et al. (92). Unilateral adrenal cyst was reported by Tuffli and Laxova (93) in a 15-year-old boy with ectodermal dysplasia syndrome (aplasia cutis verticis, hypohidrosis, nipple/breast hypoplasia, onychodysplasia, and tooth anomalies with delayed dental eruption).

EDITORIAL COMMENT

Congenital adrenal hyperplasia (CAH) is one of the most fascinating diseases in medicine, and although not specifically a morphologic condition involving the adrenal, its importance in clinical medicine mandates additional comments. CAH is the leading cause of intersex abnormalities in the newborn. Ambiguous genitalia characterize female pseudohermaphrodites, who are normal female children whose adrenal hyperplasia has produced the excessive amounts of androgen necessary to cause masculinization of the external genitalia during fetal development. CAH is transmitted as

an autosomal recessive gene, and homozygous infants lack certain enzymes which are necessary for the conversion of adrenal cholesterol to cortisol and/or aldosterone. Excessive amounts of adrenal androgen "pile up," and lead to virilization of the fetal external genitalia in the female, and usually to salt wasting when aldosterone production is blocked. Males with the condition lack ambiguous genitalia but may present with salt wasting. These patients have enzymatic defects in the biosynthesis of cortisol and can form normal amounts of cortisol only at the expense of the elevated levels of circulating ACTH. The high ACTH levels, in turn, cause hyperplasia of the adrenal cortex and excessive production of steroids found just prior to the enzyme block. Several enzymatic defects in the biosynthesis of cortisol exist; however, the most common is a defect in 21-hydroxylation, which involves the conversion of 17-hydroxyprogesterone to 11-deoxycortisol and of progesterone to deoxycorticosterone. 17-Hydroxyprogesterone is present in elevated amounts in the blood of patients with the most common defect, 21-hydroxylase deficiency, and laboratory measurement may be helpful in diagnosis. Other enzymatic defects may be present but are far rarer than the 21-hydroxylase deficiency and may not cause virilization.

A previous family history of CAH or neonatal death of unknown cause should alert the physician to the possibility of CAH. As CAH is the most common cause of genital ambiguity in the newborn, its presence should be expected when a virilized female is encountered. CAH has been treated in utero and the virilization prevented (94). Unfortunately, this will be possible only when the condition is anticipated, and most new cases are diagnosed when there is no previous family history.

Replacement therapy is complex. Patients who lose salt require therapy with cortisol and mineralicortcoid agents. The problem is that too much cortisol will depress growth and too little will allow excessive production of androgen, which leads to premature closure of the growth plates and therefore short stature. Surgical correction of the ambiguous genitalia is obviously part of the overall program of management, and is usually undertaken at around 2 to 3 months of age. Reduction of the size of the clitoris and flap vaginoplasty are required in the majority of cases (95). More severly masculinized cases require more extensive vaginal reconstruction; however, this too can be performed at an early age (96, 97) *(TSP)*.

REFERENCES

1. Wiesel J. Beiträge zur Anatomie und Entwicklung der menschlichen Nebenniere. Anat Hefte 1902;19:481–522.
2. Zuckerkandl E. The development of the chromaffin organs and of the suprarenal bodies. In: Keibel F, Mall FP, eds. Manual of human embryology. Philadelphia: JB Lippincott, 1912.
3. Kern H. Ueber den Umbau der Nebenniere im extrauterinen Leben. Deutsch Med Wschr 1911;37:971–974.
4. Lewis RW, Pappenheimer AM. A study of the involutional changes which occur in the adrenal cortex during infancy. J Med Res 1916;34:81–93.

5. Keene MFL, Hewer EE. Observations on the development of the human suprarenal gland. J Anat 1927;61:302–324.
6. Uotila UU. Early embryological development of the fetal and permanent adrenal cortex in man. Anat Rec 1940;76:183–203.
7. Crowder RE. The development of the adrenal gland in man, with special reference to the origin and ultimate location of cell types and evidence for the "cell migration" theory. Contrib Embryol Carnegie Inst Wash 1957;36:193–210.
8. Sucheston ME, Cannon MS. Development of zonular patterns in the human adrenal gland. J Morphol 1968;126:477–492.
9. Katznelson ZS. Die Entwicklung du Nebenniere des Rindes. Mikr Anat Forsch 1966;75:245–269.
10. Barbet JP, Houette A, Barres D, Durigon M. Histological assessment of gestational age in human embryos and fetuses. Am J Forensic Med Pathol 1988;9(1):40–44.
11. Hata K, Hata T, Kitao M. Ultrasonographic identification and measurement of the human fetal adrenal gland in utero: clinical application. Gynecol Obstet Invest 1988;25(1):16–22.
12. Davies J. Anatomy, microscopic structure, and development of the human adrenal gland. In: Scott HW Jr, ed. Surgery of the adrenal glands. Philadelphia: JB Lippincott, 1990:17–38.
13. Monkhouse WS, Khalique A. The adrenal and renal veins of man and their connections with azygos and lumbar veins. J Anat 1986;146:105–115.
14. Hubbard MM, Kulayat MM, Abumrad NN. Adrenocorticoids: physiology, regulation, function, and metabolism. In: Scott HW Jr, ed. Surgery of the adrenal glands. Philadelphia: JB Lippincott, 1990:39.
15. Benner MC. Studies on the involution of the fetal cortex of the adrenal glands. Am J Pathol 1940;16:787–798.
16. Swinyard CA. Growth of the human suprarenal gland. Anat Rec 1943;87:141–150.
17. Kangarloo H et al. Sonography of adrenal glands in neonates and children: changes in appearance with age. J Clin Ultrasound 1986;14(1):43–47.
18. Ashley DJB, Mostofi FK. Renal agenesis and dysgenesis. J Urol 1960;83:211–230.
19. Fortune CH. The pathological and clinical significance of congenital one-sided kidney defect, with the presentation of three new cases of agenesis and one of aplasia. Ann Intern Med 1927;1:377–399.
20. Potter EL. Pathology of the fetus and the newborn. Chicago: Year Book Medical Publishers, 1952.
21. Cywes S. Hemoperitoneum in the newborn. S Afr Med J 1967;41:1063–1073.
22. Siegel BS et al. Adrenal hemorrhage in the newborn. JAMA 1961;177:263–265.
23. Tank WS et al. Mechanisms of trauma during breech delivery. Obstet Gynecol 1971;38:761.
24. Brock CE, Ricketts RR. Hemoperitoneum from spontaneous rupture of neonatal neuroblastoma. Am J Dis Child 1982;36:370–371.
25. Murthy TVM, Irving IM, Lister J. Massive adrenal hemorrhage in neonatal neuroblastoma. J Pediatr Surg 1978;13:31–34.
26. Pizzo PA, Poplack DG. Principles and practice of pediatric oncology. New York: JB Lippincott, 1989.
27. Campbell AN, Chan HSL, O'Brien A, Smith CR, Becker LE. Malignant tumors in the neonate. Arch Dis Child 1987;62(1):19–23.
28. Welch KC, Randolph JG, Ravitch MM, O'Neill JA, Rowe MI. Pediatric surgery. Chicago: Year Book Medical Publishers, 1986.
29. Scriver CR et al. Clinical and community studies: feasibility of chemical screening of urine for neuroblastoma case finding in infancy in Quebec. Can Med Assoc J 1987;136(9):952–956.
30. Woods WG, Tuchman M. Neuroblastoma: the case for screening infants in North America. Pediatrics 1987;79(6):869–873.
31. Hayashi Y, Inaba T, Hanada R, Yamamoto K. Chromosome findings and prognosis in 15 patients with neuroblastoma found by vanillylmandelic acid mass screening. J Pediatr 1988;112(4):567–571.
32. Look AT, Hayes FA, Nitschke R, McWilliams NB, Green AA. Cellular DNA content as a predictor of response to chemotherapy in infants with unresectable neuroblastoma. N Engl J Med 1984;311(4):231–235.
33. Weinblatt ME, Heisel MA, Siegel SE. Hypertension in children with neurogenic tumors. Pediatrics 1983;71:8–12.
34. Kosloske AM, Bhattacharyya N, Duncan MH. "Incidental" neuroblastoma. Lancet 1987;2(8558):565.
35. Evans AE, D'Angio GJ, Randolph J. A proposed staging system for children with neuroblastoma. Cancer 1971;27:374–378.
36. O'Neill JA et al. The role of surgery in localized neuroblastoma. J Pediatr Surg 1985:708–712.
37. Moss TJ et al. Delayed surgery and bone marrow transplantation for widespread neuroblastoma. Ann Surg 1987;206(4):514–520.
38. Hayes FA et al. Surgicopathologic staging of neuroblastoma: prognostic significance of regional lymph node involvement. J Pediatr 1983;102:59–64.
39. Chan VTW, McGee JOD. Cellular oncogenes in neoplasia. J Clin Pathol 1987;40(9):1055–1063.
40. Seeger RC et al. Association of multiple copies of the N-myc oncogene with rapid progression of neuroblastoma. N Engl J Med 1985;313(10):1111–1116.
41. Slamon DJ et al. Identification and characterization of the protein encoded by the human N-myc oncogene. Science 1986;232(4751):762–772.
42. Quierke P, Dyson JED. Flow cytometry: methodology and applications in pathology. J Pathol 1986;149:79–87.
43. Sawada T et al. Screening for disease: mass screening for neuroblastoma in infants in Japan. Lancet 1984;2(8397):271–273.
44. Kerenyi N. Congenital adrenal hypoplasia: report of a case with extreme adrenal hypoplasia and neurohypophyseal aplasia, drawing attention to certain aspects of etiology and classification. Arch Pathol 1961;71:336–343.
45. Pinner-Poole B. The endocrine glands in anencephaly [Thesis]. Dublin: University of Dublin, Ireland, 1965.
46. Winquist PG. Adrenal hypoplasia. Arch Pathol 1961;71:324–329.
47. Blizzard RM, Alberts M. Hypopituitarism, hypoadrenalism and hypogonadism in the newborn infant. J Pediatr 1956;48:782.
48. Benirschke K, Bloch E, Hertig AT. Concerning the function of the fetal zone of the human adrenal gland. Endocrinology 1956;58:598–625.
49. Tuchman-Duplessis H, Mercier-Parot L. Ètude comparative de la structure de l'hypophyse et de la surrénale des anencéphales et des hydrocéphales humains. C R Soc Biol (Paris) 1963;157:977–981.
50. Schonenberg H, Radermacher EH, Frank M, Klemm W. [Phenyketonuria associated with Rubinstein-Taybi syndrome, spondylic dysplasia, left vascular shrinking of adrenal gland (author's trans).] Klin Padiatr 1977;189(6):482–489.
51. Turner M, O'Herlihy C. Adrenal hypofunction and trisomy 18. Obstet Gynecol 1984;63(3 Suppl):84S–85S.
52. Newman NM, Welch E, Challis DR. Adrenal hypoplasia and pituitary agenesis in a normocephalic infant, with a review of the literature. Aust Paediatr J 1988;24(5):300–303.
53. Fonkalsrud EW. The adrenal glands. In: Welch KJ, Randolph JG, Ravitch MM, O'Neill JA, Rowe MI, eds. Pediatric surgery. Chicago: Year Book Medical Publishers, 1986:1114.
54. Coupland RE. Observations on the size distribution of chromaffin granules and on the identity of adrenaline- and noradrenaline-storing chromaffin cells in vertebrates and man. In: Heller H, Lederis K, eds. Subcellular organization and function in endocrine tissues: symposium proceedings. University of Bristol, April 5-11, 1970. Soc Endocrinol Mem 1971;19:611–635 (serial).

55. Klebs E. Handbuch der pathologischen Anatomie, Vol 1. Berlin: A Hirschwald, 1876.

56. Weller CV. Heterotopia of the adrenal in liver and kidney. Am J Med Sci 1925;169:696–718.

57. Holtz F. Renal-adrenal heterotopia: case report and review of the literature. Univ Mich Bull 1955;21:400–404.

58. Kohn A. Die Nebenniere der selachier nebst Beiträgen zur Kenntnis der morphologie der Wirbelthiernebenniere im Allgemeinen. Arch Mikr Anat 1899;53:281–312.

59. Meyer AW. A congenital intra-cranial, intra-dural adrenal. Anat Rec 1917;12:43–50.

60. Wiener MF, Dallgaard SA. Intracranial adrenal gland: a case report. Arch Pathol 1959;67:228–233.

61. Graham LS. Celiac accessory adrenal glands. Cancer 1953;6:149–152.

62. Skandalakis JE, Vincenzi R, Rand EO, Poer DH. Extra-adrenal retroperitoneal "nonfunctioning" paraganglioma: report of a case and review of the literature. South Med J 1959;52(11):1368–1370.

63. Olson JR, Abell MR. Nonfunctional nonchromaffin paragangliomas of the retroperitoneum. Cancer 1969;23:1358.

64. Glenner GG, Grimley PM. Tumors of the extra adrenal paraganglion system. In: Atlas of tumor pathology, 2nd series. Washington, DC: Armed Forces Institute of Pathology, 1974.

65. Pack GT, Tabah EJ. Primary retroperitoneal tumors, a study of 120 cases. Int Abstr Surg 1954;99:313.

66. Pack GT, Ariel IM. Tumors of the soft somatic tissues. New York: Paul B Hoeber, 1958:641.

67. Stout AP. Primary retroperitoneal tumors, a study of 120 cases. Int Abstr Surg 1954;99:313.

68. Ganem EJ, Cahill GF. Pheochromocytomas coexisting in adrenal gland and retroperitoneal space, with sustained hypertension: report of a case with surgical cure. N Engl J Med 1948;238:692–697.

69. Block MA, Dockerty MB, Waugh JM. Non-chromaffin paraganglioma: report of a case. Cancer 1955;8:97.

70. Scott HW Jr, ed. Surgery of the adrenal glands. Philadelphia: JB Lippincott, 1990.

71. Marchand F. Ueber accessorische Nebennieren im Ligamentum latum. Virchow Arch [A] 1883;92:11–19.

72. Morgagni JB. The seats and causes of disease: investigated by Anatomy. Alexander B (transl). New York: Hafner, 1960.

73. Nelson AA. Accessory adrenal cortical tissue. Arch Pathol 1939;27:955–965.

74. Brites G. Encore les surrénales accessoires dans le vein de l'homme. Folia Anat Univ Conimb 1935;10:1–8.

75. Falls J. Accessory adrenal cortex in the broad ligament: incidence and functional significance. Cancer 1955;8:143–150.

76. Bret J, Brodi L. Les cortico-surrénales accessoires au niveau de l'appareil génital féminin. Rev Franç Gynecol 1959;54:451–458.

77. Aichel O. Vergleichende Entwicklungsgeschichte und Stammesgeschichte der Nebennieren: Ueber ein neues normales Organ des Menschen und der Säugethiere. Arch Mikr Anat 1900;56:1–80.

78. Dahl EV. Aberrant adrenal cortical tissue near the testis in human infants. USAF Sch Aerospace Med 1961;61:1–10.

79. Finkbeiner AE, DeRidder PA, Ryden SE. Splenic-gonadal fusion and adrenal cortical rest associated with bilateral cryptorchism. Urology 1977;10(4):337–340.

80. Hamazaki M, Saito A. Beckwith-Wiedemann's syndrome: a report of an autopsied case. Acta Pathol 1979;29(1):99–107.

81. Wolloch Y, Ziv Y, Dintsman M. Accessory adrenal: an incidental finding during orchiopexy. Panminerva Med 1986;28(1):47–49.

82. Kageyama T, Doke Y, Takahashi M, Kaneko M. Computed tomography of myelolipoma in the accessory adrenal gland. Urol Radiol 1989;11(3):153–155.

83. Kenney PJ, Robbins GL, Ellis DA, Spirt BA. Adrenal glands in patients with congenital renal anomalies: CT appearance. Radiology 1985;155(1):181–182.

84. Hadar H, Gadoth N, Gillon G. Computed tomography of renal agenesis and ectopy. J Comput Tomogr 1984;8(2):137–143.

85. Jaffe HL. The effects of bilateral suprarenalectomy on the life of rats. Am J Physiol 1926;78:453–461.

86. Glowniak JV et al. Familial extra-adrenal pheochromocytoma: a new syndrome. Arch Intern Med 1985;145(2):257–261.

87. Gualtieri T, Segal AD. Case of adrenal type tumor of spermatic cord: review of aberrant adrenal tissues. J Urol 1949;61:949–955.

88. Culp OS. Adrenal heterotopia: a survey of the literature and report of a case. J Urol 1939;41:303.

89. McDougal WS, Lorenz RA, Burr IM. Congenital adrenal hyperplasia. In: Scott HW Jr, ed. Surgery of the adrenal glands. Philadelphia: JB Lippincott, 1990:277.

90. Larrea F, Ulloa-Aguirre A, Perez-Palacios G. [Congenital adrenal hyperplasia as a cause of female pseudohermaphroditism.] Rev Invest Clin 1986;38(2):209–217.

91. Heyns CF, Rimington PD, Kurger TF, Falck VG. Benign prostatic hyperplasia and uterine leiomyomas in a female pseudohermaphrodite: a case report. J Urol 1987;137(6):1245–1247.

92. Oochi N, Rikitake O, Maeda T, Yamaguchi M. [A case of Laurence-Moon-Biedl syndrome associated with bilateral adrenal lipomas and renal abnormalities.] Nippon Naika Gakkai Zasshi 1984;73(1):89–93.

93. Tuffli GA, Laxova R. Brief clinical report: new, autosomal dominant form of ectodermal dysplasia. Am J Med Genet 1983;14(2):381–384.

94. Shapiro E, Santiago J, Crane J: Prenatal fetal adrenal suppression following in utero diagnosis of congenital adrenal hyperplasia. J Urol 1989;142:663.

95. Bauer SB. Management of congenital adrenal hyperplasia. Dial Pediatr Urol 1982;5(6):2–8.

96. Passarini-Glazel G. A new 1-stage procedure for clitorovaginoplasty in severely masculinized femal pseudohermaphrodites. J Urol 1989;142:565.

97. Parrott T, Woodard J. Abdominoperineal approach to the high short vagina in adrenogenital syndrome. J Urol 1991;146:647.

CHAPTER 20

THE OVARY AND TESTIS

John Elias Skandalakis / Stephen Wood Gray / Thomas S. Parrott / Richard R. Ricketts

The beginnings of all genotypic diseases of man are established at conception.
Without prejudice to the romantic relationship of the honeymoon, it is a truism
that the penetration of the sperm into the ovum will often result in offspring
stigmatized by a wide variety of heredital disorders.
—DAVID SEEGAL, JOURNAL OF PEDIATRICS (1963;63:685)

DEVELOPMENT

The Indifferent Stage

Although the sex of an individual human (as well as that of most other animals) normally is determined at conception by the sex chromosomes, the developing gonad shows no morphologic sex differentiation until the seventh week (stage XVIII). During this period, the future ovary or testis is in the indifferent stage and can only be termed a *gonad*.

Three primordia combine to form the gonad: the primary germ cells, which migrate into the genital ridge; the mesenchyme of the ventromedial aspects of the mesonephroi adjacent to the root of the mesentery; and the celomic epithelium overlying this mesenchyme. The last two components make up the genital ridge (Fig. 20.1). The best descriptions of the primitive gonad are those of Gillman (1), Pinkerton and his colleagues (2), and van Wagenen and Simpson (3).

PRIMORDIAL GERM CELLS

Human germ cells are first recognizable among the endodermal cells of the caudal portion of the yolk sac, near the allantoic stalk (Fig. 20.2, *A*). From 30 to 50 such cells may be seen in embryos of 2 to 3 mm (stage X) at about the 24th day.

It is probable that these cells are segregated early in cleavage, such as is the case with many invertebrates, but the details of this process are unknown. It has been suggested from studies on amphibia that segregation may occur later and that all early endoderm cells may be totipotent (4), but more evidence is needed.

During the fifth week the germ cells migrate dorsally in the wall of the yolk sac and gut, increasing in number by mitosis. By the middle of the fifth week they have reached the angle of the mesentery and the mesonephros, and by the end of the week well over 10,000 cells are present at the site of the gonad (Fig. 20.2, *B*). Migration of the cells is ameboid; no specific paths seem to be followed (5, 6).

The germ cells may be recognized by their cytoplasmic alkaline phosphatase reaction (2, 7) (Fig. 20.3).

Although the extragonadal origin of mammalian germ cells was described early in this century by Füss (8, 9) and by Felix (10), two factors delayed the recognition of the true situation. One was the weight of Waldeyer's belief in the origin of the germ cells *in situ* from the "germinal" epithelium of the genital ridge (11, 12), and the other was the difficulty in recognizing the germ cells once they had entered the genital ridge. These factors led Felix (10) to state:

> All the primary genital cells disappear in amniotes; whether they pass through a latent period to become manifest later as secondary genital cells, though possible, has not been proved.

The origin, location, and journey of the germ cells may be appreciated by Table 20.1.

The final demonstration of the early segregation of germ cells and their migration into the future gonad awaited the experimental destruction of these cells by Humphrey (13) and Dantschakoff (14), the transplantation experiments of Willier (15), the tissue cultures of Martinovitch (16) and the histologic observations of Witschi (5), Chiquoine (17), and Pinkerton and his colleagues (2). Mancini and his colleagues (18) completed the story by following the germ cells in the late fetus and in children from birth to puberty, finding them present in all stages.

The migratory stimulus, which appears before differentiation at the site of the gonad, remains unknown. It has been shown that in amphibians the presence of either the wolffian ducts or the notochord is necessary for genital ridge formation and the normal migration of the germ cells. Germ cells from an embryo with the dorsal mesoderm and neural tube removed will migrate into the gonadal site of a normal parabiotic twin embryo (19, 20).

The primordial cells are responsible for the differentiation of the gonads to testes and ovaries. If for some rea-

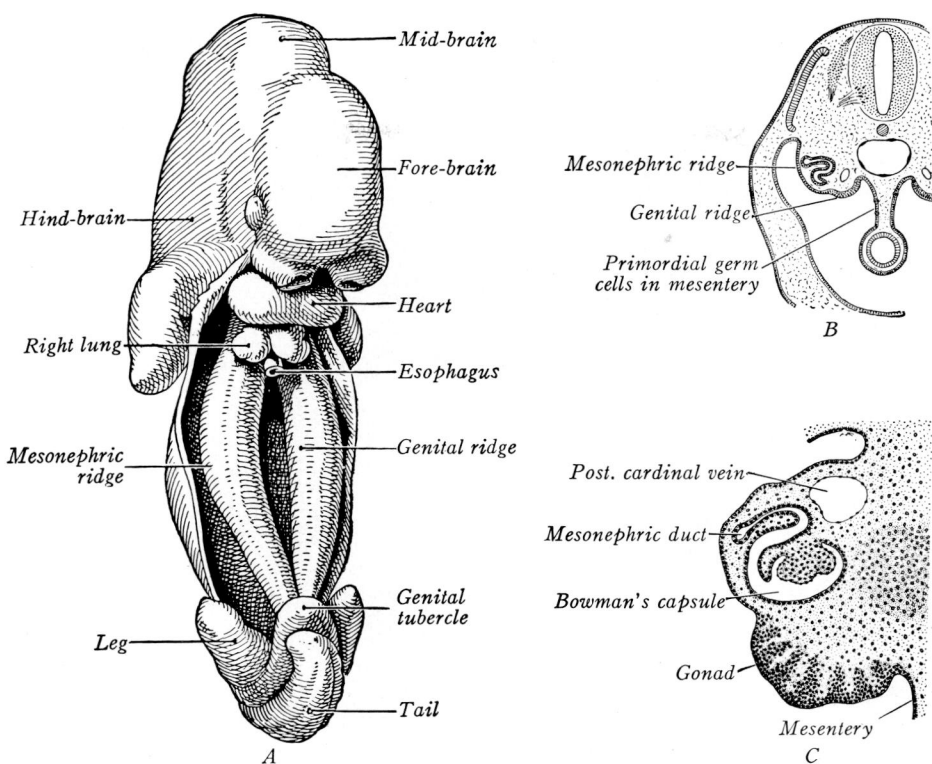

Figure 20.1. The relationship of the genital ridge to the mesonephric ridge. **A,** 9-mm human embryo with ventral body wall removed. **B** and **C,** Cross-sections through embryos of 7 mm and 10 mm. (From Arey LB. Developmental anatomy, 7th ed. Philadelphia: WB Saunders, 1965.)

son they do not reach the indifferent gonads, then testicular or ovarian agenesis takes place or perhaps gonadal indifferentiation continues.

Another interesting question is the formation of neoplasms originating from the various germ cells.

King (21) discussed and demonstrated the origin of germ cell neoplasms (Fig. 20.4).

GENITAL RIDGE

Although it has been thought the primitive germ cells migrating into the medial mesenchyme stimulate the formation of the genital ridge and eventually of the gonad, there is some contrary evidence (22). There is a slight independent differentiation of the genital ridge tissue without germ cells in the hypoplastic "streak" ovaries of women with Turner's syndrome. Ectopic germ cells do not induce ectopic gonads in amphibians (23) or in chick embryos (24).

On the other hand, agar blocks impregnated with mesodermal homogenate, when implanted on the endoderm of toad embryos with dorsolateral mesoderm removed, attract migrating germ cells (25). When 6-day-old chick gonads, labeled with tritiated thymidine, are incubated on the germinal epithelium of 3-day-old chicks, the germ cells migrate from the donor gonads to the host

genital ridge (26). The implication is that formation of the gonad attracts the germ cells rather than the gonad being induced by the germ cells after they arrive at the site.

In the sixth week the genital ridge is thickened, raised, and demarcated laterally and medially by grooves. The celomic epithelium, with a well-defined basement membrane, is present except over the ridge (2). By the seventh week the ridge has become an elongated structure protruding into the celom and connecting with the mesonephros by a thick mesentery.

Development of the epithelium over the genital ridge, called the "germinal epithelium" by earlier writers, is still controversial. The superficial cells of the ridge do not differ from the cells of the underlying mesenchyme and do not have a basement membrane until the seventh week. Pinkerton and his colleagues (2) contended that there is no true epithelium present until after the 10th week. Others are less rigorous in their definitions.

DEVELOPING GONAD (FIG. 20.5)

With the arrival of the primitive germ cells toward the end of the sixth week, the epithelial cells covering the gonad grow as cords of cells into the mesenchyme. Proliferation is from the epithelial side, so as the gonad grows peripherally, the oldest portion of the epithelial cords are the

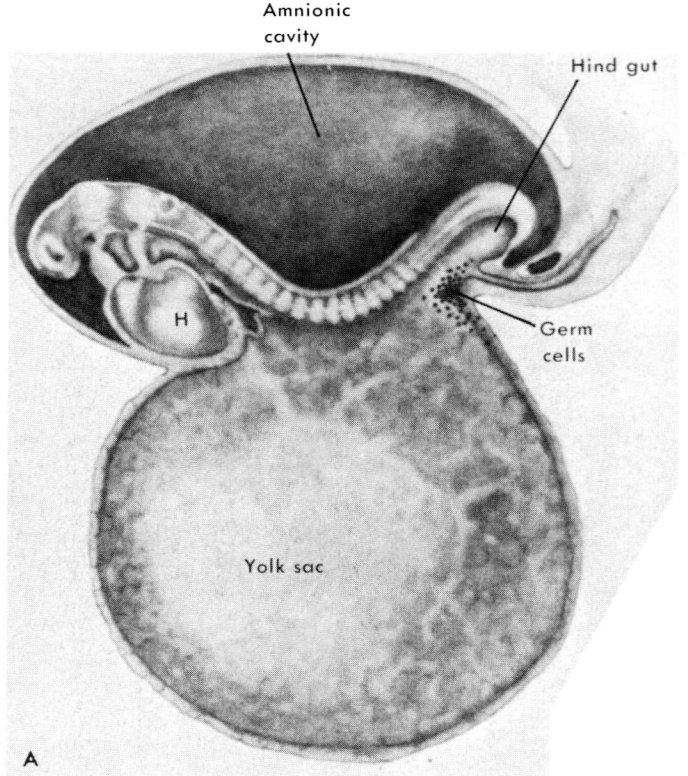

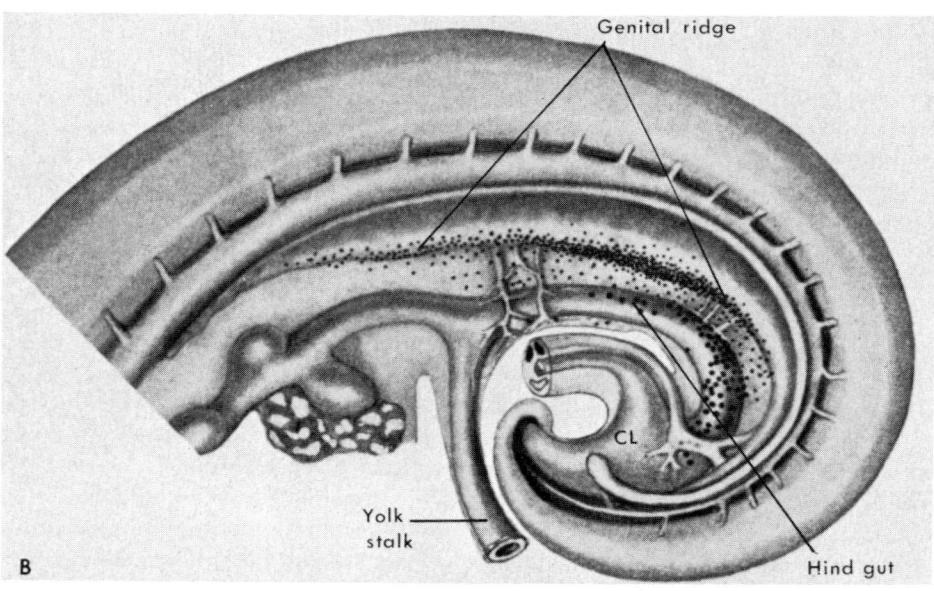

Figure 20.2. Migration of germ cells to the genital ridge. **A,** At 16 somites (3 mm). The germ cells may be seen in the yolk sac and the wall of the hindgut. **B,** At 32 somites (4.2 mm). Most of the germ cells have reached the genital ridge. A few *(large dots)* are still in the endoderm of the gut. **C,** At 7.4 mm. Migration has

deepest. These are the primary or medullary sex cords. Between the cords lie the germ cells and the gonadal mesenchyme.

Early in the eighth week, visible sex differentiation starts. In the male the sex cords continue to develop into seminiferous tubules and rete testis; in the female the sex

cords regress while the other components develop. Witschi (27) believed that hormonal activity of the testis at this time controls the masculinization of the external genitalia. If the hormone level is too low, a male pseudohermaphrodite results.

According to Friedman and Van de Velde (28), failure

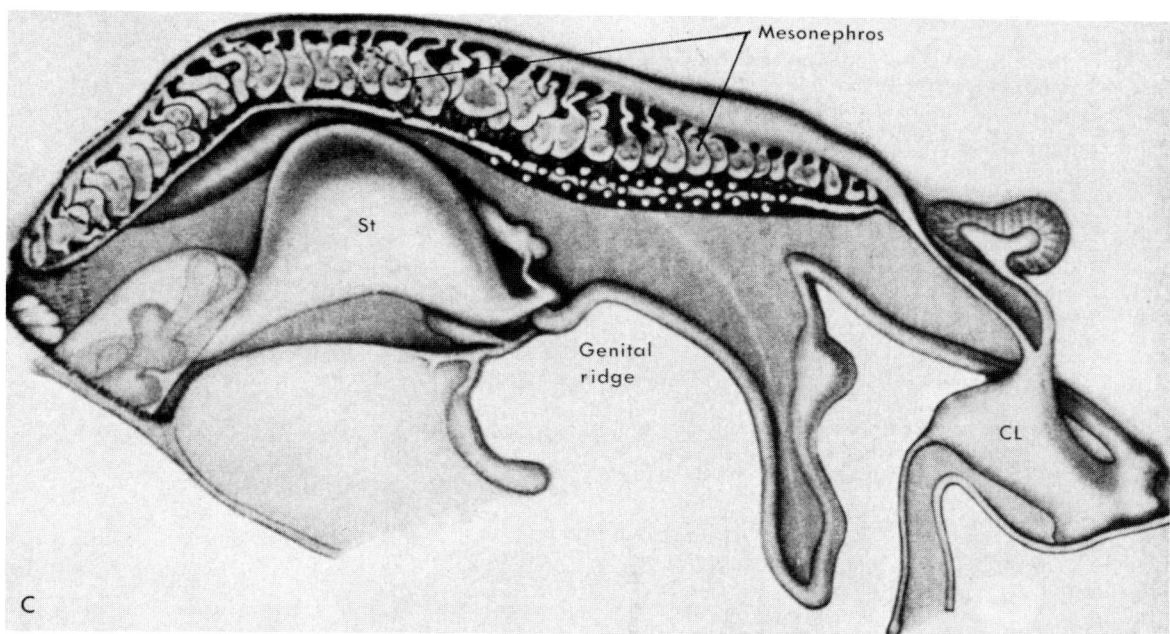

been completed. The size of the germ cells in the drawing is exaggerated and their number is reduced for clarity. *CL,* Cloaca; *St,* stomach. (From Witschi E.

Migration of the germ cells of human embryos from the yolk sac to the primitive gonadal folds. Contrib Embryol Carnegie Inst Wash 1948;32:67–80.)

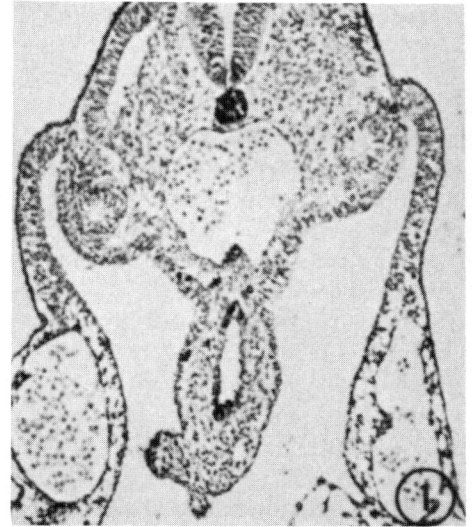 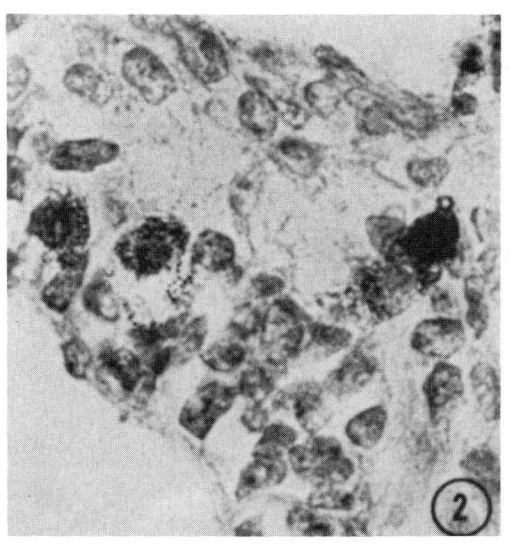

Figure 20.3. Migrating germ cells in a 3.7-mm embryo, stained by PAS for glycogen. **1,** Germ cells may be seen in gut endoderm, the splanchnic mesenchyme, the dorsal mesentery and mesoderm below, and to the left of the aorta. **2,** High-power view of the celomic angle on the left. Coarse glycogen granules

identify the germ cells. (From Pinkerton JHM et al. Development of the human ovary: a study using histochemical techniques. Obstet Gynec 1961;18:152–181.)

of the primordial cell to reach the genital ridge may cause the development of another type of cell by degeneration or differentiation and, later, it may produce extragonadal germ cell tumors.

Despite the facts that seminiferous cord-like formations appear around the 6th and 7th weeks and that histologically the fetal gonad becomes the fetal testis, the histologist will be able to determine the fetal gonad and fetal ovary around the sixth month of gestation by the forma-

tion of ovarian follicles when oocytes divide and are surrounded by granulosa cells (29).

Mittwoch (30) stated that perhaps a Y chromosome within germ cells gives the signal for differentiation to the testis or ovary. Silvers and Wachtel (31) and Ohno (32) believe that H-Y antigen is perhaps responsible for such an action. These authors attempted to explain the enigma of the Y chromosome for the differentiation of a gonad to a testicle. In 1982 Silvers et al. (33) suggested that

Table 20.1.
Origin, Location, Journey and Differentiation of Germ Cells

Week	Location
1	Human blastocyst produces primordial germ cells
3	Primordial germ cells are located in the wall of the yolk sac close to the allantois
5-6	Primordial germ cells migrate along the mesentery of the hindgut towards the genital ridge
	Multiplication of germ cells
	Genital ridge formed by mesodermal epithelium and mesenchyme
	Invasion of genital ridge by germ cells
	Possible pathology:
	1) Progenitors of extragonadal germ cell tumors may be formed
	2) Failure of germ cells to reach the genital ridge is *gonadal agenesis*
6-7	Formation of the primitive sex cords. Gonad is termed *indifferent*

	Influence of Y chromosome	*No Y chromosome*
	Seminiferous cords	Primitive granulosa cell
	↓	and oocytes = follicle
7	Testicle	↓
8		Ovary

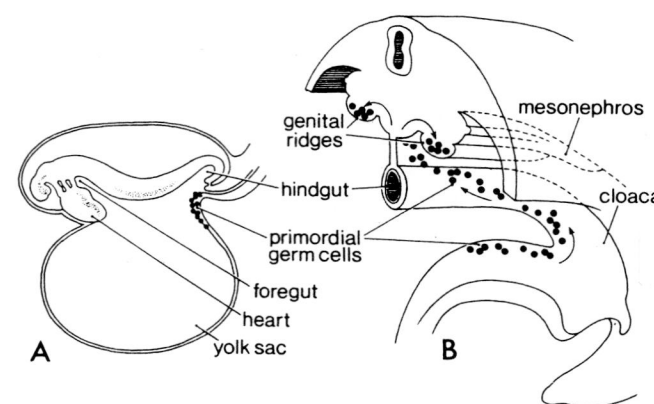

Figure 20.5. **A,** Schematic drawing of a 3-week-old embryo, showing site of origin of germ cells in wall of yolk sac. **B,** Migration path of primordial germ cells along wall of yolk sac and of dorsal mesentery into genital ridge. (From Griffin JE, Wilson JD. Disorders of the testes and male reproductive tract. In: Wilson JD, Foster DW, eds. Textbook of endocrinology. Philadelphia: WB Saunders, 1992:800.)

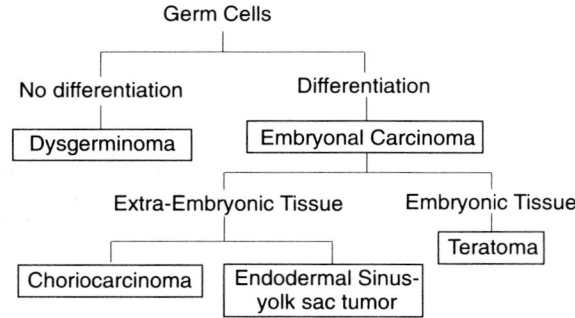

Figure 20.4. The developmental relationships of the various germ cell neoplasms (schema initially proposed by Tellum G. Classification of endodermal sinus tumor [meloblastoma vitellinum] and so-called embryonal carcinoma of the ovary. Acta Pathol Microbiol Scand 1965;64:407.) (From King DR. Ovarian cysts and tumors. In: Welch KJ et al.eds. Pediatric surgery. Chicago: Year Book Medical Publishers, 1986:1347.)

other male-specific antigens may play a role in the development of the testis.

However, the formation of testicle or ovary depends on the genetic presence of an XY or XX sex chromosome. If Y is present, its influence on the indifferent gonad will produce testicular tissue, but the absence of Y will produce ovarian tissue. Sadler demonstrates this phenomenon very well (Table 20.2). However, a continuous process is taking place, with the influence of testis or ovary, for further sex determination (Table 20.3).

Androgeny action at the cellular level is discussed by George and Wilson (35); their drawing (Fig. 20.6) is simple and easy to understand.

The Testis

PRENATAL DIFFERENTIATION

Testicular development after the indifferent stage is manifest by continued growth of the sex cords (Fig. 20.7, *A* to *D*). The cords, which are more clearly marked centrally than peripherally, become separated from the surface epithelium by smaller cells, which will produce the tunica albuginea by fiber formation (Fig. 20.7, *C*). The cords are widely separated by the proliferation of the mesenchyme, and the germ cells become incorporated into the cords. The cord cells themselves will become the Sertoli cells of the seminiferous tubules (3).

Not all primitive germ cells survive. Mancini and his colleagues (18) described more than one type of spermatogonia in the testis at birth. Only one type appears to survive; the remainder degenerate.

Although the cords will form the seminiferous tubules, they remain solid until the fifth and sixth months. Coiling as a result of elongation starts late in the third month, and connective tissue appears between tubules. This connective tissue will later join the tunica albuginea to form the septa (Fig. 20.7, *C* and *D*).

Tubules of the rete testis form in the medulla and join the persistent mesonephric tubules (ductuli effertes) by the ninth week. The older, more central portion of the epithelial cords become the tubuli recti (Figs. 20.7, *A*, and 20.8).

Gillman (29) described a remarkable transitory increase in the size and number of cells of the mesenchymal component between the third and sixth fetal months (Fig. 20.7, *C*); by the eighth month, the volume of interstitial tissue is reduced by extensive cellular degeneration

Table 20.2.
Influence of Primordial Germ Cells on Indifferent Gonad[a]

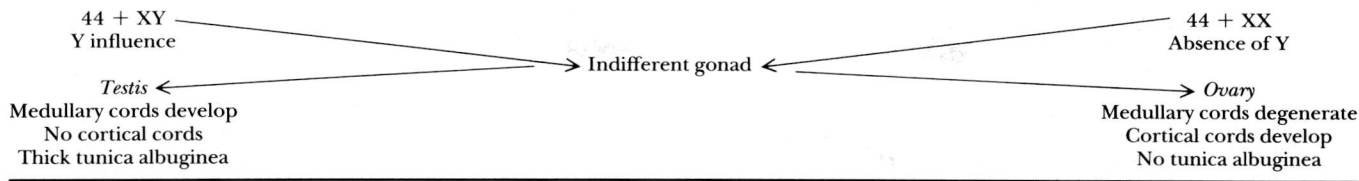

44 + XY				44 + XX
Y influence		Indifferent gonad		Absence of Y
Testis				*Ovary*
Medullary cords develop				Medullary cords degenerate
No cortical cords				Cortical cords develop
Thick tunica albuginea				No tunica albuginea

[a]From Sadler TW. Langman's medical embryology, 6th ed. Baltimore: Williams & Wilkins, 1990.

Table 20.3.
Influence of Sex Gland on Further Sex Differentiation[a]

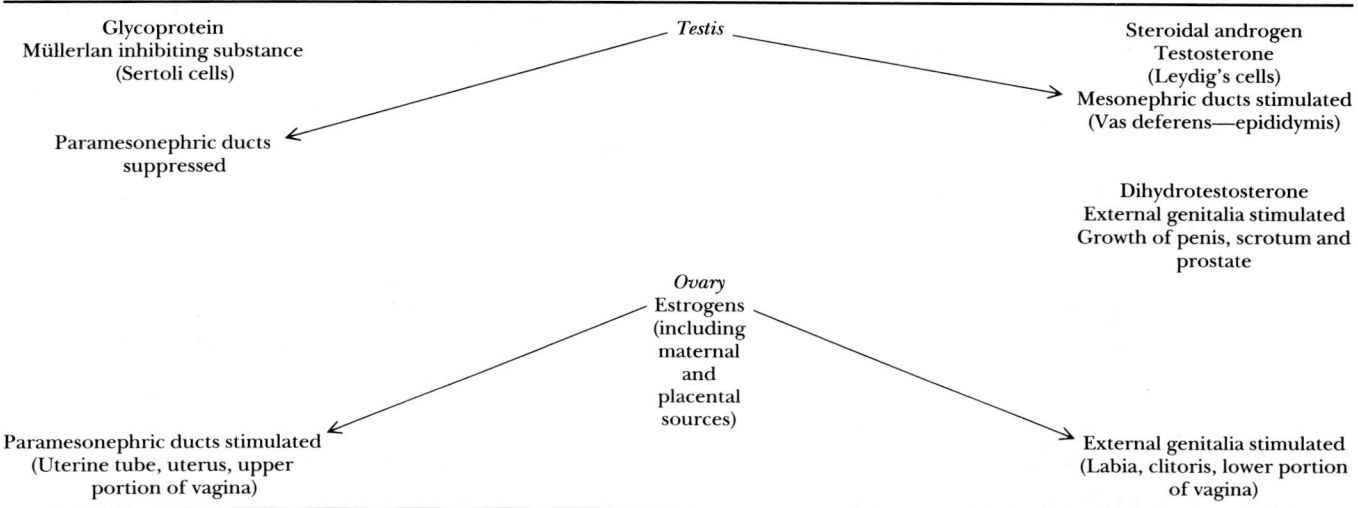

Glycoprotein
Müllerlan inhibiting substance
(Sertoli cells)

Testis

Steroidal androgen
Testosterone
(Leydig's cells)
Mesonephric ducts stimulated
(Vas deferens—epididymis)

Paramesonephric ducts
suppressed

Dihydrotestosterone
External genitalia stimulated
Growth of penis, scrotum and
prostate

Ovary
Estrogens
(including
maternal
and
placental
sources)

Paramesonephric ducts stimulated
(Uterine tube, uterus, upper
portion of vagina)

External genitalia stimulated
(Labia, clitoris, lower portion
of vagina)

[a]Modified from Sadler TW. Langman's medical embryology, 6th ed. Baltimore: Williams & Wilkins, 1990.

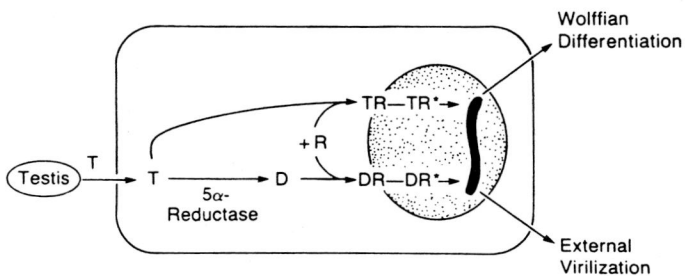

Figure 20.6. Schematic representation of androgen action at the cellular level. Receptor complexes with testosterone *(T)* and dihydrotestosterone *(D)* interact with DNA to control differentiation of the wolffian duct and the external genitalia, respectively. *R,* Androgen receptor; *R*,* transformed androgen receptor-hormone complex. (From George FW, Wilson JD. Sex determination and differentiation. In Knobil E et al., eds. The physiology of reproduction. New York: Raven Press, 1988:3–26.)

(Fig. 20.7, *D*). The Leydig cells are recognizable by the end of the third month (36).

ASSOCIATED STRUCTURES

Between the eighth and eleventh weeks, the testis, which, earlier as the genital ridge, reached from the diaphragm to the site of the internal inguinal ring, shortens and broadens. Degeneration of the mesonephros leaves a cranial diaphragmatic fold, a mesorchium, and a caudal inguinal fold. At the beginning of the seventh week (13.5 mm), the gubernaculum testis is first visible in the free edge of the inguinal fold (Fig. 20.9, *D*). The discovery of this remarkable structure has been assigned to von Haller (37), although Wells (38) was unable to confirm this. The

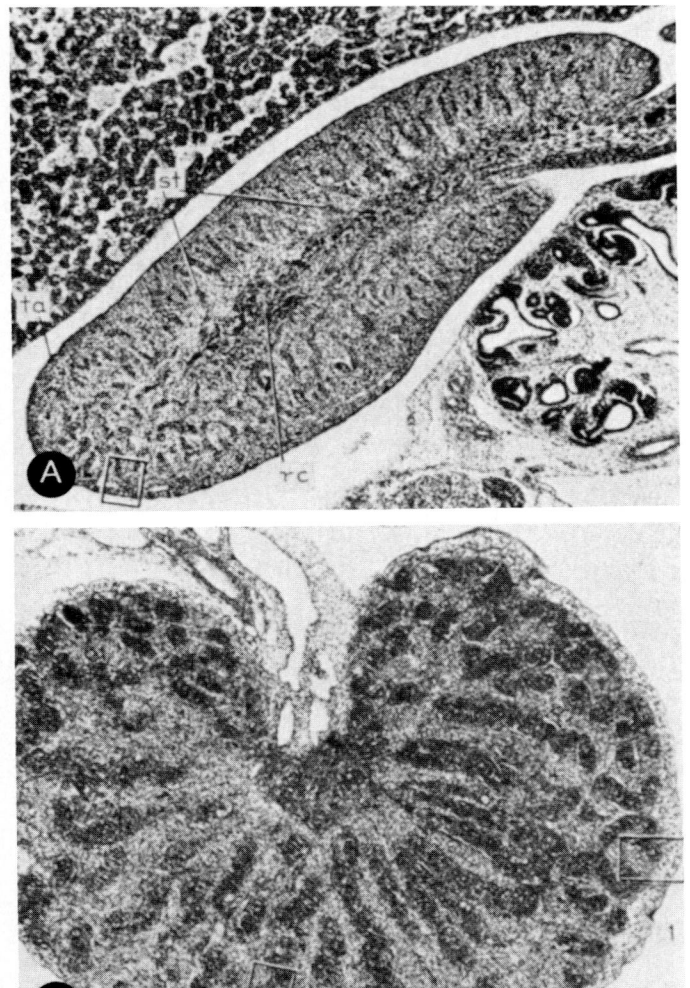

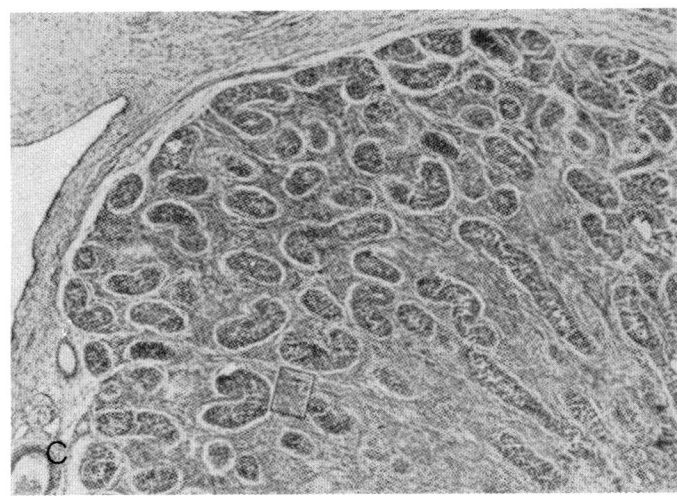

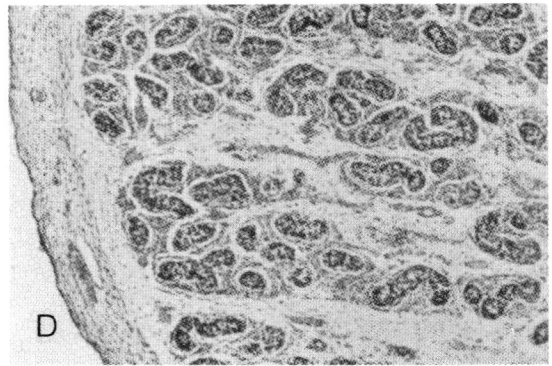

Figure 20.7. Stages in the maturation of the embryonic human testis. **A,** At 27 mm (week 8). Short straight testicular tubules are connected in part with the rete testis; connective tissue is growing between the tubules (*rc*, rete cords; *st*, straight tubules; *ta*, undifferentiated tunica albuginea). **B,** At 132 mm (16th week). Testicular cords are becoming convoluted. The rete is the dark tissue at the hilus. **C,** At 187 mm (about 22 weeks). Maximum development of interstitial tissue. The tubules are convoluted and the tunica albuginea is becoming defined. **D,** At 286 mm

(about 30 weeks). There is reduction in the mass of interstitial tissue between the tubules; the tunica albuginea and the septal connective tissue are well defined. (From Gillman J. The development of gonads in man, with a consideration of the role of fetal endocrines and the histogenesis of ovarian tumors. Contrib Embryol Carnegie Inst Wash 1948;32:83–131.) The small numbered squares indicate high power fields shown in Gillman's original plates.)

name and description belong to John Hunter, whose original report and drawing were reprinted by Wells.

The vaginal processes from the caudal end of the abdominal cavity appear about the beginning of the third month (39) (Fig. 20.9, *E*). They herniate through the abdominal wall and into the already formed scrotal swellings to produce the inguinal canal. The layers of the wall remain intact over the herniation and form the scrotal coverings. Within the canal and extending up to the testis is the thick gubernaculum (Fig. 20.9, *A* to *C*).

The testis, which is at first parallel to the long axis of the body, becomes nearly transverse by the 50-mm stage.

The so-called internal descent is the result of elongation of the lumbar region of the embryo, which carries the mesonephros up, but leaves the testis behind. There is no decrease in the distance between the testis and the site of the internal ring (39, 40). Growth of the testis is steady up to the fifth month, after which the rate declines, only to recommence at the beginning of the seventh month, just preceding the final descent (39).

DESCENT OF THE TESTIS

Just prior to descent during the seventh month, the testis lies at the level of the anterior iliac spine. The epididymis

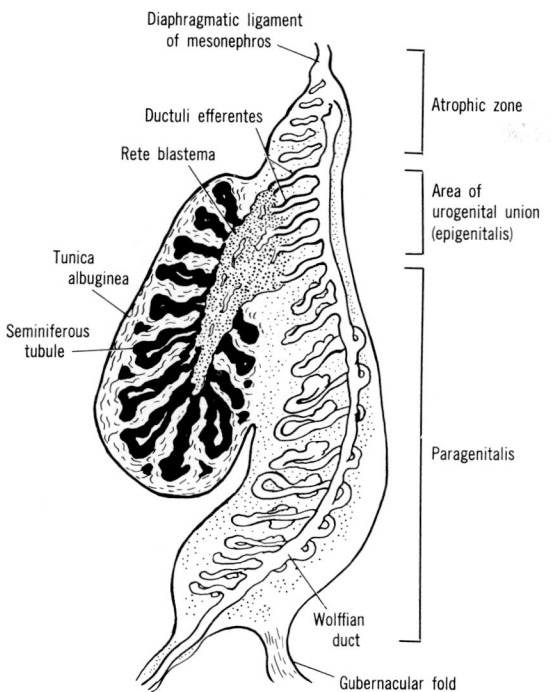

Figure 20.8. Relationship of the mesonephros to the developing testis. Only a few tubules will join the rete testis and become efferent ducts. Some tubules above and below the testes will persist as the blind-ending aberrant ductules. The caudal portion of the mesonephros will join the gubernaculum to form the inguinal ligament. (From Davies J. Human Developmental Anatomy. New York: The Ronald Press, 1963.)

is posterolateral. The gubernaculum is about 1.8 cm long and as large around as the testis and epididymis. The peritoneum dips into the inguinal canal ahead of the testis but less than halfway down the gubernaculum (Fig. 20.9, *A* and *B*). The testis and gubernaculum lie obliquely, with the end of the gubernaculum extending into the canal. There appears to be no firm attachment between the end of the gubernaculum and the scrotum: The "scrotal ligament" of Lockwood (41) fails to qualify as a ligament.

The best description of testicular descent is that of Scorer (42), who dissected the bodies of 48 fetuses who had died during the seventh to ninth months of gestation.

As the testis enters the internal ring, the gubernaculum emerges from the lower ring. As soon as it reaches the bottom of the scrotal sac, it begins to shorten until its lower two-thirds have completely disappeared (Fig. 20.9, *C*). Descent through the canal is accomplished in a few days. About 4 weeks more is required for the testis to pass from the external ring to the bottom of the scrotum. Descent does not start before the 230-mm stage (28th week) (39). It may be complete as early as 240 mm, or it may be still incomplete at birth. Among the premature births studied by Scorer (43), testes were undescended in 50% or more of infants weighing less than 4 lb and were descended in 50% or more of the larger infants. Follow-

ing emergence of the testis through the external ring, the latter contracts; after descent is complete, the entire processus vaginalis closes (Figs. 20.9, *G*, and 20.10). Scorer believed he could recognize this closure by palpation of the spermatic cord about the time of birth. Closure is complete by birth in from 50 to 75% of infants. The defects of closure of the processus vaginalis may be studied in Figure 20.11, but more details are presented in Chapter 16, "The Anterior Body Wall." The descent of the testis is illustrated in Figure 20.12.

Much has been hypothesized but little is known of the mechanical causes of testicular descent. The hormonal role in descent was demonstrated in 1930 by Shapiro (44); subsequently, Engle (45) induced premature descent of testes in the macaque with anterior pituitary hormone. Martins (46) was able to control the descent of paraffin masses simulating testes in rats and monkeys injected with testosterone. Wislocki (47) suggested that maternal chorionic gonadotropin stimulates androgen production in the adrenal cortex of the fetus, which leads to normal descent. Failure of normal androgen production in ordinary cryptorchidism is not always demonstrable, but the high frequency of retained testes in various types of pseudohermaphroditism indicates that it is an important factor in descent.

In spite of our knowledge that hormones probably regulate descent, we can only speculate about the actual mechanics. The role of intraabdominal pressure has perhaps not been sufficiently emphasized. If the testis and gubernaculum together form a cylindric plug in the inguinal canal, this plug will be forced downward at each rise of pressure in the abdomen, such as from uterine pressure in prenatal life or from crying or straining in postnatal life. If the lower end of the gubernaculum is progressively destroyed, perhaps by hormonal action, the gubernaculum may serve to lower the testis slowly into the scrotum under the pressure of the abdomen, thus acting as a brake rather than as the positive traction force, such as was originally proposed. Backhouse and Butler (48), from their studies on the gubernaculum of the pig, believed final descent results from invasion of the remaining gubernaculum by the growing cauda epididymis.

In summary, the descent of the testicle is an enigma. The forces responsible for the descent are not only poorly understood but are highly hypothetic.

1. The downward pull of the testis by the gubernaculum as a mechanical cause is not accepted. We agree with Arey (49) that the gubernaculum prepares the way as well as the space for the testicular journey.
2. Increase or decrease of intraabdominal pressure may contribute to the descent of the testicle or to the fact that the testis may remain somewhere high or low in the retroperitoneal space.
3. Frey et al. (50) speculated that this phenomenon was

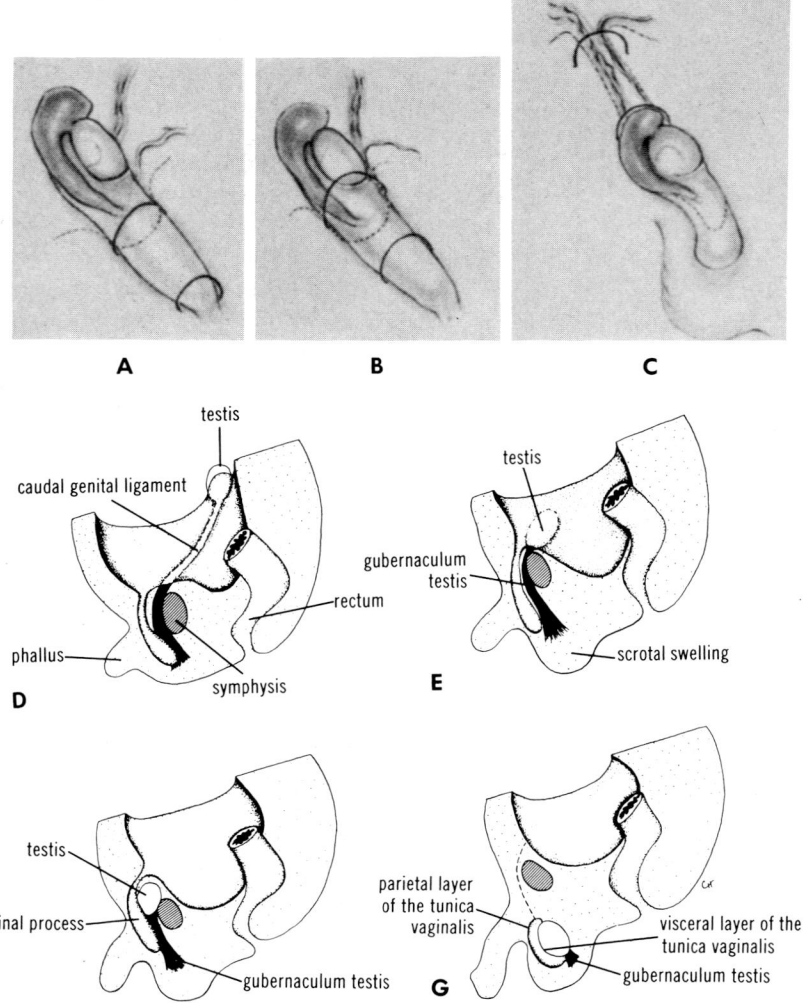

Figure 20.9. Descent of the testis. **A,** The testis before descent. The guber- | ticular descent. **D,** During the second month. **E,** During the third month. **F,** During
naculum is about twice the length of the testis and of the same diameter as the testis | the seventh month. **G,** Shortly after birth. Note that the processus vaginalis
and epididymis together. The *broken line* marks the peritoneal attachment. **B,** The | descends with the testis. (**A** to **C,** From Scorer CG. The anatomy of testicular
testis entering the internal inguinal ring. All the structures, including the peritoneal | descent, normal and incomplete. Br J Surg 1962;49:352–367; **D** to **G,** from
sac, move as a unit. **C,** The testis emerging from the external inguinal ring; the | Langman J. Medical embryology, 2nd ed. Baltimore: Williams & Wilkins, 1969.)
gubernaculum is beginning to disappear. **D** to **G,** Schematic representation of tes-

perhaps a synergistic action of abdominal pressure and androgens. Other authors, such as Roberts (51), believed it is a result of the presence of congenital defects of the anterior abdominal wall which are associated with urinary tract abnormalities.

4. There has been much written about the relationship of androgen action and testicular descent. Frey et al. (50) were able to produce testicular descent in rats using dihydrotestosterone. However, Wilson et al. (52) reported that approximately 50% of patients with androgen resistance are cryptorchid.

Sloan and Walsh (53) write about the müllerian-inhibiting hormone, which is a peptide formed in the seminiferous tubules. The müllerian-inhibiting substance may play a role keeping the testicle retroperitoneally due to persistent müllerian duct syndrome.

In other words, the müllerian-inhibiting substance, which is produced by the Sertoli cells, is responsible for the regression of the müllerian or paramesonephric duct (54). The Leydig cells are responsible for the production of testosterone which is responsible for the change of the mesonephric duct in wolffian entities (55).

Scott (56) states that a müllerian-inhibiting substance is most likely responsible for the abdominal phase of testicular descent.

Although we do not understand the strategy of testicular descent, we know the tendency of the organ to locate itself in cold climates. The testicle does not like the warmth of the retroperitoneal space. It is a warrior and does not want to have a fireplace chat with other retroperitoneal fellows, but fighting, constantly alone, practically destroys the lower abdominal wall and gloriously makes its home at the cold climate of the scrotum, a climate which will permit it to fulfill its physiologic destiny by producing spermatozoa, avoiding malignancies and calming the anxious reaction of the parents as well as of the patient.

Syndromes associated with undescended testes are

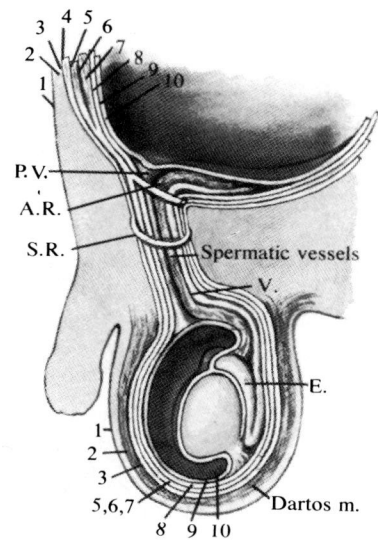

Postnatal

Abdominal Wall Layers	Scrotum Layers
1. Skin	1. Skin
2. Superficial fascia (Camper's and Scarpa's)	2. Dartos fascia and muscle
3. Fascia of external oblique	3. External spermatic fascia
4. External oblique	
5. Fascia of internal oblique	5. Middle spermatic fascia
6. Internal oblique	6. } Cremasteric muscle
7. Transverse abdominis	7.
8. Transversalis fascia	8. Internal spermatic fascia
9. Extraperitoneal fat	9. Extraperitoneal fat
10. Peritoneum	10. Tunica vaginalis testis

A.R. = abdominal inguinal ring
S.R. = subcutaneous inguinal ring
P.V. = processus vaginalis (funicular portion)
V. = vas deferens
E. = epididymis

Figure 20.10. The relationship of the fully descended testis to the inguinal rings and the elements of the scrotal wall. (From Healey JE. A synopsis of clinical anatomy. Philadelphia: WB Saunders, 1969.)

numerous. Sheldon (57) presents some of them in the form of a table (Table 20.4).

The Ovary

PRENATAL DIFFERENTIATION

The primary sex cords that formed in gonad primordia of both male and female at the end of the indifferent stage continue to develop in the future testis, but they begin to lose their configuration in the future ovary, although they are said to remain recognizable up to the eighth month (58). The cells of the sex cords enlarge and the germ cells increase in number, while the cords themselves become smaller. There is no increase in mesenchyme between the cords, as occurs in the testis (Fig. 20.13, A and B).

With the presence of the two X chromosomes, the gonads change to ovaries (Table 20.2).

Proliferation of germ cells (oogonia), especially those in the cortical region, continues to about the 15th week. Development of the oogonia into primary oocytes begins in the deepest germ cells and spreads later to peripheral cells. During this stage the germ cells lose most of their glycogen and their alkaline phosphatase activity (2). It is this change that suggested their disappearance to earlier workers. No oogonia remain after the fourth postnatal month (3).

The first primary follicles become visible in the fourth month. Oogonia, which have entered into prophase of the first maturation division, become enclosed by granulosa cells from the cortical epithelial cords (59) (Fig. 20.13, C and D). Subsequently, mesenchyme cells become flattened around the granulosa cells to form the theca. The follicle therefore comprises the three components of the ovary: the oocyte from the primitive germ cells, the granulosa cells from the epithelium, and the theca cells from the mesenchyme.

By the 36th week, the ovary is filled with primary follicles, although some oogonia are still present. Both follicular enlargement and atresia now take place. Developing follicles reach a larger size (before becoming atretic in the peritoneal period) than they will until puberty. The enlargement is probably a response to chorionic gonadotropins (2). Loss of follicles in the central part of the organ and increase in connective tissue results in a cortical shell of primary follicles at puberty.

King (21) stated that, at the time of birth, the ovaries have 400,000 follicles, but only 400 oocytes will be used during the 30 to 40 years of fertility.

According to Zamboni et al. (60) and Byskov (61), the granulosa cells in mice and sheep are formed by cells of mesonephric origin.

Mitotic divisions and proliferation are characteristic of the germ cells which produce approximately 600,000 oogonia by the eighth week and 6 to 7 million by the 20th

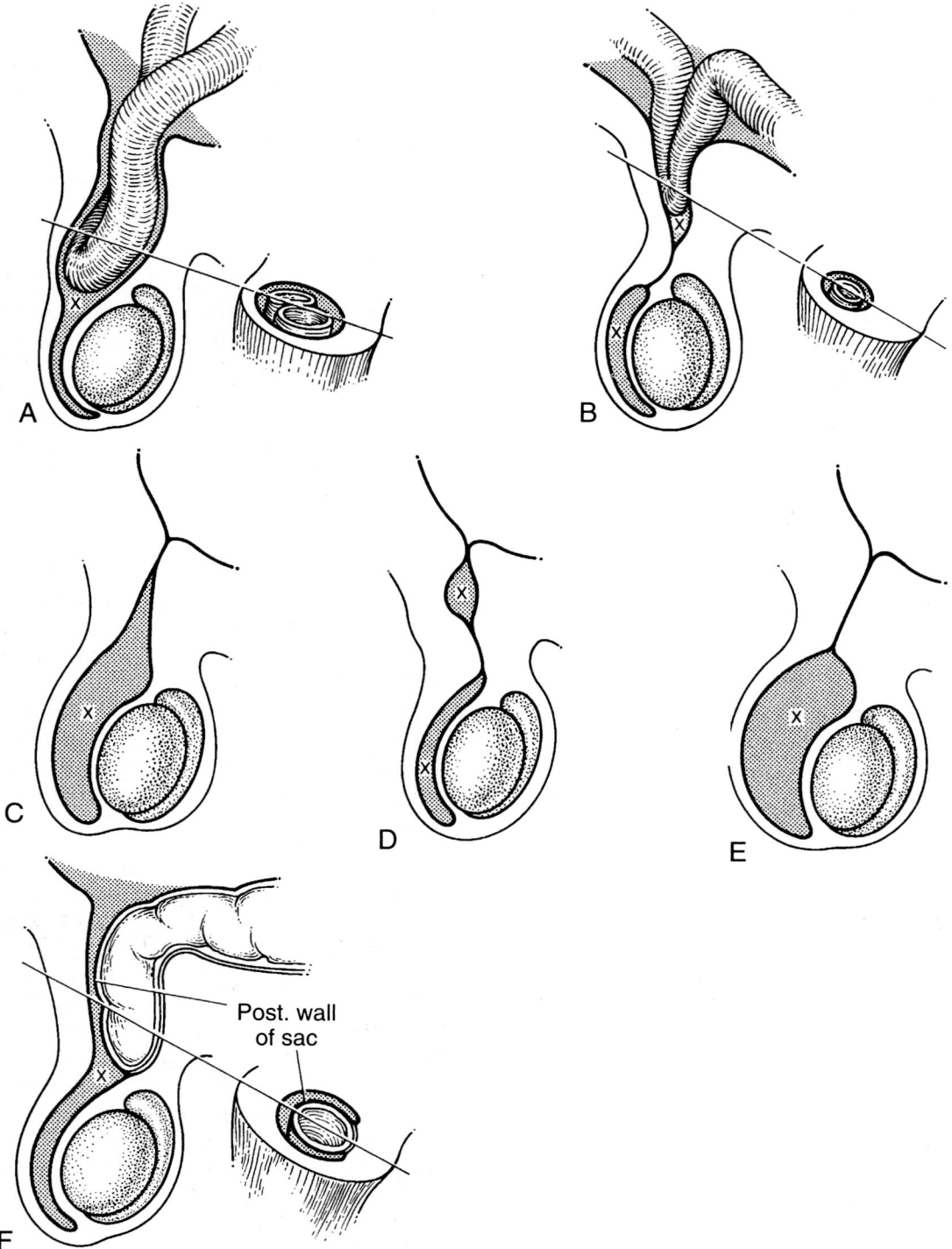

Post. wall
of sac

Figure 20.11. Defects of closure of the processus vaginalis. *Inset* shows appearance in cross-section. *X*, Processus caginalis. **A,** Completely unclosed processus. An intestinal loop or omentum may follow the testis into the scrotum (congenital indirect hernia). **B,** The cranial (funicular) portion of the processus remains unclosed. Herniation may occur later in life (acquired indirect hernia). **C,** All but the cranial portion is unclosed. Serious fluid accumulates to form an infantile hydrocele.

D, The midportion of the processus is unclosed, forming a cyst (cystic hydrocele). **E,** Normally closed processus. Fluid may accumulate in the tunica vaginalis (adult hydrocele). **F,** Sliding indirect inguinal hernia. The descending viscus, usually colon, remains retroperitoneal. The sac (processus vaginalis) remains unclosed. (From Skandalakis JE, Gray SW, Rowe JS Jr. Anatomical complications in general surgery. New York: McGraw-Hill, 1983:284.)

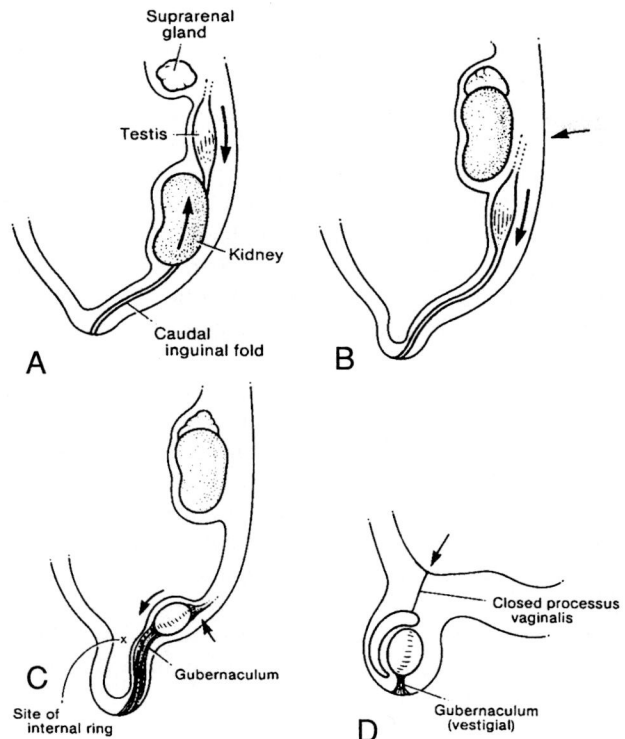

Figure 20.12. Descent of the testis. **A,** Fifth week. The spindle-shaped testis is beginning its primary descent; the kidney is ascending. **B,** Eighth to ninth weeks. The kidney has reached its adult position. **C,** Seventh month. The testis is at the internal inguinal ring; the gubernaculum in the inguinal fold is thickening and shortening. **D,** Postnatal life. The testis is in the scrotum; the processus vaginalis has closed, and the gubernaculum is vestigial. (From Skandalakis JE, Gray SW, Rowe JS Jr. Anatomical complications in general surgery. New York: McGraw-Hill, 1983:286.)

Table 20.4.
Some Syndromes Associated with Undescended Testes[a]

Chromosomal		
Sex chromosomes	XXY	XYY
	XXYY	XO/XY
	XXXXY	XX male
Autosomal Trisomy 13,		
18, 21, 9, 14		
4p−, 4q+, 5p−,		
18q−, 21q−		
Nonchromosomal		
Prader-Willi		Rubinstein-Taybi
Noonan		Seckel
Cornelia de Lange		Smith-Lemli-Opitz
Aarskog		Meckel-Gruber
Kallmann		Dubowitz
Carpenter		Cockayne
Fraser		Silver-Russell
Oculocerebrorenal		Laurence-Moon-Biedl

[a]From Sheldon CA. Undescended testis and testicular torsion. Surg Clin North Am 1985;65(5):1307.

week, as reported by Baker (62). This author also stated that 2 million will survive in follicles after birth.

Upadhyay and Zamboni (63) concluded that ectopic germ cells do not incorporate into follicles and disappear.

The origin of the germ cell neoplasm may be appreciated in Figure 20.4.

DESCENT OF THE OVARY

Ovarian descent normally ceases after the 12th week, at which time the ovary is at the pelvic brim. Lateral rotation subsequently brings it to its final position. The gubernaculum attaches to the uterus and does not shorten, as in the male; eventually the caudal part becomes the round ligament, extending from the uterus toward the inguinal canal and to the labia majora, and the cranial part becomes the ligament of the ovary. The canal of Nuck, extending into the labium major, corresponds to the processus vaginalis of the male. It is normally obliterated by the eighth month.

Vestigial Organs of the Testis and Ovary

All the vestigial remnants associated with the testis, epididymis, and vas are of mesonephric (wolffian) origin, except the appendix testis, which is a paramesonephric (müllerian) remnant (Fig. 20.14).

All the vestigial remnants associated with the ovary, tube, and broad ligaments are of mesonephric (wolffian) origin (Fig. 20.15). The reason is that the mesonephric duct in the male is responsible for the genesis of the sex organs under the influence of androgenic hormones. Epididymis, paradidymis, vas deferens, seminal vesicles, and ejaculatory ducts are organs produced by the male sex duct (mesonephric or wolffian).

In the female the mesonephric duct disappears partially, and its remnants produce vestigial structures such as epoophoron, paroophoron, and Gartner's duct.

The paramesonephric duct (müllerian) in the female produces the uterus, uterine tube, and upper vagina. In the male its most cranial end remains as a vestigial organ, the appendix testis, and the rest degenerates.

The four vestigial organs in the male are of cyst-like formation with a pedicle, which can twist and produce a clinical picture almost similar to testicular torsion.

In the female, for all practical purposes, some vestigial entities are well-developed cystic structures with a clinical significance. Some, such as the paroophoron, because of their rarity and their minute size, do not produce problems of clinical significance.

Confusion surrounds the so-called paradidymis. Most likely, it represents wolffian remnants in the male, such as the organs of Giraldès (an upper part) and perhaps, according to Told and as stated in McGregor, a lower part which is located behind the epididymal head (64). The authors, however, are not sure about the embryogenesis or the homologues of these vestigial remains (Table 20.5).

Critical Events in Ovarian and Testicular Development

The migration of the sex cells to the genital ridge in the fifth week might be expected to be a hazardous journey with many possibilities for failure. This does not seem to be the case; examples of failure are very rare indeed.

The descent of the testes in the perinatal period is the source of more trouble than is any other event in the gonadal development. If, as seems probable, failure of the testis to descend results from intrinsic inadequacy of the organ, we know little of the nature of the inadequacy and nothing of the stage in development at which it occurs.

ANOMALIES OF THE GONADS (TABLE 20.6 AND FIGURE 20.16)

Congenital Absence of One or Both Testes without Feminization

ANATOMY AND EMBRYOGENESIS

Unlike phenotypic males with Klinefelter's syndrome who are genetically female, or genetic males with Turner's syndrome who are phenotypically female, patients with simple anorchia show no chromosome anomalies and are not feminized (Table 20.7).

Some cases of monorchia represent complete unilateral agenesis of the nephrogenic mesoderm; the kidney, as well as the testis and its ducts, is absent (65). Presumably there was no potential genital ridge on the affected side, and the migrating germ cells all came to rest at the site of the contralateral gonad (see Table 17.1).

Absence of germ cells would be expected to result in aplasia of the gonads on both sides, but the fact that experimental castration of embryos before sex differentiation leads to feminization of the external genitalia (66) suggests that atrophy of previously formed testes has occurred in most cases. Some writers prefer the terms *atrophy* or *extreme dysgenesis* to *absence* (67, 68).

In the majority of cases surgically explored, the ductus deferens is present, and occasionally some epididymis tissue is found (69, 70).

A remarkable case of bilateral agenesis was reported by Amelar (71), in which the patient had normal libido and was not eunuchoid. Epididymal tissue and islands of Leydig cells, but no seminiferous tubules, were found in the scrotum on one side. The ductus deferens was present on each side and entered the scrotum. Amelar reminds us that the earliest report of confirmed anorchia (72) was based on the autopsy of a man hanged for rape.

HISTORY

Absence of one or both testes would seem to be an obvious anomaly, but the frequency of undescended testes makes surgical or necropsy confirmation necessary. The first confirmed case of which there is a record was reported in 1564 by Cabrol (72); both testes were absent.

Fisher of Boston, according to Gould and Pyle (73), reported a patient with bilateral absence of the testicles in the *American Journal of Medical Science* in 1839. Also, the same authors cite a patient of Gruber's in whom the right testicle, right epididymis, and right vas were absent from the scrotum.

In 1878 Gruber (74) was able to find and verify only 23 unilateral and 7 bilateral cases. Rea (75) and Counseller and his colleagues (76) in 1940 collected the cases in the literature. The latter authors found 24 unilateral cases (monorchia) and 11 bilateral cases (anorchia). Gross (77) added 24 unilateral cases and 6 bilateral cases in 1953, and Tibbs (67) added 13 unilateral and 1 bilateral case in 1961. These, with a few other reports, bring the total to 82 unilateral and 18 bilateral cases of absence of the testis. By a far more conservative estimate, only 15 acceptable cases have been published (78).

INCIDENCE

Among 722 patients with apparently undescended testes, Gross (77) found 30 in which one or both testes appeared to be congenitally absent. Taking Campbell's (79) estimate of 1% as the incidence of undescended testes toward the end of childhood, we can assign a startling high incidence of about 0.04% to anorchia and monorchia. This is probably too high.

Unilateral absence is twice as common on the left side, but failure of descent is more common on the right at birth.

Mercer (80) reported the occurrence of agenesis or atrophy of the testis and vas deferens in nine patients, or 3.4% of patients with ipsilateral agenesis of the vas and testicle in 237 cases of undescended testicles. Renal agenesis was found in three of the nine cases: two ipsilateral, and one contralateral. Testicular agenesis alone was found in three patients and atrophy also in three patients. Mercer thought that atrophy is the result of the intrauterine torsion. None of these reported patients had renal agenesis.

SYMPTOMS

No symptoms will arise from unilateral absence of the testis; the patient will merely complain of undescended testis. That the majority of such patients are not further examined accounts for the possible high frequency of unrecognized anorchism.

In older boys with bilateral anorchia, the presenting complaint may be delayed puberty. With few exceptions,

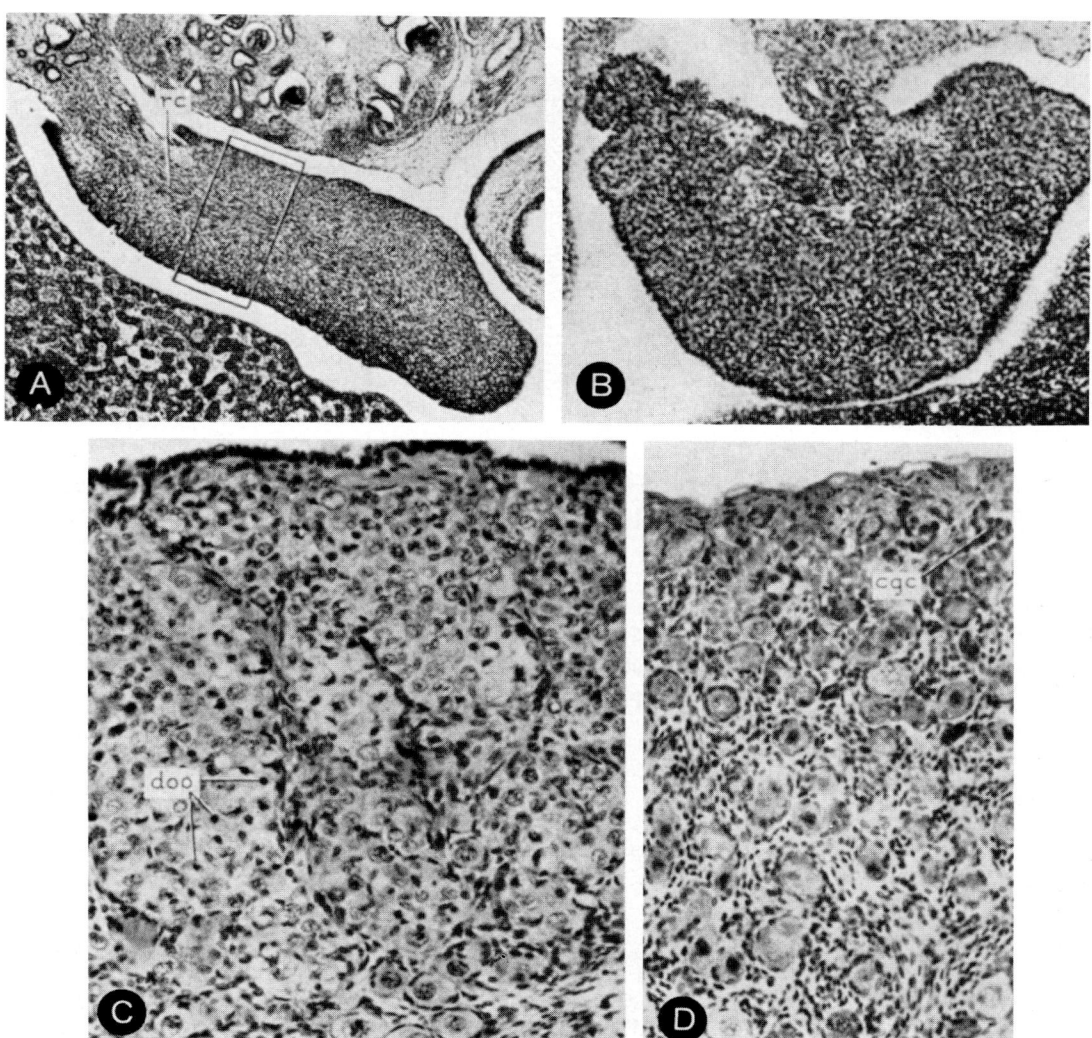

Figure 20.13. Stages in the maturation of the embryonic human ovary. **A,** At 25 mm (eighth week). A cellular cortex and an ill-defined rete *(rc)* are visible. Compare with Figure 20.7, A. **B,** At 31.5 mm (ninth week). Cortex and medulla are indicated. **C,** At 190 mm (about 22 weeks). Fetal stroma appears in the medulla where germ cells are becoming surrounded by granulosa cells, forming primordial follicles. Some germ cells *(doo)* are already degenerating in advance of the invading stroma. **D,** at 272 mm (about 30 weeks). Fetal stroma has nearly filled the cortex. Oogonia deeper in the cortex are larger than more superficial germ cells *(cgc,* cords of follicular cells not associated with germ cells). (From Gillman J. The development of the gonads in man, with a consideration of the role of fetal endocrines and the histogenesis of ovarian tumors. Contrib Embryol Carnegie Inst Wash 1948;32:83–131.) The rectangle in **A** indicates a high-power field shown in Gillman's original plate.)

such as Amelar's (70) patient, such boys remain eunuchoid but not feminized.

DIAGNOSIS

The absent testis must be distinguished from the undescended testis to support a diagnosis of anorchia. It has frequently been pointed out that complete proof of testicular absence can be obtained only at necropsy (78): a surgical search can never be exhaustive. Intravenous pyelogram (IVP) and sonography should be included to determine the diagnosis of renal agenesis.

The presence of the ductus deferens and spermatic vessels serve as a guide to the site of the testis. In most cases of anorchia or monorchia, these may be traced into the inguinal ring, where the ductus ends as a small bulb. Tibbs (67) considers that failure to find the testis at the end of the ductus is sufficient to establish its absence. Most authors now believe the spermatic vessels, not the spermatic cord, must be traced to their endpoint to be certain that the testis is absent. Diagnostic laparoscopy has proved to be useful in this regard. A search for an apparently undescended testis is desirable since the incidence of malignancy in retained testes is about 50 times that of normal, descended testes. In one patient gonad-

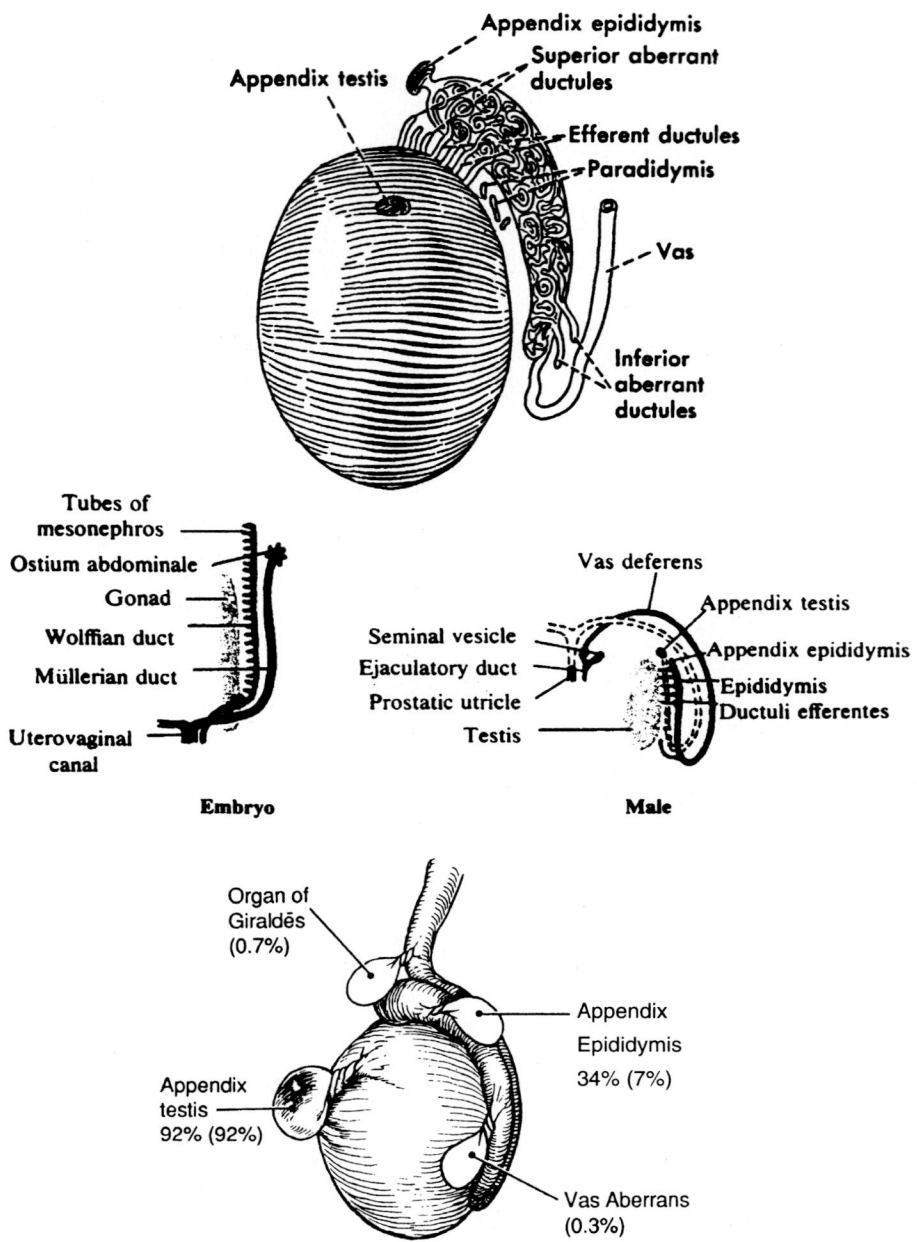

Figure 20.14. Vestigial remnants of testis, epididymis, and vas. Location and incidence of intrascrotal appendages. Number in parenthesis indicate the relative contribution of each appendage to intrascrotal appendiceal torsion. (Adapted from Rolnick D et al. Anatomical incidence of testicular appendages. J Urol 1968;100:755–756; Skoglund RW, McRoberts JW, Radge H. Torsion of testicular appendages: presentation of 43 new cases and a collective review. J Urol 1970;104:598–600; and Healy JE Jr, Hodge J. Surgical anatomy. Philadelphia: BC Decker, 1990.)

otropins were of normal levels, but there was decreased 17-ketosteroid and increased estrogen excretion (81). In a presumptive male patient the buccal smear was chromatin positive (female), but neither gonads nor female genitalia were found at laparotomy (78).

Raffensperger (82) stated that, if during exploration for undescended testicle, the vas deferens has a "nubbin scar tissue," certainly the testicle is absent.

No treatment for unilateral absence is necessary or indeed possible. Suitable hormone therapy is indicated when both testes are absent. If the affected testis is present but hypoplastic or atrophic, it should be removed.

Congenital Absence of One or Both Ovaries (Excluding Turner's Syndrome)

ANATOMY

Morgagni (83) described the body of a middle-aged woman in whom the left uterine tube was solid and short and had no associated ovary. So rare is the condition,

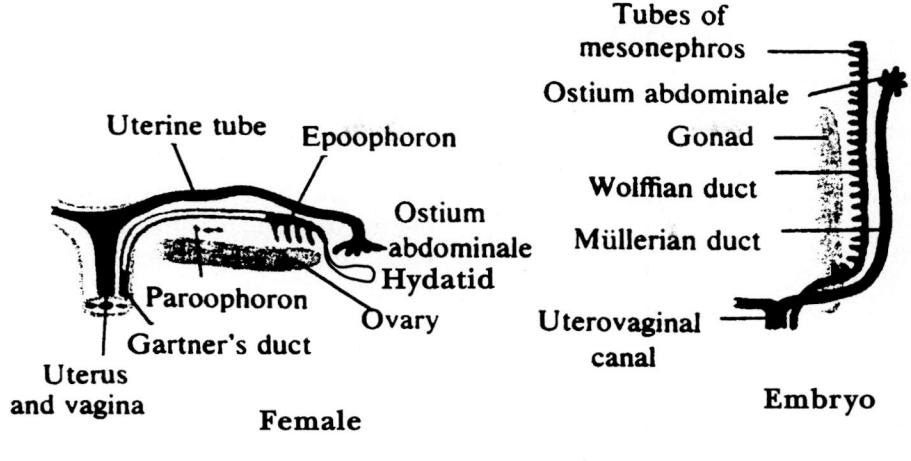

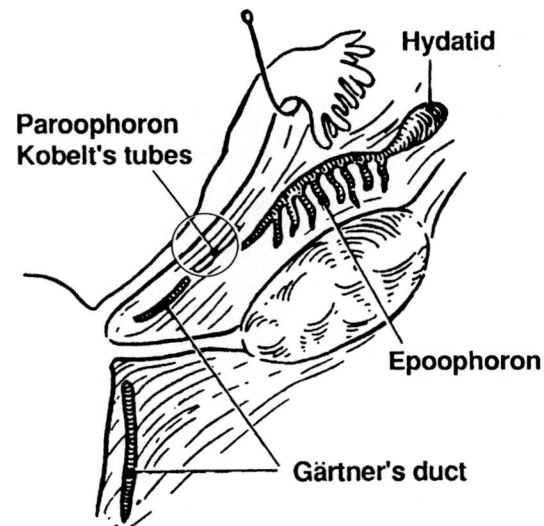

Figure 20.15. The vestigial remnants of the ovary, tube, and broad ligament. (Adapted from Hollinshead WH. Anatomy for surgeons: the thorax, abdomen and pelvis. New York: Hoeber-Harper 1958; Healy JE Jr, Hodge J. Surgical anatomy. Philadelphia: BC Decker, 1990.)

however, that by 1935 only 17 cases could be collected. By 1948 Kurcz and Sharp (84) were able to find 40 cases. Guizzetti and Pariset (85) estimated that it occurred as often as once in 2000 autopsies, but this figure seems high (Table 20.8).

As in unilateral absence of the testis, absence of an ovary usually is associated with renal agenesis and absence of the uterine tube on the same side (65). In Morgagni's case and in a more recent case (84), the kidney and a hypoplastic uterine tube were present. Kent (85) described a patient with an ectopic pregnancy in the intramural portion of an incomplete tube. There was no ovary, ovarian ligament, or mesosalpinx on that side.

A few cases are known in which no follicles are present in either ovary. Primary amenorrhea, as in Turner's syndrome, occurs, but there is no reduction in stature or other associated anomalies (see Chapter 23, "Sex Determination"). A biopsy will show normal female chromatin positive cells. Stilbestrol therapy has been successful in relieving all the symptoms except sterility (87).

HISTORY

Gould and Pyle (73) stated that Hunter, Violal, and Chanssia reported ovarian absence, and Thudium collected 21 cases "of this nature."

EMBRYOGENESIS

When nephric structures are absent on one side, the ovarian agenesis is primary and the germ cells have migrated to the normal side. In some cases the solitary ovary is larger than normal (see Table 17.1).

When no other anomalies are present, either a primary absence of germ cells or secondary atrophy is possible. The latter explanation seems the more probable (Table 20.8).

Table 20.5.
Derivation of Reproductive Tract Structures from Wolffian and Müllerian Primordia

Male	Female
Genital ridges	
Testis	
Seminiferous tubules (medulla)	Ovary
Rete testis	Pfluger's tubules[a]
Gubernaculum testis	Rete ovarii[a]
	Round ligament of uterus
	and ovary
Ligament of testis	Ligament of ovary
Mesorchium	Mesoovarium
Wolffian derivatives	
Mesonephric tubules	
Ductuli efferentes	Epoophoron[a]
Ductuli abberantes[a]	Ductuli aberrantes (Haller)[a]
Paradidymis (tubules)[a]	Paroophoron[a]
Paradidymis collecting duct	?
Mesonephric duct	
Ureter, pelvis, and collecting	Ureter, pelvis, and collecting
tubules of kidney	tubules of kidney
Trigone of bladder	Trigone of bladder
Proximal ductus epididymis	Duct of the epoophoron[a]
Distal ductus epididymis	?
Proximal ductus deferens	?
Ductus deferens	Gartner's duct[a]
Ejaculatory duct	?
Seminal vesicle	?
Appendix epididymis[a]	Appendix vesiculosa
	epoophoron[a]
Müllerian derivatives	
Appendix testis[a]	Uterine tube distal (fimbria)
	Hydatid of Morgagni?[a]
?	Oviduct
?	Uterus
?	Cervix and upper vagina
Prostatic utricle[a]	Lower vagina
Colliculus seminalis	Hymen?
Urogenital sinus derivatives	
Bladder	Bladder
Prostatic urethra above colliculus	Urethra
seminalis	
Urethra below colliculus	Lower vagina and vestibule
seminalis	
Membranous urethra	Lower vagina and vestibule
Cavernous urethra	Lower vagina and vestibule
Corpus cavernosum urethra	Vestibule of bulb
Corpus cavernosum penis	Corpus cavernosum clitori
Bulbourethral glands (Cowper's)	Vestibular glands (Bartholin's)
Urethral glands (Littré)	Minor vestibular glands
Prostate gland	Paraurethral glands of Skene?
Urethral crest & colliculus	Hymen
seminalis	
External genitalia	
Glans penis	Glans clitoris
Floor of penile urethra	Labia minora
Scrotum	Labia majora
Processus vaginalis testis	Canal of Nuck

[a]Vestigal structures.

SYMPTOMS AND DIAGNOSIS

Unilateral ovarian agenesis is not symptomatic. Genital anomalies should be expected and investigated in all patients with unilateral absence of the kidney. Conversely, discovery of gonadal or tubal anomalies should turn attention to the kidneys.

Vasilev et al. (88) reported a case of absence of ovarian parenchyme with absence of the uterine horn and tube (Slotnik-Goldfarb syndrome). They advised the use of dynamic γ-camera excretory scintigraphy for diagnosis, a procedure also advised by Peshev et al. (89) for determining the topographic anatomy of the ovaries. Rock et al. (90) reported ovarian malposition with uterine anomalies.

TREATMENT

In the rare bilateral cases, only hormonal treatment is possible. When ovariectomy is indicated for other reasons, the surgeon should verify the presence of a contralateral ovary since loss of secondary sex characteristics as well as sterility will otherwise result.

Supernumerary Testes

ANATOMY

Supernumerary testes usually lie proximal to the normal testis and often are smaller. They may have a separate or a common epididymis and ductus deferens. In Darrow and Humes' case (91), both the normal and the accessory testes were descended and had a common tunica vaginalis. They had separate spermatic cords and active spermatogenesis was seen in both testes. In Kay and Coleman's case (92), one testis with its ductus deferens was at the level of the fourth lumbar vertebra, while the other was in the inguinal canal. They were connected by the spermatic cord, but the lower testis did not open into the ductus deferens. No spermatogonia were present and both testes were less than 1 cm in length (Fig. 20.17).

Jichlibnski and Ward-McQuaid (93) reported that 50% of cases of polyorchidism are associated with cryptorchidism, 30% with indirect hernia, and the remaining with hydrocele, varicocele, epididymitis, torsion, or infertility.

EMBRYOGENESIS

The embryonic origin is from an anteroposterior division of the genital ridge, which formed two separate organs instead of one. Similar splitting of the ovarian primordium has been observed and is equally rare (page 755). The presence of two spermatic cords in some cases suggests a lateral pairing of the upper end of the wolffian duct, with fusion of the two branches at a lower level. Such duplication would involve formation of two sets of pronephric tubules and two pronephric ducts during the fourth week. While such splitting of the wolffian duct primordium is not inconceivable, it must be considered hypothetical. More probably, the already separated testicular primordia induced development of separate epi-

Table 20.6.
Anomalies of the Gonads

Anomaly	Origin of Defect	First Appearance (or Other Diagnostic Clues)	Sex Chiefly Affected	Relative Frequency	Remarks
Congenital absence of one or both testes without feminization	Atrophy after 4th week	In childhood	Male	Rare	
Congenital absence of one or both ovaries (excluding Turner's syndrome)	Atrophy after 4th week	At menarche, if bilateral; otherwise discovery is accidental	Females	Very rare	
Congenital absence of one gonad and homolateral kidney and ureter	4th week	In childhood	Both	Rare	Uterine and tubal anomalies in female
Supernumerary testes	4th week	In childhood, or accidental	Male	Very rare	Spermatic cord may or may not be duplicated
Testicular fusion	4th week	In childhood	Male	Very rare	Associates with fused kidney
Failure of union of testis and epididymis	9th week or later	In childhood (nondescent); at maturity (causes infertility if bilateral)	Male	Rare(?)	No impairment of fertility if unilateral
Undescended testes	Around birth	In childhood	Male	Very common	
Maldescended testes	Around birth	In childhood	Male	Rare	
Inguinal herniation and ectopia of ovary	Around birth	In childhood or later	Female	Rare	Some cases are acquired, not congenital

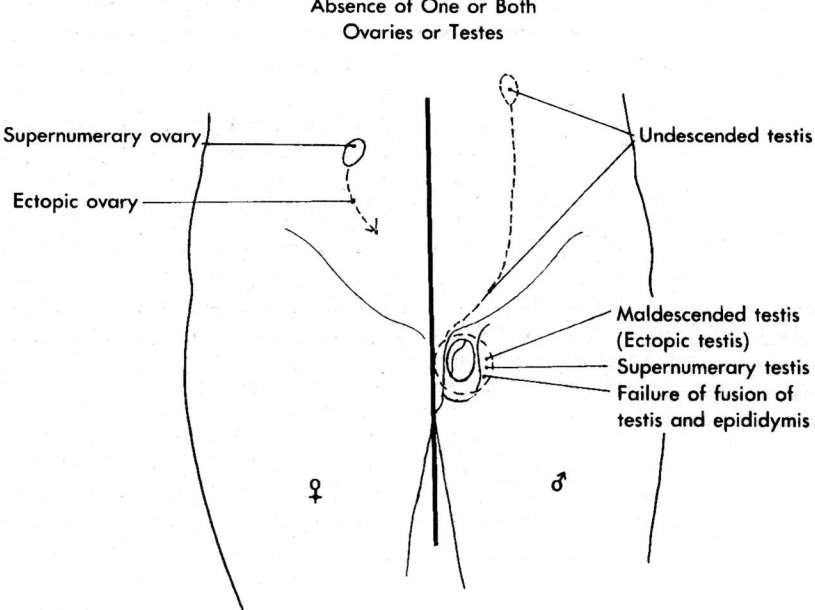

Figure 20.16.   Anomalies of the ovaries and testes.

Table 20.7.
Apparent and True Absence of the Testes

	Sex Chromosomes	Germ Cells	Nephrogenic Ridge	Testis
Phenotypic males				
Normal	XY	Present	Present	Present in scrotum
Apparent anorchia	XY	Present	Present	Present, but nondescended or maldescended; unilateral or bilateral; common
True Anorchia	XY	*Absent* on affected side	*Absent*	*Absent* (agenesis)[a]; unilateral; rare
	XY	*Absent*	Present	*Absent* (secondary dysgenesis); bilateral or unilateral; very rare
Phenotypic females				
True anorchia (Turner's syndrome)	XO	*Absent*	Present	*Absent* (primary dysgenesis); bilateral; uncommon

[a]Associated with absence of kidney and ureter on the affected side.

Table 20.8.
Absence of the Ovaries

	Sex Chromosomes	Germ Cells	Nephrogenic Ridge	Ovary
Phenotypic females				
Normal	XX	Present	Present	Present
Anovarism	XX	*Absent* on affected side	*Absent*	*Absent* (agenesis)[a]; unilateral, rare
	XX	*Absent*	Present	*Absent* (secondary dysgenesis); bilateral or unilateral, very rare
Turner's syndrome	XO	*Absent*	Present	*Absent* (primary dysgenesis); bilateral, uncommon

[a]Associated with absence of the kidney, ureter, uterine tube and hemiuterus on the affected side.

didymides at two levels of the degenerating mesonephros, and at each level a ductus epididymis elongated from a common wolffian stem. No actual evidence for either hypothesis exists (Fig. 20.18).

Lambrecht and Babayan (94) reported polyorchidism in a 4-year-old boy with maldescent of the left testicle who, at operation, was found to have a third atrophic testicle. They collected 60 cases from the literature.

HISTORY

Although it was alluded to in early mythology, supernumerary testis was first documented by Blasius (95), who found it at autopsy in 1670. According to Gould and Pyle (73), Russel reported a monk with three testicles who was so "salacious" that his great passion did not help him to keep his vows of chastity. Haller (74) collected cases of three testicles. The first histologically proven case was reported in 1895 by Lane (96). Kay and Coleman (92) were able to find only 26 authentic cases by 1956. Darrow

and Humes (91), reviewing 23 cases, found an almost equal incidence on the two sides and reported no bilateral case. Angulo and Caballero (97) reported the 28th case in 1957.

Butz and Croushore (98) stated that perhaps the reported larger size of the left testicle may be the reason supernumerary testicle is thought of as occurring more on the left than on the right side—something which does not agree with our previous edition. They (98) suggest this phenomenon occurs because of subdivision of the large testicle and bifurcation of its vessels.

SYMPTOMS AND DIAGNOSIS

There are no symptoms from supernumerary testes; discovery is usually accidental or at autopsy. In diagnosing the nature of a scrotal mass, one must distinguish among this and hydrocele (page 578 and Fig. 16.56), ectopic scrotal spleen (page 338), and crossed or transverse testicular ectopia, in which both testes lie in the same scrotal

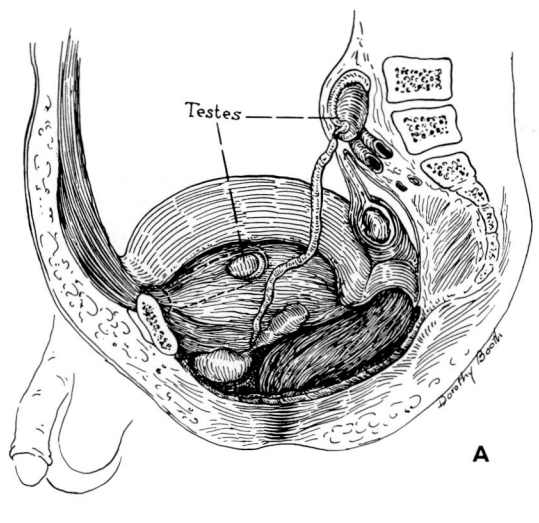

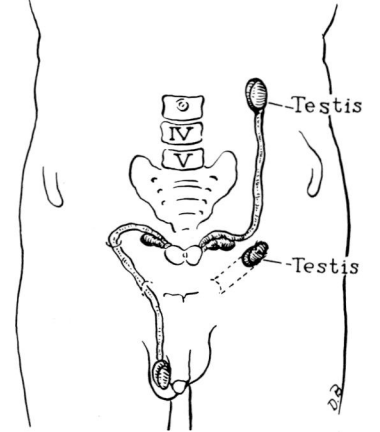

Figure 20.17. *Supernumerary testis. Patient with a normally descended testis in the left scrotum and two testis on the right, one of which was completely undescended, while the other was near the internal inguinal ring. The latter had no connection with the ductus deferens.* **A,** *Parasagittal view.* **B,** *Anterior view. (From Kay S, Coleman FP. Duplication of left undescended testicle. J Urol 1956;75:815–818.)*

pouch (page 766). All of these, except hydrocele, are as rare as is testicular duplication itself.

TREATMENT

Treatment, if necessary, consists in removal of the proximal, smaller testis, with ligation of its ductus. Biopsy of the lower testis is recommended to determine its functional state.

Medicolegal problems may arise after vasectomy. It is always advisable to explain the situation *in writing* to the patient.

Supernumerary and Accessory Ovarian Tissue

ANATOMY

True Ovarian Duplication. We have seen only one report of true duplication of the ovaries (99). Two uteri, each with a pair of uterine tubes and ovaries, were found. Duplication of the genital ridge had occurred on each side, each forming an ovary and a müllerian duct (see Fig. 22.19).

Supernumerary Ovaries. Wharton (100) described a patient with a supernumerary ovary on the right pelvic wall, lateral to the ureter. This, as well as the normal ovaries, was removed and proved histologically to be an ovary. Over a year later, a cystic mass in the same patient—which also proved to be ovarian tissue (Fig. 20.19)—was removed from retroperitoneal tissue at the base of the sigmoid mesocolon. In a second patient, who died of chorioepithelioma, an ectopic supernumerary ovary was found, without adnexa, on the left. Wharton (100) was able to find only two other cases in the literature. Winckel (101) in 1890 described a supernumerary ovary with an ostium and rudimentary tube branching from the normal right uterine tube. During the following year, Falk (102) reported a patient who had a third ovary which had no connection with the normal reproductive

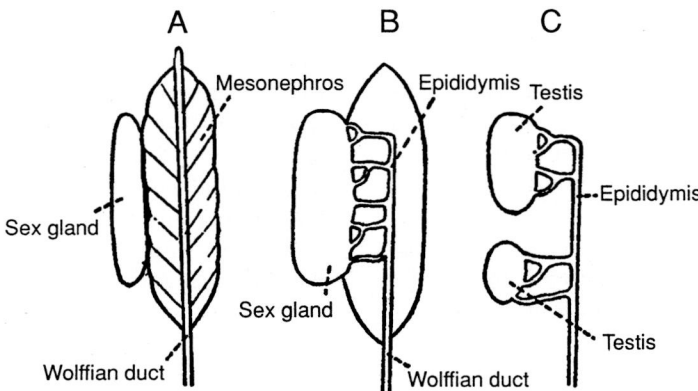

Figure 20.18. *Diagrammatic representation of the genesis of polyorchidism.* **A,** *The undifferentiated sex gland.* **B,** *A further stage of development—the testis, vasa efferentia, epididymis, and ductus deferens can be distinguished.* **C,** *Owing* to failure of atrophy of the anterior tubules, two testes are formed. (From Boggon RH. Polyorchidism. Br J Surg 1933;20:630–639.)

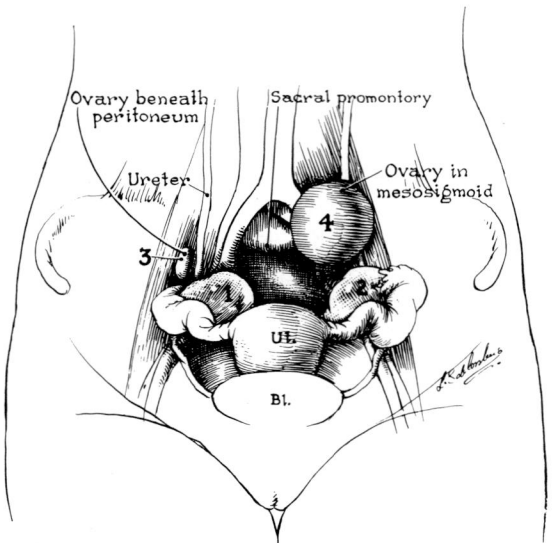

Figure 20.19. Supernumerary ovaries. Patient with four ovaries which were removed and their identity proved by microscopic examination. (From Wharton LR. Two cases of supernumerary ovary and one of accessory ovary with an analysis of previously reported cases. Am J Obstet Gynecol 1959;18:1101–1119.)

organs and which was attached to the omentum. A small segment of fallopian tube, cystic and closed at both ends, was attached to it.

Heller et al. (103) presented a case of accessory ovary with a Brenner tumor.

Mercer (104) reported two cases of benign tumors in supernumerary ovaries. Accessory ovary and atretic fallopian tube was reported by Bialer et al. (105). The patient was a 22-year-old female with several other congenital anomalies.

Accessory and Lobulated Ovaries. Wharton (100) defines an accessory ovary as excess ovarian tissue near the normal ovary. It may be connected with it and has developed from it. In contrast, a supernumerary ovary is entirely separate and appears to have arisen from a separate anlage.

The first reported case of accessory ovary was that of Grohe (106). A total of 23 cases had been reported when the literature was reviewed in 1970. Accessory or bifid fallopian tubes or ostia were associated with five of the cases. In addition to these cases with proven ovarian tissue, there have been 22 other reports of tumors in which the tumor was ovarian in type, but in which no indisputable ovarian tissue was demonstrated. Accessory ovaries have been reported in apes, baboons, monkeys, and frogs. Lobulation of the ovary, which represents the mildest degree of separation, is more common than is accessory ovary.

A number of reported cases of menstruation and one of pregnancy (107) following bilateral oophorectomy may represent the activity of accessory or supernumerary ovaries.

EMBRYOGENESIS

The migration of germ cells from the yolk sac to the hindgut and thence to the mesenchyme of the genital ridge takes place during the fifth week. That all these reach the site of a single pair of gonads is more remarkable than that they occasionally fail to do so. Supernumerary ovaries and testes occur when two groups of primary germ cells in the genital ridge fail to coalesce and, in this manner, induce the formation of separate organs.

SYMPTOMS AND DIAGNOSIS

Supernumerary or accessory ovaries produce no symptoms. Such structures can be diagnosed only on histologic section. Grossly, they may be mistaken for lymph nodes. Sonography and CT scan is a must for diagnosis and location.

Embryonal carcinoma of the ovary was reported by Abdel-Dayem et al. (108) in a 17-year old Saudi female with total situs inversus. According to these authors, 16 cases of cancer associated with situs inversus have been reported since 1936, and their case was the first case of embryonal carcinoma.

Testicular Fusion

Fusion of the testes into a single mass having two epididymides has been known to occur. Such fusion may be associated with fused kidneys (109), suggesting there may have been a deformity of the urogenital ridges themselves.

Failure of Union of Testis and Epididymis

ANATOMY

Failure of the testis to unite with those mesonephric tubules that normally form the ductuli efferentes results in a functional discontinuity of the reproductive tract. Spermatozoa are unable to pass from the seminiferous tubules into the epididymis.

In most reported cases of the defect, the testes were undescended. The epididymis may be descended, while the testis remains in the inguinal canal. If both organs are in the canal, the epididymis may lie lower than the testis (Fig. 20.20). The nondescent is probably less important than it appears to be; most cases of failure of union are discovered only because of the obvious failure of descent. Hanely and Hodges (110), directing their attention to patients with azoospermia, also found failure of union in normally descended testes.

In a few cases all or part of the epididymis may be absent (Fig. 20.21, *D* and *E*). In one such case, studied by Campbell (109), there was no epididymis, but the efferent ducts joined to form the ductus deferens (Fig. 20.21, *C*).

The failure to unite may be only partial (Fig. 20.21, *A*

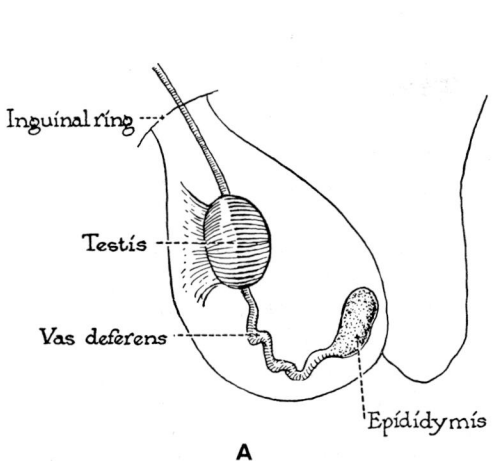

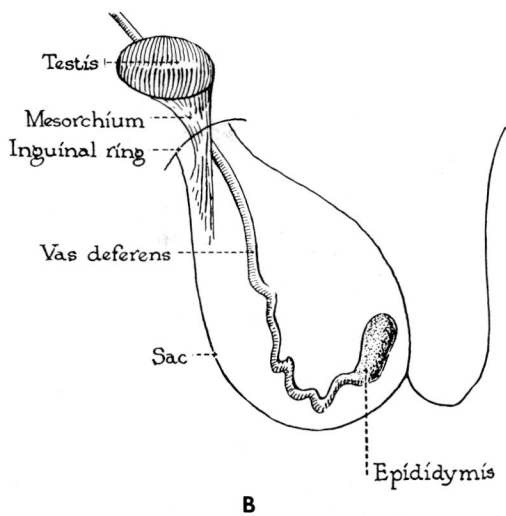

Figure 20.20. Failure of fusion of the testis and epididymis. **A,** Completely descended right epididymis with incompletely descended testis. **B,** Completely descended right epididymis with intraabdominal testis. (From Badenoch AW. Failure of the urogenital union. Surg Gynecol Obstet 1946;82:471–474.)

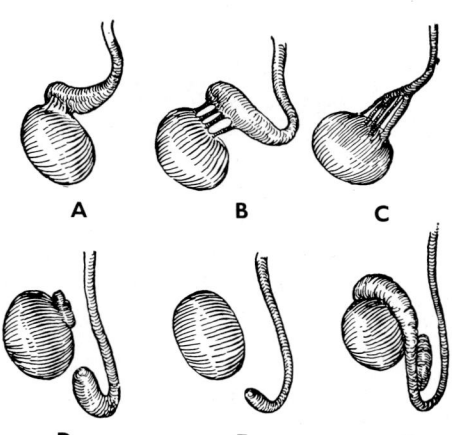

Figure 20.21. Anomalies in fusion of the testis and epididymis. **A,** Epididymis almost completely detached from the testis. **B,** Elongated efferent ductules bridging the separation between the testis and epididymis. **C,** Absence of the epididymis; the efferent ductules unite to form the ductus deferens. **D** and **E,** Partial and complete absence of the epididymis; the testis has no connection with the ductus deferens. **F,** Accessory epididymis. (From Campbell MF, Harrison JH. Urology, ed 3. (3 vol). Philadelphia: WB Saunders, 1970.)

and *B*); it may involve only one side; or it may be complete and bilateral (111). As long as some tubules connect the testis with the epididymis, the patient may be fertile.

Faulty union of testis and epididymis may leave blind-ending ductule efferentia that fill with spermatozoa and become dilated. Such tubules form spermatoceles. They may arise from *(a)* defective ducts, *(b)* from normal vestigial mesonephric tubules, such as the ductule aberrantes superior and which are connected only with the rete testis (Fig. 20.22), or *(c)* from the ductule aberrantes inferior, which are attached only to the ductus epididymis (page 775).

Normal scrotal anatomy and some congenital varia-

tions may be appreciated from a radiologic standpoint (Figs. 20.23 and 20.24).

Gracey et al. (112) reported atretic vas deferens in cystic fibrosis of the pancreas. Holsclan et al. (113) reported genital abnormalities in male patients with cystic fibrosis. Bilateral aplasia of the vas deferens was reported by Young (114).

The implication of vas deferens in cystic fibrosis was reported by Viidik and Marshall (115) as well as by Valman and France (116). Anguiano et al. (117) concluded that some, if not all, otherwise healthy men with congenital bilateral absence of the vas deferens represent a primary genital phenotype of cystic fibrosis. These authors recommend that cystic fibrosis mutation analysis should be done prior to sperm aspiration to remedy infertility.

Histologic changes of the testicle were reported by Gorenstein et al. (118) in children with varicocele. Right varicocele indicates a retroperitoneal tumor or situs inversus.

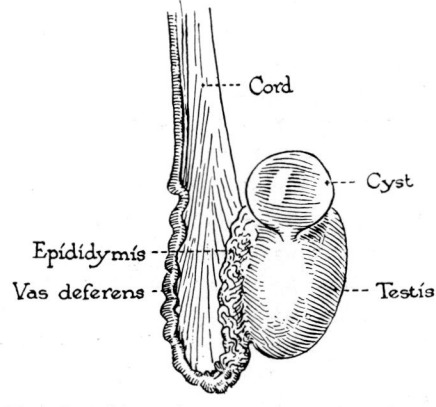

Figure 20.22. Cyst of the mediastinum testis (spermatocele). (From Badenoch AW. Failure of the urogenital union. Surg Gynecol Obstet 1946;82:471–474.)

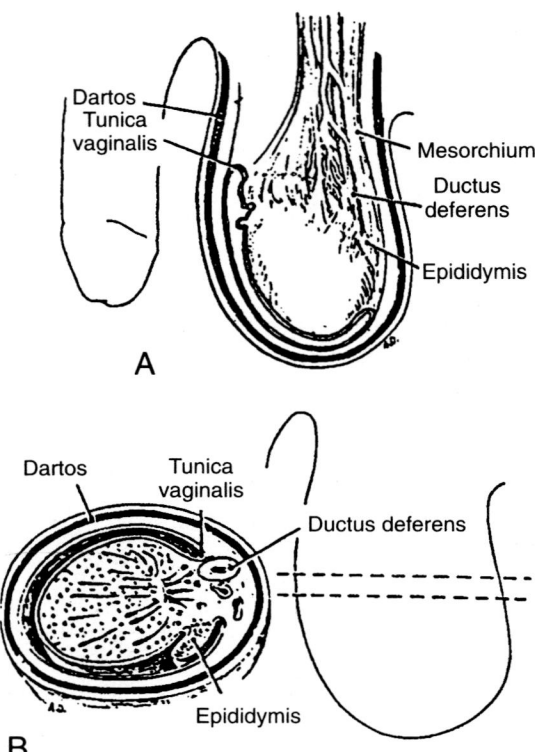

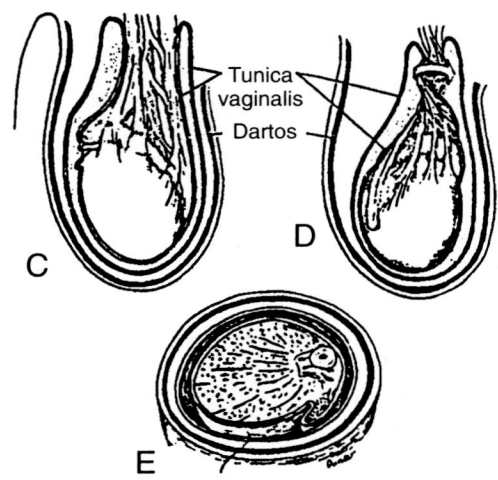

Figure 20.23. Normal scrotal anatomy and some congenital variations from a radiologic standpoint. **A** and **B,** Normal scrotal anatomy. **A,** Posteriorly, the tunica vaginalis does not prevent fixation of the testis and epididymis to the scrotal wall. **B,** Cross-section. **C** to **E,** Congenital variation. "Bell-clapper" abnormality. **C,** The tunica vaginalis completely separates the testis and the epididymis section from the scrotal wall. **D,** Cross-section. **E,** Lack of fixation allows torsion. (**A** and

B From Holder LE, et al. Testicular radionuclide angiography and static imaging: anatomy, scintigraphic interpretation, and clinical indications. Radiology 1977;125:739. Used with permission. **C** to **E,** From Holder LE et al. Testicular radionuclide angiography and static imaging: anatomy, scintigraphic interpretation, and clinical indications. Radiology 1977;125:739. Used with permission.)

EMBRYOGENESIS

Some six to twelve cranial mesonephric tubules are normally involved in the formation of the epididymis. Rete cords extend into the stroma of the wolffian body as early as the sixth week and reach the mesonephric tubules during the ninth week. The junction between the rete cords and the tubules is distal to the glomeruli, which degenerate.

At first the rete tubules are solid; they subsequently become canalized (1) (Fig. 20.8). The connection that will form the ductuli efferentes is complete by birth in the male, but in the female the connection may never be formed or, if it is formed, will break down again before birth (119).

Failure of fusion of gonadal and mesonephric elements is the normal condition in the female. In the male, however, its association with undescended testes lends weight to the argument that testes fail to descend because they are atrophic. The lead taken during descent by the epididymis and ductus deferens under these circumstances may suggest new views on testicular descent.

HISTORY AND INCIDENCE

First reported in 1851 by Follin (120), there were only 29 cases of failure of union in the literature by 1961 (121). The condition probably is more common than this figure indicates since Dean and his colleagues (111) found three cases among 245 patients with undescended testes examined at operation or at autopsy. Hanley and Hodges (110) found four examples in 300 men with azoospermia.

Badenoch (122) believed that small spermatoceles might be present in as many as 1% of males. They appear before puberty and are asymptomatic. Larger cysts usually are seen in later middle age; being painless, they often are of long standing (123) (Fig. 20.22).

SYMPTOMS

The presenting complaint may be maldescent of one or both testes in children. In adults, it may be infertility.

DIAGNOSIS

If spermatozoa can be demonstrated on testicular biopsy and the continuity of the ductus deferens can be estab-

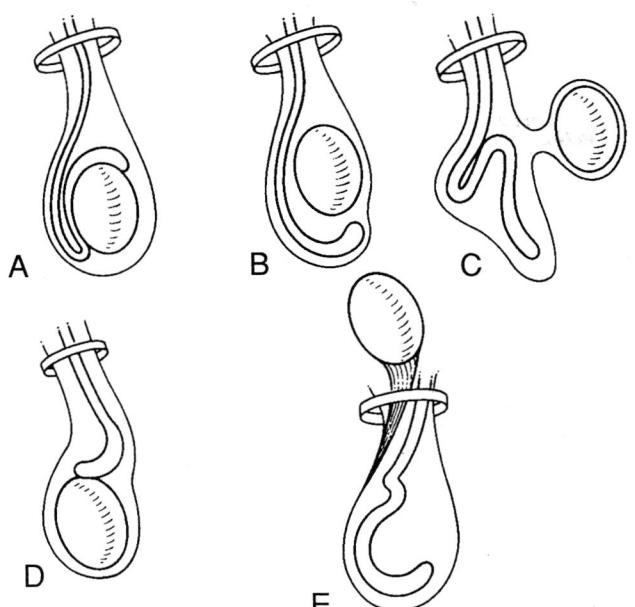

Figure 20.24. *Varieties of separation of testis and epididymis.* **A,** *Normal relations.* **B** *to* **E,** *One or both structures are maldescended. In* **E,** *the epididymis has descended normally, whereas the testis has remained above the internal ring. (From Skandalakis JE, Gray SW, Rowe JS Jr. Anatomical complications in general surgery. New York: McGraw-Hill, 1983.)*

lished, azoospermia must be caused by stenosis of the ductus epididymis or of the ductuli efferentes. Hanley and Hodges (110) believe that, in many cases, one can distinguish by inspection an epididymis containing spermatozoa from an empty epididymis. In the former case there is an obstruction in the tail of the epididymis; in the latter case there is failure of fusion with the efferent tubules.

TREATMENT

Orchidopexy should be performed if the testis can be brought down; orchidectomy is recommended if descent is not feasible. Spermatoceles should be excised. Lythgoe (121) warned that, if the condition is not recognized, the epididymis may be mistaken for an atrophic testis and removed by itself, leaving the testis still in the inguinal canal.

Hanley and Hodges (110) suggested that, when the head of the epididymis contains spermatozoa, it should be possible to bypass the obstruction and restore continuity of the spermatic channel. If spermatozoa cannot reach the epididymis, there is no present hope of restoring the connection. How often the condition is bilateral is not known; if it is unilateral, fertility may be unaffected.

Anomalies of Testicular Descent

Either or both testes may fail to descend or may descend only partially, remaining temporarily or permanently at some point along the normal path of descent. This condition (*undescended* testes) is common. Occasionally the testes may descend and deviate from the normal path of descent to become lodged in any of various abnormal locations. These are the true *ectopic* or *maldescended* testes. The distinction between the various types of retained testes is attributed to Browne (124).

UNDESCENDED TESTES

Anatomy. Testicular descent may never commence, or it may be arrested at any stage along its normal path. About 25% of undescended testes remain in the abdomen and about 75% lie in the inguinal canal. About 5% are ectopic or completely absent. Among 275 infants with undescended testes, Campbell (109) found 26% to be abdominal, 8% to be at the internal inguinal ring, 62% to be in the inguinal canal, and 4% to be at the external ring (Fig. 20.25). In another 40 cases, the testes could not be located and were either ectopic or absent. The frequency of arrest in the inguinal canal is in striking contrast to the short time it usually takes for passage through the canal to occur (43).

Embryogenesis. Since the mechanics of normal testicular descent are obscure, the causes of failure of descent are largely speculative. The explanations that have been put forward fall into three groups: insufficient androgen production, anatomic interference, and inflammatory adhesions.

That the administration of hormones can produce testicular descent both prematurely (45) and after failure of normal descent (44) has been demonstrated (page 742). Anterior pituitary extracts, chorionic gonadotropins, and androgens are all effective. The high frequency of retained testes in various types of pseudohermaphroditism (page 854) indicates that hormonal imbalance can

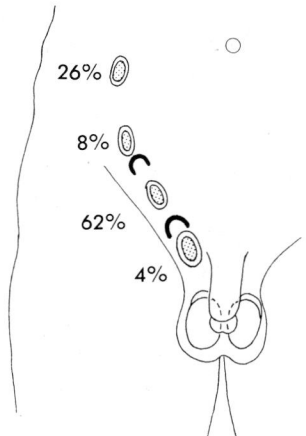

Figure 20.25. *Proportions of undescended testes arrested at various stages of descent. By far the greatest number are halted in the inguinal canal. (Data from Campbell MF, Harrison JH. Urology, 3rd ed. Philadelphia: WB Saunders, 1970.)*

inhibit normal descent. It is less clear to what extent hormonal insufficiency accounts for ordinary cryptorchidism.

A converse view—that the hormonal balance is normal, but that the testis is defective and incapable of responding to the hormone—could well be put forward by those who hold the view that testicular atrophy is the cause and not the result of failure to descend.

Testicular descent induced by hormone injection leaves open the processus vaginalis, which must then be closed surgically. To emphasize the therapeutic drawbacks to hormone therapy, some surgeons have denied the influence of androgens and have contended that only those testes that would eventually have descended spontaneously can be brought down by hormone treatment. Clinical and experimental evidence does not support this view.

Anatomic interference with testicular descent has been attributed to (a) failure of the gubernaculum testis to shorten during development; (b) weakness of the cremaster muscle, (c) insufficient length of the spermatic cord; (d) insufficient length of the spermatic artery; and (e) malformation of the internal inguinal ring or of the inguinal canal (see previous summary on the descent of the testis).

Using electronmicroscopy, Hadziselimovic and Herzug (125) observed atrophy of the Leydig cells in cryptorchid human testes. Raffensperger (82) emphasized that, if this is correct, most likely the product of the normal Leydig cell, androgen, may be responsible for testicular descent. The role of pituitary's luteinizing hormone and its relationship to testosterone (hypothalamic-pituitary-testicular axis) is well known, but the unilateral or bilateral undescended testicle is not explained by such endocrinologic action.

The theory that shortening of the gubernaculum testis serves to pull the testis into the scrotum (41) has long been abandoned. The scrotal attachment is too weak to resist any traction (126). In addition, Lemeh (40) measured the gubernaculum in 19 embryos and concluded that there is no relative shortening of that structure until the 28th week, just before the final descent of the testes, although both smooth and striated muscle fibers may be present.

Defects of the cremaster muscle have been suggested (127) and confirmed experimentally in the rat (128), but there is no reason to believe that such defects are the primary cause of cryptorchidism in man.

In older patients with undescended testes, the spermatic artery is often too short to permit placement of the testis in the scrotum; this is the result, rather than the cause, of the failure of testicular descent. The vessel has grown long enough to serve the testis where it is. Had normal descent occurred, the artery would have elongated sufficiently to serve it at the proper location.

Disproportion between the size of the inguinal ring and the size of the testis, a wide mesorchium which permits excessive freedom of movement of the testis, and deformation of the inguinal canal account for some examples of undescended testes, but they are clearly demonstrable only in extreme cases.

When testicular descent is arrested within the inguinal canal, adhesion of the testis to the surrounding tissue is frequently found at surgery. Whether the adhesions prevented descent or formed later is not always clear. Only occasionally is there a history of inflammation.

In summary, we can say that the cause of most cases of cryptorchidism is still obscure and will remain so until normal testicular descent is better understood.

Abnormalities of the epididymis and vas deferens associated with undescended testicle were summarized by Levitt et al. (129) and modified by Sheldon (57) (Table 20.9).

Associated Pathology
Threat of Malignancy.
In 1940 Gilbert and Hamilton (130) investigated 7000 malignant tumors of the testis and found 840 (12%) in undescended testes. More were in abdominal than in inguinal testes. Campbell in 1942 (131) found 165 undescended testes among 1422 testes with malignancy (11.6%). Because the incidence of undescended testes among United States military recruits was 0.23%, we can conclude that malignancy is approximately 50 times as frequent in the undescended as in the normally descended testis. The validity of this conclusion has been denied (132), but Campbell (133) refuted that argument and confirmed the greater danger of malignancy occurring in the retained testis.

According to Griffin and Wilson (134), between 5 and 12% of testicular tumors occur in cryptorchidism, despite the fact that only 0.7% of adult men have undescended testicles. We agree with the authors: A man with cryptorchidism is more likely to develop malignancies than one with a normal scrotal testis.

Fonger et al. (135) reported that the other normal testis has a risk of tumor development in approximately 11.3% of cases of tumors associated with cryptorchidism.

Associated Scrotal Anomalies.
Diebold et al. (136) reported the presence of a supernumerary spleen within the scrotum of an 81-year-old man with an atrophic testicle, a condition which belongs to the class of splenogonadal fusion disorders.

Vranjesevic et al. (137) reported a 9-year-old child with Prader-Willi syndrome (hypotonic musculature, mental retardation, obesity with gynecomastia and hypogonadism with minute penis, hypoplastic scrotum, and cryptorchidism).

Meinecke et al. (138) reported hypoplastic scrotum with cryptorchidism in a newborn infant with multiple other anomalies.

Table 20.9.
Abnormalities of Epididymis and Vas Deferens Associated with Undescended Testes

Investigator(s)/Year	Abnormality	Incidence
Michelson, 1949	Absent vas, fully descended testes	0.5–1%
Young, 1949		
Dean et al., 1952	Separation of vas and epididymis	1.2% (3/245)
Scorer and Farrington, 1971		3% (9/256)
Badenoch, 1946	Wide separation	5 cases
Lazarus and Marks, 1947	Intraabdominal testes, blind epididymis in or below canal	
Dean et al., 1952		
Lythgoe, 1961		
Nowak, 1972		
Marshall and Shermeta, 1979	Epididymal agenesis	2.4% (1/42)
	Epididymal atresia	19% (8/42)
	Elongated, looped epididymis	14% (6/42)
Whitehorn, 1954	No epididymis or vas, testes in renal fossa, testes below kidney	1 case
Dickinson, 1973		1 case

[a]Modified from Levitt SB et al The impalpable testis: a rational approach to management. J Urol 1978;120:515.

Shawl scrotum was reported in connection with anomalies in a four-generation family by Morris et al. (139).

Coupris and Bondonny (140) reported two cases of accessory scrotum, and were able to collect 13 other cases. All were located in the perineal area, most at the midline. Both testes were located at the normal scrotum, but no testes were found in the accessory scrotum. Bifid scrotum also was present.

Inguinal Hernia.

Failure of the testis to enter the internal inguinal ring leaves the inguinal canal open and unguarded, with little to prevent other abdominal contents from entering during periods of increased intraabdominal pressure, such as occur in coughing, crying, or straining. In about 90% or more of patients with undescended testes, intermittent, indirect inguinal hernia takes place (see Fig. 16.53). Orchiopexy and herniorrhaphy should be done at the same time, according to Fonkalsrud (141).

Discussion of inguinal hernia will be found in Chapter 16, "The Anterior Body Wall," in the section "Incomplete Closure of the Processus Vaginalis: Inguinal Hernia and Hydrocele."

Impaired Fertility.

Although spermatogenesis may occur in some retained testes (142) and in many testes brought down surgically, Hunter's (143) dictum that undescended testes are defective is essentially correct. Modern endocrinology emphasizes that the cryptorchid testis functions poorly in spermatogenesis and androgen secretion (134).

Does malfunction precede maldescent, or is it the opposite? We need more clinical evidence to answer this question, despite the fact that Scorer and Farrington (144) believe malfunction is the predecessor. They (144) also speculate that cryptorchidism is not a genetic phenomenon.

Growth of the seminiferous tubules in the cryptorchid testis lags behind that of the normal testis after age 5 years

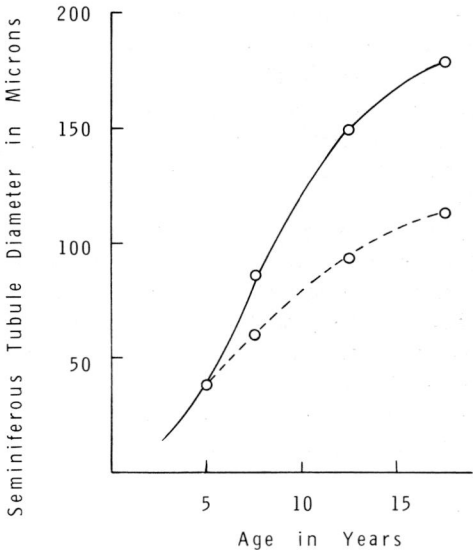

Figure 20.26. Diameter of seminiferous tubules from testes of boys of various ages. Normally descended testes are indicated by the *solid line*; undescended testes are indicated by the *broken line*. (Data from Robinson JN, Engle ET. Some observations on the cryptorchid testis. J Urol 1954;71:726–734.)

(Fig. 20.26). Spermatogenesis does not occur, but the general appearance of the retained testis is that of the normal testis of a child. Robinson and Engle (145) studied normal and cryptorchid testes and concluded that the retained testes fail to develop past the stage reached by the normal testes of boys between ages 6 and 10 years. The diameter of the seminiferous tubules reaches only 63% of the normal at age 16 years and older. As puberty progresses, there is continued degeneration of the retained testis, with little evidence that the stage of sperm formation is ever reached (Fig. 20.27). If the cryptorchid testis is not inherently abnormal, it becomes so before puberty. Robinson and Engle (145) found one normal

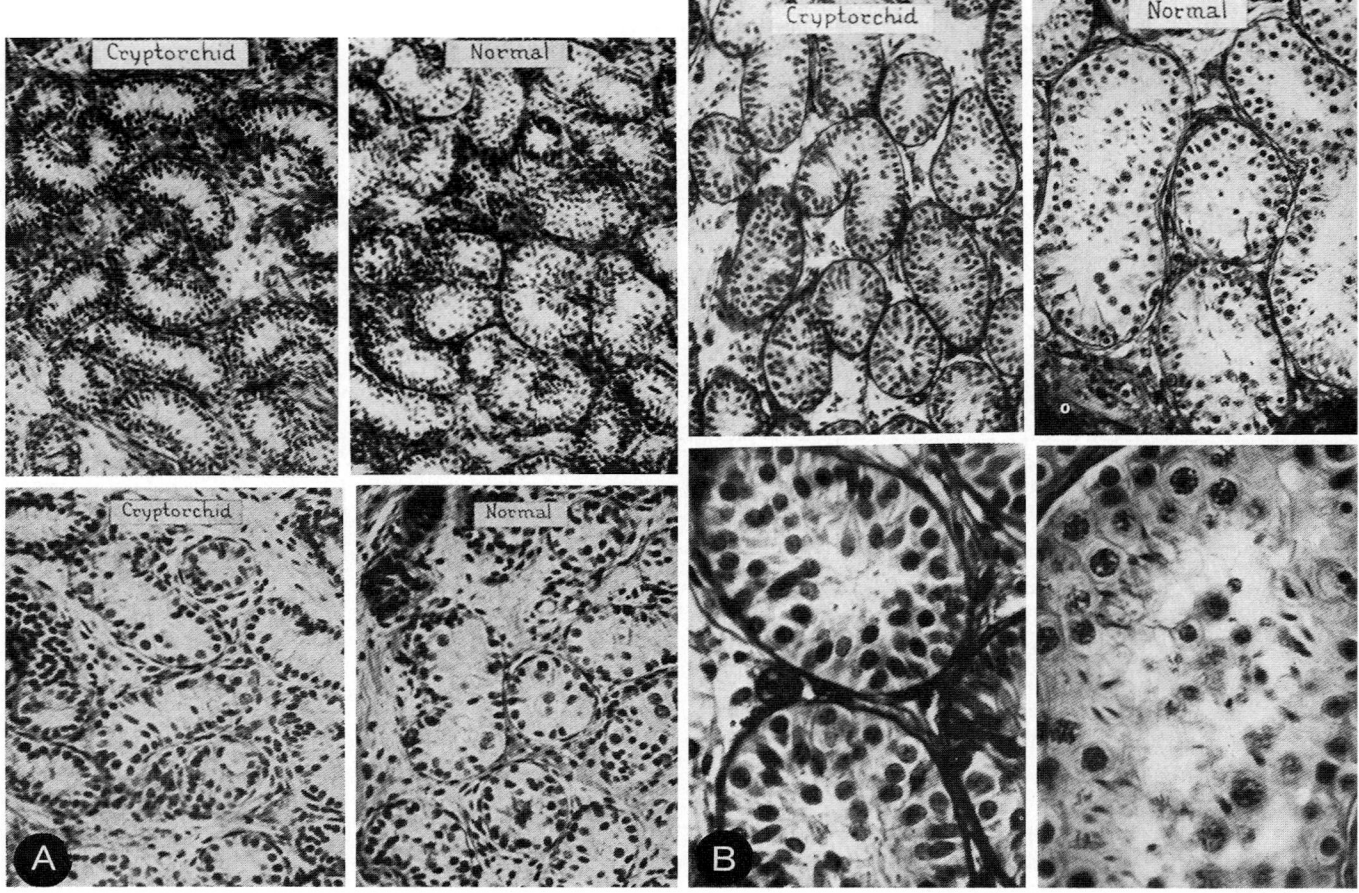

Figure 20.27. **A,** Microscopic appearance of the cryptorchid testis and the contralateral normal testis from two 5-year-old patients. Little if any difference between the cryptorchid and the normal testis can be observed. **B,** Microscopic appearance of cryptorchid and normal testis from a 15-year-old patient. The dif-

ference in tubular size is obvious at low magnification *(above)* and the absence of sperm on the cryptorchid side may be at seen higher magnification *(below).* (From Robinson JN, Engle ET. Some observations on the cryptorchid testis. J Urol 1954;71:726–734.)

testis among 20 organs 9 years after they were brought down surgically in late childhood.

Endocrine function of undescended testes remains unimpaired even when spermatogenesis is absent. There has been one report of reduced hormone activity (146), but physiologic (endocrine) deficiency does not occur even in bilateral cryptorchidism.

The ductus deferens is long enough to permit descent, so that it appears redundant for the testis in the abdomen or inguinal canal. The blood vessels, on the contrary, are only long enough to reach the testis at its actual location; in these there is no redundancy. The means by which the spermatic artery may effectively be lengthened so that the testis may lie in the scrotum was developed by Gross (77). The principle is illustrated in Figure 20.28 (147).

Over 50 years ago, MacCollum (148) reported that 80% of patients with corrected bilateral cryptorchidism were fertile. In spite of other equally good results (149), the prognosis today is much more conservative. There is little evidence that a change in location will arrest or

reverse the processes of deterioration. Testes brought into the scrotum by surgery in patients after 5 years of age develop little better than do testes left in the undescended state (150, 151). It is possible that the prognosis varies with the specific cause of maldescent, but this has not been proved. It is reasonable to believe that a testis blocked mechanically might be capable of normal functioning if helped surgically in its descent, whereas an abdominal testis which had not begun to descend spontaneously might never function normally. Whether the retained testis is abnormal or not, there is no conceivable profit in delaying surgical intervention after the age of 5 years.

The other, descended testis of patients with one undescended testis has usually been considered to be normal; hence, unilateral cryptorchidism should not impair fertility. Scott (152) suggested that even the descended testis in such patients may not be normal. He found azoospermia or subfertile sperm counts among 24 of 34 patients with untreated unilateral cryptorchidism. However, since

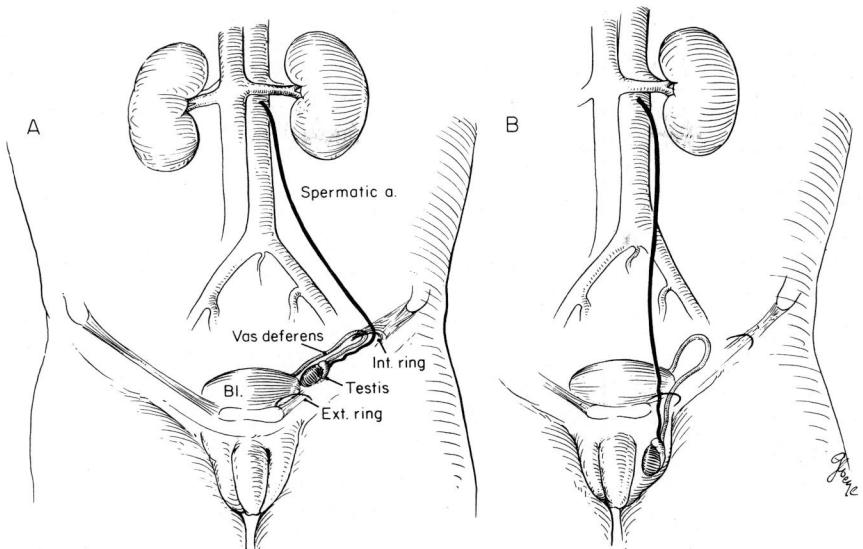

Figure 20.28. Procedure for releasing the effective length of the spermatic artery to the undescended testis. **A,** The course of the artery before surgery. **B,** The internal inguinal ring has been transported medially, and the spermatic artery will not permit testis to be placed in the scrotum. (From Fonkalsrud EW. Current concepts in the management of the undescended testis. Surg Clin North Am 1970;50:847–852.)

these were patients attending a subfertility clinic, the evidence was only suggestive. Subsequently, Hecker and Hienz (153) reported normal development and maturation in only 33% of normally descended testes of a series of patients with unilateral undescended testes.

History. Although inguinal hernia has been known and treated since antiquity, the associated undescended testis received little attention until Hunter described the normal descent of the testis from the dissection of fetuses in 1756 (143). Hunter first proposed the view that the testis was undescended because it was defective and that surgical placement of the testis in the scrotum would not restore function. This view, with modifications, persists today.

The alternative view, that the undescended testis might function normally if brought into the scrotum, became popular around the turn of the century. This theory, which was proposed by Eccles (154) as early as 1902, stimulated surgical efforts to place the undescended testis in the scrotum. Although attempts to accomplish this began in 1820 (155), the credit for designing the modern operation belongs to Bevan (156) in 1903 and Torek in 1909 (157).

Incidence. Testes usually are descended at birth, but the proportion increases markedly with birth weight. Scorer (43, 158, 159) found complete descent in almost all infants with a birth weight of over 8 lb. Testes were undescended in 21% of 300 premature infants and in 2.7% of 3312 full-term infants (Fig. 20.29).

Of infants with testes undescended at birth, descent takes place within the first month in 56% of those born prematurely and in 50% of those born at term. By the end

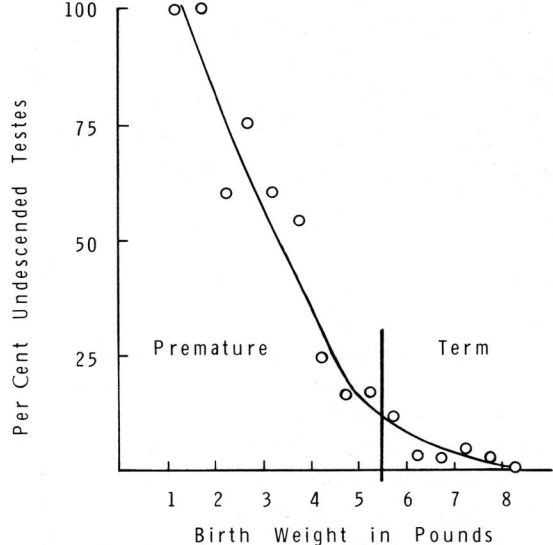

Figure 20.29. The frequency of undescended testes by birth weight of infant. (Data from study of 1642 infants by Scorer. Reported in Scorer CG. The incidence of incomplete descent of the testicle at birth. Arch Dis Child 1956;31:198–202.)

of the first year of life only 0.8% of infants have testes still undescended (159).

The question of testicular descent during childhood has still not been satisfactorily settled. Johnson (160) reported that, of 544 testes undescended by age 7 years, 300 descended later, the majority between the ages of 11 and 13 years. These figures are open to question in view of the known frequency with which the cremaster muscle retracts the testes in young boys. This undoubtedly accounts for the increase in reported cryptorchidism in schoolboys, compared with that found in younger boys and in boys at puberty. Ward and Hunter (161) found about twice as many apparently undescended testes among 8-year-old boys than among 5-year-old boys. In older boys, the frequency declined again. From such figures, one concludes that this descent at puberty is apparent rather than real (158).

The incidence of undescended testes in young adults is better known as a result of the large numbers of military recruits who have been examined. Campbell (133) collected the records of 12,535,824 men examined for U.S., British, French, and Austrian armies from 1828 to 1947 and found an incidence of undescended testes of 0.28%, with a range of 0.11 to 0.52%. The higher figures are for drafted recruits and are probably more nearly correct than are the lower figures, which apply to older, volunteer, and professional armies.

At birth, nearly twice as many right testes as left are undescended (1.8:1); in the young adult, the ratio has shifted so that fewer right than left testes are undescended (0.6:1). Among premature infants, testicular retention is more often bilateral than unilateral; among full-term infants, about 25% are bilateral; whereas among adults, only 20% or fewer are bilateral.

Symptoms. Absence of one or both testes in the scrotum, with an undeveloped appearance of the latter, requires a search for the missing organ.

Torsion of the undescended testicle was reported by Hand (162) and by Riegler (163).

Diagnosis. *Retraction of the testis* by cremasteric reflex is the commonest cause of absence of the testes from the scrotum in boys. Parents should be queried and previous examination records consulted to determine if the testis was ever present in the scrotum. Warming of the examiner's hands before any attempt at palpation is made will eliminate many cases of cremasteric retraction! Retracted testes return to the scrotum and will eventually remain there as the patient becomes older.

Sonographic studies and CT should be done. If in doubt, selective arteriography or venography should be performed. Plasma testosterone determination is another method to indicate the presence or absence of active Leydig cells. The best test, however, is diagnostic laparoscopy or exploration with the hope that the anomaly may be corrected. Also, IVP to rule out renal anomalies is a must.

Testicular ectopia (Fig. 20.30) should be considered in the differential diagnosis, the perineum should be examined; and in unilateral cases, the normal scrotal half should be palpated.

Also, anomalies of the epididymis and vas should be evaluated in the operating room. Fertility will not take place with these types of anomalies.

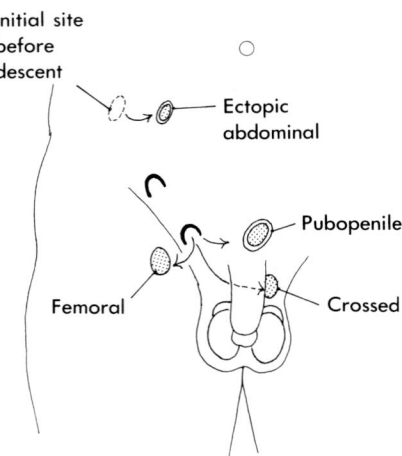

Figure 20.30. Sites of testicular ectopia. Perineal ectopia is not shown. All of these ectopias are rare.

Pseudohermaphroditism also should be considered in bilateral cryptorchidism or if any other unusual genital finding is present.

True congenital absence (page 748) of the testis cannot be distinguished from abdominal retention without surgical exploration or laparoscopy.

Even if no testis can be palpated at the external ring or in the inguinal canal, the diagnosis should be reserved until findings have been negative after several examinations at different times. The presence of any easily reducible hernia suggests that the testis is still in the abdomen.

Treatment. Surgical correction of undescended testes almost always involves repair of an indirect inguinal hernia as well. The objectives of treatment are:

1. Preservation of testicular function
2. Cosmetic improvement
3. Removal of risk of trauma to partially descended or ectopic testes
4. Perhaps lessening the risk of malignant change in the retained testis (making self-examination possible)
5. Repair of the associated inguinal hernia

In the past, it was thought that every opportunity should be given for the testis to descend normally and that no harm resulted from the testicular retention until puberty, unless the associated hernia demanded earlier surgical intervention. This viewpoint can no longer be defended.

Studies of testicular histology (145, 164, 165) argue strongly against the policy of "watchful waiting." There is little doubt that, if there is a functional testis, its preservation requires early treatment. If the testis is brought down before the patient reaches the age of 5 years, it may be functional; if it brought down later, it will almost certainly be nonfunctional. After the patient reaches the age of 5 years, surgery must be considered for cosmetic effect or for the prevention of possible future malignancy. "Late spontaneous testicular descent is therefore neither to be expected nor desired" (166). Most surgeons now perform orchiopexy when the patient is between the ages of 1 and 2 years.

Knowledge of the blood supply of the testicle is a must for a successful orchiopexy.

Figure 20.31 presents the anastomosis of the three arteries of the spermatic cord which are "co-responsible" (if the term is permissible) for the blood supply of the testes.

Salman and Fønkalsrud (167) found that division of the main spermatic artery in rats produced testicular atrophy with spermatogenic arrest and interstitial cell dysfunction. Although collateral blood flow to the testes was demonstrated, tissue perfusion was inadequate for normal spermatogenesis and endocrine function.

Huang et al. (168) reported the effects of temporary and permanent arterial, venous, and arteriovenous ischemia of the testes of young rats using histologic and enzymatic criteria of testicular injury. The authors stated that the damage was severe with either venous or arterial obstruction, and recommended rapid relief in cases of incarcerated inguinal herniae and careful detorsion in cases of testicular torsion.

Kelly et al. (169), experimenting with rats, studied the effects of Fowler-Stephens orchiopexy (FSO) on fertility in males, using the following:

1. Fowler-Stevens orchiopexy (FSO)
2. Fowler-Stevens orchiopexy and concurrent contralateral orchiectomy (FSO/OR)
3. Unilateral orchiectomy (OR)
4. Sham operation (control group)

The above authors reported the following:

1. No pregnancy from FSO/OR males
2. 81% pregnancy rate reported in the FSO group
3. 64% pregnancy rate reported in the OR group
4. 92% pregnancy rate in the control group
5. No fertility in the FSO/OR group
6. 86% male fertility reported in the unilateral orchioectomies
7. Ligation of the spermatic artery and vein for orchiopexy facilitation often is followed by ispilateral sterility

MALDESCENDED TESTES

Ectopic Sites (Fig. 20.30)

Perineal Ectopia.

An ectopic perineal testis will be found lateral to the raphe, anterior to the anus, and posterior to the root of the scrotum. It is freely movable, in contrast to a traumatically produced perineal testis, which has formed adhesions. A congenital perineal testis may be atrophic in an adult, but is usually normal in a child (75). No other

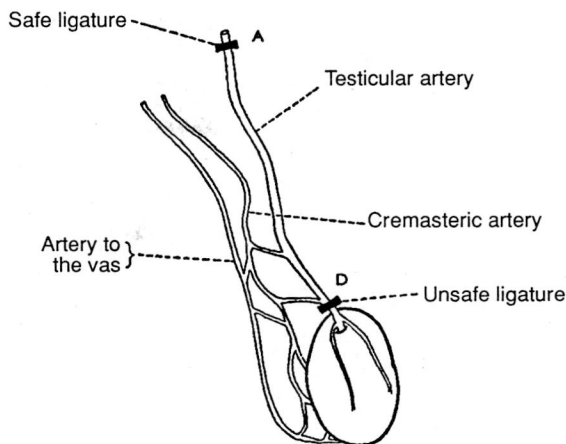

Figure 20.31. The anastomoses of the testicular artery. Ligature of testicular artery at A conserves the blood supply to the testis. Ligature at D imperils this supply. (From Fowler R, Stevens FD. The role of testicular vascular anatomy in the salvage of high undescended testes. Aust NZ Surg 1959;29:92–106.)

Table 20.10.
Review of Cases of Penopubic and Penile Testes[a]

Investigator	Patient Age	Side	Location
Popow	Postpubertal	Left	Penopubic
Poupart	20	Left	Penopubic
Moynihan	Unknown	Left	Penopubic
Forsyth	30	Unknown	Penopubic
Bernhard	24	Left	Penopubic
Kaufman	21	Right	Penopubic
Raspall	5	Right	Penile
Collins	16	Left	Penopubic
	25	Right	Penile
Campbell	10	Bilateral	Penopubic
Albin	12	Left	Penile
Middleton	3	Right	Penile
Concodora	18	Right	Penopubic
McLoughlin	45	Right	Penopubic
Redman	7	Left	Penopubic

[a]From Redman JF, Golladay ES. Penopubic and penile testicular ectopia. South Med J 1991; 84(4): 535–536.

anomalies are associated with the condition. At least one bilateral case has been reported (170).

Coplan and his colleagues (171) collected 112 cases from the literature up to 1952, starting with Hunter's (143) case in 1786. The incidence has been placed as high as 2% of imperfectly descended testes (172).

Treatment requires freeing the gubernaculum from the perineal skin and transferring the testis to the scrotum. The first reported attempt at correction of the condition (173) ended fatally; the first successful operation was reported in 1879 (174).

Pubopenile Ectopia.

Very rarely, a testis comes to rest on the dorsal surface of the penis or over the pubic bone at the base of the penis. Only nine cases were reported by 1959 (175) (Fig. 20.30).

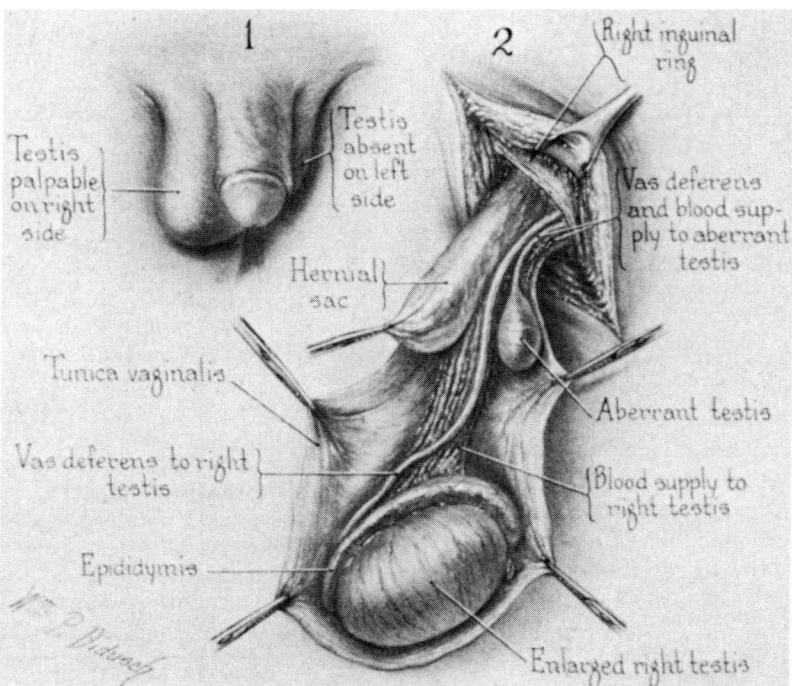

Figure 20.32. Crossed testicular ectopia. The small left testis without an epididymis lay in the right scrotum above the enlarged right testis. The ectopic testis contained a malignant tumor. (From Lowsley OS, Kerwin TJ. Clinical urology, 3rd ed. Baltimore: Williams & Wilkins, 1956.)

Freeing the testis and placing it in the scrotum is all that is required.

According to Redman and Golladay (176), in 1888 Popow (177) reported the first case of penopubic ectopia. Redman reviewed the literature and collected 10 cases of penopubic testicular ectopia and four cases of penile testicular ectopia in 1991 (Table 20.10).

Crossed (Transverse) Ectopia.
In this defect, both testes descend on the same side and lie in the same scrotal compartment (Fig. 20.32). In some cases the ductus deferentia are separate and enter the prostate on opposite sides. In other cases the ductus join above the internal ring and continue as a single tube. In one such case only a single seminal vesicle was present (178).

Kimura (179) suggested that, in cases in which the ductus were fused, one might assume that the two testes arose from the same genital ridge and that true crossing of the testes occurred only where a separate ductus deferens served each testis. While it is not impossible to assume that the primordial germ cells all migrated to the same side of the body and that the genital ridge then formed two distinct gonads, the extreme rarity of two separate anomalies counts against the theory. It assumes that there is a congenital absence of one testis, which is very rare (page 748), associated with a supernumerary testis on the other side, which is equally rare (page 752). The situation does not resemble that of the supernumerary kidney, with

which it has been compared; testicular formation, unlike kidney formation, is not induced by the duct system. We prefer the explanation put forth by Gupta and Das (180) that adherence and fusion of the developing wolffian ducts takes place early in their development and that descent of one testis causes the second testis to follow it. Where the two ductus remain separate, a crossing over appears to have occurred later. In most cases the blood supply is bilateral, but in a single case (181) two testes in the left inguinal canal were supplied by the right spermatic artery.

It is noteworthy that, in two cases quoted by Kimura (179) and in Hertzler's case (182), a rudimentary uterus and tubes were found herniated into the scrotum. This places these patients in the class of masculinized male pseudohermaphrodites (page 860).

A single case of malignancy in a crossed ectopic testis has been reported by Lowsley and Kerwin (183). It was much smaller than a normal testis and had a separate ductus deferens, but no epididymis (Fig. 20.32).

The earliest example of crossed ectopia was found at autopsy in 1845 (184). Hertzler (182) collected 14 cases up to 1916. No recent assembly of cases has been made, but examples have been reported (180, 181, 185). Both sides appear to be affected with equal frequency.

Crossed ectopia may be distinguished from unilateral duplication by the fact that the testes are usually of the same size. Hydrocele or indirect inguinal hernia, together

Highly Diagramatic Drawing of the Three Anchors

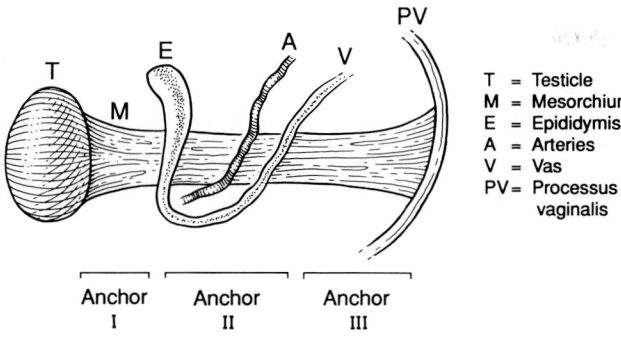

Figure 20.33.   Highly diagramatic drawing of the three anchors.

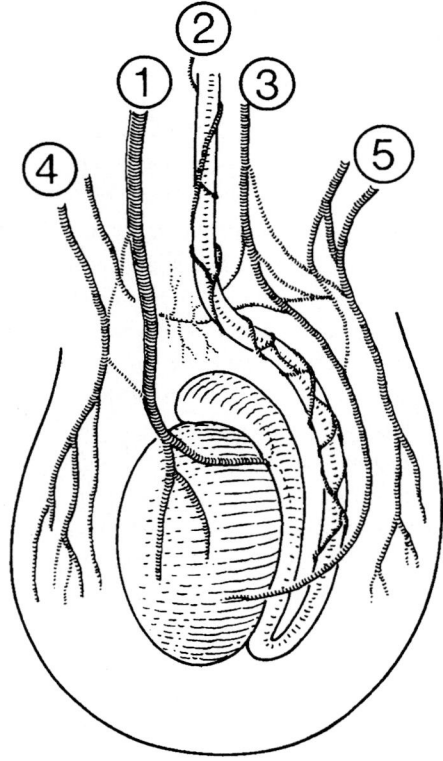

Figure 20.34.   The arterial supply of the testis and epididymis. The testicular artery is the chief source of blood to the testis, but four other arteries anastomose with the testicular artery and each other to form a collateral circulation. *1*, Testicular artery; *2*, deferential artery; *3*, cremasteric artery; *4*, posterior artery; *5*, anterior artery hanging from the vessels. Here the arteries are only demonstrated. (From Skandalakis JE, Gray SW, Rowe JS Jr. Anatomical Complications in General Surgery. New York: McGraw-Hill, 1983.)

with contralateral undescended testis, is the usual incorrect diagnosis.

Other Ectopic Sites.
Interstitial ectopia occurs when the testis lies external to the aponeurosis of the external oblique muscle.

Crural or femoral ectopia has been reported (186), in which both testes failed to enter internal inguinal ring and lay in the lower part of the pelvis, on either side of the rectum.

Lowsley and Kerwin (183) reported a case in which the left testis lay at the hilum of the kidney below the renal vessels. This is reminiscent of the position of the testis in some cases of complete absence of the kidney.

Prognosis. Maldescent, as opposed to nondescent, is more favorable to future testicular function. The ectopic testis may be a normal organ that has been deflected from its natural pathway by an anatomic peculiarity; it is more likely to function normally.

Testicular Torsion

ANATOMY OF TESTICULAR TORSION

The normal scrotal testicle is anchored by two bands of tissue, one to the epididymis and the other connecting the epididymis to the vas and to the posterior lateral wall of the processus vaginalis. The absence of a proper and sound fixation or anchoring of the testis to the epididymis (in other words, the mesorchium-thin peritoneal fold is long or absent, a rare form of torsion) and an epididymis that is also not well fixed with the processus vaginalis (a very common cause of torsion) is a predisposing anatomic etiology of testicular torsion. One or both of these "loose" fixations may be enough for the production of this clinical entity. In such a case the testicle hangs onto the processus vaginalis by three anatomic structures: *(a)* the covering of the cord, *(b)* the vas, and *(c)* the vessels (Fig. 20.33).

Additional predisposing factors for testicular torsion are the undescended testicle and the so-called superiorly inverted testicle when the epididymis is fixed to the posterior border of a testis tipped forward and the upper and lower pole are located in a transverse (horizontal) line, rather than vertical (Fig. 20.34).

Another rare congenital anomaly involving the testicle is splenogonadal fusion (see Chapter 10, "The Spleen.")

Ovarian Ectopia and Inguinal Hernia in the Female

ANATOMY

In 1941, Mayer and Templeton, attempting to classify inguinal defects in the female, proposed the term *ovarian hernia* for the presence of the ovary only (i.e., not of other associated structures) in the inguinal canal or the labium. This, they believed, corresponded to the descent of the testicle in the male. When the herniated ovary was accompanied by the uterine tube, and sometimes by the uterus as well, they preferred the term *ovarian ectopia.*

While this distinction has a sound embryologic basis, it is not easy to apply it in practice because, if the descended ovary remains undetected for a long period of time, other abdominal organs are likely to herniate. It is significant that, in reviewing the literature, Mayer and Templeton (187) found 57 questionable and 138 acceptable cases.

EMBRYOGENESIS

Herniation of the ovary is homologous to normal descent of the testis. Failure of the ovarian gubernaculum to unite with the uterus probably permits subsequent shortening, with descent of the ovary. A temporary hormone imbalance may be involved, but this has not been demonstrated.

Perhaps one should postulate that the same theories for the descent of the testis may be apply to the ovaries.

HISTORY

The earliest cases attracted attention because of pregnancy in the herniated uterus. In 1531 Pol performed a cesarean section on a pregnant patient with a right inguinal herniated uterus (188). The second example was reported by Doringius in 1778; the hernia was femoral rather than inguinal (189). Andrews (189) was able to collect 76 reported cases of herniation of the uterus, 46 cases of herniation of the uterine tube, and 82 cases of herniation of tube and ovary. He found 167 cases in which hernia of the ovary alone was mentioned but believed that, in many of these, the presence of the tube might have been overlooked.

INCIDENCE

Among 50 inguinal uterine herniae in Andrew's (189) series, 5 were acquired, 33 were definitely congenital, and the remainder were of uncertain origin. The two sides were equally involved, and in six patients the lesion was bilateral.

Uterine or vaginal anomalies were present in about 50% of Andrew's (189) collected cases. In seven, one horn of a unicornuate uterus was herniated. Fewer anomalies are found when the tube and ovary are only herniated.

Malposition of the ovaries associated with uterine anomalies was reported by Rock et al. (190).

SYMPTOMS

A mass in the inguinal canal or the labium indicates the presence of a hernia. In many cases medical advice is not sought until pregnancy occurs. In about 20% of affected patients, torsion and strangulation of the herniated ovary or tube takes place.

DIAGNOSIS

Vaginal examination will detect the lateral displacement of the uterus. The possibility of a bicornuate uterus with herniation of one horn must be kept in mind. Rectal examination will reveal a band-like structure passing from the uterus to the inguinal canal. This will be the ectopic uterine tube. In the absence of these vaginal and rectal findings, omentum or intestine, rather than reproductive organs, are in the canal. An irreducible mass without symptoms of strangulation suggests a cyst of the canal of Nuck.

Sonogram or CT scan occasionally is indicated for the diagnosis of ovarian ectopia. Dynamic γ-camera scintigraphy helps distinguish the normal ovaries medially from the large iliac vessels; they appear as a clear, oval, homogeneous accumulation of radionuclide, as reported by Peshev et al. (89).

TREATMENT

Simple reduction of the hernia and closure of the canal is the procedure of choice.

EDITORIAL COMMENTS

Problems related to maldescent of the testis constitute some of the more common problems seen in a pediatric surgical practice. Congenital abnormalities of testicular descent should first be divided into those testes that are undescended but remain palpable and those that are nonpalpable. Of palpable testes thought to be cryptorchid, there will be a subset of merely retractile testes that do not impair eventual fertility and should be considered a normal variant. Ectopic testes somehow leave the normal path of descent but remain palpable, and may reside in the superficial inguinal pouch (Denis-Browne's pouch), the perineum, the femoral canal, or the penopubic area. An interesting variant of this group is the ascended testis, which is found is boys who, on initial evaluation, appear to have testes that can be mobilized into the scrotum and remain there for a reasonable interval, but who later present for reexamination because the testis is no longer in the scrotum. Evaluation at this time reveals that the testis indeed will not stay in the scrotum on manipulation. This condition does not respond to gonadotropin administration, and surgery is necessary. The truly cryptorchid testis has never resided in the scrotum, may be palpable or nonpalpable, and invariably requires operative intervention.

There are two main potentially harmful effects of the cryptorchid state—increased potential for tumor formation, and impaired spermatogenesis with resultant infertility. Clearly there is an increased incidence of testicular cancer in men whose cryptorchidism is untreated prior to puberty. The relative increased risk is based on the observation that cryptorchid testes account for 7.3% of testis tumors, while the estimated incidence of cryptorchidism at 1 year of age is 0.8%. Thus, cryptorchid patients are overrepresented ten-fold. Orchiopexy after puberty does not decrease this risk, whereas there is some suggestion that early (prior to 24 months age) surgery may be beneficial.

Controversy exists as to whether early orchiopexy will give better fertility results when compared to similar surgery performed later but still prepuberty. What is clear is that interstitial fibrosis in undescended testes is progressive after 2 years of life, and orchiopexy before this time is beneficial in preventing this change. The only clinical data that support the importance of early orchiopexy with regard to infertility comes from Ludwig and Potepma (191) who, in a limited number of patients, have documented a definite decrease in fertility potential as the age at which orchiopexy is carried out increases.

Based on available data, one must conclude that (a) most cryptorchid testes that are repaired beyond the first few years of life produce little or no sperm; (b) in spite of reduced sperm counts, most men with unilateral cryptorchidism are fertile; and (c) men with bilaterally undescended testes have poor fertility prognosis. The surgeon who must make decisions regarding timing of orchiopexy must take all of these points into consideration (TSP).

REFERENCES

1. Gillman J. The development of the gonads in man, with a consideration of the role of fetal endocrines and the histogenesis of ovarian tumors. Contrib Embryol Carnegie Inst Wash 1948;32:83–131.
2. Pinkerton JHM, McKay DG, Adams EC, Hertig AT. Development of the human ovary: a study using histochemical techniques. Obstet Gynecol 1961;18:152–181.
3. van Wagenen G, Simpson ME. Embryology of the ovary and testis in *Homo sapiens* and *Macaca mulatta*. New Haven, CT: Yale University Press, 1965.
4. Picheral B. Capacités des noyaux cellules endodermiques embryonnaires à organiser un germe viable chez l'urodèle, Pleurodeles waltlii Michac. C R Acad Sci (Paris) 1962;255:2509–2511.
5. Witschi E. Hormones and embryonic induction. Arch Anat Microsc Morphol Exp 1965;54:601–611.
6. Jirasek JE. Die Verteilung der Urgeschlechtzellen in den Keimdrüsen menschlicherg Feten. Eine histoenzymologische Studie. Acta Histochem (Jena) 1962;13:220–225.
7. McKay DG, Pinkerton JMH, Hertig AT, Danzinger S. The adult human ovary: a histochemical study. Obstet Gynecol 1961;18:13–39.
8. Füss A. Ueber extraregionäre Geschlechtszellen bei einem menschlichen Embryo von 4 Wochen. Anat Anz 1911;39:407–409.
9. Füss A. Ueber die Geschlechtszellen des Menschen und der Säugetiere. Arch Mikr Anat 1912;81(2 Abt):1–23.
10. Felix W. The development of the urinogenital organs. In: Keibel F and Mall FP, eds. Manual of Human Embryology. Philadelphia: JB Lippincott, 1912.
11. Waldeyer W. Eierstock und Ei. Leipzig, 1870.
12. Stieve H. Die Entwicklung der Keimzellen und der Zwischenzellen in der Hodenanlage des Menschen. Z Mikr Anat Forsh 1927;10:225–285.
13. Humphrey RR. Extirpation of the primordial germ cells of *amblystoma;* its effect upon development of gonad. J Exp Zool 1927;49:363.
14. Dantschakoff W. Les cellules genitales et leur continuité. Rev Gen Sci Pures Appl 1932;43:295.
15. Willier BH. Experimentally produced sterile gonads and the problem of the origin of germ cells in the chick embryo. Anat Rec 1937;70:89–112.
16. Martinovitch PN. The development *in vitro* of the mammalian gonad, ovary and ovogenesis. Proc R Soc Biol 1938;125:232–249.
17. Chiquoine AD. The identification, origin and migration of primordial germ cells in the mouse embryo. Anat Rec 1954;118:135–146.
18. Mancini RE, Narbaitz R, Lavieri JC. Origin and development of the germinal epithelium and Sertoli cells in the human testis. Anat Rec 1960;136:477–490.
19. Gipouloux JD. Les tissues mésodermiques dorsaux exercent—ils une action attractive sur les gonocytes primordiaux situés dans l'endoderme, chez l'embryon du Crapaud commun Bufo bufo L. (Amphibien anoure)? C R Acad Sci (Paris) 1962;255:2179–2181.
20. Gipouloux JD. Influence de la corde dorsale et des uretères primaires sur l'édification des crêtes génitales et la migration des gonocytes primordiaux: démonstration expérimentale sur le Crapaud commun (Bufo bufo L). C R Acad Sci (Paris) 1963;257:1150–1152.
21. King DR. Ovarian cysts and tumors. In: Welch KJ et al., eds. Pediatric surgery. Chicago: Year Book, 1986:1347.
22. Mintz B. Embryological phases of mammalian gametogenesis. J Cell Comp Physiol 1960;56(Supp):31–48.
23. Witschi E. Genes and inductors of sex differentiation in amphibians. Biol Rev 1934;9:460–488.
24. Willier BH. Potencies of the gonad-forming area in the chick as tested in chorio-allantoic grafts. Arch Entw Roux Arch 1933;130:616–649.
25. Gipouloux JD. Une substance diffusible émanée des organes mésodermiques dorsaux attire les cellules germinales situées dans l'endoderm. C R Acad Sci (Paris) 1964;259:3844–3847.
26. Dubois R. Sur l'attraction exercée par le jeune épithélium germinatif sur les gonocytes de l'embryon de poulet en culture in vitro. C R Acad Sci (Paris) 1965;260:5885–5887.
27. Witschi E. Hormones and embryonic induction. Arch Anat Microsc Morphol Exp 1965;54:601–611.
28. Friedman NB, Van de Velde RL. Germ cell tumors in man, pleiotropic mice and continuity of germplasm and somatoplasm. Hum Pathol 1981;12:772–776.
29. Gillman J. The development of the gonads in man, with a consideration of the role of fetal endocrines and the histogenesis of ovarian tumors. Contrib Embryol Carnegie Inst Wash 1948;32:83–131.
30. Mittwoch U. How does the Y chromosome affect gonadal differentiation? Philos Trans R Soc Lond (Biol) 1970;259:113–117.
31. Silvers WK, Wachtel SS. H-Y antigen: behavior and function. Science 1977;195:956–960.
32. Ohno S. The role of H-Y antigen in primary sex determination. JAMA 1978;239:217–220.
33. Silvers WK, Gasser DL, Eicher EM. H-Y antigen, serologically detectable male antigen and sex determination. Cell 1982;28:439–440.
34. Sadler TW. Langman's medical embryology, 6th ed. Baltimore: Williams & Wilkins, 1990:273, 278.
35. George FW, Wilson JD. Sex determination and differentiation. In Knobil E et al., eds. The physiology of reproduction. New York: Raven Press, 1988:3–26.
36. Kitahara Y. Ueber die Entstehung der Zwischenzellen der Keimdrüsen des Menschen und der Säugetiere und über deren physiologische Bedeutung. Arch Entw Organ 1923;52:550–615.
37. Eberth CJ. Die mannlichen Geschlechtsorgane. Bardeleben's Hndbk Anat Mensch (Jena) 1904;7:1–310.
38. Wells LJ. Descent of the testes: anatomical and hormonal considerations. Surgery 1943;14:436–472.
39. Wyndham NR. A morphological study of testicular descent. J Anat 1943;77:179–188.
40. Lemeh CN. A study of the development and structural relation-

ships of the testis and gubernaculum. Surg Gynec Obstet 1960;110:164–172.

41. Lockwood CB. The development and transition of the testicles, normal and abnormal. Br Med J 1887;1:444–446.

42. Scorer CG. The anatomy of testicular descent, normal and incomplete. Br J Surg 1962;49:357–367.

43. Scorer CG. The incidence of incomplete descent of the testicle at birth. Arch Dis Child 1956;31:198–202.

44. Shapiro B. Kann man mit Hypophysenvorderlappen den unterentwickelten männlichen Genitalapparat bein Menschen zum Wachstum Anregen? Deutsch Med Wschr 1930;56:1605.

45. Engle ET. Experimentally induced descent of the testis in the Macacus monkey by hormone from the anterior pituitary and pregnancy urine. Endocrinology 1932;16:513–520.

46. Martins T. Mechanism of descent of testicle under action of sex hormones. In: Essays in Biology in Honor of Herbert M. Evans. Berkley: University of California Press, 1943;387–397.

47. Wislocki GB. Observations on descent of testes in macaque and in chimpanzee. Anat Rec 1933;57:133–148.

48. Backhouse KM, Butler H. The gubernaculum testis of the pig (Sus scropha). J Anat 1960;94:107–120.

49. Arey LB. Developmental anatomy, 7th ed. Philadelphia: WB Saunders, 1965.

50. Frey HL, Peng S, Rajfer J. Synergy of abdominal pressure and androgens in testicular descent. Biol Reprod 1983;29:1233–39.

51. Roberts P. Congenital absence of the abdominal muscles with associated abnormalities of the genito-urinary tract. Arch Dis Child 1965;31:236–239.

52. Wilson JD et al. The androgen resistance syndromes: 5a-reductase deficiency, testicular feminization, and related disorders. In: Stanbury JB et al., eds. The metabolic basis of inherited disease, 5th ed. New York: McGraw-Hill, 1983:1001–1026.

53. Sloan WR, Walsh PC. Familial persistent müllerian duct syndrome. J Urol 1976;115:439–61.

54. Blanchard MG, Josso N. Source of the anti-müllerian hormone synthesized by the fetal testis: müllerian-inhibiting activity of fetal bovine Sertoli cells in tissue culture. Pediatr Res 1974;8:968.

55. Jost A. A new look at the mechanisms controlling sex differentiation in mammals. Johns Hopkins Med J 1972;130:38.

56. Scott JE. The Hutson hypothesis: a clinical study. Br J Urol 1987;60(1):74–76.

57. Sheldon CA. Undescended testis and testicular torsion. Surg Clin North Am 1985;65(5):1307.

58. Forbes TR. On the fate of the medullary cords of the human ovary. Contrib Embryol Carnegie Inst Wash 1942;30:9–15.

59. Sauramo H. Histology and function of ovary from embryonic period to fertile age. Acta Obstet Gynecol Scand 1954;33(Supp 2):1–163.

60. Zamboni L, Bezard L, Mauleon P. The role of the mesonephros in the development of the sheep fetal ovary. Ann Biol Anim Biochem Biophys 1979;19:1153–1178.

61. Byskov AG. The anatomy and ultrastructure of the rete system in the fetal mouse ovary. Biol Reprod 1978;19:720–735.

62. Baker TG. A quantitative and cytological study of germ cells in human ovaries. Proc R Soc [B] 1963;158:417–433.

63. Upadhyay S, Zamboni L. Ectopic germ cells: natural model for the study of germ cell sexual differentiation. Proc Natl Acad Sci USA 1982;79:6584–6588.

64. Decker GAG, du Plessis DJ. Lee McGregor's synopsis of surgical anatomy, 12th ed. Bristol: John Wright & Sons, 1986.

65. Ashley DJB, Mostofi FK. Renal agenesis and dysgenesis. J Urol 1960;83:211–230.

66. Jost A. Recherches sur le contrôle hormonal de l'organogenese sexuelle du lapin et remarques sur certaines malformations de l'appareil génital humain. Gynecol Obstet (Paris) 1950;49:44–60.

67. Tibbs DJ. Unilateral absence of testis: eight cases of true monorchism. Br J Surg 1961;48:601–608.

68. Teter J, Janozewski Z, Wigura A, Melicow MM. Congenital anorchism with anomalous external genitalia: a report of two cases. J Urol 1962;87:964–971.

69. Kawaichi GK, Cooper P, O'Donnell HF. Monorchism: a report of two cases. N Engl J Med 1949;240:334–335.

70. Pearman RO. Congenital absence of the testicle: monorchism. J Urol 1961;85:599–601.

71. Amelar RD. Anorchism without eunuchism. J Urol 1956;76:174–178.

72. Cabrol B. Quoted by Amelar RD. Anorchism without eunuchism. J Urol 1956;76:174–178.

73. Gould GM, Pyle WL. Anomalies and curiosities of medicine. New York: Bell Publishing, 1896:319.

74. Gruber W. Ueber Congenitaler Anorchie beim Menschen. ZKK Gesellsch Aerzte Wien 1878;15:42.

75. Rea CE. The perineal testis. Am Surg 1938;108:1083–1087.

76. Counseller VS, Nichols DR, Smith HL. Congenital absence of testis: a report of seven cases of monorchidism. J Urol 1940;44:237–241.

77. Gross RE. The surgery of infancy and childhood. Philadelphia: WB Saunders, 1953.

78. Burns E, Segaloff A, Carrera GM, Colbert DW. Congenital absence of gonads: report of 2 cases. Trans Am Assoc Genitourin Surg 1962;54:53–58.

79. Campbell M. Undescended testicle and hypospadias. Am J Surg 1951;82:8–17.

80. Mercer S. Agenesis or atrophy of the testis and vas deferens. Can J Surg 1979;22:245–246.

81. Bartkowiak K, Maciejewski J, Rucki T. Agonadyzm u 12-letniego chlopca. Endokr Pol 1964;15:335–338.

82. Raffensperger JG, ed. Swenson's pediatric surgery, 5th ed. New York: Appleton & Lange, 1990.

83. Morgagni JB. The seats and causes of disease investigated by anatomy. Alexander B (transl). New York: Hafner Publishing, 1960.

84. Kurcz JA, Sharp MS. Congenital absence of one ovary associated with contralateral tubal pregnancy. Am J Obstet Gynecol 1948;55:1065–1067.

85. Guizzetti P, Pariset F. Beziehungen zwischen Missbildungen der Nieren und der Geschlechtsorgane. Virchow Arch [A] 1911;204:372–392.

86. Kent BK. Ectopic pregnancy in a congenitally defective tube with absence of the ipsolateral ovary. Am J Obstet Gynecol 1956;72:1150–1151.

87. Hoffenberg R, Jackson WPU. Gonadal dysgenesis in normal-looking females: a genetic theory to explain variability of the syndrome. Br Med J 1957;1:1281–1284, 2:1457–1461.

88. Vasilev D et al. Dynamic gamma-camera excretory scintigraphy in the diagnosis of a rare anomaly in the development of the internal genitalia (the Slotnik-Goldfarb syndrome with uterus unicornis). Akush Ginekol (Sofiia) 1989;28(4):38–40.

89. Peshev N et al. Dynamic gamma-camera scintigraphy as a method for evaluating the function of the ovarian parenchyma. Akush Ginekol (Sofiia) 1989;28(3):39–42.

90. Rock JA, Parmley T, Murphy AA, Jones HW Jr. Malposition of the ovary associated with uterine anomalies. Fertil Steril 1986;45(4):561–563.

91. Darrow RP, Humes JJ. Polyorchidism: a case report. J Urol 1954;72:53–56.

92. Kay S, Coleman FP. Duplication of left undescended testicle. J Urol 1956;75:815–818.

93. Jichlibnski D, Ward-McQuaid N. Duplication of the testis and infertility. J Urol 1963;90:583.

94. Lambrecht W, Babayan R. Polyorchidism. Klin Padiatr 1983;195(6):430–432.

95. Blasius G. Observata anatomica in homine, simia, equo, (etc.): accedunt extraordinaria in homine reperta praxin medicam aeque ac anatomen illustrantia. Amsterdam: Gaasbeeck, 1674.

96. Lane WA. A case of supernumerary testis. Trans Clin Soc Lond 1895;28:59.

97. Angulo R, Caballero L. Polyorchism and cryptorchism: report of a case. J Urol 1957;77:850–852.

98. Butz RE, Croushore JH. Polyorchidism. J Urol 1978;119:289.

99. Rowley WN. Uterine anomaly: duplication of uterus, three tubes and three ovaries. Ann Surg 1948;127:676–680.

100. Wharton LR. Two cases of supernumerary ovary and one of accessory ovary with an analysis of previously reported cases. Am J Obstet Gynecol 1959;78:1101–1119.

101. Winckel F. Lehrbuch der Frauenkrankheiten, 2nd ed. Leipzig: S Hirzel, 1890.

102. Falk E. Über überzählige Eileiter und Eierstöcke (Berlin). Klin Wschr 1891;28:1069–1071.

103. Heller DS, Harpaz N, Breakstone B. Neoplasms arising in ectopic ovaries: a case of Brenner tumor in an accessory ovary. Int J Gynecol Pathol 1990;9(2):185–189.

104. Mercer LJ, Toub DB, Cibils LA. Tumors originating in supernumerary ovaries: a report of two cases. J Reprod Med 1987;32(12):932–934.

105. Bialer MG, Wilson WG, Kelly TE. Apparent Ruvalcaba syndrome with genitourinary abnormalities. Am J Med Genet 1989;33(3):314–317.

106. Grohe F. Ueber den Bau und des Wachsthum des menschlichen Eierstocks, und über einige Krankhafte Störungen desselben. Virchow Arch [A] 1863;26:271–306.

107. Doran A. Pregnancy after removal of both ovaries for cystic tumor. J Obstet Gynaecol Br Commw 1902;2:1–10.

108. Abdel-Dayem HM, Motawi S, Jahan S, Kubasik H. Liver metastasis from embryonal carcinoma of the ovary with complete situs inversus: first reported case and review of literature. Clin Nucl Med 1984;9(10):558–560.

109. Campbell M. Urology, 2nd ed. Vol 1-3. Philadelphia: WB Saunders, 1963.

110. Hanley HG, Hodges RD. The epididymis in male sterility: a preliminary report of microdissection studies. J Urol 1959;82:508–520.

111. Dean AL Jr, Major JW, Ottenheimer EJ. Failure of fusion of the testis and epididymis. J Urol 1952;68:754–758.

112. Gracey M, Campbell P, Noblett H. Atretic vas deferens in cystic fibrosis. N Engl J Med 1969;280:276.

113. Holsclan DS et al. Genital abnormalities in male patients with cystic fibrosis. J Urol 1971;106:568.

114. Young D. Bilateral aplasia of the vas deferens. Br J Surg 1949;36:417.

115. Viidik T, Marshall DG. Direct inguinal hernias in infancy and early childhood. J Pediatr Surg 1980;15:646.

116. Valman HB, France NE. The vas deferens in cystic fibrosis. Lancet 1969;2:566.

117. Anguiano A et al. Congenital bilateral absense of the vas deferens: a primarily genital form of cystic fibrosis. JAMA 1992;267:1794–1797.

118. Gorenstein A, Katz S, Schiller M. Varicocele in children: to treat or not to treat—venographic and manometric studies. Pediatr Surg 1986;21(12):1046.

119. Wilson KM. Origin and development of the rete ovarii and the rete testis in the human embryo. Contrib Embryol Carnegie Inst Wash 1926;17:69–88.

120. Follin E. Organes genitaux: sur les corps de wolf. Arch Gen Med 1851;25:329–330.

121. Lythgoe JP. Failure of fusion of the testis and epididymis. Br J Urol 1961;33:80–81.

122. Badenoch AW. Failure of the urogenital union. Surg Gynecol Obstet 1946;82:471–474.

123. Abell I. Cysts of the testicle. Ann Surg 1936;103:941–948.

124. Browne D. The diagnosis of undescended testicle. Br Med J 1938;2:168–171.

125. Hadziselimovic F, Herzug B. The meaning of the Leydig cell in relation to the etiology of cryptorchidism: an experimental electron-microscopic study. J Pediatr Surg 1976;11:1.

126. Hunter RH. The etiology of congenital inguinal hernia and abnormally placed testes. Br J Surg 1926;14:125–130.

127. Moore NS, Tapper SM. Cryptorchidism: a theory to explain its etiology—modifications in surgical technique. J Urol 1940;43:204–207.

128. Lewis LG. Cryptorchism. J Urol 1948;60:345–356.

129. Levitt SB et al. The impalpable testis: a rational approach to management. J Urol 1978;120:515.

130. Gilbert JB, Hamilton JB. Incidence and nature of tumors in ectopic testes. Surg Gynecol Obstet 1940;71:731–743.

131. Campbell HE. Incidence of malignant growth of the undescended testicle. Arch Surg 1942;44:353–369.

132. Carroll WA. Malignancy in cryptorchidism. J Urol 1949;61:396–404.

133. Campbell HE. The incidence of malignant growth of the undescended testicle: a reply and re-evaluation. J Urol 1959;81:663–668.

134. Griffin JE, Wilson JD. Disorders of the testes and male reproductive tract. In: Wilson JD and Foster DW, eds. Textbook of endocrinology. Philadelphia: WB Saunders, 1985.

135. Fonger JD et al. Testicular tumors in maldescended testes. Can J Surg 1981;24:353–355.

136. Diebold J, Le Blaye O, Le Tourneau A, Marichez P. Intrascrotal supernumerary spleen: a long silent case of discontinuous splenogonadal fusion. Ann Pathol 1990;10(3):174–176.

137. Vranjesevic D, Jovic N, Brankovic S. Case report of a boy with Prader-Willi syndrome and focal epilepsy. Srp Arh Celok Lek 1989;117(5–6):351–359.

138. Meinecke P, Menzel J, Froster-Iskenius U. Knee pterygium syndrome in a newborn infant. Monatsschr Kinderheilkd 1989;137(4):228–230.

139. Morris CA, Palumbos JC, Carey JC. Delineation of the male phenotype in craniofrontonasal syndrome. Am J Med Genet 1987;27(3):623–631.

140. Coupris L, Bondonny JM. The accessory scrotum: apropos of 2 cases. Chir Pediatr 1987;28(1):61–63.

141. Fonkalsrud EW. Undescended testes. In: Welch KJ et al., eds. Pediatric surgery. Chicago: Year Book Medical Publishers, 1986.

142. Connolly NK. Maldescent of the testis. Am Surg 1959;25:405–420.

143. Hunter J. In: Palmer JF, ed. Works of John Hunter (1786), Vol 4. London: Longman, 1839.

144. Scorer CG, Farrington GH. Congenital anomalies of the testes: cryptorchidism, testicular torsion and inguinal hernia and hydrocele. In: Harrison JH et al., eds. Campbell's urology, 4th ed. Philadelphia: WB Saunders, 1979:1549–1565.

145. Robinson JN, Engle ET. Some observations on the cryptorchid testis. J Urol 1954;71:726–734.

146. Engberg H. Investigations on the endocrine function of the testicle in cryptorchidism. Proc R Soc Med 1949;42:652–658.

147. Fonkalsrud EW. Current concepts in the management of the undescended testis. Surg Clin North Am 1970;50:847–852.

148. MacCollum DW. Clinical study of the spermatogenesis of undescended testicles. Arch Surg 1935;31:290–300.

149. Gross RE, Jewett TC Jr. Surgical experiences from 1222 operations for undescended testis. JAMA 1956;160:634–641.

150. Charney CW, Conston AS, Meranze DR. Testicular developmental histology. Ann NY Acad Sci 1952;55:597–608.

Page 772

151. Charney CW. The spermatogenic potential of the undescended testes before and after treatment. J Urol 1960;83:697–705.
152. Scott LS. Unilateral cryptorchidism: subsequent effects on fertility. J Reprod Fertil 1961;2:54–60.
153. Hecker WC, Hienz HA. Cryptorchidism and fertility. J Pediatr Surg 1967;2:513–517.
154. Eccles WM. Anatomy, physiology and pathology of the imperfectly descended testis. Br Med J 1902;1:503–505, 570–578.
155. Wershrub LP. The human testis: a clinical treatise. Springfield, IL: Charles C Thomas, 1962.
156. Bevan AD. Surgical treatment of undescended testicle: further contribution. JAMA 1903;41:718–724.
157. Torek F. Orchiopexy for undescended testicle. Ann Surg 1931;94:97–110.
158. Scorer CG. Undescended testicle. Br Med J 1960;1:1359.
159. Scorer CG. The descent of the testis. Arch Dis Child 1964;39:605–609.
160. Johnson WW. Cryptorchidism. JAMA 1939;113:25–27.
161. Ward B, Hunter WA. The absent testicle: a report on a survey carried out among schoolboys in Nottingham. Br Med J 1960;1:1110–1111.
162. Hand JR. Treatment of undescended testis and its complications. JAMA 1985;164:1185.
163. Riegler HC. Torsion of intra-abdominal testis. Surg Clin North Am 1972;52:371.
164. Pappalepore N, Belloli GP. Studio istopathologico del testicolo ectopico. I. Concetti fondamentali sui quadri istologici del testicolo normalmente desceso, dal periodo prenatale alla puberta. Chirurgia 1962;147–172.
165. Cohn BD. Histology of the cryptorchid testis. Surgery 1967;62:536–541.
166. Johnston JH. The undescended testis. Arch Dis Child 1965;40:113–122.
167. Salman ET, Fønkalsrud EW. Effects of the spermatic vascular division for correction of the high undescended testis on testicular function. Am J Surg 1990;160:506–510.
168. Huang EJ et al. Deleterious venous occlusion in young rats. Surg Gynecol Obstet 1990;171:382–387.
169. Kelly RE Jr, Phillips JD, Fonkalsrud EW, Dindar H. Fertility after simulated Fowler-Stephens orchiopexy in rats. Am J Surg 1992;163:270–272.
170. Lucas RC. Case of displacement of both testicles in perineo. Rep Soc Study Dis Child 1902;2:274.
171. Coplan MM, Woods FM, Melvin PB. The perineal testis. South Med J 1957;50:1338–1346.
172. Jones AE, Lieberthal F. Perineal testicle. J Urol 1938;40:658–665.
173. Curling TB. A practical treatise on the diseases of the testis, and of the spermatic cord and scrotum. Philadelphia: Blanchard & Lea, 1856.
174. Annandale T. Case in which a testicle congenitally displaced into the perinaeum was successfully transplanted to the scrotum. Br Med J 1879;1:7.
175. Collins CD. Two cases of pubopenile testis. Br Med J 1959;2:225.
176. Redman JF, Golladay ES. Penopubic and penile testicular ectopia. South Med J 1991;84(4):535–536.
177. Popow W. Ectopic testiculature peno-pubienne anterieure. Bull Soc Anat Paris 1888;63:655.
178. Marsh F. Two testicles on one side. Br Med J 1911;2:1354.
179. Kimura T. Transverse ectopy of the testis, with masculine uterus. Ann Surg 1918;68:420–425.
180. Gupta RL, Das P. Ectopia testis transversa. J Indiana Med Assoc 1960;35:547–549.
181. Mukerjee S, Amesur NR. Transverse testicular ectopia with unilateral blood supply. Indian J Surg 1965;27:547–550.
182. Hertzler AE. Ectopia testis transversa with infantile uterus. Surg Gynecol Obstet 1916;23:597–601.
183. Lowsley OS, Kerwin TJ. Clinical urology, 3rd ed. Baltimore: Williams & Wilkins, 1956.
184. Lenhossek M. Ectopia testis transversa. Anat Anz 1886;1:376–381.
185. Appleby B. Pseudo-duplication of testis. Med J Anat 1961;2:215.
186. Hunt RW. Ectopic testis: report of a case of bilateral ectopia testis pelvicis and its surgical correction. J Urol 1940;44:325–332.
187. Mayer V, and Templeton FG. Inguinal ectopia of the ovary and fallopian tube: review of the literature and report of the case of an infant. Arch Surg 1941;43:397–408.
188. Adams SS. Hernia of the pregnant uterus. Am J Obstet 1889;22:225–246.
189. Andrews FT. Hernias of the uterus. Trans Am Gynecol Soc 1906;31:407–426.
190. Rock JA, Parmley T, Murphy AA, Jones HW Jr. Malposition of the ovary associated with uterine anomalies. Fertil Steril 1986;45(4):561–563.
191. Ludwig G, Potempa J. Der optimale Zeitpunkt der Behandlung des Kryptorchismus. Dtsch Med Wochenschr 1975;100(13):680–683.

CHAPTER 21

THE MALE REPRODUCTIVE TRACT

John Elias Skandalakis / Stephen Wood Gray / Bruce Broecker

Man is the measure of all things, of the things that are, that (or how) they are,
and the things that are not, that (or how) they are not.
—*PROTAGORAS OF AVDERA*
TRUTH OR REFUTATORY ARGUMENTS BY PRESTON H. EPPS

DEVELOPMENT

Both male and female reproductive duct systems are formed during early embryonic development. After the third month, the müllerian system regresses in the male, leaving only vestiges to indicate its earlier presence. Its history in the female is discussed in Chapter 22.

The wolffian duct system begins with the appearance of the pronephric duct of the primitive kidney. The development of that portion which forms the definitive excretory passages is discussed with the upper urinary tract in Chapter 17. Anomalous persistence of its lower portion as an ectopic ureter is discussed in Chapter 18.

Development of the male reproductive tract itself may be said to begin in the sixth week (10 mm), when the rete cords of the developing testis (Chapter 20) begin to fuse with six to fifteen of the mesonephric tubules to form the ductuli efferentes (1, 2) (Fig. 21.1). Felix (3) considered these to be tubules numbers 58 to 70, but subsequent workers have not agreed on exactly which tubules are involved.

With these connections, the distal portion of the wolffian duct becomes part of the male reproductive tract. Degeneration of the mesonephros has already started by the time the testis makes its connection, and by the tenth week most of the tubules caudal and cranial to the ductuli efferentes have degenerated. In the immediate vicinity of the ductuli, some mesonephric tubules persist to remain as vestigial structures associated with the epididymis (2) (Fig. 21.2). As to the hormonal action of the fetal hormones and the role they play in the formation of male and female reproductive tract, George and Wilson (4) recorded the androgen action as follows: "Testosterone enters the special cell and is changed to dihydrotestosterone by action of 5a-reductase enzyme. Both hormones bind to a specific protein which later binds to DNA, and this final concept will be responsible, not only for the differentiation of the Wolffian duct, but also for external virilization" (see Fig. 20.6).

The above work supports the concept of Jost (5) who reported:

1. Orchiectomy in XY fetuses before the indifferent stage will produce a primitive female tract.
2. Oophorectomy in XX fetuses does not hamper the feminine destiny of the tract.

The presence and action of testosterone is a must for masculinization and therefore for the production of the future reproductive organs. However, estradiol from fetal ovaries is not essential for the production of the female reproduction organs.

We strongly advise the reader to study the excellent paper of Williams-Ashman in *Perspectives in Biology and Medicine* (6).

Epididymis and Ductus Deferens

The transformation of the mesonephric duct into the ductus epididymis and ductus deferens has not been adequately described. The ductuli efferentes and the cranial portion of the wolffian duct form the epididymis. During the fourth month the ductuli elongate and coil to form the coni vasculosa. Fusions and cross-connections mask the original number of tubules involved (3). Grossly, these coiled ductuli and the cranial wolffian duct are visible as the head of the epididymis by the 12th week (50 mm) (7).

The ductus deferens, which has become separated from the ureter (page 671), terminates at the müllerian tubercle in the posterior wall of that part of the urogenital sinus, which will become the prostatic urethra. In the fourth month the region of the ductus proximal to the müllerian tubercle becomes dilated to indicate the ampulla. The epithelium of the ductus deferens does not acquire cilia before the fourth month.

Male Urethra

The male urethra is composed of two portions. The upper prostatic urethra, above the level of the colliculus seminalis at the site of the müllerian tubercle, is derived from

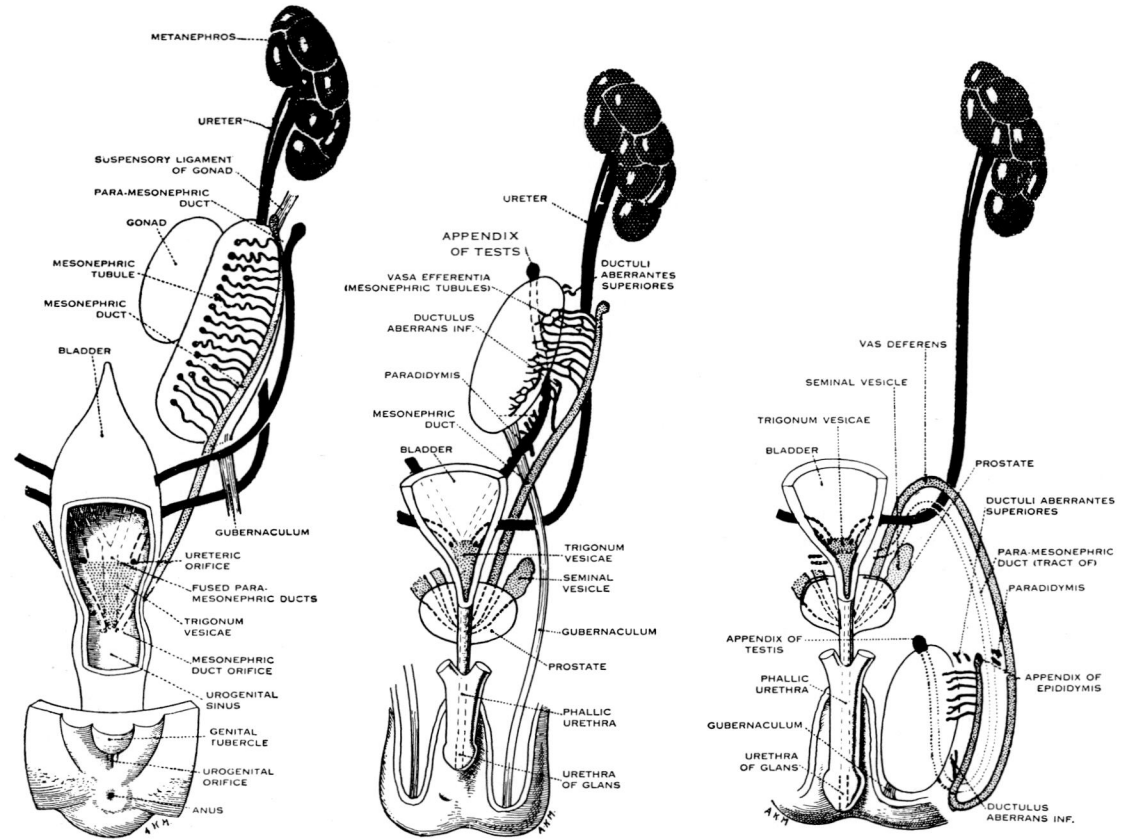

Figure 21.1. Schematic diagrams of the transformation of the indifferent stage of genital tract to the definitive male tract. (From Hamilton WJ, Boyd JD, Mossman HW. Human embryology, 3rd ed. Baltimore: Williams & Wilkins, 1962.)

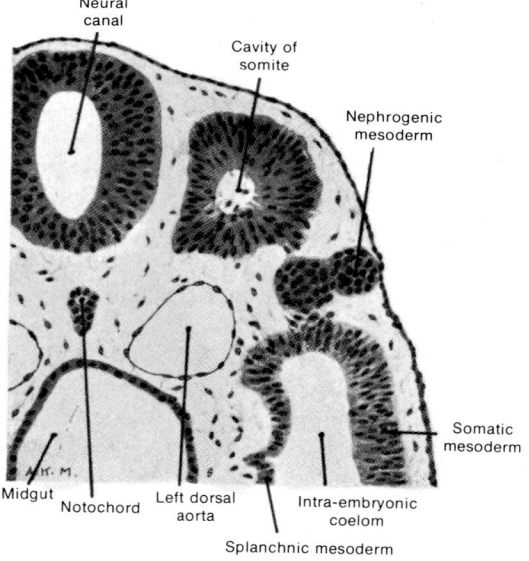

Figure 21.2. A section through a 14-mm human embryo at the level of the 10th somite. The lateral mesoderm appears dorsally as the somite and ventrally as splanchnic and somatic mesoderm, separated by the celom. Between these, a solid mesodermal region, the nephrotome or nephrogenic mesoderm, appears. The future mesonephric capsule and tubular area lie medially, the future wolffian duct, laterally. (From Hamilton WJ, Boyd JD, Mossman HW. Human embryology, 3rd ed. Baltimore: Williams & Wilkins, 1962.)

the vesicular portion of the primitive cloaca and corresponds to the female urethra.

Below this level the lower half of the prostatic urethra and the membranous urethra are derived from the pars pelvina of the urogenital sinus (8). The penile urethra is derived from pars phallica of the sinus and will be described with the penis. Endoderm forms the epithelium and splanchnic mesoderm is responsible for the connective tissue and smooth muscle formation around the urethra.

Prostate Gland

By the 12th week of development the müllerian ducts have regressed so that only the fused caudal portion retains its lumen, which ends abruptly at the epithelial plate closing the entrance to the urogenital sinus. This müllerian remnant and its closing plate flanked by the terminal portions of the wolffian ducts project into the urogenital sinus as the müllerian tubercle. The tubercle is subsequently overgrown by epithelium from the wolffian duct orifices, according to Glenister (9).

The urogenital sinus caudal to this region is the future prostatic urethra; it is lined with epithelium of endodermal origin, into which projects the müllerian tubercle (the future colliculus seminalis, or the verumontanum of the urologist). The hollow müllerian remnant within the tubercle forms the prostatic utricle, while the terminal wolffian ducts become the ejaculatory ducts of the adult.

The original account of the development of the prostate by Lowsley (10) described the appearance of five embryonic lobes, of which four persisted to form the adult gland. The studies of le Duc (11), Franks (12), and Glenister (9) suggested that the prostate has a dual origin. The true prostatic glands of the outer zone, the lateral and posterior lobes of Lowsley, are formed in the 12th week as epithelial buds from the wall of the urethra lateral to the colliculus and, hence, are of endodermal origin (Figs. 21.3 and 21.4). The submucous glands and the prostatic glands of the median lobe make up the inner zone and form later than the other glands from the epithelium of the colliculus, which contains müllerian and wolffian epithelium of mesodermal origin. This difference in the origin of the glands of the inner and outer zones is said to account for their different responses to estrogen (12).

Therefore proliferative buds of epithelium from the prostatic urethra form the prostatic gland. Zondek and Zondek (13) reported that squamous metaplasia of the glandular epithelium is common.

Norman et al. (14) reported that perhaps an embryonic prostatic indicator is the cause of participation as epithelial cells of the adult prostate. The authors hypothesize that human benign prostatic hyperplasia may result from this type of reactivation of embryonic growth potential in the adult prostate.

Latent and dormant prostatic cancer raises one of the enigmatic problems confronting the medical profession. Questions arise about this organ and its unknown biologic mechanisms.

Carcinoma of the prostate is the second highest cause of death in the U.S. male population. The factors responsible for prostatic growth are not well known. Is the urogenital sinus more carcinogenic (periphery) than the wolffian duct (central area)? Why does prostatic carcinoma flourish at the periphery (70 to 80%) and not centrally (5 to 10%)? Does embryology play any role? The reader should consult the interesting papers of McNeal and Drago (15–18). I wonder what Herophilos of Chalkedon would say today about the organ he described in 300 BC.

Seminal Vesicles

The seminal vesicles appear as lateral outpouchings of the wolffian ducts at about the 13th week. Branching becomes evident by the end of the fourth month (19). The prepubertal state is not reached until the seventh month (Fig. 21.4, *E*). We have found no detailed studies of these structures in humans. In the rat, development is only completed after birth (20).

Bulbourethral Glands of Cowper

Cowper's glands appear as buds from the posterior wall of the urogenital sinus as early as the 10th week. Their site of origin is in the proximal end of future urethra; they grow backward to terminate within the musculature of the urogenital diaphragm, where secretory bulbous structures are located (Fig. 21.3).

Remnants of the Mesonephros and the Wolffian Duct

APPENDIX EPIDIDYMIS (PEDUNCULATED HYDATID)

This structure is lined with columnar and sometimes ciliated epithelium and has been considered at various times to be of pronephric, müllerian, or wolffian origin. The present consensus is that it represents the blind cranial end of the mesonephric (wolffian) duct. Zuckerman and Krohn (21) concluded that there is no adequate proof of its specific origin. The appendix epididymis is histologically identical with the appendix testis and somewhat more constant in its occurrence. Both vary in structure from cysts to small, fimbriated funnels, and both may contain small ducts communicating with the ductus epididymis (Fig. 21.5). Both respond to estrogen but not to gonadotropins, progesterone, or male hormones.

APPENDIX TESTIS (SESSILE HYDATID)

This structure is of müllerian rather than wolffian origin and represents the cranial end of the müllerian duct (Fig. 21.5).

DUCTULI ABERRANTES

Aberrant ducts lie both cranially and caudally to the functional ductuli efferentia. The cranial group are usually connected with the rete testis, while the caudal duct (organ of Haller) is a blind diverticulum of the ductus epididymis. These ducts represent mesonephric tubules that have not completed the connection between the rete testis and the ductus epididymis, nor have they completely regressed (Fig. 21.5).

PARADIDYMIS (ORGAN OF GIRALDÈS)

These tubules, which lie superior to the head of the epididymis, are coiled and may contain chromaffin tissue (22). They are vestigial mesonephric tubules that correspond to the paroophoron of the female (Fig. 21.5) (see page 823).

The persistent and vestigial structures, together with their derivation, are shown in Table 20.5. The table corresponds approximately with wolffian and müllerian primordia for both sexes, but many embryologic questions still remain unanswered.

A

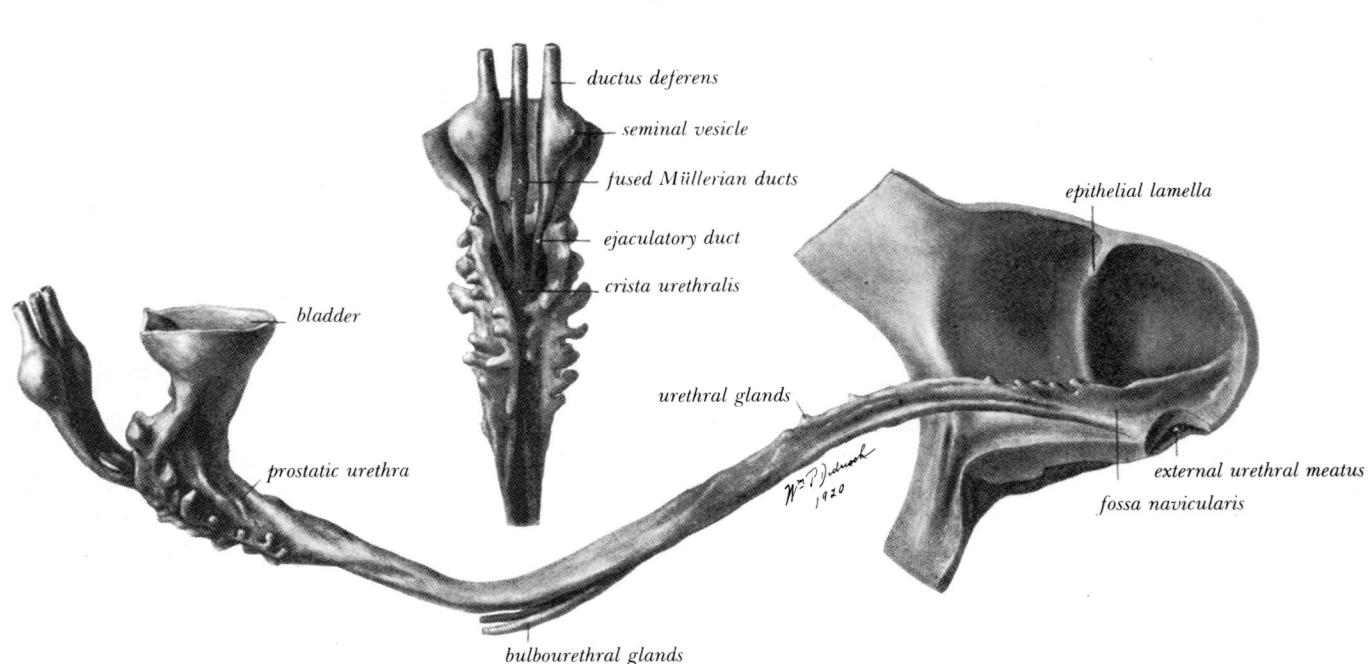

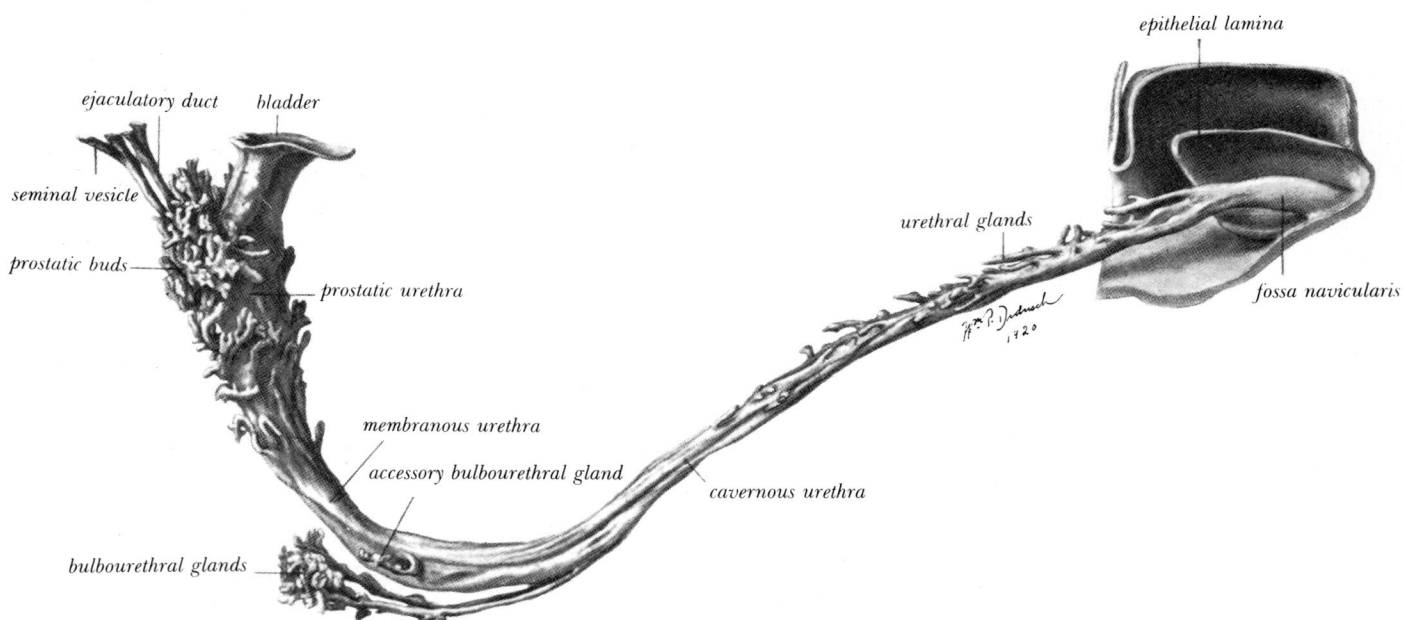

Figure 21.3. **A,** Anterior and lateral views of reconstructions of epithelial structures of the male reproductive tract at 65 mm (11 weeks). **B,** Lateral view at 130 mm (4 months). (From Johnson FP. The later development of the urethra in the male. J Urol 1920;4:447–501.)

EXTERNAL GENITALIA

Early in the fourth week at the beginning of somite formation, the site of the external genitalia is represented externally by a rhomboidal cloacal membrane, which extends cranially nearly to the umbilicus and caudally to the tail bud. Anterolateral to the margins of the membrane are two genital swellings; posterolateral are two smaller anal swellings (Fig. 21.6, *A*).

By the sixth week (8-mm stage), a median genital tubercle is present. It occupies almost all of the space between the umbilical stalk and the tail bud. The cloacal membrane has become a longitudinal groove that starts near the tip of the tubercle and extends to the site of the anus. A transverse bar separates the anal orifice from the remainder of the groove, which may now be designated as the urethral groove. The groove is bound by the urethral folds, which extend posteriorly to the end in the paired anal tubercles (Fig. 21.7, A).

Felix (3) considered the genital tubercle to be a paired structure formed by fusion of the paired genital swellings. This view has been supported by Patten and Barry (23). Spaulding (24) considered the tubercle to be unpaired, with the paired swellings being separate and forming the labioscrotal folds only. The disagreement seems to depend on how one defines the genital tubercle rather than on specific facts.

Spaulding denied the existence of an indifferent stage in the development of the genitalia, but his criteria for distinguishing gender before the end of the second month are not easy to describe or apply. He did not have the advantage of cytologic methods for sex determination based on the presence of the sex chromatin to confirm his judgments. For practical purposes, the distinction becomes apparent externally in most cases only during the third month.

During the eighth week the labioscrotal swellings lateral to the phallus move caudally. In the male the urethral groove begins to close by fusion of the edges of the urethral folds from the base toward the tip of the phallus (Fig. 21.8). Closure of the folds up to the glans is almost complete by the 45-mm stage (Fig. 21.7, B).

Johnson (8) conceived the penile urethra as resulting from simple closure of the urethral groove; Glenister (25) described a more complicated series of events. The phallic portion of the urogenital sinus extends only part way along the phallus. Its urogenital folds form the primary urethral groove. From the cloacal epithelium, a sagittal plate of endoderm cells (the urethral plate) grows into the phallus, extending to the tip in both sexes. The plate is in contact ventrally with the roof of the primary groove in the proximal part of the phallus (Fig. 21.9, B) and with the ventral ectoderm in the distal portion (Fig. 21.9, A). Beyond the end of the urogenital sinus, the urethral folds are prolonged by ventral mesenchymal proliferation on either side of the urethral plate. Splitting of the urethral plate forms the secondary urethral groove, now continuous with the primary groove in the proximal part of the phallus (Fig. 21.9, D). Subsequent fusion of the urethral folds along the entire shaft of the phallus forms the definitive urethra of the male (Fig. 21.9, E).

The glans produces a separate ectodermal plate, which grows in to meet the endodermal urethral plate (26, 27). It splits and recloses to extend the urethral passage to the tip of the penis by the 16th week (8, 28, 29) (Fig. 21.10).

In summary, the proximal penile urethra is formed from endoderm of the phallic portion of the urogenital sinus, the distal urethra from endoderm of the urethral plate, and the fossa terminalis from ectodermal ingrowth from the surface of the glans. There is still a question about whether the urethral floor is endodermal or ectodermal from the lips of the urethral folds (30).

The position of the coronary sinus is indicated by the 25-mm stage. By 57 mm, the preputial fold is present, interrupted on the inferior surface. The skin at the distal margin overgrows the glans, leaving an epithelial plate of fusion between glans and prepuce. The prepuce covers the glans by the 135-mm stage (31).

The preputial space forms by breakdown of the fused epithelial surfaces from the deepest portion outward (29). The process is complete, and the prepuce is retractable in 4% of infants at birth, in 50% at 1 year of age, and in 92% by 5 years of age (32). Phimosis is thus physiologic during the first year of life. Williams-Ashman (6) is right when he talks about the enigmatic features of penile development and functions.

Critical Events in Development

In the fourth week, the nephrogenic ridge may fail to form. As no mesonephric duct appears, the ductus epididymis, ductus deferens, and their associated structures are absent. The kidney and ureter are also absent.

Accessory urethral canals seem to be related to disturbance in penile formation in the 10th to 14th weeks. The specific error is obscure.

Arrested closure of the urethral folds during the eighth week results in hypospadias of varying severity, depending on the exact time of the arrest.

Failure of all or part of the ventral infraumbilical body wall to form completely produces a spectrum of defects, ranging from the mildly embarrassing partial epispadias with a urethral opening on the dorsum of the glans penis to the crippling exstrophy of the bladder and exstrophy of the cloaca.

ANOMALIES OF THE MALE REPRODUCTIVE TRACT (TABLE 21.1 AND FIG. 21.11)

Müllerian and Mesonephric Remnants in the Male

Two structures normally occurring in the male represent vestiges of the two ends of the müllerian ducts of the female. One, the appendix testis, lies at the upper pole of the testis; the other is embedded in the prostate gland. Both may be the site of disease. The appendix epididymis and the mesonephric tubular remnants are occasionally affected.

TORSION OF THE APPENDIX TESTIS OR OF THE APPENDIX EPIDIDYMIS

Anatomy and Embryogenesis. Despite its name of "sessile hydatid," the appendix testis may be a stalked nodule or

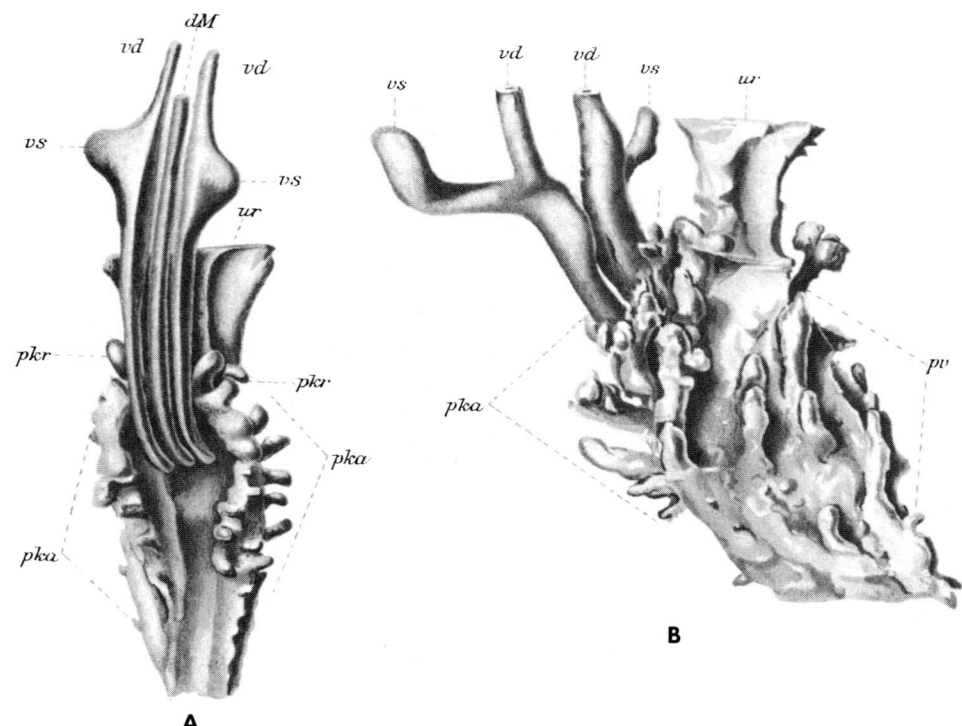

Figure 21.4. Reconstruction of the developing prostate gland and seminal vesicles from male human embryos. **A,** Anterior view at 60 mm (11 weeks). **B,** Anterolateral view at 90 to 115 mm (fourth month) vs. seminal vesicle. *vd*, Ductus deferens; *dM*, müllerian duct; *pka*, caudal posterior prostate gland; *pkr*, cranial posterior prostate gland; *pv*, anterior prostate gland; *um*, prostatic utricle; *ur*, urethra. **C,** Anterior view at 140 to 160 mm (early fifth month). **D,** Seminal vesicles

it may resemble the fimbriated end of a miniature fallopian tube. It is highly vascular and may contain ducts, which open into the tunica vaginalis (22). It usually occurs on the upper portion of the testis, beneath the visceral layer of the tunica vaginalis. The appendix testis represents the upper end of the müllerian duct and probably corresponds to the ostium tubae of the oviduct (page 816). The condition is of considerable interest to embryologists; its chief clinical importance, however, is its tendency to undergo painful torsion with inflammation necrosis secondary to occlusion of blood vessels (Fig. 21.12). Why torsion occurs in a few individuals and not in most cannot be explained anatomically, although it seems certain that a long peduncle would favor twisting.

Much more rarely, the appendix epididymis undergoes torsion.

History. Torsion of the appendix testis was mentioned as early as 1913 by Ombrédanne (33). It was first described as an entity by Colt (34) in 1922, and in the same year a case was operated upon by Walton (35). In France, Mouchet (36) called attention to the lesion by reporting a number of cases. In 1931 Dix (37) reviewed 53 cases of torsion, including several of his own and Mouchet's. By 1939 Randall (38) was able to find 68 cases of torsion of the appendix testis, two of the appendix epididymis, two of the aberrant duct of Haller, and one of

the paradidymis. Seidel and Yeaw (39) counted 107 cases of all types and added eight of their own.

Incidence. In spite of their late discovery, the conditions are not rare. We have seen four cases of torsion in a single year at St. Joseph's Infirmary (Atlanta) among 12,443 admissions (40). Among 25 consecutive pediatric patients evaluated for acute scrotal pain at Egleston Children's Hospital (Atlanta) during an 8-month period, 11 proved to have torsion of the appendix epididymis or appendix testis (41). Torsion of appendix testis or epididymis may happen at any time during childhood. The majority of the patients at Egleston are 5 to 10 years of age. Torsion of the testis (spermatic cord) rarely happens before puberty other than in neonates.

The majority of cases occur during adolescence, although they have been reported in middle age. They are very rare in infancy (42). Randall (38) suggests that the left side is more commonly afflicted than is the right, but the difference, if one exists, is not marked. In at least one case the torsion was bilateral (43). In another case the affected testis was in the inguinal canal (44). At least 150 cases have been reported in the literature (45).

Symptoms. Sudden onset of scrotal pain followed by increased swelling and inflammation is the presenting complaint in torsion of either of the appendices. The pain ranges from moderate to severe. Early on the pain may be

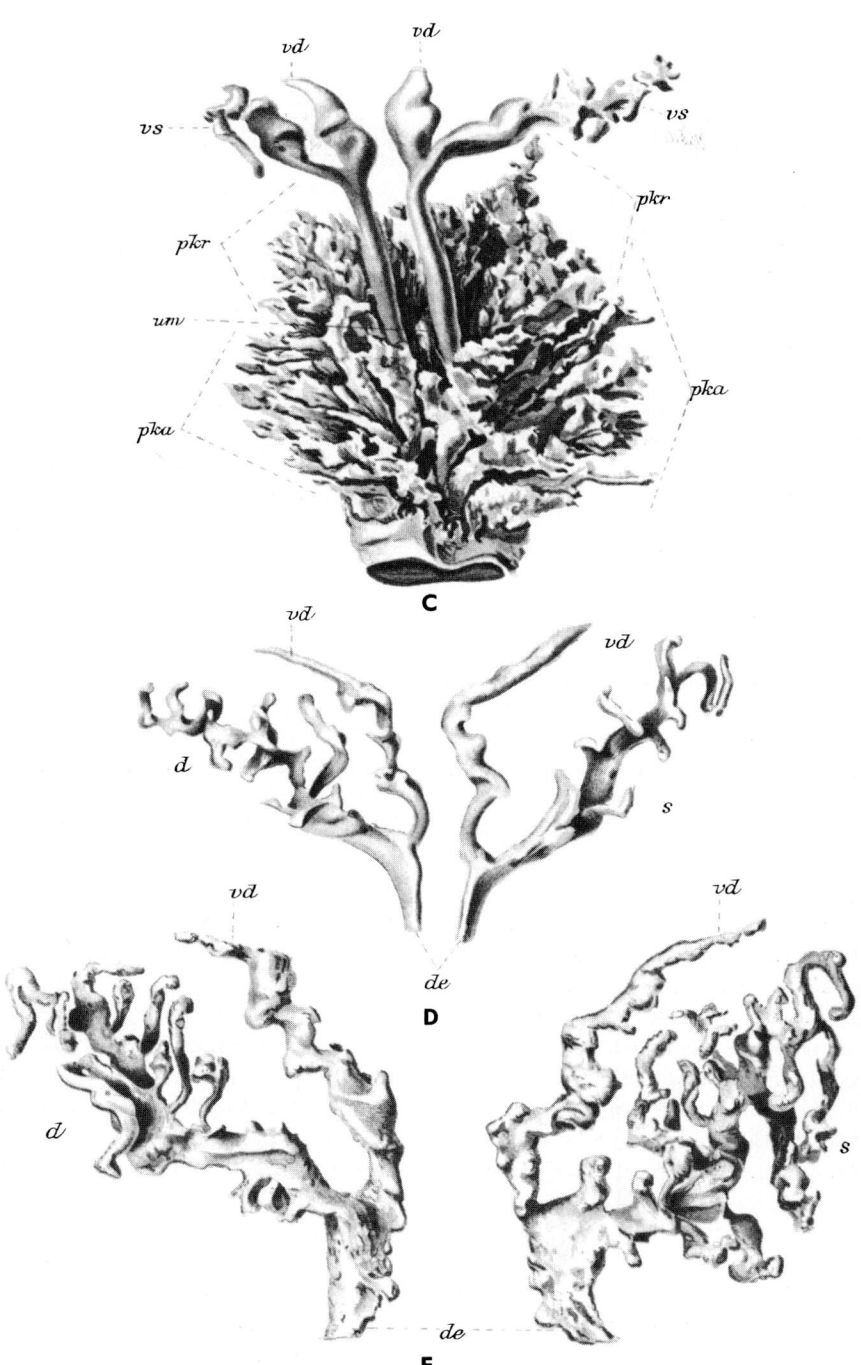

at 155 to 170 mm (late fifth month). **E,** Seminal vesicle at 200 to 260 mm (seventh month). *de,* Ejaculatory duct; *d,* right side; *s,* left side. (From Pallin G. Beiträge zur Anatomie und Embryologie der Prostata und der Saminblasen. Arch Anat Enter 1901;135–176.)

localized to the superior aspect of the testis, but as time passes and the inflammation progresses, the entire testicle and epididymis becomes swollen and painful. Fever, nausea, and prostration or urinary symptoms are unusual. If untreated the pain may persist for several weeks. Spontaneous detorsion with subsequent attacks

has been reported; one patient suffered 14 episodes over 16 years (46).

Diagnosis. Early in the course of the condition the examiner may feel the affected appendage as a small, firm mass attached to the anterosuperior pole of the testis or epididymis. Occasionally, the bluish discoloration of the

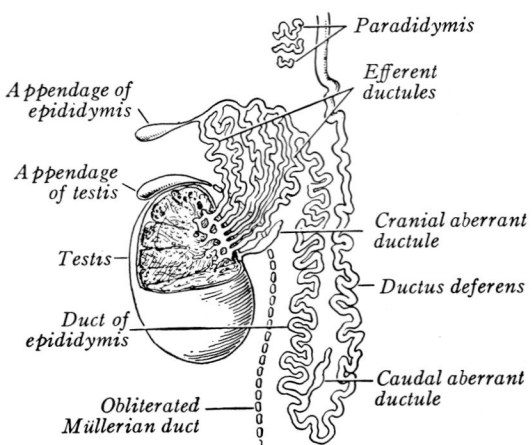

Figure 21.5. Mesonephric and müllerian vestigial structures in the vicinity of the testes of the adult male. There is great variability among these structures, and not all may be present in a single individual. (From Arey LB. Developmental anatomy, 7th ed. Philadelphia: WB Saunders, 1965.)

torsed appendage may be visible through the thin translucent scrotal skin, the so-called blue dot sign. Later in the clinical course of the condition, the examiner will find the entire testis and epididymis indurated, erythematous, and tender; the physician will be unable to discern a discrete appendix amid the generalized inflammation.

Acute epididymitis, orchitis, torsion of the spermatic cord, and incarcerated inguinal hernia are the conditions to be considered in the differential diagnosis. The absence of evidence of urinary tract infection (by urinalysis or urine culture) makes a clinical diagnosis of epididymitis unsupportable. Orchitis (viral) in the absence of mumps or other viral disease is unlikely. It should be possible to palpate a normal testis, separating it from the remaining tender swollen scrotal mass in a child with an incarcerated inguinal hernia. In addition, reduction of the hernia is usually possible and confirms this diagnosis. It may, however, be difficult to differentiate torsion of the appendix testis/epididymis from torsion of the spermatic

cord by physical examination alone in the more advanced stages of these conditions. Evaluation of testicular perfusion by scintigraphy, color Doppler sonography, or both may be quite helpful in distinguishing between inflammatory conditions with increased blood flow (epididymitis, appendiceal torsion) and ischemic conditions (torsion of the spermatic cord). In all cases, if doubt exists as to the true nature of the condition, scrotal exploration is indicated to exclude or treat torsion of the spermatic cord.

Treatment. If pain is minimal, symptomatic treatment may be all that is necessary. Pain and swelling will eventually resolve as the appendage atrophies. In most cases, however, excision of the torsed appendage will result in more rapid resolution of symptoms and is the most appropriate management. If surgery is performed, it is this surgeon's practice to remove the contralateral normal appendices although there is no conclusive evidence that they have an increased risk of subsequent torsion. Their removal adds little or no morbidity to the procedure and ensures that this event will not take place.

CYSTS OF THE PROSTATIC UTRICLE (MÜLLERIAN DUCT CYSTS)

Anatomy. The prostatic utricle, or uterus masculinus, is a median, epithelium-lined sinus, 4 to 6 mm long, which opens into the prostatic urethra between the orifices of the ejaculatory ducts on the colliculus seminalis (verumontanum).

The epithelium may be columnar, cuboidal, or flattened; in some cases it is absent. In one example (47) the epithelium was described as transitional, casting some doubt on its müllerian origin. The walls are fibrous, with some smooth muscle, and the contents are usually old blood, pus, or cellular debris. Spermatozoa are not found. Occasionally, there is no opening into the urethra; the proximal end is represented by a fibrous cord. The cavity is occasionally dilated to form a cyst that extends between the seminal vesicles and behind the bladder.

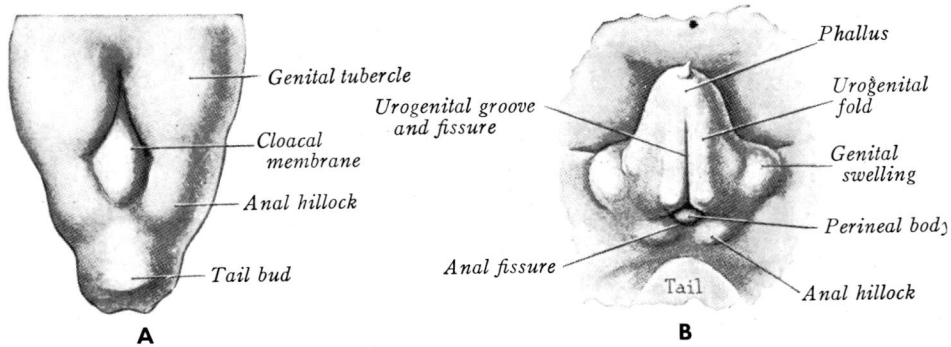

Figure 21.6. The cloacal region of the human embryo in ventral view. **A,** At 3 mm (fourth week). The cloacal membrane is intact. **B,** At 21 mm (eighth week). The cloacal membrane has ruptured and the perineal body, dividing the anus from the urogenital sinus, has reached the exterior. (From Arey LB. Developmental anatomy, 7th ed. Philadelphia: WB Saunders, 1965.)

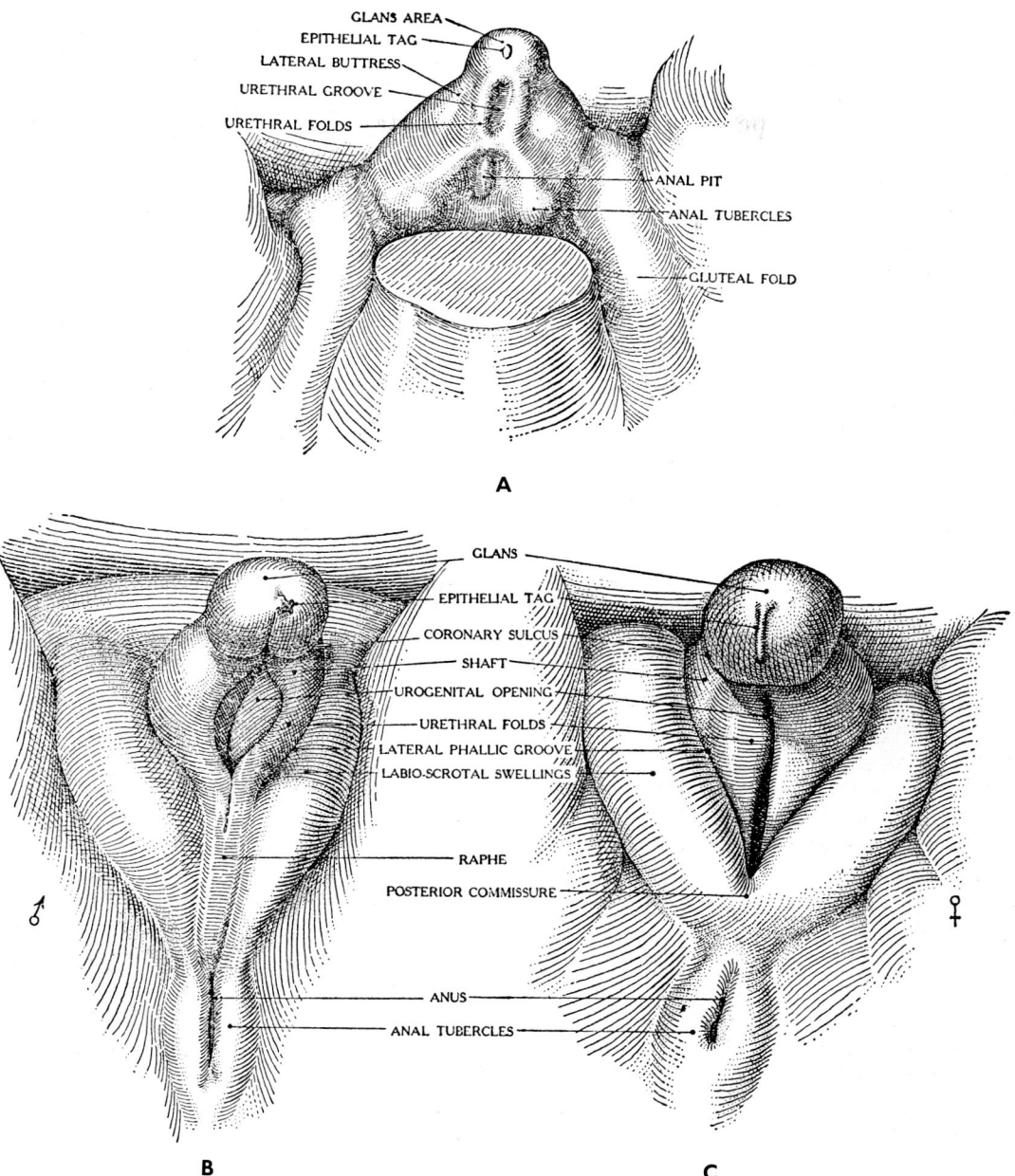

Figure 21.7. Developing external genitalia of the human embryo. **A,** At 16.8 mm (end of seventh week). No sexual differentiation is visible. The tip of the tail has been cut to reveal the genitalia. **B,** Male embryo at 45 mm (10th week). **C,** Female embryo at 49 mm (11th week). Sexual differentiation has just begun. (From Spaulding MH. The development of the external genitalia in the human embryo. Contrib Embryol Carnegie Inst Wash 1921;13:67.)

Such a cyst may have diverticula representing the uterine tubes (Fig. 21.13). The cysts vary in size from negligible enlargement to one that reached 31 × 26 × 19 cm (47).

Embryology. The utricle represents the caudal end of the fused müllerian ducts, corresponding to the vaginal and cervical portions of the ducts. It does not include that portion which becomes the body of the uterus in the female (Fig. 21.14, *A*). The relationship of the utricle and the ejaculatory ducts, which are of wolffian origin, is essentially that which existed in the embryo at the time of the greatest development of the müllerian ducts in the male.

Intrinsic enlargement of the prostatic utricle may result from more extensive conservation of the caudal portion of the müllerian ducts. In such cases the homologue of the uterine body or even the uterine tubes may be preserved (48) (Fig. 21.14, *B* and *C*). No sharp line can be drawn between enlargement of the utricle in normal males and the persistence of rudimentary but complete müllerian structures found in some pseudohermaphrod-

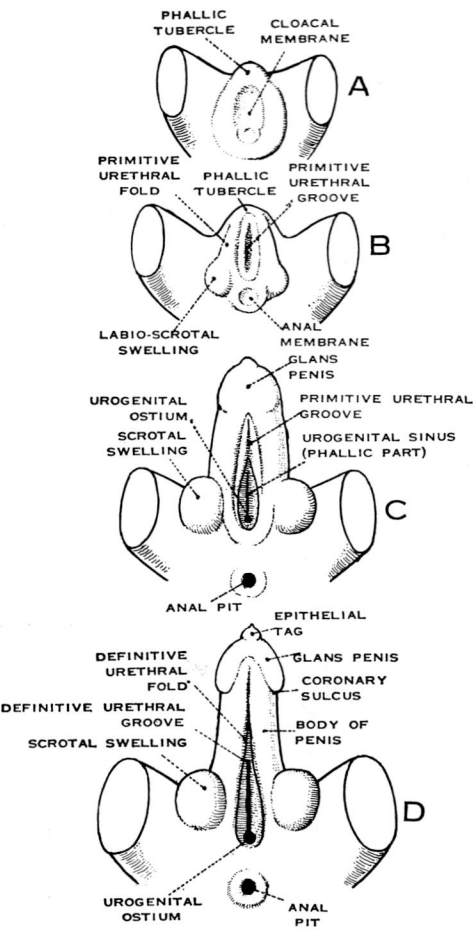

Figure 21.8. Four stages in the development of the penis and scrotum in the human male embryo and fetus as seen from below. Closure is still incomplete in stage **D.** (From Hamilton WJ, Boyd JD, Mossman HW. Human embryology, 3rd ed. Baltimore: Williams & Wilkins, 1962.)

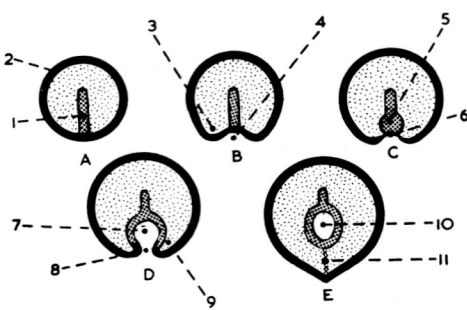

Figure 21.9. Schematic transverse sections through the shaft of the developing human penis. *1,* Endodermal urethral plate; *2,* ectodermal surface epithelium; *3,* primitive urethral fold; *4,* primitive urethral groove; *5,* thickened portion of the endodermal urethral plate; *6,* retrogressing ectodermal epithelium lining the roof of the primitive urethral groove; *7,* secondary urethral groove (lined with endodermal epithelium), produced by the breakdown of the thickened portion of the urethral plate *(5); 8,* primary urethral groove (lined with ectodermal epithelium), which is deepened by the secondary groove *(7)* to form the definitive urethral groove *(7* and *8); 9,* definitive urethral folds; *10,* endoderm-lined penile urethra; *11,* raphe produced by the fusion of the portions of the urethral folds covered by ectodermal epithelium. (From Glenister TW. A correlation of the normal and abnormal development of the penile urethra and of the intraabdominal wall. Br J Urol 1958;30:117–126.)

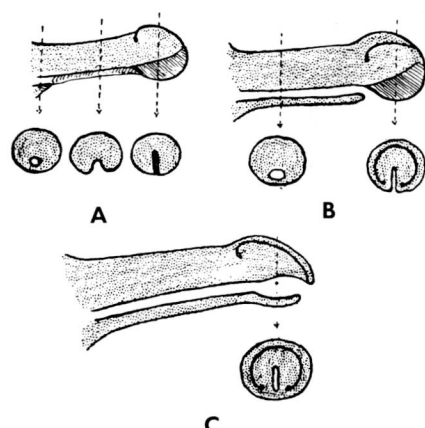

Figure 21.10. Development of the glandular urethra and its fusion with the penile urethra. **A,** The penile urethra is an open groove; a solid epithelial plate is present in the glans. **B,** The penile urethra is a tube; the glandular epithelial plate is split. **C,** Closure of the glandular portion and completion of the definitive urethra. (From Johnson FP. Urethral anomalies. J Urol 1930;23:693–699.)

ites (49) or in patients with complete hypospadias (50) (see page 805). In a few cases a slight, perhaps transitory, endocrine imbalance may stimulate hypertrophic enlargement of a normal müllerian remnant.

Functional enlargement of the utricle may result from high pressure at voiding urine. The utricle becomes filled and has no contracting force to expel the urine.

History. In 1742 Morgagni (De Sedibus XLIV:19) found a cystic cavity as large as a "middle-sized grape" in the prostate of an old man. This is the earliest reference we have seen to a possible cystic remnant of the müllerian duct in the male. Englisch (51) in 1875 described five cysts of the prostatic utricle and is usually credited with being the discoverer of the anomaly (52). In 1915 Klotz (53) reported the first example in a living patient. Lubash (54) reviewed the early literature in 1929. Slocum (55) was able to find only 49 cases in the literature in 1954, to which he added two.

Whether the enlargement is hypoplastic, hypertro-

phic, or functional, cystic dilation is caused by obstruction of the orifice of the utricle into the urethra. The orifice may be congenitally stenosed, or it may be obstructed by epithelial hypertrophy from hormonal stimulation.

Incidence. Enlarged utricles have been reported in 4% of newborn male infants and in 1% of adult males (55).

In the absence of data on the normal variation in utricular size, the true incidence of utricular enlargement is unknown. In the otherwise normally developed male, it is certainly uncommon. It is most likely to be encountered in males with penoscrotal or perineal hypospadias (56–58) or in phenotypic males with an intersex condition.

Symptoms. Utricular cysts may present with irritative or obstructive symptoms of the lower urinary tract. Epididymitis may occur as a result of the vas deferens opening directly into the cyst cavity. Complete urinary retention due to compression of the bladder neck by the enlarged cyst has been reported by Feldman and Weiss (59). Hematuria, urinary incontinence, oligospermia, and a palpable abdominal mass are all occasionally modes of presentation. Endometrial carcinoma arising from the müllerian duct cyst has been reported by Deming and Berneike (60).

Diagnosis. The enlarged prostatic utricle is readily palpated on rectal examination. It is palpable as a cystic mass cephalad to the prostate, between the bladder and rectum. Pelvis sonography or computed tomography (CT) will also readily demonstrate the cystic abnormality. Cystourethroscopy and urethrography will usually demonstrate the cyst but are not generally necessary for purposes of making a diagnosis. Müllerian duct cysts may be differentiated from seminal vesicle cysts by their midline—rather than lateral—location.

Table 21.1.
Anomalies of the Male Reproductive Tract

Anomaly	Origin of Defect	First Appearance (or Other Diagnostic Clues)	Sex Chiefly Affected[a]	Relative Frequency	Remarks
Müllerian and mesonephric remnants in the male:					
Torsion of the appendix testis or appendix epididymis		In adolescence	Male	Uncommon	Predisposing factors not known
Cysts of the prostatic utricle	12th week	In adulthood	Male	Uncommon (clinically significant)	
Absence of wolffian derivatives in the male:					
Complete absence	4th week	At birth	Male	Rare	Associated with absence of kidneys and uterus: lethal if bilateral
Partial absence	After the 4th week	In adulthood	Male	Uncommon	Bilateral absence causes infertility; unilateral absence is asymptomatic
Duplications of the ductus deferens	Late 4th week	None	Male	Rare	
Absence of the seminal vesicle	3rd month or earlier	Adulthood only if bilateral	Male	Unknown	Sterility if bilateral
Duplication of the seminal vesicle	3rd month	Never	Male	Unknown	Asymptomatic
Anomalies of the prostate gland:					
Absence of the prostate	12th week	In adulthood	Male	Rare	Associated with infantile genitalia and pituitary insufficiency
Other anomalies	?	At any age	Male	Rare	May produce urethral obstruction
Agenesis of the penis	4th week	At birth	Male	Very rare	
Agenesis of the glans penis	4th month	At birth	Male	Very rare	
Defects of the corpus spongiosum and corpora cavernosa	3rd month?	At birth	Male	Very rare	
Duplication of the penis	Various times	At birth	Male	Very rare	Similar duplication of the clitoris is even rarer
Transposition of the penis and scrotum	9th week	At birth	Male	Very rare	
Duplications of the penile urethra	10th to 14th weeks	At any age	Male	Uncommon	
Atresia and stenosis of the urethra	?	In infancy	Male	Common	Present in females also
Hypospadias	8th week or later	At birth	Male	Rare	Very rare in females; familial tendency suggested

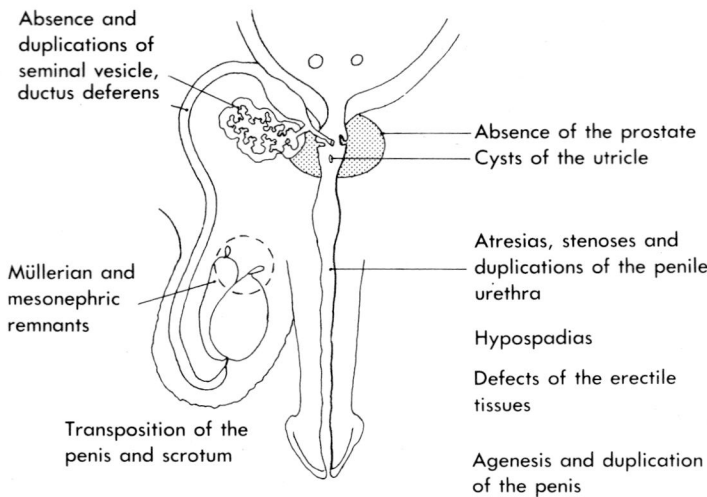

Figure 21.11.   Sites of developmental anomalies of the male reproductive tract.

Treatment. Surgical excision is indicated when the cyst is large, symptomatic, or both. A cyst which is both small and asymptomatic may be left in place with periodic reexamination. Complete excision is generally preferred to transurethral unroofing of the cyst, which does not usually provide adequate drainage and risks damage to the ejaculatory ducts. A suprapubic approach is employed if the cyst is quite large with intraabdominal extension. The origin of the cyst may be traced extravesically or by splitting the posterior bladder wall/trigone. Smaller cysts may be approached either by a suprapubic or posterior parasacral approach.

Congenital Absence of Wolffian Derivatives in the Male

ANATOMY

In the most extreme form of this defect, the testis, epididymis, ductus deferens, seminal vesicle, ureter, and kidney may be absent (61, 62) (Fig. 21.2).

More frequently, only the epididymis, ductus deferens, and seminal vesicles are absent (Fig. 21.15, *E*), and even more frequently, only the ductus epididymis and proximal portion of the ductus deferens are missing (63) (Fig. 21.15, *B* to *D*). Because the anomaly is usually found while examining patients who complain of infertility, the defect has been stated to be bilateral as often as unilateral. From its nature, this is improbable, and the figures of Michelson (61), who collected 40 cases of absence of either the epididymis or ductus deferens, of which only four were bilateral, seems closer to the real distribution. According to Rubin and Taylor (64), the anomaly occurs at the left side; however, these authors stated that there is no embryologic basis for this finding. Charney and Gillenwater (65) reported 37 cases of absence of the vas defer-

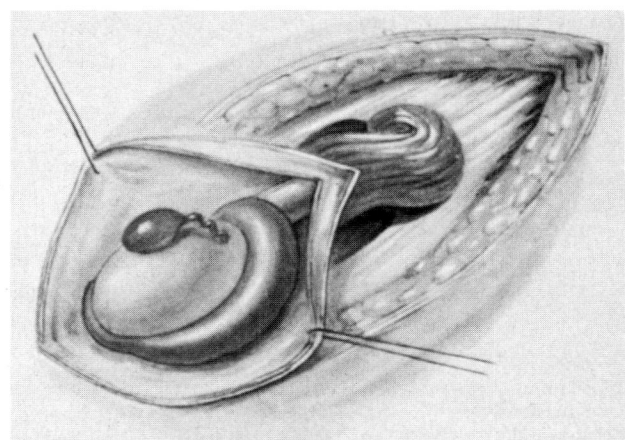

Figure 21.12.   Torsion and infarction of the appendix testis at the upper pole of an otherwise normal testis. (From Gross RF. The surgery of infancy and childhood. Philadelphia: WB Saunders, 1953.)

ens, with two cases of only ipsilateral renal agenesis and anomalies, in 12,000 infertile patients.

EMBRYOGENESIS

Complete agenesis of the genital ducts and the upper urinary tract implies failure of the mesonephros as well as of the definitive kidney to form. No wolffian duct developed, and hence, all later formed structures are absent. If both sides are involved, postnatal survival is impossible (see the section on "Bilateral Renal Agenesis" in Chapter 17).

While absence of nephric structures results in failure of duct formation, the gonad, which is formed largely from cells migrating from another part of the body, rarely is affected. Absence of the testis as well as of the ducts is only occasionally reported (61, 66). In the absence of the normal mesonephric fold, which contributes to the gubernaculum testis, the testis rarely descends. In one patient the testis lay at the site of the absent kidney and was served by short straight vessels from the aorta and vena cava (62).

The cases of partial absence of the wolffian structures may be considered an entirely different anomaly. The presence of normal ureter and kidney imply that the wolffian duct formed normally (to produce a normal ureteric bud) and that it subsequently atrophied. The fact that the upper (testicular) end of the ductus deferens is often absent, while the more proximal portion, together with the seminal vesicle, is present indicates that involution begins cranially. Only rarely does this involution extend to the seminal vesicles.

Complete agenesis of wolffian structures is a major defect of organogenesis early in development (fourth week or earlier), while partial agenesis, resulting from resorption of wolffian elements, must take place after the

caudally growing wolffian duct has reached the cloaca (end of the fourth week), and it probably occurs much later. It is tempting to consider this wolffian regression related to that which begins about the 12th week in normal females. Some have suggested that, in the absence of a testis, placental estrogens promote wolffian duct regression in normal females (67), but this does not explain regression in the presence of functioning testes. No persistence of abnormal müllerian structures has been reported in patients with wolffian agenesis. In summary, absence of the vas deferens is due to a partial or total agenesis of the right or left mesonephric duct.

HISTORY AND INCIDENCE
Hunter (29) first described atresia of the ductus epididymis and the ductus deferens in 1755. Since then, a number of cases, showing all degrees of wolffian agenesis, have been reported. Nelson (66) in 1950 reviewed 40 cases in the literature and added three cases of his own.

Among 900 subfertile men with normal testes, Michel-

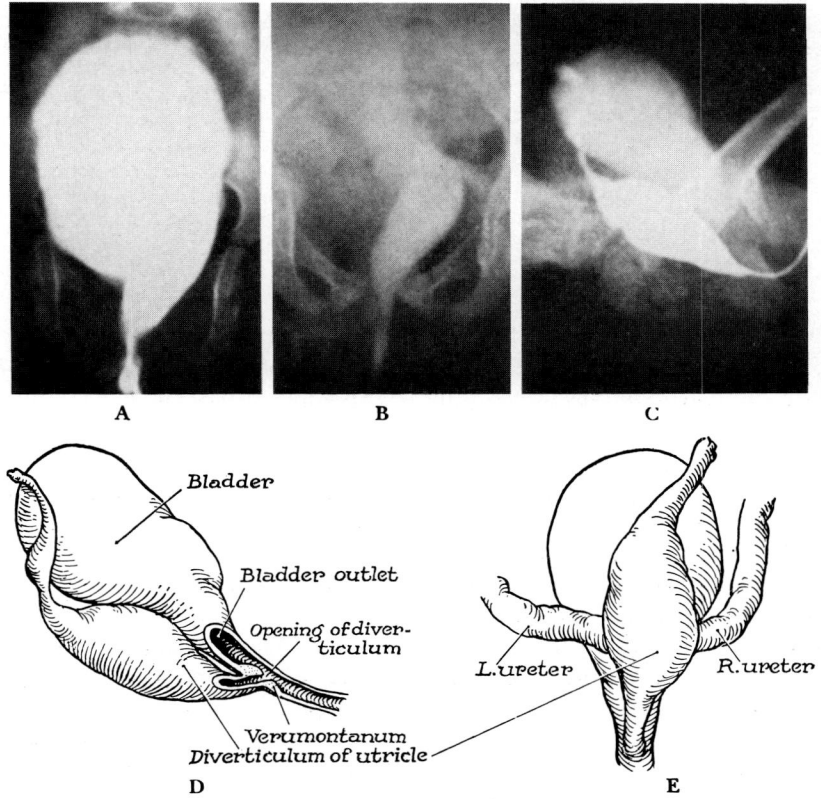

Figure 21.13. Congenital diverticulum of the utricle in an 18-month-old boy with penoscrotal hypospadias. **A,** The distended bladder and utricle are clearly shown. The dilated left upper urinary tract is feebly outlined by exstrographic reflux. Urinary distension of the diverticulum caused pressure on the lower ureters and on the urethra, thus producing obstruction. **B,** Anteroposterior view of utriculogram in **A. C,** Lateral view of combined utriculogram and cystogram, a medium of lighter density being injected into the bladder. A curious fallopian tube-like termination of the utricle is notable. **D** and **E,** Schema of local pathology. (From Campbell MF. Urology, 2nd ed. Philadelphia: WB Saunders, 1963.)

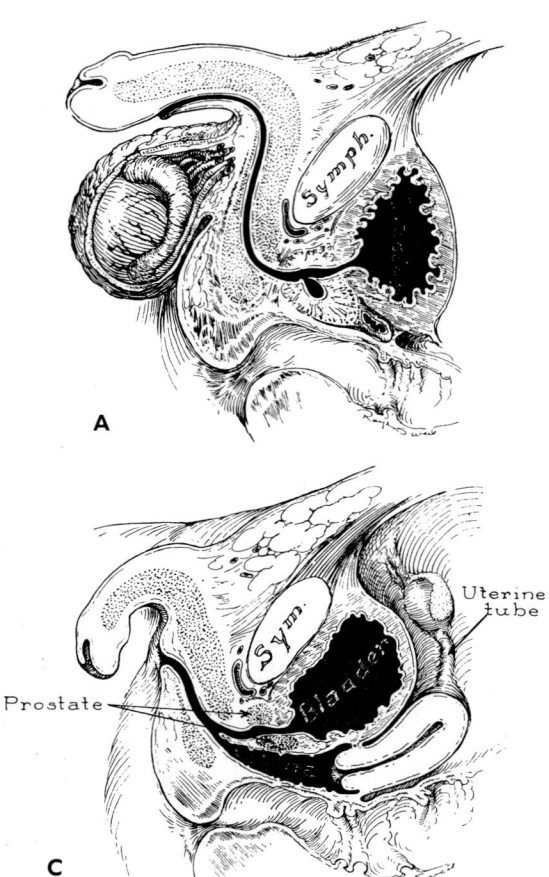

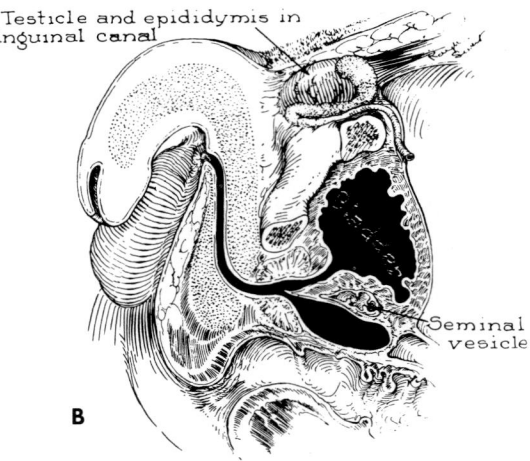

Figure 21.14. The prostatic utricle in patients with hypospadias. **A,** Normal utricle opening into the prostatic urethra. Mild hypospadias is present. **B,** An enlarged utricle in a patient with undescended testes and penoscrotal hypospadias. **C,** Extreme feminization. The utricle, which normally represents only the vaginal and cervical portions of the müllerian ducts, has developed into complete uterus and uterine tubes. The testis is undescended; the seminal vesicle and ductus deferens are absent; and perineal hypospadias is present. (From Howard FS. Hypospadias with enlargement of the prostatic utricle. Surg Gynec Obstet 1948;86:307–316.)

son (61) found 12 with absence of the ductus deferens or lower epididymis. About 6% of infertile males were found to have absence of all or part of the ductus in two other reported series (68, 69).

The small number of published cases cannot be taken to indicate that the unilateral condition is rare.

SYMPTOMS

Infertility is the chief complaint of patients with bilateral agenesis of the epididymis or ductus deferens. One patient, with agenesis of the right kidney and an undescended testis, complained of pain in the right lower quadrant. Removal of the ectopic testis relieved the symptoms (62).

DIAGNOSIS

A complete diagnosis can usually be made only by exploration or at autopsy. When sterility is the presenting complaint, palpation of the scrotum may reveal absence of the epididymis. If the testis is present in the scrotum, failure to palpate the epididymis and ductus deferens implies their absence. The ducts, if present, descend with the testis and may descend even though the testis does not do so.

The absence of fructose in the semen of azoospermic patients indicates absence of the seminal vesicles and probably absence of the ductus deferentia. This will distinguish some cases of congenital aplasia from cases of primary infertility or of ductal obstruction (70). Intravenous pyelogram (IVP) is mandatory in these cases to rule out ipsilateral or contralateral anomalies of the urinary tract. Feigelson and Pecau (71) advised that all patients with azoospermia should be investigated for cystic fibrosis.

TREATMENT

In some cases vasoepididymal anastomosis, either to the same or to the contralateral side, may bridge the gap in the reproductive tract. Artificial insemination with spermatozoa from the epididymis might be effective in some cases.

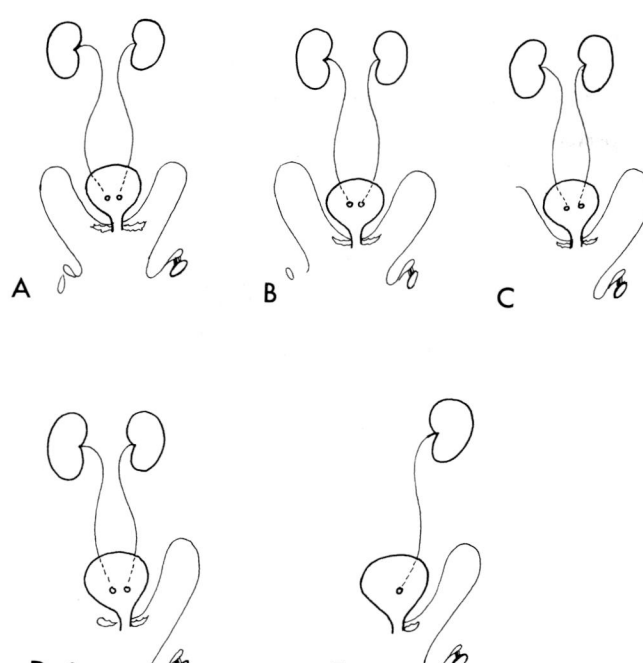

Figure 21.15. *Absence of wolffian duct derivatives.* **A,** *Absence of the ductuli efferentes only.* **B,** *to* **D,** *Progressively increasing extent of absence of the ductus deferens.* **E,** *Complete unilateral absence of wolffian duct derivatives, with abdominal testis. The kidney and ureter are usually absent as well.*

Anomalies of the Vas Deferens

For all practical purposes the anomalies of the vas deferens are congenital absence (bilateral-unilateral), congenital atresia, duplication, ectopia, anomalous pathway, and associated anomalies.

ABSENCE

Bilateral. Ochsner et al. (72) reported four cases with ipsilateral renal agenesis.

Donohue and Fauver (73) reported 26 patients with unilateral agenesis of the vas deferens, with 22 patients missing the ipsilateral renal unit and with contralateral anomalies in 33% of those patients. The same authors stated that 90 patients have been noted to have unilateral absence of the vas deferens, and 71 (79%) of these patients have had ipsilateral renal agenesis (74). Similar results were reported by Deane and May (75) and Patrick (76).

DUPLICATION OF THE DUCTUS DEFERENS

Duplication of the ductus deferens implies duplication of the wolffian duct during its earliest appearance as the pronephric duct. In most reported cases attention was

called to the anomaly by the presence of two testes on one side, each having its own ductus deferens (page 752.)

One patient had an anomalous undescended duct not associated with testicular tissue, but which was joined to a normal, descending ductus deferens at the seminal vesicle. The authors (77) considered it to be of wolffian origin, but it is more convincingly explained as a blind-ending ureter having an ectopic opening into the seminal vesicle.

Gravgaard et al. (78) reported a retroperitoneal duplication of the vas deferens and epididymis and failure of development of the ipsilateral kidney and ureter in a 26-year-old man. This extraordinary case simulated, on working diagnosis, an ectopic ureter entering the seminal vesicle.

Johnson and Perlmutter (79) reported single system ectopic ureteroceles with anomalies of the heart, testis and vas deferens in children with ureteroceles. Characteristically, one of the patients had bilateral atresia of the vas deferens.

OTHER ANOMALIES OF DUCTUS DEFERENS

At the lateral pelvic wall, the ureter is located medially to the obturator neurovascular bundle, and for all practical purposes, its downward continuation is posterolateral. The vas deferens crosses the ureter medially when the ureter approaches the seminal vesicle and the lateral side of the urinary crossing. This normal anatomy, however, occasionally becomes abnormal when the crossing becomes abnormal or when the vas is ectopic or drains into the ureter.

Anomalous crossing of the ureter by the vas deferens was reported by Rocha-Brito et al. (80). Insertion of the vas into a retroileac ureter was reported by Radhkrishnan et al. (81).

Hicks et al. (82) reported two patients with ectopic vas deferens associated with an imperforate anus and hypospadias. They stated that 19 more cases were reported, 5 of which were bilateral; in one of their cases, the ectopic vas had the highest reported insertion (Fig. 21.16).

Anomalies of the Seminal Vesicles

The anomalies of the seminal vesicles are not well documented. Campbell (48) found seminal vesicle, prostate gland, and testis absent in four of 10,919 autopsies of male infants. Unilateral absence of the ductus deferens and seminal vesicle (Fig. 19.15, *E*) is, of course, asymptomatic. Bilateral absence usually involves the ductus and results in complete sterility. Duplication and cysts of the seminal vesicles, and cysts and diverticula of the lower ductus deferens are known (Fig. 21.17). There is no information as to their frequency. Unless the cysts produce

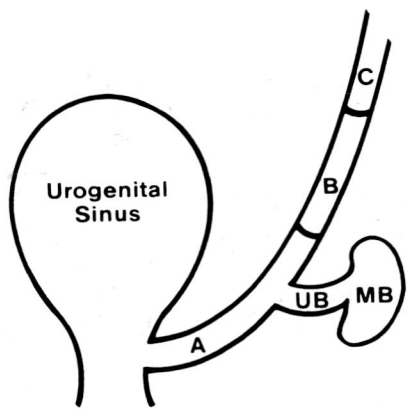

Figure 21.16. Embryology of ectopic vas deferens depicts three zones of wolffian duct (**A** to **C**). Ureteral bud *(UB)* will normally develop from common mesonephric duct *(A)*. If ureteral bud arises from proximal vas precursor *(B)*, then ectopic vas will drain into ipsilateral ureter or renal collecting system. *C*, Upper mesonephric duct; *MB*, metanephric blastema. (From Hicks CM, Skoog SJ, Done S. Ectopic vas deferens, imperforate anus and hypospadias: a new triad. J Urol 1989;141:586–588.)

obstruction of the urethra, such anomalies are asymptomatic.

Furtado (83) reported three cases of cystic seminal vesicle with ipsilateral renal agenesis. Fuselier and Peters (84) reported a case of seminal vesicle cyst associated with ipsilateral renal agenesis and ectopic ureter.

Sheih et al. (85) reported six cases of seminal vesicle cysts which were located laterally or posterior to the bladder wall. Lobel et al. (86) reported hypospermia and asthenospermia with seminal vesicle anomalies. Linseymeyer and Freidland (87) reported duplicated urethra communicating with the seminal vesicle.

Malatinsky et al. (88) reported anomalies of the seminal vesicles associated with anomalies of the vas deferens, ejaculatory ducts, and utricle in 14 patients (8.8%) after investigating 158 patients for sterility.

Several cases of seminal vesicle cyst with ipsilateral renal agenesis have been reported by Tanikawa et al. (89), Oyen et al. (90), and Kaneti et al. (91).

Complete absence of the seminal vesicle was reported by Kenney and Leesoy (92). The same authors reported seminal vesicles in the solid stage.

Dholakia et al. (93) reported ectopic ureter ending in a seminal vesicle, which also was associated with renal agenesis.

Anomalies of the Prostate Gland

ABSENCE OF THE PROSTATE GLAND

Partial or complete absence of the prostate is rare and has received little attention. Lisser (94) in 1923 reported 18 cases, all with infantile genitalia, eunuchoid habitus, and

pituitary insufficiency. Since all were diagnosed by rectal palpation, it is probable that the absence was due to atrophy rather than to agenesis. Partial absence of the prostate may occur when a unilateral absence of the ductus deferens is present.

PERSISTENCE OF THE ANTERIOR LOBE

Formed with the other four lobes, the anterior prostatic lobe normally regresses in fetal life, persisting only as small, solid epithelial outgrowths representing the atrophied tubules. Lowsley and Venero (95) found 18 instances in which the anterior lobe failed to regress and underwent hypertrophy in the adult (Fig. 21.18). Usually appearing as pea-sized structures in the ventral portion of the sphincter, they are asymptomatic. In four cases there was benign hypertrophy of this anomalous lobe alone, rather than a general prostatic enlargement. A previous prostatectomy in one patient failed to relieve the obstruction. In the three operated cases removal of the anterior lobe relieved the symptoms.

ENLARGEMENT OF THE PROSTATIC UTRICLE

This structure, the homologue of the vagina and cervix of the female, opens into the urethra at the colliculus seminalis. Although it is anatomically a part of the prostate gland, it is derived from the distal ends of the müllerian ducts, while the remainder of the prostate is of wolffian origin. Anomalies of the utricle are described on page 780.

Polse and Edelbrook (96) reported prostatic utricular enlargement as a cause of vesical outlet obstruction in children.

Morgan et al. (97) reported that obstruction of the prostatic utricle may form a utricular cyst, which may be palpated on bimanual pelvic examination on intersex patients.

HETEROTOPIC PROSTATE

Butterick et al. (98) reported ectopic prostatic tissue in the urethra.

Louw and Marsden (99) reported heterotopic prostatic tissue as a pedunculated mass within the urinary bladder.

MARION'S DISEASE

Marion's disease is a poorly understood fibrous dysplasia of the prostate gland that causes bladder neck obstruction in infants. It is discussed with other congenital causes of urethral obstruction in Chapter 18, "The Bladder and Urethra".

PROSTATE AND PRUNE BELLY SYNDROME

Deklerk and Scott (100) stated that the embryologically anomalous prostate has some normal epithelial elements

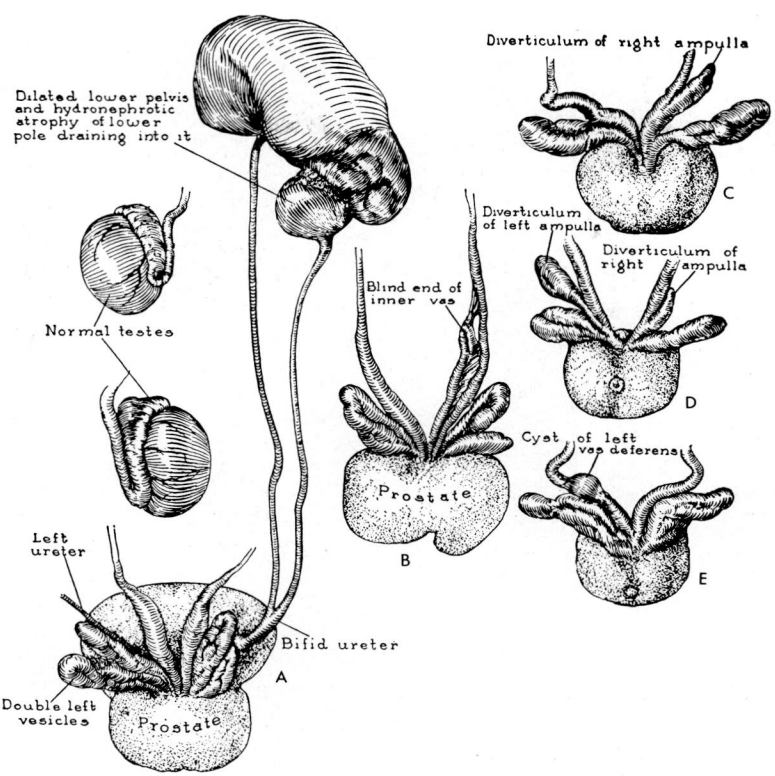

Figure 21.17. Anomalies of the seminal vesicle and ductus deferens. **A,** Double seminal vesicles, with bifid contralateral ureter. **B,** Double seminal vesicles, with blindly ending duplication of the ductus deferens. **C** and **D,** Diverticula of the ampulla of the ductus deferens. **E,** Cystic enlargement of the ductus deferens. All these anomalies are asymptomatic. (From Campbell MF. Urology, 2nd ed. Philadelphia: WB Saunders, 1963.)

in prune belly Syndrome. Stephens (101) stated that he found prostatic tubules to be small in number in only one of seven specimens.

Agenesis of the Penis

ANATOMY

In this condition, there is no external evidence of a penis. Usually, the scrotum is normal, and the testes may be descended (102) or undescended (103).

In 13 reported cases the urethra opened into the rectum (Fig. 21.19), and in 8 it opened on the perineum just anterior to the rectum. One patient had two urethral openings, one at each location (104) (Fig. 21.20). In two patients the opening was in front of the scrotum at the approximate site of the absent penis (103). Incontinence is never present; in one case the orifice within the rectum even required dilation to relieve bladder distension (105).

In at least three patients a small amount of erectile tissue was present at the urethral meatus. In one the meatus and erectile tissue were at the pubis (103); another patient had a perineal urethral meatus and a 10-cm erectile body under the skin from the perineum up to, and over, the scrotum. The testes were descended and live

spermatozoa were produced. The author reported the case under the name "concealed penis" (106).

EMBRYOGENESIS

Absence of the penis, together with the presence of a normal scrotum, supports the view that the genital tubercle and the labioscrotal swellings are independent structures. Because of the displacement of the urethra to the rectum or perineum in most cases, one must conclude that the genital tubercle never formed and that there was no pars phallica to the urogenital sinus. Such failure must have occurred as early as the fourth week. In patients in whom the urethra was located anterior to the scrotum, a later developmental failure with regression of the genital tubercle seems to be the only explanation (107).

The existence of penile agenesis without exstrophy of the bladder weakens the argument of Felix (3) and of later workers that the mesoderm of the genital tubercle is a necessary bar to the forward extension of the cloacal membrane.

HISTORY AND INCIDENCE

It is difficult to understand why so striking an anomaly was apparently first recorded as late as 1854 (108). An

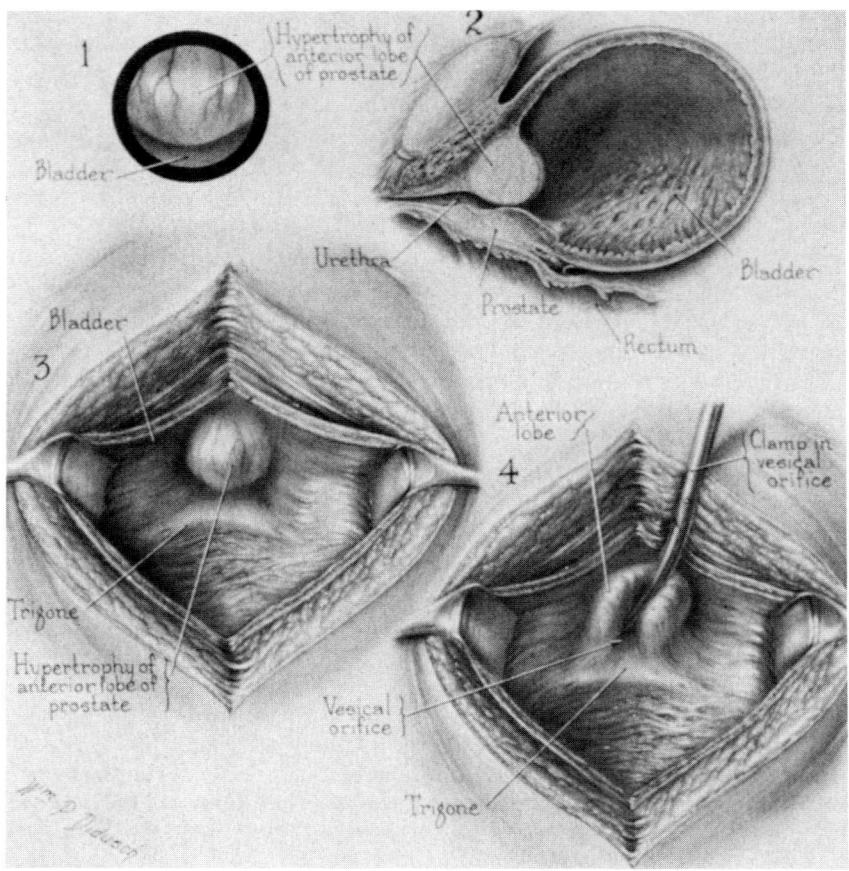

Figure 21.18. Adenomatous hypertrophy of a persistent anterior lobe of the prostate gland in a 30-year-old man. *1,* Cystoscopic view. *2,* Sagittal view of the lesions, showing obstruction to bladder emptying. *3* and *4,* Suprapubic exposure of the hypertrophic lobe. (From Lowsley OS, Venero AP. Persistent anterior lobe of the prostate gland. J Urol 1954;71:469–474.)

earlier report, by Saviard (109) in 1702, tells of a case of exstrophy of the bladder, but whether or not the penis was absent is not clear. Drury and Schwarzell (102) were able to find seven acceptable cases by 1935, and Richart and Benirschke (104) reported what they considered to be the 28th case in 1960. They did not include acardiac and sirenoid monsters, although 11 patients in their collected series had other congenital defects and died shortly after birth. The most recent review of the subject was by Gantier (110). He reported 50 cases in the literature, adding 2 from his own practice. Kessler and McLaughlin (111) reported the incidence to be between 1:10 million and 1:30 million. In a few cases no other anomalies are present (112). However, Ruprrecht et al. (113) stated that the incidence is 1:16,000 necropsies.

Several cases of penile agenesis have been recently reported, including those of Kraus (114); Dusmot et al. (115), whose work was in association with VATER syndrome; Oesch et al. (116), who reported six cases; and Berry et al. (117), who reported penile agenesis in one identical male twin.

TREATMENT

A penis was surgically constructed in one patient (103). Gender reassignment with rearing as a female is most appropriate for those children seen in infancy. Surgical reconstruction in this situation would include bilateral orchiectomy, preferably at an early age to prevent testosterone imprinting, and vaginoplasty and labial reconstruction. Those children seen at a later age who have been reared as males should probably continue in this role. Reconstruction of a phallus, utilizing various pedicle grafts and an inflatable penile prosthesis, though arduous, is feasible and can provide a satisfactory result (118).

Agenesis of the Glans Penis

Two cases have been reported in which the glans penis was absent (119, 120). In both patients the prepuce was present, but there was no preputial sulcus, and the shaft ended as a rounded stump. In de la Peña's case, a plastic reconstructive operation was performed to improve the

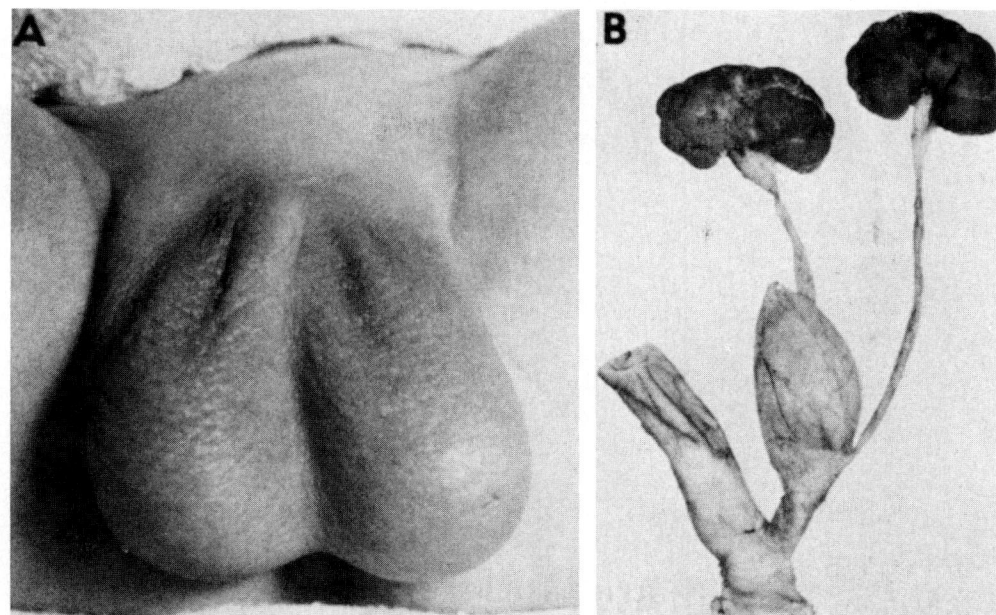

Figure 21.19. Agenesis of the penis. **A,** External view. **B,** Specimen showing urethrorectal communication. (From Potter EL. Pathology of the fetus and the newborn. Chicago: Year Book Medical Publishers, 1952.)

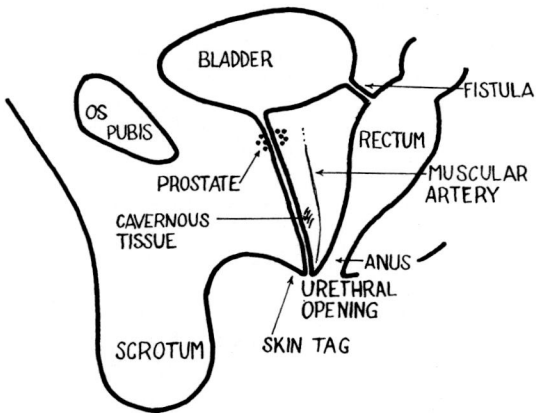

Figure 21.20. Agenesis of the penis. In this patient the urethra reached the outside, although a vesicorectal fistula was also present. (From Richart R, Benirschke K. Penile agenesis: report of case, review of the world literature, and discussion of pertinent embryology. Arch Pathol 1960;70:252–260. Copyright 1960, American Medical Association.)

patient's sexual performance, but the patient's difficulty may have been psychogenic.

As dissection of such a penis has never been described, no conclusions about the embryogenesis of the defect are possible.

Phimosis

This congenital anomaly is an overproduction of the skin of the prepuce with a stenotic preputial opening and inability to retract the redundant prepuce over the glans penis.

The treatment is neonatal circumcision, which avoids infections secondary to poor hygiene (including urinary tract infection, veneral disease, and balanitis), penile carcinoma, and paraphimosis.

Gillenwater and Grayhack (121) reported that 52% of patients with carcinoma of the penis gave a history of phimosis. The debate continues about whether the presence of the foreskin is responsible for the genesis of penile cancer.

Wolbarst (122) and Dean (123) stated that penile cancer was not reported in U.S. Jews. Dean stated that "prophylactic treatment of cancer of the penis consists in circumcising all male infants a few days after birth." Schoen (124), who recommends circumcision for the prevention of cancer, reported that the American Academy of Pediatrics favors neonatal circumcision for prevention of penile cancer. Shoen, however, advises the physician to inform parents of the advantages and disadvantages of the procedure.

The interested reader will find a very good summary of information in the publication of Lago (125).

Paraphimosis is a complication of phimosis when foreskin is forcefully turned back, forming a very tight dermal ring. The treatment consists of a small incision dorsally, long enough for the glans penis to be freed and the skin to be pulled forward. The patient must undergo circumcision as soon as the dorsal slit heals completely.

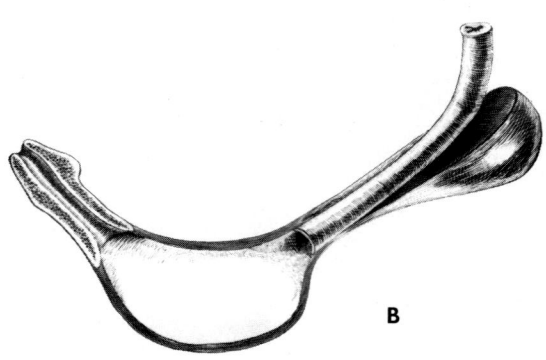

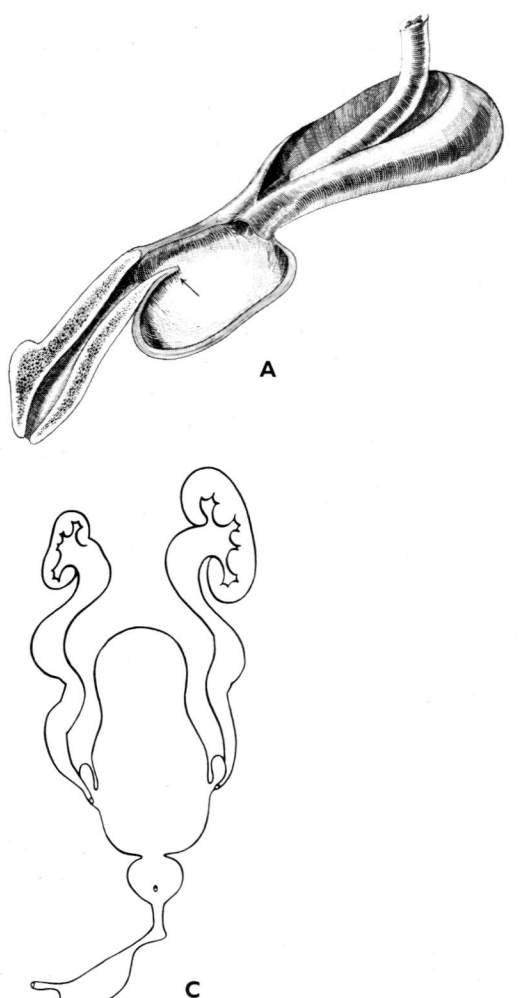

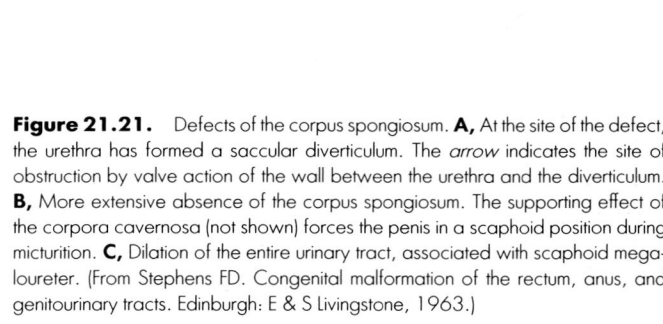

Figure 21.21. Defects of the corpus spongiosum. **A,** At the site of the defect, the urethra has formed a saccular diverticulum. The *arrow* indicates the site of obstruction by valve action of the wall between the urethra and the diverticulum. **B,** More extensive absence of the corpus spongiosum. The supporting effect of the corpora cavernosa (not shown) forces the penis in a scaphoid position during micturition. **C,** Dilation of the entire urinary tract, associated with scaphoid megaloureter. (From Stephens FD. Congenital malformation of the rectum, anus, and genitourinary tracts. Edinburgh: E & S Livingstone, 1963.)

Defects of the Corpus Spongiosum and the Corpora Cavernosa

A few cases have been reported of partial agenesis of the penile erectile tissue, resulting in dilation of the penile urethra (126, 127). Three degrees of severity have been described.

1. The absence of a localized region of the corpus spongiosum permits a saccular diverticulum of the penile urethra to develop. After a certain size is reached, the diverticulum contained within the tunica albuginea compresses and obstructs the urethra (Fig. 21.21, *A*).
2. A more extensive agenesis of the corpus spongiosum produces megalourethra. Because the normal corpora cavernosa are present, the penis takes a scaphoid shape during urination (Fig. 21.21, *B*).
3. Extensive agenesis of the corpora cavernosa as well as the corpus spongiosum in the shaft of the penis permits fusiform enlargement of the urethra (Fig. 21.22). Some normal erectile tissue is present at the base and in the glans of the penis.

All three conditions are rare; patients with anomalies of the second and third degrees also have other anomalies of the urinary tract. Lowe et al. (128) reported vascular congestion of the corpus spongiosum in children with urethral prolapse.

Duplication of the Penis and Clitoris and Other Anomalies

ANATOMY

Double penis is not a single defect with uniform anatomy or etiology. The duplication may be bilateral or sagittal; there may be two distinct penes, or they may arise from a common base. A urethra may be present in one, both, or neither.

Bilateral duplications may be found in patients with duplication of all midline structures of the caudal part of the body (pages 248 and 681), and they may exist in exstrophy of the cloaca (page 693). We are not concerned here with these anomalies (Fig. 21.23, *F*).

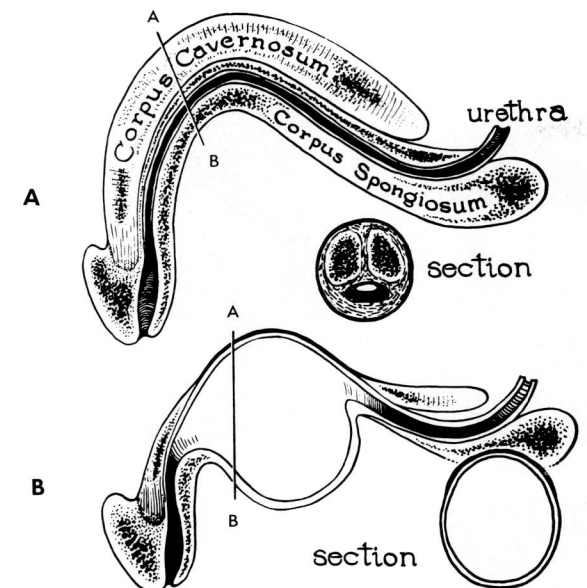

Figure 21.22. Absence of the corpora cavernosa and corpus spongiosum in the midportion of the penis. Fusiform expansion of the penile urethra has occurred. **A,** Normal penis, for comparison with **B,** penis with absence of erectile tissue. (From Stephens FD. Congenital malformations of the rectum, anus, and genito-urinary tracts. Edinburgh: E & S Livingstone, 1963.)

Simple bilateral duplications vary from a double but fused penis with a single prepuce (129) (Fig. 21.23, *E*) to a complete duplication with both members normal and usable (52) (Fig. 21.23, *B* and *C*). The scrotum is nearly always bifid; in one case it was trifid, with an empty median pouch (130).

The urethra may be doubled, as in Pendino's (52) patient, or it and the corpus spongiosum may be present in one penis and absent in the other (131). In some cases the urethra opens at the penoscrotal junction (129) or even at the perineum (132). Epispadias and exstrophy of the bladder were present in several cases (133). An intrapelvic duplicated phallus, which lay lateral to the prostate and protruded into the bladder, was discovered at cystoscopy in an adult (134).

Among midline duplications, the most striking was that reported by Davis (135), in which four peniform structures were present. The structure at the normal site was a normal penis with urethra. The second structure had a glans, prepuce, and corpora cavernosa but no urethra. The third contained only an epithelial sinus, and the fourth proved, on sectioning, to be a teratoma (Fig. 21.23, *A*).

In one patient the two midline penile shafts were convergent, having widely separated bases but a single glans. The organ was thus triangular. Only a single urethra was present (136).

Bonney et al. (137) reported clitoral hypertrophy in a girl with complete duplication of the urethra and vaginal

stenosis. Belis and Hrabovsky (138) reported clitoromegaly in a neonate with idiopathic female intersex.

A female infant with obliquely placed but normal genitalia and a midline skin cleft with a second clitoris has been reported (139). The urethra was not duplicated, although there were other defects and the child was mentally retarded (Fig. 21.23, *D*).

CONGENITAL ANOMALIES OF CLITORIS

Of the three congenital anomalies of the clitoris (agenesis, hypoplasia, and hyperplasia) agenesis of clitoris (as well as penile agenesis) is an extremely rare phenomenon. In hypoplasia, also rare, the clitoris is very small, and it is difficult to say if it is hypoplastic or "small normal."

In hyperplasia, or clitoromegaly, the clitoris is anatomically a small penis without urethra. Dehner (140) stated that it measures 2 to 3 cm in length. Clitoromegaly could be a congenital anomaly secondary to pseudo- or true hermaphroditism or the end results of abnormal hormone secretions which are responsible for the genesis of adrenogenital syndrome and so on. According to Gross et al. (141) congenital adrenal hyperplasia was responsible for the 62% of abnormalities of the clitoris.

ASSOCIATED ANOMALIES

Imperforate anus is often present (133, 142). Sacral meningocele or spina bifida, absence of one kidney (131), and separation of the pubic bones (139, 143) have been observed. In one patient a duplicated colon opened into an anus on the left and into a hemibladder on the right (144). Johnson et al. (145) reported penile duplication with other anomalies. Hollowell et al. (146) reported two cases (one adult and one infant) with duplication of the penis associated with multiple other anomalies; they studied 46 cases, dividing them in two groups: (a) complete duplication (29 cases) and (b) incomplete duplication (15 cases).

HISTORY AND INCIDENCE

The earliest reported case was seen and mentioned by two authors, Schenk (129) and Wecker (147), both writing in 1609. Neugebauer in 1898 (52, 148) was able to collect 28 cases, and Nesbit and Bromme described what they considered to be the 45th case in 1933. To these, Cochrane and Saunders (149) added nine in 1942. Pendino (52) considered his case to be the 53rd, but Vilanova and Raventós (150), whose own case was not a penile duplication, counted it as the 60th. Jeffcoate (143) collected four cases of bifid or double clitoris and added one of his own in 1957. The condition of penile duplication in animals and humans has been reviewed by Messier and Gagnon (151). Hollowell et al. (146) stated that penile duplication occurs at an approximate rate of 1:5 million live births.

Duplication of the penis is an extremely rare congeni-

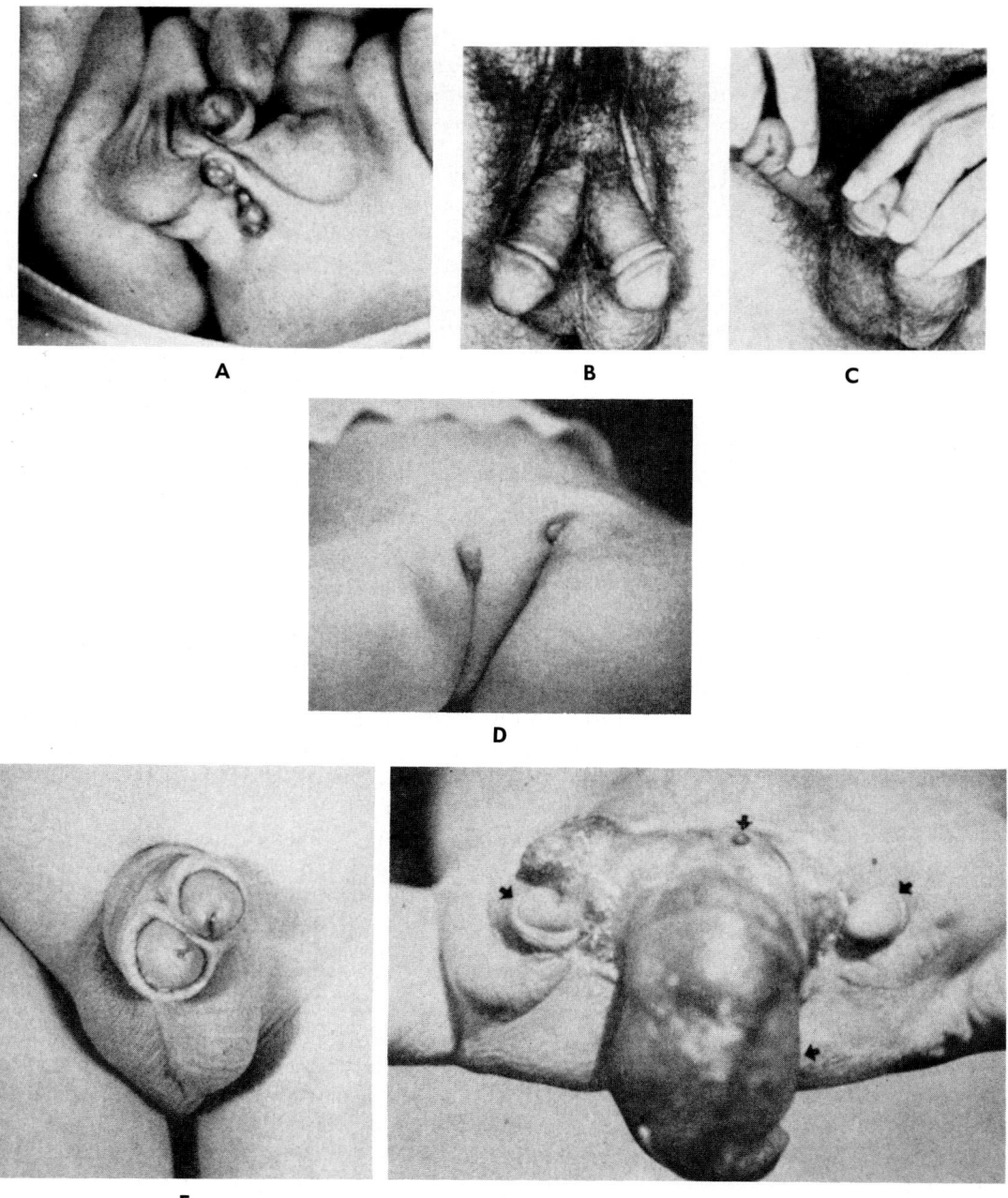

Figure 21.23. Phallic duplication. **A,** Midline triplication of the penis. The most anterior structure is a normal penis; the next two structures were incomplete penes; and the most posterior structure is a teratoma. **B,** and **C,** Bilateral penes each separate and normal except for the absence of the prepuce. Each had a normal urethra. **D,** Double clitoris. The thighs are asymmetric, and the left vulva is placed obliquely. In the cleft on the right is a clitoris with no associated urethra or introitus. **E,** Bilateral penes separated for about half the length of the shaft. Each urethra communicated with a separate hemibladder. **F,** Doubling of the penis in exstrophy of the cloaca *(lateral arrows)*. (**A,** From Davis DM. A case of double, triple or quadruple penis associated with dermoid of the perineum. J Urol 1949;61:111–115; **B** and **C,** from Pendino JA. Diphallus (double penis). J Urol 1950;64:156–157; **D,** from Kurth ME. Incomplete duplication of the female external genitalia or double clitoris. Am J Surg 1958;96:596–599; **E** and **F,** from Lattimer JK, Uson AC, Melicow MM. The male genital tract. In: Benson CD, Mustard WT, Ravitch MM, Snyder WH Jr, Welch KJ, eds. Pediatric surgery, Vol 2. Chicago: Year Book Medical Publishers, 1962.)

tal anomaly. Landy et al. (152) reported a case; they were able to collect from the literature fewer than 75 cases. They estimated the incidence at approximately 1:5.5 million live male births.

DIAGNOSIS

Diagnosis is by inspection and palpation. Normally, the deformity is recognized at birth or by the parents during infancy. However, in Fowler's patient (136), no abnormality was suspected until coitus was attempted. The urethra should always be traced by catheter or by radiography to evaluate the condition of the two organs.

TREATMENT

Because of the variations encountered, it is difficult to set any rules for treatment. Many reported cases have remained untreated. When the penis or clitoris is completely doubled, excision of the less well-formed organ should be undertaken. Where separation is incomplete, each case must be evaluated separately. Fowler (136) removed the inferior shaft and transplanted the ureter to the superior shaft without incising the glans in his patient.

It is not within the scope of this book to present details, but the interested reader will find valuable information and advice in papers of Johnston (153), Schmeller and Scherrmer (154), Westenfelder (155), and Wirtshafter (156).

Transposition of the Penis and Scrotum

ANATOMY

A dozen or more cases in which the penis lay behind the scrotum, rather than in front, have been reported since the first case was discovered by Broman (157) in 1911 (48, 158, 159) (Fig. 21.24). In two females with multiple anomalies, the clitoris was located at the posterior end of the labia (160, 161).

Three patients had no other anomalies. Two were adults and had fathered children in spite of their abnormalities (162, 163). The remainder had defects ranging from hypospadias to absence of the urethra (158, 164), absence of the entire urinary tract (165), and Fanconi syndrome (166).

Two additional cases have been reported, in which one scrotal sac was located in front and the other behind the penis. In one case the right scrotal sac was prepenile and the right kidney was absent; the penis had slight hypospadias, chordee, and an accessory glans (167). In the other case the left scrotum was misplaced and the left kidney was absent, but the penis was normal; in addition, the left foot was clubbed and the left thumb was absent (168) (Fig. 19.25). Ectopic penis was reported by Stachow and Masowski (169) and by Sanvitale (170). Kernaban (171) as

well as Ehrlich and Scardino (172) studied scrotal transposition.

EMBRYOGENESIS

As epispadias is not present in these cases, it may be assumed that the penis arose in its normal position and that the scrotal swellings were abnormally placed. Spaulding (24) believes that the presumptive scrotal swellings are first cranial to the phallus (genital tubercle) and shift caudad at about the 38-mm stage (ninth week). Failure of the shift results in formation of the scrotum in front of the penis (Fig. 21.26).

TREATMENT

Forshall and Rickham (173) undertook repair of the deformity in their patient in three operations. The penis was straightened and brought forward, producing hypospadias. In the second operation, the hypospadias was repaired, leaving a contracture, which in turn was relieved by the third operation. Campbell (48) was able to divide the scrotum, bring the penis forward and suture the scrotum behind it.

Duplications of the Penile Urethra

ANATOMY

Within the penis, the urethra may bifurcate; it may also have diverticula, or there may be blind canals extending inward from the skin. The accessory meatus may be on the glans (Fig. 21.27), on the dorsum (Fig. 21.28), or on the ventrum (Fig. 21.29). All may be called accessory urethrae. These structures are of different embryonic origin from the duplications of the proximal urethra described on page 709.

Accessory urethrae may occasionally be epispadiac. They may arise from the normal urethra below the prostate gland (Fig. 21.30, B) or from the bladder, independently of the normal urethra (173). In this latter case there is a suggestion of partially suppressed midline duplication of the penis (Fig. 19.27, C). Campbell (48) illustrated a case in which an accessory, epispadiac urethra ended blindly without reaching the bladder (Fig. 21.30, A).

Williams and Kenawi (175) classified male urethral duplications as follows:

Sagittal duplication
  Y-duplication: preanal or perineal accessory channel
  Spindle urethra: urethra splits into two and then reunites
  Epispadias: dorsal penile accessory urethra
  Hypospadias: both urethrae ventral to corpora
    Complete: two channels leave the bladder separately
    Bifid or incomplete: urethra divides below the bladder
    Abortive: accessory urethra is a blind sinus

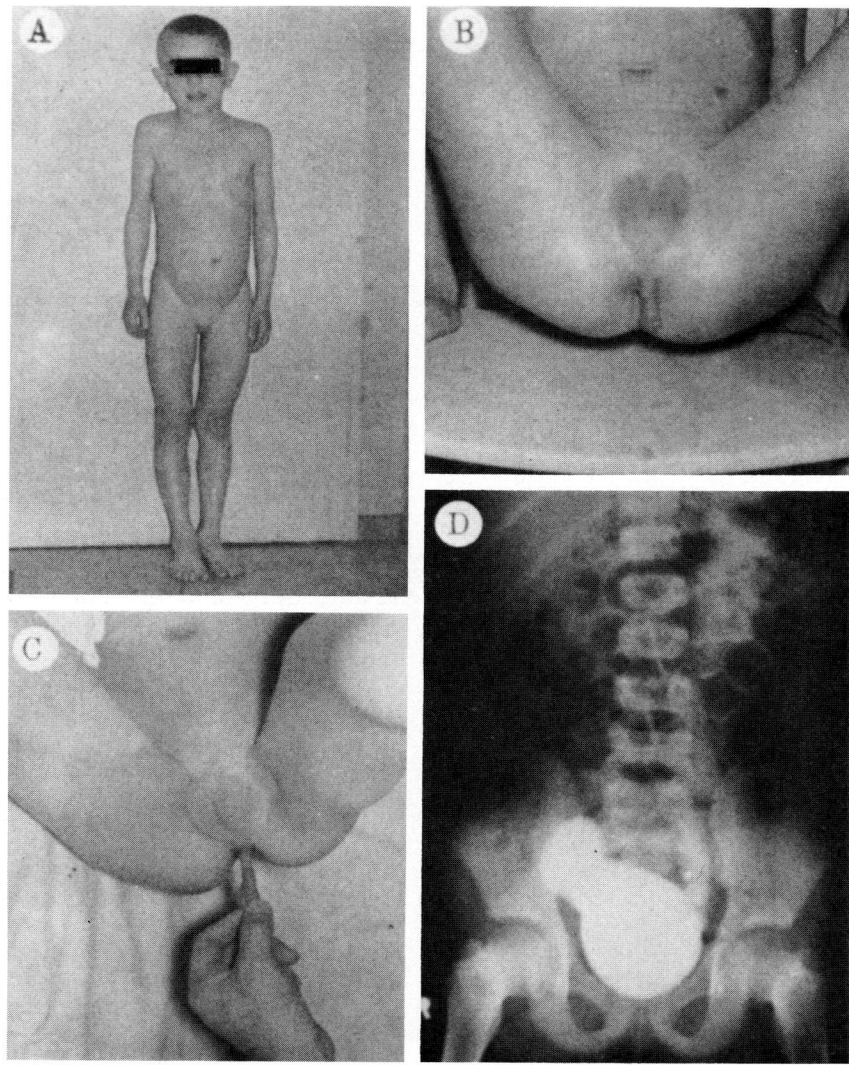

Figure 21.24. Transposition of the penis and scrotum in an 11-year-old boy. **A,** Scrotum below pubis; no penis could be seen. **B,** Child in lithotomy position; penis is behind scrotum. **C,** View of genital organs. **D,** Gravity cystogram shows large diverticulum on right side, reflux to left ureter and kidney. (From Remzi D. Transposition of penis and scrotum. J Urol 1966;95:555–557.)

   Collateral duplication
      Complete with diphallus
      Abortive: one urethra is a blind sinus

EMBRYOGENESIS

Ventral duplications, diverticula, and accessory canals are all formed by the creation of two channels, one above the other, during the closure of the penis and the formation of the raphe during the 10th to 14th weeks. Several views of the details of this process have been advanced.

Johnson (176) considered that faulty union of the genital ridges might sequester two parallel channels: one of endoderm, which would be the normal urethra, and one of the ectoderm, lying nearer the raphe. Neff (177) considered that more than one endodermal canal might be formed.

Lowsley (178) suggested that two channels are formed by the persistence of the urogenital closing plate, which extends the length of the penis, having the urogenital sinus above it and the urethral gutter below. If the plate fails to rupture and be resorbed, two channels will result.

Neither of these views is consistent with the description of the splitting of the urethral plate put forward by Glenister (9) (Fig. 19.9).

Johnson (176) offered an additional explanation for cysts and diverticula. He found duct and glandular tissue from embryonic glands of Littré isolated in the suburethral penile tissues in a fetus and suggested that they might produce epithelial cysts of the raphe. Similarly, dilation of Cowper's glands and ducts may produce canals resembling urethral diverticula, although they are not in the midline.

Accessory urethrae opening on the dorsum of the penis are less common and less easily explained (179).

HISTORY AND INCIDENCE

Aristotle is said to have seen a duplication of the urethra (174), and Vesalius apparently saw a complete duplication in a male. Although there were a few cases mentioned by 16th and 17th century writers, such as Donatus (180) and Hildanus (181), Morgagni makes no mention of them. Baillie (182) in 1797 clearly described a blind-ending duplication.

The first classification to bring order to the isolated observations was proposed by Taruffi (183) in 1891. Five years later, Le Fort (184) collected 75 cases from the literature up to that time, but not all of these have been considered satisfactory. Chauvin (185) reviewed the litera-

ture in 1927 and discussed the condition at length. Lowsley (178) collected 42 cases of blind-ending duplications in 1939. Gross and Moore (174) in 1950 collected 19 complete and 1 incomplete case of double urethrae arising from the bladder, 12 cases of urethral bifurcation, and 51 cases of blind canals from the skin of the penis. No estimates of incidence have been made.

Naparstek et al. (186) stated that only approximately 50 cases have been reported.

SYMPTOMS

Urethral bifurcations lead only to the problem associated with an ectopic meatus. Patients often habitually occlude the accessory channel during micturition.

Blind openings from the skin are asymptomatic and are rarely noticed by the patient unless they become infected (187). Lowsley (178) found 26 of 42 patients to have gonorrheal infection; 15 had the infection in the blind canal only. Nonvenereal infections may also be found (188).

Diverticula from the bladder or urethra may be asymptomatic and remain undetected, or they may be revealed by their progressive enlargement. Perineal swelling during voiding, with extra urine produced by pressure on the swelling, is pathognomonic, but Gross and Bill (189) have described patients in whom no swelling was evident. Rarely, the enlarged diverticulum ruptures, with extravasation of urine into the scrotum, groin, and lower abdominal wall. At least two such catastrophes have had a fatal outcome (190, 191). The observation of two urinary streams or urinary tract infection is usually the presenting symptom. Infection may be the result of a partially stenotic lumen of the accessory urethra. These

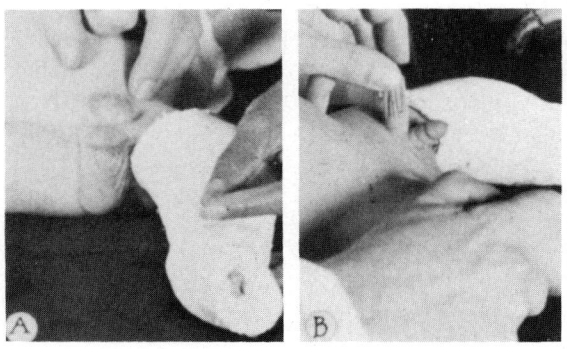

Figure 21.25. Two views of a patient with unilateral (left) transposition of the penis and scrotum. (From Flanagan MJ, McDonald JH, and Keifer JH. Unilateral transposition of the scrotum. J Urol 1961;86:273–275.)

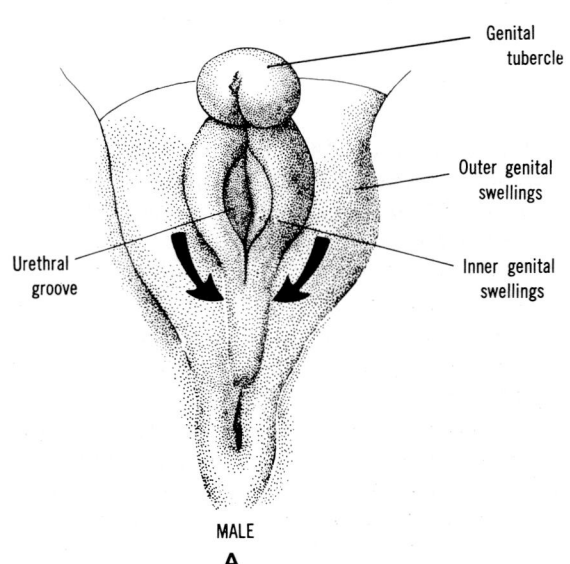

MALE

A

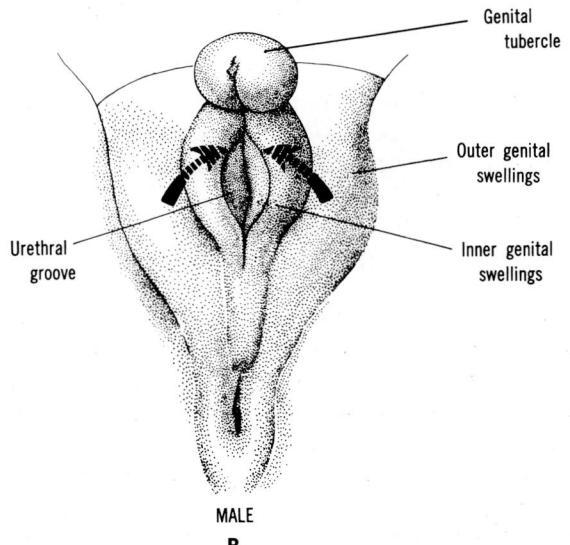

MALE

B

Figure 21.26. Development of transposition of the penis and scrotum. **A,** Normal development. The outer genital swellings, primordia of the scrotum move caudal to the phallus as the urethral groove closes. **B,** Failure of the caudal shift

of the swelling will produce transposition. (Outlines from Davies J. Human developmental anatomy. New York: Ronald Press, 1963.)

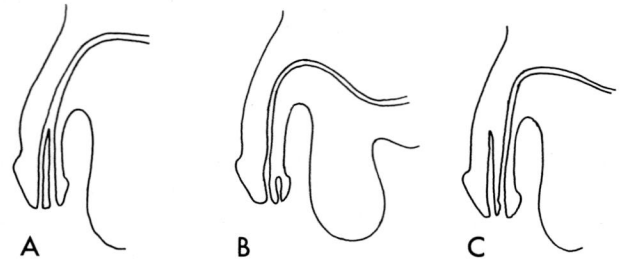

Figure 21.27. *Varieties of accessory, blind urethrae opening on the glans penis.*

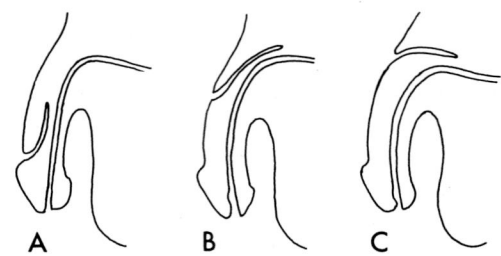

Figure 21.28. *Varieties of accessory, blind urethrae opening on the dorsum of the penis. These, perhaps, represent incipient epispadias.*

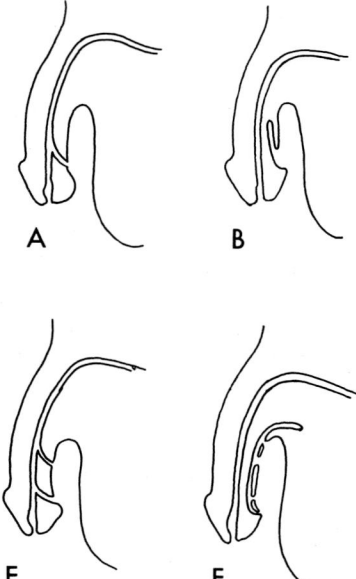

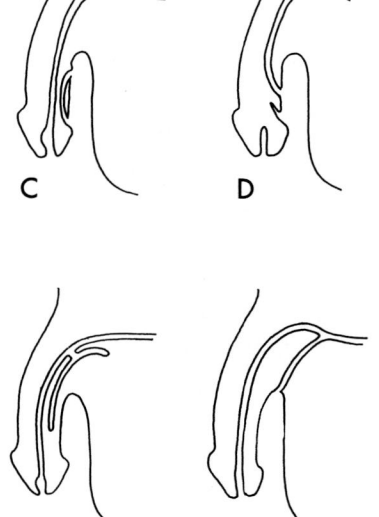

Figure 21.29. *Varieties of accessory urethrae opening on the ventral surface of the penis. Such accessory urethrae may join the normal urethra (**A, E,** and **H**); they may end blindly (**B**); or they may have multiple openings without communication with the normal urethra (**C** and **F**). **D,** Both the functional urethra and the*

*blind accessory urethra are hypospadiac. **H,** Both a normal and a penoscrotal hypospandic urethra are present. **G,** The accessory urethra has no exterior opening and must be considered to be a diverticulum.*

symptoms are likely to occur only if the accessory urethra communicates with the bladder. Blind-ending duplications of the urethra are almost always asymptomatic.

DIAGNOSIS

When accessory canals are of normal diameter, catheterization will provide the necessary information about the anatomic arrangement. A point of bifurcation can usually be detected by feeling the contact between two metal sounds. Voiding cystourethrograms have been used in some cases (192). Manual occlusion of one channel during voiding is usually helpful.

Physical examination will reveal two apparent urethral meatuses. Observation of two urinary streams, one from each meatus, confirms the diagnosis. Cystourethroscopy and urethrography are necessary to delineate the anatomy of the duplication and to establish the diagnosis of a blind-ending duplication.

TREATMENT

Blind-ending urethral duplications without symptoms need no treatment. The remaining types of urethral duplication are generally best managed by excision of the more atretic accessory channel.

Atresia and Stenosis of the Urethra

ANATOMY

Atresia. Urethral atresia may be extensive, or more rarely, it may be a simple diaphragm. Any part of the urethra may be involved. In males the most frequent condition is absence of the entire penile urethra, followed by absence of the glandular urethra. The prostatic and membranous portions are rarely involved. In females, diaphragmatic atresia is more frequent (193).

Because of the damage to the kidneys resulting from

atresia, about 33% of affected infants are stillborn. In many of the living infants an alternative urinary pathway is open. In most the urachus is patent (Fig. 18.10, *E*); in others there is a penile or a scrotal fistula (194) or a vesicovaginal fistula (195).

Valves and Strictures. Diaphragmatic atresias of the urethra may be incomplete or may become secondarily perforated. In the posterior male urethra, they are represented by Young's type 3 valves (page 706). While they are rare, their occurrence is not limited to the posterior urethra or to the male (193). Cases of valves of the cavernous urethra have been described (196, 197). If hydronephrosis does not supervene, a diverticulum may be formed proximal to the valve.

Strictures are ring-like constrictions that may represent incipient or abortive diaphragm formation. Little is known about their formation or occurrence. Most are the result of infection, but a few are of congenital origin. Amsler (198) examined 38 cases of urethral stricture in adult men and believed 5 to be of congenital origin. Harshman et al. (199) as well as Kaplan and Brock (200) discussed the subject of strictures in detail. Dodat et al. (201) reported 1.5-cm atresia of the bulbomembranous urethra. Grosse-Hokamp and Muller (202) reported atresia associated with prune belly syndrome.

Meatal Stenosis. This condition occurs almost exclusively in boys who have been circumcised, presumably secondary to episodes of meatitis which occur because of the loss of protection of the glans provided by the foreskin.

The diagnosis, while it may be suspected from observation of a small meatus on physical examination, can only be made conclusively by observation of the voided urinary stream. The stenotic meatus will produce a narrow caliber, often deflected stream.

EMBRYOGENESIS

Failure of canalization of the urethral plate to form the secondary urethral gutter of the penis is the most probable cause of atresia of the penile urethra. Absence of the entire penile urethra may imply an earlier failure of the urethral plate to develop or possibly a developmental failure of the pars phallica of the urogenital sinus itself. The latter possibility seems the least likely since one would expect it to lead only to hypospadias. Glandular atresia is present in the mildest degree of hypoplasia and probably represents a failure of the independently formed distal urethral segment to appear. It is easier to explain the atresia than to explain the absence of a hypospadiac opening. One might speculate that pressure from urine

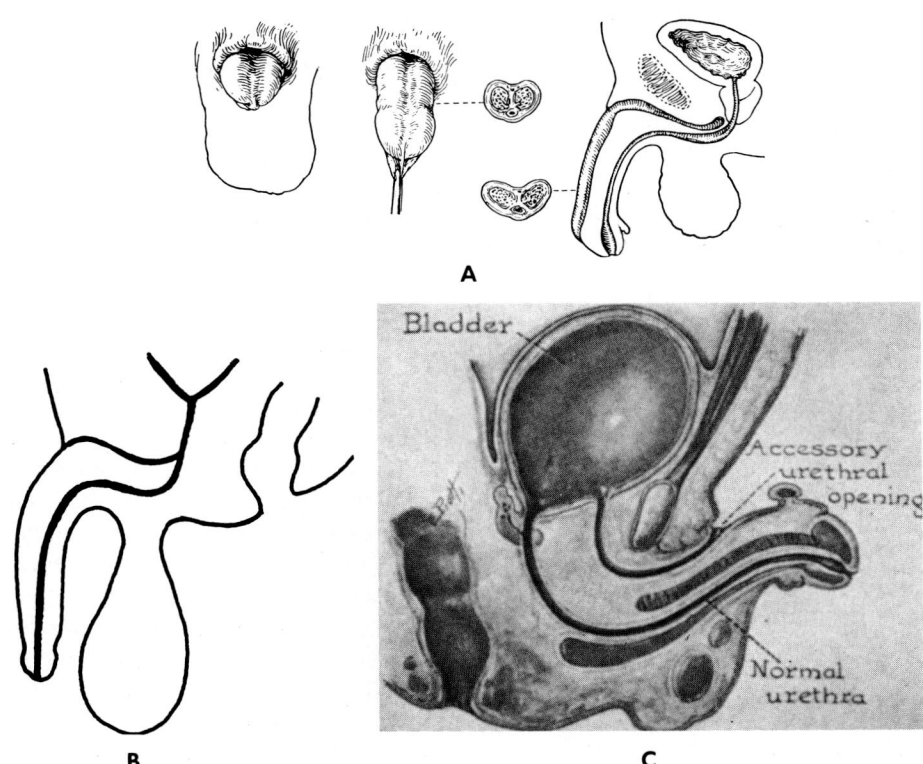

Figure 21.30. Epispadiac accessory urethrae. **A,** Blind-ending epispadiac urethra associated with a normal urethra. **B,** Epispadiac urethra arising from the normal urethra below the prostate. **C,** An epispadiac urethra arising from the bladder independently of the normal urethra. (From Gross RE, Moore TC. Arch Surg 1950;60:749–761. Copyright 1950, American Medical Association; **A,** from Campbell MF. Urology, 2nd ed. Philadelphia: WB Saunders, 1963.)

normally prevents complete closure of the urethral gutter in the absence of a meatus and that complete closure of the gutter in these cases occurred when excretory activity was abnormally low. Possibly a reduction in fetal blood pressure for a few hours at the right moment might produce the effect.

In the female, meatal stricture and atresia has been related to persistence of the urogenital membrane by Stevens (193). This explanation is reasonable.

HISTORY OF INCIDENCE

In 1550 Cabrol encountered an 18-year-old girl who urinated from her umbilicus as a result of congenital urethral occlusion. Cannulation of the urethra and ligation of the umbilical protrusion restored normal function. Cabrol's description of the case is quoted in Ménégaux and Boidot (203).

In spite of this early discovery and effective treatment, reports of the condition are rare. Ménégaux and Boidot (203) reviewed 42 cases, of both live and stillborn patients, in 1934. Dourmashkin (195) was able to collect only 87 cases by 1943, of which 50 were in live born infants. Only 11 of the 87 were female. Dourmashkin found only eight U.S. cases in 100 years. In contrast to this apparent rarity, he found four cases in 6 months at one hospital. He mentioned no familial relationships.

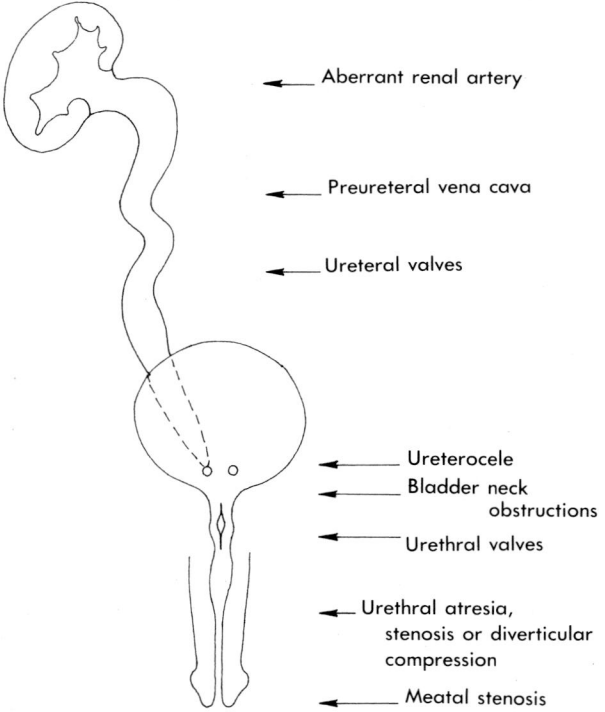

Figure 21.31. The locations in which congenital anomalies produce urinary obstruction. Three of the eight locations are in the penile urethra.

SYMPTOMS

Unless there is an alternate opening for the escape of urine, the symptoms of atresia are those of complete lower urinary tract obstruction. Hydroureter and hydronephrosis are the inevitable sequelae. All infants having a patent urachus should be suspected of having urethral atresia. Hydronephrosis secondary to meatal stenosis is rare. Most patients with this acquired condition will have it corrected due to voiding symptoms long before it leads to upper tract damage.

DIAGNOSIS

When the meatus is patent, catheterization with palpation will reveal the distal limit of the atresia. Palpation may aid in determining the length of the atretic portion. In the majority of cases the meatus is absent. Obstruction elsewhere in the urinary tract may present and must not be ruled out (Fig. 21.31). Cystourethroscopy and urethrography are the most effective means to establish the diagnosis.

TREATMENT

A simple meatotomy is sufficient for those boys with meatal stenosis. More extensive degrees of urethral atresia must be managed by urethral reconstruction or urethral replacement.

Epispadias

ANATOMY.

Epispadias is an anterior dislocation of the urethral meatus. In the male the urethra may emerge on the dorsum of the glans (balanic epispadias), on the dorsum of the shaft of the penis (penile epispadias), or on the body wall at the base of the penis (penopubic or complete epispadias). The complete form is the most frequently encountered clinically, although balanic epispadias is probably more common (Fig. 21.32, A to C).

The three degrees of the defect may also be found in females. The mildest is a bifid clitoris, with an enlarged urethral orifice; the intermediate type includes most of the urethra but not the internal sphincter; and the complete state affects the whole of the urethra, including the sphincter (Fig. 21.33, A to C). Complete epispadias in either sex is accompanied by urinary incontinence.

In the male with complete epispadias, the penis is drawn upward against the abdominal wall. The glans and the penile shaft have a dorsal groove, which passes backward to enter a tunnel beneath the pubic symphysis (Fig. 21.32, C). This groove is the roofless urethra and is lined with mucosa. The prepuce of the penis is redundant below and absent above the glans. The corpora cavernosa are loosely attached to one another, and the corpus spongiosum is absent (Fig. 21.34).

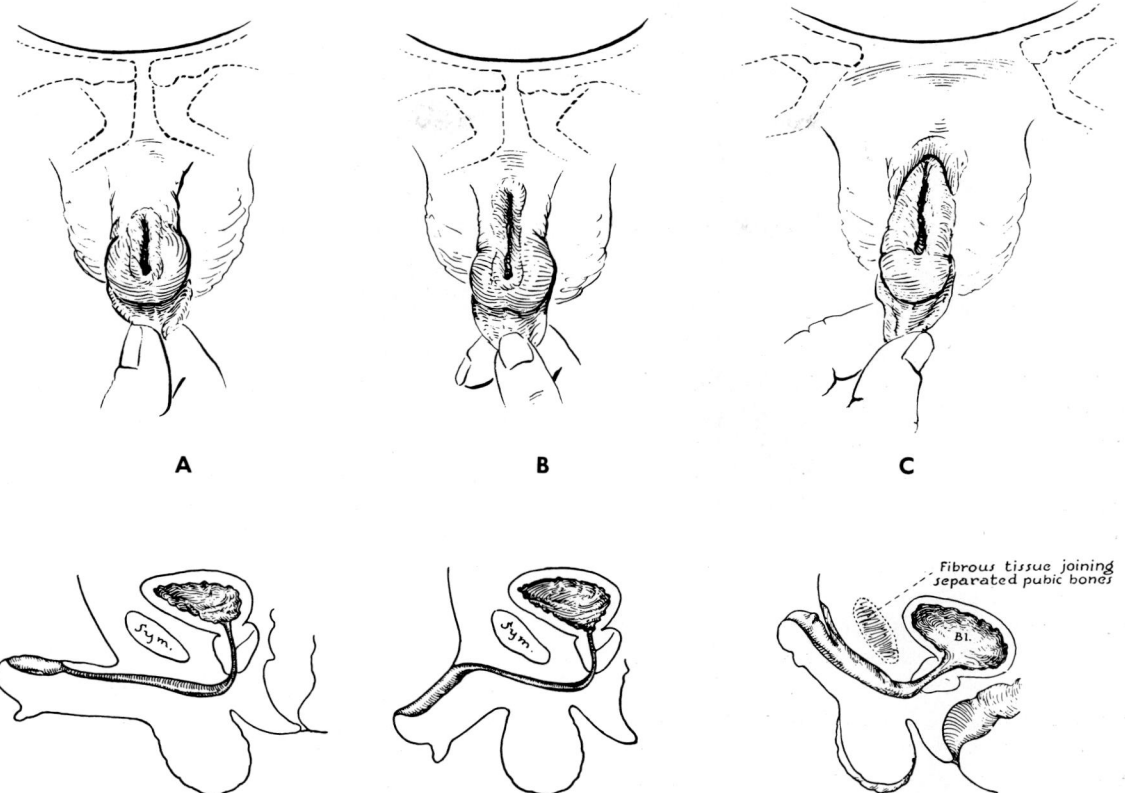

Figure 21.32. Three degrees of epispadias in the male. **A,** Balanic. **B,** Penile. **C,** Penopubic (complete). *Broken lines* indicate public bones; they are widely separated in complete epispadias. (Anterior views from Welch KJ. Hypo-spadias. In: Benson CD, Mustard WT, Ravitch WH, Synder WH Jr, Welch KJ, eds. Pediatric surgery. Chicago: Year Book Medical Publishers, 1962. Lateral views from Campbell MF. Urology, 3rd ed. Philadelphia: WB Saunders, 1970.)

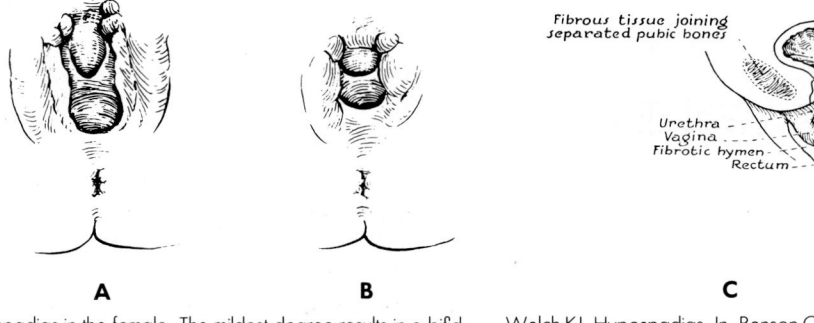

Figure 21.33. Epispadias in the female. The mildest degree results in a bifid clitoris only and requires no surgery. **A,** Second degree of epispadias. **B,** Complete epispadias (anterior view). **C,** Complete epispadias (lateral view). As in the male, the pubic bones are separated in complete epispadias. (**A** and **B,** From Welch KJ. Hypospadias. In: Benson CD, Mustard WT, Ravitch WH, Synder WH Jr, Welch KJ, eds. Pediatric surgery. Chicago: Year Book Medical Publishers, 1962; **C,** from Campbell MF. Urology, 3rd ed. Philadelphia: WB Saunders, 1970.)

The public symphysis may be normal in the milder forms of epispadias, but in the complete form, the pubic bones are widely separated and are joined by a stout connective tissue band.

The bladder is small, and the urethra is large, with a widely dilated internal sphincter. The scrotum is normal, and the testes are usually descended. In the female the labia are separated anteriorly (Fig. 21.34, *B*).

Jeffs and Masterson (204) gave the following classification: male epispadias (glandular, penile, subsymphyseal); female epispadias (bifid clitoris, subsymphyseal); epispadias with exstrophy; and epispadias with urethral duplication.

Johnston and Kogan (205) believe that epispadias is an abnormal embryologic phenomenon and not a developmental arrest.

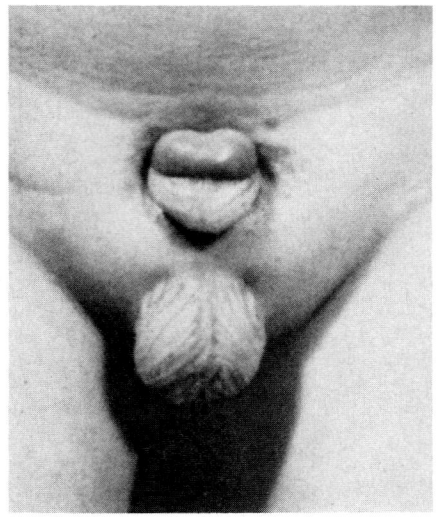
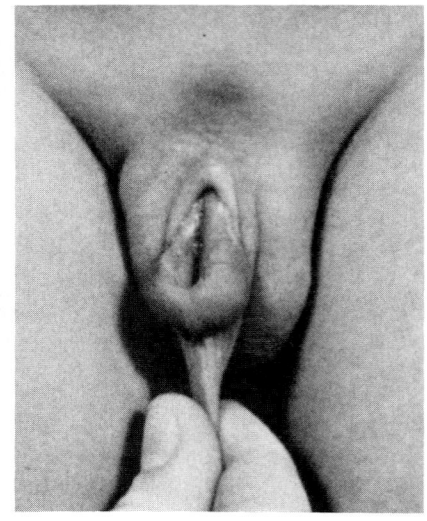

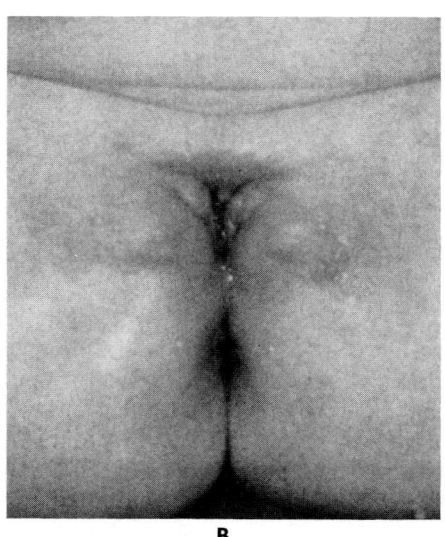

Figure 21.34. Epispadias. **A,** Penile epispadias in a male child. The sphincter of the bladder was not affected. **B,** Second degree epispadias in a female child. There was some incontinence. (From Gross RE. The surgery of infancy and childhood. Philadelphia: WB Saunders, 1953.)

Marshall and Muecke (206) and Muecke (207) reported that, perhaps, the cloacal membrane overextends cephalically, and therefore does not permit fusion of the midline of the right and left genital tubercles. Failure to fuse the paired genital tubercles with separation of the symphysis pubis, cleft glans penis, separated corpora cavernosa, and division of clitoris in half is perhaps an acceptable embryologic theory. Perhaps this upward overextension of the cloacal membrane with rupture and persistence is responsible for the abnormal communication of the amniotic cavity and the cloaca.

EMBRYOGENESIS.

Little was known about the origin of this series of defects until the normal development of the genitalia and of the infraumbilical wall was coherently described by Felix (3) in 1912. Felix and later Johnson (28) and Patten and

Barry (23) postulated a caudal shift of the lateral anlage of the genital tubercle during the fourth week. Patten and Barry conclude from their studies that "the initial departure from normal is believed to be the formation of these primordia too far caudally with reference to the proctodeum, so they are located at the level at which the urorectal fold will present externally." As a result, the urethra forms from the penopubic angle above the corpus cavernosa and produces epispadias (Figs. 21.35 and 21.36).

HISTORY.

In 1761, Morgagni (208) described a patient with incomplete epispadias and without incontinence, who was said to have fathered a child (LXVII:5,6), and he also cited another case of Salzmann (XLV:8).

Thiersch (209) is usually given credit for the first effective repair in 1869, while Young (210) in 1918 devised the modern operation of choice.

INCIDENCE.

Dees (211) found reports of 45 males and 11 females with complete epispadias among over 5 million patients seen at eight hospitals. This gives an incidence of approximately 1:118,000 for males and 1:480,000 for females. Campbell (48) found four cases among 19,046 autopsies (1:4,760) and estimates the true incidence at about 1:30,000. Males are afflicted about four times as often as are females.

SYMPTOMS.

Incontinence is the chief complaint in complete epispadias. Sterility may be mentioned by adult patients with complete epispadias, but balanic and penile forms are not always a bar to fertility. Incontinence may accompany partial epispadias in women (212).

DIAGNOSIS.

Diagnosis is by external inspection, but the following procedures should be used for evaluation *in toto* of the remaining urinary systems: IVP, cystourethrogram, cystoscopy, artificial erection with or without saline infusion

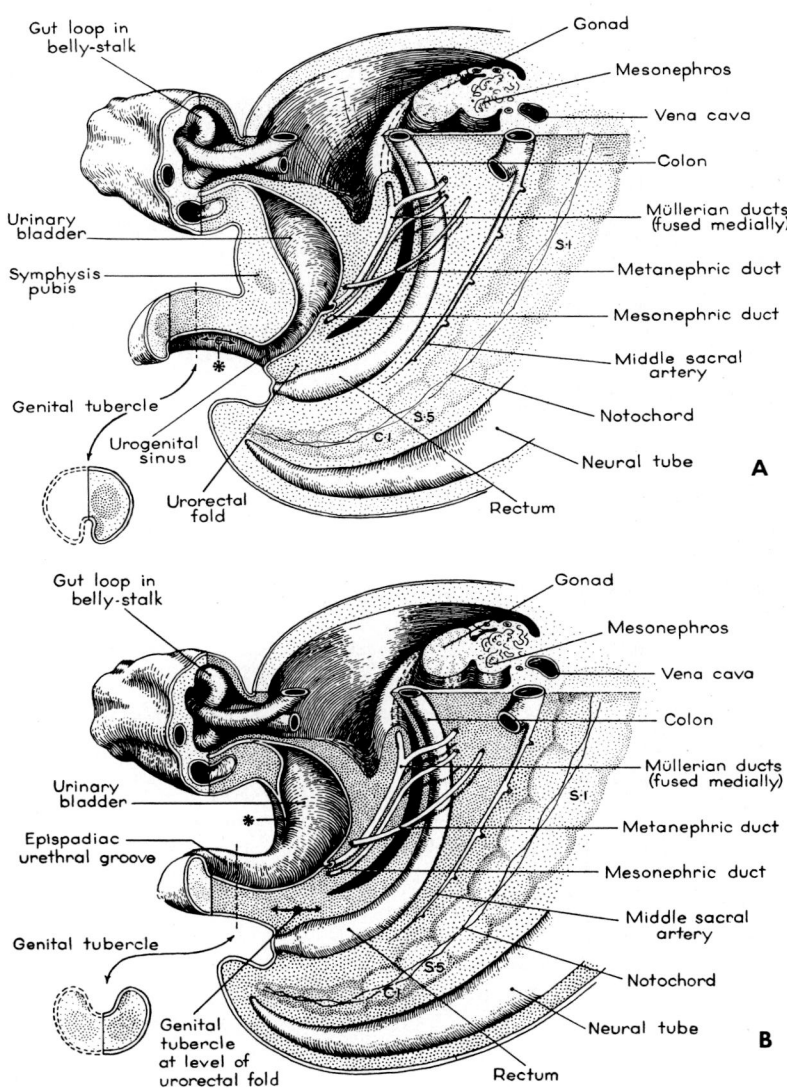

Figure 21.35. Genesis of epispadias and exstrophy of the bladder. **A,** Normal relationships of developing penis in an embryo of 8 weeks' gestation. Note that the urethral groove (marked by *asterisk*) is directly in line with the urogenital orifice. In the schematic cross-section of the genital tubercle *(lower left)*, the developing corpus cavernosum and the corpus spongiosum flanking the urethral groove are indicated by *heavier stippling.* **B,** Hypothetic stage in the genesis of exstrophy of the bladder and epispadias. Compare with **A.** Note that the belly wall in the midline (see *asterisk*) is composed of a thinning plate of ectoderm and entoderm unreinforced by mesoderm (From Patten BM, Barry A. Genesis of exstrophy of bladder and epispadias. Am J Anat 1952;90:35–57.)

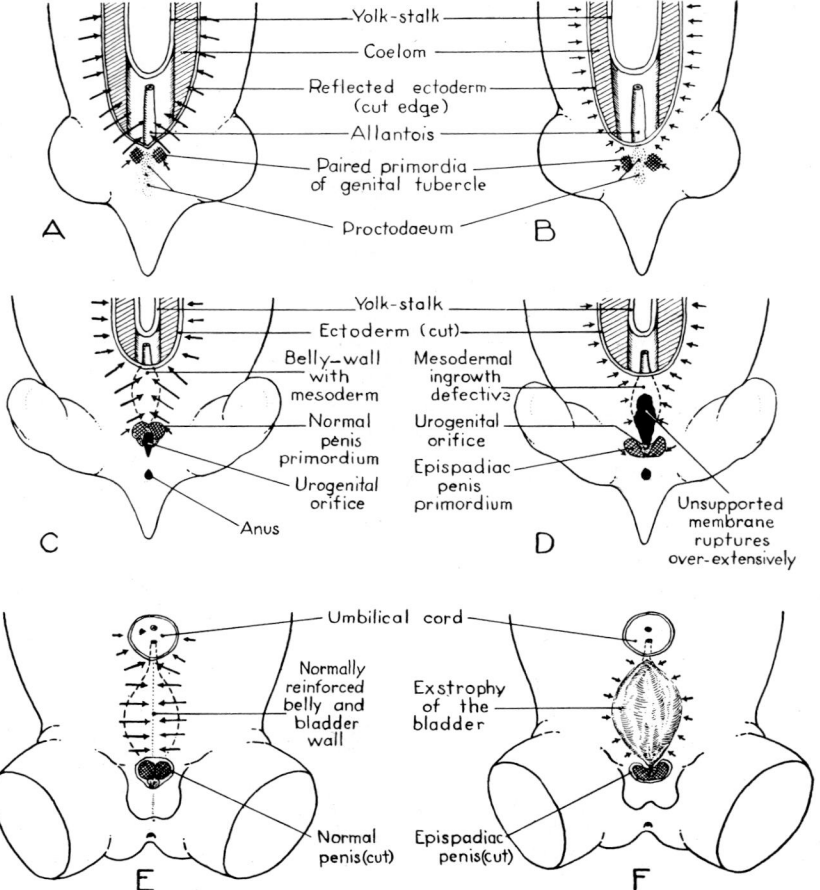

Figure 21.36.   Schematic diagrams contrasting normal with hypothetic abnormal changes in the relationships of the primordium of the genital tubercle to the cloacal membrane and the urogenital orifice. **A, C,** and **E,** Normal stages. **B, D,** and **F,** Stages in the genesis of exstrophy and epispadias. (From Patten BM, Barry A. Genesis of exstrophy of bladder and epispadias. Am J Anat 1952;90:35–57.)

into couch corpus cavernosum, and urodynamic assessment (206).

TREATMENT.

Thiersch (209) in 1869 achieved the first reasonably successful repair. He extended the urethra with skin flaps and provided the patient with a mechanical device to control the incontinence. Cantwell (213) in 1895 reconstructed the urethra, placed it between the corpora cavernosa under the skin of the ventral surface, and reapproximated the corpora cavernosa. This operation, adapted by Young (210), became the basis of modern surgical repair.

Cure for the incontinence of epispadias was first undertaken in 1880 by Duplay (214), who partially resected the bladder neck and reapproximated the edges. From dissections, Boiffin (215) showed that the muscular tissue of the sphincter was present and that tightening the sphincter by surgery was feasible. Trendelenburg (216) emphasized the importance of reuniting the symphysis with silver wire sutures, although today this is not considered necessary. Young (217) tightened the internal sphincter by a wedge-shaped excision of the roof of the prostatic urethra and anterior vesical orifice. He excised the anterior portion of the external sphincter and the roof of the urethral bulb. The combination of Cantwell's (213) urethral reconstruction and Young's sphincter repair is still the operation of choice.

During the years in which these techniques were being developed, many surgeons solved the problem by transplanting the ureters to the sigmoid colon. This procedure is no longer advocated unless reconstruction has been attempted and been unsuccessful. The modern treatment of epispadias depends on the severity of signs and symptoms of this anomaly (206). In severe cases the surgical treatment may be accomplished by three steps: (a) penile reconstruction, (b) urethral reconstruction, and (c) bladder neck reconstruction. In females, however, the treatment is repair of the paired clitoris and anterior midline approximation of the labia.

PROGNOSIS.

By 1937 Young (218) had obtained complete urinary control in 12 patients and almost complete control in a 13th. Among 13 patients with incontinence, Gross (219) achieved complete control in 11 and nearly complete control in 2. Two of his patients underwent a second operation for tightening the neck of the bladder.

Hypospadias

In both males and females the urethra is a perfect canal, but in the congenital anomaly of hypospadias, the canal becomes a gutter. This phenomenon is easily seen in males but not in females since, for all practical purposes, hypospadias does not exist in females. However, when the urethral meatus in the female is close and proximal to the hymen, we agree with Belman and Kass (220) that this situation may be considered an anomaly of the urogenital sinus.

Anatomy

The abnormal termination of the male urethra on the underside of the penis, on the scrotum, or on the perineum is termed *hypospadias*.

Meatal Location. The anatomic description of this pathology depends on the topography and location of the meatus. Belman and Kass (220) presented the following classification: glanular, coronal, distal shaft, midshaft, proximal shaft, penoscrotal, scrotal, and perineal.

Chordee. The same authors classify the chordee as mild, moderate, and severe, stating that, most likely, severe chordee are located in the coronal sulcus.

The condition is classified as glanular (i.e., of the glans penis, or balanic), with penile, penoscrotal, and perineal hypospadias corresponding to the location of the meatus.

Glanular Hypospadias. The urethra opens between the normal site on the glans and the coronal sulcus. There may be a ventral furrow, which is lined with mucosa in the glans. The glans itself may be flat and curved downward, and the orifice may be slit-like or very small. In the latter case, there is usually a dimple or a blind pouch at the site of the normal meatus. The prepuce is absent below and redundant above (hypospadiac prepuce). Balanic hypospadias is at once the mildest and the most common form of the defect (Fig. 21.37).

Penile Hypospadias. Penile hypospadias may result from the termination of the urethra on the penile shaft or from a fistulous opening, with the urethra continuing forward to open at the normal meatus or terminating blindly. The portion of the urethra beyond the orifice is usually an open gutter lined with mucosa (Figs. 21.14, *A*, and 21.38, *A* and *B*).

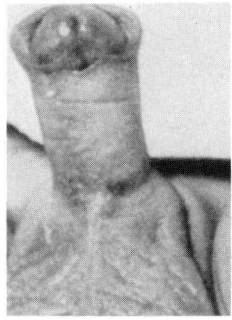

Figure 21.37. The mildest form of hypospadias in which the urethral meatus is slightly displaced ventrally on the glans. (From Potter EL. Pathology of the fetus and the newborn. Chicago: Year Book Medical Publishers, 1952.)

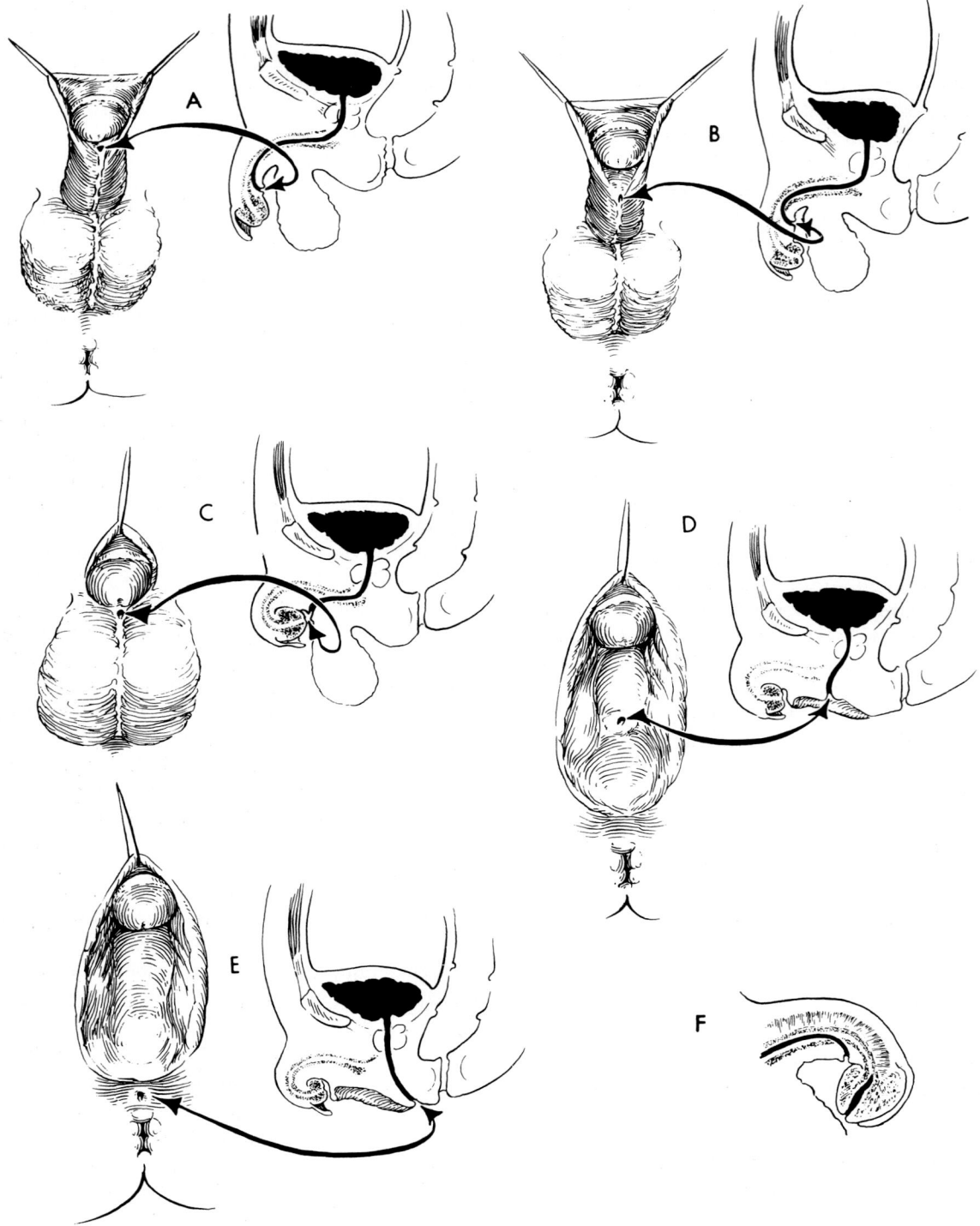

Figure 21.38. Hypospadias. **A,** and **B,** Penile hypospadias. **C,** Penoscrotal hypospadias with testes descended. **D,** Scrotal hypospadias with undescended testes. **E,** Perineal hypospadias. **F,** Penile hypospadias with a well-developed glandular urethra that may be used in surgical repair. Compare with Figure 21.14.

(From Welch KJ. Hypospadias. In: Benson CD, Mustard WT, Ravitch WH, Synder WH Jr, Welch KJ, eds. Pediatric surgery. Chicago: Year Book Medical Publishers, 1962.)

An atypical form of penile hypospadias has been reported in which the urethra reached the tip of the glans although both the urethra and the corpus spongiosum were short, as compared with the corpora cavernosa, resulting in marked chordee (221). This defect represents a partial agenesis of the corpus spongiosum. Freeing the urethra and corpus spongiosum results in a typical penile hypospadias, which may then be repaired as usual.

Penoscrotal Hypospadias. The opening of the urethra is at the junction of the penis and scrotum.

Penoscrotal hypospadias is usually accompanied by a short, flattened penis with marked chordee. It is frequently attached to the scrotal raphe by a web. The scrotum is empty in about 33% of patients and may be bifid. The corpus spongiosum is replaced by a fibrous band, which produces the chordee (Fig. 21.38, *C* and *D*). The prostatic utricle may be enlarged (Fig. 21.38, *B*).

Perineal Hypospadias. This variety, often termed *pseudovaginal*, is the most extreme form of the defect. The patient may have female internal genital structures as well as testes (Figs. 21.14, *C*, and 21.39, *E*). The penis may be rudimentary, but it is usually of normal size, with marked ventral curvature; it is covered by the hooded prepuce. The empty bifid scrotum resembles the labia of the female. The general appearance of the genitalia is feminine; it may be necessary to confirm the sex of the patient.

Hypospadias in the Female. Opening of the urethra posterior to its normal site, or into the anterior wall of the vagina, has been termed *female hypospadias.* Only a few cases are known. Cecil (222) collected 47 cases from the literature and accepted only 36 as congenital. Most have been recognized only in adults. An enlarged clitoris and meatal stenosis are often present.

The condition probably represents a mild degree of persistence of the urogenital sinus. Since the urethral opening of the female may be said to be normally hypospadiac when compared to that of the male, female hypospadias corresponds most nearly to perineal hypospadias in the male.

ETIOLOGY

Bauer et al. (223) discussed the genetic aspects of hypospadias. They reported that 21% of patients have affected other family members, such as the father (7%). Fourteen percent of the families had two male infants with hypospadias. Bauer also stated that a family without history of hypospadias has a 12% risk of having male infants with the anomaly.

Chung and Myriasthopoulous (224) reported that there is some increased risk of hypospadias in Caucasians.

Belman (225) stated that failure of timely or adequate hormone production or an inability to convert testosterones to dihydrotestosterone may produce congenital anomalies of the genital system.

ASSOCIATED ANOMALIES

About 25% of patients with hypospadias have other urinary tract anomalies. In addition, cryptorchidism and an enlarged prostatic utricle frequently accompany penoscrotal and perineal hypospadias, but not glanular hypospadias (Fig. 21.14, *B* and *C*). Patients with both hypospadias and cryptorchidism should be evaluated by karyotype for an intersex condition.

Khuri et al. (226) reported 10% incidence of undescended testicles in hypospadiac males, and Fallon et al. (227) reported urinary anomalies. Similar cases were reported by Ikoma et al. (228).

According to Mininberg et al. (229), the following syndromes are associated with hypospadias: Smith-Lemli-Opitz, Silver-Russell, and Pterygium syndromes; Lenz microphtahalmia; G syndrome and hypertelorism in males only; Down's syndrome; 4p syndrome; Klinefelter syndrome (47,XXY); gonadal dysgenesis (47,XYY); true hermaphroditism; and states of intersexuality.

Autosomal dominant chromosomal abnormalities play a peculiar and ambiguous part in all these embryologic anomalies.

EMBRYOLOGY

There are three embryologic entities that, by participation, form the external genitalia of the male: the genital tubercle, urogenital folds, and labioscrotal swelling.

The genital tubercle appears about the fifth week of intrauterine life and is responsible for the formation and site of the penis, which becomes longer and longer with the help of the fetal testicle and its androgenic secretion. During the penile formation, the two urogenital folds are united progressively and form the lateral walls of the urethra on the ventral area of the penis; therefore the urethra is situated under the genital tubercle. The labioscrotal swelling surrounds not only the urogenital fold by progressive closing below but also the genital tubercle partially (Fig. 21.39).

The formation of the spongy urethra takes place by fusion of the urogenital folds on the ventral surface of the penis. Perhaps with this phenomenon we can explain the slow movements of the external urethral opening towards the glans penis. These procedures take place around the 14th week. The formation now of the scrotum is *ad portas* with the union of the genital labioscrotal swelling.

An epithelial formation is responsible for the production of the glanular meatus at the fossa navicularis. The external genitalia is completed and present around the 12th to 14th weeks. If the urethral folds will not unite and fuse at the ventral area of the penis, the congenital anomaly of hypospadias takes place.

Chordee is a ventral curving of the penis secondary to a shortening of the ventral skin without dortos fascia and without formation *in toto* of the corpus spongiosum

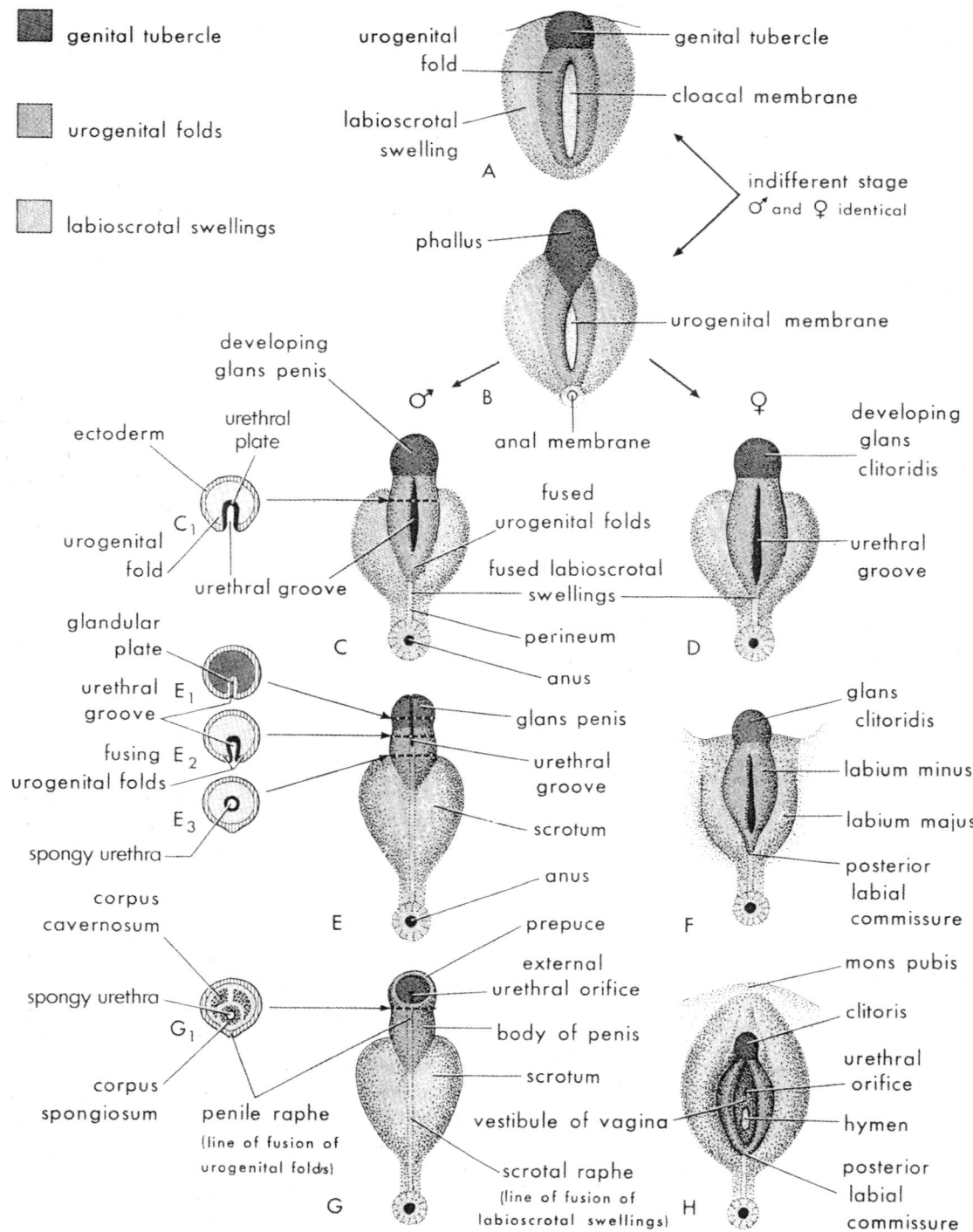

Figure 21.39. **A,** and **B,** Development of the external genitalia during the indifferent stage (fourth to seventh weeks). **C, E,** and **G,** Stages in the development of male external genitalia at 9, 11, and 12 weeks, respectively. To the left are schematic transverse sections (C_1, E_1 to E_3, and G_1, through the developing penis, illustrating formation of the spongy urethra. **D, F,** and **H,** Stages in the development of female external genitalia at 9, 11, and 12 weeks, respectively. (From Moore KL. The developing human: clinically oriented embryology, 4th ed. Philadelphia: WB Saunders, 1988.)

which, in some cases, is replaced by a fibrous band that is just a chordee. Characteristically, the prepuce forms a hood-like deformation on the dorsum of the penis. Sweet et al. (230) stated that 35% of hypospadiac infants have severe chordee. Chordee without hypospadias was reported by Devine and Horton (231), who classified these phenomena in three groups.

1. Missing spongiosum with urethra fixed to the skin of the ventral area of the penis
2. Urethra well developed but without the protection of Buck's fascia and dartos
3. Only the ventral skin responsible for chordee formation

EMBRYOGENESIS

Hypospadias results from the failure of the urethral folds to form throughout their normal length, or their failure to close distally if they have formed. The extent of the closure determines the position of the urethral orifice.

A number of writers have suggested that hypospadias represents a mild form of intersexuality. Willis (232) considered hypospadias to be one end of a series, the other of which is a completely feminized male. In penoscrotal and perineal hypospadias, the utricular enlargement and the frequent presence of the uterus and tubes, together with undescended testes, make this suggestion convincing. Balanic and penile hypospadias that show no other genital deformity may well form separate entities.

When the urethral folds have formed but not closed, a groove lined with mucosa lies on the ventral surface of the penis. Paul and Kanagasuntheram (30) consider this mucosal gutter to be the primary urethral groove lined with skin ectoderm and not deepened by the secondary groove, which forms within the endodermal urethral plate. When the urethra ends at the frenum (balanic hypospadias), the defect resulted from the failure of the separate, ectodermal glandular portion of the urethra to form.

Because the raphe of the penis is formed by the fusion of the urethral folds, it is absent distal to the urethral orifice, as is the corpus spongiosum, which becomes an inelastic band of fibrous tissue in the absence of the urethra.

A familial tendency to hypospadias has been reported in some cases. Campbell (48) mentions its occurrence in three generations of one family and in six generations of another.

HISTORY

Hypospadias is a common defect which is readily observed, and hence it has been recognized since the dawn of history. Aristotle (233) mentions its existence. Morgagni (XLVI:8,9) described three cases and doubted the infertility ascribed to these individuals by earlier writers. He compared the uncovered urethral gutter with the penile groove that occurs in turtles and concluded that insemination is possible.

Cabot (234) stated that the first repair was attempted in 1836. In 1874 Anger and Mettaver (235) first satisfactorily corrected both the chordee and the meatal ectopia. A wide variety of tubal grafts were attempted with varying degrees of success or failure before the need for autografts was understood.

INCIDENCE

Hypospadias does occur in females, but it is primarily an anomaly of males. Estimates of incidence range from 1 to 3 per 1000 births. Malpas (236) found 16 cases among 13,964 consecutive births (1:870), and Campbell (48) found a frequency of 1:420 among autopsies of male children. There is some evidence in Malpas's data that first-born children are more often affected (1:535) than are later children (1:1890). Sweet et al. (230) reported that glanural and coronal defects constitute 87%, penile 10%, penoscrotal 3%.

SYMPTOMS

In balanic hypospadias, the complaint is usually only about the appearance of the penis. In this type, standing urination is usually feasible. Constriction of the meatus, with symptoms of partial obstruction, is sometimes present. In penile hypospadias, urination often requires a sitting position, and the cosmetic problem is more pronounced. Chordee interferes with erection, and coitus may be hampered. In penoscrotal and perineal hypospadias, the disabilities are even more pronounced.

DIAGNOSIS

Hypospadias may be diagnosed by inspection. The existence of a urethral channel anterior to an orifice on the shaft should be sought.

Perineal hypospadias may require careful examination to determine the sex of an infant with this deformity. Examination of the "urethra" by urethroscopy or by radiopaque injection and radiography will determine the existence of a vagina. By palpation through the rectal wall, it may be possible to detect the presence of a uterus. Elevated 17-ketosteroid excretion in the urine will suggest the adrenogenital syndrome and the masculinization of a genetic female. A karyotype from peripheral lymphocytes should be done if there is any concern about sexual ambiguity. Psychologic evaluation of the patient and of his parents should be undertaken in the case of older children. All of these procedures should be employed before laparotomy is considered. If laparotomy is necessary, a biopsy of both gonads should be done. Of 100 of Gross's patients (219) with severe hypospadias, 32 had undescended testes. Thirteen patients underwent surgical

Table 21.2.
Procedures for Hypospadias Repair[a]

Procedure	Author	Experience	Fistulae (%)	Stenoses (%)
Single-Stage Technique				
Glanular-coronal				
MAGPI	Duckett (1981)	200	1 (0.5)	0
Urethral	Mills et al. (1981)[1]	8	0	0
advancement	Koff (1981)[2]	10	0	1 (10)
Distal shaft without chordee				
Mathieu	Wacksman (1981)	20	1 (5)	1 (5)
	Gonzales et al. (1983)	63	3 (5)	1 (1.5)
Distal shaft with or without chordee				
Flip flap	Devine and Horton (1976)	55	6 (10.9)	?
	Shubailat and Ajlumi (1978)[3]	62	1 (1.6)	1 (1.6)
	Woodard and Cleveland (1982)[4]	76	8 (10.5)	9 (12)
Mustardé	Kim and Hendren (1981)	50	0	2 (4)
	Belman (1981)[5]	30	1 (3.3)	3 (10)
Midshaft with skin chordee				
King	Sadlowsky et al. (1974)[6]	85	3 (3.5)	1 (1.2)
	Marshall et al. (1978)[7]	102	3 (3.0)	2 (2.0)
Island flap techniques				
Hodgson I	Hodgson (1975)[8]	38	3 (7.8)	4 (10.5)
Hodgson II	Hodgson (1975)	93	0	1 (1.1)
Hodgson III	Kroovand and Perlmutter (1980)[9]	47	3 (6.0)	10 (22.7)
Duckett	Duckett (1980)	100	10%[b]	
Free-graft techniques				
Devine and Horton	Devine and Horton (1977)[10]	20	4 (20)	?
	Woodard and Cleveland (1982)	28	8 (29)	5 (17.9)
Bladder mucosa	Li et al. (1981)	64	12 (18.8)	7 (10.9)
Multistage Techniques				
Denis Browne	Kelalis et al. (1977)[11]	23	(25)	?
	Gearhart and Witherington (1979)[12]	64	11 (17.1)	4 (6.2)
	Bailen and Howerton (1980)[13]	40	2 (50)	1 (2.5)
	Donnelly and Prenderville (1981)[14]	72	4 (5.5)	5 (6.9)
Crawford (modified)	Marberger and Paner (1981)[15]	183	34 (18.6)	?
	Yarbrough and Johnston (1977)[16]	96	9 (9.3)	3 (3.1)
Byars	Wray et al. (1976)[17]	253	54 (21.3)	17 (6.7)
Cecil	Kelalis (1981)[18]	135	4 (3.0)	9 (6.6)
Belt-Fuqua	Hensle and Mollitt (1981)[19]	30	2 (6.6)	1 (3.3)
	Hendren (1981)[20]	140	2 (1.4)	4 (2.8)
Smith	Smith (1980)[21]	210	6 (2.9)	7 (3.3)

[a]Modified from Kelalis P et al., eds. Clinical pediatric urology. Philadelphia: WB Saunders, 1976.
[b]Specific details not given regarding fistulae, stenoses, flap breakdown.
[1]Mills C et al. J Urol 1981; 125:701.
[2]Koff SA. J Urol 1981; 125:394.
[3]Shubailat GF, Ajlumi NJ. Plast Reconstr Surg 1978; 62:546.
[4]Woodard JR, Cleveland R. J Urol 1982; 127:1155.
[5]Belman AB. Urol Clin North Am 1981; 8:483.
[6]Sadlowski RW, Belman AB, King LR. J Urol 1974; 112:677.
[7]Marshall M Jr et al. J Urol 1978; 120:229.
[8]Hodgson NB. In Glenn JF, ed. Urologic surgery, 2nd ed. Hagerstown, MD: Harper & Row, 1975.
[9]Kroovand RC, Perlmutter AD. J Urol 1980; 124:530.
[10]Devine CJ Jr, Horton CE. J Urol 1977; 118:108.

exploration; eight had female gonads; and one was a true hermaphrodite, with mixed gonads.

TREATMENT

The ideal surgical repair of hypospadias should achieve the following:

1. Relieve the chordee and prevent its recurrence
2. Avoid urethral strictures and fistulae, which will require later correction
3. Provide a satisfactory urinary stream without dribbling or spraying
4. Convey the ejaculate to the tip of the penis
5. Provide a reasonably normal appearing penis in both the flaccid and erect positions

These ideals usually may be achieved in one surgical procedure although two stages may be required. The first stage is directed toward release of the chordee and shifting the preputial skin to a position that will facilitate subsequent urethroplasty. The formation of a new, distal urethral segment is accomplished in the second stage. The distal, glandular portion of the urethra may be present and should be used in second-stage repair (Fig. 21.38, *F*).

Table 21.2 summarizes the numerous procedures described in the literature.

Treatment of female hypospadias should be limited to enlarging the urethral orifice if it is obstructed. In rare cases reconstruction of the urethra may be necessary to eliminate incontinence.

EDITORIAL COMMENTS

It seems that the marked changes in diagnosis and rapid progress in surgical correction of the last two decades, seen in work with other parts of the genitourinary system, have been less prominent in the male reproductive tract. An exception to this concept is in correction of epispadias and hypospadias. In general, it has been my experience that surgical attempts to correct many of these defects can be performed in a single stage, rather than by multiple planned operations, such as was routine 20 years ago. Indeed, epispadias, even in its most severe forms, can reliably be corrected by lengthening the penis and dividing the urethral plate, then creating a urethra from prepuce in a single stage. Correction of the urinary incontinence, of course, must await a later date. Hypospadias is routinely corrected in a single stage, usually by using the prepuce as urethral replacement for the more severe forms or by advancing a meatal-based flap for the less involved cases. The routine use of optical magnification, delicate ophthalmic instruments, and fine-suture material have made possible significant advances in the management of these conditions.

There is a clinical distinction between torsion of the appendix testis and appendix epididymis. The so-called blue-dot sign is seen with torsion of the testicular appendage only. The resultant hemorrhagic structure can be clearly seen through the scrotal skin because there is no reason to have inflammatory changes in the skin to obscure this finding. These changes occur with epididymitis and with torsion of the epididymal appendix, which causes a reactive epididymitis and which causes changes essentially indistinguishable from the former condition. One does not encounter reactive epididymitis with torsion of the testicular appendix—hence, the clearly seen pathognomonic sign *(TSP)*.

REFERENCES

1. Wilson KM. Correlation of external genitalia and sex glands in the human embryo. Contrib Embryol, Carnegie Inst Wash 1926;18:23–30.
2. Gillman J. The development of the gonads in man, with a consideration of the role of fetal endocrines and the histogenesis of ovarian tumors. Contrib Embryol Carnegie Inst Wash 1948;32:81–131.
3. Felix W. The development of the urinogenital organs. In: Keibel F, Mall FP, eds. Manual of human embryology, Vol 2. Philadelphia: JB Lippincott, 1912.
4. George FW, Wilson JD. Sex determination and differentiation. In: Knobil E, ed. The physiology of reproduction. New York: Raven Press, 1988:3–26.
5. Jost A. A new look at the mechanisms controlling sex differentiation in mammals. Johns Hopkins Med J 1972;130:38–53.
6. Williams-Ashman HG. Enigmatic features of penile development and function. Perspect Biol Med 1990;33:335–374.
7. Blechschmidt E. The stages of human development before birth. Philadelphia: WB Saunders, 1961.
8. Johnson FP. The later development of the urethra in the male. J Urol 1920;4:447–501.
9. Glenister TW. The development of the utricle and of the so-called "middle" or "median" lobe of the human prostate. J Anat 1962;96:443–455.

[11] Kelalis PP, Benson RC Jr, Culp OS. J Urol 1977; 118:657.
[12] Gearhart JP, Witherington R. J Urol 1979; 127:66.
[13] Bailen J, Howerton LW. J Urol 1980; 123:754.
[14] Donnelly BJ, Prenderville JB. J Urol 1981; 125:706.
[15] Marberger H, Paner W. J Urol 1981; 125:698.
[16] Yarbrough WJ, Johnston JH. J Urol 1977; 117:782.
[17] Wray RC, Ribando JM, Weeks PM. Plast Reconstr Surg 1976; 58:329.
[18] Kelalis PP. J Urol (Paris) 1981; 87:93.
[19] Hensle TW, Mollitt DC. J Urol 1981; 125:703.
[20] Hendren WH. Urol Clin North Am 1981; 8:431.
[21] Smith ED. In Holder TM, Ashcraft KW eds. Pediatric surgery. Philadelphia: WB Saunders, 1980.

10. Lowsley OS. The development of the human prostate gland with reference to the development of other structures at the neck of the urinary bladder. Am J Anat 1912;13:299–350.

11. le Duc IE. The anatomy of the prostate and pathology of early benign hypertrophy. J Urol 1939;42:1217–1241.

12. Franks LM. Benign nodular hyperplasia of the prostate: a review. Ann R Coll Surg 1954;14:92–106.

13. Zondek LH, Zondek T. The foetal and neonatal prostate in congenital malformation of the urinary tract. Virchows Arch 1971;354:197.

14. Norman JT, Cunha GR, Sugimura Y. The induction of new ductal growth in adult prostatic epithelium in response to embryonic prostatic inductor. Prostate 1986;8:209–220.

15. McNeal JE. Origin and development of carcinoma in the prostate. Cancer 1969;23:24.

16. McNeal JE. The prostate and prostatic urethra: a morphologic synthesis. J Urol 1972;107:1008.

17. McNeal JE. Zonal anatomy of the prostate. Prostate 1981;2:35.

18. Drago JR. The role of new modality in the early detection and diagnosis of prostate cancer. Cancer J Clin 1987;39:326–336.

19. Pallin G. Beiträge zur Anatomie und Embryologie der Prostata und der Samenblasen. Arch Anat Entw 1901:135–176.

20. Price D. Normal development of the prostate and seminal vesicles of the rat with a study of experimental postnatal modification. Am J Anat 1936;60:79–128.

21. Zuckerman S, Krohn PL. The hydatids of Morgagni under normal and experimental conditions. Phil Trans R Soc 1938;228:147–151.

22. Murnaghan GF. The appendages of the testis and epididymis: a short review with case reports. Br J Urol 1959;31:190–195.

23. Patten BM, Barry A. Genesis of exstrophy of bladder and epispadias. Am J Anat 1952;90:35–57.

24. Spaulding MH. The development of the external genitalia in the human embryo. Contrib Embryol Carnegie Inst Wash 1921;13:67.

25. Glenister TW. A correlation of the normal and abnormal development of the penile urethra and of the infraabdominal wall. Br J Urol 1958;30:117–126.

26. Tourneaux F. Sur le développement et l'evolution du tubercle genital chez le foetus humain dans les deux sexes, avec quelques remarques concernant le development des glandes prostatiques. J Anat Physiol 1889;25:229.

27. Wood-Jones F. The development and malformation of the glans and prepuce. Br Med J 1910;1:137–138.

28. Johnson FP. Urethral anomalies. J Urol 1930;23:693–699.

29. Hunter J. Observations of certain parts of the animal economy. London, 1786.

30. Paul M, Kanagasuntheram R. The congenital anomalies of the lower urinary tract. Br J Urol 1956;28:64–74, 118–125.

31. Glenister TW. A consideration of the processes involved in the development of the prepuce in man. Br J Urol 1956;28:243–249.

32. Gairdner D. The fate of the foreskin: a study of circumcision. Br Med J 1949;2:1433–1437.

33. Ombrédanne L. Torsions testiculaires chez les enfants. Bull Mem Soc Chir 1913;38:779–791.

34. Colt GH. Torsion of hydatid of Morgagni. Br J Surg 1922;9:464–465.

35. Walton AJ. Torsion of the hydatid of Morgagni. Br J Surg 1922;10:151.

36. Mouchet A. Sur une variété d'orchite aigue de l'enfance due a une torsion de l'hydatide de Morgagni. Presse Med 1923;31:485–486.

37. Dix VW. Über Torsion des Hodenanhanges. Z Urol Chir 1931;33:486–494.

38. Randall A. Torsion of the appendix testis (hydatid of Morgagni). J Urol 1939;41:715–725.

39. Seidel RF, Yeaw RC. Torsion of the appendix testis and appendix epididymis: a report of eight cases. J Urol 1950;63:714–716.

40. Ambrose SS, Skandalakis JE. Torsion of the appendix epididymis and testis: report of six episodes. J Urol 1957;77:51–58.

41. Atkinson G, Broecker BH. Color doppler ultrasound evaluation of acute scrotal pain in children. Presented at the 55th annual meeting of the Southeastern Section of the American Urological Association, Atlanta, March 1991.

42. Scott RT. Torsion of the appendix testis. J Urol 1940;44:755–758.

43. Shattock CE. A case of torsion of the hydatids of Morgagni. Lancet 1922;1:693.

44. Moncalvi L. Torsion de l'hydatide dans un testicle ectopique. J Urol (Paris) 1933;35:501–504.

45. Khan TA. Torsion of hydatid of Morgagni. Br J Urol 1965;37:437–439.

46. Rolnick HC. Torsion of the hydatid of Morgagni. J Urol 1939;42:458–462.

47. Rhame RC, Harvard BM, Glenn JF. Giant müllerian duct cyst. JAMA 1961;177:212–214.

48. Campbell MF. Urology, 2nd ed. Philadelphia: WB Saunders, 1963.

49. Young H, Cash JR. A case of pseudohermaphroditismus masculinus, showing hypospadias, greatly enlarged utricle, abdominal testis and absence of seminal vesicle. J Urol 1921;5:405–430.

50. Howard FS. Hypospadias with enlargement of the prostatic utricle. Surg Gynecol Obstet 1948;86:307–316.

51. Englisch J. Über Cysten an der hinteren Blasenwand bie Männern. Med Jahrb 1975.

52. Pendino JA. Diphallus (double penis). J Urol 1950;64:156–157.

53. Klotz HG. Endoscopic studies on vegetations, polypi, angeioma, membranous and diphtheritic urethritis, suppuration from the ejaculatory ducts, cyst of colliculus seminalis, etc. NY Med J 1915;61:99–106.

54. Lubash S. Cyst of the prostatic utricle: a causative factor in producing impotency. Am J Surg 1929;7:123–125.

55. Slocum RC. Müllerian duct cysts. Trans South East Sect Am Urol Assoc 1954;18:26–33.

56. Kaplan GW, Piconi JR, Schuhrke DD. Posterior approach to müllerian duct and seminal vesical cysts. Birth Defects 1977;13:241.

57. Devine CL, Gonzales-Serva L, Stecks JF. Utricular configuration in hypospadias and intersex. J Urol 1980;123:407.

58. Monfort G. The transvesical approach to utricular cysts. J Pediatr Surg 1982;17:406.

59. Feldman RA, Weiss RM. Urinary retention secondary to müllerian duct cyst in a child. J Urol 1972;108:647.

60. Deming CL, Berneike RR. Müllerian duct cysts. J Urol 1944;51:563.

61. Michelson L. Congenital anomalies of the ductus deferens and epididymis. J Urol 1949;61:384–395.

62. Whitehorn CA. Complete unilateral wolffian duct agenesis with homolateral cryptorchism: a case report, its explanation and treatment, and the mechanism of "testicular descent." J Urol 1954;72:685–692.

63. Pearman RO. Congenital absence of the testicle: monorchism. J Urol 1961;85:599–601.

64. Rubin GP, Taylor I. Congenital absence of the vas deferens. Br J Surg 1976;63:464.

65. Charney CW, Gillenwater JY. Congenital absence of the vas deferens. J Urol 1965;93:399–401.

66. Nelson RE. Congenital absence of the vas deferens: a review of the literature and report of three cases. J Urol 1950;63:176–182.

67. Preisler O. On involution of the wolffian ducts in female fetuses by placental estrogens. Arch Gynaek 1962;196:475–480.

68. El-Itreby AA, Girgis SM. Congenital absence of vas deferens in male sterility. Int J Fertil 1961;6:409–416.

69. Lazebnik Y, Kamhi D. Le rôle de l'agénésie du canal déferent dans la stérilité masculine. Urol Int 1958;6:168–173.

70. Amelar RD, Hotchkiss RS. Congenital aplasia of the epididymides and vasa deferentia: effects on semen. Fertil Steril 1963;14:44–48.

71. Feigelson J, Pecau Y. Anomalies of the sperm, vas deferens, and epididymis in cystic fibrosis. Presse Med 1986;15:523–525.

72. Ochsner MA, Brannan W, Goodier EH. Absent vas deferens associated with renal agenesis. JAMA 1912;222:1055–1056.

73. Donohue RE, Fauver HE. Unilateral absence of the vas deferens: a useful clinical sign. JAMA 1989;261:1180–1182.

74. Emery CB, Goldstein AMB, Morrow JW. Congenital absence of vas deferens with ipsilateral urinary anomalies. Urology 1974;4:201–203.

75. Deane AM, May RE. Absent vas deferens in association with renal abnormalities. Br J Urol 1982;54:298–299.

76. Patrick JK. Congenital absence of the vas deferens. Am Fam Physician 1982;26:147–149.

77. Mathé CP, Dunn G. Double vas deferens associated with solitary kidney. J Urol 1948;59:461–465.

78. Gravgaard E, Garsdal L, Miller SH. Double vas deferens and epididymis associated with ipsilateral renal agenesis simulating ectopic ureter opening into the seminal vesicle. Scand J Urol Nephrol 1978;12:85–87.

79. Johnson DK, Perlmutter AD. Single system ectopic ureteroceles with anomalies of the heart, testis, and vas deferens. J Urol 1980;123:81–83.

80. Rocha-Brito R, Borges HJ, Albuquerque J. Anomalous crossing of the ureter by the vas deferens. Rev Paul Med 1966;69:107–114.

81. Radhkrishnan J, Vermillion CD, Hendren WH. Vasa deferentis inserting into retroiliac ureters. J Urol 1980;124:746–747.

82. Hicks CM, Skoog SJ, Done S. Ectopic vas deferens, imperforate anus and hypospadias: a new triad. J Urol 1989;141:586–588.

83. Furtado AJL. Three cases of cystic seminal vesical associated with unilateral renal agenesis. Br J Urol 1973;45:536.

84. Fuselier HA, Peters DH. Cyst of seminal vesicle with ipsilateral renal agenesis and ectopic ureter: case report. J Urol 1976;116:833.

85. Sheih CP, Hung CS, Wei CF, Lin CY. Cystic dilations within the pelvis in patients with ipsilateral renal agenesis or dysplasia. J Urol 1990;144:324–327.

86. Lobel B, Cipolla B, DeLannou D, Guille F. Hypofertility in males due to a secretion anomaly of the seminal vesicles and its treatment. Acta Urol Belg 1989;47:59–62.

87. Linseymeyer TA, Freidland GW. Duplicated urethra communicating with the seminal vesicle. Urol Radiol 1988;10:210–212.

88. Malatinsky E, Labady F, Lepies P, Zajac R, Jancar M. Congenital anomalies of the seminal ducts. Int Urol Nephrol 1987;19:189–194.

89. Tanikawa K, Nishizawa K, Kawamura N. Seminal vesicle cyst associated with ipsilateral renal agensis. Hinyokika Kiyo 1987;33:1474–1479.

90. Oyen R, Gielen J, van Poppel H, Baert L. Seminal vesicle cyst and ipsilateral renal agenesis: case report. Eur J Radiol 1988;8:122–124.

91. Kaneti J, Lissmer L, Smailowitz Z, Sober I. Agenesis of kidney associated with malformation of the seminal vesicle: various clinical presentations. Int Urol Nephrol 1988;20:29–33.

92. Kenney PJ, Leeson MD. Congenital anomalies of the seminal vesicles: spectrum of computed tomographic findings. Radiology 1983;149:247–251.

93. Dholakia S, Bijjani B, Elist J, Edson M. Ureteral seminal vesicle anomaly: gross hematuria as presenting symptom. Urology 1983;21:604–607.

94. Lisser H. Absence of the prostate associated with endocrine disease, notably hypopituitarism. Endocrinology 1923;7:225–255.

95. Lowsley OS, Venero AP. Persistent anterior lobe of the prostate gland. J Urol 1954;71:469–474.

96. Polse S, Edelbrook H. Prostatic utricular enlargement as a cause of vesical outlet obstruction in children. J Urol 1968;100:329.

97. Morgan RJ, Williams DI, Pryor JP. Müllerian duct remnants in the male. Br J Urol 1979;51:488.

98. Butterick JA, Schnitzer B, Abell MR. Ectopic prostatic tissue in urethra: a clinicopathologic entity and a significant cause of hematuria. J Urol 1971;105:97.

99. Louw JX, Marsden ATH. Heterotopic prostatic tissue: a report of an unusual cause of haematuria in a Bontu youth. S Afr Med J 1969;43:1082.

100. Deklerk DP, Scott WW. Prostatic maldevelopment in the prune belly syndrome: a defect in prostatic stromal epithelial interaction. J Urol 1978;120:341.

101. Stephens FD. Congenital malformation of the urinary tract. New York: Praeger, 1983.

102. Drury RB, Schwarzell HH. Congenital absence of the penis. Arch Surg 1935;30:236–242.

103. Gilles H, Harrison RJ. Congenital absence of the penis. Br J Plast Surg 1948;1:8–28.

104. Richart R, Benirscke K. Penile agenesis: report of a case, review of the world literature, and discussion of pertinent embryology. Arch Pathol 1960;70:252–260.

105. Roy KS. A case of complete absence of the penis. Indian Med Gaz 1932;67:518–519.

106. Attie J. Congenital absence of the penis: a report of a case with congenital concealed penile agenesis and congenital absence of left kidney and ureter. J Urol 1961;86:343–345.

107. Carter JP, Isa NN, Hashem N, Raasch FO Jr. Congenital absence of the penis: a case report. J Urol 1968;99:766–768.

108. Nealton. Absence de penis chez un enfant nouveau-né. Gas Hop 1854;27:45.

109. Saviard. Nouveau recueil d'observations chirurgicales. Paris: Jacques Collombat, 1702:518.

110. Gantier T, Salient J, Pena S. Testicular function in two cases of penile agenesis. J Urol 1981;126:556.

111. Kessler WO, McLaughlin AP III. Agenesis of the penis: embryology and management. Urology 1973;1:226.

112. Hanafy M, Khalil M, Eli-Khateeb S. Congenital absence of the penis: report of a case. Alexandria Med J 1962;8:582–586.

113. Ruprrecht T, Deeg KH, Bohles HJ, Stehr K. Penis agenesis. Klin Padiatr 1989;201:409–411.

114. Kraus J. Penis agenesis, persistent cloaca and anorectal agenesis. Monatsschr Kinderheilkd 1988;136:384–386.

115. Dusmot M, Fete F, Crusi A, Cox JN. VATER association: report of a case with three unreported malformations. J Med Genet 1988;25:57–60.

116. Oesch IL, Pinter A, Ransley PG. Penile agenesis: a report of six cases. J Pediatr Surg 1987;22:172–174.

117. Berry SA, Johnson DE, Thompson TR. Agenesis of the penis, scrotal raphe, and anus in one of monoamniotic twins. Teratology 1984;29:173–176.

118. Horton C, Dean J. Reconstruction of traumatically acquired defects of the phallus. World J Surg 1990;14:757.

119. Atkinson IE. Congenital absence of the glans penis. NY Med J 1898;68:668.

120. de la Peña A. Absence of glans penis. Urol Cutan Rev 1932;36:684–685.

121. Gillenwater J, Grayhack J. Adult and pediatric urology textbook. Chicago: Year Book Medical Publishers, 1987:1454–1455, 1585–1586.

122. Wolbarst AL. Circumcision and penile cancer. Lancet 1932;1:150–153.

123. Dean AL Jr. Epithelioma of the penis. J Urol 1935;33:252–283.

124. Schoen EJ. The status of circumcision of newborns. N Engl J Med 1990;322:1308–1312.

125. Lago CP. Neonatal circumcision. Surg Rounds 1991; Oct:927.

126. Dorairajan T. Defects of spongy tissue and congenital diverticula of the penile urethra. Aust N Z J Surg 1963;32:209–214.

127. Stephens FD. Congenital malformation of the rectum, anus and genito-urinary tracts. Edinburgh: E & S Livingstone, 1963.

128. Lowe FC, Hill GS, Jeffs RD, Brendler CB. Urethral problems in children: Insights into etiology and management. J Urol 1986;135:100–103.

129. Nesbit RM, Bromme W. Double penis and double bladder. AJR 1933;30:497–502.

130. Kimura H. On double penis and its complications. Jpn Med World 1930;10:63–66.

131. Donald C. A case of human diphallus. J Anat 1930;64:523–526.

132. Trenkler R. Ueber einen fall vorkommener angeborener penis-spaltung (doppelpenis). Wein Med Wsch 1914;64:1079–1082.

133. Becker H. Angeborene Fehlbildungen und Anomalien. IX. Zwei Beobachtungen von Diphallie mit weiteren Urogenitalmissbildungen. Med Mschr 1966;20:85–89.

134. Zichka-Konorsa W, Bibus B. A diphallus bifidus partly protruding into the bladder. Zentralbl Allg Pathol 1965;107:166–169.

135. Davis DM. A case of double, triple or quadruple penis associated with dermoid of the perineum. J Urol 1949;61:111–115.

136. Fowler MF. Double penis: report of a case with surgical management. Am Surg 1963;29:555–556.

137. Bonney WW, Young HH Jr, Levin D, Goodwin WE. Complete duplication of the urethra with vaginal stenosis. J Urol 1975;113:132–137.

138. Belis JA, Hrabovsky EE. Idiopathic female intersex with clitoromegaly and urethral duplication. J Urol 1979;122:805–808.

139. Kurth ME. Incomplete duplication of the female external genitalia or double clitoris. Am J Surg 1958;96:596–599.

140. Dehner LP. Female reproduction system. In: Dehner LP, ed. Pediatric surgical pathology. Baltimore: Williams & Wilkins, 1987.

141. Gross RE, Randolph J, Crigler JF Jr. Clitorectomy for sexual abnormalities: indications and technique. Surgery 1966;59:300.

142. Mogg R. A case of diphallus with vesica duplex and rectal agenesis. Acta Urol Belg 1962;30:533–536.

143. Jeffcoate TNA. Case of diphallus in female. J Obstet Gynaecol Br Commw 1957;59:406–407.

144. Cohen SJ. Diphallus with suplication of colon and bladder. Proc R Soc Med 1968;61:305.

145. Johnson CF, Carlton CE Jr, Powell NB. Duplication of the penis. Urology 1974;4:722–725.

146. Hollowell JG Jr, Witherington R, Ballagas AJ, Burt JN. Embryologic considerations of diphallus and associated anomalies. J Urol 1977;117:728–732.

147. Wecker JJ. Obs. med. rar. admirab. et monst. Lib 4, Departibus genitalibus. Pene gemino visus guidam. Francofurti 1609:577.

148. Neugebauer FL. Diphallus (double penis). Mschr Geburtsh Gynak 1898;7:550, 645.

149. Cochrane WJ, Saunders RL deCH. A rare anomaly of the penis associated with imperforate anus. J Urol 1942;47:810–817.

150. Vilanova X, Raventós A. Pseudodiphallia, a rare anomaly. J Urol 1954;71:338–346.

151. Messier B, Gagnon R. Complete diphallus in a rat. Rev Can Biol 1967;26:317–321.

152. Landy B, Signer R, Oetjey L. A case of diphalia. Urology 1984;28:48–49.

153. Johnston JH. The genital aspects of exstrophy. J Urol 1975;113:701.

154. Schmeller NT, Scherrmer HK. Trifurcation of the urethra: a case report. J Urol 1982;127:545.

155. Westenfelder M. Diphallus and bladder exstrophy: a case report. Monogr Pediatr 1981;12:50.

156. Wirtshafter A. Complete trifurcation of the urethra. J Urol 1980;123:431.

157. Broman I: Normale und abnorme Entwicklung des menschen: ein Hand- und Lehrbuch der Ontogenie und Teratologie, speziell für praktische Aerzte und Studierende der Medizin. Wiesbaden: JF Bergmann, 1911.

158. Burkitt D. Transposition of the scrotum and penis. Br J Surg 1961;48:460.

159. Remzi D. Transposition of penis and scrotum. J Urol 1966;95:555–557.

160. Meyer R. Dislocation of the phallus, penis and clitoris following pelvic malformations in the human fetus. Anat Rec 1941;79:231–242.

161. Gualtieri T, Segal A. Prepenile scrotum in a double monster: teratological considerations—the hazards of radiation. J Urol 1954;71:488–496.

162. Appleby LH. An unusual arrangement of the external genitalia. Can Med Assoc J 1923;13:514–515.

163. McGuire NC. Prepenile scrotum. Br J Surg 1954;42:203–205.

164. Huffman LF. A case of prepenile scrotum. J Urol 1951;65:141–143.

165. Francis CC. A case of prepenile scrotum (marsupial type of genitalia) associated with absence of urinary system. Anat Rec 1940;76:303–308.

166. Kuroda T, Kamiya T, Nozoe N. Two cases of Fanconi syndrome including a case with transposition of the penis and scrotum. Ann Paediatr Jpn 1967;13:53–54.

167. Adair EL, Lewis EL. Ectopic scrotum and diphallia. J Urol 1960;84:115–117.

168. Flanagan MJ, McDonald JH, Kiefer JH. Unilateral transposition of the scrotum. J Urol 1961;86:273–275.

169. Stachow J, Masowski T. Perineal transposition of the penis. Z Kinderchir 1988;43:119–121.

170. Sanvitale L. Ectopia penis associated with pubic agenesis. Riv Anat Patol Oncol 1965;28:886–898.

171. Kernaban DA. Congenital abnormalities of the scrotum. In: Horton CE, ed. Plastic and reconstructive surgery of the genital area. Boston: Little, Brown, 1973:175–181.

172. Ehrlich RM, Scardino PT. Scrotal transposition and correction of perineal hypospadias. Urol Clin North Am 1981;8:531.

173. Forshall I, Rickham PP. Transposition of the penis and scrotum. Br J Urol 1956;28:250–252.

174. Gross RE, Moore TC. Duplication of the urethra: report of two cases and summary of literature. Arch Surg 1950;60:749–761.

175. Williams DI, Kenawi MM. Urethral duplication in the male. Eur Urol 1975;1:209.

176. Johnson FP. Diverticula and cysts of the urethra. J Urol 1923;10:295–310.

177. Neff JH. Congenital canals and cysts of the genitoperineal raphe. Am J Surg 1936;31:308–315.

178. Lowsley OS. Accessory urethra: report of two cases with review of literature. NY State J Med 1939;39:1022–1031.

179. Reidy JP. A case of duplication of the penile urethra. Br J Plast Surg 1965;18:199–203.

180. Donatus M. De medica historia mirabili libri sex. Mantua, 1586.

181. Hildanus F. Opera omnia. Frankfurt am Main: J Beyeri, 1646.

182. Baillie M. The morbid anatomy of some of the most important parts of the human body, Vol 36. London: J Johnson, 1797.

183. Taruffi C. Sui canali anomali del pene. Boll Sci Med Bologna 1891;2:275–301.

184. Le Fort LC. Sur le développement de l'urétre et ses anomalies. Ann Malad Org Gen Urin 1896;618, 694, 792, 912, 1095.

185. Chauvin E. A propos des uretres doubles, en particulier de leurs variétés postérieures. J Urol Med Chir 1927;23:289–310.

186. Naparstek S. Complete duplication of male urethra in children. Urology 1980;16:391.

187. Watsell C. Congenital penile sinus. Postgrad Med J 1964;40:95–97.

188. Rinker JR. Accessory urethra in a boy. J Urol 1943;50:331–334.

189. Gross RE, Bill AA Jr. Concealed diverticulum of the male urethra as a cause of urinary obstruction. Pediatrics 1948;1:44–51.

190. Ternovsky S. Congenital urethral diverticula. Urol Cutan Rev 1930;34:478–581.

191. Geiringer D, Zucker MO. Diverticulum of the anterior urethra in a male child. Am J Surg 1939;44:463–466.

192. Arnold MW, Kaylor WM. Double urethra: case report. J Urol 1953;70:746–748.

193. Stevens WE. Congenital obstruction of the female urethra. JAMA 1936;106:89–92.

194. Tseng HC. Congenital diaphragm and fistula of penile urethra. J Urol 1951;65:590–594.

195. Dourmashkin RL. Complete urethral occlusion in living newborn: report of five cases. J Urol 1943;50:747–755.

196. Hope JW, Jameson PJ, Michie AJ. Diagnosis of anterior urethral valve by voiding urethrography: report of two cases. Radiology 1960;74:798–801.

197. Watterhouse K, Scordamaglia LJ. Anterior urethral valve: a rare cause of bilateral hydronephrosis. J Urol 1962;87:556–559.

198. Amsler E. Rétrécissements congenitaux de l'urethre caverneux chez l'homme. Helv Chir Acta 1961;28:99–107.

199. Harshman MW. Urethral stricture disease in children. J Urol 1981;126:650.

200. Kaplan GW, Brock WA. Urethral strictures in children. J Urol 1983;129:1200.

201. Dodat H, Sellem C, Pouillaude JM, Bouvier R, Takvorian P. Extensive congenital stenosis of the bulbo-membranous urethra in a child. Chir Pediatr 1987;28:125–128.

202. Grosse-Hokamp H, Muller KM. Prune belly syndrome and female pseudohermaphroditism. Pathol Res Prac 1983;177:77–83.

203. Ménégaux G, Boidot M. Des oblitérations congénitales du méat et de la portion balanique de l'uretre (hypospadias excepté). J Chir (Paris) 1934;43:641–666.

204. Jeffs RD, Masterson JST. Epispadias. In: Welch KJ, Randolph JG, Ravitch MM, O'Neil JA Jr, Rowe MI, eds. Pediatric surgery, Vol 2. Chicago: Year Book Medical Publishers, 1986:1302–1314.

205. Johnston JH, Kogan SJ. The exstrophic anomalies and their surgical reconstruction. In: Current problems in surgery. Chicago: Year Book Medical Publishers, 1974.

206. Marshall VF, Muecke EC. Variations in exstrophy of the bladder. J Urol 1962;88:766.

207. Muecke EC. The role of the cloacal membrane in exstrophy: the first successful experimental study. J Urol 1964;92:659.

208. Morgagni JB. The setas and causes of disease investigated by anatomy. B. Alexander (transl). New York: Hafner Publishing, 1960.

209. Thiersch K. Ueber die Enstekungsweise und operative 96 Behandlung der Epispadie. Arch Homoop Heilk 1869;10:20.

210. Young HH. Excision of vesical diverticula after intravesical invagination by suction: a new method. Surg Gynecol Obstet 1918;26:125–132.

211. Dees JE. Congenital epispadias with incontinence. J Urol 1949;62:513–522.

212. Stanley KE Jr., Symmonds RE, Greene LF. Partial epispadias in a girl. J Urol 1963;89:439–441.

213. Cantwell FV. Operative treatment of epispadias by transplantation of the urethra. Ann Surg 1895;22:689–694.

214. Duplay S. Sur le traitement chirurgical de l'épispadias. Bull Mem Soc Chir Paris 1880;6:169–174.

215. Boiffin A. Epispadias complet penopubien; reconstruction du col de la vessie après symphysiotomie. Franç Chir Proc Verb Paris 1895;9:576.

216. Trendelenburg F. The treatment of ectopia vesical. Ann Surg 1906;44:281–289.

217. Young HH. An operation for the cure of incontinence associated with epispadias. J Urol 1922;7:1–32.

218. Young HH. Genital abnormalities, hermaphroditism, and related adrenal disease. Baltimore: Williams & Wilkins, 1937.

219. Gross RE. The surgery of infancy and childhood. Philadelphia: WB Saunders, 1953.

220. Belman AB, Kass EJ. Hypospadias repair in children less than one year old. J Urol 1982;128:1273.

221. McIndoe A. Deformities of the male ureter. Br J Plast Surg 1948;1:29–47.

222. Cecil AB. Destructive lesions of the female urethra: a differential diagnosis from female hypospadias. Trans Am Assoc Genitourin Surg 1925;18:1–36.

223. Bauer SB, Retik AB, Colodny AH. Genetic aspects of hypospadias. Urol Clin North Am 1981;8:559.

224. Chung CS, Myriasthopoulos NC. Racial and prenatal factors in major congenital malformations. Am J Hum Genet 1968;20:44.

225. Belman AB. Hypospadias. In: Welch KJ, Randolph JG, Ravitch M, O'Neil JA Jr, Rowe MI, eds. Pediatric surgery, Vol 2. Chicago: Year Book Medical Publishers, 1986:1286–1302.

226. Khuri FJ, Hardy BE, Churchill BM. Urologic anomalies associated with hypospadias. Urol Clin North Am 1981;8:565.

227. Fallon B, Devine CJ Jr, Horton CE. Congenital anomalies associated with hypospadias. J Urol 1976;116:585.

228. Ikoma HS, Terakawa T, Satoh Y. Developmental anomalies associated with hypospadias. J Urol 1979;122:619.

229. Mininberg DT, Bingol N, Wasserman E. In: Bergsma D, ed. Birth defects compendium, 2nd ed. New York: National Foundation–March of Dimes, Alan R. Liss, 1979.

230. Sweet RA, Schrott HG, Kurland R. Study of the incidence of hypospadias in Rochester, MN, 1940–1970, and a case control comparison of possible etiologic factors. Mayo Clin Proc 1974;49:52.

231. Devine CJ Jr., Horton CE. Chordee without hypospadias. J Urol 1973;110:264.

232. Willis RA. Pathology of tumors. London: Butterworth, 1948.

233. Aristotle. Generation of animals. AL Peck (transl). The Loeb classical library. Cambridge: Harvard University Press, 1943.

234. Cabot H. Modern urology, Vol 1. Philadelphia: Lea & Febiger, 1936.

235. Anger T. Hypospadias peno-scrotal, complique de coudure de la verger; redressment du penis et urethroplastic par inclusion cutaneé; guerison. Bull Mem Soc Chir Paris 1875;1:179–194.

236. Malpas P. The incidence of human malformation and the significance of changes in the maternal environment in their causation. J Obstet Gynaecol Br Commw 1937;44:434–454.

CHAPTER 22

THE FEMALE REPRODUCTIVE TRACT

Stephen Wood Gray / John Elias Skandalakis / Bruce Broecker

"A knowledge of anatomy and physiology is just as essential to the gynecologist as a familiarity with the general principles of surgery; indeed, the very foundation stones of successful work are laid in envisaging the relations of the parts to be dealt with so clearly that the operator divides layer from layer almost as if the coverings of the body were transparent. Without this accurate knowledge of the component parts of the pelvis and abdomen and their mutual relations, to be gained only by actual dissections, surgery is not an art, but at best a haphazard procedure guided by luck; without a knowledge of physiology an operator will often ruthlessly sacrifice organs or parts of organs whose functional activity is essential to the happiness and well-being of the patient."
—*HOWARD A. KELLY, OPERATIVE GYNECOLOGY, 1898*

DEVELOPMENT

During the first three months of embryonic life, the primordia of both the male and the female reproductive tracts are present and develop together. At the end of this time, the wolffian ducts of the female regress, while the müllerian ducts continue their development.

Müllerian Ducts

The müllerian (paramesonephric) ducts are first indicated in embryos of both sexes at the 10-mm stage (late in the sixth week) by a characteristic thickening of the anterior lateral celomic epithelium covering the wolffian body. By 10.5 mm, a slight groove lined with distinctive epithelial cells is present, and soon afterward a tube is formed by fusion of the lips of the groove (Fig. 22.1). The exact position of the primordium is variable both from one embryo to another and on the two sides of the same embryo (1). The origin of the müllerian ostium from a pronephric nephrostome has been suggested (2), but little evidence is available. Faulconer (1) considers that the duct arises at the level of mesonephric rather than pronephric tubules. Actually, the specialized epithelium from which the ostium appears implies that the ostium arises independently and not from a previously formed structure.

Regardless of the origin of the ostium, the development of the duct is closely linked with that of the duct of the mesonephros (see Chapter 17). Gruenwald (3) showed that the caudally growing tip of the müllerian duct lies within the basement membrane of the mesonephric duct epithelium: "At each particular level we find the Mullerian duct first as a solid wedge between the epithelium and the basal membrane of the Wolffian duct, then acquiring a lumen, and finally we see it being separated from the Wolffian duct by basal membranes and an increasing amount of mesenchyme." The dependence of the müllerian on the wolffian duct is further demonstrated by the failure of the former to progress beyond an experimental interruption of the latter (4).

The elongating müllerian ducts lie lateral to the wolffian ducts until they reach the caudal end of the mesonephros. Here they become medial to the wolffian ducts and in contact with each other. By 30 mm (ninth week), the müllerian ducts reach the urogenital sinus and invaginate into its wall to form the müllerian tubercle, but no actual opening takes place. By 48 mm (third month), the two ducts have completely fused into a single tube (Figs. 22.2 and 22.3, C).

At about this stage, müllerian duct development in the male comes to an end; the ducts eventually regress and are marked only by vestiges at either end of their course (page 775).

In the female the wolffian ducts begin to regress a little later; by 56 mm, their openings into the urogenital sinus become closed (Fig. 22.3, D and E). Their persisting remnants are described in Chapter 21. Scheib (5) described acid phosphatase in degenerating wolffian ducts and suggested that the cells undergo autolysis.

Although the fused tips of the müllerian ducts reach the urogenital sinus, the elongation of the pelvic region carries the sinus away from the point at which the müllerian ducts fused with one another. This elongation causes the lumen of the fused ducts to recede, drawing out a solid epithelial cord between the end of the tubular por-

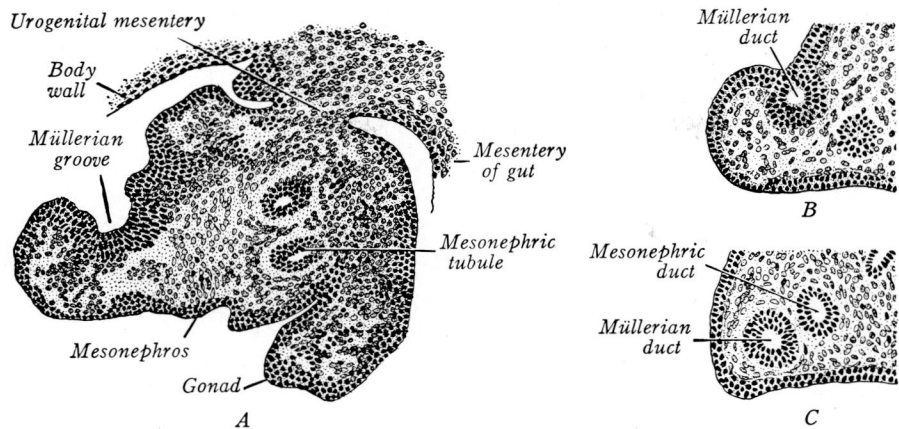

Figure 22.1. Sections through the nephrogenic ridge of a 12-mm (6 weeks) embryo to show the formation of the müllerian duct. **A,** Near the cephalic end, the duct is at first an open groove. **B** and **C,** In more caudal sections, the duct lies just lateral to the mesonephric duct. (From Arey LB. Developmental anatomy, 7th ed. Philadelphia: WB Saunders, 1965.)

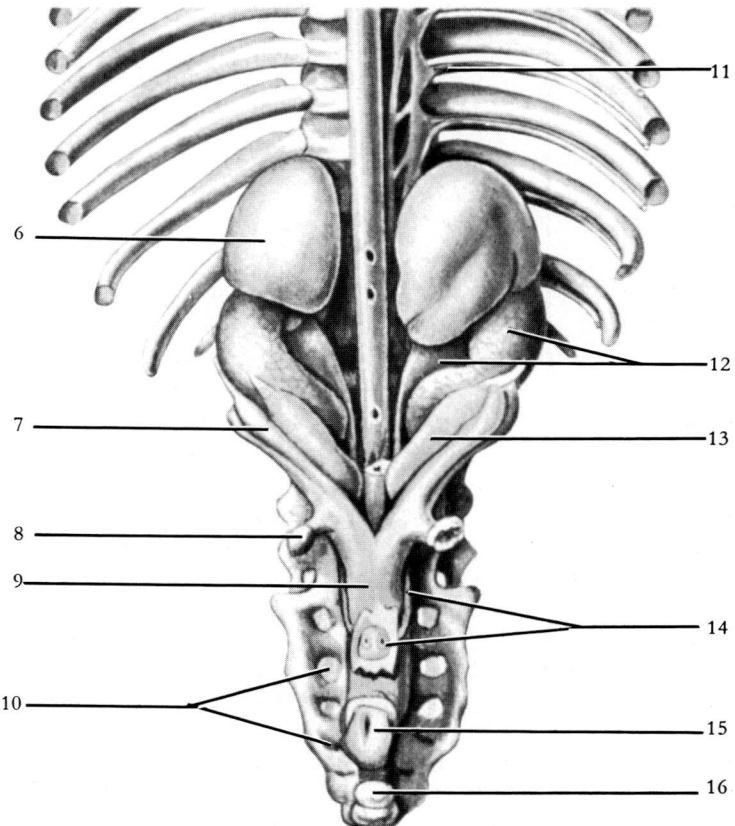

Figure 22.2. Relative positions of suprarenal glands, kidneys, ovaries, and developing müllerian ducts in a 30-mm embryo. *6,* Suprarenal gland; *7,* müllerian duct; *8,* round ligament; *9,* uterus; *10,* sacral foramina; *11,* ramus communicans; *12,* kidney; *13,* ovary; *14,* ureter; *15,* anus; *16,* coccyx. (From Blechschmidt E. The stages of human development before birth. Philadelphia: WB Saunders, 1961.)

tion and the müllerian tubercle on the wall of the sinus. This is the origin of the "solid stage" of the vagina (Fig. 22.4).

There is general agreement over events up to this point of development; however, although the subsequent development has been studied by many workers, they are somewhat less than unanimous in their views. The parts played by müllerian, wolffian, and urogenital sinus epithelium in the canalization of this solid vaginal primordium are subject to several interpretations.

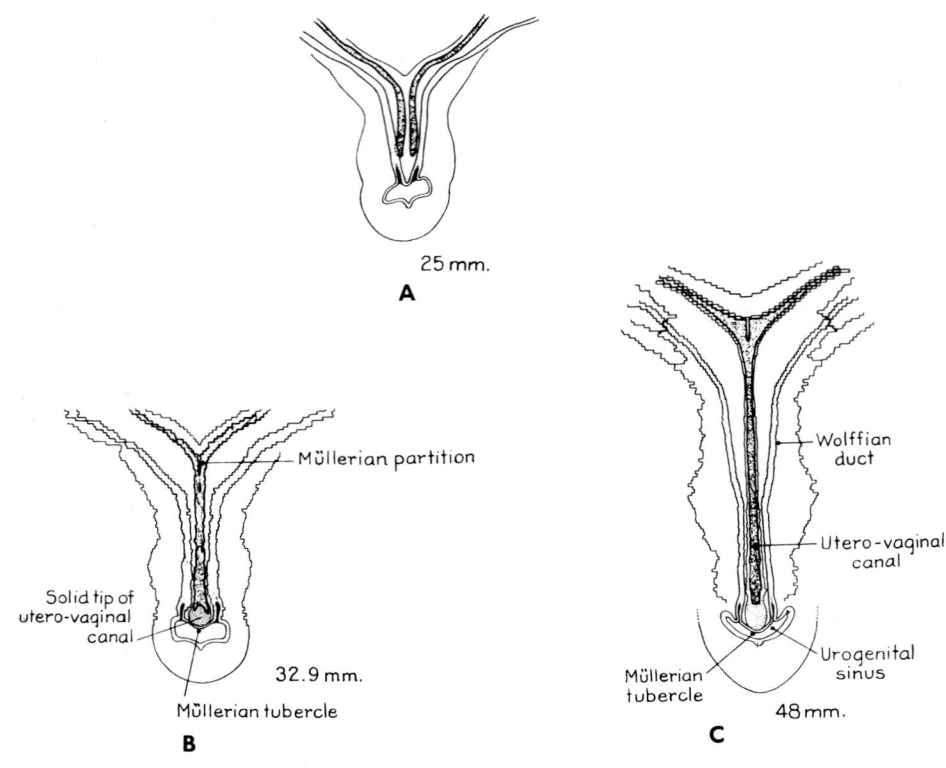

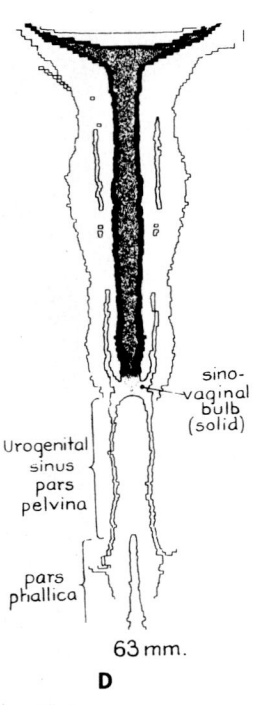

Figure 22.3. Development of the human uterus and vagina. **A,** The müllerian ducts have not reached the urogenital sinus. **B,** The müllerian ducts have reached the sinus and formed the müllerian tubercle. The paired ducts have begun to fuse. **C,** Fusion of the müllerian ducts is nearly complete. **D,** The wolffian ducts are degenerating and the solid epithelial sinovaginal bulb is enlarging. **E** and **F,** Further development of the solid epithelial mass in the vagina. According to Koff (1933),

the epithelium above the **V**-*shaped broken line* is of müllerian duct origin, while that below is derived from the urogenital sinus. The lateral bulges in the cervical region are at the site of the fornices of the vagina. The position labeled upper uterine segment *(F)* will form most of the uterine body. (From Koff AK. Development of the vagina in the human foetus. Contrib Embryol Carnegie Inst Wash 1933;24:61–90.)

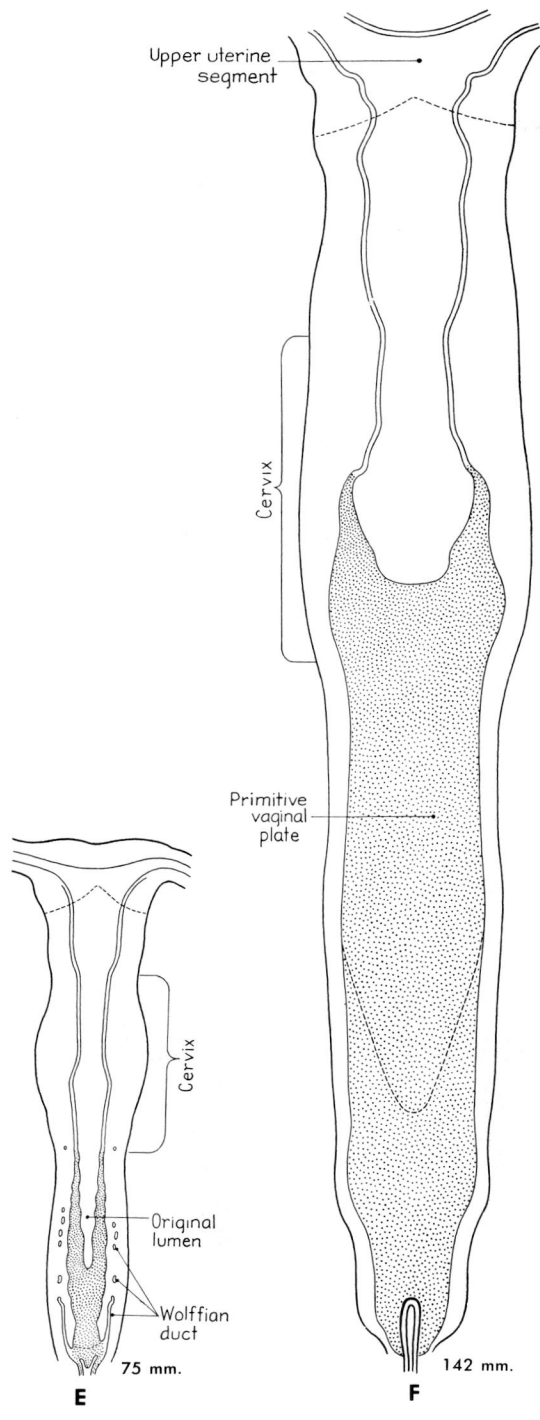

Upper uterine
segment

Cervix

Primitive
vaginal
plate

142 mm.

F

Cervix

Original
lumen

Wolffian
duct

75 mm.

E

The actual events are not complicated. The solid vaginal cord enlarges from the 142-mm stage onward by proliferation and stratification of epithelial cells and by irregular invasion of the surrounding mesenchyme (6). By the 150-mm stage, lacunae appear in the center of the cord, and by 212-mm stage (seventh month), the vagina has

become a hollow organ. At the level of the junction with the primitive urogenital sinus, the hymen remains as a partial septum (Fig. 22.5).

The source of the vaginal epithelium has been under debate. The chief views may be stated as follows:

1. *Müllerian origin:* The view that the entire vagina is formed from the lower end of the fused müllerian ducts was proposed by Felix (7) and Hunter (6) (Fig. 22.5).
2. *Wolffian origin:* While it has been suggested that the entire vagina is of wolffian origin (8), the more accepted form of this theory is that of Mijsberg (9), who believed the upper two-thirds of the canal was müllerian, but the lower one-third grew from the epithelium of the wolffian duct.
3. *Urogenital sinus origin:* This is perhaps the oldest view. Retterer (10) and Koff (11), as well as earlier writers, considered the cells of the lower portion of the solid vagina to be derived from the wall of the urogenital sinus. More recent is the view that the whole vagina is of urogenital sinus origin. Bulmer (12, 13) and a number of other investigators (14–16) have supported this view. Basing his argument on histologic grounds, Bulmer contends that epithelium from the dorsal wall of the sinus invades the müllerian epithelium and completely replaces it by the 140 mm-stage.

Forsberg (17) reexamined this "invasion" of sinus epithelium using tritiated thymidine in the developing mouse vagina. His results indicate that only the caudal portion of the vaginal epithelium is of sinus origin, whereas the cranial portion is of müllerian origin. His work indicates a metaplasia of the müllerian epithelium rather than an invasion of sinus epithelium (Fig. 22.3, *E* and *F*).

This last view supports Koff's (11) idea of a dual origin of the vagina based on the frequent presence of a normal caudal segment with complete atresia of the cranial portion. In spite of the attention this region has received from embryologists, it is possible that the last word has not yet been said.

Because of the problems posed by the formation of the vagina, the nature of the hymenal membrane has long been the subject of debate. Most authorities have considered the hymen to represent the remains of the solid epithelium at the junction of the vagina and urogenital sinus. Kanagasuntheram and Dassanayake (18) argued for an origin from the urogenital portion of the cloacal membrane, but this seems improbable.

Knowledge of the origin of the structure, however, does not indicate the source of its upper and lower epithelium. The older view was that the vaginal surface of the hymen, like the vagina itself, was covered with müllerian epithelium, while its outer surface was derived from the urogenital sinus. Hunter (6) contended that vaginal (müllerian) epithelium spreads over the external surface of the hymen and that no sinus epithelium is present. To

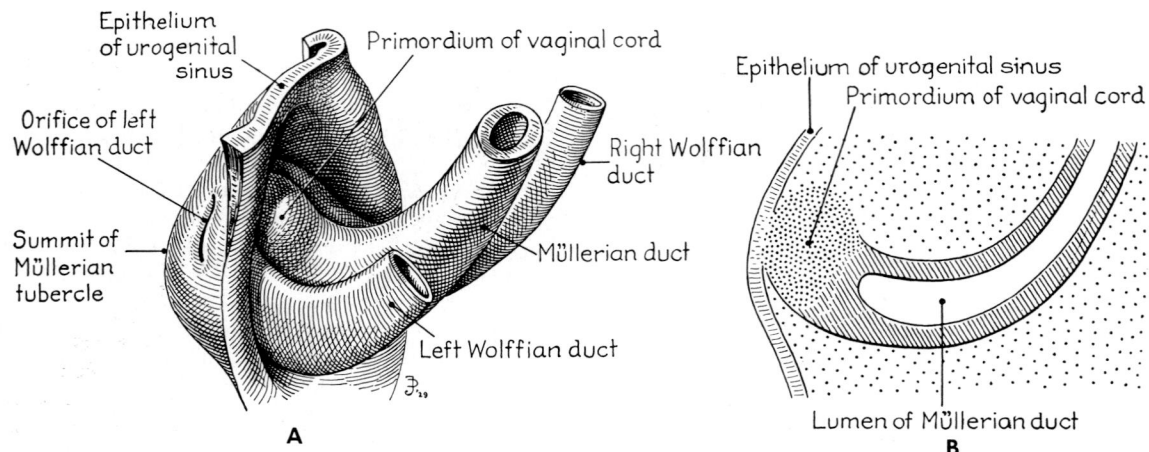

Figure 22.4. The müllerian tubercle of a 48-mm human embryo. **A,** Waxplate reconstruction. **B,** Schematic longitudinal section. (From Hunter RH. Observations on the development of the human female genital tract. Contrib Embryol Carnegie Inst Wash 1930;22:91–108.)

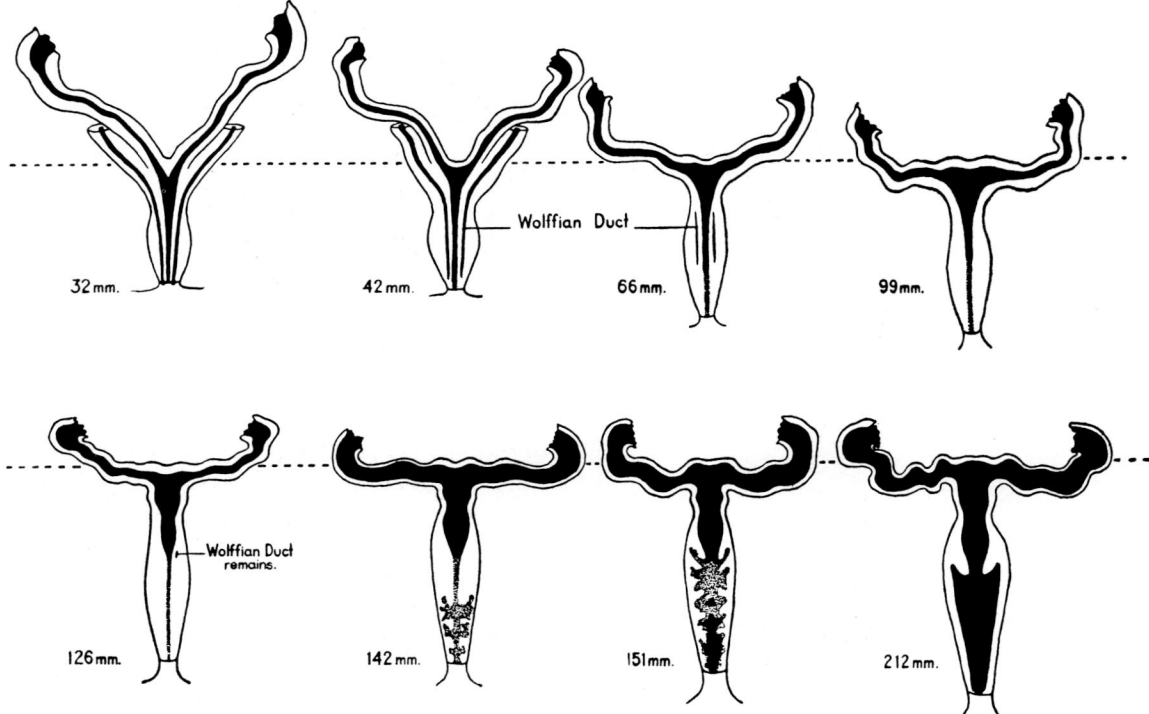

Figure 22.5. Various stages in the development of the human vagina. (From Hunter RH. Observations on the development of the human female genital tract. Contrib Embryol Carnegie Inst Wash 1930;22:91–108.)

those who, with Koff (11), believed the sinus epithelium invades the vagina, both surfaces of the hymen must be covered with epithelium of sinus origin.

Remember that the vagina is formed by participation of the uterine canal (upper part of vagina) and by the urogenital sinus, which is responsible for the genesis of the lower part. This theory of dual genesis is supported by the work of Cunha (19), O'Rahilly (20), and George and Wilson (21).

The development of the uterus and the cervix from the tubular portion of the fused müllerian ducts poses no such problems as those associated with development of the vagina. By 100 mm, the V-shaped fusion of the müllerian ducts has flattened out to a T shape, with the tubular stem of the T representing the future uterine body and cervix (Fig. 22.6, *A* and *B*). Below the tubular portion extends the solid vaginal segment. A slight constriction indicates the division between the body of the uterus and

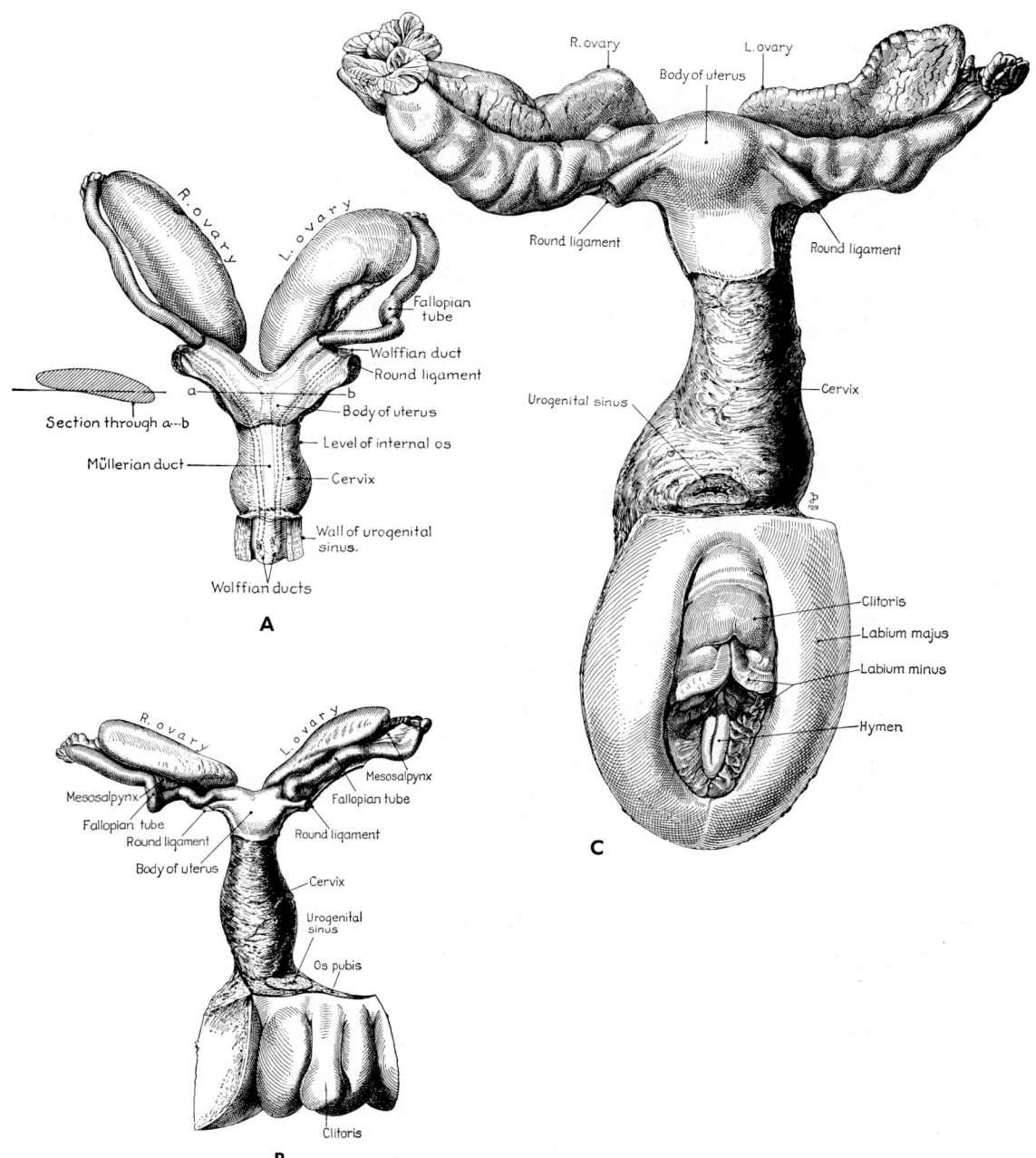

Figure 22.6. External views of the developing female genital tract. **A,** At 43 mm. **B,** At 139 mm. **C,** At 227 mm (fifth month). Note the relative sizes of the body and cervix at this stage. The proportions will not change materially until puberty.

(From Hunter RH. Observations on the development of the human female genital tract. Contrib Embryol Carnegie Inst Wash 1930;22:91–108.)

the cervix. During fetal life, the latter is larger with respect to the body. Growth is relatively slow until the vaginal epithelium becomes canalized, at which point the cervix begins to enlarge rapidly. By birth it is more than twice the length of the uterine body (Fig. 22.6, *C*). After birth—and consequently, after removal of the influence of maternal hormones—both structures decrease in size: the cervix by 66% and the body by 33%. At the same time, desquamation reduces the hypertrophic vaginal epithe-

lium from 20 or more cell layers to the normal atrophic epithelium of the infant vagina (22).

The uterine and cervical epithelium is at first columnar and becomes increasingly higher in the last few weeks before birth. The columnar uterine epithelium at the os cervix is replaced by stratified squamous vaginal epithelium after birth (6).

Spindle-shaped cells are visible in the mesenchyme around the uterus and vagina by the 11th week, but true muscle cells appear later. Two longitudinal muscular layers, with a circular layer between, are usually said to exist. These are, in turn, divided into a uterine and cervicovaginal group of muscles. In the body of the uterus the circular fibers are formed first. In the vagina the longitudinal fibers are the first to appear. The musculature is not complete until the seventh month.

It should be noted that fusion of the müllerian ducts occurs shortly after their formation, and at no time is double uterus present in normal human development. The fundic notch, which constitutes the last trace of the fusion, is not obliterated until the seventh month, according to Hunter (6).

The cranial unfused portion of the müllerian ducts becomes more prominent as the mesonephros and its ducts regress. With the increasing width of the pelvis, the ducts—which may now be called uterine tubes—course more transversely. For a short while the developing uter-

ine body encroaches on the unfused segments, but between 215 and 295 mm (eighth month), uterine growth slows and the tubes elongate, becoming slightly coiled. Unlike the uterus, they do not become smaller after birth.

The tubal musculature is indicated in the third month, with the middle circular layer appearing first and the inner and outer longitudinal layers later. At the same time the lumen loses its circularity in cross-section, and four primary longitudinal folds appear, forming first at the ostial end. Secondary folds form subsequently, and by birth the folds are almost as well developed as at maturity.

For all practical purposes, the paramesonephric duct is transformed into the female genital part. The uterine tubes are formed from its cranial vertical and horizontal parts and the uterus is developed from the right and left caudal vertical parts of the paramesonephric duct. These fuse together to form the uterine canal, which in time will become the corpus and the cervix of the uterus. The uter-

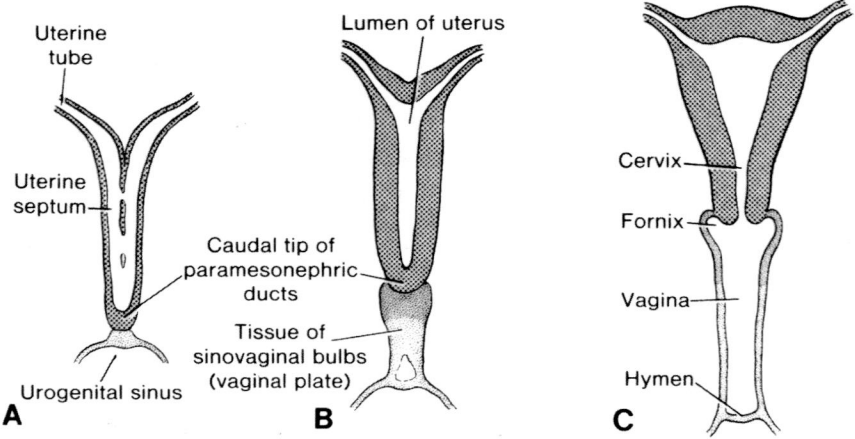

Figure 22.7. Schematic drawing showing the formation of the uterus and vagina. **A,** At 9 weeks. Note the disappearance of the uterine septum. **B,** At the end of the third month. Note the tissue of the sinovaginal bulbs. **C,** Newborn. The upper portion of the vagina and the fornices are formed by vacuolization of the paramesonephric tissue and the lower portion by vacuolization of the sinovaginal bulbs. (From Sanders RC, Blakemore K. Lethal fetal anomalies: sonographic demonstration. Radiology 1989;172:1–6.)

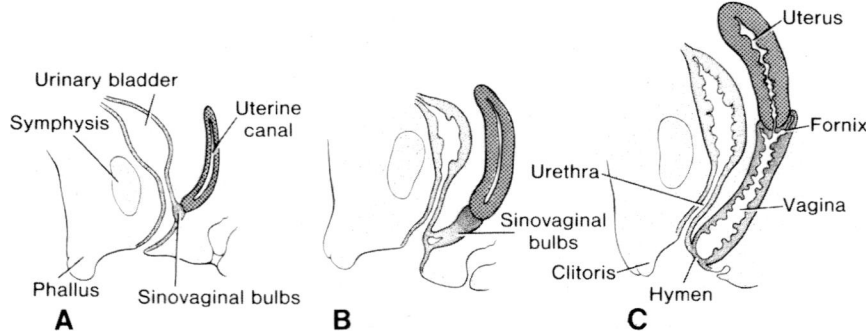

Figure 22.8. Schematic sagittal sections showing the formation of the uterus and vagina at various stages of development. (From Sanders RC, Blakemore K. Lethal fetal anomalies: sonographic demonstration. Radiology 1989;172:1–6.)

ine canal is enveloped by mesenchymal tissue. Again, in time, it will form the perimetrium and myometrium (Figs. 22.7 and 22.8).

Mesonephric Remnants in the Female

With the decline of the mesonephros, the wolffian duct and its tubules in the female lose their primary function and regress. Regression does not, however, proceed as far as complete disappearance, and the embryologist, like the archaeologist, is faced with a number of vestiges of former structures to explain. As with the archaeologist's material, most of it is in ruins; some has been converted to new use; and much has vanished.

The course of the obliterated mesonephric duct in the adult female begins near the ostium of the uterine tube and runs in the broad ligament. It enters the uterine wall above the cervix and continues downward in the cervical and vagina walls to end near the vaginal orifice (23). Along this tract are found remnants of the system (Fig. 22.9).

PEDUNCULATED HYDATID OF MORGAGNI

This structure, associated with the ostia fimbriae, is usually considered to be of müllerian origin, although there have been advocates of a wolffian or even pronephric origin (24).

APPENDIX VESICULOSA (SESSILE HYDATID)

This cystic structure usually is not associated with the fimbriae, nor is it always present. It usually is considered to represent the blind head of the wolffian duct.

EPOOPHORON (ROSENMÜLLER'S ORGAN)

This structure consists of a portion of mesonephric duct with a variable number (eight to thirteen) of tubules entering it. The tubules lie in the lateral third of the mesovarium and pass through the most lateral mesosalpingeal portion of the broad ligament. The duct lies close and parallel to the uterine tube. According to Gardner (24) and his colleagues, the duct is lined with low cuboidal epithelium without cilia. It has an inner longitudinal and an outer circular layer of smooth muscle. The tubules are convoluted and lined with both ciliated and nonciliated cells. The epoophoron is the homologue of the epididymis in the male. There is no evidence of secretory activity of the epithelium in either fetus or adult (25).

PAROOPHORON (TUBES OF KOBELT)

This is a group of mesonephric tubules more caudal than those of the epoophoron and having no duct connecting them. Felix (7) described them as lying caudal to the lateral half of the ovary and medial to the free edge of the broad ligament. Little is known of them, and they appear to be present only in infants.

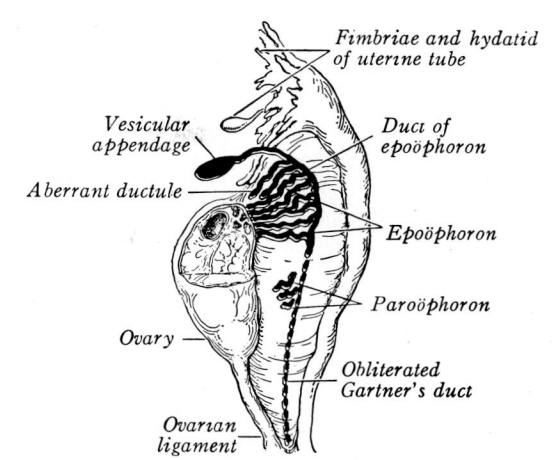

Figure 22.9. Remnants of the mesonephric (wolffian) duct system in the female. The hydatid of the uterine tube (pedunculated hydatid of Morgagni) probably represents the cranial end of the müllerian duct. These structures are quite variable and may even be absent. (From Arey LB. Developmental anatomy, 7th ed. Philadelphia: WB Saunders, 1965.)

OTHER CYSTIC REMNANTS

Gardner and his colleagues found 65 cystic structures in routine sections of 598 adult broad ligaments. From the histologic appearance, they concluded 5 were remnants of mesonephric duct and 33 were of tubular origin. The remainder they believed to be of müllerian origin (Fig. 22.10). An anomalous cord found arising from the superior portion of the uterine fundus (26) is not readily explained.

GARTNER'S CANAL (DUCTUS EPOOPHORI LONGITUDINALIS)

The distal portion of the wolffian duct in the female begins to degenerate from the 10th week onward. Remnants remaining in the cervical and vaginal walls are referred to as Gartner's canal (or duct). There is some question as to how much regression is normal. Meyer (27) thought development continued nearly to birth in those individuals in whom remnants were found. Before the duct regresses, an enlargement occurs in the lower part of the supravaginal cervical wall. This enlargement, termed the *ampulla*, becomes branched, and the branches become coiled tubules in the substance of the cervix. These tubules do not have the muscular wall typical of the rest of the canal. They are distinguishable from cervical glands by their low cuboidal epithelium, which shows no mucicarmine reaction. Szamborski (28) suggested that mesonephric derivatives in the uterus may be distinguished from glandular adenocarcinoma by a positive reaction to Lillie's allochrome stain and a negative reaction to alcian blue.

Gartner's canal rarely is detected unless pathologic changes develop. It is assumed to be present in about 20%

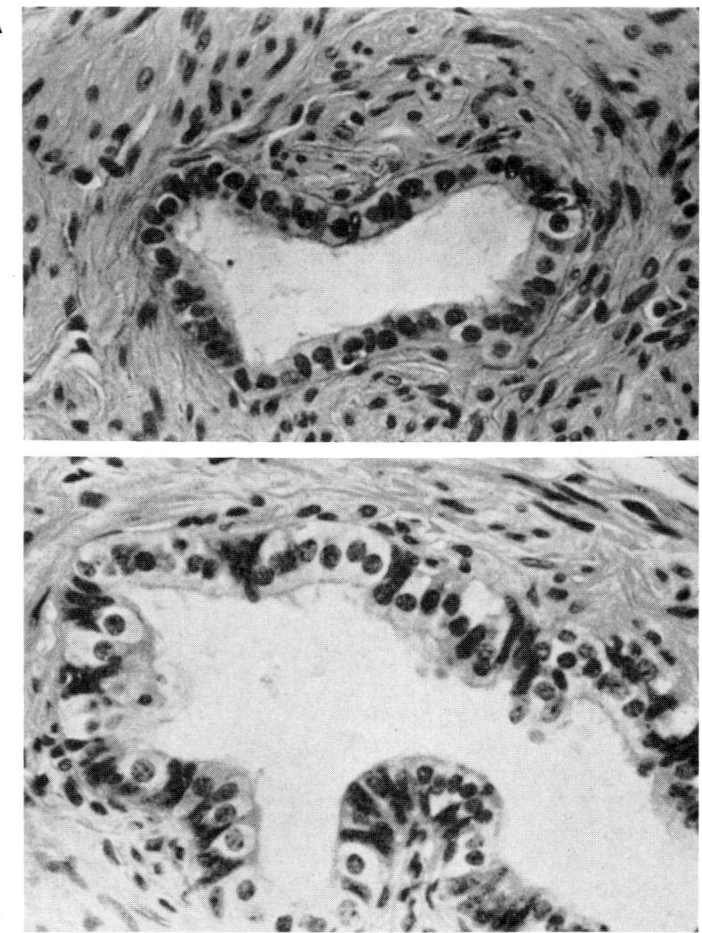

Figure 22.10. **A,** Mesonephric (wolffian), and **B,** müllerian tubules from the same broad ligament and at the same magnification. Note the greater size of cells and nuclei in the müllerian tubule. (From Gardner GH, *et al.* Normal and cystic structures of the broad ligament. Amer J Obstet Gynecol 1948;55:917–937.)

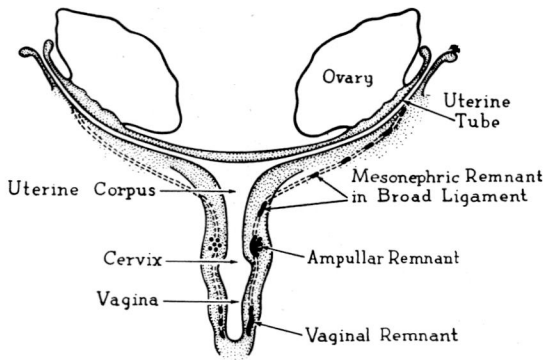

Figure 22.11. The course of Gartner's duct (wolffian duct) and the chief sites in which remnants have been reported. (From Huffman JW. Mesonephric remnants in human female. Q Bull Northwest Univ Med School 1951;25:25–38.)

of adult women, based on a small series of Rieder (29). Sneeden (30) found cervical remnants in 15 of 216 hysterectomies, but he believed many more were undetected (Fig. 22.11).

Occasionally, the canal retains its urinary function. When a ureter fails to make its normal connection with the bladder, it may retain its connection with the wolffian duct, and hence Gartner's canal may become an ectopic ureter opening into the vagina or the vestibule (page 696).

Table 20.5 shows the relationships of various vestigial structures of both male and female reproductive tracts.

External Genitalia

The development of the external genitalia proceeds almost indistinguishably in the two sexes up to the end of the second month. This series of events is described with the male genitalia on page 776 (see Fig. 21.8, A).

Those portions of the urogenital sinus below the müllerian tubercle become progressively reduced in the female, forming the vestibule. The urovaginal septum descends to the level of the urorectal septum (perineum) bringing the site of the müllerian tubercle to the level of the hymen. This development may be seen in Figure 22.12. At birth the urethra and vagina open separately at the same level on the floor of the shallow vestibule.

In the female the phallus grows more slowly than in the male. Only the posterior ends of the urogenital folds fuse in front of the anus. The remaining portions form the labia minora, which are covered with ectoderm on the outer surface and with endodermal urogenital sinus epithelium on the inner surface. They unite with the clitoris anteriorly. The labial folds remain smaller than do the homologous scrotal folds of the male. They fuse posteriorly, and their free portions form the labia majora (see Fig. 21.8, C).

The clitoris, like the penis, contains two corpora cavernosa of erectile tissue, which arise as right and left crura, joined anteriorly to form the body of the clitoris. The corpus spongiosum in the body of the clitoris is vestigial, but the posterior (bulbar) portion is divided into two vestibular bulbs of erectile tissue lying on either side of the vagina.

Remember the following:

1. Absence of the Y chromosome is responsible for the genesis of the ovary from the indifferent organ.
2. Estrogens (maternal and placental) stimulate the paramesonephric ducts, causing the genesis of the uterine tube, uterus, and upper vagina to take place.
3. Again, estrogenic stimulation of the external genitalia may cause the labiae, clitoris, and lower portion of the vagina to form (see Tables 20.2 and 20.3).

Critical Events in Development

Between the ninth and twelfth weeks, the paired müllerian ducts fuse posteriorly to form the primordium of the

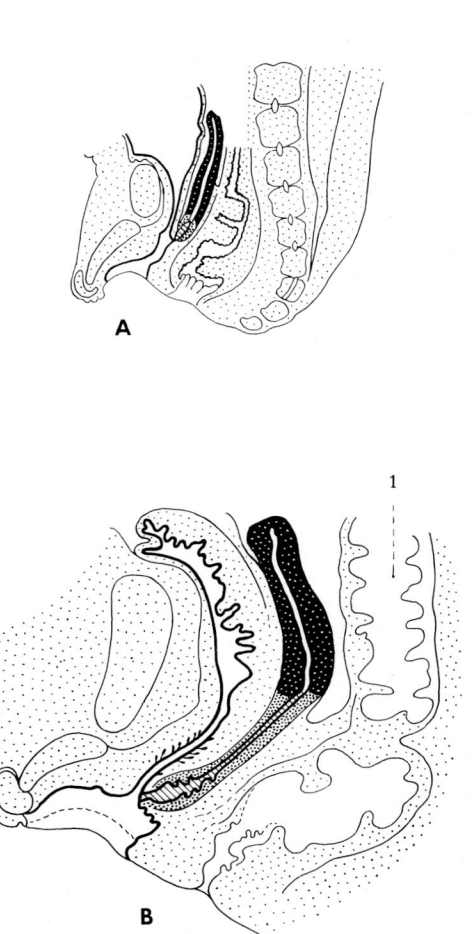

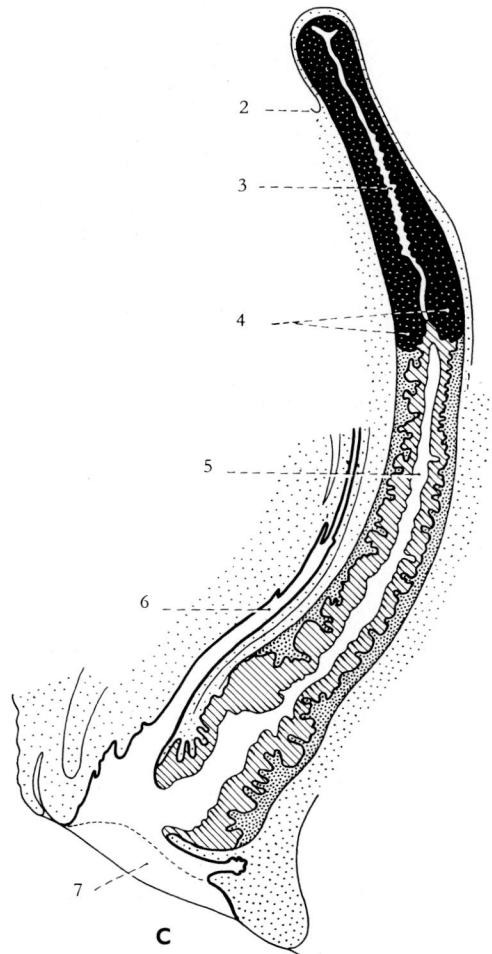

Figure 22.12. Descent of the vaginal opening at the site of the müllerian tubercle. This descent is brought about by decreased growth of the urogenital sinus. **A,** At 70 mm (12th week). **B,** At 131 mm (16th week). **C,** At 162 mm (about 18th week). There will be a further descent of the urethrovaginal septum before birth. *1,* Rectum; *2,* peritoneum; *3,* uterus; *4,* cervix; *5,* vagina; *6,* urethra; *7,* vestibule (labium minus). (From Blechschmidt E. The stages of human development before birth. Philadelphia: WB Saunders, 1961.)

Table 22.1.
Anomalies of the Female Reproductive Tract

Anomaly	Origin of Defect	First Appearance (or Other Diagnostic Clues)	Sex Chiefly Affected[a]	Relative Frequency	Remarks
Aplasia and atresia of the uterus and vagina					
Complete absence of uterus and vagina	8th week	At birth	Female	Rare	Familial tendency suggested
Absence of vagina	9th week	At birth	Female	Uncommon	Familial tendency suggested
Rudimentary, solid uterus, and vagina	17th week	At birth	Female	Rare	
Imperforate hymen	5th month	In infancy or childhood	Female	Common	
Duplication of the uterine tubes	6th to 7th weeks	Found only with ectopic pregnancy	Female	Very rare	Small asymptomatic duplications may be more frequent
Incomplete fusion of the müllerian ducts:					
Separate hemiuteri	3rd week?	At birth	Female	Very rare	Two separate vaginae
Uterus didelphys	9th week			Uncommon	May have septate vagina
Uterus unicornis	9th week			Rare	
Uterus duplex	9th week	Asymptomatic until pregnancy occurs	Female	Common	May have single or double cervix and septate vagina
Uterus septus	12th week			Uncommon	
Uterus arcuatus	7th month			Common?	
Fusion of the labia	?	Infancy	Female	Rare	May not be congenital

[a]Although these conditions may occur in males with anomalous or vestigial female structures, these anomalies all occur chiefly in females.

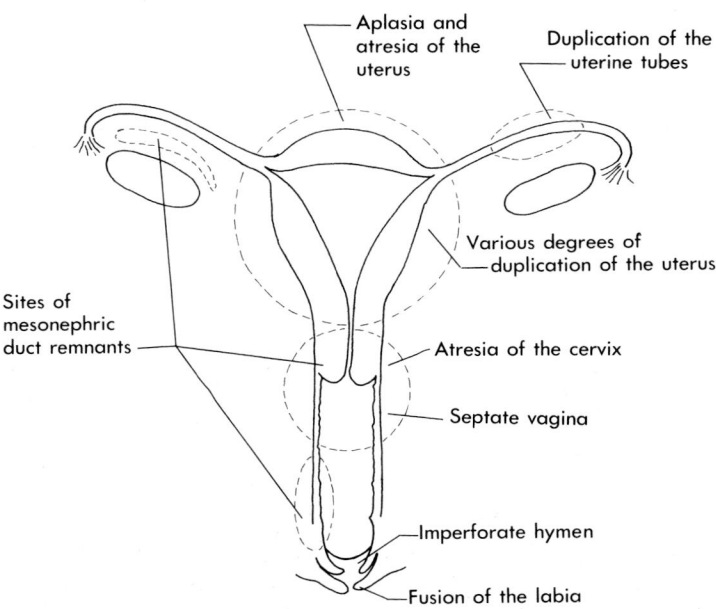

Figure 22.13. Sites of developmental anomalies of the female reproductive tract.

uterus and vagina. Incomplete fusion in varying degrees at that time produces uterine anomalies, of which uterus didelphys with septate vagina is the most extreme and uterus arcuatus the mildest form.

During the sixth and seventh month, the vagina becomes hollow by recanalization of its previous solid epithelial plug. Failure of this to occur results in vaginal atresia.

According to Rock and Azziz (31) in 1987, a survey of 50,882 children revealed that one child in every 8300 presented with malformations of the external genitalia.

One year later Ashton et al. (32) reported the incidence of congenital anomalies of the uterus as 1 to 10%.

ANOMALIES OF THE FEMALE REPRODUCTIVE TRACT (FIG. 22.13 and TABLE 22.1)

Disorders Associated with Mesonephric Vestiges in the Female

TORSION OF THE HYDATID OF MORGAGNI

This structure, associated with the fimbria of the ostium (Fig. 22.9), may undergo spontaneous torsion in females, as may the homologous structure in the males (page 777). In males the torsion usually occurs before puberty; in females it occurs during the reproductive span (33).

The frequency of torsion is impossible to judge, but it is not common. Reis and DeCosta (33) found only 26 reported cases between 1906 and 1947.

Colicky pain in the lower quadrant of the abdomen is the most common symptom. Nausea and vomiting are frequent but not always present. Torsion has been associated with dysmenorrhea in four cases and with pregnancy in five. In 11 cases, appendicitis was diagnosed; two patients were thought to have ectopic pregnancy; and six cases were correctly diagnosed before operation. In each case a gangrenous hydatid of 5 to 25 mm in diameter on a 10- to 25-mm pedicle was removed.

CYSTS OF THE BROAD LIGAMENT

While remnants of the wolffian duct are common in the broad ligament, only rarely do they become cystic. A patient with multiple large cysts was described by Bisca

(34). Such parovarian cysts may be confused on physical examination with true ovarian cysts (Fig. 22.14, B).

DILATION OF PERSISTENT GARTNER'S CANAL

Gartner's canal (Fig. 22.10) may retain a ureteral connection and form an ectopic ureter (page 696). If it is associated with a poorly functioning superior calyx of a double kidney, the flow of urine may be small and the canal may become infected. Occasionally, its distal end may be closed, resulting in dilation (35). Since this ureteral termination bypasses the bladder entirely, whatever urine is produced by the poorly functioning renal tissue will empty directly and continuously into the vagina. These patients may then present with urinary incontinence characterized by constant dampness.

Dilation with blood has been reported in a 14-year-old patient with an absent right kidney, a double uterus, and a connection between the right uterine tube and the right Gartner's duct. The Gartner's duct had become tremendously dilated (36).

Aplasia and Atresia of the Vagina and Uterus

ANATOMY

Aplasia and atresia of the female reproductive tract may be segmental or membranous, or an entire organ may be involved.

Absence and Aplasia of the Uterus and Uterine Tubes. Complete absence of the uterus is rare and always is coupled with absence of the vagina. More often, the uterus is hypoplastic or represented by a small, solid mass (Fig. 22.15), *A* and *B*). Brews (37) found nine examples of rudi-

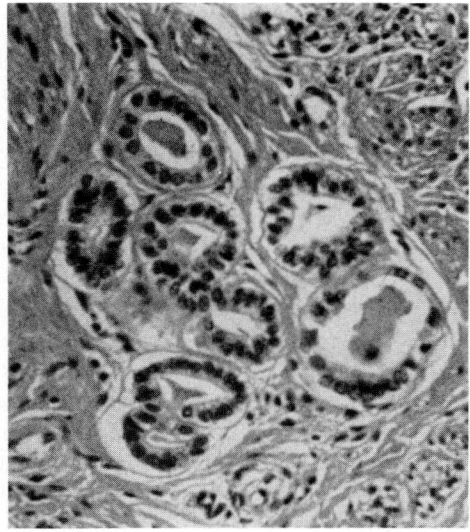
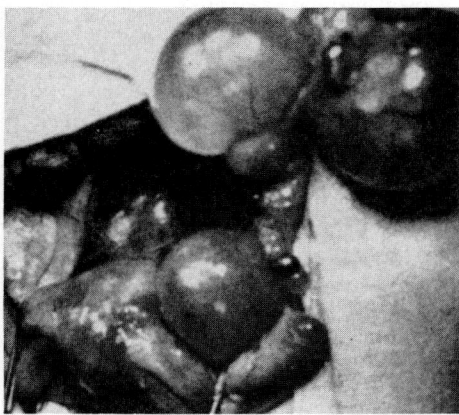

Figure 22.14. Mesonephric remnants. **A,** Tubules in the cervix lined by simple low cuboidal epithelium. **B,** Cysts in the broad ligament from mesonephric tubular remnants. (From Bisca BV. Mesonephric remnants in the adult female. Obstet Gynecol 1956;8:265–269.)

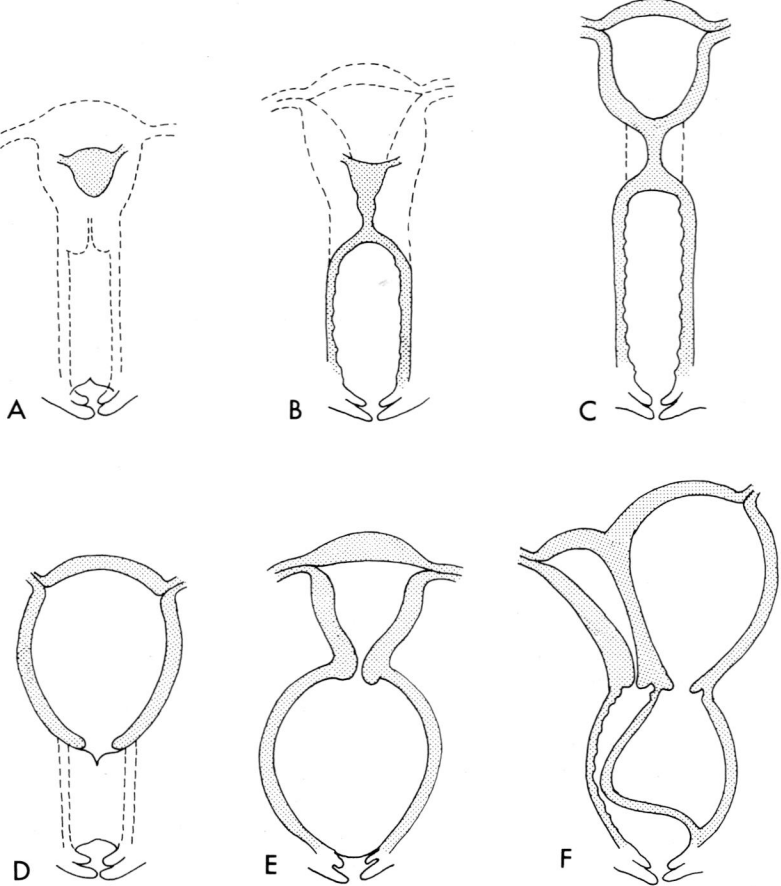

Figure 22.15. Diagrams of the varieties of aplasia and atresia of the vagina and the uterus. **A,** Hypoplastic, solid uterus with absence of the vagina. **B,** Hypoplastic uterus with normal vagina. **C,** Atresia of the cervix and upper vagina. The body of the uterus is normal. **D,** Vaginal atresia with normal uterus. **E,** Imperforate hymen with distension of the vagina. **F,** Double uterus and vagina with one vagina occluded by the septum and distension of the uterus and vagina on the occluded side.

mentary uterus in a 60-year hospital series. Pfleiderer (38) found 14 cases of solid uterus and vagina among 93 uterine anomalies. A solid, double uterus has been reported (39). Aplastic uteri may be more frequent than the reported cases would indicate because most anomalies are reported by obstetricians, who rarely see patients with nonfunctional uteri.

The uterine tubes may be well-developed even though the uterus and vagina are absent (40), or they may be aplastic. Tubal aplasia with a normal uterus is rare (41). Hypoplasia of the ovaries usually is accompanied by hypoplasia of the tubes.

Cervical and Upper Vaginal Atresia. Atresia of the cervix with normal uterine body and adnexa is rare. Eleven cases have been reported since the first one by Ludwig in 1900 (42, 43). In some cases no cervix was visible on vaginal examination; in others the cervix was rudimentary and imperforate. In each case the body of the uterus was normal (Fig. 22.15, *C*).

Upper vaginal atresia is also rare. Flemming and Kava (44) found 20 cases in the literature, and a few more have been reported since.

Vaginal Atresia. This is the classic condition of congenital absence of the vagina in which there is no müllerian duct tissue below the cervix. The uterus may or may not be present. In most individuals, there is no external trace of a vagina, but in three of McIndoe's 61 cases (45) and in nine of the 30 cases reported by Jones and Scott (46), there was a shallow invagination of the skin at the normal site of the vaginal orifice (Fig. 22.15, *A* and *D*).

The presence or absence of the uterus usually must be deduced from palpation and from whether or not periodic pain occurs. In 100 cases collected by Bryan and his colleagues (47), some upper reproductive tract structures could be palpated in 39 and periodic pain occurred in 34. The majority showed no evidence of a functional uterus.

Imperforate Hymen. The hymen represents a normally occurring membranous atresia of the vagina, which is usually perforated. It may be absent; its aperture may be large, small, or multiple; or there may be complete closure of the vagina. Complete closure is the most common and most readily cured of the forms of vaginal atresia (Fig. 22.15, *E*).

Suprahymenal Membranes. Membranous occlusion at other levels may occur and may be mistaken for imperforate hymen. Bell (48) emphasized the distension in 1912. Brews (37) found seven of 69 distal occlusions resulting from the presence of other membranes. Kanagasunteram and Dassanayake (18) discussed these suprahymenal membranes and pointed out that they contain a core of connective tissue and muscle and are not simply epithelial in nature. They usually lie just above the hymenal level and frequently are lined on the upper surface with columnar epithelium (49). The membrane may be complete or perforated; it may be as low as 1 cm below the site of the hymen (50), but usually it is higher.

EMBRYOGENESIS

Complete absence of the uterus and vagina results from failure of the distal ends of the müllerian ducts to form. Failure to progress beyond the stage reached by 23 mm (eighth week) will result in absence of both the uterus and vagina (group I defects, page 830). Failure at the 25-mm stage—after the müllerian ducts have made contact with each other, but before their ends have made contact with the urogenital sinus (Fig. 22-3, A)—will result in absence of the vagina only (group II defects) (11, 6). When the vagina and uterus are rudimentary and solid, developmental arrest has occurred at about the 126-mm stage (17th week) (Fig. 22.5). Failure of the urogenital sinus epithelium to invade the vagina (page 819) may be responsible for persistence of the solid state.

Hymenal and suprahymenal membranous occlusions must occur after the 150- to 180-mm stages (fifth month) when the then solid vagina begins to be recanalized. In this view, vaginal membranes are similar to membranous atresias appearing in the duodenum. Presumably, failure of the hymen to perforate represents a failure of the very end of the recanalization process. Kanasaguntheram and Dassanayake (18) place suprahymenal septa at the 34-mm stage, during which, they contend, the solid vaginal cord is invaded by villus-like processes of mesoderm, which may meet across the vagina and fuse. They consider that the hymen represents a portion of the cloacal membrane and that the imperforate hymen, like the imperforate anus, results from abnormal invasion of primitive streak mesoderm between the ectoderm and endoderm of the cloacal membrane. Attractive though this theory is, we believe the hymen represents the boundary between the embryonic vagina and the urogenital sinus rather than the external limit of the sinus.

A high familial incidence has been suggested by findings in several families in which sisters suffered from uterine atresia (51). McKusick and his colleagues (52) sug-

gested a hereditary basis for the more common vaginal atresia (Fig. 22.16, *A*). No abnormality in sex chromosomes is known (53).

ASSOCIATED ANOMALIES

Unilateral absence of the kidney is found in 12 to 16% of patients with absence of the vagina. Other urinary tract anomalies are common (49, 54).

HISTORY

Although Columbus (55) is credited with the first description of congenital absence of the vagina and uterus in 1559, in the second century Soranus of Ephesus mentioned cervical atresia, suprahymenal membranes, and imperforate hymen—although, oddly enough, he used the existence of these atresia to argue against the existence of a hymenal membrane in normal females. Aristotle (De Generatione IV; iv 773a) also mentions cervical atresia.

Aristotle describes the incision of the mildest form of atresia, imperforate hymen. The procedure is simple and must have been performed long before Aristotle's time. How often an operator encountered an extensive atresia or absence of the vagina rather than a simple membrane can only be guessed. Morgagni (56) tells us (XLVI:12) that Naboth in 1707 attempted to incise such a patient, but was forced to desist. Morgagni also describes his own experience (XLVI:11,12) with two patients, one of whom was referred to him with a narrow vagina that had resisted the efforts of other physicians to dilate it. On inspection he discovered that the vagina was absent and that the others had been trying to dilate the urethra. Since neither of these patients had experienced periodic pain, he concluded that their uteri also were absent. Morgagni therefore "persuaded both these women placidly to suffer a marriage, which was improperly contracted, to be dissolved rather than imprudently submit themselves to the incision" (De Sedibus XLVI:12).

The second operator, DeHaen (57) in 1761 attempted to relieve a woman with menstrual retention, but he pierced the bladder and the patient died. The first successful operation was by Amussat (58) in 1832; he forced a passage by the use of his fingers alone. In 1872 Heppner (59) designed the first of many plastic operations for the construction of a functional vagina. Marshall (57) considered that he had delivered the first live-born infant through an artificial vagina in 1897; still-born deliveries had been reported as early as 1847.

INCIDENCE

Vaginal atresia is said to have accounted for 15% of uterine anomalies seen at Tubingen over a period of 20 years (38). Bryan and his colleagues (47) estimated its frequency as 1:4000 patients. In Brews' 60-year records at

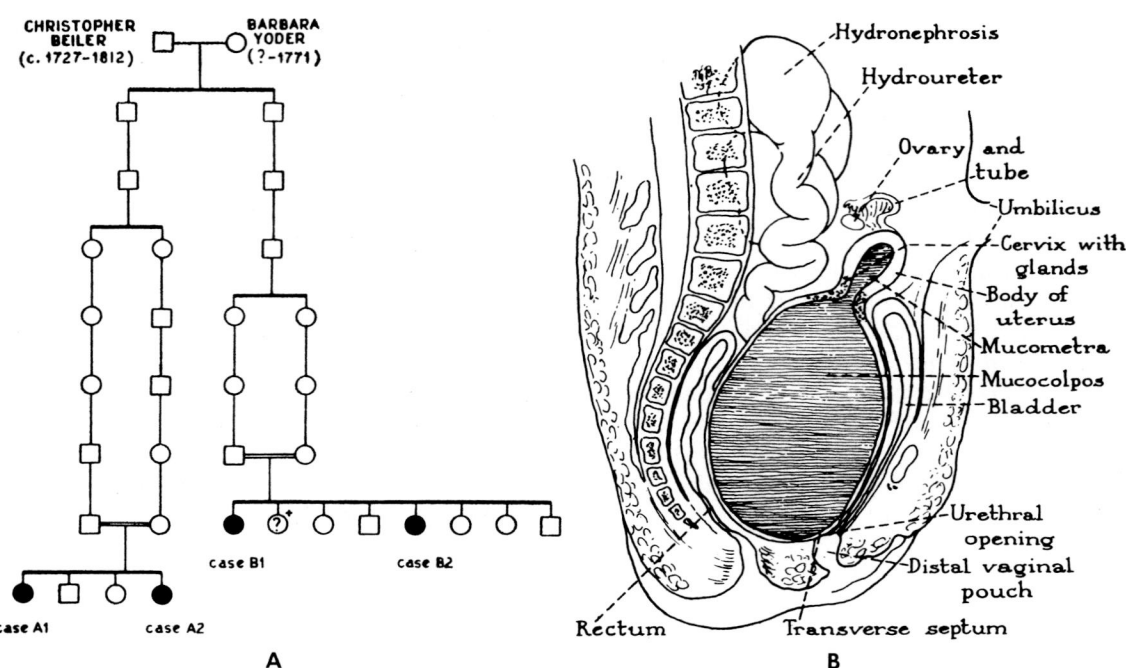

Figure 22.16. Hydrometrocolpos. **A,** Lineage of a family having four affected members appearing after two consanguineous marriages. **B,** Diagram showing the compression of colon, bladder, and urethra produced by the disten-sion. (From McKusick VA, *et al.* Hydrometrocolpos as a simple inherited malfor-mation. JAMA 1964;189:813–816.)

the London Hospital (37), there were 62 cases of imper-forate hymen, 10 cases of occlusion above the hymen, and 9 cases of absence of the vagina. Cali and Pratt (60) found 175 cases recorded at Mayo Clinic between 1920 and 1966.

CLINICAL CLASSIFICATION AND DIAGNOSIS

Group I: Absent Vagina and Uterus or Only Solid Rudiments Present. The absence of the vagina usually is noticed at birth and may come to the surgeon's attention again after puberty. There is no complaint of periodic pain, and the uterus is not palpable. Imaging with computed tomogra-phy (CT) may establish the diagnosis, or a presumptive diagnosis may be confirmed by laparoscopy or laparotomy.

In the cases reported by Leduc and his colleagues (54), the uterus was represented by a solid bud more often than it was entirely absent (Fig. 22.15, *A*).

Group II: Absent Vagina with Functioning Uterus. The absence of the vagina may be noticed at birth. Hydro-metra may be present at birth or appear in childhood (61). With puberty, hematometra, periodic pain, and occasionally vicarious menstruation will appear (47, 51). In infants, a distended bladder, urachal cyst, and lower intestinal obstruction must be ruled out (Fig. 22.15, *D*).

Although there is complete amenorrhea, secondary sex characteristics are normal, and there is a monthly temperature fluctuation, indicating a normal ovarian cycle (40).

A remarkable case that belongs in this group is that of a child having a colonic duplication, one limb of which opened at the site of the vaginal orifice. The vagina was represented by a cyst communicating with a functional uterus. The right kidney, ureter, uterine tube, and ovary were absent. In a three-stage operation, the upper part of the colonic duplication was resected, and an anastomosis of the rudimentary vagina and the lower part of the colonic duplication formed a "vagina" which drained the menstrual flow and which might in time become sexually functional (62) (Fig. 22.17).

Group III: Occluded Vagina with Functioning Uterus. Imper-forate hymen is the most common form of this condition (Fig. 22.15, *E*). Hydrocolpos in infancy or childhood may call attention dramatically to the defect (Fig. 22.18); hematocolpos shortly after menarche invariably will. Cer-vical occlusion or atresia of the upper one-third of the vagina may delay diagnosis and require more than inci-sion of a membrane (Fig. 22.15, *C*). Amenorrhea with periodic pain should direct attention to the cervix.

In the most dramatic form of this condition, an abdominal mass may be present at birth. It may fill the entire abdomen, obstructing the intestines and ureters within a few days after birth. The distended vagina may extend above the umbilicus and produce respiratory embarrassment (52). Emergency treatment is required (Fig. 22.16, *B*).

Group IV: Double Vagina with One Occluded Functioning Uterus. The vagina in these patients is septate, with one side completely closed and the other appearing normal. The uterus is usually double (Fig. 22.15, *F*). Periodic acute pain without complete amenorrhea and the presence of a palpable, tense swelling on the lateral vaginal wall are diagnostic. Palpation of a double uterus and pyelographic evidence of absence of the kidney on the affected side are suggestive.

Group V: Normal Vagina with Aplastic Uterus. The complaint is amenorrhea and sterility. The cervix may be rudimentary (Fig. 22.15, *B*). The condition must be distinguished from infantile uterus, in which a lumen is present and in which response to endocrine therapy is seen.

In 1988 Weaver (63) presented 44 tables in an effort to survey prenatal diagnosed disorders.

TREATMENT

The objectives of treatment of these defects is: *(a)* To provide adequate and separate drainage of urinary, fecal,

and menstrual products, thus reducing or eliminating the risk of infection, and *(b)* creation of a cosmetically normal and functioning vagina.

Drainage. Only those patients with functioning uterine tissue will need drainage of menstrual products. However, pooling of urine in a distended vagina may lead to infection in patients with or without functioning uterine tissue. Generally, adequate drainage through the introitus may be established by dilation, incision, or flap vaginoplasty. Only rarely will vaginostomy or hysterectomy be required to provide adequate drainage or prevent infections. If there is a vaginal duplication and only one is obstructed, the surgeon may incise the vaginal septum (64) or remove the less developed obstructed uterus (65).

Vaginal Construction. Patients with vaginal occlusion or hemiocclusion require surgery to make an existing vagina usable. Patients with an atretic vagina and functioning uterus require vaginal construction to provide both

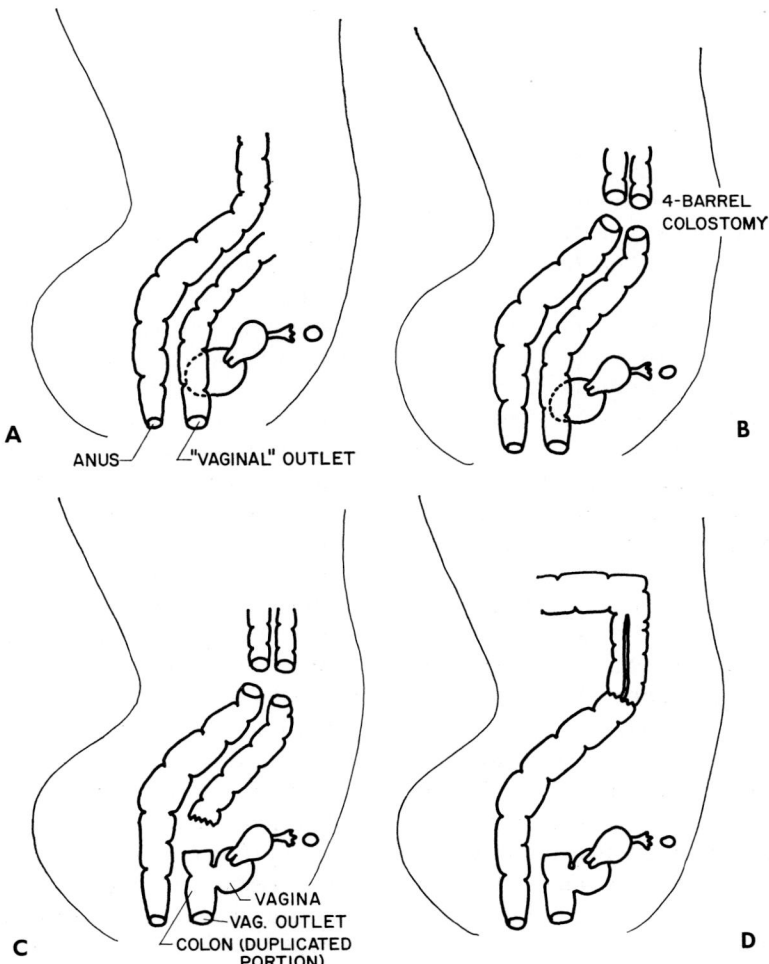

Figure 22.17. Rudimentary, cystic vagina with functioning uterus and colonic duplication opening at the site of the normal vaginal orifice. **A,** Anatomic findings before operation. **B,** First stage of repair: colostomy. **C,** Second stage of repair: opening formed between cystic vagina and lower end of colonic duplication. **D,** Third stage of repair: distal colonic duplication above vaginal anastomosis removed and double proximal colon anastomosed to single distal colon. (From Cook WH, et al. Duplication of distal colon. Report of a case and its surgical correction. AMA Arch Surg 1960;80:650–654.)

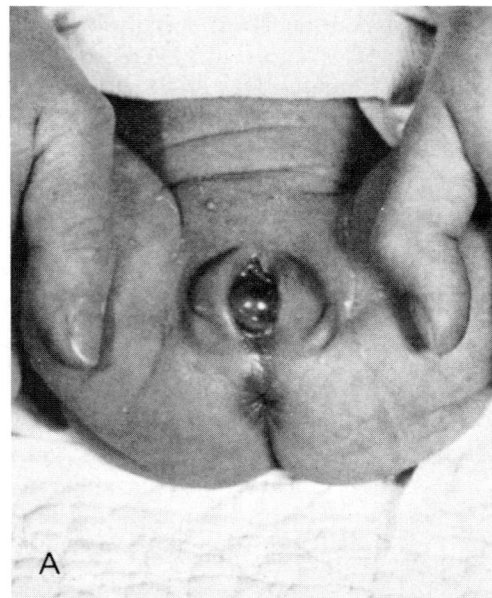
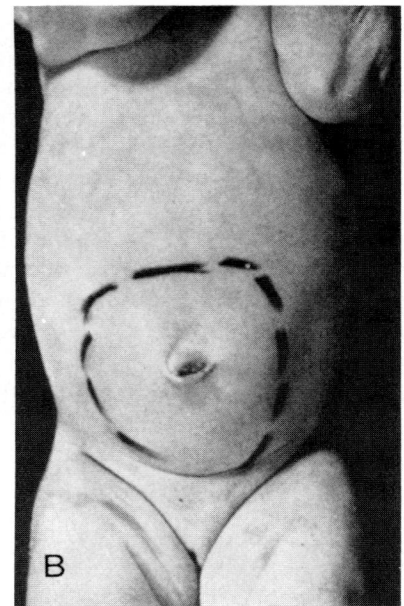

Figure 22.18. Hydrometrocolpos. **A,** The bulging vaginal membrane in an 18-day-old baby. **B,** Outline of the palpable and enormously distended uterus in a 2-week-old baby. (From Gross RE. The surgery of infancy and childhood. Philadelphia: WB Saunders, 1953.)

drainage and functional use. Patients without a vagina or uterus are candidates for vaginoplasty to provide a vagina which can function for sexual intercourse.

Marshall (57) gave a detailed history of reconstruction methods from 1872, when Heppner made free grafts of skin from the thigh to line the artificial canal. This method, modified by McIndoe (45), is still used. Pedunculated flap grafts were employed by Graves in 1921 (66). McIndoe reported results of 63 operations, for which he claimed excellent results in 50, satisfactory results in 6, and failure or poor results in 7. There were no deaths.

The oldest method is simple incision and repeated dilation, with eventual epithelization from below. Continual dilation must be employed if contracture by scar tissue is not to reduce the lumen to an inadequate size.

In 1904 Baldwin (67) introduced the ideal transplant in which a double, inverted U-shaped segment of ileum was placed in the space prepared for the vagina. The walls between the double tube were cut through at a later date. Among 14 Baldwin operations collected by Bryan and his colleagues (47), 8 were satisfactory cases and 4 operative deaths. This mortality rate is too high to justify the procedure.

Frank and Grist (68) advocated formation of the vagina without surgery by continued pressure, a tedious method requiring great cooperation by the patient.

In summary, vaginal reconstruction can be divided into three basic techniques, each of which has numerous modifications espoused by a multitude of surgeons: (a) skin grafts around a vaginal mold to line the canal of the neovagina; (b) full-thickness vascularized myocutaneous

flaps; and (c) isolated intestinal segments. Each of these techniques has advantages and disadvantages. Split-thickness skin grafts provide a very pleasing cosmetic result but are dry and insensate. Myocutaneous flaps are also dry and somewhat bulkier. Therefore, they are not as cosmetically satisfactory, yet they do provide some level of sensation. They are also less prone to perforation than the much thinner split-thickness grafts. Isolated intestinal segments have lubrication due to intestinal secretion; however, these secretions are constant (not just in response to sexual stimulation) and ultimately prove bothersome and unpleasant to many. They also have limited sensation.

A modified technique to create a neovagina with an isolated segment of sigmoid colon was reported by Freundt et al. (69). The interested reader also will find useful information in Tolhurst and van der Helm's *The Treatment of Vaginal Atresia* (70).

Indications for Surgery. If hydrocolpos or hematocolpos is present, drainage must be established at once. It is no longer necessary to wait until adulthood or even adolescence to reconstruct the vagina in patients with hydrocolpos or hematocolpos. It can be safely and successfully done during infancy. Those patients with hydrocolpos and imperforate anus often undergo the vagina reconstruction at the same time as the anal pull-through (at approximately 1 year of age). Total vaginal reconstruction should probably wait until adolescence or adulthood (in those patients with vaginal agenesis). The difference between feasibility and desirability must be clear in the surgeon's mind.

Table 22.2.
Prognosis in Five Types of Atresia of the Uterus and Vagina

Normal Sexual Function	Lesion Group	Possibility of Pregnancy
By surgery	I	None
By surgery	II,III,IV	Reasonable
Present	V	None

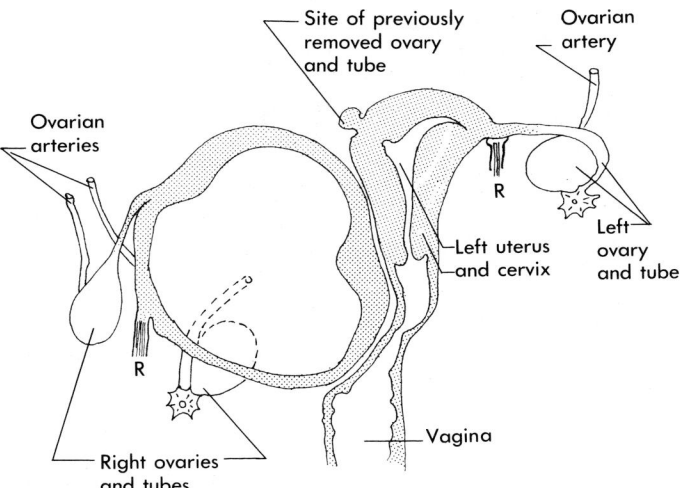

Figure 22.19. *Diagrammatic sketch of complete bilateral true duplication of ovaries, tubes, and uterus with a single vagina. The left uterus and tubes are nearly normal and communicate with the vagina; the medial left ovary and tube were surgically removed at a previous operation. The right uterus has two uterine tubes with two ovaries. There is no cervix and no communication with the single vagina that is compressed by the distended right uterus. There appear to be only two round ligaments (R). (Redrawn from a sketch of the fresh surgical specimen by Rowley WN. Uterine anomaly: duplication of uterus, three tubes and three ovaries: report of a case. Ann Surg 1948;127:676–680.)*

PROGNOSIS

The prognosis following treatment of the various lesions is summarized in Table 22.2.

Duplication of the Müllerian Ducts

ANATOMY

Unlike duplication of the uterus and vagina, which arises from failure of fusion of the paired müllerian ducts, müllerian duct duplication implies a doubling of the ducts on one or both sides. This condition is extremely rare. Complete bilateral doubling of ovaries, uterine tubes, and uterus, but not of vagina, has been reported by Rowley (71) (Fig. 22.19). In a case reported by Kelso (72), the müllerian ducts were doubled to produce a uterus unicornis on one side, in addition to a complete but septate uterus and vagina (Fig. 22.20, *A*).

Tubal duplications not involving the uterus have occasionally been reported. Thorek and his colleagues (73) found a patient with uterus duplex unicollis who had two uterine tubes, each with fimbriae, arising from the left horn. A single tube on the right was gravid (Fig. 22.20, *B*).

A lesser degree of duplication was found in a hysterectomy specimen described by Curtis and Anson (74). The infundibulum on both sides was duplicated for about 1.5 cm, and it merged with the normal tube at both ends. In 1911 Walthard (75) warned that some so-called abdominal pregnancies might be in accessory tubes, traces of which subsequently were obliterated by the developing trophoblast. He cited one case of accessory tubal pregnancy.

Accessory tubes and accessory ostia are frequently reported (76), but most of the tubes are portions of the epoophoron, which is a wolffian duct remnant (pages 775 and 823).

EMBRYOGENESIS

All of these duplications result from a splitting of the müllerian duct during its development in the seventh week. The splitting was extensive and bilaterally in Rowley's (71) patient and short and reanastomosing in Curtis and Anson's patient (74). Kelso's (72) case represented a unilateral doubling extending to the cervix. In neither Rowley's nor Kelso's case it is clear whether the two horned uteri were composed of ipsilateral or contralateral pairs of müllerian ducts. The anatomic evidence in both points to ipsilateral pairing. In Rowley's patient the kidneys were not described, but the presence of four ovaries suggests there was a splitting of the genital ridge on each side, and there might well have been a duplication of wolffian ducts preceding the müllerian duplication.

Anomalies of Incomplete Fusion of the Uterine and Vagina Primordia

The varieties of uterine anomalies are well known, but their classification and terminology are subject to some disagreement. Much of the difficulty arises from the fact that the most common malformations result from varying degrees of fusion of the embryonic müllerian ducts. Examples may be found of all degrees of fusion, and in attempting to supply a terminology, we are, in fact, trying to give names to arbitrary stages of what is essentially a continuous series. Under these circumstances, precision is difficult.

With some modification, the classification of Jarcho (77) is the most simple and useful. Yet neither Jarcho's terminology nor the scheme of Monie and Sigardson (78) is completely satisfactory.

TRUE DUPLICATION OF THE UTERUS

These rare cases have unilateral or bilateral duplication of the müllerian ducts with consequent doubling of reproductive structures on one or both sides. They are not hemiuteri. Halal (79) presented a complete duplication of

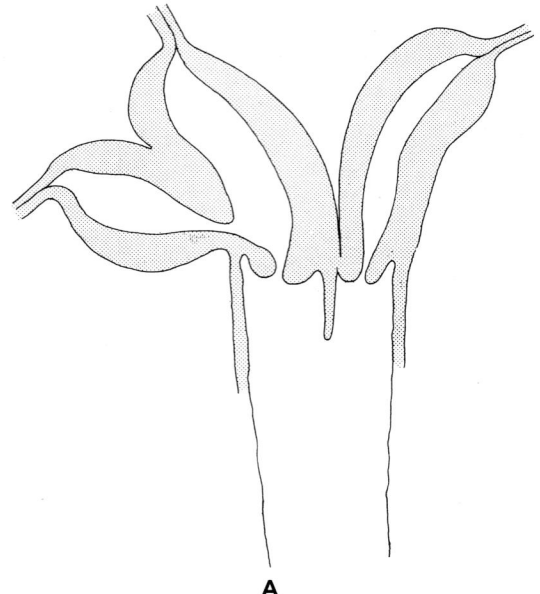

A

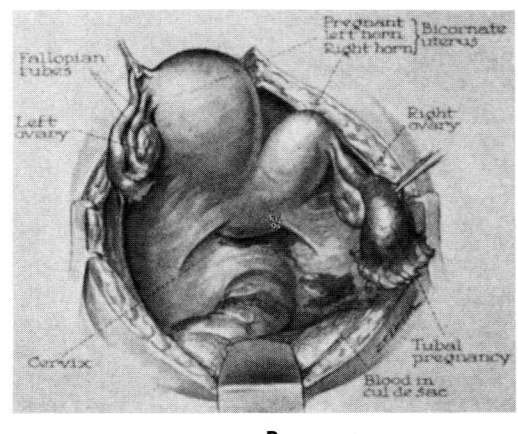

B

Figure 22.20. Duplication of uterus and uterine tubes. **A,** Bicornuate uterus with a third uterine horn on one side. There were three uterine tubes; the number of ovaries was not determined. **B,** Bicornuate uterus with duplication of the left uterine tube; the left ovary was not duplicated. The patient had a pregnancy in the left uterine horn and another in the right uterine tube. (**A,** Drawing from radiographs

from Kelso JW. Unusual malformation of the uterus. Am J Obstet Gynecol 1956;72:922–923; **B,** from Thorek P, et al. Simultaneous pregnancies in a fallopian tube and bicornate uterus associated with three fallopian tubes: a first world case report and review of the literature. Am J Surg 1950;79:512–523.

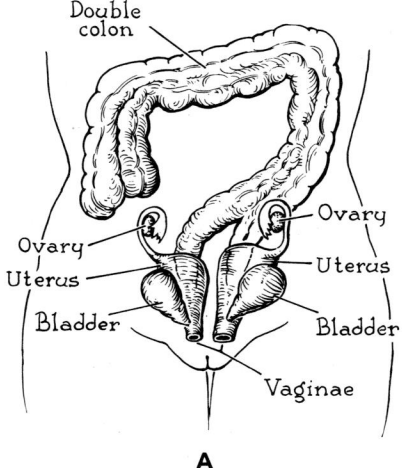

A

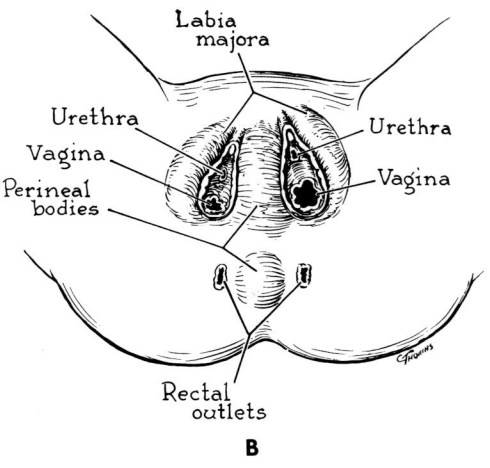

B

Figure 22.21. Separate hemiuteri with separate vaginae. **A,** Anterior view. **B,** Perineal view. This condition is associated with hemibladders and with duplication of the urethra, the colon, and sometimes the lower vertebrae. The patient illustrated here had normal functioning on both sides; the left vagina was used for

intercourse. One pregnancy ended in abortion of twins. (From Beach PD et al. Duplication of the primitive hindgut of the human being. Surgery 1961;49:779–793.)

the uterus and vagina with severe upper limb hypoplasia in a French-Canadian family with several other congenital anomalies to both male and female relatives.

INCOMPLETE FUSION OF THE MÜLLERIAN DUCTS

Anatomy. In contradistinction to the true duplications, all of these "duplications" represent degrees of separation of lateral halves of the uterus and vagina.

Separate Hemiuteri with Separate Vaginae.
This rare condition is associated with duplication of some or all postumbilical viscera; colon and anus (page 248) and urethra and bladder (page 681). Vaginal openings are widely separated and the entire vulva may be duplicated (Fig. 22.21). One such patient was delivered of a living child from the right hemiuterus and, in a subsequent pregnancy, from the left hemiuterus (80).

Table 22.3.
Etiology of Palpable Abdominal Masses in 115 Patients Reported by Several Authors

Site and Cause	Number of Patients	Site and Cause	Number of Patients
Kidney		**Gastrointestinal tract**	
Hydronephrosis	33	Duplications	5
Multicystic kidney	35	Giant cystic meconium	2
Polycystic kidney	2	peritonitis	
Renal vein thrombosis	3	Mesenteric cyst	1
Solid tumors	2	Volvulus of ileum	1
Retroperitoneum		Teratoma of stomach	1
Neuroblastoma	7	Leiomyoma of colon	1
Teratoma	2	*Hepatic or biliary tract*	
Hemangioma	1	Hemangioma of liver	2
Bladder		Solitary cyst of liver	1
Urethral valves	1	Hepatoma	1
Female genital tract		Distended gallbladder	1
Hydrocolpos	7	Choledochal cyst	1
Ovarian cyst	5		

Modified from Woodard JR. Neonatal and perinatal emergencies. In: Harrison JR et al, eds. Campbell's urology. Philadelphia: WB Saunders, 1979.

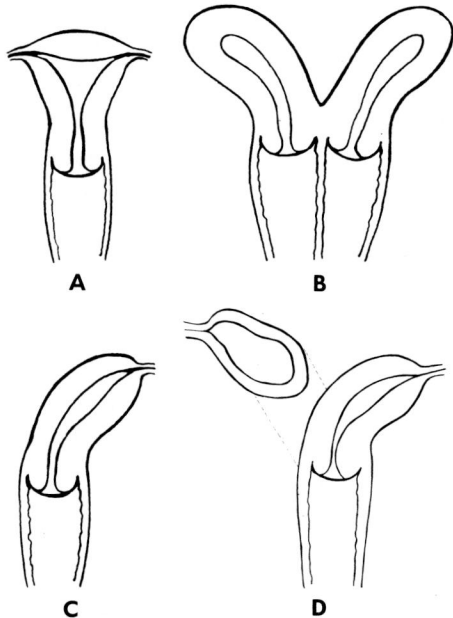

Figure 22.22. Fusion anomalies of the uterus. **A,** Normal uterus (uterus simplex). **B,** Uterus didelphys, with septate vagina. **C,** Uterus unicornis. **D,** Uterus unicornis with rudimentary contralateral hemiuterus. (**A, B,** and **C,** From Jarcho J. Malformations of the uterus. Am J Surg 1946;71:106–166.)

Uterus Didelphys with Septate Vagina.
The uterine cavities are completely separate. The fundi are externally separate, but the two cervices are externally united. One cervix may be larger than the other. In about 75% of cases of uterus didelphys, the vagina is septate (Fig. 22.22, *B*). Very rarely, the vaginal septum is asymmetric and completely closes one portion of the vagina. This conformation results in hydrocolpos and hematocolpos (Fig. 22.15, *F*). Brews (37) found eight cases among 83 cases of hematocolpocele. About 20

other examples have been reported (64, 81, 82). The kidney on the side of the hematocolpocele usually is absent.

Frequently associated with the didelphic uterus is a peritoneal fold, which extends from the posterior surface of the bladder, between the uterine horns, to the anterior surface of the rectum. This rectovesical fold contains a branch of the superior hemorrhoidal artery and is a remnant of the ventral mesentery (83, 84). A continuation of this fold also may extend from the bladder to the anterior abdominal wall (page 195).

The interested reader will find useful information about uterine and vaginal malformations in the following publications:

1. Beekhuis and Hage (85) reported a double uterus associated with an obstructed hemivagina and ipsilateral renal agenesis in two patients.
2. Burbige and Hensle (86) reported two cases of uterus didelphys and vaginal duplication with unilateral obtrusion as a newborn abdominal mass.
3. Whitaker and Woodard (87) presented the etiology of palpable abdominal masses in a table (Table 22.3).
4. Flieguer (88) discussed unusual problems of the double uterus and emphasized that overlooking patients with uterine malformation is not the best treatment for the patient.
5. Tolete-Velcek et al. (89) emphasized that uterovaginal malformations may produce a trap for the unsuspecting surgeon.
6. Morgan et al. (90) reported uterus didelphys with unilateral hematocolpos, ipsilateral renal genesis, and menses in a 13-year-old girl. These authors collected 115 similar cases from the literature.

Uterus Unicornis.
A single-horned uterus resembles one half of a uterus didelphys. An asymmetric uterus having only a single uterine tube opens into a normal vagina (Fig. 22.22, *C*).

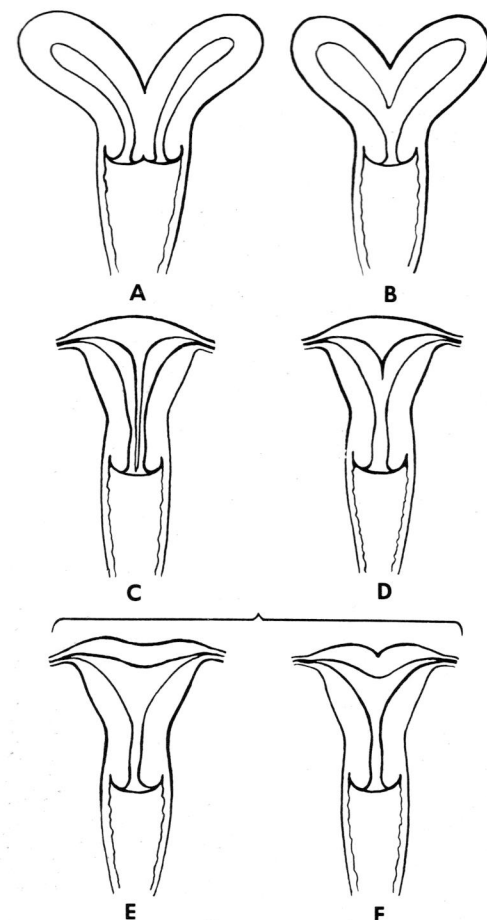

Figure 22.23. Fusion anomalies of the uterus. **A,** Uterus duplex bicollis. **B,** Uterus duplex unicollis. Both bicollis and unicollis forms are often lumped together as "bicornuate." **C,** Uterus septus. **D,** Uterus subseptus. **E** and **F,** Uterus arcuatus. The fundus is flattened or notched. (From Jarcho J. Malformations of the uterus. Am J Surg 1946;71:106–166.)

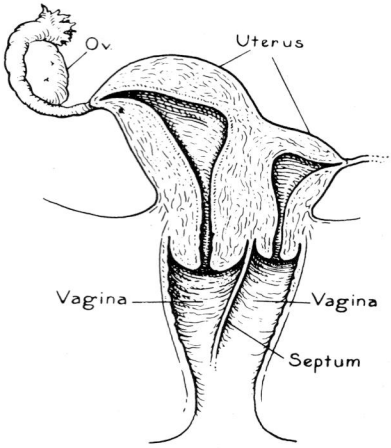

Figure 22.24. Schematic drawing of an example of uterus duplex bicollis with asymmetric uterine horns and a deviated vaginal septum. *Ov.,* ovary. (From Jarcho J. Malformations of the uterus. Am J Surg 1946;71:106–166.)

The other hemiuterus and tube are absent, or the hemiuterus is a closed structure without connection with the vagina or the other uterine horn (Fig. 22.22, *D*). Absence of the kidney on the side of the defective uterine horn is not unusual in this condition. Beernick et al. (91) presented five patients with uterine unicornis in uterus solidaris.

Uterus Duplex Bicollis (Bicornuate Uterus).

In this condition the uterine cavities are separate and the fundus is deeply notched. Two cervices are present, and the dividing septum may be perforated (92). The vagina is sometimes septate (Fig. 22.22, *B*), but usually it is normal (Fig. 22.21, *A*). The two hemiuteri may be unequal (Fig. 22.24).

Shenker and Brickman (93) reported the ultrasonographic diagnosis of a bicornuate uterus with incomplete vaginal septum and unilateral renal genesis in two patients. Aragona et al. (94) reported a bicornuate uterus

with several other multiple anomalies. According to Golan et al. (95) bicornuate uterus is the most common congenital uterine anomaly.

Uterus Duplex Unicollis (Bicornuate Uterus).

Externally, this form resembles the bicollis type, but internally, the septum does not reach the cervix, which is single (Fig. 22.23, *B*).

Uterus Septus.

The uterus in this condition is externally normal but contains a septum dividing it into lateral halves and reaching the cervix. A uterus with a partial septum is sometimes designated as uterus subseptus. Twins seem to occur about three times more often than in normal uteri (96) (Fig. 22.23, *C* and *D*). The septum may deviate so that one uterine cavity is closed (97).

Beyer et al. (98) reported uterus septus with adenocarcinoma of one-half of the uterus. They considered the case coincidental.

Assaf et al. (99) reported 17 cases with intrauterine septum treated under vision using CO_2 hysteroscopy and/or optical scissors.

Uterus Arcuatus.

In this type, the uterus is normal and without a septum, but the fundus is flatter than usual and may display a midline notch (Fig. 22.23. *E* and *F*).

Embryogenesis. Failure of the müllerian primordia to fuse completely during the ninth to twelfth weeks accounts for uterus didelphys, duplex, and septus. In no sense, however, can the anomalous uterus be considered to result from an arrested developmental stage; fusion or failure of fusion takes place before the uterus and vagina are differentiated. Uterus didelphys is not a normal embryonic stage of uterine development in humans.

Uterus arcuatus, on the other hand, may be considered an "infantile" or arrested uterus since the final obliteration of the funic notch takes place only in the seventh month, after the uterus is differentiated.

Uterus unicornis represents the failure of the müllerian duct to form on one side, or its failure to reach the urogenital sinus with its partner.

Absence of one uterine half frequently indicates absence of the kidney on the same side. When unilateral uterine and renal agenesis exist, the underlying defect is the failure of the wolffian duct and, hence, of the müllerian duct to form.

If the ovary is also absent, the defect includes the whole of the mesonephric and genital ridges on that side (100) (see Table 17.1).

Although wolffian and müllerian ducts may have formed, the kidney may be absent because the ureteric bud failed to develop. The large number of symmetric, but septate or arcuate uteri associated with kidney agenesis suggests the mesonephric duct, which is adequate to form a ureter, also may fail to induce complete müllerian duct fusion. Only the final fusion process seems to be affected. Uterus didelphys, representing maximum fusion failure, is not associated with renal agenesis.

History. Inexplicably, the bicornuate uterus was considered in antiquity to be the normal form of the human uterus. Although Galen probably knew that the cavity was undivided, it remained for daCarpi (100) in 1522 to first illustrate the single cavity (Fig. 22.25). A true bicornuate uterus was seen by Catti in 1557 (Morgagni, III:21) (56) and by Schenck von Grafenberg in 1595 (101). Purcell (102) described a double vagina with a double uterus, gravid on one side, in 1773–1774. The first unicornuate uterus is said to have been described in 1794 (101). Surgical excision of the septum of a double uterus was first performed by Ruge (103) in 1884. In 1903 Strassmann (104) first removed the septum from above.

An excellent bibliography of the earlier literature on uterine anomalies can be found in Weintrob's paper (105).

INCIDENCE

The general incidence of uterine anomalies has been placed at 0.16% by Semmens (106), at 0.15% by Fenton and Singh (107), and at 0.13% by Blair (108). Much higher incidences, 0.3 and 0.39%, were reported by Baker and his colleagues (109) and by Thomas and Langley (110). The differences depend largely on the number of cases of uterus arcuatus included. In a general series of uterine anomalies, many such cases must remain undetected. Falls (111), who was looking specifically for arcuate uteri, found 155 cases among 7553 obstetric patients, an incidence of over 2%. Whether all such cases deserve the rank of anomaly may be questioned: Some are merely variations.

It is surprising how easily uterine anomalies can be

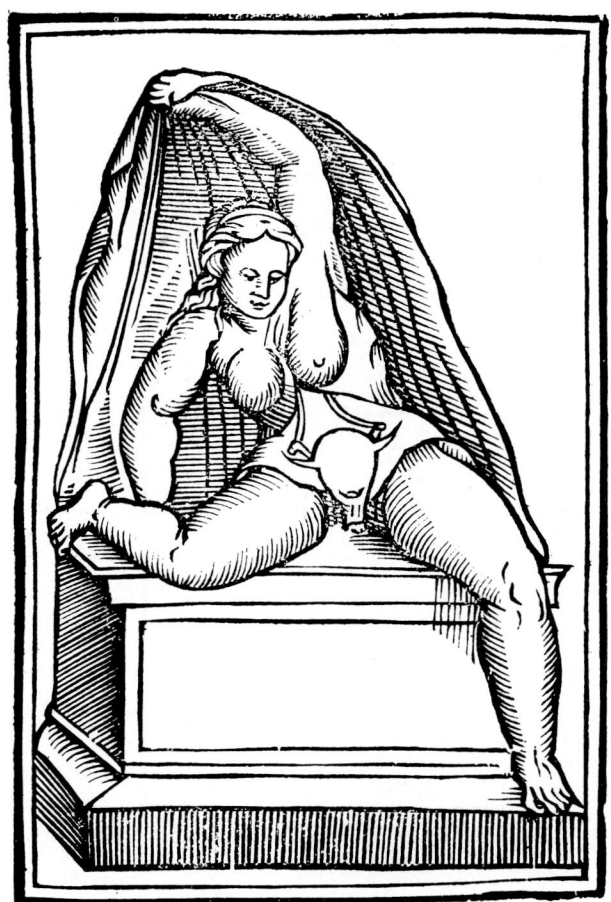

Figure 22.25. The earliest known picture of the human uterus in its normal, undivided form. (From daCarpi JB. Isagogae breves: a short introduction to anatomy, 1522. Lind LR (transl). Chicago: University of Chicago Press, 1959.)

overlooked. Between 1954 and 1962 Zabriskie (112) found 0.31% of uteri malformed. In the last 20 months of the study the rate had risen to 0.93%.

It must be remembered that the quoted figures are usually from obstetric series. In these, anomalies that cause sterility will be under-estimated, while those predisposing the patients to obstetric difficulties will be over-estimated. Symptoms rarely occur in the absence of pregnancy. An estimate of 0.15% (113) may not be too high.

The relative frequency of types of uterine anomalies in several large series is shown in Table 22.4.

It is noticeable from the table that uterus didelphys was found much more frequently in the three U.S. series (107, 109, 110). Conversely, fewer cases of arcuate uterus are reported in the United States than abroad. We know of no organized search for geographic and racial variations.

Symptoms. Except when an isolated, rudimentary uterine horn or a closed septate vagina results in menstrual retention, incomplete uterine fusion anomalies rarely cause symptoms unless pregnancy occurs.

Table 22.4.
Percentage of Uterine Anomalies Reported in Six Series

	Thomas and Langley (1959)	Fenton and Singh (1952)	Baker et al. (1953)	Pfleiderer (1929)	Hay (1958)	Blair (1960)
Number of Cases	63	77	128	79	65	68
Uterus didelphys	23.8	37.6	39.0	—	—	2.9
Uterus duplex bicollis	50.9	6.5	1.6	19.0	4.6	11.8
Uterus duplex unicollis		32.4	46.0	19.0		30.8
Uterus unicornis	4.8	—	3.1	7.6	1.5	—
Uterus septus	11.1	7.8	4.7	20.2	6.2	1.5
Uterus subseptus	7.9	6.5	4.7		83.1	11.8
Uterus arcuatus	1.6	9.1	0.8	34.2	4.6	25.0

Table 22.5.
Complications of Pregnancy in Women with Anomalous and Normal Uteri

	Anomalous Uterus	Normal Uterus
Abortion rate	14.7%	6.0%
Prematurity	31.2	12.0
Cesarean section	27.6	5.4
Perinatal mortality	13.7	9.9
Antepartum hemorrhage	17.2	3.9
Postpartum hemorrhage	21.4	4.0
Manual removal of placenta	45.2	2.4

COMPLICATIONS OF PREGNANCY

Uterine anomalies do not preclude successful pregnancy, but they increase the danger to both mother and child.

Blair (108) compared the pregnancy histories of 68 patients having uterine anomalies with those of patients having normal uteri. In all aspects, prospects were unfavorable for those with anomalies (Table 22.5). Blair's series contained slightly fewer cases of uterus didelphys and slightly more cases of uterus arcuatus than most U.S. series (Table 22.4).

The fact that there is increased frequency of breech presentations should be added to these unfavorable results. Thomas and Langley (110) reported an incidence of 14.1% in contrast to 3.8% for normal patients, at one hospital.

Uterus Didelphys. Only about 40% of pregnancies in patients with didelphic uteri can be expected to terminate in spontaneous delivery (83). Several cases of simultaneous pregnancy in both uterine halves have been reported. In some, deliveries have been separated by as much as 3 to 9 weeks (114-116). Twins are said to be more frequent (77).

Uterus Duplex, Septus, and Subseptus. Falls (111) reported the results of 46 pregnancies in bicornuate uteri without distinguishing between those with single and double cer-

vix. Twenty-seven infants were born alive, four were still-born, and fifteen were aborted. Of those born alive, nine were premature. Two cases of double pregnancy have been reported (117, 118). The prognosis for pregnancy in patients with a double uterus and double cervix appears to be better than in those with double uterus and one cervix (Fig. 22.23, *A* and *B*).

Way (119), grouping uterus duplex unicollis and uterus septus and subseptus together, reported that abortion occurred in 26%, the fetus presented transversely in 27%, and the placenta required manual removal in 15%. Jarcho (77) and Thomas and Langley (110) described cases in which the septum was fenestrated; the breech presented at one cervix and the feet at the other (Fig. 22.26).

Uterus Arcuatus. Although the deformity seems small, Falls (111) found cesarean delivery to have been performed in 13.5% of pregnancies in arcuate uteri. Three mothers and fourteen infants died.

Uterus Unicornis. Improbable as it may appear, pregnancy in an isolated, rudimentary uterine horn does occur. Rolen and his associates (120) collected 65 cases in the English language literature and added five of their own. In 80% of these cases, there was no communication between the rudimentary horn and the remainder of the uterus or the vagina (Fig. 22.22, *D*). Transperitoneal migration of either sperm or fertilized ova must have taken place (121). Curiously, pregnancy in the "normal" horn of such uteri is only slightly more frequent; Rolen and his colleagues (120) could find only 168 cases, of which 90 went to term.

Without surgical intervention, a pregnant rudimentary uterine horn will rupture, often with a fatal outcome. In one case such a rupture resulted in a secondary abdominal pregnancy. Both mother and infant survived (122).

Obstetric Prognosis. In general, fetal loss is greatest in mothers with uterus didelphys and unicornis and bicornis unicollis than with other anomalies (123, 124), although

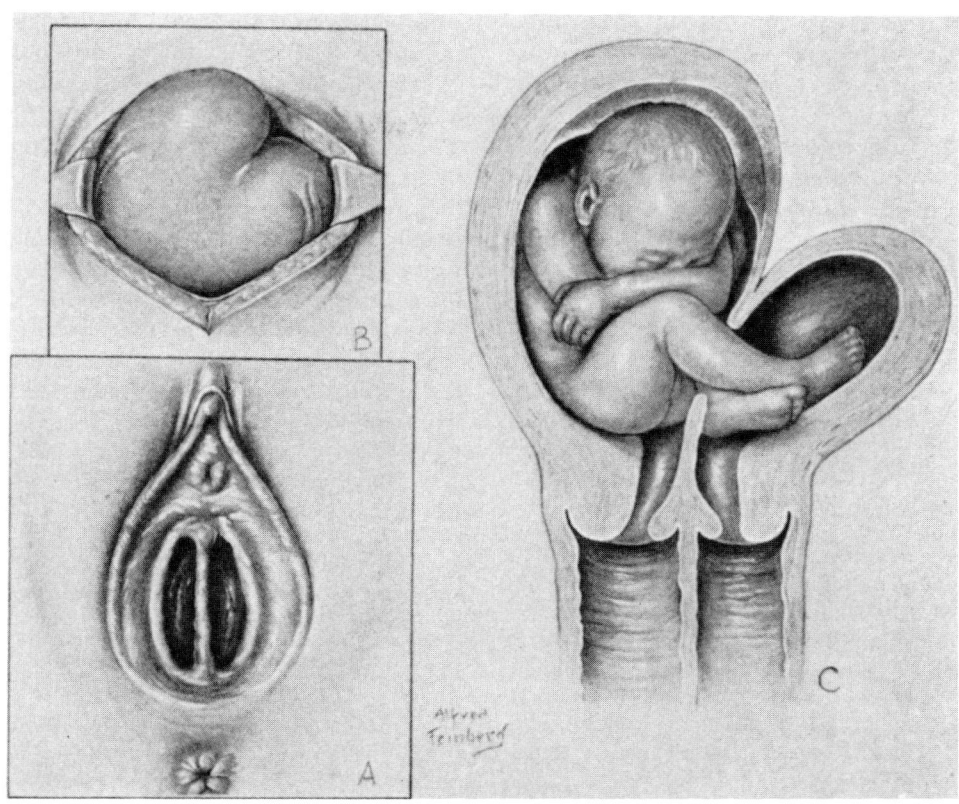

Figure 22.26. Pregnancy in a patient with a double uterus and vagina. The uterine septum was incomplete. **A,** The appearance of the genitalia. **B,** The unopened uterus at laparotomy. **C,** Schematic drawing of the position of the fetus. The body of the fetus was in the right horn and the feet in the left horn. Delivery was by cesarean section. (From Jarcho J. Malformations of the uterus. Am J Surg 1946;71:106–166.)

not all authorities agree about the relative rank of the specific anomalies (125). The high abortion rate in septate uteri occurs because the ovum often implants on the septum, which is too thin to provide an adequate blood supply to the growing fetus. The difficulty in delivery of a didelphic uterus is caused by obstruction from the enlarged, nongravid half. It is not clear why uterus arcuatus, the mildest form of fusion failure, should be responsible for obstetric complications. Hay (126) suggested that many uteri diagnosed as arcuate are actually subseptate.

Semmens (106) proposed a clinical classification of anomalous uteri. He divided all of the anomalies into two groups on the basis of whether the functional (gravid) portion of the uterus was of one-sided origin (uterus didelphys, uterus bicornis unicollis, uterus septus, or uterus arcuatus), or whether it was essentially fused (uterus bicornis unicollis, uterus septus, or uterus arcuatus). While this division is simple to recognize, the prognosis in the two groups is not strikingly different.

Carey and Steinberg (127) reported vaginal dystocia in a patient with a double uterus and a longitudinal vaginal septum. Salat-Baroux (128) studied recurrent spontaneous abortions in patients with septate uterus. Ben-Rafael (129) reported an association of pregnancy-induced hypertension and uterine malformations. Pennes et al. (130) advised that, when dilation and curettage fails to produce embryonic tissue, sonography is indicated to rule out ectopic gestation or uterine anomalies. Fetoscopy without complications was recommended by Petrikovsky (131) as an aide for diagnosis of congenital anomalies of the fetus.

Diagnosis. Examination of patients complaining of habitual abortion, sterility, dysmenorrhea, and dyspareunia may lead to a diagnosis of uterine anomaly. The presence of a vaginal septum is highly suggestive, and the visualization of two cervices confirms the diagnosis of uterus didelphys or uterus duplex bicollis. The diagnosis of other anomalies requires the use of flexible probes (114) or of uterosalpingography to determine the extent of the dividing septum.

Palpation may reveal the external form of the uterus, but in pregnancy a double uterus may be distinguished from a tumor and from extrauterine pregnancy or pregnancy with a tumor. Some obstetricians consider the position of the fetus to be diagnostic (Fig. 22.27).

Actual diagnoses were recorded in Blair's (108) 68 mothers with anomalous uteri. Seventeen were diagnosed before parturition, nine during labor, twelve at cesarean section, and sixteen during manual delivery of the placenta. Discovery of the condition in the remainder was not associated with pregnancy.

B. Walton Lillehei stated once that "what mankind can dream, research and technology can achieve." We have witnessed this with the diagnosis of congenital anomalies of the genitourinary system, including fetal abnormalities, in the last 15 years:

1. The role of the sonography presented by Fleisher and Shanker (132)
2. Vaginal evaluation with magnetic resonance imaging (MRI) reported by Hricak et al. (133)
3. Ultrasound examination for fetal congenital anomalies reported by Sollie et al. (134)
4. The report of Nicotra et al. (127) on congenital anomalies in spontaneous abortions reaching 25.5 and 5.3% in infertility, using hysterosalpingographies
5. The diagnosis by Bondonny et al. (136) of multiple anomalies using a combination of diagnostic modalities, such as vaginoscopic examination and ultrasound
6. Prenatal diagnosis of congenital anomalies was analyzed by Suzumori (137) who studied the use of technical advances for *in utero* diagnosis of genetic disorders
7. Sanders and Blakemore's (138) demonstration of lethal fetal anomalies by sonography
8. The diagnosis of müllerian anomalies with MRI during pregnancy by Kelley et al. (139)
9. The use of transvaginal sonography by Lewit et al. (140) to study the normal and abnormal uterus
10. Hydrometrocolpos was diagnosed with ultrasound by Sawhney et al. (141)

The brotherhood of science and technology continues. For instance, Levine et al. (142) successfully removed a teratoma originating in the oropharynx by a perinatal approach.

However, science and technology have also produced a system of multiple syndromes with multiple clinical pictures and innumerable combinations of signs and symptoms. The authors decided to bypass these problematic conditions, such as Fryns (143, 144), Mayer-Rokitansky (145), and Rokitansky-Kustner syndromes (146).

Treatment and Surgical Prognosis. Excision of a vaginal septum is a simple and necessary precaution in all cases. When one side of the vagina is incomplete and leads to a rudimentary horn, a hemihysterectomy should be performed.

Excision of the uterine septum may be through the vagina or from the outside. The Strassmann (104) approach through the top of the uterus has been evaluated by Steinberg (147), who was able to report the outcome of 107 operations from the literature. Dysmenorrhea was relieved in 31 patients; there were 51 live births,

of which 14 were cesarean. In addition, there were eight abortions and stillbirths, and one postoperative death. No pregnancies occurred in the remaining patients. In 1966 Strassmann's son reported 205 living children from 170 mothers among 263 patients who underwent Strassmann's metroplasty (148).

Jones and his colleagues (149) compared pre- and postoperative fecundity in patients with excised uterine septa. Before surgery, 22% of the pregnancies resulted in living children; after septal excision, 72% of pregnancies were successful. Septal excision will permit many patients to carry a pregnancy to term. The only alternatives to suffering repeat abortions from a divided uterus are effective contraception and hysterectomy.

Ectopic Endometrium

TUBAL ENDOMETRIUM

In about a dozen reported cases, the mucosa of the uterine tube had the characteristics of uterine endometrium (150). Typically, the tube is thickened and sealed at the ostium. The mucosa may be partially or entirely altered. The usual folds of the tubal mucosa are absent, and the muscularis may be hyperplastic. Dysmenorrhea may occur, or there may be no symptoms. Diagnosis may be made only by histologic section.

Whether this represents a congenital anomaly or a secondary heteroplasia is not known. Because both tube and uterus arise from the müllerian ducts, the alternatives are equally possible. The relationship of tubal pregnancy to possible areas of endometrium in the tube comes at once to mind, but evidence of such a relationship is lacking.

ECTOPIC ENDOMETRIUM

The origin of endometrium on the peritoneal surface of the ovary or of other pelvic and abdominal organs has been debated, sometimes fiercely, for 75 years (151).

One view is that endometriosis represents metaplasia of celomic cells or, more specifically, that it is an expression of a normally suppressed embryonic potentiality of such cells to form reproductive tissue (152–155).

In contrast to the metaplastic view first put forward by Sampson (156, 157), in this view endometriosis results from regurgitation of menstrual blood containing viable endometrial cells. Such cells become seeded on pelvic peritoneal surfaces and grow into patches of endometrium. Desquamated endometrial cells are alive and can be cultured in vitro (158, 159) and in vivo (160). The supporters of this view explain the rare appearance of endometriosis outside the peritoneal cavity—in the lung (161), or the umbilicus (162)—as benign metastases traveling by venous or lymphatic channels.

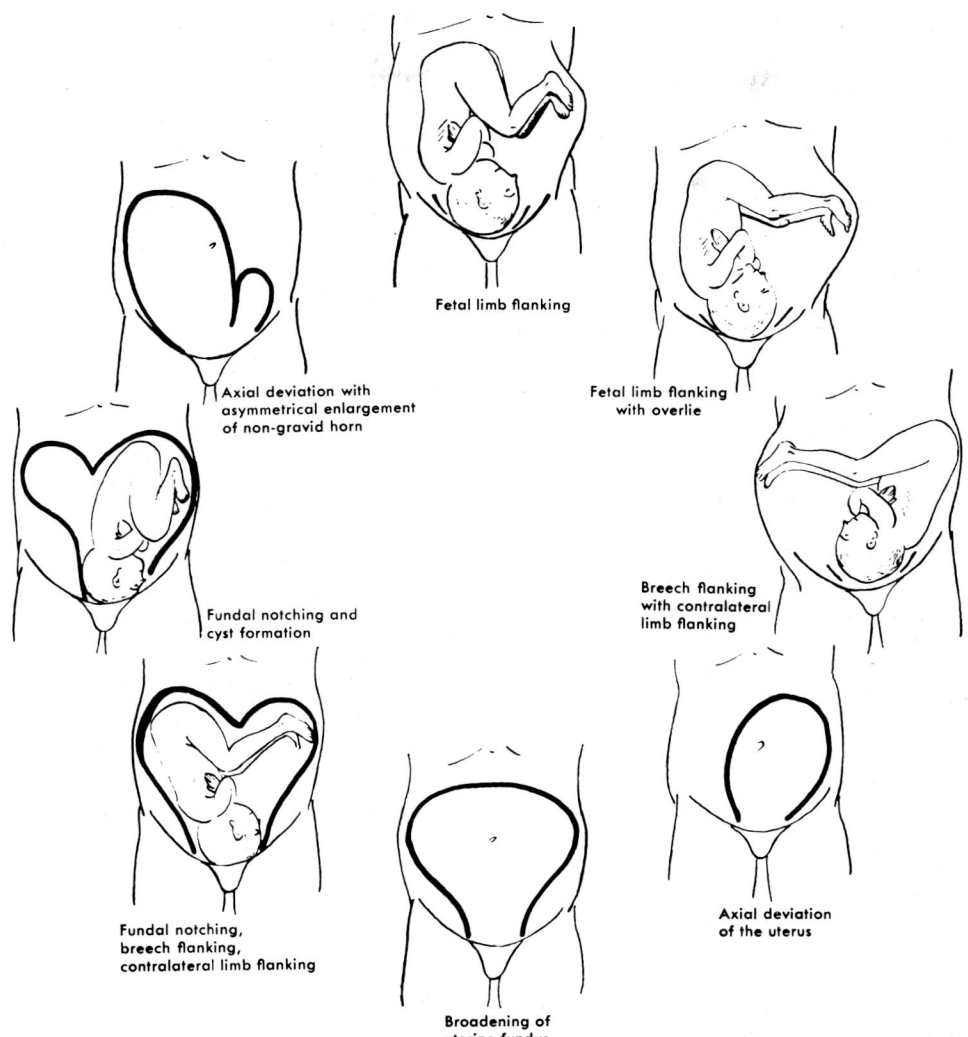

Figure 22.27. Diagnostic signs which suggest the presence of uterine anomalies. Where the uterine outline is shown, the position of the uterus is significant; in the others, the position of the fetus is significant. (From Semmens JP: Congenital anomalies of female genital tract: functional classification based on review of 56 personal cases and 500 reported cases. Obstet Gynecol 1962;19:328–350; after Hay D. The diagnosis and significance of minor degrees of uterine abnormality in relation to pregnancy. Obstet Gynaecol Br Commw 1958;65:557–582.)

At present, the migration view appears to have positive evidence in its favor, but there remain a few cases that are not easily explained. Madding and Kennedy (163) described an endometrial tumor on the left ovary of a woman with absence of the vagina and paired rudimentary uteri. Her left tube had been surgically removed 5 years before the tumor appeared.

A curious example of ectopic endometrium lying within a leiomyoma, which was attached—perhaps secondarily—to the omentum, has been reported (164).

Jenkins et al. (165) reported the following location of ectopic endometrium in 182 patients with infertility and endometriosis:

Ovary unilateral or bilateral	54.9%
Posterior broad ligament	35.2%
Anterior cul-de-sac	34.6%
Posterior cul-de-sac	34.0%
Uterosacral ligament	28.0%

The above authors did not find any endometriosis of the cervix or vagina. Adhesion formation followed the same anatomic pathway. They believe that the Sampson (156, 157) hypothesis of retrograde menstruation is most likely the cause of endometriosis.

Finkel et al. (166) reported the first case of endometrial cyst of the liver. Plawner and Sabattini (167) reported endometrial carcinoma of the prostate. Ombe-

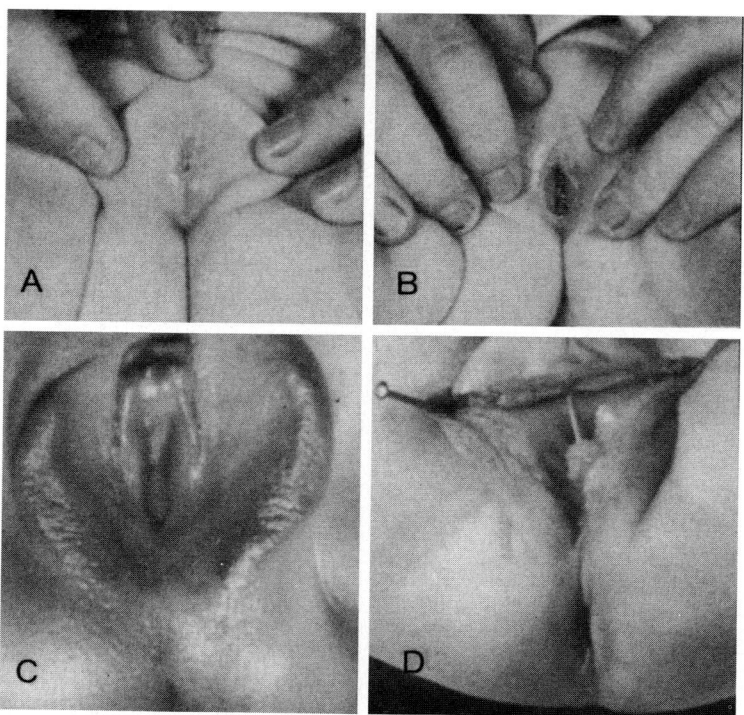

Figure 22.28. *Anomalies of the female genitalia in which the vaginal orifice appears to be absent. **A,** Fusion of the labia minora, showing a small aperture for urination. The orifices of the urethra and vagina are covered. **B,** Normal introitus following separation of the fused labia. **C,** Agenesis of the vagina and urethra associated with the absence of the uterus and both kidneys. **D,** A perineal fold extending anteriorly over the vaginal and urethral orifices (the probe is in the vagina). This malformation may be associated with hyperadrenalism. (**A** and **B,** From Campbell MF. Anomalies of the genital tract. In Harrison JH, Campbell MF, eds. Urology, 3rd ed. Philadelphia: WB Saunders, 1970; **C** and **D,** from Potter EL. Pathology of the fetus and the newborn. Chicago: Year Book Medical Publishers, 1952.)*

let (168) reported endometrial ossification in a case in which ectopic bony endometrial tissue was found in a woman with infertility.

Heterotopic Cartilage in the Uterus

Cartilage islands have been reported in the endometrium, in the myometrium, beneath the serosa, and in an endometrial polyp from both fundus and cervix of the uterus. All have occurred in women of childbearing age, both nulligravida and multigravida.

There is no reason to consider these structures, which are asymptomatic, to be of embryonic origin, nor is there evidence they are neoplastic. They appear instead to represent metaplasia of connective tissue elements. Roth and Taylor (169) described nine cases and collected an additional 24 cases from the literature.

Gronroos et al. (170) reported five cases of glial tissue in the uterus, islands of cartilage, bone, and keratinizing squamous epithelium. The authors postulated that these tissue are most likely of fetal origin.

In 1988, Remmele et al. (171) presented two cases of heterotopic cartilage in the uterus. They stated that fewer than 50 cases had been published and that this is a phenomenon of displacement and retention of fetal tissue or perhaps metaplasia.

Fusion of the Labia Minora and Other Anomalies

Congenital fusion of the labia minora is occasionally encountered in children. The fusion is not complete; a small orifice remains at the anterior end of the vulva (Fig. 22.28, *A* and *B*).

This condition has been said to represent minimal pseudohermaphroditism, but the clitoris is not enlarged, nor are there other suggestive signs. Intrauterine inflammation also has been suggested as a cause. Other genital anomalies are rarely present.

Urinary obstruction and inflammation from retained urine are the chief symptoms. Because the unfused orifice may resemble the urethral meatus, the parents of the patient may confuse the condition with vaginal atresia (Fig. 22.28, *C*).

Treatment is by division of the labia in the line of

fusion. Fusion of the labia minora in infancy was reported by Craig (172), by Frizzi and Morelli (173), Melzer and Rotem (174), and several other authors.

Fernández-Larrañaga and Comesaña-Dávila (175) reported urethrovaginal reflux secondary to fusion of labia minora and Corroy et al. (176) reported dysuria due to "synechia" fusion of the labia minora.

Defects of the Clitoris and Labia

Congenital anomalies of the clitoris are included in Chapter 21 in the section on "Duplication of the Penis and Clitoris and Other Anomalies."

Duplication of the clitoris originates similarly to duplication of the penis, although it is more rarely reported. One case from the literature is mentioned on page 793 and illustrated in Figure 21.24, D.

Transposition of the clitoris to a position posterior to the labia has been described. This condition is homologous to transposition of the penis and scrotum in the male (page 795).

Bruneteau et al. (177) reported two cases with pure gonadal dysgenesis with an XY chromosomal constitution. One of them had infantile but otherwise normal external genitalia, and the other had an underdeveloped labia majora and clitoris. Both patients responded well to hormonal treatment.

Forest et al. (178) presented the case of an aunt and niece with clitoridomegaly, absence of labia minora, and other anomalies. Arya et al. (179) reported a case of hypertrophic labia majora and clitoris in a lethal case of a G syndrome in a female. Chen et al. (180) reported on members of a Nicaraguan family the males of which had small penes and scrotums and the females of which had aplasia of the labium majus and small clitorides. All had multiple other anomalies.

Singer et al. (181) describe a 46XY newborn infant with Smith-Lemli-Opitz syndrome and multiple congenital anomalies including female external genitalia, a testis palpable in each labium majus, a cone-shaped cervix, and normal vagina.

EDITORIAL COMMENTS

Several malformations involving the internal genitalia in females are of interest to the surgeon. For classification purposes, they may be thought of as those presenting primarily in infancy and those in which the diagnosis is usually made at adolescence or later. An excellent presentation of these anomalies can be found in the leading textbook on pediatric urology by Kelalis, King, and Belman (182). Urogenital sinus anomalies (UGS), and the more severe cloacal abnormalities, although rare, constitute challenging technical problems for which a number of unique surgical procedures have been devised. In less complicated cases of UGS, the diagnosis

may not be immediately apparent unless unsuccessful attempts are made to catheterize the urethra. Very mild forms are classified as "female hypospadias" and require no special therapy. More severe forms can be associated with urinary retention and necessitate intermittent catheterization. Special forms of UGS are encountered in severely masculinized females with adrenogenital syndrome in whom the high short vagina enters the sinus above the external urethral sphincter. Extensive operations have been devised in which the vagina is detached from the sinus, allowing the sinus to serve as urethra. The vagina is then exteriorized by mobilizing and attaching clitoral shaft skin (183) or multiple perineal skin flaps (184). Some infants with UGS may also have complete occlusion of the vagina and present with an abdominal mass, representing accumulation of vaginal and uterine secretions, a product of maternal hormonal stimulation. These conditions are the result of an incomplete canalization of the vagina that occurs during the fifth month of gestation. An imperforate hymen can result in distension of the vagina leading to hydrocolpos or in distension of both the vagina and uterus (hydrometrocolpos). A pull-through operation has been devised by Ramenofsky and Raffensburger (185), which can be employed in infancy, in which the UGS then serves as the urethra.

Even more challenging are the cloacal abnormalities associated with imperforate anus. These very complex anomalies are characterized by a common vestibule for the gastrointestinal, genitourinary, and gynecologic tracts, and the infant presents with a single opening in the perineum (as opposed to two openings in the child with UGS). Surgical procedures for correction of these severe anomalies have been devised by Hendren (186) and Peña (187).

Surgically-important abnormalities of the female reproductive tract presenting in adolescence center around varying degrees of stenosis, atresia, or agenesis of the vagina. Often there is an associated urological anomaly. The constellation of vaginal agenesis, varying degrees of uterine maldevelopment, normal ovaries, and unilateral renal agenesis has been given the name of the Mayer-Rokitansky-Hauser syndrome. This condition may be discovered at birth if the vagina is noted to be absent, but more commonly presents later in life as amenorrhea. The labia, clitoris, and urethra are normal, whereas the uterus may vary from normal to the more characteristic rudimentary bicornuate structure without a lumen. Surgical treatment invariably involves construction of a vagina. The use of a short segment of sigmoid colon for replacement, as reported by Hensle and Dean (188), seems to offer the best chance of a good result, with little chance of stricture and without unpleasant mucous production *(TSP)*.

REFERENCES

1. Faulconer RJ. Observations on the origin of the müllerian groove in human embryos. Contrib Embryol Carnegie Inst Wash 1951;34:159–164.
2. Brachet A. Traité d'embryologie des vertébrés. 2nd ed. Paris: Masson et Cie, 1935.

3. Gruenwald P. The relation of the growing müllerian duct to the wolffian duct and its importance for the genesis of malformations. Anat Rec 1941;81:1–19.

4. Gruenwald P. Zur Entwicklungsmechanik des Urogenital systems beim Huhn. Arch Entw 1937;136:786–813.

5. Scheib D. Sur la régression du canal de Müller mâle de l'embryon de poulet: localisation de la phosphatase acide au microscope électronique. C R Acad Sci (Paris) 1965;261:5219–5221.

6. Hunter RH. Observations on the development of the human female genital tract. Contrib Embryol Carnegie Inst Wash 1930;22:91–108.

7. Felix W. The development of the urogenital organs. In: Keibel F, Hall FP, eds. Manual of human embryology, Vol 2. Philadelphia: JB Lippincott, 1912.

8. Hart DB. Adenoma vaginae diffusum (adenomatosis vaginae) with a critical discussion of present views of vaginal hymenal development. Edinb Med J 1911;6:577–590.

9. Mijsberg WA. Uber die Entwicklung der Vagina, des Hymen und des Sinus urogenitalis beim Menschen. Z Anat Entw 1924;74:684–760.

10. Retterer E. Sur l'origine du vagin de la femme. C R Soc Biol (Paris) 1891;3:291–293.

11. Koff AK. Development of the vagina in the human foetus. Contrib Embryol Carnegie Inst Wash 1933;24:61–90.

12. Bulmer D. The early stages of vaginal development in the sheep. J Anat 1956;90:123–134.

13. Bulmer D. The development of the human vagina. J Anat 1957;91:490–509.

14. Vilas E. Über die Entwicklung der menschlichen Scheide. Z Anat Entw 1932;98:263–292.

15. Kempermann CT. Beiträge zur Entwicklung des Genitaltraktus der Säuger; das Schicksal der kaudalen Enden der Wolffschen Gänge beim Weibe und ihre Bedeutung für die Genese der Vagina. Morphol Jahrb 1935;75:151–179.

16. Zuckerman S. The histogenesis of tissues sensitive to oestrogens. Biol Rev 1940;15:231–271.

17. Forsberg JG. Mitotic rate and autoradiographic studies on the derivations and differentiation of the mouse vaginal anlage. Acta Anat (Bassel) 1965;62:266–282.

18. Kanagasuntheram R, Dassanayake AGS. Nature of the obstructing membrane in primary cryptomenorrhea. J Obstet Gynaecol Br Commw 1958;65:487–492.

19. Cunha GR. The dual origin of vaginal epithelium. Am J Anat 1975;143:387.

20. O'Rahilly R. The development of the vagina in the human. In: Blandau RJ, Bergsma D, eds. Morphogenesis and malformation of the genital systems. New York: Alan R Liss, 1977;123–136.

21. George FW, Wilson JD. Sex determination and differentiation. In Knobil E et al, eds. The physiology of reproduction. New York: Raven Press, 1988:3–26.

22. Fraenkel L, Papanicolaou GN. Growth, desquamation and involution of the vaginal epithelium of human fetuses and children, with a consideration of the related hormonal factors. Am J Anat 1938;62:427–451.

23. Sorkness J, Swenson JA, Woodward RS, Saiki AK. Mesonephroma: a urologic problem. J Urol 1958;79:183–189.

24. Gardner GH, Greene RR, Peckham BM. Normal and cystic structures of the broad ligament. Am J Obstet Gynecol 1948;55:917–937.

25. Beltermann R. Elektronenmikroskopische Untersuchungen am Epoophoron des Menschen. Arch Gynak 1965;200:275–284.

26. Dunnihoo DR. An anomaly of the mesovarium. Obstet Gynecol 1961;18:103–105.

27. Huffman JW. Mesonephric remnants in cervix. Am J Obstet Gynecol 1948;56:23–40.

28. Szamborski J. Mesonephric derivatives in the female genital tract with special reference to a staining method. Obstet Gynecol 1963;21:375–378.

29. Rieder C. Ueber die Gartner'schen (Wolff'schen) Kanäle beim menschlichen Weibe. Virchow Arch [A] 1884;96:100–130.

30. Sneeden VD. Mesonephric lesions of the cervix. Cancer 1958;11:334–336.

31. Rock JA, Azziz R. Genital anomalies in childhood. Clin Obstet Gynecol 1987;30;3:682–696.

32. Ashton D, Amin HK, Richart, RM. The incidence of asymptomatic uterine anomalies in women undergoing transcervical tubal sterilization. Obstet Gynecol 1988;72(1):28–30.

33. Reis RA, De Costa EJ. Torsion of the hydatid of Morgagni. Am J Obstet Gynecol 1948;56:770–776.

34. Bisca BV. Mesonephric remnants in the adult female. Obstet Gynecol 1956;8:265–269.

35. Bleier W. Gartnersche-Gang-Zysten der Scheide als Hinweis auf weitere Missbildungen im Urogenitalsystem. Z Geburtsch Gynak 1955;143:71–86.

36. Verhaeghe A, Libersa C, Herbeau J, Dubois R, Dupont J. Hematometra in a double uterus communicating with a Gärtner's duct and renal agensis. Lille Chir 1960;15:59–66.

37. Brews A. Some clinical aspects of developmental anomalies of the female genito-urinary tract. Proc R Soc Med 1957;50:199–206.

38. Pfleiderer A. Ueber Gebärmuttermissbildungen. Mschr Geburtsh Gynak 1929;82:401–420.

39. Schmidt F. A rare anomaly of the female genitalia. Zentralbl Gynak 1965;87:233–236.

40. Müller P. Le syndrome atrésie vaginale et utérus bifide rudimentaire: considérations étiopathogéniques et cliniques. Bull Fed Gynecol Obstet Franc 1961;13(suppl):502–504.

41. Kent BK. Ectopic pregnancy in a congenitally defective tube with absence of the ipsilateral ovary. Am J Obstet Gynecol 1956;72:1150–1151.

42. Zarou GS, Acken HS, Brevetti RC. Surgical management of congenital atresia of the cervix. Am J Obstet Gynecol 1961;82:923–928.

43. Maliphant RG. Gynatresia: report of three uncommon clinical types. Br Med J 1948;2:555–558.

44. Flemming EA, Kava HL. Congenital atresia of the upper two-thirds of the vagina and cervical os with hematometria. Am J Obstet Gynecol 1940;40:296–301.

45. McIndoe A. Treatment of congenital absence and obliterative conditions of the vagina. Br J Plast Surg 1950;2:254–267.

46. Jones HW, Scott WW. Hermaphroditism, genital anomalies and related endocrine disorders. Baltimore: Williams & Wilkins, 1958.

47. Bryan AL, Nigro JA, Counseller VS. One hundred cases of congenital absence of vagina. Surg Gynecol Obstet 1949;88:79–86.

48. Bell WB. Further investigation into the chemical composition of menstrual fluid and the secretions of the vagina, as estimated from an analysis of hematocolpos fluid, together with a discussion of the clinical features associated with hematocolpos, and a description of the character of the obstructing membrane. J Obstet. Gynaecol Br Commw 1912;1:209–215.

49. White AJ. Vaginal atresia: high transversus septum. Obstet Gynecol 1966;27:695–698.

50. Rea E, Theron HF. Hydrometrocolpos. S Afr Med J 1957;31:1013–1015.

51. Novak E. Congenital absence of the uterus and vagina: with report of six cases. Surg Gynecol Obstet 1917;25:532–537.

52. McKusick VA, Bauer RL, Koop CE, Scott RB. Hydrometrocolpos as a simple inherited malformation. JAMA 1964;189:813–816.

53. Azoury RS, Jones HW. Cytogenetic findings in patients with congenital absence of the vagina. Am J Obstet Gynecol 1966;94:178–180.

54. Leduc B, Van Campenhout J, Simard R. Congenital absence of the vagina: observations on 25 cases. Am J Obstet Gynecol 1968;100:512–520.

55. Columbus R. De re anatomica, libri XV. Venice, 1559.

56. Morgagni JB. The seats and causes of disease investigated by anatomy. Alexander B (transl). New York: Hafner Publishing, 1960.

57. Marshall GB. Artificial vagina: a review of the various operative procedures for correcting atresia vaginae. J Obstet Gynaecol Br Commw 1913;23:193–212.

58. Amussat JZ. Observation sur une operation de vagin artificiel pratiquee avec succes par un nouveau procédé, suive de quelques reflexions sur les vices de conformation du vagin. Gaz Med 1832:785.

59. Paunz A. Über die Bildung einer kunstlichen Vagina bei angeborenen volkommenen Defekt derselben. Zentralbl Gynak 1923;47:883–888.

60. Cali RW, Pratt JH. Congenital absence of the vagina. Am J Obstet Gynecol 1968;100:752–763.

61. Dennison WM, Bacsich P. Imperforate vagina in the newborn: neonatal hydrocolpos. Arch Dis Child 1961;36:156–159.

62. Cook WH, Singer B, Frank LJ Jr. Duplication of distal colon: report of a case and its surgical correction. AMA Arch Surg 1960;80:650–654.

63. Weaver DD. A survey of prenatally diagnosed disorders. Clin Obstet Gynecol 1988;31:253–269.

64. Macdonald CR. Unusual forms of gynatresia. J Obstet Gynaecol Br Commw 1960;67:848–852.

65. Embrey MP. A case of uterus didelphys with unilateral gynatresia. Br Med J 1950;1:820–821.

66. Graves WP. Method of constructing artificial vagina. Surg Clin North Am 1921;1:611–614.

67. Baldwin JE. The formation of an artificial vagina by an intestinal transplantation. Ann Surg 1904;40:398–403.

68. Frank RT, Geist SH. Additional reports on the satchel handle operation for artificial vagina ("The formation of artificial vagina by a new plastic technic"). Am J Obstet Gynecol 1932;32:256–258.

69. Freundt I, Toolenaar TAM, Huikeshoven FJM, Drogendijk AC, Jeekel H. A modified technique to create a neovagina with an isolated segment of sigmoid colon. Surg Gynecol Obstet 1992;174:11–16.

70. Tolhurst DE, van der Helm TWJS. The treatment of vaginal atresia. Surg 1991;172:407–414.

71. Rowley WN. Uterine anomaly: duplication of uterus, three tubes and three ovaries—report of a case. Ann Surg 1948;127:676–680.

72. Kelso JW. Unusual malformation of the uterus. Am J Obstet Gynecol 1956;72:922–923.

73. Thorek P, Moses J, Wong J. Simultaneous pregnancies in a fallopian tube and bicornate uterus associated with three fallopian tubes: a first world case report and review of the literature. Am J Surg 1950;79:512–523.

74. Curtis AH, Anson BJ. Bilateral double infundibulum of the uterine tube. Anat Rec 1938;71:177–179.

75. Walthard M. Ueber ein junges menschliches Ei im Mesosalpingiolum einer Nebentube. Z Geburtsh Gynäk 1911;69:553–580.

76. Zólcínski A, Robaczyski J, Ziólkowski M. Über die Bebentuben und akzessorischen Tubenostien. Zentralbl Gynak 1964;86:548–559.

77. Jarcho J. Malformations of the uterus. Am J Surg 1946;71:106–166.

78. Monie SW, Sigardson LA. A proposed classification for uterine and vaginal anomalies. Am J Obstet Gynecol 1950;59:696–698.

79. Halal F. A new syndrome of severe upper limb hypoplasia and müllerian duct anomalies. Am J Med Genet 1986;24:119–126.

80. Gemmell JE, Paterson AM. Duplication of bladder, uterus, vagina and vulva with successive full time pregnancy and labour in each uterus. J Obstet Gynaecol Br Emp 1913;23:25–32.

81. Semmens JP. Uterus didelphys and septate vagina. Obstet Gynecol 1956;8:620–626.

82. Milne HA. Double uterus with unilateral haematocolpos and absence of ipsilateral kidney. Proc R Soc Med 1965;58:238.

83. Miller NF. Clinical aspects of uterus didelphys. Am J Obstet Gynecol 1922;4:398–407.

84. Hunter W. Recto-vesical ligament in association with double uterus. J Obstet Gynaecol Br Commw 1960;67:429–433.

85. Beekhuis JR, Hage JC. The double uterus associated with an obstructed hemivagina and ipsilateral renal agenesis. Eur J Obstet Gynecol Reprod Biol 1983;16:47–52.

86. Burbige KA, Hensle TW. Uterus didelphys and vaginal duplication with unilateral obstruction presenting as a newborn abdominal mass. J Urol 1984;132:1195–1198.

87. Whitaker RH, Woodard JR. Paediatric urology. London: Butterworth, 1985.

88. Flieguer JR. Uncommon problems of the double uterus. Med J Aust 1988;145:510–512.

89. Tolete-Velcek F et al. Utero vaginal malformations: a trap for the unsuspecting surgeon. J Pediatr Surg 1989;24:736–740.

90. Morgan MA, Thurnau GR, Smith ML. Uterus didelphys with unilateral hematocolpos, ipsilateral renal agenesis and menses: a case report and literature review. J Reprod Med 1987;32:47–58.

91. Beernink FJ, Beernink HE, Chinn A. Uterus unicornis with uterus solidaris. Obstet Gynecol 1976;47:651–653.

92. Hadden D. Double uterus and vagina. Am J Obstet Gynecol 1922;3:526–527.

93. Shenker L, Brickman FE. Bicornuate uterus with incomplete vaginal septum and unilateral renal agenesis. Radiology 1979;133:455–457.

94. Aragona F, Glazel GP, Zaramella P, Zorzi C, Talenti E. Agenesis of the bladder. Urol Radiol 1988;10:207–209.

95. Golan A et al. Cervical cerclage: the role in the pregnant anomalous uterus. Int J Fertil 1990;35:164–170.

96. Miller MC. Twin pregnancy in a septate uterus. J Obstet Gynaecol Br Commw 1961;68:673–675.

97. Connell EB. Uterus didelphys presenting as leukorrhea: report of a case. Obstet Gynecol 1961;18:495–497.

98. Beyer WF, Freissler G, Schlotter CM, Kuhn H. Uterus septus with adenocarcinoma of one half of the uterus. Geburtshilfe Frauenheilkd 1984;44:513–515.

99. Assaf A, Serour G, Elkady A, el Agizy H. Endoscopic management of the intrauterine septum. Int J Gynaecol Obstet 1990;32:43–51.

100. daCarpi JB, Isagogae Breves: a short introduction to anatomy, 1522. LR Lind (transl). Chicago: University of Chicago Press, 1959.

101. Ricci JV. The geneology of gynaecology, 2nd ed. Philadelphia: Blakiston, 1950.

102. Purcell J. Description of double uterus and vagina. Phil Trans 1773/1774;64:474.

103. Ruge P. Über einen Fall von Schwangerschaft bei Uterus septus. Z Geburtsh Gynäk 1884;10:141–143.

104. Strassmann P. Die operative Vereinigung eines doppelton Uterus. Zentralbl Gynak 1907;31:1322.

105. Weintrob M. Abnormalities of the female genitalia. J Int Coll Surg 1944;7:381–397.

106. Semmens JP. Congenital anomalies of female genital tract: functional classification based on review of 56 personal cases and 500 reported cases. Obstet Gynecol 1962;19:328–350.

107. Fenton AN, Singh BP. Pregnancy associated with congenital abnormalities of the female reproductive tract. Am J Obstet Gynecol 1952;63:744–755.

108. Blair RG. Pregnancy associated with congenital malformations of the reproductive tract. J Obstet Gynaecol Br Emp 1960;67:36–42.

109. Baker WS et al. Congenital anomalies of the uterus associated with pregnancy: an analysis of 118 cases from the literature with a report of nine additional cases. Am J Obstet Gynecol 1953;66:580–597.

110. Thomas M, Langley II. Congenital anomalies of the uterus. West J Surg 1959;67:339–343.

111. Falls FH. Pregnancy in the bicornuate uterus. Am J Obstet Gynecol 1956;72:1243–1254.

112. Zabriskie JR. Pregnancy and the malformed uterus. West J Surg 1962;70:293–296.

113. Dunselman GAJ. Congenital malformation of the uterus: results of Strassmann's metroplasty [Thesis]. Utrecht: Madlener-Sittard, 1959.

114. Dorgan LT, Clarke PE. Uterus didelphys with double pregnancy. Am J Obstet Gynecol 1956;72:663–666.

115. Drucker P, Finkel J, Savel LE. Sixty-five day interval between the births of twins. Am J Obstet Gynecol 1960;80:761–763.

116. Green QL, Schanck GP, Smith JR. Normal living twins in uterus didelphys with 38 day interval between deliveries. Am J Obstet Gynecol 1961;82:340–342.

117. Barrett AB. Bicornate uterus with pregnancy in each horn. Am J Obstet Gynecol 1934;28:612–614.

118. Braze A. Bicornate uterus with pregnancy in each horn. JAMA 1943;123:474–476.

119. Way S. A further contribution to the study of the influence of failure of müllerian duct fusion in pregnancy and labour. J Obstet Gynaecol Br Commw 1947;54:469–476.

120. Rolen AC, Choquette AJ, Semmons JP. Rudimentary uterine horn: obstetric and gynecologic implications. Obstet Gynecol 1966;27:806–813.

121. Nokes JM. Pregnancy in an atretic uterine horn. Am J Obstet Gynecol 1934;28:250–253.

122. O'Leary JL, O'Leary JA. Rudimentary horn pregnancy. Obstet Gynecol 1963;22:371–375.

123. Jones WS. Obstetric significance of female genital anomalies. Obstet Gynecol 1957;10:113–127.

124. Greiss F Jr, Hampton MC. Genital anomalies in women: an evaluation of diagnosis, incidence and obstetric performance. Am J Obstet Gynecol 1961;82:330–339.

125. Chastrusse L, Dubecq JP, Parneix M. Forty-four cases of congenital uterine malformations. Rev Franc Gynecol Obstet 1961;56:429–441.

126. Hay D. The diagnosis and significance of minor degrees of uterine abnormality in relation to pregnancy. J Obstet Gynaecol Br Commw 1958;65:557–582.

127. Carey MP, Steinberg LH. Vaginal dystocia in a patient with a double uterus and a longitudinal vaginal septum. Aust N Z J Obstet Gynaecol 1989;29:74–75.

128. Salat-Baroux J. Recurrent spontaneous abortions. Reprod Nutr Dev 1988;28:1555–1568.

129. Ben-Rafael Z. The association of pregnancy-induced hypertension and uterine malformations. Gynecol Obstet Invest 1990;30:101–104.

130. Pennes DR, Bowerman RA, Silver TM, Smith SJ. Failed first trimester pregnancy termination: uterine anomaly as etiologic factor. J Clin Urol 1987;15:165–170.

131. Petrikovsky BM. Intrapartum fetoscopy: technique and indications. Endoscopy 1988;20:142–143.

132. Fleisher AC, Shawker TH. The role of sonography in pediatric gynecology. Clin Obstet Gynecol 1987;30:735–746.

133. Hricak H, Chang, YC, Thurnher S. Vagina: evaluation with MR imaging. I. Normal anatomy and congenital anomalies. Radiology 1988;169:169–174.

134. Sollie JE, vanGeijn HP, Arts NF. Validity of a selective policy for ultrasound examination of fetal congenital anomalies. Eur J Obstet Gynecol Reprod Biol 1988;27:125–132.

135. Nicotra M et al. Hysterosalpingographic abnormalities in infertile women: radiological and clinical interpretation. Acta Eur Fertil 1988;19:79–82.

136. Bondonny JM, Boissinot F, Vergnes P, Diard F, Sandler B. The association of a dysplastic kidney with a single vaginal ectopic ureter and a homolateral genital abnormality in a girl. Chir Pediatr 1988;29:273–80.

137. Suzomori K. Prenatal diagnosis of congenital anomalies: present status and future problems. Nippon Sanka Fujinka Gakkai Zasshi 1988;40:1027–1032.

138. Sanders RC, Blakemore K. Lethal fetal anomalies: sonographic demonstration. Radiology 1989;172:1–6.

139. Kelley JL III, Edwards RP, Wozney P, Vaccarello L, Laifer SA. Magnetic resonance imaging to diagnose a müllerian anomaly during pregnancy. Obstet Gynecol 1990;75:521–523.

140. Lewit N, Thaler I, Rottem S. The uterus: a new look with transvaginal sonography. J Clin Urol 1990;18:331–336.

141. Sawhney S, Gupta R, Berry M, Bhatnagar V. Hydrometrocolpos: diagnosis and follow-up by ultrasound. Aust Radiol 1990;34:93–94.

142. Levine AB, Alvarez M, Wedgwood J, Berkowitz RL, Holzman I. Contemporary management of a potentially lethal fetal anomaly: a successful perinatal approach to epignathus. Obstet Gynecol 1990;76:962–966.

143. Ayme S et al. Fryns syndrome: report on 8 new cases. Clin Genet 1989;35:191–201.

144. Schwyzer U, Briner J, Schinzel A. Fryns syndrome in a girl born to consanguineous parents. Acta Paediatr Scand 1987;76:167–171.

145. Ogawa O, Hashimoto K, Taniguchi T, Nakagawa T, Nishimura Y. A case of Mayer-Rokitansy syndrome. Hinyokika Kiyo 1988;34:1461–1467.

146. Kords H. Rokitansky-Kustner syndrome. Geburtshilfe Frauenheilkd 1976;36:672–677.

147. Steinberg W. Strassmann's metroplasty in the management of bipartite uterus causing sterility or habitual abortion. Obstet Gynecol Surv 1955;10:400–430.

148. Strassmann EO. Fertility and unification of double uterus. Fertil Steril 1966;17:165–176.

149. Jones HW, Delfs E, Jones GES. Reproductive difficulties in double uterus: the place of plastic reconstruction. Am J Obstet 1956;72:865–883.

150. Marchetti AA. Endometrium-like mucosa lining the fallopian tube. Am J Obstet Gynecol 1940;40:69–79.

151. Ridley JH. The histogenesis of endometriosis: a review of facts and fancies. Obstet Gynecol Surg 1968;23:1–35.

152. Gardner GH, Greene RR, Ranney B. Histogenesis of endometriosis: recent contributions. Obstet Gynecol 1953;1:615–637.

153. Gardner GH, Greene RR, Ranney B. The histogenesis of endometriosis. Am J Obstet Gynecol 1959;78:445.

154. Willis RA. The borderland of embryology and pathology. London: Butterworth, 1958.

155. Witschi E. Embryology of the uterus, normal and experimental. Ann NY Acad Sci 1959;75:412–435.

156. Sampson JA. Perforating hemorrhagic (chocolate) cysts of the ovary, their importance and especially their relation to pelvic adenomas of the endometrial type. Arch Surg 1921;3:245–323.

157. Sampson JA. Peritoneal endometriosis due to the menstrual dissemination of endometrial tissue into the peritoneal cavity. Am J Obstet Gynecol 1927;14:422–469.

158. TeLinde RW, Scott RB. Experimental endometriosis. Am J Obstet Gynecol 1960;60:1147–1173.

159. Keettel WC, Stein RJ. The viability of the cast-off menstrual endometrium. Am J Obstet Gynecol 1951;61:440–442.
160. Ridley JH, Edwards IK. Experimental endometriosis in the human. Am J Obstet Gynecol 1958;76:783–789.
161. Lattes R, Shepard F, Tovell H, Wylie R. A clinical and pathologic study of endometriosis of the lung. Surg Gynecol Obstet 1956;103:552–558.
162. Cullen TS. Embryology, anatomy and diseases of the umbilicus together with diseases of the urachis. Philadelphia: WB Saunders, 1916.
163. Madding GF, Kennedy PA. Endometriosis: case supporting coelomic metaplasia as possible cause. JAMA 1963;183:686–688.
164. Chabon J, Sedlis A. An "accessory uterus": a case report. West J Surg 1963;71:6–8.
165. Jenkins S, Olive DL, Haney AF. Endometriosis: pathogenetic implications of the anatomic distribution. Obstet Gynecol 1986;67:335–338.
166. Finkel L, Marchevsky A, Cohen B. Endometrial cyst of the liver. Am J Gastroenterol 1986;81:576–578.
167. Plawner J, Sabattini M. Endometrial carcinoma of prostate: differentiation with ectopic prostatic tissue in elderly male. Urology 1987;29:117–118.
168. Ombelet W. Endometrial ossification, an unusual finding in an infertility clinic. J Reprod Med 1989;34:303–6.
169. Roth E, Taylor HB. Heterotopic cartilage in the uterus. Obstet Gynecol 1966;27:838–844.
170. Gronroos M, Meurman L, Kahra K. Proliferating glia and other heterotopic tissues in the uterus. Obstet Gynecol 1983;61:261–6.
171. Remmele W, Schmidt-Wontroba H, Kaiser E, Piroth H. Heterotopic cartilage tissue in the uterus. Geburtshilfe Frauenheilkd 1988;48:184–188.
172. Craig DS. Fusion of the labia minora in infancy. Practitioner 1966;196:424–426.
173. Frizzi V, Morelli L. On an uncommon cause of dysuria in children: fusion of the labia minora. Minerva Urol 1967;19:189–194.
174. Melzer M, Rotem Y. Fusion of labia minora. Harefuah 1970;78:387–388.
175. Fernández-Larrañaga A, Comesaña-Dávila E. Urethro-vaginal reflux caused by fusion of the labia minora. Acta Urol Esp 1985;9(2):183–184.
176. Corroy JS, Girot V, Amicabile C, Guillemin P. Synechia of the labia minora as a cause of dysuria. Ann Urol (Paris) 1989;23:504–505.
177. Bruneteau DW, Sipahiogle IB, Byrd JR, Greenblatt RB. Pure gonadal dysgenesis with an XY chromosomal constitution. Am J Obstet Gynecol 1976;124:55–59.
178. Forest MG, dePerretti E, Campo-Paysaa A. Familial case of male pseudohermaphroditism due to 17-ketoreductase defect. Ann Endocrinol (Paris) 1979;40:545–546.
179. Arya S, Viseskul C, Gilbert EF. The G syndrome. Am J Med Genet 1980;5:321–324.
180. Chen H, Chang CH, Misra RP, Peters HA, Grijalva NS, Opitz JM. Multiple pterygium syndrome. Am J Med Genet 1980;7:91–102.
181. Singer LP, Marion RW, Li JK. Limb deficiency in an infant with Smith-Lemli-Opitz syndrome. Am J Med Genet 1989;32:380–383.
182. Merguerian P, Mclorie G. Disorders of the female genitalia. In: Kelalis PP, King LR, Bellman AB, eds. Clinical pediatric urology, vol 2, 3rd ed. Philadelphia: WB Saunders, 1992.
183. Paserini-Glazel G. A new one-stage procedure for clitorovaginoplasty in severely masculinized female pseudohermaphrodites. J Urol 1989;142:565.
184. Parrott T, Woodard J. Abdominoperineal approach to management of the high short vagina in the adrenogenital syndrome. J Urol 1991;146:647.
185. Ramenofsky ML, Raffensburger JG. An abdomino-perineal-vaginal pull-through for definitive treatment of hydrocolpos. J Pediatr Surg 1971;6:381.
186. Hendren WH. Repair of cloacal anomalies: current technics. J Pediatr Surg 1986;21:1159.
187. Peña A. The surgical management of persistent cloaca: results in 54 patients treated with a posterior sagittal approach. J Pediatr Surg 1989;24:590.
188. Hensle TW, Dean GE. Vaginal replacement in children. J Urol 1992;148:677.

CHAPTER 23

SEX DETERMINATION

John Elias Skandalakis / Stephen Wood Gray / Thomas S. Parrott

"In a sense, man begins his existence as a hermaphrodite."
—STEPHEN S. WACHTEL, 1983

INTRODUCTION

It is not within the scope of this chapter to present genetic disorders in toto, congenital anomalies associated with genes, or the multiple syndromes which have been described so well by genetic scientists. Nadler et al. (1) stated that a single mutant human gene is responsible for approximately 4000 disorders.

Table 23.1 gives the single-gene disorders and Table 23.2 single-gene inheritance.

The terms *malformation, deformation, disruption,* and *dysplasia* produce confusion, and many times these words are used the wrong way. Spranger et al. (2) summarized the nomenclature recommended by an international working group as follows:

Malformation: A morphologic defect of an organ, part of an organ, or larger region of the body resulting from an intrinsically abnormal developmental process
Disruption: A morphologic defect of an organ, part of an organ, or a larger region of the body resulting from the extrinsic breakdown of, or an interference with, an originally normal developmental process
Deformation: An abnormal form, shape, or position of part of the body caused by mechanical forces
Dysplasia: Abnormal organization of cells into tissue(s) and the morphologic result(s)

Rosenbaum (3) gives a number of well-known syndromes by malformation:

Biliary atresia
  Trisomy 18
  Arteriohepatic dysplasia (Alagille syndrome)
Diaphragmatic hernia
  Trisomy 18
  Trisomy 21
Tracheoesophageal fistula
  Trisomy 18
  Trisomy 21
  VATER association
Hirschsprung's disease
  Trisomy 21
  Smith-Lemli-Opitz syndrome
  Waardenburg syndrome

Hypospadias
  Trisomy 13
  13q-
  Aniridia (Wilms' tumor)
  Cryptophthalmos syndrome
  Hypertelorism-hypospadias syndrome (BBB syndrome, G syndrome)
  Robinow syndrome
  Smith-Lemli-Opitz syndrome
Imperforate anus
  Trisomy 18
  Trisomy 22
  Cat-eye syndrome (partial trisomy 22)
  13q-
  Cryptophthalmos syndrome
  Kaufman-McKusick syndrome
  Laurence-Moon-Biedl syndrome
  Meckel syndrome
  VATER association
Inguinal hernia
  Aarskog-Scott syndrome
  Ehlers-Danlos syndrome
  Marfan syndrome
  Mucopolysaccharidoses
Malrotation
  Trisomy 13
  Trisomy 18
  Trisomy 21
  Cat-eye syndrome (partial trisomy 22)
  de Lange syndrome
  Meckel syndrome
  Zellweger syndrome
Omphalocele
  Trisomy 13
  Trisomy 18
  Trisomy 21
  Beckwith-Wiedemann syndrome
  Meckel syndrome
Pyloric stenosis
  Trisomy 18
  Turner syndrome
  de Lange syndrome
  Smith-Lemli-Opitz syndrome
  Zellweger syndrome

848

Table 23.1.
Single-Gene Disorders[a]

Autosomal Dominant	Autosomal Recessive	X-Linked	Total
934[b]	588[b]	115[b]	1,637[b]
(893)	(710)	(128)	(1,731)
1,827	1,298	243	3,368

[a]From Rosenbaum KN. Genetics and dysmorphology. In: Kelalis PP, King LR, Belman AB, eds. Clinical pediatric urology, 3rd ed. Philadelphia: WB Saunders, 1992.
[b]Denotes inheritance proved. Parentheses denote inheritance not proved but suspected.

Table 23.2.
Single-Gene Inheritance

A. Autosomal dominant
    Aa = affected heterozygote
    aa = normal
    Parental genotypes   Aa × aa
    Offspring genotypes   Aa(½) or aa(½)
B. Autosomal recessive
    AA = normal
    Aa = heterozygote (carrier)
    aa = homozygote (affected)
    Parental genotypes   Aa × Aa
    Offspring genotypes   AA(¼);Aa(½);aa(¼)
C. X-linked recessive
    XY = normal male
    X′Y = affected male (hemizygote)
    XX = normal female
    X′X = carrier female
    Parental genotypes   XX × X′Y
    Offspring genotypes   X′X(½);XY(½)

[a]From Rosenbaum KN. Genetics and dysmorphology. In: Kelalis PP, King LR, Belman AB, eds. Clinical pediatric urology, 3rd ed. Philadelphia: WB Saunders, 1992.

NORMAL DEVELOPMENT OF SEXUALITY

Early in the seventh week of development, the previously indifferent gonad begins to differentiate into an ovary or a testis, and the sex of an embryo may be determined by histologic section (see Fig. 20.7). At about the same time or a few days later, a difference in the external genitalia is apparent to the experienced observer, but not until the 12th week is the difference evident on casual inspection (see Fig. 21.8 and page 825). However, long before these stages, primary determination of sex has taken place.

Reindollar and McDonough (4) presented a beautiful timetable of the events in utero of normal male and female sexual differentiation (Fig. 23.1 and 23.2).

Genetic Sex Determination

In the human, the cells of the adult body contain 46 chromosomes, which can be arranged in 23 pairs. For many years it was thought that humans, like lower primates, had 24 pairs of chromosomes. The haploid number of 23

chromosomes in man observed by Ford and Hamerton (5) confirmed the diploid number of 46 found by Tjio and Levan (6). The karyotype of the 23 bivalents from human testicular material was demonstrated by Chen and Falek (7).

The pairs of chromosomes are distinguished from each other, falling naturally into groups, and have been numbered from 1 to 22 according to centromere location and decreasing order of size (8). These 22 pairs are known collectively as autosomes. The remaining 23rd pair are the sex chromosomes (Fig. 23.3).

The sex chromosomes in the female are similar in size and shape, but those in the male are dissimilar. The two sex chromosomes of the female, and the larger of the two sex chromosomes of the male, are designated the X chromosomes, while the smaller of the male pair is known as the Y chromosome. The complement of chromosomes in a given cell nucleus, defined by chromosome number and morphology, is termed the *karyotype;* that of the normal female may be expressed as 46,XX (Fig. 23.3, *A*) and that of the male as 46,XY (Fig. 23.3, *B*). The presence of either two X chromosomes (female) or of an X and a Y chromosome (male) determines the genetic sex of the individual.

This genetic sex is established at conception by the chromosome complement of the egg and of the sperm that fertilizes it. In both oogenesis and spermatogenesis, the gametes are formed by reduction of the diploid number of chromosomes present in the oogonia or spermatogonia to the haploid number present in the ovum and sperm, by a series of meiotic divisions. A single representative of each pair of autosomes and sex chromosomes is present in each sex cell. The karyotype of the ovum normally is always 23,X; however, because the sex chromosomes of the male are dissimilar, two types of spermatozoa are formed: 23,X and 23,Y.

The union of sperm and ovum restores the diploid number of chromosomes and results in a female karyotype of 46,XX or a male karyotype of 46,XY. As a result of replication of the chromosomes at each cell division, all the cells of the entire body receive the chromosome complement of the original fertilized ovum.

Prior to the late blastocyst stage, there is no way of recognizing sex in the embryonic cells (9, 10). After that stage, cells having the female sex chromosomes (XX) display the typical heterochromatin characteristic of the female. This *sex chromatin,* or *Barr, body* represents one of the two X chromosomes possessed by the cell (Fig. 23.4). It has been suggested that either the maternal or the paternal X chromosome may form the Barr body, depending on the particular cell (11); whichever it is, the same one forms the Barr body in every one of its daughter cells. If, as in some anomalous karyotypes, there are more

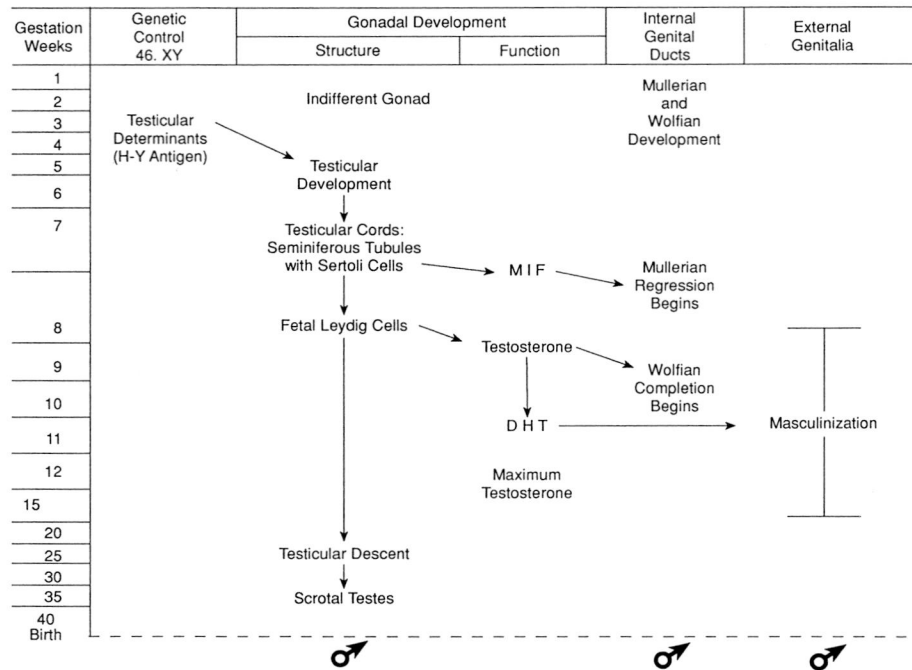

Figure 23.1. Schematic timetable of events for in utero normal male sexual differentiation. (From Reindollar RH and McDonough PG. The child with ambiguous genitalia. In: Lavery JP, Sanfilippo JS, eds. Pediatric and adolescent obstetrics and gynecology. New York: Springer-Verlag, 1985:38–60.)

than two X chromosomes, all but one will form heterochromatin bodies, so that the X complement of a cell is always one plus the number of heterochromatin bodies.

Although Lyon (11, 12) suggested that the normal heterochromatic X chromosome has little subsequent genetic effect on the cell, it has been found that supernumerary heterochromatic X chromosomes in Klinefelter's syndrome suppress testicular function and the 49,XXXXY karyotype inhibits testicular descent. Additional X chromosomes in the female do not affect reproductive function, but in both males and females, supernumerary X chromosomes appear to decrease mental ability (see Fig. 23.13).

Role of the Sex Chromosomes in Development

The presence of at least one X chromosome appears to be necessary for the survival of the mammalian organism and probably for the survival of its individual cells. Chromosome complements with no sex chromosomes, or with only Y chromosomes, are not known to occur.

The specific role of the X chromosome appears to be that of stimulating development of the female reproductive organs. A single X suffices for the müllerian ducts and their derivatives, but the evidence from Turner's syndrome indicates that two X chromosomes are required for ovarian development. However, Bahner and his colleagues (13) reported a woman of XO karyotype who had a child.

Testicular development depends on the presence of a Y chromosome, and testicular stroma and tubules will form even though germ cells are absent. The presence of testicular tissue in true hermaphrodites having an XX karyotype is at present explained by assuming that some cells, which happened not to be included in the biopsy, contain Y chromosomes.

The presence of a gonad depends, then, on the existence of two sex chromosomes; if neither a Y nor a second X chromosome is present, only a fibrous streak will indicate the site of the gonad.

In the male, the testis formed under the influence of the Y chromosome stimulates the wolffian duct derivatives and masculine genitalia and suppresses further development of the müllerian duct derivatives. The relationships among chromosomes, gonad development, and reproductive tract development are illustrated in Table 23.3.

Removal of the testes from an embryo results in regression of wolffian ducts and normal development of müllerian ducts as well as of feminine genitalia (14). Removal of the ovaries at the same stage produces identical results. Evidently, masculine differentiation requires the presence of the testis, while feminine differentiation will occur in the absence of any gonads. The müllerian

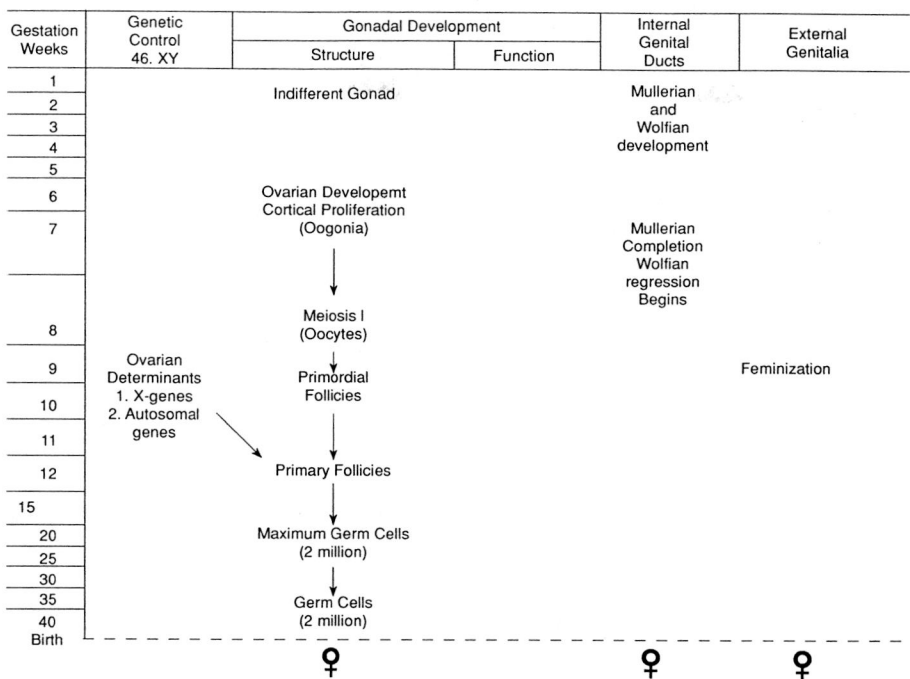

| Gestation Weeks | Genetic Control 46. XY | Gonadal Development | | Internal Genital Ducts | External Genitalia |
		Structure	Function		
1		Indifferent Gonad		Mullerian and Wolfian development	
2					
3					
4					
5					
6		Ovarian Developemt Cortical Proliferation (Oogonia)		Mullerian Completion Wolfian regression Begins	
7					
8		Meiosis I (Oocytes)			
9	Ovarian Determinants 1. X-genes 2. Autosomal genes	Primordial Follicles			Feminization
10					
11					
12		Primary Follicies			
15					
20		Maximum Germ Cells (2 million)			
25					
30					
35		Germ Cells (2 million)			
40					
Birth					
		♀		♀	♀

Figure 23.2. Schematic timetable of events for in utero normal female sexual differentiation. (From Reindollar RH and McDonough PG. The child with ambiguous genitalia. In: Lavery JP, Sanfilippo JS, eds. Pediatric and adolescent obstetrics and gynecology. New York: Springer-Verlag, 1985:38–60.)

structures develop to maturity, whereas the wolffian structures regress with the remainder of the mesonephros in the presence of an X chromosome, regardless of the presence or absence of an ovary. Stimulation of the wolffian structures and suppression of müllerian structures are the result of activity of a testis formed in the presence of a Y chromosome. In this sense, wolffian ducts are not "suppressed" in the female.

Jones and Scott (15) postulated the presence of two masculinizing hormones from the fetal testis: (a) an agent that stimulates development of male genitalia and wolffian duct derivatives and (b) an agent that suppresses müllerian duct derivatives.

Testosterone fulfills the requirements of the first hypothetic agent (16), but it does not accomplish normal müllerian regression. Bruner and Witschi (17) found that both androgens and estrogens stop the growth of the female reproductive tract, but that maturation rather than atrophy of the inhibited structures takes place. Müllerian ducts of mouse male embryos regress when grown in vitro with testes, but they develop further if the testis is not present (18). In the chick embryo, a testicular graft does not produce müllerian regression before the eighth day, regardless of the age of the donor (19). Separate elaboration of the two agents must be postulated to account for the suppression of female structures without masculinization in feminized male pseudohermaphrod-

ites (page 860) and for the normal masculinization without complete suppression of uterus and tubes in masculinized male pseudohermaphrodites (page 860).

The second hormone important in sexual differentiation has been called, at various times, müllerian-inhibiting substance (MIS), müllerian regression factor (MRF), and anti–müllerian hormone (AMH). It is secreted by embryonic testicular Sertoli cells, and inhibits the development of müllerian ducts in the male. An enzyme-linked immunoassay (ELISA) test for MIS was used to investigate infants with intersex states by Harbison and associates (20). They believe that this test is a valuable tool in studying precise genetic error and in making correct clinical diagnoses in intersex states.

Virilization due to excessive androgen production by either the fetus or the mother is another example of an incomplete masculinizing effect.

In summary, the following conclusions may be stated:

1. Genetic (chromosomal) sex is determined at conception.
2. Testis formation depends on the presence of the Y chromosome.
3. Ovary formation depends on the presence of two X chromosomes.
4. Female reproductive structures other than the ovaries will form in the presence of one X chromosome; fetal male structures, on the other hand, will regress.
5. Male reproductive structures other than the testes will

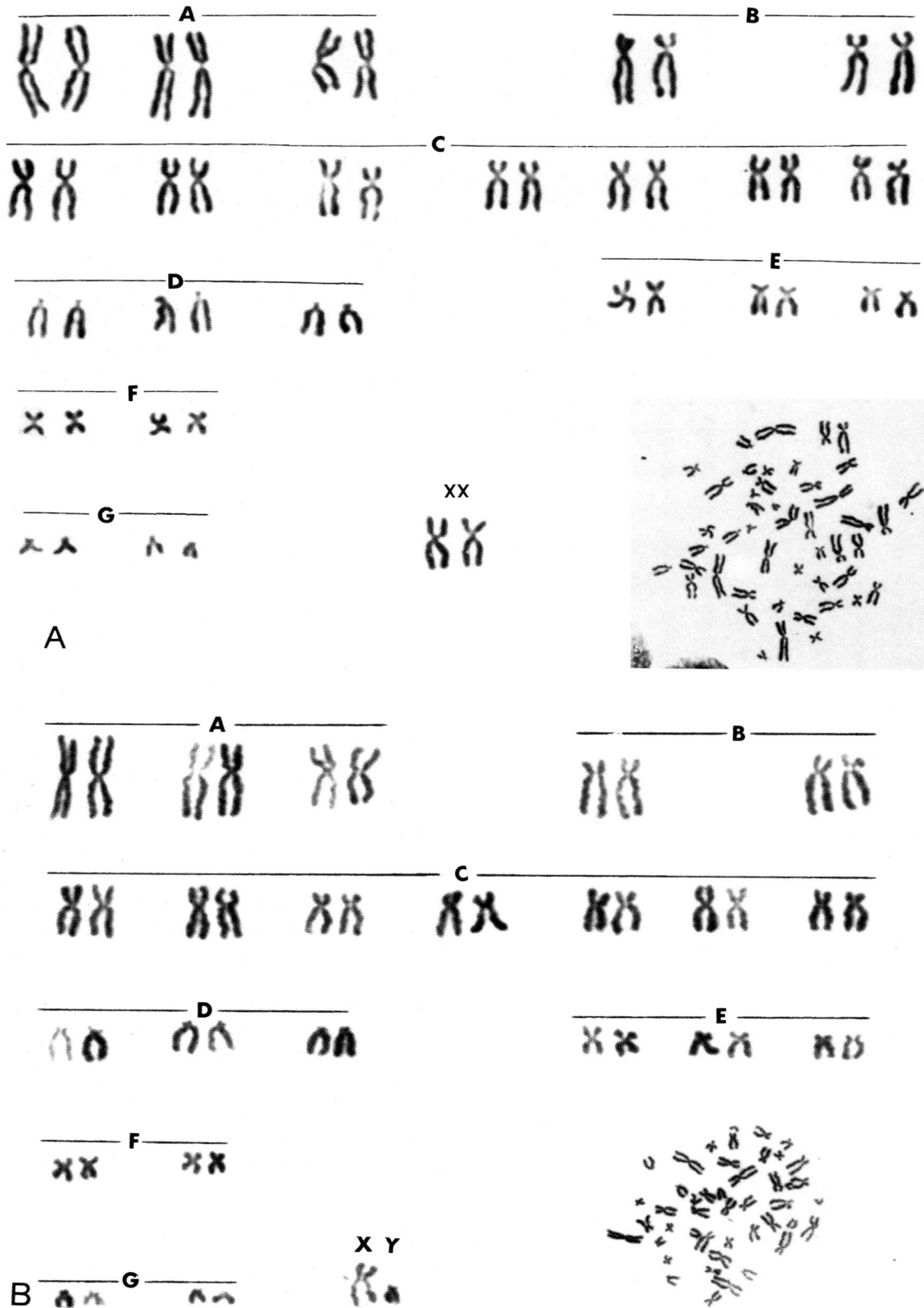

Figure 23.3. **A,** Normal female human chromosome complements. **B,** Normal male chromosome complements. (Courtesy of Dr. Arthur Falek, Division of Human Genetics, Georgia Mental Health Institute, and Department of Psychiatry, Emory University, Atlanta, GA.)

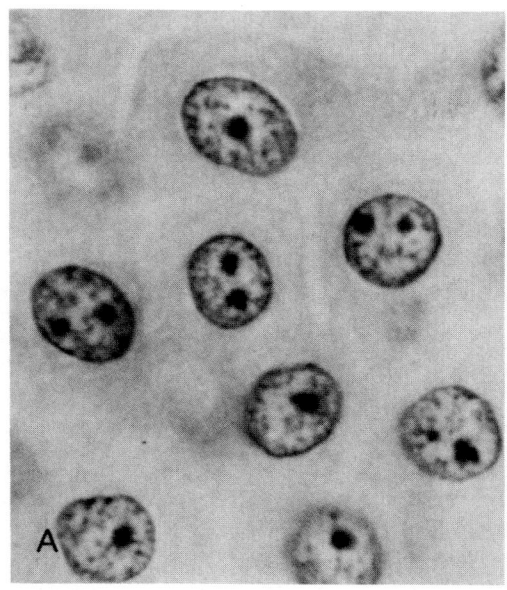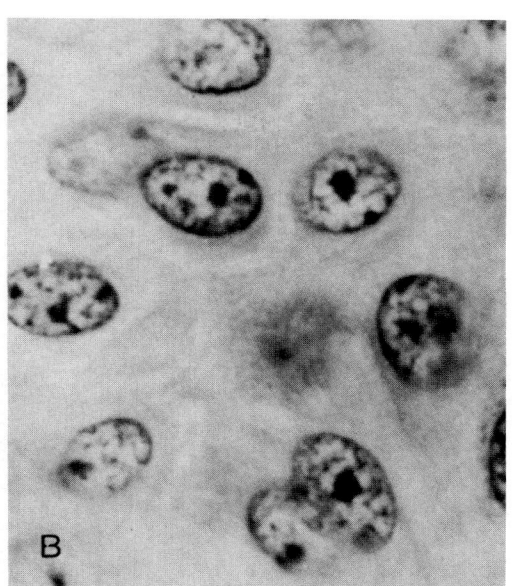

Figure 23.4. Sex chromatin (× 1800). Photomicrographs of sections of skin from a male subject **(A)** and from a female subject **(B).** In nuclei of three cells in **B,** a peripherally placed mass of sex chromatin, the Barr body, may be seen.

(From Bloom W, Fawcett DW. A textbook of histology, 9th ed. Philadelphia: WB Saunders, 1968.)

Table 23.3.
Sex Determination Tables

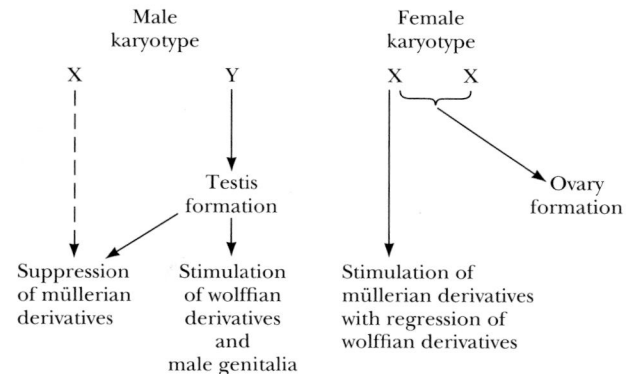

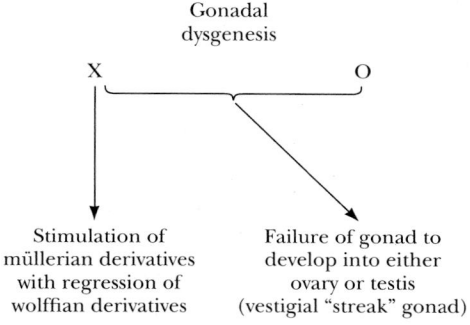

form in the presence of testicular steroid hormones. Female structures will be suppressed in the presence of the testes, presumably by different testicular hormones.

Critical Events in Development

The most critical event in normal sex determination occurs at conception, when the chromosome complement is established. Some errors of sexual development (Turner's and Klinefelter's syndromes) are determined even earlier, during the formation of the gametes themselves. During the first few cleavages of the embryo, mosaicism may lay the foundation for sexual anomalies.

In later embryonic life, disturbances in the development of the suprarenal glands may result in malformed female genitalia. Other genital anomalies associated with apparently normal chromosome patterns and normal suprarenal glands cannot be related to specific times in development.

Reindollar and McDonough (4) reminded their readers that some defects will not be identified until puberty, with perhaps aberrant external maturation or sexual infantility.

ANOMALIES OF SEXUALITY (TABLE 23.4, FIG. 23.5)

Hermaphroditism, Pseudohermaphroditism, and Sexual Ambiguity

Individuals whose sex is in doubt have always attracted attention, both lay and medical. Superstition, mythology,

Table 23.4.
Anomalies of Sexuality

Anomaly	Origin of Defect	First Appearance (or Other Diagnostic Clues)	Sex Chiefly Affected	Relative Frequency	Remarks
Female pseudohermaphrodites of adrenocortical origin					
Congenital suprarenal hyperplasia	Anytime after 3rd month	At birth or later, depending on severity	Female	Uncommon	Genetically determined
Extrinsic androgenic influence	Later half of gestation	At birth	Female	Very rare	From maternal ovarian arrhenoblastoma, or testosterone therapy during pregnancy
Female pseudohermaphrodites of nonsuprarenal origin					
Idiopathic	?	At birth	Female	Very rare	
Nonspecific	4th week or later	At birth	Female	Rare	Associated with severe urogenital anomalies
Male pseudohermaphrodites					
Feminized form	12th week?	At puberty, if at all	Male (but appear female)	Rare?	Genetically determined; may never be recognized
Masculinized form	12th week?	At puberty, if at all	Male	Uncommon?	May never be recognized
True hermaphrodites	Possibly at conception?	At birth or later	?	Rare	Individuals may appear to be of either sex
Klinefelter's syndrome	At conception (genetic)	Undiscovered except when sought for	Male	Uncommon	Associated with sterility
Turner's syndrome	At conception (genetic)	At puberty	Female	Uncommon	Associated with coarctation, Klippel-Feil syndrome and primary amenorrhea with sterility
Noonan's syndrome	At conception (genetic)	In infancy	Male	Rare	Associated with undescended testes, Klippel-Feil syndrome and sterility

and even science have contributed to the mystery and confusion of the subject.

The condition has been known since antiquity, with the term *hermaphrodite* having been used—and perhaps coined—by Theophrastus, who wrote in the fourth century before the Christian era. Young (21), whose 1937 book is a great landmark in the field, includes an illustration of a statue of a reclining nude hermaphrodite of about the same period, attributed to an Athenian named Polycles. Plato (22) in the *Symposium* (speech of Aristophanes) speaks in a comic vein of a primitive hermaphroditic state of man to illustrate the nature of love, but Pliny a few centuries later appears to have accepted the existence of an actual race of "androgyni."

In the modern Greek language of today "androgynos" means husband and wife. In addition, the use of the term *hermaphroditique* at large means an upside down situation, similar to the Greek words *klafsigelos* (cry and laugh) and *tragelafos* (goat and deer).

By "hermaphrodite," the ancient writers meant an individual with the appearance and function of both sexes. Under the influence of platonic idealism, they assumed that such individuals would combine the perfec-

tion and beauty of both. The classic hermaphrodite was not neuter.

The reality, alas, does not conform to the platonic ideal. Far from displaying the attributes of both sexes, most display an ambiguous condition or "intersex," with gradation from slightly masculinized females through slightly feminized males. In addition, there exist functional neuters who are completely without gonads.

CLASSIFICATION OF INDIVIDUALS OF DOUBTFUL SEX

Classifications of the varieties of intersex have been based on anatomic, histologic, cytologic, and psychiatric criteria. Throughout the history of most of these endeavors, investigators have implicitly assumed that the individual must belong to one sex or the other and that the problem is one of identification. In contrast to this, Freud proposed the theory of a dual innate and constitutional sexuality present in all individuals, although each is predominantly masculine or feminine. We shall see that recent discoveries of the presence of more than one karyotype in the same individual (mosaicism) also throws doubt on the theory of a simple dichotomy of sex.

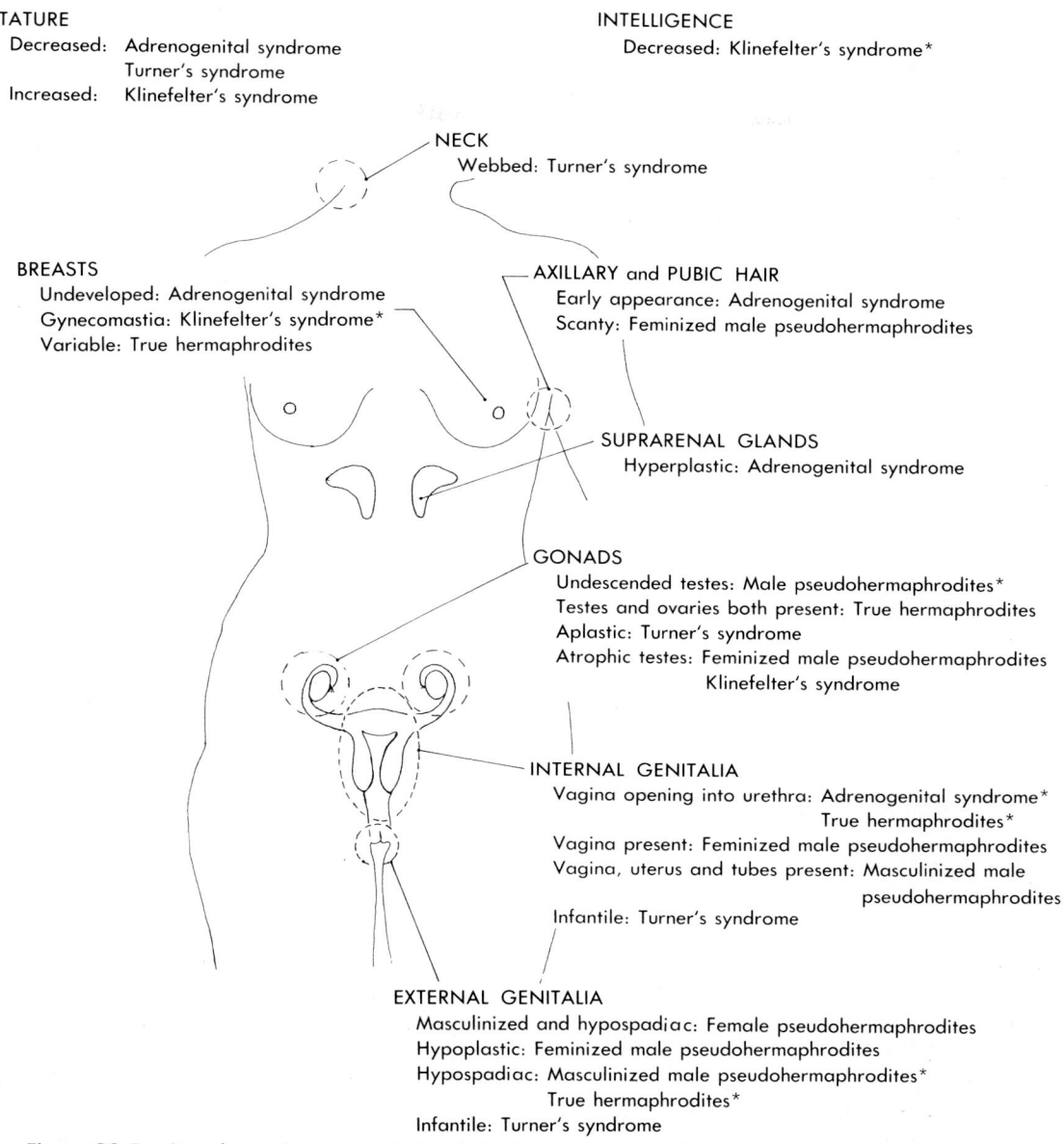

STATURE
  Decreased: Adrenogenital syndrome
              Turner's syndrome
  Increased: Klinefelter's syndrome

INTELLIGENCE
  Decreased: Klinefelter's syndrome*

NECK
  Webbed: Turner's syndrome

BREASTS
  Undeveloped: Adrenogenital syndrome
  Gynecomastia: Klinefelter's syndrome*
  Variable: True hermaphrodites

AXILLARY and PUBIC HAIR
  Early appearance: Adrenogenital syndrome
  Scanty: Feminized male pseudohermaphrodites

SUPRARENAL GLANDS
  Hyperplastic: Adrenogenital syndrome

GONADS
  Undescended testes: Male pseudohermaphrodites*
  Testes and ovaries both present: True hermaphrodites
  Aplastic: Turner's syndrome
  Atrophic testes: Feminized male pseudohermaphrodites
                   Klinefelter's syndrome

INTERNAL GENITALIA
  Vagina opening into urethra: Adrenogenital syndrome*
                               True hermaphrodites*
  Vagina present: Feminized male pseudohermaphrodites
  Vagina, uterus and tubes present: Masculinized male
                                    pseudohermaphrodites
  Infantile: Turner's syndrome

EXTERNAL GENITALIA
  Masculinized and hypospadiac: Female pseudohermaphrodites
  Hypoplastic: Feminized male pseudohermaphrodites
  Hypospadiac: Masculinized male pseudohermaphrodites*
               True hermaphrodites*
  Infantile: Turner's syndrome

Figure 23.5. Sites of anomalies associated with sexual ambiguity. An *asterisk* indicates that the anomaly may or may not be present in a specific syndrome.

The earliest practical classification is that of Klebs (23), who in 1876 divided individuals on the basis of the histology of the gonads and, within groups, on anatomic features. His basic divisions were: male pseudohermaphrodites (with true testes), female pseudohermaphrodites (with true ovaries), and true hermaphrodites (with ovary and testis or with ovotestis).

In this system, pseudohermaphrodites may be further subdivided into internal, external, or complete, depending on what portion of the genital system is in disagreement with the histologic gonadal sex.

With the discovery by Barr and Bertram (24) in 1949 of the sex chromatin in female cat neurons—and eventually in nearly all resting female somatic cells, including blood neutrophils—it became possible to establish a cytologic criterion for determination of sex. More recently, it has become possible to visualize and identify specific sex chromosomes in somatic cells.

Not the least important aspect of the problem of classification is the desire of many clinicians—those who must deal directly with patients and their families, for example—for a simple set of rubrics that will have as few emotional overtones as possible and that will agree with the results which may be expected from surgical recon-

Table 23.5.
Two Classifications for Patients with Abnormalities of Sexual Differentiation.[a]

Original Classification	New Classification
Male pseudohermaphroditism	I. Deletion syndromes without Y cell lines
	II. Deletion syndromes with Y cell lines (45,X/46,XY)[b]
	III. 46,XY
	A. Gonadal dysgenesis (Swyer's sydrome)
	B. Empty pelvis; agonadia[b]
	C. Enzyme deficiencies
	1. 17-Ketoreductase deficiency[b]
	2. 17α-Hydroxylase deficiency[b]
	3. 5α-Reductase deficiency[b]
	D. Testicular feminization
	1. Complete[b]
	2. Incomplete[b]
	E. Nonendocrine/non–sex chromosome defects[b]
	F. 46,XY true hermaphrodite[b]
True hermaphroditism	IV. 46,XX/46,XY true hermaphrodite[b]
Female pseudohermaphroditism	V. 46,XX
	A. 46,XX true hermaphrodite[b]
	B. 46,XX sex reversed male
	C. Congenital adrenal hyperplasia
	1. 21-Hydroxylase deficiency forms[b]
	2. 11β-Hydroxylase deficiency[b]
	3. 3β-Ol-dehydrogenase deficiency[b]
	D. Maternal androgen
	1. Drug[b]
	2. Tumors of pregnancy[b]
	E. Nonendocrine/non–sex chromosome defects[b]
	VI. 47,XXY

[a]From Reindollar RH, McDonough PG. The child with ambiguous genitalia. In Lavery JP, Sanfilipo JS, eds. Pediatric and adolescent obstetrics and gynecology. New York: Springer-Verlag, 1985:38–60.
[b]Syndromes presenting with sexual ambiguity.

struction. We sympathize with this desire for what might be called a "therapeutic classification of intersexuality," but we do not believe it is useful in understanding the condition.

We do not deny the logic of the classification of Reindollar and McDonough (4) who compared the "old" with the "new" philosophy for patients with sexual differentiation (Table 23.5).

There is plenty of merit and logic in both classifications. The student will benefit from the study of both, but we prefer to follow the classification presented in our first edition (Table 23.6).

In the following discussion we divide individuals of ambiguous sex into six groups:

1. Female pseudohermaphrodites (ovaries present), whose condition results from adrenocortical disturbances of fetal, maternal, or extrinsic origin
2. Female pseudohermaphrodites (ovaries present), whose condition is of nonsuprarenal origin
3. Male pseudohermaphrodites (testes present), who may appear either masculine or feminine
4. True hermaphrodites (both ovarian and testicular tissue present)
5. Phenotypic males with defective testes (Klinefelter's syndrome)
6. Phenotypic females with defective ovaries (Turner's syndrome)

Female Pseudohermaphrodites of Adrenocortical Origin
Congenital Suprarenal Hyperplasia (Adrenogenital Syndrome).

The earliest case history is that of a patient born in Naples in 1820, whose complete history and autopsy findings were described by Crecchio (25) in 1865. This history is repeated at some length in Jones and Scott's monograph (15). Crecchio observed the suprarenal hyperplasia but did not recognize its significance. It remained for Apert (26) in 1910, who examined several patients, to notice the constancy of the hyperplasia and suggest the term *hypernephric syndrome.*

The extent of the masculinization depends on the time of onset of the disease. If it occurs early in development, the vagina opens into the urethra at the colliculus seminalis, or, embryologically speaking, both vagina and urethra open into a persistent urogenital sinus. This is the most common form of the anomaly (Fig. 23.6).

If the condition does not arise until later in development, the sinus is reabsorbed as usual, and the vagina and urethra open separately (Fig. 23.6, *A*). Postnatal onset will result in masculinization of secondary sex characteristics but will not affect the genitals.

Table 23.6.
Classification of Individuals of Ambiguous Sex

Type of Sexual Ambiguity	Apparent Sex	Sex Chromatin	Karyotype	Gonad	External Genitalia	Type of Breasts	Menstruation	Usual Time of Discovery	Remarks
Adrenogenital syndrome, female pseudohermaphrodite	Male	Positive	46 (XX)	Ovaries	Penis-like hypospadiac phallus; undescended gonads	Male	No	Infancy	Elevated 17-ketosteroid output; retarded growth after puberty
Nonsuprarenal female pseudohermaphrodite	?	Positive	46 (XX)	Ovaries	May resemble genitalia of adrenogenital syndrome	Female	Yes	Infancy	Other anomalies present, usually urinary and rectal
Feminized male pseudohermaphrodite	Female	Negative	46 (XY)	Atrophic testes	Hypoplastic phallus; cryptorchidism	Male	No	Infancy	Uterus and tubes absent; vagina present
Masculinized male pseudohermaphrodite	Male or ambiguous	Negative	46 (XY)	Testes	Normal, or perineal hypospadias with chordee and cryptorchidism	Male	No	At any age, depending on severity	Uterus and tubes present or rudimentary; vagina normal or shallow; grades into mild hypospadias
True hermaphrodite	Male or female	Positive or negative	Variable	Ovary and testis or ovotestis	Genitalia variable; phallus often hypospadiac	Frequently female	Often	Any age	Vagina normal or opening into urethra
Turner's syndrome (gonadal dysgenesis)	Female	Negative	45 (XO) and variations	Trace of ovaries or none	Infantile female	Male	No	Childhood or puberty	Usually with webbed neck, cubitus valgus and short stature
Klinefelter's syndrome	Male	Positive	47 (XXY) and variations	Atrophic testes	Normal male	Frequent gynecomastia	No	Accidentally, in maturity	Azoospermia; often mental retardation

Regardless of the gross appearance, the gonads are ovaries and are undescended. The female internal organs are well-developed, and the phallus is large, and usually hypospadiac, although occasionally there is a complete penile urethra (27, 28) (Figs. 23.6, *D,* and 23.7).

In late infancy and early childhood, precocious skeletal development and early appearance of pubic hair mark the disease. The early increase in growth rate results in epiphysial closure at a much earlier age than is usual, and the patient remains shorter than the normal adult female. Menarche does not take place, and breast development does not occur. The habitus is usually female or ambigu-

ous. Most untreated individuals live as females, but a few, such as Crecchio's original patient, successfully assume a masculine role.

The suprarenal hyperplasia is marked. Jones (29) found suprarenal glands that weighed up to 90 gm, compared with a normal 5 gm for the same age. This hyperplasia is largely of the adult zona reticularis, which occupies over 50% of the thickness of the cortex. The zona glomerulosa may be reduced in infants with electrolyte imbalance, or it may be normal. The zona fasciculata tends to be reduced, and its lipid content is below normal. The indications at present are that the zona fasciculata is

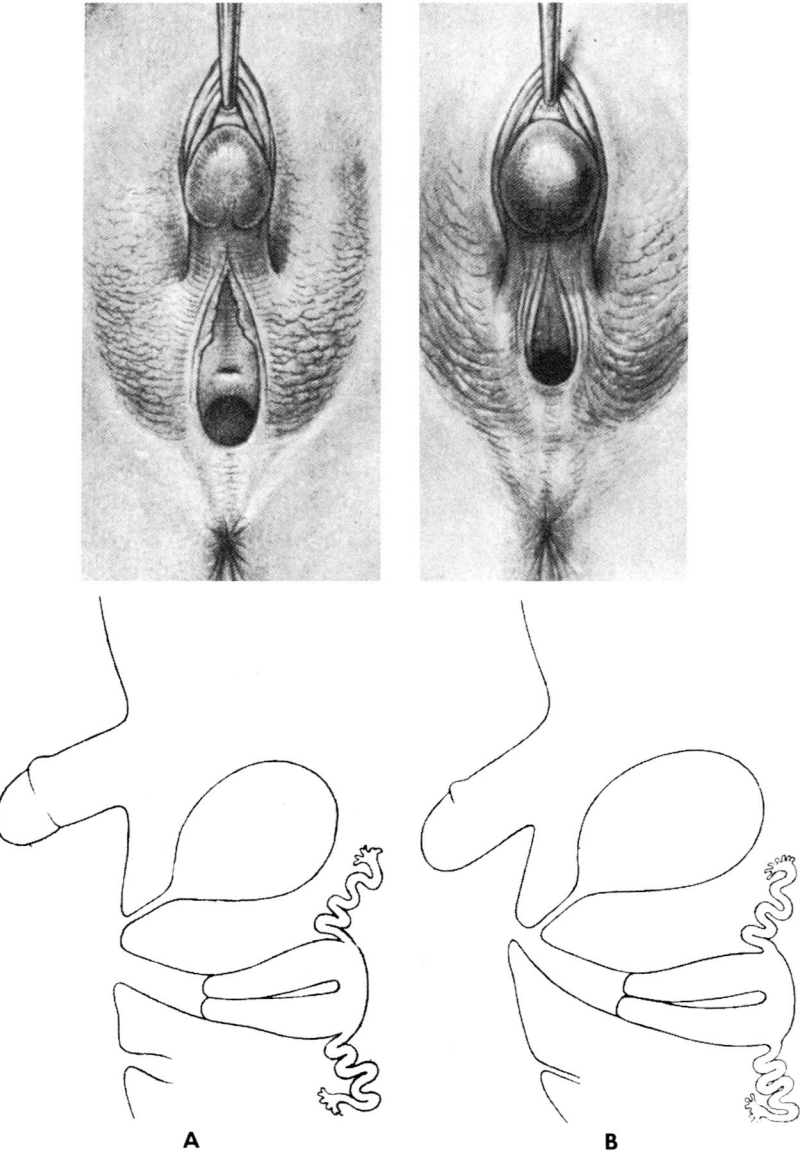

A   **B**

Figure 23.6. The spectrum of masculization of the external genitalia found in female pseudohermaphrodites of adrenocortical origin. Clitoromegaly is present in all. **A,** Minimal labial fusion with separate urethral and vagina orifices. **B** and **C,** Progressive labial fusion forming a funnel-shaped urogenital sinus into which the

unable to synthesize glucocorticoids, and hence, intermediate androgenic steroids accumulate. Pituitary ACTH production rises because it is not inhibited by the presence of glucocorticoids in the blood. The ACTH stimulates the formation of more androsteroids and induces further cortical hyperplasia. These, in turn, suppress pituitary gonadotropin production; hence, no ovarian or uterine cycle takes place (15, 30). The synthesis of androgens by the embryonic suprarenal cortex has been denied by some workers (31).

About 50% of patients with the adrenogenital syndrome show other symptoms of adrenocortical distur-

bance associated with zona glomerulosa deficiency. Vomiting, dehydration, and cyanosis resembling addisonian crises result from electrolyte disturbances with low sodium and high serum potassium levels. This has been termed the *salt-losing* form.

Two other forms of the disease have been described. In one, hypertension is the predominant clinical manifestation; in the other, the infant fails to thrive, and the condition is accompanied by minimal virilization in the female and genital hypoplasia in the male (32). The differences in the adrenocortical biochemistry of these four forms of the disease are outside the scope of this book,

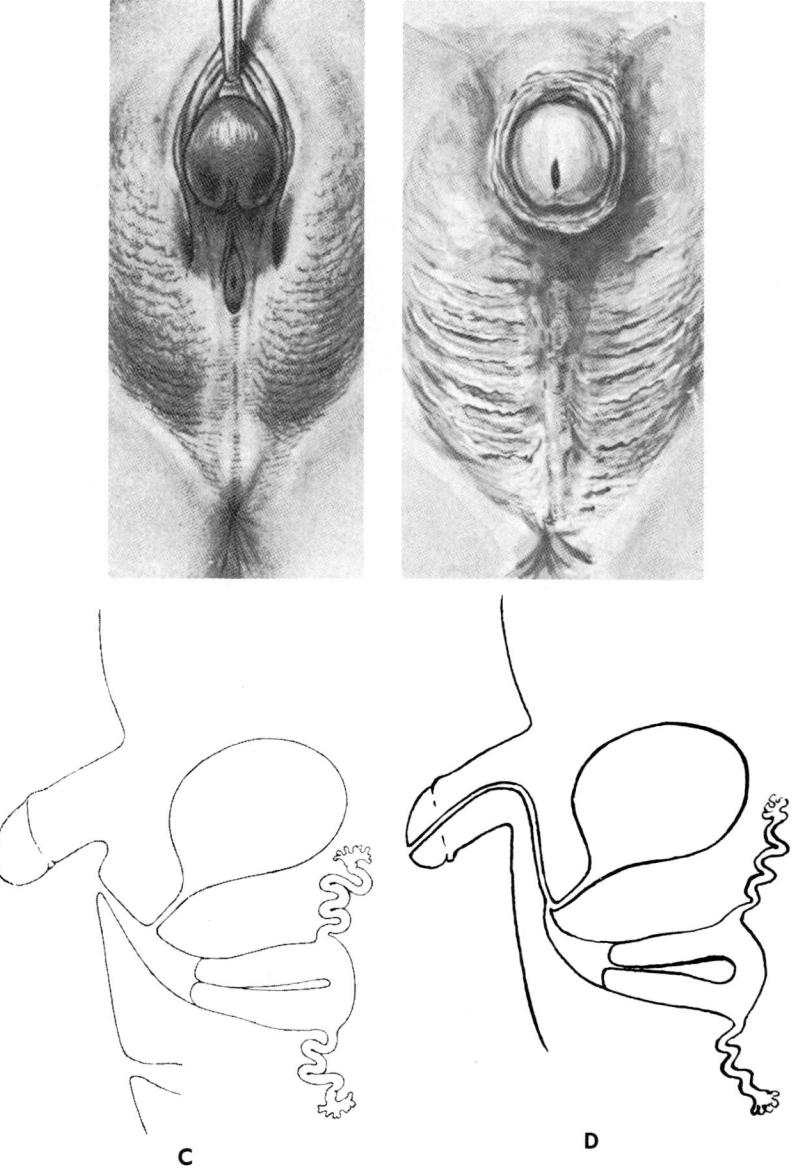

C

D

cervix and urethra open. **D,** Complete masculization, with complete labial fusion and a phallic urethra. (Wilkins L. The diagnosis and treatment of endocrine disor-ders in childhood and adolescence, 3rd ed. Springfield, IL. Charles C. Thomas, 1965.) (**A, C,** From Wilkins 1965; **D,** from Federman 1967.)

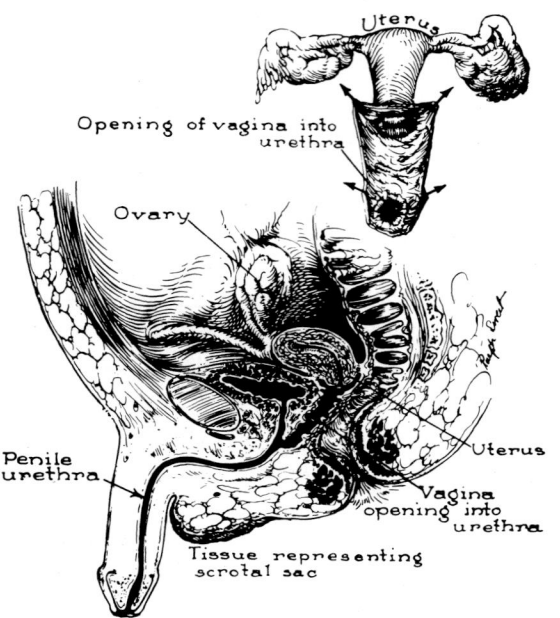

Figure 23.7. Details of internal anatomy of a female pseudohermaphrodite of adrenocortical origin. Internal structures are unequivocally female, but externally, the genitalia exactly duplicate those of a boy with undescended testes. This is the rarest form of the adrenogenital syndrome in the female. (From Bentinck RC et al. Female pseudohermaphroditism with penile urethra, masquerading as precocious puberty and cryptorchidism. J Clin Endocrinol 1956;16:412–418.)

but the interested reader may consult Federman (33) for more details and for a pertinent bibliography.

The adrenogenital syndromes appear to be transmitted as autosomal recessive traits. One of four offspring will be themselves carriers (heterozygous). The simple virilizing form and the salt-losing form are separate but related entities, occurring in different pedigrees (34). No sterility, reduction in family size, or increase in miscarriage rate appears in families with affected offspring. A slight increase in pregnanetriol excretion following ACTH administration has been observed in the parents of patients with the adrenogenital syndrome, but the difference is too small to be diagnostic for heterozygosity (35). The adrenogenital syndrome appeared once in 67,000 births in Maryland, from which Childs et al. (35) estimated that the incidence of heterozygous individuals was about 1:128.

Extrinsic Androgenic Influences.

Effects similar to those of fetal suprarenal hyperplasia may be seen in the female infants of mothers with ovarian arrhenoblastoma (36, 37) and those of mothers who have had testosterone or progestin therapy during pregnancy. Wilkins (38) reviewed 70 such cases in 1960 and observed that this condition should now be of historic interest only.

Female Pseudohermaphrodites of Nonsuprarenal Origin

Idiopathic Group.

This group is composed of a small number of cases in which the condition resembles that produced by the adre-

nogenital syndrome, except that it is not progressive and no suprarenal pathologic condition, either fetal or maternal, can be found. Jones and Scott (15) collected some 16 cases under the rubric "nonvirilized female pseudohermaphrodites."

Nonspecific Group.

This group, originally separated from other types of female pseudohermaphroditism by Carpenter and Potter (30), is distinguished by the presence of other severe congenital malformations, such as renal agenesis, uterine anomalies, and imperforate anus (39). The clitoris is enlarged and the gonads are undescended. This group represents true anomalous, arrested genitalia without masculinization.

Male Pseudohermaphrodites.

Feminized Forms.

These individuals have feminine external genitalia with a shallow vagina. Müllerian derivatives are rudimentary or absent. Breasts usually develop at puberty, but axillary and pubic hair is scanty (40). The testes are abdominal or inguinal and seminiferous tubules are immature, but Leydig cells are present (Fig. 23.8). The karyotype is 46,XY. Morris (41), and Morris and Mahesh (42) characterized these individuals as showing "testicular feminization" and reviewed a large number of cases. In spite of their XY karyotype, some of these patients are attractive women who are happily married. The vagina, although ending blindly, may be of adequate length, and the patient's only complaint is primary amenorrhea and sterility (43).

There is a familial tendency, with about 50% of the male children affected (44). The trait is a sex-linked recessive or a sex-limited autosomal dominant; we cannot make the distinction because the affected individuals are infertile. Transmission is through the mother, who may show decreased body hair or who may have had delayed menarche (45).

Masculinized Forms.

The varieties of masculinized male pseudohermaphrodites do not form a coherent group. Probably all represent chromosomal disorders, but the number and types of these is as yet obscure.

Examples range from individuals with poorly developed male genitalia to apparently normal males, but all have a uterus, tubes, and vagina as well as testes and one or both ductus deferentia (46). Some of these men may be unaware of their anomaly and may marry and beget children; their persistent müllerian derivatives may be discovered only on surgery. Nilson (47) reviewed 35 cases in which the female organs were found in inguinal herniae; he designated this condition "herniae uteri inguinalis of the male." Failure of the testes to descend is not uncommon among these individuals, and the retained testes seem as susceptible to malignant change as do those of cryptorchid males who are otherwise normal (48).

In other individuals, the testes are rudimentary or are

represented by a streak of tissue. These belong to the "mixed gonadal dysgenesis" group of Federman (33). They are usually chromatin negative, but mosaics of karyotypes 45,XO/48,XXXY (49) and 46,XX/45,XO from skin, together with 46,XY/45,XO from blood (50), have been described. Still other mosaic types have been reported (51, 52).

True Hermaphrodites. By definition, a true hermaphrodite possesses both ovarian and testicular tissue. Young (21), accepting only cases with histologic proof, found 20 cases reported from 1900 to 1936. Overzier (53) found 55 cases in 1950, and Merrill and Ramsey (54) collected 114 cases in 1963.

Anatomically, these individuals vary widely. The phallus may resemble a penis or a clitoris and is usually, but not always, hypospadiac. A normal vagina may be present, or it may open into the urethra. Menses may or may not occur, and breasts may be well or poorly developed. Body habitus may be masculine, feminine, or indeterminate. About 66% are phenotypic male.

Young (21) divided the true hermaphrodites into *(a)* lateral hermaphrodites, in whom one gonad was an ovary and the other a testis; *(b)* unilateral hermaphrodites, in whom one gonad was of mixed type; and *(c)* bilateral hermaphrodites, in whom both gonads were mixed. He found the unilateral type to be the most common. In the lateral type, a ductus deferens is present only on the testicular side, and a round ligament only on the ovarian

side. The ovarian and testicular tissues in the ovotestis are not always completely segregated. Bunge and Bradbury (55) showed sections in which oocytes were visible in seminiferous tubules (Fig. 23.9). In a 1963 count (54), there were 22 lateral (more often with the ovaries on the left), 41 unilateral, 26 bilateral, and 25 undetermined cases.

Two reports of true hermaphrodites with XY/XO mosaicism are known (56, 57). In Hirshhorn's (56) patient, the mosaicism was discovered in the bone marrow tissue. Several other examples of XY/XO mosaicism are known (58), but these patients had either rudimentary testes or ovaries and were not hermaphrodites. Most are phenotypically female. The fourth case of mosaicism was said to have XY/XO karyotype in blood cells and XX/XO karyotype in the skin. One ovary and one testis were present, but both a ductus deferens and a uterine tube were present on each side (50).

Federman (33) collected cytologic reports on 37 hermaphrodites. Seventeen had a 46,XX pattern, but in most cases only blood cells were examined. Two had a 46,XY complement and three were mosaics of 46,XX/46,XY, which one might intuitively expect to be the usual situation (59). Eight were mosaics of a variety of karyotypes.

An interchange of chromosomal material between the X and the Y chromosomes during meiosis leaves the possibility that one X chromosome of an XX hermaphrodite might contain the genes of the normal Y chromosome (60). Double fertilization of an ovum and its polar body,

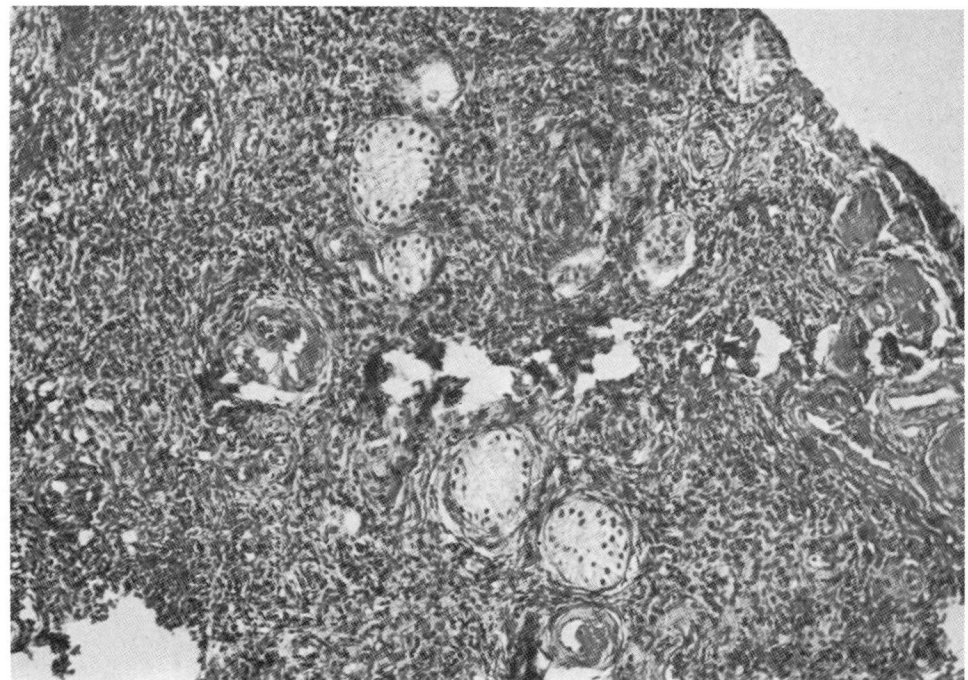

Figure 23.8. *Feminized male pseudohermaphroditism. Section of testis from an adult patient with female habitus, breasts with little glandular tissue, and a shallow, blind vagina. The testes were undescended and had a few immature seminiferous tubules and abundant Leydig cells. No trace of follicle formation is evident. (From Federman DD. Abnormal sexual development: a genetic and endocrine approach to differential diagnosis. Philadelphia: WB Saunders, 1967.)*

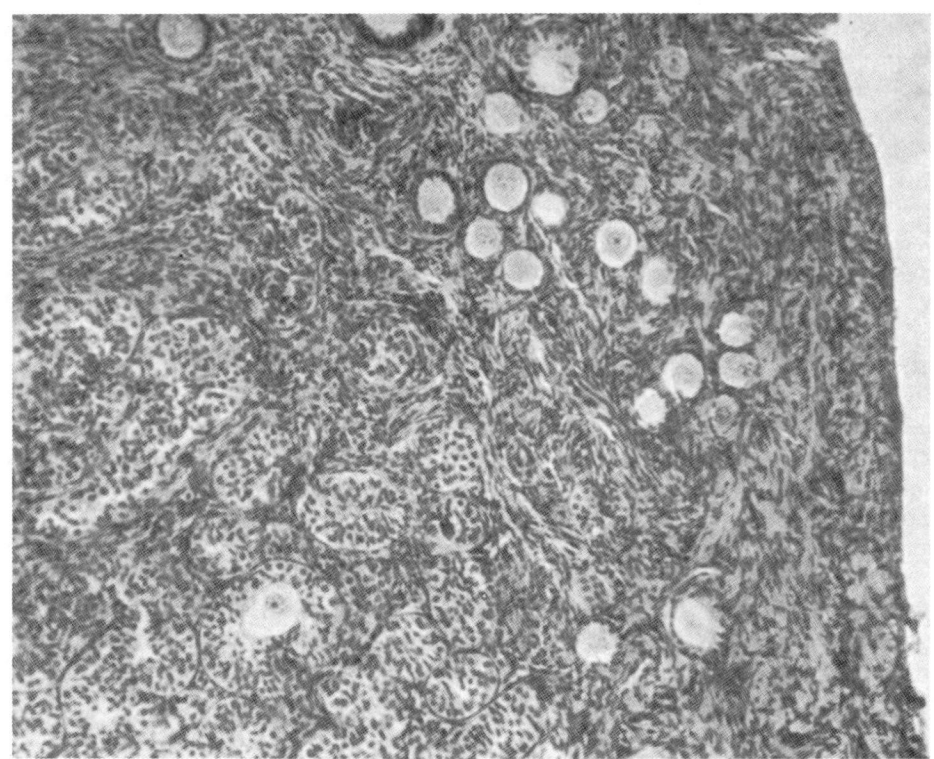

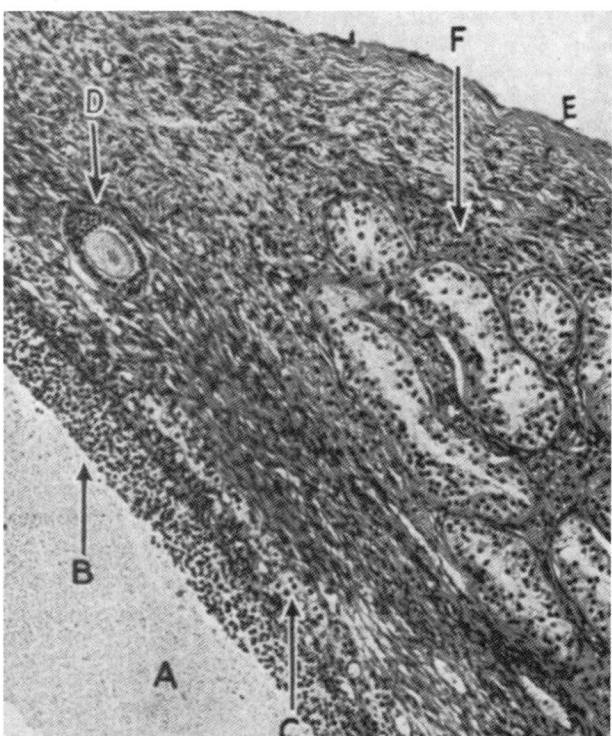

Figure 23.9. True hermaphroditism. Two sections through ovotestes. **Top,** Section showing intermingled ovarian and testicular tissue. An oocyte clearly occupies the lumen of a seminiferous tubule at the lower left. **Bottom,** Section from the gonad of an 18-year-old patient with female habitus. *A,* Central cavity of a mature Graffian follicle; *B,* granulosa cells; *C,* theca layer; *D,* small ovarian follicle with normal ovum; *E,* germinal epithelium at surface of ovary; *F,* seminiferous tubules with mature sperm and interstitial cells. **Top,** From Bunge RG, Bradbury JT. Oocytes in seminiferous tubules. II. A case report of bilateral ovotestes. J Clin Endocrinol 1959;19:1661–1666; **Bottom,** from Brewer JI et al. True hermaphroditism. JAMA 1952;148:431–435.)

with the subsequent contribution of both to form a genetically mosaic embryo, has been suggested (61). Gartler and his colleagues (62) described a phenotypic female with an ovary and an ovotestis, an XX/XY chromosome complement, and heterochromia iridis. They interpreted these findings—together with blood group studies—as the result of double fertilization of two egg nuclei by two genetically different sperm.

Most recently the search for an exact locus on the chromosome for testis determination (testis-determining factor, or TDF), has been identified in the sex-determining region on the short arm of the Y chromosome (SRY). Analysis of SRY in true hermaphrodite patients has led to some confusion about its role, or at least its place as the sole determining factor for testis determination. Tho et al (63) failed to find the SRY locus in five patients with 46,XX true hermaphroditism, despite the presence of biopsy-proven testicular tissue. Conversely, 22 of 24 individuals with 45,X/46,XY mosaicism tested positive for SRY. In a study from Paris only three of thirty patients with 46,XX true hermaphroditism were found to have the SRY locus (64). Autosomal or X-linked mutations elsewhere in the sex-determining pathway were thought to be possible explanations for the phenotype observed in the 27 SRY-negative cases. This concept was supported by the work of Berkovitz and associates from Johns Hopkins, whose analysis of five subjects with 46,XX and true hermaphroditism demonstrated that this condition is a genetically heterogeneous condition, with some subjects having TDF sequences but most not (65). The 46,XX subjects without SRY were thought to have a mutation of an autosomal gene that permits testicular determination in the absence of TDF.

Phenotypic Males with Defective Testes (Klinefelter's Syndrome). Though this syndrome (as such) was first described in 1942 by Klinefelter and his colleagues (66), its occurrence can be traced as far back as 1812. It has been called "testicular dysgenesis," "primary microorchidism," "medullary gonadal dysgenesis," and "chromatin-positive microorchidism." The components of the syndrome are: *(a)* small testes with hyalinization of the seminiferous tubules and normal Leydig cells; *(b)* azoospermia; and *(c)* high urinary gonadotropin (FSH) output (67).

Extensive efforts have recently been made to quantitate the exact histologic abnormality found in the testes of patients with Klinefelter's syndrome (68). Gynecomastia is common, and mental retardation is not infrequent. Although the syndrome may be recognized before puberty by the small testes, gynecomastia, and mental dullness (69), it is usually detected later in life, often during examination for infertility.

The testes are small (1 to 2 cm), and the number of Leydig cells appears to be increased as a result of the decrease in tubular tissue. Ejaculation is normal, but the ejaculate is without spermatozoa. That these individuals are not physiologically eunuchoid is suggested by the report of a patient with benign prostatic hypertrophy, a condition that does not occur in eunuchs (70). The endocrinologic aspects of Klinefelter's syndrome are still obscure. Yet, the association of such genital abnormalities as partial penoscrotal transposition (71) and cryptorchidism with chordee (72) suggest that there might be some disordered hormonal production during embryogenetic genital development.

Patients with Klinefelter's syndrome may have a predisposition for the development of neoplasia, particularly extragonadal germ-cell tumors. Hasle and colleagues (73) reported the association of a mediastinal germ cell tumor with Klinefelter's syndrome and reviewed the literature. Dysmorphic supracellar tumors were found in two patients with Klinefelter's syndrome by Hamed et al (74). One of the two had bilateral optic atrophy and decreased vision.

In 1956 Plunkett and Barr (75) described sex chromatin-positive cells in patients with Klinefelter's syndrome and suggested, among other possibilities, that this might indicate the presence of an extra X chromosome. Three years later Jacobs and Strong (76) found 47 chromosomes in cells from patients with Klinefelter's syndrome, rather that the normal 46. The karyotype was 47,XXY. In addition, patients have been found with 48,XXYY (77); 48,XXXY (78, 79), and 49,XXXYY (80), as well as with mosaic chromosome complements of 46,XX/47,XXY, 46,XY/47,XXY, 47,XXY/48,XXXY, and 48,XXXY/49,XXXXY (80–89).

A "Klinefelter personality" has begun to emerge with the increasing numbers of patients being discovered. The limited intelligence is associated with low ambition and continual failure to persist in school, job, or marriage. Excessive talkativeness is common. Increasing severity of mental retardation and testicular damage appears to be related to the increasing number of X chromosomes. On the other hand, individuals with Klinefelter's syndrome as well as those with the XYY and XXYY complements seem to show aggressive, often delinquent behavior (85, 86). A plea for early detection of this abnormality is made by Mandoki and Sumner, who believe that many of the developmental, behavioral, and emotional problems associated with an additional X chromosome are amenable to psychiatric, endocrinologic, and surgical treatment (87).

In an examination of the oral mucosa of 1911 male infants born in Winnipeg, Moore (88) found five with sex chromatin-positive nuclei or about 1:400 males (0.26%). Ferguson-Smith (69) found an incidence of 1.2% among 663 mentally handicapped male children in Glasgow. In neither series was sex chromatin reversal seen in females.

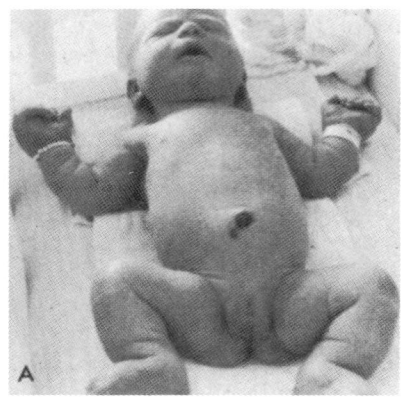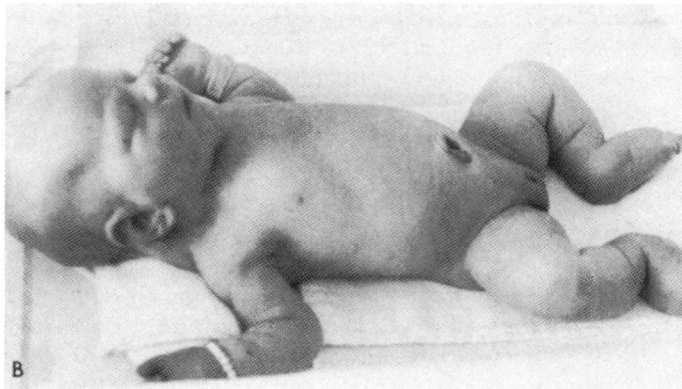

Figure 23.10. Female infant with Turner's syndrome. Note the webbed neck. The edema of the hands and feet is transitory. (From Mehan DJ. The role of the urologist in the evaluation and treatment of patients with ambiguous external genitalia. Southern Med J 1963;56:828–833.)

A survey of over 70,000 U.S. Air Force recruits gave an incidence of 1:3600 men (89), a figure much lower than that suggested by the Winnipeg data. However, the low frequency of mentally defective persons among military recruits may account for the lower incidence of Klinefelter's syndrome in that population.

It cannot yet be said with certainty that all infants with this condition will grow up to be sterile. An allegedly fertile male with Klinefelter's syndrome has been reported (90). However, certain studies of male infertility suggest that more than 10% of azoospermic males may be chromatin positive (33).

A few patients with the clinical picture of Klinefelter's syndrome have the chromatin-negative (male) type of nuclei. They have been designated as having "false Klinefelter's syndrome," "chromatin-negative Klinefelter's syndrome," or "Del Castillo syndrome" (91). In some of these patients spermatogenesis may occur. Mothers of both chromatin-positive and chromatin-negative Klinefelter's syndrome patients tended to be significantly older than mothers of normal children (92). Simpson (93) reported that, during gametogenesis, maternal and paternal nondisjunction with abnormal karyotypes was documented by Xq blood typing.

Phenotypic Females with Defective Ovaries (Turner's Syndrome). In 1749 Morgagni (94) dissected the body of a woman with ovarian dysgenesis and described the typical characteristics of Turner's syndrome. The woman was very small, the external genitalia were infantile, and the vagina was rudimentary and without rugae. The uterus was smaller than that of an infant's, and the cervix was larger than the fundus. The tubes were normal, but there was no trace of ovaries. Morgagni failed to mention only the underdeveloped and widely spaced breasts.

The syndrome, as originally described by Turner (95) in 1938, was characterized by primary amenorrhea, webbed neck, cubitus valgus, and short stature (Fig. 23.10). Because the somatic anomalies had earlier been noted by Ullrich (96), his name is sometimes also given to the syndrome. Sharpey-Schafer (97) in 1941 associated the syndrome with ovarian dysgenesis, and in 1954 Polani and his colleagues (98) showed that such women were chromatin negative and suggested they had only 45 chromosomes. This was confirmed in 1959 by Ford and his colleagues (99). Since that time "Turner's syndrome" has been used to designate phenotypic females who lack one sex chromosome (45,XO). Somatic anomalies without ovarian dysgenesis may also occur with normal sex chromosome, but with triplication (trisomy) of autosome 18 (47,XX,E18+). This condition is now called "Edward's syndrome." Women with this condition are fertile and can transmit the somatic stigmata to their offspring (100). The relationship between sex chromosome constitution and phenotype in these patients was reviewed by Morishima and Grumbach (101).

There is some evidence that deletion of the short arm of one X chromosome results in the phenotype of Turner's syndrome. When the long arm is deleted, normal stature with streak gonads and no other anomalies are seen (102). Three related syndromes may thus be distinguished (103).

In women with Turner's syndrome, the external genitalia are infantile, but the clitoris is enlarged. The labia do not become pigmented. The vagina is short, and the uterus and tubes are hypoplastic, but there is no unusual persistence of wolffian duct derivatives. The gonads may

Table 23.7.
Chromosomal Syndromes

Syndrome	Gonads	Typical Somatic Anomalies
Turner's	Streak	Present
Edward's	Normal	Present
"Pure" gonadal dysgenesis	Streak	Absent

have a few primary follicles, or they may be represented by wavy connective tissue (streak ovaries) in the broad ligament (Fig. 23.11). Gonadotropin excretion is normal or high, and 17-ketosteroid excretion is low.

While as a rule the gonads are represented by a connective tissue streak, oogonia have been seen (104), menstruation has been reported (105, 106), and in one case a woman with XO karyotype produced a child (13).

Familial Turner's syndrome has been reported in mosaics (107) and in association with a deletion of the short arm of the X chromosome (108). In the former, phenotypic implications of the cytogenetic findings in the patients are discussed, and literature data on fertility in Turner's syndrome is reviewed. Researchers at Boston Children's Hospital (109) reported on the absence of

"Turner" stigmata in a 46,XYp-female with streak gonads and a large deletion of the Yp chromosome which included chromosomal gene SRY. The patient did not display any Turner's syndrome stigmata, such as webbing of the neck or cardiac or other abnormalities. The findings were thought to be consistent with a role for SRY in testis differentiation in humans.

Most patients are short in stature, with a webbed neck and a low hairline. Fusion of cervical vertebrae may occur (110). These signs are also those of the Klippel-Feil syndrome, which occurs in both sexes and which is not necessarily associated with primary amenorrhea in the female. We reviewed the published cases of the Klippel-Feil syndrome elsewhere (111) and believe that chromosome examination of female patients with these cervical

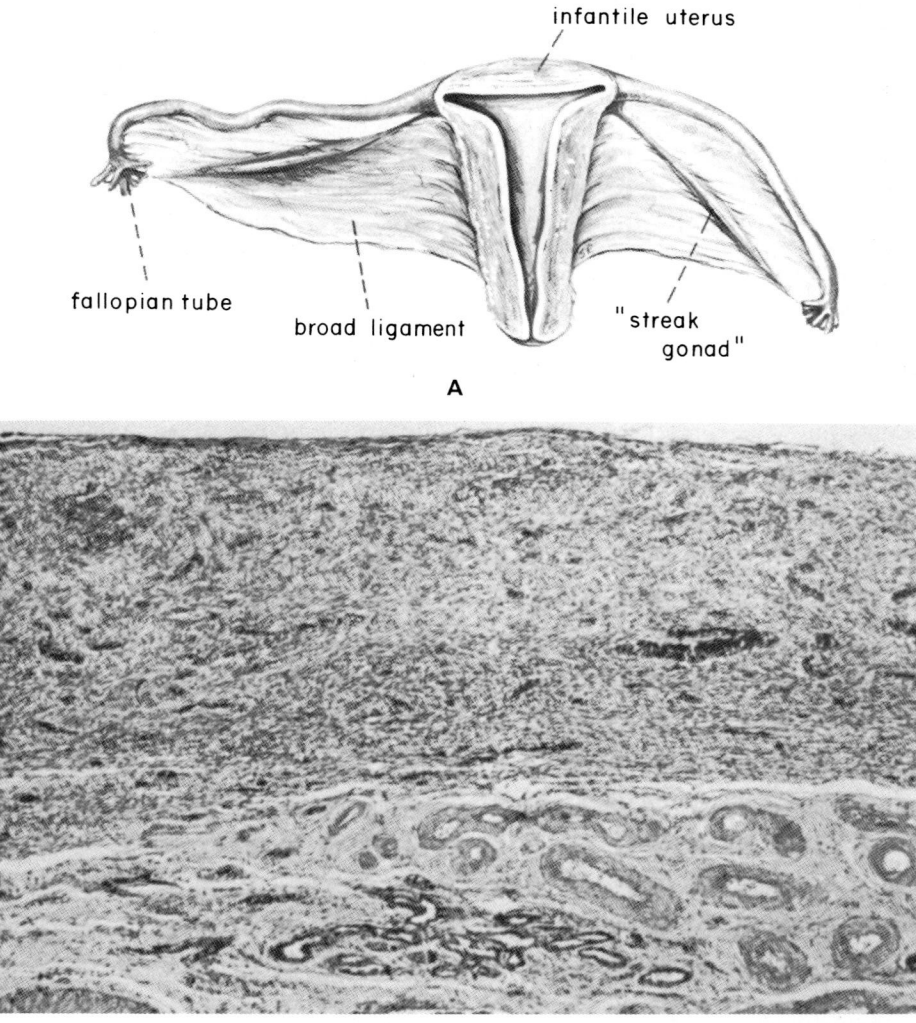

Figure 23.11. Turner's syndrome, gonadal dysgenesis. **A,** The internal genitalia, showing the infantile uterus and the "streak" gonads. **B,** Section through the "streak" gonad. The connective tissue suggests the theca of follicles, but no follicles, cells, or ova are present. The darker staining structures perhaps represent rete tubules. (From Federman DD. Abnormal sexual development: a genetic and endocrine approach to differential diagnosis. Philadelphia: WB Saunders, 1967.)

vertebral defects would show that many, but not all, were chromatin negative.

An altered angle between carpal and metacarpal bones has been reported (112) and bony changes similar to osteoporosis have been observed (110). Coarctation of the aorta and red-green color blindness frequently accompany Turner's syndrome; also, renal malformations, usually horseshoe kidney or anomalies of rotation, occur in about 25% of cases (113–116). Oral anomalies have been described (117). Unlike patients with Klinefelter's syndrome, those with Turner's syndrome do not seem to be mentally retarded. Pigmented nevi may appear in childhood and suggest the diagnosis.

In addition to the XO karyotype, mosaics have been reported, some of which show Turner's syndrome (118). Harden and Jacobs (84) list 45,XO/46,XY, 45,XO/46,XX, and 45,XO/47,XYY as having been found. A mosaic 45,XO/46,XX was a typical case of Turner's syndrome (119). The individuals with 45,XO/46,XY (52, 120), 45,XO/49,XXXXY (49), and XO/XxY (51) were male pseudohermaphrodites, while 46,XX/47,XY/45,XO (50) was a true hermaphrodite.

Unilateral gonadal agenesis (streak ovary) with a contralateral testis in phenotypic females with 45,XO/46,XY karyotype has been reported by Greenblatt and his colleagues (121), who suggest that these patients represent a link between Turner's syndrome and male pseudohermaphroditism. This is the "mixed gonadal dysgenesis" of Federman (33).

Growth hormone treatment of short stature in Turner's syndrome patients has been promising (122). In combination with anabolic steroids, studies show a synergistic effect that does not cause an undue increase in bone age. Rosenfeld and associates reported the results of treatment of a large number of girls with karyotype-proven Turner's syndrome with human growth hormone (hGH) alone or combined with oxandrolone (123). When compared with the anticipated growth rate in untreated patients, the growth rate after treatment with hGH, both alone and in combination with oxandrolone, showed a sustained increase for at least 6 years. The authors concluded that therapy with hGH alone or in combination with oxandrolone, can result in a sustained increase in growth rate and a significant increase in adult height for most prepubertal girls with Turner's syndrome. Similar good results in the treatment of short stature with the use of recombinant hGH were reported from a multicenter study (124).

Noonan's Syndrome in the Male.
In 1943 before the discovery of the chromosomal aberration, Flavell (125) described a young man with gonadal infantilism, short stature, cubitus valgus, and webbed neck. Through 1968 about 100 cases appeared in the literature (126–131). Clinical details of 151 individuals with Noonan's syndrome were recently reported (132). Polyhydramnios complicated one-third of the pregnancies. Common cardiac anomalies included pulmonic stenosis and hypertrophic cardiomyopathy, with a normal echocardiogram present in only 12.5% of all cases. Significant feeding difficulties during infancy were present in three-fourths. The children were short and underweight but with median head circumferences. Motor depression, abnormal vision, and abnormal hearing were common; however, most were attending normal primary or secondary schools. Other associations included undescended testicles in over three-fourths, hepatosplenomegaly in one-half, and evidence of abnormal bleeding in many.

The testes are hypoplastic and often are undescended; pubic and axillary hair are scanty. Leydig cells may be absent (128). Skeletal anomalies are common and at least four patients have had cervical vertebral defects that would assign them to the Klippel-Feil syndrome as we have described it (111). Mental retardation and cardiovascular defects, including coarctation of the aorta, are common.

All cases examined have been chromatin negative, and in at least nine cases the karyotype was determined to be 46,XY, as in normal males (117, 133). This implies that the somatic characters of Turner's syndrome may be carried on autosomes.

It is well known that patients with Turner's syndrome have 45,X karyotype; mosaicism; and 45,X cell line and 46,X,i (Xq) or 46XX.

However, Reindollar and McDonough (4) believe that the most important factor is the deletion of the X-located ovarian genes.

ORIGIN OF ANOMALIES OF PRIMARY SEX DETERMINATION

We have seen (page 856) that sexual ambiguity may arise from either hormonal imbalance in embryonic life or from chromosomal aberrations at conception. Most female pseudohermaphrodites clearly are examples of the effect of excess adrenocortical hormones. Women with Turner's syndrome are likewise the victims of abnormal chromosome distribution at conception. In many other intersexual states, however, the relative roles of hormones and chromosomes are not clear.

Aberrations of sex chromosomes are of two kinds. In one, there is an addition or a deletion of sex chromosomes throughout the cells of the body. The individual has a single but abnormal karyotype. In the other kind, cells from different parts of the body may be of different karyotypes; one, and frequently both, of which are abnormal. These individuals are said to be mosaics.

Aberrations of the first type originate not in the cells of the affected individuals but in the gonads of the parents before conception.

Meiotic nondisjunction during spermatogenesis

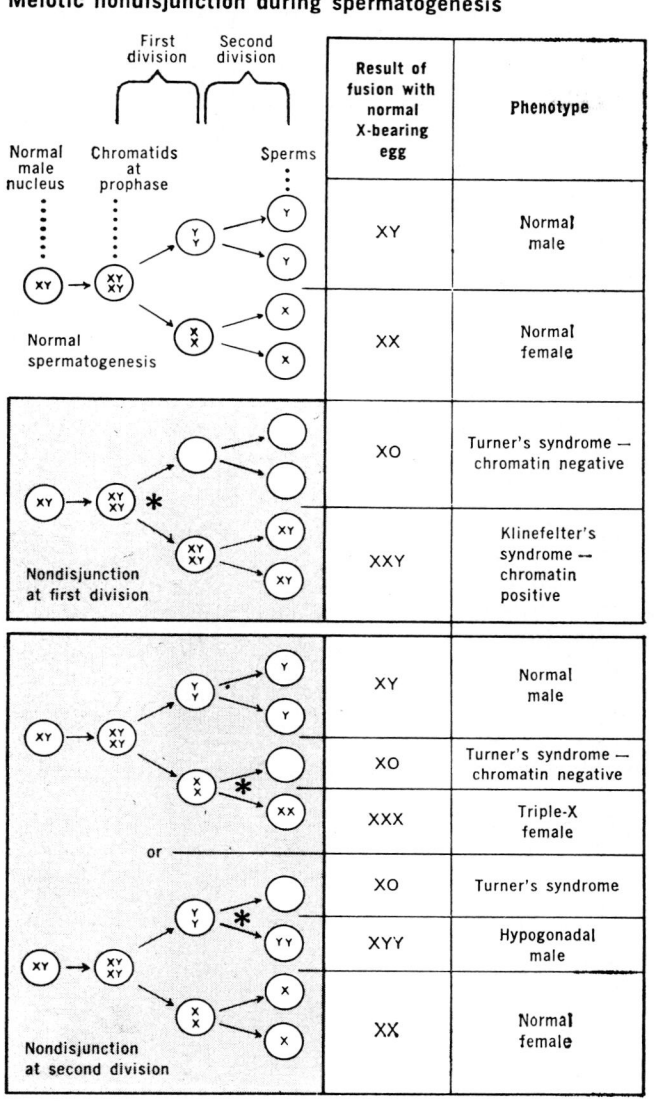

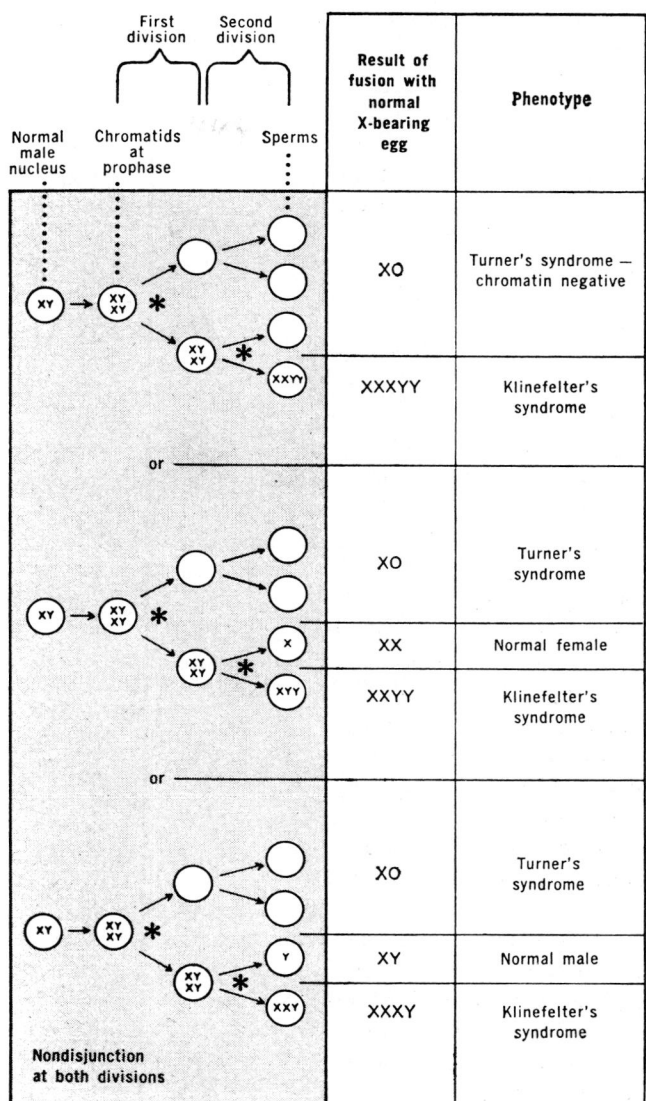

*point of nondisjunction

*point of nondisjunction

Figure 23.12. The effects of nondysjunction during spermatogenesis, assuming union with a normal ovum. (Courtesy of Mrs. Audrey Bishop. From Gordon RR. et al. Chromosome abnormalities. Modern Med 1963;31:104–114.)

The specific error is the failure of chromosomes to separate (nondisjunction) and move toward opposite poles of the spindle during either or both of the meiotic divisions of gametogenesis. As a result, of the ova or sperm that are produced, some have two, three, or four sex chromosomes, and some have none. It was thought at first that nondisjunction during spermatogenesis would account for the observed anomalous karyotypes (Fig. 23.12), but with the discovery of karyotypes such as XXXX, it became apparent that the ovum must also be involved.

Assuming abnormal sex chromosome complements in either of both gametes, there are 91 possible karyotypes among the resulting zygotes, as shown in Table 23.8. Two are, of course, normal; six others cancel out their deletions or additions to produce XX or XY zygotes with one sex chromosome from each parent (N). In seven other combinations (n), both sex chromosomes come from a single parent but form a normal complement. Twelve, with YY, YO, and OO karyotypes, are lethal. Nine other karyotypes may exist but have not been seen. Ten combinations will result in an XO (Turner's syndrome) karyotype or XXXY (Klinefelter's syndrome) karyotype. In 16 combinations, superfemales (XXX+) will be formed, and in four, supermales (XYY, XXYY). This distribution does not, of course, represent the actual frequency of occur-

Table 23.8.
Results of Chromosomal Nondisjunction During Gametogenesis

Meiosis	Normal		1 or 2			3		
	Egg Sperm	X	XX	O	XXX	X	XXXX	O
Normal	X	N	sf	t	sf	N	sf	t
	Y	N	k	L	K	N	k	L
1	XY	k	k	n	k	k	?	n
	O	t	n	L	sf	t	sf	L
2	XX	sf	sf	n	sf	sf	?	n
	YY	sm	k	L	k	sm	?	L
	O	t	n	L	sf	t	sf	L
3	XXY	k	k	k	?	k	?	k
	Y	N	k	L	k	N	k	L
	XYY	k	k	sm	k	k	?	sm
	X	N	sf	t	sf	N	sf	t
	XXYY	k	?	k	?	k	?	k
	O	t	n	L	sf	t	sf	L

Key:
1, Nondisjunction at first meiotic division.
2, Nondisjunction at second meiotic division.
3, Nondisjunction at first and second meiotic divisons.
N, XX, XY; normal complement, one sex chromosome from each parent, 1 ♂ :1 ♀.
n, XX, XY; normal complement, both sex chromosomes from one parent,
  2 ♂ :5 ♀.
k, XXY, XXYY, XXXY, XXXYY, XXXXY, XXXXYY; Klinefelter's syndrome
sf, XXX → XXXXX; "super females."
t, XO; Turner's syndrome.
sm, XYY; "super males."
?, Not reported, various karyotypes; possibly lethal.
L, YY, YO, OO; probably lethal.

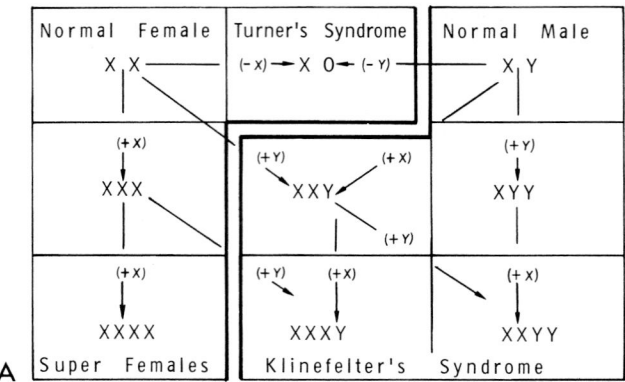

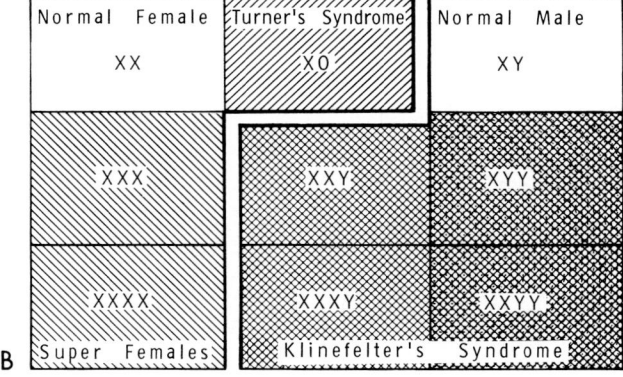

Figure 23.13. **A,** Additions and deletions to the normal male or female sex chromosome complements. The complements to the left of the *heavy line* are phenotypically female; those to the right are phenotypically male. **B,** Some of the major effects of altered sex chromosome complements. Intelligence tends to decrease with added sex chromosomes. (**A,** Modified from Federman DD. Abnormal sexual development: a genetic and endocrine approach to differential diagnosis. Philadelphia: WB Saunders, 1967.)

rence of these anomalies; XXY and XO are the most common.

A general pattern of the effects of sex chromosome anomalies may be seen in Figure 23.13. The deletion of one sex chromosome (whether X or Y) results in an infertile, short, phenotypic female (XO). The addition of X chromosomes to the normal female complement (XX) reduces intelligence but affects neither stature nor fertility. The addition of X chromosomes to the normal male complement (XY) reduces intelligence but affects neither stature nor fertility, while the addition of extra Y chromosomes reduces intelligence and fertility and increases stature.

Aberrations of the second type result from errors in one or more mitoses at early cleavage of the fertilized ovum. As in meiosis, nondisjunction of sex chromosomes may occur in mitosis. The result is an individual with two cell lineages of differing karyotypes. If an X chromosome in a female is involved, the result is an XO, and an XXX cell line. If a Y chromosome in a male is involved, an XO and an XYY cell line results. Nondisjunction of an X chromosome in a male does not produce mosaicism; only the XXY line survives since the YO cells are not viable. If the nondisjunction takes place during the second or later cleavage divisions, there will be normal cell line in addi-

tion, giving a triple mosaicism: XX/XO/XXX. See Table 23.9 for the mechanisms producing these mosaics.

In addition to nondisjunction, one chromosome may lag behind the others at anaphase. Such a chromosome will be lost at telophase, resulting in a chromosome deletion in one of the two daughter cells. In this case only two cell lineages will result, whether the anaphase lag takes place in the first or in subsequent cleavage divisions. If the single X chromosome of the male is lost, the YO cell line will disappear; if the zygote survives, all cells will be

Table 23.9.
Production of Mosaicism Following Nondisjunction of Sex Chromosomes in Early Cleavage of the Ovum

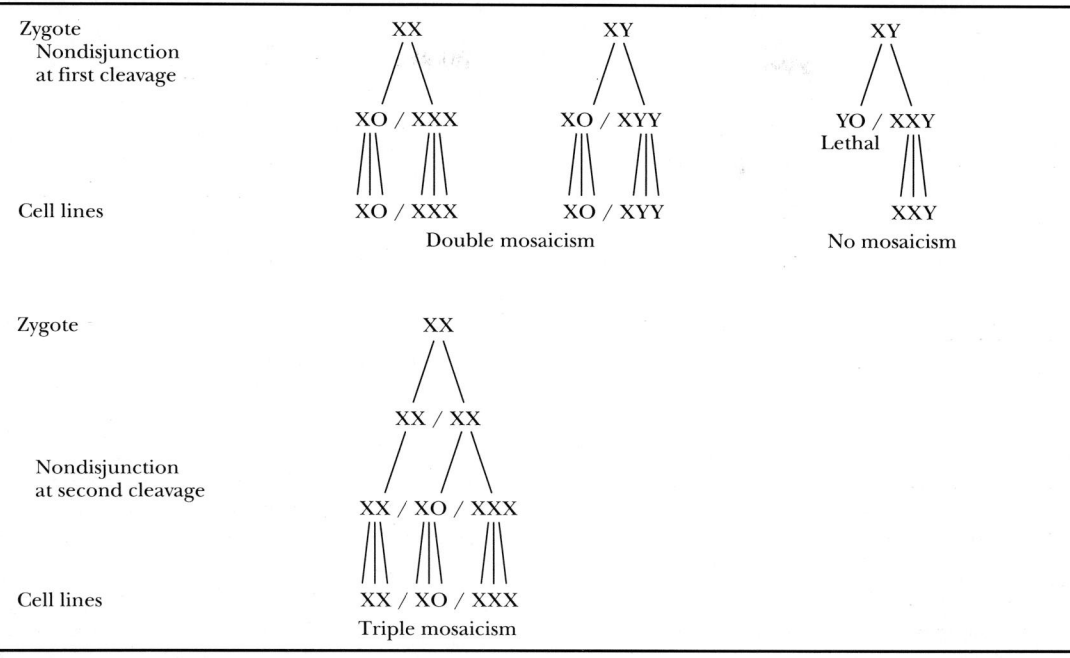

Table 23.10.
Production of Mosaicism Following Anaphase Lag of a Sex Chromosome in Early Cleavage of the Ovum

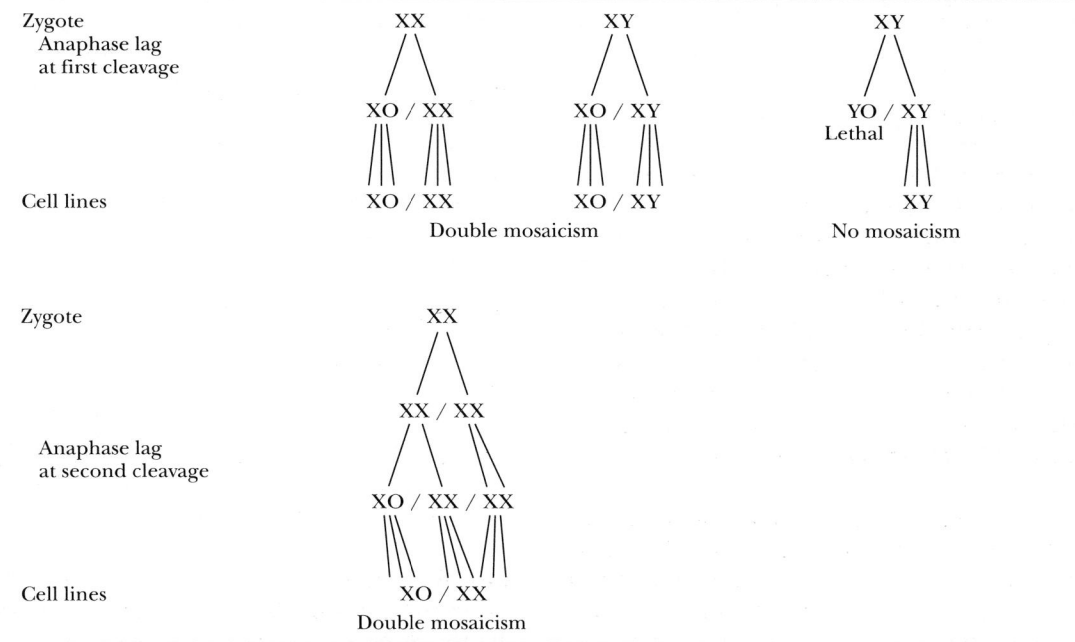

XY (Table 23.10). Anaphase lag may also occur during gamete formation, but its effects will hardly be distinguishable from those of nondisjunction.

While examples of anaphase lag and the subsequent loss of an autosome have been recognized (134, 135), most such cases must be lethal to one of the daughter cells. When one sex chromosome is lost, an XX/XO or XY/XO mosaicism results. These are not infrequently encountered. A pair of monozygous twins of opposite sex, the male having an XY and the female an XO karyotype, has been reported (136). It was assumed that one Y chromosome was lost during the first cleavage division,

Table 23.11.
Distribution of Types of Pseudohermaphrodites and Hermaphrodites

	Money (1895–1950)	Wilkins, 1936–1954 (1955)	Gross and Meeker (1955)	TOTAL	
				Number	Percentage
Female (adrenogenital)	122	46	28	196	44.8
Female (nonsuprarenal)	8	1	9	18	4.1
Male	129	22	26	177	40.5
True hermaphrodites	39	1	6	46	10.5
TOTALS	298	70	69	437	99.9

and two discordant individuals developed, rather than a single individual with XY/XO mosaicism.

Although it has been known in insects for many years (137), chromosomal mosaicism was first found in adult humans in 1959 (99). There is reason to believe that the condition is not uncommon and that not all such mosaicisms produce phenotypic abnormalities.

RELATIVE INCIDENCE OF TYPES OF HERMAPHRODITISM AND PSEUDOHERMAPHRODISM

Female pseudohermaphrodites with the adrenogenital syndrome are the most frequently encountered group of patients of doubtful sex, and female pseudohermaphrodites of nonsuprarenal origin are the least commonly seen. Without doubt, because of the nature of the defects involved, large numbers of afflicted individuals never come to medical attention. Money (138) collected the cases in the English language literature from 1895 to 1950; Wilkins and his colleagues (139) reported 70 cases from Johns Hopkins Hospital; and Gross and Meeker (140) reported 69 cases of their own. The distribution of types in these series is shown in Table 23.11.

The proportion of true hermaphrodites is probably misleadingly high as a result of more frequent reporting of such interesting cases. Table 23.10 does not include the chromosomal gonadal dysgeneses, which are probably the most common of all, but which rarely were recognized until recently.

DIAGNOSIS

The diagnostic procedures in cases of doubtful sex should be devoted to:

1. Identifying or eliminating the adrenogenital syndrome, which requires immediate treatment
2. Identifying or eliminating the chromosomal aberration syndromes of either sex that are not amenable to surgical treatment
3. Identifying the remaining cases to establish the basis for sound surgical correction

Recognition of Suprarenal Hyperplasia. All cases of doubtful sex should be suspected of resulting from suprarenal hyperplasia. Early diagnosis is necessary to forestall possible metabolic disorders.

Diagnosis is by determination of 24-hour output of 17-ketosteroids in the urine. Output in infants with suprarenal hyperplasia is 2 to 5 mg/day and may rise to 100 mg in adult (normal values are 6 to 18 mg/day for males and 4 to 13 mg/day for females). Cortisone will produce a marked decrease in 17-ketosteroid output in suprarenal hyperplasia, but not when a suprarenal tumor is present. The absence of genital deformity, of course, suggests a suprarenal tumor, rather than congenital suprarenal hyperplasia.

In modern times, a more accurate and better diagnosis of congenital suprarenal hyperplasia in the vertebrate may be established by elevation of 17-hydroxyprogesterone, as well as of 4-androstenedione, testosterone, and dehydroepiandrostenedione-sulfate, according to Bercovici et al. (141). Since the most frequent enzyme deficiency with this problem is 21-hydroxylase, repeated electrolytes will indicate the salt-wasting form which is produced by deficiencies of 21-hydroxylase (4). Early diagnosis is a must.

Suprarenal hyperplasia resulting from maternal therapeutic hormone administration may be distinguished from the adrenogenital syndrome only in that virilization does not continue after birth. A history of progesterone or testosterone therapy to the mother during pregnancy may usually be elicited.

Cells of these patients obtained at biopsy will be sex chromatin positive.

Recognition of Chromosomal Aberrations. In the male, Klinefelter's syndrome shows little morphologic evidence to suggest that the individual is not sexually normal. Azoospermia discovered after a complaint of sterility may be the only evidence. A testicular biopsy and the finding of sex chromatin-positive cells in the apparent normal male are confirmatory.

Turner's syndrome in the female is usually suggested by the short stature, webbed neck, and cubitus valgus. These may not have been associated with sexual dysfunction by the parents so that the child may not be examined until menarche fails to take place. The finding of sex chromatin-negative cells at biopsy confirms the diagnosis.

Evidence for mosaicism rests on chromosome counts of a large number of cells and, when possible, on cells from more than one tissue. Harden (84) warned against errors arising from increasing deletion of sex chromosomes with age.

Vincent et al. (142) studied 26,950 amniocenteses and found cytogenetic abnormalities in 416 cases (1.54%) with termination of pregnancy in 276 (73.02%). Most of the terminated pregnancies were cases with chromosomal autosomal abnormality—81.91% (in comparison to 42.35%) were affected with a sex chromosomal abnormality. Pregnancies with autosomal trisomies were terminated in about 92 to 95% of cases.

Recognition of Other Conditions. Elimination of the two previous categories leaves female pseudohermaphrodites of nonsuprarenal origin, male pseudohermaphrodites, and true hermaphrodites.

Female pseudohermaphrodites without suprarenal pathology are rare and usually have other marked malformations of the urinary tract and rectum, which require early surgical intervention. If these procedures are successful, they may also provide sufficient information to facilitate evaluation of the malformation of the genitalia.

The male pseudohermaphrodites of the masculinizing type may have a normal vagina, a shallow vagina, or none at all. The external genitalia are masculine, but there is usually hypospadias with chordee. One or both testes are undescended. The cells are sex chromatin negative, or there may be bizarre mosaicism.

The feminizing male pseudohermaphrodite, like the masculinizing type, has sex chromatin-negative cells. The external genitalia are feminine, but there is no corresponding müllerian development. If reared as girls, these patients may appear at puberty with a complaint of delayed menarche. Exploratory laparotomy may be undertaken to determine sex or to discover the true abnormality. Diagnosis by elimination and through chromosome studies should make exploratory surgery unnecessary in most cases.

The true hermaphrodites are among the most difficult of the types of intersex conditions to diagnose. Habitus, external genitalia and breasts may appear fundamentally masculine or feminine. Chromosomal examination and sex chromatin determinations give no unequivocal answer. Diagnosis is often incidental to surgery or exploratory laparotomy. Confirmation is made only when histologic evidence shows the presence of both ovarian and testicular tissue.

TREATMENT

The strategy of treatment of those complicated conditions depends on the good cooperation of the gynecologist who will first see the anomaly; the geneticist who will recommend conservative or surgical treatment upon evaluation and diagnosis, and finally the pediatric surgeon who, with the help of the pediatrician, will operate

after the team explains the situation to the family. Polin (143) advised that the parents can be told that there are four general etiologic categories for malformations: mendelian disorders, multifactorial disorders, environmental disorders, and chromosomal disorders. As Polin states, this is one of the easiest explanations as to the cause of malformations until a specific diagnosis is determined.

Of the varieties of intersex conditions, only those resulting from suprarenal hyperplasia involve specific therapy directed toward nongenital symptoms. Many of these patients must be treated for water and electrolyte imbalance. Treatment with cortisone and desoxycorticosterone acetate, together with added salt in the diet, will usually control such imbalances during critical periods of illness.

Following diagnosis of the specific condition and the repair of incidental associated anomalies, the problem of treatment becomes twofold:

1. Toward the approximation of which sex should the surgeon direct his efforts?
2. What specific procedures should be employed?

Choice of Sex. As with most other problems involving sex, this has been debated at great length over many years. Among the factors involved are: *(a)* the sex of rearing; *(b)* the histology of the gonad; *(c)* the anatomy of the genitalia; and *(d)* the effects of changing an already "assigned" sex, regardless of anatomic considerations.

The morphologic school, which emphasized the gonadal sex, is the oldest. It has been backed by legal and theological views, which have in turn been based on the idea that there is a true sex, which must be discovered and to which each individual must conform as nearly as is possible. Several tragic instances of the conflict between individuals of ambiguous sex and authorities are recounted in Young's monograph (21).

A second school of thought, which may be designated "environmentalist," has urged that all efforts be directed toward maintaining the sex of original rearing. Adherents of this theory have felt that the establishment of sexuality during the formative childhood years is more important than the genetic sexuality present at birth. This view, of course, does not apply to the problem when diagnosis must be made at birth.

Both the morphologic and the environmental schools have the advantage of supplying readily defined sex dichotomies—to one of which the individual must be assigned. In the one view the person's sex is thought to be predetermined. In the other it is assigned by the parents. However, in both instances the ambiguity can be resolved.

A third view, which has arisen only since the recent development of reconstructive surgery, may be called the "pragmatic" view. In essence, this view holds that normal

appearing external genitalia are of much greater significance to the individual than is the invisible presence of
seminiferous tubules or ovarian follicles. The sex of
choice depends on whether surgical reconstruction can
achieve relatively normal male genitalia or female genitalia more readily. With increasing recognition of pseudohermaphroditism and hermaphroditism at birth and
during infancy, and with increasing improvement of
reconstructive surgery, this view will doubtless become
more universally accepted.

In general, feminization will be surgically feasible
more often that will masculinization. Wilkins (144) found
only 20 of 242 pseudohermaphrodites in whom the genitalia were suitable for reconstruction as males.

Female pseudohermaphrodites with suprarenal hyperplasia have normal female internal organs and require
only clitoridectomy and separation of the fused labia.

Masculinized male pseudohermaphrodites have been
divided by Jones (29) and Wilkins (144) into three groups:

1. Those in whom internal female structures are normal;
   removal of the phallus is all that is necessary to feminize
   them
2. Those in whom postpubertal elongation of the vagina will
   be required in addition to phallectomy
3. Those in whom tubes, uterus, and vagina all are lacking.
   (If the phallus is suitable for masculine reconstruction
   this should be done; if not, phallectomy and vaginal construction will be necessary.)

Feminized male pseudohermaphrodites have no internal müllerian structure, except a vagina, but their external genitalia are essentially feminine.

In both types of male pseudohermaphrodites, the
undescended testes should be removed before the age of
20 years, if the patient is feminized, because of the danger
of malignant changes.

Suitable hormone therapy to maintain the desired secondary sex characters must be instituted in cases in which
the gonads have been removed or are inactive.

EDITORIAL COMMENTS

Sexuality is not a single identifiable entity but the end result of a
cascade of events, each step largely dependent on the previous
event and responsible for those that follow. Usually this process is
orderly and results in an individual whose sexual determinants are
appropriate to the "true sex" of that person. In intersex states,
incongruities in the orderly progression of sex determination occur,
and the concept of "true sex" must be re-defined.

There are basically seven determinants of what we call the sex
of an individual: five morphologic and two psychologic. Easiest
perhaps for the lay public to understand is the chromosomal component: There are male chromosomes (e.g., 46,XY) and there are
female chromosomes (46,XX). The chromosomal component

determines whether the undifferentiated gonad becomes testis or
ovary. Simplistically, if the Y chromosome is present, the undifferentiated gonad becomes a testis; if absent, an ovary. Early evidence localized the exact site on the Y chromosome responsible
for this differentiation to the H-Y antigen on the short arm. Lately,
however, doubt has been cast on the concept that the testis determining factor and the H-Y antigen are identical. It appears that not
only is a gene on the short arm of the Y chromosome necessary for
testicular differentiation, but that there must also be interaction with
certain genes on the autosome as well.

Gonadal status constitutes the next determinant of sex. Males
have testes and females have ovaries. Problems in sexual determination can occur when both gonadal structures occur in the same
individual, such as in true hermaphrodites. Individuals with Turner's
syndrome have only streaks for gonads, but are they any less
"female" than people with normal ovarian complement? As the
chromosomal determination is responsible for gonadal status, the
basic hormonal composition of an individual depends on the predominant gonad. Testes elaborate testosterone; ovaries make
estrogen. Testosterone is substantially responsible for the appearance of the external genitalia; however; there are "females" with
very high serum levels of testosterone whose end organs (i.e.,
external genitalia) are unresponsive to the masculinizing effects of
androgenic substances. The interaction of chromosomes, gonads,
and hormones meld together to determine the appearance of the
external genitalia, and constitute what an individual looks like from
a sexual standpoint, the phenotype. In certain intersex states, an
individual may possess many of the external characteristics one
considers typical of maleness or femaleness, yet have inconsisten-
cies in any of the other four morphologic sex-determining features.
Additionally, confusion can exist when the sex of rearing, or an
individual's gender role (how the person perceives himself or herself) is found, on investigation, to be inappropriate to any of the
morphologic determinants.

Efforts to classify accurately and manage these complex
abnormalities of sexual differentiation have been hampered in the
not too distant past by a lack of understanding of the basic pathophysiology involved. Certain hallmark studies have, however,
increased our knowledge of this potential for disordered sexual
development and have allowed us to formulate a rational scheme
of classification, to plan an orderly workup when sexual ambiguity
is encountered, and to execute a proper surgical experience
designed to bring the observed abnormalities of the external and
internal genitalia into line with the other determinants of sexual
development. Such a study is that of Jost (145, 146), as outlined in
an article by Hendren and Crawford (147). Jost showed, in the
male rabbit embryo, that removal of the fetal testes before the
19th day of gestation resulted in female differentiation. Such
embryos showed formation of uterus, fallopian tubes, and female
external genitalia, with no development of the wolffian primordia.

Gonadectomy soon after maturation of the wolffian ducts into seminal vesicles and vasa had no retroactive influence on these structures but blocked further male development. This resulted in animals with male internal structures but female external genitalia. Castration of female embryos, no matter at what stage, resulted in no change in the development of internal or external structures. Unilateral removal of the fetal testis produced ipsilateral female duct development but not failure of external virilization. Removal of both fetal testes and administration of testosterone gave normal development of wolffian primordia, but there was failure of regression of the müllerian ducts. These classic experiments showed that maleness is an active developmental process, depending on two products of the fetal testis. One is testosterone, which causes male differentiation of the external genitalia and wolffian structures. The other is müllerian inhibiting substance (MIS), which does just that. External development always is along female lines if androgen is absent.

The classification scheme that I have found most helpful in clinical practice, in sorting out these complex intersex problems, has been that which is outlined in the classic treatise by Allen (148), based on gonadal histology:

I. Female pseudohermaphrodite (ovary + ovary)
   A. Secondary to endogenous androgens (adrenogenital syndrome or congenital adrenal hyperplasia)
   B. Secondary to maternal androgens
      1. Exogenous, administered progestogen
      2. Endogenous, virilizing tumors
II. True hermaphrodite (ovary + testis)
III. Male pseudohermaphrodite (testis + testis)
   A. Secondary to inadequate androgen production
   B. Secondary to inadequate androgen utilization
      1. Incomplete (Reifenstein, Gilbert-Drefus, Lub's syndromes)
      2. Complete (testicular feminization syndrome)
   C. Secondary to inadequate conversion of testosterone to dihydrotestosterone (5-α-reductase deficiency)
   D. Secondary to deficient MIS (hernia uteri inguinalis)
   E. Secondary to dysgenetic testis
IV. Mixed gonadal dysgenesis (testis + streak)
V. Pure gonadal dysgenesis (streak + streak)
   A. Turner's syndrome
   B. XX type
   C. XY type

The interested reader is referred to Allen's excellent monograph for further discussion of the various entities listed in the preceding. The principle advantage of the scheme is that the histology of the gonads is subject to less uncertainty in interpretation than dependence on other parameters such as karyotype or morphology of the external genitalia. Its major disadvantage is that it fails to emphasize the relationship which seems to exist between certain patients in different categories who have dysgenetic gonads.

Any infant with ambiguous genitalia must be thoroughly examined as soon after birth as feasible so that proper sex assignment can be made. The need for pelvic laparotomy and gonadal biopsy can be determined after the results of chromosomal, biochemical, and radiographic evaluations are complete. In general, if neither gonad is palpable, with the prominent exception of congenital adrenal hyperplasia, laparotomy and biopsy are necessary (TSP).

REFERENCES

1. Nadler HC, Sacks AJ, Evans MI. Genetics in surgery and prenatal diagnosis. In: Raffensperger JG, ed. Swenson's pediatric surgery, 5th ed. Norwalk, CT: Appelton & Large, 1990.
2. Spranger J, Benirschke K, Hall JG. Errors of morphogenesis: concepts and terms. J Pediatr 1982;100:160.
3. Rosenbaum KN. Genetics and dysmorphology. In: Welch KJ, Randolph JG, Ravitch MM, O'Neill JA Jr, Rowe MI. Pediatric surgery, 4th ed. Chicago: Year Book Medical Publishers, 1986:3–8.
4. Reindollar RH, McDonough PG. The child with ambiguous genitalia. In: Lavery JP, Sanfilippo JS, eds. Pediatric and adolescent obstetrics and gynecology. New York: Springer-Verlag, 1985:38–60.
5. Ford CE, Hamerton JL. The chromosomes of man. Nature 1956;178:1020–1023.
6. Tjio JH, Levan A. The chromosome number of man. Hereditas 1956;42:1.
7. Chen ATL, Falek A. Centromeres in human meiotic chromosomes. Science 1969;166:1008–1010.
8. Denver Study Group. A proposed standard system of nomenclature of human mitotic chromosomes. Am J Hum Genet 1960;12:384–388. JAMA 1960;174:159–162. Lancet 1960;1:1063. Chicago Conference: Standardization in human cytogenetics. Birth Defects Original Article Series II: 2, 1966. The National Foundation, New York.
9. Park WW. The occurrence of sex chromatin in early human and macaque embryos. J Anat 1957;91:369–373.
10. Melander Y. Chromosome behavior during the origin of the sex chromatin in the rabbit. Hereditas 1962;48:645–661.
11. Lyon MF. Sex chromatin and gene action in the mammalian X-chromosome. Am J Hum Genet 1962;14:135–148.
12. Lyon MF. Gene action in the X-chromosome of the mouse (Mus musculus L.). Nature 1961;190:372–373.
13. Bahner F et al. A fertile female with XO sex chromosome constitution. Lancet 1960;2:100–101.
14. Jost A. Recherches sur la différenciation sexuelle de l'embryon de lapin. III. Rôle des gonads foetales dans la différenciation sexuelle somatique. Arch Anat Microsc Morphol Exp 1947;36:271–315.
15. Jones HW, Scott WW. Hermaphroditism, genital anomalies and related endocrine disorders. Baltimore: Williams & Wilkins, 1958.
16. Greene RR. Hormonal factors in sex inversion: the effects of sex hormones on embryonic sexual structures of the rat. Biol Symp 1942;9:105–123.
17. Bruner JA, Witschi E. Testosterone-induced modifications of sex development in female hamsters. Am J Anat 1946;79:293–320.
18. Weniger J. Régression de canal de müller d'embryon de souris mâle sourmis in vitro á l'action de l'hormone testiculaire. C R Acad Sci (Paris) 1964;259:1899–1901.
19. Stoll R, Couland H. Action de la greffe testiculaire sur les canaux

de Müller de l'embryon de poulet. C R Soc Biol (Paris) 1966;160:964–966.

20. Harbison MD, Magid ML, Josso N, Mininberg DT, New MI. Anti-müllerian hormone in three intersex conditions. Ann Genet 1991;34:226–232.

21. Young HH. Genital abnormalities, hermaphroditism and related adrenal diseases. Baltimore: Williams & Wilkins, 1937.

22. Plato. The symposium. In: The dialogues of Plato, Vol 1. B. Jowett (transl). New York: Charles Scribner's, 1871.

23. Klebs I. Handbuch der pathologischen Anatomie. Berlin: August Hirshwald, 1876:1–2, 718.

24. Barr ML, Bertram EG. A morphological distinction between neurons of the male and female, and the behavior of the nucleolar satellite during accelerated nucleoprotein synthesis. Nature 1949;163:676–677.

25. Crecchio L. Ann d'Hyg 1865;25:178.

26. Apert E. Bull Soc Pediatr (Paris) 1910;12:33.

27. Bentinck, RC, Lisser H, Reilly WA. Female pseudohermaphroditism with penile urethra, masquerading as precocious puberty and cryptorchidism. J Clin Endocrinol 1956;16:412–418.

28. Rook GD, Green M, Sard JT. Adrenogenital syndrome with phallic urethra. Am J Dis Child 1961;101:645–649.

29. Jones WS. Congenital anomalies of female genital tract. Trans N Engl Obstet Gynecol Soc 1953;7:79–94.

30. Carpenter PJ, Potter EL. Nuclear sex and genital malformation in 48 cases of renal agenesis with especial reference to nonspecific female pseudohermaphroditism. Am J Obstet Gynecol 1959;78:235–258.

31. Levina SE. Role of adrenals and ovaries in morphogenesis of external genitalia during human fetal development. Fed Proc 1963;22(Suppl):260–261.

32. Bongiovanni AM. Adrenogenital syndrome with deficiency of 3B-hydroxysteroid dehydrogenase. J Clin Invest 1962;41:2086.

33. Federman DD. Abnormal sexual development: a genetic and endocrine approach to differential diagnosis. Philadelphia: WB Saunders, 1967.

34. Prader A, Anders GJPA, Habich H. Zur Genetik des kongenitalen Syndromes (virilisierende Nebennierenhyperpasic). Helv Paediatr Acta 1962;17:271–284.

35. Childs B, Grumbach MM, Van Wyk JJ. Virilizing adrenal hyperplasia: a genetic and hormonal study. J Clin Invest 1956;35:213–222.

36. Brentnall CP. A case of arrhenoblastoma complicating pregnancy. J Obstet Gynaec Brit Comm 1945;52:235–240.

37. Trousier. Tumeur virilisante de l'ovarie découvert au cours de la grossesse et ayant entraîné la virilisation du foetus. Bull Soc Chir (Paris) 1962;52:252–256.

38. Wilkins L. Masculinization of female fetus: due to use of orally given progestins. JAMA 1960;172:1028–1032.

39. Franks RC, Northcutt R. Female pseudohermaphroditism and renal anomalies. Am J Dis Child 1963;105:490–496.

40. Sibilla A, Coghi I. Considerations of two cases of "feminizing cryptorchidism." Riv Ostet Ginec 1962;17:540–555.

41. Morris JM. The syndrome of testicular feminization in male pseudohermaphrodites. Am J Obstet Gynecol 1953;65:1192–1211.

42. Morris JM, Mahesh, VB. Further observations on the syndromes "testicular feminization." Am J Obstet Gynecol 1963;87:731–748.

43. Roberts EAB, Horwitz A. Testicular feminization: report of a case. Am Surg 1967;33:480–482.

44. Grumbach MM, Barr ML. Cytologic tests of chromosomal sex in relation to sexual anomalies in man. Recent Progr Horm Res 1958;14:255–334.

45. Puck TT, Robinson A, Tjio JH. Familial primary amenorrhea due to testicular feminization: a human gene affecting sex differentiation. Proc Soc Exp Biol Med 1960;103:192–196.

46. Alexander DS, Ferguson-Smith MA. Chromosomal studies in some variants of male pseudohermaphroditism. Pediatrics 1961;28:758–763.

47. Nilson O. Hernia uteri inguinalis beim Manne. Acta Chir Scand 1939;83:231–249.

48. Taub J. Malignant testis tumor, cryptorchidism and polyorchidism in a pseudohermaphrodite. J Urol 1954;71:475–482.

49. Warkany J, Chu EHY, Kauder E. Male pseudohermaphroditism and chromosomal mosaicism. Am J Dis Child 1962;104:172–179.

50. Schuster J, Motulsky AG. Exceptional sex-chromatin pattern in male pseudohermaphrodititsm with XX/XY/XO mosaicism. Lancet 1962;1:1074–1975.

51. Miles CP, Luzzatti L, Storey SK, Peterson CD. A male pseudohermaphrodite with a probable XO/XxY mosaicism. Lancet 1962;2:455.

52. Bottura C, Ferrari I. Male pseudohermaphroditism with XO chromosomal constitution on bone marrow cells. Br Med J 1962;2:110–111.

53. Overzier C. Hermaphroditismus versus. Acta Endocrinol 1955;20:63–80.

54. Merrill JA, Ramsey JE. True hermaphroditism: a report of a case and review of the literature. Obstet Gynecol 1963;22:505–512.

55. Bunge RG, Bradbury JT. Oocytes in seminiferous tubules. II. A case report of bilateral ovotestes. J Clin Endocrinol 1959;19:1661–1666.

56. Hirschhorn K, Decker WH, Cooper HL. Human intersex with chromosome mosaicism of type XY/SO: report of a case. N Engl J Med 1960;263:1944–1948.

57. Miller OJ. Sex determination: the sex chromosomes and the sex chromatin pattern. Fertil Steril 1962;13:93–104.

58. Willemse CH, van Brink JM, Los PL. XY/XO mosaicism. Lancet 1962;1:488–489.

59. Waxman SH, Kelley BC, Gartler SM, Burt B. Chromosome complement in a true hermaphrodite. Lancet 1962;1:161.

60. Ferguson-Smith MA. X-Y chromosomal interchange in the aetiology of true hermaphroditism and of XX Klinefelter's syndrome. Lancet 1966;2:475–476.

61. Zuelzer WW, Beattie DM, Reisman LE. Generalized unbalanced mosaicism attributable to dispermy and probable fertilization of a polar body. Am J Hum Genet 1964;16:38–51.

62. Gartler SM, Waxman SH, Giblett E. An XX/XY human hermaphrodite resulting from double fertilization. Proc Nat Acad Sci USA 1962;48:332–335.

63. Tho SP et al. Absence of the testicular determining factor gene SRY in XX true hermaphrodites and presence of this locus in most subjects with gonadal dysgenesis caused by Y aneuploidy. Am J Obstet Gynecol 1992;167:1794–1802.

64. McElreavey K et al. A minority of 46,XX true hermaphrodites are positive for the Y-DNA sequence including SRY. Hum Genet 1992;90:121–125.

65. Berkovitz GD et al. The role of the sex-determining region of the Y chromosome (SRY) in the etiology of 46,XX true hermaphroditism. Hum Genet 1992;88:411–416.

66. Klinefelter HF, Reifenstein EC Jr., Albright F. Syndrome characterized by gynecomastia, aspermatogenesis without A-leydigism, and increased excretion of follicle-stimulating hormone. J Clin Endocrinol 1942;2:615–627.

67. Klinefelter HF Jr. Klinefelter's syndrome. In: HW Jones HW, Scott WW, eds. Hermaphroditism, genital anomalies and related endocrine disorders. Baltimore: Williams & Wilkins, 1958.

68. Martin R, Santamaria L, Nistal M, Fraile B, Paniagua R. The peritubular myofibroblasts in the testes from normal men and men

with Klinefelter's syndrome. A quantitative, ultrastruactural, and immunohistochemical study. J Pathol 1992;168:59–66.

69. Ferguson-Smith MA. The prepubertal testicular lesion in chromatin-positive Klinefelter's syndrome (primary microorchidism) as seen in mentally handicapped children. Lancet 1959;1:219–222.

70. Miller HC, McDonald DF. Klinefelter's syndrome and benign prostatic hypertrophy. JAMA 1963;186:215–218.

71. Fuse H, Sumiya H, Takahara M, Shiseki Y, Shimazaki J. Klinefelter's syndrome with prepenile scrotum. Urology 1992;40:438–440.

72. Sasagawa I et al. Klinefelter's syndrome associated with unilateral cryptorchidism and chordee without hypospadia. Urol Int 1992;48:428–429.

73. Hasle H, Jacoabsen BB, Asschenfeld P, Andersen K. Mediastinal germ cell tumour associated with Klinefelter syndrome. A report of case and review of the literature. Eur J Pediatr 1992;151:735–739.

74. Hamed LM, Maria BL, Quisling R, Fanous MM, Mickle P. Suprasellar tumors of maldevelopmental origin in Klinefelter's syndrome. A report of two cases. J Clin Neuroophthalmol 1992;12:192–197.

75. Plunkett ER, Barr ML. Testicular dysgenesis affecting the seminiferous tubules principally, with chromatin positive nuclei. Lancet 1956;2:853–856.

76. Jacobs PA, Strong JA. A case of human intersexuality having a possible XXY sex-determining mechanism. Nature 1959;183:302–303.

77. Takai S, Sasaki T, Hikita M. Klinefelter's syndrome with XXYY complex [Japanese]. Jpn J Urol 1965;56:616–621.

78. Ferguson-Smith MA, Johnston AW, Handmaker SD. Primary amentia and micro-orchidism with an XXXY sex-chromosome constitution. Lancet 1960;2:184–187.

79. Day RW, Levinson H, Larson W, Wright SW. XXXXY sex chromosome in males. J Pediatr 1963;65:589–598.

80. De la Chapelle A, Hortling H, Niemi M, Wennstrom J. XX-sex chromosomes in a human male. Acta Med Scand 1964;412(suppl):25–38.

81. Crooke AC, Hayward MD. Mosaicism in Klinefelter's syndrome. Lancet 1960;1:1198.

82. Finley WH, Finley SC, Pittman CS. Phenotypic male with mosaic sex chromosomes. JAMA 1964;188:758–760.

83. Lubs HA. Testicular size in Klinefelter's syndrome in men over fifty: report of a case with XXY/XY mosaicism. N Engl J Med 1962;267:326–331.

84. Harden DG, Jacobs PA. Cytogenetics of abnormal sexual development in man. Br Med Bull 1961;17:206–212.

85. Muldal AS, Ockey CH, Thompson M, White LLR. Double male: a new chromosome constitution in the Klinefelter's syndrome. Acta Endocrinol 1962;39:183–203.

86. Baker D, Telfer MA, Richardson CE, Clark GR. Chromosome errors in men with antisocial behavior: comparison of selected men with Klinefelter's syndrome and XYY chromosome pattern. JAMA 1970;214:869–878.

87. Mandoki MW, Sumner GS. Klinefelter syndrome: the need for early identification and treatment. Clin Pediatr 1991;30:161–164.

88. Moore KL. Sex reversal in newborn babies. Lancet 1959;1:217–219.

89. Kaplan NM, Norfleet RG. Hypogonadism in young males (with emphasis on Klinefelter's syndrome). Ann Intern Med 1961;54:461–481.

90. Warburg E. Fertility in Klinefelter's syndrome. Acta Endocrinol (Kobenhavn) 1963;43:12–26.

91. Nelson WO. Sex differences in human nuclei with particular ref-

erence to the Klinefelter syndrome, gonadal agenesis and other types of hermaphroditism. Acta Endocrinol 1956;23:227–245.

92. Ferguson-Smith MA, Mack WS, Ellis PM, Dickson M. Chromosome analysis and parental age in the del Castillo syndrome. Lancet 1963;2:1121.

93. Simpson JL. Klinefelter syndrome. In: Simpson JL, ed. Disorders of sexual differentiation. New York: Academic Press, 1976:303–322.

94. Morgagni JB. The seats and causes of disease investigated by anatomy. Alexander B (transl). New York: Hafner Publishing, 1960.

95. Turner HH. Syndrome of infantilism, congenital webbed neck and cubitus valgus. Endocrinology 1938;23:566–574.

96. Ullrich O. Über typische Kombinationsbilder multipler Abartungen. Z Kinderheilk 1930;49:271–276.

97. Sharpey-Schafer EP. Case of pterygo-nuchal infantilism (Turner's syndrome), with post-mortem findings. Lancet 1941;2:559–560.

98. Polani PE, Hunter WF, Lennox B. Chromosomal sex in Turner's syndrome with coarctation of the aorta. Lancet 1954;2:120.

99. Ford CE, Jones KW, Polani PE, de Almeida JC, Briggs JH. A sex chromosome anomaly in a case of gonadal dysgenesis. Lancet 1959;1:711–713.

100. Nora JJ, Sinha AK. Direct familial transmission of the Turner phenotype. Am J Dis Child 1968;116:343–350.

101. Morishima A, Grumbach MM. The inter-relationship of sex chromosome constitution and phenotype in the syndrome of gonadal dysgenesis and its variants. Ann NY Acad Sci 1968;155:695–715.

102. Ferguson-Smith MA. Karyotype-phenotype correlations in gonadal dysgenesis and their bearing on the pathogenesis of malformations. J Med Genet 1965;2:142–155.

103. Sohval AR. The syndrome of pure gonadal dysgenesis. Am J Med 1965;38:615–625.

104. Greenblatt RB. Oogonia in rudimentary gonads in a case of Turner's syndrome with male sex chromatin pattern. J Clin Endocrinol 1958;18:227–230.

105. Hoffenberg R, Jackson WPU, Muller WHP. Gonadal dysgenesis with menstruation: report of two cases. J Clin Endocrinol 1957;17:902–907.

106. Monardo A. Gonadal dysgenesis in a woman after seventeen years of regular menses. Am J Obstet Gynecol 1965;91:106–109.

107. Verschraegen-Spae MR, Depypere H, Speleman F, Dhondt M, De-Paepe A. Familial Turner syndrome. Clin Genet 1992;41:218–220.

108. Massa G, Vanderschueren-Lodeweyckx M, Fryns JP. Deletion of the short arm of the X chromosome: a hereditary form of Turner syndrome. Eur J Pediatr 1992;151:893–894.

109. Muller U, Kirkels VG, Scheres JM. Absence of "Turner" stigmata in a 46, XYp-female. Hum Genet 1992;90:239–242.

110. Haddad HM, Wilkins L. Congenital anomalies of gonadal aplasia. Pediatrics 1959;23:885–902.

111. Gray SW, Romaine CB, Skandalakis JE. Congenital fusion of the cervical vertebrae. Surg Gynecol Obstet 1964;118:373–385.

112. Kosowicz J. The carpal sign in gonadal dysgenesis. J Clin Endocrinol 1962;22:949–952.

113. Polani PE. Turner's syndrome and allied conditions: clinical features and chromosome abnormalities. Br Med Bull 1961;17:200–205.

114. Jeune M, Bertrand J, Deffrenne P, Forget H. Fréquence des malformations de l'arbre urinaire au cours du syndrome de Turner: etude de 24 cas. Pediatrie 1962;17:897–907.

115. Aubertin E et al. Syndrome Turner avec malformation rénale inhabituelle. J Med Bordeaux 1963;140:1113–1118.

116. Hung W, LoPresti JM. Urinary tract anomalies in gonadal dysgenesis. AJR 1965;95:439–441.

117. Gorlin RJ, Redman RS. Chromosomal abnormalities and oral anomalies. Am J Surg 1964;108:370–379.

118. Sohval AR. Sex chromatin, chromosomes, and male infertility. Fertil Steril 1963;14:180–207.

119. Ferrier P, Garler S, Mahoney CP, Shepard TH II, Burt B. Study of a case of gonadal dysgenesis with positive chromatin pattern. Am J Dis Child 1961;102:581–582.

120. Cukier J, Job J-C, De Grouchy J, Nezelof C. Hypospadias périnéal révélateur d'une forme rare d'état intersexuel. J Urol Nephrol (Paris) 1963;69:467–478.

121. Greenblatt RB, Dominquez H, Mahesh VB, Demos R. Gonadal dysgenesis intersex with XO/XY mosaicism. JAMA 1964;188:221–224.

122. O'Shea D, Powell D: Growth hormone therapy in Turner's syndrome. Ir Med J 1992;85:68–69.

123. Rosenfeld RG et al: Six-year results of a randomized, prospective trial of human growth hormone and oxandrolone in Turner's syndrome. J Ped 1992;121:49–55.

124. Takano K, Shizume K, Hibi I. Treatment of 46 patients with Turner's syndrome with recombinant human growth hormone (YM-17798) for three years: a multicenter study. Acta Endocrinol (Copenh) 1992;126:296–302.

125. Flavell G. Webbing of neck with Turner syndrome in male. Br J Surg 1943;31:150–153.

126. Morishima A, Grumbach MM. Karyotypic analysis in a case of Turner's syndrome in a phenotypic male. Am J Dis Child 1961;102:585–586.

127. Steiker DD, Mellman WJ, Bongiovanni AM, Eberlein WR, Leboef G. Turner's syndrome in the male. J Pediatr 1961;58:321–329.

128. Morishima A, Grumbach MM. Karyotypic analysis in a case of Turner's syndrome in a phenotypic male. Am J Dis Child 1961;102:585–586.

129. Heller, RH. The Turner phenotype in the male. J Pediatr 1965;66:48–63.

130. Noonan JA. Hypertelorism with Turner phenotype. Am J Dis Child 1968;116:373–380.

131. Kaplan MS, Opitz JM, Gossett FR. Noonan's syndrome. Am J Dis Child 1968;116:359–366.

132. Sharland M, Burch M, Mckenna WM, Paton MA. A clinical study of Noonan's syndrome. Arch Dis Child 1992;67:178–183.

133. Court Brown WM, Jacobs PA, Doll R. Interpretation of chromosome counts made on bone marrow cells. Lancet 1960;1:160–163.

134. Lejeune J et al. Monozygotisme heterocaryote: jumeau normal et jumeau 21 trisomique. C R Acad Sci (Paris) 1962;254:4404–4406.

135. Bruins J, van Bolhius J, Biijlsma A, Nijenhuis L. Discordant monozygotic twins. In: Proceedings of the Ninth International Congress of Genetics. The Hague, Netherlands, 1963.

136. Turpin R, Lejeune J, Lafourcade J, Chigot PL, Salmon C. Presumption of monozygotism in spite of a sexual dimorphism: XY male subject and haploid X neuter subject. C R Acad Sci (Paris) 1961;252:2945–2946.

137. Morgan TH, Bridges CB. The inheritance of a fluctuating character. J Gen Physiol 1919;1:639–643.

138. Money J. Hermaphroditism: an inquiry into the nature of a human paradox [Thesis]. Harvard University, 1952.

139. Wilkins L, Grumbach MM, VanWyk JJ, Shepard TH, Papadatos C. Hermaphroditism: classification, diagnosis, selection of sex and treatment. Pediatrics 1955;16:287–302.

140. Gross RE, Meeker IA. Abnormalities of sexual development: observations from 75 cases. Pediatrics 1955;16:303–324.

141. Bercovici JP et al. Hormonal profiles of heterozygotes in humans for 21-hydroxylase deficiency defined by HLA B typing. J Steriod Biochem 1981;14:1049–1054.

142. Vincent VA, Edwards JG, Young SR, Nachtigal M. Pregnancy termination because of 26,950 amniocenteses in the southeast. South Med J 1991;84:1210–1213.

143. Polin R. Congenital anomalies. In: Schwartz MW, ed. Principles and practice of clinical pediatrics. Chicago: Year Book Medical Publishers, 1987.

144. Wilkins L. Abnormalities of sex differentiation. Classification, diagnosis, selection of gender of rearing and treatment. Pediatrics 1960;26:846–857.

145. Jost A. Problems in fetal endocrinology: the gonadad and hypophyseal hormones. Recent Prog Hormone Res 1953;8:379.

146. Jost A. Hormond factors in the development of the fetus (Cold Springs Harbor Symposium). Quant Biol 1954;19:167.

148. Hendren WH, Crawford JD. The child with ambiguous genitalia. Curr Probl Surg 1972;11:1–64.

149. Allen TD. Disorders of sexual differentiation. Urology 1976;7(suppl):1–32.

CHAPTER 24

THE LYMPHATIC SYSTEM

John Elias Skandalakis / Stephen Wood Gray / Richard R. Ricketts

*If we mistake not, in proper time, it (the lymphatics) will allow to the greatest
discovery both in physiology and pathology that anatomy has suggested since the
discovery of circulation.*
—*WILLIAM HUNTER*

DEVELOPMENT

Two paired and two unpaired endothelial sacs which
appear during the third and fourth months form the primordia of the lymphatic system:

1. Two jugular sacs in the neck, one on each side.
2. One sac at the mesenteric root.
3. The cisterna chyli, composed of one sac.
4. Two posterior sacs, each along the sciatic veins.

One may support the idea that there are only five
points of origin and not six, by combining the mesenteric
and cisterna chyli sacs to one appearing at the eighth week
of development. Both opinions are right.

The paired jugular lymph sacs appear late in the sixth
week (10-mm stage) in the lateral angle between the internal jugular veins (precardinal veins) and the subclavian
veins (Fig. 24.1). By the 17-mm stage, extensions into the
upper limbs are visible. The retroperitoneal sac consists
of a plexus of capillaries at the root of the mesentery by
the 20-mm stage and is an identifiable structure by the
end of the eighth week (23 mm). At about the same time
the cisterna chyli, dorsal to the aorta at about the same
level as that of the retroperitoneal sac, makes its appearance. Very shortly afterward, the paired posterior sacs
appear at the bifurcation of the femoral and sciatic veins.
These lymphatic sacs become linked with one another by
endothelial channels by the end of the ninth week (30
mm) (Fig. 24.2).

Linkage of the jugular lymph sacs with the cisterna
chyli produces a bilateral system of lymphatic trunks, connected with one another across the midline by numerous
anastomoses. Of these trunks, the inferior portion of the
right trunk and the superior portion of the left trunk,
together with a diagonal anastomosing channel at the
level of the fourth to sixth thoracic segments, will form
the definitive thoracic duct. Discontinuous segments or
secondary channels represent the other portions of the
originally paired system (1). After the ninth week, the jug-

ular lymph sacs and cisterna chyli cease to enlarge and
eventually become mere dilations of the thoracic duct.

Controversy over the mode of formation of the lymph
sacs and the lymphatic vessels draining into them began
with the discovery of the jugular lymph sacs in 1896 by
Saxer (2). The widely held view of William His (1863–
1934) that the vascular system was formed by an orderly
invasion of proliferating blood vessels originating from
the yolk sac led at once to the idea that lymphatic vessels
were similarly formed by further proliferation of the
venous system. The specific description of this process
was contained in the work of Sabin (3, 4). By means of delicate India ink injections, she traced the developing lymphatics and concluded that the jugular and posterior
lymph sacs arose from the neighboring veins, while lymphatic vessels were subsequently formed by outgrowths
of endothelium into the surrounding mesenchyme. In
1905 Lewis (5) added to this picture, showing that the
lymph sacs become separated from the parent veins at the
16- to 20-mm stage and make new connections with them
at about 30 mm. The view of lymphatic development
based on the work of Sabin and Lewis has been termed
the *centrifugal theory.*

In 1910 Huntington and McClure (6) contended that
the lymphatics did not form by proliferation from previously existing lymph sacs but by the formation of mesenchymal spaces that subsequently coalesced into a system
of vessels, which eventually joined the venous system.
Huntington (7) contended that the jugular sac and its
extension toward the limb bud taps mesenchymal hemopoietic tissue and contains primitive blood cells, which
are emptied into the venous circulation, after which the
vessels revert to the lymphatic system proper (Fig. 24.1).
The view that lymphatics are formed by coalescence of
mesenchymal spaces has been termed the *centripetal
theory.*

In still a third view, Kampmeier (8, 9) describes venous
precursors of the lymphatic and the lymph sacs. The

EMBRYOLOGY FOR SURGEONS

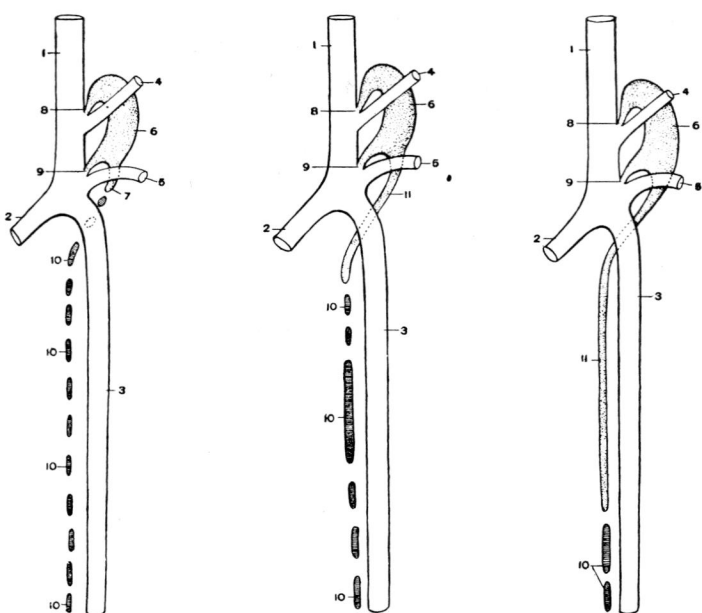

Figure 24.1. Stages in the development of the thoracic duct from the jugular lymph sac. *1,* Precardial vein; *2,* duct of Cuvier; *3,* postcardinal vein; *4,* external jugular-cephalic vein; *5,* subclavian vein; *6,* jugular lymphsac; *7,* thoracic duct approach of jugular lymphsac; *8,* common jugular lymphaticovenous tap; *9,* jugulosubclavian lymphaticovenous tap; *10,* thoracic duct analages; *11,* thoracic duct. (From Huntington GS, McClure CFW. The anatomy and development of the jugular lymph sac in the domestic cat. Am J Anat 1910;10:177–311.)

definitive lymph vessels form as perivascular spaces around the veins, which subsequently degenerate. The transient veins arise from the parent veins, and after their degeneration, the new, enveloping lymph sac forms new connections with the subclavian veins.

Controversy between proponents of the centrifugal and centripetal theories was heated and even rancorous for a few years. Interest eventually waned before agreement could be reached, and the subject has been almost ostentatiously neglected for many years. There is no lack of exhaustive studies on lymphatic development in fish, amphibians, birds, and mammals. An excellent bibliography is that of Kampmeier (9). A new approach with new methods will be required to determine the true developmental story.

According to Sabin (10), the lymph nodes appear to start within the neck around the ninth week by invasion of connective tissue into small lymphatic sacs. Another invasion by lymphocytes takes place and lymph vessels and lymph follicles are formed later within the lymph nodes.

Critical Events in Development

The development of the lymphatic vessels is poorly understood and the true origin of many of the apparent anomalies is obscure.

One known critical event is the connection of the downward growing thoracic duct with the cisterna chyli.

Clark (11) observed a case of failure of connection. The thoracic duct did not extend below the diaphragm. All the abdominal lymphatics coursed downward, over the inguinal ligament and upward beneath the skin of the side, to empty finally into the subclavian vein. Pick and his colleagues (12) reported a case of communication of the lumbar lymphatics with the renal veins. Experimental evidence for other lymphaticovenous pathways has been described by Pressman and Simon (13). Such communications, which occur regularly in certain species, are of interest in diagnostic lymphangiography. The subject has been reviewed by Roddenberry and Allen (14).

From early researchers such as Gasparo Aselli (1581–1626), Thomas Bartholin (1616–1680), and Olaf Rudbeck (1630–1702) to contemporary investigators such as H. Rouviere, C.D. Haagensen, and Leonard Weiss (to name just a few), the work on lymphatics continues. Despite the fact that we now know more about lymphatics today, there is still a great deal of work to be done.

Parke et al. (15) described a subserous lymphatic plexus coursing longitudinally in association with the tenial coli traveling up and down (proximally and distally) before draining into regional mesocolic lymphatics. Perhaps this is the orthodox way of lymphatic draining of the colon, or it may be a variation. The future will tell. Natsugoe et al. (16), in their work on lymphatic anastomosis of the G-E junction, emphasized that proximal and distal drainage is accomplished by intramural anasthemoses.

ANOMALIES OF THE LYMPHATIC SYSTEM (TABLE 24.1 and FIG. 24.3)

Variations of the Thoracic Duct

ANATOMY

The thoracic lymph channels, originally paired, arise embryonically from the cisterna chyli at the level of the third and fourth lumbar vertebrae and ascend on either side of the vertebral column to enter the subclavian arteries on either side. Numerous cross-anastomoses occur between the two trunks.

In the usual condition in the adult, the right embryonic trunk persists up to the level of the fourth to sixth thoracic vertebrae, where the definitive duct crosses to the left embryonic trunk to ascend and enter the left subclavian vein. Because the available pathways were originally bilateral, there are many variations in the final course of the duct (Fig. 24.4).

Variations in Origin (Fig. 24.5). Right and left lumbar lymphatic trunks arise from several roots and converge to form the thoracic duct. The junction lies between the second lumbar and the twelfth thoracic vertebrae. A cisterna chyli is present when the junction is low (Fig. 22.5, *C*). When it is higher, there may be dilation of both lumbar trunks, which perhaps represents the unfused lateral primordia of the cisterna (Fig. 22.5, *D*), or there may be no trace of a cisterna (Fig. 22.5, *A* and *B*) (17). A cisterna is present in about 50% of adults examined (1, 18, 19).

Variations in Course. A number of variant courses are known for the thoracic duct. The "usual" course described above is found in 60 to 70% of bodies examined. The next most frequent condition is doubling of the lower part of the duct by the persistence of both right and left trunks below the crossing, at the fourth to sixth thoracic vertebrae. Davis (1) found a number of such examples, but van Pernis (20) found far fewer, although in the absence of diagrams his data are difficult to interpret.

Even when a single trunk has formed the path of the thoracic duct, the contralateral trunk usually is not absent, but merely is interrupted into short segments connected with the main trunk by numerous cross-anastomoses. In addition, the thoracic duct may itself break up into a plexus of lymphatic vessels, which reunite to form a single channel higher in the thorax (17).

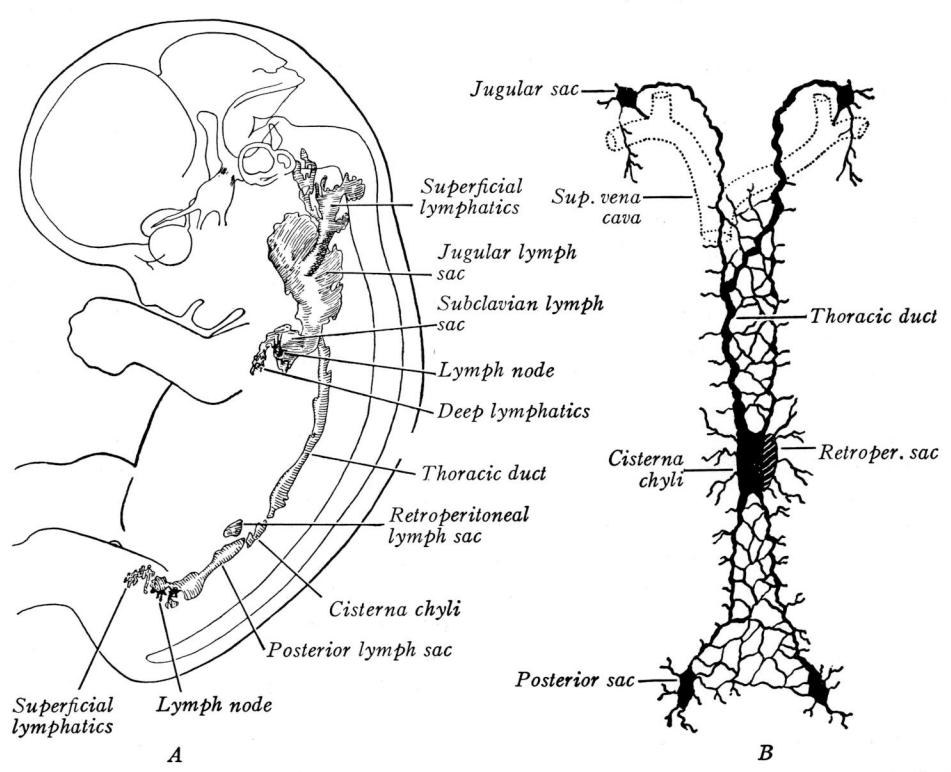

Figure 24.2. Development of the lymphatic vessels. **A,** Human embryo at 9 weeks, showing the primitive lymph sacs and the developing vessels. **B,** Ventral view of the formation of the single thoracic duct from the primitive paired lymphatic plexus. (From Arey LB. Developmental anatomy, 7th ed. Philadelphia: WB Saunders, 1965; **A,** after Sabin FR. The development of the lymphatic system. In: Keibel F, Mall FP, eds. Manual of human embryology. vol 2. Philadelphia: JP Lippincott, 1912.)

Table 24.1.
Anomalies of the Lymphatic System

Anomaly	Origin of Defect	First Appearance (or Other Diagnostic Clues)	Sex Chiefly Affected	Relative Frequency	Remarks
Variations in the course of the thoracic duct	2nd month	No pathologic structures	Equal	Common	
Cystic hygroma (cystic lymphangioma)	6th to 9th weeks?	At birth or in infancy	Equal (neck); male (groin)	Uncommon	Invasive growth; may be a neoplasm
Primary lymphedema: Milroy's disease	3rd month?	At birth	Equal?	Rare	Familial tendency
Lymphedema precox	3rd month?	At any age	Equal?	Rare	
Mesenteric, omental and retroperitoneal lymphatic cysts	?	In infancy to middle age	Male (children); female (adults)	Uncommon	

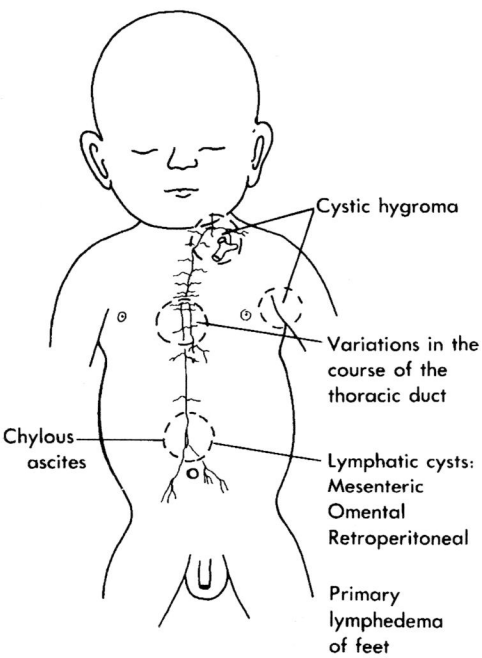

Figure 24.3. Location of anomalies of the lymphatic system.

Patterns of the variations of the thoracic duct are shown in Figure 24.6, from Davis (1). Many of the original descriptions of these variations date back to the late 18th century, when interest in the anatomy of the lymphatic system was at its height. Most of the references to these descriptions are found in Rouvière (17).

Variations in Termination. Termination of the thoracic duct is typically by one or more channels into the left subclavian vein (Fig. 24.7, *B* and *C*). Zhdanov (19) found that only 27% of thoracic ducts end as a single trunk (Fig. 24.7, *A*). In most cases the main duct breaks into a number of branches before entering the venous system. In some cases, however, the branches reunite just before entrance. Almost 25% enter at three or more vessels.

In more than 50% of the population, the thoracic duct opens into the subclavian vein just above its junction with the internal jugular. Opening into the angle between the two vessels is common, but openings also are found into the internal jugular vein, the innominate vein, or the vertebral vein (Fig. 24.7, *C*). Frequently, a dilation exists near the end of the duct, which may represent the remains of the embryonic jugular lymph sac.

When the thoracic duct terminates normally on the left, a short right thoracic trunk, usually only a few millimeters long, may enter the right subclavian artery. Usually no trunk is present; the jugular and subclavian tributaries enter the veins separately, without joining (21).

When the thoracic duct itself enters the venous system on the right (Fig. 24.7, *D*), there is frequently but not always an anomalous retroesophageal right subclavian artery (17). Hollinshead (22) suggests that pressure from the anomalous vessel on the left side of the vertebral column exerts pressure on the developing left thoracic duct and forces the main flow into the right lymphatic trunk.

Cystic Hygroma (Cystic Lymphangioma)

Cystic hygroma belongs to the group of lesions known as lymphangiomas. Lymphangiomas are characterized by the presence of fluid-filled, endothelium-lined spaces derived from lymphatic vessels. Three forms of the disease have been distinguished, on the basis of size of the fluid-filled spaced:

1. Simple lymphangioma: Capillary-sized, thin-walled lymph channels
2. Cavernous lymphangioma: Dilated lymph channels with fibrous adventitia
3. Cystic lymphangioma (cystic hygroma): Cysts from a few millimeters to a few centimeters in diameter, with thick fibrous walls

Although there is no sharp distinction among the three types and although all may be found together in the same lesion (23), there is a difference in their distribution. For example, the great majority of cystic hygromas are found in the neck.

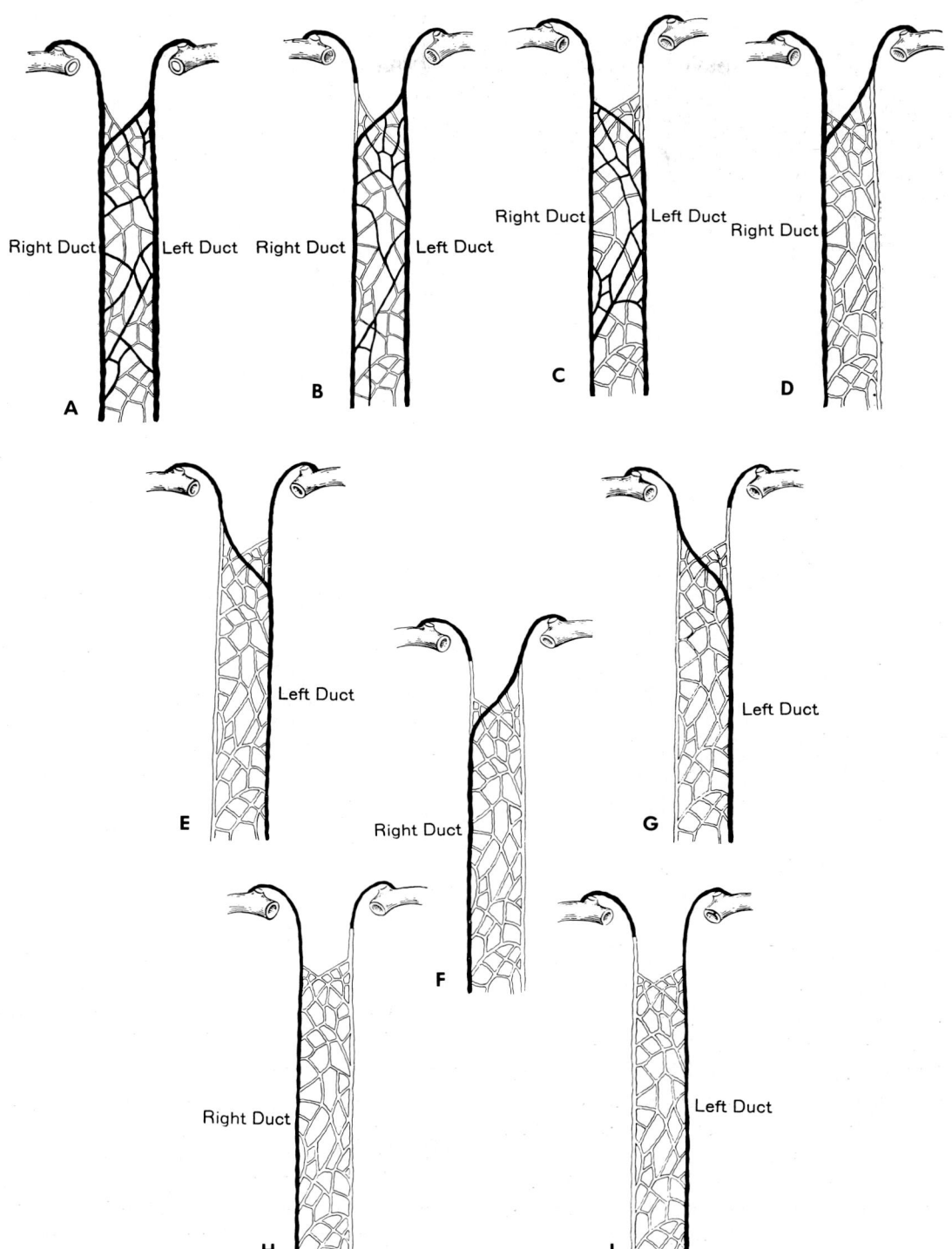

Figure 24.4. Variations in the development of the thoracic duct. **A,** Primitive paired thoracic ducts. **B** to **I,** Possible configurations of the duct in the adult. **F** is the most common pattern. (From Davis HK. A statisical study of the thoracic duct in man. Am J Anat 1915;17:211–244.)

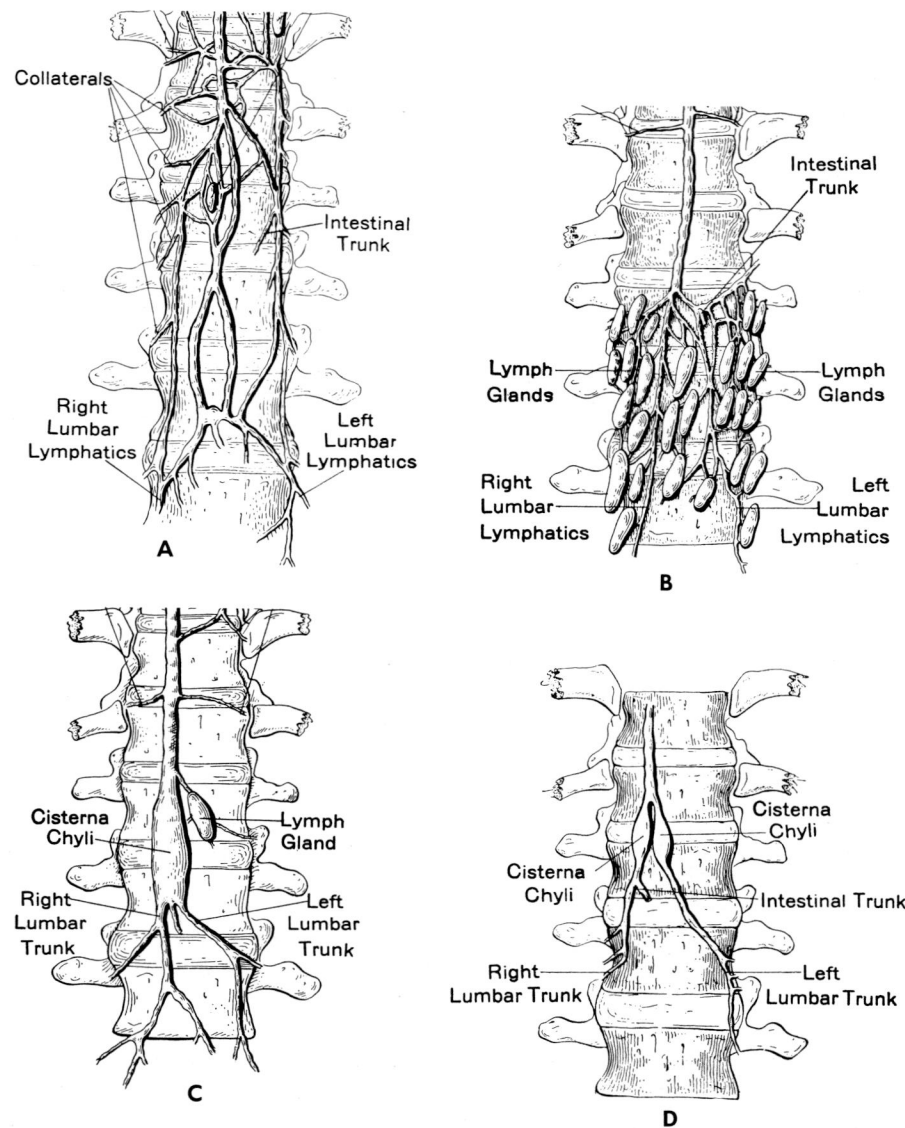

Figure 24.5. Variations in the origin of the thoracic duct. In **A,** the duct forms at the level of the third lumbar vertebra, while in **D,** it starts at the level of the 12th thoracic vertebra. The cisterna chyli is absent in **A** and **B;** it is present in **C** and doubled in **D.** (From Davis HK. A statistical study of the thoracic duct in man. Am J Anat 1915;17:211–244.)

The reader should not confuse these with lymphangiomyomatosis which is not congenital and most likely is of hormonal etiology (24).

ANATOMY

In cystic hygroma, the cysts are numerous and large, and they may communicate with one another. Young cysts are thin walled, whereas older cysts have thick, fibrous walls. Muscle bundles and blood vessels occasionally appear to traverse the cyst, but they lie outside the cyst lining of flat hexagonal cells. Lymphoid tissue may be found in the walls. The contents of the cyst are clear and straw colored, unless infection has occurred. The cystic mass is not encapsulated.

LOCATION

More than 80% of reported cases of cystic hygroma occur in the neck. The oral cavity, mediastinum, axilla, and groin are affected in most of the remaining cases. Figure 24.8 shows the distribution of 112 cases (25). Other, less commonly affected sites are also indicated.

In the neck, the lesion may affect either side, or it may be bilateral. The left posterior triangle is the most frequent single location (25). The lesion may extend upward into the tongue and floor of the mouth or downward into the mediastinum (Fig. 24.9).

Mediastinal cystic hygroma, whether it is an extension from a cervical lesion or confined to the thorax, is the most serious form of the disease. Cervicomediastinal hygroma may occupy the posterior and superior mediastinum, displacing the trachea and esophagus forward, or it may enter the anterior mediastinum (26, 27). Cystic hygroma arising in the thorax may occupy any part of the mediastinum, but there is a predilection for the anterior costophrenic angle, and expansion into the right hemithorax is more usual than into the left (28).

Cystic hygroma of the groin consists of multiple cysts overlying the inguinal canal and the femoral vessels. It frequently involves the scrotum or labia and the thigh. It may extend upward into the abdomen beneath the skin, or it may lie beneath the peritoneum (29, 30).

Cystic hygroma usually is present at birth, but it may sometimes manifest only in later life. The structure may grow slowly or extremely rapidly, and fluctuations in size may occur; sudden enlargement is not uncommon.

Feins and Raffensperger (31) presented the following distribution: neck, 75%; axilla, 20%; and trunk or extremities, 5%.

PATHOGENESIS

Lymphangiomas usually are considered to be hamartomas—excessive local developments of lymphatic tissue.

Bill and Sumner (23) argued that the particular form of the lesion depends on the tissue surrounding it. When muscle fibers are present to limit dilation of the lymph spaces, such as in the lips and tongue, the lymphangioma remains cavernous. In fatty tissue and along fascial planes, the lesion takes the cystic form.

Others, such as Gross (25) and Ward and his colleagues (32), believed that cystic hygroma of the neck and axilla are specific malformations of lymphatic development in the region of the primitive jugular lymph sac.

EDITORIAL COMMENT

Since more than 95% of congenital cystic lymphangiomas occur in the neck, axilla, or groin, the obvious conclusion is that there is a related developmental anomaly of the lymphatic system in these areas. Since these are the exact sites for the junction of developing primitive jugular lymph sacs, it is logical to assume that these represent congenital anomalies in development and occur where one would expect at the site of embryonic junction. The controversy regarding a congenital anomaly versus a true neoplasm is probably best resolved by recognizing that the apparent invasion of normal structures by the lymphangioma is probably more likely due to the formation of these ectopic segments of the lymphatic system in

primordial mesenchymal tissue which subsequently forms muscle and other soft tissues. There is certainly no evidence that there is increased mitotic activity of congenital lymphangiomas; therefore, any suggestion that this represents a malignant neoplasm is not histologically sound (JAH, CNP).

These spaces may arise as pinched off buds of the sac (centrifugal theory of Sabin [3, 4] and Lewis [5]) or as mesenchymal clefts that failed to establish connection with the developing main lymphatic channels (centripetal theory of Huntington and McClure [6]). This sequestration presumably takes place between the sixth week, when the jugular lymph sacs form, and the ninth week, when the lymphatic channels are complete. Similarly, cystic hygroma may form the tributaries of the iliac lymph sacs in the groin.

Cystic hygroma is not produced by the mere enlargement of a few congenitally sequestered endothelial-lined lymphatic spaces; instead, active growth of the endothelium results in the invasive process which characterizes the lesion. This growth, first described by Goetsch (33), proceeds by the formation of endothelial sprouts from the walls of cysts at the margin of the lesion. These sprouts insinuate themselves along fascial planes between organs and subsequently develop lymph-filled cavities, which are either new cysts or extensions of the parent cyst. Continued enlargement takes place by slow dissection and sometimes by pressure atrophy of normal structures.

It is curious that these endothelial cysts do not, in the course of their extension, reestablish contact with the normal lymphatic channels and thus provide drainage. Failure of such communications to form suggests that the cystic endothelium is not merely normal, although isolated, lymphatic vascular tissue, but that it has undergone changes which make it incompatible with the endothelium of normal, functional lymph channels.

The majority of workers consider cystic hygroma to be a sequestration defect of the lymphatic vessels and, hence, a development anomaly (23, 25, 34).

In spite of this, the failure of anastomosis between normal and pathologic vessels, together with its mode of growth, suggests strongly that cystic hygroma is a congenital, benign neoplasm.

Smith and Jones (35) support the theory that failure of communications, accumulation of lymph fluid, and distension are the phenomena responsible for the genesis of this anomaly (Fig. 24.10).

HISTORY

First described in 1828 by Redenbacher (36), cystic hygroma was named by Wernher in 1843 (37). Wernher, supported later by Virchow, viewed the lesion as a neo-

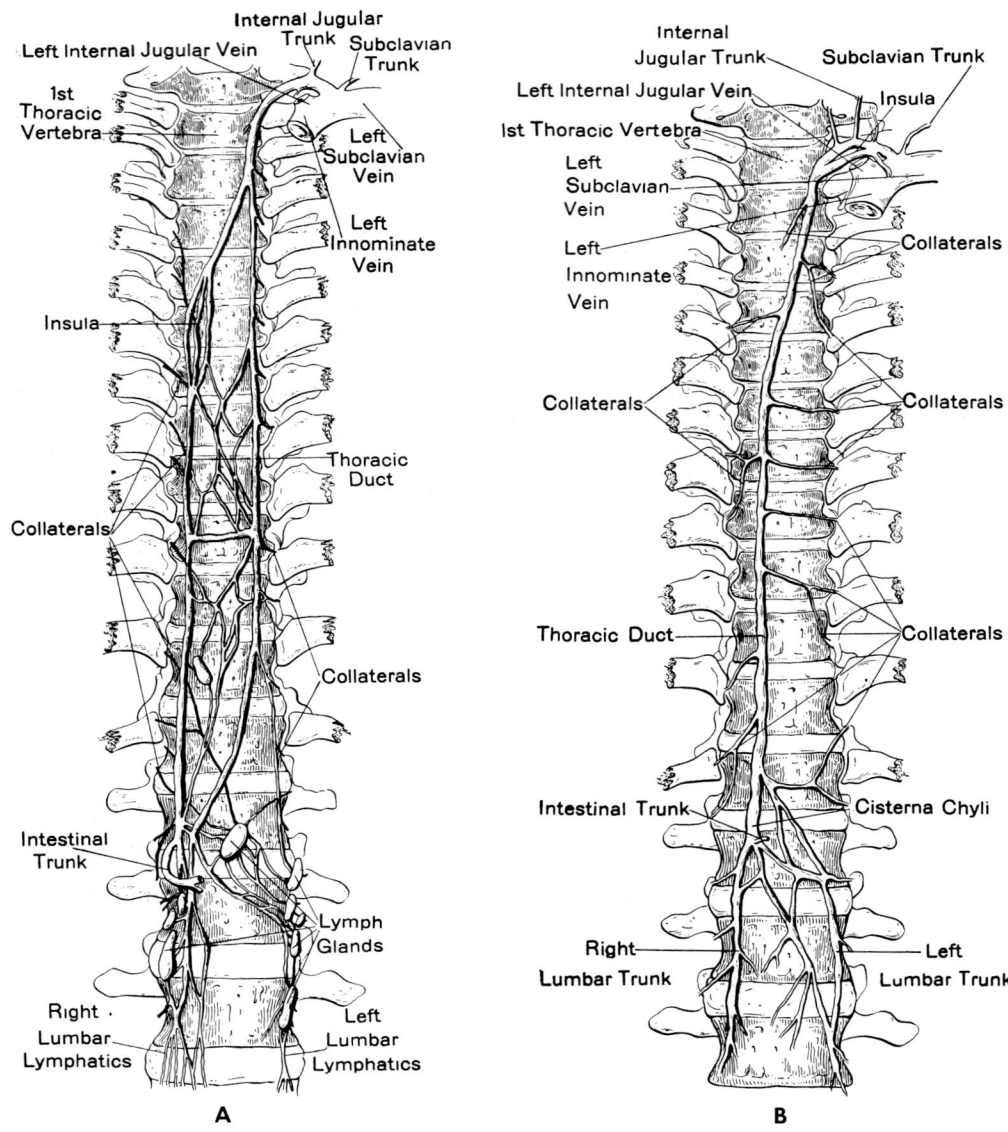

Figure 24.6. Variations in the course of the thoracic duct. **A,** The primitive paired ducts are retained along most of the course. **B** and **C,** The more usual pattern, with some caudal left-sided elements persisting. **D,** Persistence of the left duct only; at the level of the 10th thoracic vertebra. (From Davis HK. A statistical study of the thoracic duct in man. Am J Anat 1915;17:211–244.)

plasm. Arnold (38) in 1865 and Koester (39) in 1872, who demonstrated the typical endothelial lining of the cysts, considered it to be a congenital malformation (32).

In 1913 Dowd (40) collected 137 cases from the literature, beginning with that of Sandifort before 1781. He emphasized the congenital origin of the cysts, in accordance with the embryologic studies of the origin of lymphatic vessels by Huntington and McClure (6). The work of Goetsch (33) in 1938 on the invasive properties of the cysts served to revive the older view of their neoplastic nature.

ASSOCIATED SYNDROMES

Cystic hygromas, according to Romero et al. (41), are associated with chromosomal aberrations such as Turner's and other syndromes (Table 24.2).

EDITORIAL COMMENT

There have been several reports of prenatal diagnosis by sonography of cystic lymphangioma masses in the cervical region. These masses have been noted to disappear in the course of further fetal development and be replaced by fibrosis with subsequent webbing of the neck. Webbed neck is characteristic of Turner's syn-

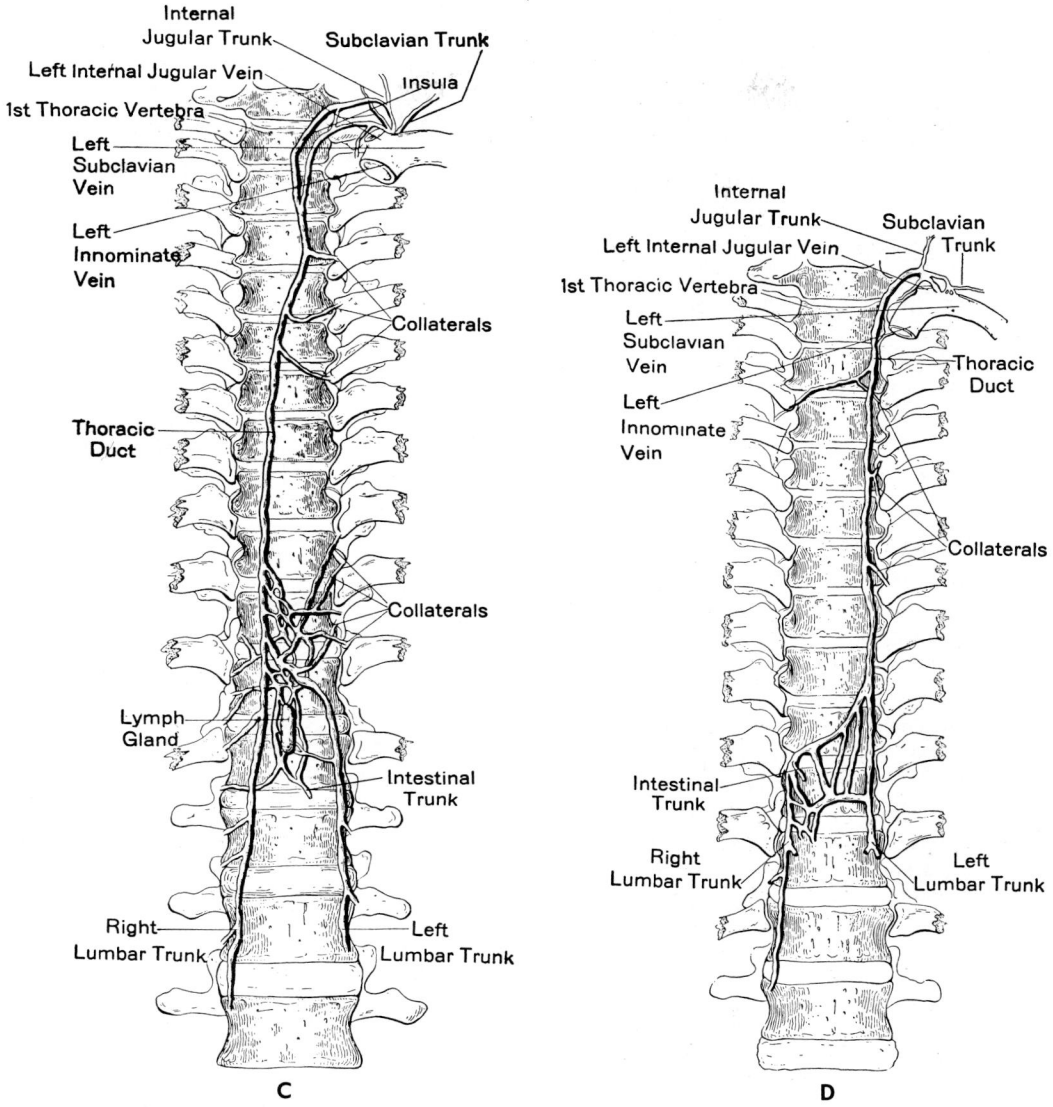

drome, and good evidence exists that webbed neck may be a fetal healing process of earlier cystic lymphangioma masses in the neck. Further documentation of this remarkable transformation must be forthcoming before this can be definitely verified, but it seems likely that the webbed neck present in many syndromes results from earlier abnormalities of a cystic lymphangioma-like tissue in the cervical area (JAH, CNP).

INCIDENCE

In our own experience (42), there were 21 cases of cervical cystic hygroma among 2519 patients with neck masses in Atlanta hospitals from 1954 through 1963. These represented 0.44% of all neck masses seen during the period and 1:6800 (all) surgical admissions. Later, with 19 years' experience and 7748 neck masses, we found only 32 cases of cystic hygroma in the neck (43) (see the discussion under "Rule of Seven").

Among Gross's 112 patients, the lesion was present at birth in 65% and was recognized within the first 2 years in 90%, but its appearance as late as the third and fourth decades of life has been reported (32, 44). Fifty-six cases in the groin or the scrotum were reported up to 1955 (29). Hundreds of cases of cervical cystic hygroma can be found in the literature.

There is no evidence of an unequal sex ratio in cystic hygroma of the neck, but in lesions of the groin, five times as many males as females are affected.

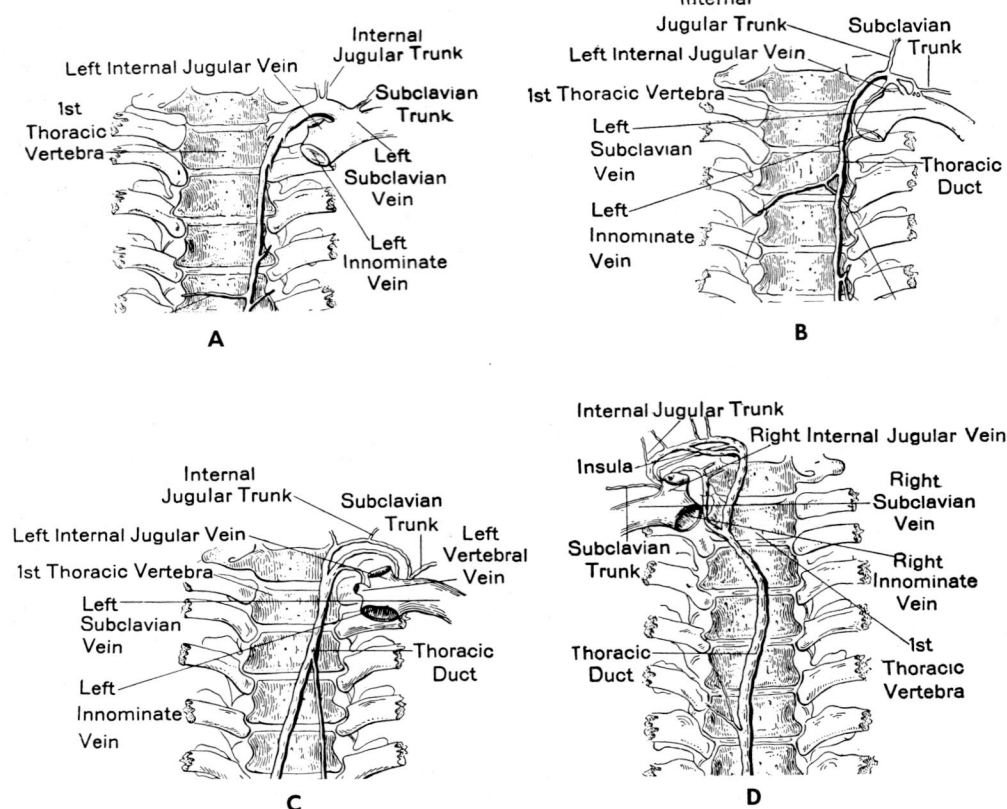

Figure 24.7. Variations in the termination of the thoracic duct. **A,** Single channel entering the subclavian vein. **B,** Quadruple channels entering the vein. **C,** Triple channels entering the subclavian and vertebral veins. **D,** Termination by the three branches into the right jugular vein. (From Davis HK. A statistical study of the thoracic duct in man. Am J Anat 1915;17:211–244.)

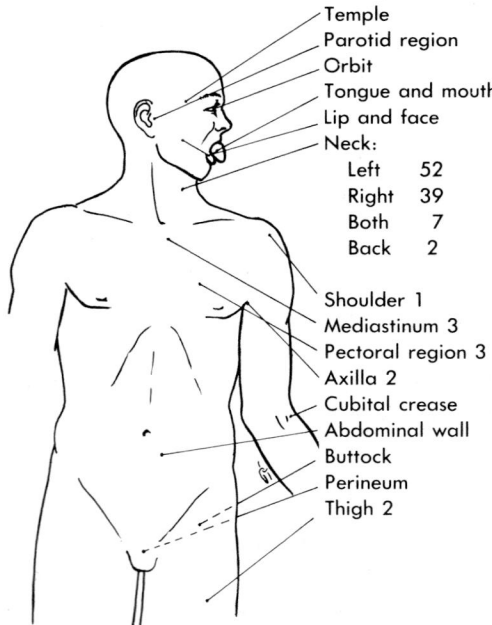

The overall incidence of cystic hygroma in fetuses has been reported by Byrne and her colleagues (45). Of 3500 miscarriages, these researchers found a cystic hygroma in 1:200 miscarried fetuses greater than 3 cm in crown-rump length.

SYMPTOMS

In spite of the striking deformity of cystic hygroma of the neck, pain and discomfort are rare unless infection has occurred. If the mediastinum is involved, dyspnea, wheezing, fever, and cyanosis may be produced by obstruction. Death from tracheal encirclement also has been observed (27, 36). Many mediastinal cysts are asymptomatic and are discovered only accidentally.

Figure 24.8. Sites of 112 cases of cystic hygroma reported by Gross. *Numerals* refer to the number of cases in each location in his series. Cystic hygroma has also been reported from other sites (*without numerals*); most of these are rare. (From Gross RE. The surgery of infancy and childhood. Philadelphia: WB Saunders, 1953.)

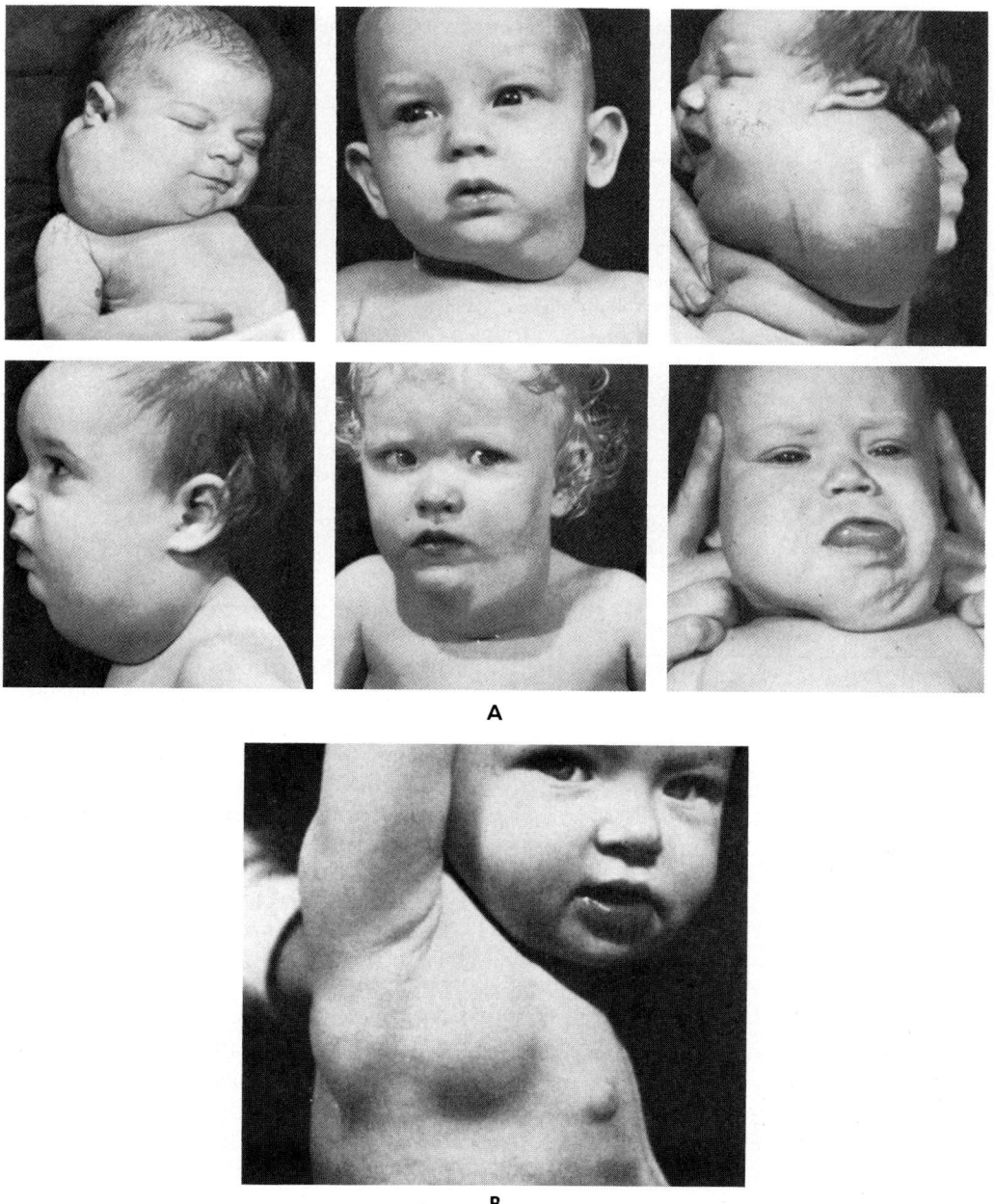

Figure 24.9. Cystic hygroma. **A,** Photographs of six patients with cystic hygroma of the neck. **B,** Patient with cystic hygroma of the axilla. (From Gross RE. The surgery of infancy and childhood. Philadelphia: WB Saunders, 1953.)

DIAGNOSIS

Cystic hygromas are fluctuant rather than tense; they are not fixed to the overlying skin, but they are not movable over the underlying structures. Unlike other tumors of the neck, cystic hygromas are readily transilluminated by bright light. Radiography is rarely helpful in identifying the tumor, although it may aid in determining the extent of mediastinal invasion in cervicomediastinal hygromas.

For the localization and extension of the cystic mass, computed tomography (CT) especially of the neck and thorax, should be used.

Treatment

Spontaneous regression of cystic hygroma has been reported (44), but it is too rare to justify expectant treatment. Infection with fatal sepsis is far more likely to result.

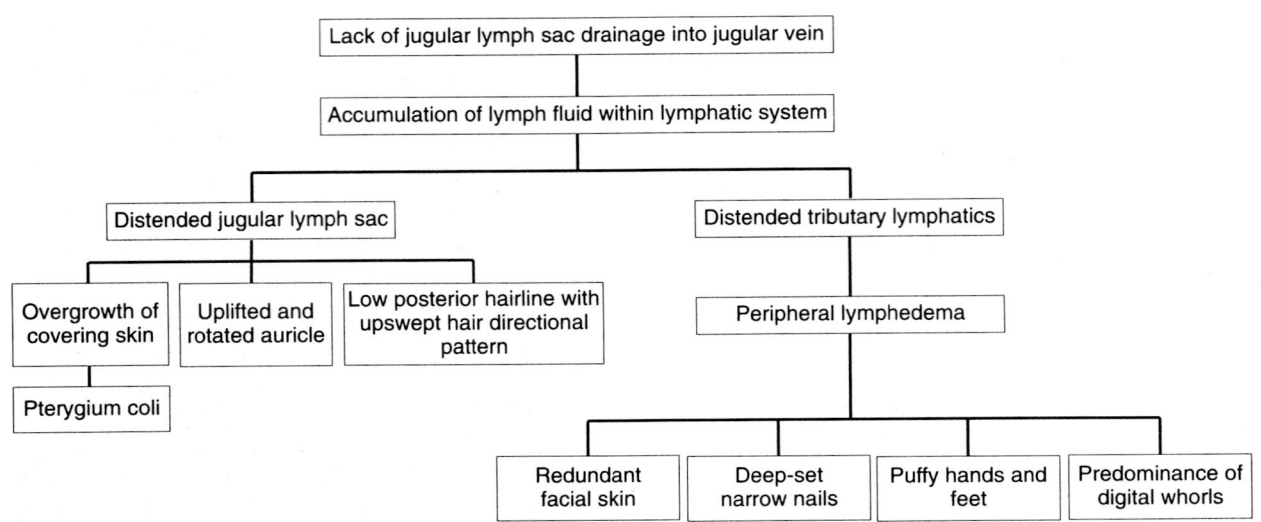

Figure 24.10. Lymphatic obstructive sequence. (Reproduced with permission from Smith DW, Jones KL. Recognizable patterns of human malformation: genetic embryologic and clinical aspects, 3rd ed. Philadelphia: WB Saunders, 1982:472.)

Table 24.2.
Karyotype in 60 Cases of Fetal Cystic Hygroma[a]

Karyotype	No. of Cases (%)
Abnormal karyotype	
Turner's syndrome	
45 XO	30 (50)
Mosaic	1 (1.6)
Trisomy 21	4 (6.6)
Trisomy 18	3 (5)
Trisomy 13	2 (3.3)
47,XXY	1 (1.6)
Total	41 (68)
Normal karyotype	11 (18)
Karyotype not available	8 (13)

[a]Data derived from Bluth et al. South Med J 1984; 77:1335; Chervenak et al. N Engl J Med 1983; 309:822; Garden et al. Am J Obstet Gynecol 1986; 154:221; Greenberg et al. Clin Genet 1983; 24:389; Pearce et al. Prenat Diagn 1984; 4:371; Redford et al. Prenat Diagn 1984; 4:327; and from cases collected by the authors.

Aspiration of the cysts is useless except to remove pressure temporarily from underlying structures. The cysts refill rapidly, and repeated aspiration eventually leads to infection.

Sclerosing solutions have been used in the past, but they are dangerous because of the proximity of great vessels to the thin-walled cysts. Gross (25) warned that the possibility of lymphaticovenous anastomoses may permit the sclerosing fluid to enter the circulation.

Irradiation has resulted in a few cures (46), but it too has been considered dangerous because it results in increased susceptibility to infection and in cosmetic disfiguration. However, irradiation has been used effectively to reduce the size of the lesion prior to surgical treatment (44).

Surgical dissection of the cysts is the treatment of choice. The surgeon must be prepared to follow the course of the cysts into the deepest planes of the neck. While no definite harm is done in opening the cysts, they are easier to dissect intact than collapsed. If any portion of a cyst is allowed to remain, the tumor will recur.

When the lesion extends into the mediastinum, the mediastinal component may be removed through a neck incision, or a thoracotomy may be required. Of nine such patients treated at the Mayo Clinic, six survived, and the five of these who could be followed were cured. Sclerosing solutions have been used to extirpate the mediastinal portion of the lesion (44).

PROGNOSIS

Cystic hygroma diagnosed *in utero* generally carries a poor prognosis (47, 48, 49) although a few cases of spontaneous resolution have been reported (50, 51).

The surgical mortality reported in Dowd's (40) 1913 review was 43.5%. This was reduced to about 4% or less (25, 45) at mid-century. According to Ravitch and Rush (52) in 1986, the mortality should be none, but the mortality of cervicothoracic lesions is about 2 to 5%. About 10% recurrence rate can be expected as a result of incomplete excision. Recurrence is more frequent in cavernous lymphangioma of the tongue, floor of the mouth, and face.

Renal Hygroma

Encapsulated cystic formation can occur within the renal paranchyma without evidence of invasion. According to Joost et al. (53), Henshel reported the first case.

According to Mullins et al. (54), renal hygroma is very rare; only 24 cases have been reported. The Mullins researchers studied two 25-year-old sisters who had renal hygroma. We agree with Singer (55) who suggested that, most likely, this is a congenital anomaly caused by disruption of lymphatic vessels producing abnormal communications. Supporting this theory, Mullins et al. (54) reported that 29.2% of their patients were less than 18 months of age. Pyelonephritis was suggested by Heptinstall (56), but many patients with renal hygroma did not have any evidence of pyelonephritis.

Excision of the hygroma is the treatment of choice of both surgeons and pathologists when malignancy does not exist. However, since the diagnosis of benignity is extremely difficult to make prior to surgery, nephrectomy should be performed.

Mullins et al. (54) noted that 22 of 24 patients underwent nephrectomies.

Primary Lymphedema

Leriche (57) maintains that the ''treatment of lymphedema will only improve if radiography of lymphatic vessels has demonstrated the pathophysiology.''

Many terms have been used to designate an early appearing, spontaneous, self-originating edema. Among these are *Milroy's disease, idiopathic edema,* and *lymphedema praecox.*

In 1892 Milroy (58) reported a case of lymphedema, restricted largely to the feet. The condition was apparent at birth, and Milroy was able to trace the disease through six generations of a family with 97 individuals, of whom 22 were affected. Accordingly, Milroy's disease is both congenital and familial.

A similar condition, however, can occur at any age. The majority of cases, usually designated as ''lymphedema praecox,'' occur in patients between the ages of 10 and 35 years.

Allen and his colleagues (59) discussed the possible cause of lymphedema and first suggested that the entire explanation might rest on a congenital underdevelopment of the lymphatics. The extensive lymphangiograms performed on a large series of patients of different ages by Kinmonth and his associates (60) indicate a single entity: primary lymphedema due to faulty development of lymphatic vessels (Fig. 24.11). In the Kinmonth series, 14% of patients showed absence of lymph trunks in affected areas. Aplasia was a frequent finding in cases of congenital and severe lymphedema. Fifty-five percent fell into a group in which lymph trunks were deficient in both size and number (hypoplasia). Twenty-four percent showed dilated and tortuous (varicose) lymphatics. In this latter group, concomitant complications included chylous reflux to the lower limb, chylous ascites, chyluria, and lymphatic fistulae. Associated vascular anomalies are more common among such patients than they are in a

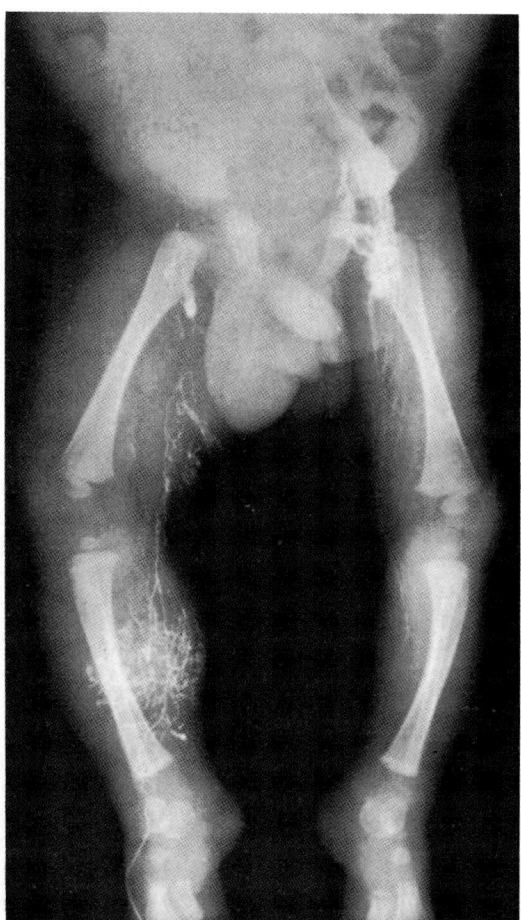

Figure 24.11.   Lymphogram of child. The patient exhibited chylous ascites, right inguinal hernia, and lymphedema of right lower extremity. There is hypoplasia of the lymphatics in the upper thigh and inguinal region, with distension of the distal part of the lymphatic tree. (Photograph courtesy of Professor J. B. Kinmonth, St. Thomas's Hospital Medical School, London.)

normal population. This might be expected since arteries, veins, and lymphatics are closely associated during fetal development.

Kinmonth et al. (60) stated:

> Where the deformity is sufficiently severe, edema is present at birth, whereas in others with less marked deformity drainage is adequate to avoid edema until some extra load is thrown on the lymphatics in some way or other. This may be caused by the formation of an inflammatory or traumatic exudate, pregnancy, the onset of menstruation, or in other ways. The subnormal lymphatics are then found unable to cope with the extra demand on their function and permanent edema results.

Servelle (61) presented 642 cases of lymphedema and claimed that it was he who performed the first lymphography in 1943. He quotes Leriche, (57) saying that the treatment of lymphedema will only improve if cardiography of lymphatic vessels has demonstrated the pathophysiology!

Chylous ascites may occur during the first 6 months of life as the result of aplasia, hypoplasia, or failure of the mesenteric lymphatics to connect with the thoracic duct. Chylous ascites also may be part of generalized hypoplasia of the lymphatic system, with backflow into intestinal lymphatics, which in turn rupture into the intestinal lumen, causing loss of protein and fat. Chyluria may result from lymphatic backflow and rupture into the kidney pelvis (62, 63).

As might be expected, maldevelopment of the lymphatic system has its counterpart in animals. Herbertson and Wallace (64) observed chylous ascites in 17% of the newborn mice in a Cambridge strain. The affected mice appeared normal at birth, but after suckling, milky fluid accumulated in the peritoneal cavity. The mesenteric lymph vessels were distended, tortuous, and exuded chyle. Many animals recovered, but the more severely affected became too weak to suckle and died. Primary lymphedema also has been studied in dogs and sheep.

Chavez (65) provided an extensive review of diagnosis and treatment of lymphatic defects in 1964 and stated:

> From the recent reports, we have come to realize the complexity of the problem, and find that primary or idiopathic cases of chyluria, chylous ascites, intestinal lymphangiectasis and lymphedema are associated either with concomitant alterations of the lymphatics in other areas of the body or with other congenital malformations, usually of the vascular system. These lymphatic abnormalities may therefore be con-

sidered as parts of a single entity having different manifestations.

The anomalies of the lymphatic system are plentiful and poorly understood. For instance, can we explain an angiofollicular lymph node hyperplasia causing a neck mass (66), and how can we explain heterotopic tissue in lymph nodes in relation to metastatic disease (67)? The association of lymphatic anomalies with other anomalies is also still an enigma. Miller and Motolsky (68) studied genetic lymphedema syndromes, and presented nine in a table (Table 24.3).

We present a few examples of the many anomalies, not to discuss the subject in toto but to mention the innumerable possible combinations.

Lymphangiomas in several solid organs, intestinal lymphangiectasia, and generalized lymphangiomatosis have been reported, but the subject is too large for the scope of this book. Not only in the tonsils, the thymus, and the spleen (the primary lymphatic organs) but all over the human body, lymphatic congenital anomalies will find a mysterious way to develop. Rynlin and Foajaco (69) reported pulmonary lymphangiectasia, and Asch et al. (70) discussed the rarity of hepatic and splenic similar lesions. Murphishi et al. (71) reported generalized lymphangiomatosis.

Hereditary congenital lymphedema in a newborn girl with pseudosexual ambiguity was reported by Sarda (72). The karyotype was 46XX, both lower extremities were involved, and the mother's family confirmed a non–Milroy disease.

Table 24.3.
Genetic Lympedema Syndromes[a]

Condition	Inheritance	Age of Onset	Associated Clinical Features[b]
Milroy's disease	Autosomal dominant	Congenital	Pleural effusion, chylous ascites
Meige's disease	Autosomal dominant	Puberty and later	One pedigree suggestive of autosomal recessive inheritance reported
Yellow nail syndrome	Autosomal dominant	Adults	Dystrophic, yellow nails,[c] pleural effusions
Distichiasis—lymphedema syndrome	Autosomal dominant	Puberty and later	Extra row eyelashes,[c] partial ectropion lower lid, vertebral anomalies, webbed neck, spinal extra dural cysts
Noonan syndrome	Autosomal dominant	Puberty and later	Facial dysmorphia, congenital heart disease, webbed neck, atrophic testes, short stature, mental deficiency
Lymphedema associated with cerebrovascular malformation	Autosomal dominant	Puberty and later	Cranial bruit frequent, primary pulmonary hypertension
Lymphedema and cholestasis	Autosomal recessive	Congenital or early childhood	Recurrent cholestatic jaundice[c] described in Norwegian families
Turner's syndrome	Chromosomal-XO	Newborn period	Edema of dorsum of hands and feet—usually resolves in months or years, coarctation of aorta, short stature, small chin, webbed neck
Lymphedema associated with ptosis[d]	Autosomal dominant	Puberty	Ptosis[c]

[a]From Miller M, Motulsky AC Noonan syndrome in an adult family presenting with chronic lymphedema. Am J Med 1978; 65:382.
[b]Not all clinical features are present in each case of a given syndrome.
[c]Constant feature of syndrome.
[d]This condition may be an expression of Noonan syndrome.

We do not know how to classify the Klippel-Trenaunay-Weber syndrome which may be associated with lymphatic anomalies such as lymphedema and lymph vessel malformations. Klippel and Trenaunay presented this syndrome in 1900 with the following involvement:

1. Nevi of the involved extremity
2. Varicosities in the same limb, which started in childhood
3. Hypertrophy of bones and all soft tissues in the involved extremities

The interested reader will find an excellent review of this syndrome in the paper of Servelle (73) in which he reported 768 operated cases.

Witt et al. (74) discussed lymphedema in Noonan's syndrome (multiple congenital anomalies). Because of the number of cases reported the suggestion was made that lymphedema is a much more frequent concomitant with Noonan's syndrome. A similar case was reported by White (75). Also, testicular lymphogiomatosis in Noonan's syndrome was reported by Nistal et al. (76).

Voight et al. (77) reported fetal neck edema in eight patients in association with Down and Turner's syndrome.

Crowe and Dickerman (78) discussed the possibility of a genetic association between microcephaly and lymphedema. Similar cases were reported by Leung (79). A family with lymphedema praecox and cleft palate was discussed by Figueroa et al. (80).

Dahlberg et al. (81) reported two brothers with congenital lymphedema, hypoparathyroidism and several other somatic anomalies. The pleiotropic effect of autosomal or X-linked recessive gene was suggested as the cause.

Tudose and Rada (82) reported extensive fibrosis and lipomatosis of lymph nodes of the inguinoiliac area in patients with primary lymphoedema. The authors raised the question of whether these are genetic or developmental anomalies.

Treatment of lymphedema is usually conservative; however, the massive deformity resulting from edema with subcutaneous fibrous tissue proliferation has stimulated many surgical efforts. Among the procedures tried were massive tissue resection, skin grafting, and the insertion of skin and nylon threads (83).

As a second year student, I (JES) witnessed Condoleon, himself, perform the Condoleon operation for elephantiases on one of the lower extremities (I do not remember whether the patient was female or male or the age of the patient). He made a long elliptical incision at the lateral aspect of the lower extremity, starting from the iliac crest and ending above the external malleolus. Subcutaneous tissue and fascia were incised corresponding to the skin incision. Heavy continuous catgut was used to close the incision, and a heavy dressing was applied tightly. I do not remember the results of this case, but it makes me feel good today to know that I saw the master performing.

EDITORIAL COMMENT

It should be emphasized that the Condoleon operation was introduced for the treatment of *acquired* lymphoedema or elephantiasis secondary to filarial infection and was occasionally used also for the lymphoedema secondary to deep venous insufficiency due to thrombophlebitis and recanalization of the veins of the lower extremities. This type of interstitial edema is quite different from that seen with congenital lymphedema or Milroy's disease. Congenital lymphatic obstruction resulting from abnormal development and connections of the lymphatics especially in the lower extremity are usually so extensive that there are no available collateral lymphatic channels, which are necessary for a successful Condoleon operation. The results of extensive excision and skin grafting for Milroy's disease have been disappointing. Nevertheless, because it occurs so frequently in young adolescent girls and is cosmetically so distressing, many plastic surgical procedures have been introduced in an attempt to correct the obvious deformity. The lymphoedema secondary to deep venous incompetence has a different pathophysiology and will often respond to interrupting connecting venous channels, which have no valves, and to allowing venous return exclusively through the deep system, which is protected by the overlying muscle. This is not true for congenital lymphoedema; therefore, attempts to improve venous return are misguided because congenital lymphoedema results from an anomaly in lymphatic development and is not related to venous incompetence (JAH, CNP).

Mesenteric, Omental, and Retroperitoneal Lymphatic Cysts

Although we discuss mesenteric, omental, and retroperitoneal cysts under lymphatic anomalies, we recognize that their lymphatic origin is not beyond question and that some retroperitoneal cysts are almost certainly of nonlymphatic origin. It will be convenient, however, to consider them at this time and to point out the doubtful and exceptional cases.

ANATOMY

Location. Burnett and his colleagues (84), reviewing 185 cases of abdominal lymphatic cysts in 1950, found the following distribution:

Mesentery of small intestine	50.3%
Mesentery of sigmoid colon	16.2%
Mesocolon	11.9%
Mesentery of cecum	8.7%
Mesentery of descending colon	2.7%
Mesentery of appendix	1.6%

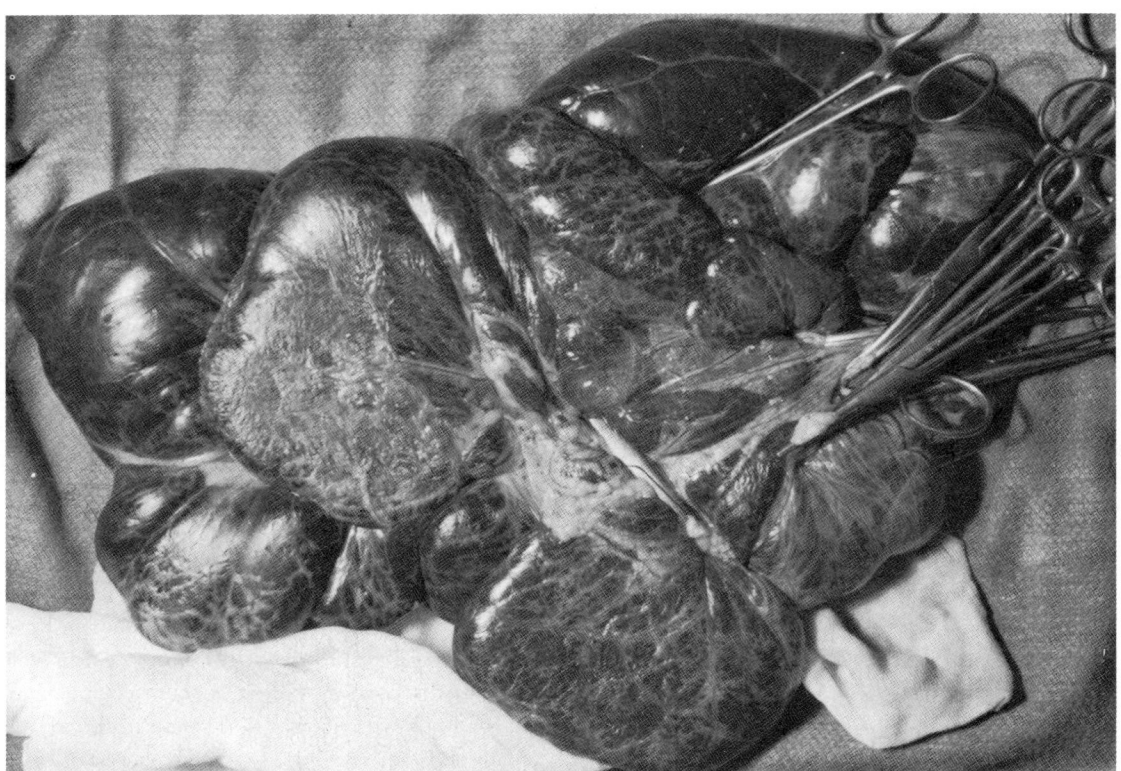

Figure 24.12.   Multilocular omental cyst from a 3-year-old child. The cyst contained 1300 cc of fluid. (From Gross RE. The surgery of infancy and childhood. Philadelphia: WB Saunders, 1953.)

Omentum	2.2%
Gastrohepatic mesentery	0.5%
Duodenum	0.5%
Retroperitoneal	5.4%

Possibly related to mesenteric cysts are the instances of spherical cysts found lying free in the abdomen. Lined and covered with epithelium, these curious cysts have no blood vessels in the connective tissue. The first case was reported by Plaut (85) in 1928, and at least six have been found since then. All were in adults, and all but one of the seven patients were women. Hinshaw (86) reviewed the series and suggested that the cysts arise from mesothelial cell metaplasia. This explanation must be considered tentative; the origin of these cysts is completely obscure.

Structure of the Cysts. Mesenteric cysts may be single, multiple, or loculated (Fig. 24.12 and 24.13). The walls are usually thin, often with a lining of squamous, cuboidal, or columnar epithelium. In three cases in our own experience (87), no epithelium was present, having been presumably destroyed during expansion of the cyst. Smooth muscle fibers may be found in the connective tissue wall, but they are not arranged as true muscularis such as occurs in an enteric cyst. Inflammatory cells are frequently present. The leaves of the mesentery form a serosa on the outer surface. At least two calcified cysts have been described (84, 85).

The contents of the cysts may be serous, sanguineous, or chylous (Fig. 24.13). The chylous cysts are less frequently encountered than are the serous. Various circumstances may alter the contents of a chylous cyst. The content, therefore, is not a reliable means of ascertaining the origin of the cyst (89, 90) (Fig. 24.13, *C*). However, Gerster (91) believed the chylous milky appearance results from fatty degeneration of the cyst wall and cites examples of chylous cysts elsewhere in the body.

Retroperitoneal cysts are similar in structure to cysts within the leaves of the mesentery. If tubular and glomerular remnants can be demonstrated (92), they are of nephrogenic rather than lymphatic origin.

Size. Mesenteric cysts vary in size from microscopic to immense. One was the size of an orange when discovered and had attained a volume of 13 liters when operated on 24 days later (93). Another patient had a 5000-cc cyst that produced several more liters of fluid during 2 weeks' postoperative drainage. Such huge cysts usually fill the entire abdomen, adhering to all viscera. They are not tense and therefore readily accommodate themselves to the irregularities of the visceral contours (94).

Retroperitoneal cysts may be almost as large as mesenteric cysts. From one, over 4 liters of fluid was aspirated; the cyst filled the abdominal cavity from the ribs to the pubic symphysis (95). Omental cysts may be equally large (96).

EMBRYOGENESIS

Various origins have been suggested for these cysts. The majority, being lined with endothelium, are considered to arise from lymphatic spaces associated with the embryonic retroperitoneal lymph sac. Their origin is thus similar to that of cystic hygromas of the neck, which are associated with embryonic jugular lymph sac.

Gerster (91) viewed mesenteric cysts as lymphangiomas arising from new growth of lymph vessels. If such is their origin, they may not be present at birth. Among nondevelopmental causes, trauma and lymphatic obstruction have been advanced. The late onset and rapid enlargement of some cysts encourage belief in the possibility of an acquired origin. Experimental obstruction of

lymphatics in dogs has failed, however, to produce cysts (97).

Cysts formed in the mesocolon have been attributed to local failure of fusion of the mesocolon and the parietal peritoneum during the final stages of intestinal rotation and fixation. They would thus be lined with mesothelium rather than endothelium (98). They may be formed in the peritoneal wall and bulge into the mesentery by later extension. Similar sequestration of celomic epithelium in the lungs has been described. A few retroperitoneal cysts with columnar epithelium are not of the intestinal type; they are without a muscular layer and arise from mesonephric remnants (98, 99). They represent the remains of an aplastic kidney. It must be concluded that there is no single, common origin of nonenteric mesenteric cysts.

HISTORY

Early descriptions of mesenteric cysts do not often distinguish between intestinal duplications and cysts of congenital, parasitic, or tubercular origin. The Florentine

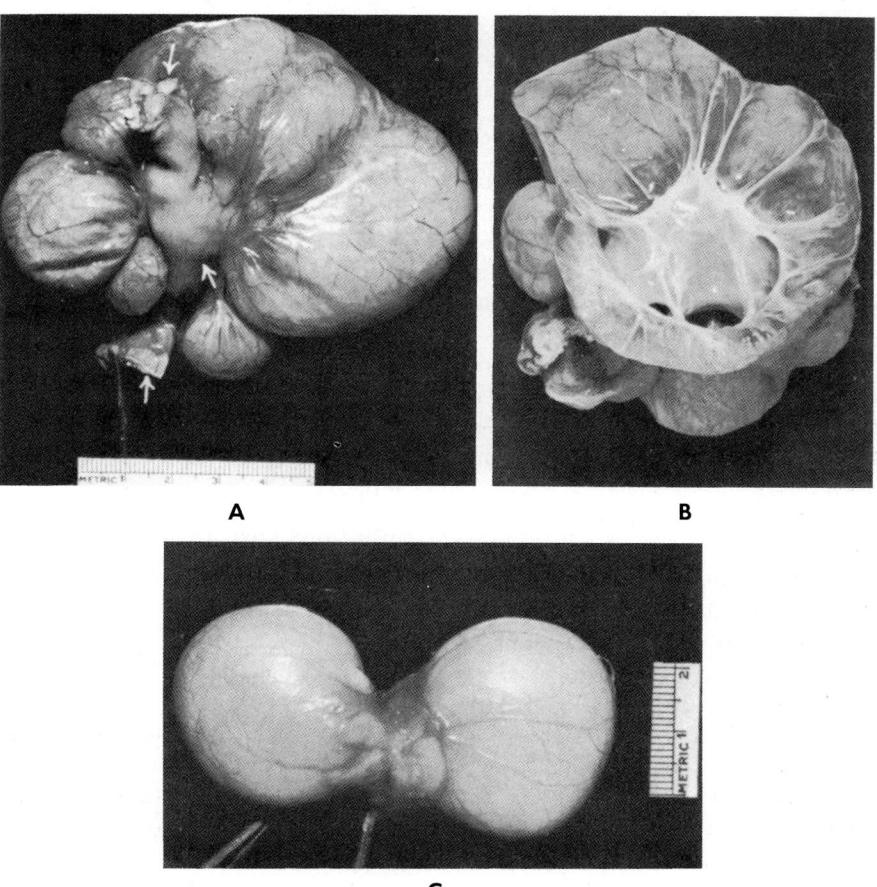

Figure 24.13. Mesenteric lymphatic cysts. **A,** Serous cyst from a 4-year-old child. A segment of ileum (*arrows*) had to be removed with the cyst. **B,** The same cyst opened to show loculation. **C,** Chylous cyst from the mesentery of a 7-week-old infant. The cyst is dumbbell-shaped and bulged from both sides of the mesentery. (From Gross RE. The surgery of infancy and childhood. Philadelphia: WB Saunders, 1953.)

Benivieni (100) usually is credited with having described a mesenteric cyst from the autopsy of an 8-year-old boy in 1507, although the lesion seems to have been solid rather than cystic (101). In 1842 Rokitansky (102) provided the first good description. Tillaux (103) performed the first operation in 1880 by excising a pedunculated cyst. In 1883 Pean first successfully marsupialized a mesenteric cyst (104).

Dowd (105) in 1900 provided an adequate classification of cysts, separating the enteric, lymphatic, and acquired infectious cysts. From this date on, there is little excuse for confusion of terminology.

Gerster (91) reviewed the literature up to 1939, supplying an annotated bibliography. Burnett and his colleagues (84) collected 200 true lymphatic cysts of the mesentery from the literature up to 1950, although Beahrs and his colleagues (106) estimated that there were then about 600 cases. Engel and his colleagues (90) reviewed 23 chylous cysts from the Mayo Clinic in 1961. Sprague (98) provided a good review of the lesions in 1960.

INCIDENCE

Mesenteric cysts occur in about 1:140,000 hospital admissions (0.0007%). Seven were found in 1 million admissions to the Mayo Clinic (94), and 21 were found in a total of almost 3 million hospital admissions, compiled from various sources by Sprague (98).

Age and Sex. Burnett et al. (84) found 27.1% of reported cases to occur in the first decade of life and 12 to 18% to occur in each of the next four decades. Fewer than 13% were reported in patients over age 50 years. Among 82 pediatric patients, 14 were under 1 year and 35 were under 5 years of age (107).

Among children, more males than females have been reported (1.7:1) (107), but in a series including adults, there were many fewer males than females (1.1:6) (84). Most of the retroperitoneal cysts have been found in females.

SYMPTOMS

Pain is present in about 80% of patients, nausea and vomiting in about 50%; and constipation in about 25%. Gradual distension of the abdomen without rigidity often is seen in children (108). The pain may be due to obstruction of the intestine through pressure, leakage of cyst contents into the peritoneum, or traction on the mesentery (109).

A mass is palpable in only about 25% of the cases because these cysts are not tense. In two elderly patients, a nontender, freely movable mass was the only sign of the disease except for chronic constipation (87).

DIAGNOSIS

Preoperative recognition of the condition is rare, although mesenteric cysts should be considered when

symptoms of obstruction exist. Plain roentgenograms may show a shadow displacing the intestine, while fluoroscopy may demonstrate mobility of the mass. Excretory urograms eliminate retroperitoneal tumors, and a barium radiographic series may outline the position of the mass (107). Lowman and his colleagues (104) believe careful elimination of other possibilities can result in a positive radiologic diagnosis.

TREATMENT

Enucleation of the mesenteric cyst is the treatment of choice unless the blood supply to the intestine is involved. Segmental resection, with end-to-end anastomosis, will then be necessary (110). Omental cysts may be removed by omentectomy.

Marsupialization has been considered obsolete by a number of authors, but it is probably the only possible treatment for huge cysts that adhere to all abdominal viscera, such as those described by Beahrs and Judd (94) and Ford (93). It must be kept in mind that large cysts are usually loculated.

Drainage or aspiration are therapeutically ineffective, although they may be a necessary step when removing the cysts. No untoward effects of rupture of the cyst during excision have been reported (90).

MORTALITY

The mortality for all procedures up to 1950 was 12.4% (84), but where enucleation, resection, or marsupialization was employed, only 14 of 139 patients died. Currently, mortality from treatment of mesenteric cysts should not occur (111, 112).

Congenital Chylothorax

For further consideration of this anomaly, see Chapter 13, "The Trachea and Lungs."

DEFINITION

Effusion of chyle in one or both pleural cavities.

ANATOMY

The right pleural cavity is most involved but bilateral accumulation was reported by Doolittle et al. (113).

EMBRYOLOGY

Overproductivity of chyli, failure of communications of the lymphatic vessels, minimal reabsorption of lymph, and perhaps abnormalities of the pulmonary lymphatics, all are responsible synergetically (or by solitary action) for the genesis of this embryologic phenomenon.

PATHOLOGY

Pulmonary hypoplasia secondary to compression, mediastinal shift, congestive heart failure, or hydrops may be present.

ASSOCIATED ANOMALIES

The following anomalies may be associated with congenital chylothorax: trisomy 21, congenital pulmonary lymphangiectasia, T-E fistula, extralobar pulmonary sequestration, and polyhydramnios.

DIAGNOSIS

If plural effusion is present, chylothorax should be suspected. Remember that the lymph at birth has a serous fluid appearance. According to Benacerraf and Frigoletto (114) and Van Aerde et al. (115), a level of more than 60% lymphocytes present in the fluid is perhaps diagnostic for chylothorax. Brodman (116) reported respiratory distress in 40% of newborns, which may be present within 24 hours or within the first week of life. Prenatal diagnosis is not difficult.

TREATMENT

Repeated thoracocentesis, continuous thoracic drainage, and special diet (medium chain triglycerides) are recommended. If this therapy does not bring good results, ligation of the thoracic duct as reported by Andersen et al. (117) should be considered.

The Lymphatic System and Cancer

In 1992 Heys and Eremin (118) theorized that involvement of regional lymph nodes is a prognostic index of survival for carcinoma and an indicator of distant metastases. They report that, while regional lymphatics may play an ameliorating role in early-stage cancer, their role diminishes with progressive tumor growth, and they may in fact produce a biological environment for carcinoma cell multiplication and dissemination to distal targets.

Japanese researchers have reported good results with extended lymphadenectomy (119, 120); the non–Asian experience has not been as promising (121–123).

REFERENCES

1. Davis HK. A statistical study of the thoracic duct in man. Am J Anat 1915;17:211–244.
2. Saxer F. Über die Entwicklung und den Bau der Lymphdrüsen und die Enttehung der roten und weissen Blutkörperchen. Anat Hefte 1896;6.
3. Sabin FR. On the origin of the lymphatic system from the veins, and the development of the lymph hearts and thoracic duct in the pig. Am J Anat 1902;1:367–389.
4. Sabin FR. The development of the lymphatic system. In: Keibel F, Mall FP, eds. Manual of human embryology, Vol 2. Philadelphia: JB Lippincott, 1912.
5. Lewis FT. The development of the lymphatic system in rabbits. Am J Anat 1905;5:95–111.
6. Huntington GS, McClure CFW. The anatomy and development of the jugular lymph sac in the domestic cat. Am J Anat 1910;10:177–311.
7. Huntington GS. The development of the mammalian jugular lymph sac, of the tributary primitive ulnar lymphatic and of the thoracic ducts from the viewpoint of recent investigations of vertebrate lymphatic ontogeny, together with a consideration of the genetic relations of lymphatic and haemal vascular channels in the embryos of amniotes. Am J Anat 1914;16:259–316.
8. Kampmeier OF. Ursprung und Entwicklungsgeschichte des Ductus thoracicus nebst Saccus lymphaticus jugularis und Cysterna chyli beim Menshen. Morphol Jahrb 1931;67:157–234.
9. Kampmeier OF. The development of the jugular lymph sacs in the light of vestigial provisional and definitive phases of morphogenesis. Am J Anat 1960;107:153–176.
10. Sabin FR. The lymphatic system in human embryos with consideration of the morphology of the system as a whole. Am J Anat 1909;9:43.
11. Clark ER. An anomaly of the thoracic duct with a bearing on the embryology of the lymphatic system. Contrib Embryol Carnegie Inst Wash 1915;3:45–54.
12. Pick JW, Anson BJ, Burnett HW. Communications between lymphatic and venous systems at renal level in man. Q Bull Northwest Univ Med School 1944;18:307–316.
13. Pressman JJ, Simon MB. Experimental evidence of direct communications between lymph nodes and veins. Surg Gynecol Obstet 1961;113:537–541.
14. Roddenberry H, Allen L. Observations on the abdominal lymphaticovenous communications of the squirrel monkey (Saimiri sciureus). Anat Rec 1967;159:147–158.
15. Parke WW, Settles HE, Bunger PC, Neufeld DA. Longitudinal lymphatic plexuses of the teniae coli and their probable clinical significance. Clin Anat 1991;4:341–347.
16. Natsugoe S, Aikou T, Shimazu H, Tabata M. Lymphatic anastomoses between the distal esophagus and gastric cardia in dogs. Clin Anat 1991;4:357–365.
17. Rouvière H. Anatomy of the human lymphatic system. Tobias MJ (transl). Ann Arbor: Edwards Bros., 1938.
18. Jossifrow GM. Der Anfang des Ductus thoracicus und dessen Erweiterung. Arch Anat Physiol Anat Abt 1906;68.
19. Zhdanov DA. General anatomy and physiology of the lymphatic system. Lennigrad: Medgiz, 1952.
20. van Pernis PA. Variations of the thoracic duct. Surgery 1949;26:806–809.
21. Zhdanov DA. The right lymphatic duct and its roots [Sb. Materialy k. anatomii linfaticheskih sosudov i uzlov.] Gorky, 1942.
22. Hollinshead WH. Anatomy for surgeons, Vol 2. The thorax, abdomen, and pelvis. New York: Hoeber-Harper, 1956.
23. Bill AH Jr, Sumner DS. A unified concept of lymphangioma and cystic hygroma. Surg Gynecol Obstet 1965;20:79–86.
24. Burlew BP, Shames JM. Lymphangiomyomatosis: hormonal implications in etiology and therapy. South Med J 1991;84:1247–1249.
25. Gross RE. The surgery of infancy and childhood. Philadelphia: WB Saunders, 1953.
26. Divertie MB, Lim RA, Harrison EG, Bernatz PE, Burger TC. Mediastinal cystic hygroma. Proc Mayo Clin 1960;35:460–466.
27. Lim RA, Divertie MB, Harrison EG, Bernatz PE. Cervicomediastinal cystic hygroma. Dis Chest 1961;40:265–275.
28. Childress ME, Baker CP, Samson PC. Lymphangioma of the mediastinum: report of case with review of literature. J Thorac Surg 1956;31:338–348.
29. Gueukdjian SA. Lymphangioma of the groin and scrotum. J Int Coll Surg 1955;24:159–170.
30. Gueukdjian SA. Cystic lygroma of the groin and scrotum. Br J Urol 1956;28:279–282.
31. Feins NR, Raffensperger JG. Cystic hygroma, lymphangioma, and lymphedema. In: Raffensperger JG (ed.) Swenson's pediatric surgery, 5th ed. Norwalk, CT: Appelton & Lange, 1990.
32. Ward GE, Hendrick JW, Chambers RG. Cystic hygroma of neck. West J Surg 1950;58:41–47.
33. Goetsch E. Hygroma colli cysticum and hygroma axillare: patho-

logical and clinical study and report of twelve cases. Arch Surg 1938;36:394–479.

34. Willis RA. Pathology of tumors, 2nd ed. London: Butterworth, 1960.

35. Smith DW, Jones KL. Recognizable patterns of human malformations: genetic embryologic and clinical aspects, 3rd ed. Philadelphia: WB Saunders, 1982:4.

36. Galofré M, Judd ES, Pérez PE, Harrison EG. Results of surgical treatment of cystic hygroma. Surg Gynecol Obstet 1962;115:319–326.

37. Wernher A. Die angeborenen Kysten-Hygrome und die ihnen verwondten Geschwulste in anatomischer, diagnostischer und therapeutischer Beiziehung: Dankschrift zur Feier des 50 jährigen Doctor Jubiläums des Dr. Wilhelm Nebel. Giessen: GF Heyer, Vater; 1843.

38. Arnold J. Zwei Fälle von Hygroma colli cysticum congenitum und deren fraglich Beziehung zu dem Ganglion intercaroticum. Virchow Arch [A] 1865;33:209.

39. Koester K. Ueber hygroma cysticum congenitum. Verh Phys Med Gesellsch Wurzb 1872;3:44–61.

40. Dowd CN. Hygroma cysticum colli: its structure and etiology. Ann Surg 1913;58:112–132.

41. Romero R, Pilu G, Jeanty P, Ghidini A, Hobbins JC. Prenatal diagnosis of congenital anomalies. Norwalk, CT: Appelton & Lange, 1988:115–118.

42. Skandalakis JE, Gray SW, Takakis NC, Godwin JT, Poer DH. Tumors of the neck. Surgery 1960;48:375–384.

43. Skandalakis JE, Gray SW, Androvlakis JE. Swelling of the neck: a statistical analysis of 7,748 cases with emphasis on differential diagnosis of nonthyroid tumors. Volume in honour of BG Kourias. (Private printing) Athens (Greece), 1975.

44. Fuller FW, Conway H. Cystic hygroma. Surg Gynecol Obstet 1959;108:457.

45. Byrne J, Blanc WA, Warburton D. The significance of cystic hygroma in fetuses. Hum Pathol 1984;15:61.

46. Briggs JD, Leix F, Snyder WH, Chaffin L. Cystic and cavernous lymphangioma. West J Surg 1953;61:499–506.

47. Thomas RL. Prenatal diagnosis of giant cystic hygroma: prognosis, counselling, and management—case presentation and review of the recent literature. Prenat Diagn 1992;12(11):919–923.

48. Suchet IB, van der Westhuizen NG, Labatte MF. Fetal cystic hygromas: further insights into their natural history. Can Assoc Radiol J 1992;43(6):420–424.

49. Tannirandorn Y et al. Fetal cystic hygromata: insights gained from fetal blood sampling. Prenat Diagn 1990;10(3):189–193.

50. Hill LM, Macpherson T, Rivello D, Peterson C. The spontaneous resolution of cystic hygromas and early fetal growth delay in fetuses with trisomy 18. Prenat Diagn 1991;11(9):673–677.

51. Baccichetti C, Lenzini E, Suma V, Benini F, Marini A. Spontaneous resolution of cystic hygroma in a 46,XX normal female. Prenat Diagn 1990;10(6):399–403.

52. Ravich MM, Rush BF. Cystic hygroma. In: Welch KJ, Randolph JG, Ravich MM, O'Neil JA Jr, Rowe MI, eds. Pediatric surgery, 4th ed. Chicago: Year Book Medical Publishers, 1986.

53. Joost J, Schaefer R, Altwein JE. Renal lymphangioma. J Urol 1977;118:22–24.

54. Mullins JR, Shield CF, Porter MG. Hygroma renalis: two cases within a family and a literature review. Surgery 1992;111:339–342.

55. Singer DR, Miller JD, Smith G. Lymphangioma of the kidney. Scott Med J 1983;28:293–294.

56. Heptinstall RH ed. Pathology of the kidney, 3rd ed. Boston: Little, Brown, 1983.

57. Leriche as quoted in Servelle M. Surgical treatment of lymphedema: a report on 652 cases. Surgery 1987;101:485–495.

58. Milroy WF. An undescribed variety of hereditary edema. NY Med J 1892;56:505.

59. Allen EV, Barker NW, Hines EA. Peripheral vascular diseases. Philadelphia: WB Saunders, 1946.

60. Kinmonth JB, Taylor GW, Tracy GD, Marsh JD. Primary lymphedema, clinical and lymphangiographic studies of a series of 107 patients in which the lower limbs were affected. Br J Surg 1957;43:1–10.

61. Servelle M. Surgical treatment of lymphedema: a report on 652 cases. Surgery 1987;101:485–495.

62. Kelley ML Jr., Butt HR. Chylous ascites: an analysis of its etiology. Gastroenterology 1960;39:161–165.

63. Pomerantz M, Waldman TA. Systemic lymphatic abnormalities associated with gastrointestinal protein loss secondary to intestinal lymphangiectasia. Gastroenterology 1963;45:703–711.

64. Herbertson BM, Wallace ME. Chylous ascites in newborn mice. J Med Genet 1964;1:10–23.

65. Chavez CM. Lymphangiography. Am J Med Sci 1964;248:225–245.

66. Wright TE, Duvall AJ. Angiofollicular lymph node hyperplasia causing a neck mass in nail-patella syndrome. Am J Dis Child 1983;137:498.

67. Sawicki MP, Howard TJ, Passaro E Jr. Heterotopic tissue in lymph nodes: an unrecognized problem. Arch Surg 1990;125:1394–1398.

68. Miller M, Motulsky AC. Noonan Syndrome in an adult family presenting with chronic lymphedema. Am J Med 1978;65:382.

69. Rynlin AM, Fojaco RM. Congenital pulmonary lymphangiectasis associated with a blind common pulmonary vein. Pediatrics 1968;41:931.

70. Asch MJ, Cohen AH, Moore TC. Hepatic and splenic lymphangiomatosis with skeletal involvement: report of a case and review of the literature. Surgery 1974;76:334.

71. Murphishi G, Arcivue EL, Kause JR. Generalized lymphangioma in infancy with chylothorax. Pediatrics 1970;46:566.

72. Sarda P, Jalaguier J, Montoya F, Bonnet H. Hereditary congenital lymphedema with pseudosexual ambiguity. J Genet Hum 1988;36:353–360.

73. Servelle M. Klippel and Trenaunay's syndrome: 768 operated cases. Ann Surg 1984;201:365–373.

74. Witt DR et al. Lymphedema in Noonan syndrome: clues to pathogenesis and prenatal diagnosis and review of the literature. Am J Med Genet 1987;27:841–856.

75. White SW. Lymphedema in Noonan's syndrome. Int J Dermatol 1984;23:656–657.

76. Nistal M, Paniagua R, Bravo MP. Testicular lymphangiectasis in Noonan's syndrome. J Urol 1984;131(4):759–761.

77. Voight HJ, Claussen U, Ulmer R. Fetal neck edema: early sonographic indications of a chromosome abnormality. Geburtshilfe Frauenheilkd 1986;46:879–882.

78. Crowe CA, Dickerman LH. A genetic association between microcephaly and lymphedema. Am J Med Genet 1986;24:131–135.

79. Leung AK. Dominantly inherited syndrome of microcephaly and congenital lymphedema. Clin Genet 1985;27:611–612.

80. Figueroa AA, Pruzansky S, Rollnick BR. Meige disease (familial lymphedema praecox) and cleft palate: report of a family and review of the literature. Cleft Palate J 1983;20:151–157.

81. Dahlberg PJ, Borer WZ, Newcomer KL, Yutuc WR. Autosomal or X-linked recessive syndrome of congenital lymphedemia, hypoparathyroidism, nephropathy, prolapsing mitral valve, and brachytelephalangy. Am J Med Genet 1983;16:99–104.

82. Tudose N, Rada O. Structural and ultrastructural changes of lymph nodes in primary lymphoedema. Morphol Embryol (Bucur) 1984;30:29–31.

83. Zieman SA. Lymphedema: causes complications, and treatment of the swollen extremity. New York: Grune & Stratton, 1962.

84. Burnett WE, Rosemond GP, Bucher RM. Mesenteric cysts: report of 3 cases, in one of which a calcified cyst was present. Arch Surg 1950;60:699–706.

85. Plaut A. Multiple peritoneal cysts and their histogenesis. Arch Pathol 1928;5:754.

86. Hinshaw JR. Unattached cysts in the peritoneal cavity. Ann Surg 1957;145:138–143.

87. Skandalakis JE. Mesenteric cyst: a report of three cases. J Med Assoc GA 1955;44:75–80.

88. Vaughn AM, Lees WM, Henry JW. Mesenteric cysts: a review of the literature and report of a calcified cyst of the mesentery. Surgery 1948;23:306–317.

89. Gross JI, Goldenberg VE, Humphries EM. Venous remnants producing neonatal chylous ascites. Pediatrics 1961;27:408–414.

90. Engel S, Clagett OT, Harrison EG Jr. Chylous cysts of the abdomen. Surgery 1961;50:593–599.

91. Gerster JCA. Retroperitoneal chyle cysts: with especial reference to the lymphangiomata. Ann Surg 1939;110:339.

92. Maury JM. Retroperitoneal cysts of wolffian origin. Surg Gynecol Obstet 1918;26:663.

93. Ford JR. Mesenteric cysts: review of the literature with report of an unusual case. Am J Surg 1960;99:878–884.

94. Beahrs OH, Judd ES Jr. Chylangiomas of the abdomen. Proc Mayo Clin 1947;22:297–304.

95. Hadley MN. The origin of the retroperitoneal cystic tumors. Surg Gynecol Obstet 1936;22:174.

96. McLaughlin JS, Mansberger AR, Lyon JA, Green K. Giant omental cyst: case report with emphasis on radiological diagnosis. Am Surg 1964;125–128.

97. Lee FC. Large retroperitoneal chylous cyst: report of a case with experiments on lymphatic permeability. Arch Surg 1942;44:61–71.

98. Sprague NF Jr. Mesenteric cysts (2 cases). Am Surg 1960;26:42–49.

99. Hansmann GH, Budd JW. Massive unattached retroperitoneal tumors. JAMA 1932;98:6–10.

100. Benivieni A. De abiditis nonnullis ac marandis morborum et sanationem cousis. Florence, Italy, 1507.

101. Miller IA. Rarity of congenital mesenteric cysts. Am J Dis Child 1935;50:1196.

102. Rokitansky C. Lehbuch I. Pathologie und Anatomie. Vienna, 1842.

103. Millard P, Tillaux P. Kyste du messenitere chez un homme. Bull Acad Med Paris 1880;17:831.

104. Lowman RM, Walters II, Stanley HW. Mesenteric chylous cysts: associated diagnostic and surgical problems. J Int Coll Surg 1952;18:265–290.

105. Dowd CN. Mesenteric cysts. Ann Surg 1900;32:515.

106. Beahrs OH, Judd ES Jr, Dockerty MB. Chylous cyst of the abdomen. Surg Clin North Am 1950;30:1081–1096.

107. Arnheim EE, Schneck H, Norman A, Preizin DH. Mesenteric cysts in infancy and childhood. Pediatrics 1959;24:469–476.

108. Stahl WM Jr, Joy RC. Chylous cysts of the mesentery in infants. J Pediatr 1961;58:373–376.

109. Handelsman JC, Ravitch MM. Chylous cysts of the mesentery in children. Ann Surg 1954;140:185.

110. Amos JA. Multiple lymphatic cysts of the mesentery. Br J Surg 1959;46:588–592.

111. Hebra A, Brown MF, McGeehin KM, Ross AJ III. Mesenteric, omental, and retroperitoneal cysts in children: a clinical study of 22 cases. South Med J 1993;86(2):173–176.

112. Chung MA, Brandt ML, St Vil D, Yazbeck S. Mesenteric cysts in children. J Pediatr Surg 1991;26(11):1306–1308.

113. Doolittle WM, Ohmart D, Egan EA. Congenital bilateral pleural effusions: a cause for respiratory failure in the newborn. Am J Dis Child 1973;125:435.

114. Benacerraf BR, Frigoletto FD. Mid-trimester fetal thoracentesis. J Clin Ultrasound 1985;13:202.

115. Van Aerde J, Campbell AN, Smyth JA. Spontaneous chylothorax in newborns. Am J Dis Child 1984;138:961.

116. Brodman RF. Congenital chylothorax: recommendations for treatment. NY State J Med 1975;75:553.

117. Andersen EA, Hertel J, Petersen SA, Sorensen HR. Congenital chylothorax: management by ligature of the thoracic duct. Scand J Thorac Cardiovasc Surg 1984;18:193–194.

118. Heys SD, Eremin O. The relevance of tumor draining lymph nodes in cancer. Surg Gynecol Obstet 1992;174:533–540.

119. Shiu MH et al. Influence of the extent of resection on survival after curative treatment of gastric carcinoma: a retrospective multivariate analysis. Arch Surg 1987;122:1347–1351.

120. Noguchi Y et al. Radical surgery for gastric cancer: a review of the Japanese experience. Cancer 1989;64:2053–2062.

121. McNeer G, Bowden L, Booher RJ, McPeak CJ. Elective total gastrectomy for cancer of the stomach. Ann Surg 1974;180:252–256.

122. Douglass HO, Nave HR. Gastric adenocarcinoma: management of the primary disease. Semin Oncol 1985;12:32–45.

123. Fielding JWL et al. Clinioopathological staging of gastric cancer. Br J Surg 1984;71:677–680.

CHAPTER 25

THE PERICARDIUM

Willis H. Williams / Stephen Wood Gray / John Elias Skandalakis

" . . . a smooth tunic envelops the heart and contains a small amount of fluid resembling urine."
—HIPPOCRATES, 460 B.C.

DEVELOPMENT

Early in the fourth week, at the beginning of somite formation, clefts appear in the embryonic mesoderm. These clefts occupy a horseshoe-shaped area lateral to the neural plate and pass across the midline anterior to the developing head fold of the embryo (Figs. 25.1 and 25.2). They are the beginning of the intraembryonic celom that separates the mesoderm into somatic and splanchnic layers. The individual mesenchymal clefts soon coalesce to form a continuous cavity extending backward beside the head to communicate with the celomic spaces of the rapidly forming myotomes. The bend of the horseshoe represents the future pericardial cavity, while the lateral arms represent the pleural canals and, later, the pleural cavities (Fig. 25.1).

In the floor of the pericardial cavity, splanchnopleure cells form the cardiogenic plate, from which will develop the myocardium and the visceral pericardium or epicardium. Beneath this layer (between it and the underlying endoderm) is the angioblastic layer that will form the endocardial tube. Both layers bulge into the pericardial cavity to form the tubular heart attached to the splanchnic layer by a mesocardium. Ventrally, in origin with the continued overgrowth of the head fold and the closure of the midgut, this mesocardium becomes dorsal, suspending the heart from the splanchnopleure, which has turned almost 180 degrees, to lie beneath the ventral surfaces of the foregut. Further development of the heart itself is discussed in Chapter 26.

By the rotation of the pericardium under the pharynx, the lateral prolongations of the cavity (the arms of the horseshoe) become dorsal, extending above the septum transversum and lying on either side of the foregut. Ventrally, two corresponding prolongations, the ventral parietal recesses, end blindly (1, 2) (Fig. 25.2).

All of these changes take place during the third week of gestation. The pericardial cavity is very large; the future pleural cavities are narrow and lead into a small peritoneal cavity. The opening of the pleural canals into the pericardial cavity is bound laterally by the ducts of Cuvier (common cardinal veins), which drain the primitive venous system into the sinus venosus at the cranial side of the transverse septum. The bulge of the ducts into the pleural canal is called the pulmonary ridge of Mall (Figs. 25.3, *A*, and 25.4, *A*, and *B*).

By the end of the fourth week the lung buds have begun to bulge into the pleural canals from the medial mesenchymal mass that lies between the two canals. With the subsequent enlargement of the pleural canal in this region, the ducts of Cuvier do not move laterally, but develop mesentery-like folds of tissue from the lateral wall. These are the pleuropericardial membranes. At about the 10-mm stage (end of the sixth week), the membranes fuse with the medial mesenchyme, first on the right and subsequently on the left, obliterating the openings between the pericardial and pleural spaces (Figs. 25.3, *B*, and 25.4, *C*).

With the development of the lungs, the pleural cavities begin to enlarge faster than does the pericardial cavity (Fig. 25.4, *D*), expanding cranially into the somatic mesoderm beyond the cranial limits of the pericardium. That portion of the pericardial wall formed by the pleuropericardial membrane continues to enlarge until it forms the whole of the lateral walls of the adult pericardium. The remainder of the pericardium forms from those portions attached to the anterior and posterior mediastinum, the superior mediastinum, and the diaphragm.

Critical Events in Development

Failure of the normally transitory ventral parietal recesses to become absorbed in the fourth week results in pericardial cysts and diverticula.

Defective formation of the pleuropericardial membranes, which separate the future pleural and pericardial cavities, may take place in the fifth week. A defect in the pericardium—usually on the left—results from such failure.

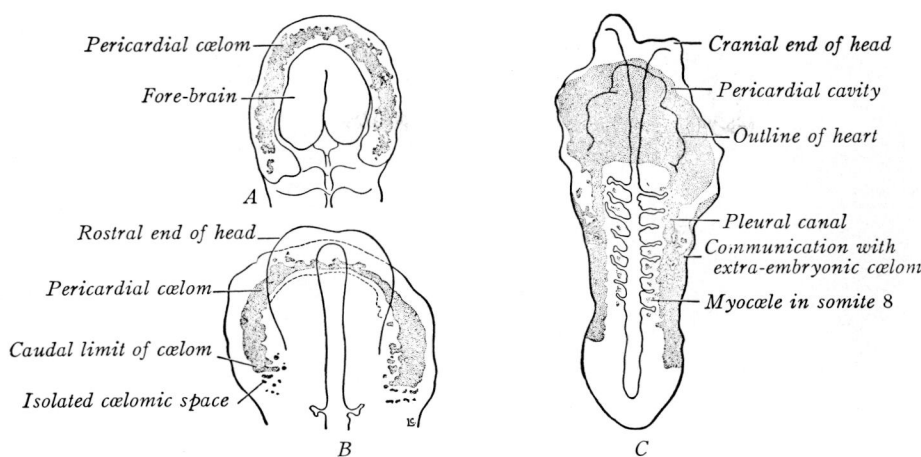

Figure 25.1. Development of the embryonic celom early in the fourth week **A,** At the one-somite stage. **B,** At two somites. **C,** At nine somites. (From Arey LB. Developmental anatomy. Philadelphia: WB Saunders, 1965.)

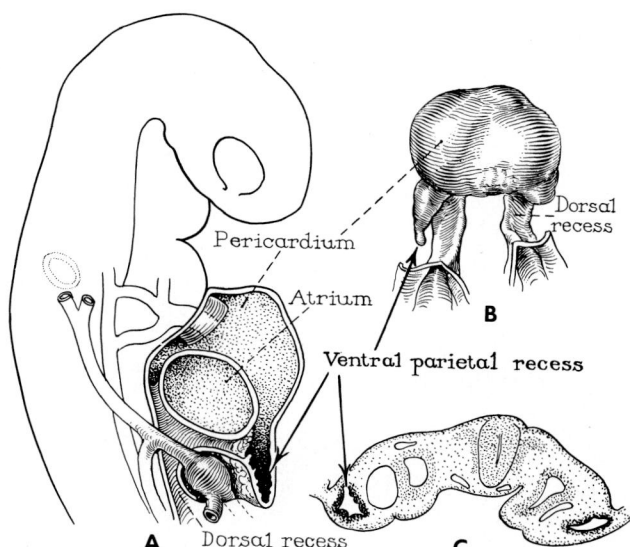

Figure 25.2. The ventral parietal recesses of the pericardium. **A,** Parasagittal section through the pericardium of a rabbit embryo, 9 days old. **B,** Ventral view of a cast of the pericardium of a human embryo of 20 somites. **C,** Cross-section of a 10-somite rabbit embryo. (From Lillie WI, McDonald JR, Clagett OT. Pericardial celomic cysts and pericardial diverticula: Concept of etiology and report of cases. J Thorac Surg 1950;20:494.)

ANOMALIES OF THE PERICARDIUM (TABLE 25.1 AND FIGURE 25.5)

Congenital Defects of the Pericardium

ANATOMY

The pericardial cavity surrounding the heart is lined with a simple squamous epithelium (mesothelium) on a layer of connective tissue. The heart and great vessels are invaginated within this cavity so that, strictly speaking,

there is a visceral pericardium (epicardium) covering the heart itself and a parietal pericardium forming the outer surface of the pericardial cavity. The visceral and parietal layers are continuous with one another at the pericardial reflections where the great veins and arteries enter and exit. The parietal layer alone usually is termed the *pericardium*. Hippocrates would have been right about his definition of the pericardium if he would have added that it envelops the beginning and the end of the great vessels (Fig. 25.6 and 25.7).

Anteriorly, the pericardium lies over the anterior mediastinum, separating the anterior surface of the heart from the posterior surface of the sternal periosteum. Superiorly, the thymus extends downward between the anterior pericardium and the posterior surface of the manubrium. Posteriorly, the pericardium rests on the posterior mediastinum, within which lie the esophagus and the thoracic aorta. Inferiorly, the base of the pericardium rests on the central portion of the diaphragm. Laterally and anterolaterally, the pericardium and the parietal pleura lie in contact with one another, forming a single, tough, fibrous membrane, the pleuropericardium—covered on both sides by mesothelium.

Ellis and colleagues (3) classified 85 cases from the literature into groups suggested by Moore (4) and Fanfani and deBiase (5) (Table 25.2).

Right-sided defects are rare (3.5%). The majority are left-sided pleuropericardial (group A) defects (78%). The pleural and pericardial cavities are in communication. When the defect is large, the heart may be almost wholly in the left pleural cavity (Fig. 25.8). When the defect is smaller, a portion of the heart—usually the auricular appendage—may herniate during each cardiac cycle (6–9). Death has been documented after herniation of the

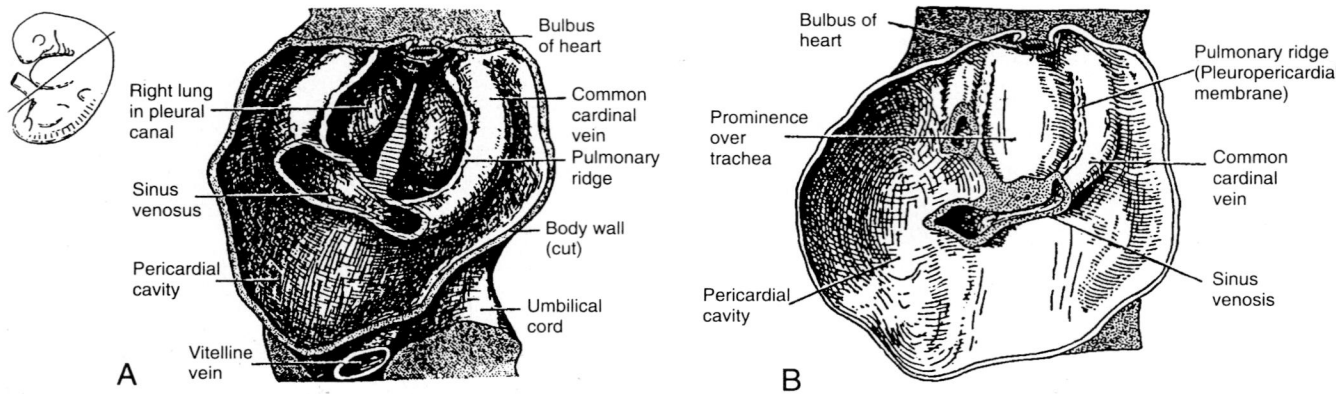

Figure 25.3. Models of the human pericardial cavity opened ventrally. **A,** At 5 mm. **B,** At 10 mm. The plane of section is shown at the left. (From Arey LB. Developmental anatomy. Philadelphia: WB Saunders, 1965.)

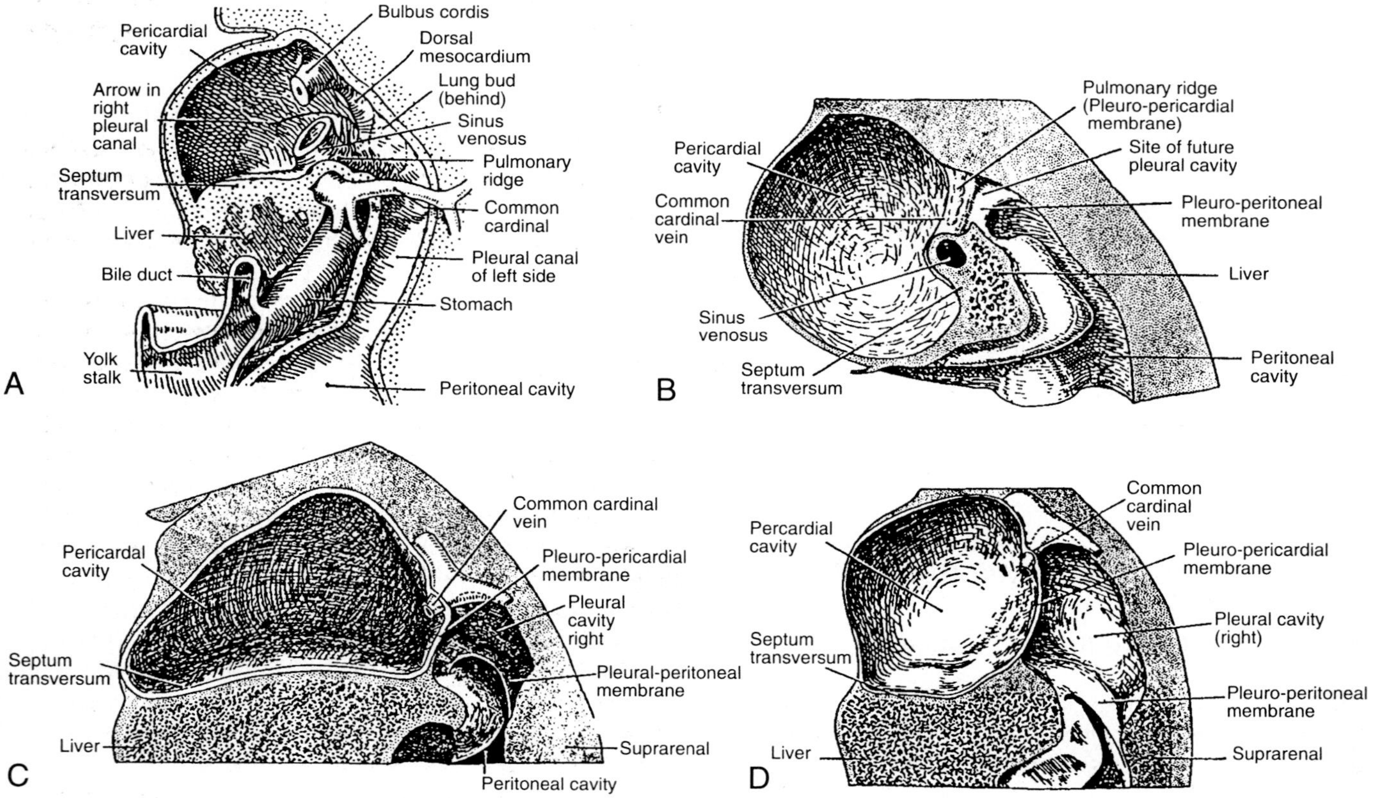

Figure 25.4. Models of the right side of the human pericardial cavity. **A,** At 3 mm. **B,** At 5 mm. **C,** At 13 mm. **D,** At 16 mm. (From Arey LB. Developmental anatomy. Philadelphia: WB Saunders, 1965.)

Table 25.1.
Anomalies of the Pericardium

Anomaly	Origin of Defect	First Appearance (or Other Diagnostic Clues)	Sex Chiefly Affected	Relative Frequency	Remarks
Congenital defects of the pericardium	5th-6th weeks	At any age, if at all	Male	Rare	Usually asymptomatic; more frequent on left
Pericardial cysts and diverticula	4th week	Adolescence or later	Male	Rare	Rarely symptomatic

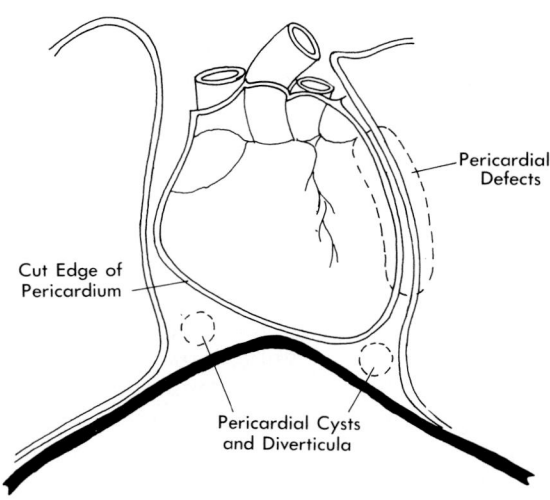

Figure 25.5. Sites of congenital anomalies of the pericardium.

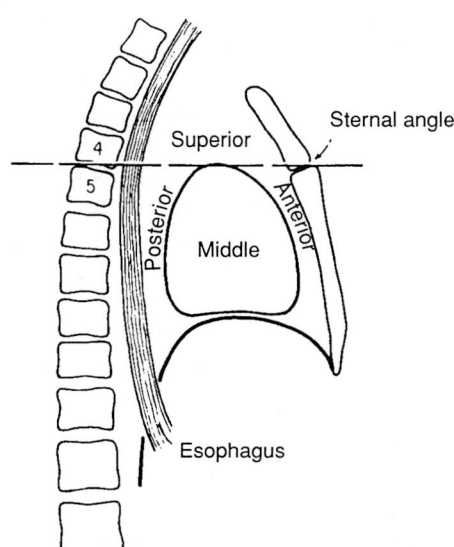

Figure 25.6. Diagrammatic lateral view of the thorax indicating the divisions of the mediastinum. The *dashed line* forming the lower boundary of the superior mediastinum also marks the division between the ascending aorta and the aortic arch anteriorly and that between the arch and the descending aorta posteriorly. (From Skandalakis JE, Gray SW, Rowe JS Jr. The anatomy of the human pericardium and heart. In: Bourne GH, ed. Hearts and heart-like organs. New York: Academic Press, 1980.)

left atrium and left ventricle through the defect with subsequent strangulation by the unyielding fibrous edges of the defect (10). The entire heart may remain within the pericardial cavity if the defect is small. In at least one documented case, the lung herniated into the pericardial cavity (11), indicating that the defect is not always a "one-way street."

The fibrous component of the pericardium is absent, but a thin-walled mesothelial layer (parietal pleura) separates the heart and lung in the relatively rare group B defects (3%).

The phrenic nerves can be anticipated to lie anterior to partial defects and may lie quite close to the anterior midline when defects are large (12), an important surgical consideration.

Defects of group C involving the diaphragmatic pericardium are discussed with defects of the diaphragm (page 515).

EMBRYOGENESIS

Pericardial defects lie in that area of the pericardium formed by the embryonic pleuropericardial membrane. There is general agreement that such defects result from failure of the membrane to form or from its atresia after formation (13).

Separation of the pericardial cavity and the future pleural cavities occurs by the medial migration of the pulmonary ridge of Mall overlying the duct of Cuvier during the fifth week. This ridge, fusing with the transverse septum, forms the pleuropericardial membrane (Fig. 25.3, B). Premature regression of the left duct of Cuvier, coupled with growth of the heart and pericardial cavity, leaves an unclosed orifice, the iter venosum, which will increase rather than decrease in size with later growth. Bulging of the heart into the pleural canal may prevent later closure, thus producing a large or "complete" defect. Smaller defects result from failure of the closing membrane to grow fast enough to compensate for the enlarging pericardial cavity. In rare instances, the growth forces are balanced so that the pleural mesothelium closes the opening, but the mesenchymal portion and the pericardial mesothelium do not. Theories of closure are discussed in detail by Sunderland and Wright-Smith (10).

There is some evidence that the developing lung occa-

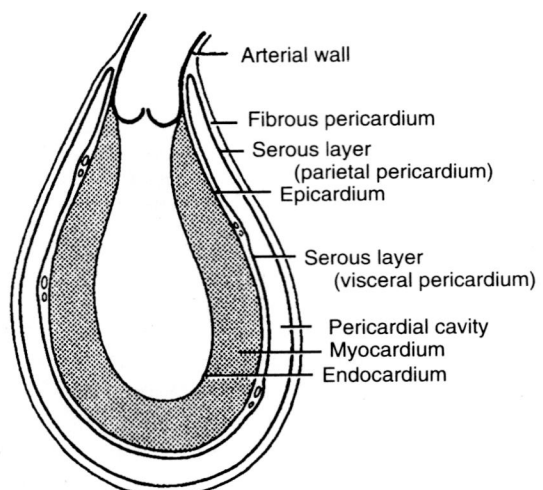

Figure 25.7. Diagrammatic representation of the pericardium and its relation to the heart. (From Skandalakis JE, Gray SW, Rowe JS Jr. The anatomy of the human pericardium and heart. In: Bourne GH, ed. Hearts and heart-like organs. New York: Academic Press, 1980.)

Table 25.2.
Congenital Defects of the Pericardium

Location of Defect		Percentage of 85 Cases
A. Defects of the pleuropericardium		85
1. Left side only		78.0
a. Foramen-like partial defects	21.0	
b. Large or complete defects	57.0	
2. Right side only		3.5
a. Partial defects	2.3	
b. Large or complete defects	1.2	
3. Both sides (complete absence)		3.5
B. Defects of the pericardium with normal parietal pleural membrane		3
C. Defects of the diaphragmatic pericardium		12
TOTAL		100

sionally may herniate through the unclosed pleuropericardial opening. Normal expansion of the lung is lateral to the duct of Cuvier, but in one patient a bronchogenic cyst was found with a pedicle closing the pericardial defect (6). This cyst almost certainly represented a sequestered portion of developing lung which had passed through the unclosed orifice.

ASSOCIATED ANOMALIES

Among the collected cases of Ellis and his associates (14), 31% had other congenital anomalies, usually involving the heart, lungs, peritoneum, pleural cavities, or the kidneys. Bronchial cysts were present in two cases and an enteric cyst in one. Kapouleas et al. (15) reported successful repair of a Bochdalek's hernia and an intrathoracic solitary hepatic cyst in a 3.4-kg infant girl with peri-

cardial agenesis which did not complicate recovery or normal cardiac function 1 year after operation.

Matsuoka et al. (16) described a 43-year-old patient with cough, dyspnea, and hemoptysis who, following detailed investigation, was shown to have an anomalous inferior vena cava with azygous vein continuation, dysgenesis of the lung, and probable, but not proven, absence of the left pericardium. This association is interesting, since it is during the 33rd to 36th embryonal days that fusion of the inferior vena cava is known to occur, as is lobulation of the lung and formation of the left pericardium from the embryonic pleuropericardial membrane. Persistence, in this case, of the right superior vena cava derived from the right duct of Cuvier probably assured normal development of the right-sided pericardium. An unknown teratogenic effect occurring between day 33 and 36 of embryonic development could thus account for this interesting triad of anomalies.

Associated intracardiac defects may dominate the clinical presentation. They include tetralogy of Fallot, atrial septal defect, patent ductus arteriosus, mitral valve stenosis, tricuspid valvular regurgitation, mitral valve prolapse (the "billowing mitral valve syndrome"), Eisenmenger physiology (increased pulmonary vascular resistance), and the rare and fatal bifid heart. Diaphragmatic defects may be combined into a pentalogy with abdominal wall defects, lower sternal defects, deficiency of the anterior diaphragm, and congenital intracardiac defects (17).

HISTORY

Columbus (18) mentioned a case of absence of the pericardium in 1559. Its authenticity has been questioned, as has that of some later cases, but because we have not seen the original statement of Columbus, we are unable to judge.

The first unequivocal case was that of Baillie in 1788 (19). By 1910 Ebstein (20) collected 32 cases, all from autopsied cadavers. The first case to be recognized in life was that of Ladd (21) in 1936. This was discovered accidentally during repair of a diaphragmatic hernia. Ellis and his colleagues (14) collected and analyzed 99 cases up to 1959 and evaluated the possible diagnostic procedures. By 1964, 113 cases were found in the literature (11).

INCIDENCE

Since absence of symptoms is common, published reports undoubtedly do not reflect the true frequency of pericardial defects. Significant abnormalities are rare. A pathologic review of 74 cases found at autopsy revealed that all individuals had led normal, active lives; absence of the pericardium had not contributed to the causes of death (22). Prevalence based on large autopsy series varies from 1:14,000 (23) to 2:13,000 (24).

Taysi et al. (25) described two relatives, each having absence of the left pericardium. Study of the pedigree suggested a multifactorial determination of congenital absence of the pericardium despite the known male predilection. The majority of affected patients have been men (male/female, 3:1). Since discovery of the defect is usually accidental, it may occur at any age.

Pericardial defects of group A (pleuropericardial type) have been reported in an orangutan (26), a cat (27), and a dog (4).

SYMPTOMS

Most pericardial defects are asymptomatic, coming to attention incidentally on routine chest x-ray examination. Most defects discovered at autopsy had not contributed to death (22). When symptoms do occur, they may include chest pain, dyspnea, palpitation, dizziness, syncope, hemoptysis, and shortness of breath. Sudden death has been described as due to herniation and strangulation

of the heart within the edges of the defect (10, 28, 29).

Gehlmann and van Ingen (29) reported the first documented patient requiring operation for relief of chest pain caused by total absence of the left pericardium with strangulation of the heart between the left pulmonary ligament, the diaphragm, and the left anterior chest wall. A computed tomographic (CT) scan suggested the diagnosis, confirmed by thoracoscopy, in a 44-year-old man complaining for 16 hours of acute, continuous left-sided chest pain. The heart was freed and the defect repaired through a left thoracotomy using an allograft of porcine pericardium; the pain was relieved and did not recur during 1 year of follow-up.

Auch-Schwelk and colleagues (30) described four categories of chest pain syndromes associated with pericardial defects based on a review of cases reported in the literature. Group one patients were asymptomatic, attracting attention only by abnormal electrocardiographic or roentgenographic findings or by incidental

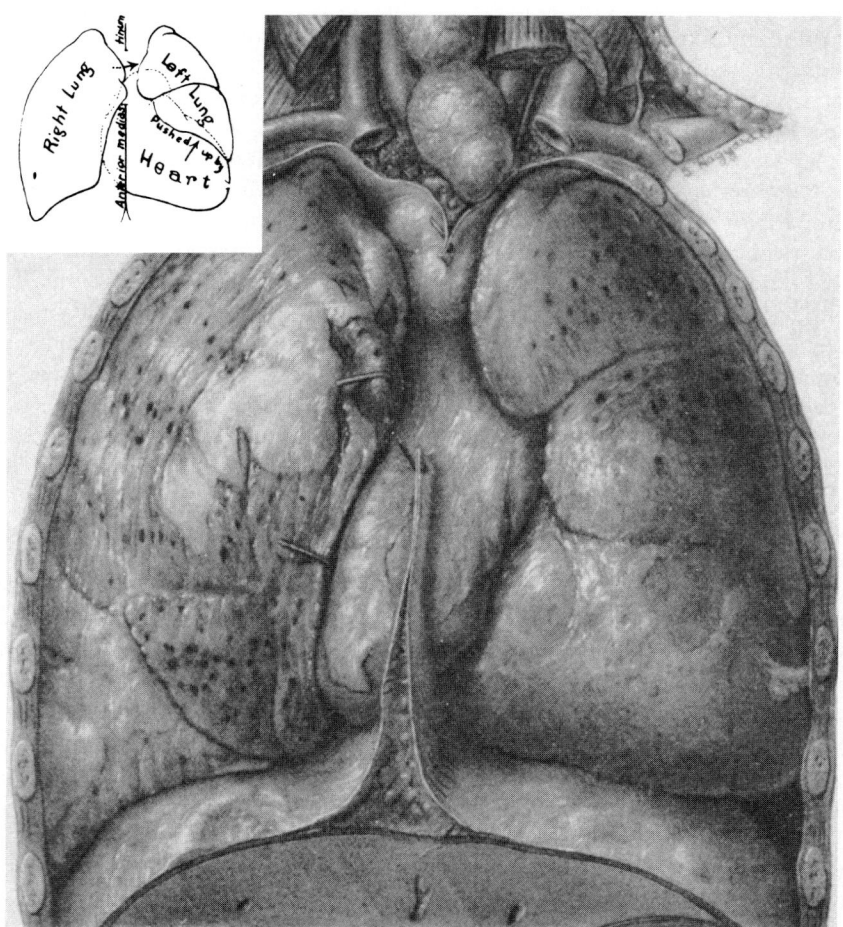

Figure 25.8. Absence of part of the anterior mediastinum and entire left half of the pericardium. Here is a window between the two pleural cavities and the heart is in the left cavity. (From Southworth H, Stevenson CS. Congenital defects of the pericardium. Arch Int Med 1938;61:223–240.)

recognition during operations for unrelated problems. Thirty-three such patients were reviewed. Group two patients complained of vague chest pain of short duration (seconds), inconsistently inducible by changes in body position or exertion. Seventeen such patients were reviewed. Group three patients had severe sharp or dull chest pain on the side of the pericardial defect with repeated attacks associated with dyspnea, palpitations, arrhythmias, and/or syncope. A parahilar mass usually was present on chest x-ray examination. The typical cause of the chest pain was atrial herniation and strangulation through the pericardial defect. Almost all of the nine reviewed cases required operation. Group four included five children, all of whom were admitted with acute and severe chest pain and arrhythmias or acute heart failure; they died within hours. Strangulation of the left ventricle through a partial pericardial defect was confirmed at autopsy. The latter two groups obviously emphasize the importance of considering the diagnosis of partial pericardial defects in the differential diagnosis of acute or recurrent chest pain and, when indicated, expeditious operation to either excise the pericardium widely or repair the defect with a pericardial substitute (31, 32).

Hoorntje and colleagues (33) described herniation of the left atrium through a partial congenital pericardial defect associated with short periods of syncope that were not related to the presence of an incidental type II Wenckebach block. The diagnosis was confirmed by intravenous digital subtraction angiography (DSA). The pericardial defect was closed surgically in a 20-year-old man using a bovine pericardial patch. No symptoms recurred during more than 3 years of follow-up although the conduction abnormalities persisted, suggesting that left atrial herniation was indeed the cause of the syncopal episodes.

Right-sided defects, though very rare, have presented as caval obstruction due to herniation of the right lung into the pericardium or as pleuritic inspiratory right-sided chest pain (34).

Beppu et al. (35) demonstrated significantly greater left and right ventricular volumes as determined by CT in patients with absence of the left pericardium, as compared with normal control subjects, while both groups lay in the left lateral position. Greater differences in right ventricular volumes were noted between the two groups. No such differences were observed when the subjects were lying in the right lateral position. Preload is greater in the left lateral position, thus suggesting that the ventricles—particularly the right ventricle—are more compliant or distensible in those with congenital absence of the left pericardium than in those individuals having an intact pericardium. There is evidence that persons with pericardial defects have the same life expectancy as the general population (24). The presence of adhesions, postmortem evidence of pleuropericarditis, and the frequent finding of pneumonia as the cause of death in the pre–

antibiotic era suggest that there may be some danger from the spread of pleural infection.

DIAGNOSIS

Abbott (36) suggested that pericardial defects might be diagnosed in life by radiography; De Garis (26) proposed pneumothorax as a diagnostic measure. The diagnosis of partial pericardial defects can be subtle and difficult. Ellis et al. (3) first described the electrocardiographic clues which subsequently proved more reliable in the diagnosis of complete defects than for diagnosis of the clinically more important partial defects. Right axis deviation, incomplete right bundle branch block, a leftward-shifted transition zone in the precordial leads, and occasionally, sinus bradycardia suggest a pericardial defect. When defects causing right ventricular volume overload have beeen excluded (37), these electrocardiographic findings associated with leftward and posterior displacement of the apical impulse and levoposition or elevation of the cardiac apex on chest x-ray examination are virtually diagnostic of a pericardial defect. The heart is hypermobile in most cases of pericardial defects; hence, chest fluoroscopy during inspiration and expiration may be helpful.

Physical examination may reveal a systolic murmur, wide splitting of the second heart sound, and leftward and posterolateral displacement of the apical cardiac impulse (PMI). Morgan (38) described a syndrome of absent left pericardium that included left ventricular enlargement and hypertrophy, a systolic ejection murmur at the base of the heart, right axis deviation, and levoposition of the heart. Additional radiographic features include elongation of the heart's left border; prominent aortic knob and pulmonary artery; radiolucent bands between either the aortic knob and main pulmonary artery segment or between the diaphragm and base of the heart caused by interposed lung; prominence of the left atrial appendage; an unusual left-sided convexity seen with herniation of the left atrial appendage; and an obscured right border of the heart.

In addition to right axis deviation; the electrocardiogram may reveal incomplete right bundle branch block, right ventricular hypertrophy, clockwise displacement of the QRS transition zone in the precordial leads, or tall peaked P waves in the precordial leads.

Postural changes in the vectorcardiogram occurring in four patients with defects of the left pericardium were believed to be due to the hypermobility of the unrestrained heart (39).

The importance of the M-shaped pattern of the jugular phlebogram as a useful physical and phonocardiographic indicator of congenital absence of the pericardium was demonstrated by Matsuhisa et al. (40). The characteristic features of the pattern include decreased depth of the x-descent and a tall v-wave followed by a deep y-descent caused by loss of decrease in pericardial pressure during ventricular ejection and altered cardiac position as a result of absence of the pericardium. The pattern was more pronounced with complete absence of the pericardium but nonetheless characteristic in partial absence.

Dimond et al. (41) reported the first case of partial left-sided defect associated with herniation of the left atrial appendage that was demonstrated by cineangiography. Levo follow-through angiography or DSA after pulmonary arterial contrast medium injection is advocated to demonstrate herniation of the left atrium (42). Lajos and colleagues (43) first demonstrated a localized stenosis of the left anterior descending coronary artery caused by the edge of a pericardial defect.

Cross-sectional two-dimensional echocardiography is a simple and accurate method for diagnosis of congenital aneurysms of the left atrium (44) which also must prompt consideration of herniation of the left atrium through partial pericardial defects (45–47) or expansion of the left atrium (48). Limitations of the M-mode, two-dimensional, and contrast-enhanced echocardiography in these conditions are summarized by Nicolosi et al. (49).

Left-sided pericardial defects may mimic volume overload of the right ventricle causing dilation of the right ventricle and paradoxic anterior motion of the septum in systole.

Vargas-Barron and colleagues (50) described the differential diagnosis of partial absence of the left pericardium and congenital left atrial aneurysm as first described by Semans and Taussig (51), emphasizing the superior accuracy of CT and magnetic resonance imaging (MRI) compared to the less specific cardiac angiography and M-mode or two-dimensional echocardiography. CT is advocated for identification of both partial and total pericardial defects and for evaluation of atypical chest pain which might be associated with such defects (52–54). The diagnostic value of MRI in the delineation of total and partial pericardial defects has been confirmed by Gutierrez et al. (55) and Schiavone and O'Donnell (56).

Radionuclide perfusion scans demonstrate a wedge of lung between the heart and the left hemidiaphragm when a left pericardial defect is present (57).

Rodgers and colleagues (58) demonstrated the value of thoracoscopy for early diagnosis of cardiac herniation following radical pneumonectomy, suggesting that this method also would be useful in identification of congenital pericardial defects.

TREATMENT

Surgical treatment of pericardial defects is controversial and is, of course, not offered to those who remain asymptomatic and undiagnosed (32). Complete defects probably do not justify surgery since they pose little if any potential morbidity. On the other hand, partial defects—

particularly those associated with herniation of the left atrium or part of the left ventricle—can and probably should be treated by surgical enlargement of the defect (pericardiectomy) or closure of the defect with prosthetic or allograft pericardial substitute.

Bernal and colleagues (59) used angiocardiography to confirm left atrial and partial left ventricular herniation through a partial left-sided pericardial defect in a previously healthy 44-year-old man who complained of palpitation and nonspecific chest pain. Symptoms were relieved by pericardiotomy—that is, simply enlarging the defect to prevent strangulation.

Amiri and associates (60) reported their treatment of a 43-year-old man with partial absence of the left pericardium, a 2-year history of angina pectoris, and coronary arterial occlusions of more than 90% in both the right coronary artery and the left anterior descending coronary artery but no positive risk factors for coronary arterial disease. Intraoperative assessment proved that the coronary arterial occlusions were exactly at the sites of stricture caused by the edges of the pericardial defect through which the heart had partially herniated. A relaxing incision in the pericardium and two coronary bypass grafts relieved symptoms. Angiography 1 year later showed patent grafts and no further cardiac strangulation. This case suggests the importance of including partial absence of the pericardium in the differential diagnosis of chest pain, particularly angina pectoris in the young patient or the patient without significant coronary arterial disease risk factors. MRI or CT should define this rare cause of chest pain.

Chapman et al. (61) described relief of atypical angina pectoris in a 29-year-old woman by a polytetrafluoroethylene prosthetic patch repair of a partial left pericardial defect through which the left atrium and a portion of the left ventricle had herniated.

Finally, Savage and Nolan (62) reported successful vaginal delivery of a normal 41-week-old (gestational) male infant to a 22-year-old woman who had refused elective repair of a known left atrial herniation through a partial left pericardial defect. The feared potential complications which might have accompanied the Valsalva maneuvers of vaginal delivery did not occur. Even under these stressful circumstances, the natural history—and thus the indications for operation—remains unpredictable. Expectant observation is justified in asymptomatic cases.

Pericardial Cysts and Diverticula

ANATOMY

In the anterior part of the angle formed by the pericardium and the diaphragm, diverticula of the pericardium or cystic sequestrations of the pericardium are occasionally encountered. They are lined with simple squamous epithelium (mesothelium) and are filled with a clear limpid fluid, from the presence of which they are sometimes called "springwater cysts." Pericardial cysts, occasionally multilocular, may attain a capacity of 1000 cc, but they are not tense and rarely produce symptoms of compression.

Almost all lie in the cardiophrenic angle, more often on the right side, but as many as 30% are found in other locations (63). Some cysts are located higher in the mediastinum, and a few cross the midline beneath the sternum, in front of the pericardium (64, 65).

Diverticula also are usually found on the right side, and a few are anterior or posterior. Two cases with multiple diverticula have been reported. These structures are usually from 5 to 8 cm long (66).

EMBRYOGENESIS

Most cysts and diverticula of the pericardium represent persistence of the ventral parietal recesses of the pericardium, which appear in the fourth week and usually are obliterated in the human embryo without a trace (67) (Fig. 25.2). Multiple cases of the association between thoracic cysts of foregut origin (e.g., mediastinal esophageal duplication cysts) and defects of the pericardium have been reported (68), suggesting that these abnormal thoracic masses of several morphologic types have a similar embryogenesis.

If the recess fails to undergo regression, a diverticulum results; if the distal portion alone persists, a cyst remains. A pedicle may or may not be present to indicate the former connection of the cyst with the pericardium proper. Mazer (69) mentioned a minute communication between an apparent cyst and the pericardial cavity. Recognition of such a communication depends upon the care with which it is sought.

Derivation of these structures from the persistence of blindly ending ventral pericardial recesses derived from the mesodermic celom was first suggested by Lillie and his colleagues (67). An alternative theory, put forward by Lambert (70), attributed the cysts to mesenchymal clefts that failed to coalesce with others in the initial formation of the pericardial cavity very early in embryonic life. It seems unlikely that such small vesicles would persist or that they would be so uniformly located.

Viikari (71) suggested that mesothelial cysts on the diaphragm to the right of the pericardium should be attributed to the infracardiac bursa. This is a remnant of the embryonic pneumatoenteric recess of the peritoneum. It becomes isolated in the posterior mediastinum to the right of the esophagus when the diaphragm is formed (Fig. 25.9). It may persist even in adults. This structure may account for pericardial cysts situated posteriorly and on the right. Cysts lying more anteriorly must be attributed to the ventral parietal recesses.

The development of a pericardial cyst 10 years after acute pericarditis suggests that not all pericardial cysts are congenital in origin but perhaps represent organization of a loculated inflammatory process in some cases (72). Most pericardial diverticula appear to be acquired rather than congenital, and their etiology is obscure (73). They arise through herniation of the serous layer between the fibers of the dense connective tissue layer. They are not limited to the pericardiophrenic angle.

HISTORY AND INCIDENCE

Although pericardial cysts were known as early as 1869 (64), they received little attention in the United States until 1940 when Lambert (70) discussed them in his presidential address to the American Association for Thoracic Surgery. Over 200 cases of pericardial cysts were described in the literature by 1990, but undoubtedly, the incidence is much higher since this benign anomaly is probably not reported very often (74).

Le Roux (65), examining 300,000 mass x-rays from the general population of Edinburgh, found three pericardial cysts. Among 101 patients at Edinburgh with mediastinal tumors, two had pericardial cysts. There were 20 cysts, all discovered accidentally, in the Edinburgh series (65).

McAllister and Fenoglio (75) found 82 pericardial cysts (15.4%) and seven bronchogenic cysts (1.3%) in a massive review of 533 tumors and cysts of the heart and pericardium in the collection of the Armed Forces Institutes of Pathology. Among the 89 infants and children in the review, there were only two (2.2%) pericardial cysts and one (1.1%) bronchogenic cyst, emphasizing the relative infrequency with which cysts are either symptomatic or identified in infants and children (76).

The anatomic distribution of the 82 pericardial cysts from the Armed Forces Institute of Pathology series (75, 76) was as follows: right costophrenic angle, 57 (70%); left costophrenic angle, 18 (22%); anterior and superior mediastinum, 4 (4%); and posterior mediastinum, 3 (4%). Twice as many cysts are found on the right side of the body as on the left; about 10% are multilocular. They may be recognized at any age. About 60% occur in males. Pericardial cysts account for 7% of all primary tumors of the mediastinum (77) and 15.4% of all tumors of the heart and pericardium (75).

Pericardial cysts range in size from 1 to 15 cm in diameter. The majority are unilocular but the cyst lining (collagen with scattered elastic fibers covered by a single layer of mesothelial cells) may be trabecular, giving an external appearance of multilocularity. Foci of hyperplastic mesothelial cells, calcification, and accumulations of lymphocytes and plasma cells are sometimes present in the cyst wall (76). Cysts may communicate with the pericardial cavity; if the communication is significant, the term *diver-*

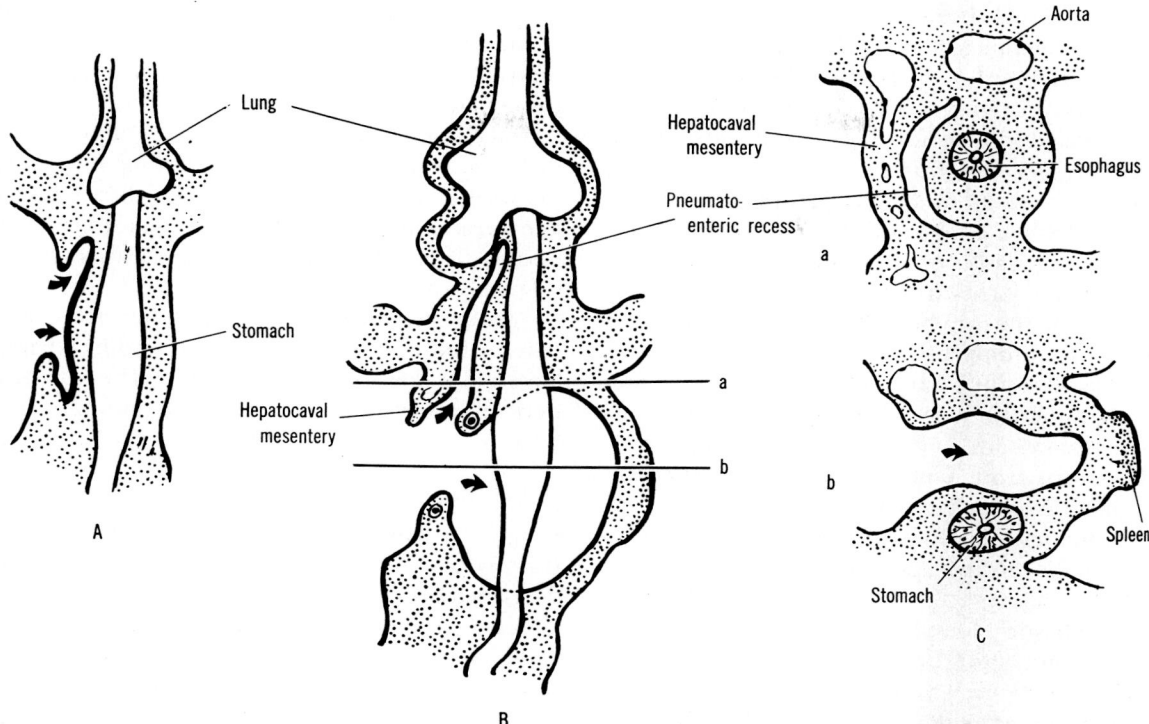

Figure 25.9. The development of the omental and infracardiac bursae in the sixth week. **A,** The bursa begins as an excavation of the right side of the mesentery at the level of the stomach. **B,** An extension craniad on the right side of the esophagus forms the pneumatoenteric recess. Subsequent loss of communication with the abdominal cavity forms the infracardiac bursa of the adult. **C,** Cross sections at levels *a* and *b* in B. (Modified after Frazer JE. A manual of human embryology. London: Bailliere, Tyndall & Cox, 1940.)

ticulum is more appropriate. Cysts and diverticula are microscopically identical.

A review of 34 atypical upper mediastinal pericardial cysts (separated from the diaphragm) (75) published in 1986 revealed a greater left-sided incidence (34%) and a greater likelihood for confusion with more ominous mediastinal masses including thymoma, lymphoma, mesenchymal tumor, or extragonadal germ cell tumor.

Proven congenital pericardial diverticula are found much less often than are cysts. Maier in 1946 considered his case to be the first one reported in this country (73). Ware and Conrad (79) accepted 15 cases in the literature and added one of their own. Fell and his colleagues (66) tabulated 29 cases in 1959, but not all of these could be considered to be congenital. None were in infants or children.

SYMPTOMS

In the great majority of cases, patients with cysts or diverticula of the pericardium have no symptoms related to the anomaly. Slightly more than one-third of the 82 patients with pericardial cysts in the Armed Forces Institute of Pathology series were symptomatic (76), usually complaining of precordial or substernal chest pain. Cysts usually present in mid-adult life as an incidental mass found on a routine chest x-ray examination. Symptoms, when present, typically include substernal chest discomfort or pressure, dyspnea, or a nonspecific cough (74). Only occasionally are the symptoms relieved by removal of the cyst.

A unique exception to the harmless nature of these structures is a report by Davis and his associates (80) of a large, right-sided diverticulum that compressed the right bronchus and right pulmonary artery. The heart and trachea were displaced to the right, and the right lung was atelectatic. The patient, first seen at age 7 years, had cyanotic episodes and failed to grow or gain weight during the next 3 years before surgery. The obstructed lung returned to normal upon removal of the diverticulum.

Complications of pericardial cysts include rupture (rare) (81) and progressive enlargement (78). One case of apparent spontaneous resolution of a pericardial cyst has been reported (82), and in another case a cyst resolved after apparent spontaneous or perhaps iatrogenic rupture (81).

DIAGNOSIS

Cysts and diverticula appear on radiography as smooth, rounded masses below the hilum or in the cardiophrenic angle. Occasionally, they lie across the midline and appear in both cardiophrenic angles. Pericardial cysts may be confused clinically and radiographically with other tumors of the pericardium including lipoma, hemangioma, and lymphangioma (83). Other anomalies that have been confused with pericardial cysts include middle mediastinal thymoma (84), foreign body granuloma (85), and bronchogenic cysts (86). MRI, CT, and M-mode and two-dimensional echocardiography can usually help in differentiating among masses of pericardial origin.

Because of their location, it is necessary to rule out herniation through the foramen of Morgagni. This can be done by injecting air into the peritoneal cavity or by performing a gastrointestinal barium x-ray series. Le Roux (65) found eight such herniae, together with two dermoid cysts, one thymic cyst, one aneurysm of the right ventricle, one metastasis from a uterine carcinoma, and one unusual projection of the liver, all of which had been considered on radiologic diagnosis to be pericardial cysts or diverticula. Angiocardiography excludes ventricular aneurysm.

The characteristic pointed appearance of benign mediastinal cysts, including bronchogenic and pericardial cysts, on CT (87) helps to differentiate these benign masses from the potentially malignant solid mediastinal masses including lymphoma and lymph node metastases. Other CT characteristics include a sharply defined oval or tubular mass without infiltration of contiguous anatomy, a uniformly thin wall, homogeneous attenuation near water density (0-20 HU), and absence of contrast enhancement (absence of internal vascularization) (87). Bronchogenic cysts usually have a higher density (20-130 HU).

The symptoms of most intrathoracic masses identified by plain chest x-ray examination are usually nonspecific. Imaging techniques useful in management of such masses, including pericardial cysts, ideally should (a) define the exact location, size, and extent of the mass and its hemodynamic and respiratory consequences; (b) suggest histopathology (benign versus malignant, primary versus secondary); and (c) guide optimal treatment. MRI probably comes closest to the ideal diagnostic modality (88). Solid, fatty, and fluid-filled "tumors" are easily identified and distinguished from one another and from the simple unilocular fluid-filled pericardial cyst. Calcified tumors, in contrast to fibrous tumors, may be more easily identified by CT. Concomitant use of an intravenous contrast agent during MRI or CT is helpful in ambiguous cases.

Meloni and colleagues (89) demonstrated the value of two-dimensional echocardiography for the differentiation of pericardial cysts from solid tumors, diaphragmatic and hiatal herniae, left ventricular aneurysms, aneurysms of the descending aorta, hematomas, echinococcal cysts, and pleural effusions. Two-dimensional echocardiogra-

phy and CT accurately diagnosed a large clot-containing pericardial cyst causing severe respiratory distress in a newborn, allowing for successful early surgical removal (90).

MRI is particularly useful in the diagnosis of pericardial cysts in atypical locations, including the posterior cardiophrenic angle, subcarinal area, left hilus, or right laterotracheal region, and in separating mediastinal masses from normal adjacent mediastinal structures of relatively similar density (91).

Mediastinal cystic hygromas differ from pericardial cysts in that they incorporate surrounding structures and have a well-developed blood supply. The vessels serving a pericardial cyst are rarely large enough to require ligation.

TREATMENT

Surgery usually is necessary only to confirm the diagnosis. In only one case (that of Davis and his colleagues [80] described previously) have pericardial cysts or diverticula affected respiratory or cardiac function. No case of malignancy is known.

Removal is not difficult. Cysts shell out readily without the necessity of ligating blood vessels; diverticula require simple ligation and removal. No operative deaths have been reported. Braude and colleagues (74) recently reported excision of the largest pericardial cyst yet described—a 28 × 28 × 18 cm cystic mass identified by CT occupying the left inferior hemithorax and causing gross upward displacement of the left lower lobe bronchus and extrinsic compression of the segmental bronchi. The cyst was firmly adherent to the pericardium anteriorly, but there was no communication with the pericardial space. Histology revealed a single layer of flattened mesothelial cells.

Pericardial cysts were successfully excised in 78 of the 82 patients in the Armed Forces Institute of Pathology series; all patients were alive and well without evidence of recurrence or symptoms at least 2 years after surgery (76). The four other cysts were found incidentally at autopsy.

Two cases of epicardial cysts (92, 93) have been reported, both of which were treated by resection of the free wall while avoiding injury to the subjacent coronary arteries. Such cysts are symptomatic only when large enough to cause significant cardiac compression or displacement.

Sarin (94) first described the diagnosis and aspiration of what was thought to be a pericardial cyst anterior to the right mainstem bronchus. This may, of course, have been a bronchogenic cyst. Nonetheless, the safety of this method and the freedom from recurrence after aspiration, preceded by contrast medium injection if necessary, in this and other patients (95) treated by aspiration indicates that this conservative approach is an alternative to thoracotomy in an otherwise poor-risk surgical candidate. Although cysts have been treated by aspiration under fluoroscopic guidance without recurrence for up to 3 years (95), thoracotomy with complete surgical excision allows full histologic examination and reduces the risk of aspirating an unrecognized hydatid cyst (96).

Aspiration for diagnosis and as treatment of pericardial and other fluid-filled cysts and soft tissue densities within the mediastinum remains controversial. Stoller and colleagues (78) described up to 3 years of follow-up without recurrence after aspiration of cysts in six patients. Westcott (97) advocated aspiration of mediastinal masses for diagnosis before resection because this strategy has proved to be safe, accurate, and useful for ablation of cystic masses.

EDITORIAL COMMENT

Recent advances with video-assisted thorascopic surgery have allowed the surgeon to perform intrathoracic procedures through small intercostal incisions (without rib retraction) with the assistance of specialized instruments, video cameras, and double–lumen endotracheal tubes for elective lung collapse on the side of interest. Localized pericardiectomy and resection of pericardial cysts have been reported with excellent results (cm).

REFERENCES

1. His W. Mittheilungen zur Embryologie der Säugetheire und des Menschen. Arch Anat Leipzig Anat Abt 1881;303–329.
2. Elliott RA. A contribution to the development of the pericardium. Am J Anat 1931;48:355–390.
3. Ellis FH, Kirklin JW, Swan HJC, DuShane JW, Edwards JE. Diagnosis and surgical treatment of common atrium (cor triloculare-biventriculare). Surgery 1959;45:160–172.
4. Moore RL. Congenital deficincies of the pericardium. Arch Surg 1925;11:765.
5. Fanfani M, de Biase G. Le agenesie del pericardio. Arch "deVecchi" Anat 1954;22:1003–1063.
6. Rusby NL, Sellors TH. Congenital deficiency of the pericardium associated with a bronchogenic cyst. Br J Surg 1945;32:357–364.
7. Chang CH, Leigh TF. Congenital partial defect of the pericardium associated with herniation of the left atrial appendage. AJR 1961;86:517–522.
8. Kavanagh-Gray D, Musgrove E, Stanwood D. Congenital pericardial defects. N Engl J Med 1961;265:692–694.
9. Duffie ER Jr, Moss AJ, Maloney JF Jr. Congenital pericardial defects with herniation of the heart into the pleural space. Pediatrics 1962;30:746–748.
10. Sunderland S, Wright-Smith RJ. Congenital pericardial defects. Br Heart J 1944;6:167–175.
11. Hipona FA, Crummy AB Jr. Congenital pericardial defect associated with tetralogy of Fallot; herniation of normal lung into the pericardial cavity. Circulation 1964;29:132–135.
12. Orellana J, Aberdeen E, Baron MG. Anomalous phrenic nerves in a patient with congenital absence of the left pericardium. Mt Sinai J Med 1981;48:443–445.
13. Perna G. Sopra un arresto di sviluppo della sierosa pericardica nell'uomo. Anat Anz 1909;35:323.
14. Ellis K, Leeds NE, Himmelstein A. Congenital deficiencies in the parietal pericardium: a review with two new cases including successful diagnosis by plain roentgenography. AJR 1959;82:125–137.
15. Kapouleas GP, Keramidas DC, Soutis M. Bochdalek's hernia combined with agenesis of the pericardium and intrathoracic solitary cyst of the liver. Z Kinderchir 1989;44:377–378.
16. Matsuoka T, Kimura F, Sugiyama K, Nagata N, Takatani O. Anomalous inferior vena cava with azygos continuation, dysgenesis of lung, and clinically suspected absence of left pericardium. Chest 1990;97:747–749.
17. Spitz L et al. Combined anterior abdominal wall, sternal, diaphragmatic, pericardial, and intracardiac defects: a report of five cases and their management. J Pediatr Surg 1975;10:481.
18. Columbus R. De Re Anatomica. Venetüs, 1559.
19. Baillie M. On the want of a pericardium in the human body. Trans Soc Improvement Med Chir Knowledge (London) 1793; 1:91.
20. Ebstein E. Bemerkungen zur Klinik der Herzbeuteldefekte. München Med Wschr 1910;57:522–524.
21. Ladd WE. Congenital absence of the pericardium. N Engl J Med 1936;214:183–187.
22. Ronka EKF, Tessmer CF. Congenital absence of pericardium: report of case. Am J Pathol 1944;20:1944.
23. Verse M. Fall von kongenitalem Defekt des Herzbeutels. Muenchn Med Wochenschr 1909;56:2667.
24. Southworth H, Stevenson CS. Congenital defects of the pericardium. Arch Int Med 1938;61:223–240.
25. Taysi K, Hartmann AF, Shackelford GD, Sundaram V. Congenital absence of left pericardium in a family. Am J Med Genet 1985;21:77–85.
26. DeGaris CF. Pericardial patency and partial ectocardia in a newborn orangutan. Anat Rec 1934;59:69–82.
27. Walker WF, Zessman JE. A case of an incomplete pericardial cavity in the cat. Anat Rec 1952;113:459–465.
28. Saiato R, Hotta F. Congenital pericardial defect associated with cardiac incarceration: case report. Am Heart J 1980;100:866–870.
29. Gehlmann HR, van Ingen GJ. Symptomatic congenital complete absence of the left pericardium: case report and review of the literature. Eur Heart J 1989;10:670–675.
30. Auch-Schwelk W et al. Differential diagnosis of chest pain and diagnostic findings in pericardial defects combined with coronary artery disease. Clin Cardiol 1988;11:650–657.
31. Siderys H, Bowers WD, Schumacher R. Congenital absence of the right pericardium: a rare cause of clinical confusion. J IN State Med Assoc 1979;72:121–123.
32. Nasser WK, Helmen C, Tavel ME, Feigenbaum H, Fisch C. Congenital absence of the left pericardium: clinical, electrocardiographic, radiographic, hemodynamic and angiographic findings in six cases. Circulation 1970;41:469–478.
33. Hoorntje JC, Mooyaart EL, Meuzelaar KJ. Left atrial herniation through a partial pericardial defect: a rare cause of syncope. Pace 1989;12:1841–1845.
34. Moene RJ, Dekker A, Harten H. Congenital right-sided pericardial defect with herniation of part of the lung into the pericardial cavity. Am J Cardiol 1973;31:519–522.
35. Beppu S, Naito H, Matsuhisa M, Miyatake K, Nimura Y. The effects of lying position on ventricular volume in congenital absence of the pericardium. Am Heart J 1990;120:1159–1166.
36. Abbott M. Congenital cardiac disease. In: Osler W, ed. Osler's modern medicine, Vol 4. Philadelphia: Lea & Febiger, 1927.
37. Inoue H, Fujii J, Mashima S, Murao S. Pseudo right atrial overloading pattern in complete defect of the left pericardium. J Electrocardiol 1981;14:413–418.
38. Morgan JR. Congenial absence of the left pericardium. Ann Intern Med 1971;74:370.

39. Inoue H et al. Postural changes of vectorcardiogram in defect of the left pericardium. J Electrocardiol 1981;14:21–24.
40. Matsuhisa M, Shimomura K, Beppu S, Nakajima K. Jugular phlebogram in congenital absence of the pericardium. Am Heart J 1986;112:1004–1010.
41. Dimond EG, Kittle CF, Voth DW. Extreme hypertrophy of the left atrial appendage: the case of the giant dog ear. Am J Cardiol 1960;5:122–125.
42. Rogge JD, Mishkin ME, Genovese PD. Congenital partial defect with herniation of the left atrial appendage. Ann Intern Med 1966;64:137–141.
43. Lajos TZ, Bunnell IL, Colokathis BP, Schimert G. Coronary artery insufficiency secondary to congenital pericardial defect. Chest 1970;58:73–76.
44. Foale RA et al. Congenital aneurysms of the left atrium: recognition by cross-sectional echocardiography. Circulation 1982;66:1065–1069.
45. Candan I, Erol C, Sonel A. Cross-sectional echocardiographic appearance in presumed congenital absence of the left pericardium. Br Heart J 1986;55:405–407.
46. Burrows PE et al. Partial absence of the left parietal pericardium with herniation of the left atrial appendage: diagnosis by cross-sectional echocardiography and contrast-enhanced computed tomography. Pediatr Cardiol 1987;8:205–208.
47. Rowland TW, Twible EA, Norwood WI Jr, Keane JF. Partial absence of the left pericardium: diagnosis by two-dimensional echocardiography. Am J Dis Child 1982;136:628–630.
48. Ruys F, Paulus W, Stevens C, Brutsaert D. Expansion of the left atrial appendage is a distinctive cross-sectional echocardiographic feature of congenital defect of the pericardium. Eur Heart J 1983;4:738–741.
49. Nicolosi GL et al. M-mode and two-dimensional echocardiography in congenital absence of the pericardium. Chest 1982;81:610–613.
50. Vargas-Barron J et al. The differential diagnosis of partial absence of left pericardium and congenital left atrial aneurysm. Am Heart J 1989;118:1348–1350.
51. Semans JH, Taussig HB. Congenital "aneurysmal" dilatation of the left auricle. Bull Johns Hopkins Hosp 1939;63:404.
52. Salem DN, Hymanson AS, Isner JM, Bankoff MS, Konstam MA. Congenital pericardial defect diagnosed by computed tomography. Cathet Cardiovasc Diagn 1985;11:75–79.
53. Moncada R et al. Diagnostic role of computed tomography in pericardial heart disease: congenital defects, thickening, neoplasms, and effusions. Am Heart J 1982;103:262–282.
54. Baim, RS, MacDonald IL, Wise DJ, Lenkei SC. Computed tomography of absent left pericardium. Radiology 1980;135:127–128.
55. Gutierrez FR, Shackelford GD, McKnight RC, Levitt RG, Hartmann A. Diagnosis of congenital absence of left pericardium by MR imaging. J Comput Assist Tomogr 1985;9:551–553.
56. Schiavone WA, O'Donnell JK. Congenital absence of the left portion of parietal pericardium demonstrated by nuclear magnetic resonance imaging. Am J Cardiol 1985;55:1439–1440.
57. D'Altoria RA, Caro JY. Congenital absence of the left pericardium detected by imaging of the lung: case report. N Engl J Med 1977;18:267.
58. Rodgers BM, Moulder PV, DeLaney A. Thoracoscopy: new method of early diagnosis of cardiac herniation. J Thorac Cardiovasc Surg 1979;78:623–625.
59. Bernal JM et al. Angiocardiographic demonstration of a partial defect of the pericardium with herniation of the left atrium and ventricle. J Cardiovasc Surg 1986;27:344–346.
60. Amiri A, Weber C, Schlosser V, Meinertz TH. Coronary artery disease in patient with a congenital pericardial defect. Thorac Cardiovasc Surg 1989;37:379–381.
61. Chapman JE Jr, Rubin JW, Gross CM, Janssen ME. Congenital absence of pericardium: an unusual cause of atypical angina. Ann Thorac Surg 1988;45:91–93.
62. Savage RW, Nolan TE. Pregnancy in a woman with partial absence of the left pericardium: a case report. J Reprod Med 1988;33:385–386.
63. Feigin DS, Fenoglio JJ, McAllister HA, Madewell JE. Pericardial cysts: a radiologic-pathologic correlation and review. Radiology 1977;125:15–20.
64. Bristowe JS. Diverticulum from the pericardium. Trans Pathol Soc Lond 1869;20:101.
65. Le Roux BT. Pericardial coelomic cysts. Thorax 1959;14:27–35.
66. Fell SC, Schein CJ, Bloomberg AE, Rubinstein BM. Congenital diverticula of the pericardium. Ann Surg 1959;149:117–125.
67. Lillie WI, McDonald JR, Clagett OT. Pericardial celomic cysts and pericardial diverticula: concept of etiology and report of cases. J Thorac Surg 1950;20:494.
68. Kassner EG, Rosen Y, Klotz DH Jr. Mediastinal esophageal duplication cyst associated with a partial pericardial defect. Pediatr Radiol 1975;4:53–56.
69. Mazer ML. True pericardial diverticulum. AJR 1946;55:27–29.
70. Lambert AVS. Etiology of thin-walled thoracic cysts. J Thorac Surg 1940;10:1–7.
71. Viikari SJ. A study of the bursa infracardia: development, anatomy and surgical pathology. Ann Chir Gyn Fenniae Supp 1950;39:1.
72. Peterson DT, Zatz LM, Popp RL. Pericardial cyst ten years after acute pericarditis. Chest 1975;67:719–721.
73. Maier HD. Diverticulum of the pericardium with observations on the mode of development. Circulation 1957;16:1040–1045.
74. Braude PD, Falk G, McCaughan BC, Rutland J. Giant pericardial cyst. Aust N Z J Surg 1990;60:640–641.
75. McAllister HA, Fenoglio JJ. Tumors of the cardiovascular system. In: Firminger HI, ed. Atlas of tumor pathology. Washington, DC: Armed Forces Institute of Pathology, 1978 (fasc 15, 2nd series).
76. McAllister HA Jr. Primary tumors and cysts of the heart and pericardium. Curr Probl Cardiol 1979;4:1–51.
77. Nelson TG, Shefts LM, Bowers WF. Mediastinal tumors: an analysis of 141 cases. Dis Chest 1957;32:123.
78. Stoller JK, Shaw C and Matthay RA. Enlarging, atypically located pericardial cyst: recent experience and literature review. Chest 1986;89:402–406.
79. Ware GW, Conrad HA. Pericardial coelomic cysts. Am J Surg 1954;88:272–279.
80. Davis WC, German JD, Johnson NJ. Pericardial diverticulum causing pulmonary obstruction. Arch Surg 1961;82:285–289.
81. King JF, Crosby I, Pugh D, Reed W. Rupture of pericardial cyst. Chest 1971;60:611–612.
82. Kruger SR, Michaud J, Cannon DS. Spontaneous resolution of a pericardial cyst. Am Heart J 1985;109:1390–1391.
83. Wychulis AR, Connolly DC, McGoon DC. Pericardial cysts, tumors and fat necrosis. J Thorac Cadiovasc Surg 1971;62:294–300.
84. Adebonojo SA, Grillo IA, Falase AO, Aghadiuno PU. Middle mediastinal thymoma simulating pericardial cyst. Int Surg 1977;62:343–345.
85. Uflacker RP, Duarte DL. A foreign body granuloma simulating a pericardial cyst: an unusual case report. Br J Radiol 1977;50:522–523.
86. Kwak DL, Stork WJ, Greenberg SD. Partial defect of the pericardium associated with bronchogenic cyst. Radiology 1971;101:287–288.
87. Demos TC, Budorick NE, Posniak HV. Benign mediastinal cysts: pointed appearance on CT. J Comput Assist Tomogr 1989;13:132–33.

88. Rienmuller R, Tiling R. Evaluation of paracardiac and intracardiac masses in children. Semin Ultrasound CT MR 1990;11:246–250.

89. Meloni L, Ruscazio M, Versace R, Mela Q, Cherchi A. Unusual pericardial cyst location: value of two-dimensional echocardiography in diagnosis. J Ultrasound Med 1988;7:519–522.

90. Bini RM, Nath PH, Ceballos R, Bargeron LM Jr, Kirklin JK. Pericardial cyst diagnosed by two-dimensional echocardiography and computed tomography in a newborn. Pediatr Cardiol 1987;8:47–50.

91. Boisserie LM, Martigne C, Laurent F, Drouillard J, Grelet P. A pleuropericardial cyst in an unusual location: the value of magnetic resonance. Comput Med Imaging Graph 1988;12:277–280.

92. Edwards MH, Ahmad A. Epicardial cyst: a case report. Thorax 1972;27:503–506.

93. Komeda M et al. Epicardial cyst: report of a case with successful resection. Jpn Circ J 1985;49:1201–1205.

94. Sarin CL. Pericardial cyst in the superior mediastinum treated by mediastinoscopy: a case report. Br J Surg 1970;57:232–233.

95. Klatte EC, Yune HY. Diagnosis and treatment of pericardial cysts. Radiology 1972;104:541–544.

96. Le Roux BT, Kallichurum S, Shama DM. Mediastinal cysts and tumours. Curr Probl Surg 1984;21:49–54.

97. Westcott JL. Percutaneous needle aspiration of hilar and mediastinal masses. Radiology 1941;141:323–329.

CHAPTER 26

THE HEART

Jane L. Todd / Mark E. Silverman /
Margaret L. Kirby / Stephen Wood Gray / John Elias Skandalakis

*"A surgeon who tries to suture the heart deserves to lose the
esteem of his colleagues."*
—BILLROTH, 1883

DEVELOPMENT

Early Development of the Heart

Most of our knowledge of the earliest development of the heart and the derivation of tissues involved in heart development has been obtained from experimental studies on amphibian and chick embryos. Much of this work has been ably reviewed by DeHaan (1).

Four groups of cells are necessary for development of the heart to proceed normally. These are the myocardial, endocardial, epicardial, and neural crest-derived ectomesenchymal cells. Each of these cells types is derived from a different area of the early embryo and is reviewed prior to a discussion of the process of heart development.

Prior to the appearance of the primitive streak, most of the cells of the embryonic disc have a limited ability to form cardiac muscle in culture (2, 3). Using marking techniques, Rosenquist (4) mapped the presumptive myocardium-forming areas of the blastodisc. Presumptive myocardium-forming cells were found in the primitive streak stage of the chick embryo located in the epiblast about midway along the length of the streak. The cells extend laterally from the midline to halfway to the edge of the embryonic disc. The cells are spatially ordered during invagination so that the cells which will form the myocardium of the outflow tract migrate through the primitive streak first, followed by presumptive ventricular, atrial, and finally sinus venosus cells. Having completed this ectodermal to mesodermal transformation, the cells continue to migrate to form the crescent-shaped cardiogenic plate, which is a portion of the splanchnic mesoderm located cranial to the oropharyngeal membrane. The paired areas of presumptive cardiac mesoderm remain as an intact epithelial sheet that forms the myocardial sheaths of the heart-forming tubes. These tubes move ventrally and medially to fuse across the midline in the late neurula stage (Fig. 26.1) (3, 5–9). No histologic differentiation of this region can be seen at this stage, but the presence of cardiac myosin has been shown (10), and there are periodic acid-Schiff positive granules not found elsewhere in the mesoderm (11).

While the origin of the myocardium has been clearly shown, the derivation of the atrial and ventricular endocardium is unclear. The endocardium of the atria and ventricles may be derived from the cardiogenic plate. However, initial studies have not identified cardiogenic plate cells seeding any part of the embryo other than myocardium, so it is possible that atrial and ventricular endocardium are not derived from the cardiogenic plate (12). The endocardium of the outflow region has been mapped to the cephalic paraxial and lateral mesoderm underlying and slightly rostral and lateral to the otic placode (13). These cells become interspersed with the atrial and ventricular endocardium during the initial stages of cardiogenesis.

These studies support evidence that has accumulated indicating that the cardiogenic plate itself forms only the myocardium of the future heart. Earlier references to a epimyocardial sheath have been shown to be incorrect, and it is now known that the epicardium grows later in development as protrusions of the dorsal mesocardium on the right ventral wall of the sinus venosus. The epicardium seeds the myocardium with mesenchymal cells that form a cardiac vascular plexus and ultimately become the adult coronary vessels.

The actual formation of the heart tissue from the presumptive cardiac mesoderm appears to be under the positive influence of the foregut endoderm (14, 15) and the negative influence of the neural plate (16, 17). Explanted cardiac mesoderm from amphibian embryos rarely forms a heart tube; the presence of endodermal tissue is necessary (18). After the tail bud stage, heart formation becomes independent of the presence of either gut or neural plate tissue (19). It is probable, although it has not been demonstrated, that foregut endoderm plays a similar role in induction of the mammalian heart.

The final group of cells needed for heart formation arrive much later and are derived from the neural crest.

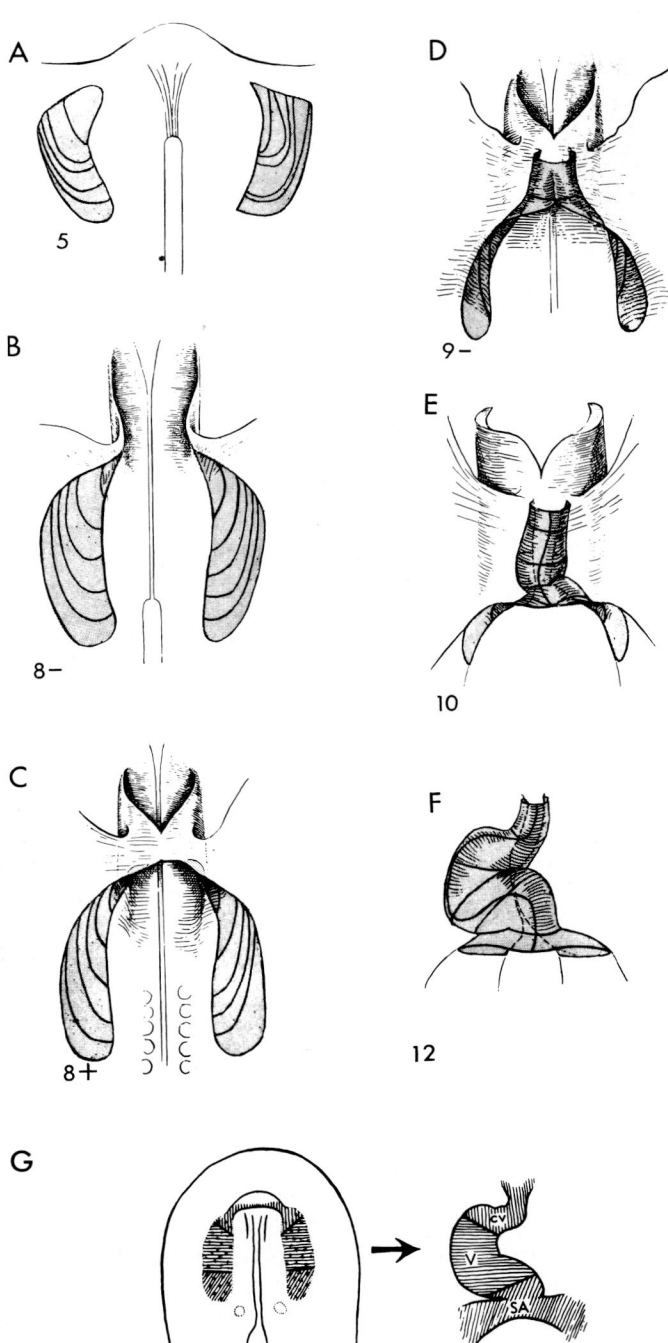

Figure 26.1. Heart formation in the chick embryo. **A** to **F,** Movements of the cardiogenic mesoderm have been mapped from stage 5 (19 to 22 hours of incubation) to stage 12 (26 to 29 hours of incubation). Arbitrary boundary lines permit the movement of specific areas to be traced through all stages. (From Stalsberg H, DeHaan RL. The precardiac areas and the formation of the tubular heart in the chick embryo. Develop Biol 1969;19:128–159.) **G,** Recapitulation showing the origins of the primary heart segments. *V,* Ventricular region; *cv,* conoventricular region: *SA,* sinoatrial region (From De Haan RL. Morphogenesis of the vertebrate heart. In: De Haan RL, Ursprung H, eds. Organogenesis. New York: Holt, Rinehart & Winston, 1965.)

These cells originate in the neural fold located between the mid-otic placode and the caudal level of somite 3. These cells migrate first to the circumpharyngeal region located dorsal to the presumptive pharyngeal arches 3, 4, and 6 and then populate the pharyngeal arches as they form (20). Somewhat later, the cells continue their migration into the outflow region of the heart where they participate in septation of the aortic sac and truncus arteriosus (21). Proper septation of the aortic sac and truncus arteriosus is necessary for septation of the conus arteriosus. Therefore these three areas will be referred to as the outflow tract.

Neural crest cells are necessary for septation of the outflow tract, but they also support cardiovascular development in the pharyngeal arches. The aortic arch arteries develop in the pharyngeal arches, and neural crest cells support their formation and maintenance. Since the aortic arch arteries are downstream from the developing heart, they are especially important in defining the hemodynamic characteristics of the region. As the definitive aortic arch artery derivatives develop—arch of the aorta, brachycephalic, common carotid, and subclavian arteries—neural crest cells become organized as the tunica media of these vessels (21, 22).

At the end of the third week of human development (stage 9), the mesoderm, cranial and craniolateral to the neural plate, begins to split into somatic (dorsal) and splanchnic (ventral) layers. The space thus formed is the embryonic celom. The splitting first appears as a series of vesicles, which soon become confluent in a horseshoe-shaped region about the time the first somite is forming (23). The cranial and medial portion of the celom will become the pericardial cavity, while the lateral prolongation will become the pleural and peritoneal cavities (see Chapter 25, "The Pericardium") (Fig. 26.2, *A* to *C*).

During the splitting of the mesoderm, the cardiogenic cells are segregated in the splanchnic layer where they form the cardiogenic plate (5). In the chick embryo the presumptive epimyocardial mesoderm behaves as a coherent sheet, and it retains, in spite of folding and deformation, its continuity with the remainder of the splanchnic mesoderm. It does not break up into cell clusters (24) (Fig. 26.1).

During the formation of the celomic cavity, the head of the embryo overgrows the portion of the embryonic disc containing the cardiogenic region. As this development proceeds, a pocket of endoderm, the foregut, is formed, and the splanchnic mesoderm, together with the cardiogenic plate, is folded over beneath this floor, rotated 180 degrees from its previous position (Fig. 26.2, *D* to *F*).

On its endodermal side, another layer of cells, the

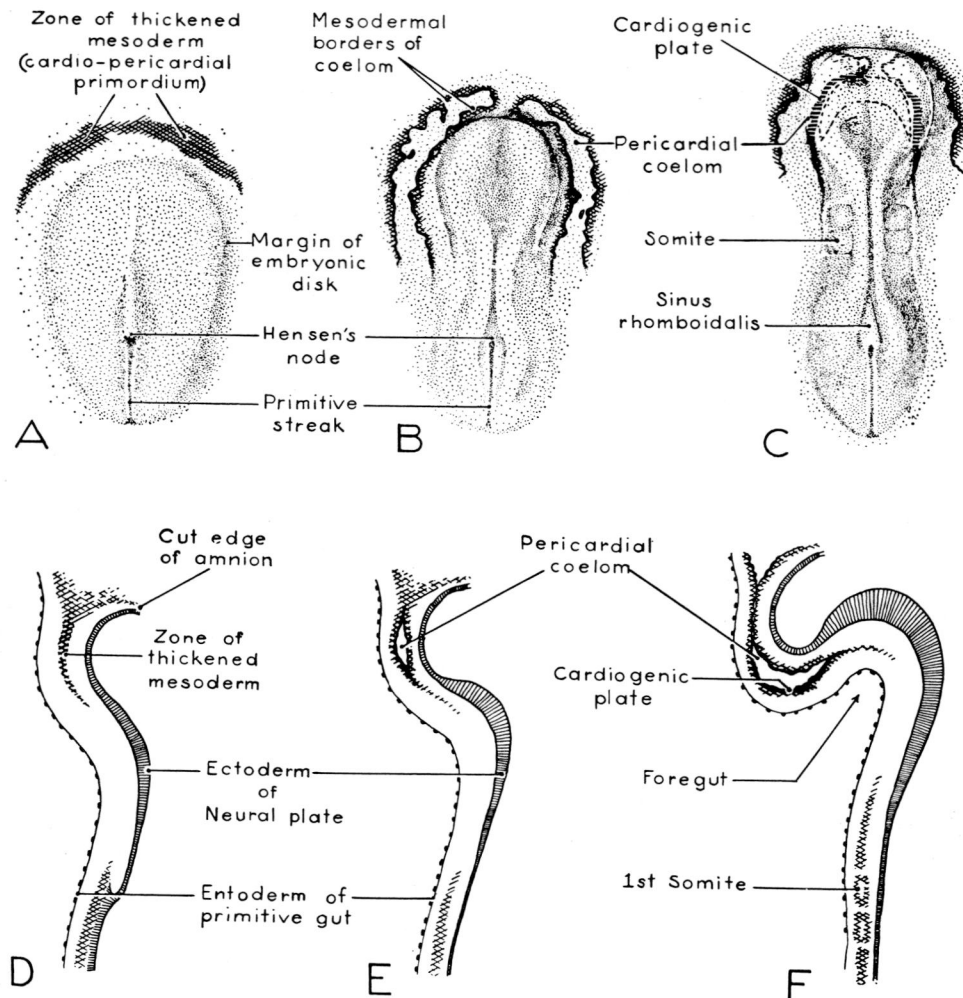

Figure 26.2   The development of the cardiac and pericardial mesoderm and the celom in the third week of development. **A** to **C,** Dorsal view of the mesoderm. The overlying ectoderm is represented as *semitransparent.* The *broken lines* in **C** indicate the margins of the foregut and the anterior intestinal portal. **D** to **F,** Long sections of the same embryonic stages, showing the rolling movement of the cardiac primordium that places it ventral to the foregut. Compare with Figure 26.3. (From Patten BM. Human embryology, 3rd ed: New York: McGraw-Hill Book Company, 1968.)

angioblasts, appears to form the endocardium (Fig. 26.3, *A*). These cells are continuous with similar cells formed by the blood islands of the yolk sac. These latter will form the vitelline veins, which will connect the blood islands of the yolk sac with the developing heart (25). The heart at this stage may be considered to be a pair of blood islands, larger than those farther out on the splanchnic mesoderm, and differing from them in having potential myocardial cells (Fig. 26.3, *A*).

The angioblasts form as a sheet of cells containing cysts, which join to create a network of channels. In the cardiac region, these channels become two main endothelial tubes by the 4- to 6-mm stage (Fig. 26.3, *B*). Anteriorly, the tubes are fused in the future bulbar region (Fig. 26.3, *C*), but posteriorly, they are separate or have only small cross connections (23). Subsequent caudad

fusion of the tubes takes place as the foregut elongates by ventrolateral infolding of the endoderm and the splanchnic mesoderm. The space between the endocardial angioblasts and the myocardial mesoderm is at first occupied by a gelatinous acellular layer of mucopolysaccharides that is laid down by the myocardium and called the "cardiac jelly." The cardiac jelly is important in maintaining anterograde blood flow, as well as shape, in the avalvular heart. It also provides a medium for transfer of signals from myocardium to endocardium and vice versa. The cardiac jelly in the atrioventricular and conotruncal regions is permeated by endothelial cells undergoing transformation to mesenchyme (26, 27). These cells will be involved in septation and valve formation in these regions (Fig. 26.4).

Almost as soon as the paired endothelial channels have

formed, they fuse with one another to create the primary tubular heart. The endothelial tube is surrounded by the myocardial layer, which then secretes the cardiac jelly. The cardiac jelly has been referred to as a thick basement membrane (28). Because of the thickness of the jelly layer, the capacity of the embryonic heart is much smaller than the size of the myocardial structure would suggest (Fig. 26.5).

During the early somite stages (early fourth week) the primitive myocardium is roughly demarcated by several lateral infoldings or sulci. The fate of these areas has been differently interpreted by Davis (29) and by DeVries and Saunders (30). Although we agree with the interpretation of the latter, the views of Davis have been incorporated in a number of embryology texts and are given below for comparison.

In amphibians, which have a single ventricle, a normal heart may form from each of the cardiac primordium (31). Interestingly, the left half forms a heart with normal situs, while the right half usually forms a heart with situs inversus.

In birds and mammals, the two ventricles are in serial arrangement and do not form from equivalent right and left halves of the primitive cardiac tube. The left side of the fused primordia, however, contributes most of the left ventricle, while the right side contributes most of the right ventricle (Fig. 26.6).

The asymmetry of the heart is established as early as the seventh somite stage. The right atrioventricular sulcus and the left interventricular sulcus are deeper than their contralateral partners, so that the primordium of the left ventricle is displaced to the left and that of the right ventricle is displaced to the right. The dorsal mesentery of the heart disappears between the 7- and 16-somite stages, leaving the heart attached to the pericardium at the venous and arterial ends only, defining the boundaries of the transverse pericardial sinus. By the fifth week, at the 25- to 30-somite stage (stages 12 and 13), the primary cardiac tube forms a loop forward and to the right, with four roughly right-angled bends. This is the normal "D loop" of Van Praagh and his colleagues (32). If the loop turns to the left instead of the right, while

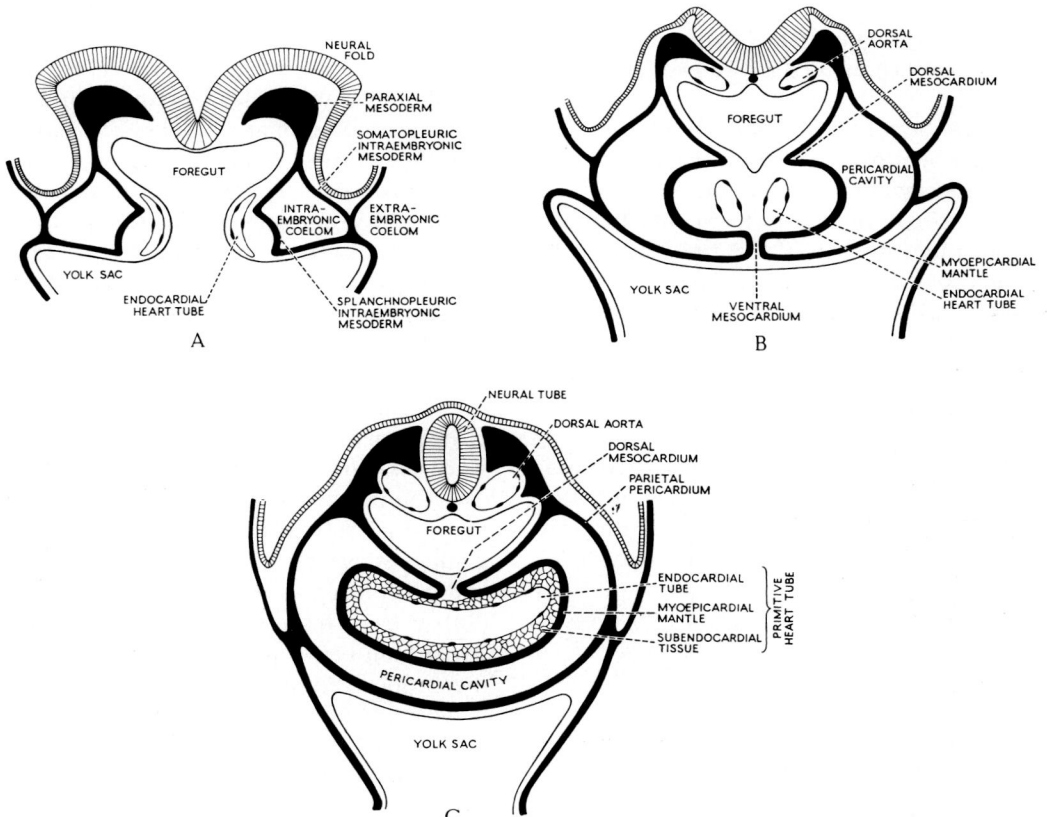

Figure 26.3. Three stages in the development of the heart from paired endocardial heart tubes during the early somite period in the fourth week. The intraembryonic celom becomes the pericardial cavity, while the local splanchnopleure becomes the myocardium. The ventral mesocardium has disappeared and the endocardial tubes have fused in the stage shown at **C** (10 somites). (From Harrison RG. A textbook of human embryology, ed 2. Philadelphia: WB Saunders Co., 1963.)

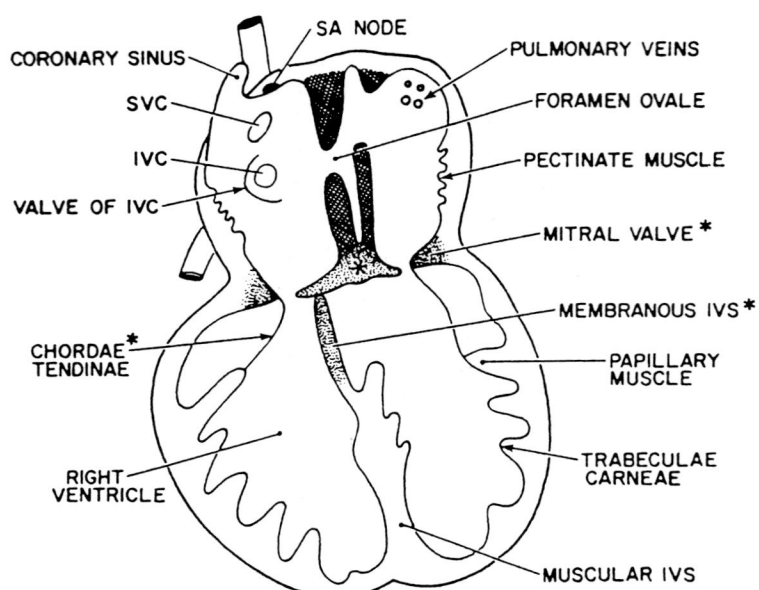

Figure 26.4. Generalized mammalian heart following organogenesis. The *asterisks* denote derivatives of endocardial cushion tissue. (From Markwald RR, Runyan RB, Kitten GT, Funderburg FM, Bernanke DH, Brauer PR. Use of collagen gel cultures to study heart development: proteoglycan and glycoprotein interactions during the formation of endocardial cushion tissue. In: Trelstad RL, ed. The role of extracellular matrix in development. New York: Alan R. Liss, Inc. 1984.)

the visceral situs remains normal, inversion of the ventricles results (see page 964). The normal loop and resulting disposition of the heart chambers are shown in Figures 26.6 and 26.7.

The studies of Stalsberg and DeHaan (24) on the chick embryo suggest that bending of the heart is not the passive response of an elongating tube in a limited pericardial space. Their measurements indicate that bending results from more rapid growth of the right side at the cranial end of the tube and more rapid growth of the left side of the caudal end. Although it has been thought that hydration of the hyaluronic acid in the cardiac jelly might be associated with normal looping, Baldwin and Solursh (33) showed that degradation of hyaluronic acid by *Streptomyces* hyaluronidase does not prevent normal looping. This and the fact that blood flow is not necessary for normal looping support the idea that looping is an intrinsic and active mechanism of the myocardium. Cell death in the heart tube is not likely to play any role in cardiac looping (34). At any rate, looping is an especially important event in that it defines the inflow and outflow portions of the tube until the heart has been partitioned by septa.

In this early loop, sometimes referred to as the bulboventricular loop, the sinus venosus, atrium, atrioventricular canal, and presumptive left ventricle all form in a series the inflow tract, while the bulbus cordis (presumptive right ventricle, conus cordis, truncus arteriosus) and aortic sac form the outflow tract. In this configuration, the bulboventricular fold demarcates the inflow from the outflow and acts roughly as a valve. The regression of the bulboventricular fold is extremely important as the

mature inflow and outflow portions of the heart form. In the mature heart the inflow consists of the atria and atrioventricular valves. The outflow tract includes the infundibulum and vestibule, semilunar valves, and base of the aorta and pulmonary trunks. The infundibulum/vestibule are derived from the conus cordis, the semilunar valves from the truncus arteriosus and the base of the aorta and pulmonary trunk from the aortic sac.

The question of the influence of the bloodstream on the morphogenesis of the heart becomes important with the establishment of circulation. Grant (35) attributes to von Baer the first suggestion that hemodynamic factors influence morphogenesis. Bremer (36) observed that the earliest movement of blood through the embryonic heart is the form of two confluent streams from the horns of the sinus venosus. The shape of the heart at this stage is such that the two streams would spiral about one another to the left as they pass from atrium to truncus arteriosus. Bremer suggested that the spiral stream guided the formation of this portion of the heart. DeVries and Saunders (30) agree with this interpretation, arguing that the spiral stream impresses itself on the gelatinous layer between the endocardium and the myocardium.

That blood flow can and does influence vascular patterns is well known. Simons (37) has shown that tadpoles deprived of lungs at the 12-mm stage have an absolute decrease in left atrial size, although the atrial septum develops normally. It has been pointed out by several authors that the atrial septum is the only part of the heart that develops perpendicular to the flow of blood rather than parallel to it.

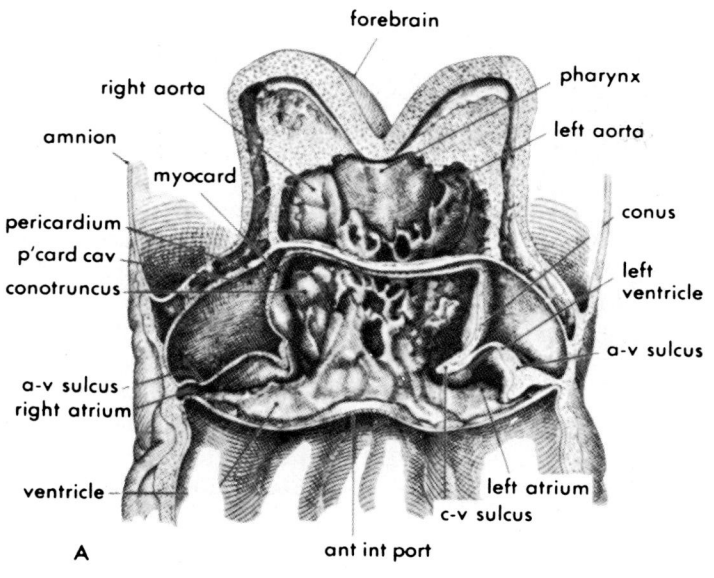

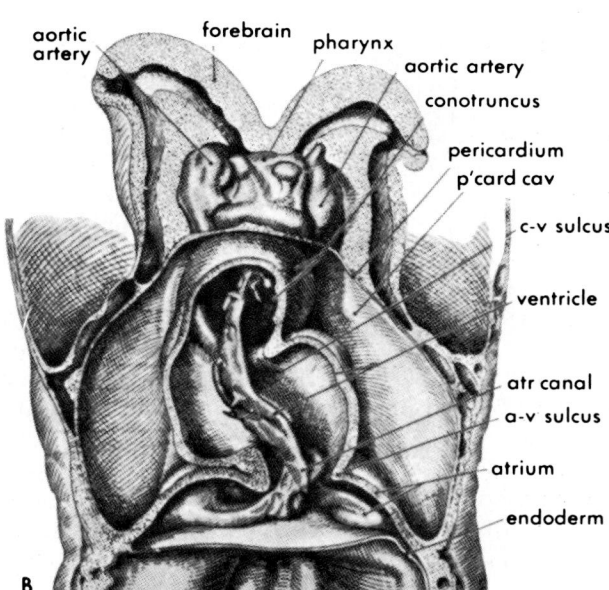

Figure 26.5. Two stages in the formation of the human heart during the fourth week. The myocardium has been dissected away to reveal the endocardial channels. Note the discrepancy in size between the exterior and the interior of the heart. **A,** At four somites. **B,** At eight somites. (From DeHaan RL. Morphogenesis of the vertebrate heart. In: DeHaan RL, Ursprung H, eds. Organogenesis. New York: Holt, Rhinehart & Winston, 1965.)

This discussion of the spiral streams may be pertinent to the problems of transposition of the great vessels (see page 944). Rychter (38) produced the simulacrum of corrected transposition in chick embryos by clamping the bulboventricular groove during the third day of development. It should be noted that Rychter did not document the pattern of blood flow through the heart after the clamp was placed on the heart and thus the transpositions that resulted are not necessarily due to an altered blood flow pattern.

By stage 14, at the end of the fifth week, the major tor-

sions of the heart are complete, and the sinus venosus, the atria, the ventricles, and the truncus arteriosus are demarcated (Fig. 26.6). The spiral division of the truncus is suggested, and the atrioventricular canal has begun to divide into two channels. The next series of steps involves the partitioning of the heart. Two great landmarks in our understanding of these steps are the detailed anatomic study of the heart in the seventh week (stages 17 and 18) by Vernall (39) and a similar study of the heart in the ninth week (stages 22 and 23) by Licata (40). Study Figures 26.8 and 26.9 to appreciate the dilations and con-

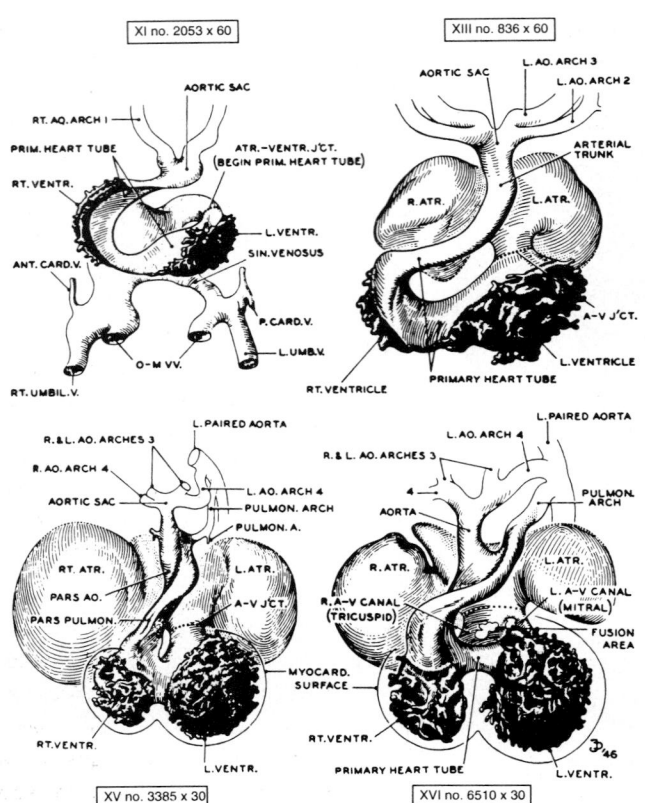

Figure 26.6. Ventral views of the endothelial portion of the developing human heart. Note the two trabeculated areas that will become the left and right ventricles. (From Streeter GL. Developmental horizons in human embryos: description of age groups XIX, XX, XXI, XXII, and XXIII. Contrib Embryol Carnegie Inst Wash 1951;34:165–196.)

strictions of the primitive cardiac tube and the mechanism of septation of the heart.

DIVISION OF THE ATRIOVENTRICULAR CANAL

The atrioventricular canal at the end of the fourth week is a laterally elongated, slit-like opening. On the ventral (anterior) and dorsal (posterior) edges of the slit, thickenings of connective tissue form the endocardial cushions. These cushions come into contact and fuse with another during the sixth week (stage 16), dividing the atrioventricular canal into left and right orifices (Fig. 26.10).

In addition to dividing the canal, the endocardial cushions contribute to the formation of the atrioventricular valves (Fig. 26.11, *E*). The area of fusion of the cushions will form the adjacent portions of the annuli fibrosi surrounding the atrioventricular orifices and probably the right trigone of the cardiac skeleton. It is to this area that the atrial septum from above, and the ventricular septum from below, will attach when the partitioning of the heart is complete (Fig. 26.11, *F*).

The embryologic entities responsible for the develop-

ment of the atrioventricular valves are: the internal layer of the muscular ventricle wall (major contribution) and mesenchymal tissue derived from the endocardium (very small contribution). Abnormal fusion of the endocardial cushion, perhaps secondary to changes of the extracellular matrix, is most likely responsible for atresias of the mitral and tricuspid valves. However, the role of the atrioventricular endocardial cushion still is debated by many scholars.

THE PARTITION OF THE ATRIUM

The sequence of events that lead to the division of the primitive atrium were first set forth by Born (41) and Tandler (42). Subsequent studies by Odgers (43), Licata (40), Patton (44), and Vernall (39) have added details.

Separation of the atria begins in the fifth week (stage 13). A crescentic ridge of the dorsocranial atrial wall indicates the first (septum primum) (Fig. 26.11, *A* and *B*) of the two septa that will form the definitive atrial partition. This septum is formed largely of muscle, but its free edge contains a band of connective tissue. The edge is directed toward the atrioventricular canal, where the endocardial cushions are developing.

Atrial septal formation and junction of the endocardial cushions are separately controlled events. Fusion of the cushions may take place without completion of septum primum formation, or the septum may form normally but fail to find normal anchorage if the cushions are not fused.

Early in the seventh week (stage 17), the edge of the septum primum reaches the fused endocardial cushions, closing the communication between the atria, which is known as the ostium (foramen) primum. Just before the ostium primum closes (stage 16), an aperture appears in the cranial portion of the septum forming a new opening, the ostium (foramen) secundum (Fig. 26.11, *C*). This opening is usually attributed to local resorption and tissue breakdown; Odgers (43) considered it to be a primary hiatus left during growth of the septum.

This new opening permits blood from the right atrium to reach the left atrium, which would otherwise receive only the small venous return from the developing lungs if the atrial septum were intact. The atria cannot be completely separated during fetal life, but the necessary preparations for rapid closure at birth must be made (Fig. 26.11, *D*).

By the middle of the seventh week, after the obliteration of the ostium primum and the appearance of the ostium secundum, a second interatrial septum begins to form as a ridge of the atrial wall to the right of the septum primum. Also crescent shaped, it is oriented toward the opening of the sinus venosus instead of toward the atrioventricular canal. The dorsal limb of this crescent reaches and fuses with the left sinoatrial valve, while the ventral limb reaches the fused endocardial cushions at their junction with the septum primum (Fig. 26.12).

The time of the appearance of the septum secundum seems to be variable. Vernall (39) found no trace of it in four of six hearts of embryos between 14 and 15 mm in length. Odgers (43) found it present in 17.5 and 19-mm embryos.

The septum secundum never becomes complete. Growth slows and stops about the end of the sixth month, leaving an arc-like aperture, the foramen ovale. This aperture, however, does not coincide with the foramen secundum in the septum primum (Fig. 26.11, *F*). Since it is thicker than the septum primum, the foramen ovale forms the seat of the atrial valve (fossa ovalis), while the thinner septum primum forms the flexible flap (valvula).

The passage left through the two septa permits blood to pass from right to left but—because of the flap-valve action of the septum primum—not from left to right. In the normal fetal circulation, the umbilical return maintains a higher pressure in the right atrium. As late as the ninth week, the ostium secundum is still large and the interatrial communication is greater than at term (40). With the development of the lungs, there is a decrease in the amount of systemic blood passing through the communicating foramen.

Functionally, the foramen ovale closes when the left atrial pressure exceeds the right atrial pressure. Until birth, the pulmonary return is too small to raise left atrial pressure high enough to close the valve. With expansion of the lungs and closure of the ductus arteriosus, the valve of the foramen closes functionally. By the sixth postnatal week, functional closure is complete in about 90% of infants, and, by 3 months, closure is complete in nearly all normal infants.

Following functional closure, there is fibroblastic hypertrophy of the valvula of the septum primum and eventual adhesion of the flap with the septum secundum. This stage is termed *anatomic closure*. General agreement exists that adhesion stops short of completion in 17 to 25% of individuals. These individuals have a slit-like tunnel through the atrial septum that persists into adult life. This is not a physiologic handicap. At autopsy, a probe may be passed through this tunnel, but in life little or no blood passes. Gassendi (45) first described such probe patency in 1640, but he did not appreciate its significance as a vestige of the foramen ovale.

EDITORIAL COMMENT

The septum primum forms and descends in a superior to inferior direction and joins with the atrial portion of the endocardial cushions. The superior portion of the septum primum then resorbs, leaving an opening that is eventually closed by downward descent of the septum secundum. Failure of the septum primum to develop results in an ostium primum defect, often with associated mitral valve cleft of the anterior leaflet. Failure of the septum secundum

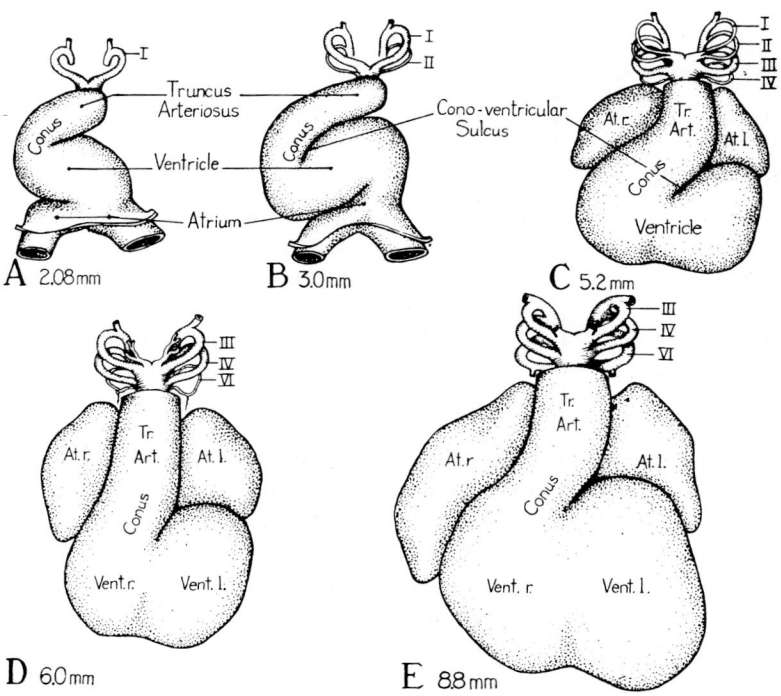

Figure 26.7. Ventral views of the exterior of the developing human heart. Compare with Figure 26.6. (From Kramer TC. The partitioning of the truncus and conus and the formation of the membranous portion of the interventricular septum in the human heart. Am J Anat 1942;71:343–370.)

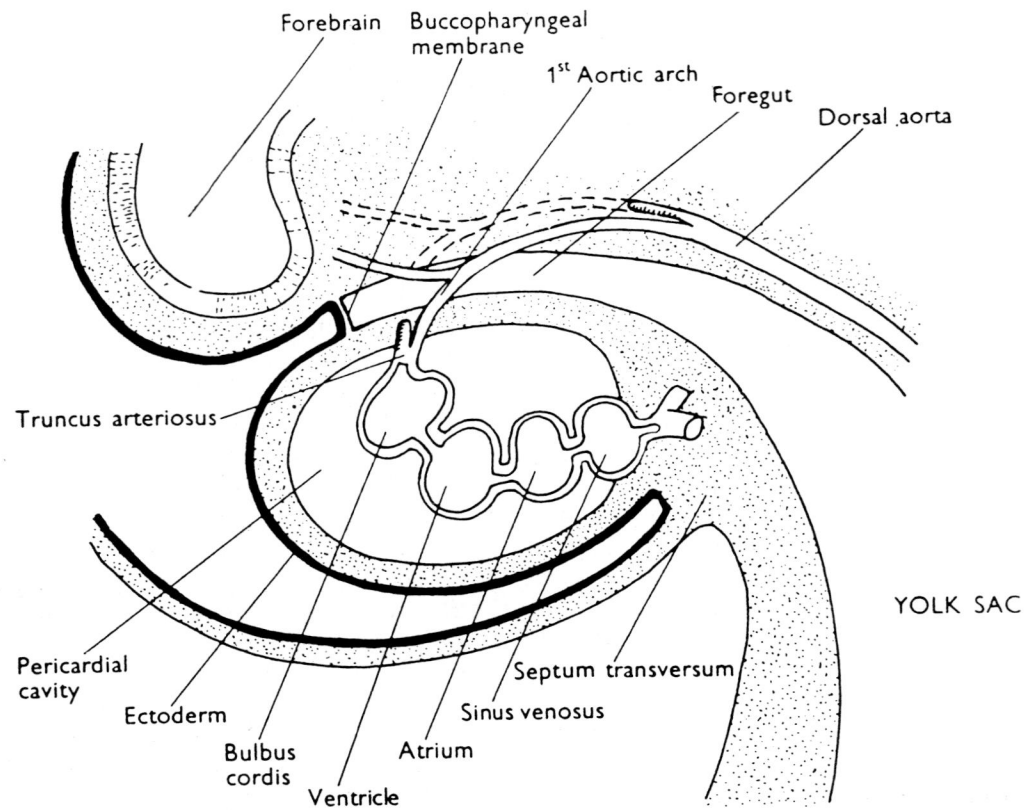

Figure 26.8. The heart tube becomes subdivided into a number of chambers. From its cranial end, a pair of aortic arches pass, one on either side of the foregut, to form the paired dorsal aortae. These fuse more caudally to form a single dorsal aorta. (From Beck F, Moffat DB, Lloyd JB. Human embryology and genetics. Oxford: Blackwell Scientific, 1973.)

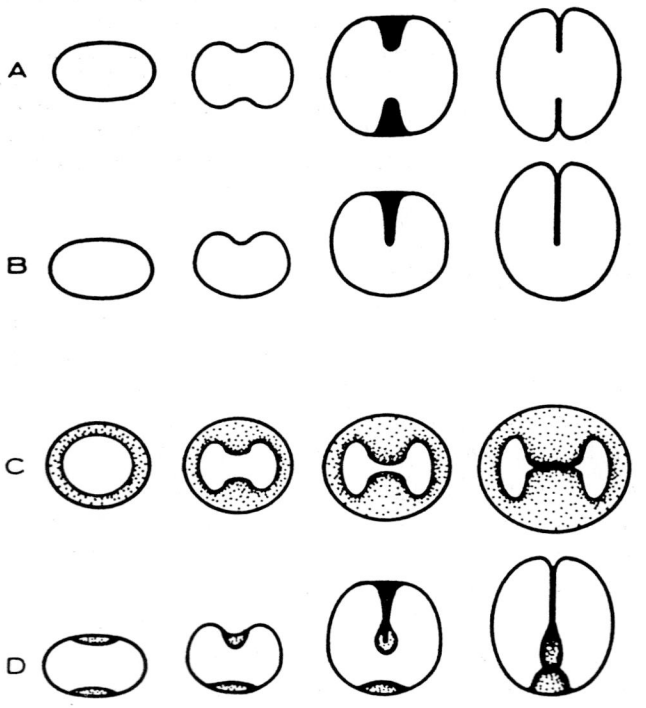

to develop results in an ostium secundum defect. Failure of the septum primum and septum secundum to develop results in a single atrium (CM).

ATRIAL ABSORPTION OF THE SINUS VENOSUS

The primitive sinus venosus receives the anterior cardinal veins from the upper part of the body and the posterior cardinal veins from the posterior part of the body. It opens distally into the future atrial region of the primary heart tube and is, at first, the most symmetric part of the developing heart (Fig. 26.13, *A* to *C*).

In the fifth week, the atrial septal complex begins to form to the left of the opening of the sinus venosus into the primitive atrium so that all blood from the sinus enters the right atrium (Fig. 26.13, *D*).

In the seventh week, the superior and inferior venae cavae replace the cardinal system; these open into the

Figure 26.9. Mechanism of cardiac septation. **A** and **B,** Passively formed septum. **C,** Actively formed septum. **D,** Combination of **B** and **C.** (Van Mierop LHS: Morphological development of the heart. In: Berne RM, ed. Handbook of physiology: the cardiovascular system, vol 1. The Heart. Bethesda, MD: American Physiological Society, 1979:1. Reproduced with permission from the American Physiological Society.)

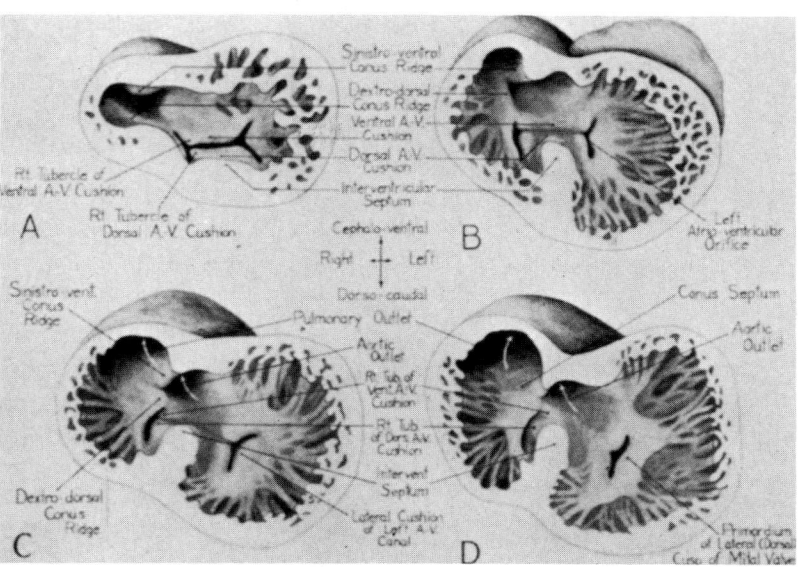

Figure 26.10. Four stages in the partitioning of the atrioventricular canal. The ventricular apex was removed and the heart is viewed from below. Observe the relationship of the two conus ridges to the interventricular septum. **A,** 8.8 mm. **B,** 11 mm. **C,** 13 mm. **D,** 14.5 mm. (From Kramer TC. The partitioning of the truncus and conus and the formation of the membranous portion of the interventricular septum in the human heart. Am J Anat 1942;71:343–370.)

right horn of the sinus venosus. The left horn now receives only the vestigial oblique vein of Marshall, a remnant of the anterior cardinal vein and the coronary venous drainage. It is represented in the adult by a venous enlargement on the posterior surface of the heart, the coronary sinus (Fig. 26.13, *F*).

Although the major somatic venous drainage is to the right horn, its growth does not keep up with that of the atrium. During the sixth and seventh weeks, the right horn of the sinus venosus becomes incorporated in the growing atrial wall (Fig. 26.13, *E*). It receives the superior vena cava cranially and the inferior vena cava caudally; its boundary with the original atrial wall on the right is marked by the sulcus terminalis. Although it is blended into the atrial wall, the sinus venosus tissue retains its phylogenetic and ontogenetic function as the pacemaker of the heart. The sinoatrial node is the controlling tissue of the heart beat in its position at the most proximal portion of the old primary heart tube.

Cor triatriatum dexter is total persistence of the right sinus valve of the embryonic heart which produces in the right atrium a septum partitioning the intercaval part from the atrial body, producing at the same time a very small opening. Savas et al. (46) recently presented such a case which was corrected by percutaneous balloon.

Persistent left superior vena cava is a persistence of the left sinus horn and left anterior cardinal vein (47).

ATRIAL ABSORPTION OF THE PULMONARY VEINS

The pulmonary veins entering the left atrium are increased from a single vein at the 6-mm stage to four veins as the atrium absorbs two orders of branching into its wall. This is discussed with the embryogenesis of the vascular supply to the lungs (Chapter 14), but the following comments by Van Mierop and Kutsche (48) are in order.

1. Overresorption of the septum primum will produce a large ostium secundum with or without septum secundum. If both septa primum and secundum are absent, a persistent atrioventricular canal may be present.
2. Total anomalous pulmonary venous return may develop if the common pulmonary vein is not absorbed into the true left atrium. This may be due to early involution or failure of the common pulmonary vein to develop. A form of partial anomalous return may occur if only some of the pulmonary veins become part of the left atrium.

EDITORIAL COMMENT

Total anomalous pulmonary venous return, by necessity, requires some pulmonary venous connection to the systemic venous circulation and an atrial septal defect. Failure of pulmonary venous absorption into the left atrium results in absorption to (*a*) the left cardinal vein (total anomalous pulmonary venous return, supracardiac); (*b*) the left horn of the sinus venosus or coronary sinus (total anomalous pulmonary venous return, intracardiac); (*c*) the vitelline vein (total anomalous pulmonary venous return, infracardiac); and (*d*) mixed-type with a combination of the preceding. Complete repair requires direct left atrial to common pulmonary vein anastomosis in the supracardiac and infracardiac types and coronary sinus to left atrial baffling in the intracardiac type (CM).

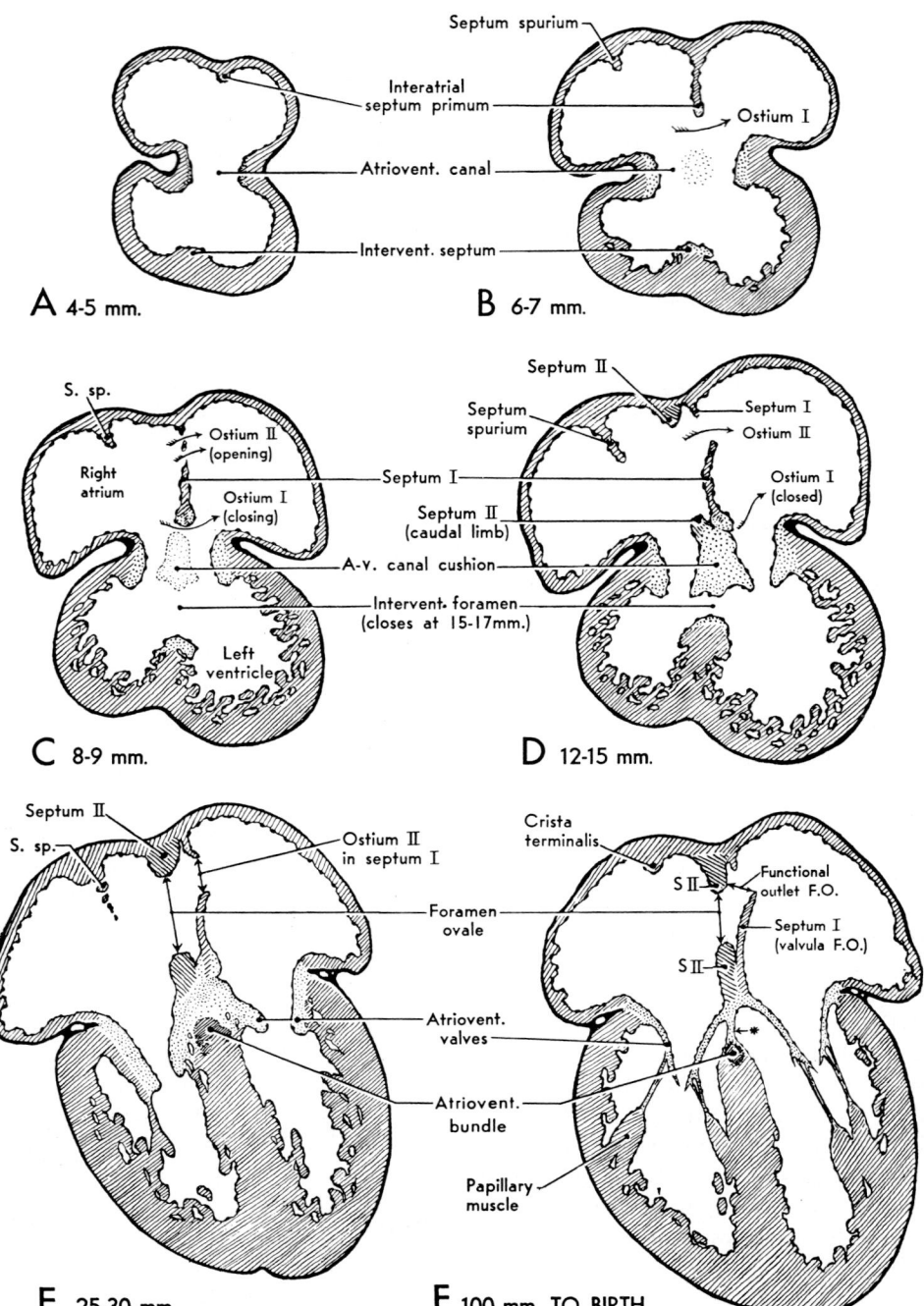

Figure 26.11. Diagrammatic frontal sections through the heart at six different stages, showing the partitioning of the atrioventricular canal, the partitioning of the atria, and the development of the ventricular septum. *Stippled areas* indicate endocardial cushion tissue; *diagonal hatching* indicates myocardium. The *asterisk* in F indicates the membranous portion of the ventricular septum. (From Patten BM. Human embryology, 3rd ed. New York: McGraw-Hill, 1968.)

3. Cor triatriatum sinister results from incomplete absorption of the common pulmonary vein into the true left atrium. This results in a horizontal septum separating the venous inflow portion from the mitral valve and the left atrial appendage. There may be only a narrow ostium between the two chambers.

EDITORIAL COMMENT

The clinical severity of cor triatriatum sinister depends on the size of the opening between the confluence of pulmonary veins and the lower left atrium. This defect has a wide anatomic presentation, ranging from a small opening in the intraatrial membrane to a dia-

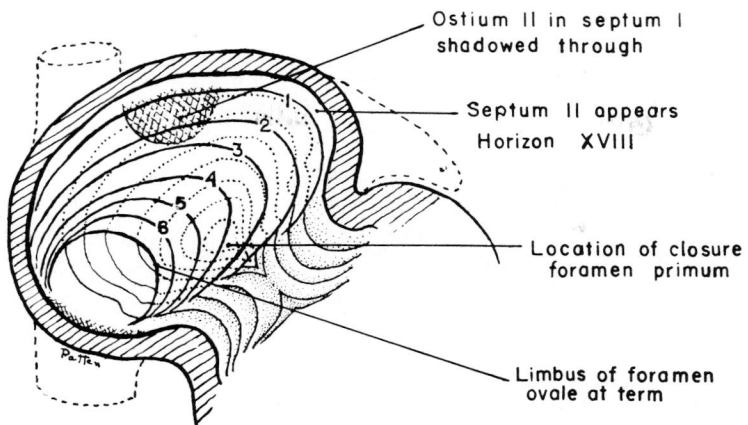

Ostium II in septum I
shadowed through

Septum II appears
Horizon XVIII

Location of closure
foramen primum

Limbus of foramen
ovale at term

Figure 26.12. Diagram of the progress of growth of septum primum *(dotted contour lines)*, septum secundum *(solid contour lines)*, and endocardial cushions *(stippled area)*. The difference in the direction of growth of the two septa is appar- ent. (From Patten BM. Persistent interatrial foramen primum. Amer J Anat 1960;107:271–280.)

phragm upstream to the mitral valve. Prompt diagnosis and timely operation to relieve the obstruction is curative (CM).

THE PARTITION OF THE VENTRICLES

In a strict sense, the right and left ventricles of the embryonic heart arise separately, and the concept of the partitioning of an originally common ventricular chamber is false.

The primary heart tube of Streeter (49) extends from the presumptive atrioventricular opening to the truncus arteriosus. It is continuous, although sharply angulated. The first indication of the future ventricles is the appearance of two rapidly growing "trabeculated" regions (Fig. 26.6). In these regions, the endocardial tube loses its smooth walls and irregular outpouchings appear in the wall. Here, the cardiac jelly between the endocardium and potential myocardium is reduced or becomes cellular (49). Ninety percent of the ventricular mass will arise from these trabeculated areas (35). The two ventricular primordia are at this time in series; the future left is proximal and the future right is distal.

The interventricular portion of the primary heart tube retains its position, while the two trabeculated ventricles descend and approach each other to form the muscular portion of the future interventricular septum (35, 49). The septum is thus formed by fusion of the two primordia, not by invagination or appositional growth. The septum reaches the already fused endocardial cushions by the seventh week (stages 17 and 18) (39). The conduction system becomes established before the septum fuses with the cushions (Fig. 26.14).

The fate of the interventricular canal, the portion of the heart tube connecting the two ventricles, has been interpreted in two ways. The older view is that the mus- cular septum does not close the canal. The canal is finally obliterated, partly by connective tissue from the conus ridges and partly by continuations of the developing spiral truncus ridges and the right margin of the endocardial cushions (Fig. 26.14). This connective tissue becomes the membranous portion of the ventricular septum (50).

In the view put forward by Grant (35, 51), the truncus ridges align with the muscular interventricular septum, and the membranous septum is formed as described above. Grant believes that this represents closure of only part of the interventricular canal. Growth of that part not involved in the left ventricular outflow tract fails to keep up with the growth of the ventricles themselves. By stage 22 it is reduced to a small channel at the upper end of the septum (Fig. 26.15). At its midportion, this canal is never more than 0.5 mm in diameter. Much of the wider left end of the canal is added to the left ventricle as the infundibulum. Grant believes that the contribution of this canal to the left ventricle forms the angulation of the left ventricular outflow tract and explains why the aortic orifice faces the right ventricle and apparently "overrides" the crest of the muscular septum in some types of interventricular septal defects.

EDITORIAL COMMENT

Overriding of the aorta in some ventricular defects, such as those associated with tetralogy of Fallot, is thought to be due to anterior deviation of the infundibular septum, resulting in malalignment with the muscular septum. The anterior migration of the infundibular septum takes the aorta with it, resulting in the overriding aorta that straddles the muscular septum. This anterior migration also presumably causes pulmonary stenosis, which of course is part of the tetralogy of Fallot (CM).

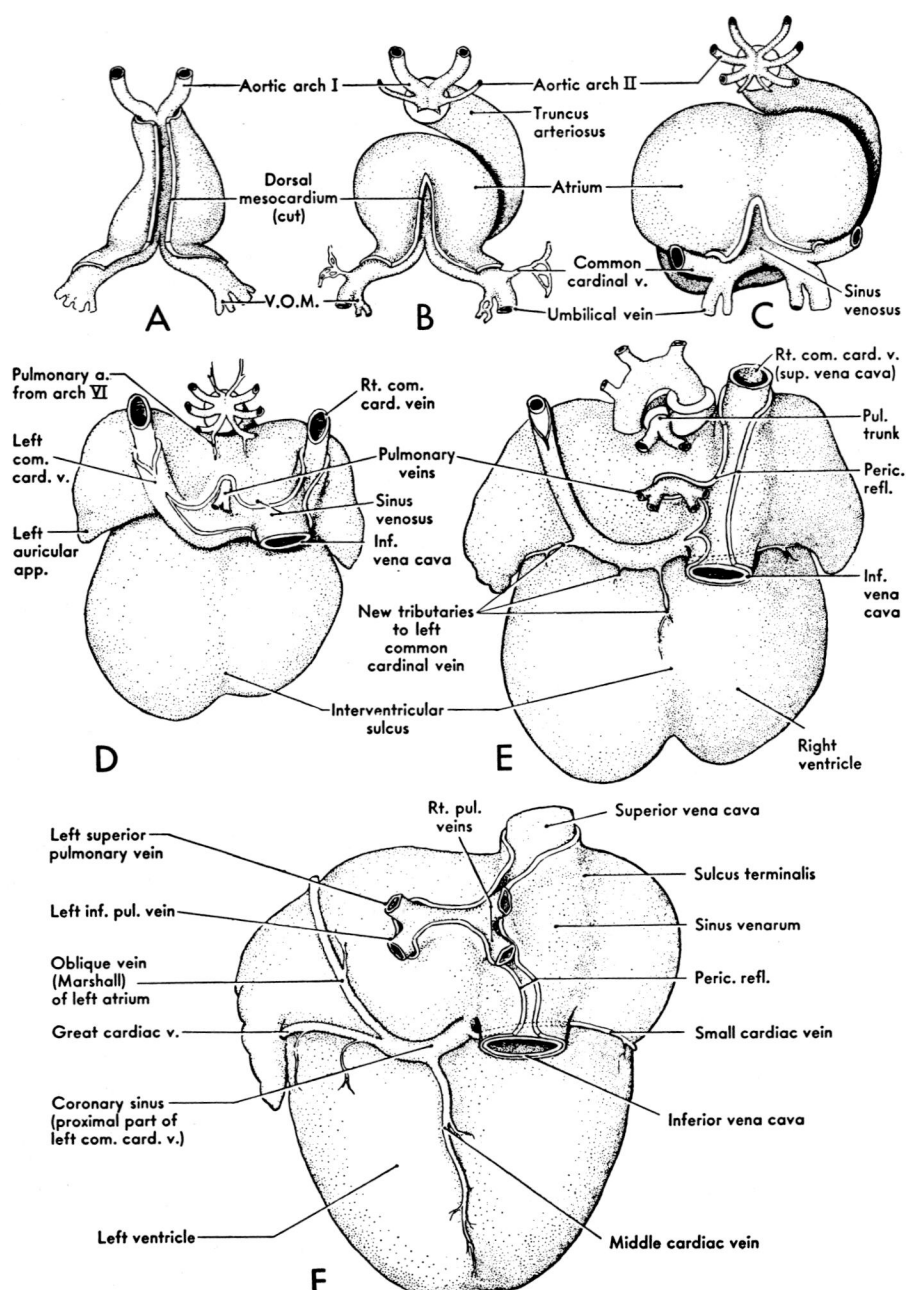

Figure 26.13. Dorsal aspect of the developing heart, showing the fate of the sinus venosus and changes in the venous drainage into the heart. **A,** 8 to 10 somites. **B,** 12 to 14 somites. **C,** 17 to 19 somites. **D,** 6 to 8 mm. **E,** About 25 mm. **F,** About 60 mm. The oblique vein of Marshall in **F** is the remnant of the left common cardinal vein. (From Patten BM. Human embryology, 3rd ed. New York: McGraw-Hill, 1968.)

The membranous septum is not evident in embryos of the seventh week (stage 18) (Fig. 26.11, *D*). It is complete but not histologically mature in embryos of the ninth week (40). Closure appears to be slow and variable.

PARTITION OF THE OUTFLOW TRACT (AORTIC SAC, TRUNCUS ARTERIOSUS, AND CONUS CORDIS)

The bases of the aorta and pulmonary trunk are remnants of the aortic sac. The partition of the aorta and pulmo-

nary sac arises as a ridge in the dorsal part of the aortic sac between the origins of the fourth and sixth aortic arch arteries. This "aorticopulmonary septum" is formed from neural crest cells. Once this partition has formed its lateral margins, it connects with the spiraling truncal ridges which also are populated by neural crest cells that have migrated via the pharyngeal arches into the truncus. These ridges divide the future aortic and pulmonary trunks at the level of the semilunar valves. The truncus arteriosus is compressed almost entirely into the region of the semilunar valves. The truncal ridges are thickenings of the subendocardial tissues (Fig. 26.16). The spiral ridges of the truncus appear to continue as the "conus ridges," which will divide the right and left ventricular outflow tracts. The conal ridges are not populated by neural crest cells but by endocardially-derived mesenchyme, such as in the atrioventricular endocardial cushions. Kramer (50) and DeVries and Saunders (30) have shown that the spiral truncal ridges end at the site of the semilunar valves and that the "conus [bulbar] ridges" are not continuations of them. The right conus ridge becomes the aorticopulmonary ligament, the lowest level of the separation of aortic and pulmonary vessels. From this structure and from the connective tissue of the right tubercle of the dorsal endocardial cushion, the membranous part of the interventricular septum is formed (Fig. 26.10)

Persistent truncus arteriosus occurs if partition of the components of the outflow septum—aortic sac, truncus, and conus—does not take place due to hypoplasia and failure to fuse. The genesis of persistent truncus arteriosus is probably related to neural crest and mesenchymal tissue migration.

EDITORIAL COMMENT

Experimental studies in chick embryos have shown that ablation of the neural crest results in persistent truncus arteriosus. The neural crest also develops into the pharyngeal pouches, then the thymus and parathyroids. This association explains the prevalence of truncus arteriosus with the DiGeorge syndrome (CM).

Aorticopulmonary septal defect (AP window) is due to malalignment and/or failure of fusion between the distal part of the truncal septum and the aorticopulmonary septum. There is a communication between the ascending aorta and the pulmonary trunk (47).

The proper relationship of the aorta and pulmonary artery to the left and right ventricles depends on the correct approximation of the truncal septation and the ventricular septum. If there is incorrect meeting of the two

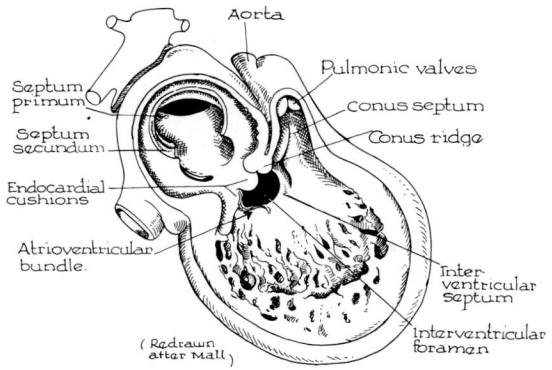

Figure 26.14. The fetal heart before closure of the interventricular foramen, showing the position of the atrioventricular conducting bundle along the postero-inferior margin of the foramen. (From Reemtsma et al. The cardiac conduction system in congenital anomalies of the heart. Surg 1958;44:99–108.)

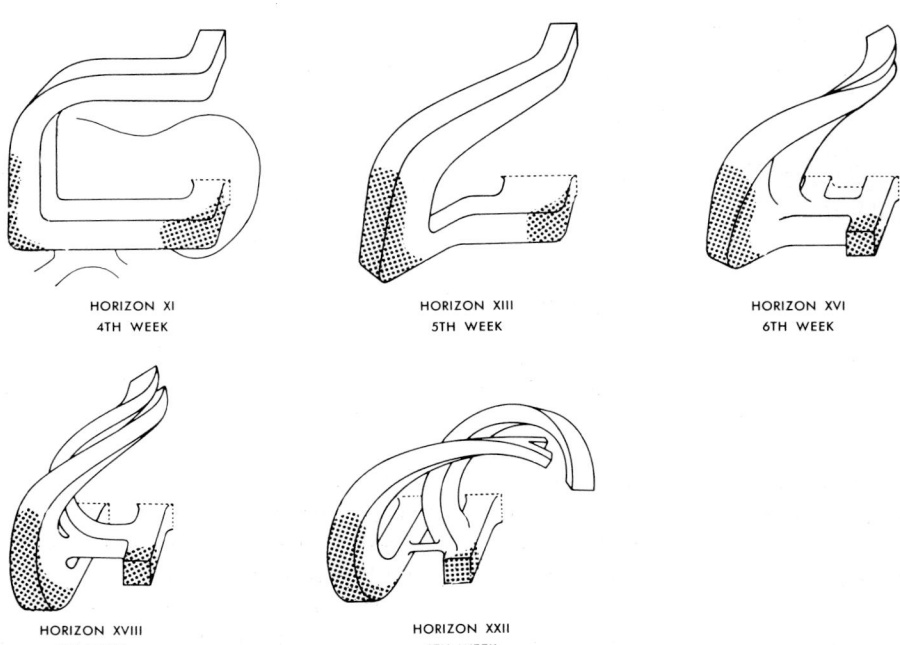

HORIZON XI
4TH WEEK

HORIZON XIII
5TH WEEK

HORIZON XVI
6TH WEEK

HORIZON XVIII
7TH WEEK

HORIZON XXII
8TH WEEK

Figure 26.15. Geometric schemata of the development of the primary heart tube. Only the endothelial surfaces are shown; atria are indicated only in the earliest stage. The trabeculated regions (future right and left ventricles) are *stippled*. The remnant of the interventricular canal is shown in stage 22. (From Grant RP. The embryology of the ventricular flow pathways in man. Circulation 1962;25:756–779.)

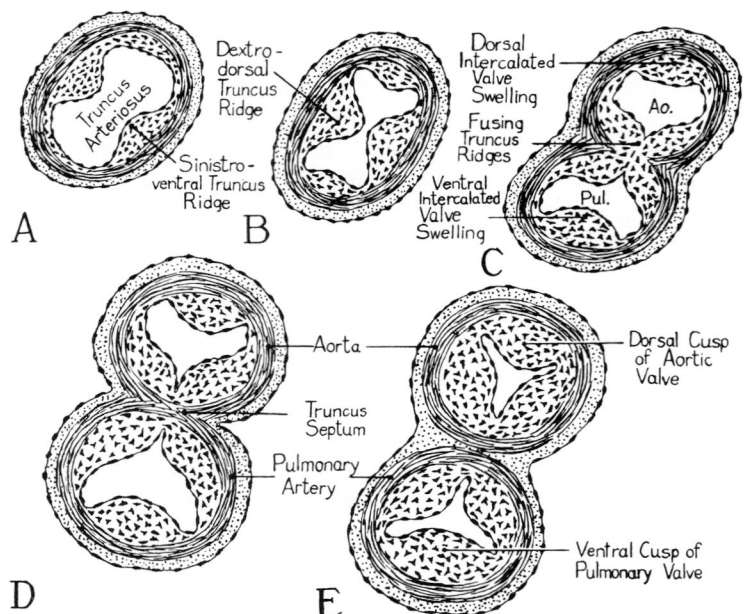

Figure 26.16. Diagrammatic cross-sections through the truncus arteriosus at the level of the primordia of the semilunar valves. Division of the truncus and demarcation of the valve cusps is shown. (From Kramer TC. The partitioning of the truncus and conus and the formation of the membranous portion of the interventricular septum in the human heart. Am J Anat 1942;71:343–370.)

components, various types of transposition of the great vessels will result. A number of writers have analyzed these relationships in geometric terms. Their explanations are beyond the scope of this book and require detailed study; the interested reader should consult Lev and Saphir (52), Spitzer (53), Pernkopf and Wirtinger (54), and de la Cruz and associates (55, 56).

EMBRYOGENESIS OF THE CONDUCTING SYSTEM OF THE HEART

Wenink (57) reported that four rings of specialized myocardia which separate the primitive chambers of the heart are perhaps responsible for the formation of the conducting system:

1. Sinoatrial: Between the atrium and the sinus venosus
2. Atrioventricular: Between inlet and atrium
3. Primary: Between inlet and outlet
4. Arterial: Between truncus arteriosus and outlet

Near the crux of the heart, three of these rings are brought into apposition because of the looping and septation of the heart. When the sinus venosus is incorporated within the right atrium, the sinoatrial node is formed close to the opening of the inferior vena cava. Specifically, the invaginated sinus venosus brings the sinoatrial ring into the base of the atrial septum, where it takes part in the formation of the superficial part of the atrioventricular nodes. The deep portion of the node is formed by the posterior part of the atrioventricular ring.

All these events take place with the help from cells in the left wall of the sinus venosus and from cells originating from the atrioventricular canal, both of which are responsible not only for the atrioventricular node formation, but also for the right and left bundle of His.

EDITORIAL COMMENT

The conduction system that links the atria and ventricles is normally at the atrioventricular node and extends to the bundle of His. During embryonic life, however, many atrioventricular conduction pathways usually resorb. Failure of this process leads to persistent atrioventricular pathways and may result in Wolff-Parkinson-White syndrome and other forms of atrial tachycardias caused by accessory pathways. These pathways can be mapped by electrophysiologic techniques and can be ablated either surgically or by transcatheter radiofrequency techniques (CM).

Critical Events In Cardiac Development

The critical events in cardiac development are numerous, and deviation from the normal pattern at any one time may have several results, some of which appear only in postnatal life.

1. Bending of the heart to the right or to the left occurs in the third week. If the tube bends to the left, inversion of the ventricles will result. This is one component of "corrected" transposition of the great vessels.

2. Septation of the truncus and conus begins in the fifth week. Improper division of these structures accounts for some aortic and pulmonary stenoses, including tetralogy of Fallot.

3. Fusion of the endocardial cushions of the atrioventricular canal occurs in the sixth week. Arrest of this process before fusion is complete leads to septal and valvular anomalies in addition to the basic defect.

4. Formation of the two septa that will partition the atria takes place in the sixth and seventh weeks. This correct formation will, of course, only be tested after birth.

5. During the eighth and ninth weeks, the membranous portion of the ventricular septum forms, completing the partition of the ventricles. Most ventricular septal defects result from developmental arrest of this process.

Clark (58) postulated that four developmental mechanisms are responsible for the genesis of cardiac malformations: mesenchymal tissue migration, cardiac hemodynamics, cellular death, and abnormal extracellular matrix. However, the same author wisely stated that phylogenesis cannot explain the etiology and pathogenesis of human malformations because we do not know how the hearts of our ancestors and the hearts of amphibians and reptiles has changed. Clark also stated that developmental arrest cannot explain the responsible mechanism for human cardiac malformation.

The timing and sequence of events in the development of the human heart have been carefully documented by O'Rahilly (59).

ANOMALIES OF THE HEART

Congenital dysmorphologies of the heart and great vessels are among the most complex, as well as the most thoroughly studied, of human malformations. Although one might expect so complicated a dynamic system to be rendered ineffective by the smallest malfunction, in actuality the cardiovascular system has great powers of compensation. It is intriguing that many heart defects result from an attempt by the early heart loop to compensate for a hemodynamic abnormality at some distant site in the cardiovascular system. For instance, in hearts that will ultimately have persistent truncus arteriosus, the looped heart becomes unlooped as a result of dilation to maintain cardiac output at or above the normal level (60). Many of the most serious defects result not in death but merely in impaired functioning. It is this fact that permits corrective surgery in infancy and sometimes even in maturity. The compensatory responses frequently confused early embryologists; it was not always easy to determine which defects were primary embryonic failure and which were secondary adaptations. In some cases a defect, such as a patent ductus arteriosus or an open foramen ovale, is vitally necessary to preserve the life of an individual who has other cardiovascular abnormalities.

Table 26.1.
Pathogenetic classification of congenital cardiovascular malformations[a]

I. Ectomesenchymal tissue migration abnormalities
 Conotruncal septation defects
  Increased mitral aortic separation (a clinically silent, forme fruste)
  Subarterial, type I ventricular septal defect
  Double outlet right ventricle
  Tetralogy of Fallot
  Pulmonary atresia with ventricular septal defect
  Aorticopulmonary window
  Truncus arteriosus communis
 Abnormal conotrucal cushion position
  Transposition of the great arteries (dextro-)
 Branchial arch defects
  Interrupted aortic arch type B
  Double aortic arch
  Right aortic arch with mirror-image branching
II. Abnormal intracardiac blood flow
 Perimembranous ventricular septal defect
 Left heart defects
  Bicuspid aortic valve
  Aortic valve stenosis
  Coarctation of the aorta
  Interrupted aortic arch type A
  Hypoplastic left heart, aortic atresia:mitral atresia
 Right heart defects
  Bicuspid pulmonary valve
  Secundum atrial septal defect
  Pulmonary valve stenosis
  Pulmonary valve atresia with intact ventricular septum
III. Cell death abnormalities
 Muscular ventricular septal defect
 Ebsteins malformation of the tricuspid valve
IV. Extracellular matrix abnormalities
 Endocardial cushion defects
  Ostium primum atrial septal defect
  Type III, inflow ventricular septal defect
  Atrioventricular canal
  Dysplastic pulmonary or aortic valve

[a]From Clark EB. Growth, morphogenesis and function: the dynamics of cardic vascular development. In Moller JM, Neal WA, Lock JA, eds. Fetal, neonatal ar infant heart disease. New York: Appleton-Century-Crofts, 1989:1–14.

Current research is centered on the cellular an molecular basis of cardiovascular morphogenesis. Thi includes the study of extracellular matrix, cell migratio and interaction, and physiology of the developing hear Additional investigation involves the epidemiology an genetics of various forms of congenital heart disease (61 62). From research perspectives, Clark (63) proposes a innovative pathogenic classification of congenital hear disease (Table 26.1).

Incidence Of Congenital Heart Disease

The incidence of congenital heart disease ranges betwee 5 and 10 per 1000 live births (64). Mitchell and his co leagues (65) found an incidence of 8.14:1000 total birth 7.67:1000 live births and 27.53:1000 stillbirths. Tabl

Table 26.2.
Incidence of Specific Congenital Heart Defects[a]

Defect	Percentage of Cases[b] Averaged
Ventricular septal defect	28.3
Pulmonary stenosis	9.5
Patent ductus arteriosus	8.7
Ventricular septal defect with pulmonary stenosis[c]	6.8
Atrial septal defect, secundum	6.7
Aortic stenosis	4.4
Coarctation of aorta	4.2
Atrioventricular canal[d]	3.5
Transposition of great arteries	3.4
Aortic atresia	2.4
Truncus arteriosus	1.6
Tricuspid atresia	1.2
Total anomalous pulmonary venous connection	1.1
Double outlet right ventricle	0.8
Pulmonary atresia without ventricular septal defect	0.3

[a]From Nugent EW, Plauth WH, Edwards JE, Williams WH. The pathology, abnormal physiology, clinical recognition, and medical and surgical treatment of congenital heart disease. In Hurst JW, Schlant RC, Sononenblick EH, Wenger NK, eds. The heart, 7th ed. New York: McGraw-Hill, 1990.
[b]Total number of cases = 103,590.
[c]Includes tetraology of Fallot.
[d]Includes partial and complete.

26.2 summarizes the current incidence of specific defects as compiled by Nugent and her colleagues (66).

Familial tendencies are evident in some forms of congenital heart disease. The more common defects such as ventricular septal defects recur more frequently than do more complex lesions (67). The risk for affected children is greater when the mother, rather than the father, has congenital heart disease. The recurrence rate is 4 to 18% in children of affected mothers and 1 to 5% in children of affected fathers (67).

In the 1960s, about 40% of children with congenital heart disease died before their fifth birthday (68). Advance in diagnostic techniques, nursing care, and medical and surgical intervention have reduced the mortality from congenital heart disease. For example, in Sweden, Esscher and Michelson (69) found the death rate attributable to congenital heart disease in children in their first year of life to be 1.6:1000. Half of the deaths occurred in the first month of life.

A sizable proportion (7 to 20%) of patients with congenital heart disease have other congenital anomalies (70) (Table 26.3).

For convenience, we discuss in this chapter only anomalies of the heart chambers and their valves. Anomalies of the coronary arteries are considered in Chapter 27 and anomalies of the pericardium in Chapter 25.

The major blood vessels also are treated in specific chapters; the aorta in Chapter 28, the venae cavae in Chapter 29, and the pulmonary vessels, both venous and arterial, in Chapter 14.

The close association of congenital cardiac anomalies and gastrointestinal malformations is summarized beautifully by Rosenthal (71). Tables 26.4 and 26.5 are presented without further comments.

Atrial Septal Defects

DEFINITION

Three defects of the atrial septum are discussed in this section: sinus venosus atrial septal defects, ostium secundum atrial septal defects, and coronary sinus atrial septal defects (Fig. 26.17). Ostium primum atrial septal defect and common atrium are included in the section on complete atrioventricular canal.

EMBRYOLOGY

Embryologically, an ostium secundum defect occurs because the septum primum (valve of the foramen ovale) fails to close the foramen ovale, allowing a left to right shunt (Fig. 26.11). This may be secondary to incomplete development of the septum secundum or excessive resorption of the septum primum (72, 73). In 25 to 30% of adult hearts, the flap of the septum primum does not fuse with the septum secundum although it is functionally closed.

Sinus venosus atrial septal defects (also called subcaval defects) lie outside the region of the fossa ovalis. They are thought to represent abnormal attachment of the right pulmonary veins to either the superior or inferior vena cava. An atrial septal defect occurs when the wall between the pulmonary veins and vena cava is absorbed (72).

A coronary sinus defect occurs at the site of the entrance of the coronary sinus into the left atrium. It is caused by an opening in the wall between the coronary sinus and the left atrium. The opening may be complete (unroofed coronary sinus) or may be represented by fenestrations in the wall between the coronary sinus and the left atrium (74).

CLINICAL ASPECTS

Clinically, ostium secundum atrial septal is one of the most common congenital heart defects (7%) (73). The incidence is twice as common in females as in males. Usually no other defects occur, although an atrial septal defect may be part of a more complex cardiac defect. In the Holt-Oram syndrome, an atrial septal defect is associated with an absent or deformed radius. This is inherited as an autosomal dominant trait although sporadic cases may occur.

Most patients with an atrial septal defect are not detected until after infancy. However, an infant may uncommonly develop heart failure and fail to thrive because of an atrial septal defect (75). A child is sometimes found to have cardiac enlargement on a chest x-ray

Table 26.3.
Syndromes Featuring Congenital Heart Disease[a]

Name of Syndrome	Clinical Features	Cardiac Lesion	Etiological Factors: Chromosomal Abnormalities
Asymmetric crying facies	Asymmetric facies on crying (usually right sided) ? due to agenesis of anguli oris muscle. There may also be other congenital defects	Septal defect or other abnormality	
Bonnevie-Ullrich	More usually applied to Turner's syndrome with special features in the newborn. Prominence of redundant skin over back of neck; migratory edema and lymphangiectasia of hands and feet. Deep-set nails	See Turner's syndrome	See Turner
Cri-du-chat	Physical and mental regardation. Cat-like cry. Microcephaly. Hypertelorism. Epicanthic folds. Downward slant of palpebral fissures. Cleft palate	Variable	Partial deletion of short arm of chromosome 5
De Lange	Physical and mental retardation. Small hands and feet. Bushy eyebrows. Thin lips with midline break in upper and notch in lower	Variable. Ventricular septal defect	Sporadic. ?Mutant gene
DiGeorge 3rd and 4th branchial arch syndrome	Aplasia of thymus gland impairs cellular immunity causing susceptibility to infections. Parathyroid hypoplasia causes hypocalcemia with tetany and convulsions. Physical and mental retardation. Choanal atresia	Septal defects. Truncus arteriosus. Anomalies of great vessels; double aortic arch; interrupted arch	Sporadic. Males/females: 2/1. Failure of 3rd and 4th branchial arch development
Down	Mongoloid facies. Mental retardation. Hypotonia. Short metacarpals and phalanges	Atrioventricular canal. Septal defect. Patent ductus. Tetralogy of Fallot	21 Trisomy (94%). 21 Trisomy/normal mosaicism (2.4%). Translocation (3.3%)
Ebstein	Excessive breathlessness, cyanosis, syncope but many are symptom-free. Death sudden or from congestive heart failure	Displacement of tricuspid valve into right ventricle. Large right atrium. Arrhythmia. Associated congenital heart lesions in one-third	Sporadic
Ehlers-Danlos	Hypermobility of joints, hyperelasticity of skin	Atrial septal defect, atrioventricular septal defect, tetralogy of Fallot	Autosomal dominant
Ellis-van Creveld Chondroectodermal	Growth retardation. Short extremities. Genu valgus. Polydactyly, small thorax, hypoplasia of teeth and nails. Early cardiac or respiratory death in some	Atrial septal defect (50%)	Autosomal recessive
Holt-Oram	Hypoplasia of thumb, radius, clavicles with narrow shoulders. Phocomelia may occur. Scoliosis	Variable. Atrial, ventricular septal defect. Arrhythmia (frequent)	Autosomal dominant
Hurler Gargoylism Mucopolysaccharidosis	Characteristic facies with hypertelorism, protruding tongue. Physical and mental retardation later in first year. Kyphosis. Corneal opacities. Hepatosplenomegaly	Infiltration of coronary arteries (narrowing) and valves (mitral incompetence) causes heart failure	Autosomal recessive
Infantile hypercalcaemia (see Williams syndrome)	Mental and physical retardation. Characteristic facies: epicanthic folds, hypertelorism, snub nose, carp mouth. Vomiting. Diarrhea, hypercalcemia inconstant (role uncertain)	Supravalvar aortic stenosis. Pulmonary artery branch stenoses. Coarctation of aorta. Systemic hypertension	Sporadic. Dietetic ?excess maternal vitamin D intake
Ivemark	A syndrome associated with isomerism	Anomalies of venous drainage. Endocardial cushion defects. Conotruncal abnormalities	Sporadic
Kartagener	Situs inversus. Absent frontal sinus in some. Bronchiectasis. Upper and lower airway infections frequent: pansinusitis, otitis, pneumonia	Anomalies of venous return, endocardial cushions, septation, and great vessels. Dextrocardia	Autosomal recessive
Laurence-Moon-Biedl-Bardet	Mental retardation, obesity, hypogenitalism, retinitis pigmentosa	Tetralogy of Fallot	?
Leopard, multiple lentigines	Multiple dark spots on skin present at birth. Physical and mental retardation (mild). Hypogonadism	Pulmonary stenosis. Prolonged P-R interval and QRS complex. Aortic stenosis	Autosomal dominant

Table 26.3. *continued*

Name of Syndrome	Clinical Features	Cardiac Lesion	Etiological Factors: Chromosomal Abnormalities
18 Long arm deletion	Mental and physical retardation. Narrow or atretic auditory canal. Cleft palate. Long hands; tapering fingers. Undescended testicles	Variable	Long arm deletion of chromosome 18
Marfan	Connective tissue defect resulting in tall stature, thin limbs, hypotonia, scoliosis, narrow palate, lens subluxation and lung malformation	Dilation or aneurysm of aorta or pulmonary artery. Aortic valve and mitral valve incompetence (50%)	Autosomal dominant
Noonan, Male Turner's	Physical and some mental retardation. Characteristic facies with epicanthic folds; ptosis of eyelids; low-set ears. Webbed neck. Cubitus valgus. Pectus excavatum. Small penis. Undescended testicles. Occurs in male and female	Pulmonary stenosis. Septal defect. Left ventricular obstruction or nonobstructive myopathy	Sporadic. No chromosomal abnormality
Osteogenesis imperfecta	Fragile bones, blue sclera	Weakness of the media of arteries, aneurisms, valvular incompetence	Autosomal dominant
Pseudo-Hurler, Polydystrophy, Mucolipidosis III	Physical and mental retardation. Similar to Hurler syndrome but milder	Aortic stenosis and incompetence	Autosomal recessive
Radial aplasia thrombocytopenia	Absent or hypoplastic radius and sometimes other limb defects. Thrombocytopenia. Eosinophilia	Variable; 25%	Autosomal recessive
Rubella	Mental and physical retardation. Deafness, cataract, anemia, thrombocytopenia. Hepatosplenomegaly. Obstructive jaundice. Osteolytic trabeculation in metaphyses with subperiosteal rarefaction. Interstitial pneumonia	Patent ductus. Pulmonary artery branch stenoses. Septal defect. Carditis. Lesions may cause heart failure	Rubella virus transmitted from mother. May persist in excretions of infant for months
13 Trisomy	Gross mental retardation. Microcephaly. Cleft lip and palate. Widespread skeletal abnormality. Single umbilical artery. Early death	Ventricular and atrial septal defects. Patent ductus. Other gross defects 80%	Trisomy for large part of D group (13 to 15) chromosome
18 Trisomy	Mental and physical retardation. Small mouth and palpebral fissures. Short sternum. Limb abnormalities. Hirsutism. Single umbilical artery. Early death	Ventricular and atrial septal defects. Patent ductus and other lesions	Extra 18 chromosome
Turner Gonadal dysgenesis	Female with short stature. Ovarian dysgenesis. Lymphedema of hands and feet. Prominent ears. Web neck. Broad chest. Widely spaced nipples. Cubitus valgus. Horseshoe kidney. Buccal smear shows no female sex chromatin (Barr bodies)	Cardiac defect in over 20% and of these 70% have coarctation of the aorta	Sporadic. Chromosome pattern 45,XO (or mosaics XX/XO,XY/XO or part of X missing)
VATER	*VATER* describes the main anomalies: Vertebral anomalies; vascular anomalies including ventricular septal defect and single umbilical artery; anal atresia; tracheoesophageal fistula and atresia; radial dysplasia; polydactyly; syndactyly; renal anomaly; single umbilical artery. Physical and mental retardation (but not in all)	Ventricular septal defect and other lesions	Sporadic
Williams (see Infantile hypercalcemia syndrome)	Physical and mental retardation. Coarse hair. Hypoplastic nails. Hypercalcemia occasionally found	Supravalvar aortic stenosis. Peripheral pulmonary artery stenosis. Pulmonary valve stenosis. Ventricular septal defect	Sporadic
Wolff-Parkinson-White	Paroxysmal tachycardia which may cause heart failure, ECG: short P-R interval and slurred upstroke of QRS may be found between attacks	Usually heart otherwise normal	Accessory atrioventricular node and conducting bundle of Kent. Sporadic

[a]From Arnold R. Heart disease in the neonate. In: Lister J, Irving IM, eds. Neonatal surgery, 3rd ed. London: Butterworths, 1990.

Table 26.4.
Distribution of Selected Gastrointestinal Abnormalities in Infants with Congenital Heart Disease Enrolled in the New England Regional Infant Cardiac Program (8/23/83)[a]

	No.	Percent
Imperforate anus	38	13.5
Esophageal atresia/tracheoesophageal fistula	34	12.1
Diaphragmatic hernia	27	9.6
Omphalocele	21	7.5
Duodenal atresia	19	6.8
Intestinal obstruction/malrotation	15	5.3
Pyloric stenosis	15	5.3
Others	112	39.9
TOTAL	281	100.0

From Rosenthal A. Congenital cardiac anomalies and gastrointestinal malformations. In: Pierpont ME, Moller JH, eds. Genetics of cardiovascular disease. Boston: Martinus Nijhoff, 1986.

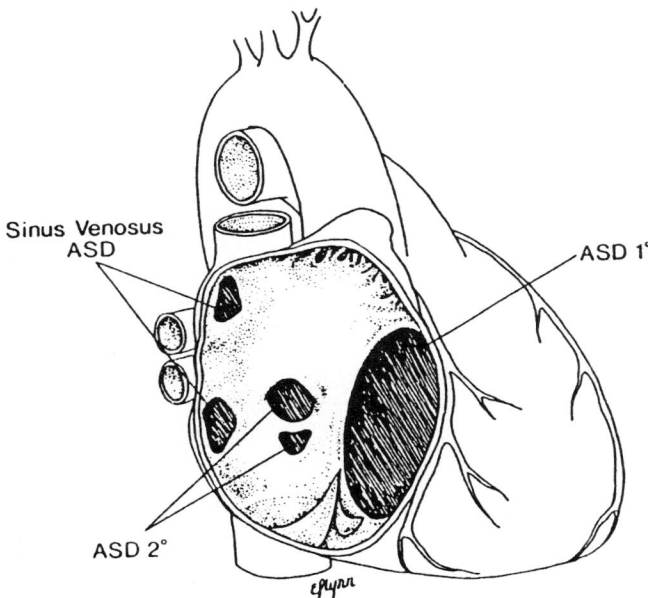

Figure 26.17. Diagram of the atrial septum showing several types of atrial septal defects. An ostium primum defect *(ASD 1°)* is located immediately adjacent to the mitral and tricuspid valves. Ostium secundum defects *(ASD 2°)* are located near the fossa ovalis in the center of the septum. Sinus venosus defects are located in the area derived from the embryologic sinus venosus. (From Fyler DC, ed. Nadas' pediatric cardiology. Philadelphia: Hanley & Belfus, 1992.)

examination done for frequent pulmonary infections, and an atrial septal defect is subsequently found.

On physical examination prominence of the left precordium may be secondary to cardiac enlargement. The first heart sound may be split or accentuated (72, 73). The second heart sound is widely split. If a significant left-to-right shunt is present, an S3 will be heard at the left lower sternal border. A systolic murmur is heard at the upper left sternal border. This is caused by the increased pulmonary blood flow secondary to the left-to-right shunt at the atrial level. With a significant shunt, a diastolic rumble secondary to increased tricuspid valve flow may be heard at the lower left sternal border. Tachycardia, intercostal retractions, flaring of the nares, and hepatomegaly may be seen if there is congestive heart failure. Pulmonary vascular obstructive disease is uncommon in childhood and adolescence although it may occur in later life (76). In older patients the condition may not be discovered until atrial arrhythmias bring them to medical attention. Years of left-to-right shunting at the atrial level causes atrial enlargement, which is thought to predispose these patients to atrial flutter and fibrillation.

DIAGNOSIS

Diagnosis is made by clinical and chest x-ray examinations and electrocardiograms (ECGs). An rSr' is often seen in lead V_1. In children, two-dimensional echocardiography clearly displays the atrial septum and demonstrates the defect (77). In older patients, cardiac catheterization may be necessary if there is doubt about the diagnosis. In these patients the subcostal echo window is usually not available because of patient size.

EDITORIAL COMMENT

Most large atrial septal defects can be diagnosed by physical examination and confirmed by transthoracic or transesophageal echocardiography without cardiac catheterization. The shunt is mostly left-to-right but often can be bidirectional and result in "paradoxic" emboli, which are emboli from the venous system that travase the atrial septal defect and cause systemic arterial obstructions (CM).

TREATMENT

Small defects are well tolerated and do not require surgery. Some atrial septal defects close or get smaller. Larger defects that persist require surgery (77). The long-term outlook for such patients is excellent although the best results occur in patients operated on by age 25 years (78). Some patients, particularly adult women, develop pulmonary vascular obstructive disease. Recommendations have been made regarding the feasibility of surgical repair in such patients (76).

Ventricular Septal Defects

DEFINITION

A ventricular septal defect is an opening in the ventricular septum which permits communication between the two ventricles.

ANATOMY

Several classifications for ventricular septal defects exist. One well-established classification is divided into four cat-

Table 26.5.
Distribution of Major Gastrointestinal Malformations in Infants with Cardiac Abnormality Registered in the New England Regional Infant Cardiac Program (8/28/83)[a]

Cardiac Diagnoses	No. with Gastrointestinal Malformation										
	Diaphragmatic Hernia	Hirschsprung's Disease	Esophageal Atresia/TEF	Omphalocele	Imperforate Anus	Duodenal Stenosis/Atresia	Pyloric Stenosis	Annular Pancreas	Biliary Atresia	Other GI Malformations[b]	TOTAL
Ventricular septal defect	3	0	9	3	9	6	5	2	1	10 + (3)	51
D-transposition	0	0	0	1	2	0	0	0	1	5 + (4)	13
Tetralogy of Fallot	5	3	6	7	7	0	0	1	0	5 + (4)	38
Patent ductus arteriosus	1	1	1	1	2	3	2	1	0	5 + (2)	19
Hypoplastic left heart	1	0	2	0	0	1	0	1	0	2	7
Coarctation	1	0	5	0	1	0	0	0	0	7 + (3)	17
Endocardial cushion defect	0	3	1	0	3	5	0	1	0	7 + (1)	21
Malposition	4	0	3	4	3	2	2	1	2	3 + (2)	26
Pulmonary stenosis	2	0	1	0	0	0	2	0	0	(3)	8
Single ventricle	0	0	1	0	1	1	0	0	0	0	3
Pulmonary atresia (IVS)	0	0	1	0	0	0	0	0	0	1	2
Anomalous pulmonary venous return	0	0	0	0	1	0	0	0	0	2	3
Aortic stenosis	0	1	0	0	1	0	0	0	0	0	2
Truncus arteriosus	0	0	3	0	2	0	0	0	0	3	8
Atrial septal defect (II)	1	0	0	1	1	0	0	0	0	7 + (1)	11
Myocarditis	0	0	0	0	0	0	0	0	0	1	1
Tricuspid atresia	0	0	1	0	0	0	0	0	0	7	8
DORV	0	0	0	0	1	0	1	0	0	2	4
L-transposition	0	0	0	0	0	0	0	0	0	0	0
Lung disease	7	0	2	1	0	0	1	0	0	4 + (3)	18
Miscellaneous	2	1	2	3	4	1	2	0	0	5 + (1)	21
TOTAL	27	9	38[c]	21	38	19	15	7	4	103	281[d]

[a]From Rosenthal A. Congenital cardiac anomalies and gastrointestinal malformations. In: Pierpont ME, Moller JH, eds. Genetics of cardiovascular disease. Boston: Martinus Nijhoff, 1986.

[b]Gastrointestinal anomalies here include cleft lip and palate ($N = 25$), gastrointestinal reflux ($N = 31$), intestinal obstruction or malrotation ($N = 15$), Meckels diverticulum ($N = 8$), and others ($N = 24$). No. in brackets in this column are infants with insufficient data on the gastrointestinal anomaly.

[c]Includes three infants with associated omphalocele and one with omphalocele and malrotation.

[d]Includes 34 infants with chromosomal anomaly.

egories. Type I represents the supracristal defect, which also is called a subpulmonic defect. This ventricular septal defect is positioned beneath the pulmonic valve and is associated with a high incidence of aortic insufficiency. The most common membranous defect is called type II. Type III defects occur beneath the septal leaflet of the tricuspid valve and are associated with left axis deviation. They also are called ventricular septal defects of the atrioventricular canal type. Type IV defects are found entirely in the muscular septum.

EDITORIAL COMMENT

Another rare type of ventricular septal defect is the left ventricular-to-right atrial defect (Gerbode type of VSD) that occurs when the membranous portion of the VSD is absent. The tricuspid valve annulus is slightly lower than the mitral valve annulus, leaving a small potential opening from the left ventricle to the right atrium (CM).

With the advent of high-resolution two-dimensional echo imaging and color Doppler interrogation of the ventricular septum, an alternate classification came into common usage (79, 80). Since membranous defects are surrounded partially by muscular tissue, they are subdivided into three types: perimembranous inlet, perimembranous trabecular, and perimembranous outlet. Perimembranous inlet defects lie posterior to the septal leaflet of the tricuspid valve. They are called defects of the atrioventricular canal type in the other classification. Muscular defects also are classed into three types: inlet, trabecular, and infundibular. Defects in the outlet septum may occur beneath the pulmonic valve "subpulmonic" and also beneath the aortic valve. Aortic insufficiency may occur with these defects because of prolapse of a coronary cusp into the defect (Fig. 26.18).

EMBRYOLOGY

The embryology of the ventricular septum is succinctly summarized by Gumbiner and Takeo (79) and is reproduced here.

> The embryologic formation of the normal ventricular septum has been described in a number of elegant studies [81–84]. After cardiac looping at 23 to 25 days' gestation, the primitive left ventricle, formed from the ventricular portion, and the primitive right ventricle, formed from the proximal portion of the bulbus cordia, are connected by the primary interventricular foramen. Growth and trabeculation of the ventricles accounts for formation of the major portion of the muscular septum as the medial walls of the ventricles become apposed and fuse together [83, 84]. While the ventricles enlarge, the atrioventricular canal moves rightward, such that the atria communicate with the primitive right ventricle. As this happens, the plane of the primary interventricular foramen shift leftward, and, as the interventricular foramen II, it gives access from the left ventricle to the posteromedial portion of the conus cordis. The conus swellings appear at approximately the same time as the truncal swellings and the atrioventricular cushions. They ultimately merge to form the conus septum, separating the conus cordis into the anterolateral and posteromedial portions. . . . The conus septum also separates the interventricular foramen (now foramen III) from the AV canal. Completion of the interventricular septum is accomplished by fusion of the endocardial cushion tissue from the conus septum, with the superior portion of the muscular septum and a portion of the right superior endocardial cushion [80, 81]. With this fusion, the interventricular foramen III is closed. Later, this portion of the septum thins to become the membranous interventricular septum. . . . The formation of the membranous and peri-

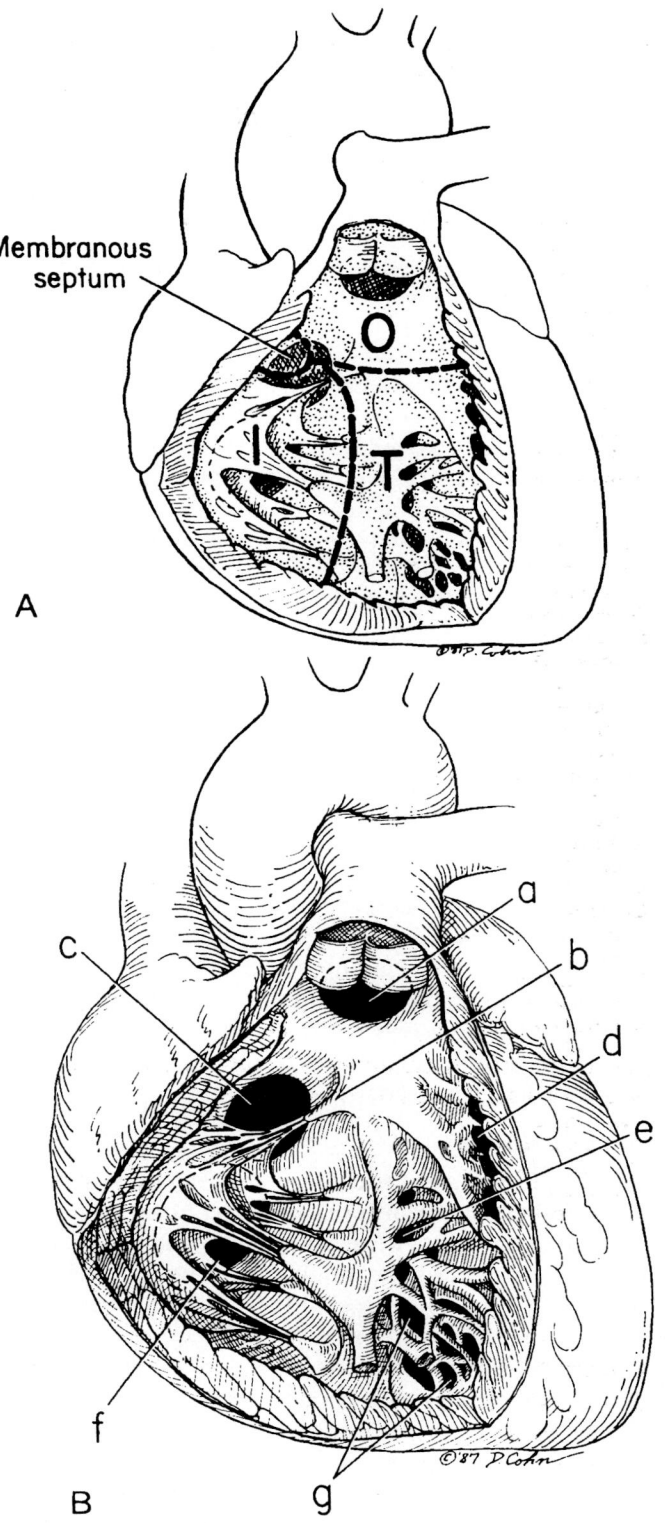

Figure 26.18. **A,** Ventricular septum viewed from right ventricular side is made up of four components: *I,* inlet component extends from tricuspid annulus to attachments of tricuspid valve; *T,* trabecular septum extends from inlet out to apex and up to smooth-walled outlet; *O,* outlet septum or infundibular septum, which extends up to pulmonary valve, and membranous septum. **B,** Anatomic position of defects. *a,* Outlet defect; *b,* papillary muscle of the conus; *c,* perimembranous defect; *d,* marginal muscular defects; *e,* central muscular defects; *f,* inlet defect; *g,* apical muscular defects. (From Graham TP, Bender HW, Spach MS. Ventricular septal defects. In: Adams FH, Emmanouilides GC, Riemenschneider TA, eds. Moss' Heart diseases in infants, children, and adolescents, 4th ed. Baltimore: Williams & Wilkins, 1989.)

membranous septum is a late and multifaceted developmental event and is subject to numerous aberrations that may manifest later as perimembranous ventricular septal defect [85]. Defects of the outlet septum are felt to represent failure of fusion of portions of the conus septum [82]. Inlet defects may represent failure or complete fusion of the right superior endocardial tissue with the muscular septum. Muscular defects, particularly in the trabecular septum, are probably due to excessive excavation of the septum during the growth of the ventricle, or inadequate merger of the medial walls of the ventricles.

INCIDENCE

In the majority of published series, ventricular septal defect ranks as the most common congenital cardiac malformation if bicuspid aortic valve is excluded. Ventricular septal defects were present in 62 of Abbott's 1000 autopsied cases of congenital heart disease (85). Hoffman and Rudolph (86) estimated the incidence at 0.95:1000 live births at term and at 4.51:1000 live premature births, a total of about 2:1000 live births. Approximately 20% of patients seen in large pediatric cardiology clinics are said to have an isolated ventricular septal defect (79, 87).

SYMPTOMS

A small defect is not associated with symptoms and is compatible with a normal life unless endocarditis occurs. These defects frequently close spontaneously. Moderate-sized defects are usually well tolerated but frequently cause congestive heart failure in infancy. Surgical closure may be required to allow the child to thrive. When a large defect is present, congestive heart failure usually occurs during infancy. These infants are short of breath, develop respiratory infections, and demonstrate poor growth and development. Excessive sweating due to increased sympathetic tone and fatigue with feeding are common. Surgery is usually required.

DIAGNOSIS

The diagnosis of a ventricular septal defect is usually easily made by the appearance of a harsh holosystolic murmur along the mid-left sternal border. The murmur may not be heard until the pulmonary vascular resistance starts to fall in the first weeks of life. Heart failure occurs with a large defect or a moderate defect with high pulmonary blood flow. Cyanosis does not appear unless there is associated pulmonic stenosis or the development of pulmonary vascular obstructive disease. Cyanosis also may be present when a ventricular septal defect is part of a complex cyanotic congenital heart defect. The chest x-ray film may demonstrate increased pulmonary vascularity when the shunt is large. In patients with small defects the x-ray film findings often are normal. An electrocardiogram is less helpful in a small infant but may show signs of left and right ventricular hypertrophy later in the

course. The diagnosis is usually established clinically, and a semiquantitative analysis of the size of the shunt determined by color-flow Doppler (80). Cardiac catheterization is obtained to determine the shunt size, to measure pulmonary pressure, and to calculate pulmonary vascular resistance. This information is helpful in determining the timing of surgery.

PROGNOSIS

Up to 50% of small ventricular septal defects will close in the first year of life and a few more will close later (88). Large- or moderate-sized defects often become smaller and also may close.

The infant in the first year of life with congestive heart failure will require surgery (89). If surgery is not done at the appropriate time the infant may seem to be doing better as pulmonary hypertension becomes fixed and left to right shunting decreases. As the pulmonary vascular resistance rises, right to left shunting appears and the patient becomes cyanotic. When the pulmonary hypertension is so elevated, as measured in the catherization laboratory, the patient is said to have Eisenmenger's syndrome. Surgery cannot be safely performed on such patients, due to the increased perioperative mortality.

All patients with a ventricular septal defect are at risk for bacterial endocarditis. Patients with a subpulmonic ventricular septal defect may develop aortic insufficiency secondary to prolapse of an aortic leaflet into the defect. This also is seen in patients with a membranous ventricular septal defect.

TREATMENT

Antibiotic prophylaxis for dental and other procedures is the only treatment indicated for a small ventricular septal defect. Surgical closure of the ventricular septal defect is indicated for a large defect associated with symptoms of heart failure or when a moderate-sized defect persists with a shunt exceeding 2:1. Repair of isolated perimembranous ventricular septal defects is accomplished with low mortality (90). Good results also are seen in the repair of other ventricular septal defects (91, 92).

EDITORIAL COMMENT

The indications for surgical closure of VSDs have been liberalized as the result of significantly improved results. Type I (supracristal, subarterial, conal) defects should be closed without regard to the left-to-right shunt because of the almost certain development of aortic valve prolapse and insufficiency in these patients. Surgical closure halts this development. Bacterial endocarditis must also be considered to be a significant problem in patients with small VSDs. Many centers currently close VSDs with left-to-right shunts of 1.5:1 or greater (CM).

Atrioventricular Canal and Related Endocardial Cushion Defects

DEFINITION

Endocardial cushion defects include hearts with a deficiency in the lower part of the atrial septum (an ostium primum atrial septal defect) occurring alone or with a ventricular septal defect. There is always a "scooped out" portion of the ventricular septum, reflecting the deficiency of the atrioventricular septum. This is true whether or not there is a ventricular septal defect. Variable deformities of the mitral and tricuspid valves occur. There is a disproportionate relationship between the inlet and outlet dimensions of the heart in comparison to a normal heart (Fig. 26.19). The aortic valve is superior to its normal position, causing a narrowing of the left ventricular outflow tract.

CLASSIFICATION OF DEFECTS

Defects are classified as complete or partial. An ostium primum atrial septal defect is classified as a partial endocardial cushion defect. A deficiency exists in the lowermost portion of the atrial septum. A cleft in the anterior leaflet of the mitral valve is commonly found. A ventricular septal defect is not present; however, there is a deficiency in the atrioventricular septum, giving a scooped-out or concave appearance angiographically (93, 94).

Common atrium also is classified as a partial form of an endocardial cushion defect. Most of the septum is absent. This deformity frequently is associated with complex forms of congenital heart disease (93).

Complete endocardial cushion defects (also called atrioventricular canal defects) are classified in a graded

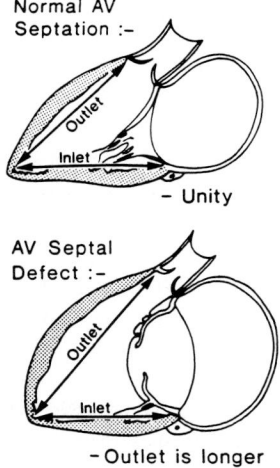

Normal AV
Septation :-

Outlet

Inlet

– Unity

AV Septal
Defect :-

Outlet

Inlet

– Outlet is longer

Figure 26.19. This diagram illustrates the morphology of normal atrioventricular septation and atrioventricular septal defect. (From Anderson RH, Ho SY. The developmental anatomy of atrioventricular septal defects. In: Clark EB, Takao A, eds. Developmental morphogenesis and function . New York: Mount Kisco, 1990.)

series from mild to severe (93). An ostium primum atrial septal defect is present. There is a ventricular septal defect of varying size. A common atrioventricular valve is present. It usually has five leaflets and commissures. There are two major bridging leaflets. The posterior leaflet may be attached by chordae to the crest of the ventricular septum and may obliterate the interventricular communication. The attachments of the anterior leaflet to the ventricular septum and papillary muscles are variable. Several classifications have been proposed (95, 96). A widely used classification is that of Rastelli and colleagues (97) (amplified by Piccoll et al. [98, 99]) who described types A, B, and C—differentiating them by the variations in the anterior bridging leaflet. In type A, most commonly seen in Down syndrome, the anterior leaflet is committed predominantly to the left ventricle. There may be chordal attachments to the ventricular septum. In type B, the anterior bridging leaflet is larger and attaches to papillary muscles in the right ventricle. There is no chordal attachment to the interventricular septum, and free interventricular communication may occur. In type C, there is a freely movable overhanging large anterior bridging leaflet that has no attachment to the ventricular septum or to a papillary muscle. An intermediate form of an atrioventricular canal is said to occur when fibrous tissue connected to the crest of the ventricular septum joins the two bridging leaflets, forming two separate valves (100). Not all agree with this terminology, believing that these forms also should be classed as partial defects (94).

EMBRYOLOGY

The single communication between the atrial and ventricular regions of the embryonic heart is divided into left and right atrioventricular canals by swellings of the endocardium, which arise from the dorsal and ventral walls of the primitive passage. These swellings, the endocardial cushions, fuse to partition the canal and provide anchorage for the atrial and ventricular septa. Their contribution to formation of the valves themselves remains controversial (101). Currently, they are though to provide the "glue" needed for delineation of the valves (Fig. 26.20). Partial endocardial cushion defects encompass abnormalities of the lower atrial septum without an accompanying ventricular septal defect. Complete endocardial cushion defects also have a ventricular septal defect.

The embryology of endocardial cushion defects remains controversial. It has been thought that the primary deformity results from failure of the endocardial cushions to form the septum and atrioventricular valves (93). Others (94, 102) believe that the primary deficiency is in the atrioventricular septum, causing the uniformly seen "scooped out" ventricular septum. The failure of

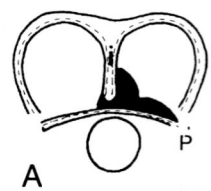

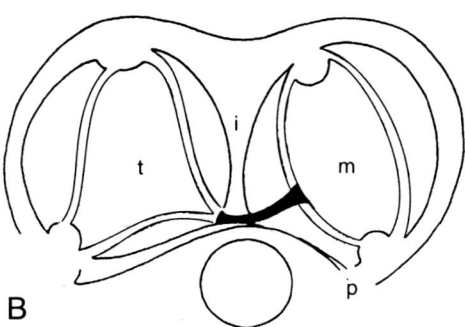

Figure 26.20. Diagrammatic view of the cardiac base. **A,** Before valve formation. **B,** After valve formation. The aortic leaflet of the mitral valve *(m)* derives from inlet septum *(i)* as well as primary fold *(p)*. The cushion mass (in *black*) keeps the two together. In the right ventricle, at the site of the cushion mass, a commissure is formed between the septal and anterosuperior leaflets of the tricuspid valve *(t)*. Note that the relative size of the cushion mass diminishes with the growth of the heart. (From Wenink ACG, Gittenberger-de Groot AC. Embryology of the mitral valve. Int J Cardiol 1986;11:75–84.)

the cushions to fuse is thought to be secondary to the deficiency of the atrioventricular septum.

INCIDENCE

Complete atrioventricular canal occurs infrequently, but over 50% of the patients have Down syndrome. There is an equal gender distribution. Ostium primum atrial septal defects do not occur more frequently in patients with Down syndrome (93, 103).

SYMPTOMS

Children with an endocardial cushion defect develop symptoms within the first year of life (93, 104, 105). Symptoms are rare, however, in the first month of life before the pulmonary vascular resistance has fallen. The manifestations include recurrent respiratory infections, congestive heart failure, and failure to thrive. Cyanosis does not appear until later when pulmonary hypertension has developed.

DIAGNOSIS

Children with this condition are small with poor development. The features of Down syndrome are present in over 50% of patients. Auscultatory findings include a murmur of mitral insufficiency at the apex, a murmur

from a ventricular septal defect at the lower left sternal border, a diastolic flow rumble, and a widely split second heart sound. The heart is enlarged on x-ray examination and pulmonary vascular markings are increased. The ECG is characteristic with a prolonged PR interval, left axis deviation, and a right ventricular conduction delay. The diagnosis is confirmed by characteristic findings on the echocardiogram. Cardiac catheterization is used for measurement of pulmonary artery pressure and calculation of pulmonary vascular resistance.

TREATMENT

Surgical correction of an endocardial cushion defect usually is done early in life before pulmonary vascular obstructive disease develops. The repair consists of closure of the atrial and ventricular septal defects and reconstruction of the mitral and tricuspid valves. The abnormality of the left-sided atrioventricular valve in partial defects has been stressed and the "cleft" in the anterior leaflet of the mitral shown to represent a commissure in a trileaflet valve. Anatomic left-sided obstructive lesions may occasionally occur in atrioventricular septal defects and affect the surgical repair (106).

PROGNOSIS

Without surgery, patients suffer from congestive heart failure and frequent pulmonary infections. Elevated pulmonary vascular resistance invariably develops and may have an early onset in these patients (106). With improved surgical technique, operative surgical mortality has fallen. A prosthetic mitral valve is sometimes required following repair of a complete atrioventricular canal because of unacceptable residual mitral insufficiency. Postoperatively, these patients also may manifest left ventricular outflow obstruction, requiring additional surgery (103).

Anomalies of the Tricuspid Valves

TRICUSPID ATRESIA

Anatomy. In tricuspid atresia, the site of the right atrioventricular canal is marked by a connective tissue scar without evidence of valve leaflets. Blood from the right atrium passes through an atrial septal defect to the left atrium. The right ventricle is hypoplastic or rudimentary, and the pulmonary artery is proportionately smaller than normal. There may or may not be a ventricular septal defect. If no defect is present, the right ventricle is reduced to a slit in the myocardium, and the pulmonary artery is atretic.

Tricuspid atresia occurs with normally related great vessels and with dextrotransposition (d-transposition) of the great vessels. Levotransposition (l-transposition) and other malpositions of the heart also may occur with tricuspid atresia (107, 108). When normal great vessels are present, tricuspid atresia can occur with pulmonary atresia and an intact ventricular septum. When a small ventricular septal defect is present, pulmonary stenosis usually also is present. When a large ventricular septal defect is present, there is usually no pulmonary stenosis. The same relationship between the presence or absence of a ventricular septal defect and pulmonary stenosis or atresia also exists when the great vessels are transposed.

Embryology. The tricuspid leaflets, as well as the tendinous chords and papillary muscles, originate from undermining of the ventricular myocardium with minimal, if any, contributions of the endocardial cushions (109) (Fig. 26.21). It has been noted that the tricuspid dimple is located above the posterior part of the ventricular septum in patients with tricuspid atresia (40). It is thought that the tricuspid atresia may be the result of a malalignment between the ventricular loop and the atria. Such a malalignment would not allow the undermining of the septum needed for leaflet formation.

Incidence. Although uncommon (1.1 to 2.4% in clinical series), tricuspid atresia is the third most common cyanotic congenital heart defect (107, 108, 110). There is no gender predilection except when d-transposition of the great arteries is present. In these cases there is a slight increase in the number of males.

Symptoms and Diagnosis. Cyanosis is present from birth due to the obligatory right-to-left shunting across the atrial septal defect. Dyspnea, easy fatigue with feeding, respiratory infections, perspiration, and decreased growth are common, depending on the size of the atrial septal defect, the relationship of the great vessels, and the

presence or absence of a ventricular septal defect and pulmonary stenosis. Brain abscess is a known complication (111).

Treatment. Surgery is required to improve hypoxemia, regulate pulmonary blood flow, and correct associated anomalies. Palliative operations are done in the neonatal period to increase pulmonary blood flow utilizing a Blalock-Taussig shunt or a central shunt. In older children, the right atrium is connected directly or indirectly to the pulmonary artery (Fontan or modified Fontan procedure). Commonly a bidirectional cavopulmonary shunt is done prior to the Fontan procedure to decrease the work of the left ventricle (112, 113).

Prognosis. The outlook for patients with tricuspid atresia has improved greatly with the use of the bidirectional cavopulmonary shunt and with modifications in the Fontan procedure (114). In the early postoperative period, problems with ventricular dysfunction and increased pulmonary vascular resistance may occur. Some centers have used a fenestrated baffle with delayed closure of the atrial septum to treat this problem (115). Late right sided failure and protein-losing enteropathy may occur (114).

EDITORIAL COMMENT

Patients with tricuspid atresia have a favorable outlook after the Fontan operation as long as the pulmonary bed has been treated with a systemic-to-pulmonary artery shunt in the case of severe pulmonary stenosis or atresia or with a pulmonary artery band in the case of unobstructed pulmonary flow. Other favorable anatomic considerations are a single left rather than right ventricle and strong likelihood of competent valves (CM).

EBSTEIN'S ANOMALY OF THE TRICUSPID VALVES

Definition. In Ebstein's anomaly of the tricuspid valve, the septal and posterior leaflets are displaced toward the apex of the right ventricle and do not originate from the true annulus. Only the anterior leaflet originates from the annulus, but it is abnormal functionally and structurally.

Anatomy. The basic defect in Ebstein's anomaly is the displacement of the tricuspid valve toward the apex of the right ventricle. The anterior leaflet is the most nearly normal with at least part of its base attached to the annulus fibrosis. It is larger than normal and may be the only functional leaflet. The medial and posterior leaflets arise from the ventricular septum and the wall of the right ventricle below the annulus. They may be wholly or partially fused to the ventricular wall or bound down by short chordae tendinea, and they are usually deformed to the point of being nonfunctional. There is a great variation in the number, length, and position of the chordae tendinea and the papillary muscles. The valvular tissue may appear normal, or it may be fleshy; fenestrated leaflets are common (Fig. 26.22).

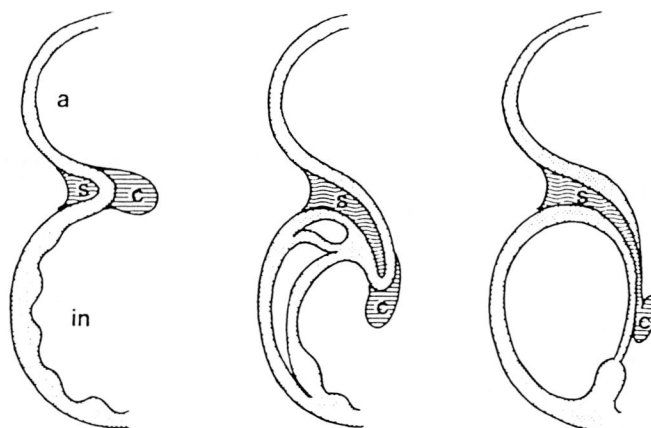

Figure 26.21. Diagram to show the general principle of invagination of sulcus tissue(s) and myocardial undermining which leads to the formation of valves between atrium *(a)* and inlet segment *(in)* and their tension apparatus. Note that the endocardial cushion tissue *(c)* initially forms a conspicuous mass, but that in the final stage it does not contribute to the material of the valve. (From Wenink ACG, Gittenberger-de Groot AC, Brom AG. Developmental considerations of mitral valve anomalies. Int J Cardiol 1986;11:85–98.)

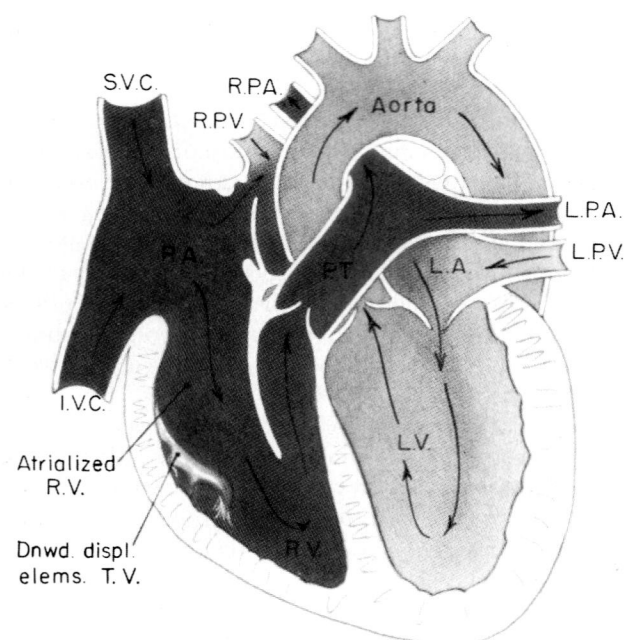

Figure 26.22. Cardiac circulation in Ebstein's anomaly. The incompetent and displaced tricuspid valve increases right atrial pressure above the left so that the foramen ovale does not close. (From Kanjuh VI, Edwards JG. A review of congenital anomalies of the human heart and great vessels according to functional categories. Pediat Clin N Amer 1964;11:55–105.)

The portion of the right ventricle above the anomalous valve is thin and resembles atrial rather than ventricular myocardium ("atrialization" of the ventricle). It contracts, however, with the remainder of the ventricle and not with the atrium. The resulting paradoxic contraction of the atrium and atrialized ventricle produces atrial dilation and gives a globular appearance to the heart.

Ebstein's anomaly of the left-sided atrioventricular valve may occur in l-transposition of the great vessels. The ventricles are inverted in this disorder, and the left-sided atrioventricular valve is a tricuspid valve.

Embryogenesis. Ebstein's anomaly of the tricuspid valve is thought to occur because of incomplete delamination of the right ventricular myocardium. Maternal ingestion of lithium has been cited as one possible cause. The posterior and medial leaflets are displaced into the right ventricle. These leaflets are formed in the third and fourth gestational months. The anterior leaflet is formed much earlier and usually is more completely undermined arising closer to the true annulus (116, 117).

Symptoms and Diagnosis. Cyanosis may be the presenting symptom in infancy. This usually will regress as the pulmonary vascular resistance falls and pulmonary blood flow increases. Later in life, dyspnea on exertion, fatigue, and palpitations may be experienced (118, 119). Left ventricular dysfunction has been reported (120, 121).

On examination of the older patient, cyanosis may or may not be present. Classic findings include a prominent early systolic click related to the tricuspid valve ("sail sound") (122), a widely split second heart sound, and a systolic murmur related to tricuspid regurgitation or right ventricular outflow obstruction. Loud atrial and or ventricular gallops may be present. The ECG is very useful, showing a prolonged PR interval, right bundle branch block of various duration, and sometimes evidence of the Wolff-Parkinson-White syndrome (123). The chest x-ray film also may be characteristic with a globular cardiac silhouette and a small vascular pedicle (124). The diagnosis usually is easily made by echocardiography, which shows apical displacement of one or more leaflets and tethering of the valve to the right ventricular wall (125). Tricuspid regurgitation can be seen with color-flow Doppler scan. Cardiac catheterization rarely is necessary because of the accuracy and safety of echocardiography and Doppler imaging.

Treatment and Prognosis. The newborn infant may be intensely cyanotic at birth and require prostaglandin E to maintain ductal patency. The prostaglandin can usually be weaned as the pulmonary vascular resistance falls. Occasionally, an infant cannot be weaned and requires a systemic pulmonary shunt (126). For the older patient, therapy is limited to treatment of arrhythmias and prevention of bacterial endocarditis. The risk of endocarditis is small. A plastic repair of the tricuspid valve with closure of the atrial septum can be performed in some patients. At times, a tricuspid valve replacement becomes necessary (127).

The prognosis is highly dependent on the severity of the defect, which may range from mild to severe. The most common cause of death is congestive heart failure. Sudden death from arrhythmia may occur (128).

EDITORIAL COMMENT

In some infants the Ebstein's tricuspid valve is so severely malformed and insufficient that simple palliation is not feasible. Under these circumstances the surgeon may wish to close off the right ventricular cavity with a pericardial patch and perform a systemic-to-pulmonary artery shunt. The resultant physiology eliminates the severe tricuspid regurgitation to prepare the patient for a Fontan univentricular repair. Surgical therapy for infants who are otherwise stable and have a reasonably well-developed right ventricle can be delayed well into adolescence when symptoms of tricuspid regurgitation and cyanosis occur. Under these circumstances, atrial septal defect closure, tricuspid valvuloplasty, and if present, surgical ablation of Wolff-Parkinson-White syndrome can be performed (CM).

OTHER TRICUSPID VALVE DEFECTS

Tricuspid Stenosis. Tricuspid stenosis usually is associated with a hypoplastic right ventricle and either atresia or severe stenosis of the pulmonary valve. It also may exist uncommonly as an isolated defect (129).

The valve may be hypoplastic or severly deformed, with poor leaflet formation and abnormal papillary muscle attachments. The leaflets are at the annulus of the valve and are not displaced to the right ventricle, such as in Ebstein's anomaly. Such valves are called dysplastic (130, 131). The disorder is highly associated with pulmonary valve obstruction.

Clefts of the Tricuspid Valve. Clefts in the tricuspid valve may occur in partial or complete endocardial cushion defects. A cleft in the septal leaflet of the tricuspid valve also may be seen in patients with a membranous ventricular septal defect. This allows a left ventricle to right atrial (LV-RA) shunt. The LV-RA shunt also may be due to tricuspid insufficiency caused by the proximity of the defect to the valve (132).

Duplication of the Tricuspid Valve. Duplication of the tricuspid valve has been reported (133). There are two separate valves, each with its own set of papillary muscles. Other anomalies do not usually co-exist. In addition, a heart with six separate valve cusps, all inserted on the valve ring, was reported (134).

Uhl's Malformation (Parchment Heart). This is similar to Ebstein's anomaly. The characteristics of this disease are atrophic right ventricular wall, dilated right ventricle, and a normal tricuspid valve (135, 136).

Anomalies of the Pulmonary Valve and Right Ventricular Outflow Tract

PULMONARY STENOSIS AND ATRESIA

Anatomy. The primary lesion is a fusion, partial or complete, of the three cusps of the pulmonary semilunar valves (137–143). The lines of fusion may remain, or they may be obliterated. If fusion is complete, a diaphragm forms completely across the pulmonary artery, and the valve is said to be atretic.

Pulmonary Stenosis with Intact Ventricular Septum. The stenosis may be valvular with partial fusion of the cusps of the semilunar valve. A domed valve occurs most frequently, but the cusps also may be bicuspid, unicommissural, or dysplastic (thickened, unfused leaflets) (144). A hypoplastic pulmonary annulus with stiff hypoplastic leaflets also occurs (145).

The right ventricle proximal to the stenosis may be reduced in size, but the walls are hypertrophied. In valvular stenosis, the pulmonary artery above the valve is thin walled and dilated. The right atrium may be hypertrophied if the tricuspid valve is incompetent. Often the foramen ovale is patent. Atrial septal defects may be present. The ductus arteriosus usually is closed.

The degree of obstruction is variable. Mild pulmonary valve stenosis is defined as a catheterization pressure gradient across the valve of less than 40 mm Hg. Moderate stenosis is seen when the gradient across the valve is between 40 and 80 mm Hg and the right ventricular pressure is greater than half, but not at left ventricular levels. Severe stenosis exists when the gradient across the valve is greater than 80 mm Hg and right ventricle pressure equals or exceeds left ventricle pressure (137).

Critical pulmonic stenosis can be an emergency in the newborn. Less critical obstruction is followed medically until intervention becomes necessary. Currently, balloon pulmonary valvuloplasty is the initial treatment for valvar stenosis (146). However, valvuloplasty usually is not successful for a dysplastic pulmonary valve or in the neonate with critical pulmonary stenosis. If balloon valvuloplasty is unsuccessful or unsuitable, a surgical valvotomy can be performed. At times the valve has to be resected and a transannular patch placed to relieve obstruction caused by a small valve annulus (147).

Pulmonary Atresia with Intact Ventricular Septum. In this defect, the cusps of the pulmonary valve are completely fused with one another, forming a diaphragm across the pulmonary artery. Pulmonary circulation is provided through a patent ductus arteriosus or through bronchial collateral vessels. The foramen ovale is patent. An atrial septal defect also may be present. The right ventricle and tricuspid valve are of variable size. Right ventricular coronary sinusoids exist. The size of the ventricle and the extent of the coronary sinusoids significantly effect the clinical course.

The infant appears normal except for cyanosis. The second heart sound is single. A systolic murmur due to tricuspid regurgitation and/or a patent ductus arteriosus can be present. In some cases no murmur is heard. The ECG shows a normal or rightward mean QRS axis. The prominence of the P waves and QRS complexes varies with the size of the right ventricle (139). In patients with a small hypoplastic right ventricle, posterior left ventricular forces are prominent and there is evidence of right atrial hypertrophy. The x-ray examination findings can vary from being relatively normal at birth to cardiomegaly due to right atrial and left ventricular enlargement (148). The diagnosis is made by echocardiography. The imperforate valve can be imaged, and the size of the right ventricle and tricuspid valve assessed (149). Forward flow across the valve can be evaluated with Doppler ultrasound (150).

Embryology. Pulmonary stenosis and atresia with intact ventricular septum are thought to share a common etiology. It is postulated that the abnormality occurs after cardiac septation since the ventricular septum is intact (151). The ductus arteriosus is also in a normal position, suggesting that fetal blood flow was once normal (152). An infection is thought to occur after the normal development of the valve (141). (Whether the valve becomes stenotic or atretic depends on the timing and extent of the purported infectious insult.)

EDITORIAL COMMENT

Pulmonary stenosis and atresia with intact ventricular septum is thought to occur late in embryologic development for the reasons stated in this text. Since the advent of accurate fetal echocardiography, this defect has been identified in the second trimester of gestation and progression of severe stenosis to atresia has been documented with concomitant thickening of the right ventricle. Recent developments with fetal cardiopulmonary bypass in lambs have demonstrated that simple intracardiac interventions are possible. If human fetal surgery is to become a reality, pulmonary stenosis and atresia with intact ventricular septum will be the disease for which the most could be accomplished. A decompressed right ventricle in fetal life would have a greater chance at growth with a lesser possibility of sinusoidal development, which would eventually result in a biventricular repair (CM).

Anomalies of the Mitral Valve

EMBRYOLOGY

The formation of the mitral valve and its tension apparatus occurs by undermining of ventricular myocardium and invagination of the atrioventricular junction (153). Endocardial cushion tissue facilitates valve formation but does not comprise the bulk of the tissue mass.

Valve formation depends on normal septation (Fig. 26.23). Lesions such as double-orifice mitral valve and parachute valve occur in hearts with normal septation but with incomplete undermining of the ventricular wall. More complex lesions such as straddling mitral valve and atrioventricular canal defects occur when there is a deficiency in the ventricular septum. The precise embryologic reason for mitral atresia has not been elucidated (154).

MITRAL ATRESIA

An atretic mitral valve shows no trace of valvular tissue at the normal site. Instead, there is only the suggestion of a membrane or a dimple where the valve is expected (155).

In mitral atresia the normal flow of fetal vena caval blood to the left atrium through the foramen ovale, and from there to the left ventricle and aorta, is interrupted (156). Secondary anatomic changes result from the obstruction of blood flow to the left ventricle (157). The right atrium is large and dilated. The atrial septal opening is often restrictive. The septum primum may herniate through the foramen ovale into the right atrium, forming an aneurysm of the atrial septum. Pulmonary lymphangiectasia may occur when the atrial septum is intact and there is no outlet for returning pulmonary venous blood.

Alternately, anomalous pulmonary venous connections may occur, or there may be a left atrial-coronary sinus connection through an unroofed coronary sinus.

Infants present in cardiogenic shock and low cardiac output. These signs are accentuated after the patent ductus arteriosus closes. The diagnosis is easily made by two-dimensional echocardiography.

Treatment. Mitral atresia usually is associated with aortic atresia and a slit-like or nonexistent left ventricle as part of the hypoplastic left heart syndrome (157). Mitral atresia also may occur with a ventricular septal defect, in which case the left ventricle is larger. Norwood (158) devised a procedure (now named for him) for the treatment of hypoplastic left heart syndrome. Since then, this surgical approach (Norwood I) has been expanded, to be followed by a cavopulmonary shunt (112) and finally to include the Fontan procedure (174). A 52% 4-year survival rate has been reported among 76 patients who underwent a Fontan procedure after surviving the previous two surgeries (159).

EDITORIAL COMMENT

Another treatment for hypoplastic left heart syndrome is infant orthotopic cardiac transplantation with extended arch reconstruction. This represents replacement therapy instead of palliative therapy associated with the Norwood-Fontan approach. Donor availability and immunosuppression complications, however, have prevented the universal application of this therapy. In the future, both of these therapies will be evaluated in the light of earlier fetal diagnosis and pregnancy termination for those families who elect to do so (CM).

MITRAL STENOSIS

Congenital mitral stenosis limits blood flow from the left atrium to the left ventricle. The obstruction may be caused by abnormalities in the mitral annulus, leaflets, chordae tendinea, or papillary muscles—often in combination (160). Classical mitral stenosis consists of thickened leaflets, shortened chordae tendinea, and decreased intrachordal spaces (161).

Incidence. This is an uncommon congenital malformation. It occurs in less than 0.42% of patients with congenital heart disease (162). There is a male preponderance (162).

Diagnosis. Congenital mitral stenosis often presents during the first year of life with dyspnea, cough, and evidence of pulmonary edema. The first heart sound may or may not be accentuated. Pulmonic closure is increased in intensity. A diastolic murmur is heard at the apex. The ECG usually shows a P wave abnormality and rightward QRS configuration (161). The abnormal valve can be imaged by two-dimensional echocardiography and the

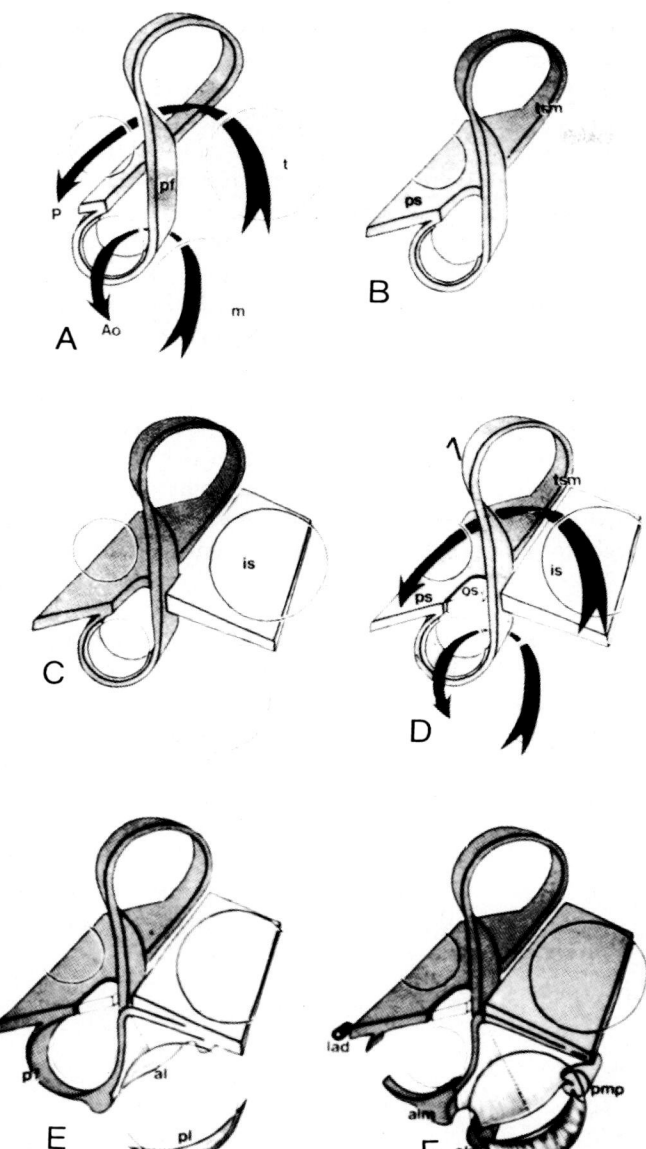

Figure 26.23. **A,** Schematic view of the cardiac base. The cardiac apex is situated to the right and above in this figure. Although this drawing represents an early embryonic stage, the atrioventricular valve annuli (*m* and *t*) and the attachments of the arterial valves have already been drawn as separate structures. The basal part of the primary fold *(pf)* is seen to separate the atrioventricular and arterial valve attachments (i.e., it finds itself between inlet segment [to the right] and outlet segment [to the left]). The *arrows* indicate the bloodstreams from mitral annulus *(m)*, passing the primary fold, to the aortic valve *(Ao)*, and from tricuspid annulus *(t)*, passing the primary fold to the pulmonary valve *(P)*. **B,** Diagram in the same orientation as **A.** Expansion of inlet and outlet segments has caused development of the primary septum *(ps)* from the intervening primary fold. The apical part of this fold remains recognizable as the septomarginal trabeculation (= moderator band, *tsm*) of the mature right ventricle. **C,** The inlet septum *(is)* has developed within the inlet segment. **D,** The outlet septum *(os)* has developed within the outlet segment to complete septation. All septal structures, including the primary septum *(ps)*, inlet septum *(is)*, and septomarginal trabeculation *(tsm)* are there, but valve formation has still to occur. The *arrows* indicate the separate bloodstreams as in **A.** For further orientation, the *asterisk* indicates the position of the left anterior descending coronary artery. Note the part of the primary fold encircling the aortic

root, giving very narrow boundaries to the outlet portion of the left ventricle. **E** and **F,** Diagrams to show development of the mitral valve. **E,** Mitral valve formation in progress, with formation of aortic *(al)* and parietal *(pl)* leaflets. The left ventricular part of the primary fold *(pf)* is thinning out. **F,** Completion of the mitral valve. The *dotted line* indicates the dual composition of the aortic leaflet. Part of the left ventricular portion of the primary fold has persisted as the anterolateral muscle bundle *(alm)* which is wedged between aortic and mitral orifices. *alp,* Anterolateral papillary muscle; *pmp,* posteromedial papillary muscle; *lad,* left anterior descending coronary artery. (From Wenick ACG, Gittenberger-de Groot AC, Brom AG. Developmental consideration of mitral valve anomalies. Int J Cardiol 1986;11:85–98.)

gradient across the valve measured with Doppler interrogation.

Treatment. The urgency of treatment depends on the severity of symptoms. With significant symptoms medical management is unsuccessful and surgery is required. Valve replacement in infants and young children is unattractive (163, 164). Anticoagulation is required. It may be difficult to find an appropriate valve size for a tiny child. Once a valve is placed, the mitral annulus growth is limited, although some believe that growth does occur (163). For these reasons, increased attention is being given to balloon angioplasty of the valve (165).

Prognosis. The prognosis depends on the severity of the symptoms and the age at which intervention is first required.

DOUBLE-ORIFICE MITRAL VALVE

Two papillary muscles are present when a double-orifice mitral valve occurs. Each orifice has its own set of chordae tendinea that insert into one papillary muscle. This has been thought of as a double-parachute mitral valve (166). Mitral valve function is usually normal, but stenosis and insufficiency may occur (154). Stenosis may be significant in the setting of an atrioventricular canal. The lesion has been described in association with ventricular septal defect, coarctation of the aorta, endocardial cushion defect, and other congenital cardiac lesions (161).

Conotruncal Abnormalities

PULMONARY STENOSIS WITH VENTRICULAR SEPTAL DEFECT (TETRALOGY OF FALLOT) AND PULMONARY ATRESIA WITH VENTRICULAR SEPTAL DEFECT

Anatomy. These defects differ substantially from pulmonary stenosis and atresia with intact ventricular septum. A large ventricular septal defect is present. There is malalignment of the ventricular septum reflecting the conotruncal abnormality. The pulmonary valve is atretic or stenotic. The pulmonary arteries are small. In pulmonary atresia with ventricular septal defect, the pulmonary arteries may be completely absent. The only blood supply provided to the lungs may be by collateral vessels (167, 168).

PULMONARY STENOSIS WITH VENTRICULAR SEPTAL DEFECT—TETRALOGY OF FALLOT

The components of tetralogy of Fallot are: (a) pulmonary stenosis; (b) a large ventricular septal defect; (c) displacement of the aorta to the right, allowing it to override the ventricular septal defect; and (d) hypertrophy of the right ventricle. The aorta is enlarged, and the pulmonary artery is reduced in diameter. The foramen ovale usually is patent. A right-sided aortic arch occurs in about 20% of affected patients.

Obstruction to pulmonary flow may be produced by the narrowing of the right ventricular outflow tract (infundibular stenosis), by malformed pulmonary valves (valvular stenosis), or by both. Obstruction also may occur distal to the pulmonary valve and affect the main and branch pulmonary arteries (169).

The clinical presentation of tetralogy of Fallot depends primarily on the severity of the right ventricular outflow tract obstruction. If severe, the right-to-left shunting through the ventricular septal defect is great, and symptoms appear early. Intense cyanosis may be the presenting sign in the newborn. In others, cyanosis may not appear for weeks or months. Right-to-left shunting increases as obstructive infundibular hypertrophy increases. The diagnosis is made by two-dimensional echocardiography, which shows the ventricular septal defect and outlines the narrowing of the right ventricular outflow tract (170). Angiography is important to the surgeon. With it, the right ventricular outflow tract can be profiled, and the main pulmonary artery and its branches clearly shown (171). Areas of distal stenosis can be seen. The size and position of the ventricular septal defect can be visualized.

The intensely cyanotic newborn can be given prostaglandin E_1 to maintain ductal patency and ensure a pulmonary blood supply. If the anatomy for primary total correction is unfavorable, a systemic to pulmonary shunt can be performed and the complete repair carried out at a later time. Complete repair includes closing the ventricular septal defect and enlarging the right ventricular outflow tract (172, 173). Late problems following surgery include sudden death due to ventricular arrhythmias (174).

PULMONARY ATRESIA WITH VENTRICULAR SEPTAL DEFECT (FIG. 26.24)

The anatomy in this defect is the same as that in tetralogy of Fallot except that the pulmonary valve is atretic. A sig-

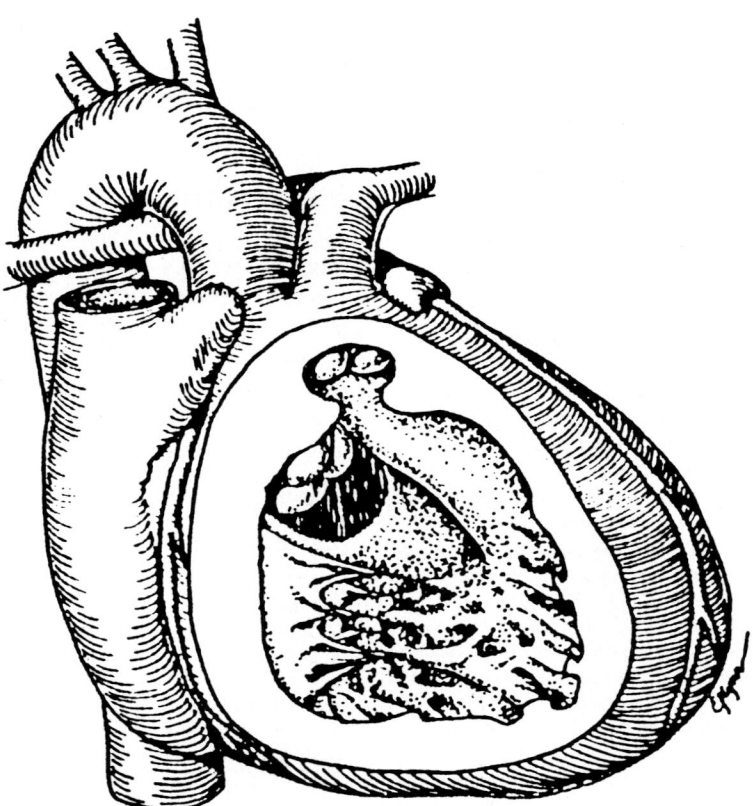

Figure 26.24.   Drawing of the anatomy of tetralogy of Fallot. There is infundibular obstruction, a ventricular septal defect (through which the aortic leaflets can be seen), and a right aortic arch. (From Fyler DC. Tetralogy of Fallot. In: Fyler DC, ed. Nadas' pediatric cardiology. Philadelphia: Hanley & Belfus, 1992.)

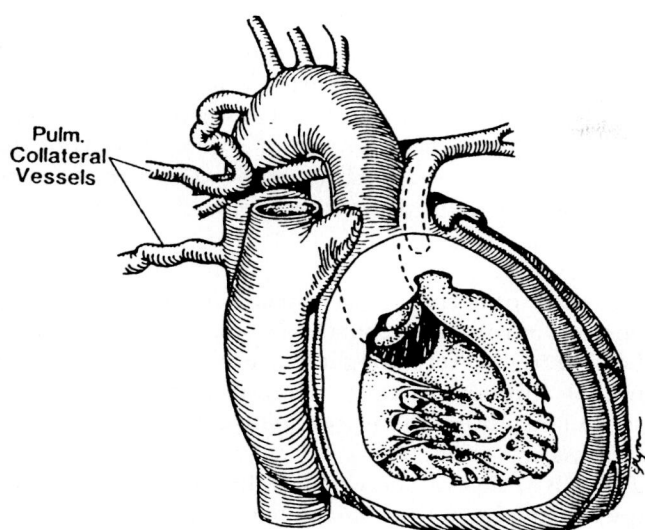

Figure 26.25. Drawing of the anatomy of tetralogy of Fallot with pulmonary atresia. There is no outflow from the right ventricle because of pulmonary atresia. The entire right ventricular output passes through the ventricular defect into the left ventricle and aorta. The main pulmonary artery is small (sometimes only a remnant exists). There are bizarre vessels supplying the lung collaterals) which arise from the descending aorta. (From Fyler DC, ed. Nadas' pediatric cardiology. Philadelphia: Hanley & Belfus, 1992.)

nificant difference is in the source of pulmonary blood supply (169, 175). The main pulmonary artery may be atretic. Right and left pulmonary arteries may be confluent, or they may be discontinuous, each supplied by a separate ductus arteriosus. One pulmonary artery may be supplied by collateral vessels. In some cases the collateral flow is profuse and congestive heart failure occurs (176).

Infants with pulmonary atresia are cyanotic at birth (Fig. 26.25). Acidosis and cardiogenic shock can occur when the ductus arteriosus closes. After stabilizing with prostaglandin and correction of the acidosis, the diagnosis can be made with echocardiography. Angiography can delineate the pulmonary blood supply (168). The surgical approach will depend on the anatomy and the patient's clinical condition. A modified Blalock-Taussig shunt or central shunt can be done. This may be a palliative procedure or may represent the first step in a staged repair (177). Because there may be discontinuity of the pulmonary arteries, a "unifocalization procedure" may be necessary to establish a contiguous blood supply (178, 179). Pulmonary enlargement can be encouraged by a shunt procedure or by placing a conduit between the right ventricle and the pulmonary artery (180).

TETRALOGY OF FALLOT WITH ABSENT PULMONARY VALVE

In this lesion the pulmonary annulus is restrictive and the pulmonary valve functionally absent (181, 182). In some cases, remnants of connective tissue are seen at the annu-

lus (183). There is a ventricular septal defect and infundibular stenosis. Massive dilation of the pulmonary arteries due to pulmonary insufficiency is present. At birth a distinctive "to-and-fro" murmur of pulmonary insufficiency is heard. X-ray films show dilated pulmonary arteries. The infant is stressed by respiratory problems caused by the dilated pulmonary arteries (184). Abnormally branching pulmonary arteries also may occur, exacerbating the clinical problem (185).

Embryology. The influence of the neural crest on outflow tract septation has received increasing research attention (21, 186). Tetralogy of Fallot is a cardiac defect that occurs after neural crest cell ablation in experimental animals. The relationship between the experimental work and morphogenesis in the human infant has not been elucidated. Nonetheless, the research is intriguing.

The malalignment of the ventricular septum seen in the tetralogy occurs because of failure of the trabecular septum and infundibular septum to unite (169, 187). As a result, the aorta overrides the septum. In addition, unequal division of the bulbus, together with decreased spiraling of the bulbotruncal ridges, alters the right ventricular outflow tract, narrowing it. The degree of narrowing may be to the point of atresia.

The cause of the tetralogy with absent pulmonary valve is less clear. The pulmonary valve annulus is small. The massively dilated pulmonary arteries are thought to be secondary to pulmonary insufficiency occurring in utero. The cause of the damage to the valve in utero is speculative.

EDITORIAL COMMENT

The dilated pulmonary arteries most likely are due to the increase in utero right ventricular–to–pulmonary artery regurgitant fraction. The massive pulmonary artery dilation then causes severe bronchotrachial compression, leading to severe tracheomalacia (CM).

ANOMALIES OF THE AORTIC VALVE AND LEFT VENTRICULAR OUTFLOW TRACT

Aortic Atresia
Definition.

There is no opening at the aortic valve area. The atretic part is located proximal to the origin of the coronary arteries (188). This may occur as part of the hypoplastic left heart syndrome and may be associated with mitral atresia and a hypoplastic left ventricle and ascending aortic arch (189, 190).

Anatomy.

The ascending aorta is greatly reduced and provides blood by retrograde flow to the coronary arteries only (Fig. 26.26). The aortic valve cusps may be fused into a diaphragm, or there may be a membranous septum across the aortic orifice with no trace of valvular structure (188).

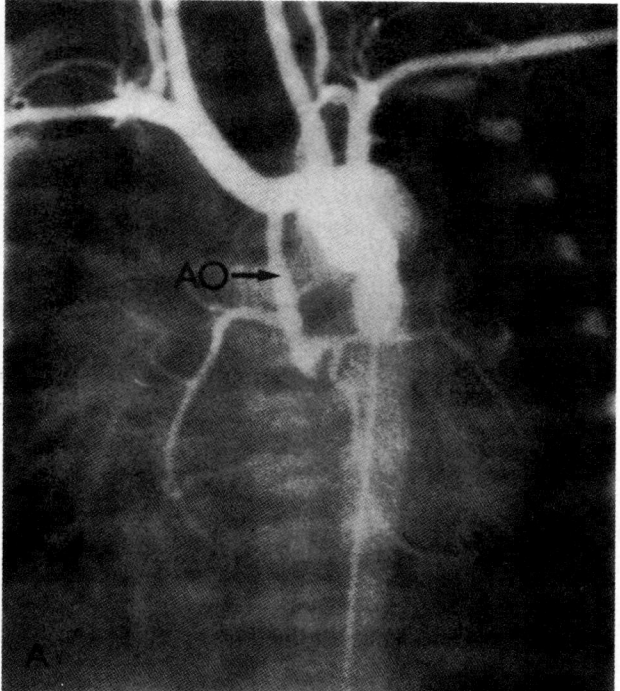

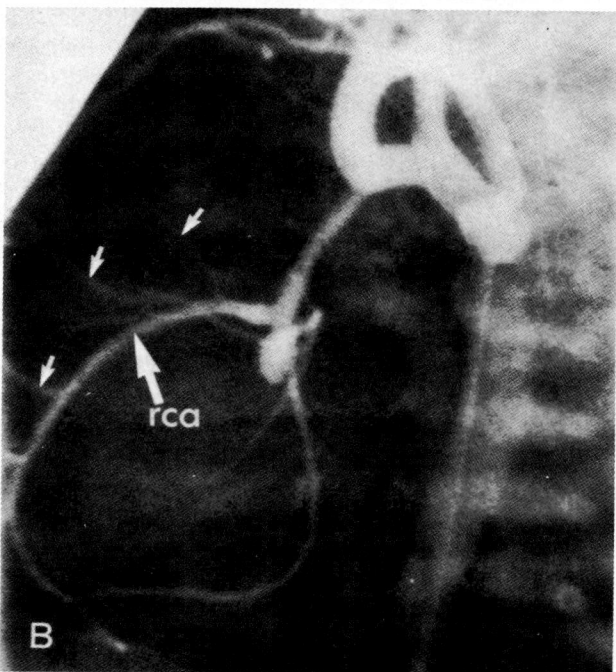

Figure 26.26.   A, Frontal and, **B,** lateral retrograde aortogram in a neonate with necrospy-proven aortic atresia. **A,** Note the diminutive ascending aorta *(AO)* that seems to terminate in the coronary arteries. **B,** This lateral aortogram opacifies the atretic aortic root and the dominant right coronary artery *(rca)* with enlarged infundibular or conal branches *(small white arrows)*. (From Adams RM. Hypoplastic left heart syndrome. In: Adams FH, Emmanouilides GC, Reimenschneider TA eds. Moss' heart disease in infants, children, and adolescents, 4th ed. Baltimore: Williams & Wilkins, 1989.)

The descending aorta is of nearly normal size, supplied by the patent ductus arteriosus arising from the enlarged pulmonary trunk. The superficial appearance is of an aorta arising from the pulmonary artery. There is a high association with mitral atresia or severe stenosis of the mitral valve and entire mitral arcade (191). An atrioventricular canal defect also can be seen with mitral and aortic atresia.

Embryology.

The cause of aortic atresia remains uncertain. The flow-dependent rule (192) equates the size of a vessel with the flow through it. It is thought that an event in utero effects outflow through the aortic valve, resulting in aortic atresia and hypoplasia of the ascending aorta (191).

Incidence.

There is a slightly increased male incidence. The frequency of the lesion ranges between 7 and 9% in a population of children with congenital heart disease (191).

Symptoms and Diagnosis.

Babies with aortic atresia usually appear normal at birth (193). They become symptomatic when the ductus closes and the systemic circulation is dramatically reduced. Acidosis and cardiogenic shock ensue. Prostaglandin E$_1$ can open the ductus and stabilize the baby's condition. The baby may then undergo a cardiac transplant (189) or the first stage of a Norwood procedure (158). It is significant to note that Norwood's aggressive surgical approach to this problem in the early 1980s changed the clinical approach to these babies. They now are considered surgical candidates, whereas previously, medical management was the standard.

Aortic Stenosis

Anatomy.

Congenital obstruction of the left ventricular outflow tract may occur at the supravalvular, valvular, or subvalvular levels.

Supravalvular aortic stenosis (Fig. 26.27). Obstruction is produced by a narrowing of the ascending aorta above the aortic semilunar valves. Three categories are described (194, 195). There is a discrete hourglass deformity, a membranous type, and the diffuse hypoplastic type. The coronary arteries arise proximal to the obstruction and are enlarged and tortuous.

Clinically this deformity may occur sporadically or be familial (194). Patients with both the familial and nonfamilial forms may have normal intelligence and normal facies. However, a nonfamilial form also exists in which facies and intelligence are abnormal. Williams syndrome is characterized by elfin facies, psychomotor and growth retardation, peripheral pulmonary arterial stenosis, idiopathic hypercalcemia, craniosynostosis, dental anomalies, and inguinal hernia. The patients are memorable because of their distinctive facies.

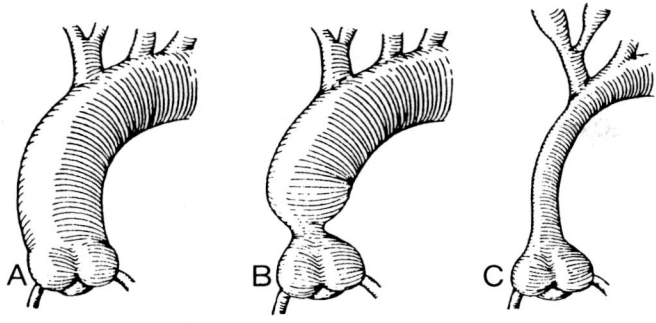

Figure 26.27. The anatomic types of supravalvar aortic stenosis. **A,** normal; **B** and **C,** Two forms of supravalvar stenosis. The difference between these two forms is in the length of the obstruction, which sometimes involves virtually all of the ascending aorta. Note the obstructions in the innominate and common carotid arteries as they arise from the aortic arch. Other obstructions, such as coarctation of the aorta, renal artery stenosis, and pulmonary artery stenosis, are found in some patients. (From Fyler DC. Aortic outflow abnormalties. In: Flyer DC, ed. Nadas' pediatric cardiology. Philadelphia: Hanley & Belfus, 1992:506.)

A recent retrospective surgical review (196) highlighted the fact that patients with the localized form of obstruction do better surgically than do those with diffuse disease. Endarterectomy may be one way to approach the patient with diffuse disease.

Valvular aortic stenosis. The cusps of the semilunar valves may be partially fused to form a perforated, dome-shaped diaphragm, such as is seen in pulmonary stenosis (197). More frequently, fusion occurs along only two commissures so that the stenotic opening is eccentric. The cusps are thickened and irregular. Calcification of the deformed valve is common in older patients (198).

Subvalvular (subaortic) stenosis. Three types of obstruction occur below the aortic valve (199). There is a discrete type with a thin obstructing membrane. A second type has a thicker membrane with a muscular base forming a "collar." Finally, a diffuse tunnel type exists. It is of note that this latter form of left ventricular obstruction is progressive and has a high association with other congenital cardiac deformities, such as a ventricular septal defect (200, 201).

Embryogenesis.
The aortic leaflets are formed from fusion of the truncus swellings in the truncus with tissue from the intercalated disc (202). The leaflets then form from undermining of left ventricular tissue. The most common deformity is a bicuspid valve. In the larger leaflet a raphe can usually be seen, suggesting fusion of two smaller leaflets (198). A unicommissural valve also can be seen. The etiology of fusion of primitive valve leaflets or the failure to form clearly defined leaflets has not been elucidated. Alterations in intrauterine blood flow have been suggested (195, 203).

The cause of supravalve aortic stenosis is unclear (196).

Subvalvular aortic stenosis is not thought to be the primary cardiac problem. Rather, it is thought to develop in response to stress generated in the heart secondary to other obstructive forces in the left heart (200, 201).

Incidence.
Aortic stenosis appeared in 2.3% of Abbott's 1000 cases of major congenital heart lesions (85). Recent work (136) estimates that 7% of infants and children with clinical congenital heart disease will have aortic stenosis. Valvular stenosis is the most common type, accounting for 60% of all aortic stenosis. Supravalvular aortic stenosis is the least common type (197). The preponderance of males has been emphasized. All or most of this preponderance is found in patients with valvular aortic stenosis. A bicuspid aortic valve is considered the most common congenital heart deformity (198).

Symptoms.
Patients with aortic stenosis can be divided into two classes. Neonatal critical aortic stenosis is a medical emergency similar to that posed by infants with hypoplastic left heart syndrome (204). In other patients the symptoms evolve. Generally, the classic triad for aortic stenosis—syncope, shortness of breath, and chest pain—is not seen until the fourth decade of life or later. However, congestive heart failure, syncope, and sudden death have been observed in childhood.

Diagnosis.
Children with Williams syndrome have a classic facial appearance (195, 202, 204). The features include a broad forehead, large mouth, upturned nose, curved upper lip, widely spaced teeth, and low set ears. This face has been referred to as an "elfin-like" appearance. With supravalvular aortic stenosis, a harsh systolic murmur is located high along the right sternal border, and there may be a notable difference between the amplitude and the rate of rise of the right and left carotid pulses. With valvular aortic stenosis, a systolic click is best appreciated along the left sternal border near the apex. There may or may not be a harsh systolic murmur at the right upper sternal border. Sometimes only a diastolic murmur is present. The carotid pulses are equal and may decrease when severe left ventricular outflow is present. With discrete, subaortic stenosis the harsh systolic murmur is loudest along the mid-left sternal border. The ECG in each of these conditions is helpful only when the obstruction is severe and left ventricular hypertrophy has occurred. With valvular aortic stenosis, poststenotic dilation of the ascending aorta may be seen. An echocardiogram correctly identifies the site and severity of the left ventricular obstruction and has significantly decreased the need for cardiac catheterization.

Treatment.
The newborn with critical aortic stenosis represents a medical emergency. These infants have been treated sur-

gically with variable results (205). Recently, attention has been focused on attempts to open the severely stenotic valves with balloon angioplasty (106).

In older children and adults, treatment of valvular aortic stenosis is indicated when the left ventricular obstruction is moderately severe to severe (207). Balloon valvuloplasty can be done in many of these patients (208). A surgical valvulotomy is a low-risk procedure which has excellent results but an incidence of recurrence (209).

A subaortic membrane is resected, even when the obstruction is only moderately severe, to prevent progressive trauma to the aortic leaflets from the jet of blood (210). This can result in aortic insufficiency.

Supravalvular aortic stenosis may be difficult to manage because the coronary arteries also can be involved in the medial hypertrophy of their walls. Resection of the narrowed segment (197), with or without coronary bypass surgery, can be done.

Prognosis.

The newborn with critical aortic stenosis has a higher risk of death than the older child or adult (205, 211–213). Children with moderately severe to severe valvular aortic stenosis are followed and referred for surgery as indicated. Otherwise, patients often do quite well until the fourth or fifth decade (198) when symptoms develop. Once symptoms begin, the mortality without surgery increases. Mild aortic stenosis may progress to severe aortic stenosis over many years due to hemodynamic stresses on the aortic valve.

TRANSPOSITION OF THE GREAT ARTERIES (FIG. 26.28)

Definition. A number of terms describing alterations in the relationships of various parts of the heart to each other and to other organs are extant. The special meanings of these terms in cardiac anatomy must be kept in mind.

The normal asymmetric arrangement of the viscera, with the liver and the systemic atrium on the right side of the body, is known as *situs solitus;* its mirror image, in which the symmetry is reversed, is *situs inversus.*

Atrial situs usually corresponds with that of the abdominal viscera, although there are cases in which the abdominal situs is indeterminate. These cases are usually accompanied by absence of the spleen (214). All of the transposition and inversion anomalies also may occur in situs inversus, with the venous atrium being on the left.

Dextrotransposition (D-Transposition) of the Great Arteries.
Transposition of the great arteries is one of the most common forms of cyanotic congenital heart disease. In this malformation the atria and ventricles are normally related. The ventriculoarterial connections are abnormal. The pulmonary artery arises from the left ventricle and the aorta arises from the right ventricle. The aorta is anterior to the pulmonary artery—a reversal of the usual

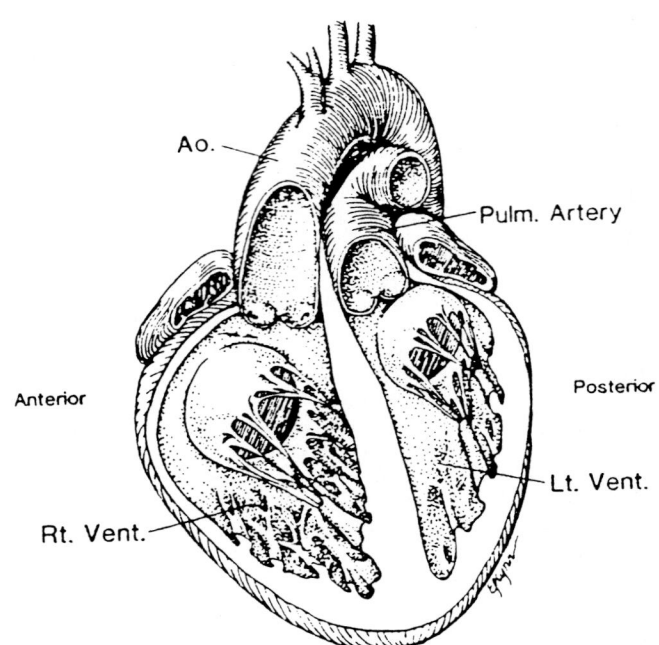

Figure 26.28. Transposition of the great arteries, lateral view. The aorta arises anteriorly from the right ventricle; the pulmonary artery arises posteriorly from the left ventricle. As diagrammed, there is no communication shown between the pulmonary and systemic circulations, a situation not compatible with life. For survival there must be communication between the two circuits, usually as a patent ductus arteriosus, ventricular defect, or atrial opening. (From Fyler DC, ed. Nadas' pediatric cardiology. Philadelphia: WB Saunders, 1992.)

relationship. This has been called simple transposition. Complex transposition is present when there is an associated large ventricular septal defect with or without significant pulmonary stenosis.

Embryology. Peacock (215) in 1866 suggested that transposition was the result of defective development of the septum dividing the truncus arteriosus into the aorta and pulmonary artery. In 1875 Rokitansky (216) carried this idea of an abnormal truncus further and explained the overriding aorta and the pulmonary stenosis of tetralogy of Fallot on the basis of unequal division of the truncus. Intraventricular septal defects were seen as resulting from failure of bulbar and ventricular septa to unite properly.

A most remarkable explanation was proposed by Spitzer (217) in 1923 as part of a phylogenetic explanation of the development of the heart. Pernkopf and Wirtinger (218) described torsion of the embryonic heart occurring at three levels and at different times. Theories of septal malrotation were proposed by Lev and Saphir (52) and by de la Cruz and her associates (55, 56). Shaner (219) attributed the lack of twisting of the aorticopulmonary septum to delay in its formation.

A transfer of the roles of the septal ridges and the valvular primordia of the truncus was suggested by Van

Mierop and Wiglesworth (220). In normal development, the sinistroinferior truncus swelling appears and joins the sinistroanterior conus swelling, while the dextrosuperior ridge joins the dextroposterior swelling. In cases of transposition, it is suggested that the valvular swellings arise earlier and become the septal ridges so that sinistrosuperior truncal ridges join the dextroposterior conus swellings. In each case the earliest appearing pair forms the septum, and the later appearing pair forms the valve.

Bartelings and Gittenberger-de Groot (221) succinctly reviewed current historical thought about the embryology of transposition. They speculate that "mirror image formation of the columns of the aortopulmonary septum," which "grow out" of the truncal ridges, could explain the ventriculoarterial abnormalities in transposition but could not explain all the morphologic ramifications in this entity. The trigger for the aorticoseptal deviation remained hypothetic. Transposition of the great arteries "continues to be somewhat of an enigma."

Recent work has emphasized the role of neural crest cells in truncal septation (21, 187, 222). Experimental neural crest work in the chick embryo has produced transposition of the great vessels. Future research may show that the transposition complexes are the result of perturbations in normal neural crest migration or perhaps represent alterations in biochemical substrates that could alter flow patterns in the embryonic heart.

Diagnosis. Infants with transposition of the great arteries and an intact ventricular septum are cyanotic at birth. When there is an associated large ventricular septal defect, the cyanosis may be more difficult to perceive and the correct diagnosis delayed.

Transposition in an otherwise normal heart would be fatal at birth: the pulmonary and systemic circulations would be completely separated and no oxygenated blood would reach the aorta after the placenta was detached. All live born infants with transposition have one or more shunts. An atrial septal defect or a patent foramen ovale may be combined with a ventricular septal defect, a patent ductus arteriosus or both. In this way deoxygenated blood can reach the lungs and oxygenated blood can be pumped to the systemic circulation.

Treatment and prognosis. After a newborn is referred to a tertiary care center, prostaglandin E_1 therapy can be started to ensure ductal patency and allow mixing of the two circulations. A balloon atrial septostomy may be done to enlarge the foramen ovale to allow mixing at the atrial level (223). Surgery is then planned. Currently, the procedure of choice at most centers is the arterial switch procedure which is done in the immediate newborn period (224). This procedure is thought to be preferable to atrial redirection procedures because the left ventricle is the systemic ventricle and because arrhythmias are less com-

mon (225). Patients selected for this operation must have a left ventricle capable of supporting the circulation and coronary arteries amenable to the required transfer procedure (226). A contraindication to this procedure may be fixed left ventricular outflow obstruction.

EDITORIAL COMMENT

The arterial switch operation for neonates with transposition of the great arteries and intact ventricular septum can now be performed with an operative mortality of between 3 and 8%, which has been established at many centers. Accomplishing both anatomic and physiologic correction appears to offer great potential for excellent long-term results. Postoperative complications associated with the atrial baffle operations, such as atrial arrhythmias, atrioventricular valve insufficiency, and ventricular dysfunction, have not emerged. Moreover, the incidence of anastomotic narrowing and neoaortic insufficiency are quite low. Preliminary intermediate results indicate that the arterial switch operation performed in the first few weeks of life is the procedure of choice for neonates with transposition of the great arteries and intact ventricular septum (CM).

Many patients have undergone atrial redirection procedures, the Mustard or Senning procedures. Late arrhythmias (227), particularly atrial flutter and late right ventricular failure, have made these operations less attractive then previously (228, 229). It is hoped that the long-term follow-up for arterial switch patients will be more favorable.

Levotransposition (L-Transposition) of the Great Vessels (Congenitally Corrected Transposition of the Great Vessels)

Definition. In this malformation the ventricles are inverted. Blood flows from the morphologic right atrium through the mitral valve to the inverted left ventricle and then out to the pulmonary artery through the pulmonary valve. Blood returns from the lungs to the anatomic left atrium and enters the inverted right ventricle through the tricuspid valve. Blood then enters the aorta through the aortic valve. Therefore blood flow is physiologically correct. The great vessels are transposed, the aorta being anterior to the pulmonary valve. The aorta makes up the left border of the heart and creates a distinctive x-ray picture (Fig. 26.29).

Embryology. The ventricles are identified by their morphology rather than by their position (230). A reversal of this relationship is called "inversion" rather than "transposition," which is reserved for the position of the great arteries.

While the right and left atria arise from the right and left sides of the primitive paired heart tube, the two ventricles arise in tandem, after fusion of the paired primor-

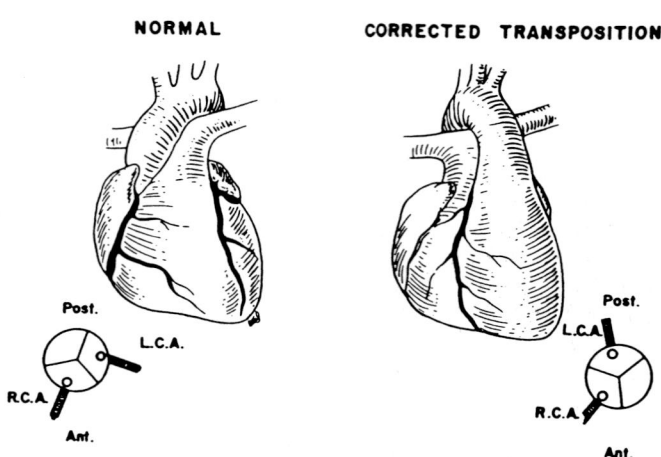

Figure 26.29.   External view of the heart and great vessels in a normal person and in one with corrected transposition of the great arteries. Note that the left border of the heart in the patient with corrected transposition is occupied by the aorta, not the pulmonary artery. Note also the anterior position of the aorta. The origin of the coronary arteries is illustrated in the insert. The left coronary originates from the posterior sinus and the right coronary from the right anterior sinus. (From Nadas AS, Fyler DC. Pediatric cardiology. Philadelphia: WB Saunders. 1972:702. with permission.)

dia, and their formation bears no relationship to the paired origin of the primordial heart tube.

At the end of the second week, the bulboventricular loop of the primitive heart tube turns to the right (the D-loop of Van Praagh) (32, 231, 232). The bend thus formed is the primordium of the right ventricle, while that of the left ventricle rises from the proximal portion nearer the midline. This establishes the relative positions of the two ventricles. Should the bulboventricular loop turn to the left (the L-loop of Van Praagh), the morphologic right ventricle will lie to the left of the left ventricle, thus reversing their normal relationships without affecting the proximal atrial relationships or the distal truncal relationships (Fig. 26.30). This reversal of the loop is not related to situs of the viscera and atria and is not associated with changes elsewhere in the heart or the body.

Diagnosis.   This is an uncommon congenital defect (231, 232). Patients with l-transposition may be asymptomatic and the problem only incidentally found. However, there is a high frequency of associated ventricular septal defect and pulmonary stenosis which brings the patient to medical attention. Dextrocardia is not infrequent. There also is a high incidence of "ebsteinization" of the left-sided atrioventricular valve (the tricuspid valve). The associated atrioventricular valve insufficiency can be hemodynamically significant requiring surgery. There also is a high incidence of congenital complete heart block which evolves over time.

The diagnosis is made based on clinical suspicion, perhaps suggested by an x-ray examination, auscultation, or

ECG. The ECG shows absence of a septal q wave in lead V_6 and a septal q in lead V_1 because of the direction of depolarization in these hearts. Heart block also may be seen. Two-dimensional echocardiography (233) and angiography (234) confirm the diagnosis. The morphology of the coronary arteries also can be visualized angiographically, demonstrating their course in the inverted ventricle.

Prognosis and Treatment.   Patients may have a long survival with this congenital defect (235). The usual course, however, involves patients with atrioventricular valve insufficiency due to a dysplastic or Ebstein valve or with right ventricular outflow tract obstruction. Heart block also occurs as part of the natural history of the disease. A recent review (236) recommended early surgery for patients with congestive heart failure to prevent right ventricular dilation. Those with pulmonary outflow obstruction could undergo surgery safely at a later time. Surgery can be accomplished with low hospital morbidity (237, 238).

Duplication of the Heart

Although the two primordial endocardial tubes of salamanders may be experimentally induced to form separate, complete hearts (239), duplication of the heart is usually found only in double monsters. Two observations in humans in supernumerary cardiac chambers without other evidence of twinning has been made by Barnard and Brink (240). These may represent independent development of partially unfused cardiac tubes. In the most striking case there was a large "atrium" and a small "ventricle" attached to the left atrial and ventricular walls. The demarcation between the two anomalous chambers was continuous with the atrioventricular sulcus of the normal heart. The "atrium" opened into the "ventricle" without valves, and the "ventricle" opened into the normal left ventricle. This curious case seems to admit no other explanation than that of incipient embryonic duplication (Fig. 26.31).

Aiello et al. (241) reported the case of a 3-day-old boy who was admitted to the hospital with cyanosis and tachydyspnea and who died 2 days later. At autopsy two "half-hearts" were found, each totally separated from the other, with each half having the following anomalies: a single atrium and ventricle, two trunci, double superior and inferior venae cavae, anomalous pulmonary venous drainage, and common pericardium. Several other anomalies were not splenic. Aiello and her colleagues believe that perhaps the explanation for this defect was a lack of fusion of the primitive cardiac tubes (Fig. 26.32).

Tausig has proposed that isolated cardiac malformations have an evolutionary origin. In 1988 she provided an excellent review of the literature on the duplication of

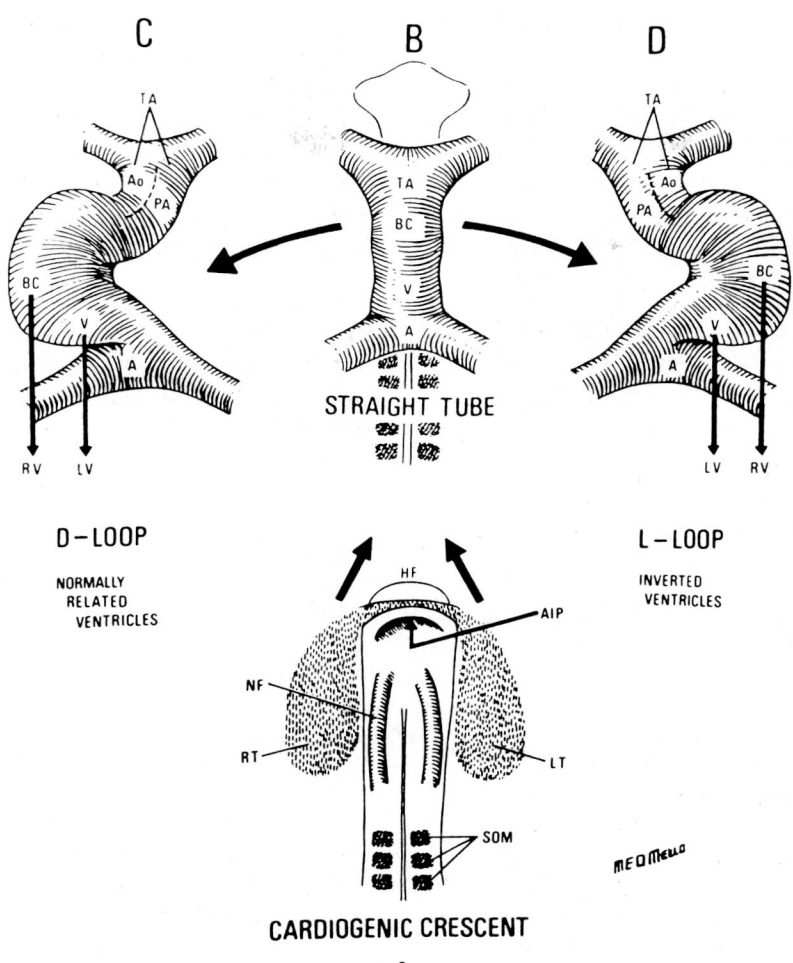

Figure 26.30. Cardiac loop formation. D-loop formation results in solitus (noninverted) ventricles, with solitus right ventricular (RV) sinus to the right, solitus left ventricular (LV) sinus to the left. L-loop formation results in "inverted" ventricles, with "inverted" RV sinus to the left and "inverted" LV sinus to the right. A, Atrium; AIP, anterior intestinal portal; Ao, aorta; BC, bulbus cordis; HF, head fold; LT, left; LV, morphologically left ventricle; NF, neural fold; PA, pulmonary artery; RT, right; RV, morphologically right ventricle; SOM, somites; TA, truncus arteriosus; V, ventricles. (From Van Praagh R. The segmental approach to understanding complex cardiac lesions. In: Eldrege WJ, Lemele GM, Goldberg H (eds). Current Problems in Congenital Heart Disease. New York: Spectrum, 1979.)

the heart. The same author reported the existance of only one authentic case of duplicate hearts in a human (242).

Diverticula of the Heart

ANATOMY

A cardiac diverticulum is a rare and striking anomaly. It arises, usually from the anterior surface of the ventricle, as a tubular myocardial process lying within a tube of pericardium. The diverticulum extends anteriorly and inferiorly and often passes through a diaphragmatic defect and an upper abdominal wall defect, ending near the umbilicus (Fig. 26.33). If the diverticulum does not reach the diaphragm, the latter is intact (243–245) (see

also Chapter 16, "The Anterior Body Wall," Defects of the Anterior Thoracic Wall and Figure 16.25).

HISTORY

The earliest case is that of O'Bryan (1837), which is mentioned by Peacock (246).

ETIOLOGY

A ventricular diverticulum arises from a failure of the cardiac loop to separate from the structures of the septum transversum during the fifth week. A transitory adhesion produces a small diverticulum without a diaphragmatic defect, whereas a more persistent attachment leaves a

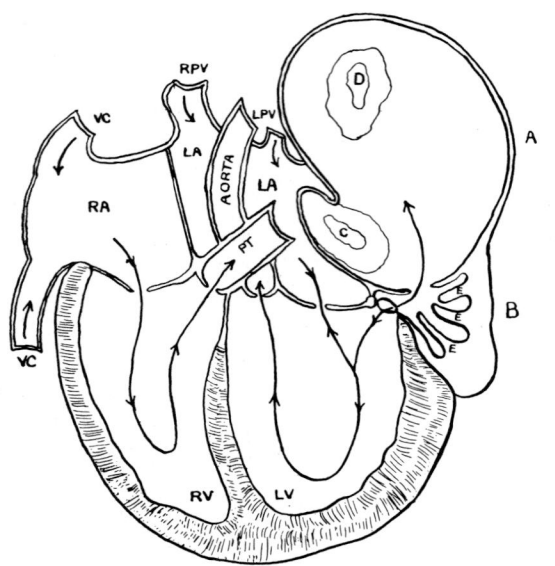

Figure 26.31. Duplication of the heart. **A,** Upper compartment. **B,** Lower compartment of the accessory heart. **C** and **D,** Fibrin-coated pockets. **E,** Trabeculae carnae (one of two known cases). (From Barnard PJ, Brink . Supernumerary chambers to the left heart. Brit Heart J 1956;18:309–319.)

defect in the portion of the diaphragm derived from the transverse septum. The presence of the large diverticulum prevents subsequent closure of the abdominal wall above the umbilicus.

According to Gowitt and Zaki (247), the diverticulum arises early in embryogenesis from an outpouching of the endomyocardium through a weak region in the left ventricular wall. Its exact etiology, however, remains unclear.

INCIDENCE

Congenital cardiac diverticuli are rare. They usually occur as part of a malformation syndrome that affects the medial thoraco-abdominal line (248). There have been approximately 80 cases of congenital cardiac diverticulum in the literature to 1988 (247). This, however, does not include the findings of Sanada et al. (249). These authors reported in 1989 that they had found 20 cases of left ventricular diverticula from 4300 consecutive angiocardiographic records (13 males and 7 females whose age ranged from 17 to 78 years with a mean of 52 ± 16 years).

ASSOCIATED ANOMALIES

Congenital diverticulum of the heart is often associated with thoracic or abdominal midline alterations and also

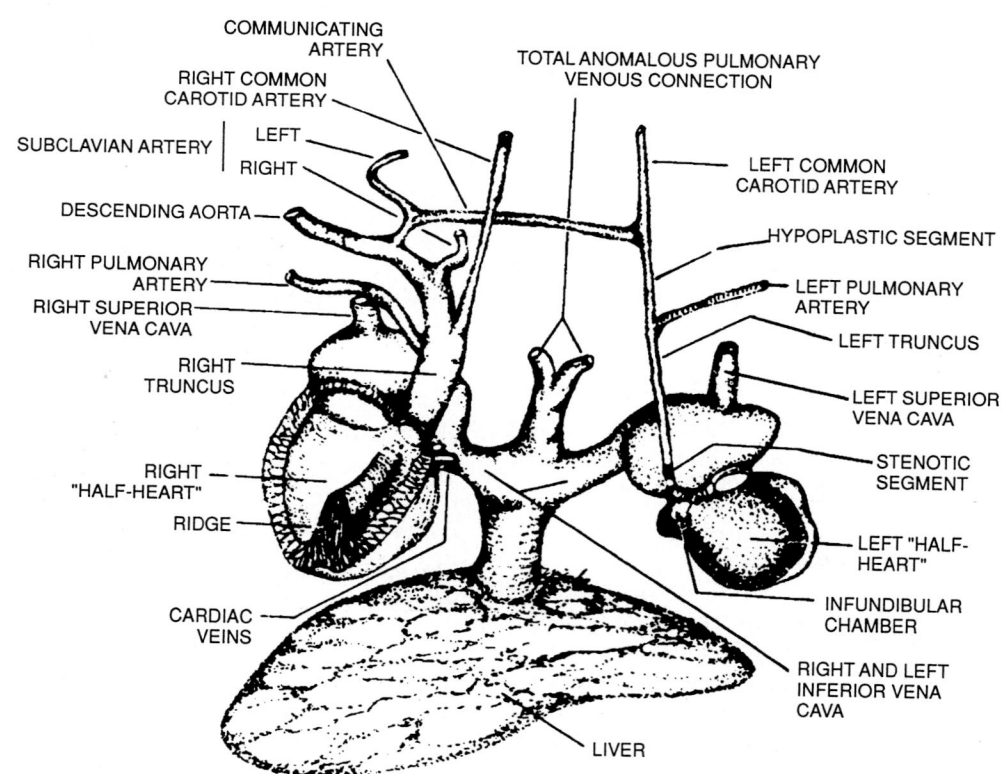

Figure 26.32. Schematic drawing of malformations. (From Aiello VD, deMorais CF, Ribeiro IG, Savaia N, Ebaid M. An infant with two "half-hearts" who survived for five days: a clinical and pathological report. Pediatr Cardiol 1987;8:181–6.

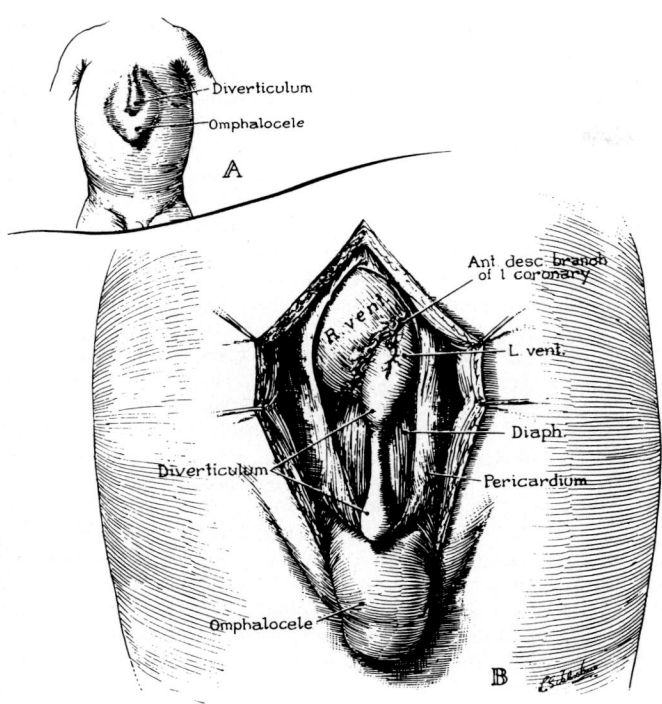

Figure 26.33. Diverticulum of the left ventricle with accompanying upper abdominal wall defect and omphalocele. (From Taussig HB. Congenital malformations of the heart, vol 2. Cambridge, Mass: Harvard University Press, 1960.)

with various types of cardiac and extracardiac malformations.

DIAGNOSIS

In most cases there is an umbilical hernia and a visible epigastric pulsation. The absence of a sternal defect, together with heart sounds in the normal location, will rule out ectopia cordis. The diagnosis may be made by cardiac catheterization and confirmed by magnetic resonance imaging. Angiography, scintigraphic imaging, or two-dimensional echocardiography also are recommended.

TREATMENT

Resection of the diverticulum, either as an isolated operation or at the time of correction of accompanying malformations, is the treatment indicated.

SOME OVERALL COMMENTS

Clark (personal communication, 1992) is right in stating that it is impossible to classify all defects due to etiologic heterogeneity and phenotypic variability. A genetic basis most likely plays a great role in congenital cardial anomalies; and, perhaps Taussig's theory of the evolutionary origin of isolated cardiac malformation is a sound pro-

posal. Clark states that there is increased evidence as to the genetic basis of congenital cardiovascular malformations. He cites that particular left-sided obstructive defects likely are single gene abnormalities with variable phenotypic expression.

The overall multiplicity of congenital anomalies with their pathologic physiology produce several syndromes which confuse the reader. The asplenia and polysplenia syndromes are vivid examples. The associated anomalies produce a cross fire of symptoms and signs in such a way that the reader, if unaware of the normal embryology, anatomy, and physiology of the heart, will find himself or herself in a terra incognita unable to understand the pathologic physiology of the problem. Names and syndromes test daily the neonatal cardiologist as well as the pediatric surgeon.

Without any further comments, we refer our readers again to the excellent table of Arnold on syndromes associated with congenital heart disease (Table 26.3).

The chapter of Neill (250) in the book *Genetics of Cardiovascular Disease,* edited by Pierpont and Moller, is excellent; and *Developmental Cardiology,* edited by Clark and Takao (62), is an excellent storehouse of information.

The multiplicity of cardiac malformations in the same newborn baby will occasionally dictate heart transplantation. We refer the reader to the paper of Chartrand et al. (251) and the paper of Chiavarelli et al. (252). The latter reported that neonatal transplantation of the heart is effective and durable for uncorrectable heart disease. There are excellent intermediate-term results: Of a total of 52 newborns who underwent heart transplantation, 90% survived the operation and 85% were late survivors.

REFERENCES

1. DeHaan RL. Morphogenesis of the vertebrate heart. In: DeHaan RL, Ursprung H, eds. Organogenesis. New York: Holt, Rinehart & Wiston, 1965.
2. Olivio OM. Précoce détermination de l'ébauche du coeur dans 1 embryon de poulet et sa différenciation histologique et physiologique in vitro. C R Assoc Anat (Prague) 1928;23:357–374.
3. Spratt NT. Location of organ-specific regions and their relationship to the development of the primitive streak in the early chick blastoderm. J Exp Zool 1942;89:69–101.
4. Rosenquist GC. Location and movements of cardiogenic cells in the chick embryo: the heart-forming portion of the primitive streak. Dev Biol 1970;22:461–475.
5. Mollier S. Die erste Anlage des Herzens bein den Wirbelteiren. In: Handbuch der Vergleichenden und experimentellung Entwickslungslehre der Wirbeltiere. O. Hertwig, ed. Jena: Gustav Fisher, 1906.
6. Butler E. The developmental capacity of regions of the unincubated chick blastoderm as tested in chorioallantoic grafts. J Exp Zool 1935;70:357–389.
7. Rawles ME. A study of the localization of the organ-forming areas in the chick blastoderm of the head-process stage. J Exp Zool 1936;72:271–315.
8. Rawles ME. The heart-forming areas of the early chick blastoderm. Physiol Zool 1943;16:22–43.

9. Rudnick O. Differentiation in culture of pieces of early chick blastoderm. I. Definitive primitive streak and head process stages. Anat Rec. 1938a;70:351–368. II. Short primitive streak stage. J Exp Zool 1938b;79:399–425.

10. Ebert JD. Analysis of the synthesis and distribution of the contractile protein, myosin, in the development of the heart. Proc Natl Acad Sci USA 1953;39:333.

11. Chiquoine AD. The distribution of polysaccharides during gastrulation and embryogenesis in the mouse embryo. Anat Rec 1957;129:495–515.

12. Mikawa T, Borisov A, Brown AMC, Fischman DA. Clonal analysis of cardiac morphogenesis in the chick embryo using a replication-defective retrovirus. I. Formation of the ventricular myocardium. Dev Dynamics 1992;193:11–23.

13. Noden DM. Origins and patterning of avian outflow tract endocardium. Development 1991;111(4):867–876.

14. Orts-Llorca F. Influence of the endoderm on heart differentiation during the early stages of development of the chicken embryo. Roux Arch Entw Org 1963a;154:533–551.

15. Orts-Llorca F. Influence de l'entoblaste dans la morphogénèse et la differenciation tardive du coeur du poulet. Acta Anat (Basel) 1963b;52:202–214.

16. Amano H, Fautrez J. Le rôle de la masse entoblastique dans la formation du coeur de l'urodèle. Arch Biol (Liege) 1962;73:193–204.

17. DeHaan RL. Organization of the cardiogenic plate in the early chick embryo. Acta Embryol Morphol Exp (Palermo) 1963;6:26–38.

18. Jacobsen AG. Influences of ectoderm and endoderm on heart differentiation in the newt. Develop Biol 1960;2:138–154.

19. Jacobson AG. Heart determination in the newt. J Exp Zool 1961;146:139–151.

20. Kuratani SC, Kirby ML. Initial migration and distribution of the cardiac neural crest in the avian embryo: an introduction to the concept of the circumpharyngeal crest. Am J Anat 1991;191(3):215–227.

21. Kirby ML, Waldo KL. Role of neural crest in congenital heart disease. Circulation 1990;82(2):332–340.

22. Le Lievre CS, Le Douarin NM. Mesenchymal derivatives of the neural crest: analysis of chimaeric quail and chick embryos. J Embryol Exp Morphol 1976;34(1):125–154.

23. Davis CL. Development of the human heart from its first appearance to the stage found in embryos of twenty paired somites. Contrib Embryol Carnegie Inst Wash 1927;19:245–284.

24. Stalsberg H, DeHaan RL. The precardiac areas and the formation of the tubular heart in the chick embryo. Develop Biol 1969;19:128–159.

25. Sabin FR. Studies on the origin of blood-vessels and of red blood-corpuscles as seen in the living blastoderm of chicks during the second day of incubation. Contrib Embryol Carnegie Inst Wash 1920;9:213–264.

26. Markwald RR, Mjaatvedt CH, Krug EL. Induction of endocardial cushion tissue formation by adheron-like, molecular complexes derived from the myocardial basement membrane. In: Clark EB, Takao A, eds. Developmental cardiology: morphogenesis and function. Mount Kisco, NY: Futura, 1990.

27. Markwald RR, Mjaatvedt CH, Krug EL, Sinning AR. Inductive interactions in heart development: role of cardiac adherons in cushion tissue formation. Ann NY Acad Sci 1990;588:13–25.

28. Markwald RR, Krug EL, Runyan RB, Kitten GT. Proteins in cardiac jelly which induce mesenchyme formation. In: Ferrans FJ, Rosenquist G, Weinstein C, eds. Cardiac morphogenesis. New York: Elsevier, 1985:60–69.

29. Davis CL. Development of the human heart from its first appear-

30. DeVries PA, Saunders JB de C H. Development of the ventricles and spiral outflow tract in the human heart: a contribution to the development of the human heart from age group IX to age group XV. Contrib Embryol Carnegie Inst Wash 1961;37:87–114.

31. Fales DE. A study of double hearts produced experimentally in embryos of Amblystoma punctatum, J Exp Zool 1946;101:281–298.

32. Van Praagh R, Ongley PA, Swan HJC. Anatomic types of single or common ventricle in man. Am J Cardiol 1964;13:367–386.

33. Baldwin HS, Solursh M. Degredation of hyaluronic acid does not prevent looping of the mammalian heart in situ. Dev Biol 1989;136(2):555–559.

34. Colvin EV. Cardiac embryology. In: Garson A Jr, Bricker JT, McNamara DG, eds. The science and practice of pediatric cardiology. Philadelphia: Lea & Febiger, 1990:88.

35. Grant RP. The embryology of the ventricular flow pathways in man. Circulation 1962;25:756–779.

36. Bremer JL. Presence and influence of two spiral streams in the heart. Am J Anat 1932;49:409–440.

37. Simons JR. Pulmonary return as an agent in the fetal development of the atrium in Rana temporaria. J Embryol Exp Morphol 1957;5:250–255.

38. Rychter Z. Experimental morphology of the aortic arches and the heart loop in chick embryos. Adv Morphol 1962;2:333–371.

39. Vernall DG. The human embryonic heart in the seventh week. Am J Anat 1962;111:17–24.

40. Licata RH. The human embryonic heart in the ninth week. Am J Anat 1954;94:73–125.

41. Born G. Beiträge zur entwicklungsgeschichte des säugetierherzens. Mikrosc Anat 1889;33:284–378.

42. Tandler J. The development of the heart. In: Keibel F, Mall FP, eds. Manual of human embryology. Philadelphia: JB Lippincott, 1912.

43. Odgers PNB. Formation of the venous valves, foramen secundum, and septum secundum in the human heart. J Anat 1936;69:412–422.

44. Patten BM. Persistent interatrial foramen primum. Am J Anat 1960;107:271–280.

45. Gassendi P. Elegans de septo cordis pervio observatio. Tallmadge GK (transl). Bull Hist Med 1939;7:429–457.

46. Savas V, Samyn J, Schreiber TL, Hauser A, O'Neill WW. Cor triatriatum dexter: recognition and percutaneous transluminal correction. Cathet Cardiovasc Diagn 1991;23:183–186.

47. Van Mierop LH. Introduction to congenital heart disease. Ann NY Acad Sci 1990;588:8–12.

48. Van Mierop LHS, Kutsche LM. Embryology of the heart. In: Hurst JW, Schlant RC, Sonnenblick EH, Wenger NK, eds. The Heart, 7th ed. New York: McGraw-Hill, 1990.

49. Streeter GL. Developmental horizons in human embryos: descriptions of age groups XV, XVI, XVII, and XVIII, being the third issue of a survey of the Carnegie collection. Contrib Embryol Carnegie Inst Wash 1948;32:133–203.

50. Kramer TC. The partitioning of the truncus and conus and the formation of the membranous portion of the interventricular septum in the human heart. Am J Anat 1942;71:343–370.

51. Grant RP. The morphogenesis of transposition of the great vessels. Circulation 1962;26:819–840.

52. Lev M, Saphir O. A theory of transposition of the arterial trunks based on the phylogenetic and ontogenetic development of the heart. Arch Pathol 1945;39:172–183.

53. Spitzer A. The architecture of normal and malformed hearts: a phylogenetic theory of their development. Springfield, I: Charles C Thomas, 1951.

54. Pernkopf E, Wirtinger W. Das wesen der transposition im gebiete des herzens, ein versuch der erklärung auf entwicklunsgeschichtlicher grundlage. Virchow Arch [A] 1935;295:143–174.

55. de la Cruz MV et al. An embryologic explanation for the corrected transposition of the great vessels. Am Heart J 1959;57:104–117.

56. de la Cruz MV, de Rocha JP. An ontogenetic theory for the explanation of congenital malformations involving the truncus and conus. Am Heart J 1956;51:782–805.

57. Wenink ACG. Embryology of the heart. In: Anderson RM, Macartney FJ, Shinebourne EA, Tynan M, eds. Pediatric cardiology. Edinburgh: Churchill Livingstone, 1987.

58. Clark EB. Cardiac embryology: its relevance to congenital heart disease. Am J Dis Child 1986;140:41–44.

59. O'Rahilly R. The timing and sequence of events in human cardiogenesis. Acta Anat 1971;79:70–75.

60. Tomita H, Connuck DM, Leatherbury L, Kirby ML. Relation of early hemodynamic changes to final cardiac phenotype and survival after neural crest ablation in chick embryos. Circulation 1991;84(3):1289–1295.

61. Kirby ML. Overview of problems and approaches in heart development. NY Acad Sci 1990;588:1–7.

62. Clark EB, Takao A. Overview: a focus for research in cardiovascular development. In: Clark EB, Takao A, eds. Developmental cardiology: morphogenesis and function. Mount Kisco, NY: Futura, 1990;3–12.

63. Clark EB. Growth, morphogenesis and function: the dynamics of cardiovascular development. In: Moller JM, Neal WA, Lock JA, eds. Fetal, neonatal and infant heart disease. New York: Appleton-Century-Crofts, 1989:1–14.

64. Hoffman JIE, Christianson R. Congenital heart disease in a cohort of 10,502 births with long-term follow up. Am J Cardiol 1978;42:641–647.

65. Mitchell SC, Sellman AH, Wesphal MC, Park J. Etologic correlates in a study of congenital heart disease in 56,109 births. Am J Cardiol 1971;28(6):653–657.

66. Nugent EW, Plauth WH, Edwards JE, Williams WH. The pathology, abnormal physiology, clinical recognition, and medical and surgical treatment of congenital heart disease. In: Hurst JW, Schlant RC, Sonnenblick EH, Wenger NK, eds. The heart, 7th ed. New York: McGraw-Hill, 1990.

67. Nora JJ, Nora AH. Etiology of congenital heart diseases revisted: genetic core lesions, genetic-environmental interactions, developmental mechanisms, and chance. In: Clark EB, Takao A, eds. Developmental cardiology: morphogenesis and function. Mount Kisco, Futura. 1990:549–556.

68. Hamilton DI. The surgery of congenital heart defects. In: Lister J, Irving M, Rickham PP, eds. Neonatal surgery, 3rd ed. London: Butterworths, 1990:319.

69. Esscher E, Michaelson B. Cardiovascular malformations in infant death: ten year clinical and epidemiological study. 1975;37:824–829.

70. Arnold R. Heart disease in the neonate. In: Lister J, Irving M, Rickham PP, eds. Neonatal surgery, 3rd ed. London: Butterworths, 1990:281.

71. Rosenthal A. Congenital cardiac anomalies and gastrointestinal malformations. In: Pierpont ME, Moller JH, eds. Genetics of cardiovascular disease. Boston: Martinus Nijhoff, 1986:113.

72. Vick GW, Titus J. Defects of the atrial septum including the atrioventricular canal. In: Garson A, Bricker JT, McNamara DG, eds. The science and practice of pediatric cardiology. Philadelphia: Lea & Febiger, 1990:1023–1054.

73. Feldt RH, Porter CJ, Puga FJ, Seward JB. Defects of the atrial septum and the atrioventricular canal. In: Adams FH, Emmanouilides GC, Riemenschneider TA, eds. Heart disease in infants, children

and adolescents, 4th ed. Baltimore: Williams & Wilkins, 1989:170–189.

74. Soto B, Pacifico AD. Angiography in congenital heart malformations. Mount Kisco, NY: Futura, 1990.

75. Mahoney LT, Truesdell SC, Krzmarzick TR, Lauer RM. Atrial septal defects that present in infancy. Am J Dis Child 1986;140(11):1115–1118.

76. Steele PM, Fuster V, Cohen M, Ritter DG, McGoon DC. Isolated atrial septal defect with pulmonary vascular disease: long-term follow-up and prediction of outcome after surgical correction. Circulation 1987;76(5):1037–1042.

77. Sneider AR, Serwer G. Echocardiography in pediatric heart disease. Chicago: Year Book Medical Publishers, 1990.

78. Murphy JG et al. Long-term outcome after surgical repair of isolated atrial septal defect. N Engl J Med 1990;323:1634–1650.

79. Gumbiner CH, Takao A. Ventricular septal defect. In: Garson A, Bricker JT, McNamara DG, eds. The science and practice of pediatric cardiology. Philadelphia: Lea & Febiger, 1990:1002–1019.

80. Snider AR, Serwer GA. Echocardiography in pediatric heart disease. Chicago: Year Book Medical Publishers, 1990:140–150.

81. Goor DA, Edwards JE, Lillehei CW. The development of the interventricular septum of the human heart: correlative morphogenetic study. Chest 1970;58:453.

82. Van Mierop LHS, Kutsche LM. Development of the ventricular septum of the heart. In: Lue H, Takao A, eds. Subpulmonic ventricular septal defect. Proceedings of the Third Asian Congress of Pediatric Cardiology. Tokyo: Springer-Verlag, 1986.

83. Langman J. Medical embryology, 3rd ed. Baltimore: Williams & Wilkins, 1975.

84. Mitchell SC, Berendes HW, Clark WM. The normal closure of the ventricular septum. Am Heart J 1967;73:334.

85. Abbott M. Atlas of congenital cardiac diseases. New York: American Heart Association, 1936.

86. Hoffman JIE, Rudolph AM. The natural history of ventricular septal defects in infancy. Am J Cardiol 1965;16:634–653.

87. Graham TP, Bender HW, Spach MS. Ventricular septal defect. In: Adams FH, Emmanouilides GC, Riemenschneider TA, eds. Heart disease in infants, children and adolescents. Baltimore: Williams & Wilkins, 1989:189–207.

88. Fyler DC. Ventricular septal defect. In: Fyler DC, ed. Nadas' pediatric cardiology. Philadelphia: Hanley & Belfus, 1992:435–457.

89. Weintraub RG, Menahem S. Early surgical closure of a large ventricular septal defect: influence on long-term growth. J Am Coll Cardiol 1991;18(2):552–558.

90. Moller JH, Patton C, Varco RL, Lillehei CW. Late results (30 to 35 years) after operative closure of isolated ventricular septal defect from 1954 to 1960. Am J Cardiol 1991;68(15):1491–1497.

91. Serraf A et al. Surgical management of isolated multiple ventricular septal defects. J Thorac Cardiovasc Surg 1992;103(3):437–443.

92. Backer CL, et al. Surgical management of the conal (supracristal) ventricular septal defect. J Thorac Cardiovasc Surg 1991;102:288–296.

93. Feldt RH, Porter C, Edwards WD, Puga FJ, Seward JB. Defects of the atrial septum and the atrioventricular canal. In: Adams FH, Emmanouilides GC, Riemenschneider TA, eds. Heart disease in infants, children and adolescents. Baltimore: Williams & Wilkins, 1989:170–189.

94. Becker AE, Anderson RH. Atrioventricular septal defects: what's in a name? J Thorac Cardiovasc Surg 1982;83:461–469.

95. Van Mierop LHS, Alley RD, Kausel HW, Stranhan A. The anatomy and embryology of endocardial cushion defects. J Thorac Cardiovasc Surg 1962;43:71–83.

96. Omeri MA, Bishop M, Oakley C, Bentall HH, Cleland WP. The

mitral valve in endocardial cushion defects. Br Heart J 1965;27:161–176.

97. Rastelli GC, Kirklin JW, Titus JL. Anatomic observations on complete atrioventricular canal with special reference to atrioventricular valves. Mayo Clin Proc 1966;41:296.

98. Piccoli GP et al. Morphology and classification of complete atrioventricular defects. Br Heart J 1979;42:621–632.

99. Piccoli GP, Wilkinson JL, Macartney FJ, Gerlis LM, Anderson RL. Morphology and classification of complete atrioventricular defects. Br Heart J 1979;42:633–639.

100. Soto B, Pacifico AD. Angiocardiography in congenital malformations. Mount Kisco, NY: Futura, 1990:163.

101. Wenink ACG, Gittenberger de Groot AC. The role of atrioventricular endocardial cushions in the septation of the heart. Int J Cardiol 1985;8:25–44.

102. Anderson RH, Ho SY. The developmental anatomy of atrioventricular septal defect. In: Clark EB, Takao A, eds. Developmental cardiology: morphogenesis and function. Mount Kisco, NY: Futura, 1990:575–592.

103. Vick WG, Titus JL. Defects of the atrial septum including the atrioventricular canal. In: Garson A, Bricker JL, McNamara DG, eds. The science and practice of pediatric cardiology. Philadelphia: Lea & Febiger, 1992:1023–1054.

104. Barber G, Chin AJ. Volume loads expect TAPVD. In: Long WA, ed. Fetal and neonatal cardiology. Philadelphia: WB Saunders, 1990:445–454.

105. Piccoli GP et al. Left-sided obstructive lesions in atrioventricular septal defects: anatomic study. J Thorac Cardiovas Surg 1982;83:453–460.

106. Newfeld EA et al. Pulmonary vascular disease in complete atrioventricular canal defect. Am J Cardiol 1977;39(5):721–726.

107. Driscoll DJ. Tricuspid atresia. In: Garson A, Bricker JT, McNamara DG, eds. The science and practice of pediatric cardiology. Philadelphia: Lea & Febiger, 1990:1118.

108. Rao PS. Tricuspid atresia. In: Long WA, ed. Fetal and neonatal cardiology. Philadelphia: WB Saunders, 1990:526.

109. Wenick ACG, Gittenberger-de Groot AC, Brom AG. Developmental considerations of mitral valve anomalies. Int J Cardiol 1986;11:85–98.

110. Rosenthal A, Dick M. Tricuspid atresia. In: Adams FH, Emmanouilides GC, Riemenschneider TA, eds. Heart disease in infants, children and adolescents, 4th ed. Baltimore: Williams & Wilkins, 1989:348.

111. Phornphutkul C, Rosenthal A, Nadas AS, Berenborg W. Cerebrovascular accidents in infants and children with cyanotic congenital heart disease. Am J Cardiol 1973;32:329.

112. Trusler GA et al. The cavopulmonary shunt: evolution of a concept. Circulation 1990;82(5):131–138.

113. Kobayashi J et al. Hemodynamic effects of bidirectional cavopulmonary shunt with pulsatile pulmonary blood flow. Circulation 1991;5(3):219.

114. Driscoll DJ et al. Five-to-fifteen-year follow-up after Fontan operation. Circulation 1992;82:469–496.

115. Bridges ND, Lock JE, Castenada AR. Baffle fenestration with subsequent transcatheter closure: modificarton of the Fontan operation for patients at increased risk. Circulation 1990;82:1681–1689.

116. Porter CJ. Ebstein's anomaly of the tricuspid valve. In: Garson A, Bricker JT, McNamara DG, eds. The science and practice of pediatric cardiology. Philadelphia: Lea & Febiger, 1990:1134–1144.

117. Van Mierop LHS, Kutsche LM, Victoria BE. Ebstein anomaly. In: Adams FH, Emmanouillides GC, Riemenschneider TA, eds. Heart disease in infants, children and adolescents, 4th ed. Baltimore: Williams & Wilkins, 1989:361–371.

118. Radford DJ, Graff RF, Neilson GH. Diagnosis and natural history of Ebstein's anomaly of the tricuspid valve in childhood and adolescence. Br Heart J 1985;54:517–522.

119. Watson H. Natural history of Ebstein's anomaly of the tricuspid valve in childhood and adolescence: an international cooperative study of 505 cases. Br Heart J 1974;36:417–427.

120. Benson LN, Child JS, Schwaiger M, Perloff JK, Schelbert HR. Left ventricular geometry and function in adults with Ebstein anomaly of the tricuspid valve. Circulation 1987;75:353–359.

121. Monibi AA et al. Left ventricular anomalies associated with Ebstein's malformation of the tricuspid valve. Circulation 1978;57:303–306.

122. Fontana ME, Wooley CF. Sail sound in Ebstein's anomaly of the tricuspid valve. Circulation 1972;46:155–164.

123. Lowe KG, Emslie-Smith D, Robertson PGC, Watson H. Scalar, vector, and intracardiac electrocardiograms in Ebstein's anomaly. Br Heart J 1968;30:617–629.

124. Amplatz K et al. The roentgenologic features of Ebstein's anomaly of the tricuspid valve. AJR 1959;81:788–794.

125. Shiina A et al. Two-dimensional echocardiographic spectrum of Ebstein's anomaly: detailed anatomic assessment. J Am Coll Cardiol 1984;3:356–370.

126. Rao SP. Other tricuspid valve anomalies. In: Long WA, ed. Fetal and neonatal cardiology. Philadelphia: WB Saunders, 1990:541–550.

127. Mair DD et al. Surgical repair of Ebstein's anomaly: selection of patients and early and late operation results. Circulation 1985;72:(Suppl 2):70–76.

128. Smith WM et al. The electrophysiologic basis and management of symptomatic recurrent tachycardia in patients with Ebstein's anomaly of the tricuspid valve. Am J Cardiol 1982;49:1223–1234.

129. Rao SP. Other tricuspid valve anomalies. In: Long WA, ed. Fetal and neonatal cardiology. Philadelphia: WB Saunders, 1990:548–548.

130. Lang D et al. Pathologic spectrum of malformations of the tricuspid valve in prenatal and neonatal life. J Am Coll Cardiol 1991;17(5):1161–1167.

131. Sharland GK, Chita SK, Allan LD. Tricuspid valve dysplasia or displacement in intrauterine life. J Am Coll Cardiol 1991;17(4):944–949.

132. Soto B, Pacifico AD, eds. Angiocardiography in congenital heart malformations. Mount Kisco, NY: Futura, 1990:339–343.

133. Cabrera A et al. Duplicación de la válvula tricúspide. Rev Esp Cardiol 1988;41:443–445.

134. Ikegaya T, Kutura C, Hayashi H, Muro H, Yamazaki N. A case of congenital tricuspid valve abnormality showing six leaflets. Eur Heart J 1991;12:94–95.

135. Child JS. Uhl's anomaly (parchment right ventricle): clinical echocardiographic, radionuclear, hemodynamic and angiocardiographic features. Am J Cardiol 1984;53:653.

136. Nugent EW, Plauth WH, Edwards JE, Williams WH. The pathology, abnormal physiology, clinical recognition, and medical and surgical treatment of congenital heart disease. In: Hurst JW, Schlant RC, Sonnenblick EH, Wenger NK, eds. The heart, 7th ed. New York: McGraw-Hill, 1990:655–794.

137. Cheatham JP. Pulmonary stenosis. In: Garson A, Bricker JT, McNamara DG, eds. The science and practice of pediatric cardiology. Philadelphia: Lea & Febiger, 1990:1394.

138. Gutgesell HP. Pulmonary valve abnormalities. In: Long WA, ed. Fetal and neonatal cardiology. Philadelphia: WB Saunders, 1990:551–560.

139. Riopel DA. Pulmonary valve atresia with intact ventricular septum. In: Garson A, Bricker JT, McNamara DG, eds. The science and practice of pediatric cardiology. Philadelphia: Lea & Febiger, 1990:1108–1117.

140. Rocchini AP, Emmanouilides GC. Pulmonary stenosis. In: Adams

FH, Emmanouilides GC, Riemenschneider TA, eds. Heart disease in infants, children and adolescents, 4th ed. Baltimore: Williams & Wilkins, 1989:308–338.

141. Maron BJ, Hutchins GM. The development of the semilunar valves in the human heart. Am J Pathol 1974;74:331–344.

142. Moore GW, Hutchins GM, Brito JC, Kemp H. Congenital malformations of the semilunar valves. Human Pathol 1980;11:367–372.

143. Oka M, Angrist A. Mechanism of cardiac valvular fusion and stenosis. Am Heart J 1967;74:37–47.

144. Gikonyo BM, Lucas RV, Edwards JE. Anatomic feature of congenital pulmonary valvular stenosis. Pediatr Cardiol 1987;8:109–115.

145. Soto B, Pacifico AD. Angiocardiography in congenital heart malformations. Mount Kisco, NY: Futura, 1990:507.

146. Caspi J et al. Management of neonatal critical pulmonic stenosis in the balloon valvotomy era. Ann Thorac Surg 1990;49(2):273–278.

147. Kirklin JW, Barratt-Boyes BG. Cardiac surgery. New York: John Wiley & Sons, 1986:829–832.

148. Kiefer SA, Lewis SC. Radiologic aspects of pulmonary atresia with intact ventricular septum. Br Heart J 1963;25:655–662.

149. Leung MP, Mok CH, Hui PW. Echocardiographic assessment of neonates with pulmonary atresia and intact ventricular septum. J Am Coll Cardiol 1988;12:719–725.

150. Smallhorn JF et al. Noninvasive recognition of functional pulmonary atresia by echocardiography. Am J Cardiol 1984;54(7):925–926.

151. Kutsche LM, Van Mierop LHS. Pulmonary atresia with and without ventricular septal defect: a different etiology and pathogenesis for the atresia in the 2 types? Am J Cardiol 1983;51:932–935.

152. Santos MA et al. Development of ductus arteriosus in right ventricular outflow tract obstruction. Circulation 1980;62:818–822.

153. Wenick ACG, Gittenberger-de Groot AG. Embryology of the mitral valve. Int J Cardiol 1986;11:75–84.

154. Wenick ACG, Gittenberger-de Groot AC, Brom AG. Developmental consideration of mitral valve anomalies. Int J Cardiol 1986;11:85–98.

155. Gittenberger-de Groot AC, Wenink ACG. Mitral atresia: morphological details. Br Heart J 1984;51:252–258.

156. Rudolph AM. Congenital diseases of the heart. Chicago: Year Book Medical Publishers, 1974:1–16.

157. Freedom RF. Hypoplastic left heart syndrome. In: Adams FH, Emmanouilides GC, Riemenschneider TA, eds. Heart disease in infants, children, and adolescents, 4th ed. Baltimore: Williams & Wilkins, 1989:515–517.

158. Norwood W, Lang P, Hansen D. Physiological repair of aortic atresia-hypoplastic left heart syndrome. N Engl J Med 23–26 1983;308:23–26.

159. Farrell PE et al. Outcome and assessment after the modified Fontan procedure for hypoplastic left heart syndrome. Circulation 1992;85:116–122.

160. Ruckman R, Van Praagh R. Anatomic types of congenital mitral stenosis: report of 49 autopsy cases with consideration of diagnosis and surgical implications. Am J Cardiol 1978;42:592–601.

161. Strasburger JF. Cor triatriatum pulmonary vein obstruction, supravalvar mitral stenosis, and congenital mitral valve disease. In: Garson A, Bricker JT, McNamara DG, eds. The science and practice of pediatric cardiology. Philadelphia: Lea & Febiger, 1990:1308–1315.

162. Nugent EW, Plauth WH, Edwards JE, Williams WH. The pathology, abnormal physiology, clinical recognition, and medical and surgical treatment of congenital heart disease. In: Hurst JW, Schlant RC, Sonnenblick FH, Wenger NK, eds. The heart, 7th ed. New York: McGraw-Hill, 1990:720–721.

163. Zweng TN et al. Mitral valve replacement in the first 5 years of life. Ann Thorac Surg 1989;47:720–724.

164. Almeida R et al. Surgery for congenital abnormalities of the mitral valve at the Hospital for Sick Children, London, from 1969–1983. J Cardiovasc Surg 1988;29:95–99.

165. Grifka RG, O'Loughlin MP, Nihill MR, Mullins CE. Double-trans-septal, double-balloon valvuloplasty for congenital mitral stenosis. Circulation 1992;85:123–129.

166. Sneider AR, Serwer GA. Echocardiography in pediatric heart disease. Chicago, Year Book Medical Publisher, 1990:224–228.

167. Haworth SG, Macartney FJ. Growth and development of pulmonary circulation in pulmonary atresia with ventricular septal defect and major aortopulmonary collateral arteries. Br Heart J 1980;44:14–24.

168. Shimazaki Y, Maehara T, Blackstone EH, Kirklin JW, Bargeron LM Jr. The structure of the pulmonary circulation in tetralogy of Fallot with pulmonary atresia: a quantitative cineangiographic study. J Thorac Cardiovasc Surg 1988;95(6):1048–1958.

169. Neches WH, Park SC, Ettedgui JA. Tetralogy of Fallot and tetralogy of Fallot with pulmonary atresia. In: Garson A, Bricker JT, McNamara DG, eds. The science and practice of pediatric cardiology. Philadelphia: Lea & Febiger, 1990:1073–1078.

170. Snider AR, Serwer GA. Echocardiography in pediatric heart disease. Chicago: Year Book Medical Publisher, 1990:150–153.

171. Soto B, Pacifico AD. Angiocardiography in congenital heart malformations. Mount Kisco, NY: Futura, 1990:353–376.

172. Groh MA et al. Repair of tetralogy in infancy: effect of pulmonary artery size on outcome. Circulation 1991;84(Suppl 5):206–212.

173. Kirklin JW et al. Morphologic and surgical determinants of outcome events after repair of tetralogy of Fallot and pulmonary stenosis: a two institution study. J Thorac Cardiovasc Surg 1992;103(4):706–723.

174. Gillette PC, Garson A Jr. Sudden cardiac death in the pediatric population. Circulation 1992;85(Suppl 1):64–69.

175. Mair DD, Edwards WD, Julsrud PR, Hagler DJ, Puga FJ. Pulmonary atresia and ventricular septal defect. In: Adams FH, Emmanouilides GC, Riemenschneider TA, eds. Heart disease in infants, children, and adolescents, 4th ed. Baltimore: Williams & Wilkins, 1989:289–301.

176. Benson LN et al. Surgical correction of pulmonary atresia and ventricular septal defect with large systemic-pulmonary collaterals. Ann Thorac Surg 1984;38:522–525.

177. Di Donato RM et al. Neonatal repair of tetralogy of Fallot with and without pulmonary atresia. J Thorac Cardiovasc Surg 1991;101(1):126–137.

178. Puga FJ, Leoni FE, Julsrud PR, Mair DD. Complete repair of pulmonary atresia, ventricular septal defect, and severe peripheral aborization abnormalities of the central pulmonary arteries. J Thorac Cardiovasc Surg 1989;98:1018–1029.

179. Sawatari K, Imai, Kurosawa H, Isomatsu Y, Momma K. Staged operation for pulmonary atresia and ventricular septal defect: new techniques for unifocalization. J Thorac Cardiovasc Surg 1989;98:738–750.

180. Haas GS, Laks H, Milgarter E. Pulmonary atresia with ventricular septal defect. In: Cardiac surgery: state of the art reviews. Philadelphia: Hanley & Belfus, 1989:425–443.

181. Fouron JC et al. Prenatal diagnosis and circulatory characteristics in tetralogy of Fallot with absent pulmonary valve. Am J Cardiol 1989;64(8):547–549.

182. Momma K, Ando M, Takao A. Fetal cardiac morphology of tetralogy of Fallot with absent pulmonary valve in the rat. Circulation 1990;82(4):1531–1532.

183. Emmanouides GC, Thanopoulos B, Siassi B, Feishbein M. "Agenesis" of the ductus arteriosus associated with the syndrome of

tetralogy of Fallot and absent pulmonary valve. Am J Cardiol 1976;73:403–409.

184. Lakier JR, Stanger P, Heymann MA, Hoffman JIE, Rudolph AM. Tetralogy of Fallot with absent pulmonary valve: natural history and hemodynamic considerations. Circulation 1974;50:167–175.

185. Rabinovitch M et al. Compression of intrapulmonary bronchi by abnormally branching pulmonary arteries associated with absent pulmonary valves. Am J Cardiol 1982;50:804–813.

186. Kirby ML, Turnage KL, Hays BM. Characterization of conotruncal malformations following ablation of "cardiac" neural crest. Anat Rec 1985;213:87–93.

187. Clark EB, Van Mierop LHS. Development of the cardiovascular system. In: Adams FH, Emmanouilides GC, Riemenschneider TA, eds. Heart disease in infants, children, and adolescents, 4th ed. Baltimore: Williams & Wilkins, 1989:9–10.

188. Roberts WC et al. Aortic valve atresia: a new classification based on necropsy study of 73 cases. Am J Cardiol 1976;37:753–756.

189. Bailey LL, Gundry SR. Hypoplastic left heart syndrome. Pediatr Clin North Am 1990;37(1):137–150.

190. Barber G. Hypoplastic left heart syndrome. In: Garson A, Bricker JT, McNamara DG, eds. The science and practice of pediatric cardiology. Philadelphia: Lea & Febiger, 1990;1316–1318.

191. Freedom RM. Hypoplastic left heart syndrome. In: Adams FH, Emmanouilides GC, Riemenschneider TA, eds. Heart disease in infants, children, and adolescents. Baltimore: Williams & Wilkins, 1989:515–517.

192. Ursell PC, Byrne JM, Fears TR, Strobino BA, Gersony WM. Growth of the great vessels in the normal human fetus with cardiac defects. Circulation 1991;84(5):2028–2033.

193. Kiel EA. Aortic valve obstruction. In: Long WA, ed. Fetal and neonatal cardiology. Philadelphia: WB Saunders, 1990:471–476.

194. Friedman WF. Aortic stenosis. In: Adams FH, Emmanouilides GC, Riemenschneider TA, eds. Heart disease in infants, children, and adolescents, 4th ed. Baltimore: Williams & Wilkins, 1989:224–243.

195. Shaner RF. Abnormal pulmonary and aortic semilunar valves in embryos. Anat Rec 1963;147:5–13.

196. Sharma BK et al. Supravalvar aortic stenosis: a 29-year review of surgical experience. Ann Thorac Surg 1991;51:1031–1039.

197. Doty DB. Supravalvar aortic stenosis. Ann Thorac Surg 1991;51:886–887.

198. Roberts WC. The congenitally bicuspid aortic valve: a study of 85 autopsy cases. Am J Cardiol 1970;26:72–83.

199. DeLeon SY et al. Conal enlargement for diffuse subaortic stenosis. J Thorac Cardiovasc Surg 1991;102:814–820.

200. Gewillig M, Daenen W, Dumoulin M, Van Der Hauwaert L. Rheologic genesis of discrete subvalvular aortic stenosis: a Doppler echocardiographic study. J Am Coll Cardiol 1992;19:818–24.

201. Borow KM, Glagov S. Discrete subvalvular aortic stenosis: is the presence of upstream complex blood flow disturbances an important pathogenic factor? J Am Coll Cardiol 1992;19:825–827.

202. Latson LA. Aortic stenosis: valvular, supravalvular, and fibromuscular subvalvular. In: Garson A, Bricker JT, McNamara DG, eds. The science and practice of pediatric cardiology. Philadelphia: Lea & Febiger, 1990:1334–1352.

203. Sans-Coma V et al. Bicuspid aortic and pulmonary valves in the Syrian hamster. Int J Cardiol 1992;34:249–254.

204. Fyler DC. Aortic outflow abnormalities. In: Fyler DC, ed. Nadas' pediatric cardiology. Philadelphia: Hanley & Belfus, 1992:493–512.

205. Rhodes LA, Colan SD, Perry SB, Jonas RA, Sanders SP. Predictors of survival in neonates with critical aortic stenosis. Circulation 1991;84(6):2325–2335.

206. Zeevi B, Keane JF, Castaneda AR, Perry SB, Lock JE. Neonatal critical valvar aortic stenosis: a comparison of surgical and balloon dilatation therapy. Circulation 1989;80(4):831–839.

207. DeBoer DA, Robbins RC, Maron BJ, McIntosh CL, Clark RE. Late results of aortic valvotomy for congenital valvar aortic stenosis. Ann Thorac Surg 1990;50(1):69–73.

208. Sullivan ID et al. Balloon dilatation of the aortic vavle for congenital aortic stenosis in childhood. Br Heart J 1989;61(2):186–191.

209. Brown JW et al. Surgical spectrum of aortic stenosis in children: a thirty-year experience with 257 children. Ann Thorac Surg 1988;45(4):393–403.

210. Douville EC, Sade RM, Crawford FA Jr, Wiles HB. Subvalvar aortic stenosis: timing of operation. Ann Thorac Surg 1990;50(1):29–33.

211. Freedom RM. Balloon therapy of critical aortic stenosis in the neonate - The therapeutic conundrum resolved? Circulation 1989;80:1087–1088.

212. Shaddy RE, Boucek MM, Sturtevant JE, Ruttenberg HD, Orsmond GS. Gradient reduction, aortic valve regurgitation and prolapse after balloon aortic valvuloplasty in 32 consecutive patients with congenital aortic stenosis. J Am Coll Cardiol 1990;16(2):451–456.

213. Turley K et al. Neonatal aortic stenosis. J Thorac Cardiovasc Surg 1990;99(4):679–683.

214. Putschar WGJ, Manion WC. Congenital absence of the spleen and associated anomalies. Am J Clin Pathol 1956;26:429–470.

215. Peacock TB. Malformations of the human heart, 2nd ed. London: J Churchill & Sons, 1866.

216. Rokitansky C. Doie Defecte der Schedewande des Herzens. Vienna: W Braumuller, 1875.

217. Spitzer A. Über den bauplan des normalen und missgebildeten Herzens: Versuch einer phylogenetischen Theorie. Virchow Arch [A] 1923;243:81–201.

218. Pernkopf E, Wirtinger W. Das Wesen der Transposition im Gebiete des Herzens, ein Versuch der Erklärung auf entwicklungsgeschictlicher Grundlage. Virchow Arch [A] 1935;295:143–174.

219. Shaner RF. Anomalies of the heart bulbus. J Pediatr 1962;61:233–241.

220. Van Mierop LHS, Wiglesworth FW. Pathogenesis of transposition complexes. II. Anomalies due to faulty transfer of the posterior great artery. Am J Cardiol 1963a;12:226–232.

221. Bartelings MM, Gittenberger-de Groot AC. Morphogenetic considerations on congenital malformation of the outflow tract. II. Complete transposition of the great arteries and double outlet right ventricle. Int J Cardiol 1991;33:5–26.

222. Kirby ML, Gale TF, Stewart DE. Neural crest cells contribute to normal aorticopulmonary septation. Science 1983;220:1059–1061.

223. Rashkind WJ, Miller WW. Creation of an atrial septal defect without thoracotomy: a palliative approach to transposition of the great arteries. JAMA 1966;96:991–992.

224. Wernovsky G, et al. Results of the arterial switch operation in patients with transposition of the great arteries and abnormalities of the mitral or left ventricular outflow tract. J Am Coll Cardiol 1990;16(6):1446–1456.

225. Menahem S, Ranjit MS, Brawn WJ, Mee RBB, Wilkerson JL. Cardiac conduction abnormalities and rhythm changes after neonatal anatomical correction of transposition of the great arteries. Br Heart J 1992;67:246–249.

226. Mayer JE, Sanders SP, Jonas RA, Castaneda AR, Wernovsky G. Coronary artery pattern and outcome of arterial switch operation for transposition of the great arteries. Circulation 1990;82(Suppl 5):139–145.

227. Braunstein PW, Sade RM, Gillette PC. Life-threatening postop-

erative junctional ectopic tachycardia. Ann Thorac Surg 1992;53:726–728.

228. Gewillig M, Cullen S, Mertens B, Lesaffre E, Deanfield J. Risk factors for arrhythmia and death after Mustard operation for simple transposition of the great arteries. Circulation 1991;84:(suppl 3):187–192.

229. Morris CD, Menashe VD. Twenty-five-year mortality after surgical repair of congenital heart defect in childhood. JAMA 1991;266(24):3447–3458.

230. Lev M. Pathologic diagnosis of positional variations in cardiac chambers in congenital heart disease. Lab Invest 1954;3:71–82.

231. Mullins CE. Ventricular inversion. In: Garson A, Bricker JT, McNamara DG, eds. The science and practice of pediatric cardiology. Philadelphia: Lea & Febiger, 1990:1233–1245.

232. Fyler DC. "Corrected" transposition of the great arteries. In: Fyler DC, ed. Nadas' pediatric cardiology. Philadelphia: Mosby–Year Book. 1992:701–706.

233. Snider AR, Serwer GA. Abnormalities of ventricular connection. In: Echocardiography in pediatric heart disease. Chicago: Year Book Medical Publishers, 1990:186–190.

234. Soto B, Pacifico AD. Atrioventricular discordant connection. In: Angiocardiography in congenital heart malformations. Mount Kisco, NY: Futura, 1990:239–271.

235. Ikeda U, Kimura K, Suzuki O, Furuse M, Natsume T. Long-term survival in "corrected transposition" [Letter]. Lancet 1991;337(8734):180–181.

236. Lundstrom U, Bull C, Wyse RKH, Somerville J. The natural and "unnatural" history of congenitally corrected transposition. Am J Cardiol 1990;65:1222–1229.

237. Di Donato RM, et al. Corrected transposition in situs inversus: biventricular repair of associated cardiac anomalies. Circulation 1991;84(Suppl 3):193–199.

238. Ilbawi MN et al. An alternative approach to the surgical management of physiologically corrected transposition with ventricular septal defect and pulmonary stenosis and atresia. J Thorac Cardiovasc Surg 1990;100:410–415.

239. Fales DE. A study of double hearts produced experimentally in embyros of *Amblystoma punctatum*. J Exp Zool 1946;101:281–298.

240. Barnard PJ, Brink AJ. Supernumerary chambers to the left heart. Br Heart J 1956;18:309–319.

241. Aiello VD, deMorais CF, Ribeiro IG, Savaia N, Ebaid M. An infant with two "half-hearts" who survived for five days: a clinical and pathological report. Pediatr Cardiol 1987;8:181–186.

242. Taussig HB. Evolutionary origin of cardiac malformations. J Am Coll Cardiol 1988;12:1029–1086.

243. Skapinker S. Diverticulum of the left ventricle of the heart. Arch Surg 1951;63:629–634.

244. Potts WJ, DeBoer A, Johnson FR. Congenital diverticulum of the left ventricle. Surgery 1953;33:301–307.

245. Lowe JB, Williams JCP, Robb D, Cole D. Congenital diverticulum of the left ventricle. Br Heart J 1959;21:101–106.

246. Peacock TB. Malformations of the human heart, 2nd ed. London: J Churchill & Sons, 1866.

247. Gowitt GT, Zaki SA. Rupture of a cardiac diverticulum resulting in sudden death. Am J Forens Med Pathol 1988;9:155–158.

248. Maroto C et al. Diverticulo cardiaco congenito con origen en ambos ventriculos. Rev Esp Cardiol 1991;44(5):351–354.

249. Sanada H et al. Two-dimensional echocardiographic and left ventriculographic evaluations of left ventricular diverticula. J Cardiol 1989;19:1107–1116.

250. Neill CA. Congenital cardiac malformations and syndromes. In: Pierpont MEM, Moller JM, eds. The genetics of cardiovascular disease. Boston: Martinus Nijhoff, 1987.

251. Chartrand C, Guerin R, Kangah M, Stanley P. Pediatric heart transplantation: surgical considerations for congenital heart diseases. J Heart Trans 1990;9:608–616.

252. Ciavarelli M, et al. Neonatal cardiac transplantation: intermediate-term results and incidence of rejection. Arch Surg 1992;127(a):1072–1076.

CHAPTER 27

THE CORONARY VESSELS

John Elias Skandalakis / Stephen Wood Gray / Mark E. Silverman

"Moreover, just as there are two arteries carrying blood to supply the heart with food and heat, so are there two veins, also called coronary from their roundabout course, which serve to bring the blood back again."
—RICHARD LOWER, TRACTATUS DE CORDE, 1669

DEVELOPMENT

As late as 1904 Lewis (1) stated that "nothing is known of the development of the coronary arteries." Lewis' own description of the contribution of the intramyocardial sinusoids to the coronary circulation, together with Bianchi's (2) description of coronary vessels in nonmammalian vertebrates, marked the beginning of understanding of the anatomy and embryology of these vessels. Grant (3) studied the formation of the coronary vessels in the rabbit and observed that the coronary veins appear before the coronary arteries. Most of our information rests on this work, that of Bennett (4) and that of Goldsmith and Butler (5) on pig embryos (Figs. 27.1 and 27.2).

The vascular system of the heart has three components. The first to appear is phylogenetically the oldest. In the fourth week, ridges in the ventricular walls develop into a system of muscular trabeculae, between and behind which are extensions of the ventricular cavity. These intertrabecular spaces or sinusoids of Minot reach the bulbus cordis anteriorly and the atria posteriorly; in depth, they extend nearly to the epicardium (Fig. 27.3, A). They increase in number, but decrease to little more than capillary size by the third month. Their small, persistent communications with the chambers of the heart are the thebesian veins.

About the middle of the sixth week, the middle cardiac vein appears as a outgrowth from the sinus venosus (coronary sinus). Veins spread over the epicardium from the right and left atrioventricular grooves and the posterior interventricular furrow. Branches spread over the myocardium and enter it to communicate with the intertrabecular spaces (Fig. 27.3, B).

By the end of the sixth week, the coronary arteries appear as endothelial sprouts from the left and right posterior quadrants of the bulbus cordis, as yet undivided into aortic and pulmonary trunks. Subsequent branching makes the arterial systems complete by the second month. The arterial branches tap the epicardial plexus of capillaries already formed by the veins, thus completing the coronary circulation (Figs. 27.3, C, and 27.4, A).

The coronary arteries and veins are essentially epicardial, with the myocardial vessels being derived from the primitive intertabecular spaces. Only in the interventricular septum do coronary arteries and veins penetrate deeply into the myocardium (Fig. 27.4, C).

Goor and Lillehei (6) stated that, in early embryologic development, vascular spaces are formed by consolidation of other intertrabecular spaces which are lined by endothelium and which are entrapped and form subendocardial and endocardial vascular plexus. The vascular plexus are connected with the aorta and also form sinusoids within the myocardium.

Suzuki et al. (7) believe that the formation of the truncal valve is independent of the formation of the coronary orifices—the reason being that among 22 hearts with four leaflets, there was a high incidence of coronary artery orifices in opposite sinuses (17:22, or 77.3%) and a low incidence of coronary arteries orifices in adjacent sinuses (2:22, or 9.1%).

The interested student will find useful information about major anomalies of coronary arteries in adulthood in a paper by Roberts (8). Landolt et al. (9) emphasized the importance of coronary artery anomalies in operations for congenital heart disease.

After studying 4250 patients without associated congenital heart disease, Engel et al. (10) reported major variations in anatomic origin of the coronary arteries which were discovered by angiography. The interested student will find very useful informations in this excellent paper.

Critical Events in Development

The single critical event in the formation of the coronary arteries occurs during the sixth week, with the partitioning of the truncus arteriosus. Deviations from the normal

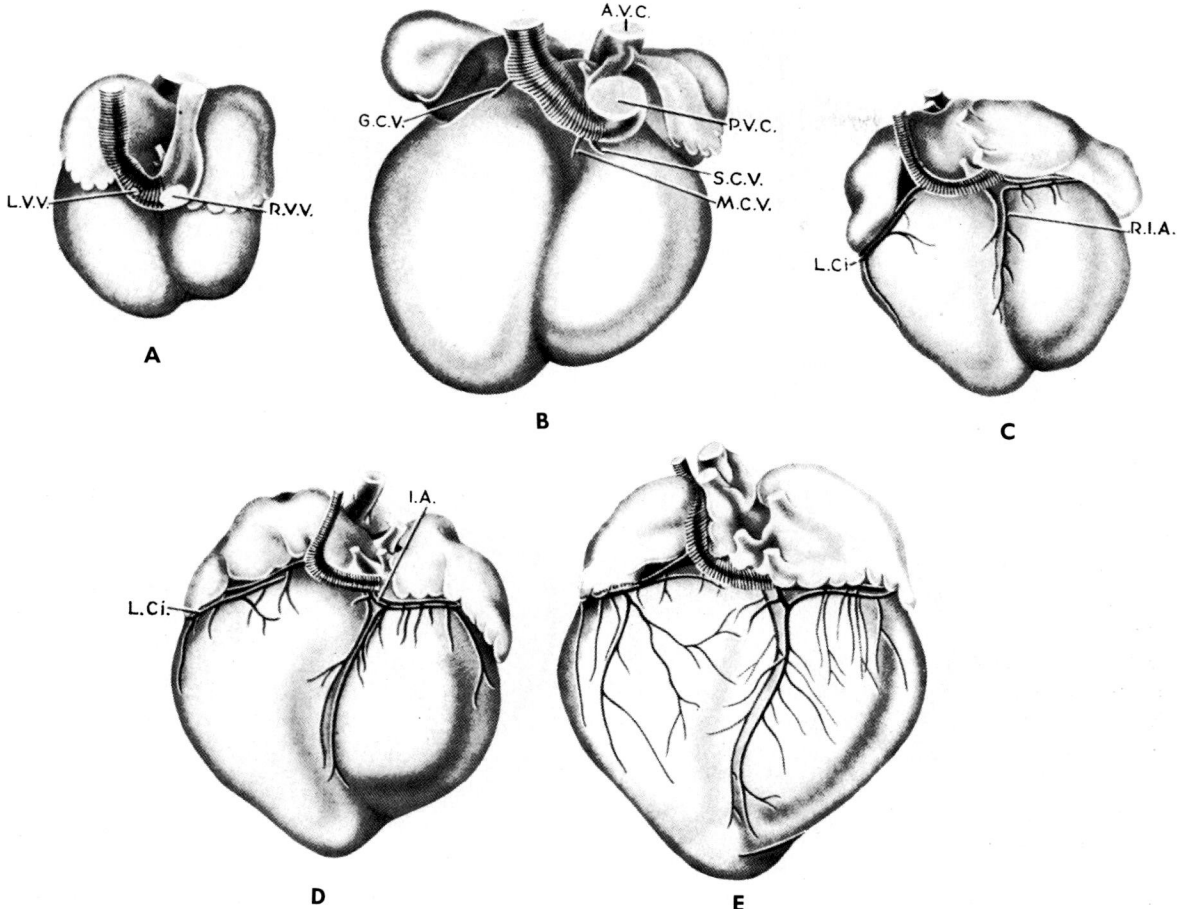

Figure 27.1. Development of the coronary vessels (posterior view, embryonic pig). **A,** The common cardinal veins; but no coronary veins are present (7-mm embryo). **B,** Left atrium displaced to expose the great cardiac vein; the origin of the great, middle, and small veins is apparent (12-mm embryo). **C,** The right coronary artery has reached the midline of the posterior surface and formed the posterior descending artery; from the left, the circumflex artery has extended to the posterior surface (20-mm embryo). **D,** Further development of the posterior descending branch of the right coronary artery (30-mm embryo). **E,** Almost complete adult pattern of coronary vessels (45-mm embryo). *LVV,* Left vitelline vein; *RVV,* right vitelline vein; *AVC,* anterior vena cava; *GCV,* great cardiac vein; *PVC,* posterior vena cava; *SCV,* small cardiac vein; *MCV,* middle cardiac vein; *LCi,* left circumflex artery; *RIA,* right interventricular (posterior descending) artery; *IA,* interventricular artery. (From Goldsmith, JB, Butler HW. The development of the cardiac-coronary circulatory system. Am J Anat 1937;60:185–201.)

pattern of partitioning may cause one of both coronary arteries to arise from the pulmonary trunk or may lead to the suppression of one of the two coronary arteries.

Coronary Circulation

Coronary circulation, arterial as well as venous, has been studied extensively since the first edition of this book. Coronary arteriography in newborns and adults presented new information about the anatomy of the coronary vessels, their origin, and their variations. About 30 years ago, Sones (11) presented selective coronary arteriography. It is now more than 60 years since Forssman (12) performed the first catheterization of the human heart. Fifteen years have passed since Gruentzig and colleagues (13, 14) reported on percutaneous transluminal coronary angioplasty.

ANOMALIES OF THE CORONARY VESSELS

The overall anomalies of coronary vessels and their circulation may be studied in Tables 27.1 and 27.2 and in Figure 27.5.

Variations of the Coronary Arteries

According to Davidson and Bashore (15), who reviewed the reports of coronary arteriography by Engel et al. (10)

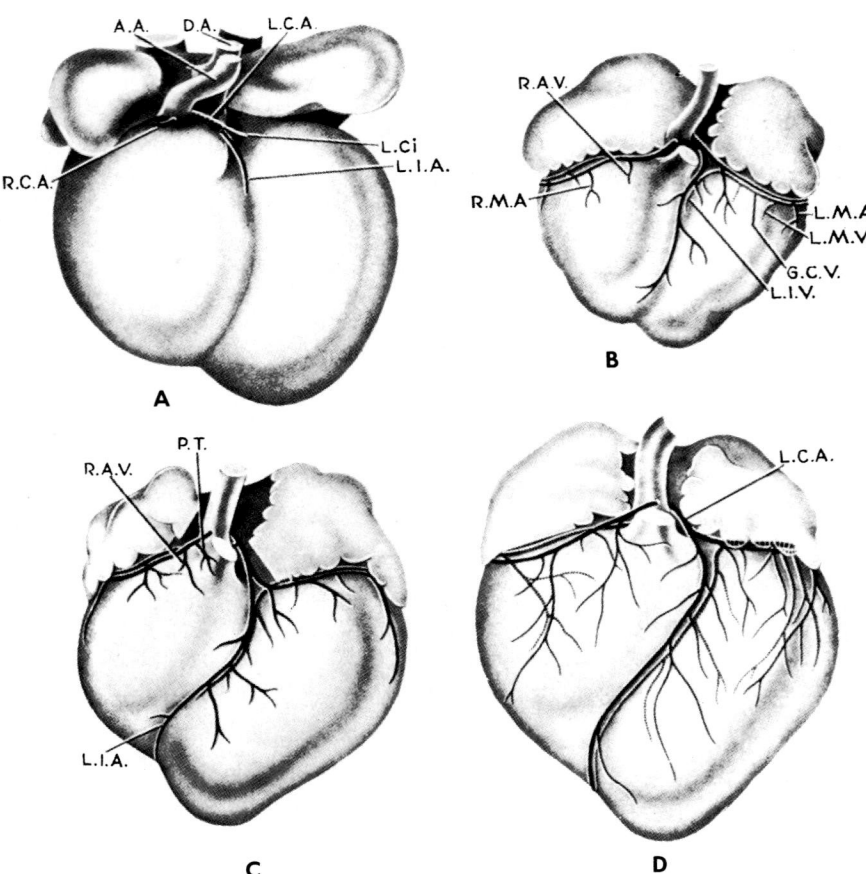

Figure 27.2. Development of the coronary vessels (anterior view, embryonic pig). **A,** Both coronary arteries are present; the left has branched to form the circumflex and anterior descending branches (12-mm embryo, same heart as Fig. 27.1, **B**). **B,** Further development of the coronary arteries; the great cardiac vein has reached the anterior surface and formed the left interventricular vein (20-mm embryo, same heart as Fig. 27.1, **C**). **C,** The anterior descending artery has reached the apex of the heart (30-mm embryo, same heart as Fig. 27.1, **D**). **D,** Almost complete adult pattern of coronary vessels (45-mm embryo, same heart as

Fig. 27.1, **E**). *AA,* Ascending aorta; *DA,* ductus arteriosus; *LCA,* left coronary artery; *RCA,* right coronary artery; *LCi,* left circumflex artery; *LIA,* left interventricular (anterior descending) artery; *RAV,* right anterior ventricular artery; *RMA,* right marginal artery; *LMA,* left marginal artery; *LMV,* left marginal vein; *GCV,* great cardiac vein; *LIV,* left interventricular vein; *PT,* pulmonary branch. (From Goldsmith JB, Butler HW. The development of the cardiac-coronary circulatory system. Am J Anat 1937;60:185–201.)

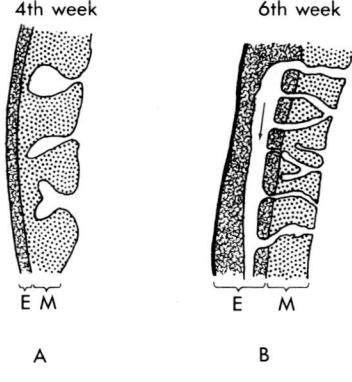

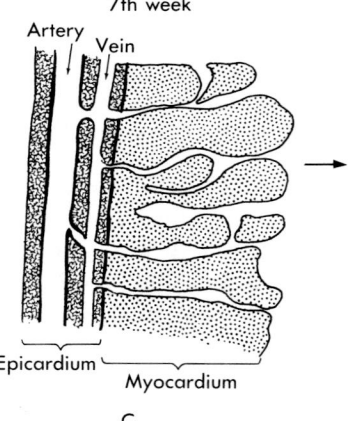

Figure 27.3. Development of the coronary vessels. **A,** Myocardial trabeculae and sinusoids, fourth week. **B,** Appearance of the coronary veins communicating with the greatly-narrowed sinusoids, sixth week. **C,** Appearance of the coronary arteries which tap the already established venous capillary plexus. Drainage is now either into the coronary sinus by way of the veins or into the ventricular lumen through the capillary-like sinusoids (thebesian veins).

Table 27.1.
Anomalies of the Coronary Vessels

Anomaly	Origin of Defect	First Appearance (or Other Diagnostic Clues)	Sex Chiefly Affected	Relative Frequency	Remarks
Accessory coronary artery	6th week	None	Equal	Common	
Single coronary artery	6th week	None	Equal	Rare?	
Pulmonary origin of both coronary arteries	6th week	At birth	?	Very rare	Fatal within days
Pulmonary origin of one coronary artery:					
Early phase, poor collateral circulation		At birth	?	Rare	May be fatal within weeks
Late phase, good collateral circulation		None	?	Very rare	May be suddenly fatal in childhood or in adulthood
Congenital coronary artery fistula	2nd month	None	?	Uncommon	

Table 27.2.
Congenital Anomalies of Coronary Circulation

Arterial	Venous
I. Anomalous origin	Enlargement of coronary sinus
A. From the aorta	Absence of coronary sinus
1. From contralateral sinus of Valsalva	Atresia of right ostium
Stenosis	Stenosis
2. Single coronary artery	Hypoplasia
3. Stenosis	
4. Atresia	
B. From the pulmonary artery	
II. Coronary arterial fistula	
III. Coronary artery aneurysm	
IV. Muscle bridge	

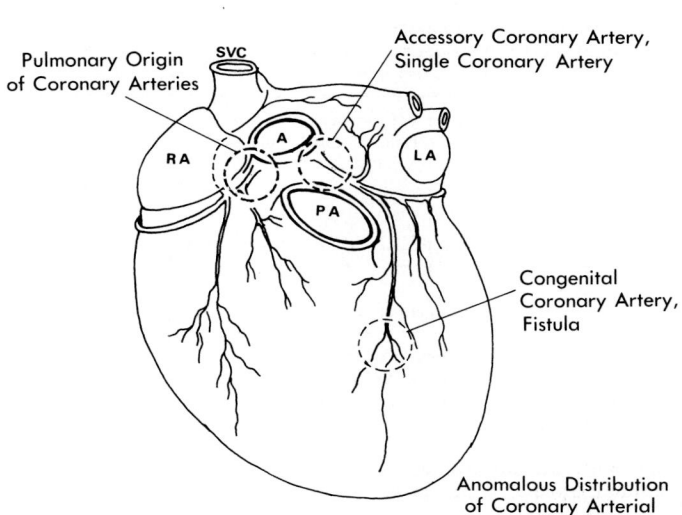

Figure 27.5. Sites of coronary artery anomalies.

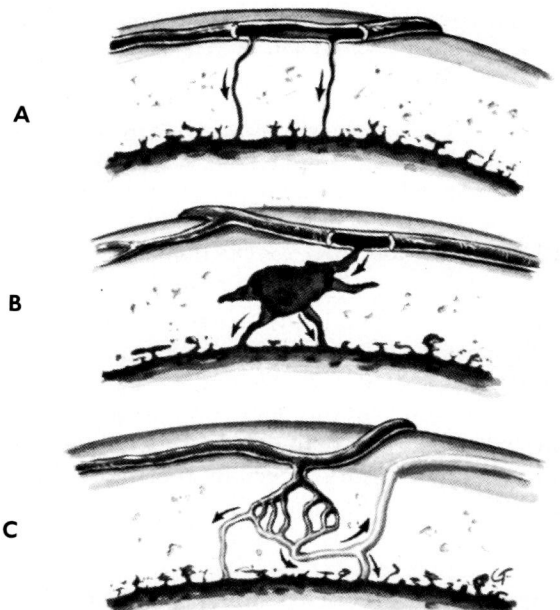

Figure 27.4. Types of coronary artery endings. **A,** Arterioluminal (directly through thebesian veins). **B,** Arteriosinusoidal (into remnants of the primitive sinusoids and thence through thebesian veins). **C,** In a capillary plexus, with drainage into either coronary or thebesian veins. (From Blake HA, Manion WC, Mattingly TW, Baroldi G. Coronary artery anomalies. Circulation 1964;30:927–940.)

and Chaitman et al. (16) consisting collectively of 8000 reported cases, the incidence of coronary anomalies is approximately 1%. The same authors classified coronary anomalies into two categories: minor and major (Table 27.3).

A very interesting work presented by Ogden (17) reports numerically the congenital variations of coronary arteries in 224 patients (Table 27.4).

An anomalous coronary artery may be totally asymptomatic or may produce symptoms if lack of coronary perfusion is present. An example is that of coronary arteries originating from the pulmonary artery.

Normally the left coronary artery arises from the left aortic sinus of Valsalva and divides into an anterior descending branch and a circumflex branch. The right coronary artery arises from the right sinus of Valsalva and passes to the right to anastomose with the circumflex artery and continues as the posterior descending branch, which anastomoses near the apex with the anterior

Table 27.3.
Anomalies of the Coronary Arteries[a]

Minor Anomalies
    Circumflex artery from the right coronary artery or right sinus of
       Valsalva
    Left anterior descending artery from the right coronary artery or
       right sinus of Valsalva
    Left main coronary artery from the right sinus of Valsalva
    Right coronary artery from the left sinus of Valsalva
    Right coronary artery from the posterior (noncoronary) sinus of
       Valsalva
    Single coronary artery
    Multiple coronary ostia
Major Anomalies
    Coronary artery fistulas
    Anomalous origin of the left or right coronary artery from the pul-
       monary artery
    Coronary artery atresia
    Coronary artery hypoplasia
    Congenital coronary artery aneurysms
    Congenital coronary artery stenosis

[a]From Davidson CJ, Bashore TM. Coronary arteriography. In: Sabiston DC Jr,
Spencer FC, eds. Surgery of the chest. Philadelphia: WB Saunders, 1990.

Table 27.4.
Congenital Variations of the Coronary Arteries in 224 Patients[a]

Congenital Variations	No. of Cases
Major coronary anomalies (75 cases)	
Coronary "arteriovenous" fistula[b]	31
Anomalous origin from the pulmonary artery	44
Left coronary artery	39
Right coronary artery	4
Both coronary arteries	1
Minor coronary variations (63 cases)	
High takeoff	2
Multiple ostia	6
Anomalous circumflex artery origin	14
Anomalous anterior descending artery origin	11
Absent proximal ostium/single ostium in other aortic sinus	10
Absent proximal ostium/multiple ostia in other aortic sinus	10
Hypoplastic proximal coronary artery	5
Congenital proximal stenosis	2
Congenital distal stenosis	1
Coronary artery from the posterior aortic sinus	1
Ventricular origin of an accessory coronary artery	1
Second coronary anomalies (86 cases)	
Secondary coronary "arteriovenous" fistula	3
Variations in transposition of the great vessels	65
Variations in truncus arteriosus	6
Variations in tetralogy of Fallot	4
Ectasia of coronary arteries in supravalvular aortic stenosis	5
Mural coronary artery	3

[a]Adapted from Ogden JA. Congenital anomalies of the coronary arteries. Am J
Cardiol 1970; 25:474.
[b]This category does not include cases of adult anomalous origin of the right or left
coronary artery from the pulmonary artery.

descending branch from the left. The first thorough study
of variations in this pattern was made in 1921 by Gross
(18).

Blake and his colleagues (19) found some variation of
the coronary orifice within the sinus of Valsalva.

Table 27.5.
Variations of the Coronary Orifice

Variation	Right (%)	Left (%)
Orifice at level of cusp margin	71	48
Orifice above level of cusp margin	19	34
Orifice below level of cusp margin	10	18

From Blake HA, Manion WC, Mattingly TW, Baroldi G. Coronary artery anomalies. Circulation 1964; 30:927–940.

The orifice has been said to be higher in cases of persistent truncus arteriosus and in some transpositions of
the great vessels. The superficial appearance of a coronary artery arising from the aortic arch is actually a
greatly reduced ascending aorta with aortic valvular stenosis. Such an aorta supplies only the coronary arteries
by retrograde flow from the patent ductus arteriosus (Fig.
27.6 and 27.7) (19).

In their compendium of human anatomic variations,
Bergman et al. (20) reported several interesting variations
of coronary vessels from the literature. A few examples
are the following:

1. A conus artery arising from the aorta was found in 50%
   of 651 subjects.
2. In 50% of hearts the right coronary artery supplied the
   sinoarterial and atrioventricular nodes. In 7% of hearts
   the left coronary artery supplied these nodes, and in 43%
   one artery (right or left) supplied one node or the other.
   The same authors quoted Spalteholz who stated that the
   sinoarterial node was supplied by the right coronary
   artery in 68%, by the left in 32%, and very rarely by an
   extracarotid artery.
3. "Large and direct" anastamosis of right or left coronary
   artery occurred in 9%. In most hearts, smaller anastomoses take place, and in 3% of hearts there is no communication between the right and left coronary artery.

ACCESSORY CORONARY ARTERIES

These are normal branches of the coronary arteries,
which arise independently from the aortic sinuses.
Strictly speaking, these arteries are not "accessory"; only
the openings from the sinus are accessory.

The first branch of the right coronary artery, the right
conus branch, may leave the aortic sinus independently to
form a right accessory artery in about 50% of human
hearts (21) (Fig. 27.8, A). Other normal branches may
also arise separately, usually on the right (22) (Fig. 27.8,
B).

The circumflex branch may arise independently of the
anterior (left) descending branch, from the same aortic
sinus, or even from the sinus giving rise to the right coronary artery (21) (Fig. 27.8, C).

From the statistics of Engel (10) and Chaitman (16),
one finds that the most common congenital variation is of

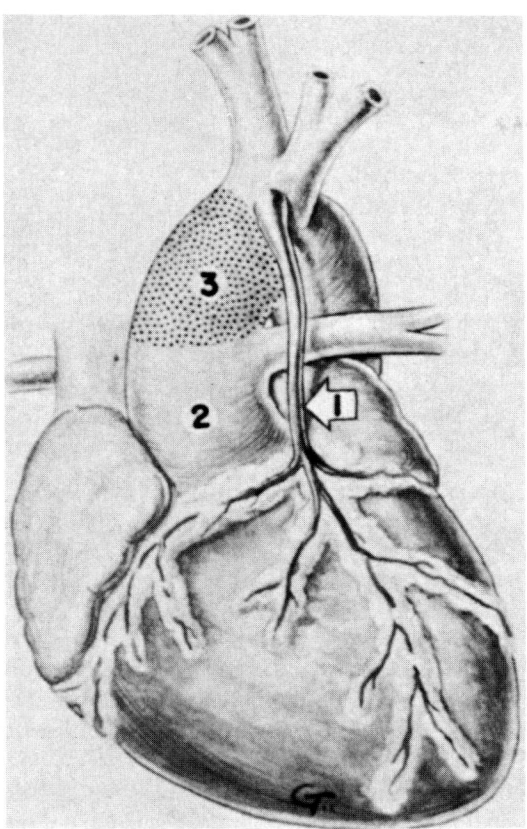

Figure 27.6. *Apparent high origin of a coronary artery. The vessel (1) is actually a partially transposed ascending aorta, with atresia of the aortic valve. The large vessel is composed of the pulmonary trunk (2) and the ductus arteriosus (3). Flow in the hypoplastic aorta is retrograde and supplies the coronary arteries only. (From Blake HA, Manion WC, Mattingly TW, Baroldi G. Coronary artery anomalies. Circulation 1964;30:927–940.)*

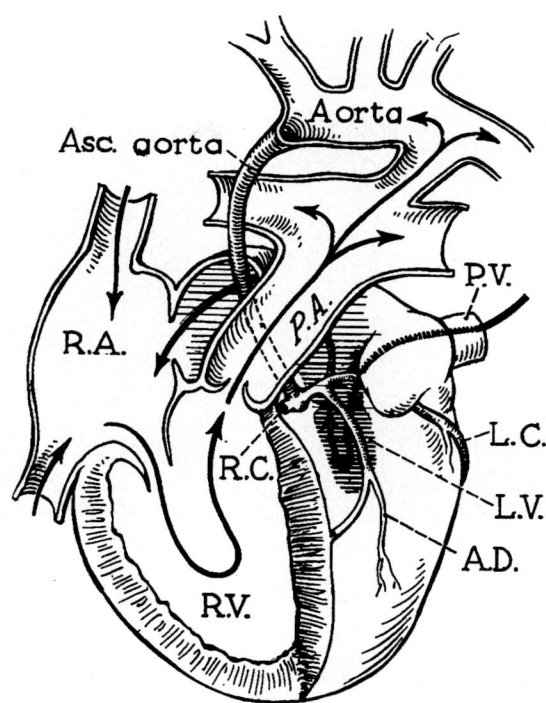

Figure 27.7. *Cardiac circulation in aortic valvular atresia. The left ventricle and the mitral valve are hypoplastic. L.C., Left coronary artery; A.D., anterior descending coronary branch; R.C., right coronary artery. (From Neufeld HN, Adams P, Edwards, JE, Lester RG. Diagnosis of aortic atresia by retrograde aortography. Circulation 1962;25:278–280.)*

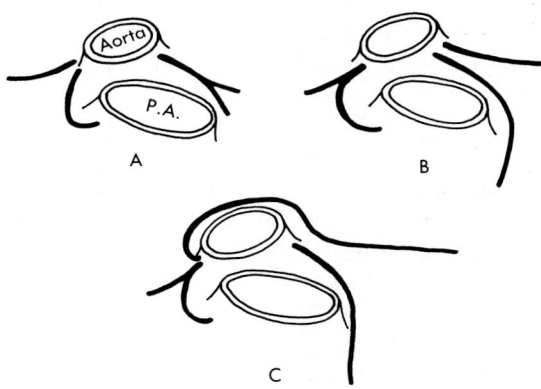

Figure 27.8. *"Accessory" coronary arteries. A, The right artery and its first branch (right conus artery) arise separately from the same aortic sinus. B, The circumflex and anterior descending arteries arise separately from the same aortic sinus. C, The circumflex artery arises from the same sinus as does the right artery. The left artery is represented by the descending branch only.*

the circumflex artery (0.5%), originating from the right coronary artery or the right coronary sinus (Figs. 27.9).

Liberthson et al. (21) reported aberrant coronary artery patterns in 21 cases (Fig. 27.10).

"SINGLE CORONARY ARTERY"

The first description of a single coronary artery was attributed to Thebesius (24) in 1716 by Smith (25). Three separate types of "single coronary artery" must be distinguished: fusion of right and left arteries; absence of right or left artery; and atypical single arteries.

According to Sharbaugh and White (26), both coronaries originate from a single ostium in 0.04% of cases and characteristically, the singularity is equal for the right or left coronary artery. In 40% of the cases there are other cardiac anomalies, and by the age of 40 years, 15% of cases with no other defects will have severe cardiac problems. Joswig et al. (27) reported that the occurrence between right and left coronary single artery is equal.

Patients with a single coronary artery may be asymp-

tomatic and have a normal prognosis. Sudden death due to myocardial ischemia or infarction has been reported (28, 29).

Fusion of Right and Left Arteries. In the mildest form of the anomaly, both right and left arteries arise from the same sinus of Valsalva by separate orifices (30) (Fig. 27.11, *A*). In other cases there is a common orifice leading to the

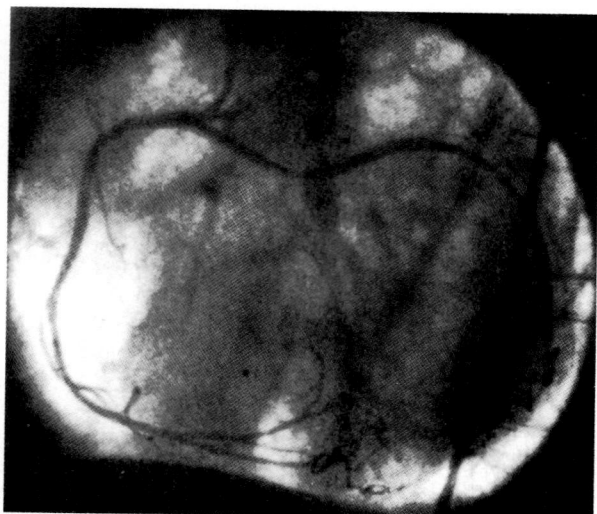

Figure 27.9.   Coronary arteriogram and diagram of the most common anomaly, which is in the left circumflex coronary artery *(LCX)* arising from the right sinus of Valsalva and coursing between the aorta and main pulmonary artery. *RCA,*

Right coronary artery. (From Davidson CJ, Bashore TM. Coronary arteriography. In: Sabiston DC Jr, Spencer FC, eds. Surgery of the chest. Philadelphia: WB Saunders, 1990.)

two vessels. Either the right or the left artery arises normally from the aorta and the other arises as a branch from it (Fig. 27.11, *B*). More often the left arises as a branch from the right. Smith (25) collected 17 cases. At least one surgical death has resulted from inadvertent sectioning of such an anomalous left coronary artery during ventriculotomy (31).

This type of single coronary artery has been found in 15% of rats from folic acid–deficient mothers (32).

Absence of Right or Left Artery.   This is an extreme case of right or left artery preponderance described later in this chapter. A single artery, usually the left, serves the entire heart, with the other vessel entirely lacking. There were 10 cases in Smith's series (25), all in adults (Fig. 27.11, *C*).

Atypical Single Arteries.   Smith (25) collected 15 cases in which a single coronary artery did not follow the pattern of either the normal right or the normal left coronary artery. Three cases occurred with cor biloculare and several with other cardiac malformations, but in three adults the heart was otherwise normal.

RIGHT OR LEFT CORONARY PREPONDERANCE

There is considerable individual variation in the extent of myocardium served by the two coronary arteries. Usually the right artery serves the right ventricle and part of the posterior surface of the left ventricle, while the left artery serves the remainder of the left ventricle (33) (Fig. 27.12). Schlesinger (34) classified the distribution into right preponderance (48%), left preponderance (18%), and "balanced" (34%). In right preponderance, the right artery extends past the crux to the left ventricle; in left preponderance, the left artery serves the entire left ventricle (Fig. 27.13). An earlier study by Gross (18) indicated a

larger percentage in the balanced group and fewer in the extreme groups. Schlesinger's autopsy studies suggest that the balanced group of individuals will suffer the least from the effects of coronary arteriosclerosis, while those with left coronary preponderance will suffer the most.

According to Bergman et al. (20) coronary artery preponderance occurs in about 30% of cases, with left coronary in 12% and right coronary in 18%. The same authors stated that left coronary artery dominance is eight times more frequent in males (18.2%) than in females (2.6%), while the right coronary artery preponderance is almost twice as common in females (23.1%) as in males (14.6%).

ORIGIN FROM THE CONTRALATERAL SINUS OF VALSALVA

Such an artery, to reach its anatomic territory and to fulfill its physiologic destiny, has to travel a long way from its origin, as follows: *(a)* cross over the base of the heart; and *(b)* pass the aorta or pulmonary artery anterior, posterior, or between, according to Kimbiris et al. (35) and Liberthson et al. (36).

Harrison and Baim (37) reported acute angulation of the proximal portion and compression between the great vessels.

Sudden death may take place from acute occlusion of the left main coronary artery due to compression between the aorta and pulmonary artery with exercise because of elevation of cardiac output (hypothetized by Libertson et al. [23]). Cheitlin et al. (38) reported a 27% sudden death rate in young patients when the left coronary artery originated from the right sinus of Valsalva. Kimbiris et al. (35) stated that the course is more benign with patients who have right coronary artery originating from the left sinus of Valsalva. According to Harrison and Baim (37), stenosis or atresia of the coronary ostium is a very rare anomaly, and only 7 cases are reported. The authors quote Levin et al. (39) and Byrum et al. (40).

MUSCLE (MYOCARDIAL) BRIDGE

This congenital anomaly was reported by Noble et al. (41) and Grondin et al. (42) as a myocardial bridging of the left anterior descending coronary artery. Anatomically, this is a muscular cord compressing the artery and producing a systolic compression, or "milking," as the above group of investigators reported.

The mural coronary artery, as Geiringer (43) called the intracardiac segments, is present in approximately 20% of autopsied hearts. According to Harrison and Baim (37), myocardial ischemia may be revealed by exercise. Symp-

toms do not start in early life but usually develop at middle age with angina pectoris.

Diagnosis. Diagnosis is made by angiography and thallium-210 myocardial perfusion scanning.

Treatment. Treatment is conservative, with oral propranolol therapy or surgery by bridge release or coronary bypass.

CONGENITAL CORONARY ARTERY ANEURYSM

Glickel et al (44) stated that this condition may occur in 1.5% of patients, with diagnosis by autopsy or coronary angiography. Number, size, or topography vary, but according to Befeler et al. (45), these anomalies occur more on the right coronary artery than the left. If not atherosclerotic, the patient is asymptomatic.

Treatment. Treatment consists of ligation and aortacoronary bypass.

MISCELLANEOUS ANOMALIES

The pattern and distribution of coronary arteries in hearts with complete transposition of the great vessels and with levocardia has been described in detail by Lev and his colleagues (46) and by Rowlatt (47). Absence of the atrial septum, or a defect of either the atrial or the ventricular septum, does not affect the normal pattern. The presence of a common ventricle or mixed levocardia produces a characteristic alteration of the coronary arterial pattern (see Fig. 27.14).

The origin of the right coronary artery from the descending thoracic aorta was diagnosed by angiographic studies and reported by Cheatham et al. (48). Gerlis et al. (49) reported three distinct coronary arterial anomalies: aneurysm of the left coronary artery; origin of the right

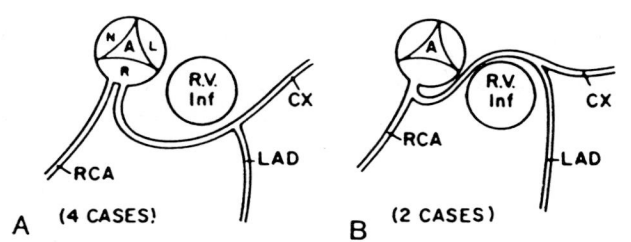
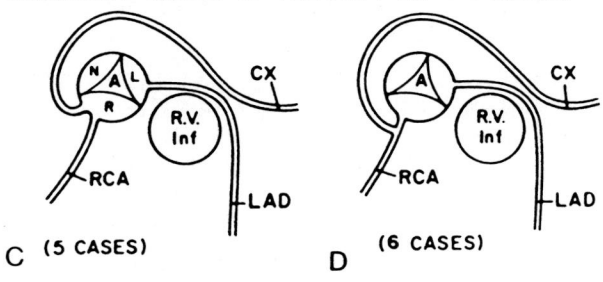
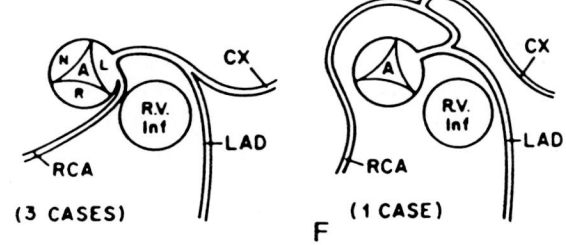

Figure 27.10. Schematic representation of aberrant coronary artery patterns. (A, Aorta; R.V. Inf, right ventricular infundibulum; R, right sinus of Valsalva; L, left sinus of Valsalva; N, noncoronary sinus.) *Numbers in parentheses* indicate the frequency of the aberrant pattern in this series of 21 cases. (From Liberthson RR et al. Aberrant coronary artery origin from the aorta. Circulation 1974;50:774.

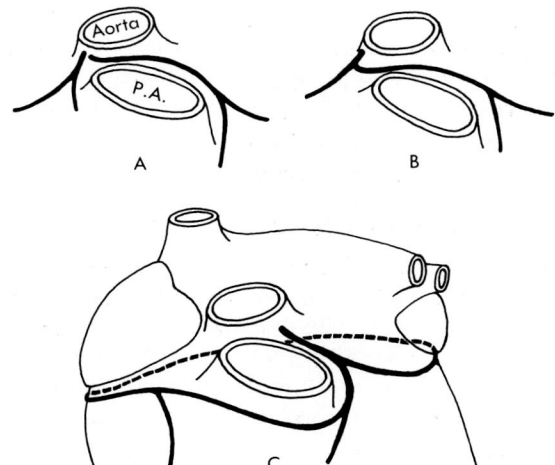

Figure 27.11. Types of "single" coronary artery. **A,** Fusion of right and left arteries. Each arises separately, but from the same aortic sinus. **B,** As in **A,** but with a common orifice. **C,** True absence of the right coronary artery. The entire blood supply is from the left artery.

coronary artery from the pulmonary artery; and a supernumerary coronary artery arising from the right ventricle.

EDITORIAL COMMENT

Increased application of the arterial switch operation to infants with transposition of the great arteries has resulted in an heightened awareness of coronary artery distribution because of the coronary transfer stage, which is critical for a successful operation. It is of great interest that transposition patients have favorably faced aortic and pulmonary artery sinuses of Valsalva no matter what the anteroposterior rotational relationship. This allows potential coronary transfer to the corresponding pulmonary artery (neoaorta) in virtually every case. There is, however, an embryologic consequence that causes an intramural course of a coronary artery. This type of coronary arises from the aorta; it makes an abrupt 90 degree turn within the wall of the aorta and exits as a well-formed coronary artery at some distance downstream from the internal orifice. These arteries are highly variable and may indeed traverse commissures. Embryologic developmental significance remains unclear (CM).

Pulmonary Origin of the Coronary Arteries

ANATOMY

During development of the truncus arteriosus, one or both coronary arteries may arise normally but communicate with a third artery. The left coronary artery is more commonly affected than is the right. Only eight cases were found in which both arteries arose anomalously (50). When both arteries originated from the pulmonary trunk, none of the affected infants lived more than a few days.

If collateral circulation from the normal artery does not reach the area served by the anomalous artery, myocardial ischemia occurs and death may result. This has been called the "infantile" type of the anomaly (51) (Fig. 27.15, A). If the collateral circulation is good, the myocardium is not ischemic; however, a left-to-right shunt may exist with retrograde flow in the artery arising from the pulmonary trunk (52) (see the discussion under "Congenital Coronary Artery Fistula," on page 967). This is designated the "adult" type (Fig. 27.15, B). Edwards (53) showed that these two conditions are not anatomic types, but instead are successive phases of the anomaly. If the patient survives the infantile ischemic phase, collateral circulation will develop, and the anomaly will become the adult type.

Ehren et al. (54) reported an association between common origin of the carotid arteries with anomalous origin of the left coronary artery from the pulmonary artery.

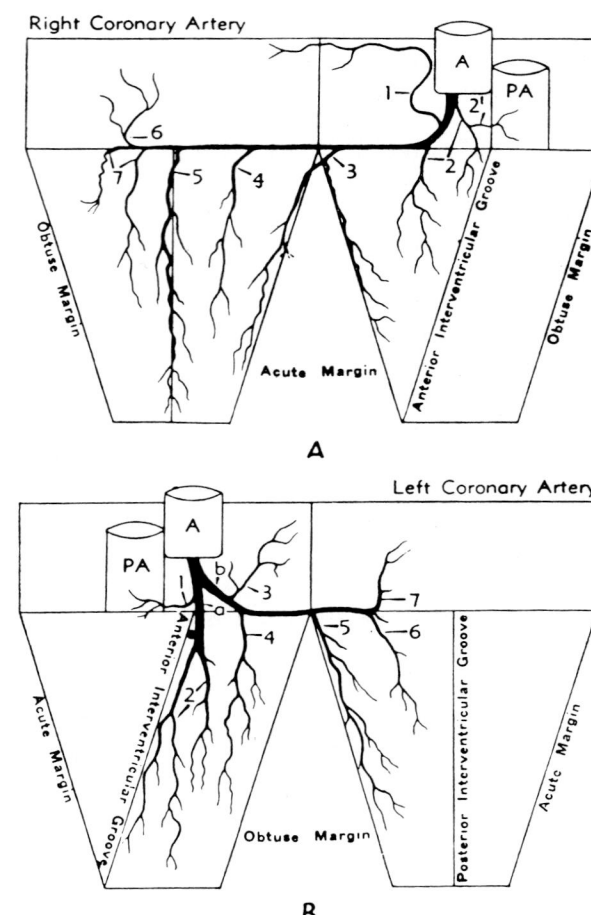

Figure 27.12. "Balanced" distribution of the right and left coronary arteries to the two ventricles. **A,** The right coronary artery and its branches. *1,* Anterior branch to the right atrium; *2,* anterior branches to the right ventricle—the first gives off the right conus branch (*2'*); *3,* branch to the acute margin; *4,* posterior branch to the right ventricle; *5,* posterior interventricular branch; *6,* posterior branch to the right atrium; *7,* posterior branches to the left ventricle. **B,** The left coronary artery and its branches. *1,* Left conus branch; *2,* left branches; *3,* anterior branch to the left atrium; *4,* anterior branch to the left ventricle; *5,* branch to the obtuse margin; *6,* posterior branch to the left ventricle; *7,* posterior branch to the left atrium; *A,* aorta; *PA,* pulmonary artery; *a,* anterior interventricular branch; *b,* circumflex branch. (From di Guglielmo L, Guttadauro M. Anatomic variations in the coronary arteries: an arteriographic study in living subjects. Acta Radiol (Stockh) 1954;11:393–416.)

EMBRYOGENESIS

The coronary arteries sprout from the left and right sides of the truncus arteriosus, before the aortic and pulmonary trunks become separated. If either artery arises more posteriorly than usual, or if the septum forms abnormally, one or both may be included in the pulmonary artery rather than in the aorta (55).

An alternative view was offered by Hackensellner (51). He stated that coronary arterial anlagen form behind each of the presumptive semilunar valve cusps in both pulmonary and aortic portions of the truncus, and all but two aortic primordia normally disappear. This view does not seem well supported by the evidence.

A third theory was proposed by Blake and his colleagues (19). They suggested that, because of the spiral form of the truncus septum, a vertical displacement of the coronary artery primordium might shift the origin of the vessel from the aorta into the pulmonary artery.

As there is no difference in the oxygen content of the pulmonary artery and the aorta before the lungs begin to function, the heart is not affected by this anomaly until after birth.

HISTORY AND INCIDENCE

Brooks in 1886 (57) described a right coronary artery arising from the pulmonary artery, and Abbott (58) described first the anomalous origin of the left coronary artery from the pulmonary. Abrikossoff (55) in 1911 reported a similar anomaly on the left. Not until 1934 did

Grayzel and Tennant (59) describe an anomalous origin of both arteries. Seventy-five infantile and sixteen adult cases were reported up to 1962 (60). Blake and his associates (19) reviewed all the anomalies of the coronary arteries.

It has been estimated that a coronary artery arises from the pulmonary artery once in 300,000 births and accounts for 0.5% of congenital cardiovascular disease (56).

SYMPTOMS

In the rare situation in which both coronary arteries originate from the pulmonary artery, the infant will develop cyanosis and dyspnea and will die within a few days unless pulmonary hypertension is present. Heifetz et al. (62) reviewed 25 infants in whom right and left coronary arteries originate from the pulmonary artery, reporting a survival rate of 9 hours to 7 years (63). When the right coronary artery alone originates from the pulmonary

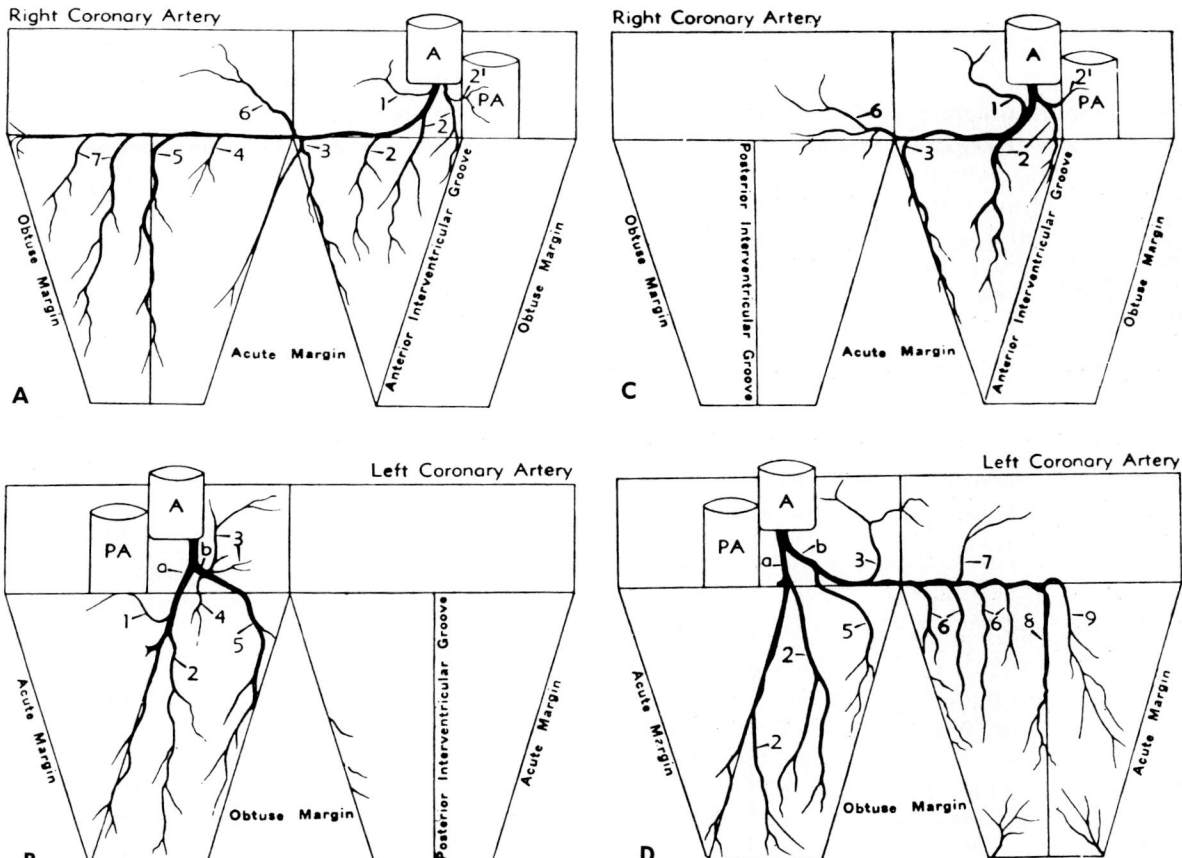

Figure 27.13. **A** and **B,** Preponderance of the right coronary artery. **A,** Distribution of the right artery. **B,** Distribution of the left artery. **C** and **D,** Preponderance of the left coronary artery. **C,** Distribution of the right artery. **D,** Distribution of the left artery. See Figure 27.11 for identification of symbols *1-7*. *8,* Posterior interventricular branch; *9,* posterior branch to the right ventricle. (From diGuglielmo L, Guttadauro M. Anatomic variations in the coronary arteries: an arteriographic study in living subjects. Acta Radiol (Stockh) 1954;41:393–416.)

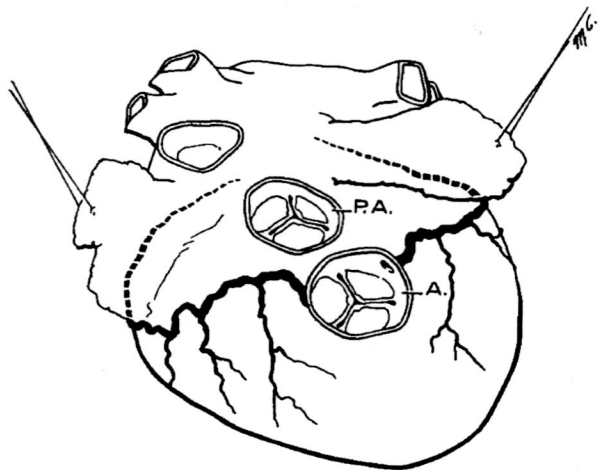

Figure 27.14. A single ventricle in which the septum has failed to form frequently exhibits a characteristic pattern of coronary arteries. There is no main anterior or posterior descending artery; numerous short descending branches are present anteriorly and laterally. A "bald" cardiac apex is highly suggestive of a single ventricle. The presence of transposition of the great vessels is incidental. (From Sherman FE. An atlas of congenital heart disease. Philadelphia: Lea & Febiger, 1963.)

artery, no symptoms usually occur. An anomalous origin of the left coronary artery from the pulmonary trunk is a more common malformation. This often presents in the first few months of life with paroxysmal attacks of distress, pallor, or sweating or evidence of heart failure. The anomaly may be silent until later in life when sudden death or myocardial infarction can occur.

DIAGNOSIS

Mitral regurgitation, secondary to papillary muscle dysfunction, is a common sign. Continuous murmurs may be present from collateral circulation. The diagnosis is usually made by an electrocardiogram which shows an anterolateral ST segment elevation or infarction. Echocardiography may be diagnostic.

TREATMENT

In the adult phase of the lesion, in which good collateral circulation has developed, ligation of the anomalous vessel will end the left-to-right shunt and increase the blood flow to the myocardium (Fig. 27.15, C). Heart failure in this phase is less the result of low oxygen tension in the artery than the result of low perfusion pressure. Ligation has been successful in nine infants, six children, and one adolescent. In all but one, a left-to-right shunt existed. Eleven infants have died following ligation (64).

In the infantile phase, with inadequate collateral circulation, the amount of shunted blood is small, and the difficulty lies in the lack of sufficiently oxygenated blood

to part of the myocardium. Ligation of the anomalous artery will merely produce ischemia and heart failure (60). Transplantation of the anomalous artery to the aorta or attachment of a systemic artery to the aorta or attachment of a systemic artery to the anomalous coronary artery appears to hold the greatest promise for effective treatment of these cases (61).

To summarize treatment, various surgical approaches have been tried when the left coronary artery rises from the pulmonary trunk. Ligation of the artery at its origin and a graft between the aorta and left coronary circulation is the most common approach (65, 66).

EDITORIAL COMMENT

The clinical significance of a pulmonary artery origin of a left or right coronary artery depends on the degree of intramyocardial collateralization to the contralateral artery. If diagnosed early, both the right and left coronary can be reimplanted to the aorta or connected to the systemic arterial circulation by a number of methods. Late diagnosis, especially in the case of a poorly collateralized anomalous pulmonary artery origin of the left main coronary artery, will result in myocardial infarction and severe dysfunction and will necessitate cardiac transplantation. Occasionally, an anomalous pulmonary artery origin of a coronary artery may be life-sustaining. I recently performed corrective surgery on a 12-year-old child with tetralogy of Fallot and acquired pulmonary atresia in which the only pulmonary artery flow came from left coronary collaterals to the right coronary artery, which arose anomolously from the pulmonary artery. She was kept alive by right coronary artery retrograde flow through capillaries and collaterals from the left coronary artery. As noted by the authors in the next section, coronary artery fistula can also act as a source of pulmonary artery flow in cyanotic patients with pulmonary atresia (CM).

Anatomy of the Abnormal (Fig. 27.16)

Origin of the Left Coronary Artery from the Pulmonary Artery. When the left coronary artery originates from the pulmonary artery, the right coronary artery arises from the aorta. The three courses of the left coronary artery are: (*a*) between aorta and pulmonary artery; (*b*) posterior to the aorta; and (*c*) anterior to the right ventricular outflow (Fig. 27.17).

Wesselhoeft et al. (67) studied 140 cases (67 of their own) both pathologically and pathophysiologically.

Treatment should establish good perfusion of the left coronary arterial territory. This may be accomplished by anastomosing the left coronary artery to internal mammary or subclavian artery. A synthetic graft or autologous vein between the aorta and the left anomalous coronary

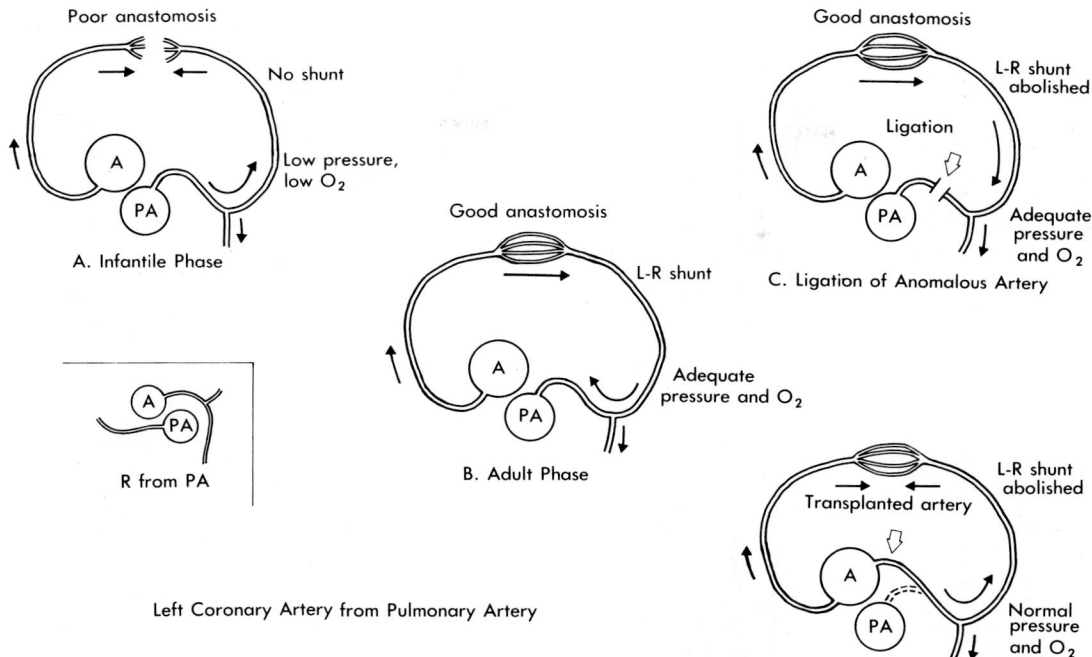

Left Coronary Artery from Pulmonary Artery

Figure 27.15. Pulmonary origin of the left coronary artery. **A,** *Infantile phase,* characterized by poor distal anastomosis, low pressure and poor oxygen supply to left ventricle, no shunt. **B,** *Adult phase,* with good distal anastomosis established resulting in a left-to-right shunt; pressure and oxygenation in left ventricle are adequate but below normal. **C,** Repair of the lesion by ligation of the anomalous left coronary artery. The shunt is abolished, but pressure and oxygen supply to the left ventricle are still below normal. **D,** Transplantation of the anomalous artery to the aorta; normal function is restored. *Inset,* A similar anomaly, with the right coronary artery arising from the pulmonary artery.

artery with subsequent ligation was reported by Arciniegus et al. (68). Older patients have a better prognosis than infants.

Origin of the Left Coronary Artery from the Right Aortic Sinus. The same treatment is suggested as stated above.

Origin of the Right Coronary Artery from the Pulmonary Artery. It is extremely rare for the left coronary artery to arise from the aorta. Treatment consists of implantation of the right coronary artery into the ascending aorta.

Origin of Both Right and Left Coronary Artery from the Pulmonary Artery. Total anomalous origin of the coronary arteries from the pulmonary artery is the rarest form of anomalies of the coronary arteries (62). There have been approximately 26 cases reported in the literature. None of the known attempts at surgical correction have been successful (62, 69).

Congenital Atresia of the Left Coronary Arteries. This condition was reported by Byrum et al. (40). The artery was hypoplastic. Mullins et al. (70) reported repair using saphenous vein graft.

Origin of the Circumflex Artery from the Right Aortic Sinus or Right Coronary Artery. According to Nugent et al. (71), this condition occurs in less than 0.5% of the general population. Conservative follow-up is the treatment of choice.

Anterior Descending Artery Originating from the Right Sinus of Valsalva by a Separate Ostium or from the Right Coronary Artery. This anomaly is associated with tetrology of Fallot (2%). It is a benign process but must be recognized and protected during surgical correction of tetralogy of Fallot.

Precapillary Fistula. A precapillary fistula may connect the right or left coronary artery with the coronary sinus, a cardial chamber, the superior vena cava, or the pulmonary artery (39).

Congenital Coronary Artery Fistula

ANATOMY

Blood from the coronary arteries normally passes through myocardial capillaries before draining into the coronary veins or through the thebesian veins into the heart. By developmental error, a branch of a coronary artery may open directly into the pulmonary artery or into a chamber of the heart. Such openings have been termed *coronary arteriovenous fistulae,* although the term is a misnomer when the opening is into the left chambers of the heart.

Either the right or the left coronary artery may be

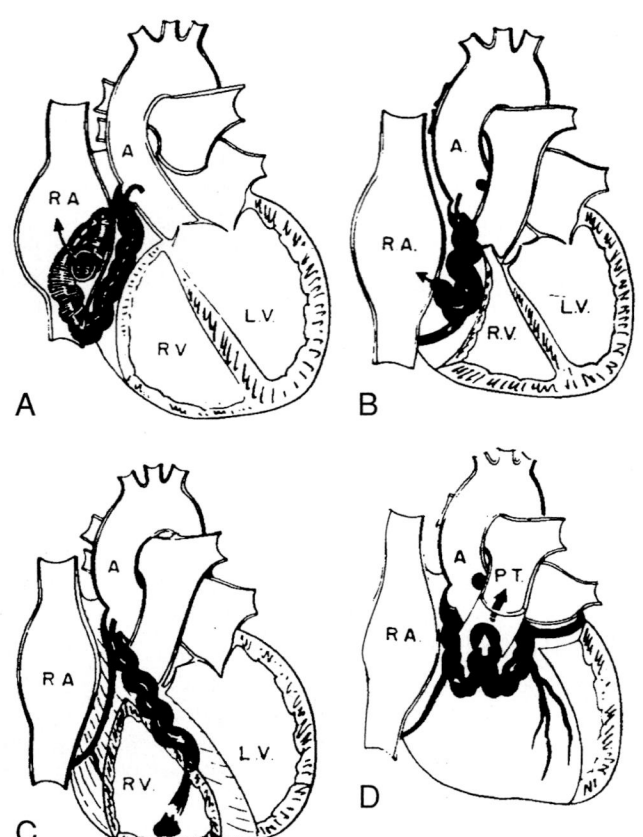

Figure 27.16. Anomalous communications of coronary arteries. **A,** Right coronary artery communicates with coronary sinus. **B,** Right coronary artery communicates with right atrium *(RA)*. **C,** Anomalous communication of right coronary artery with right ventricle *(RV)*. **D,** Two coronary arteries arise from the aorta *(A)* and make collateral communication with accessory coronary artery arising from pulmonary trunk *(PT)*. *LV,* left ventricle (From Nugent EW, Plauth WH, Edwards JE, Williams WH. Congenital heart disease: the pathology, abnormal physiology, clinical recognition, and medical and surgical treatment of congenital heart disease. In: Hurst, JW, ed. The heart. New York: McGraw-Hill, 1990.)

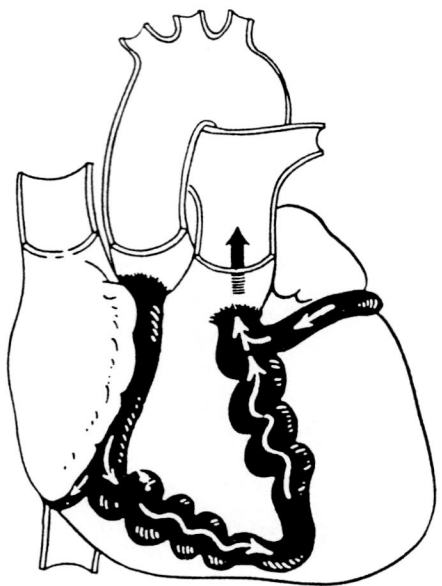

Figure 27.17. Anomalous origin of the left coronary artery from the pulmonary trunk. With time, wide collaterals develop between the two coronary systems, so that right coronary arterial blood is shunted into the left coronary system and thence into the pulmonary trunk (From Nugent EW, Plauth WH, Edwards JE, Williams WH. Congenital heart disease: The pathology, abnormal physiology, clinical recognition, and medical and surgical treatment of congenital heart disease. In Hurst JW, ed. The heart. New York: Mc Graw-Hill, 1990.)

involved, and the fistula may empty into any chamber of the heart, the coronary sinus, or the pulmonary artery. Figure 27.18 shows the location of fistulae from the series of Neufeld and his colleagues (72). Lowe et al. (73) studied the involvement of the arteries and the site of fistulous communication in 286 patients with congenital coronary artery fistulae. According to Dehner (74), the fistula is an uncommon anomaly, but fistulae between the right coronary artery and right ventricle occur more often. Cases have been reported by Lucas (75) and by Perry et al. (76). The incidence of bilateral fistulae was reported by Baim et al. (77) as 4 to 5% of all cases.

The most common coronary artery involved with a congenital coronary fistula is the left (56% of the cases), according to Lowe and colleagues (78) (Tables 27.6 and 27.7).

Harrison and Baim (37) presented the following statistics after tabulating the data from Levin et al. (39) and Roberts' (8) publications.

Right ventricle	41%
Right atrium	26%
Pulmonary artery	17%
Coronary sinus	7%
Superior vena cava	1%
Left atrium	5%
Left ventricle	3%

The most common communication is a solitary one, but rare cases of multiple communications have been reported by McNamara and Gross (79).

Pulmonary atresia with ventricular septal defect and coronary artery fistula were reported by Vigneswaran and Pollock (80), who stated that most of the blood reaching the lungs came through the fistulae.

Fistulous communications between a solitary coronary artery and the pulmonary arteries are the primary source of pulmonary blood supply in tetralogy of Fallot with pulmonary valve atresia, as reported by Pohl et al. (81).

Coronary artery fistula as a source of pulmonary circulation in pulmonary atresia and ventricular septal defect was reported by Bogers et al. (82).

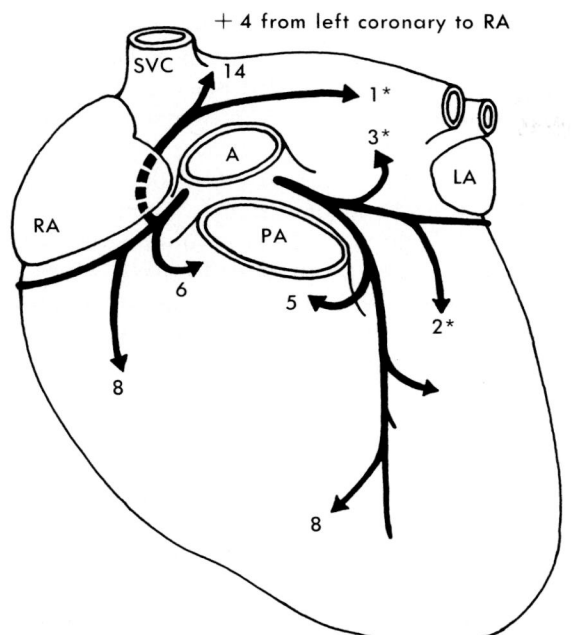

Figure 27.18. Sites of 51 coronary artery fistulae from the literature. Those occurring at sites marked with an *asterisk* produce an effect similar to aortic valve incompetence. At the other sites, a left-to-right shunt is produced.

Table 27.6.
Congenital Coronary Artery Fistulas—Involved Coronary Artery in 286 Patients[a]

	Percentage
Right coronary artery	56
Left coronary artery	36
Both right and left coronary arteries	5
Single coronary artery	3

[a]From Lowe JE, Oldham HN Jr, and Sabiston DC Jr. Surgical management of congenital coronary artery fistulas. Ann Surg 1981; 194:371.

Table 27.7.
Congenital Coronary Artery Fistulas—Site of Fistulous Communication in 286 Patients[a]

	Percentage
Right ventricle	39
Right atrium (coronary sinus, superior vena cava)	33
Pulmonary artery	20
Left atrium	6
Left ventricle	2

[a]From Lowe JE, Oldham HN Jr, Sabiston DC Jr. Surgical management of congenital coronary artery fistulas. Ann Surg 1981; 194:371.

Functional Complications. Coronary flow into the right heart (e.g.: both atrium and ventricle) or into the pulmonary artery acts as a left-to-right shunt. Liberthson et al. (36) reported 13 cases from the literature that indicated significant left-to-right shunt. The majority of fis-

tulae are of this type. Steinberg and his colleagues (83) measured the flow by catheterization in four patients and found that fistulae carried from 26 to 55% of the left ventricular output. "Coronary steal" is present when diastolic intracoronary pressure is low. There is no concrete evidence that it plays a role in myocardial ischemia.

The less common fistula to the left heart produces the effect of an incompetent aortic valve, increasing the work of the left ventricle. When the fistula opens into the left ventricle, the coronary run-off occurs only during diastole.

A fistula between the right coronary artery and the left atrium has been described by Augusti and his colleagues (84), who made a preoperative diagnosis by cineangiocardiography. Fistulae to a pulmonary vein (85) and to a persistent left superior vena cava (86) have also been reported.

The fistulous artery is tremendously dilated (up to 3.5 cm in one patient) and tortuous. It may have a saccular aneurysm, which occasionally reaches an immense size. The left ventricle is hypertrophic, and the aorta may be dilated. Depending on the size and duration of the shunt, the right ventricle may be dilated as well.

EMBRYOGENESIS

When the fistula is in a chamber of the heart, the anomaly results from the persistence of one or more large intertrabecular spaces, which would normally have become reduced to capillary diameter. This is a developmental arrest at the stage in which these spaces are large and communicate with the coronary arteries and with the chambers of the heart (about the second month). At least two cases are known in which the defect was not localized. The intertrabecular spaces remained large and in open communication with the heart chambers throughout the myocardium (87, 88). One infant so affected lived 14 months.

A different anomaly with a similar effect is represented by a fistula between the coronary and pulmonary circulation through an artery arising from the pulmonary trunk. Retrograde flow from the normal through the anomalous artery into the pulmonary artery provides the shunt (52) (see the section on "Pulmonary Origin of the Coronary Arteries").

HISTORY AND INCIDENCE

Krause (89) described the first coronary artery fistula, according to Lowe and Sabiston (78), who stated that approximately 400 more cases have been reported in the literature. In 1911 Trevor (90) described a coronary fistula to the right ventricle vein. In 1958 Steinberg and his colleagues (83) were able to find only 22 cases in the literature. As a result of their review—and that of Gasul and his associates, who collected 45 cases in 1960 (91)—

an increasing number of cases have been recognized. Coronary artery fistula can no longer be considered an anatomic rarity. Indeed, Hallman and his colleagues (92) considered it to be the most common of coronary artery anomalies.

The first successful closure of a fistula was performed in 1947 by Biorck and Crafoord (93). By 1961 there were at least 19 cases of operative repair in the literature (94).

Liberthson et al. (36) stated that 53% of such patients were 20 years of age or younger at the time of diagnosis.

SYMPTOMS

Patients are typically asymptomatic. If a large shunt is present, the patient may experience dyspnea, fatigue, or heart failure. Myocardial ischemia or infarction and sudden death have been described (95-98). Potentially, symptoms might arise from pulmonary hypertension or myocardial ischemia. Rupture of the aneurysm, when present, remains a threat throughout life.

Daniel et al. (99) presented manifestations of coronary fistula without any other cardiac anomalies in the form of a table (Table 27.8).

DIAGNOSIS

The diagnosis is entertained when a continuous murmur is noted along the right or left sternal border in an acyanotic, asymptomatic person. The best site for auscultation will vary depending on the location of the chamber into which the fistula drains (95, 98). X-ray examination and electrocardiogram are of little help. The echocardiogram may show the course, and site of drainage of fistula (98). An angiographic examination is usually the definitive diagnostic procedure.

TREATMENT

Treatment is often indicated because of the size of the shunt, the risk of endocarditis, or the possibility of rupture. The fistula is usually corrected by ligation.

Table 27.8.
Major Presenting Clinical Manifestations of Coronary Artery Fistulas when Present as Sole Cardiac Anomaly[a]

	No. of Cases	Percentage of Total
Asymptomatic murmur	67	45
Dyspnea on exertion; fatigue	34	22
Congestive heart failure	21	14
Angina or nonspecific chest pain	10	7
Bacterial endocarditis	9	6
Frequent upper respiratory tract infections	9	6
TOTAL	150	100

[a]From Daniel TM, Graham TP, Sabiston DC Jr. Coronary artery-right ventricular fistula with congestive heart faiure: surgical correction in the neonatal period. Surgery 1970; 67:985.

Ligation and division of the artery as close to the fistula as possible is the treatment of choice. Hallman and his colleagues (92) recommended placing mattress sutures between the artery and the ventricular wall to close the fistula. If an aneurysm is present, it should be excised. Temporary occlusion of blood flow before ligation will determine the extent of the myocardial ischemia produced by the ligation. Unless the shunt is very large, the operation should be considered elective (100).

Urrutia et al. (101) obliterated the fistula under the coronary artery with obliterating mattress sutures. They reported 58 cases with good results.

Anomalies of the Coronary Veins

The normal anatomy and variation of the coronary veins have not been extensively investigated. Coronary venography in humans by Gensini et al. (102) increased our knowledge of the anatomy, variations, and perhaps the pathophysiology of the coronary venous system.

Twenty years later, Hutchins et al. (103), using angiography, reported that the heart has more veins than arteries. The same authors think that, if cardiac ischemia is present, this plethora of veins will prevent metabolic end products. It is probable that in the absence of other cardiac malformations, no disability arises from venous anomalies alone.

The oblique vein of the left atrium represents the proximal portion of the left superior vena cava. In the presence of a persistent left superior vena cava, it may be said to receive the great cardiac vein before entering the coronary sinus (see Chapter 29). Atresia of the coronary sinus may force the coronary drainage through a persistent left superior vena cava to the innominate artery and into the systemic venous return (104) or, more directly, into the left atrium (105).

Variations of the thebesian valves at the orifice of the coronary sinus appear to affect the ease with which the sinus may be reached by an intracardiac catheter. In about 50% of hearts examined, catheterization should be easy; in 25%, the valve structure renders it impossible. A relationship between heart failure and a large coronary sinus orifice has been claimed (106).

The congenital anomalies of the coronary sinus, such as enlargement, absence, atresia, or hypoplasia as reported by Mantini et al. (107), are anomalies associated very closely with those of the superior vena cava and inferior vena cava, with the most common cause being persistent superior vena cava converted to the coronary sinus (Table 27.9).

Coronary sinus septal defect associated with tricuspid atresia was reported by Rumisek et al. (108). Two of ten patients with tricuspid atresia who underwent the Fontan procedure were noted to have coronary sinus septal

Table 27.9.
Coronary Sinus Anomalies

Absence	Left superior vena cava communicating with the left atrium or with the left side of the common atrium
Atresia	Blood to the persistent left superior vena cava or by multiple connection to the atria
Enlargement	Persistent left superior vena cava connected to the coronary sinus (most common) or left vena cava continuous with left superior vena cava by way of hemizygous
Hypoplasia	

defects in the early postoperative period. The authors suggest recognition prior to surgery and selective closure during the operation.

REFERENCES

1. Lewis F T. The intra-embryonic blood-vessels of rabbits from 8½ to 13 days. Am J Anat 1904;3:12–13.
2. Bianchi A. Morphologia della arteriae coronariae cordis. Arch Ital Anat Embriol 1903;3:89.
3. Grant RT. Development of the cardiac coronary vessels in the rabbit. Heart 1926a;13:261–271.
4. Bennett HS. The development of the blood supply to the heart in the embryo pig. Am J Anat 1936;60:27–53.
5. Goldsmith JB, Butler HW. The development of the cardiac-coronary circulatory system. Am J Anat 1937;60:185–201.
6. Goor DA, Lillehei CW. Congenital malformations of the heart: embryology, anatomy and operative considerations. New York: Grune & Stratton, 1975.
7. Suzuki A, Ho SY, Anderson RH, Deanfield JE. Coronary arterial and sinusal anatomy in hearts with a common arterial trunk. Ann Thorac Surg 1989;48:792–797.
8. Roberts WC. Major anomalies of coronary arterial origin seen in adulthood. Am Heart J 1986;5:941–963.
9. Landolt CC, Anderson JE, Zorn-Chelton S, Guyton RA. Importance of coronary artery anomalies in operations for congenital heart disease. Ann Thorac Surg 1986;41:351–355.
10. Engel HJ, Torres C, Page HL. Major variations in anatomical origin of the coronary arteries. Cathet Cardiovasc Diagn 1975;1:157.
11. Sones FM Jr, Shivey EK, Proudfit WL, Westcott RN. Cinecoronary arteriography [Abstract]. Circulation 1959;20:773.
12. Forssman W. The catheterization of the right side of the heart. Klin Wochenschr 1929;8:2085.
13. Gruentzig AR et al. Coronary transluminal angioplasty [Abstract]. Circulation 1977;56:11.
14. Gruentzig AR, Senning A, Siegenthaler WE. Nonoperative dilation of coronary artery stenosis: percutaneous transluminal coronary angioplasty. N Engl J Med 1979;301:61.
15. Davidson CJ, Bashore TM. Coronary arteriography. In: Sabiston DC Jr, Spencer FC, eds. Surgery of the chest, 5th ed. Philadelphia: WB Saunders, 1990.
16. Chaitman BR, Lesperance J, Saltiel J, Bourassa MG. Clinical, angiographic, and hemodynamic findings in patients with anomalous origin of the coronary arteries. Circulation 1976;53:122.
17. Ogden JA. Congenital anomalies of the coronary arteries. Am J Cardiol 1970;25:474.
18. Gross L. The blood supply to the heart in its anatomical and clinical aspects. New York: Paul B Hoeber, 1921.
19. Blake HA, Manion WC, Mattingly TW, Baroldi G. Coronary artery anomalies. Circulation 1964;30:927–940.
20. Bergman RA, Thompson SA, Afifi AK, Saadeh FA. Compendium of human anatomic variation. Baltimore: Urban & Schwarzenberg, 1988.
21. Schlesinger MJ, Zoll PM, Wessler S. The conus artery: a third coronary artery. Am Heart J 1949;38:823–836.
22. Symmers W. Note on accessory coronary arteries. J Anat Physiol 1907;41:141–142.
23. Liberthson RR et al. Aberrant coronary origin from the aorta: diagnosis and clinical significance. Circulation 1974;50:774.
24. Thebesius AC. Dissertatio medica de circulo sanguinis in cordo. Ludg. Batav.: JA Langerak, 1716.
25. Smith JC. Review of single coronary artery with report of two cases. Circulation 1950;1:1168–1175.
26. Sharbaugh AH, White RS. Single coronary artery: analysis of the anatomic variation, clinical importance, and report of five cases. JAMA 1974;230:243.
27. Joswig BC et al. Transmural myocardial infarction in the absence of coronary arterial luminal narrowing in a young man with single coronary arterial anomaly. Cathet Cardiovasc Diagn 1978;4:297.
28. Murphy ML: Single coronary artery. Am Heart J 1967;74:557.
29. Newton MC, Burwell LR: Single coronary artery with myocardial infarction and mitral regurgitation. Am Heart J 1978;95:126.
30. Jokl E, McClellan JT, Ross GD. Congenital anomaly of left coronary artery in a young athlete. JAMA 1962;182:573–574.
31. Friedman S, Ash R, Klein D, Johnson J. Anomalous single coronary artery complicating ventriculotomy in a child with cyanotic congenital heart disease. Am Heart J 1960;59:140.
32. Monie IW, Nelson MM. Abnormalities of pulmonary and other vessels in rat fetuses from maternal pteroylglutamic acid deficiency. Anat Rec 1963;147:397–405.
33. de Guglielmo L, Guttadauro M. Anatomic variations in the coronary arteries: an arteriographic study in living subjects. Acta Radiol (Stockh) 1954;41:393–416.
34. Schlesinger MJ. The relation of anatomical pattern to pathologic conditions of the coronary arteries. Arch Path 1940;30:403–415.
35. Kimbiris D, Iskandrian AS, Segal BL, Bemis CE. Anomalous aortic origin of coronary arteries. Circulation 1978;58:606.
36. Liberthson RR et al. Congenital coronary arteriovenous fistula. Circulation 1979;59:849.
37. Harrison DC, Baim DS. Nonatherosclerotic causes of coronary heart disease. In: Hurst JW, ed. The heart, 7th ed. New York: McGraw-Hill, 1990.
38. Cheitlin MD, McAllister HA, DeCastro CM. Myocardial infarction without atherosclerosis. JAMA 1975;231:951.
39. Levin DC, Fellows KE, Abrams HL. Hemodynamically significant primary anomalies of the coronary arteries. Circulation 1978;58:25.
40. Byrum CJ et al. Congenital atresia of the left coronary ostium and hypoplasia of the left main coronary artery. Am Heart J 1980;99:354.
41. Noble J et al. Myocardial bridging and milking effect of the left anterior descending coronary artery: normal variant or obstruction. Am J Cardiol 1976;37:993.
42. Grondin P et al. Successful course after supra-arterial myotomy for myocardial bridging and milking effect of the left anterior descending artery. Ann Thorac Surg 1977;24:422.
43. Geiringer E. The mural coronary artery. Am Heart J 1951;41:359.
44. Glickel SZ, Maggs PR, Ellis FH. Coronary artery aneurysm. Ann Thorac Surg 1978;25:372.
45. Befeler B et al. Coronary artery aneurysms: study of the etiology, clinical course and effect on left ventricular function and prognosis. Am J Med 1977;62:597.
46. Lev M, Alcalde VM, Baffes TG. Pathologic anatomy of complete transposition of the arterial trunks. Pediatrics 1961;28:293–306.

47. Rowlatt UF. Coronary artery distribution in complete transposition. JAMA 1962;179:269–278.

48. Cheatham JP, Ruyle NA, McManus BM, Gammel GE. Origin of the right coronary artery from the descending thoracic aorta: angiographic diagnosis and unique coronary artery anatomy at autopsy. Cathet Cardiovasc Diagn 1987;13:321–324.

49. Gerlis LM, Ho SY, Milo S. Three anomalies of the coronary arteries co-existing in a case of pulmonary atresia with intact ventricular septum. Int J Cardiol 1990;29:93–95.

50. Roberts WC. Anomalous origin of both coronary arteries from the pulmonary artery. Am J Cardiol 1962;10:595–600.

51. Gouley BA. Anamalous left coronary artery arising from pulmonary artery (adult type). Am Heart J 1950;40:630.

52. Sabiston DC, Neill CA, Taussig HB. The direction of blood flow in anomalous left coronary artery arising from the pulmonary artery. Circulation 1960;22:591.

53. Edwards, JE. The direction of blood flow in coronary arteries arising from the pulmonary trunk. Circulation 1964;29:163.

54. Ehren H, Wells TR, Landing BH. Association of common origin of the carotid arteries with anomalous origin of the left coronary artery from the pulmonary artery. Pediatr Pathol 1985;7:59–66.

55. Abrikossoff A. Aneurysma des linken Herzventrikels mit abnormer Abgangsstelle der linken Koronararterie von der Pulmonalis bei einem fünfmonatlichen Kinde. Virchow Arch [A] 1911;203:413–420.

56. Hacksensellner HA. Akzessorische Kranzgefässanlagen der Arteria pulmonalis unter 63 menschlichen Embryonenserien mit einer grössten Länge von 12 bis 36 mm. Z Mik Anat Forsch 1956;62:153.

57. Brooks H St J. Two cases of an abnormal coronary artery of the heart arising from the pulmonary artery. J Anat Physiol 1886;20:26–29.

58. Abbot ME. Congenital cardiac disease. In: Osler W, ed. Modern medicine, Vol 4. Philadelphia: Lea & Febiger, 1908.

59. Grayzel DM, Tennant R. Congenital atresia of the tricuspid orifice and anomalous origin of the coronary arteries from the pulmonary arteries. Am J Pathol 1934;10:791.

60. Agustsson MH et al. Anomalous origin of left coronary artery from pulmonary artery. JAMA 1962;180:95–101.

61. Keith JD. The anomalous origin of the left coronary artery from the pulmonary artery. Br Heart J 1959;21:149–161.

62. Heifetz SA, Robinowitz M, Mueller, KH, Virmani R. Total anomalous origin of the coronary arteries from the pulmonary artery. Pediatr Cardiol 1986;7:11.

63. Fisher EA, Sepehri B, Lendrum B, Luken J, Levitzky S: Two-dimensional echocardiographic visualization of the left coronary artery in anomalous origin of the left coronary artery from the pulmonary artery: pre- and postoperative studies. Circulation 1981;63:698.

64. Likar E, Criley JM, Lewis KB. Anomalous left coronary artery arising from the pulmonary artery in an adult: a review of the therapeutic problem. Circulation 1966;33:727–732.

65. Perry LW, Scott LP: Anomalous left coronary artery from pulmonary artery: report of 11 cases—review of indications for and results of surgery. Circulation 1970;41:1043.

66. Midgley FM et al. Repair of anomalous origin of the left coronary artery in the infant and small child. J Am Coll Cardiol 1984;4:1231.

67. Wesselhoeft H, Fawcett JS, Johnson AL. Anomalous origin of the left coronary artery from the pulmonary trunk: its clinical spectrum, pathology, and pathophysiology based on a review of 140 cases with seven further cases. Circulation 1968;38:403.

68. Arciniegas E, Farooki ZQ, Haimi M, Green EW. Management of anomalous left coronary artery from the pulmonary artery. Circulation 1980;62(Suppl 1):168.

69. Lloyd TR, Mervin WJ Jr, Lee J. Total anomalous origin of the coronary arteries from the pulmonary artery in an infant with aorticopulmonary septal defect. Pediatr Cardiol 1987;8:153–154.

70. Mullins CE et al. Atresia of the left coronary ostium: repair by saphenous vein graft. Circulation 1972;46:989.

71. Nugent EW, Plauth WH Jr, Edwards JE, Williams WH. The pathology, abnormal physiology, clinical recognition, and medical and surgical treatment of congenital heart disease. In: Hurst JW, ed. The heart. New York: McGraw-Hill, 1990.

72. Neufeld JN et al. Congenital communication of a coronary artery with a cardiac chamber or the pulmonary trunk ("coronary artery fistula"). Circulation 1961;24:171–179.

73. Lowe JE, Oldham HN Jr, Sabiston DC Jr. Surgical management of congenital coronary artery fistulas. Ann Surg 1981;194:371.

74. Dehner LP. Pediatric surgical pathology. Baltimore: Williams & Wilkins, 1987.

75. Lucas RV Jr. Anomalous venous connections, pulmonary and systemic. In: Adams FH, Emmanouilides GC, eds. Moss' heart disease in infants, children and adolescents. Baltimore: Williams & Wilkins, 1983.

76. Perry LW, Scott LP III, McClenathan JE. Congenital coronary artery fistulae. Clin Proc Children's Hosp 1974;30:114.

77. Baim DS, Kline H, Silverman JF. Bilateral coronary-pulmonary artery fistulae: report of five cases and review of the literature. Circulation 1982;65:810.

78. Lowe JE, Sabiston DC Jr. Congenital malformations of the coronary circulation. In: Sabiston DC Jr, Spencer FC, eds. Surgery of the chest, 5th ed. Philadelphia: WB Saunders, 1990.

79. McNamara JJ, Gross RE. Congenital coronary artery fistula. Surgery 1969;65:59.

80. Vigneswaran WT, Pollock JC. Pulmonary atresia with ventricular septal defect and coronary artery fistula: a late presentation. Br Heart J 1988;59:387–388.

81. Pohl E, Fong L, Anderson RH, Park SC, Zuberbuhler JR. Fistulous communications between a solitary coronary artery and the pulmonary arteries as the primary source of pulmonary blood supply in tetralogy of Fallot with pulmonary valve atresia. Am J Cardiol 1989;63:140–143.

82. Bogers AJ, Rohmer J, Wolsky SA, Quaegebeur JM, Huysmans HA. Coronary artery fistula as source of pulmonary circulation in pulmonary atresia with ventricular septal defect. Thorac Cardiovasc Surg 1990;38:30–32.

83. Steinberg I, Baldwin JS, Dotter CT. Coronary arteriovenous fistula. Circulation 1958;17:372.

84. Augusti R et al. Congenital right coronary artery to left atrium fistula. Am J Cardiol 1967;19:428–433.

85. Dedichen H, Skalleberg L, Cappelen C. Congenital coronary artery fistula. Thorax 1966;21:121–128.

86. Hipona FA. Congenital coronary arterial fistula to a persistent left superior vena cava. AJR 1966;97:355–358.

87. Grant RT. An unusual anomaly of the coronary vessels in the malformed heart of a child. Heart 1926b;13:273–277.

88. Soloff LA. Anomalous coronary arteries arising from the pulmonary artery: report of case in which left coronary artery arose from pulmonary artery. Am Heart J 1942;24:118–127.

89. Krause W. Z Rationelle Med 1865;24.

90. Trevor RS. Aneurysm of the descending branch of the right coronary artery, situated in the wall of the right ventricle and opening into the cavity of the ventricle, associated with great dilatation of the right coronary artery and nonvalvular infective endocarditis. Br J Child Dis 1911;8:546–549.

91. Gasul BM et al. Congenital coronary arteriovenous fistula. Pediatrics 1960;25:531–560.

92. Hallman GL, Cooley DA, Singer DB. Congenital anomalies of the coronary arteries: anatomy, pathology, and surgical treatment. Surgery 1966;59:133–144.

93. Biorck G, Crafoord G. Arteriovenous aneurysm on the pulmonary artery simulating patent ductus arteriosus botalli. Thorax 1947;2:65.

94. Engle MA, Goldsmith EI, Holswade GR, Goldberg HP, Glenn F. Congenital coronary artriovenous fistula. N Engl J Med 1961;264:856–858.

95. McNamara JJ, Gross RE. Congenital coronary artery fistula. Surgery 1969;65:59.

96. Eie H, Hillestad L. Arteriovenous fistulas of coronary arteries. Scand J Thorac Cardiovasc Surg 1971;5:34.

97. Hobbs RE, Millit HD, Raghavan PV, Moodie DS, Sheldon WC. Coronary artery fistulae: a 10 year review. Cleve Clin Q 1982;49:191.

98. Liberthson RR, Sagar K, Berkoben JP, Weintraub RM, Levine FH: Congenital coronary arteriovenous fistula. Circulation 1979;59:849.

99. Daniel TM, Graham TP, Sabiston DC Jr. Coronary artery-right ventricular fistula with congestive heart failure: surgical correction in the neonatal period. Surgery 1970;67:985.

100. Reidy JF, Anjus RT, Quereshi SA, Baker EJ, Tynan MJ. Transcatheter embolization in the treatment of coronary artery fistulas. Am College Cardiol 1991;18:187.

101. Urrutia-S CO, Falaschi G, Ott DA, Cooley DA. Surgical management of 56 patients with congenital coronary artery fistulas. Ann Thorac Surg 1983;35:300.

102. Gensini GG et al. Anatomy of the coronary circulation in living man: coronary venography. Circulation 1965;31:778.

103. Hutchins GM, Moore W, Hatton, EV. Arterial-venous relationships in the human left ventricular myocardium: anatomic basis for countercurrent regulation of blood flow. Circulation 1986;74:1195.

104. Prows MS. Two cases of bilateral superior venae cavae, one draining a closed coronary sinus. Anat Rec 1943;87:99.

105. Fieldstein LE, Pick J. Drainage of the coronary sinus into the left auricle. Am J Clin Pathol 1942;12:66.

106. Hellerstein HK, Orbison JL. Anatomic variations of the orifice of the human coronary sinus. Circulation 1951;3:514–523.

107. Martini E et al. Congenital anomalies involving the coronary sinus. Circulation 1966;33:317.

108. Rumisek JD, Piggott JD, Weinberg PM, Norwood WI. Coronary sinus septal defect associated with tricuspid atresia. J Thorac Cardiovasc Surg 1986;92:142–145.

CHAPTER 28

THE THORACIC AND ABDOMINAL AORTA

John Elias Skandalakis / Stephen Wood Gray / Panagiotis Symbas

*Most wise Asclepiad, if you knew anatomy, you would teach us
that the artery differs from the vein not only in thickness,
but also in the number and quality of the coats. Despite the fact
that you do not know anything with accuracy, you dare to express
your opinion like a specialist, you who ignore and scorn the anatomical
research of Herophilos, you who undergrade Erasistratos,
and you who give not too much attention to Hippocrates.*
—GALEN, (KÜHN, 1882; III:467)

DEVELOPMENT

The earliest blood vessels of the embryo form from the mesoderm of the yolk sac and the body stalk as anastomosing cords of angioblasts, which subsequently become endothelial tubes. These angioblastic cords grow into the embryonic body to form the primitive blood vessels (Fig. 28.1).

The "angioblast" theory of His (1) holds that this is the only way in which blood and lymph vessels form. An alternative view, the "local origin" theory, proposed originally by Rückert and Mollier (2), holds that some vessels arise secondarily from mesenchymal clefts, which later coalesce to form vessels. The argument was based on studies conducted chiefly on the developing lymphatic vessels. Sabin (3) supported the angioblast theory, whereas McClure (4) defended local origin. The controversy ended in exhaustion and indifference rather than in agreement, and there has been little concern with it in recent years.

In spite of the lack of certainty as to the origin of the primitive vessels themselves, there is little doubt that later development is by the outgrowth of a capillary net from existing vessels and subsequent formation of preferred paths through the net (5, 6).

It is not within the scope of this book to discuss congenital malformations secondary to teratogenic agents, but we want to mention the work of Bindber (7). He studied the possible relationship of aortic arch anomalies and DiGeorge syndrome and suggested that this syndrome is of truncated pharyngeal arch development with two general forms:

1. Agenesis or incomplete development of the sixth pharyngeal arch with pulmonic circulation through the fifth arch
2. Agenesis or incomplete development of the fifth and sixth pharyngeal arches with pulmonic circulation through the fourth arch with the possibility of descent of the third arch into the thorax

Bindber (7) experimented with hamsters using fertilizer (bis[dichloroacetyl]diamine) as a teratogenic agent and produced malformations of the aortic arches and several other anomalies.

Aortic Arches

The systemic arterial system of mammals is first laid down according to the plan that originated in ancestral, water-dwelling vertebrates. From the heart, lying ventral to the foregut, pairs of arteries (aortic arches) pass laterally around the gut and caudad as the dorsal aortae, which subsequently fuse to form a single vessel dorsal to the gut. Between the pairs of arteries are paired evaginations of the skin (branchial clefts). This arrangement is fundamental for oxygen transfer from water to blood in gill-breathing animals. In mammals, no gills are formed, and the primitive system of paired aortic arches becomes almost unrecognizably rearranged during later development.

At the end of the third week, the paired dorsal aortae and the first aortic arch are represented by the medial marginal vessels of the angioblast net, which has invaded the embryonic body. Ventrally, the arch connects with the anterior ends of the unfused cardiac primordia (6, 8). Soon afterward, the heart tubes fuse, and the lateral angioblast net regresses to leave the aortae and arches as definitive vessels. These arise from the anterior end of the heart, passing around the foregut and extending caudally on either side of the notochord (Fig. 28.2). All that remains of the more ventral portion of the angioblast net are a number of branches from the aortae to the yolk sac (the vitelline arteries). Anteriorly, the vitelline veins from the yolk sac enter the posterior end of the heart. Circulation of blood has almost certainly begun by this time.

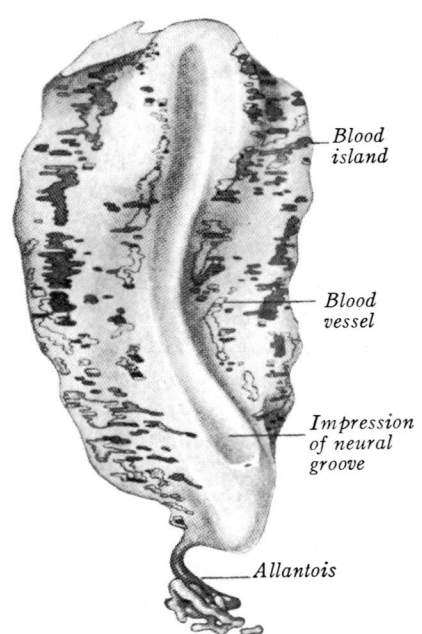

Figure 28.1. The origin of the vascular system. Model of a human embryo of two somites (3 weeks) showing only mesoderm with blood islands. *Dark masses* indicate solid islands; *light areas* indicated primordia of vessels. (From Arey LB. Developmental Anatomy, 6th ed. Philadelphia: WB Saunders, 1959.)

Our knowledge of subsequent aortic arch development rests on the stages beautifully worked out in human embryos by Congdon (9) and in cat (10) and pig (11) embryos. During the late fourth and fifth weeks (3- to 7-mm stage), a total of six pairs of aortic arches are formed. Some are present for a short time only; at no one time are more than four arches present (Fig. 28.3).

Although most textbook descriptions speak of arches "appearing" and "dropping out," the appearance of a definitive aortic arch is preceded by a capillary plexus, and a regressing arch breaks up into a similar multiplicity of channels (12). In addition, the development and size of embryos are not exactly correlated. Table 28.1 may be taken as a rough guide to the sequence of development of the arches.

No true ventral aorta exists in the human embryo. The truncus arteriosus terminates in a broad dilation termed the *aortic sac,* from the lateral borders of which emerge the ventral limbs of the aortic arches. With the decrease in the number of arches, the sac decreases in size and loses its identity in the truncus.

The two dorsal aortae are at first separated by the neural tube and the notochord, which is in contact with the roof of the gut. With separation of the gut from the over-

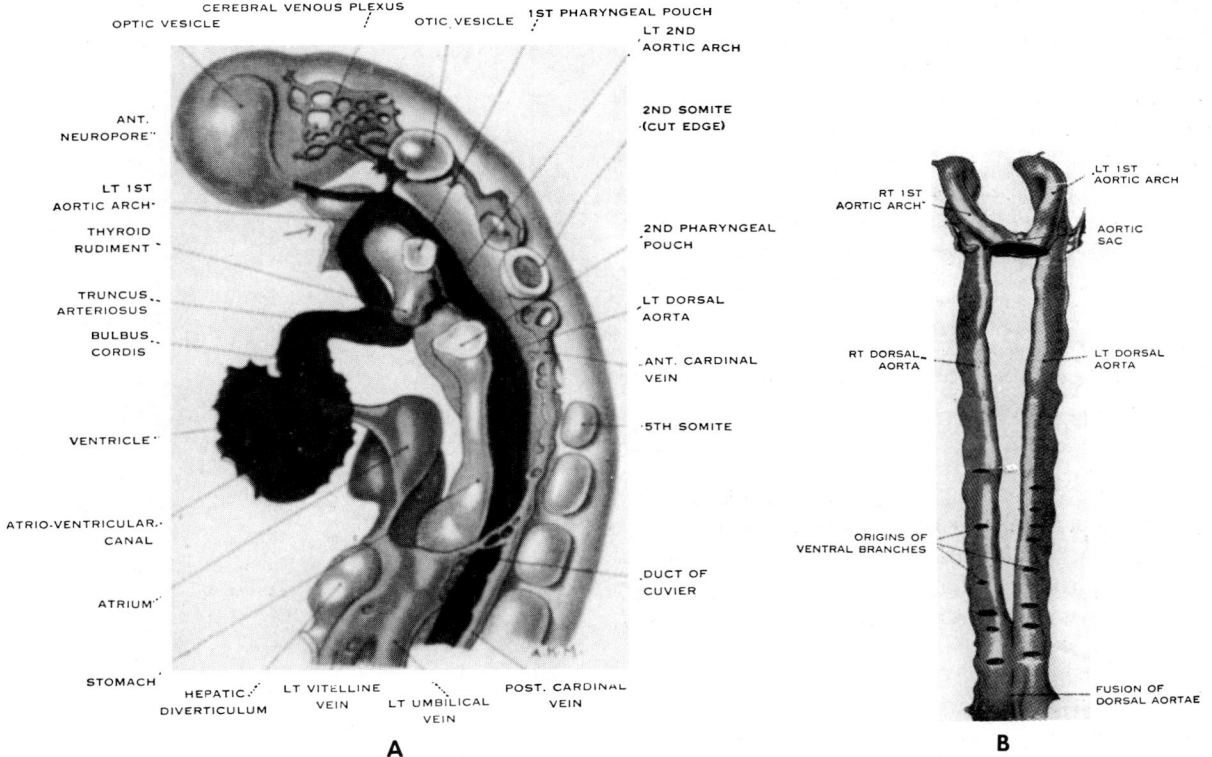

Figure 28.2. The heart and aortic arch system of a 22-somite human embryo. The first arch is at the peak of its development, and the second arch is forming. **A,** Lateral view. **B,** Ventral view. (From Hamilton WJ, Boyd JD, Mossman HW. Human embryology, 3rd ed. Baltimore: Williams & Wilkins, 1962.)

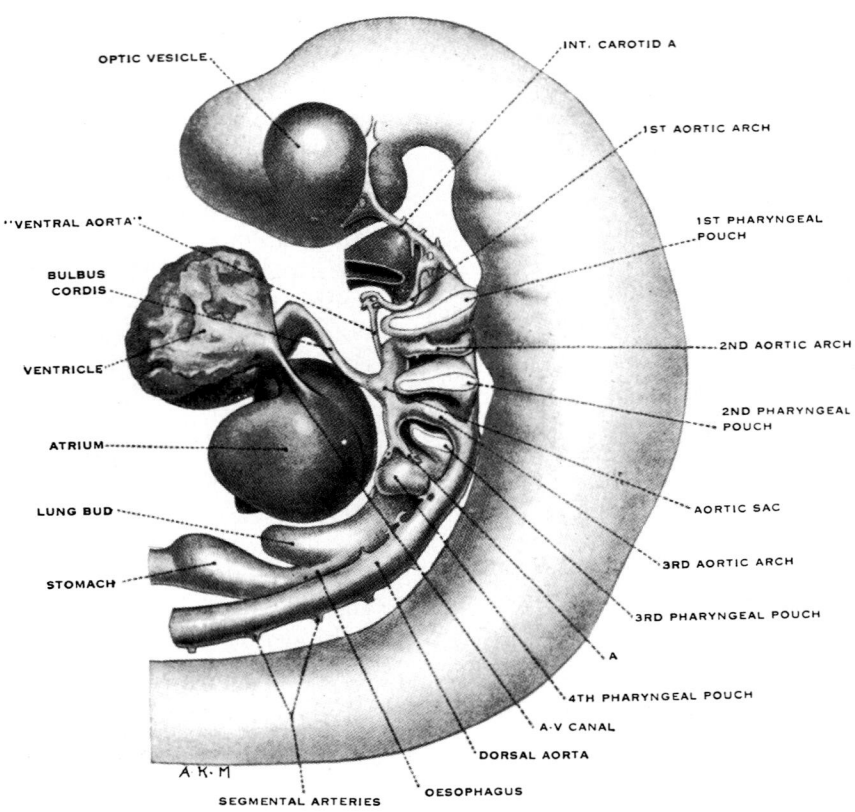

Figure 28.3. The heart and aortic arch system of a 4-mm human embryo. The first arch is regressing; the second and third arches are well-developed; and the ventral and dorsal twigs of the fourth arch have not yet joined at A. (From Hamilton WJ, Boyd JD, Mossman HW. Human embryology, 3rd ed. Baltimore: Williams & Wilkins, 1962.)

Table 28.1.
Sequence of Development of the Aortic Arches

Aortic Arches	Crown-Rump Length, mm.	Streeter Horizon	Age
1	3	X	4th week
1 2	3.5	XI	4th week
1 2 3	4	XII	5th week
- 2 3	5	XIII	5th week
- - 3 4 5 6	5.5	XIV	5th week
- - 3 4 6	7	XVI	6th week
- - 3 4 6L	13	XVII	7th week
- - - 4 6L	14	XVIII	7th week
- - - 4L 6L	16	XVIII	7th week

lying structures, cross-connections develop between the aortae until they form a plexus of vessels. This plexus breaks down to produce a single aorta posteriorly. By the 15-mm stage, fusion is complete up to the level of the 10th somite (13).

The first and second arches disappear by losing their connection with the aortic sac and becoming small local branches of the cranial dorsal aorta. The first becomes the mandibular, and the second the hyoid artery (12) (Fig. 28.4).

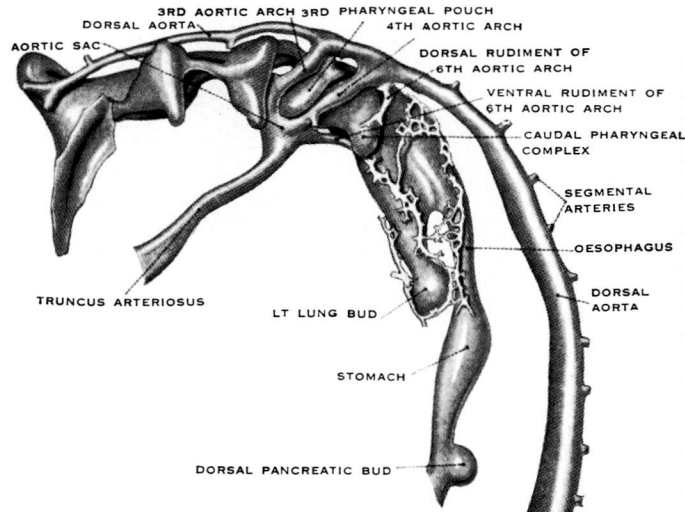

Figure 28.4. The aortic arch system of a 5-mm human embryo. The first and second arches have disappeared. The third and fourth arches are complete, and the sixth arch is nearly formed. The pulmonary artery is developing from the foregut plexus and is connected with both dorsal and ventral twigs of the sixth arch. (From Hamilton WJ, Boyd JD, Mossman HW. Human embryology, 3rd ed. Baltimore: Williams & Wilkins, 1962.)

The third arch itself persists, but the dorsal aortae (ductus caroticus) between the third and fourth arches disappear, so that blood passing through the third arch travels only to the head of the embryo. This pathway, composed of the third arch and the dorsal aorta cranial to it, becomes the internal carotid artery (Fig. 28.5).

Experimental ligation of aortic arches in chick embryos suggests the existence of two groups of arches. Arches 1, 2, and 5 cannot be made to persist even as necessary channels. The portions of arches 3, 4, and 6 that normally disappear, as well as the left aortic arch, can be forced to persist if they are necessary to the circulation (14–16). A familiar example is the persistence of the distal left sixth arch (ductus arteriosus) in preductal aorta interruption (Fig. 28.6). Warkany and his colleagues (17) also

were unable to influence the disappearance of the first two arches in the rat by vitamin A–deficiency experiments. The right arch and dorsal aorta, on the other hand, could be forced to persist where necessary for circulation. In day-old chicks, the percentage of persistent left aortic arches varies with the strain and with the individual parents, suggesting a genetic basis for arch formation (18).

While these changes have been taking place in the aortic arch system, the heart and the arches have been moving caudally. The arches, when first formed, lie at the level of the occipital segments, and the heart lies almost directly ventral to the arches. The caudad movement comprises two phases. During formation of the caudal arches and regression of cranial ones, the aortic sac

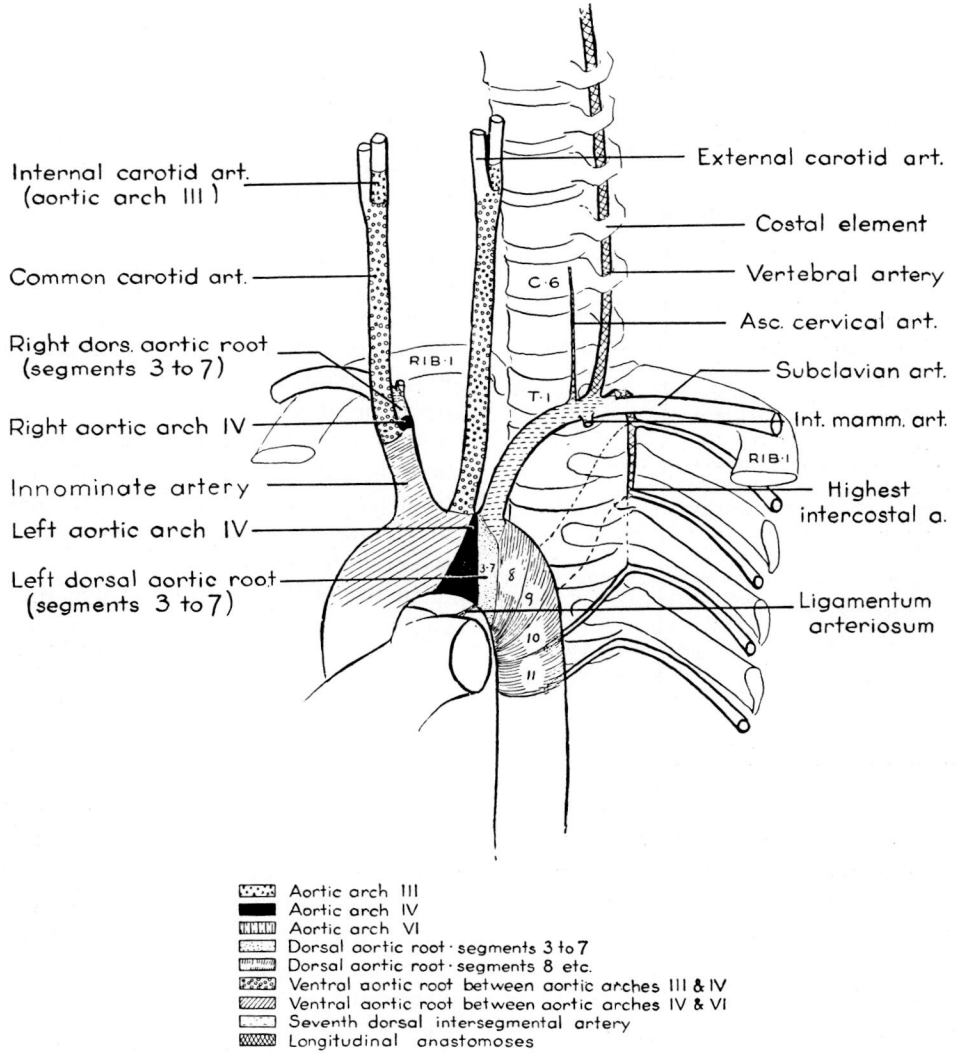

Figure 28.5. Diagram of the adult aorta and its main branches, with the location and extend of the vessels derived from the various embryonic aortic arch components, indicated by use of the same schematic analysis employed in Figure 28.7. (From Barry A. Aortic arch derivatives in the human adult. Anat Rec 1951;111:221–228.)

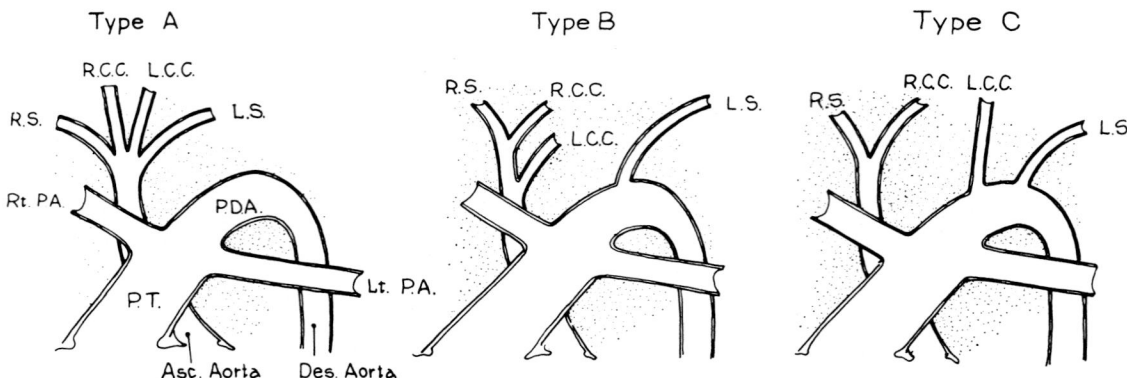

Figure 28.6. Diagrammatic illustrations of the three principal anatomic types of complete interruption of the aortic arch. *P.T.,* Pulmonary trunk; *P.D.A.,* ductus arteriosus; *PA,* pulmonary artery; *R.S.,* right subclavian artery; *R.C.C.,* right com- mon carotid artery; *L.C.C.,* left common carotid artery; *L.S.,* left subclavian artery. (From Roberts WC, Morrow AG, Braunwald E. Complete interruption of aortic arch. Circulation 1962;26:39–59.)

Table 28.2.
Fate of the Embryonic Aortic Arches[a]

Embryonic Vessel	What It Becomes
1. Truncus arteriosus	Aortic and pulmonary roots
2. Aortic sac	Ascending aorta, brachiocephalic artery, and aortic arch up to the origin of the left common carotid artery
3. First arches	Parts persist as components of the maxillary arteries
4. Second arches	Parts persist as the stapedial arteries
5. Third arches	Common carotid arteries and proximal segment of the internal carotid arteries
6. Fourth arches	
a. Right	Most proximal segment of the right subclavian artery
b. Left	Aortic arch segment between the left common carotid and left subclavian arteries
7. Fifth arches	No known derivations; transient and never well developed
8. Sixth arches	
a. Right	Proximal part becomes proximal segment of the right pulmonary artery; distal part disappears early
b. Left	Proximal part becomes proximal segment of the left pulmonary artery; distal part persists, until birth, as ductus arteriosus
9. Right dorsal aorta	Cranial portion becomes part of the right subclavian artery; remainder disappears
10. Left dorsal aorta	Distal aortic arch
11. Right seventh intersegmental artery	Part of the right subclavian artery
12. Left seventh intersegmental artery	Left subclavian artery

[a]From Van Mierop LHS, Kutsche LM. Embryology of the heart. In: Hurst JW et al., eds. The heart, 7th ed. New York: McGraw-Hill, 1990.

moves back along the floor of the pharynx, which is itself elongating craniad. In the second phase, with the disappearance of the first two arches and the separation of the caudal pharyngeal derivatives from the pharynx, the caudad movement of the heart and arches increases. The fourth arch descends four and one-half segments relative to the pharynx and 13 segments relative to the neural tube (9). The heart and aorta reach their normal thoracic position late in the seventh week (18-mm stage). By the end of the following week, the developing upper ribs have joined the sternum and the thoracic cavity has separated from the neck. The most striking evidence of this migration of the arch system is in the position of the laryngeal branches of the vagus nerves. These nerves, which pass caudally to the sixth arch, are carried downward under the ductus arteriosus on the left and under the subclavian artery on the right.

In summary, at various times during fetal development, six pairs of aortic arch vessels form connections between the dorsal and ventral aorta, which practically exists only as a sac (Table 28.2).

Definitive Thoracic Aorta

While it is usual to say that the right fourth arch drops out, leaving the left arch as the definitive aorta, the actual processes are more complex than this statement suggests (13). Although the right fourth arch decreases in size, it is only that portion of the right dorsal aorta between the seventh intersegmental artery (the right subclavian artery) and the point of fusion of right and left dorsal aortae that disappears. The right arch and the proximal segments of the right dorsal aorta form the proximal right subclavian artery (Fig. 28.7).

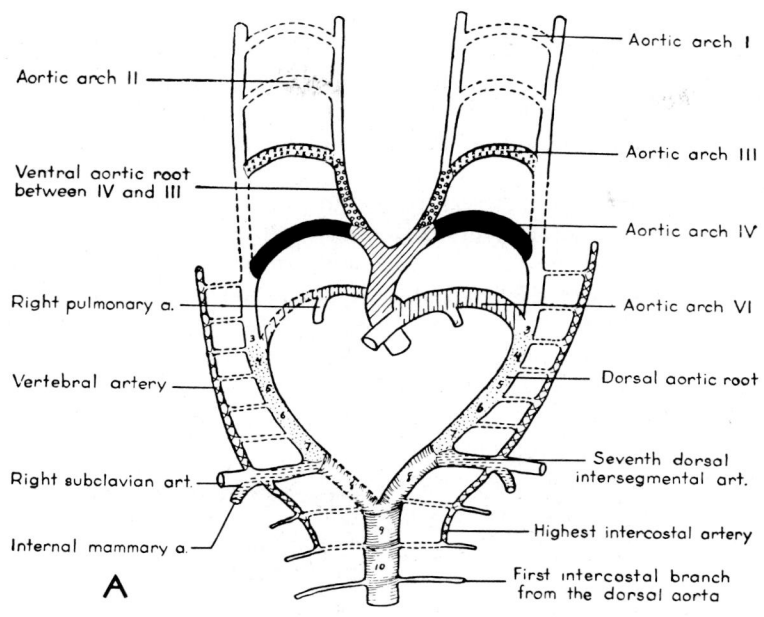

Aortic arch II

Ventral aortic root between IV and III

Right pulmonary a.

Vertebral artery

Right subclavian art.

Internal mammary a.

A

Aortic arch I

Aortic arch III

Aortic arch IV

Aortic arch VI

Dorsal aortic root

Seventh dorsal intersegmental art.

Highest intercostal artery

First intercostal branch from the dorsal aorta

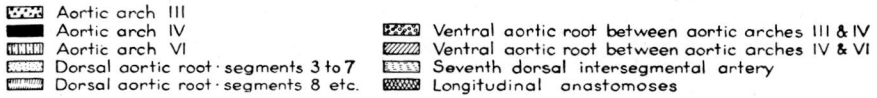

Aortic arch III
Aortic arch IV
Aortic arch VI
Dorsal aortic root · segments 3 to 7
Dorsal aortic root · segments 8 etc.

Ventral aortic root between aortic arches III & IV
Ventral aortic root between aortic arches IV & VI
Seventh dorsal intersegmental artery
Longitudinal anastomoses

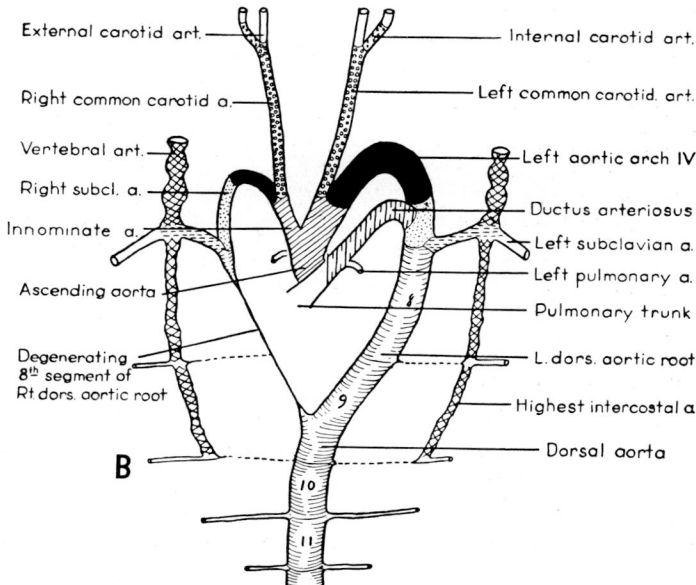

External carotid art.

Right common carotid a.

Vertebral art.

Right subcl. a.

Innominate a.

Ascending aorta

Degenerating 8th segment of Rt dors. aortic root

B

Internal carotid art.

Left common carotid art.

Left aortic arch IV

Ductus arteriosus

Left subclavian a.

Left pulmonary a.

Pulmonary trunk

L. dors. aortic root

Highest intercostal a

Dorsal aorta

Figure 28.7. Schematic diagrams indicating the various components of the aortic arch complex in the human embryo. **A,** Basic plan. Those components that do not normally persist in the adult are indicated by *broken outlines*. Since the fifth arch appears only in rudimentary form, if present at all, it has been omitted from the diagram. **B,** Extent of alteration of the basic plan that has occurred in embryos of 15 mm (seventh week). (From Barry A. Aortic arch derivatives in the human adult. Anat Rec 1951;111:221–228.)

The ascending and proximal portions of the arch of the adult aorta, as well as the brachiocephalic trunk, are derived from the aortic sac and the dorsal part of the truncus arteriosus. The remainder of the arch is derived from the embryonic left fourth arch and the left dorsal aortic root down to the junction with the obliterated right aortic root. Segments three to eight of the dorsal aortic root extend from the fourth arch to the junction; the subclavian is the seventh and only persisting intersegmental artery in this region (13). The descending thoracic aorta is formed by the unpaired aorta caudal to the level of fusion of the paired aortic roots (Fig. 28.5).

Up to the third prenatal month, the wall of the aorta increases in thickness faster than the lumen increases in diameter. During the second trimester, the lumen increases relative to wall thickness. From the sixth month onward, the thickness of the wall again slowly increases relative to the diameter of the lumen. This trend is reversed again in old age (19).

Definitive Pulmonary Trunk

The primitive pulmonary arteries form as caudal extensions from the aortic sac at the time of the appearance of

the fourth arches (4 mm). The sixth arches, themselves, form as twigs from the dorsal aorta. These twigs grow ventral to join the primitive pulmonary arteries. In one sense the sixth arch may be said to arise from the pulmonary artery, not the artery from the arch (6, 9, 20) (Fig. 28.4).

By the end of the sixth week (11 mm) (Figs. 28.8 and 28.9), the left proximal pulmonary channel and the left sixth arch are larger than the corresponding vessels on the right. Early in the seventh week (13 mm), the right sixth arch degenerates and the right proximal segment becomes absorbed into the left proximal segment. Soon afterward, the right dorsal aortic root below the right subclavian artery disappears (21). The subsequent development of the pulmonary artery has been discussed in the chapter on "Pulmonary Circulation."

Separation of Aortic and Pulmonary Trunks

At the junction of the truncus arteriosus and the aortic sac, enlargement early in the fifth week is confined to the ventral wall. The openings of the pulmonary arteries, which at first are lateral, come to lie close together on the posterior wall. Late in the week (5 to 6 mm), two longitudinal ridges appear in the truncus, extending from just

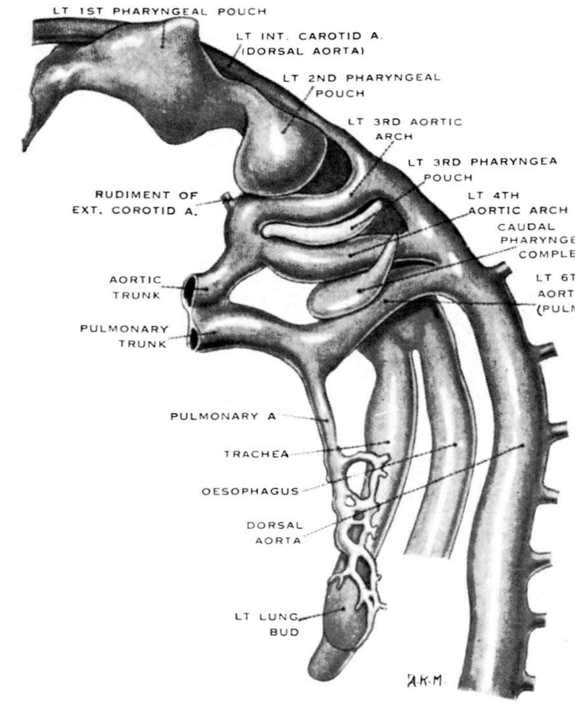

Figure 28.8. The aortic arch system of an 11-mm human embryo. The third, fourth, and sixth arches are well developed, and the pulmonary artery serves the tracheal plexus, at this stage separated from the esophageal plexus. The cranial aortae will remain paired and form the common and internal carotid arteries. (From Hamilton WJ, Boyd JD, Mossman HW. Human embryology, 3rd ed. Baltimore: Williams & Wilkins, 1962.)

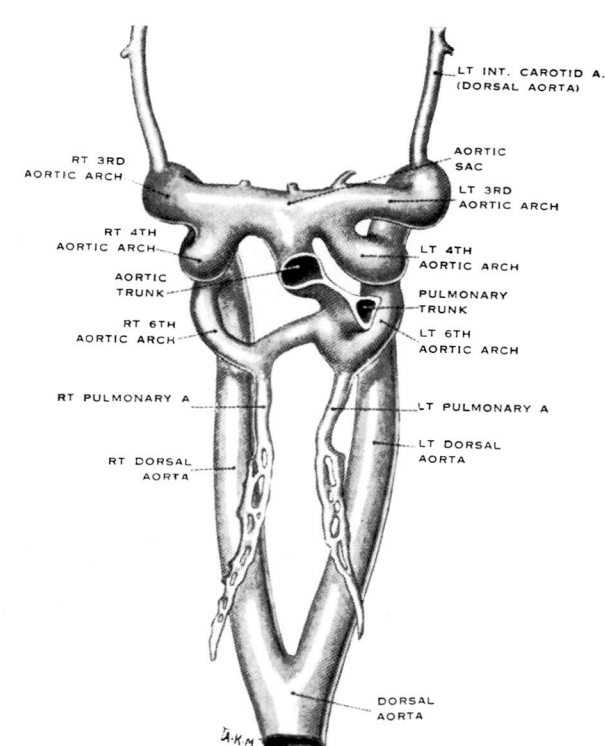

Figure 28.9. Ventral view of the aortic system shown in Figure 28.9. (From Hamilton WJ, Boyd JD, Mossman HW. Human embryology, 3rd ed. Baltimore: Williams & Wilkins, 1962.)

above the pulmonary arteries in a clockwise spiral through the truncus and conus arteriosus ("bulbus cordis" of Davis). These ridges form the aortopulmonary septum which will separate the aortic and pulmonary trunks. The spiral septum leaves the pulmonary arteries dorsally and to the right of the aorta. By the seventh week (13 mm), internal separation is complete and external division is indicated. No rotational movement occurs in the truncus, the ridges assuming this spiral position with their first appearance (22, 23). Shanner (24) seems to be one of the last to believe that the truncus actually rotates.

Marking the division between the truncus and the conus, two short, additional ridges form at 90-degree angles from the septal ridges. These, together with the locally expanded margins of the fused septal ridges, are the primordia of the aortic and pulmonary semilunar valves. Excavation of the subendothelial connective tissue from the distal end converts these swellings into functional valves.

Development of the septal ridges below this level was considered with the development of the heart (see Chapter 26).

Sadler (25) gave the following summary:

1. Septa and Twist: A pair of opposing ridges develop on the right superior and left inferior walls of the cephalic part of the truncus during the fifth week (Fig. 28.10). These ridges, truncus swellings or cushions, grow in the direction of the sac in a manner in which they twist around each other. After complete fusion, the ridges form a septum known as the aorticopulmonary septum (Fig. 28.11). Thus the truncus is divided into an aortic and a pulmonary channel.

2. The Union of the Septa: Swellings, similar to those at the truncus, develop at about the same time along the right dorsal and left ventral walls of the conus cordis (Fig. 28.11). These grow toward each other and in a distal direction to unite with the complete truncus septum.

3. The Division of the Conus by the Conus Septum Formation: The proximal extremity of the right conus swelling ends at the superior border of the right atrioventricular orifice (Fig. 28.12 and Fig. 28.13). That on the left extends proximally along the right side of the anterior limb of the muscular interventricular septum (Fig. 28.12). With the fusion of the two conus swellings, the septum divides the conus into an anterolateral portion (the outflow tract of the right ventricle) (Fig. 28.13) and a posteromedial portion (the outflow tract of the left ventricle) (Fig. 28.14).

Critical Events in Development

The most frequent developmental errors in the formation of the thoracic aorta occur at the end of the second

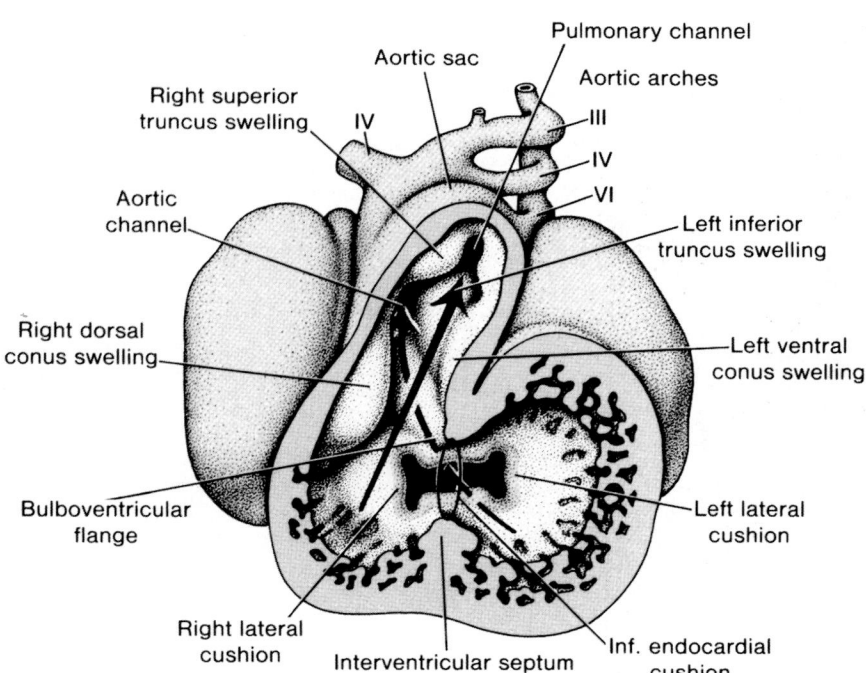

Figure 28.10. Frontal section through the heart of a 9-mm embryo. At this stage of development, blood from the atrial cavity enters the left primitive ventricle, as well as the right primitive ventricle. Note the development of the cushions in the anteriovenous (A-V) canal. The swellings in the truncus and conus are clearly visible. The right indicates the primitive interventricular foramen. *Arrows* indicate blood flow. (From Sadler TW, ed. Langman's medical embryology, 6th ed. Baltimore: Williams & Wilkins, 1990:199.)

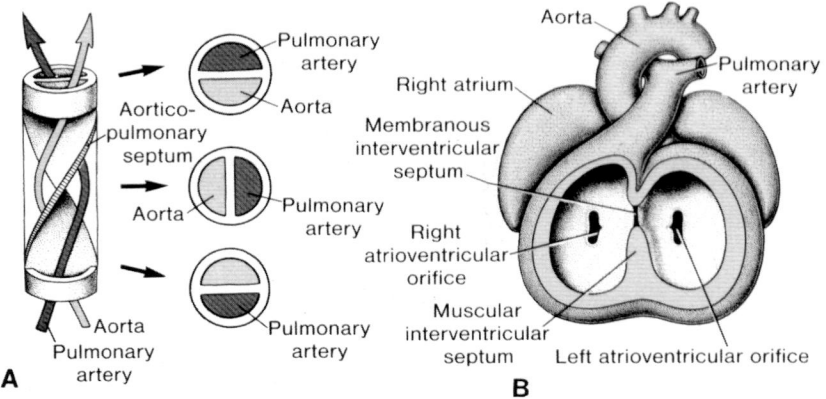

Figure 28.11. **A,** Diagram to show the spiral shape of the aorticopulmonary septum. **B,** Position of aorta and pulmonary artery at the 25-mm stage (eighth week). Note how the aorta and pulmonary artery twist around each other. (From Sadler TW, ed. Langman's medical embryology, 6th ed. Baltimore: Williams & Wilkins, 1990:197.)

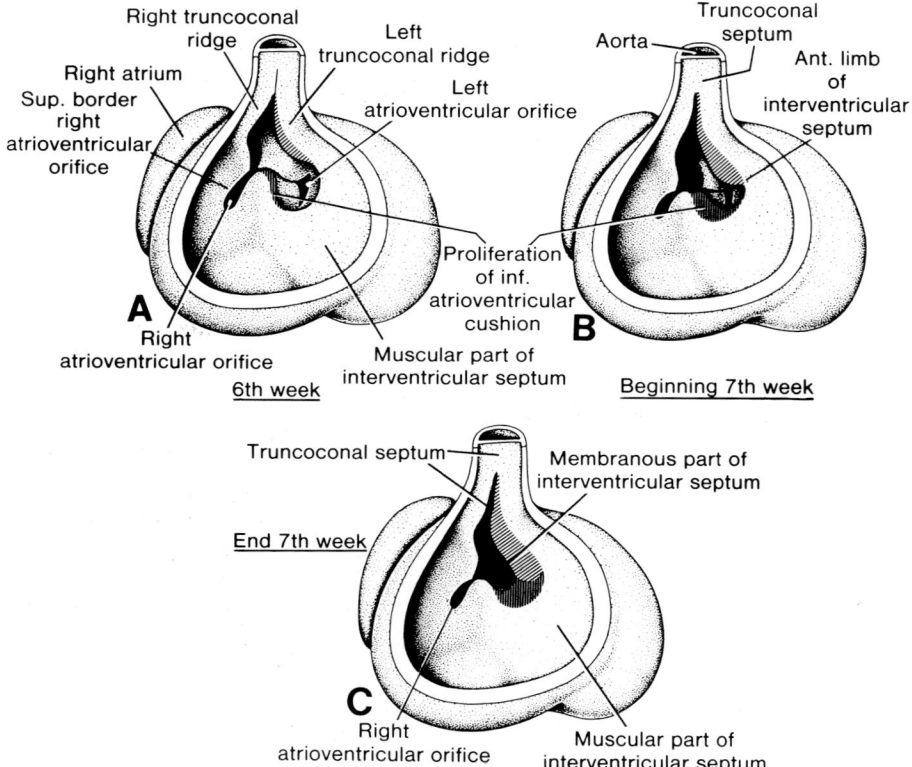

Figure 28.12. Schematic drawings showing the development of the truncoconal ridges and the closure of the interventricular foramen. The proliferations of the right and left conus swellings, combined with the proliferation of the inferior atrioventricular cushion, eventually close the interventricular foramen and form the membranous portion of the interventricular septum. **A,** At 6 weeks (12 mm). **B,** Beginning of seventh week (14.5 mm). **C,** End of seventh week (20 mm). (From Sadler TW, ed. Langman's medical embryology, 6th ed. Baltimore: Williams & Wilkins, 1990:198.)

month. In early postnatal life another developmental problem may manifest.

The definitive formation of the aortic arch takes place during the eighth week, when the right fourth arch normally disappears. If it fails to do so, a double aortic arch results; if, instead, the normal left arch regresses, a right-sided aortic arch results. At the same time, a retroesophageal subclavian artery may be created by abnormal regression of the right arch and the descending aortic limb.

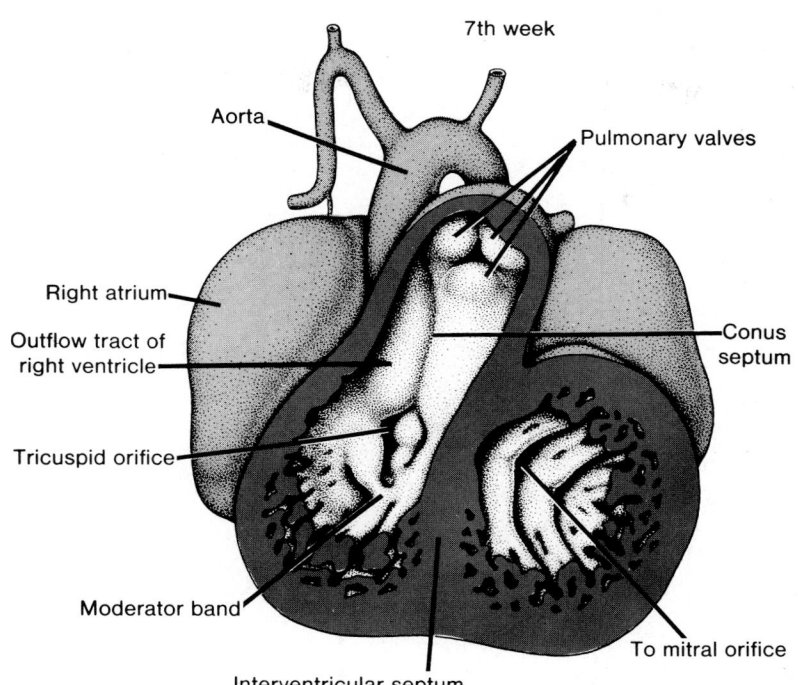

Figure 28.13. Frontal section through the heart of a 16-mm embryo. Note the conus septum and the position of the pulmonary valves. (From Sadler TW, ed. Langman's medical embryology, 6th ed. Baltimore: Williams & Wilkins, 1990:199.)

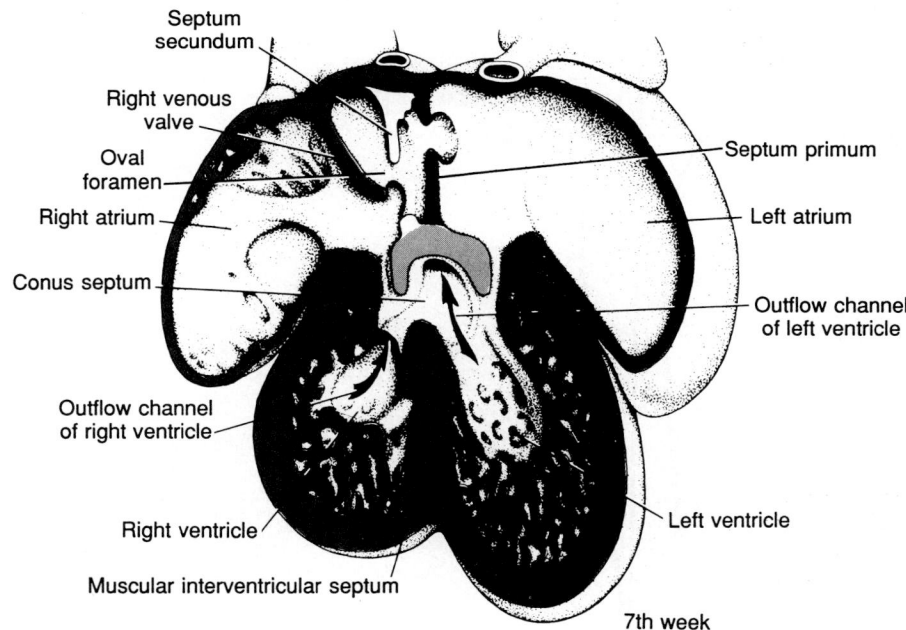

Figure 28.14. View of a frontal section through the heart of a 15-mm embryo. The conus septum is completed and blood from the left ventricle enters the aorta. Note the septa in the atrial region. (From Sadler TW, ed. Langman's medical embryology, 6th ed. Baltimore: Williams & Wilkins, 1990:200.)

Some forms of coarctation and interruption of the aorta also are formed during the eighth week by partial segmental regression of the left arch, with normal regression of the right arch.

Normal closure of the ductus arteriosus immediately after birth may fail to take place from intrinsic inadequacy of the ductus tissue or from abnormally high pressure of blood passing through it. In either case, closure will not take place later.

ANATOMY OF PEDIATRIC THORACIC AORTA WITH AND WITHOUT CONGENITAL HEART DEFECTS

It is well known that, with age, the thoracic aorta grows and the lumen of the aorta increase together with size. We know the measurements of the normal thoracic aorta in adults. Aronberg and her colleagues (26) studied the normal aortic diameters by computed tomography (CT) (Tables 28.3 and 28.4; Fig. 28.15). It also is known that the size of the aorta increases with age and body surface (27, 28, 29). Clarkson and Brandt (30) reported using cineangiographic measurements of several parts of the aorta in 18 normal children and 47 children with congenital heart disease that did not involve the aorta (Fig.

Table 28.3.
Overall Averages (Based on 84 Patients with Complete Data)[a,b]

B₁	A₁	A₂	B₂	C	THVB
3.6 (2.4–4.7)	23.51 (2.2–4.6)	2.63 (1.8–4.0)	2.48 (1.6–3.7)	2.42 (1.4–3.3)	3.44 (2.4–4.5)

[a]From Aronberg DJ et al. Normal thoracic aortic diameters by computed tomography. J Comput Tomogr 1984; 8(2):249.
[b]These numbers represent the average aortic diameters across age and sex categories. Minimum and maximum values are shown in parentheses.
THVB, Thoracic vertebral body size.

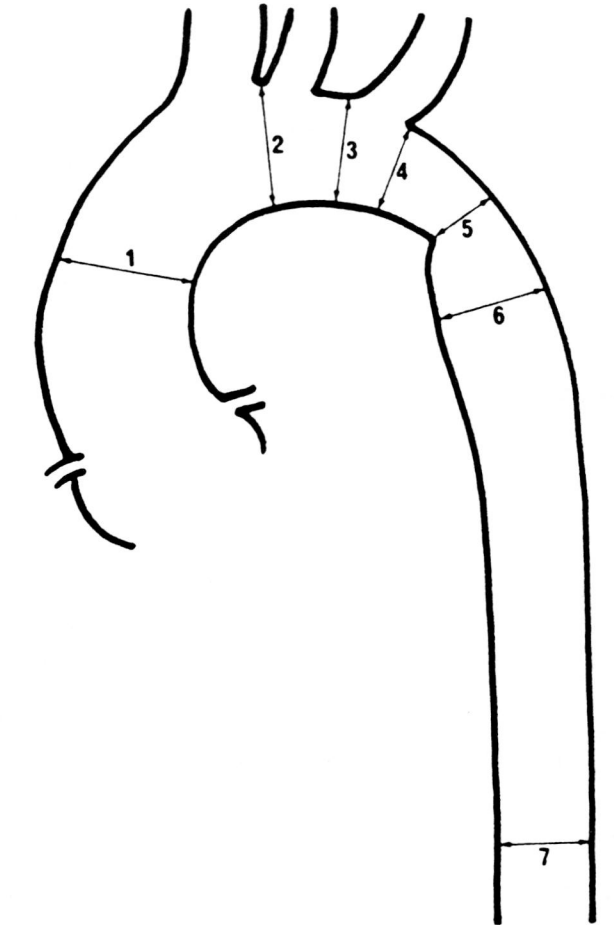

Figure 28.16. Diagram showing sites where measurements were made: *1*, Midascending aorta; *2*, between innominate and left common carotid arteries; *3*, between innominate and left common carotid arteries; *4*, distal to left subclavian artery; *5*, isthmus (i.e., region between left subclavian artery and the ductus arteriosus), the narrowest part of the upper descending aorta was measured; *6*, widest part of postisthmic region; and *7*, lower descending aorta above the diaphragm. (From Clarkson PM, Brant PWT. Aortic diameters in infants and young children: normative measurements determined with CT. Radiology 1985;61:3–6.)

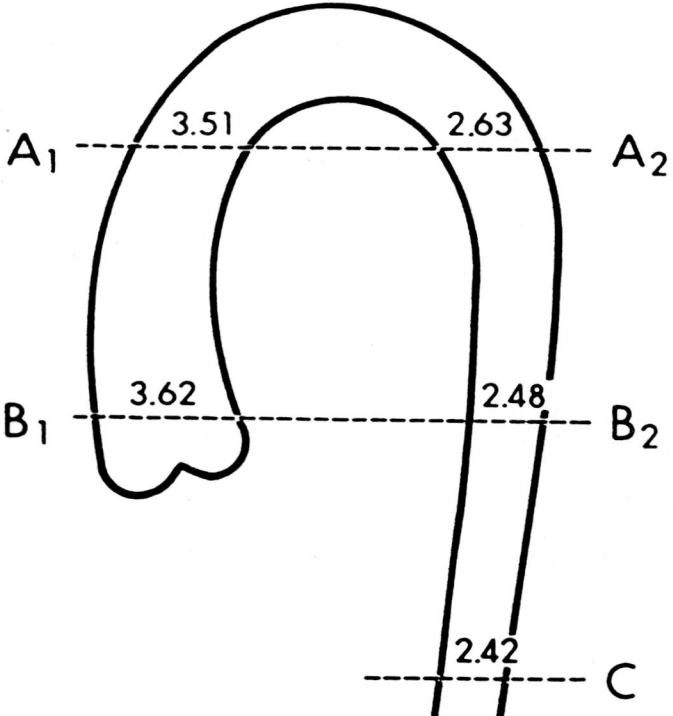

Figure 28.15. A line drawing of the lateral profile of the aorta illustrates three measurement levels: *A, B*, and *C*. The average value (in centimeters) at each level is indicated on the *dashed line*. (From Aronberg DJ et al. Normal thoracic aortic diameters by computed tomography. J Comput Assist Tomogr 1984;8:2.)

28.16). They tabulated their results according to age and body surface. Their results are presented in the following table (Table 28.5).

The normal pediatric thoracic aorta was evaluated by

Table 28.4.
Aortic Diameters: Normal Ranges (Based on 102 Patients)[a]

	Men (Years)			Women (Years)			
	21–40	41–60	⩾61	21–40	41–60	⩾61	(± 2 SD)
Centimeters							
B_1	3.47	3.63	3.91[b]	3.36	3.72	3.50[c]	(± 0.76)
A_1	3.28	3.64	3.80[b]	2.80	3.47	3.68[b]	(± 0.87)
A_2	2.21	2.64	3.14[b]	2.06	2.63	2.88[b]	(± 0.72)
B_2	2.25	2.39	2.98[b]	1.91	2.45	2.64[b]	(± 0.61)
C	2.12	2.43	2.98[b]	1.89	2.43	2.40[b]	(± 0.55)
Ratios							
A_1/A_2	1.48	1.38	1.22[b]	1.41	1.35	1.29	(± 0.31)
B_1/B_2	1.56	1.52	1.33[b]	1.78	1.55	1.38[b]	(± 0.44)
Taper							
B_1-C	1.36	1.24	0.96[b]	1.37	1.30	1.09	(± 0.91)

[a]From Aronberg DJ et al. Normal thoracic aortic diameters by computed tomography. J Comput Assist Tomogr 1984; 8(2):249.
[b]Age is a statistically significant variable (within sex) at $P < 0.01$.
[c]Age is a statistically significant variable (within sex) at $P < 0.05$.

Table 28.5.
Aortic Diameters[a]

No. Cases	Age	Asc Ao	I-LCC	LCC-LSC	Beyond LSC	Isthmus	Postisthmus	DA	LCC-LSC % DA	Isthmus % DA
4	< 1 wk	8.2[b] (0.7)[c]	6.5 (0.4)	6.2 (0.5)	5.6 (0.5)	5.5 (0.4)	7.6 (1.3)	7.0 (0.8)	90 (6)	79 (3)
6	1 wk </mo	9.1 (0.9)	—	6.5 (0.6)	5.7 (0.7)	5.2 (0.8)	7.3 (0.7)	6.0 (0.3)	108 (11)	87 (12)
16	1 < 6 mo	9.9 (1.8)	7.7 (1.4)	6.6 (0.9)	6.0 (1.0)	5.7 (0.9)	7.1 (0.9)	5.8 (0.6)	113 (15)	98 (16)
6	6 < 12 mo	12.7 (1.2)	—	8.7 (1.1)	8.0 (0.9)	7.7 (0.9)	9.2 (0.8)	7.7 (1.1)	114 (7)	101 (9)
10	1 < 2 yr	11.8 (1.0)	—	9.3 (0.9)	8.8 (0.7)	8.3 (0.7)	9.5 (1.3)	8.1 (0.9)	116 (9)	103 (5)
6	2 < 3 yr	13.7 (1.9)	—	10.4 (1.7)	10.0 (1.3)	9.7 (1.5)	11.2 (1.6)	9.2 (1.2)	113 (14)	106 (14)
6	3 < 4 yr	14.1 (2.2)	—	11.2 (1.3)	10.9 (1.5)	10.6 (1.5)	11.5 (1.7)	9.4 (0.9)	118 (7)	112 (10)
6	4 < 5 yr	15.1 (2.0)	—	10.2 (2.1)	10.2 (2.1)	9.7 (2.2)	10.5 (2.1)	8.9 (1.3)	114 (9)	108 (12)
5	5 < 6 yr	14.9 (0.9)	—	13.0 (0.6)	12.6 (1.5)	11.6 (1.3)	11.6 (1.1)	10.3 (0.8)	127 (16)	113 (10)
	BSA									
17	< 0.25	9.0 (1.0)	6.9 (1.0)	6.3 (0.6)	5.7 (0.7)	5.4 (0.7)	7.2 (1.0)	6.1 (0.7)	104 (13)	90 (16)
9	0.25 < 0.30	10.7 (1.9)	8.2 (1.1)	7.2 (0.7)	6.5 (0.7)	6.1 (0.8)	7.6 (0.6)	6.0 (0.7)	120 (11)	102 (11)
4	0.30 < 0.40	12.5 (0.9)	—	8.4 (0.5)	8.0 (0.9)	7.5 (0.7)	9.4 (0.7)	7.6 (0.5)	110 (4)	98 (6)
10	0.40 < 0.50	12.2 (1.7)	—	9.4 (1.3)	8.9 (1.0)	8.4 (1.0)	9.6 (1.4)	8.2 (1.1)	115 (13)	103 (11)
10	0.50 < 0.60	13.8 (1.7)	—	10.7 (1.3)	10.1 (1.5)	9.8 (1.6)	11.2 (1.6)	9.2 (0.9)	116 (6)	106 (10)
7	0.60 < 0.70	13.9 (2.1)	—	10.4 (2.2)	10.3 (2.0)	9.8 (1.8)	10.4 (1.6)	8.8 (1.1)	118 (14)	110 (10)
7	0.70–0.83	15.4 (1.1)	—	12.2 (1.5)	12.0 (1.6)	11.2 (1.7)	11.6 (1.7)	10.1 (0.9)	120 (8)	110 (11)

[a]From Clarkson PM, Brant PWT. Aortic diameters in infants and young children: normative angiographic data. Pediatr Cardiol 1985; 6:3–6.
[b]Diameter (mm).
[c]Figures in parentheses refer to ISD.
Asc Ao, Ascending aorta; *BSA*, body surface area; *DA*, descending aorta; *I*, innominate artery; *LCC*, left common carotid artery; *LSC*, left subclavian artery; *SD*, standard deviation.

Fitzgerald et al. (31) (Fig. 28.17 and 28.18; Table 28.6). McLoughlin et al. (32) discussed the role of CT in the evaluation of seven patients with congenital anomalies of the aortic arch and subclavian arteries. Day (33) used CT to evaluate neonates for aortic arch location with esophageal atresia.

DIAGNOSIS OF CONGENITAL ANOMALIES OF THE THORACIC AORTA

In the last 20 years, radiologic technology has reached unbelievable heights. The debt that we owe to the responsible physicians, biotechnologists, and cardiologists is great. Here, only a few anomalies are given.

Otero-Cagide et al. (34) used digital subtraction angiography in the diagnosis of vascular rings, anomalous right subclavian arteries, right aortic arch, and aberrant left subclavian artery.

Kersting-Sommerhoff et al. (35) and Gomes (36) stated that magnetic resonance imaging (MRI) is an effective, noninvasive method for the evaluation of congenital aortic arch anomalies. Kersting-Sommerhoff and colleagues evaluated 18 patients; a right aortic arch was present in 13 of these; mirror-image branching was present in 10 cases; an aberrant left subclavian artery was found in 3 cases; and a double aortic arch was present in 2 patients. The MRI diagnoses were confirmed by angiography, CT scan, surgery, and autopsy.

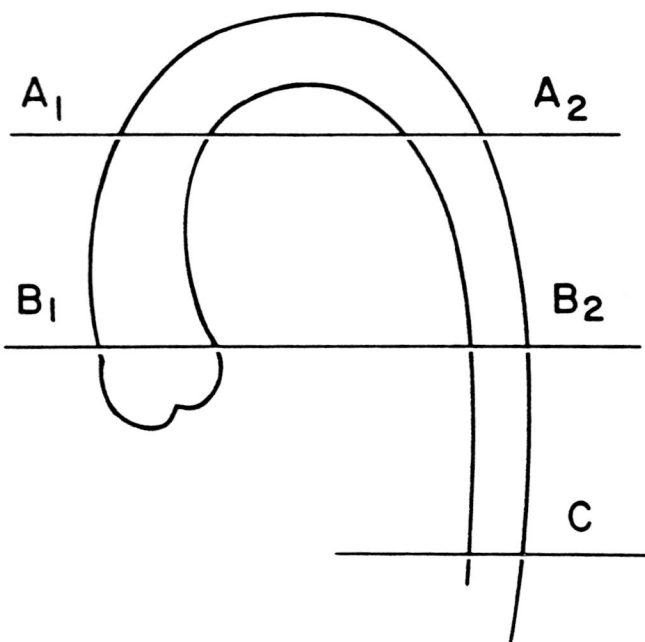

Figure 28.17. Illustration of the thoracic aorta depicting the approximate levels of aortic measurement. (From Fitzgerald SW, Donaldson JS, Poznanski AK. Pediatric thoracic aorta: normal measurements determined with CT. Radiology 1987;165:667–669.)

MRI also was shown to have high sensitivity in evaluating great vessel relationships (100%), thoracic aorta abnormalities (94%), and several other cardial and vascular anomalies (37).

Bertolini et al. (38) reported 49 infants with symptomatic compression of the trachea and/or esophagus, having the following anomalies: double aortic arch with left descending aorta (in 14); double aortic arch with right descending aorta (in 6); anomalous innominate artery (in 4); right aortic arch with aberrant left subclavian artery (in 4); left aortic arch with aberrant right subclavian artery (in 10); and aberrant left pulmonary artery (pulmonary sling) (in 2).

Fontana et al. (39) reviewed 65 patients with the origin of the right pulmonary artery from the aorta; 95% of them presented during the first year. Accurate diagnosis was made by cineangiography; associated cardiovascular anomalies were found in 85%. They reported that the right pulmonary artery originates from the ascending aorta more commonly than does the left (ratio of 8:1).

Posniak et al. (40) discussed the use of CT for diagnosis of thoracic aortic aneurysms, including aneurysms of genetic disorders (Marfan's syndrome) and other congenital anomalies. Tahernia (41) examined the role of echocardiography in the early detection of aortic dilatation associated with Marfan's syndrome and the controversial effect of β-blockers on progressive aortic dilatation.

Jaffe (42) reported the radiographic manifestations of malformations of the aortic arch, such as left, right, or double aortic arch, which produce compression of the trachea, bronchus, or esophagus, as well as several other anomalies such as coarctation and interrupted aortic arch. Diagnosis was established by chest x-ray films, esophagrams, angiographs, CT scans, and MRI.

EDITORIAL COMMENT

The diagnosis of a vascular ring starts with the plain chest radiograph. A myriad of other diagnostic procedures may be employed. The goal should be to arrive at a diagnosis with the most efficient use of the multiple tests available. These include barium esophagogram, bronchoscopy, cardiac catheterization, tracheograms, computed tomography, magnetic resonance imaging, and echocardiography. Most of the time, an esophagogram is all that is necessary for accurate diagnosis (CM).

ANOMALIES OF THE AORTA (TABLE 28.7 AND FIGURE 28.19)

Variations in the Branches of the Aortic Arch

In the "normal" arrangements of branches, the aortic arch gives off (a) the brachiocephalic artery, which divides into the right subclavian, the vertebral, and the right common carotid arteries; (b) the left common carotid artery; and (c) the left subclavian artery, from which arises the left vertebral artery. This pattern is present in about 75% of black Americans (43). Such an arrangement has been designated by Adachi (44) as type A (Fig. 28.20).

Two other branching patterns are encountered with appreciable frequency. In type B, the brachiocephalic and left common carotid arteries arise from a common trunk, and in type C, the left vertebral artery is a primary branch from the aortic arch. Types A, B, and C are the most common variations. They comprise from 92.2% (black Americans) to 98.7% (Japanese) of the branching patterns found in these populations by cadaver dissections.

The remaining varieties encountered in the cadavers examined by a number of investigators are summarized by McDonald and Anson (43). These include 14 types, none of which occurred in more than 2% of the total number examined. As many as four primary branches or as few as two may arise from the aortic arch.

All the varieties described, with the exception of those with retroesophageal right subclavian artery, may be considered normal and of purely anatomic interest. Gross (45) believes that a brachiocephalic artery arising slightly distal to its normal origin can cause tracheal compression. The thoracic surgeon must be aware, however, of the possible vascular patterns he or she may encounter.

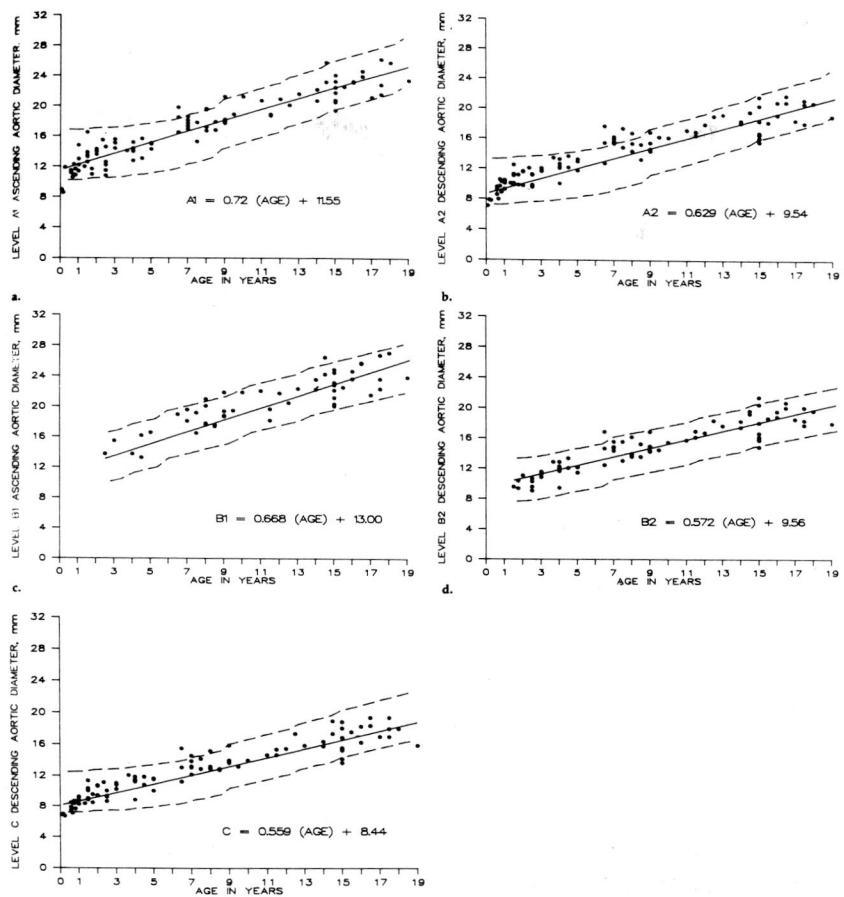

Figure 28.18. Plotted distributions of aortic diameters versus age. The *solid lines* represent linear regression lines, and the *dashed lines* represent 95% confidence bands. **A,** *A₁,* ascending aortic diameter. **B,** *A₂,* descending. **C,** *B₁,* ascending. **D,** *B₂,* descending. **E,** *C,* descending. (From Fitzgerald SW, Donaldson JS, Poznanski AK. Pediatric thoracic aorta: normal measurements determined with CT. Radiology 1987; 165:667–669.)

Table 28.6.
Aortic Diameter Correlated with Patient Ages[a,b]

Aortic Diameters	r
A_1	.94
A_2	.93
B_1	.87
B_2	.91
C	.93

[a]From Fitzerald SW, Donaldson JS, Poznanski AK. Pediatric thoracic aorta: normal measurements determined with CT. Radiology 1987; 165:667–669.
[b]Values represent linear regression coefficient. $P < .001$ for all diamters.

EDITORIAL COMMENT

Tracheal innominate artery compression is thought by some to represent abnormal medial innominate takeoff from the aorta resulting in anterior tracheal compression, which can become life-threatening. Although some have advocated reimplanting the innominate artery upstream on the aorta, most authors agree that innominate ateriopexy to the underside of the sternum provides the best results. Tracheomalacia caused by chronic innominate compression may take months to years to resolve (CM).

Aguinaga et al. (46) reported asymptomatic ectasia in the origin of the left subclavian artery associated with narrowing of the aortic arch.

Bergman (47) discusses branching and its combinations:

When there are more than three branches, the vertebral arteries are usually added or the extra branch may be the thyroid gland. A common form, with four vessels, is one in which the left vertebral arises between the left carotid and left subclavian. The following orders of branching have also been reported:

(a) Right carotid, right subclavian, left carotid, left subclavian.
(b) Right carotid, left carotid, right subclavian, left subclavian.
(c) Right carotid, left carotid, left subclavian, right subclavian (from descending aorta). This variation has an incidence of about 0.4%.

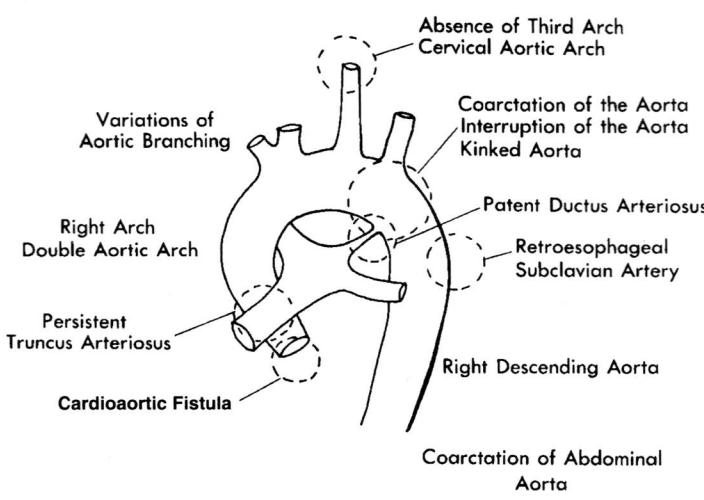

Figure 28.19. Sites of congenital anomalies of the thoracic aorta.

Table 28.7.
Anomalies of the Aorta[a]

Anomaly	Origin of Defect	First Appearance	Sex Chiefly Affected	Relative Frequency	Remarks
Kinked aorta	7th week?	None	Equal	Rare	Asymptomatic
Aortic hypoplasia	?	Young adulthood	Male	Rare	
Double aortic arch	7th week	Infancy	Equal	Uncommon	
Right aortic arch	7th week	Adulthood	Male	Uncommon	
Retroesophageal subclavian artery	7th week	Any age	Female	Common	Usually asymptomatic
Persistent third arch	7th week	Childhood	?	Very rare	
Cardioaortic fistula and aneurysm	6th week	Adulthood	Male	Rare	Some cases acquired
Coarctation of aorta	8th week or later	Childhood	Male	Common	
Interruption of aortic arch		Infancy	Male	Rare	
Coarctation of the abdominal aorta	?	Adolescence or adulthood	Equal	Rare	
Patent ductus arteriosus	At birth	Childhood	Female	Common	
Persistent truncus arteriosus	4th to 7th weeks	Childhood	Male	Rare	

[a]Coarctation of the pulmonary artery, see Chapter 14.

(d) Left carotid, right carotid, right subclavian, left subclavian.

(e) Left carotid, right carotid, left subclavian, right subclavian.

(f) Right subclavian, right carotid, left carotid, left subclavian (absence of innominate).

(g) Right brachiocephalic, left carotid, left vertebral, left subclavian.

(h) The usual branches (80% of cases)—right brachiocephalic, left common carotid, left subclavian—plus a vertebral (the left vertebral more often than the right vertebral). This variation has an incidence of about 5%.

(i) Right brachiocephalic, left carotid, left subclavian, left vertebral.

(j) Right brachiocephalic, left carotid, left subclavian, right subclavian.

(k) Right brachiocephalic, left vertebral, left subclavian, right subclavian.

(l) Right subclavian, bicarotid stem, left vertebral, left subclavian.

(m) Right innominate (with right carotid and right internal) thoracic branches), left carotid, left subclavian, right subclavian.

(n) Right brachiocephalic, left carotid, left subclavian, right vertebral.

(o) Right brachiocephalic, left internal carotid, left external carotid, left subclavian.

(p) In cases of right aortic arch: left carotid, right carotid, right subclavian, left subclavian.

(q) Right brachiocephalic, right internal thoracic, left carotid, left subclavian.

	Per Cent in U.S.	
	White	Black
	74	53
	20	38
	3	1
	<1	<0.5
	1	2
	<0.5	2
	<0.5	<0.5

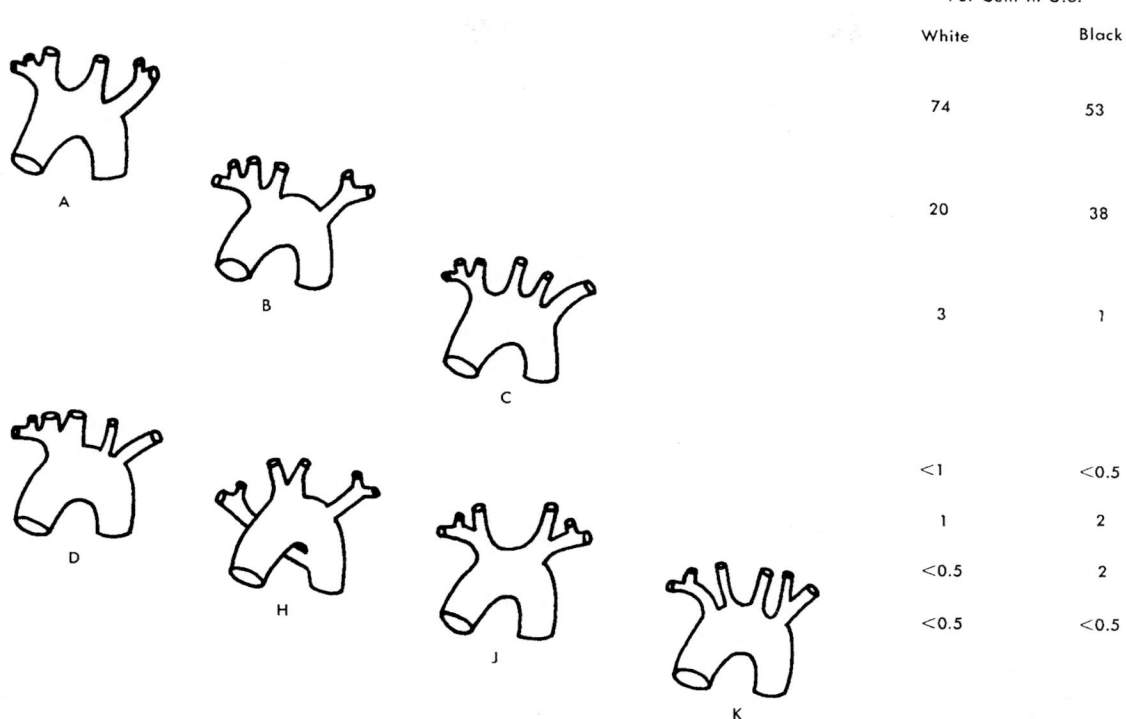

Figure 28.20. Variations in the branches of the aortic arch. The letters refer to types of Adachi as used by McDonald and Anson. The letters *E, F, G,* (not shown) and *J* are applied to rarely encountered variations; *E* has been found only among the Japanese. The letter *I* was not used in the Adachi series. (From Adachi B. Das Arteriensystem der Japaner. Kyoto, 1928; McDonald JJ, Anson BJ. Variations in the origin of arteries derived from the aortic arch in American whites and Negroes. Am J Phys Anthrop 1940;27:91–103.)

(r) Right brachiocephalic, right inferior thyroid, left carotid, left subclavian.

(s) Right brachiocephalic, left carotid, left inferior thyroid, left subclavian.

(t) Right brachiocephalic, left carotid, left superior intercostal, left subclavian.

(u) Right brachiocephalic, left thymic, left carotid, left subclavian.

When there are five arteries, the extra branches are usually the right subclavian and left vertebral. However, additions to the usual complement of three may include an internal and an external carotid in place of a common carotid, or two vertebrals. In the absence of the brachiocephalic, then the subclavian, common carotid, and one vertebral are branches of the arch. The reported order of branching follows:

(a) Right brachiocephalic, right vertebral, left carotid, left vertebral, left subclavian

(b) Right brachiocephalic, left carotid, left vertebral, left subclavian, right subclavian (from descending aorta).

(c) Right subclavian, right carotid, left carotid, left vertebral, left subclavian.

(d) Right carotid, left carotid, left vertebral, left subclavian, right subclavian (from descending aorta).

(e) Right carotid, left carotid, left subclavian, left vertebral, right subclavian (from descending aorta).

(f) Right brachiocephalic, right internal thoracic, left carotid, left vertebral, left subclavian.

(g) In cases of right arch: left carotid, right carotid, right vertebral, right subclavian, left subclavian.

(h) Also in cases of right arch: innominate with left carotid and left vertebral branches, right carotid, right vertebral, right subclavian, left subclavian.

Cases of six branches result from the separate origin for both vertebrals and both subclavians. Additional examples of branching order include the following: *(a)* with a double aortic arch, the subclavian, external carotid, and internal carotid arise successively on the right and left side; *(b)* right subclavian, right vertebral, right carotid, left carotid, left vertebral, and left subclavian; and *(c)* innominate with a thyroidea ima branch, two left vertebrals, left inferior thyroid, and left subclavian.

In about 80% of people, the branching order is right brachiocephalic, left common carotid, and left subclavian; in 11%, a common stem exists for the brachiocephalic and left common carotid, with the left subclavian arising independently from the arch.

Uncommonly, the three branches are accompanied by less significant branches: *(a)* a left thymic, *(b)* a right internal thoracic, (c) a right inferior thyroid, (d) a thyroidea ima, and (e) a left ventricular coronary.

The following arteries have been found arising from the aortic arch: external carotid, internal carotid, right vertebral, inferior thyroid, thymic, thyroidea ima, and left coronary. In rare instances, the lower parts of the lungs may receive anomalous arteries from the thoracic aorta (or the upper part of the abdominal aorta). The thoracic aorta may give rise to a right subclavian (levels T_2, T_3, T_4), a supreme intercostal, and a renal artery which descends through the aortic hiatus.

Pseudocoarctation of the Aorta ("Kinked Aorta")

ANATOMY

The normal aortic arch is an even, convex loop straightening out smoothly into the descending aorta. In the configuration called "kinked aorta," the descending portion forms an angle directed forward and downward at the level of the ligamentum arteriosum. The aorta proximal to the kink is longer than normal and the arch rises higher in the mediastinum. Distal to the angulation, the aorta may be dilated. There is no stenosis at the angulation (Fig. 28.21).

The aortic deformation may displace the left bronchus and the pulmonary artery forward, downward, and to the right. The esophagus also may be displaced forward and to the right. According to Gaynor and Sabiston (48), the term *pseudocoarctation* was first used by Dotter and Steinberg in 1952, but the first definition of this condition in adult cases was by Rosler and White (49) in 1931.

EMBRYOGENESIS

Pseudocoarctation of the aorta is a rare condition. Although usually considered to be congenital, it has generally been found in adults. Winer et al. (50) believed this condition to be due to failure of normal embryologic compression. Rather, it results from persistent growth of the normally compressed aortic segment proximal to the ligamentum arteriosum. The distance between the origin of the left common carotid and the left subclavian arteries often is increased. This portion of the aorta is derived from the fourth arch (51).

INCIDENCE

As discovery is accidental, no estimate of incidence is possible. Cases of kinked aorta are seen with equal frequency in males and females (52) and in all age groups (53).

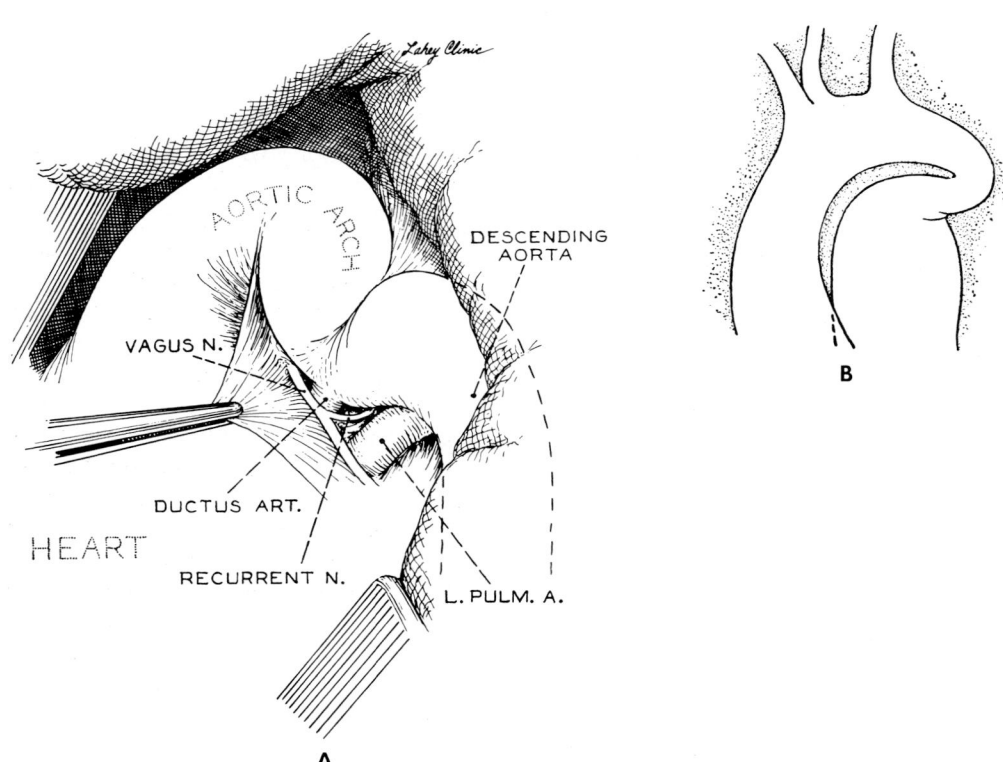

Figure 28.21. Kinked aorta. **A,** Apparent traction by the ductus arteriosus. **B,** Tracing of an angiocardiogram showing aortic deformity. It is evident that these deformities may be mistaken for coarctation of the aorta. (**A,** From Souders CR et al. An aortic deformity simulating mediastinal tumor: a subclinical form of coarctation. Dis Chest 1951; 20:35–45. **B,** After Pattinson JN, Grainger RG. Congenital kinking of the aortic arch. Br Heart J 1959;21:555–561.)

SYMPTOMS AND DIAGNOSIS

Individuals with this condition usually are asymptomatic. It may, however, be differentiated from true coarctation of the aorta by the absence of systemic hypertension, collateral circulation in the branches of the thoracic aorta, and positive pulsation of the femoral artery (52, 54). The femoral artery pulse may be weak, however, in some patients.

A chest x-ray examination shows the appearance of a mediastinal mass because of the elongation of the aortic arch. An esophageal barium x-ray examination in the left lateral or left anterior oblique position may show an S or 3 shape (55). Ruckman (56) noted, however, that an aortogram is often required to show the kinked portion of the aorta.

Although it is usually an isolated anomaly, pseudocoarctation may be associated with patent ductus arteriosus, ventricular septal defect, aortic stenosis, subaortic stenosis, transposition of the great arteries, atrial septal defect, anomalies of the aortic arch, aneurysm of the sinus of Valsalva, corrected transposition, and bicuspid aortic valve. The incidence and distribution of associated cardiac anomalies are parallel with those seen in true coarctation (54). Furthermore, it is sometimes part of a syndrome of complex malformations (e.g., Turner's, Noonan's, and Hurler's syndromes).

Aortitis syndrome (Takayasu's disease) must be taken into consideration in the differential diagnosis in children. Aneurysm formation and mediastinal mass are important alternatives in the differential diagnosis of pseudocoarctation.

TREATMENT

Surgery is generally unnecessary. If treatment is considered necessary, sectioning of the restraining ligamentum arteriosum will partially, if not completely, relieve the aortic angulation. Such relief might accompany other aortic surgery; however, surgical correction for aortic kinking alone is unwarranted. One might note that Perloff (57) warns that an aneurysm may occur in the elongated and kinked segment of the aortic knob, and for this reason he asserts that these cases should be examined regularly.

Anomalies of Complete or Partial Persistence of Right-Sided Aortic Elements

CLASSIFICATION

Attempts have been made to construct a classification that will fit all of the variations of these anomalies of the aortic arch. Edwards (58) based his system on whether the ductus arteriosus was on the left or the right. He listed 12 possible categories, of which 6 were mirror images of the

other 6. Kirklin and Clagett (59) designed an even more complicated system with 32 categories, many of them hypothetic; and Harley's system (60) contains 34 possibilities, of which 16 are as yet hypothetic combinations.

All such classifications must embrace combinations of the following:

1. Right, left, or double aortic arch
2. Descending aorta on right or left
3. Right or left ductus (ligamentum) arteriosum
4. Retroesophageal subclavian artery on right or left

The simplified classification in Table 28.8 includes combinations of three of the four variable elements. It is possible that the combinations indicated as not reported will eventually be found, but they will be very rare.

According to Idriss (61) vascular anomalies which produce tracheoesophageal obstruction can be divided as follows:

Group I:	True complete vascular ring
Subgroup Ia:	Double aortic arch
Subgroup Ib:	Right aortic arch with left ligamentum from descending aorta
Group II:	Left arch
Group III:	Pulmonary artery sling

According to Idriss, the right and left aortic arch are equal only in 7% of patients; the right or posterior are larger in 73% of patients and the left or anterior in 20% (Fig. 28.22).

EMBRYOGENESIS

The embryonic elements involved in the formation of the arch of the aorta are *(a)* a proximal segment composed of the ventral aorta (aortic sac), the fourth aortic arch, and the dorsal aortic root proximal to the seventh dorsal intersegmental artery, and *(b)* a distal segment composed of the dorsal aortic root from the seventh dorsal intersegmental artery to the junction of the left and right dorsal roots. Thus, in the primitive symmetric stage, there are right and left proximal and distal segments between the heart and the dorsal aorta.

In normal development, the right distal segment disappears in the eighth week, and the right proximal segment, together with the seventh dorsal intersegmental artery, becomes the right subclavian artery. The left proximal and distal segments, together with the seventh dorsal intersegmental artery, becomes the right subclavian artery. The left proximal and distal segments, together with the primitive ventral aorta, become compressed to form the arch of the aorta and the upper part of the descending aorta (13).

DOUBLE AORTIC ARCH (FIG. 28.23, *A* TO *D*).

Anatomy. A double aortic arch arises as a bifurcation of the ascending aorta, with both limbs passing over the

Table 28.8.
Types of Left, Right, and Double Aortic Arches

	Left Aortic Arch	Right Aortic Arch	Double Aortic Arch Both Arches Functional	Double Aortic Arch Only Posterior Arch Functional
Left descending aorta:				
Left ligamentum arteriosum	Normal *(I,J)*[a]	Rare *(G,H)*	Rare *(A)*	Uncommon *(D)*
Right ligamentum arteriosum	Not reported	Not reported	Rare *(B)*	Not reported
Right descending aorta:				
Right ligamentum arteriosum	Rare *(K)*	Uncommon *(E,F)*	Rare *(C)*	Not reported
Left ligamentum arteriosum	Not reported	Rare	Rare	Not reported

*Letters refer to Figure 28.23.

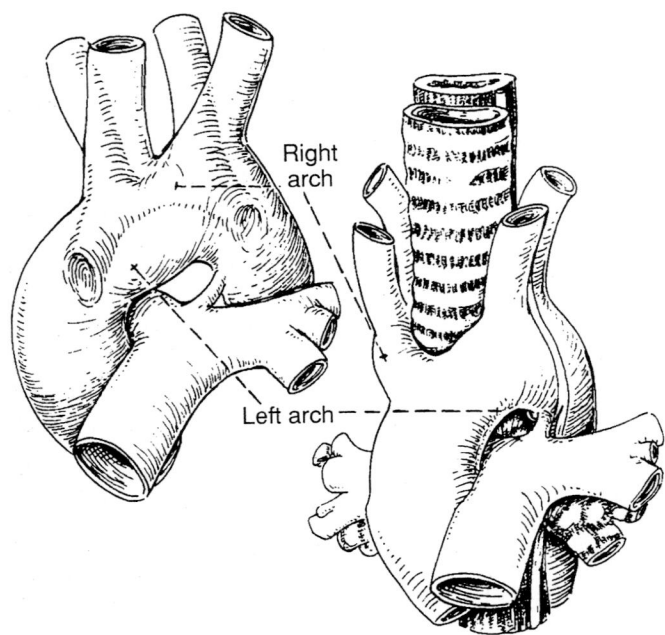

Figure 28.22. Double aortic arch with the left side dominant. **A,** Left antero-lateral view. **B,** Anterior view showing compression of trachea and esophagus. (From Idriss TS. Vascular ring. In: Raffensperger JG, ed. Swenson's pediatric surgery, 5th ed. Norwalk, CT: Appleton & Lange, 1990.)

respective bronchi and joining at a level posterior to the esophagus to form the descending thoracic aorta. Each subclavian artery and common carotid arises independently from its respective aortic arch.

The descending aorta is almost always in the normal position on the left (Fig. 28.23, *A*). The vascular ring thus formed completely surrounds the trachea and esophagus and may compress them.

Rarely are the two limbs of equal caliber (62). More often the left (pretracheal) is smaller, sometimes even represented only by a vestigial fibrous cord. The left subclavian artery may arise with the left common carotid

artery proximal to the atretic portion (Fig. 28.23, *D*), or it may arise distal to it from a diverticulum of the right (postesophageal) limb (63). This condition might better be termed *right aortic arch with retention of the left* (62, 63). The left ductus arteriosus is present, and there also may be a persistent and patent right ductus (64). The recurrent laryngeal nerves pass under both arches.

Embryogenesis. In doubling of the aorta, it is usually the right distal segment which fails to disappear. The right limb (postesophageal) thus is composed of a normally reduced proximal segment and a longer, persistent distal segment, which join the normal arch on the left to form the common descending aorta (Figs. 28.23, *A* and *B*, and 28.24, *A* to *C*). Primitive symmetry is lost because the upper descending dorsal aorta is on the left, as in the normal condition.

Where the left (anterior) limb of the double arch is narrowed, the portion derived from the fourth aortic arch is usually the affected region (Figs. 28.23, *D*, and 28.24, *D* to *F*).

History and Incidence. The first report of constriction from a double aortic arch appeared in 1837 (65). Wolman (66) reprinted an abstract of this case, with its symptoms and subsequent autopsy findings. Until 1936, only 40 examples of this anomaly were discovered, all at autopsy.

Double aortic arch is the most common type of symptomatic vascular ring (67). It has been described with other cardiac anomalies in 20% of cases. Ventricular septal defect and tetralogy of Fallot are the most common associated congenital diseases, but it also may occur with left patent arterial duct, common arterial trunk, and aortic coarctation (68, 69).

Symptoms and Diagnosis. About 75% of affected individuals are symptomatic. Symptoms range from mild to life-threatening respiratory obstruction and apnea. Those affected who are asymptomatic usually are detected accidentally as older children and young adults. Inspiratory stridor, dyspnea, and wheezing are characteristic and are accentuated with feeding, crying, or respiratory infections. Voluntary hyperextension of the neck often is observed, along with resistance to enforced flexion, which narrows the airway.

A vascular shadow to the right of the esophagus and trachea simulating an isolated right aortic arch is the usual picture on chest roentgenogram. This is due to the fact that the right arch is the larger of the two arches in between 75 and 85% of patients. The frontal view of a barium swallow or esophagram will reveal bilateral compression of the esophagus with the larger and more superior indentation indicating the dominant arch. The lateral view will show a large posterior esophageal indentation, seen as the dominant arch crosses the midline. Aortography is recommended to evaluate the relative sizes and the patency of the two arches and to identify the brachiocephalic arterial branches. Complete cardiac catheterization always is indicated if associated heart disease is suspected.

Treatment. No therapy is required for those few patients who remain asymptomatic. However, the majority of patients present within the first month or two of life with symptoms which may have been present since birth. Once present, these persist and usually progress. Surgical relief of the constricting ring is recommended as soon as possible for symptomatic patients.

EDITORIAL COMMENT

Through a left thoracotomy careful dissection in the posterior mediastinum should be performed to clearly delineate the anatomic configuration of the vascular ring. In particular, the left subclavian artery, ligamentum arteriosum, and descending aorta should be identified first. Typically, the left arch is the smaller of the two arches, and it may be atretic where it inserts into the descending aorta. In our series of patients at Children's Memorial Hospital in Chicago, the right arch (posterior arch) was dominant in 73% of the patients, the left-sided or anterior arch was dominant in 20%, and the arches were of equal size in 7%. With a dominant right arch, segments of the left arch were atretic in 40% of the patients. With a dominant left arch, segments of the right arch were atretic in 33% of the patients. The atretic area occurred most frequently in the posterior or distal end of the lesser arch. The vascular ring caused by the double aortic arch is released by dividing the lesser of the two arches, usually at the atretic area. The lesser arch is divided between clamps at a site selected to preserve brachiocephalic blood blow. After applying the vascular clamps, the anesthesiologist carefully checks the carotid and radial pulses on both the left and right sides. This ensures that the blood flow is not interrupted. Then the ring is divided and the two stumps are each oversewn. In addition, the ligamentum arteriosum is always divided, and careful dissection is performed around the esophagus and the

trachea to lyse any residual adhesive bands. The mediastinal pleura is left widely open. The recurrent laryngeal nerves and phrenic nerves are identified and protected throughout the case (CM).

RIGHT AORTIC ARCH

Anatomy. A right arch may exist together with a left arch, as described in the preceding, or it may exist independently. Three varieties of right aortic arch are known:

1. A right aortic arch as the mirror image of the normal arch is the most common (Fig. 28.23, *I*). The order of primary branches is reversed: The heart and usually other organs are reversed (situs inversus).
2. No situs inversus, but true persistence of right aortic arch and right dorsal aorta (Fig. 28.23, *E*): Cardiac anomalies, double superior venae cavae, and a retroesophageal left subclavian artery are common (Fig. 28.23, *F*).
3. Persistence of the aortic arch only on the right: Drainage occurs into a normal left-sided descending aorta by passage behind the esophagus (Fig. 28.23, *G* and *H*).

When a right arch and a left ligamentum arteriosum are present, the latter passes from the left pulmonary artery to the descending aorta or to the left subclavian artery, coursing to the left of the trachea and esophagus. These structures may be compressed by the ring formed by the aorta, the pulmonary artery, and the ligament.

Most right aortic arches are associated with situs inversus; when this is not the case, most commonly an aberrant rather than a normal left subclavian artery also is present (63).

Embryogenesis. A persistent right aortic arch may be formed as the mirror image of a normal left arch by the disappearance of the left distal segment. This is the condition that exists in situs inversus. It also may exist without inversion of other viscera (Figs. 28.23, *E*, and 28.25, *D* to *F*). In the latter case the presence of a left aberrant subclavian artery as the most distal branch from the aorta is common (Fig. 28.23, *F*).

The second variety of persistent right arch arises from the disappearance of only the proximal portion of the left distal aortic segment. The right distal segment becomes absorbed into the remaining part of the left distal segment so that the persistent right arch drains into a left-sided descending aorta (Fig. 28.23, *G*). When the left subclavian artery arises from a diverticulum of the descending aorta (70), instead of from a left brachiocephalic artery, it is the left proximal aortic segment that has vanished. The diverticulum represents the greatly shortened proximal portion of the left distal segment and the subclavian artery is "aberrant" but not retroesophageal.

History and Incidence. A persistent right arch was reported in 1793 by Abernathy (71); however, earlier writers may have mentioned other examples. Luetmer

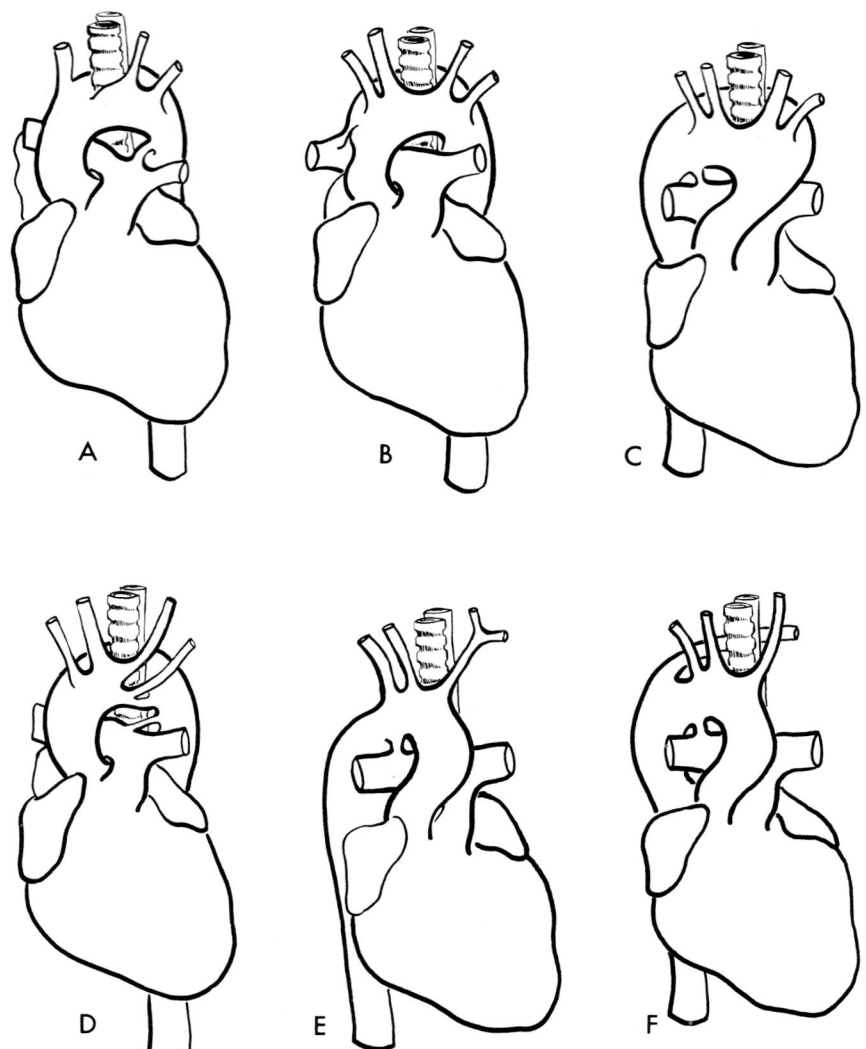

Figure 28.23. Anomalies of the arch of the aorta and its branches. **A,** Double aortic arch, both limbs functional, with left ligamentum arteriosum and left descending aorta. **B,** As in **A,** with right ligamentum arteriosum. **C,** Double aortic arch with right ligamentum arteriosum and right descending aorta. **D,** Double aortic arch with atresia of left arch, left ligamentum arteriosum, and left descending aorta.

E, Right aortic arch, with right ligamentum arteriosum and right descending aorta. **F,** As in **E,** with retroesophageal left subclavian artery. **G,** Right aortic arch with left ligamentum arteriosum, left descending aorta, and left subclavian artery from branchiocephalic artery. **H,** As in **G,** with separated left carotid and subclavian arteries. **I,** Left aortic arch with left ligamentum arteriosum and left descending

and Miller (72) presented a review of the literature on cases of right aortic arch with isolation of the left subclavian artery (Table 28.9).

This anomaly occurs in approximately 0.1 to 0.14% of the population. The incidence of congenital heart disease is 98% when there is mirror-image branching. The majority of these patients having tetralogy of Fallot. The incidence of cardiac anomalies is about 10% in the presence of an aberrant left subclavian artery. A right aortic arch is found in approximately 53% of individuals with pulmonary atresia and ventricular septal defect, 31% of those with tetralogy of Fallot, 31% of individuals with

truncus arteriosus, 20% of individuals with double-outlet right ventricle, and 5% of patients with tricuspid atresia (73).

Symptoms and Diagnosis. Individuals with a right aortic arch who do not present with heart disease or with a nonrestrictive ring are asymptomatic.

Symptoms of compression from persistent right aortic arch and left ductus arteriosus are similar to those produced by a double arch, but these develop later in infancy and are perhaps less severe. Mild symptoms may exist for many years or may begin only late in life. The fact that the aorta increases in diameter up to the age of 40 years (74)

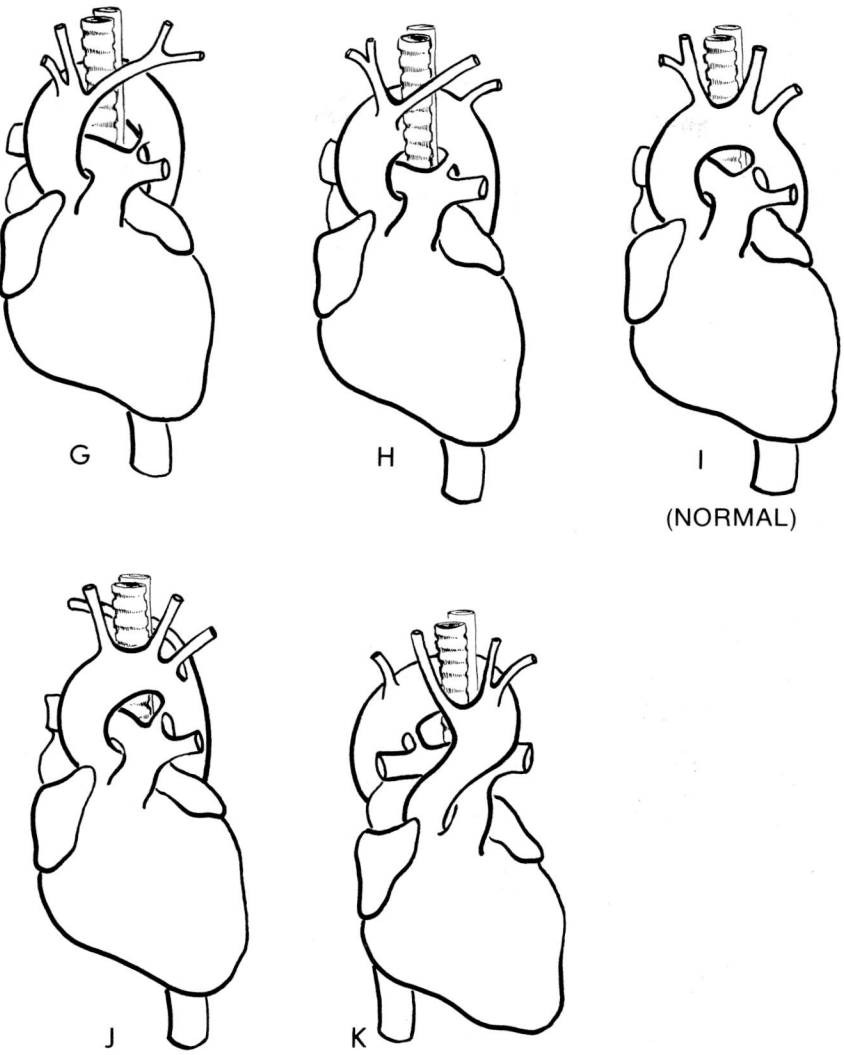

(NORMAL)

aorta. (This is the normal pattern of the arch; in situs inversus, a mirror image is present). **J,** As in **I,** with retroesophageal right subclavian artery. **K,** Left aortic arch with right ligamentum arteriosum and right descending aorta. These are 11 of the 34 possible variations of the aortic arch pattern described by Harley. Of the 34 variations that could occur, 16 have not been described. (Redrawn from Harley HRS. The development & anomalies of the aortic arch & its branches. Br J Surg 1959;46:561–573.)

may explain such cases. Right aortic arch is the next most frequent vascular ring disorder, after the double aortic arch (75).

Right aortic arch may be diagnosed by plain chest x-ray examination, two-dimensional echocardiography (from the suprasternal view), and MRI.

Treatment. Surgery is required if tracheal and esophageal compression is caused by an associated retroesophageal subclavian arterial segment and/or a left-sided ligamentum arteriosum. All forms of such compression may be relieved by division of the ligamentum arteriosum through a posterolateral left thoracotomy (76).

EDITORIAL COMMENT

For the patient with a right aortic arch and a left ligamentum, careful dissection is accomplished through a left thoracotomy with identification of the configuration of the aortic arch and the ligamentum arteriosum, which is identified as compressing the esophagus. The ligamentum is either doubly ligated and divided or doubly clamped and divided with the two stumps oversewn. Any adhesive bands are lysed and the recurrent laryngeal nerve and phrenic nerves are carefully identified and protected. In addition, patients with a right aortic arch and a left ligamentum may have a Kommerell's diverticulum at the origin of the left subclavian artery from the

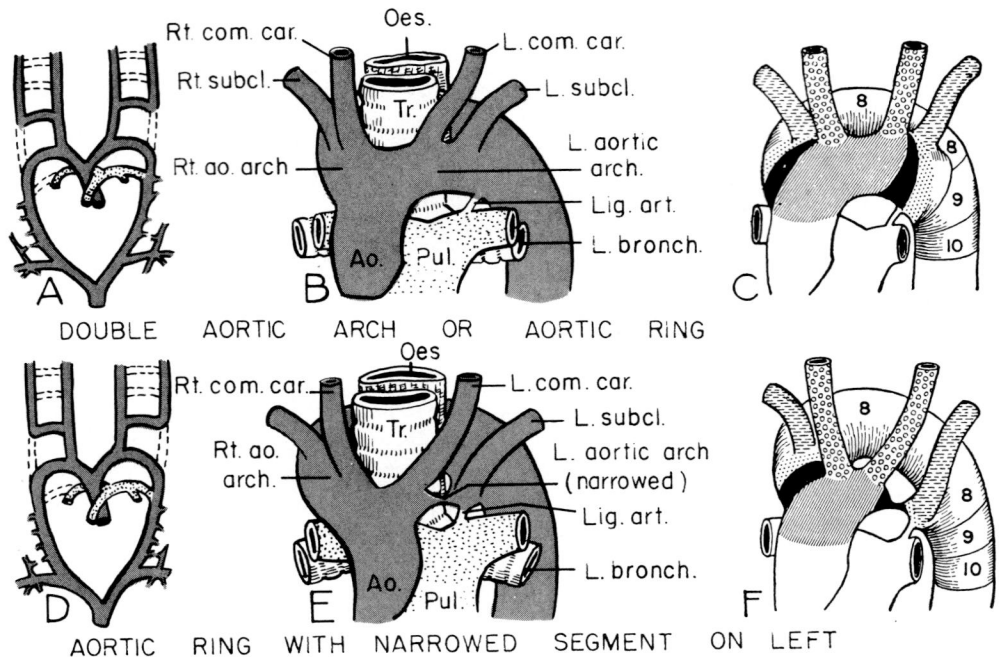

Figure 28.24. Double aortic arch with left descending aorta. **A** to **C,** Arches of approximately equal diameter. **D** to **F,** Left arch greatly narrowed at site of embryonic fourth arch. Symbols and shading are the same as in Figures 28.5 and 28.7. (**A** and **D,** From Patten BM. Human embryology, 3rd ed. New York:

McGraw-Hill, 1968; **B** and **E,** from Edwards JE. Anomalies of the derivatives of the aortic arch system. Med Clin NA 1948; 32:925–949; **C** and **F,** after Barry A. Aortic arch derivatives in the human adult. Anat Rect 1951;111:221–228.)

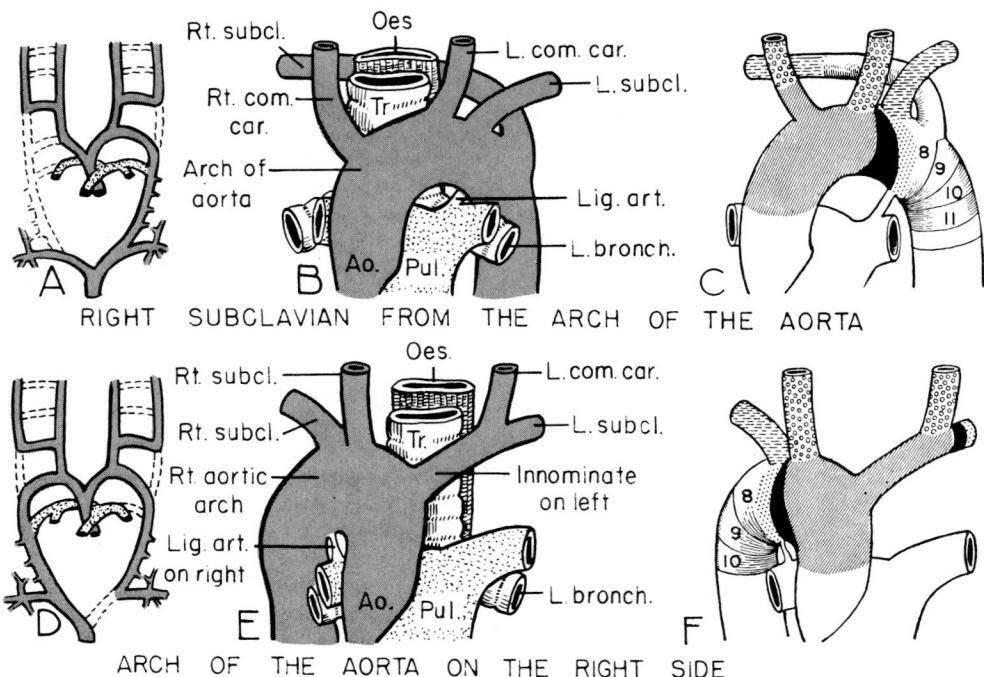

Figure 28.25. Aortic arch anomalies. **A** to **C,** Retroesophageal right subclavian artery. **D** to **F,** Right aortic arch with right descending aorta. Symbols and shading are the same as in Figures 28.5, 28.7, and 28.24). (**A** and **D,** From Patten BM. Human embryology, 3rd ed. New York: McGraw-Hill, 1968; **B** and

E, from Edwards JE. Anomalies of the derivatives of the aortic arch system. Med Clin NA 1948; 32:925–949; **C** and **F,** after Barry A. Aortic arch derivatives in the human adult. Anat Rec 1951;111:221–228.)

Table 28.9.

Summary of Reported Cases of Angiographically or Pathologically Documented Right Aortic Arch With Isolation of Left Subclavian Artery[a]

Reference	Patient Age (yr)	Symptoms of Ischemia		Congenital Heart Disease	Comment
		Vertebrobasilar	Left Upper Extremity		
Barger et al., 1956	<1	—	—	Bilat PDA	—
Massumi, 1963	6	No	No	No	R cervical arch, atretic R common carotid artery
Stewart et al., 1966	—	—	—	TOF	—
	—	—	—	Truncus arteriosus	—
D'Cruz et al., 1966	4	—	—	VSD	—
	—	—	—	DORV Mitral atresia	Persistent left SVC
Antia & Ottesen, 1966	6	No	No	No	Supravalvular aortic stenosis
Bradley, 1966	21	No	No	No	Short mod, coarctation
Gerber, 1967	8	No	No	No	Possible hypercalcemic syndrome
Maranhao et al., 1968	19	No	No	No	—
Love, 1968	30	Yes (<1 yr)	Yes (<1 yr)	No	—
Replogle, 1968	2	—	—	TOF	—
Lansing & Murphy, 1968	4	No	No	TOF	—
	<1	No	No	TOF	Persistent L SVC
Skalpe & Semb, 1969	7	No	No	TOF	—
Victorica et al., 1970	2	No	No	TOF	—
	<1	No	No	TOF	PAPVR
Shuford et al., 1970	23	No	Yes (11 yr)	No	—
	34	No	No	No	—
Pieroni et al., 1972	<1	No	No	VSD	—
Sunderland et al., 1972	<1	—	No	ASD L PDA	TAPVR Cleft mitral valve
Knight & Edwards, 1974	—	—	—	TOF	—
Borushok et al., 1974	18	No	No	No	Long coarctation
	53	Yes	—	No	—
Rodriguez et al., 1975	<1	No	No	TOF	—
	<1	No	No	VSD	—
	<1	No	No	TOF	—
	3	No	No	TOF	—
				No	—
				No	
Stanford et al., 1978	22	No	Yes (3 yr)	No	—
Roguin et al., 1981	6	No	No	TOF	—
Lakner & Lukacs, 1981	33	Yes	Yes	No	—
	48	No	Yes	No	—
	35	Yes	No	No	—
Nath et al., 1981	5	No	No	TOF	—
	2	No	No	TOF	—
	<1	No	No	DORV	—
	<1	—	—	VSD	—
Stein & Christie, 1982	34	No	No	No	—
Luetmer & Miller, 1990	52	Yes (2 yr)	No	No	—

[a]From Luetmer PH, Miller GM. Right aortic arch with isolation of the left subclavian artery. Mayo Clin Proc 1990; 65:407–413.

ASD, Atrial septal defect; *Bilat,* bilateral; *DORV,* double-outlet right ventricle; *L,* left; *mod.,* moderate; *PDA,* patent ductus arteriosus; *PAPVR,* partial anomalous pulmonary venous return; *R,* right; *SVC,* superior vena cava; *TAPVR,* total anomalous pulmonary venous return; *TOF,* tetralogy of Fallot; *VSD,* ventricular septal defect.

descending aorta. This diverticulum is embryologically a remnant of the left fourth aortic arch, which is otherwise involuted. This diverticulum may enlarge to proportions that can independently compress the esophagus or trachea. In this instance, the diverticulum or aneurysmal dilatation should either be resected or pexed to the thorax or spine to prevent its independent compression of the trachea or esophagus (CM).

Anterior aortopexy through a right thoracotomy has been used successfully to treat severe tracheal and right main stem bronchial obstruction caused by a right aortic arch without a vascular ring (77).

McNally and Rak (78) found that dysphagia lusoria caused by right aortic arch and diverticulum of Kommerell with an aberrant left subclavian artery may be satisfactorily managed by dietary modification when symptoms are mild.

LEFT AORTIC ARCH WITH RIGHT DESCENDING AORTA (FIG. 28.23, K)

Anatomy. This anomaly is the reverse of the third variety described previously.

Embryogenesis. Case reports support the pathogenic concept of the Rathke diagram of a complete double aortic primitive arch originating from the pulmonary and supraaortic vascular structures which are formed by the obliteration or disappearance of particular segments of the structure. Such a theory could explain the embryogenesis of these complex anomalies (79, 80).

Incidence. Approximately 17 cases had been reported in the literature up to 1989.

Symptoms and Diagnosis. Tracheal deviation to the right and the position of the descending aorta on the right side of the thoracic vertebral column will be revealed on routine chest roentgenogram. An esophagogram will show an indentation of the esophagus dorsally.

This anomaly may be accompanied by a right ligamentum arteriosum and may lead to formation of a symptomatic vascular ring in infancy, which most likely will result in severe respiratory distress in the infant. No ring is formed, however, if the left-sided ligamentum persists (as in approximately 67% cases).

The presence of such a ring has important ramifications for diagnosis and treatment. Ergin et al. (81) recommend barium swallow and angiography and warn against bronchoscopy and bronchography which could aggravate the airway obstruction.

Treatment. Left aortic arch and right descending aorta should be considered in any infant with congenital heart disease who develops signs of upper airway obstruction. Decision of surgical treatment rests on an exact preoperative diagnosis of the anomaly and possible associated conditions.

Minami et al. (80) assert that a right thoracotomy is required for the surgical treatment of a vascular ring formed by a left aortic arch, a retroesophageal segment, a right descending aorta, and right-sided ductus or ligamentum arteriosum.

EDITORIAL COMMENT

Most arch-ligamentum rings are approached through a left thoracotomy. In the case of left aortic arch and right descending aorta, the tensile ligamentum arteriosum is best approached from a right thoracotomy if symptoms warrant operative therapy (CM).

RETROESOPHAGEAL SUBCLAVIAN ARTERY (FIG. 28.26)

Anatomy. Although sometimes listed as a variation in the branches of the aortic arch, the aberrant retroesophageal subclavian artery must be considered to represent persistence of right arch elements.

From an otherwise normal left aortic arch, the right subclavian artery arises as the most distal, rather than as the most proximal, branch. It passes to the right, behind the trachea and esophagus, and in front of the vertebral column (Fig. 28.23, *J*). Compression of the esophagus

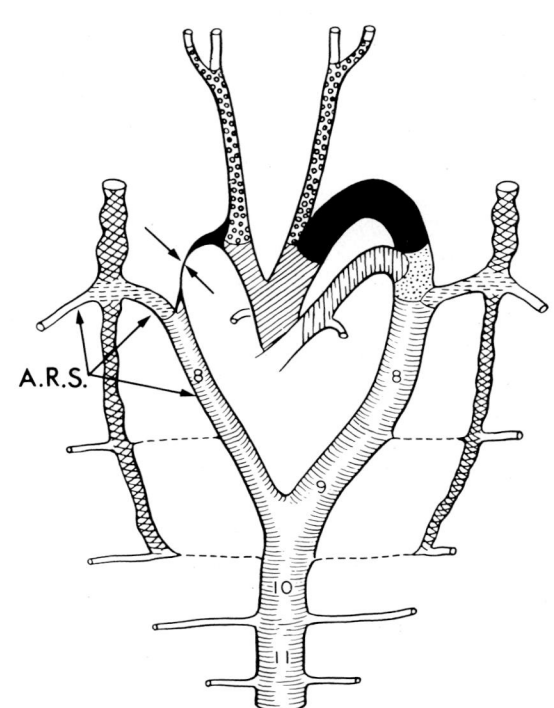

Figure 28.26. Development of an aberrant retroesophageal right subclavian artery (A.R.S.) Persistence of right segment 8 and regression of the right fourth arch is the opposite of the normal development, as seen in Figure 28.7. (From Beabout JW, Stewart JR, King OW. Aberrant right subclavian artery: dispute of commonly accepted concepts. AJR 1964;92:855–858.)

and trachea by the aberrant artery may interfere with swallowing (dysphagia lusoria).

A similar anomaly may occur when the right arch of the aorta persists. The left subclavian artery arises from the right arch and passes behind the esophagus to the left arm (Fig. 28.23, *F*). This condition is common with a persistent right arch.

The recurrent branch of the right vagus nerve normally loops under that part of the right subclavian artery derived from the right fourth arch. When the right subclavian is aberrant, the segment from the fourth arch is absent; the recurrent nerve leaves the vagus at a higher level, reaching the larynx directly or passing under the inferior thyroid artery. In a few cases it loops under a persistent right ductus arteriosus (70). When an aberrant left subclavian artery arises from a right-sided aortic arch, the nerve loops under the left ligamentum arteriosum, which passes from the left pulmonary artery to the aberrant left subclavian artery.

Frequently, but not always, the thoracic duct opens into the right subclavian vein rather than into the left in the presence of an anomalous right subclavian artery (82).

Embryogenesis. Right retroesophageal subclavian arteries arise by the disappearance of the right proximal aortic segment and the persistence of the right distal segment, which normally disappears. The subclavian artery thus is formed from the distal aortic root and the seventh dorsal intersegmental artery. Shortening of the left distal aortic root brings the origin of the aberrant right subclavian artery just distal to the normal left subclavian artery (13, 83) (Figs. 28.23, *F*, 28.25, *A* to *C*, and 28.26).

Similarly, when the right aortic arch persists and drains into a right descending aorta, the left subclavian may pass behind the esophagus to produce a mirror image of the retroesophageal right subclavian artery. When a right arch drains into a left-sided descending aorta, a similar persistence of the right distal segment produces a left subclavian artery arising from an aortic diverticulum. The aberrant artery does not pass posterior to the esophagus since the right arch has itself crossed behind it (Fig. 28.23, *H*).

History and Incidence. Interference with deglutition by an aberrant subclavian artery was described in 1794 by Bayford (84), who introduced the term *dysphagia lusoria*. Although isolated cases had been reported (85), dysphagia received little attention until 1946 when Gross (86) reawakened interest in the problem.

The right subclavian artery arises as the fourth branch of the aortic arch in approximately 0.5% of individuals with a left aortic arch.

Aberrant left subclavian artery may be associated with a right aortic arch.

Symptoms and Diagnosis. An aberrant right subclavian artery with an otherwise normal left aortic arch seldom if ever produces symptoms. The exception are the occasional cases in which it is implicated with dysphagia.

An aberrant left subclavian artery arising from a right aortic arch almost invariably is part of a loose, but complete, vascular ring. This is due to its connection with the left pulmonary artery via a persistent left patent ductus arteriosus or ligamentum arteriosum. Although this is the most common of vascular rings, it rarely produces symptoms. If the origin of the subclavian artery is aberrant, atresia or stenosis of the origin of a subclavian artery appears to be more common (67).

The aberrant right subclavian artery creates a shallow, oblique, posterior indentation of the barium-filled esophagus, slanting upward from left to right on chest roentgenogram. The aberrant left subclavian artery associated with right aortic arch and tetralogy of Fallot creates a similar shallow, oblique indentation, slanting upward from right to left.

Treatment. The retroesophageal subclavian artery rarely causes symptoms or requires surgical intervention to relieve dysphagia (86, 87).

A left thoracotomy after mobilization of the retroesophageal segment will divide the artery and thus allow the vessel to retract into the right hemithorax (67).

Cervical Aortic Arch (Persistent Complete Third Aortic Arch)

The aortic arch is displaced upwards as compared with its normal position in this rare congenital anomaly. The cervical arch usually is right-sided, passing behind the trachea and esophagus. This position may lead to respiratory distress and dysphagia. The branching pattern of the arch vessels is variable. Haughton et al. (88) classified cervical aortic arches into five morphological types based on the side of the descending aorta and the branching pattern.

Embryologically, this appears to represent persistence of the right third arch and the right ductus caroticus, with disappearance of both fourth arches (89) (Fig. 28.27, *D* to *F*). The anomaly dates from the seventh week of embryonic life; it is the result of obstruction of the fourth arches. The relation of progressive degenerative changes in the aneurysmal wall might indicated the predisposition to mediacystic necrosis or the high incidence of arch anomalies in patients with connective tissue disorders (90). Felson and Strife (91) note that the anomaly's unusual connections confirm some of the views about the maldevelopment of aortic arch.

Cervical aortic arch was first described by Reid (92) in 1914. The first clinical report of the anomaly was by Beavan and Fatti in 1947 (89). There have been approximately 57 cases reported in the literature since that time.

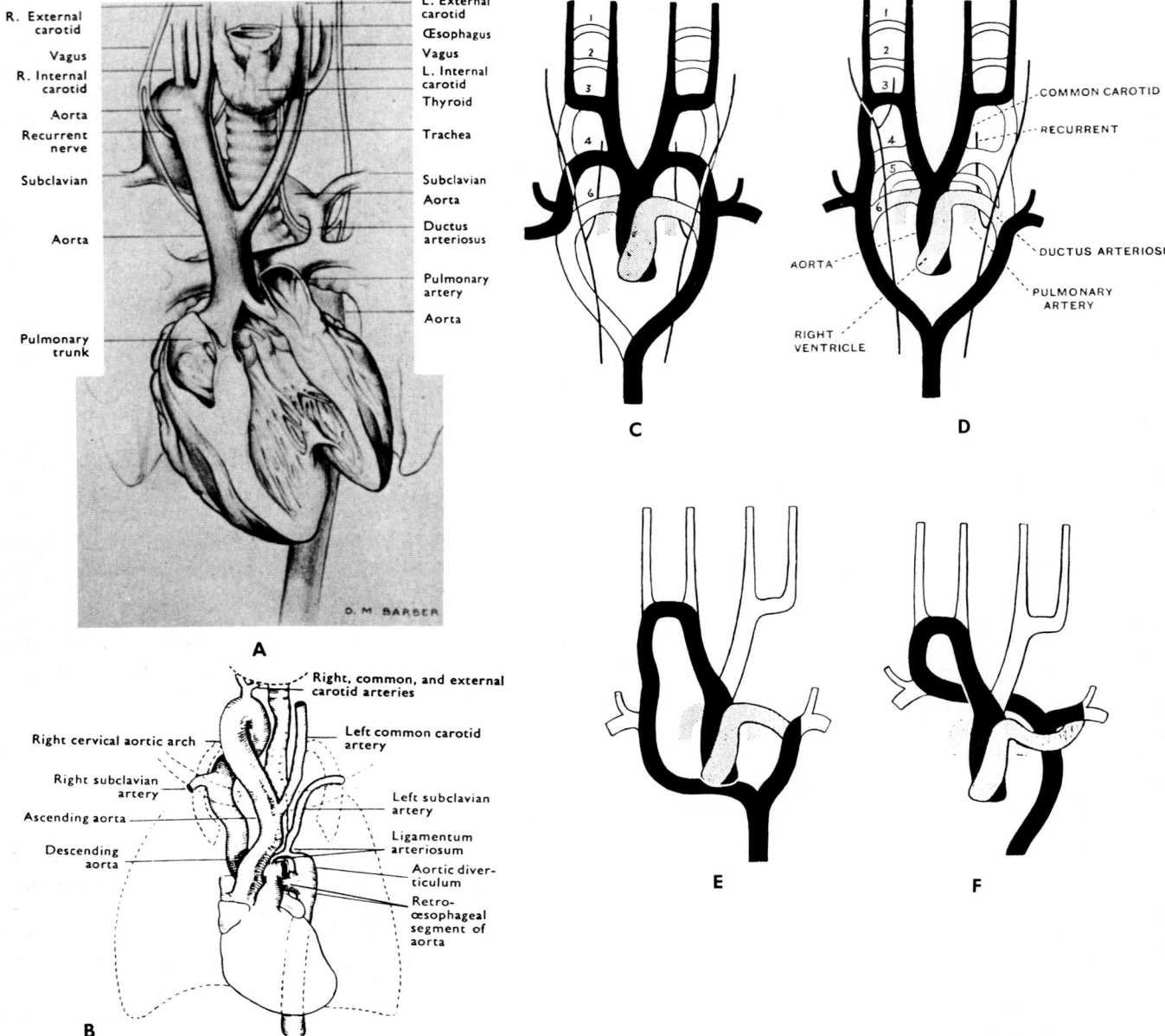

Figure 28.27. Persistent third aortic arch forming the aorta. **A** and **B,** Two nearly identical cases. The patient illustrated in **A** was assumed to have an aneurysm in the neck; the arch was ligated, with a fatal result. **B,** Constriction of trachea and esophagus in this patient was relieved by sectioning the ligamentum arteriosum.

There is no apparent sex preponderance. Many of the patients have been asymptomatic. The most common symptom is dysphagia although wheezing, coughing, stridor, choking, apneic spells, and repeated bouts of aspiration pneumonia generally caused by compression of the esophagus or trachea by a vascular ring also have been reported. Therefore, presenting features vary from a pulsatile swelling in the supraclavicular fossa to symptoms simulating a respiratory tract infection. Swallowing problems are more common in patients with documented ductus or ligamentum.

The predominant congenital heart anomaly associated with right cervical arch is ventricular septal defect (93). Left cervical aortic arch has been associated with patent ductus arteriosus, tetralogy of Fallot, and pseudotruncus. Sobrino-Marquez et al. (94) reported cases associated with pulmonary atresia with interventricular septal defect and pulmonary branch stenosis.

The diagnosis can be made on observation of an absent aortic knob at its usual site, descending aorta on the wrong side, posterior indentation of the trachea, and a large posterior defect on the mid-third of the back of the esophagus. Angiography will confirm the diagnosis; it demonstrates the abnormal sequence of the brachiocephalic vessels, the retroesophageal course of the aortic arch, and the contralateral descending aorta. Two-dimensional echocardiography, CT, and MRI have been used to describe the diagnostic features of the anomaly. Such imaging is useful should surgery be contemplated (91). Baker et al. (95) assert that aortography is necessary for a definitive diagnosis because its use prevents an erroneous clinical diagnosis, either of an aneurysm of the brachiocephalic arteries or of a neck or mediastinal neoplasm.

Absence of the Third Aortic Arch (Agenesis of an Internal Carotid Artery)

Normally, the third aortic arch, together with the cephalic portion of the dorsal root of the aorta, persists as the internal carotid artery (Fig. 28.7). Abnormal regression of these vessels results in absence of the artery.

This rare developmental anomaly occurs before the 24-mm stage of embryogenesis. The exact embryologic stage at which inappropriate involution of components of the third aortic arch occur may determine the type of collateral circulation which develops in this anomaly (96–99).

From the first report of Tode in 1787 (100) until 1980,

there were 62 cases of an absent internal carotid artery presented in the literature (96). Of the cases in the literature to 1993, there were 18 cases of bilateral agenesis (96). There is a male predominance.

Absence of one or both of the arteries may be entirely asymptomatic under usual conditions. The defect may, for instance, be found accidently at autopsy or at incidental surgery of the neck (Fig. 28.28). This type of anomaly, however, has often been associated with intracranial aneurysm. Initial symptoms may be due to subarachnoid hemorrhage from intracranial aneurysms, anomalous vasculature, or transient ischemic attacks related to atheromatous lesions (96).

Absence may be disclosed by angiography and confirmed by cavernous sinography and CT of the base of the skull (101).

The basic approaches to surgical reconstruction of vertebral artery stenosis include transsubclavian-vertebral thromboendarterectomy with or without patch angioplasty, patch angioplasty with or without endarterectomy, direct vertebral anastomosis to the subclavian or carotid artery, and bypass or interposition grafting. Cali et al. (96) note that a direct anastomosis into the ipsilateral common carotid or subclavian artery is generally preferred because it avoids the difficulties of obtaining an adequate end-point with an endarterectomy and the additional dissection and multiple suture lines with a bypass or interposition graft.

Congenital Aneurysm of the Sinus of Valsalva

ANATOMY

Congenital weakness of the wall of one of the three aortic sinuses of Valsalva may permit aneurysmal dilation and eventual rupture (Fig. 28.29). The structural defect of the sinus aneurysm has been described as a lack of continuity between the aortic annulus and aortic media which facilitates formation of the aneurysmal sac, the walls of which are composed of fibrous tissue (102, 103). Aneurysms of the sinus of Valsalva may occur in the right, left, or noncoronary sinus. These aneurysms may be single or multiple (two or more sinuses involved), although there are varying reports as to the frequency of multiple aortic sinus aneurysms (102). The most common site is on the right (75 to 90%), followed by the noncoronary sinus (10 to 25%); the remainder occur in the left coronary sinus (104). The aneurysm may originate in any of the three aortic sinuses and may protrude into any chamber of the heart. The classification in Table 28.10 indicates the known combinations and their relative frequencies.

EMBRYOGENESIS

Aneurysms of the sinus of Valsalva may be acquired or congenital. Acquired aneurysms may result from trauma,

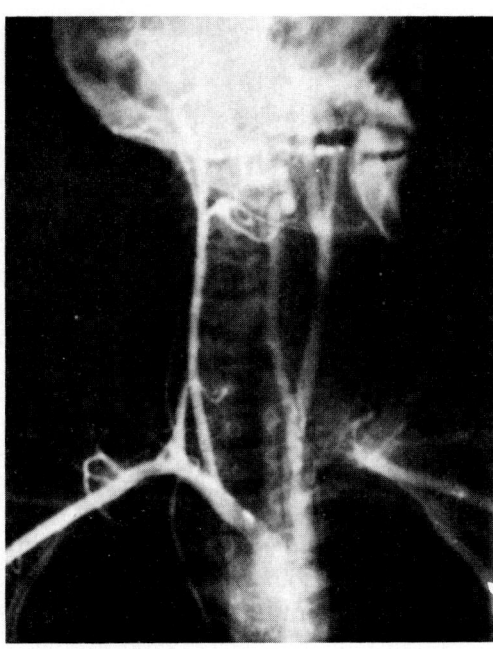

Figure 28.28. Absence of the right internal carotid artery. Arteriogram of patient in whom the anomaly was accidentally discovered following head injury. (From Hussain SA et al. Congenital absence of the internal carotid artery. J Cardiovasc Surg 1968;9:285–287.)

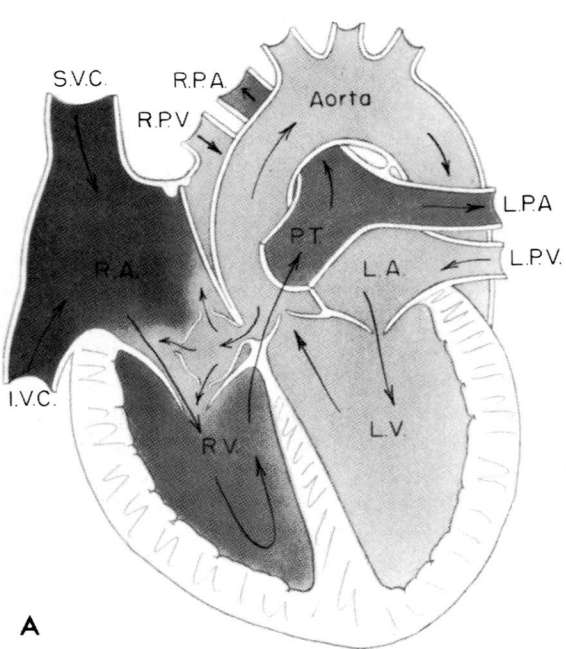

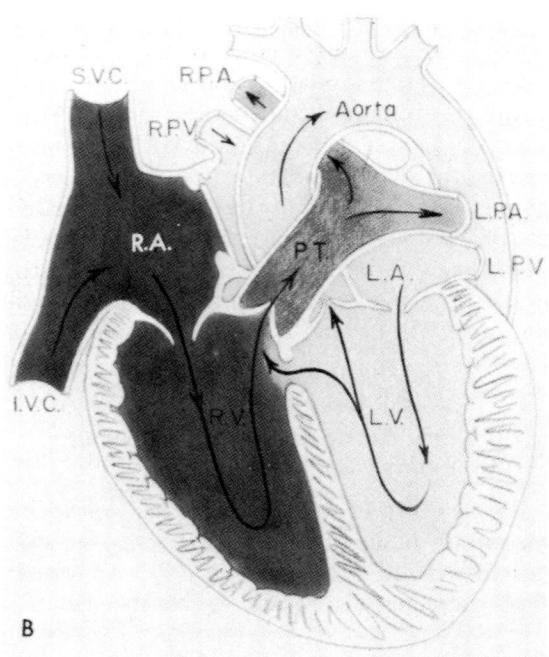

Figure 28.29. Sinus of Valsalva fistula. **A,** Aneurysm involves the posterior sinus and ruptures into the right atrium. **B,** Aneurysm involves right aortic sinus and ruptures into the right ventricle. A ventricular septal defect is commonly associated, as illustrated. *SVC,* Superior vena cava; *IVC,* inferior vena cava; *RA,* right atrium; *RV,* right ventricle; *PT,* main pulmonary arterial trunk; *RPA,* right pulmonary artery;

LPA, left pulmonary artery; *RPV,* right pulmonary vein; *LPV,* left pulmonary vein; *LA,* left atrium; *LV,* left ventricle; *Ao,* aorta. (From Edwards JE: Classification of congenital heart disease in the adult. In: Roberts WC, ed. Congenital heart disease in adults. Cardiovasc Clin Series 10/1. Philadelphia: FA Davis, 1979:1.)

Table 28.10.
Combinations and Relative Frequencies of Aneurysms[a]

From	Into	Percent Relative Frequency
Right coronary sinus	Right ventricle:	
	With ventricular	40
	septal defect	20
	Without ventricular	
	septal defect	
	Right atrium	20
Noncoronary sinus	Right atrium	20
	Right ventricle	Rare
	Left ventricle	Rare
Left coronary sinus	Right atrium	Rare
	Left atrium	Rare

[a]From Sakakibara S, Kono S. Congenital aneurysm of the sinus of Valsalva: anatomy and classification. Am Heart J 1962; 63:405–424; and from Omat A, Ersanli O, Kanuni A, Aykan TB. Congenital aortic sinus aneurysms with particular reference to dissection of the interventricular septum. Am Heart J 1966; 72:158–164.

tuberculosis, endocarditis, fungal infections, syphilis, Marfan's syndrome, and senile-type dilation in which the three sinuses dilate as a result of the normal aging process.

The aneurysm usually ruptures into the right ventricle,

the right atrium, or both into the right atrium and the ventricle (105). Rupture into the left ventricle, intrapericardial, pulmonary artery, or interventricular septum is very rare.

The aneurysm may rupture spontaneously or secondary to bacterial endocarditis (106). Rupture into the right ventricle or atrium generally causes a left-to-right shunt with cardiac failure. The aneurysm can result in aortic regurgitation (107, 108) or compression or obstruction of the adjacent structures (109, 110). Aneurysm of the right coronary sinus can cause right ventricular outflow obstruction, while a left sinus aneurysm can produce compression of the left coronary artery (110) or the left circumflex coronary artery (107).

HISTORY AND INCIDENCE

The first report of an aneurysm of the sinuses of Valsalva appeared in 1840 (111), and only 18 cases had been reported by 1940. By 1960 Sakakibara and Konno (112) collected 88 cases and in 1966, Onat et al. (113) added 77 cases. The first successful repair was performed by Morrow and his colleagues in 1956 (114) on an aneurysm protruding into the right atrium.

The congenital aneurysm, with an incidence ranging from 0.1 to 3.5% of all congenital heart defects, is more common than the acquired form. There is a 4:1 male predominance of congenital aneurysm with an age range from 11 to 67 years of age (57). Goldberg and Krasnow (102) note that a racial predominance is suggested by the finding that the incidence of these aneurysms is higher in far eastern countries than in western countries.

Unruptured coronary sinus aneurysms are less frequently reported because they usually are clinically silent. In addition, acquired aortic sinus aneurysms are reported less frequently than congenital ones. Jones and Langley (115) established criteria differentiating acquired from congenital aneurysms: They may arise from any sinus, are often extracardiac, tend to extend superiorly, rarely are associated with congenital cardiac defects or cardioaortic fistulae, and usually are associated with acquired heart disease.

SYMPTOMS AND DIAGNOSIS

Aortic sinus aneurysms usually are clinically silent until rupture. The most common age for rupture is from puberty to age 30 years. The size of the rupture, the receiving chamber, and any associated anomalies will influence the presentation of a patient. The common symptoms are the abrupt onset of dyspnea, fatigue, and paroxysmal nocturnal dyspnea with orthopnea, reflecting the sudden volume overload induced by an acute large rupture, causing a left-to-right or left-to-left shunt. Chest pain is reported less frequently (102).

Diagnosis may be made with two-dimensional echocardiography with the use of contrast echocardiography, spectral Doppler, or color-flow Doppler imaging. A rupture is generally indicated by a consistent echo dropout or discontinuity at the tip of the aneurysm. The parasternal long- and short-axis views at the base are considered best to visualize both ruptured and unruptured aneurysms from a complete two-dimensional echocardiographic study (116).

There is a high incidence of associated congenital cardiac anomalies such as ventricular septal defects, aortic regurgitation, and bicuspid aortic valve. These generally can be diagnosed by echocardiography.

TREATMENT

Unruptured aneurysms of the sinus of Valsalva without co-existing cardiac anomalies usually are closely monitored without surgical intervention.

The ruptured aneurysm of the sinus of Valsalva should be surgically corrected on diagnosis. The procedure should be tailored to the individual patient; however, the common approaches to repair are as follows: (a) through the chamber into which the aneurysm has ruptured and (b) a double approach, one in which the recipient chamber and aortic root are opened (102).

Associated anomalies should be corrected at time of

surgical intervention for the aneurysm. The operation is low risk; however, patients remain prone to the development of late valvular complications such as endocarditis or thromboembolic complications.

EDITORIAL COMMENT

Sinus of Valsalva aneurysms are quite rare and can cause many symptoms besides the physiologic consequences of an aortic to cardiac chamber fistula. Unruptured aneurysms may produce coronary artery compression and myocardial infarction. The aneurysm can also encroach on the conduction tissues and cause heart block and other arrhythmias. Other complications include valvular insufficiency, endocarditis and pulmonary vascular obstructive disease. When recognized, repair is usually straightforward, especially with modern techniques of cardiopulmonary bypass and myocardial protection (CM).

Coarctation, Atresia, and Interruption of the Aortic Arch

The term *coarctation* refers to a constriction of the lumen of the aortic arch near the entrance of the ductus arteriosus. The narrowing may be moderate, severe, or complete. If it is complete, there may be a diaphragm or a cord-like atretic segment or there may be a complete interruption of the vessel, termed congenital *absence* of the arch.

COARCTATION OF THE AORTA

Anatomy. Discrete narrowing of the distal segment of the aortic arch occurs usually near the point of entry of the ductus arteriosus. A deformity of the media of the aorta is the characteristic lesion of this anomaly.

The right ventricle via the pulmonary trunk and through the ductus to the descending aorta provides the blood supply to the lower part of the body when the constriction is proximal to the ductus. However, the vascularization of the lower part of the body becomes compromised if the ductus becomes obliterated postnatally.

A collateral circulation to the trunk and lower limbs has to develop prenatally at, or even below, the site of the constriction. Since the constriction may be located above or below the entrance of the ductus arteriosus, two types of coarctation may be distinguished, the preductal and postductal types. These categories are no longer referred to as infantile and adult types, respectively. Rather, they seem to be correlated with patency or closure of the duct (117). In the preductal type, the ductus arteriosus persists, whereas in the postductal type this channel is usually obliterated.

In this anomaly, an abnormally large expansion of ductal tissue occurs into the anterior, superior, and posterior walls of the aorta. This may exert a pull, by fibrosis, on the vessel and may interfere with subsequent growth of the aorta. This abnormal process is most likely independent of closure of the ductus (117). The abnormal infolding of the aortic wall causes the lumen to be narrowed and eccentric (118).

Embryogenesis. Controversy surrounds theories on the pathogenesis of coarctation of the aorta. Romero et al. (119) provide an overview of the three main hypotheses. In 1828 Reynaud proposed that the anomaly is a primary developmental defect of the aortic arch. Rosenberg (120) revived this theory and suggested that aortic coarctation may result from failure of connection of the fourth and sixth aortic arches with the descending aorta.

The Skodaic theory relates the anomaly to the presence of aberrant ductal tissue at the level of the aortic arch. This results in a narrowing of the vessel at the time of ductal closing.

The third hypothesis holds that coarctation is the result of decreased blood flow in the ascending aorta and increased flow in the ductus. After this hemodynamic perturbance, the major blood flow pathway occurs through the ductus arteriosus and the descending aorta. An aortic ridge opposite the ductus is formed as a result of the increased flow. The decreased flow through the isthmus creates conditions favorable for the development of narrowing.

History. Some writers have credited Morgagni (121) with being the first to see a coarctation of the aorta (De Sedibus, IVIII:6). From his description of a greatly enlarged right ventricle with an aorta "contracted to an amazing narrowness, near to the heart," we suspect that this was a case of atresia of the ascending aorta, such as described by Evans (122), rather than a typical coarctation.

The first full description was by Paris in 1791 (123). While Paris noted the characteristic dilated collateral arteries, their full development was not described in detail until Meckel's description in 1827 (124). His drawing of the collateral circulation from the dissection of a robust, active adult with coarctation is still reproduced (125). He first observed the erosion of the ribs by the intercostal arteries, a sign which was to become of diagnostic importance in 1929 through Railsback and Dock's (126) use of radiography.

By 1886 there were 88 cases in the literature (127). In 1903 Bonnet (128) showed that coarctation was not a single lesion and divided it into the infantile and adult types. Two hundred cases were reviewed by Abbott in 1928 (129).

The first successful surgical repairs, both reported in 1945, were accomplished by Crafoord and Nylin (130) and by Gross and Hufnagel (131). Reifenstein and his colleagues (132) described the findings in 104 autopsies performed between 1928 and 1947. In 1960 we reviewed the

entire literature on coarctation accompanied by aneurysms (133) and subsequently published a discussion of the embryogenesis of coarctation and the mechanics of aneurysm (134).

Incidence. Coarctation of the aorta accounts for approximately 8% of congenital heart disease in infants and children. It ranks behind only ventricular septal defect and patent ductus arteriosus in frequency. Approximately one-fifth of those infants admitted with heart failure within the first weeks of life will have coarctation without significant associated defects. The male/female ratio is approximately 3:1 for isolated coarctation, but it is only 1.1:1 for complicated coarctation (67).

Symptoms and Diagnosis. In symptomatic infants, the deformity of the media of the aorta lies either opposite the ductus or in a preductal location. In adolescents and adults the lesion is usually distal to the ligamentum arteriosum. Although rare, the lesion lies proximal to the origin of the left common carotid artery. Left ventricular hypertrophy is the principal cardiac abnormality (67). The anomaly in older children is rarely symptomatic.

Intracardiac associated anomalies are present in 87 to 90% of patients. They include abnormal communications, aortic stenosis, aortic insufficiency, ventricular septal defect, atrioseptal defect, a variety of transpositions of the great vessels, ostium primum defects, truncus arteriosus, tubular hypoplasia of the aortic arch, and double outlet right ventricle (119, 67). Coarctation of the aorta and VSD are the most common cardiac defects in Turner's syndrome.

It is extremely difficult to make a prenatal diagnosis. In fact, in some cases the anomaly is a postnatal event related to ductal closure. Furthermore the detection of symptoms in utero is a difficult task. Coarctataion of the aorta has, however, been diagnosed in the fetus (135, 136). The work of Hornberger and her colleagues (137), which presents normal values for human aortic arch growth, may facilitate the prenatal diagnosis of coarctation of the aorta.

The diagnosis of the anomaly relies on the demonstration of a narrowing of the vessel in the isthmal region. Chest roentgenogram, electrocardiogram, and echocardiogram are helpful in the diagnosis. Doppler flow studies may be useful for diagnostic confirmation although some researchers have challenged their reliability (138, 139). Some authors (67) recommend aortography in older children to demonstrate the exact site and length of the coarctation, as well as to show unusual features of the collateral circulation which may be of importance to the surgeon.

Treatment. Although it is agreed that coarctation of the aorta should be surgically corrected, there is still debate over the choice of operation, particularly for infants. Nugent et al. (67) provided an excellent section on surgical management. However, while Nugent allowed for patch aortoplasty, Rubay et al. (140) noted that this technique has a threat of aneurysm formation and has been discarded by many surgeons. Furthermore, they concluded that neither subclavian flap angioplasty nor end-to-end anastomosis showed any superiority as compared with the other in terms of morbidity and mortality. As in all cases, they correctly assert that surgical technique must be appropriate to the specific anatomy in a given case.

EDITORIAL COMMENT

Traditionally, coarctation of the aorta was managed by resection and end-to-end anastomoses. However, a significant rate of restenosis was noted in infants. Subclavian flap aortoplasty subsequently gained popularity and was heralded by some as the optimal surgical approach for coarctation in infancy. Recent studies have reported a high incidence of recoarctation in young infants after subclavian flap repair. The extended end-to-end repair, a modification of the classic end-to-end technique, was developed to address this high incidence of restenosis. Currently, there is no unaminity of opinion regarding the optimal surgical approach to coarctation in infancy. The main portion of this controversy concerns young infants less than 3 months of age with concomitant arch hypoplasia. Proponents of extended end-to-end repair contend that three deficiencies in the subclavian flap method contribute to the relatively high incidence of restenosis that some studies have reported in young infants. The first is failure of subclavian flap aortoplasty to address transverse arch hypoplasia, which often co-exists with aortic coarctation in neonates. Transverse arch hypoplasia, they point out, is specifically addressed by the extended end-to-end technique. Proponents of the subclavian flap technique respond by citing recent reports that indicate transverse arch growth after relief of the isthmic and paraductal obstruction with subclavian flap aortoplasty. As for the second deficiency, proponents of the extended end-to-end technique cite failure of resection of all ductal tissue in subclavian flap aortoplasty. Recent reports have characterized circumferential ductal tissue at the level of the ductus arteriosus or ligamentum arteriosum. Proponents of the extended end-to-end technique also emphasize the variability of ductal tissue, which can extend either downstream or upstream from the ductus arteriosus. Those who favor the subclavian flap repair claim that careful attention to surgical detail notably reduces the incidence of recurrence. As for the third deficiency, proponents of the extended end-to-end technique cite the potential occurrence of postoperative limb ischemia and late growth retardation of the left upper limb after subclavian flap aortoplasty, which is refuted by the subclavian flap protagonists. At the present time, both methods have benefits and drawbacks. Long-term follow-up should help to resolve this issue in the future (CM).

Some authors note that the recurrence of coarctation and the development of aortic valve dysfunction are relatively common after surgery for coarctation (141). Rubay et al. (140), however, conclude that this is primarily the result of faulty surgical technique. Hypertension occurs in a significant proportion of survivors (142).

INTERRUPTION OF THE AORTIC ARCH

Anatomy. This anomaly is characterized by the absence of a channel between the aortic arch and the descending aorta. The ductus arteriosus remains widely open. The descending aorta and subclavian arteries are supplied with blood of low oxygen content. The two common carotid arteries are supplied by the aortic trunk. An interrupted aortic arch is frequently combined with an abnormal origin of the right subclavian artery.

Variations may occur in the origin of branches of the arch (Fig. 28.30). Classification by site of the interruption revealed the following distribution: type A, 44%; type B, 51%; and type C, 5%. Nugent et al. noted that there are other less common patterns (67).

Embryogenesis. An interrupted aortic arch may arise when, for example, the connection between the fourth and sixth left arches disappears. The main cause, however, usually is intracardiac, such as a left-to-right shunt through an interventricular septal defect. This results in a reduced flow in the ascending aorta. A left-to-right shunt, such as that provided by an interventricular or an interatrial septal defect, is necessary for extrauterine life (117).

Extension of the conal septum into the left ventricle exaggerates this phenomenon. Narrowing of the outflow tract results and in turn causes a further increase in the left-to-right ventricular shunt and a corresponding further decrease in forward aortic blood flow. This may, in turn, lead to severe hypoplasia of the ascending aorta in addition to aortic coarctation or interruption (143).

History and Incidence. This anomaly was first described by Steidele (144) in 1778. A classification of three types was developed by Celoria and Patton (145) in 1959.

Interruption of the aortic arch accounts for about 1.3 (146) to 4% (67) of the deaths among infants with congenital heart disease. There is no sex predilection.

Symptoms and Diagnosis. Patients usually present with respiratory distress and mild to severe cyanosis, with or without decreased peripheral pulses. Cross-sectional echocardiography usually provides reliable imaging of the aortic arch in children and can accurately identify congenital anomalies (147). Some authors question the accuracy and therefore the use of Doppler ultrasound in measuring pressure gradients in coarctation (148, 149). The majority of patients with this anomaly have associated cardiovascular anomalies which significantly influence prognosis and surgical management. The most com-

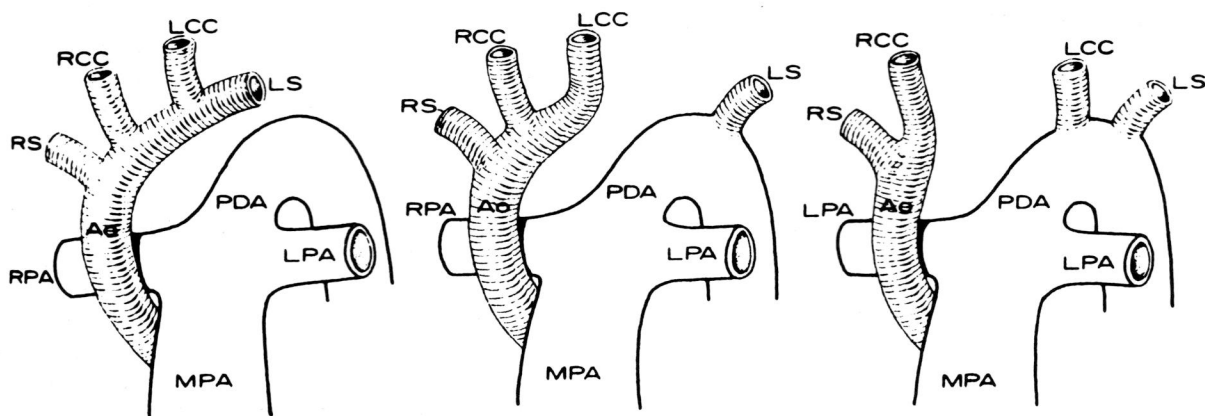

Figure 28.30. Classification of interrupted aortic arch. Type A *(left)* is interruption distal to left subclavian artery *(LS)*; type B *(middle)* is interruption distal to the innominate or right common carotid artery *(RCC)*. *Ao*, Descending aorta; *LPA*, left pulmonary artery; *MPA*, main pulmonary artery; *PDA*, patent ductus arteriosus; *RPA*, right pulmonary artery; *RS*, right subclavian artery. (From Jones EL, Plauth WH Jr, Hatcher CR Jr. A palliative operation for all types of aortic arch interruption in the neonate. J Thorac Cardiovasc Surg 1975;69:581.)

Table 28.11.
Anatomical Type and Results of Operation for Interrupted Aortic Arch[a]

Patient No.	Type of Interruption	Associated Lesions	Repair	Result
1. RF	B	Single ventricle, TGV	Left thoracotomy, graft interposition, PA band	Late death
2. GC	B	VSD	Left thoracotomy, primary anastomosis, PA band	Hospital death
3. AB	B	VSD	Left thoracotomy, primary anastomosis, PA band	Hospital death
4. SM	B	VSD	Left thoracotomy, primary anastomosis, PA band	Hospital death
5. MJ	B	VSD	Complete repair	Alive
6. CS	B	VSD	Complete repair	Alive
7. JD	A	TGV, VSD	Left thoracotomy, primary anastomosis, PA band	Late death
8. JR	A	Aortopulmonary window	Complete repair	Alive
9. TJ	B	Truncus arteriosus	Left thoracotomy, primary anasthomosis	Hospital death
10. DH	A	Aortopulmonary window	Complete repair	Alive
11. AB	B	VSD	Complete repair	Late death
12. MS	A	VSD	Complete repair	Reoperation for anastomotic stricture; alive
13. JF	B	Truncus arteriosus	Left thoracotomy, primary anastomosis, PA narrowing	Hospital death
14. TR	A	Aortopulmonary window	Complete repair	Alive
15. JF	A	TGV, single ventricle	Left thoracotomy, primary anastomosis, PA band	Hospital death
16. KM	A	Aortopulmonary window	Complete repair	Alive

[a]From Hammon JW Jr et al. Repair of interrupted aortic arch and associated malformations in infancy: indications for complete or partial repair. Ann Thorac Surg 1986; 42:17–21.
TGV, Transposition of great vessels; *PA*, pulmonary artery; *VSD*, ventricular septal defect.

mon of these are patent ductus arteriosus and ventricular septal defect. Van Mierop and Kutsche (150) reported that interrupted aortic arch and persistent truncus arteriosus were associated in 50% of the cases with DiGeorge syndrome.

Treatment. Several surgical approaches might be used in an attempt to surgically manage this anomaly. How-

ever, the increased fetal pulmonary artery blood flow caused by associated cardiac lesions makes selection of the proper operative approach more difficult (151) (Table 28.11). Primary total repair of the interrupted aortic arch complex with closure of the associated ventricular septal defect in infancy has yielded the best long-term results. A survival rate of 80% or better can be anticipated after surgery at the hands of an experienced surgeon (67).

EDITORIAL COMMENT

One stage repair of interrupted aortic arch and ventricular septal defect closure has gained popularity recently, owing to the improved results seen after repair when the resultant physiology is as close to normal as possible. Both parts of the operation can be accomplished through a median sternotomy with varying periods of deep hypothermia and circulatory arrest (CM).

Atypical Coarctation

COARCTATION OF THE ABDOMINAL AORTA

Anatomy. Two types of coarctation of the abdominal aorta occur: *(a)* stenosis of a short segment, resembling coarctation of the aortic arch (segmental) and *(b)* an abrupt narrowing of the aortic lumen which continues as far as the bifurcation (hypoplastic). In either type, the stenosis may begin above, at, or below the level of the renal arteries (152).

Collateral circulation is established through the lower intercostal and internal mammary arteries, between the superior and inferior mesenteric arteries, or through the lumbar arteries.

Embryogenesis. There is debate as to whether these lesions are congenital or acquired. Some are certainly the result of local aortitis (153), whereas others are probably congenital. Maycock (154) suggested that failure of fusion of the paired embryonic aortae with the subsequent loss of one of the pair might account for the hypoplasia. In view of the response of blood vessels to the volume of blood presented to them (e.g., pulmonized bronchial arteries), it seems improbable that hypoplasia would persist unless collateral circulation were well developed in early embryonic life.

EDITORIAL COMMENT

Atypical coarctations are thought to occur as a result of intrauterine vascular accidents that limit the development of the affected arterial wall. Numerous upstream and downstream collateral vessels develop to maintain perfusion distal to the coarctation. The best surgical results are achieved with a prosthetic bypass graft, which is associated with the least dissection, the least chance of collateral artery injury, and probably the least chance of developing perioperative paraplegia (CM).

Takayasu's aortitis, chronic nonspecific arteritis, gestational rubella, rheumatic fever, some autoimmune diseases, and fibromuscular dysplasia have been implicated as causes of acquired coarctations (155, 156).

History and Incidence. The first case was described by Quain (157) in 1847. The first successful surgical repair was by Beattie and his colleagues (158) in 1951. In a review of the literature, Graham et al. (159) reported more than 100 cases of abdominal aortic coarctations.

A rare anomaly, coarctation of the abdominal aorta accounts for only 0.5 to 2% of clinically recognized coarctations of the thoracic and abdominal aorta (160). It is usually seen in younger people; only one case was reported in an individual over 60 years of age (161).

Symptoms and Diagnosis. The lesion usually is asymptomatic during infancy and childhood. Coldness of lower extremities and claudication of buttocks and calves are usually the only complaints.

Concomitant renal artery stenosis exits in more than half the patients; thus hypertension is a leading symptom.

Vaccaro et al. (155) assert that aortography is necessary if an accurate diagnosis is to be made and an appropriate operation performed, whereas Kodama et al. (156) recommend angiography.

Treatment. Surgical intervention is the treatment of choice. Hypertension is believed to be renin mediated and is difficult to control medically. Patients, therefore, usually require renal artery revascularization combined with aortic bypass or replacement early in life. Hallett et al. (162) recommend optimizing the use of autogenous methods of renal artery reconstruction including saphenous vein aortorenal bypass, splenorenal arterial anastomosis, hepatorenal saphenous vein bypass, and renal autotransplantation.

Coarctations without renal artery involvement are most appropriately managed by aortoaortic bypass with a knitted Dacron prosthesis (155).

ASSOCIATED NONAORTIC COARCTATIONS

Coarctation of the aortic arch may be associated with atresia or stenosis of the left subclavian artery (118), or the subclavian artery alone may be coarcted (163). Levine et al. (164) reported a patient with atresia of a left brachiocephalic trunk with a right-sided arch. The left side was filled by reversal of flow in the left vertebral artery, called the "subclavian steal."

Hofbeck et al. (165) believe that a congenital subclavian steal syndrome may be caused by coarctation or interruption of the aortic isthmus or by isolation of a subclavian artery. They described a patient with D-transposition of the great arteries, a left aortic arch, and isolation of the right subclavian artery which originated from the right pulmonary artery via a right ductus arteriosus. They were able to noninvasively demonstrate a subclavian steal syndrome through the use of echocardiography and doppler sonography of the cerebral arteries.

COARCTATION OF THE PULMONARY ARTERY

Coarctation of the pulmonary artery is discussed in Chapter 14.

Patent Ductus Arteriosus (Ductus Arteriosus Galeni)

ANATOMY

Patent ductus arteriosus represents persistent patency of the vessel that normally connects the main pulmonary arterial trunk with the descending thoracic aorta in the fetus. This anomaly is the most common type of extracardiac shunt. (166).

Patients with the anomaly may be categorized according to whether the vascular resistance through the ductus itself is small, moderate, or large. Since the resistance of the ductus is related to its cross-sectional area, as well as to its length, it is difficult to define the anatomic size of the ductus in each group (67).

EMBRYOGENESIS

The ductus arteriosus, a large vessel connecting the pulmonary artery with the aorta, is a normal structure in fetal life. All humans are born with a "congenital patent ductus." Normally this vessel closes and becomes obliterated during the first year of life. Failure of closure constitutes an anomalous condition.

The prenatal ductus appears as a direct continuation of the pulmonary trunk, which is somewhat larger in diameter than the aorta, which it joins. It enters the anteromedial side of the aorta about 1 cm below the junction with the left subclavian artery, at an angle of about 32 degrees (167, 168).

Usually cylindric, the ductus is from 0.5 to 0.7 cm in diameter and from 0.7 to 1 cm in length at birth. It is occasionally funnel shaped, with the larger end toward the aorta, or it may be "aneurysmal," with a dilation between its two ends.

Histologically, the ductus resembles a muscular artery rather than an elastic artery, such as the pulmonary artery and aorta. The intima bulges slightly into the lumen; the bulges produced by local thickenings have elastic fibers and smooth muscles (169). The inner elastic membrane is continuous with that of the aorta and the pulmonary artery (170). The tunica media, which is thicker on the superior (convex) side than on the inferior side, contains more muscle fibers than does the aorta. In addition, mucoid material is found between the muscle fibers of the tunica media of the ductus, and there is no external elastic membrane (171, 172). Danesino and his associates (172) believe that the subendothelial cushions are the result of muscular shortening and constriction rather local growth.

Following active closure of the ductus, degeneration occurs through replacement of smooth muscle by collagen and elastic fibers until only a fibrous cord, the ligamentum arteriosum, remains.

NORMAL CLOSURE OF THE DUCTUS ARTERIOSUS

Closure of the ductus occurs in two phases: early functional closure by muscular contraction, followed later by anatomic obliteration.

Considerable effort has been expended on determining the normal time of both phases of closure. Although the ductus may appear open in cadavers of infants several weeks after birth, functional contraction of the lumen usually occurs early in postnatal life. Through a comparison of oxygen saturation in the hand with that in the foot, Eldridge et al. (173) concluded that the ductus is functionally closed within 3 days. Evidence of muscular closure of the ductus in newborn infants in the first 3 hours was obtained by use of 100% oxygen; the ductus could be reopened by lowering the percentage of oxygen (174, 175).

The ductus is not anatomically obliterated until relatively long after it is functionally closed. Christie (176) found anatomic closure at 2 weeks in 33% of infants examined. At the end of the second month 88% were closed, and after 1 year only 1% were still patent. Older estimates (177) suggested much slower closure: 2% by the 15th day and less than 50% by the end of the second month. Variations in the criteria for "closed" are probably responsible for these differences.

The initial closure of the ductus arteriosus results from the contraction of its own smooth musculature. Increased oxygen tension of the blood passing through it may provide the required stimulus, as held by early workers (171, 178, 179). There is some evidence that neonatal respiratory distress interferes with closure of the ductus, as would be expected if oxygen tension initiates contraction (180), but asphyxia neonatorum alone rarely produces a measurable postponement of closure (181). Other factors such as length of gestation and vasoactive substances such as prostaglandins and catecholamines also may play an important role in this process (182, 183).

Both sympathetic and parasympathetic nerve fibers are present in the wall of the ductus (184, 185), and in some cases vagal stimulation can produce ductal constriction (186). Blood pressure and presence of carbon dioxide and other metabolites in the blood have no effect (178). Postnatal respiration with the consequent rise in blood oxygen concentration is the effective cause of the contraction phase of closure of the ductus.

PATHOGENESIS OF PATENCY

Failure of the ductus arteriosus to close may result from a primary failure of the musculature contraction phase, or it may be secondary to large differences between the aortic and pulmonary pressures. Such differences create a ductal flow too great to be overcome by the ductal musculature. Preductal coarctation of the aorta, transposition of the great vessels, and pulmonary stenosis or atresia are important causes for such differences.

In certain anomalies (so-called ductus-dependent conditions such as pulmonary atresia with intact ventricular septum) persistent patency of the ductus is desirable. It does, however, tend to close at a normal rate (67).

Maternal rubella during the first 3 months of pregnancy has been implicated in the cause of multiple congenital abnormalities in various systems, including the cardiovascular system (187). The rubella virus has been directly implicated with the cause of patent ductus arteriosus.

Arterial hypoxemia induced by nonpulmonary causes, such as living in high altitudes, also has been shown to be associated with patency of the ductus arteriosus (188, 189).

The unexpanded lungs of the fetus produce an effective peripheral obstruction to pulmonary output, which raises the pressure in the pulmonary artery. Blood flow through the ductus is therefore from pulmonary artery to aorta (right-to-left shunt) (Fig. 28.31, A). With the opening of the pulmonary capillary bed at birth, the pulmonary pressure falls and the flow through the ductus halts and then reverses (left-to-right shunt) (Fig. 28.31, B). If the ventricular septum is intact, there is a left-to-right shunt through the patent ductus (Fig. 28.31, C to E); certain other lesions result in a right-to-left shunt (Fig. 28.31, F to I). Therefore, by preventing closure of the ductus, hypoxia increases pulmonary blood flow and aggravates the clinical picture (75).

There are several compensatory physiologic mechanisms (e.g., Frank-Starling mechanism, myocardial hypertrophy, and stimulation of the sympathetic adrenal system) aimed at maintaining a normal effective systemic

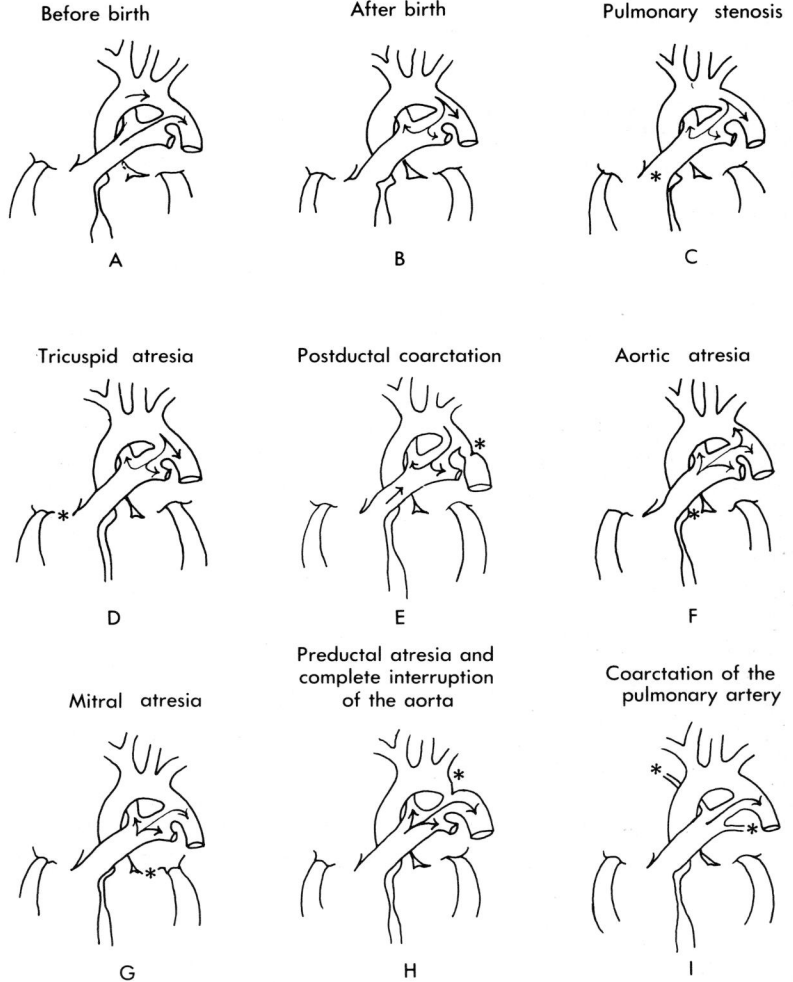

Figure 28.31. Direction of blood flow through patent ductus arteriosus. **A,** Right-to-left shunt before birth. **B,** Left-to-right shunt after birth. **C** to **E,** Cardiac malformations that may result in a left-to-right shunt through the ductus. **F** to **I,** Cardiac malformations that may result in a right-to-left shunt through the ductus. An *asterisk* marks the site of the lesion. In these flow diagrams, it is assumed that the ventricular septum is intact.

output. These mechanisms most likely are responsible for the rapid heart rate and the sweating commonly seen in infants with heart failure. Continued persistence of the volume overload will result in compensatory myocardial hypertrophy. In general, these compensatory mechanisms are well developed in older children and adults. They are not as well developed in newborns and are even less developed in preterm infants. It is therefore important to pay attention to the degree of maturity of the infant (189).

HISTORY

Although the ductus arteriosus was known to Galen and later to Fallopius (190), the name of Bottallo has become associated with it. How this occurred is unknown. Although Bottallo described a patent foramen ovale, he does not seem to have been concerned with the ductus. The duct probably should be named "ductus arteriosus (Galeni)" not "ductus arteriosus (Bottallo)." We think change should start now as Galen is one of the first author's (JES) ancestors. The term *ductus arteriosus* itself seems first to have been used by Aranzi in 1595 (191).

The first adequate description of the ductus was made in 1826 by Kilian (170). Histologic studies began with Langer (192) in 1857. Normal closure time was investigated by Billard (193) in 1828, and the first diagnosis of a patent ductus in life was subsequently confirmed at autopsy in 1845 by Chevers (194). In 1867 Gerhardt (195) described the machinery-like murmur of a patent ductus.

In spite of these advances, Wells (196) was able to collect only 41 cases of uncomplicated patent ductus arteriosus up to 1908, of which 24 were in adults. Not until 1907 was ductal ligation seriously proposed (197), and not until 1938 was it attempted (198). In 1939 Gross and Hubbard (199) reported the first successful ligation. Since then, thousands of operations have been performed, with very low mortality.

Muscular contraction was suggested as early as 1857 by Langer (192), who observed the structural differences between the wall of the ductus arteriosus and the walls of the arteries connected by the ductus. Although many other ideas were put forward, the theory of valvular closure of the aortic orifice of the ductus (200) was the only one to gain much prominence. The work of Kennedy and Clark (171) in 1942, followed by that of Born et al. (178), seemed to settle the question in favor of Langer's hypothesis.

INCIDENCE

Depending on gestational age and the presence of respiratory distress syndrome (RDS), the incidence of the anomaly in preterm infants ranges from 30 to 80%. The incidence of isolated patent ductus arteriosus is consid-

erably less (1:2000 live births) in the term infant beyond the neonatal period. The anomaly accounts for 5 to 10% of all types of congenital heart disease (189). Mouzinho et al. (201) suggest that symptomatic patent ductus arteriosus may occur in up to 50% of very low–birth-weight (≤ 1500 g) infants.

There is a much higher incidence in females, although the genders seem to be equally affected in cases associated with rubella syndrome (202). Detailed information may be found in Keith et al. (73) and in reports on a large number of patients (201–207). A seasonal fluctuation in the number of affected girls but not of boys has been suggested, with a greater number of affected girls born between May and December than between December and May (180, 203).

A number of examples of patent ductus arteriosus in siblings or in successive generations of the same family have been reported (204, 208, 209), but no genetic pattern emerges clearly. Patent ductus may occur in only one of a pair of twins; more often, if it is present at all, it will be found in both (210).

SYMPTOMS AND DIAGNOSIS

Older patients with small ductus arteriosus generally are asymptomatic. A loud continuous murmur is the only significant finding in these patients. In preterm infants, initially the heart murmur is crescendo systolic; later it becomes continuous (211).

Infants and older children with moderate or large patent ductus arteriosus become symptomatic in a manner similar to those with large ventricular septal defects— that is, with signs of left ventricular failure. Typically, there is a hyperactive precordium, bounding pulses, loud heart sounds, and a loud continuous murmur over the upper left sternal border. However, the heart murmur usually is only systolic, and in many instances no murmur is audible (silent ductus arteriosus) in preterm infants recovering from RDS (211).

The size of the shunt has an impact on the findings of the various diagnostic methods used. Nugent et al. (67) outline the findings utilizing chest roentgenogram, electrocardiogram, echocardiogram, and cardiac catheterization. Doppler echocardiography seems to be the most useful diagnostic aid currently available (211, 212).

TREATMENT

Surgical management usually is recommended. Even in the most experienced hands, nonsurgical transcatheter closure does not compare favorably with the low mortality, minimal morbidity, and likelihood of complete obliteration accomplished routinely by direct surgical intervention (67). Furthermore, Gravanis (211) notes that the use of indomethacin in the treatment of preterm infants with patient ductus arteriosus has practically eliminated the need for surgical ligation of the ductus arteriosus. In 1933 Laborde et al. (213) presented a controversial video-assisted thoracoscopic technique for interruption of patent ductus arteriosus.

Rashkind, Mullins, and Lock and their co-workers (214–216), however, support closure of the patent ductus arteriosus by nonsurgical means. Of importance is the note by Gelb and his colleagues (212) that some abnormalities (i.e., congenital intrathoracic left-to-right shunts and systemic artery-to-pulmonary fistulae or collateral vessels) might be confused with patent ductus arteriosus. They therefore recommend that all patients, particularly those with atypical findings, undergo a thorough cardiac catheterization with angiography prior to implantation of a ductal device.

EDITORIAL COMMENT

Recently, transcatheter prosthetic closure of patent ductus arteriosus has been performed with variable success rates. Long-term results must be evaluated in light of the present standards for surgery (CM).

Anomalous Ductus Arteriosus

RIGHT DUCTUS ARTERIOSUS

In situs inversus with a right aortic arch and a right descending aorta, the ductus arteriosus is on the right side.

When a persistent right arch and a left descending aorta are present, the ducts arteriosus is usually on the left. It passes from the left pulmonary artery to the descending aorta, forming the left side of a vascular ring that may compress the trachea and esophagus (Fig. 26.28, A).

Steinberg et al. (217) reported a right arch with bilateral, patent ductus arteriosus and absent left pulmonary artery.

Although interruption of the aortic arch commonly occurs with a left-sided descending aorta and left-sided patent ductus arteriosus, this anomaly may rarely exist with a right descending aorta. There was an associated right ductus arteriosus in all of the few reported cases of this latter condition (218, 219). Because of the close proximity of the right ductus arteriosus to the superior portion of the right bronchus in these cases, some surgeons have recommended that the right ductus arteriosus always be ligated and divided, rather than simply ligated (218).

DOUBLE DUCTUS ARTERIOSUS

A few cases have been reported in which the great vessels are normal. A normal left ductus arteriosus is present (obliterated or patent), and a persistent patent right ductus arises from the right subclavian or right innominate artery to join the right pulmonary artery (64, 220). Unusual configurations of the great vessels are more typical (Fig. 28.32).

PERSISTENT RIGHT OR LEFT DUCTUS ARTERIOSUS REPLACING THE PROXIMAL PULMONARY ARTERY

When one pulmonary artery is absent, the lung may be supplied by an anomalous ductus arteriosus arising from the aorta or the brachiocephalic artery. Embryologically, this anomaly consists of absence of the proximal sixth arch and persistence of the distal portion (the ductus arteriosus). These anomalies are considered with anomalies of the pulmonary arteries (see Chapter 14).

ANOMALOUS LEFT DUCTUS ARTERIOSUS

Sherman (221) illustrated a long ductus extending from the pulmonary trunk to the left subclavian artery in a case of tetralogy of Fallot (Fig. 28.33).

ABSENCE OF THE DUCTUS ARTERIOSUS

When pulmonary stenosis and ventricular septal defect co-exist, such as in tetralogy of Fallot, the ductus arteriosus may be absent. Presumably, the ductus formed but disappeared in fetal life because of the great reduction in pulmonary flow caused by stenosis.

The ductus arteriosus is absent in at least 50% of patients with persistent truncus arteriosus. Absence of significant blood flow through the ductus in the presence of the much larger aorticopulmonary connection permits the ductus to disappear early in fetal life.

Failure of Separation of Aortic and Pulmonary Trunks (Persistent Truncus Arteriosus, Aorticopulmonary Septal Defect)

PERSISTENT TRUNCUS ARTERIOSUS

Classifications. The classification systems of Collett and Edwards (222) and the subsequent reclassification by Van Praagh and Van Praagh (223) provide a uniform diagnostic approach to this anomaly (Fig. 28.34).

Van Praagh and Van Praagh (223) presented their classic study of the anatomy of the common aorticopulmonary trunk (truncus arteriosus communis) and its embryological implications in 1965. Based on a series of 57 necropsy cases and on the literature, they concluded that there are two basic types of common aorticopulmonary trunk: those with a ventricular septal defect and those without. The latter is extremely rare.

All of their cases associated with ventricular septal defect consisted of the following: (*a*) absence of the distal portion of the pulmonary infundibulum (similar to tetralogy of Fallot with pulmonary atresia); (*b*) partial or complete absence of the pulmonary valve; (*c*) complete or par-

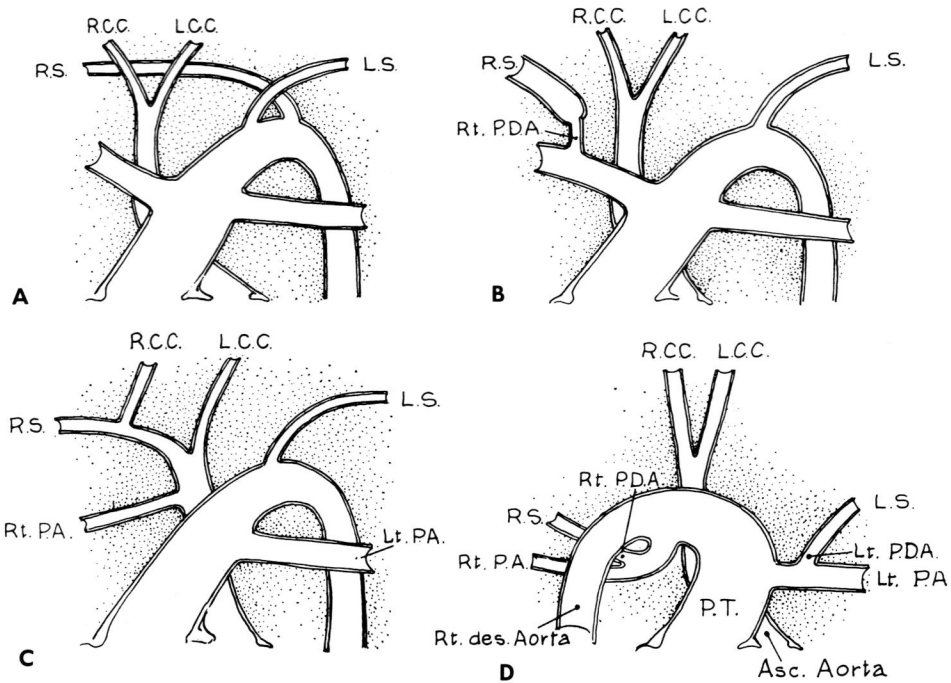

Figure 28.32. Diagrammatic illustrations of four variations of basic type B aortic arch interruption. **B** and **D,** The ductus arteriosus persists on the right, as well as on the left. *PT,* Pulmonary trunk; *PDA,* ductus arteriosus; *PA,* pulmonary artery;

RS, right subclavian artery; *RCC,* right common carotid artery; *LCC,* left common carotid artery; *LS,* left subclavian artery. (From Roberts WC, Morrow AG, Braunwald E. Complete interruption of aortic arch. Circulation 1962;26:39–59.)

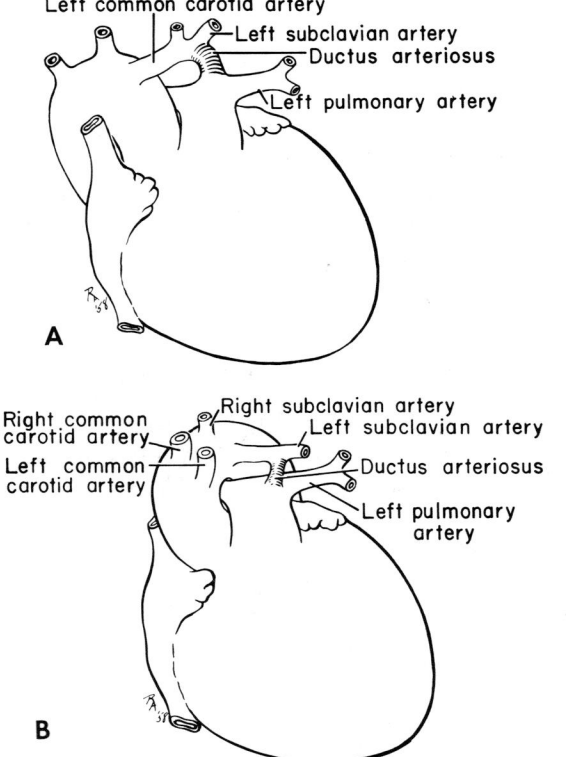

Figure 28.33. Left ductus arteriosus connecting the left subclavian artery with the pulmonary trunk. **A,** With right aortic arch. **B,** With left aortic arch. In both cases the branches of the aortic arch are abnormally placed. (From Sherman FE. An atlas of congenital heart disease. Philadelphia: Lea & Febiger, 1963.)

tial absence of the aorticopulmonary septum; and *(d)* arterial arches four and six varied inversely in their development (e.g., well-developed aortic arch without absent ductus arteriosus or interrupted aortic arch with a large patent ductus arteriosus).

They concluded that a "true" persistent truncus arteriosus does not exist because an undivided conotruncal channel is present. Although the truncus is undivided, the anomaly, at the level of the conus, represents absence of the entire distal portion of the pulmonary infundibulum (septum and free wall) and not failure of septation (223).

Yoshizato and Julsrud (224) present an excellent comparison of both classification systems, as well as an angiographic demonstration of the Van Praagh classification.

Anatomy (Fig. 28.35). Persistent truncus arteriosus is characterized by a single arterial trunk which arises from the base of the heart and gives origin to the coronary, pulmonary, and systemic arteries. Furthermore, a single semilunar valve without a remnant of a second atretic valve is present. This later feature differentiates persistent truncus arteriosus from pulmonary or aortic valve atresia, in both of which a single arterial vessel also receives the entire cardiac output (211).

Embryogenesis. In the early embryo, the truncus arteriosus lies between the conus cordis proximally and the aortic sac and aortic arch system distally. The appearance of truncal swellings, the proximal ascending aorta, and the pulmonary trunk divides the truncal lumen into two

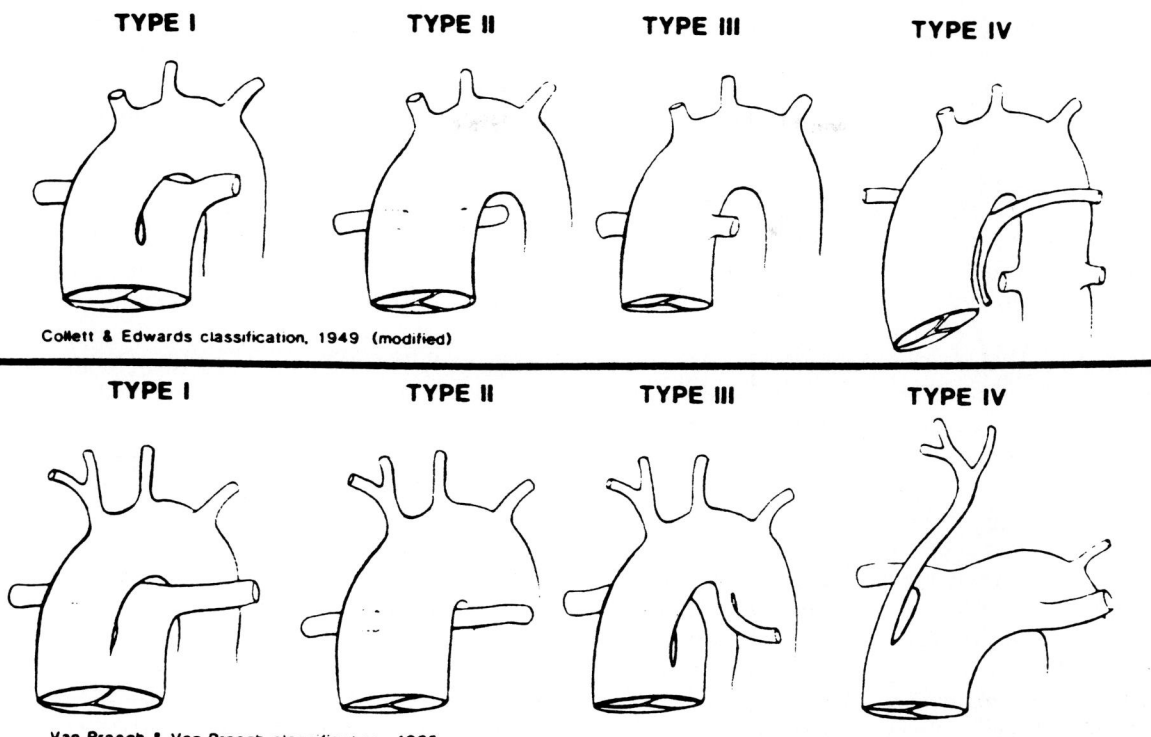

Figure 28.34. Classification of truncus arteriosus by Collett and Edwards *(top)* and Van Praagh *(bottom)*. (From Yoshizato T, Julsrud PR. Truncus arteriosus revisited: an angiographic demonstration. Pediatr Cardiol 1990;11(1):37.)

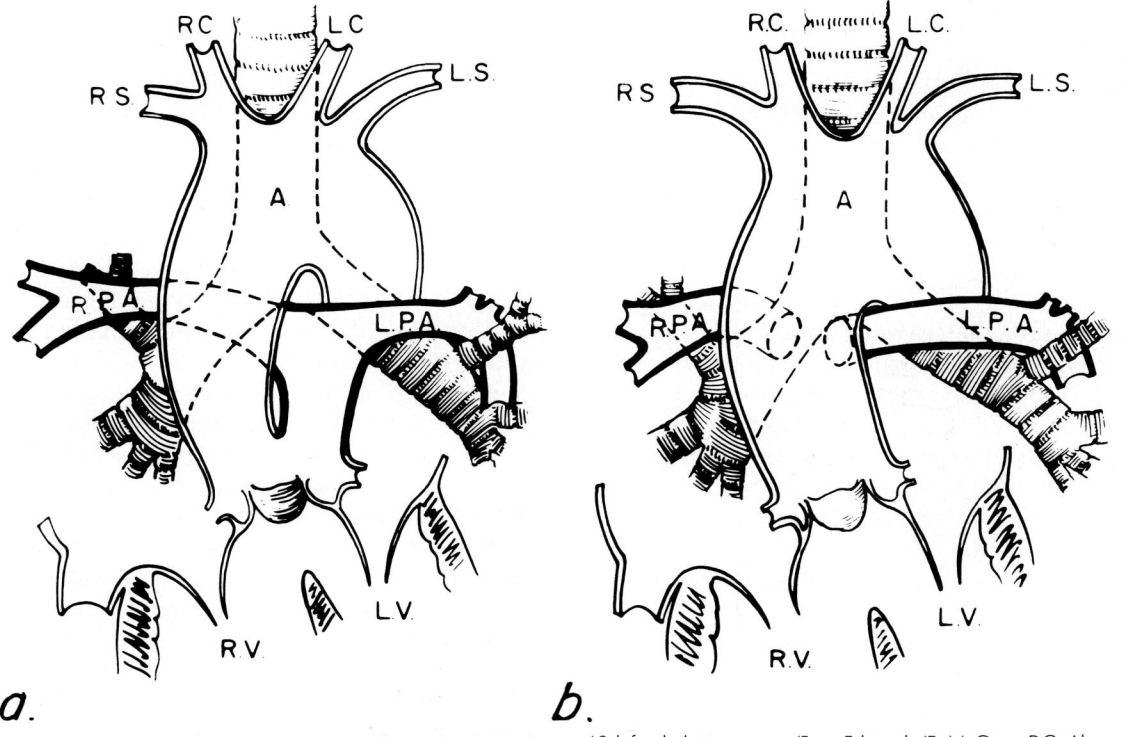

Figure 28.35. Persistent truncus arteriosus. *a,* Type 1. *b,* Type II. *RV,* Right ventricle; *LV,* left ventricle; *RPA,* right pulmonary artery; *LPA,* left pulmonary artery; *A,* aorta; *RS,* right subclavian artery; *RC,* right carotid artery; *LC,* left carotid artery; *LS,* left subclavian artery. (From Edwards JE, McGoon DC. Absence of anatomic origin from heart of pulmonary arterial supply. Circulation 1973;47:393.)

channels. The right ventricular origin of the pulmonary trunk and the left ventricular origin of the aorta are established during the process of fusion between the truncal septum and the developing conal septum. The respective semilunar valves develop from tissue swellings at the sites of conotruncal fusion. Meanwhile, the paired sixth aortic arches, along the aortic sac, migrate leftward; the paired fourth aortic arches move rightward. Concurrently, an aortopulmonary septum, which eventually fuses with the distal truncal septum, is formed by invagination of the roof of the aortic sac. As a result, the right and left pulmonary arteries originate from the pulmonary trunk, while the aortic arch is a continuation of the ascending aorta. The normal intertwining of the great arteries is a result of the spiral course of the truncoaortic partition (211).

A number of congenital ventriculoarterial anomalies, including persistent truncus arteriosus, may result from the abnormal development of the conotruncal and truncoaortic septation. A large ventricular septal defect may result from deficiency or absence of the conal (infundibulum) septum. Insufficiency (or very rarely stenosis) may be attributed to deformity of the single truncal valve. Should remnants of distal truncoaortic septation develop, the pulmonary arteries may arise together from a short pulmonary trunk; otherwise, they may arise directly and separately from the root of the common trunk (211).

History and Incidence. A type II persistent truncus arteriosus, arising from a single ventricle, was described in 1798 by Wilson (225). A type III defect was described in 1830 by Elliotson (226), and a type I was reported in 1831 by Tiedeman (227). About 32 cases of all types were on record by 1900. Humphreys (228) suggested criteria for persistent truncus arteriosus and found only 15 cases up to 1932 that appeared satisfactory. Collett and Edwards (222) collected 93 cases of all types and mentioned several others not readily classifiable. By 1964 Giordano (229) had found 105 cases of persistent truncus arteriosus in the literature, and 49 more were found in the files of the Armed Forces Institute of Pathology. Among Abbott's (125) 1000 cases, there were 21 examples of persistent truncus and 10 of aortic septal defects.

The first successful repair of a type III defect was performed by Gross (230) in 1952.

Persistent truncus arteriosus occurs in about 0.7% of patients with congenital heart disease (73) and accounts for 2 to 3% of all the cardiac anomalies found at autopsy (211).

Type I is the most frequently encountered persistent truncus arteriosus (60%), with type II being the second most common (35%). Deshpande et al. (231) present an interesting report of 16 cases of the anomaly, which they categorize using both systems.

Symptoms and Diagnosis. The volume of pulmonary blood flow and the competence of the truncal valve will largely determine the clinical features of persistent truncus arteriosus. Symptoms such as mild cyanosis or signs of heart failure may appear in the neonatal period. Most patients are diagnosed in infancy. As the pulmonary flow increases with time, the mild cyanosis present early after birth may diminish or disappear. However, there is always moderate arterial hypoxemia, a result of the mixing of the systemic and pulmonary venous return. Respiratory and feeding difficulties with failure to thrive and other signs of heart failure will appear within a few weeks, in a manner similar to that seen in infants with large ventricular septal defects or patent ductus arteriosus (211).

Two-dimensional echocardiography (specifically parasternal long-short axis views and subcostal for right or left outflow tract axis views) is most helpful in the diagnosis. Confirmation may be made by the use of pulsed Doppler ultrasonography (232). Others recommend cardiac catheterization and angiocardiography if precise diagnosis is not clear (211).

Truncus arteriosus occurs as an isolated cardiovascular anomaly in the majority of cases. Occasionally it has been reported in association with anomalies of other systems, particularly the DiGeorge syndrome (233). Rao et al. (234) report a rare case of tricuspid atresia in association with truncus arteriosus. They found only 12 similar cases in the literature. Diógenes et al. (235) reported a rare case of common arterial trunk associated with absence of right atrioventricular connexion.

Treatment. The majority of symptomatic infants die within the first year of life if they do not undergo palliative or reparative surgery. However, patients who survive infancy usually develop pulmonary vascular disease. Surgical treatment has been the only hope for infants with persistent truncus arteriosus. Primary repair of the malformation is currently offered to infants before 1 year of age with excellent results (Rastelli procedure) (211, 236).

Bove et al. (237) recommend repair in the first month of life. Based on their experience with 11 neonates and young infants with truncus arteriosus undergoing repair (mediate age of 21 days), they concluded that the operative risk is low and results are good even in neonates. Eight of nine late survivors grew normally following surgery to establish right ventricle-pulmonary artery continuity (a porcine valved conduit was used in three patients and an aortic or pulmonary homograft in eight). Their success is mirrored by that of Ebert et al. (238) who have been successful in the physiological correction of truncus arteriosus in infants under 6 months of age. These authors reported 11 operative deaths of 100 infants who underwent surgery. Of the 86 long-term survivors, 55 returned for conduit change because of either body growth or pseudointima proliferation of the conduit.

They noted that there were no mortalities at the time of conduit change, 29 of which were repaired using a straight tube between the ventricle and pulmonary trunk, while 26 had valve conduits placed.

EDITORIAL COMMENT

Recent surgical developments have given patients with truncus arteriosus an excellent chance for perioperative survival and an optimistic outlook for a long life. Patients with successful repair of truncus arteriosus must be followed closely for aortic (truncal) insufficiency and right ventricular–to–pulmonary artery conduit failure and can be expected to undergo at least two subsequent open heart procedures. Fortunately, the results of conduit replacement have been excellent thus far (CM).

AORTICOPULMONARY SEPTAL DEFECT

Classification. Three types of aorticopulmonary septal defect (APSD) may be morphologically distinguished. The first is a defect usually of moderate or small size with a more or less circular border. It is localized approximately halfway between the arterial valves and the bifurcation of the pulmonary trunk. In the second, the border is described as slightly more than one turn of a spiral. The third type represents a defect, usually large, in which no posterior (distal) border exists. These varying appearances suggest that each type is the result of different developmental mechanisms (239).

Anatomy. This rare anomaly is characterized by a communication between the ascending aorta and the pulmonary trunk. There are two discrete ventricular outflow tracts supporting separate ascending portions of the great vessels. According to Lau et al. (240), the lower margin of the communication is usually just distal to the coronary artery ostia. Kutsche and Van Mierop (239) reported that, in 72% of 106 patients, the defect was proximal and in 38%, it extended distally (i.e., there was no distal border). The ostium of the right pulmonary artery was often incorporated in the defect in patients with a distal defect.

Embryogenesis. Nonfusion of the embryonic aorticopulmonary and truncal septi may explain the first type of APSD. This may be compared pathogenetically with a small- or moderate-sized ventricular septal defect in the area of the membranous septum. The second type may be the result of malalignment of the embryonic aorticopulmonary and truncal septi. Such a mechanism has been used to explain the genesis of ventricular septal defects believed to be due to right anterior (tetralogy of Fallot) or left posterior displacement of the truncoconal (infundibular) septum (241, 242). Total absence of the embryonic aorticopulmonary septum may explain the third type (239).

History and Incidence. Until 1956, 62 patients with aortopulmonary septal defects were reported in the literature. Forty additional cases were added during the early and mid-1960s (243). In 1952 Gross successfully corrected an aortopulmonary window in a 1-year-old girl by simple ligation, a technique which he considered unsatisfactory (204). In 1956 Shumway and Lewis (244) first demonstrated the feasibility of closure of an experimentally created aortopulmonary window through the pulmonary trunk. The transaortic approach for the management of this anomaly was first suggested by Wright et al. in 1968 (245).

The anomaly occurs in less than 2% of all cases of ductus arteriosus (211). A male/female ratio of 1.8:1 was found in a review of 236 cases (239). In a series at the University of Florida, 13 patients with APSD were found among approximately 6522 children with congenital heart disease, giving an incidence of 0.2% (239).

Symptoms and Diagnosis. Kutsche and Van Mierop (239) and Blieden and Moller (246) reported an approximately 50% occurrence of associated cardiovascular anomalies with APSD.

Patients with serious associated anomalies usually present as neonates. Presentation is dominated by these other serious cardiac malformations, and the APSD may be an incidental finding. Infants between 1 and 3 months of age may present with congestive heart failure due to a large left to right shunt through the aorticopulmonary window. If associated anomalies are present, they generally are incidental findings. Older patients (3 to 15 years of age) may present with similar abnormal physical signs, except that they usually are not in heart failure (240).

Associated anomalies include the following: interruption of the aortic arch (240, 247); tetralogy of Fallot; pulmonary atresia; aortic stenosis; mitral incompetence; patent ductus arteriosus; and aortic incompetence.

Kutsche and Van Mierop (239) note that APSD has not been associated with DiGeorge syndrome. This is curious because other uncommon anomalies involving the arterial pole of the heart, such as interruption of the aortic arch (IAA) type B and persistent truncus arteriosus (TA), which some (248, 222, 223) consider to be developmentally related to APSD, occur often in the DiGeorge syndrome.

Kutsche and Van Mierop (239) conclude that APSD and truncus arteriosus appear to be pathogenetically unrelated and do not represent variants of the same anomaly.

Cardiomegaly and pulmonary plethora are present on chest radiography, cardiomegaly in the majority of patients. The presence of a right-sided aortic arch does not exclude APSD. Further, there are no particular electrocardiographic features distinguishing this anomaly

Human Embryology and Teratology

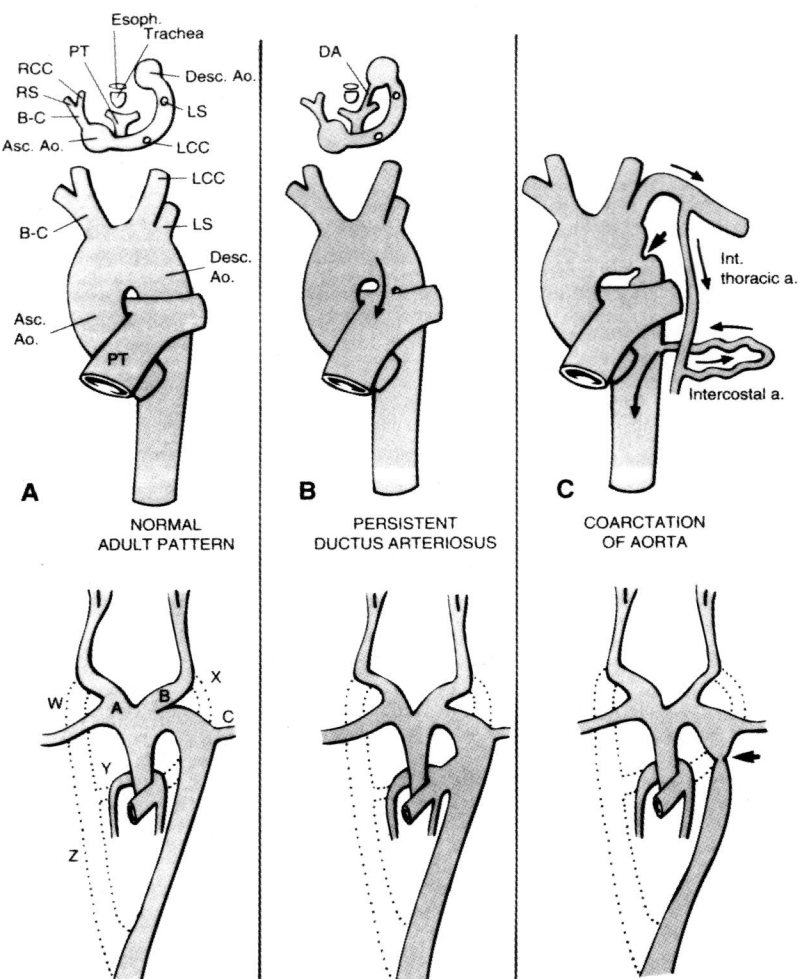

Figure 28.36. The arch of the aorta and aortic anomalies. The uppermost drawings are views from above, the middle are from in front, and the lowermost figures show the likely mode of development. **A,** Normal pattern, in which *W, X, Y,* and *Z* have disappeared, and three main branches *(a, b, c)* arise: brachiocephalic, left common carotid, and left subclavian. **B,** Persistent ductus arteriosus on the left side. **C,** Coarctation of the aorta *(arrow),* showing collateral circulation through the internal thoracic artery and one of many tortuous intercostal arteries. **D,** Right arch of the aorta with right ductus arteriosus. **E,** Double arch of the aorta, forming an aortic ring that encloses the trachea and esophagus *(uppermost draw-* *ing).* **F,** Retroesophageal right subclavian artery, showing regression of right aortic arch 4 and persistence of right dorsal aortic root *(asterisk).* **G,** Interrupted arch of the aorta, in which some way must be found to convey oxygenated blood to the lower part of the body. *Ao.,* Aorta; *B-C,* brachiocephalic trunk; *DA,* ductus arteriosus; *LCC,* left common carotid artery; *LS,* left subclavian artery; *PT,* pulmonary trunk; *RCC,* right common carotid artery; *RS,* right subclavian artery. (From O'Rahilly R, Muller F. Human embryology & teratology. New York: Wiley-Liss, 1992:126–127).

from ventricular septal defect or a large ductus arteriosus.

Treatment. Lau et al. (240) recommend the transaortic approach. They note that this method gives a clear view of the margin of the defect and permits accurate closure. The incision is made in normal aortic tissue rather than into a thin-walled pulmonary trunk which may be dilated. Furthermore, they note that the technique avoids the need for fistula dissection and should have a negligible mortality.

Abdominal Aorta

The abdominal aorta is the downward continuation of the thoracic descending aorta formed by the fusion of the paired dorsal aorta, an action starting around the fourth week.

The abdominal aorta, as well as the thoracic aorta, has lateral, ventral, and dorsal arteries, each with a specific anatomical destiny. The abdominal aorta has bilateral ventral, dorsal and segmental branches.

Cardiovascular and Lymphatic Systems

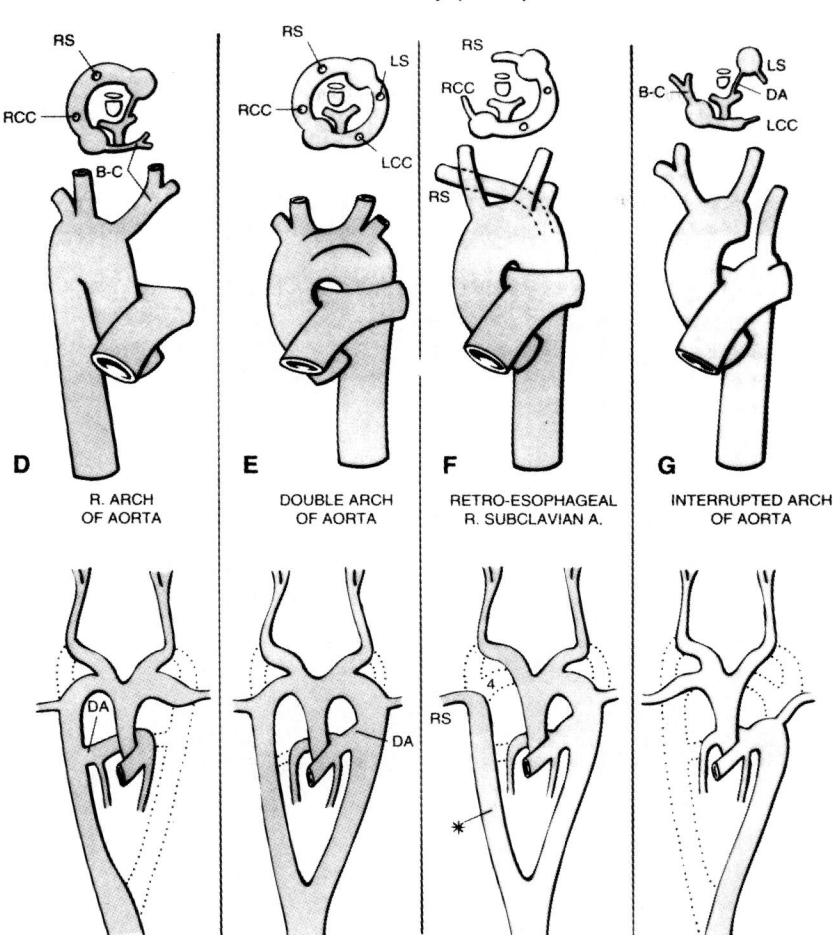

Figure 28.36.   D to G.

The four upper lumbar arteries of the abdominal aorta are paired dorsal segmental arteries. The fifth lumbar arteries are merely the right and left common iliacs. The left iliac arteries are also the products of the fifth dorsal lumbar arteries, which are united with one umbilical artery.

The vitelline arteries are the end results of the paired ventral arteries; after fusion they form the celiac axis, superior mesenteric artery, and inferior mesenteric artery.

The lateral segmental branches of the abdominal aorta are responsible for the formation of arteries, providing the blood supply to the adrenals, kidneys, and gonads and partially to the diaphragm by formation of the phrenic arteries. The middle sacral artery is a remnant of the dorsal aorta. The history of congenital anomalies of the abdominal aorta is the history of the main organ and its branches.

Table 28.12.
Incidence of Specific Congenital Heart Defects[a]

Defect	Percentage of Cases[b] Averaged
Ventricular septal defect	28.3
Pulmonary stenosis	9.5
Patent ductus arteriosus	8.7
Ventricular septal defect with pulmonary stenosis[c]	6.8
Atrial septal defect, secundum	6.7
Aortic stenosis	4.4
Coarctation of aorta	4.2
Atrioventricular canal[d]	3.5
Transposition of great arteries	3.4
Aortic atresia	2.4
Truncus arteriosus	1.6
Tricuspid atresia	1.2
Total anomalous pulmonary venous connection	1.1
Double outlet right ventricle	0.8
Pulmonary atresia without ventricular septal defect	0.3

[a]From Nugent EW et al. The pathology, abnormal physiology, clinical recognition, and treatment of congenital heart disease. In. Hurst JW, ed. The Heart, 7th ed. New York: McGraw-Hill, 1990.

Table 28.13.
Cardiac Death-Free Survival by Year of Surgery[a]

Year of Surgery	n	Median Age at Surgery, y	Proportion Surviving						
			30 d	1 y	5 y	10 y	15 y	20 y	25 y
Tetralogy of Fallot									
1958–1964	77	8.2	0.88 ± 0.04	0.87 ± 0.04	0.86 ± 0.04	0.86 ± 0.04	0.86 ± 0.04	0.84 ± 0.04	0.83 ± 0.04
1965–1969	74	5.3	0.86 ± 0.04	0.82 ± 0.04	0.82 ± 0.04	0.82 ± 0.04	0.82 ± 0.04	0.81 ± 0.05	—
1970–1974	81	2.1	0.90 ± 0.03	0.90 ± 0.03	0.89 ± 0.04	0.88 ± 0.04	0.88 ± 0.04	—	—
1975–1979	73	1.4	0.81 ± 0.05	0.81 ± 0.05	0.81 ± 0.05	0.81 ± 0.05	—	—	—
1980–1984	67	0.9	0.91 ± 0.04	0.90 ± 0.04	0.90 ± 0.04	—	—	—	—
1985–1989	53	0.8	0.98 ± 0.02	0.98 ± 0.02	—	—	—	—	—
Ventricular septal defect									
1958–1964	67	6.2	0.84 ± 0.04	0.82 ± 0.05	0.80 ± 0.05	0.80 ± 0.05	0.80 ± 0.05	0.80 ± 0.05	0.79 ± 0.05
1965–1969	43	5.3	0.95 ± 0.03	0.93 ± 0.04	0.93 ± 0.04	0.93 ± 0.04	0.93 ± 0.04	0.90 ± 0.05	—
1970–1974	57	4.6	0.93 ± 0.03	0.91 ± 0.04	0.91 ± 0.04	0.87 ± 0.04	0.87 ± 0.04	—	—
1975–1979	75	2.5	0.92 ± 0.03	0.92 ± 0.03	0.92 ± 0.03	0.92 ± 0.03	—	—	—
1980–1984	68	1.1	0.97 ± 0.02	0.97 ± 0.02	0.96 ± 0.02	—	—	—	—
1985–1989	68	0.7	0.98 ± 0.02	0.98 ± 0.02	—	—	—	—	—
Atrial septal defect									
1958–1964	42	9.6	1.0	1.0	1.0	1.0	1.0	1.0	1.0
1965–1969	67	7.5	0.97 ± 0.02	0.97 ± 0.02	0.97 ± 0.02	0.97 ± 0.02	0.97 ± 0.02	0.97 ± 0.02	—
1970–1974	88	6.8	0.98 ± 0.02	0.98 ± 0.03	0.98 ± 0.02	0.98 ± 0.02	—	—	—
1975–1979	88	5.4	1.0	1.0	1.0	1.0	—	—	—
1980–1984	81	5.2	1.0	1.0	1.0	—	—	—	—
1985–1989	106	3.5	1.0	1.0	—	—	—	—	—
Coarctation of the aorta									
1958–1964	51	7.4	0.92 ± 0.04	0.92 ± 0.04	0.90 ± 0.04	0.90 ± 0.04	0.90 ± 0.04	0.88 ± 0.05	0.81 ± 0.06
1965–1969	35	7.7	0.91 ± 0.05	0.89 ± 0.05	0.89 ± 0.05	0.86 ± 0.06	0.86 ± 0.06	0.86 ± 0.06	—
1970–1974	72	5.0	0.92 ± 0.03	0.88 ± 0.04	0.88 ± 0.04	0.86 ± 0.04	0.86 ± 0.04	—	—
1975–1979	98	3.7	0.94 ± 0.02	0.92 ± 0.03	0.92 ± 0.03	0.92 ± 0.03	—	—	—
1980–1984	115	1.4	0.93 ± 0.02	0.91 ± 0.03	0.91 ± 0.03	—	—	—	—
1985–1989	76	0.3	1.0	0.97 ± 0.02	—	—	—	—	—

Aortic stenosis									
1958–1964	11	12.6	1.0	1.0 ± 0.06	1.0	0.91 ± 0.09	0.82 ± 0.11	0.73 ± 0.13	0.73 ± 0.13
1965–1969	5	9.7	1.0	1.0	1.0	1.0	0.86 ± 0.08	1.0	—
1970–1974	21	9.3	0.90 ± 0.06	0.90 ± 0.06	0.86 ± 0.08	0.86 ± 0.08	—	—	—
1975–1979	27	9.7	0.96 ± 0.04	0.92 ± 0.05	0.92 ± 0.05	0.92 ± 0.05	—	—	—
1980–1984	27	3.6	0.82 ± 0.08	0.82 ± 0.08	0.78 ± 0.08	—	—	—	—
1985–1989	42	0.4	0.98 ± 0.02	0.93 ± 0.04	—	—	—	—	—
Pulmonic stenosis									
1958–1964	30	7.2	0.87 ± 0.06	0.87 ± 0.06	0.87 ± 0.06	0.87 ± 0.06	0.87 ± 0.06	0.87 ± 0.06	0.83 ± 0.07
1965–1969	34	5.6	1.0	1.0	1.0	1.0	0.90 ± 0.04	1.0	—
1970–1974	48	4.3	0.92 ± 0.04	0.92 ± 0.04	0.92 ± 0.04	0.92 ± 0.04	—	—	—
1975–1979	21	0.9	0.95 ± 0.05	0.95 ± 0.05	0.95 ± 0.05	0.95 ± 0.05	—	—	—
1980–1984	30	1.6	1.0	1.0	1.0	—	—	—	—
1985–1989	29	0.8	0.97 ± 0.03	0.97 ± 0.03	—	—	—	—	—
Transposition of the great arteries									
1968–1974	34	1.2	0.68 ± 0.08	0.62 ± 0.08	0.62 ± 0.08	0.56 ± 0.09	0.53 ± 0.09	—	—
1975–1979	33	0.8	0.64 ± 0.08	0.64 ± 0.08	0.57 ± 0.09	0.54 ± 0.09	—	—	—
1980–1984	42	0.5	0.83 ± 0.06	0.79 ± 0.06	0.71 ± 0.07	—	—	—	—
1985–1989	43	0.3	0.93 ± 0.04	0.93 ± 0.04	—	—	—	—	—
Patent ductus arteriosus									
1958–1964	98	4.2	1.0	1.0	0.99 ± 0.01	0.99 ± 0.01	0.99 ± 0.01	0.99 ± 0.01	0.99 ± 0.01
1965–1969	54	4.8	1.0	1.0	1.0	0.98 ± 0.02	0.98 ± 0.02	0.96 ± 0.03	—
1970–1974	98	3.1	1.0	1.0	1.0	1.0	1.0	—	—
1975–1979	85	2.5	1.0	1.0	1.0	1.0	—	—	—
1980–1984	101	1.7	1.0	1.0	1.0	—	—	—	—
1985–1989	65	1.6	1.0	1.0	—	—	—	—	—

aFrom Morris CD, Menashe VD. 25-year mortality after surgical repair of congenital heart defect in childhood: A population-based cohort study. JAMA 1991;266:3451.

Table 28.14.
Odds Ratios for the Relationship Between Each Occupation and Birth Defect Group[a]

	Ventricular Septal Defect (VSD)					Atrial Septal Defect (ASD)				
	Cases	Controls	OR	95%	C.L.	Cases	Controls	OR	95%	C.L.
Administrators, managers	80	192	0.90	0.68	1.18	54	89	1.13	0.79	1.61
Engineers, architects, draftsmen	33	58	1.24	0.80	1.93	20	31	1.23	0.69	2.17
Surveyors, geologists, prospectors	2	6	0.77	0.16	3.80	2	10	0.38	0.09	1.71
Accountants, mathematical/physical scientists	17	56	0.68	0.39	1.17	13	30	0.81	0.42	1.55
Biological scientists	2	4	1.11	0.20	6.06	1	1	2.00	0.12	32.07
Pharmacists, chemists, chemical engineers	8	23	0.67	0.30	1.51	1	4	0.44	0.05	3.73
Engineering, science technicians	7	18	0.89	0.37	2.14	4	12	0.67	0.21	2.07
Dentists	5	6	1.51	0.48	4.82	0	3	—	—	—
Physicians, surgeons	14	18	1.58	0.78	3.18	5	14	0.61	0.22	1.70
Nurses, health technicians	6	29	0.44	0.19	1.05	4	7	1.07	0.31	3.76
Teachers, librarians	30	74	0.94	0.61	1.44	10	36	0.50	0.24	1.03
Legal and social service workers	13	55	0.51	0.28	0.94	12	31	0.73	0.36	1.46
Entertainers, athletes	1	8	0.29	0.04	2.37	0	3	—	—	—
Writers, journalists	5	6	1.78	0.53	5.97	2	5	0.80	0.15	4.13
Artists	1	7	0.33	0.04	2.76	1	3	0.67	0.07	6.42
Photographers, photo processors	2	3	1.53	0.26	9.08	3	1	6.00	0.62	57.81
Printers	4	15	0.60	0.20	1.81	3	10	0.55	0.14	2.09
Salesmen	57	151	0.83	0.60	1.14	29	81	0.67	0.44	1.04
Clerks	33	82	0.85	0.56	1.29	19	40	0.91	0.52	1.60
Shippers, messengers	13	43	0.61	0.33	1.15	9	18	0.89	0.39	2.03
Electronic equipment operators	5	12	0.88	0.30	2.58	6	4	2.40	0.69	8.31
Firemen	10	10	2.37	0.98	5.70	10	4	4.75	1.36	16.55
Policemen, guards	10	45	0.49	0.24	0.98	10	28	0.66	0.32	1.36
Armed forces	25	97	0.57	0.37	0.90	16	63	0.41	0.22	0.76
Janitors	13	12	2.45	1.10	5.45	7	10	1.44	0.49	4.20
Personal service workers	4	5	1.58	0.42	5.90	3	8	0.65	0.17	2.50
Textile workers	3	6	1.17	0.29	4.67	1	0	—	—	—
Food service workers	21	22	1.67	0.89	3.16	9	9	1.94	0.77	4.94
Food processors	17	36	0.99	0.55	1.80	10	26	0.72	0.34	1.50
Farm managers and workers	30	54	1.13	0.72	1.79	16	32	0.92	0.49	1.72
Fishermen, hunters, trappers	28	32	1.16	0.65	2.08	12	12	2.05	0.87	4.83
Forestry and logging workers	85	143	1.13	0.84	1.50	54	54	2.03	1.35	3.05
Plywood mill workers	5	25	0.41	0.16	1.05	4	21	0.33	0.11	0.97
Sawmill workers	56	94	1.09	0.77	1.53	36	56	1.22	0.78	1.91
Paper workers	18	38	1.05	0.59	1.86	13	23	1.10	0.53	2.28
Stone, glass, and concrete workers	5	19	0.55	0.20	1.55	8	7	2.07	0.73	5.86
Metal miners	9	14	1.32	0.55	3.18	3	4	1.38	0.30	6.39
Foundry and smelter workers	15	34	1.05	0.57	1.95	14	24	1.27	0.52	3.07
Welders, cutters	15	31	1.13	0.61	2.10	9	14	1.21	0.52	2.85
Sheetmetal, iron, and other metal workers	46	72	1.49	1.01	2.18	32	38	1.55	0.96	2.50
Petroleum and gas workers	1	7	0.33	0.04	2.69	2	1	4.00	0.36	44.22
Chemical workers, nes[b]	9	16	1.30	0.57	2.96	7	10	1.44	0.52	3.98
Construction workers	36	91	0.84	0.56	1.26	28	36	1.41	0.85	2.32
Electricians, electrical, and electronics workers	32	66	1.11	0.73	1.71	28	34	1.57	0.94	2.60
Carpenters, wood workers	42	72	1.31	0.89	1.94	21	55	0.72	0.43	1.20
Painters	12	18	1.56	0.75	3.26	7	13	1.08	0.42	2.82
Handlers, laborers, nes[b]	28	38	1.45	0.87	2.41	11	17	1.14	0.52	2.49
Material moving equipment operators	18	55	0.74	0.43	1.27	15	32	0.86	0.45	1.62
Motor vehicle operators	91	168	1.23	0.94	1.61	40	87	0.87	0.58	1.28
Aircraft operators	4	5	1.85	0.50	6.89	4	4	1.78	0.45	7.00
Railway and other transport workers	10	30	0.72	0.35	1.50	5	16	0.53	0.18	1.53
Water transport workers	13	30	1.02	0.53	1.97	7	12	1.17	0.46	2.97
Boiler and transport firemen	9	14	1.42	0.60	3.34	7	10	1.27	0.49	3.30
Service station attendants	9	16	1.14	0.50	2.58	3	7	0.73	0.19	2.88
Vehicle mechanics	34	62	1.20	0.78	1.84	15	37	0.76	0.41	1.40
Mechanics, nes[b]	28	56	1.14	0.72	1.81	16	30	1.05	0.57	1.95
Millwrights	0	0	—	—	—	1	1	2.00	0.12	32.07
Students	11	27	0.94	0.46	1.91	3	16	0.32	0.09	1.14
TOTALS	1,081	2,272				657	1,213			

	Other Heart Defects					Patent Ductus Arteriosus (PDA)				
	Cases	Controls	OR	95%	C.L.	Cases	Controls	OR	95%	C.L.
Administrators, managers	79	171	0.94	0.71	1.25	54	102	1.18	0.84	1.67
Engineers, architects, draftsmen	18	67	0.58	0.34	0.98	13	35	0.78	0.41	1.48
Surveyors, geologists, prospectors	4	9	0.99	0.30	3.25	2	4	1.19	0.22	6.47
Accountants, mathematical/physical scientists	20	64	0.67	0.41	1.12	14	36	0.91	0.49	1.69
Biological scientists	1	3	0.74	0.08	6.88	0	6	—	—	—
Pharmacists, chemists, chemical engineers	6	15	0.90	0.35	2.32	3	8	0.72	0.18	2.92
Engineering, science technicians	9	13	1.51	0.63	3.63	7	9	1.61	0.59	4.39
Dentists	0	3	—	—	—	0	3	—	—	—
Physicians, surgeons	3	23	0.29	0.09	0.96	6	9	1.41	0.48	4.14
Nurses, health technicians	11	20	1.19	0.57	2.48	4	13	0.54	0.15	1.89
Teachers, librarians	28	69	0.91	0.58	1.42	14	46	0.68	0.37	1.25
Legal and social service workers	23	45	1.11	0.67	1.84	18	41	0.97	0.55	1.71
Entertainers, athletes	2	5	0.94	0.19	4.76	1	5	0.46	0.05	3.86
Writers, journalists	1	3	0.75	0.08	7.21	2	5	1.00	0.19	5.27
Artists	1	1	2.25	0.14	36.95	0	2	—	—	—
Photographers, photo processors	3	4	1.64	0.36	7.34	0	3	—	—	—
Printers	9	17	1.20	0.53	2.70	2	4	1.25	0.23	6.75
Salesmen	62	170	0.76	0.56	1.03	33	91	0.76	0.50	1.15
Clerks	30	91	0.70	0.46	1.06	16	51	0.64	0.36	1.13
Shippers, messengers	13	27	1.04	0.53	2.03	8	14	1.17	0.48	2.86
Electronic equipment operators	3	7	0.93	0.24	3.61	3	5	1.28	0.31	5.24
Firemen	1	14	0.16	0.02	1.23	4	9	1.06	0.32	3.49
Policemen, guards	16	58	0.61	0.35	1.07	4	20	0.44	0.15	1.30
Armed forces	32	108	0.63	0.42	0.94	17	51	0.74	0.42	1.30
Janitors	14	12	2.35	1.07	5.13	5	9	1.03	0.32	3.32
Personal service workers	4	7	1.19	0.35	4.02	5	8	1.19	0.37	3.79
Textile workers	4	8	0.86	0.27	2.72	4	1	7.60	0.84	68.58
Food service workers	14	36	0.59	0.31	1.12	9	19	0.77	0.33	1.81
Food processors	20	34	1.22	0.69	2.13	9	25	0.76	0.35	1.64
Farm managers and workers	34	64	1.03	0.67	1.58	15	34	0.97	0.51	1.83
Fishermen, hunters, trappers	26	28	1.23	0.69	2.21	12	14	1.30	0.55	3.04
Forestry and logging workers	103	131	1.50	1.14	1.98	39	67	1.29	0.85	1.95
Plywood mill workers	6	19	0.67	0.27	1.67	12	10	2.52	1.08	5.87
Sawmill workers	74	100	1.49	1.09	2.05	38	53	1.54	1.00	2.37
Paper workers	14	48	0.64	0.35	1.18	5	25	0.42	0.16	1.10
Stone, glass, and concrete workers	6	10	1.36	0.49	3.79	1	8	0.27	0.03	2.25
Metal miners	10	10	1.94	0.80	4.71	3	7	0.60	0.13	2.76
Foundry and smelter workers	23	37	1.36	0.80	2.30	6	10	1.41	0.51	3.91
Welders, cutters	11	17	1.49	0.69	3.20	8	11	1.63	0.65	4.07
Sheetmetal, iron, and other metal workers	45	70	1.42	0.97	2.09	24	36	1.45	0.85	2.49
Petroleum and gas workers	0	6	—	—	—	0	6	—	—	—
Chemical workers, nes[b]	12	21	1.20	0.58	2.48	7	14	1.07	0.43	2.67
Construction workers	42	68	1.40	0.95	2.07	23	51	0.99	0.60	1.64
Electricians, electrical, and electronics workers	31	73	0.94	0.61	1.44	17	44	0.85	0.48	1.52
Carpenters, wood workers	46	89	1.11	0.77	1.60	21	45	0.96	0.56	1.65
Painters	6	16	0.74	0.28	1.94	11	11	2.34	1.00	5.45
Handlers, laborers, nes[b]	24	63	0.76	0.47	1.24	13	19	1.27	0.59	2.70
Material moving equipment operators	29	51	1.26	0.79	2.00	8	23	0.87	0.38	2.01
Motor vehicle operators	87	179	1.06	0.81	1.39	43	94	0.93	0.63	1.38
Aircraft operators	0	5	—	—	—	2	6	0.78	0.16	3.90
Railway and other transport workers	24	35	1.48	0.87	2.51	10	13	1.90	0.81	4.48
Water transport workers	6	21	0.63	0.25	1.58	6	10	1.32	0.47	3.71
Boiler and transport firemen	8	18	0.95	0.42	2.19	5	10	1.03	0.34	3.10
Service station attendants	8	11	1.48	0.60	3.65	3	8	0.82	0.22	3.11
Vehicle mechanics	36	89	0.88	0.59	1.30	15	31	1.01	0.53	1.90
Mechanics, nes[b]	19	38	1.12	0.64	1.96	16	27	1.36	0.72	2.56
Millwrights	1	2	1.08	0.10	12.15	0	0	—	—	—
Students	13	27	1.05	0.53	2.08	8	19	0.94	0.41	2.20
TOTALS	1,125	2,309				594	1,256			

[a]From Olshan AF, Teschke K, Baird PA. Paternal occupation and congenital anomalies in offspring. Am J Ind Med 1991;20:455–456.)

[b]nes, Not elsewhere specified.

ANOMALIES AND VARIATIONS OF THE ABDOMINAL AORTA

In comparison with the thoracic aorta, the abdominal aorta has few congenital anomalies. Its branches, however, have several variations. Although the scope of this book does not permit a detailed presentation of abdominal aortic variations and anomalies, a few of the many variations of its branches are discussed here.

Kami and Morishita (249) reported a case of a double inferior vena cava, which was accompanied by atypical branches of the abdominal aorta.

Coarctation of the abdominal aorta constitutes a rare group of vascular abnormalities, including segmental stenoses and extended hypoplasia. Although hypertension usually is the only clinical finding, there are a diversity of anatomic lesions and surgical techniques used for treatment (250–252). Smith and Kelly (253) cited coarctation of the abdominal aorta with associated narrowing of the origin of major visceral arteries as a rare cause of life-threatening hypertension.

It is often difficult to determine whether the coarctation is congenital in origin or due to Takayasu's arteritis (250). Piyachon and Suwanwela (254) have observed geographic differences in sex incidence, anatomical distribution, and the type of lesion observed in association with Takayasu's arteritis.

In a case reported by Takeshita et al. (255), the abdominal aorta was divided into two abnormal vessels. One vessel was the celiac artery, while the other was considered to be the abdominal aorta. These authors present their findings and discuss the embryological basis of this rare anomaly.

Several other works are worth mentioning. Although the statistical data may no longer be valid, Michels' (256) 1955 work still represents 20 years of his work and is a storehouse of information. Nelson et al. (257) and Paz, Rak, and Rosen (258) discuss variations of the celiac axis and the mesenteric arteries. In 1992 Kornblith et al. (259) presented a work on the anatomy of the splenic circulation. This effort represents a continuation of their previous contribution to a study of celiac and superior mesenteric arteries.

Finally, Van Damme and Bonte's *Vascular Anatomy in Abdominal Surgery* (260) provides an excellent discussion of variations of the branches of the abdominal aorta.

CONCLUDING REMARKS

It is impossible to fully comprehend the embryogenesis and anatomy associated with every congenital heart defect, although a well-placed reference often is appreciated (Fig. 28.36 and Table 28.12). Despite the too numerous anomalies and the overwhelming amount of information, surgical advances made within the past 30 years have provided treatment for congenital heart defects in children who might not otherwise have lived to maturity. Significant trends of decreasing patient age at surgery, as well as decreasing operative mortality, have occurred over the past three decades.

In 1991 Morris and Menashe (261) elucidated the altered natural history of patients with congenital heart defects after surgical treatment (Table 28.13). Although surgical repair of most congenital heart defects is associated with lingering cardiac mortality, particularly for aor-

Table 28.15.
Cardiovascular Malformations: Distribution by Race and Sex Prevalence per 1000 Live Births[a]

	Female	Male	
Atrioventricular canal defect all infants	.744	.198	Black
	n = 22	n = 6	
	.414	.116	White
	n = 17	n = 5	
Atrioventricular canal defect with Down syndrome	.541	.132	Black
	n = 16	N = 4	
	.317	.093	White
	n = 13	n = 4	
Complete transposition	.169	.198	Black
	n = 5	N = 6	
	.097	.419	White
	n = 4	n = 18	
Obstructive left heart syndrome	.169	.264	Black
	n = 5	n = 8	
	.317	.652	White
	n = 13	n = 28	
Single ventricle	.068	.066	Black
	n = 2	n = 2	
	.268	.140	White
	n = 11	n = 6	
Hypoplastic left heart syndrome	.304	.396	Black
	n = 9	n = 12	
	.244	.372	White
	n = 10	n = 16	
Tetralogy of Fallot	.440	.264	Black
	n = 13	n = 8	
	.317	.396	White
	n = 13	n = 17	
Tricuspid atresia	.169	.066	Black
	n = 5	n = 2	
	.097	.186	White
	n = 4	n = 8	
Anomalous pulmonary venous return	.101	.165	Black
	n = 3	n = 5	
	.049	.140	White
	n = 2	n = 6	
Double-outlet right ventricle	.068	.033	Black
	n = 2	n = 1	
	.121	.140	White
	n = 5	n = 6	
Truncus arteriosus	.034	.033	Black
	n = 1	n = 1	
	.049	.070	White
	n = 2	n = 3	

[a]From Storch TG, Mannick EE. Epidemiology of congenital heart disease in Louisiana: an association between race and sex and the prevalence of specific cardiac malformations. Teratology 1992;46:273

tic stenosis, coarctation, and transposition, more than 8500 individuals with surgical repair of a congenital heart defect in childhood will reach adulthood each year in the United States (262).

Increasing surgical proficiency and improved operative and perioperative care undoubtedly have well served patients who undergo surgery. Furthermore, as Morris and Menashe (261) note, continued analyses of cohorts following surgical management may identify risk factors for mortality that will allow targeting of specific populations for more intensive follow-up.

Such efforts are mirrored by the work of Olshan, Teschke, and Baird (263) who explored paternal occupation as a risk factor for birth defects in offspring (Table 28.14) and by the work of Storch and Mannick (264) who demonstrated that the prevalence of a subset of cardiac malformations differs by race and sex (Table 28.15).

Current studies such as these provide the basis for future research, which will continue to provide a more complete understanding of human embryogenesis.

REFERENCES

1. His W. Lecithoblast und Angioblast: Abhandelr Math Phys KK Sachs Gesellschaft Wissenchaft 1900;25:171–328.
2. Rückert W, Mollier S. Die Entstehung der Gëfasse und des Blutes bei Wirbeltieren. In: Handbuch der Vergleichend Experimentell Entwicklungslehre dem Wirbeltiere. Hertwig Herausgeben 1906:1019.
3. Sabin FR. Origin and development of the primitive vessels of the chick and of the pig. Contrib Embryol Carnegie Inst Wash 1917;6:63–124.
4. McClure CFW. The endothelium problem. Anat Rec 1921;22:219–237.
5. Evans HM. On the development of the aorta, cardinal and umbilical veins, and other blood vessels of vertebrate embryos from capillaries. Anat Rec 1909;3:498–518.
6. Bremer JL. The development of the aorta and aortic arches in rabbits. Am J Anat 1912–13;13:11–128.
7. Bindber M. The teratogenic effects of a bis(dichloroacetyl)diamine on hamster embryos: aortic arch anomalies and the pathogenesis of the DiGeorge syndrome. Am J Pathol 1985;118(2):179–193.
8. Bremer JL. The earliest blood-vessel in man. Anat Rec 1914;8:102.
9. Congdon ED. Transformation of the aortic-arch system during the development of the human embryo. Contrib Embryol Carnegie Inst Wash 1922;14(65-71):47–110.
10. Coulter CB. The early development of the aortic arches of the cat, with especial reference to the presence of a fifth arch. Anat Rec 1909;3:578–592.
11. Heuser CH. The branchial vessels and their derivatives in the pig. Contrib Embryol Carnegie Inst Wash 1923;15:121–146.
12. Padget DH. Development of cranial arteries in human embryo. Contrib Embryol Carnegie Inst Wash 1948(207);32:205–212.
13. Barry A. Aortic arch derivatives in the human adult. Anat Rect 1951;111:221–238.
14. Stephan F. Contribution expérimentale a l'étude du développement du système circulatoire chez l'embryon de poulet. Bull Biol 1952;86:217–308.
15. Rychter Z. Cevnu soustava zaroduku kurete. II. Uvodni sdeleni k

pokusnemu uyrazovani aortalnich oblouku 4 dne zarodecneho vyvaje. Folia Morphol 1957;5:237–254.
16. Rychter Z. Experimental morphology of the aortic arches and the heart loop in chick embryos. Adv Morphogenesis 1962;2:333–371.
17. Warkany J, Roth CB, Wilson JG. Multiple congenital malformations: a consideration of etiologic factors. Pediatrics 1948;1:462–471.
18. Froud MD. Persistence of the left systemic aortic arch in the chick. J Genet 1954;52:456–465.
19. Onnis C, Giuliani B. Rilievi biometrici dell'aorta umana nelle eta pre-natale e post-natale. Riv Pat Clin Sper 1962;3:313–320.
20. Tandler J. Development of the blood, the vascular system, and the spleen. II. The development of the heart. In: Keibel F, Mall FP, eds. Manual of human embryology. Philadelphia: JB Lippincott, 1912.
21. Navaratnam V. Observations on the right pulmonary arch artery and its nerve supply in human embryos. J Anat 1963;97:569–573.
22. de la Cruz MV, da Rocha JP. An ontogenetic theory for the explanation of congenital malformations involving the truncus and conus. Am Heart J 1956;51:782–805.
23. Kramer TC. The partitioning of the truncus and conus and the formation of the membranous portion of the interventricular septum in the human heart. Am J Anat 1942;71:343–370.
24. Shaner RF. Anomalies of the heart bulbus. J Pediatr 1962;61:233–241.
25. Sadler TW. Langman's medical embryology, 6th ed. Baltimore: Williams & Wilkins, 1990.
26. Aronberg DJ et al. Normal thoracic aortic diameters by computed tomography. J Comput Assist Tomogr 1984;8(2):247–250.
27. Arvidsson H. Angiocardiographic measurements in congenital heart disease in infancy and childhood. Acta Radiol 1963;1:981–994.
28. Moss AJ, Adams FH, O'Loughlin BJ, Dixon WJ. The growth of the normal aorta and of the anastomotic site in infants following surgical resection of coarctation of the aorta. Circulation 1959;19(3):338–349.
29. Rosenberg HS, Klima T, Henderson SR, McNamara DG. Maturation of the aortic isthmus. Cardiovasc Res Center Bull 1971;10:47–56.
30. Clarkson PM, Brandt PW. Aortic diameters in infants and young children: normative angiographic data. Pediatr Cardiol 1985;6(1):3–6.
31. Fitzgerald SW, Donaldson JS, Poznanski AK. Pediatric thoracic aorta: normal measurements determined with CT. Radiology 1987;165(3):667–669.
32. McLoughlin MJ, Weisbrod G, Wise DJ, Yeung HP. Computed tomography in congenital anomalies of the aortic arch and great vessels. Radiology 1981;138(2):399–403.
33. Day DL. Aortic arch in neonates with esophageal atresia: preoperative assessment using CT. Radiology 1985;155(1):99–100.
34. Otero-Cagide M, Moodie DS, Sterba R, Gill CC. Digital subtraction angiography in the diagnosis of vascular rings. Am Heart J 1986;112(6):1304–1308.
35. Kersting-Sommerhoff BA, Sechtem UP, Fisher MR, Higgins CB. MR imaging of congenital anomalies of the aortic arch. AJR 1987;149(1):9–13.
36. Gomes AS. MR imaging of congenital anomalies of the thoracic aorta and pulmonary arteries. Radiol Clin North Am 1989;27(6):1171–1181.
37. Kersting-Sommerhoff BA et al. Magnetic resonance imaging of congenital heart disease: sensitivity and specificity using receiver operating characteristic curve analysis. Am Heart J 1989;118(1):155–161.

38. Bertolini A et al. Vascular rings and slings: diagnosis and surgical treatment of 49 patients. J Cardiovasc Surg 1987;28(3):301–312.

39. Fontana GP, Spach MS, Effmann EL, Sabiston DC Jr. Origin of the right pulmonary artery from the ascending aorta. Ann Surg 1987;206(1):102–113.

40. Posniak HV et al. CT of thoracic aortic aneurysms. Radiographics 1990;10(5):839–855.

41. Tahernia AC. Cardiovascular anomalies in Marfan's syndrome: the role of echocardiography and β-blockers. South Med J 1993;86(3):305–310.

42. Jaffe RB. Radiographic manifestations of congenital anomalies of the aortic arch. Radiol Clin North Am 1991;29(2):319–334.

43. McDonald JJ, Anson BJ. Variations in the origin of arteries derived from the aortic arch in American whites and Negroes. Am J Phys Anthrop 1940;27:91–107.

44. Adachi B. Das arteriensystem der Japaner. Kyoto, 1928.

45. Gross RE. The surgery of infancy and childhood. Philadelphia: WB Saunders, 1953.

46. Aguinaga MA et al. Ectasia in the origin of the left subclavian artery: a case report of congenital malformation of the aortic arch. Angiology 1987;38(7):568–570.

47. Bergman RA, Thompson SA, Afife AK, Saadeh FA. Compendium of human anatomic variation. Baltimore: Urban & Schwarzenburg, 1988.

48. Gaynor JW, Sabiston DC Jr. Patent ductus arteriosus coarctation of the aorta, aortopulmonary window, and anomalies of the aortic arch. In: Sabiston DC Jr, Spencer GC, eds. Surgery of the chest, 5th ed. Philadelphia: WB Saunders, 1990:1128–1172.

49. Rosler H, White PD. Unusual variations of roentgen shadow of elongated thoracic aorta. Am Heart J 1931;6:768.

50. Winer HE et al. Pseudocoarctation and mid-arch aortic coarctation. Chest 1977;72(2):519–521.

51. Pattinson JN, Grainger RG. Congenital kinking of the aortic arch. Br Heart J 1959;21:555–561.

52. Dungan WT, Char F, Gerald BE, Campbell GS. Pseudocoarctation of the aorta in childhood. Am J Dis Child 1970;119:401–406.

53. Bilgic A, Özer S, Atalay S. Pseudocoarctation of the aorta. Jpn Heart J 1990;31(6):875–879.

54. Angelini GD, Kulatilake ENP, Hayward M, Ruttley MSR. Pseudocoarctation of the aortic arch associated with bicuspid aortic valve lesion: is it a surgical entity? Thorac Cardiovasc Surgeon 1985;33(1):36–37.

55. Hoeffel JC et al. Pseudocoarctation or congenital kinking of the aorta: radiologic considerations. Am Heart J 1975;89(4):428–436.

56. Ruckman RN. Anomalies of the aortic arch complex. In: Adams FH, Emmanouilides GC, Riemenschneider TA, eds. Moss' heart disease in infants, children and adolescents, 4th ed. Baltimore: Williams & Wilkins, 1989.

57. Perloff JK. The clinical recognition of congenital heart disease, 3rd ed. Philadelphia: WB Saunders, 1987.

58. Edwards JE. Anomalies of the derivatives of the aortic arch system. Med Clin North Am 1948;32:925–949.

59. Kirklin JW, Clagett OT. Symposium on respiratory obstruction in infancy and childhood. Vascular "rings" producing respiratory obstruction in infants. Proc Mayo Clin 1950;25:360–367.

60. Harley HRS. The development and anomalies of the aortic arch and its branches. Br J Surg 1959;46:561–573.

61. Idriss TS. Vascular ring. In: Raffensperger JG, ed. Swenson's pediatric surgery, 5th ed. Norwalk, CT: Appleton & Lange, 1990:689–696.

62. Blincoe H, Lowance MI, Venable J. A double aortic arch in man. Anat Rec 1936;66:505–517.

63. Sprong DH Jr, Cutler NL. A case of human right aorta. Anat Rec 1930;45:365–375.

64. Kelsey JR Jr, Gilmore CE, Edwards JE. Bilateral ductus arteriosus representing persistence of each sixth aortic arch. Arch Pathol 1953;55:154–161.

65. Von Siebold CT. J Geburtsch Frauenz Kinderkrankh 1837;16:294.

66. Wolman IJ. Syndrome of constricting double aortic arch in infancy: report of case. J Pediatr 1939;14:527–533.

67. Nugent EW, Plauth WH Jr, Edwards JE, Williams WH. The pathology, abnormal physiology, clinical recognition, and medical and surgical treatment of congenital heart disease. In: Hurst JW, ed. The Heart, 7th ed. New York: McGraw-Hill, 1990.

68. Gnanapragasam JP, Keeton BR, Fong LV. Double aortic arch, tetralogy of Fallot with pulmonary atresia and atrioventricular septal defect. Clin Cardiol 1991;14:522–524.

69. Okuda Y et al. Double aortic arch associated with coarctation of both limbs: a case report. Angiology 1991;42(9):760–764.

70. Bahnson HT, Blalock A. Aortic vascular rings encountered in the surgical treatment of congenital pulmonic stenosis. Ann Surg 1950;131:356–362.

71. Abernathy J. Account of two instances of uncommon formation, in the viscera of the human body. Phil Trans R Soc Lond 1793;83:59–66.

72. Luetmer PH, Miller GM. Right aortic arch with isolation of the left subclavian artery: case report and review of the literature. Mayo Clin Proc 1990;65:407–413.

73. Keith JD, Rowe RD, Vlad P. Heart diseases in infancy and childhood, 3rd ed. New York: Macmillan, 1978.

74. Dotter CT, Steinberg I. The angiocardiographic measurement of the normal great vessels. Radiology 1949;52:353–357.

75. Waldhauser JA, Pae WE. Thoracic great vessels. In: Welsh KJ et al., eds. Pediatric surgery, Vol. 2. Chicago: Year Book Medical Publishers, 1986:1399.

76. Arciniegas E. Vascular rings. In: Arciniegas E, ed. Pediatric Cardiac Surgery. Chicago: Year Book Medical Publishers, 1985.

77. Gidding SS et al. Airway compression by a right aortic arch in the absence of a vascular ring. Chest 1984;85(5):703–705.

78. McNally PR, Rak KM. Dysphagia lusoria caused by persistent right aortic arch with aberrant left subclavian artery and diverticulum of Kommerell. Dig Dis Sci 1992;37(1):144–149.

79. Sanchez-Torres G, Roldan-Conesa D. Left aortic arch without a circumflex segment and a right descending aorta: a hypothetical case and a real example. Arch Inst Cardiol Mex 1989;59(2):125–131.

80. Minami K et al. Left aortic arch, retro-esophageal aortic segment, right descending aorta and right patent ductus arteriosus—a very rare "vascular ring" malformation. Thorac Cardiovasc Surg 1986;34:395–397.

81. Ergin MA, Jayaram N, LaCorte M. Left aortic arch and right descending aorta: diagnostic and therapeutic implications of a rare type of vascular ring. Ann Thorac Surg 1981;31(1):82–85.

82. Hammer Dl, Meis AM. Thyroid arteries and anomalous subclavian in the white and the Negro. Am J Phys Anthrop 1941;28:227–237.

83. Beabout JW, Stewart JR, Kincaid OW. Aberrant right subclavian artery: dispute of commonly accepted concepts. AJR 1964;92:855–864.

84. Bayford D. An account of a singular case of deglutition. Mem Med Soc Lond 1794;2:275.

85. Rendu A. Mémoire pour servir a l'historie des anomalies artérielles. Gastroenterol Med Paris 1842;10:129–135.

86. Gross RE. Surgical treatment for dysphagia lusoria. Ann Surg 1946;124:532–534.

87. Arciniegas E. Vascular anomalies compressing the trachea and esophagus. In: Ravitch MM et al., eds. Pediatric surgery, 3rd ed. Chicago: Year Book Medical Publishers, 1979.
88. Haughton VM, Fellows KE, Rosenbaum AE. The cervical aortic arches. Radiology 1975;114(3):675–681.
89. Beavan TED, Fatti L. Ligature of aortic arch in the neck. Br J Surg 1947;34:414–416.
90. Van Nooten G, Deuvaert F, De Paepe J, Primo G. Left-sided cervical aortic arch. Acta Chir Belg 1986;86:248–250.
91. Felson B, Strife JL. Cervical aortic arch: a commentary. Sem Roentgen 1989;24(2):114–120.
92. Reid DG. Three examples of a right aortic arch. J Anat Physiol 1914;48:174–181.
93. Kumar S et al. Left cervical arch and associated abnormalities. Cardiovasc Intervent Radiol 1989;12(2):88–91.
94. Sobrino-Marquez JM et al. Cervical aortic arch associated with cardiopathy. Rev Esp Cardiol 1992;45(8):537–540.
95. Baker KS et al. Cervical aortic arch: case report with a 12-year follow-up. J Can Assoc Radiol 1987;38(4):302–304.
96. Cali RL, Berg R, Rama K. Bilateral internal carotid artery agenesis: a case study and review of the literature. Surgery 1993;113(2):227–233.
97. Janicki PC, Limbacher JP, Guinto FC Jr. Agenesis of the internal carotid artery with a primitive transsellar communicating artery. AJR 1979;132(1):130–132.
98. Rosen IW et al. Angiographic demonstration of congenital absence of both internal carotid arteries. J Neurosurg 1975;42(4):478–482.
99. Servo A. Agenesis of the left internal carotid artery associated with an aneurysm on the right carotid syphon. J Neurosurg 1977;46(5):677–680.
100. Tode. Medizinisch-chirurgische Bibliothek, Copenhagen, 10, 408 (1787).
101. Handa J et al. Agenesis of an internal carotid artery: angiographic, tomographic and computed tomographic correlation. Neuroradiology 1980;19(4):207–211.
102. Goldberg N, Krasnow N. Sinus of Valsalva aneurysms. Clin Cardiol 1990;13:831–836.
103. Edwards JE, Burchell HB. The pathologic anatomy of deficiencies between the aortic root and the heart including aortic sinus aneurysms. Thorax 1957;12:125.
104. Fishbein MC, Obma R, Roberts WC. Unruptured sinus of Valsalva aneurysm. Am J Cardiol 1975;35(6):918–922.
105. Pan-Chih et al. Surgical treatment of the ruptured aneurysm of the aortic sinuses. Ann Thorac Surg 1981;32(2):162–166.
106. Meyer J. Clinical considerations and surgical treatment in 45 patients: aneurysm and fistula of the sinus of Valsalva. Ann Thorac Surg 1975;19(2):170–179.
107. Glock Y et al. Isolated aneurysm of the left sinus of Valsalva: rupture into the left atrium, left ventricle and dynamic coronary constriction. J Cardiovasc Surg 1990;31(2):235–238.
108. Varin J et al. Anéurysme calcifié non rompu du sinus de Valsalva avec angor et insuffisance aortique: cure chirurgicale. Ann Cardiol Angeiol 1990;39(7):411–415.
109. Gander M et al. Grosses Sinus-Valsalvae-Aneurysma mit dem klinischen Bild eines kombinierten Mitralvitiums. Fortsch Rontgenstr 1980;133(1):94–97.
110. Hinterauer L et al. Sinus-Valsalvae-Aneurysma mit subanulärer Ruptur in den linken Ventrikel, Kompression der linken Kranzarterie und rezidivierender Perikarditis. Fortschr Rontgenstr 1982;136(4):482–485.
111. Thurman J. On aneurysms, and especially spontaneous aneurysms of the ascending aorta and sinus of Valsalva. Med Chir Trans 1840;23:323.
112. Sakakibara S, Konno S. Congenital aneurysm of the sinus of Valsalva: anatomy and classification. Am Heart J 1962;63:405–424.
113. Onat A, Ersanli O, Kanuni A, Aykan TB. Congenital aortic sinus aneurysms with particular reference to dissection of the interventricular septum. Am Heart J 1966;72:158–164.
114. Morrow AG, Baker RR, Hanson HF, Mattingley TW. Successful surgical repair of ruptured aneurysm of the sinus of Valsalva. Circulation 1957;16:533–538.
115. Jones AM, Langley FA. Aortic sinus aneurysms. Br Heart J 1949;11:325–341.
116. Feigenbaum H. Echocardiography, 4th ed. Philadelphia: Lea & Febiger, 1986.
117. O'Rahilly R, Muller F. Human embryology & teratology. New York: Wiley-Liss, 1992.
118. Clagett OT, Kirklin JW, Edwards JE. Anatomic variations and pathologic changes in 124 cases of coarctation of the aorta. Surg Gynecol Obstet 1954;98:103.
119. Romero R et al. Prenatal diagnosis of congenital anomalies. Norwalk, CT: Appleton & Lange, 1988.
120. Rosenberg H. Coarctation of the aorta: Morphology and pathogenesis considerations. In: Rosenberg HS, Bolande RP, eds. Perspectives in Pediatric Pathology, Vol 1. Chicago: Year Book Medical Publishers, 1973.
121. Morgagni G. The seats and causes of diseases investigated by anatomy. Alexander B (transl). Mount Kisco, NY: Futura Publishing, 1980.
122. Evans W. Congenital stenosis (coarctation), atresia and interruption of the aortic arch: study of 28 cases. Q J Med 1933;2:1–31.
123. Paris M. Rétrècissement considérable de l'aorte pectorale observé à l'Hôtel Dieu de Paris. J Chir Desault 1791;2:107.
124. Jarcho S. Coarctation of the aorta (Albrecht Meckel, 1827). Am J Cardiol 1962;9:307–311.
125. Abbott ME. Atlas of congenital cardiac diseases. New York: American Heart Association, 1936.
126. Railsback OC, Dock W. Erosion of the ribs due to stenosis of the isthmus (coarctation) of the aorta. Radiology 1929;12:58–61.
127. Barie E. Du retrecissement congenital de l'aorte descendante. Rev Med (Paris) 1886;6:343, 409, 501.
128. Bonnet IM. Sur la lésion dite sténose congénitale de l'aorte dans la région de l'isthme. Rev Med (Paris) 1903;23:108,255, 335, 418, 481.
129. Abbott ME. Coarctation of the aorta, II. Statistical study and historical retrospect of 200 recorded cases with autopsy of stenosis or obliteration of the descending arch in subjects above the age of 2 years. Am Heart J 1928;3:574–618.
130. Crafoord C, Nylin G. Congenital coarctation of aorta and its surgical treatment. J Thorac Surg 1945;14:347–361.
131. Gross RE, Hufnagel CA. Coarctation of aorta: experimental studies regarding its surgical correction. N Engl J Med 1945;233:287–293.
132. Reifenstein GH, Levine SA, Gross RE. Coarctation of the aorta: a review of 104 autopsied cases of the "adult type," 2 years of age or older. Am Heart J 1947;33:146–168.
133. Skandalakis JE, Edwards BF, Gray SW, Davis BM, Hopkins WA. Coarctation of the aorta with aneurysm. Surg Gynecol Obstet 1960;111(4):307–326.
134. Edwards BF, Gray SW, Hopkins WA, Davis BM, Skandalakis JE. Coarctation of the aorta complicated by the formation of an aneurysm. Surgery 1962;52:444–450.
135. Allan LD, Crawford DC, Tynan M. Evolution of coarctation of the aorta in intrauterine life. Br Heart J 1984;52(4):471–473.
136. Ianniruberto A, Tajani E. Ecocardiografia fetale e diagnosi prenatale di malformazioni congenite. In Zulli P, Catizone FA, Ianni-

ruberto A, eds. Esperienze di Ultrasonografia in Ostetricia e Gine-cologia. Cosenza: Bios, 1983.

137. Hornberger LK et al. Echocardiographic study of the morphology and growth of the aortic arch in the human fetus. Circulation 1992;86(2):741–747.

138. Houston AB et al. Doppler ultrasound in the assessment of sever-ity of coarctation of the aorta and interruption of the aortic arch. Br Heart J 1987;57:38–43.

139. Scott PJ, Wharton GA, Gibbs JL. Failure of Doppler ultrasound to detect coarctation of the aorta. Int J Card 1990;28(3):379–381.

140. Rubay JE et al. Surgical repair of coarctation of the aorta in infants under one year of age. J Cardiovasc Surg 1992;33(2):216–222.

141. Raj Behl P, Santé P, Blesovsky A. Surgical treatment of isolated coarctation of the aorta: 18 years' experience. Thorax 1987;42:309–314.

142. Simsolo R et al. Long-term systemic hypertension in children after successful repair of coarctation of the aorta. Am Heart J 1988;115(6):1268–1273.

143. Ilbawi MN et al. Surgical management of patients with interrupted aortic arch and severe subaortic stenosis. Ann Thorac Surg 1988;45:174–180.

144. Steidele RJ. Sammig. Verschiedener in der chirug. 'prakt, Lehrs-chule Gemachten Beobb 1777–1778;2:114.

145. Celoria GC, Patton RB. Congential absence of the aortic arch. Am Heart J 1959;58:407.

146. Collins-Nakai RL et al. Interrupted aortic arch in infancy. J Pediatr 1976;88(6):959–962.

147. Huhta JC et al. Two-dimensional echocardiographic assessment of the aorta in infants and children with congenital heart disease. Cir-culation 1984;70(3):417–424.

148. Houston AB et al. Doppler ultrasound in the assessment of sever-ity of coarctation of the aorta and interruption of the aortic arch. Br Heart J 1987;57(1):38–43.

149. Scott PJ, Wharton GA, Gibbs JL. Failure of Doppler ultrasound to detect coarctation of the aorta. Int J Cardiol 1990;28(3):379–381.

150. Van Mierop LH, Kutsche LM. Cardiovascular anomalies in DiGeorge syndrome and importance of neural crest as a possible pathogenetic factor. Am J Cardiol 1986;58:133–137.

151. Hammon JW Jr et al. Repair of interrupted aortic arch and asso-ciated malformations in infancy: indications for complete or par-tial repair. Ann Thorac Surg 1986;42:17–21.

152. D'Abreau AL, Rob CG, Vollmar JF. Die Coarctatio aortal abdom-inalis. Langenbeck Arch Klin Chir 1959;290:521–546.

153. Inada K, Shimizu H, Yokoyama T. Pulseless disease and atypical coarctation of the aorta with special reference to their genesis. Surgery 1962;52:433–443.

154. Maycock Wd'A. Congenital stenosis of the abdominal aorta. Am Heart J 1937;13:633–646.

155. Vaccaro PS, Myers JC, Smead WL. Surgical correction of abdom-inal aortic coarctation and hypertension. J Vasc Surg 1986;3(4):643–648.

156. Kodama K et al. Atypical coarctation of the abdominal aorta as a cause of acute hypertensive heart failure. Jpn Heart J 1991;32(2):273–279.

157. Quain R. Partial coarctation of the abodminal aorta. Trans Pathol Soc Lond 1847;1:244.

158. Beattie EJ Jr, Cooke FN, Paul JS, Orbison JA. Coarctation of the aorta at the level of the diaphragm treated successfully with a pre-served human blood vessel graft. J Thorac Surg 1951;21:506–512.

159. Graham LM et al. Abdominal aortic coarctation and segmental hypoplasia. Surgery 1979;86(4):519–529.

160. DeBakey ME et al. Coarctation of the abdominal aorta with renal arterial stenosis: surgical considerations. Ann Surg 1967;165:830–843.

161. Bergqvist D et al. Coarctation of the abdominal aorta in elderly patients: Case report and review of the literature. Acta Med Scand 1988;223(3):275–280.

162. Hallett JW Jr et al. Coarctation of the abdominal aorta: current options in surgical management. Ann Surg 1980;191(4):430–437.

163. Grishman A, Sussman ML, Steinberg MF. Atypical coarctation of the aorta with absence of the left radical pulse. Am Heart J 1944;27:217–224.

164. Levine S, Serfas LS, Rusinko A. Right aortic arch with subclavian steal syndrome (atresia of left common carotid and left subclavian arteries). Am J Surg 1966;111:632–637.

165. Hofbeck M, Rupprecht T, Reif R, Singer H. Faulty origin of the right subclavian artery from the pulmonary artery: a rare cause of subclavian steal syndrome in childhood. Monatsschr Kinderheilkd 1991;139(6):363–365.

166. Edwards JE. Classification of congenital heart disease in the adult. In: Roberts WC, ed. Congenital heart disease in adults. Cardiovasc Clin Series 10/1, FA. Philadelphia: FA Davis, 1979.

167. Noback GJ, Rehman I. The ductus arteriosus in the human fetus and newborn infant. Anat Rec 1941;81:505–527.

168. Mancini AJ. A study of the angle formed by the ductus arteriosus with the descending thoracic aorta. Anat Rec 1951;109:535–539.

169. Jager BV, Wollenman OJ Jr. An antomical study of the closure of the ductus arteriosus. Am J Pathol 1942;18:595–613.

170. Noback GJ, Anderson FD, Cooper WG. On the presence of nerve tissue in the media of the human ductus arteriosus. Anat Rec 1951;109:331.

171. Kennedy JA, Clark SL. Observations on the physiological reac-tions of the ductus arteriosus. Am J Physiol 1942;136:140–147.

172. Danesino VL, Reynolds SRM, Rehman IH. Comparative histolog-ical structure of the human ductus arteriosus according to topog-raphy, age, and degree of constriction. Anat Rec 1955;121:801–829.

173. Eldridge FL, Hultgren HN. The physiologic closure of the ductus arteriosus in newborn infants. J Clin Invest 1955;34:987–996.

174. Barclay AE, Franklin KJ, Prichard MML. The foetal circulation and cardiovascular system and the changes that they undergo at birth. Springfield, IL: Charles C Thomas, 1945.

175. Moss AJ, Emmanouilides GC, Adams FH, Chuang K. Response of ductus arteriosus and pulmonary and systemic arterial pressure to changes in oxygen environment in newborn infants. Pediatrics 1964;33:937–944.

176. Christie A. Normal closing time of the foramen ovale and the duc-tus arteriosus: anatomic and statistical study. Am J Dis Child 1930;40:323–326.

177. Scammon RE, Norris EH. On the time of the post-natal oblitera-tion of the fetal blood-passages (foramen ovale, ductus arteriosus, ductus venosus). Anat Rec 1918;15:165–180.

178. Born GVR, Dawes GS, Mott JC, Rennick BR. The constriction of the ductus arteriosus caused by oxygen and by asphyxia in new-born lambs. J Physiol 1956;132:304–342.

179. Kovalvcíc V. The response of the isolated ductus arteriosus to oxy-gen and anoxia. J Physiol (London) 1963;169:185–197.

180. Record RG, McKeown T. Observations relating to the aetiology of patent ductus arteriosus. Br Heart J 1953;15:376–386.

181. Hellstrom B, Jonsson B. Late prognosis in asphyxia neonatorum. Acta Paediatr (Uppsala) 1953;42:398–406.

182. Heymann MA. Fetal and neonatal circulations. In: Adams FH, Emmanouilides GC, Riemenschneider TA, eds. Moss' heart dis-ease in infants, children and adolescents, 4th ed. Baltimore: Wil-liams & Wilkins, 1989.

183. Heymann MA. Patent ductus arteriosus. In Moss' heart disease in infants, children and adolescents, 4th ed. Baltimore: Williams & Wilkins, 1989.

184. Boyd JD. The nerve supply of the mammalian ductus arteriosus. J Anat 1941;75:457–468.

185. Savchenko LV. On the nerve supply of the ductus arteriosus. Mat Teor I Klin Med (Tomsk) 1963;2:6–9.

186. Barcroft J, Kennedy JA, Mason MF. The relations of the vagus nerve to the ductus arteriosus in the guinea pig. J Physiol 1938;92:1P–2P.

187. Nora JJ. Etiologic aspects of heart diseases. In: Adams FH, Emmanouilides GC, Riemenschneider TA, eds. Moss' heart disease in infants, children and adolescents, 4th ed. Baltimore: Williams & Wilkins, 1989.

188. Dexter L. Congenital defects of the heart in high altitudes. N Engl J Med 1952;247:851–852.

189. Emmanouilides GC, Gravanis MB. Pathogenesis and pathophysiology of structural congenital heart disease. In: Granvanis MB, ed. Cardiovascular disorders: pathogenesis and pathophysiology. St. Louis: Mosby, 1993.

190. Fallopius G. Medici mulenesis observations. Venice [Venetiis]: MA Ulmus, 1562.

191. Franklin KJ. Ductus venosus (Arantii) and ductus arteriosus (Botalli). Bull His Med 1941;9:580–584.

192. Langer C. Zur Anatomie der fötalen Kreislauforgane. Z Ges Aerzt Wien 1857;36:329–339.

193. Billard CM. Traité des maladies des infants nouveaux—nés et à la mamelle, fondé sur de nouvelles observations cliniques et d'anatomie pathologique faitès a l'hôpital des enfants trouvés de Paris. Paris, 1828.

194. Chevers N. Observations on the permanence of the ductus arteriosus and constriction of the thoracic aorta and the means by which the duct becomes naturally closed. Lond Med Gaz 1845;1:187–192.

195. Gerhardt C. Persistenz des ductus arteriosus Botalli. Jenaische Z Med Zaturw 1867;3:105–117.

196. Wells HG. Persistent patency of the ductus arteriosus. Am J Med Sci 1908;136:381–400.

197. Munro JC. Ligation of the ductus arteriosus. Ann Surg 1907;46:335–338.

198. Graybiel A, Strieder JW, Boyer NH. An attempt to obliterate the patent ductus arteriosus in a patient with subacute bacterial endarteritis. Am Heart J 1938;15:621–624.

199. Gross RE, Hubbard JP. Surgical ligation of a patent ductus arteriosus: report of first successful case. JAMA 1939;112:729–731.

200. Strassman P. Anatomische und physiologische Untersuchugen über den Blutkreislauf beim Neugeborenen. Arch Gynaek 1894;45:393–445.

201. Mouzinho AI, Rosenfeld CR, Risser R. Symptomatic patent ductus arteriosus in very-low-birth-weight infants: 1987–1989. Early Hum Dev 1991;27(1-2):65–77.

202. Krovetz LJ, Warden HE. Patent ductus arteriosus: an analysis of 515 surgically proven cases. Dis Chest 1962;42:46–57.

203. Polani PE, Campbell M. Factors in the causation of persistent ductus arteriosus. Am Hum Genet 1960;24:343–357.

204. Gross RE. Surgical closure of an aortic septal defect. Circulation 1952;5:858–863.

205. Kjellberg SR et al. Diagnosis of congenital heart disease: a clinical and technical study, 2nd ed. Chicago: Year Book Publishers, 1959.

206. Scott HW Jr. Closure of patent ductus by suture-ligation technique. Surg Gynecol Obstet 1950;90:91–95.

207. Ekstrom G. The surgical treatment of patent ductus arteriosus. Acta Chir Scand 1953;104:421–422.

208. Lamy M, DeGrouchy J, Schweisguth O. Genetic and nongenetic factors in the etiology of congenital heart disease: a study of 1188 cases. Am J Hum Genet 1957;9:17–41.

209. Burman D. Familial patent ductus arteriosus. Br Heart J 1961;23:603–604.

210. Uchida IA, Rowe RD. Discordant heart anomalies in twins. Am J Hum Genet 1957;9:133–140.

211. Gravanis MB. Cardiovascular disorders: pathogenesis and pathophysiology. St. Louis: Mosby, 1993.

212. Gelb BD, OLaughlin MP, Mullins CE. Prevalence of additional cardiovascular anomalies in patients referred for transcatheter closure of patent ductus arteriosus. J Am Coll Cardiol 1990;16(7):1680–1686.

213. Laborde F et al. A new video-assisted thoracoscopic surgical technique for interruption of patent ductus arteriosus in infants and children. J Thorac Cardiovasc Surg 1993;105(2):278–280.

214. Rashkind WJ et al. Nonsurgical closure of patent ductus arteriosus: clinical application of the Rashkind PDA occluder system. Circulation 1987;75(3):583–592.

215. Lock JE et al. Transcatheter umbrella closure of congenital heart defects. Circulation 1987;75(3):593–599.

216. Wessel DL et al. Outpatient closure of the patent ductus arteriosus. Circulation 1988;77(5):1068–1071.

217. Steinberg I, Miscall L, Goldberg HP. Congenital absence of left pulmonary artery with patent ductus arteriosi. JAMA 1964;190:394–396.

218. Van Hare GF et al. Interrupted aortic arch with a right descending aorta and right ductus arteriosus, causing severe right bronchial compression. Pediatr Cardiol 1988;9(3):171–174.

219. Pierpont ME et al. Interruption of the aortic arch with right descending aorta: a rare condition and a cause of bronchial compression. Pediatr Cardiol 1982;2(2):153–159.

220. Poynter CWM. Arterial anomalies pertaining to the aortic arches and the branches arising from them. Stud Zool Lab Univ Nebraska 1916;16:229.

221. Sherman FE. An atlas of congenital heart disease. Philadelphia: Lea & Febiger, 1963.

222. Collett RW, Edwards JE. Persistent truncus arteriosus: a classification according to anatomic types. Surg Clin North Am 1949;29:1245–1270.

223. Van Praagh R, Van Praagh S. The anatomy of common aorticopulmonary trunk (truncus arteriosus communis) and its embryologic implications: a study of 57 necropsy cases. Am J Card 1965;16:406–425.

224. Yoshizato T, Julsrud PR. Truncus arteriosus revisited: an angiographic demonstration. Pediatr Cardiol 1990;11(1):36–40.

225. Wilson J. A description of a very unusual formation of the human heart. Phil Trans R Soc Lond 1798;88:346–359.

226. Elliotson J. Case of malformation of the pulmonary artery and aorta. Lancet 1830;1:247–248.

227. Tiedeman F. Abweichende Anordnung der Pulsaderstämme des Herzens. Z Physiol 1831;4:287.

228. Humphreys EM. Truncus arteriosus communis persistens. Arch Pathol 1932;14:671–700.

229. Giordano A. Persistent truncus arteriosum communis: review of the literature and presentation of 49 cases of true truncus arteriosus and 18 examples of related conditions. Folia Hered Pathol Suppl 1964;4.

230. Anderson RC. Causative factors underlying congenital heart malformations. I. Patent ductus arteriosus. Pediatrics 1954;14:143–151.

231. Deshpande J, Desai M, Kinare S. Persistent truncus arteriosus: an autopsy study of 16 cases. Int J Cardiol 1992;37(3):395–399.

232. Cabrera A et al. Persistent truncus arteriosus. Echocardiographic study of 8 cases. Rev Esp Cardiol 1990;43(7):492–496.

233. Van Mierop LH, Kutsche LM. Cardiovascular anomalies in DiGeorge syndrome and importance of neural crest as a possible pathogenetic factor. Am J Cardiol 1986;58(1):133–137.

234. Rao PS et al. Tricuspid artresia: association with persistent truncus arteriosus. Am Heart J 1991;122(3 pt 1):829–835.

235. Diógenes TC, Atik E, Aiello VD. Common arterial trunk associated with absence of atrioventricular connexion. Int J Cardiol 1990;27(3):385–388.

236. Rastelli GC, Titus JL, McGoon DC. Homograft of ascending aorta and aortic valve as a right ventricular outflow: an experimental approach to the repair of truncus arteriosus. Arch Surg 1967;95:698–708.

237. Bove EL et al. Repair of truncus arteriosus in the neonate and young infant. Ann Thorac Surg 1989;47:499–506.

238. Ebert PA et al. Surgical treatment of truncus arteriosus in the first 6 months of life. Ann Surg 1984;200(4):451–456.

239. Kutsche LM, Van Mierop LHS. Anatomy and pathogenesis of aorticopulmonary septal defect. Am J Cardiol 1987;59:443–447.

240. Lau KC et al. Aorto-pulmonary window. J Cardiovas Surg 1982;23:21–27.

241. Van Mierop LHS, Gessner IH. Pathogenetic mechanisms in congenital cardiovascular malformations. Prof Cardiovasc Dis 1972;15:67–85.

242. Becker AE, Anderson RH. Cardiac Pathology: an integrated text and colour atlas. New York: Raven Press, 1982.

243. Meisner H, Schmidt-Habelmann P, Sebening F, Klinner W. Surgical correction of aorto-pulmonary septal defects. Dis Chest 1968;53:750–758.

244. Shumway NE, Lewis FJ. The closure of experimental aortic septal defects under direct vision and hypothermia. Surgery 1956;39:604–610.

245. Wright JS, Freeman R, Johnston JB. Aorto-pulmonary fenestration: a technique of surgical management. J Thorac Cardiovasc Surg 1968;55:280–283.

246. Blieden LC, Moller JH. Aorticopulmonary septal defect: an experience with 17 patients. Br Heart J 1974;36(7):630–635.

247. Fisher EA, DuBrow IW, Eckner FAO, Hastreiter AR. Aorticopulmonary septal defect and interrupted aortic arch: a diagnostic challenge. Am J Cardiol 1974;34:356–359.

248. Becker AE, Anderson RH, eds. Pathology of congenital heart disease. London: Butterworths, 1981.

249. Kami K, Morishita T. An autopsy case of double inferior vena cava accompanied by atypical lateral branches of the abdominal aorta with special consideration to the embryology. Okajimas Folia Anat Jap 1983;59(6):387–403.

250. Roques X et al. Coarctation of the abdominal aorta. Ann Vasc Surg 1988;2(2):138–144.

251. Palmaz JC et al. Male hypoplastic infrarenal aorta and premature atherosclerosis. Surgery 1983;94(1):91–94.

252. van Meurs-van Woezik H et al. Tandem coarctation of the thoracic aorta with hypoplasia of the abdominal aorta. Thorac Cardiovasc Surg 1985;33(1):44–47.

253. Smith SH, Kelly DR. Coarctation of the abdominal aorta in a child: morphometric analysis of the arterial lesion. Pediatr Pathol 1986;5:363–371.

254. Piyachon C, Suwanela N. Takayasu arteritis in Thailand. Heart Vessels Suppl 1992;7:60–67.

255. Takeshita T et al. A case of a rare anomaly of the abdominal aorta: magnetic resonance image and angiographic finding. Nippon Igaku Hoshasen Gakkai Zasshi 1990;50(3):258–261.

256. Michels NA. Blood supply and anatomy of the upper abdominal organs, with a descriptive atlas. Philadelphia: JB Lippincott, 1955.

257. Nelson TM, Pollack R, Johasson O, Abcarian H. Anatomic variants of the celiac, superior mesenteric, and inferior mesenteric arteries and their clinical relevance. Clin Anat 1988;1:75–91.

258. Paz Z, Rak Y, Rosen A. Anatomical basis for celiac trunk and superior mesenteric artery entrapment. Clin Anat 1991;4:256–264.

259. Kornblith PL, Boley SJ, Whitehouse BS. Anatomy of the splanchnic circulation. Surg Clin North Am 1992;72(1):1–30.

260. Van Damme JP, Bonte J. Vascular anatomy in abdominal surgery. New York: Thieme Medical Publishers, 1990.

261. Morris CD, Menashe VD. 25-Year mortality after surgical repair of congenital heart defect in childhood: a population-based cohort study. JAMA 1991;266(24):3447–3452.

262. Manning JA. Insurability and employability of young cardiac patients. Cardiovasc Clin 1981;11(2):117–127.

263. Olshan AF, Teschke K, Baird PA. Paternal occupation and congenital anomalies in offspring. Am J Ind Med 1991;20(4):447–475.

264. Storch TG, Mannick EE. Epidemiology of congenital heart disease in Louisianna: an association between race and sex and the prevalence of specific cardiac malformations. Teratology 1992;46(3):271–276.

CHAPTER 29

THE SUPERIOR AND INFERIOR VENAE CAVAE

John Elias Skandalakis / Stephen Wood Gray / Panagiotis Symbas

The vessels with thin wall and foul of blood are named veins, and all the great veins are named **cavae.** *Later the physicians used to name* **cava** *the vein which receives branches from the liver, kidneys. . . . Pyxagoras named this vein* **cava.** *Others however named* **cava** *the one who is passing through the diaphragm towards the heart. Others again name this vein and the previous one* **cava.** *. . . Homer used the word* **cava** *with the meaning emptying and large.*
—*ROUFOS OF EFESSOS*

DEVELOPMENT

The Primitive Venous System

The origin of the blood vessels and lymphatic vessels has been the subject of such a long and exhausting controversy that eventual indifference rather than crucial experiment has caused the topic to be dropped without being solved.

As early as 1868 His (1), observing the formation of blood islands and the network of primitive vessels formed from them in the area vasculosa of the yolk sac, suggested the existence of a specific angiogenic tissue, the angioblast. Cells of the angioblast migrate into the yolk stalk, forming first the vitelline veins and then, by ramification, all the blood vessels of the body (Fig. 29.1). This view was given authority by Minot (2), Evans (3), and Sabin (4) in their respective contributions to Keibel and Mall's *Manual of Human Embryology* in 1912 (5).

Not everyone accepted the angioblast theory. In 1906 Rückert and Mollier (6) as well as Maximow suggested that blood vessels might arise independently from the embryonic mesoderm. Bremer (7) proposed the existence of angiogenic centers in the body of the embryo as well as in the yolk sac. By 1917 Sabin (8) had abandoned the angioblast theory, and in 1921 McClure (9) became the chief exponent of the local origin theory, stating that mesenchyme anywhere in the body could bring blood vessels into being by the formation of endothelium-lined spaces, which subsequently coalesce into vascular channels.

Regardless of the means by which the earliest blood vessels are formed, establishment of the channels that become the named vessels of the body is by outgrowth from preexisting vessels. In most cases the initial vascular supply to an area is a capillary network. As the area enlarges with the growth of the embryo, certain channels of the capillary bed enlarge and eventually become the major vessels supplying or draining the area. In a few places a major vessel may grow as a sprout from another major vessel and tap a previously formed capillary plexus.

The anterior cardinal veins arise during the fourth week, after the dorsal aortae and the first aortic arch are present. From the cranial end of the first arch, the primitive internal carotid artery supplies a capillary plexus about the eye, midbrain, and hindbrain and otic vesicle. The earliest venous channel drains these capillary beds cranially as the vena capitis medialis (primary head vein) at the side of the neural tube. At the level of the first somite, the vein shifts laterally into the somites to become the anterior cardinal vein, receiving several anastomoses from the aorta. In the more caudal region, the posterior cardinal veins form by coalescence of lateral capillary beds served by the descending aorta.

The primitive cardinal system is "captured" by anastomoses with umbilical veins and the vitelline veins at the posterior end of the developing heart. The connections thus established form the ducts of Cuvier, which receive the anterior and posterior cardinal veins dorsally, the umbilical veins posteriorly, and the vitelline veins posteroventrally. The ducts unite ventrally to open into the sinus venosus of the heart. In the fourth week, when the embryo is about 4 mm long, a symmetric system of veins drains the cranial and caudal portions of the body, the yolk sac, and the placenta (Fig. 29.2).

It is beyond the scope of this book to follow the development of the veins other than the major ones entering the heart. The classic studies of the development of the venous drainage of the head are those of Streeter (10, 11). Lewis (12) and Woollard (13) described the development of the veins of the limbs.

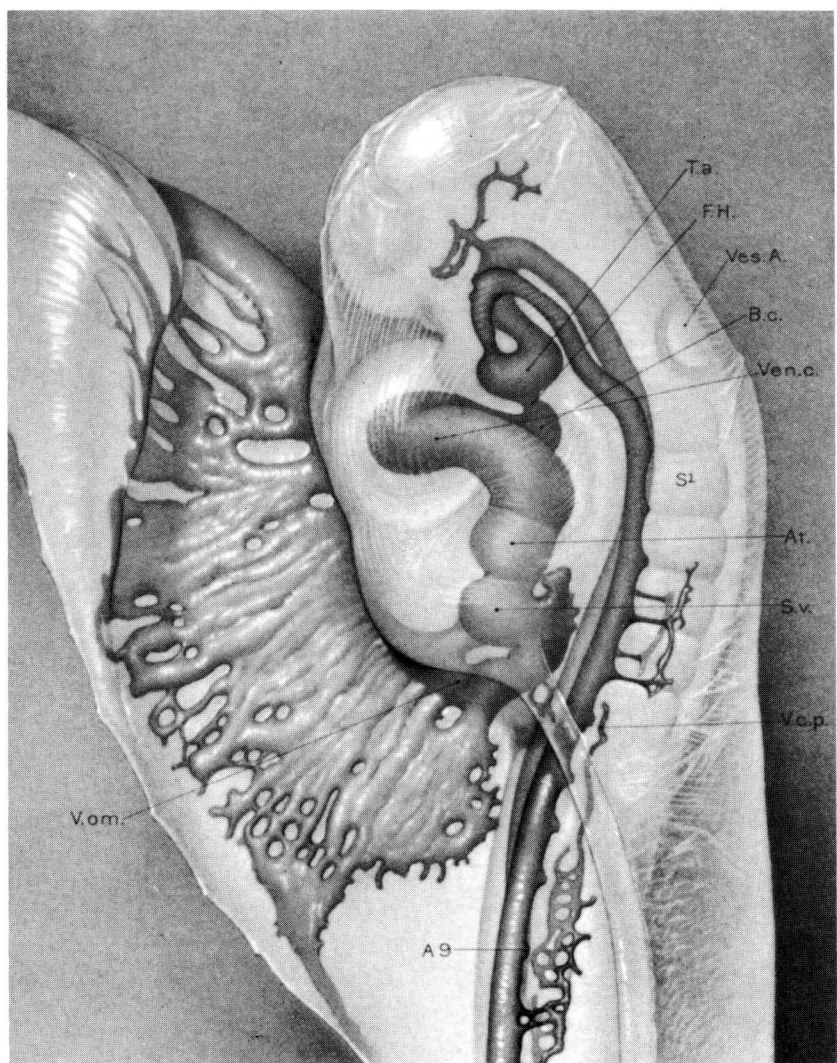

Figure 29.1. Model of a pig embryo of 14 somites. The angioblast sheet of the yolk sac has invaded the embryonic body to form the vitelline veins *(V. om.)* that join the heart at the sinus venosus *(S. v.).* The umbilical vein is shown but not labeled. *T.a.,* Truncus arteriosus; *F.H.,* arterioventricular constriction; *Ves.A.,* otic vesicle;

B.c., bulbus cordis; *Ven.c.,* primordium of ventricles; *At.,* primordium of atria; *V.c.p.,* posterior cardinal vein; S¹, first somite; *A9,* ninth segemental spinal artery. (From Sabin FR. Origin and development of the primitive vessels of the chick and of the pig. Contrib Embryol Carnegie Inst Wash 1917;6:61–124.)

Development of the Superior Vena Cava

The symmetry of the anterior system of veins becomes altered as early as the fourth week, when the sinoatrial opening moves to the right side of the yet undivided atrium. Between the sixth and eighth weeks, the ducts of Cuvier become incorporated into the sinus venosus. On the right, the sinus venosus—which receives the right anterior cardinal vein, the enlarging pars hepatica of the future inferior vena cava, and the smaller right posterior cardinal vein—will be totally absorbed into the wall of the right atrium. The transverse portion of the sinus will remain as the coronary sinus, while the left horn will atrophy completely.

Among the tributaries of the anterior cardinal veins, a pair draining the thymus on each side anastomose across the midline, between the two cardinal veins (14). These are recognizable as the left brachiocephalic vein by the eighth week (22 mm) (15). Thus, as the left duct of Cuvier and the left side of the sinus venosus atrophy, blood is shunted via this anastomosis from the left anterior cardinal vein to the right anterior cardinal vein, which is subsequently known as the superior vena cava (SVC) (Fig. 29.3). In summary, the SVC is formed by a combination

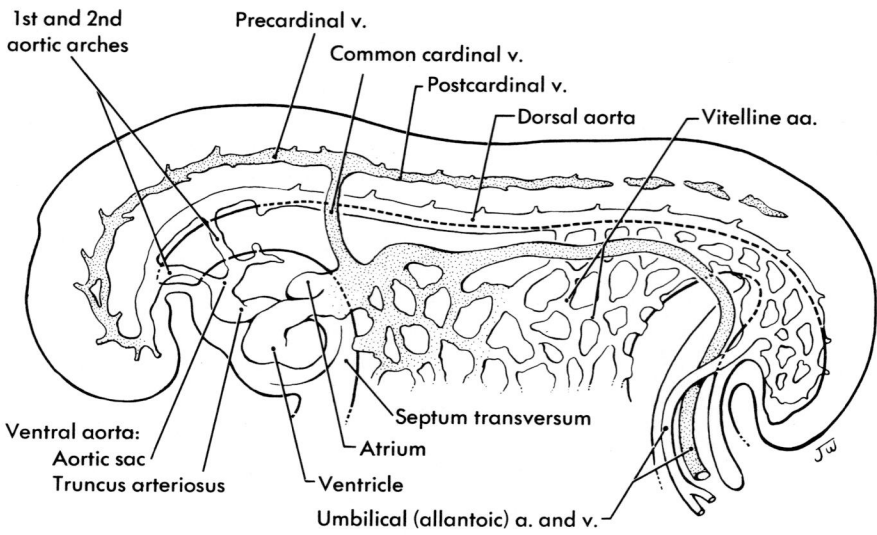

Figure 29.2. The basic vascular plan of the human embryo at the end of the first month. Paired vessels are shown only on the side toward the observer. (From Allan FD. Essentials of human embryology. New York: Oxford University Press, 1969.)

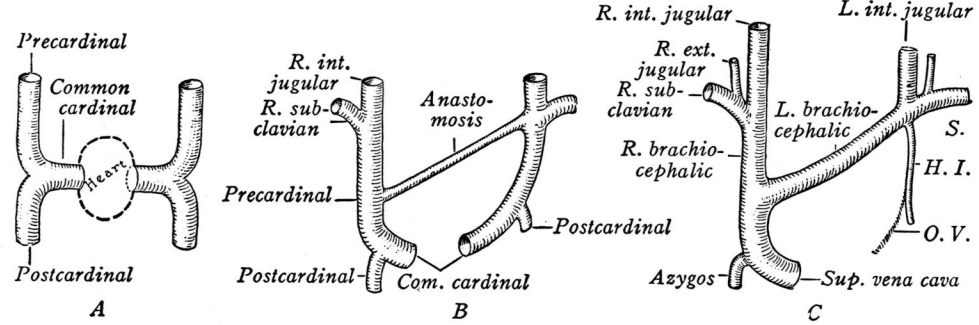

Figure 29.3. Transformation of the cardinal veins into the superior vena cava. **A,** At 6 weeks. **B,** At 8 weeks. **C,** Adult. The left brachiohepatic vein forms from anastomosing channels draining the thymus. *S,* Left subclavian vein; *H.I.,* highest intercostal vein; *O.V.,* oblique vein of the left atrium. (From Arey LB. Developmental anatomy. 7th ed. Philadelphia: WB Saunders, 1965.)

of the proximal part of the right anterior cardinal vein and the right common cardinal vein.

Of the left anterior cardinal vein below the brachiocephalic vein, the most distal remnant is a portion of the left superior intercostal vein. Proximally, a small inconstant vein from the pericardium may reach the coronary sinus by way of the pericardial (vestigial) fold of Marshall (16). Occasionally, a larger vessel in this location (oblique vein of Marshall) drains the mediastinum. Usually, the only proximal remnant is the oblique vein of the left atrium, a tributary of the great cardiac vein (Fig. 29.4, *D*). Very rarely, this channel persists and receives the right SVC (17) (Fig. 29.4, *B*).

Development of the Inferior Vena Cava

Our knowledge of the complexities of the developing venous system of the lower part of the body rests largely on the work of McClure and Butler (15), Huntington and McClure (18), and Lewis (19). Development of these veins is complicated, and the original works must be consulted for complete understanding. We are concerned here only with the formation of the inferior vena cava (IVC).

Between the fifth and eighth weeks, two sets of veins, in addition to the postcardinal vein, form in relation to the developing mesonephros. The first of these, the subcardinal veins, lie medial to the mesonephros and form a broad anastomosis with each other below the level of the entrance of the umbilical artery (Fig. 29.5, *A* and *B*). They are present as early as the fifth week. The second major set of embryonic vessels, the supracardinal or lateral sympathetic veins, are present during the seventh week, lying dorsal and medial to the postcardinal veins (Fig. 29.5, *C* and *D*). Cross-connections are frequent between the three sets of vessels.

The IVC is formed among these embryonic venous

channels much the way builders of large highways utilize existing rural road networks: Some existing channels are enlarged; others are closed off; and in some places entirely new connections are made (Fig. 29.5, *F*). Possible choices among the embryonic pathways are numerous, but in the human, variation in the pattern is unusual.

There is no clue to the causes behind the selection of channels other than that the pathways are similar among mammalian embryos.

Above the renal anastomosis, the IVC is formed from the right subcardinal vein. By the sixth week, capillaries at the cephalic end of the right subcardinal vein have

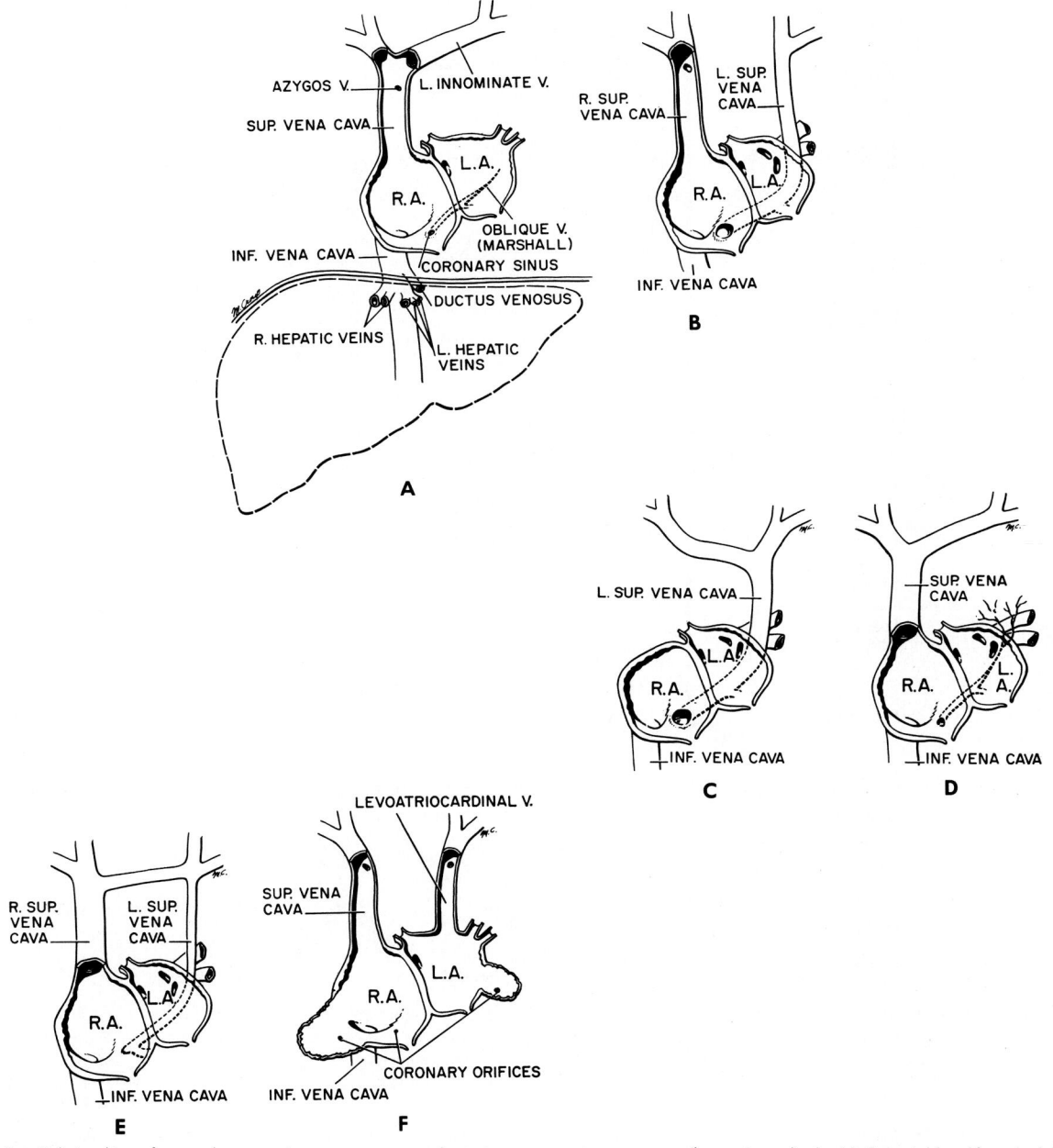

Figure 29.4. Relationships of anomalous superior venae cavae to the atria. **A,** Normal cranial and caudal systemic return. **B,** Left superior vena cava draining into the right atrium through the coronary sinus. **C,** Absent right superior vena cava. Left vein drains into right atrium. **D,** Patent oblique vein of Marshall receiving small mediastinal veins. **E,** Atresia of the coronary sinus. Blood flow is retrograde through the vein of Marshall and the persistent left superior cava. **F,** Persistent left superior vena cava (levoatriocardinal vein). Sytemic blood from the left upper part of the body drains to the left atrium. The coronary sinus and left brachiocephalic vein are usually absent. The orifices of the symmetric azygos system are indicated in each superior caval vessel. (From Sherman FE. An atlas of congenital heart disease. Philadelphia: Lea & Febiger, 1963.)

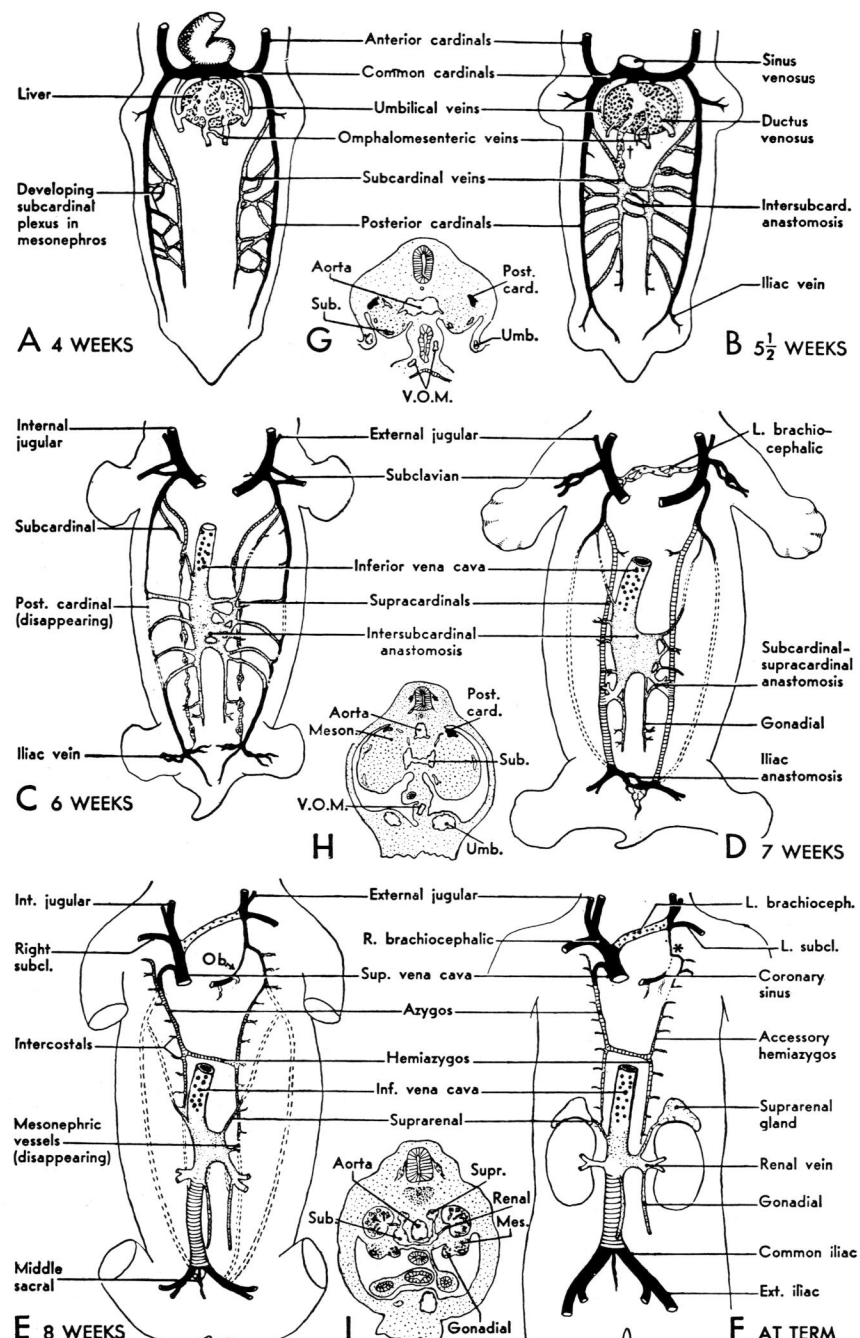

Figure 29.5. Diagrams of the stages in the development of the superior and inferior venae cavae from the symmetric cardinal venous system. **A** to **F**, Stages in ventral (anterior) view. **G** to **I**, Cross-sectional views. Cardinal veins are *black*, subcardinal veins are *stippled*, and supracardinal veins are *horizontally hatched*.

Vessels arising independently of these three systems are indicated by a pattern of *heavy dots*. The *asterisk* in **F** indicates the left superior intercostal vein. *Ob.,* Oblique vein of left atrium (vein of Marshall); *V.O.M.,* omphalomesenteric vein. (From Patten BM. Human embryology. New York: McGraw-Hill, 1968.)

extended beyond the end of the mesonephros to make contact with the liver. Through these, the hepatic portion of the vena cava is formed. It joins the old right vitelline vein to enter the sinus venosus. Of the left subcardinal vein above the renal anastomosis, only the left suprarenal vein remains (Fig. 29.5, *F*).

Below the renal anastomosis, most of the IVC is formed from the right supracardinal vein. Proximally, it connects with the cephalic portion by an anastomosis formed between the subcardinal and supracardinal veins in the seventh week. This segment, designated the renal collar, forms the renal veins on each side as well as a por-

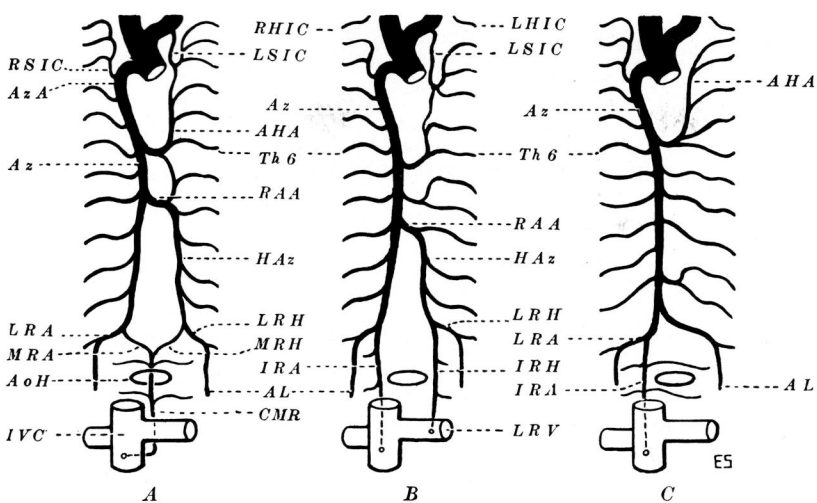

Figure 29.6. Three of the most frequently encountered patterns of the azygos veins (see also Fig. 29.5, **F**). *AL,* Ascending lumbar vein; *Az,* azygos vein; *AHA,* accessory hemiazygos vein; *AoH,* aortic hiatus of diaphragm; *AzA,* azygos arch; *CMR,* common medial root of origin of the azygos and hemiazygos veins; *HAz,* hemiazygos vein; *IVC,* inferior vena cava; *LRV,* left renal vein; *RAA,* retroaortic anastomoses; *RHIC* and *LHIC,* right and left highest intercostal veins; *RSIC* and *LSIC,* right and left superior intercostal veins; *LRA, IRA,* and *MRA,* lateral, intermediate, and medial roots of origin of the azygos vein; *LRH, IRH,* and *MRH,* lateral, intermediate, and medial roots of origin of the hemiazygos vein; *Th 6,* sixth intercostal vein. (From Seib GA. The azygos system of veins in American whites and American negroes, including observations on the inferior caval venous system. Am J Phys Anthrop 1934;19:39–164.)

tion of the vena cava on the right. The subcardinal veins below the renal collar form the veins to the gonads. The left supracardinal vein disappears.

Caudally, the right supracardinal vein joins the iliac anastomosis of the postcardinal system and thus receives drainage from the lower extremities (Fig. 29.5, *F*).

Most of the supracardinal veins above the renal level remain as the azygos on the right and the hemiazygos on the left. On the right, the azygos joins the proximal portion of the right posterior cardinal vein to enter the SVC. On the left, an accessory azygos (left azygos) frequently persists and joins the left superior intercostal vein (Fig. 29.6).

In summary, the hepatic segment of the IVC is formed by the right vitelline vein, the renal segment by the right subcardinal vein, and the sacrocardinal segment by the right sacrocardinal vein.

The channels that will form the SVC are all present by the seventh week, and the definitive channel is already larger than the alternative pathways. By the end of the eighth week, almost all of the changes have been completed although the left supracardinal vein below the renal collar has not disappeared. It is probably the last of the old channels to vanish since it persists the most frequently as an anomalous left IVC.

Critical Events in the Development of the Venae Cavae

The chief anomalies of the veins comprise the persistence of embryonic channels. For the SVC, the fifth week is

important; for the IVC, the sixth and seventh weeks are the times of definitive remodeling.

ANOMALIES OF BOTH CAVAE

Anomalies of both IVC and SVC in the same individual are rare but not uncommon. It is not possible for the authors to present all the associated anomalies involved, but for all practical purposes, the abnormal drainage of both these great vessels is peculiar and enigmatic.

Huhta et al. (20) in 1982 tested the sensitivity and specificity of cross-sectional echocardiographic diagnosis of systemic venous return in 789 children with congenital heart disease. They reported excellent diagnostic results. Only one case with absence of the suprarenal segment of the IVC was not diagnosed correctly.

Peoples et al. (21) reviewed autopsies of 146 cases of polysplenia, 41 being their own personal cases. These authors, because of their findings, contend that the condition is that of bilateral left-sidedness. They reported multiple anomalies such as the bilateral SVC, interruption of IVC with azygos continuation, and others.

Vitarelli et al. (22) evaluated three patients with total anomalous pulmonary venous drainage with cross-sectional color-flow Doppler echocardiography. Two of their three patients had supracardiac drainage to the left vertical vein or to the right SVC, and one patient had infracardiac drainage as retrograde flow to the IVC. Congenital absence of both SVCs with the superior systemic veins drained under the diaphragm into two azygos veins was reported by Hussain et al. (23).

Table 29.1.
Anomalies of the Superior and Inferior Venae Cavae

Anomaly	Origin of Defect	First Appearance (or Other Diagnostic Clues)	Sex Chiefly Affected	Relative Frequency	Remarks
Persistent left superior vena cava	5th week	Symptoms related to associated cardiac defects only	Equal	Common	Not anomalous in complete situs inversus; usually associated with cardiac defects
Absence of hepatic segment of inferior vena cava	6th week	Symptoms related to associated cardiac defects only	Equal	Uncommon	
Double inferior vena cava; left-sided inferior vena cava	7th week	None	Equal	Common	
Preureteral vena cava	7th week	At any age	Equal	Rare	Compression of ureter produces symptoms

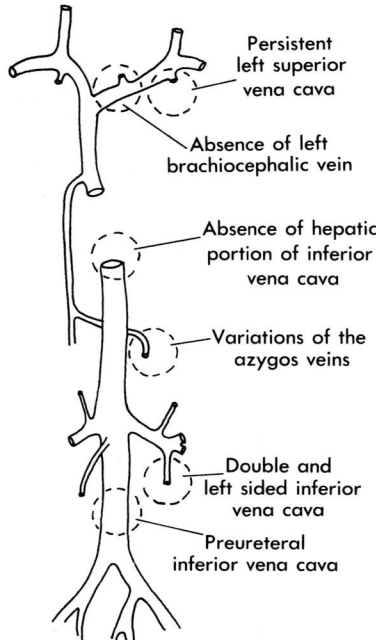

Figure 29.7. Sites of anomalies of the superior and inferior venae cavae.

ANOMALIES OF THE SUPERIOR AND INFERIOR VENAE CAVAE (TABLE 29.1 AND FIG. 29.7)

Congenital Anomalies of SVC

1. Left SVC
2. Duplication
3. Anomalous systemic draining to the heart
4. Congenital aneurysm

From all the above congenital anomalies, the one which has clinical significance, according to Smith (24), is the anomalous systemic venous return to the heart. Kabbani et al. (25) reported left single SVC draining into the left atrium, and Viart et al. (26) reported total anomalous venous draining. Oxygen desaturation is one of the car-dinal conditions if such an anomaly is present together with other intracardiac defects. A complete review of the different types of anomalous systemic venous return to the heart is provided by Mazzucco (27) et al.

EDITORIAL COMMENT

Left SVC drainage directly into the left atrium is an embryologic curiosity which can cause significant systemic arterial desaturation due to the right-to-left shunt. The usual communication of the left common cardinal vein and the left horn of the sinus venosus has obviously been altered, resulting in left SVC drainage into the left atrium. Whatever the cause, this rare anomaly of the venous system oftentimes requires correction by: (a) ligation, if small; (b) intraatrial pericardial baffle; or (c) reimplantation of the left SVC into the superior portion of the left pulmonary artery (*CM*).

For all practical purposes, left SVC, duplications, and congenital aneurysm are asymptomatic.

ANOMALIES OF THE SUPERIOR SYSTEMIC VEIN (PERSISTENT LEFT SUPERIOR VENA CAVA)

In the normal adult, blood from the right side of the head and the right arm drain by way of the SVC into the right atrium. Drainage from the left side of the head and the left arm crosses the midline as the left brachiocephalic vein to join the SVC.

This normal arrangement, derived from an initially symmetric embryonic system, may not always be found. There may be a SVC on both the left and the right sides, or there may be only a left SVC (Fig. 29.8).

Anatomy

Double Superior Vena Cava.

The most primitive condition is an undivided atrium, into which two SVCs open above and two IVCs open below. The pulmonary veins may join either of the venae cavae, or they may enter the single atrium independently. In slightly more advanced examples, the atrial septum is present, and each SVC enters the atrium on its own side (Fig. 29.4, *F*).

In both of the above arrangements, there may or may not be a left brachiocephalic vein between the two venae cavae (Fig. 29.9, *B* and *C*). In all cases there are important cardiac defects, usually of septation, in addition to the doubling of the vena cava.

More frequent than the primitive anomalies described above is the pattern in which the anomalous left SVC enters the coronary sinus and thus drains into the right atrium, as does the normal right vena cava (Fig. 29.9, *B* and *C*, and Fig. 29.4, *B*). An anastomosing brachiocephalic vein may or may not be present. Cardiac defects are present in about 33% of such cases (Fig. 29.10).

EDITORIAL COMMENT

The persistent left SVC is formed by the left anterior cardinal vein and, for the most part, communicates with the right atrium through the left horn of the sinus venosus which becomes the coronary sinus. As noted, these abnormal venous communications do not cause circulatory aberrations since the desaturated blood eventually returns to the right side of the heart and is eventually distributed to the lungs for oxygenation appropriately. Difficulties arise

when surgical interventions are performed. For instance, a left transvenous endocardial pacemaker wire cannot be placed if the patient has a persistent left vena cava to the coronary sinus. The surgeon must quickly recognize this aberrant anatomy and revise the approach. Often, patients are operated on for other intracardiac malformations without preoperative knowledge of a persistent left SVC. The absence of the innominate vein and an unusually small right SVC should signal the presence of a left SVC. The clinical significance of a left SVC during cardiopulmonary bypass is that torrential blood flow into the coronary sinus will obscure the intracardiac landmarks and pathology. In addition, uncontrolled left SVC flow into the coronary sinus will warm the heart if cardioplegic arrest is performed. The informed and alert cardiac surgeon will correctly assess the presence of a left SVC under these circumstances and take effective steps to occlude or drain it into the venous reservoir (*CM*).

Rossi et al. (28) reported bilateral SVC in a newborn with congenital atrioventricular block in right atrial isomerism (asplenia) associated with several other congenital defects. Snider and Silverman (29) reported persistent left SVC, total anomalous pulmonary venous return to

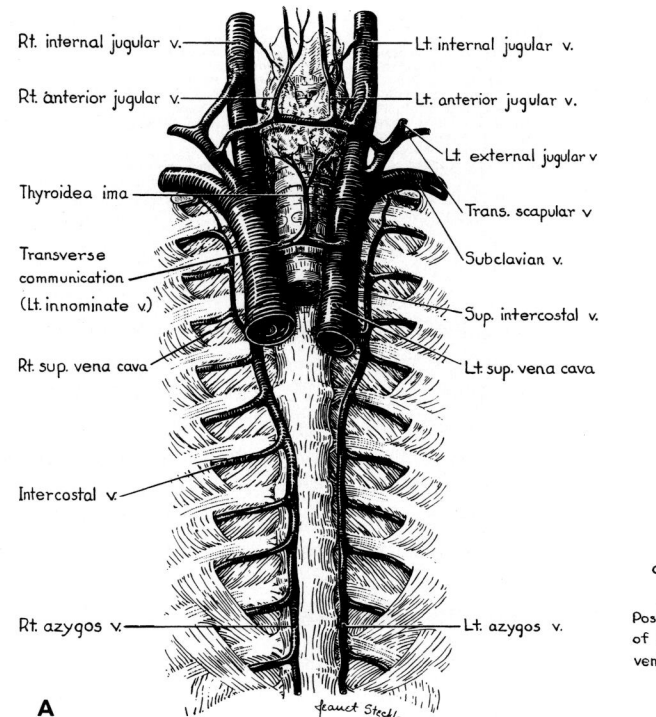

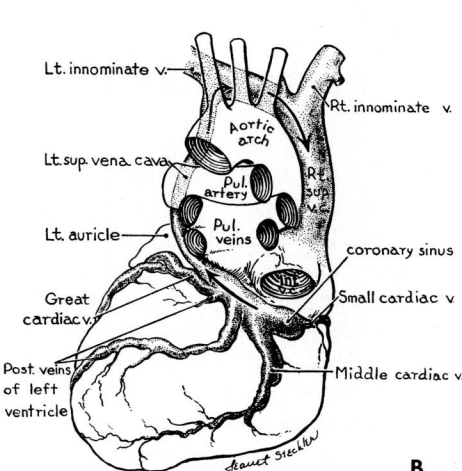

Figure 29.8.   Double superior vena cava. **A,** Almost complete symmetry of the superior venae cavae and azygos veins. There are anastomoses between the venae cavae at the levels of the thymus and thyroid gland. The former would normally become the innominate (brachiocephalic) vein and is so labeled here. **B,** Diagrammatic representation of blood flow from a closed coronary sinus through a persistent left superior vena cava. (From Prows MS. Two cases of bilateral superior venae cavae, one draining a closed coronary sinus. Anat Rec 1943;87:99–106.)

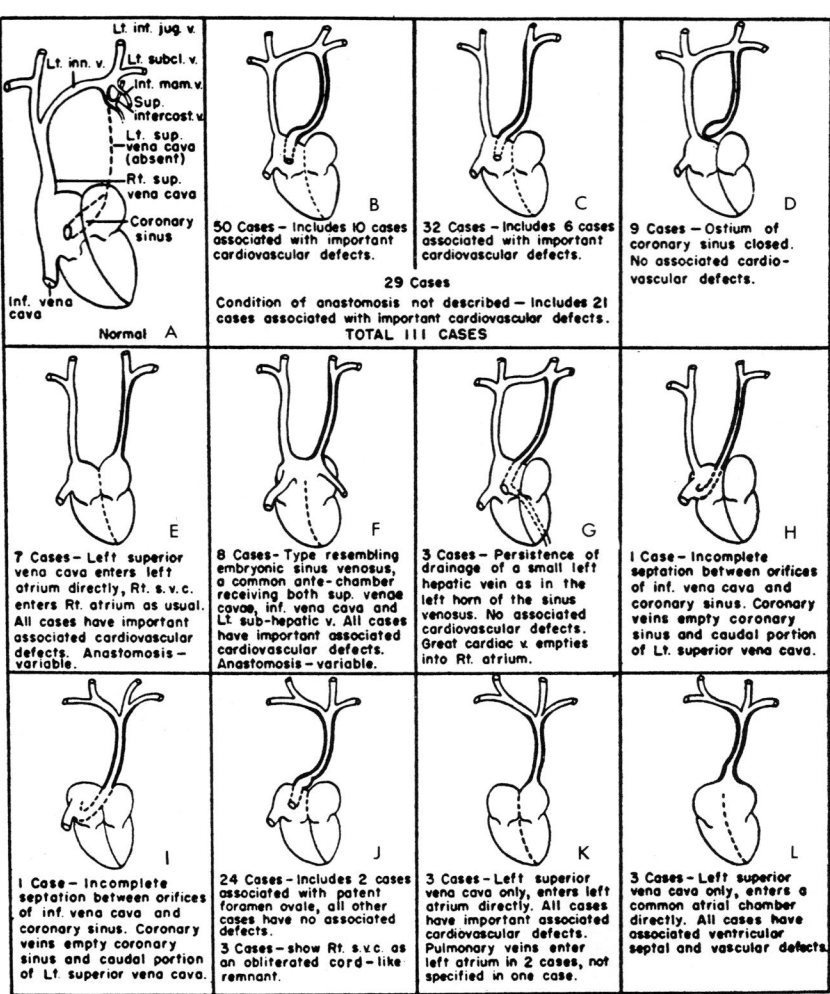

Figure 29.9. Types of persistent left or double superior venae cavae. Incidence is that among 170 cases from the world literature. *Broken septal line* indicates septal defect. (Partial persistence is illustrated in Figure 29-11, *I*, and *J*).

(From Winter FS. Persistent left superior vena cava: survey of world literature and report of thirty additional cases. Angiology 1954;5:90–132.)

the right SVC, and SVC obstruction after Mustard's operation.

Left-Sided Superior Vena Cava.

When the left SVC is the only persistent vein, there is a brachiocephalic vein carrying blood from right to left. The persistent vein enters the coronary sinus and the right atrium in the same manner as it does when both venae cavae are present (Fig. 29.4, *C*, and Fig. 29.9, *J*). As with double venae cavae, there may be an undivided atrium as well as serious septal defects (30) (Fig. 29.9, *L*).

A persistent left SVC is also present in complete transposition of the viscera (situs inversus viscerum), with dextrocardia. In such cases it empties into the left atrium, as does the coronary sinus, which comes from the right side. In situs inversus, a left SVC is part of the total mirror image rather than an anomalous vessel per se. Double

venae cavae are more common when transposition is partial than when it is complete (31).

While about 75% of both double SVC and left sided SVC result in no circulatory dysfunction, in the remainder, severe dysfunction, often incompatible with life, may exist. When developmental arrest occurs early, there is a single ventricle. In other cases there may be a large septal defect, or the left SVC may enter the left ventricle (32).

EDITORIAL COMMENT

Some patients with single ventricles and heterotaxy syndromes of "bilateral right-sidedness" or "bilateral left-sidedness" often have bilateral SVCs. These patients, if associated with favorable pulmonary vascular hemodynamics, can undergo a Fontan operation employing a total cavopulmonary artery anastomosis and lateral tunnel baffle to direct the IVC flow to the SVC. Both SVCs are transsected at their entry into the heart and the left SVC is anastomosed to the superior portion of the left pulmonary artery. The divided right SVC is anastomosed to the right pulmonary artery with the superior portion to the superior margin of the right pulmonary artery and the inferior portion to the inferior margin of the right pulmonary artery. An atrial baffle directing IVC flow to the SVC orifice completes the repair (CM).

Anomalies of the pulmonary venous drainage are often associated with anomalies of the SVC. Either the left or the right SVC may receive the pulmonary veins (17) (Fig. 29.11). In some cases only the distal portion of the left SVC persists, and drainage is through the brachiocephalic vein to the right atrium (Fig. 29.11, I). The anomalous drainage is usually but not always total. Septal defects are always present (see Chapter 14, "Pulmonary

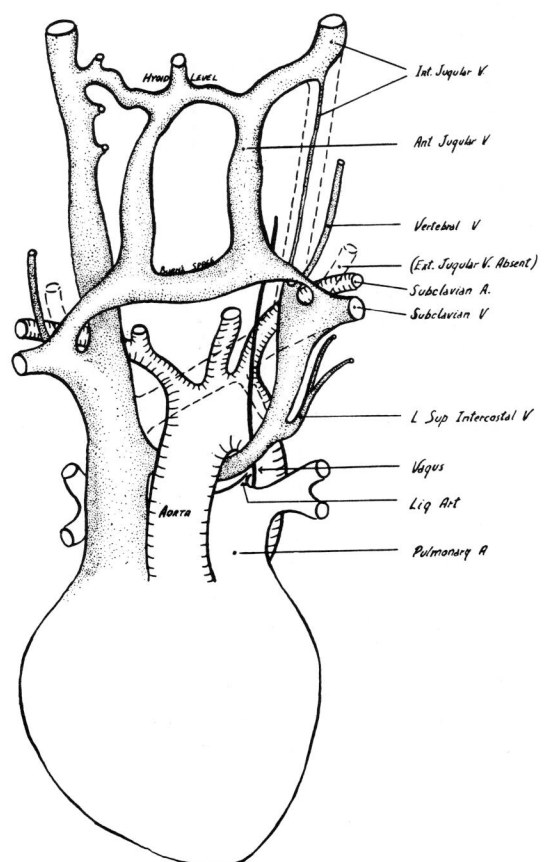

Figure 29.10. Double superior vena cava. In contrast to the case shown in Figure 29.8, the hyoid and thyroid anastomoses have persisted, while the more caudal thymus anastomosis (indicated by *broken lines*), which normally forms the left brachiocephalic vein, has dropped out. (From Friedman SM. Report of two unusual venous abnormalities (left posterior vena cava; postaortic left innominate vein). Anat Rec 1945;92:71–76.)

Circulation). The variations on this pattern are numerous (Fig. 29.11).

In a few cases the persistent left SVC receives a left azygos vein, so that the azygos system retains its primitive symmetry. Nandy and Blair (33) described a case and collected seven others from the literature. When the superior caval development is normal, a persistent left azygos vein (accessory hemiazygos vein) often enters the left superior intercostal vein, the distal portion of which is probably part of the primitive left SVC (34) (Fig. 29.6, A).

Left-sided SVC was reported by Stevenson et al. (35) in 1979 in all their patients who had total anomalous pulmonary venous return. Konstam et al. (36) reported left SVC communicating to the left atrium diagnosed by nuclear angiography and total body scan.

Bjerregaard and Laursen (37) reported persistent left SVC associated with congenital heart defects. The authors stated that most likely the anomaly is associated with pulmonary atresia and with anomalous pulmonary venous connection.

Yu et al. (38) reported left-sided SVC with anomalous aortic arch and multiple other congenital deformities. Mantagos et al. (39) reported persistent left SVC in two unrelated newborn infants with multiple other malformations and complete trisomy 9 in all cells examined. The authors advised doing chromosome studies on infants who have congenital malformations and who die in the newborn period and counseling the parents accordingly.

Yiannikas et al. (40), assessing patients with left-to-right shunts, reported associated anomalies such as a persistent left SVC, coarctation of the aorta and partial anomalous venous return.

Pulmonary agenesis and left SVC was reported by Mardini and Nyhan (41). Weisbrod and Todd (42) reported congenital left SVC with absent right SVC, which was diagnosed by computed tomographic (CT) scanning.

Rey et al. (43) reported on percutaneous balloon angioplasty in an infant with obstructed total anomalous pulmonary vein return into the left SVC. Sand et al. (44) reported seven patients with anomalous left SVC connected to the left atrium.

EDITORIAL COMMENT

As noted earlier, total anomalous pulmonary venous drainage into a left SVC which connects with the left atrium does not create any hemodynamic abnormality, provided there is not obstruction to the drainage. With obstruction, there will be significant pulmonary venous congestion leading to marked pulmonary artery hypertension and major hemodynamic abnormalities. When there is total anomalous pulmonary venous drainage into the IVC or the sinus venosus, a marked alteration in hemodynamics exists because pulmonary venous blood is being delivered to the right side of the

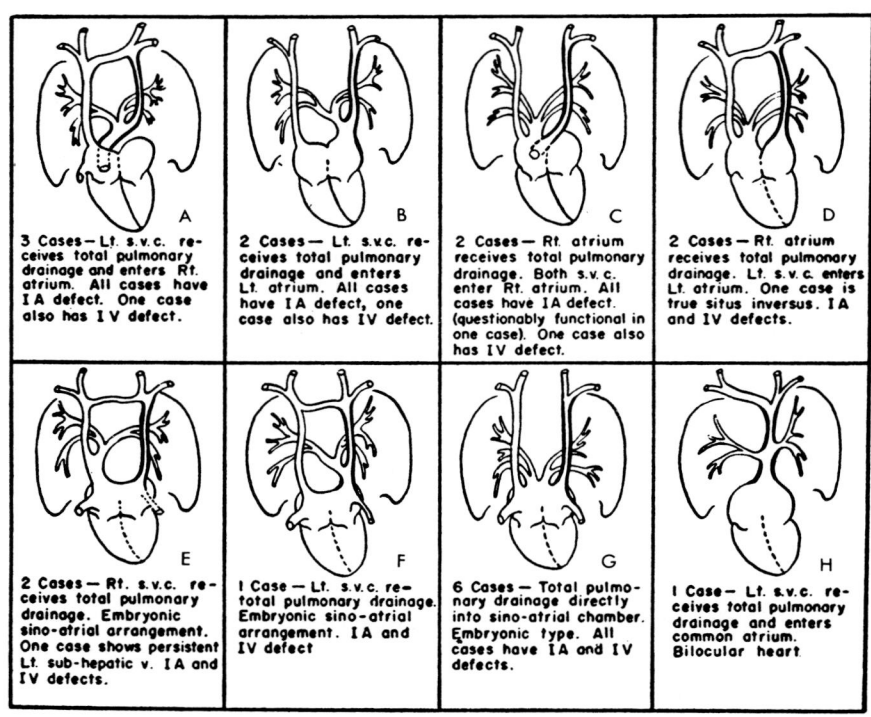

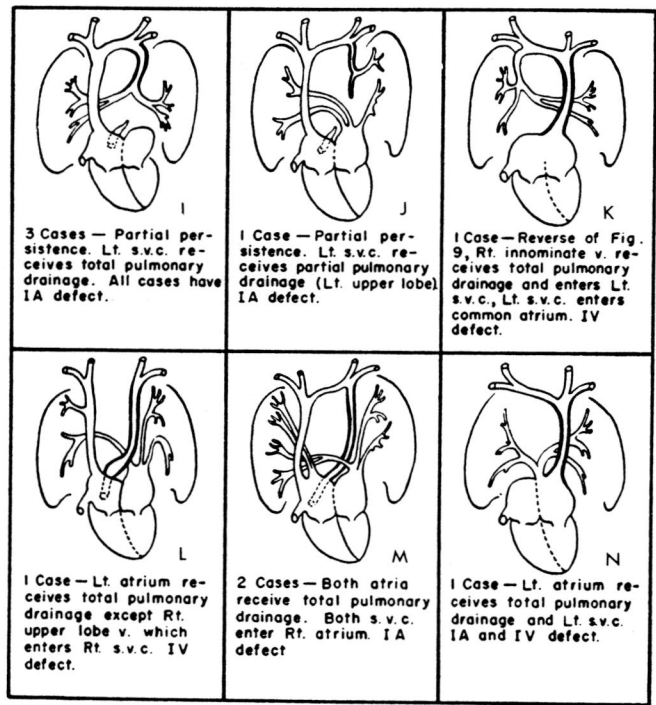

Figure 29.11. Patterns of persistent left superior vena cava associated with anomalous pulmonary drainage. (From Winter FS. Persistent left superior vena cava: survey of world literature and report of thirty additional cases. Angiology 1954;5:90–132.)

heart with a resulting very large left-to-right shunt. Even this condition can be well tolerated in a newborn infant if there is a large atrial septal defect and good communication between the two sides of the heart. It is only in those situations where the junction of the total anomalous pulmonary venous draining vein into the right-sided caval system is obstructed by a stenotic connection that there is significant obstruction to pulmonary venous drainage. The result is severe pulmonary artery hypertension and congestive heart failure (JAH/CNP).

Hofbeck et al. (45) reported coarctation of the aorta, absence of pulmonary valve, ventricular septal and other defects, and anomalous drainage of the right superior pulmonary vein into the SVC. These authors believe that there is most likely an early involution of the ductus arteriosus in syndromes with absent pulmonary artery associated with ventricular septal defects.

Choi et al. (46) reported that in 24 (0.98%) of 2457 patients with congenital heart disease, the brachiocephalic vein was in an anomalous position below the aortic arch. The authors stated that this anomaly is more common with tetralogy of Fallot or ventricular septal defects with pulmonary atresia and most likely right aortic arch.

Rodefeld et al. (47) reported cor triatriatum with persistent left SVC and several other defects. Havase et al. (48) described persistent left SVC associated with completely unroofed coronary sinus.

Suzuki et al. (49) reported hypoplastic left ventricular syndrome with premature closure of foramen ovale, total anomalous pulmonary venous return, and anomalous connection of the right upper pulmonary vein to the SVC—right atrial (SVC-RA) junction, plus several other vascular anomalies.

Embryogenesis. All varieties of persistent left SVC represent developmental arrest. The most primitive condition, in which the paired venae cavae enter an undivided atrium, can be referred to the condition existing at five weeks, when the atria have not yet expanded and the sinoatrial opening is still medially placed (Fig. 29.9, *F*).

The left brachiocephalic vein arises during the eighth week and may be present even though both venae cavae open into an atrium undivided, as a result of an earlier developmental arrest (Fig. 29.11, *E* and *F*). It is apparent that if the brachiocephalic anastomosis fails to form, the vena cava on the left must persist. The converse is not true; persistence of the left caval trunk with a functional brachiocephalic anastomosis is as common as the condition without it.

History. Double and left-sided SVCs were seen by Morgagni (50) in 1728 (De Sedibus XLVII:30) and 1736 (LVI:31), but our understanding of their development begins with the work of Marshall (51) in 1850. He identified the remnants of the left superior caval trunk (the

vein of Marshall). McCotter (52) collected 116 cases from the literature in 1916; his paper should be consulted for the earliest references. By 1954 Winter (53) had found 174 cases and diagrammed the variations. Nandy and Blair (33) estimated that, by 1965, there were 246 cases of bilateral SVC in the literature. Gensini and his colleagues (54) in 1959 reported 37 cases recognized by catheterization or angiography in living subjects. The first diagnosis by catheter was made by Cournand and his associates (55) in 1949.

Incidence. While a superior left vena cava is not a rare anomaly, its incidence is not known. It is probably close to 1:750 dissected cadavers. Not surprisingly, those cases with associated cardiac anomalies are disproportionately frequent in clinical studies (31, 32) although angiography reveals increasing numbers of asymptomatic cases.

Symptoms. Uncomplicated double or persistent left SVC is asymptomatic. In complicated cases symptoms are those of septal defects, anomalous connections with the pulmonary veins, or anomalous drainage into the left atrium.

Diagnosis. Recognition of SVC anomalies is by cardiac catheterization or angiocardiography (54, 56). Whereas a left-sided SVC will be found by angiocardiography through the right arm, the left arm must be used if double caval veins are to be demonstrated (57).

Prognosis. When septal defects co-exist, death before the age of 10 years is usual. Among 174 cases collected by Winter (53), 47% died before age 20 years. This cannot be taken as an index of mortality, however, because his series included relatively few uncomplicated cases.

ANOMALOUS DRAINAGE INTO THE RIGHT SVC

Vaquez-Perez and Frontera-Izquierdo (58) reported a right SVC draining into the left atrium. The authors stated that this is the fifth case in the literature and the first one in a male.

Shapiro et al. (59) reported right SVC receiving pulmonary venous drainage from the right lung and which drained in both atria by two channels. Park et al. (60) reported anomalous drainage of the right SVC into the left atrium.

Anomalies of the Inferior Venae Cavae

The IVC has several anomalies such as length, location, duplication, abnormal connections and draining, "absence of the IVC," and membranous obstruction.

ABSENCE OF THE HEPATIC SEGMENT OF THE INFERIOR VENA CAVA

Anatomy. Although this anomaly has been called "absence of the vena cava," this name is misleading and incorrect; it should be dropped from the literature. Only

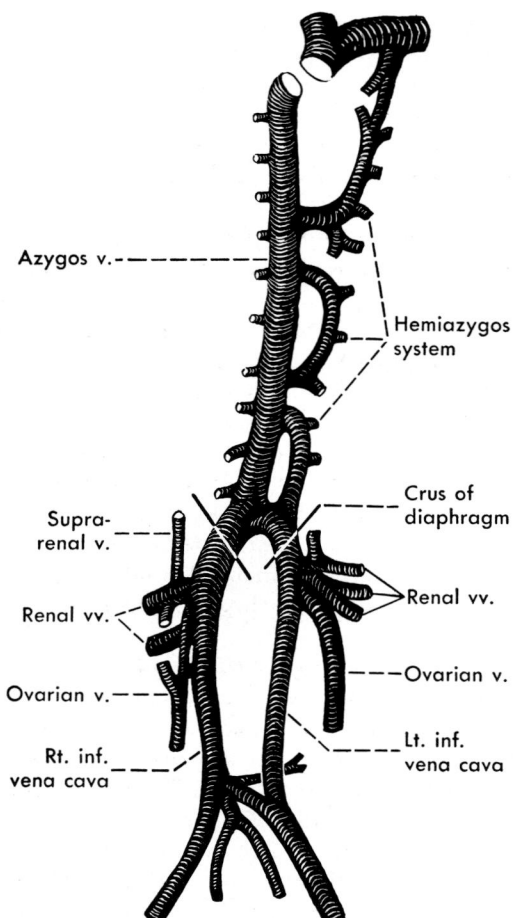

Figure 29.12. "Absence" of the inferior vena cava. Above the renal vein, the paths of the supracardinal veins have persisted as the azygos and the hemiazygos veins replacing the hepatic part of the inferior vena cava. Below the renal veins, the vena cava is doubled. (From Hollinshead WH. Anatomy for surgeons. New York: Hoeber-Harper, 1956; redrawn from Huseby RA, Boyden EA. Absence of the hepatic portion of the inferior vena cava with bilateral retention of the supracardinal system. Anat Rec 1941;81:537–544.)

the hepatic and prerenal portions of the normal vena cava are absent; continuity is by way of the azygos or the hemiazygos vein, the remnants of the embryonic supracardinal veins (Fig. 29.12). Drainage is into the right or left SVC; the hepatic veins enter the heart alone. Associated cardiac anomalies are frequent, but the anomaly may occur without other defects.

Embryogenesis. This condition results from failure of the right subcardinal vein tributaries to connect with the veins of the liver during the sixth week. The result is the persistence of either the right or the left supracardinal vein, together with a short portion of the right or left posterior cardinal vein. Rarely, the supracardinal vein persists on both sides (azygos), usually draining into a double SVC (33) (Fig. 29.13).

History and Incidence. McClure and Huntington (61)

found 33 references to "absence of the vena cava," the earliest in 1775 by Winslow. In 1941 Huseby and Boyden (62) collected 15 cases and added one of their own. Since the introduction of angiography and catheterization, many more have been found. Anderson and his colleagues (63) collected 21 cases between 1941 and 1961 and described 16 of their own. Fifteen of these were found among 2500 patients with congenital heart defects seen over a period of only 6 years at University of Minnesota hospitals. Among 40 cases, 32 were continuations on the right (azygos) and eight on the left (hemiazygos). All patients had other cardiac defects, and 17 had some transposition of the heart, abdominal viscera, or both. About 0.5% of patients with congenital cardiac defects

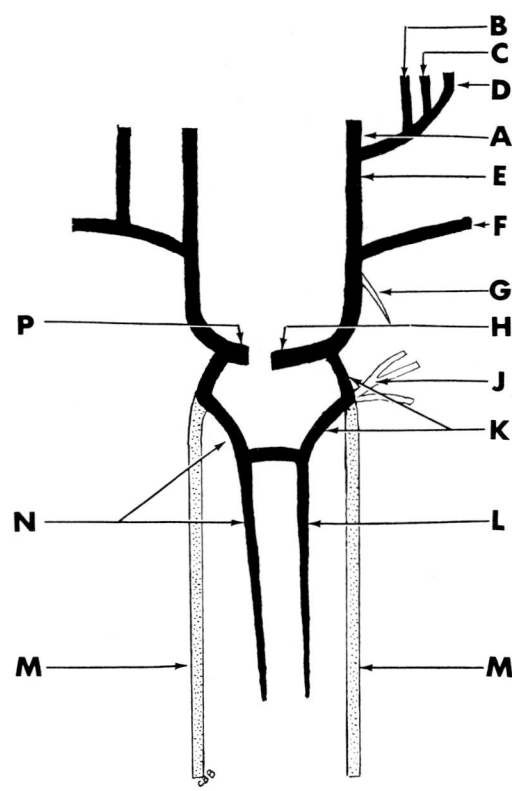

Figure 29.13. Atypical development of the superior and inferior venous drainage in the adult male cadaver. The superior vena cava is paired, and both sides receive symmetrically paired azygos vessels. The inferior vena cava was normal. A, Internal jugular vein; B, left facial vein; C, left retromandibular vein; D, left posterior auricular vein; E, "common jugular" portion of internal jugular vein; F, left subclavian vein; G, first posterior intercostal vein; H, left superior vena cava replacing typical coronary sinus; J, left superior intercostal vein with no contribution from anterior cardinal and entering left azygos instead of left brachiocephalic; K, proximal portion of left azygos vein derived from left supracardinal and persistent proximal portion of left posterior cardinal vein; L, (inferior) hemiazygos portion of left azygos vein derived in typical manner form distal portion of left supracardinal vein; M, distal portions of posterior cardinal veins lost during development; N, right azygos vein formed in typical manner; P, right superior vena cava receiving no tributary from left side of body. (From Nandy K, Blair CB Jr. Double superior venae cavae with completely paired azygous veins. Anat Rec 1965;151:1–10.)

appear to have azygos or hemiazygos continuation of the vena cava. There is no information about the frequency in individuals without associated cardiac defects.

The anomaly has been reported in a number of mammals other than humans. References may be found in McClure and Huntington (61).

Symptoms and Diagnosis. The presence of an anomalous vena cava alone produces no symptoms. Cyanosis, when present, arises from a wide variety of associated cardiac anomalies.

Diagnosis is by angiocardiography by way of a vein in the leg. The anomalous vein shows as a "candy cane," most clearly seen in lateral views.

Treatment. No treatment is required for this anomaly. If no cardiac defects are present, there will be no physiologic disturbance of circulation. The surgeon must be aware of the possibility of such a condition, however, before he or she sacrifices the azygos or hemiazygos vein during thoracic surgery. One such fatal accident has been reported (64).

EDITORAL COMMENT

The other surgical implication of an anomalous IVC draining through the azygos system is for open heart surgery repair of other congenital abnormalities. Since cannulation requires placing a catheter in the IVC through the atrium as well as the SVC for venous return to the heart lung machine, the surgeon must be aware of the absent portion of the IVC lest the inferior caval cannula be inserted too far and perforate the back wall of the hepatic vein confluence which is in direct communication with the right atrium. Once recognized, the patient can be treated appropriately with cardiopulmonary bypass by placing a larger cannula in the SVC to accommodate the increased venous return through the azygous system as well as the SVC drainage (JAH).

ANOMALIES OF THE POSTRENAL INFERIOR VENA CAVA

Anatomy

Double Inferior Vena Cava.

The presence of a right and left IVC below the renal veins is not an unusual variation (Fig. 29.12). The left vein may be smaller than the right, and it may extend for only a short distance, usually at the level of the third and fourth lumbar vertebrae (Fig. 29.14, A and C). When small, it is usually designated as a left paravertebral vein (65).

The left and right cavae join, anterior to the aorta, at or below the level of the renal veins. There may be also a lumbar anastomotic vessel between them, passing behind the aorta (66) (Fig. 29.14, A and B). Inferiorly, each cava may be formed by the junction of the iliac vein on its own side, with or without an iliac anastomosis. Both common iliac veins may join the larger of the two cavae if the smaller ends in a lumbar anastomosis with the larger (61).

Left Inferior Vena Cava.

A persistent left cava with absence of the right cava is a mirror image, below the renal veins, of the normal IVC. It occurs in situs inversus, in which the entire vena cava, as well as other abdominal organs, is affected, or in the absence of situs inversus, in which case it may be the sole anomaly (Fig. 29.14, B).

Preureteral Inferior Vena Cava.

Because its significance is primarily urologic, this anomaly is usually called "retrocaval ureter" (see Chapter 17, "The Kidney and Ureter"). The right ureter passes behind and around the vena cava to reach the bladder (Fig. 29.15). It does not occur on the left.

Persistent Renal Collar.

A rare anomaly associated with double venae cavae is the presence of a left renal vein anterior to, as well as posterior to, the aorta. Between the kidney and the aorta, these veins are connected with a left vena cava; thus, they form a complete ring around the aorta (Fig. 29.14, A). McClure and Huntington (61) mention three examples in humans.

Preaortic Iliac Anastomosis.

Normally, the iliac veins unite behind the aorta to form the IVC. Occasionally, this junction is found anterior to the aorta. While this condition is anomalous in humans and other placental mammals, it is normal in many marsupial mammals (61). Two examples have been reported in humans.

Embryogenesis

Double and Left-sided Vena Cava. (Fig. 29.16 and Fig. 29.17) The normal postrenal IVC is formed from the right supracardinal vein of the embryo (Fig. 29.5, E). The most common anomalies result from the persistence of the left subcardinal vein (left IVC) (Fig. 29.14, B) or both subcardinal veins (double IVC) (Fig. 29.14, C).

McClure and Huntington (61) concluded from their study of the embryonic veins of the abdomen that there could be 14 possible arrangements of the adult inferior systemic venous return in addition to the usual one. Only two of these, persistent left supracardinal vein and persistent left and right supracardinal veins, are at all common. A few other types have been found occasionally. At least 10 other types have been found to occur in the cat, which exhibits more variation in its venous architecture than does either the dog or human (67).

Preureteral Vena Cava.

Persistence of the right embryonic subcardinal vein, together with its anastomosis with the right postcardinal vein as the lower IVC, brings the definitive vena cava in front of, instead of behind, the right ureter (Fig. 29.18). It could occur on the left with a persistent left subcardinal vein, but this has not been reported.

Persistent Renal Collar.

The renal collar is a system of embryonic venous anastomoses. Posterior to the aorta, it is formed by anastomoses

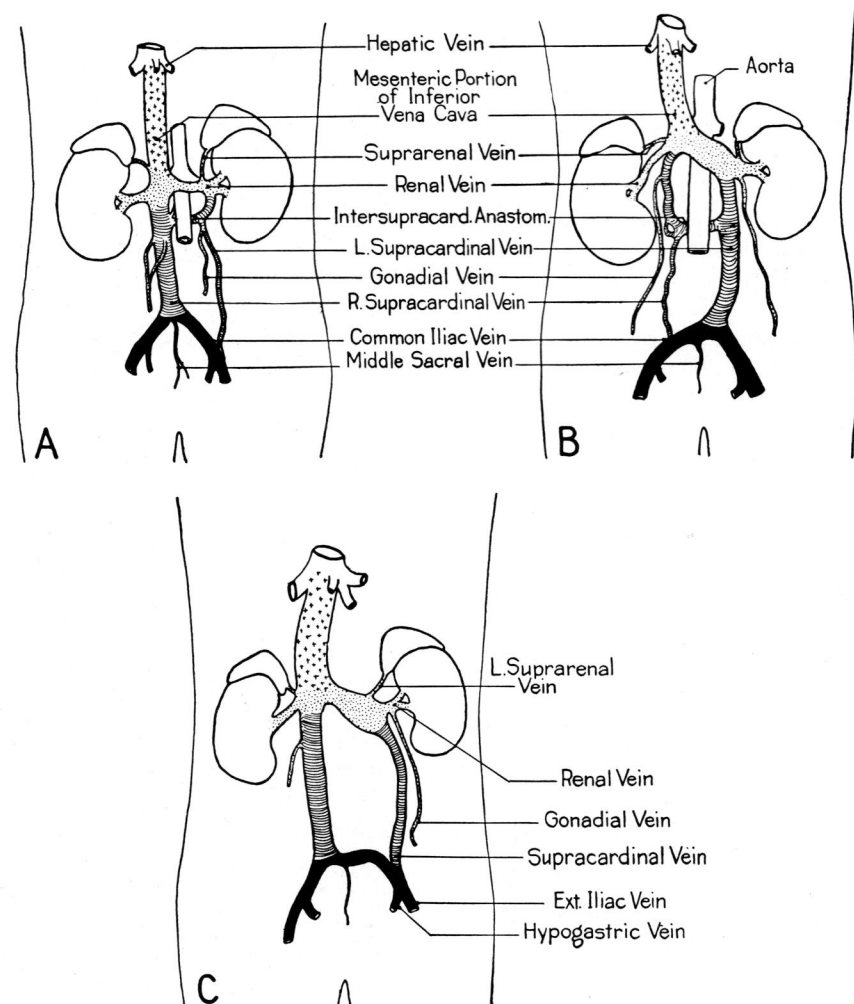

Figure 29.14. Duplication of the inferior vena cava. **A,** Renal collar formed by persisting suprapericardial anastomosis. **B,** Renal collar with main caval channel from left supracardinal vein. **C,** Double inferior vena cava with persistence of both supracardinal veins. (From Patten BM. Human embryology. New York: McGraw-Hill, 1968.)

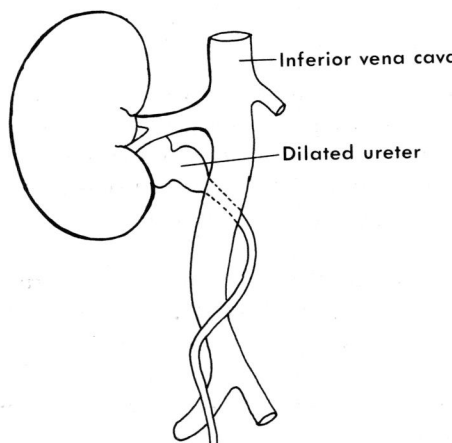

Figure 29.15. Preureteral vena cava (retrocaval ureter). The right ureter passes behind the vena cava instead of lying in front. In theory, it could occur on the left. Dilation of the upper, with hydronephrosis, may result.

between the supracardinal veins; anteriorly, it is formed by subcardinal-postcardinal anastomoses and the intersubcardinal anastomosis; and laterally, it is formed by the subcardinal-supracardinal anastomoses, which receive the renal veins. Normally, the proximal left renal vein is derived from the subcardinal-postcardinal anastomosis and represents that part of the collar in front of the aorta, while the remainder of the ring disappears. In the anomaly, the posterior and right lateral elements are also preserved to form the postaortic renal vessels (Fig. 29.14, *A*).

History and Incidence. Double venae cavae appear to have been first described in 1674 by Blasius (68). At least seven cases were seen in the 18th century; Morgagni (50) saw both the double cavae (De Sedibus XLVII:30) and the left-sided cava (De Sedibus LVI:31), which was also described in 1778 by Wrisberg (69).

Double IVCs are found in from 2 to 3% of individuals

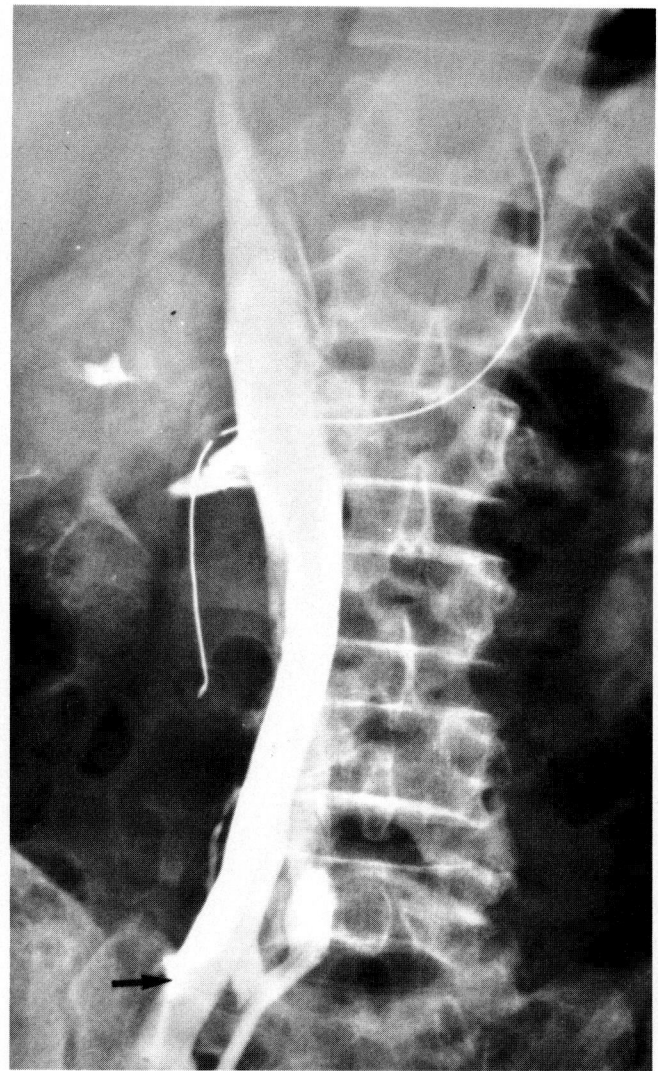

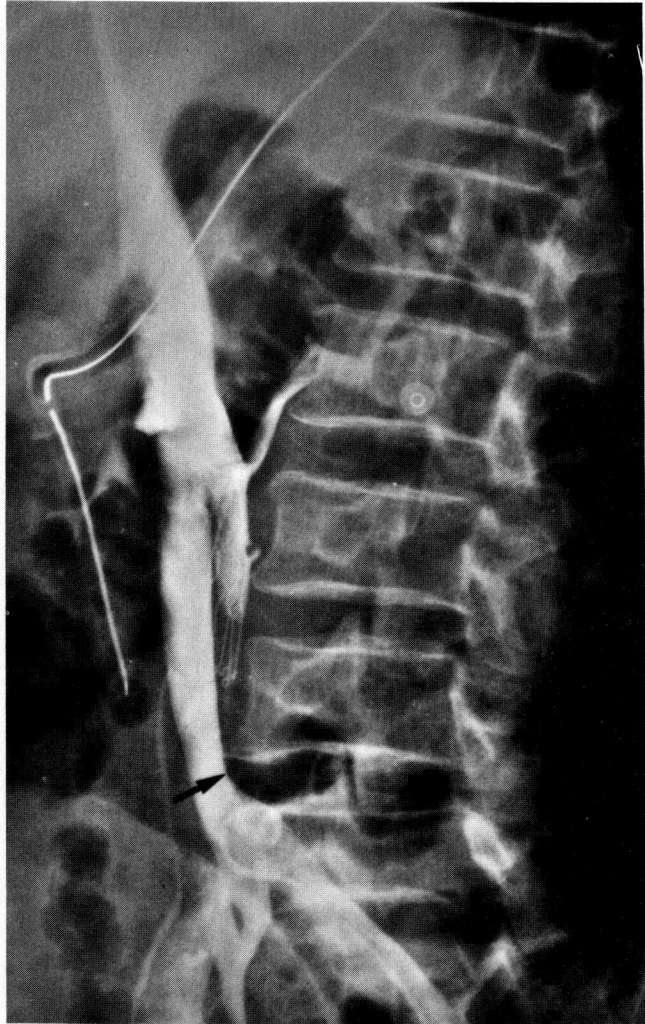

Figure 29.17. Oblique projection of left inferior venacavagram with placement of Greenfield filter in right inferior vena cava.

Figure 29.16. Inferior venacavagram in the AP projection performed from right iliac view, showing duplication of the inferior vena cava with reflux into the left inferior vena cava.

(34, 67), whereas a single left vena cava is found in 0.2 to 0.5%. In dogs, the frequency of the anomaly is similar to that in humans, whereas in cats, fully 20% have anomalous venae cavae (67).

Symptoms and Diagnosis. Anomalies of the IVC produce no symptoms and are usually discovered at surgery or on autopsy. Visualization of the vena cava by angiography occasionally reveals an anomaly (70). A review of the most common anomalies of the IVC and their appearance utilizing magnetic resonance imaging (MRI) is provided by Friedland et al (71).

Treatment. Caval anomalies, with the exception of a preureteral vena cava, do not require surgical treatment. Their presence may be, however, an important surgical consideration. Caval ligation for recurrent pulmonary embolism will be ineffective unless both limbs of the double venae cavae are ligated. In rare instances, the surgeon may find double cavae an advantage, when the normal cava must be sacrificed. Corrective treatment for preureteral vena cava is discussed in Chapter 17, "The Kidney and Ureter."

Shinohara et al. (72) presented seven cases of asplenia syndrome and three of polysplenia. Absence of IVC with azygos continuation was seen in all cases with polysplenia, and the authors raised the question of possible implications from a pathogenetic standpoint between asplenia and polysplenia. The authors also stated that each syndrome has been characterized by a tendency for symmetric development of normally asymmetric organs with some anomalies.

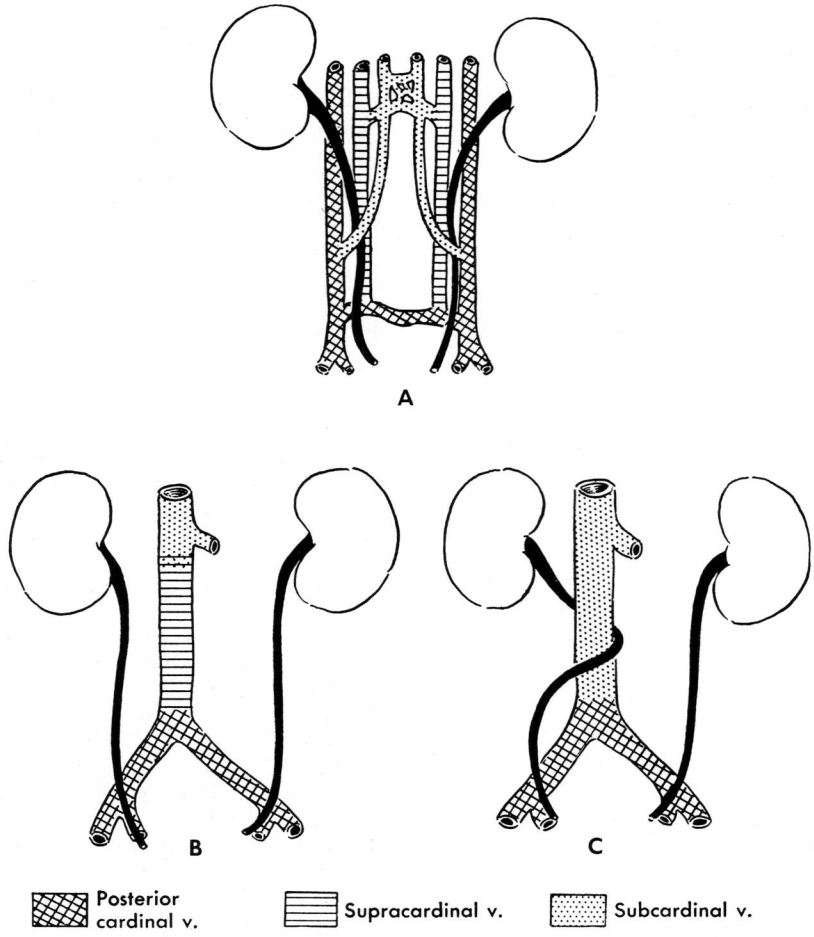

Posterior cardinal v.   Supracardinal v.   Subcardinal v.

Figure 29.18. Preureteral vena cava. **A,** The relationship of the ureter to the three primitive cardinal veins. **B,** Normal development of the inferior vena cava form the postrenal right supracardinal vein. **C,** Development of the vena cava from the postrenal right subcardinal vein. The anomaly is in caval, not ureteral, development. (From Hollinshead WH. Anatomy for surgeons. New York: Hoeber-Harper, 1956.)

Alexander et al. (73), using CT, reported six cases of IVC anomalies, one being left sided. Huhta et al. (74), using the two-dimensional echocardiographic diagnostic technique of situs, reported azygos continuation of the IVC to the right atrial connection; with right isomerism, the IVC and the aorta run together on one or the other side of the spine. They found the IVC to be anterior to the aorta, close to the diaphragm, receiving both the right hepatic veins in a normal way or one hepatic vein presenting an abnormal connection.

With left isomerism, most of the cases of the IVC have azygos continuation with the junction seen posterior to the aorta. Partial anomalous pulmonary venous return to the IVC or to the portal vein was reported by Kangarloo et al. (75), using sonography in four infants with differing extra thoracic left-to-right shunts.

Kawashima et al. (76) reported four patients with absent IVC with azygos or hemiazygos continuation and several other cardiac anomalies such as single ventricle, single atrium, common atrioventricular valve (with or without regurgitation), and pulmonary stenosis. The authors performed a total cavopulmonary shunt successfully in three of their four patients.

Currarino and Williams (77) reported 33 patients with several anomalies, as follows: nine with simple pulmonary hypoplasia; eight with anomalous venous return to the right atrium or IVC (scimitar syndrome); seven with absence of the ipsilateral pulmonary artery; seven with accessory diaphragm; and two with pulmonary sequestration adjacent to a diaphragmatic hernia.

With the help of MRI, Fisher et al. (78) reported the following venous anomalies: three cases of persistent left SVC and one case each of total anomalous venous return; left IVC to left atrium; interrupted IVC with azygos; and interrupted IVC with hemiazygos. In addition, they reported two cases of retroaortic left renal vein. Several other congenital defects were associated with the above anomalies, such as coarctation of the thoracic aorta, polysplenia, and others.

Terabayashi et al. (79) reported a 24-year-old female

with hemolytic anemia and thrombosis of the hepatic vein and IVC at the level of the diaphragm. The authors questioned if the membranous obstruction was congenital or acquired secondary to thrombosis. However, Amodeo et al. (80) reported membranous obstruction of the IVC in a child who was 5 years of age.

If one compares the above cases, one has to accept that membrane formation within the IVC is a congenital phenomenon and not an acquired one. Rossal and Caldwell (81) reported IVC obstruction due to a persistent eustachian valve, and Ohara et al. (82) and Watkins and Fortin (83) reported obstruction secondary to a suprahepatic web.

IVC with azygos continuation, left-sided liver, single right-sided spleen, and a normal left-sided heart was reported by Sacks and Rifkin (84). Total anomalous pulmonary venous return to the IVC and left-sided heart hypoplasia was reported by LeBlanc et al. (85). Placement of two Greenfield filters in a duplicated vena was reported by Rohrer and Cutler (86).

Herer et al. (87) presented a case of a right-sided pulmonary vein with normal drainage into the left atrium which was associated with an azygos continuation of the IVC.

Absent prerenal IVC with azygos continuation, biliary atresia, polysplenia, and several other anomalies was reported by Hoffman et al. (88), who advised liver transplantation in these cases.

Beedle et al. (89) reported congenital absence of the intrahepatic segment of the IVC with azygos continuation. The authors emphasized that accidental ligation of the azygos vein is fatal.

Bellah et al. (90) described anomalous portal venous connection to the suprahepatic vena cava. This portosystemic shunt was diagnosed with ultrasound.

Anomalous pulmonary venous draining into the IVC below the diaphragm was reported by Baxter et al. (91). This scimitar syndrome was evaluated by MRI and confirmed by surgery.

Ledesma-Medina et al. (92) advised in toto preoperative radiologic evaluation in patients who will undergo liver transplantation. The authors stated that vascular anomalies such as absent portal vein and/or IVC in patients with biliary atresia and polysplenia syndrome may preclude liver transplantation.

However, Woodle et al. (93) reported the first case of hepatic transplantation in a 10-year-old girl with congenital absence of the portal vein, polysplenia, and IVC anomalies.

REFERENCES

1. His W. Untersuchungen über die erste Anlage Wirbelthieleibes. Leipzig: FCW Vogel, 1868.
2. Minot CS. Development of the blood, the vascular system, and the spleen. I. The origin of the angioblast and the development of the blood. In: Keibel F, Mall FP, eds. Manual of human embryology, Vol 2. Philadelphia: JB Lippincott, 1912.
3. Evans HM. Development of the blood, the vascular system, and the spleen. III. The development of the vascular system. In: Keibel F, Mall FP, eds. Manual of human embryology, Vol 2. Philadelphia: JB Lippincott, 1912.
4. Sabin FR. Development of the blood, the vascular system, and the spleen. IV. The development of the lymphatic system. In: Keibel F, Mall FP, eds. Manual of human embryology, Vol 2. Philadelphia: JB Lippincott, 1912.
5. Keibel F, Mall FP, eds. Manual of human embryology. Philadelphia: JB Lippincott, 1912.
6. Rückert W, Mollier S. Die Entstehung der Gëfasse und des Blutes bei Wirbeltieren. Handb Vergl Expt Entw Wirbeltieren 1906:1:1019.
7. Bremer JL. The earliest blood-vessels in man. Am J Anat 1914;16:447–476.
8. Sabin, FR. Origin and development of the primitive vessels of the chick and of the pig. Contrib Embryol Carnegie Inst Wash 1917;6:61–124.
9. McClure CFW. The endothelium problem. Anat Rec 1921;22:219–237.
10. Streeter GL. The development of the venous sinuses of the dura mater in the human embryo. Am J Anat 1915;18:145–178.
11. Streeter GL. The developmental alterations in the vascular system of the brain of the human embryo. Contrib Embryol Carnegie Inst Wash 1918;8:5–38.
12. Lewis FT. The development of the veins in the limbs of rabbit embryos. Am J Anat 1906;5:113–120.
13. Woollard HH. The development of the principal arterial stems in the forelimb of the pig. Contrib Embryol Carnegie Inst Wash 1922;14:139–154.
14. Anikiew A. Zur Frage über die Entwicklung der vena anonyma sinistra. Anat Anz 1909;34:24–29.
15. McClure CFW, Butler CG. The development of the vena cava inferior in man. Am J Anat 1925;35:331–383.
16. Cameron J. A specimen showing complete remains of the left superior vena cava. J Anat Physiol 1915;49:140–147.
17. Braudo M, Beanlands DS, Trusler G. Anomalous drainage of the right superior vena cava into the left atrium. Can Med Assoc J 1968;99:715–719.
18. Huntington GS, McClure CFW. The development of the veins in the domestic cat (felis domestica) with especial reference, (1) to the shape taken by the supracardinal veins in the development of the postcava and azygos veins and (2) to the interpretation of the variant conditions of the postcava and its tributaries, as found in the adult. Anat Rec 1920;20:1–30.
19. Lewis FT. The development of the vena cava inferior. Am J Anat 1902;1:229–244.
20. Huhta JC, Smallhorn JF, Macartney FJ, Anderson RH, deLeval M. Cross-sectional echocardiographic diagnosis of systemic venous return. Br Heart J 1982;48(4):388–403.
21. Peoples WM, Moller JH, Edwards JE. Polysplenia: a review of 146 cases. Pediatr Cardiol 1983;4(2):129–137.
22. Vitarelli A, Scapato A, Sanguigni V, Caminiti MC. Evaluation of total anomalous pulmonary venous drainage with cross-sectional colour-flow Doppler echocardiography. Eur Heart J 1986;7(3):190–195.
23. Hussain SA, Chakravarty S, Chaikhouni A, Smith JR. Congenital absence of superior vena cava: unusual anomaly of superior systemic veins complicating pacemaker placement. PACE 1981;4(3):328–334.
24. Smith BM. Venous disease. In: Welch KJ, Randolph JG, Ravitch MM, O'Neill JA Jr, Rowe MI, eds. Pediatric surgery. Chicago: Year Book Medical Publishers, 1986:1518.

25. Kabbani S, Feldman M, Angelini P. Single left superior vena cava draining into the left atrium. Ann Thorac Surg 1973;16:518.

26. Viart P, LeClerc JL, Pimo G. Total anomalous systemic venous drainage. Am J Dis Child 1977;131:195.

27. Mazzucco A, Bortolotti U, Stellin G, Gallucci V. Anomalies of the systemic venous return: a review. J Card Surg 1990;5:122–133.

28. Rossi L, Montella S, Frescura C, Thiene G. Congenital atrioventricular block in right atrial isomerism (asplenia): a case due to atrionodal discontinuity. Chest 1984;85(4):578–580.

29. Snider AR, Silverman NH. Suprasternal notch echocardiography: a two-dimensional technique for evaluating congenital heart disease. Circulation 1981;63(1):165–173.

30. Fleming JS, Gibson RV. Absent right superior vena cava as an isolated anomaly. Br J Radiol 1964;37:696–697.

31. Campbell M, Deuchar D. The left sided superior vena cava. Br Heart J 1954;16:423–439.

32. Fraser RS, Dvorkin J, Rossall RE, Eiden R. Left superior vena cava: a review of associated congenital heart lesions, catheterization data and roentgenologic findings. Am J Med 1961;31:711–716.

33. Nandy K, Blair CB Jr. Double superior venae cavae with completely paired azygos veins. Anat Rec 1965;151:1–10.

34. Seib GA. The azygos system of veins in American Whites and American Negroes, including observations on the inferior caval venous system. Am J Phys Anthrop 1934;19:39–164.

35. Stevenson JG, Kawabori I, Guntheroth WG. Pulsed Doppler echocardiographic detection of total anomalous pulmonary venous return: resolution of left atrial line. Am J Cardiol 1979;44(6):1155–1158.

36. Konstam MA, Levine BW. Strauss HW, McKusick KA. Left superior vena cava to left atrial communication diagnosed with radionuclide angiocardiography and with differential right to left shunting. Am J Cardiol 1979;43(1);149–153.

37. Bjerregaard P, Laursen HB. Persistent left superior vena cava: incidence, associated congenital heart defects and frontal plane P-wave axis in a paediatric population with congenital heart disease. Acta Paediatr Scand 1980;69(1):105–108.

38. Yu CW, Chen H, Baucum RW, Hand AM. Terminal deletion of the long arm of chromosome 4: report of a case of 46,XY, del(4) (g31) and review of 4g- syndrome. Ann Genet 1981;24(3):158–161.

39. Mantagos S, McReynolds JW, Seashore MR, Breg WR. Complete trisomy 9 in two liveborn infants. J Med Genet 1981;18(5):377–382.

40. Yiannikas J et al. Intravenous digital subtraction angiography in the assessment of patients with left to right shunts before and after surgical correction. J Am Coll Cardiol 1985;3(6):1507–1514.

41. Mardini MK, Nyhan WL. Agenesis of the lung: report of four patients with unusual anomalies. Chest 1985;87(4):522–527.

42. Weisbrod GL, Todd TR. Congenital left superior vena cava with absent right superior vena cava: a cause of progressive mediastinal widening. J Can Assoc Radiol 1985;36(2):155–157.

43. Rey C, Marache P, Francart C, Dupuis C. Percutaneous balloon angioplasty in an infant with obstructed total anomalous pulmonary vein return. J Am Coll Cardiol 1985;6(4):894–896.

44. Sand ME, McGrath LB, Pacifico AD, Mandke NV. Repair of left superior vena cava entering the left atrium. Ann Thorac Surg 1986;42(5):560–564.

45. Hofbeck M, Rockelein G, Singer H, Rein J, Gittenberger deGroot AC. Coarctation of the aorta in the syndrome of absent pulmonary valve with ventricular septal defect. Pediatr Cardiol 1990;11(3):159–163.

46. Choi JY, Jung MJ, Kim YH, Noh CI, Yun YS. Anomalous subaortic position of the brachiocephalic vein (innominate vein): an echocardiographic study. Br Heart J 1990;64(6):385–387.

47. Rodefeld MD et al. Cor triatriatum: clinical presentation and surgical results in 12 patients. Ann Thorac Surg 1990;50(4):562–568.

48. Havase S et al. A case of completely unroofed coronary sinus with persistent left superior vena cava. Jpn J Thorac Surg 1991;44(2):172–175.

49. Suzuki K et al. Hypoplastic left heart syndrome with premature closure of foramen ovale: report of an unusual type of totally anomalous pulmonary venous return. Heart Vessels 1990;5(2):117–119.

50. Morgagni JB. The seats and causes of disease investigated by anatomy. Alexander B (transl). New York: Hafner, 1960.

51. Marshall J. On the development of the great anterior veins in man and mammalia, etc. Phil Trans R Soc London 1850;140:133–170.

52. McCotter RE. Three cases of the persistence of the left superior vena cava. Anat Rec 1916;10:371–383.

53. Winter FS. Persistent left superior vena cava: survey of world literature and report of thirty additional cases. Angiology 1954;5:90–132.

54. Gensini G, Caldini P, Casaccio F, Blount SG. Persistent left superior vena cava. Am J Cardiol 1959;4:677–685.

55. Cournand A, Baldwin JS, Himmelstein A. Cardiac catheterization in congenital heart disease. New York: Commonwealth Fund, 1949.

56. Pecorini J, Macchi RJ, Suarez LD, Perosio AM. Persistence of the left superior vena cava. Prensa Med Argent 1959;46:2409–2416.

57. Steinberg I, Dubilier W Jr, Lukas DS. Persistence of left superior vena cava. Dis Chest 1953;24:479–488.

58. Vaquez-Perez J, Frontera-Izquierdo P. Anomalous drainage of the right superior vena cava into the left atrium as an isolated anomaly: rare case report. Am Heart J 1979;97(1):89–91.

59. Shapiro EP et al. Drainage of right superior vena cava into both atria: review of the literature and description of a case presenting with polycythemia and paradoxical embolization. Circulation 1981;63(3):712–717.

60. Park HM et al. Anomalous drainage of the right superior vena cava into the left atrium. J Am Coll Cardiol 1983;2(2):358–362.

61. McClure CFW, Huntington GS. The mammalian vena cava posterior. Amer Anat Mem 15. Philadelphia: Wistar Institute, 1929. American Anatomical Memoirs, No. 15. Memoirs of the Wistar Institute of Anatomy and Biology.

62. Huseby RA, Boyden EA. Absence of the hepatic portion of the inferior vena cava with bilateral retention of the supracardinal system. Anat Rec 1941;81:537–544.

63. Anderson RC, Adams P Jr, Burke B. Anomalous inferior vena cava with azygous continuation (infrahepatic interruption of the inferior vena cava): report of 15 new cases. J Pediatr 1961;59:370–383.

64. Effler DB, Greer AE, Sifers EC. Anomaly of the vena cava inferior: report of a fatality after ligation. JAMA 1951;146:1321–1322.

65. Milloy FJ, Anson BJ, Cauldwell EW. Variations in inferior caval veins and in their renal and lumbar communications. Surg Gynecol Obstet 1962;115:131–142.

66. Givens MH. Duplication of the inferior vena cava in man. Anat Rec 1912;6:475.

67. Reis RH, Esenther G. Variations in the pattern of renal vessels and their relation to the type of posterior vena cava in man. Am J Anat 1959;104:295–318.

68. Blasius G. Observata anatomico-practica in homine brutisque variis. Amsterdam [Amstelodami]: Gaasbeeck, 1674.

69. Wrisberg HA. Observationes anatomicae de vena azyga duplici: alisque hujus venae varietatibus. Gottingae, 1778.

70. Hirsch DM, Chan K. Bilateral inferior vena cava. JAMA 1963;185:729–730.

71. Friedland GW, deVries PA, Nino-Murcia M, King BF, Leder RA, Stevens S. Congenital anomalies of the inferior vena cava: embryogenesis and MR features. Urol Radiol 1992;13:237–248.

72. Shinohara Y et al. Asplenia and polysplenia syndrome. Acta Pathol Jpn 1982;32(3):505–511.

73. Alexander ES, Clark RA, Gross BH, Colley DP. CT of congenital anomalies of the inferior vena cava. Comput Radiol 1982;6(4):219–226.

74. Huhta JC, Smallhorn JF, Macartney FJ. Two-dimensional echocardiographic diagnosis of situs. Br Heart J 1982;48(2):97–108.

75. Kangarloo HN et al. Sonography of extrathoracic left-to-right shunts in infants and children. AJR 1983;141(5):923–926.

76. Kawashima Y et al. Total cavopulmonary shunt operation in complex cardiac anomalies: a new operation. J Thorac Cardiovasc Surg 1984;87(1):74–81.

77. Currarino G, Williams B. Causes of congenital unilateral pulmonary hypoplasia: a study of 33 cases. Pediatr Radiol 1985;15(1):15–24.

78. Fisher MR, Hricah H, Higgins CB. Magnetic resonance imaging of developmental venous anomalies. AJR 1985;145(4):705–709.

79. Terabayashi H, Okuda K, Nomura F, Ohnishi K, Wong P. Transformation of inferior vena caval thrombosis to membranous obstruction in a patient with the lupus anticoagulant. Gastroenterology 1986;91(1):219–224.

80. Amodeo A et al. Relief of membranous obstruction of the inferior vena cava in a 5-year-old child. J Thorac Cardiovasc Surg 1986;92(6):1101–1103.

81. Rossal RE, Caldwell RA. Obstruction of inferior vena cava by a persistent eustachian valve in a young adult. J Clin Pathol 1957;10:40.

82. Ohara I, Ouchi H, Takahashi K. A bypass operation for occlusion of the hepatic inferior vena cava. Surg Gynecol Obstet 1963;117:151.

83. Watkins E, Fortin CL. Surgical correction of a congenital coarctation of the inferior vena cava. Ann Surg 1964;159(4):536.

84. Sacks LV, Rifkin IR. Mirror image arrangement of the abdominal organs with a left-sided morphologically normal heart. Br Heart J 1987;58(5):534–536.

85. LeBlanc JG, Patterson MW, Taylor GP, Ashmore PG. Total anomalous pulmonary venous return with left heart hypoplasia. J Thorac Cardiovasc Surg 1988;95(3):540–542.

86. Rohrer MJ, Cutler BS. Placement of two Greenfield filters in a duplicated vena cava. Surgery 1988;104(3):572–574.

87. Herer B, Jaubert F, Delaisements C, Huchon G, Chretien J. Scimitar sign with normal pulmonary venous drainage and anomalous inferior vena cava. Thorax 1988;43(8):651–652.

88. Hoffman MA, Celli S, Ninkov P, Rolles K, Calne RY. Orthotopic transplantation of the liver in children with biliary atresia and polysplenia syndrome: report of two cases. J Pediatr Surg 1989;24(10):1020–1022.

89. Beedle RJ, Yeo W, Morcos SK. Congenital absence of the intrahepatic segment of the inferior vena cava with azygos continuation presenting as a mediastinal mass. Postgrad Med J 1989;65(762):253–255.

90. Bellah RD, Hayek J, Teele RL. Anomalous portal venous connection to the suprahepatic vena cava: sonographic demonstration. Pediatr Radiol 1989;20(1-2):115–117.

91. Baxter R, McFadden PM, Gradman M, Wright A. Scimitar syndrome: cine magnetic resonance imaging demonstration of anomalous pulmonary venous drainage. Ann Thorac Surg 1990;50(1):121–123.

92. Ledesma-Medina J, Dominquez R, Bowen A, Young LW, Bron KM. Pediatric liver transplantation. I. Standardization of preoperative diagnostic imaging. Radiology 1985;157(2):335–338.

93. Woodle ES et al. Successful hepatic transplantation in congenital absence of recipient portal vein. Surgery 1990;107(4):475–479.

CHAPTER 30

ANOMALIES OF SITUS AND SYMMETRY

Stephen Wood Gray / John Elias Skandalakis / Richard Ricketts

"The long unmeasured pulse of time moves everything, There is nothing hidden that it cannot bring to life. Nothing once known that may not become unknown."
—SOPHOCLES, "AJAX"

DEVELOPMENT

Development of Situs

Although the human body is essentially bilaterally symmetric, the right and left sides are not identical in detail. The most marked asymmetries are found in the position or arrangement of the following: venae cavae, arch of the aorta, chambers of the heart, lobulation of the lungs, liver and gallbladder, spleen, stomach, and intestines.

The position of the organs as normally encountered is called *situs solitus;* if the asymmetries are reversed, the condition is *situs inversus.* A mixture of normal and reversed asymmetries is "partial situs inversus."

Two types of partial situs inversus have been postulated by Moller and his colleagues (1) (Fig. 30.1). In one, both sides of the body are essentially right sides (dextro-isomerism); in the other, both sides are essentially left sides (levoisomerism). There is also reason to believe that the partial and complete forms of situs inversus are separate embryonic and genetic entities.

The oldest and most persistent theory of visceral inversion is that twins are often (or always) mirror images of each other and that a single individual with situs inversus represents a survivor whose normal twin has died early in utero. "Double monsters," as they were sometimes called, in whom the organs of one half are transposed, are readily demonstrated (2); nevertheless, not all conjoined twins show inversion in one member. The original "Siamese twins," Eng and Chang, each had normal situs (3). Among monozygotic separate twins, one member may have situs inversus, while the other may have normal situs; both may have situs inversus; or both may have situs solitus (4). Although it may be related to twinning, the frequency of situs inversus is probably not significantly higher in monozygotic twins than it is in other segments of the population, nor is a real increase in twinning seen in the families of individuals with situs inversus.

Cunniff and his associates (5) in 1988 presented six pairs of conjoined twins. In three of the four dicephalous pairs, the right twin had an abnormality of laterality such as right aortic arch, reversed great vessels, bilateral right-sided isomerism of the lungs, asplenia, and situs inversus viscerum. The left twin had normal great vessel orientation and situs solitus in each case. Several other abnormalities were found, such as fusion of the hearts in three dicephalous twin pairs.

The fact that gastropod molluscs have an obvious asymmetry and that it may be reversed in nature, has made them objects of considerable interest. Dextral or sinistral symmetry in snails was shown by Crampton (6) in 1894 to be determined in the early cleavage stages; this was confirmed in 1897 by Conklin (7). Although bilateral symmetry (and asymmetry) is without doubt a very ancient phylogenetic development, its origin in the first cleavages of the molluscs (which have determinate cleavage) may not be identical with its manner of origin in vertebrates (which have indeterminate cleavage of totipotent blastomeres).

Experimentally, situs inversus has been produced in several forms. Newman (8) subjected blastulae of the echinoderm *Patiria* to low temperatures and was able to increase the reversed asymmetry from the normal 8-12% to 27% of mature individuals. Spemann (9), using the toad *Bombinator,* and Pressler (10), using *Rana,* were able to produce situs inversus by surgically removing a portion of the medullary plate from the embryo at the neurula stage and replacing it after rotating it 180 degrees. This, of course, was done long after the major axes of the embryo had been established. In the mid–20th century, von Woellwarth (11) showed that the rotation of the excised piece was not the important factor. Excision and replacement without turning produced a similar effect. He was able to demonstrate that unilateral injury alone, especially on the left, was sufficient to produce inversion.

These experiments suggest that developmental delay caused by reorganization after injury to one side is sufficient to induce reversal of symmetry. The left side of the amphibian embryo normally is the governing half. If it is injured, the right side develops the characteristics of a mirror image of the left side while the left becomes a mir-

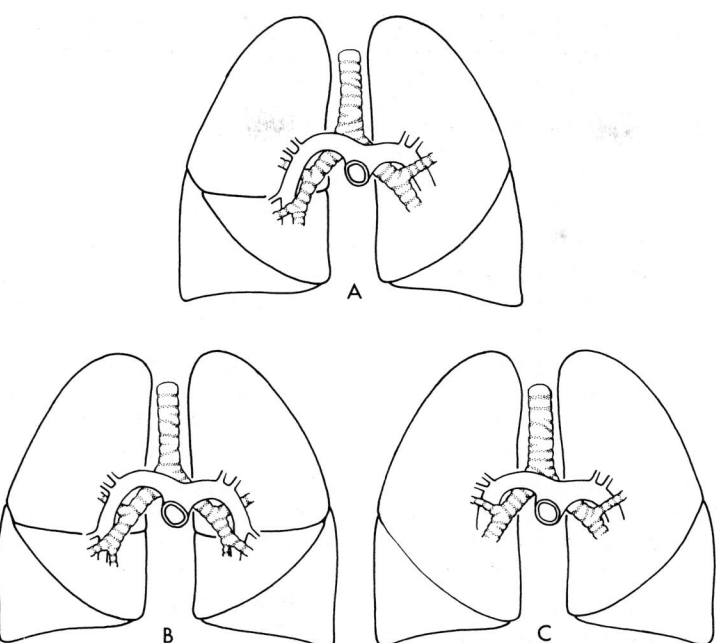

Figure 30.1. Pulmonary patterns associated with splenic anomalies. **A,** Situs solitus and normal spleen. The right lung has three lobes and the upper lobe bronchus is eparterial. The left lung has two lobes, and the upper lobe bronchus is hyparterial. In situs inversus totalis and normal spleen, the lungs form a mirror image of this pattern. **B,** Asplenia syndrome. Both lungs have three lobes and eparterial bronchi (i.e., there are two "right lungs"). **C,** Polysplenia syndrome. Both lungs have two lobes and hyparterial bronchi (i.e., there are two "left lungs"). (Redrawn from Moller JH, Nakib A, Anderson RC, Edwards JE. Congenital cardiac disease associated with polysplenia: developmental complex of bilateral "leftsidedness." Circulation 1967;36;789–799)

ror image of the right. Situs, although it is determined early in development, is not irreversible until asymmetric organs actually appear.

Critical Events in Development.

Although the origin of situs is obscure, its establishment takes place in early cleavage. Even if the theory of injury to the dominant side is correct, the effect is produced in the first 3 weeks of gestation.

To discuss the several syndromes, forms, and cases of situs and symmetry is impossible. We present only Kartagener's syndrome as an example (12).

KARTAGENER'S SYNDROME

Anatomy. Total situs inversus, bronchiectasis, and abnormal paranasal sinuses producing chronic sinusitis make up the triad named for Kartagener, who described a number of cases in 1933 (13) and 1935 (14). Torgersen (4) would add nasal polyposis to the syndrome.

Kartagener's syndrome is present in from 18 to 26% of patients with complete situs inversus (15). Varano and Merklin (16) found 159 cases reported in 15 years.

The sinuses are absent or normal in many cases and are smaller than normal in others (Fig. 30.2). The characteristic bronchiectasis has been considered by some authors

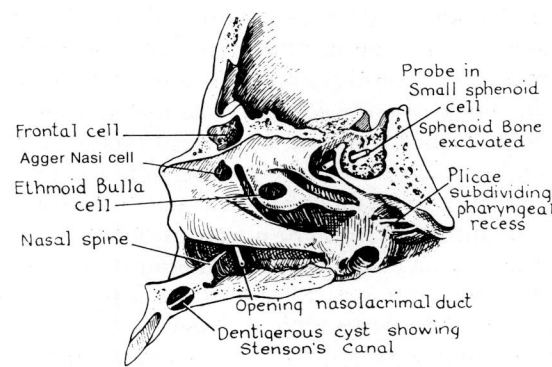

Figure 30.2. Abnormal paranasal sinuses in Kartagener's syndrome. Lateral nasal wall dissection, showing small sphenoid sinus, ethmoid bulla, and agger nasi cells, a reduced frontal sinus, and a dentigerous cyst. (From Varano NR, Merklin RJ. Situs inversus: review of the literature, report of four cases and analysis of the clinical implications. J Int Coll Surg 1960;33:131–148)

to be acquired and by others to be congenital. Varano and Merklin (16) favor a congenital origin. The condition appears to be familial: In a number of families, some members are afflicted with the entire triad, whereas others have bronchiectasis and sinusitis or bronchiectasis only (17–19). Most patients show symptoms from infancy, but the diagnosis is usually made in young adults. The sexes are equally affected.

Embryogenesis. The basic work on the familial pattern of situs inversus was done by Cockayne (20) in 1938. He investigated 58 cases, from 52 sibships. Torgersen (4) reported 29 families with more than one example of inversion. Seven of his families had three affected members. In the families of individuals with Kartagener's triad, the incidence of bronchiectasis with and without situs inversus is appreciably higher than normal (17–19).

Cockayne (20) in 1938 postulated a single autosomal recessive gene for situs inversus, but several years later Torgersen (21) realized that the condition must result from a complex of dominant genes with varying expression, depending on the presence or absence of individual genes of the complex. In a series of cases from consanguineous marriages, the respiratory elements in Kartagener's triad were more frequently encountered than was the situs inversus component. Torgersen's 1949 data (4) indicates that mothers of children with situs inversus are not significantly older than mothers of unaffected children, but that, when the inversion is associated with bronchiectasis or congenital heart disease, the mothers have been found to be slightly older.

Symptoms. Bronchiectasis and chronic sinusitis are the conditions for which the patient seeks treatment; the situs inversus by itself is asymptomatic.

Diagnosis. Diagnosis of total situs inversus has been described previously. Chest x-ray films will show the bronchiectasis, and skull x-ray films will determine the absence or malformations of the paranasal sinuses.

Treatment. The bronchiectasis is the portion of the triad that may require surgical treatment. Pulmonary lobectomy has been performed several times (22). The surgeon must keep in mind the reversed lobar anatomy of the lung. The chief danger in Kartagener's syndrome is pulmonary infection from the chronic sinusitis.

Many lesions are discovered incidentally during treatment for other diseases. Stumper and associates (23), reporting in 1990, were able to diagnose atrial situs by means of transesophageal echocardiography. Dunseath and his colleagues (24) demonstrated dextrocardia and complete abdominal situs inversus by scintigraphy. Meinecke et al. (25) in 1990 reported situs inversus associated with agnathia and holoprosencephaly. Two years later, Stoler and Holmes (26) found situs inversus totalis and agnathia with a normal central nervous system.

In our own experience, reported in 1991, a 68-year-old woman was aware of her dextrocardia from chest x-ray films but was unaware of the existence of situs inversus totalis. The diagnosis was made by ultrasound (27).

Lupin and Misco (28) and Rott (29) showed that, in some patients with Kartagener's syndrome, the cilia of the respiratory system are defective (immotile cilia syndrome). The defect appears to be the failure of the dynein arms to attach to the nine tubular doublets. The defective

cilia are found in the cells of the trachea and in the flagellated spermatozoa of the testis. It is possible, therefore, that normal ciliary function may be required for the determination of situs.

Escudier et al. (30) presented a case of a 28-year-old man with Kartagener's syndrome who was infertile despite having normal cilia and spermatozoa. The ultrastructure of ciliary and flagellar axonemes was even normal. The patient presumably had abnormal cilia of the respiratory tract in association with his Kartegener's syndrome. It was not clear why this patient had abnormal cilia in the respiratory system and normal cilia in the genitourinary system and why he was infertile.

Conraads et al. (31), on the other hand, presented a 40-year-old man with Kartagener's syndrome with respiratory symptoms who had normal axoneme in both respiratory and sperm cilia and who was fertile.

ANOMALIES OF BODY ASYMMETRY (TABLE 30.1)

Disturbances of body asymmetry and anomalies of splenic development may occur independently, but they frequently are associated. Although Chapter 10 "The Spleen" provides a complete discussion of splenic anomalies, for the sake of a complete presentation of body asymmetry, we have included splenic anomalies in Table 30.1.

Situs Inversus Viscerum (Heterotaxia)

UNCOMPLICATED SITUS INVERSUS

In total situs inversus, the heart lies to the right of the midline, with the positions of all its chambers reversed. The aorta turns to the right. There are three lobes to the left lung and two lobes to the right; the thoracic duct is on the right and empties into the right subclavian vein. The liver and stomach are transposed, with the gallbladder lying to the left of the midline. The spleen is on the right. The cecum is in the left lower quadrant; the hepatic flexure is located on the left; and the splenic flexure on the right. The sigmoid colon is appropriately reversed. In males the right scrotal half hangs lower than the left. All asymmetric blood vessels are reversed (Fig. 30.3).

In partial situs inversus, inversion may be limited to the thorax or to the arrangement of the cardiac chambers only. Transposition of the stomach only has been reported in several patients (15, 32) but some cases appear to be the result of malrotation rather than of reversed situs.

Associated Anomalies. Not all cases of situs inversus are uncomplicated. Three striking syndromes are associated with this malformation—one, Kartagener's syndrome, may accompany total situs inversus, and the other two, the asplenia syndrome and the polysplenia syndrome,

Table 30.1.
Anomalies of Body Symmetry and Associated Anomalies of the Spleen

Anomaly	Origin of Defect	First Appearance	Sex Chiefly Affected	Relative Frequency	Remarks
Total situs inversus					
Uncomplicated	At conception, or 1st	None	Equal	Uncommon	
Kartagener's syndrome	to 2nd week	Infancy	Equal	Rare	Familial
Partial situs inversus					
Asplenia syndrome	At conception, or 1st to 2nd week	Usually at birth	Male	Rare	Severe cardiac defects associated; usually fatal in 1st year of life
Polysplenia syndrome	At conception, or 1st to 2nd week	Usually at birth	Male	Rare	Severe cardiac defects associated; usuallly fatal in 1st year of life
Simple agenesis of the spleen	6th week	None	Equal	Rare ?	Usually without other anomalies
Accessory spleens	6th week	None	Unknown	Common	
Splenogonadal fusion	7th to 8th weeks	Childhood or later	Male	Very rare	

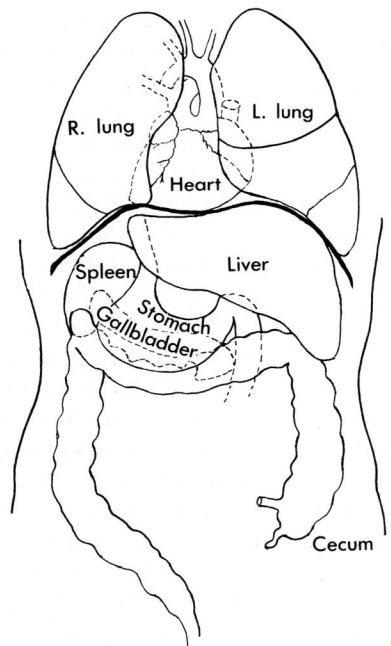

Figure 30.3. Situs inversus viscerum totalis.

accompany partial visceral inversion. These splenic syndromes are described in Chapter 10. In 1990 Tskhai (33) reported anomalies of the bile ducts with situs inversus, and Gontijo et al. (34) reported use of a polytetrafluoroethylene (PTFE) graft to correct anomalous drainage of a persistent left superior vena cava.

Embryogenesis. Just as the development of normal asymmetry is obscure, even in the simplest animals, so the causes of situs inversus are unknown. Von Woellwarth's experiments (11) suggest that some cases may arise from

early embryonic accidents. Other cases, especially partial situs inversus associated with specific malformations, appear to have a genetic basis. Hummel and Chapman (35) described a strain of mice from the Jackson Memorial Laboratories in which situs inversus resembled that found in humans (i.e., complete situs inversus was not accompanied by other anomalies, but partial situs inversus was accompanied in 80% of cases by vascular, splenic, and pulmonary anomalies). Unlike the situation in humans, however, partial inversion was more frequent than total inversion.

In 1990 Rylaarsdam et al. (36) reported four patients in whom the authors found discordance between the anatomy of the bronchial tree and the external aspect of the atrial appendages. Two of their patients had bronchial situs solitus with atrial levoisomerism. Their third patient had bronchial levoisomerism with atrial situs solitus, and the fourth was found to have inverted bronchial anatomy with levoisomerism of the atrial appendages.

History. Aristotle (37) (De Generatione IV:4) mentions the occurrence of situs inversus in animals, implying that it is uncommon but well known. The history of the subject is said to be thoroughly covered by Karishima (38) in a thesis of 1912. This thesis is not available for study, and only thirdhand mention of the earlier cases can be found. Fabricius is said to have observed liver and spleen reversal in 1600 (39), and Servius mentioned a case in 1643. Marie de Medici, Queen of France, was said to have situs inversus, and Beck (40) quotes a joking reference to the condition in Moliere's play, *The Physician in Spite of Himself,* published in 1655. In spite of Aristotle's remarks, the existence of situs inversus was not taken seriously before the middle of the 18th century. The first clinical diagnosis seems to have been made in 1824, soon after the development of percussion and auscultation as diagnostic tools. Vehsemeyer (41) is credited with the first radiologic diagnosis.

Karishima (38) in 1912 is said to have collected 200 cases; Cleveland (42) added 160 more up to 1925; Johnson (39) collected 632 total and partial cases from 1925 to 1946; and Varano and Merklin (16) found another 722 from 1946 to 1960.

Incidence. From 1910 to 1947, 76 cases of situs inversus totalis were found among 1,551,047 patients at the Mayo Clinic, an incidence of 1:20,400 (15). From 1886 to 1936, 23 cases were discovered among 232,112 patients at Massachusetts General Hospital (43), an incidence of 1:10,100. Among a number of small hospital and autopsy series, all of which had more than a single example, there were 25 cases among 222,374 individuals, or an incidence of 1:8900.

In addition to these figures, the results from a number of mass x-ray surveys for tuberculosis are known: Philippine Islands, 1936, 32:126,858 (1:4000) (44); France, 1937, 24:273,500 (1:11,400) (45); U.S. defense workers, 1945, 40:442,252 (1:11,000), male only and dextrocardia only (46); U.S. Navy examination, 1946, 12:100,000 (1:8350) (47); and Norway, 1949, 195:1,500,000 (1:7700) (4).

Whether these differences represent geographic variation or care in interpreting the x-ray films is not clear. Certainly, the frequency among Filipinos is the highest yet found, and this high frequency has been further confirmed by the finding of four cases among 10,000 autopsies in Philippine hospitals (44). Only small variations in the sex ratio have been reported; there is probably no real difference.

Signs and symptoms. A number of indicative signs exist, the presence of which should suggest situs inversus to the surgeon.

1. Lower right testicle: This is probably the most consistent sign in male patients, but Lowe and McKeown (48) reported normal lower left testicle in a patient with situs inversus.
2. Counterclockwise hair whorl: This is an inconsistent finding.
3. Left-handedness: This is frequently mentioned as an indication but has been disproved as such. There is no higher incidence of left-handedness in situs inversus (20, 49).

The presenting symptoms will be those of abdominal or thoracic disease unrelated to situs inversus. Recognition of the signs are a prerequisite to successful surgery.

Most individuals with uncomplicated total situs inversus are unaware of their condition. At least one unsuspecting woman attempted suicide without success by shooting herself in the normal location of the heart, without being aware of its dextroposition (50).

Chiu et al. (51) studied right and left atrial isomerism diagnosed as situs ambiguous (36 cases of right atrial isomerism and seven cases of left). Autopsies were performed in 18 cases. The authors stated that the most common cause of death after palliative or definitive operation was anomalous pulmonary venous connections which were not detected, pulmonary venous strictures, and uncorrected valvular disease; they emphasized that successful operation depends on the abnormal anatomy involved.

Diagnosis. Suspicion of situs inversus in a patient should lead to further physical examination. The apex beat of the heart will be found on the right instead of on the left, and abdominal percussion will reveal the transposition of the liver and stomach.

A chest x-ray film will prove the presence of true dextrocardia, in contrast to a right-sided heart resulting from a mediastinal shift. Electrocardiograms will show an inversion of lead I and a transposition of leads II and III (50).

A barium enema will establish the visceral inversion of the abdomen as well as reveal any malrotation, which may confuse the picture obtained by palpation.

In 1990 Dietz and Shanen (52) advised computed tomography (CT) preoperatively for better classification of Kartagener's syndrome. In that same year Angulo-Cuesta et al. (53) reported immotile cilia syndrome as a cause of sterility and suggested that coincidental situs inversus may be useful in making the diagnosis.

Treatment. No treatment is necessary for uncomplicated situs inversus, but if it remains unrecognized, it presents a hazard to abdominal and thoracic surgery. Blegen (54) reviewed 158 surgical operations in 144 patients: 125 with complete and 19 with partial situs inversus. In only 55% was the condition recognized preoperatively. In 32% it was recognized during surgery, and in 13% the inversion was suspected and confirmed only after the operation was unsuccessful and the incision was closed. Of the 17 operations in the last group, 10 were appendectomies.

The pain of appendicitis was localized in the left lower quadrant in 32 cases and in the right lower quadrant in 21. Blegen does not correlate these findings with the patient's knowledge of his condition. The surgical incision was made on the right in 27 cases and on the left in 30. In this connection, it should be noted that in at least one patient, situs inversus was coupled with a malrotation, which placed the cecum in the usual location, in the right lower quadrant (55).

The pain of cholecystitis seems to be localized correctly more often than is that of appendicitis, having been reported on the left in 16 cases with situs inversus and on the right in only 2 cases. Nevertheless, a right-sided incision was made in five patients. Situs inversus was recognized in 17 of 24 cholecystectomies, compared with 39 out of 73 appendectomies. The difference is probably caused by the emergency nature of acute appendicitis, which leaves little time for physical examination.

In 1990 Yamaguchi et al. (56) reported coronary artery bypass in dextrocardia with situs inversus totalis, and Dulganov and Nelip (57) reported synchronous esophageal and laryngeal carcinoma in a patient with complete situs inversus. Organ et al. (27) in 1991 reported a patient with situs inversus and with adenocarcinoma of the distal bile duct. A few years earlier Woods (58) presented a case of brain asymmetry in situs inversus.

Errors of Body Symmetry

Vertebrate animals including humans have a correspondence in size, shape, and measurement on opposite sides of a dividing line or median plane. This is bilateral symmetry. The opened abdomen and its contents seem far from symmetric at first glance. Symmetry can be determined embryologically rather than anatomically. It is based on the fact that most, if not quite all, of the embryonic viscera arise as single midline or bilaterally paired organs. When these structures are cleared away, the spleen remains the largest normally asymmetric organ. This is discussed at greater length in Chapter 10, "The Spleen." In addition to the spleen, other abdominal and thoracic organs are subject to hypertrophy, hyperplasia, hypoplasia, or aplasia.

Total Hemihypertrophy

Georgmaneanu and associates (59) in 1983 collected nine cases of hemihypertrophy. The left side was more affected (7:2), and there was no sex difference. Other congenital defects were present in all of the abnormal patients; three out of the nine also had congenital tumors.

Intrauterine Growth Retardation

Crane and Kopta (60) in 1980 divided the lesion into "symmetric" growth retardation, in which all structures are proportionately reduced in size, and "asymmetric," in which some are affected more than others.

The asymmetric deformity is the result of placental insufficiency. It is associated with chronic hypertension, preeclampsia, and diabetes (61).

Etiology of Situs

The authors suggest that rotation of the primitive heart tube initiates the process of lateralization and that the laterality defects of the viscera seen in the right twin are a result of their abnormal cardiac rotation.

Brueckner et al. (62) in 1989 reported a linkage mapping of a mouse gene (iv), that controls left-right asymmetry of the heart and viscera. Brown and associates (63) in that same year reported their experimental embryologic studies of the development of asymmetry in which the sideness of drug-induced limb abnormalities was linked with reversal of situs inversus in mice. They conclude that the maternal environment plays no role in the development of asymmetry.

Hanzlik et al. (64) reported that the murine situs inversus viscerum (iv) gene responsible for visceral asymmetry is linked tightly to the Igh-C cluster on chromosome 12.

Evidence for an adrenergic mechanism in the control of body asymmetry has been suggested by Fujinaga and Baden (65). They conclude that receptor mediated stimulation of the α-1 adrenergic pathway is involved in the control of normal body asymmetry in developing rat embryos.

According to Arey (66), a determining factor for the asymmetries of the viscera can be shown to lie in the gut of amphibians since a 180-degree rotation of the archenteron roof that corresponds to the later duodenum brings about situs inversus. Arey also believed that transposition of the viscera is an extreme type of symmetry reversal.

These ideas were published many years ago, and today we still do not know the answer to the control of the fundamental properties of heterotaxia, situs inversus, partial, or total asymmetry. Is congenital total lateral hyperplasia a severe unilateral asymmetry or is the other side severely hypoplastic? Brassett and Ellis (67) reviewed the subject in their article, entitled "Transposition of the Viscera," emphasizing the etiology, genetics, diagnostic features and concomitant disease.

REFERENCES

1. Moller JH, Nakib A, Anderson RC, Edwards JE. Congenital cardiac disease associated with polysplenia: a developmental complex of bilateral "leftsidedness." Circulation 1967;36;789–799.
2. Morrill CU. Symmetry reversal and mirror imaging in monstrous trout and comparison with similar conditions in human double monsters. Anat Rec 1919;16:265.
3. Guttmacher AF. Biographical notes on some famous conjoined twins. In: Bergsma D, ed. Conjoined twins. Birth Defects 1967;3:10–17.
4. Torgersen J. Genic factors in visceral asymmetry and in the development and pathologic changes of lungs, heart and abdominal organs. Arch Pathol 1949;47:566–593.
5. Cunniff C, Jones KL, Jones MC, Saunders B, Shepard T, Benirschke K. Laterality defects in conjoined twins: implications for normal asymmetry in human embryogenesis. Am J Med Genet 1988;31(3):669–677.
6. Crampton HE. Reversal of cleavage in a sinistral gastropod. Ann NY Acad Sci 1894;8:167.
7. Conklin EG. The embryology of crepidula. J Morphol 1897;1313:1–226.
8. Newman HH. The question of mirror-imaging in human one-egg twins. Hum Biol 1940;12:21–34.

9. Spemann H. Ueber embryonale Transplantation. Naturw Rundschau 1906;21:543.

10. Pressler K. Beobachtungen und Versuche über den normalen und inversen Situs viscerum et cordis bei Anurenlarven. Roux Arch Entw 1911;32:1–35.

11. von Woellwarth C. Experimentelle Untersuchungen über den Situs Inversus der Eingeweide und der Habenula des Zwischenhirns bei Amphibien. Roux Arch Entw 1950;144:178–256.

12. Kinney TB, DeLuca SA. Kartagener's syndrome. Am Fam Physician 1991;44(1):133–134.

13. Kartagener M. Zur Pathogenese der Bronchiektasien. I. Mitteilung: Bronchiektasien bei Situs viscerum inversus. Beitr Klin Tuberk 1933;83:489–501.

14. Kartegener M, Ulrich K. Zur Pathogenese der Bronchiektasien; Bronchiektasien und Veränderungen der Nasennebenh öhlen. Beitr Klin Tuberk 1935;86:349–357.

15. Mayo CW, Rice RG. Situs inversus totalis: statistical review of data on seventy-six cases, special reference to diseases of the biliary tract. Arch Surg 1949;58:724–730.

16. Varano NR, Merklin RJ. Situs inversus: review of the literature, report of four cases and analysis of the clinical implications. J Int Coll Surg 1960;33:131–148.

17. Bergstrom WH, Cook CD, Scannell J, Berenberg W. Situs inversus, bronchiectasis and sinusitis: report of family with 2 cases of Kartagener's triad and 2 additional cases of bronchiectasis among 6 siblings. Pediatrics 1950;6:573–580.

18. Hebel R. Familiäre Haufung der Kartegener Trias. Z Laryng Rhinol Otol 1952;31:83–90.

19. Overholt EL, Bauman DF. Variants of Kartagener's syndrome in the same family. Ann Int Med 1958;48:574–579.

20. Cockayne EA. The genetics of transposition of viscera. Q J Med 1938;7:479–493.

21. Torgersen J. Triad of Kartagener: contribution to its hereditary and developmental basis. Schweiz Med Wschr 1952;82:770.

22. Streete BG, Stull FE. Kartagener's syndrome. Arch Surg 1959;79:156–157.

23. Stumper OF, Sreeram N, Elzenga NJ, Sutherland GR. Diagnosis of atrial situs by transesophageal echocardiography. J Am Coll Cardiol 1990;16(2):447–450.

24. Dunseath R, Williams W, Patton D. A scintigraphic demonstration of dextrocardia and complete abdominal situs inversus. Clin Nucl Med 1990;15(7):501–503.

25. Meinecke P, Padberg B, Laas R. Agnathia, holoprosencephaly, and situs inversus: a third report. Am J Med Genet 1990;37(2):286–287.

26. Stoler JM, Holmes LB. A case of agnathia, situs inversus, and a normal central nervous system. Teretology 1992;46:213–216.

27. Organ BC, Skandalakis LJ, Gray SW, Skandalakis JE. Cancer of the bile duct with situs inversus totalis. Arch Surg 1991;126:1150–1153.

28. Lupin AJ, Misko GJ. Kartagener syndrome with abnormalities of cilia. J Otolaryngol 1978;7(2):95–102.

29. Rott HD. Kartagener's syndrome and the syndrome of immotile cilia. Hum Genet 1979;46(3):249–261.

30. Escudier E, Escalier D, Homasson JP, Pinchon MC, Bernaudin JF. Unexpectedly normal cilia and spermatozoa in an infertile man with Kartagener's syndrome. Eur J Respir Dis 1987;70(3):180–186.

31. Conraads VM et al. Ultrastructurally normal and motile spermatozoa in a fertile man with Kartagener's syndrome. Chest 1992;102(5):1616–1618.

32. Almy MA, Volk FH, Graney CM. Situs inversus of stomach. Radiology 1953;61:376–381.

33. Tskhai VF. [Anomaly of the bile ducts in a patient with situs inversus.] Klin Khir 1990;(9):69.

34. Gontijo B et al. The use of PTFE graft to correct anomalous drainage of persistent left superior vena cava. J Cardiovasc Surg 1990;31(6):815–817.

35. Hummel KP, Chapman DB. Visceral inversion and associated anomalies in the mouse. J Hered 1959;50:9.

36. Rylaarsdam M, Attie F, Buendia A, Munoz L, Calderon J, Zabal C. [Discordance in the anatomy of the bronchial tree and atrial appendages.] Arch Inst Cardiol Mex 1990;60(4):393–399.

37. Aristotle. Generation of animals. Peck AL (transl). The Loeb Classical Library. Cambridge: Harvard University Press, 1943.

38. Karashima I. Ein Fall von Situs inversus viscerum totalis. München: Kastner & Callwey, 1912.

39. Johnson JR. Situs inversus with associated abnormalities: review of the literature and report of three cases. Arch Surg 1949;38:149–162.

40. Beck C. A case of transposed viscera, with choleithiasis, relieved by a left-sided cholecystostomy. Ann Surg 1899;29:593–600.

41. Vehsemeyer H. Ein Fall von kongenitaler Dextrokordie, zugleich ein Beitrag zur Verwerthung der Röntgenstrahlen in Gebiete der inneren Medicin. Deutsch Med Wschr 1897;23:180.

42. Cleveland M. Situs inversus viscerum: an anatomic study. 1926;13:342–368, 1926.

43. Adams R, Churchill ED. Situs inversus, sinusitis and bronchiectasis. J Thorac Surg 1937;7:206–217.

44. Francisco SA, Ongpin C. Situs inversus totalis: case discovered by x-ray among Filipinos. J Philipp Med Assoc 1936;16:133–140.

45. Sieur M, Clenet E. Un cas exceptionnel d'heterotaxie thoraco-abdominale. J Radiol Electrol 1937;21:313–314.

46. Gould DM. Non-tuberculosis lesions found in mass x-ray surveys. JAMA 1945;127:753–756.

47. Caplan SM. Dextrocardia with situs inversus: report of eight cases with a review of literature of dextrocardia. US Navy Med Bull 1946;46:1011–1016.

48. Lowe CR, McKeown T. Dextrocardia with and without transposition of abdominal viscera, with report of case in one monozygotic twin. Ann Eurgen 1954;18:267.

49. Torgersen J. Anomalies of the spine in anomalies of the viscera and constitution. Acta Radiol 1948;29:311–320.

50. Smith HL, Horton BT. Congenital dextrocardia with complete situs transversus: production of a normal electrocardiogram by change of leads. Proc Mayo Clin 1936;11:181–184.

51. Chiu ES et al. Clinical implications of atrial isomerism. Br Heart J 1988;60(1):72–77.

52. Dietz R, Schanen G. CT in the preoperative clarification of Kartagener's syndrome. Röntgenblatter 1990;43(11):463–464.

53. Angulo-Cuesta J et al. The immotile cilia syndrome as a cause of sterility. Arch Esp Urol 1990;43(7):773–777.

54. Blegen HM. Surgery in situs inversus. Ann Surg 1949;129:244–259.

55. Boeminghaus H. Anomaly of the large intestine in connection with situs transversus. Deutsch Ztschr Chir 1920;155:174–188.

56. Yamaguchi T, Kikuchi S, Doi H, Watanabe A, Ebuoka M. [Coronary artery bypass in dextrocardia with situs inversus totalis: a case report.] Nippon Kyobu Geka Gakkai Zasshi 1990;38(9):1538–1542.

57. Dulganov KP, Nelip VE. [Synchronous early cancer of the esophagus and larynx in a patient with complete situs viscerum inversum.] Vopr Onkol 1990;36(9):1125–1125.

58. Woods RP. Brain asymmetries in situs inversus: a case report and review of the literature. Arch Neurol 1986;43(10):1083–1084.

59. Georgmaneanu M, Iagaru N, Popescu-Miclosanu S, Badulescu M. Congenital hemihypertrophy: tendency to association with other abnormalities and/or tumors. Morphol Embryol 1983;29(1):39–45.

60. Crane JP, Kopta MM. Comparative newborn anthropometric data in symmetric versus asymmetric intrauterine growth retardation. Am J Obstet Gynecol 1980;138(5):518–522.

61. Gruenwald P. Chronic fetal distress and placental insufficiency. Biol Neonate 1963;5:215.

62. Brueckner M, D'Eustachio P, Horwich AL. Linkage mapping of a mouse gene, *iv*, that controls left-right asymmetry of the heart and viscera. Proc Natl Acad Sci USA 1989;86(13):5035–5038.

63. Brown NA, Hoyle CI, McCarthy A, Wolpert L. The development of asymmetry: the sidedness of drug-induced limb abnormalities is reversed in situs inversus mice. Development 1989;107(3):637–642.

64. Hanzlik AJ et al. The murine *situs inversus viscerum* (iv) gene responsible for visceral asymmetry is linked tightly to the *Igh-C* cluster on chromosome 12. Genomics 1990;7(3);389–393.

65. Fujinaga M, Baden JM. Evidence for an adrenergic mechanism in the control of body asymmetry. Dev Biol 1991;143(1);203–205.

66. Arey LB. Developmental anatomy, 7th ed. Philadelphia: WB Saunders, 1965.

67. Brassett C, Ellis H. Transposition of the viscera: a review. Clin Anat 191;4:139–147.

CHAPTER 31

TERATOMAS

Richard Ricketts / Stephen Wood Gray / John Elias Skandalakis

"Your order shall commence with the formation of the child in the womb, saying
which part of it is formed first and so on in succession, placing its parts according
to the times of pregnancy until the birth, and how it is nourished, learning in part
from the eggs which hens make."
—*LEONARDO DA VINCI (1452Ä1519) QUARDERNI D'ANATOMIA, VOL I*

DEVELOPMENT

The most striking and bizarre structures in the human body are the tumors known as teratomas (from the Greek words τέρασ [monster] and ὄγκοσ or ὄγκομα [tumor]). A teratoma is a neoplasm of more than one cell type unrelated to the structure to which it is attached. The tumor may be cystic or solid; composed of mature cells, immature cells, or both; and show derivatives of all three embryonic germ layers: endoderm, mesoderm, and ectoderm.

Estimates that 6 and 10% of all human malformations are of teratogenic origin have been given (1) (see Chapter 1, "The Surgeon and the Problem"). However, the purpose of this chapter is not to give details about teratology nor to discuss the environmental or teratogenic agents responsible for the genesis of teratomas. We will mention only briefly the morphologic aspects of these congenital malformations.

Classification

There are several proposed classification systems based on pathology. One system (2) classifies teratomas into mature, immature, and malignant. Mature teratomas contain well-differentiated, benign, mature "adult" tissues only; these are not malignant. Immature teratomas contain "embryonic" tissues that are not frankly malignant; mature tissues can be present as well. These tumors are not malignant either. Malignant teratomas contain frankly malignant tissue in any one element of the teratoma; mature or embryonic tissues may be present as well. Malignant teratomas are further divided according to the type of malignant component: embryonal carcinoma, germinoma, yolk sac carcinoma (endodermal sinus tumor), and choriocarcinoma.

Teratomas of the ovary have been classified by Scully (3) into the following groups:

Immature teratomas: This is a malignant form of teratoma that contains immature structures resembling those of the embryo. Some mature elements are usually present.

Mature teratomas (solid): This form of teratoma is composed exclusively of mature elements. It is predominantly solid.

Mature teratoma (cystic, dermoid): This is composed largely of a cyst lined wholly or partly by an epithelium resembling the epidermis. Mesodermal, endodermal, and other ectodermal derivatives are usually present. Teeth and bones are common.

Mature teratomas (malignant transformation): This includes all cases in which a cancer has developed from one of the elements of the tumor (4).

Classification of teratomas by location has always been a problem. There has often been a sense that at least the more developed tumor somehow represents a failed twin. This idea has led some researchers to see whole limbs and organs where none exists.

Altman et al. (5) developed a classification by location for sacrococcygeal teratomas. They divide the tumors into four types. Type I tumors are almost completely external with a small presacral component. Type II tumors present externally but have significant intrapelvic extension. Type III tumors are visible externally, but the major mass is in the pelvis and abdomen. Type IV tumors are not externally visible; they are totally presacral.

Teratomas develop close to normal anatomic entities in a parasitic manner as their blood supply originates from the nearest neighboring organ by a pedicle formation or by a narrow or large basis of attachment. Teratomas of ovaries and testicles are the exception, however, because the anomaly is within the gonadal parenchyma.

Results from several series studies of location of teratomas are presented in Table 31.1. For a presentation of characteristics of teratomas at various sites, see Table 31.2.

Embryogenesis

Three theories about the genesis of teratomas have been proposed to explain the complex histology and the specific sites of these tumors.

I. During migration from the yolk sac, totipotent cells of the primitive streak may lag behind the larger mass of such cells. Some of these migratory cells, lying between the ectoderm and endoderm, may fail to develop into specified mesodermal structures. The resulting tumors are axial or paraxial (6).

II. According to Linder et al. (7), primitive germ cells arise from the yolk sac in the fifth week, migrate to the urogenital ridge, and eventually enter the presumptive gonad. Tissue from ovarian teratomas in five patients was examined and compared with "normal" tissue. The normal tissues were heterozygous for 17 chromosome polymorphisms, whereas the teratomas were uniformly homozygous. The group believes their findings indicate that "ovarian teratomas are parthenogenic tumors that arise from a single germ cell after the first meiotic division." Linder et al. (7) demonstrated parthenogenesis during migration.

III. The idea sense that at least the more developed tumors somehow represent the existence of a failed twin has stimulated speculation from the earliest observations of the tumors. This theory is most applicable to tumors of the brain, mediastinum, abdomen, and sacrococcygeal regions, all of which are known attachment sites for conjoined twins (see Chapter 32, "Conjoined Twins").

One of the strongest opponents of the twin concept has been Willis (8), who stated that "The widely promulgated belief that a gentle series of gradations exists between conjoined twins and teratomas is mistaken." Willis believed that there was strong tendency for observers to see what they wanted to see.

In spite of this statement, the possibility of such development has been confirmed by several sources (9–14). Sobis and Vandeputte (9) discovered teratomas in the exteriorized rat yolk sac, and there has been a greater acceptance of the possibility that complex structures, such as fingers complete with nails, may be found (10).

According to Damjanov et al. (11), several published papers conclude that "structures of high organizational

Table 31.1.
Distribution of Primary Site for Teratomas From Several Large Series[a]

Primary Site:	Berry[b] (N = 91)	Carney[c] (N = 58)	Mahour[d] (N = 133)	Grosfeld[e] (N = 85)	Mabougunge[f] (N = 96)	Tapper[g] (N = 254)	Total (N = 717)
Sacrococcygeal	58 (64)[h]	22 (38)	57 (43)	59 (69)	61 (64)	102 (40)	359 (57)
Ovary	10 (11)	5 (9)	51 (38)	8 (9)	8 (8)	94 (37)	176 (25)
Testis	7 (8)	3 (5)	6 (5)	2 (2)		8 (3)	26 (4)
Mediastinum	5 (5)	17 (29)	4 (3)	10 (12)	1 (1)	11 (4)	48 (7)
Retroperitoneal	1 (1)	3 (5)	6 (5)	1 (1)	5 (5)	12 (5)	29 (4)
Cervical	3 (3)		1	3 (4)	12 (13)	6 (2)	25 (3)
Central nervous system	3 (3)	7 (12)	4 (3)			9 (4)	23 (3)
Gastric	2 (2)		1		1 (1)		4 (0.5)
Oropharynx	2 (2)	1 (2)	3 (2)		3 (3)	6	15 (2)
Other			1 umbilical cord		1 chest wall 2 perineal 1 abdomen 1 liver	2 liver 1 back 1 abdomen 2 orbital	

[a]From Grosfeld JL, Billmire DF. Teratomas in infancy and childhood. Curr Probl Cancer 1985; 9(9):1–53.
[b]Berry CL, Keeling J, Hilton C. Teratomata in infancy and childhood: a review of 91 cases. J Pathol 1969; 98:241–252.
[c]Carney JA et al. Teratomas in children: clinical and pathological aspects. J Pediatr Surg 1972; 7:271–282.
[d]Mahour GH, Landing BH, Woolley MM. Teratomas in children: clinicopathologic studies in 133 patients. Z Kingerchir 1978; 23:365–380.
[e]Grosfeld JL, Ballantine TVN, Baehner RL. Benign and malignant teratomas in children: analysis of 85 patients. Surgery 1976; 80:297–305.
[f]Mabougunge OA et al. Teratomas in Nigerian children. East Afr Med J 1980; 57:461–469.
[g]Tapper D, Lack EE. Teratomas in infancy and childhood: a 54-year experience at the Children's Hospital Medical Center. Ann Surg 1982; 198:398–410.
[h]Number in parentheses represents the percentage of cases within the series.

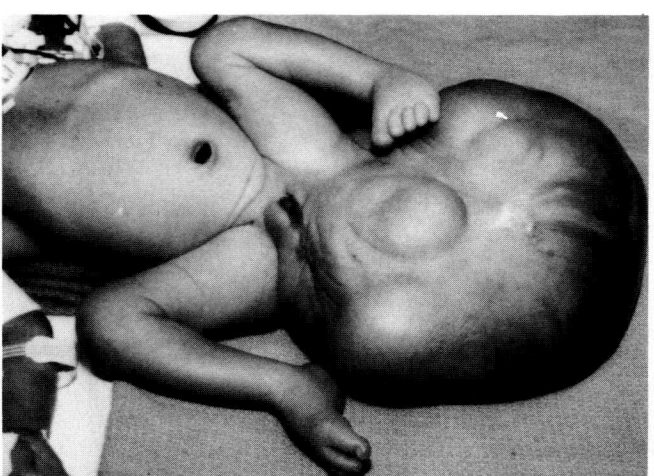

Figure 31.1. Large type I sacrococcygeal teratoma of a newborn female. Note anterior displacement of the rectum.

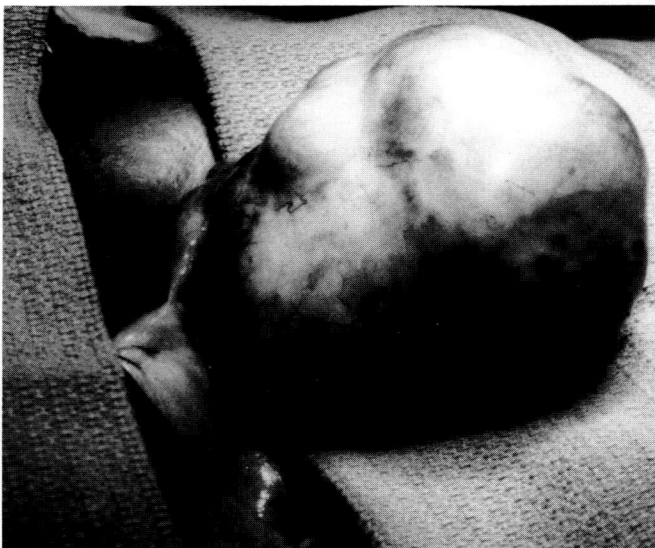

Figure 31.2. Ovarian teratoma, predominantly cystic. Note relationship to the fallopian tube and uterus.

level may occasionally be found in teratomas and that fetiform teratomas, although rare, nevertheless exist" (12–13). Hunter and Lennox (14) suggested that "If teratomata are simply ordinary tumors. . . , they should consist of tissues of the same sex as the host; if, on the other hand, they are in any sense derived from separate individuals, the sex should sometimes be independent of that of the host."

As is often the case, determining the sex of the teratomata was not always simple. After the discovery of the sex chromatin by Barr and Bertram (15), Hunter and Lennox (14) evaluated the teratomas of 12 females and 9 males. As expected, they found Barr bodies to be present in all the female teratomas. They also discovered Barr bodies in five of the male teratomas, thereby suggesting the teratoma to be of different origin than the individual to whom it was attached. Theiss et al. (16) further supported this hypothesis when they found 29 teratomas with female sex patterns in an examination of 96 testicular teratomas.

However, the discoveries of Myers (17) cast doubt on this theory. In a study of testicular teratomas, he found some regions of the teratoma in which only 5% of the cells contained Barr bodies, but in another region 66% of the cells contained Barr bodies.

History

Although a number of tumors reported before 1800 may have been teratomas, the pathology of the period was usually inadequate to be sure of the diagnosis (8). However, Virchow (18) reported "formations which not only correspond with different tissues of the body but at times

with whole regions of it, forms of which I have called teratomas," and almost 100 years later, Willis (8) defined a teratoma as a "true tumor or neoplasm composed of multiple tissues of kinds foreign to the parts in which it arises."

The earliest nonequivocal good illustration is that of Scultetus (19), who showed the mass of hair present in an ovarian teratoma. Wheeler (20) reproduced Scultetus' drawing of the specimen.

The teratoma remained a curiosity for about a century after Scultetus. According to reports, it could be very large, very heavy, with two or more types of hair, and as many as 300 teeth (20).

For a complete history of the teratoma, see Table 31.3.

SACROCOCCYGEAL TERATOMAS

Teratomas of the sacrococcygeal region are the most frequent and, because of their location, the most visible. Some types of sacrococcygeal teratomas are suggestive of a mendelian dominant pattern of inheritance (21). The inherited variety are usually presacral and may or may not be associated with congenital anomalies such as bony sacral defects, rectal wall involvement, anorectal stenosis, and abnormalities of the lower urinary tract (22).

Incidence

Sacrococcygeal teratomas are the most common tumors of the newborn and carry a malignancy rate of 10% at

Table 31.2.
Characteristics of Teratomas at Various Locations

Teratoma	Frequency	Sex and Presenting Age	Anatomy	Associated Anomalies	Malignancy
Sacrococcygeal teratoma (Fig. 32.1)	Most common; 1:40,000 live births; 40–70% of all teratomas	Female > male Newborn	I. External II. External and intrapelvic III. Pelvic IV. Presacral	Anorectal anomalies	Malignancy increases with age
Ovarian teratoma (Fig. 32.2)	50% of all ovarian masses in childhood	Female, equal right and left 6–12 yrs; rarely less than 2 yr	10 × 15 cm average; 5% bilateral	—	15% malignant; all immature lesions have some potential for metastasis
Testicular teratoma	60–80% of testicular neoplasms	Male Mostly under 2 yr	Equal right and left; rarely bilateral	Hydrocele	Malignant, from yolk sac derivatives; infantile and young adult groups
Mediastinal teratoma	20% of all mediastinal tumors of childhood	Equal Newborns to 15 yr and young adults	Mostly in anterior mediastinum	—	Occurs after 15 yr
Pericardial teratoma	Fewer than 50 cases reported	Equal 25% in newborns; 67% by 1 yr	Congenital heart failure; atrial compression and rotation of the heart	—	Two cases of malignancy known
Cervical teratoma (Fig. 32.3)	Fewer than 150 cases reported	Equal At birth, often with respiratory distress; becomes malignant in adult	Often associated with thyroid gland	Increased prematurity; respiratory distress; polyhydramnios	Benign before 15 yr; malignancy usual in adult patients
Gastric teratoma (Fig. 32.4)	Fewer than 60 cases reported	Almost all male 1st yr of life; very rare in adults[a]; all benign	15–15 cm, multicystic	—	—

[a]Gray SW, Johnson HC Jr, Skandalakis JE. Gastric teratoma in an adult: with a review of the literature. South Med J, 1964; 57:1346–1351.

birth (23, 24). The incidence of malignancy rises as the infant advances in age, reaching as high as 40 to 60% by 2 months of age (25). Sacrococcygeal teratomas are present in 1–2:40,000 live births. They are four times more common in girls, but the malignancy rate approaches equality in both sexes, perhaps leaning toward a male predominance (26).

Diagnosis

In addition to the physical examination, several diagnostic procedures should be performed when evaluating a potential sacrococcygeal teratoma. The major concern prior to surgery in these patients is the amount of intrapelvic extension. This can be determined by ultrasonography without exposing the patient to ionizing radiation or contrast-enhancing material. Magnetic resonance imaging (MRI) may be useful in differentiating a sacrococcygeal teratoma from a low-lying meningocele. α-Fetoprotein (AFP) is a useful marker for sacrococcygeal teratoma. Since AFP levels are normally elevated in newborns, it is not a useful marker initially. However, an elevated AFP following excision of the tumor may be an indication for tumor recurrence (27).

Table 31.3.
Landmarks in the History of Teratomas

Year	Author	Contribution
1658	Scultetus	Gross pathology of ovarian teratoma
1789	Baillie	Distinguished between ovarian teratoma and ovarian pregnancy
1839	Gross	1st U.S. case
1841	Stanley	1st successful surgical removal by Blizard
1843	Kohlrausch	Histologic recognition of skin
1849	Rokitansky	Fistula
1857	Lebert	Thorough histologic description
1857	Pesch	First malignant ovarian tumor
1869	Virchow	Gave the name "teratoma"
1875	Pauly	Reviewed ovarian teratomas
1935	Willis	Denies organ-forming ability
1954	Hunter and Lennox	Sex chromosome study begins
1955	Peterson et al.	Review of 1000 cases
1965	Abell et al.	Ovarian dermoid in 3-month-old infant; presence of sperm excluded

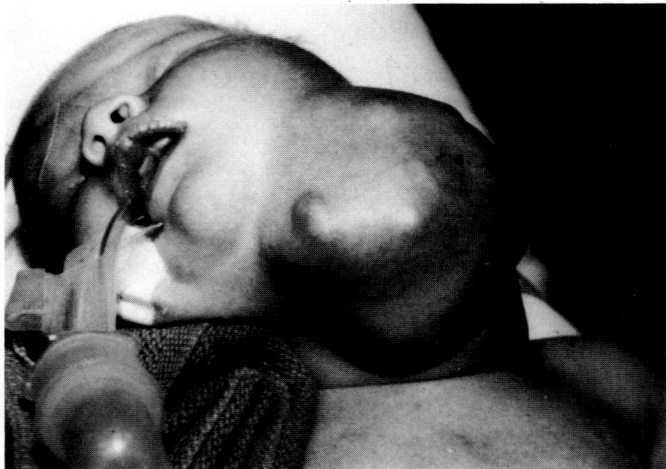

Figure 31.3. Cervical teratoma in a newborn resulting in mild respiratory distress.

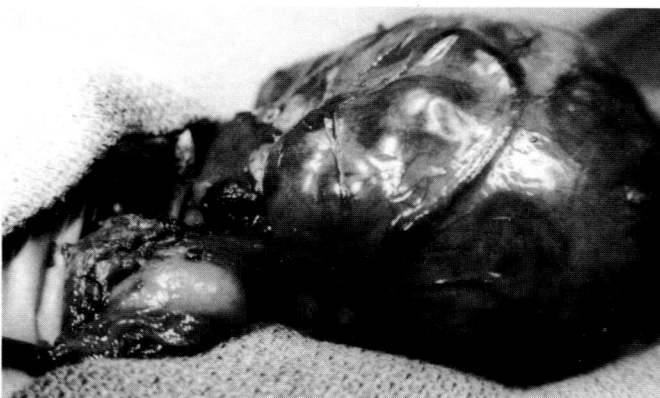

Figure 31.4. Exophytic gastric teratoma arising from the greater curvature of the stomach in an infant.

Treatment

The treatment of sacrococcygeal teratomas is complete excision, including the coccyx (21, 26). Failure to remove the coccyx is associated with a recurrence rate of 37% (27). Patients with malignant teratomas may also undergo radiation or chemotherapy following excision which results in improved survival rates when compared to excision alone (28).

EDITORIAL COMMENT

Serum α-fetoprotein is practically always significantly elevated in infants and young children with large sacrococcygeal teratomas. This, in itself, is not useful because there is no correlation with the level of α-fetoprotein with benign or malignant sacrococcygeal teratoma. Nevertheless, it is a useful baseline because, after surgical excision of the sacrococcygeal teratoma, there will be a sequential fall in α-fetoprotein levels. This should return to normal; with careful monitoring on a monthly basis, any evidence of recurrence will be manifest by a secondary rise in α-fetoprotein, which emphasizes the necessity of careful reevaluation and testing, including CT scans and/or MRI studies (JAH).

However, there are no reported cases of survival in patients who have malignant teratomas with metastatic disease (29).

REFERENCES

1. Nadler HL. Teratology. In: Welch KJ, Randolph JG, Ravitch MM, O'Neill JA, Rowe MI, eds. Pediatric surgery. Chicago: Year Book Medical Publishers, 1986:11.
2. Mahour GH. Sacrococcygeal teratomas. Cancer J Clin 1988;38:362–367.
3. Scully RE. Tumors of the ovary and maldeveloped gonads. In: Hartmann WH, Cowan WR, eds. Atlas of tumor pathology, 2nd series. Washington: Armed Forces Institute of Pathology, 1979.
4. Waxman M, Deppisch LM. Malignant alteration in benign teratomas. In: Damjanov I, Knowles BB, Solter D, eds. The human teratomas: experimental and clinical biology. Clifton, NJ: Humana Press, 1983:105.
5. Altman RP, Randolph JG, Lilly JR. Sacroccoccygeal teratoma. J Pediatr Surg 1974;9(3)389–398.
6. Grosfeld JL, Billmire DF. Teratomas in infancy and childhood. Curr Probl Cancer 1985;9(9):1–53.
7. Linder D, McCaw BK, Hecht F. Parthenogenic origin of benign ovarian teratomas. N Engl J Med 1975;292:63–66.
8. Willis RA. The borderland of embryology and pathology. London: Butterworth, 1958:430, 410–454.
9. Sobis H, Vandeputte M. Sequential morphological study of teratomas derived from displaced yolk sac. Dev Biol 1975;45:276–290.
10. Dutz W, Sadeghee S. A teratoid finger in the sigmoid colon. J Pathol Bacteriol 1968;95:289–291.
11. Damjanov I, Knowles BB, Solter D, eds. The human teratomas, experimental and clinical biology. Clifton, NJ: Humana Press, 1983:35.

12. Harris HR, Whitehouse DB. A foetiform teratoma. J Obstet Gynaecal Br Commonw 1967;74:776–778.

13. Azouri RS, Jubayli NW, Barakat BY. Dermoid cysts of ovary containing fetus-like structure. Obstet Gynecol 1973;42:887–891.

14. Hunter WF, Lennox B. The sex of teratoma. Lancet 1954;2:633–634.

15. Barr ML, Bertram EG. A morphological distinction between neurones of the male and female, and the behavior of the nucleolar satellite during accelerated nucleoprotein synthesis. Nature 1949;163(4148):676–677.

16. Theiss EA, Ashley DJB, Mostofi FK. Nuclear sex of testicular tumors and some related ovarian and extragonadal neoplasms. Cancer 1960;13:323–327.

17. Myers LM. Sex chromatin in teratomas. J Pathol Bacteriol 1959;78:585–587.

18. Virchow R. Vorlesungun uber Pathologie. Berlin: Hirschwald, 1863:96.

19. Scultetus J (Johann Scholz). Trichiasis admiranda sive morbus pilaris mirabilis observatus. Norimbergae: Enderi, 1658.

20. Wheeler JE. History of teratomas. In: Damjanov I, Knowles BB, Solter D, eds. The human teratomas: experimental and clinical biology. Clifton, NJ: Humana Press, 1983:1–22.

21. Raffensperger JG, ed. Swenson's pediatric surgery, 5th ed. Norwalk, CT: Appleton & Lange, 1990:383–391.

22. Woolley MM. Teratoma. In: Welch KJ, Randolph JG, Ravitch MM, O'Neill JA, Rowe MI, eds. Pediatric surgery, 4th ed. Chicago: Year Book Medical Publishers, 1986:265–275.

23. Flake AW, Harrison MR, Adzick NS, Laberge JM, Warsof SL. Fetal sacrococcygeal teratoma. J Pediatr Surg 1986;21:563–566.

24. Feldman M, Byrne P, Johnson MA, Fischer J, Lees G. Neonatal sacrococcygeal teratoma: multiimaging modality assessment. J Pediatr Surg 1990;25:675–678.

25. Billmire DF, Grosfeld JL. Teratomas in childhood: analysis of 142 cases. J Pediatr Surg 1986;21:548–551.

26. Schropp KP et al. Sacrococcygeal teratoma: The experience of four decades. J Pediatr Surg 1992;27:1075–1079.

27. Ein SH, Mancer K, Adeyemi SD. Malignant sacrococcygeal teratoma-endodermal sinus, yolk sac tumor, in infants and children: a 32-year review. J Pediatr Surg 1985;20:473–477.

28. Johnston PW. The diagnostic value of alpha-fetoprotein in an infant with sacrococcygeal teratoma. J Pediatr Surg 1988;23:862–863.

29. Avery GB, ed. Neonatology, 3rd ed. Philadelphia: JB Lippincott, 1987:1022–1024.

CHAPTER 32

CONJOINED TWINS

Richard Ricketts / Stephen Wood Gray / John Elias Skandalakis

"Observations on aborted conjoined twin embryos, with their intact adnexa, will supply the only reliable clues for a definite explanation of such complex developmental aberrations."
—A.A. ZIMMERMANN

EMBRYOGENESIS

A number of investigators have thoroughly studied the embryogenesis of conjoined twins (1–4). Conjoined twins are derived from a single blastocyst and are similar to monovular twins; however, according to Schnaufer (5), they "remain joined by some aberration in the duplication process that normally produces two identical twins." The embryologist's challenge is to discover why the "aberration" occurs and to reconstruct the crime of abnormal duplications.

EDITORIAL COMMENT

A recent encyclopedic review of the *etiology* of conjoined twins by Dr. Rowena Spencer (6) of New Orleans has led her to a new comprehensive explanation of the causation of conjoined twins and a new classification. If this new classification is accepted by authorities in the field of developmental anomalies, genetics, and embryology, Dr. Spencer will have contributed important information to a better understanding of the formation of conjoined twins (JAH).

Some essential terminology, needed to precede to possible embryologic explanations of this anomaly, begins with the term *monovular pregnancy*. Monovular pregnancy occurs when a single fertilized ovum divides from a single blastocyst; the infants have the same sex and the same chromosomes and are known as *monozygotic identical twins*. A *polyovular pregnancy* occurs when there is fertilization of two or more ova. A *zygote* is the fertilized ovum. A *blastocyst* is a cluster of cells of a zygote. It is composed of three parts: inner cell mass, trophoblast, and blastocele, each of which has a specific embryologic destiny. A *trophoblast* forms most of the chorion, and the inner cell mass forms the embryo.

Near the sixth day after fertilization, the blastocyst penetrates the endometrium. Monozygotic fetuses are produced from cells in the blastocyst that polarize and develop into two germinal discs which, in time, will form two monozygotic fetuses. Incomplete fission at this point may be the cause of the genesis of such extreme abnormalities. Zimmerman (7) asserts that the production of conjoined twins is due to anarchy in the morphogenesis or organogenesis processes with resulting morphologic anatomy ranging from simple to complex. Fusion of the embryonic axes after inner cell mass splitting is another theory of the genesis of conjoined twins (8).

CLASSIFICATION

There are several classification systems for conjoined twins, such as those proposed by Potter and Craig (9) and by Hirst and Piersol (10). A simple system, which is clinically useful, classifies the twinning by the most prominent sites of connection, plus the Greek root *-pagos*, meaning "that which is fixed" (11). From this system, the following classification emerges:

1. *Thoracopagus:* The junction is from the umbilicus cephalad, and the twins always face each other. This is the most common type of conjoined twinning and accounts for about 75% of the cases. The sterni, diaphragm, and livers are always fused. The pericardial sac is common in 90%, and the hearts are fused in 75%—a fatal event. The biliary tracts are fused in about 22%, and the gastrointestinal (GI) tracts are fused in about 50% of the cases.
2. *Omphalopagus (xiphopagus):* The junction is from the umbilicus to the xiphoid, and the twins face each other. There is usually a connecting bridge between the livers, and the lower GI tracts and genitourinary (GU) tracts may also be joined.
3. *Pygopagus:* The twins face away from each other and are joined at the sacrum, buttocks, and perineum. There is a complicated fusion of the lower GI and GU tracts as well as the internal and external genitalia. The spinal cords are usually separate.
4. *Ischiopagus:* The twins are joined from the umbilicus to the pelvis and either have two (bipus), three (tripus [the

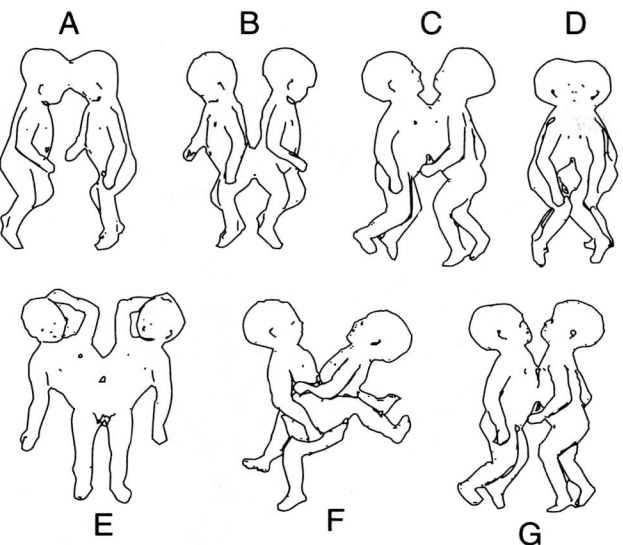

Figure 32.1. **A,** Craniopagus. **B,** Pygopagus. **C,** Thoracopagus. **D,** Cephalopagus. **E,** Parapagus. **F,** Ischiopagus. **G,** Omphalopagus. (From Arey AB. Developmental anatomy, 7th ed. Philadelphia: WB Saunders, 1965.)

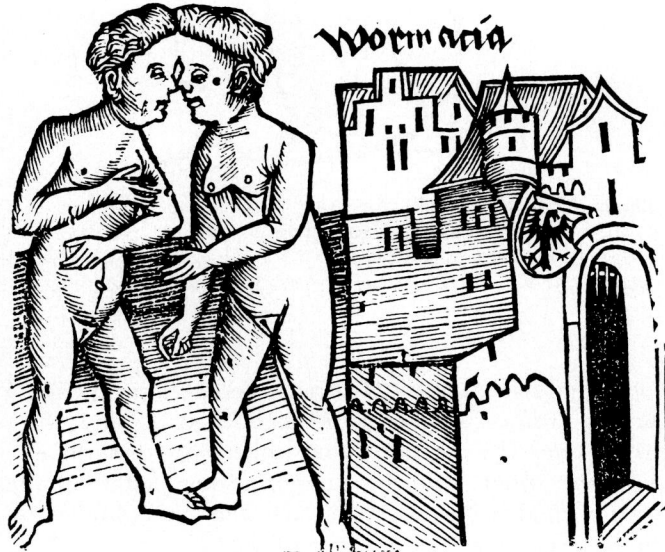

Figure 32.2. Craniopagus similar to that described by Munster. An unsigned woodcut dated 1510 in the collection of Yale Medical Historic Library. These were apparently seen in Worms, Germany, 11 years before Luther's famous trial. (Artist and publisher unknown. Reprinted with permission from Guttmacher AF, Nichols BL. Teratology of conjoined twins. In: Bergsma D, ed. Conjoined twins. New York: The National Foundation-March of Dimes BD: OAS III 1967;1:3–9.)

most common]), or four (tetrapus) lower extremities. The internal and external anatomy is quite complicated and variable and may include imperforate anus, vaginal anomalies, rectovaginal communications, fusion of the lower GI and GU tracts, and abnormal internal genitalia.

5. *Craniopagus:* The junction is at the vertex, occiput, or lateral parietal areas of the skull. This is the rarest type of conjoined twinning (accounting for about 2% of cases).

The "complete" type, with extensively fused brain tissue, is generally fatal. In the "partial" type, the brains are separated by bone or dura mater, and surgical separation of the twins is often possible.

6. *Rare and Unusual Types*
   A. Monocephalus diprosopus: single head with facial duplication
   B. Dicephalus: two distinct heads on one body
   C. Monocephalus tripus dibrachius: partial duplication of the pelvis with a third leg
   D. Monocephalus tetrapus dibrachius: partial duplication of the pelvis with four legs
   E. Dicephalus dipygus: partial duplications of both cranial and caudal regions
   F. Parasites (teratomas, fetus-in-fetu)

Another clinically useful classification system by Spencer (6) groups deformities with respect to cardiac involvement (Fig. 32.1):

Conjunction never involving the umbilicus or the heart:
   A. Craniopagus: cranial union only
   B. Pygopagus: posterior union of the rump

Conjunction always involving the umbilicus

and always involving the heart:

   C. Thoracopagus: anterior union of the upper half of the trunk
and usually involving the heart:
   D. Cephalopagus: anterior union of the upper half of the body, with two faces on *opposite sides* of a conjoined head
   E. Parapagus (formerly called dicephalus or diprosopus): lateral union of the lower half of the body, extending variable distances upward; in the extreme case there are two faces *side-by-side* on one head

but never involving the heart:
   F. Ischiopagus: anterior union of the lower half of the body
   G. Omphalopagus: anterior union of the middle of the trunk

HISTORY

The history of conjoined twins is diverse, extremely interesting, and can best be appreciated through a pictorial essay of illustrations of conjoined twins through the ages (Figs. 32.2 through 32.24). Fascination with the occurrence of this bizarre anomaly was documented as early as the 16th century (12); it is still discussed and written about today.

INCIDENCE

According to Schnaufer (5), the true incidence of conjoined twins is impossible to ascertain because the major-

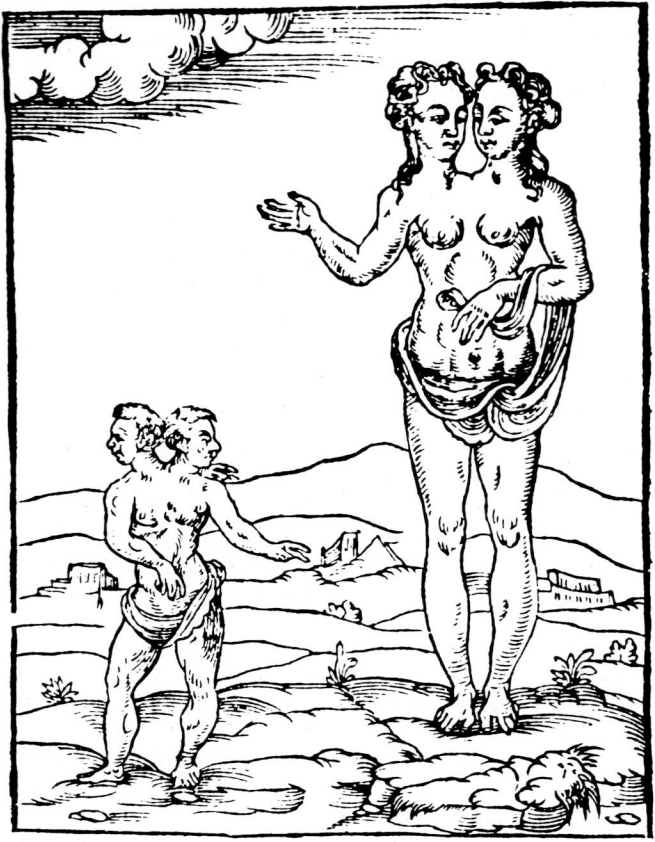

Figure 32.3. Dicephalus. Illustrations from the theologic study by Boaistuau in 1560. (Reprinted with permission from Guttmacher AF, Nichols BL. Teratology of conjoined twins. In: Bergsma D, ed. Conjoined twins. New York: The National Foundation-March of Dimes BD: OAS III 1967;1:3–9.)

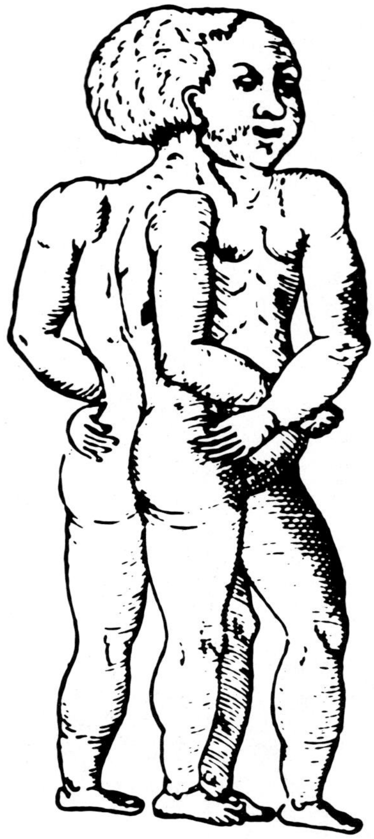

Figure 32.4. Syncephalus. These twins were illustrated in Paré's work published in 1579. (Reprinted with permission from Guttmacher AF, Nichols BL. Teratology of conjoined twins. In: Bergsma D, ed. Conjoined twins. New York: The National Foundation-March of Dimes BD: OAS III 1967;1:3–9.)

ity are either aborted or stillborn, but she suggests that perhaps an estimate of 1:50,000–60,000 births is accurate. Female conjoined twins are more common than male: 70% of conjoined twins are female. Monozygotic twinning has no racial preference, and it is not related to heredity, maternal age, or parity. However, the incidence of dizygotic twinning is, in contrast, greatly influenced by these factors (5).

In their review, Rudolph et al. (13) reported that, of 60 conjoined twins, 31 were stillborn and 6 died at delivery.

DIAGNOSIS

Presenting a clinical picture of conjoined twins is very difficult because of the greatly varying degrees of complexity in each case. The picture could be a very benign one—connection by piece of skin—to an extremely difficult one, due to multiple, severe associated anomalies.

Depending on the type of twinning present, all of the potentially conjoined organ systems must be thoroughly evaluated to determine if surgical separation is possible or not. If not, can one of the twins be saved, and, if so, which one? The decision about which twin to sacrifice to save the other must be preoperatively based on the involvement of the various organ systems and with the full understanding and acceptance of the parents.

To evaluate the brains, computed tomography (CT) and cerebral angiography is used (14). A magnetic resonance imaging (MRI) scan would also be very helpful, but its use in evaluating conjoined twins has not yet been reported. The hearts are evaluated with electrocardiography, echocardiography, and angiography; fusion of the heart (and great vessels) is generally fatal for both twins (11). The GI tracts are evaluated with upper and lower contrast-enhanced studies. The biliary tracts are evaluated with hepatobiliary iminodiacetic acid (HIDA) scintiscans, transhepatic cholangiography, or endoscopic retrograde cholangiopancreatography. The GU tracts can be evaluated by contrast-enhanced CT or urography, cystograms, nuclear scanning, and/or endoscopy. Vascular supply to the lower extremities in ischiopagus twins is

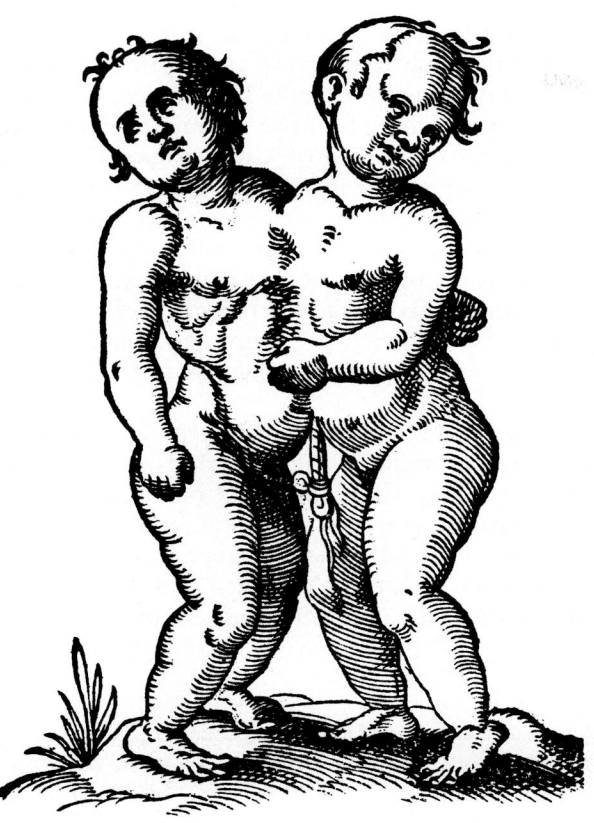

Figure 32.5. A view of the conjoined thorax and umbilicus in thoracopagus twins. (From Rueff, 1580. Reprinted with permission from Guttmacher AF, Nichols BL. Teratology of conjoined twins. In: Bergsma D, ed. Conjoined twins. New York: The National Foundation-March of Dimes BD: OAS III 1967;1:3–9.)

evaluated by selective angiography. The amount of cross-circulation or blood volume exchange between the twins can be determined by administering isotope-tagged albumin or red blood cells to one of the twins (15). Similarly, perfusion fluorometry is a useful technique to determine blood flow to the skin for planning complicated reconstructions (16).

TREATMENT

Surgical separation of conjoined twins is the treatment of choice (11). Procedures range from the very simple to the very difficult. In complex cases, multiple surgical specialties may be involved. The surgical procedure should be

Figure 32.6. Views of thoracopagus *(left)* and pygopagus *(right)* conjoined twins from the book on obstetrics by Rueff, 1580. (Reprinted with permission from Guttmacher AF, Nichols BL. Teratology of conjoined twins. In: Bergsma D, ed. Conjoined twins. New York: The National Foundation-March of Dimes BD: OAS III 1967;1:3–9.)

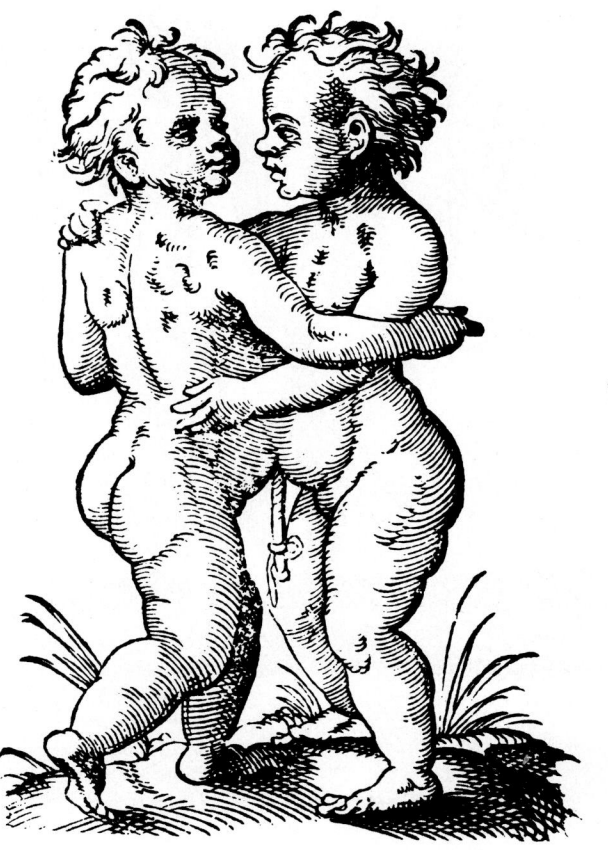

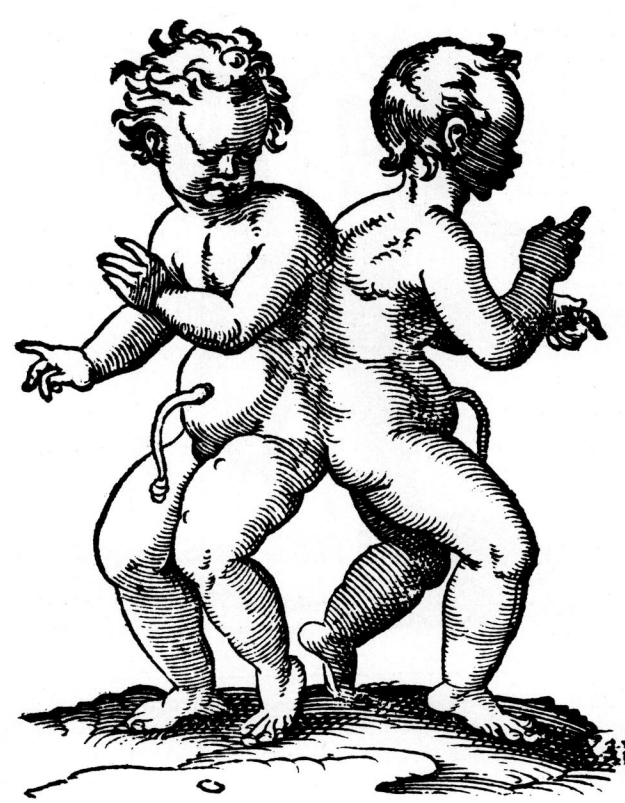

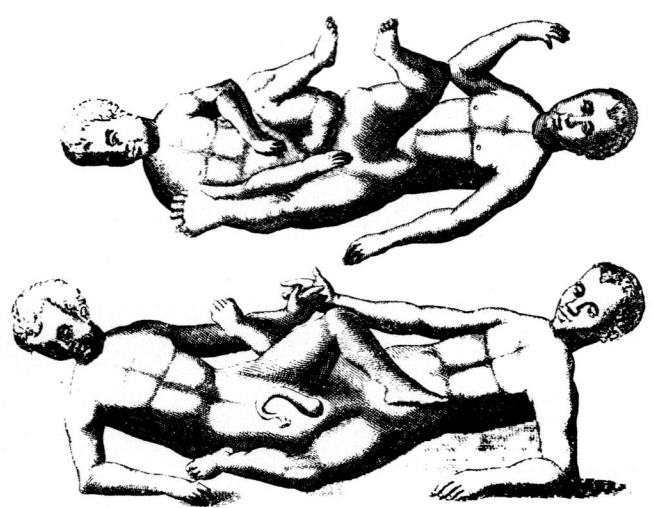

Figure 32.7. Ischiopagus cases. Illustrations from the treatise on monsters by Licetus in 1665. (Reprinted with permission from Guttmacher AF, Nichols BL. Teratology of conjoined twins. In: Bergsma D, ed. Conjoined twins. New York: The National Foundation-March of Dimes BD: OAS III 1967;1:3–9.)

delayed for 3 to 6 months if possible. This interval allows the twins to stabilize and grow, and it provides adequate time for a thorough workup to be completed and a comprehensive operative plan to be formulated. This time can also be used to expand skin or tissue to make closure after the surgical separation less complicated (14, 17–19).

There are only three indications for early ("emergency") separation: *(a)* one twin is stillborn or threatening the life of the other; *(b)* there is a congenital anomaly of one or both twins which is incompatible with life, but which can be corrected (e.g., ruptured omphalocele) (5, 20); or *(c)* there is extensive damage to the connecting bridge.

Detailed planning based on the type of twinning, the fused viscera, and the presence of other congenital anomalies is necessary for a successful outcome. Two completely separate anesthetic, surgical, and nursing teams with appropriate subspecialty support must be identified—one for each twin. The anesthetic management is complicated by the degree of cross-circulation from one

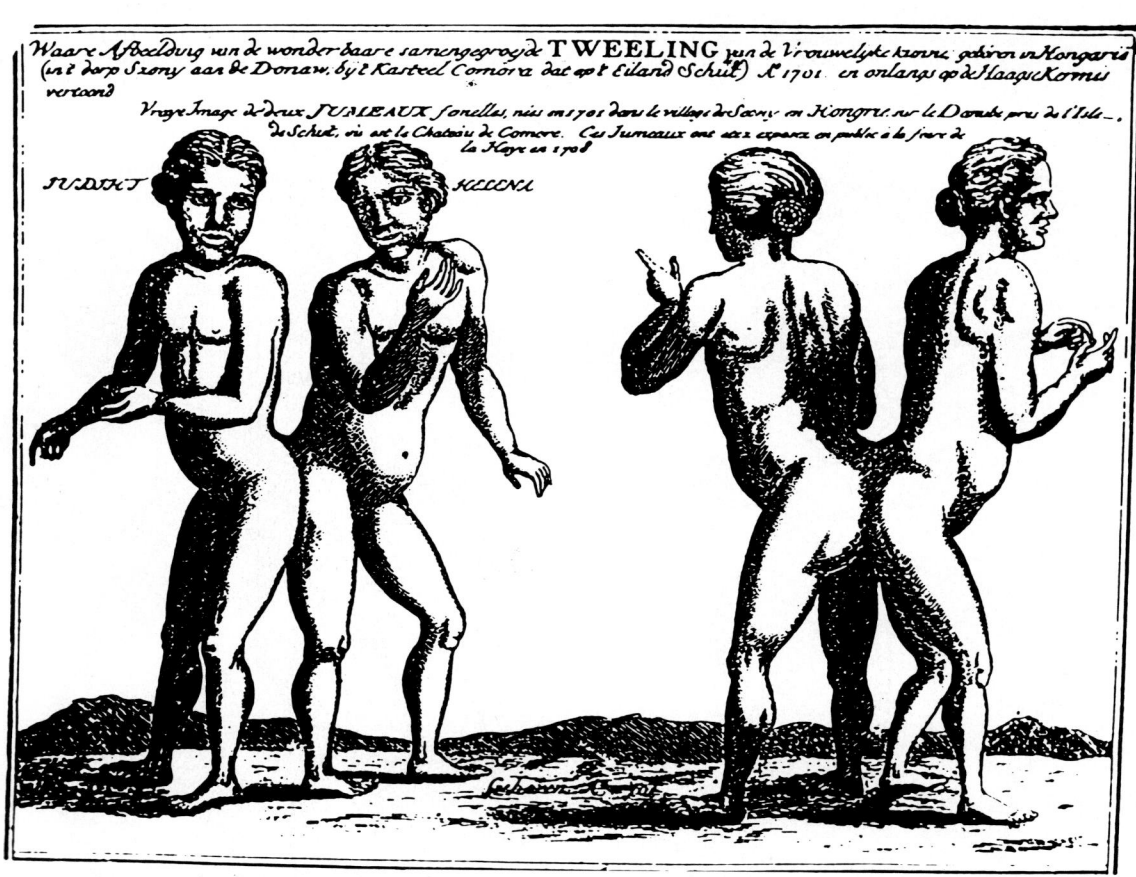

Figure 32.8. The Hungarian sisters, Helena and Judith, a poster in Yale Medical Historical Library's collection—"One urine-passage serves for both, one anus, so they tell; The other parts their numbers keep, and serve their owners well." (Reprinted with permission from Guttmacher AF. Biographical notes on some famous conjoined twins. In: Bergsma D, ed. Conjoined twins. New York: The National Foundation-March of Dimes BD: OAS III 1967;1:10–17.)

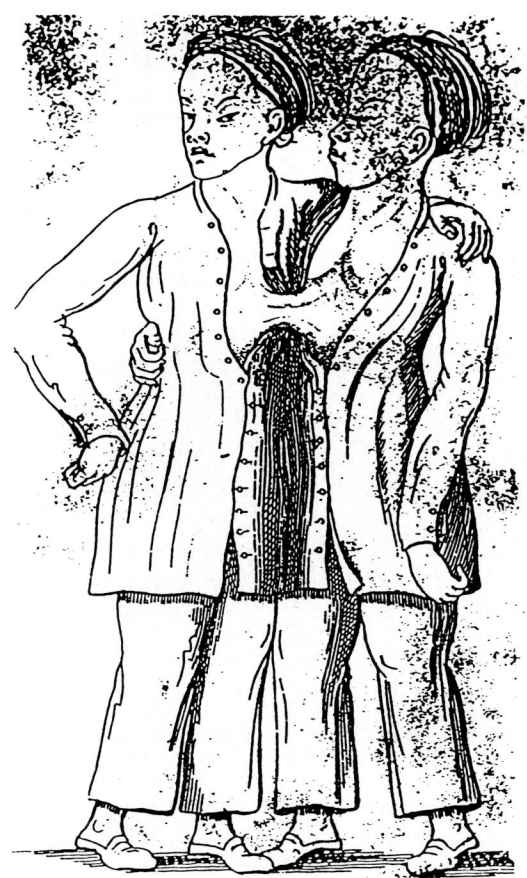

Figure 32.9.   Chang and Eng Bunker. This illustration is from an early description by J.C. Warren in 1829. (Reprinted with permission from Guttmacher AF. Biographical notes on some famous conjoined twins. In: Bergsma D, ed. Conjoined twins. New York: The National Foundation-March of Dimes BD: OAS III 1967;1:10–17.)

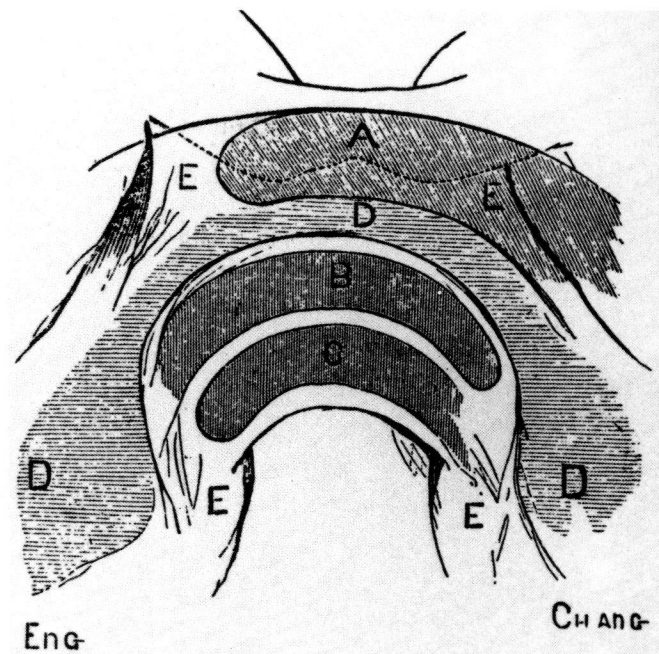

Figure 32.10.   1874 diagram illustrating the nature of the conjunction in the Bunker twins. *A,* Upper or hepatic pouch of Chang; *B,* the peritoneal pouch of Eng; *C,* the peritoneal pouch of Chang; *D,* connecting liver band; *E, E, (dotted line)* union of the ensiform cartilages; *E, E,* lower border of the band. (Reprinted with permission from Guttmacher AF. Biographical notes on some famous conjoined twins. In: Bergsma D, ed. Conjoined twins. New York: The National Foundation-March of Dimes BD: OAS III 1967;1:10–17.)

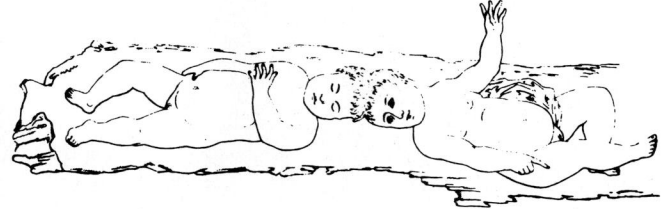

Figure 32.11.   Craniopagus. This line drawing illustrates twins studied by Baer in 1845. (Reprinted with permission from Guttmacher AF, Nichols BL. Teratology of conjoined twins. In: Bergsma D, ed. Conjoined twins. New York: The National Foundation-March of Dimes BD: OAS III 1967;1:3–9.)

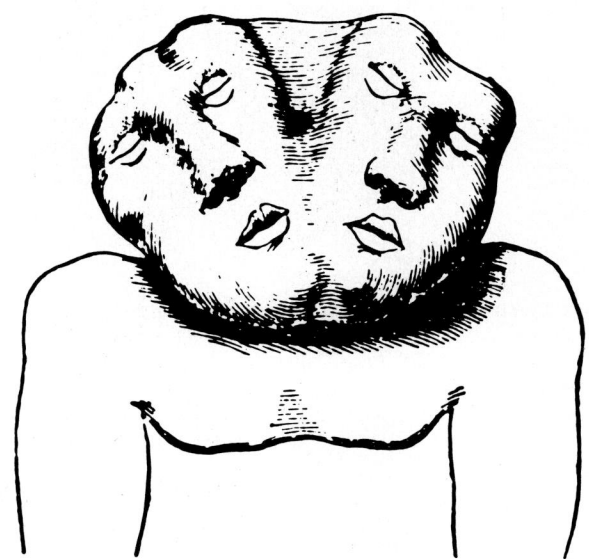

Figure 32.12.   "Case of a double headed monster which occurred in the practice of Dr. H.N. Shultz," reported by Dr. D. Gilbert in 1864, is a true case of diprosopus. (Reprinted with permission from Guttmacher AF, Nichols BL. Teratology of conjoined twins. In: Bergsma D, ed. Conjoined twins. New York: The National Foundation-March of Dimes BD: OAS III 1967;1:3–9.)

Figure 32.14. The Biddenden maids. This reproduction of an imprinted cake is from Ballantyne's book on antenatal pathology (1904). (Reprinted with permission from Guttmacher AF. Biographical notes on some famous conjoined twins. In: Bergsma D, ed. Conjoined twins. New York: The National Foundation-March of Dimes BD: OAS III 1967;1:10–17.)

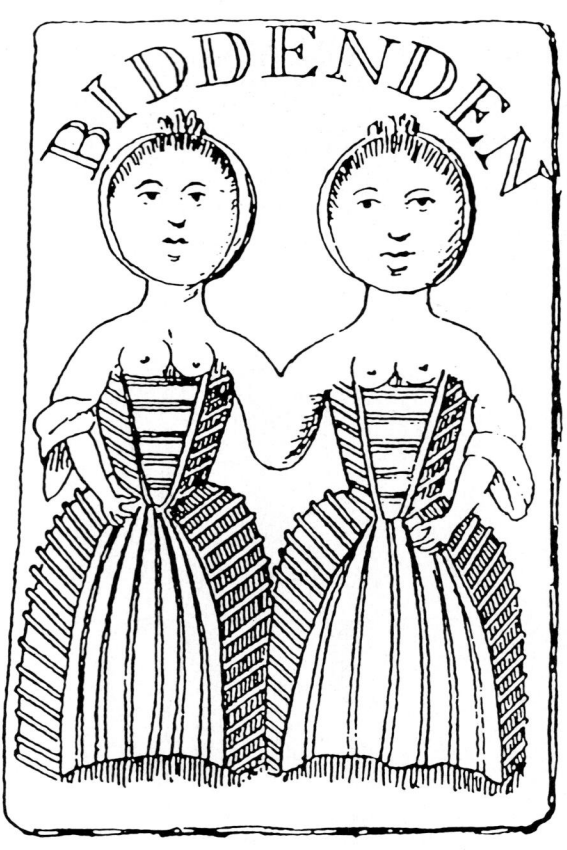

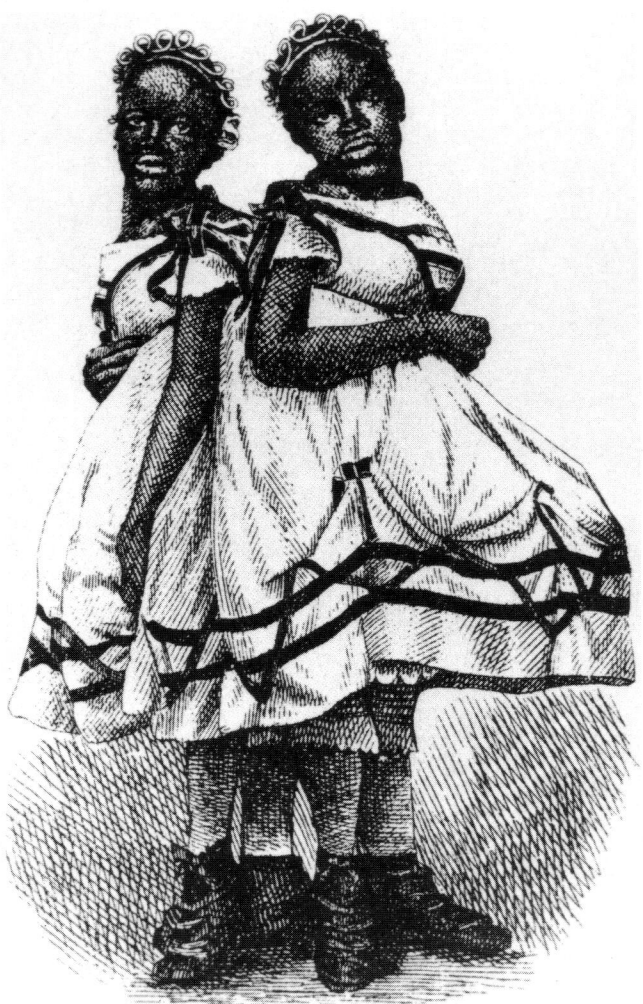

Figure 32.13. Millie and Chrissie from an 1868 medical society review. Born to slave parents in South Carolina, they were connected at the first sacral vertebra to the coccyx. The right half of the sacrum of one was joined to the left half of the other. (Reprinted with permission from Guttmacher AF. Biographical notes on some famous conjoined twins. In: Bergsma D, ed. Conjoined twins. New York: The National Foundation-March of Dimes BD: OAS III 1967;1:10–17.)

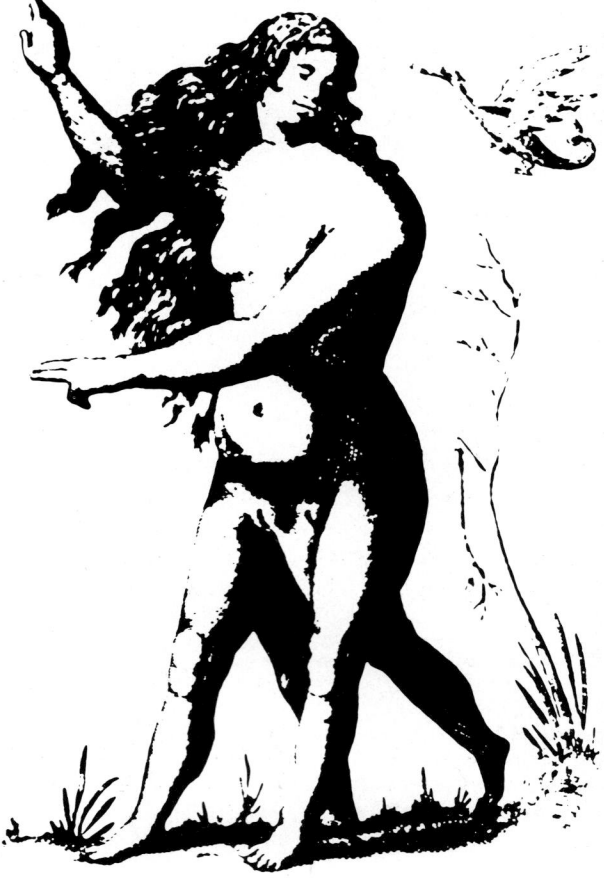

Figure 32.15. Dipygus. The heraldic decorations reveal the awe of the artist in this illustration from Licetus who emphasized the supranatural significance of conjoined twins. (Reprinted with permission from Guttmacher AF, Nichols BL. Teratology of conjoined twins. In: Bergsma D, ed. Conjoined twins. New York: The National Foundation-March of Dimes BD: OAS III 1967;1:3–9.)

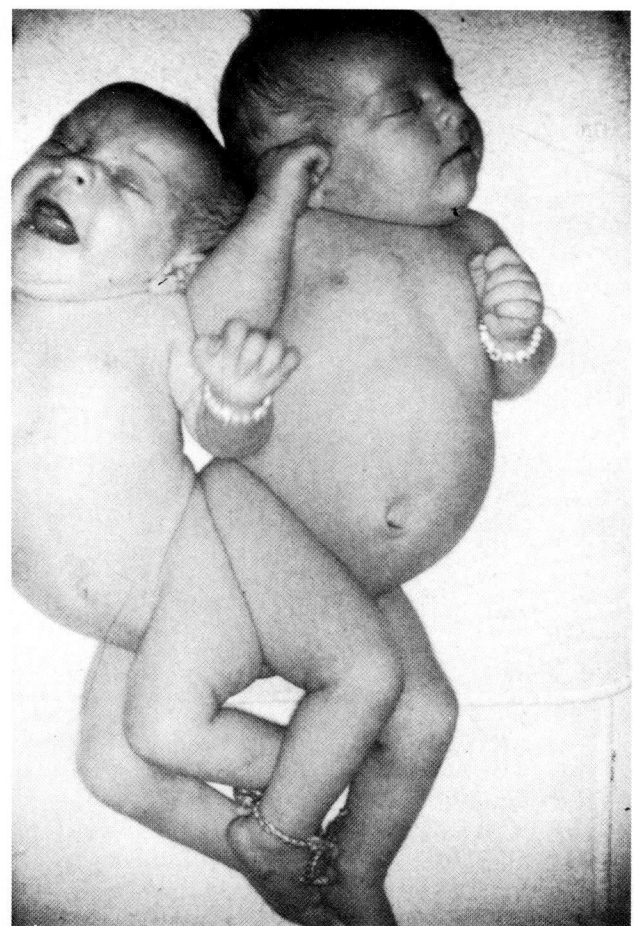 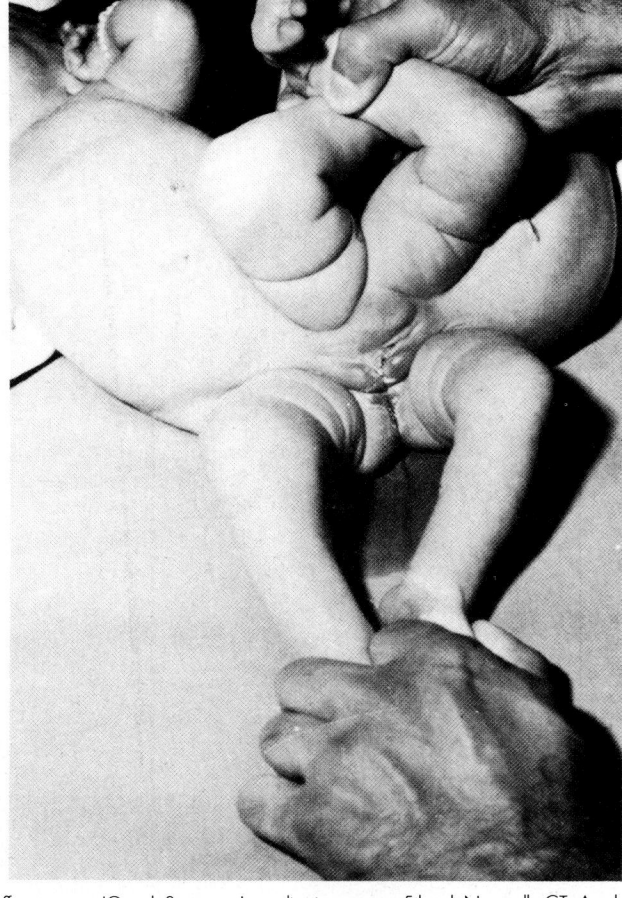

Figure 32.16. **A,** Pygopagus twins with fused sacrum and perineum. **B,** Perineal view showing single anus and vulva. (From Schnaufer L. Conjoined twins. In:

Raffensperger JG, ed. Swenson's pediatric surgery, 5th ed. Norwalk, CT: Appleton & Lange, 1990:976.)

twin to the other. Each twin requires extensive monitoring of central venous pressure, arterial pressure, electrolytes, blood gases, and urinary output. A dress rehearsal to practice positioning, prepping and draping, and movement of the twins once they are separated is useful. One designated spokesperson should be identified to impart the appropriate information to the press in these potentially highly publicized cases.

As in the case of thoracopagus twins, surgeons may be faced with some difficult moral and ethical dilemmas as circumstances may dictate that life and death decisions be made regarding the division of vital organs. Pepper (21) provides a thorough and thought-provoking discussion of these issues.

RESULTS

A thorough review of almost all reported attempts at surgical separation of conjoined twins through December 1987 was compiled by Hoyle in 1990 (11). To this list five sets can be added as "personal communication" (22) and

one set from one of the present authors (17). Other cases have undoubtedly been reported since 1987 (18, 23).

According to Hoyle's review (11), the survival rate for both twins, based on the type of twinning, was:

Thoracopagus	29%
Omphalopagus	70%
Craniopagus	33%
Ischiopagus	74%
Pygopagus	56%

The mortality rate for both twins, based on the type of twinning, was:

Thoracopagus	34%
Omphalopagus	14%
Craniopagus	37%
Ischiopagus	15%
Pygopagus	6%

In the other cases either one twin died perioperatively or was sacrificed, and one twin lived. Analysis of the results also revealed: *(a)* emergent operations resulted in an increased perioperative mortality; and *(b)* there has

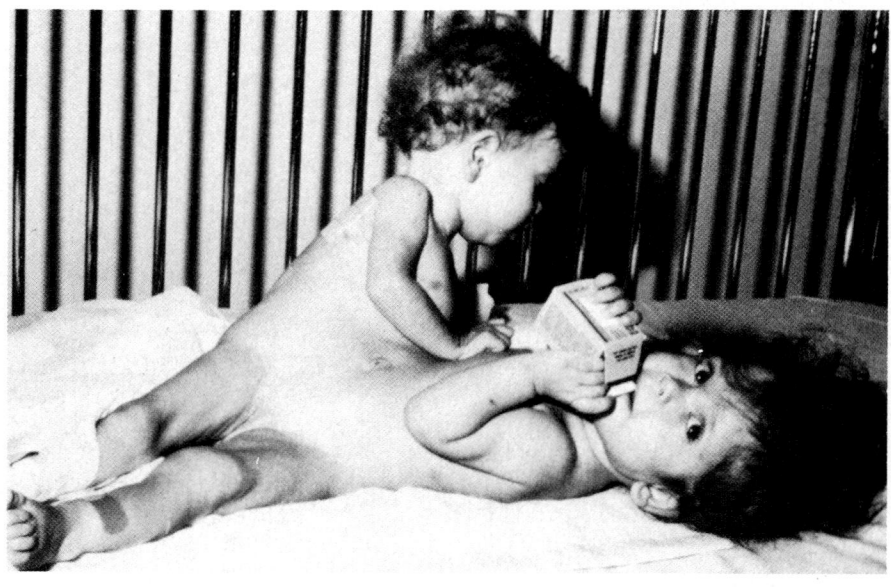

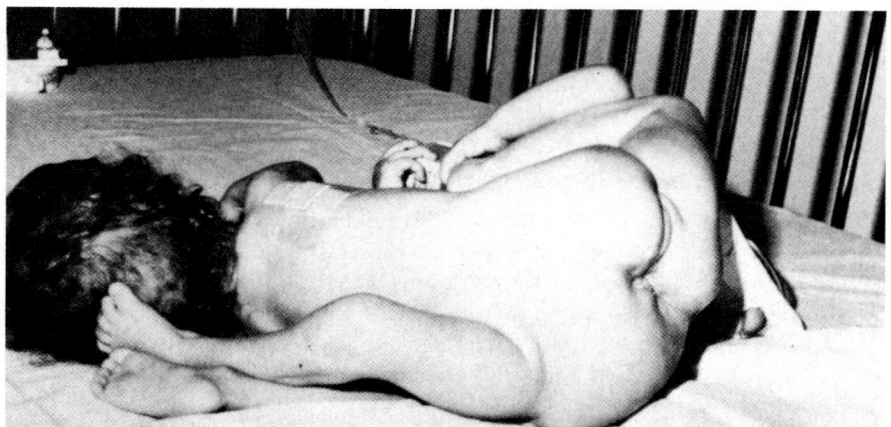

Figure 32.17. **A,** Ischiopagus twins fused from umbilicus to perineum. **B,** Perineal view showing single anus. (From Schnaufer L. Conjoined twins. In: Raffensperger JG, ed. Swenson's pediatric surgery, 5th ed. Norwalk, CT: Appleton & Lange, 1990:977.)

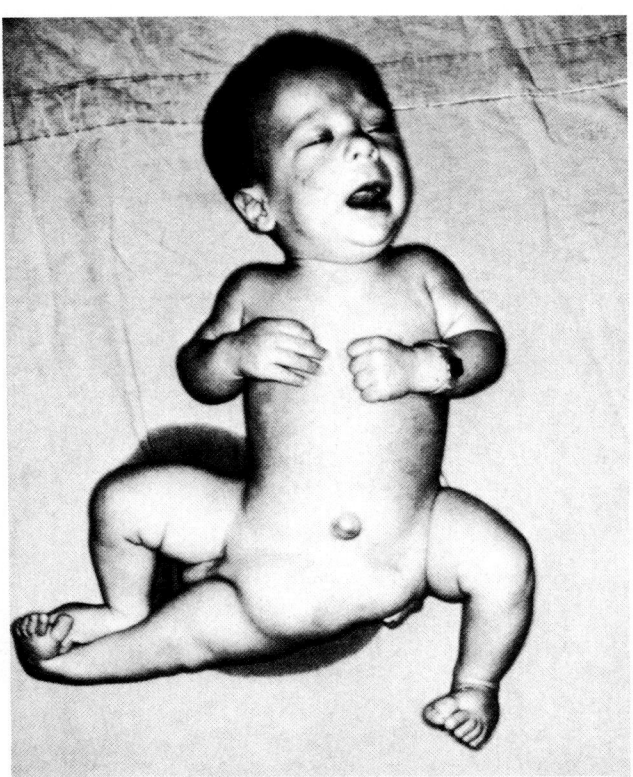

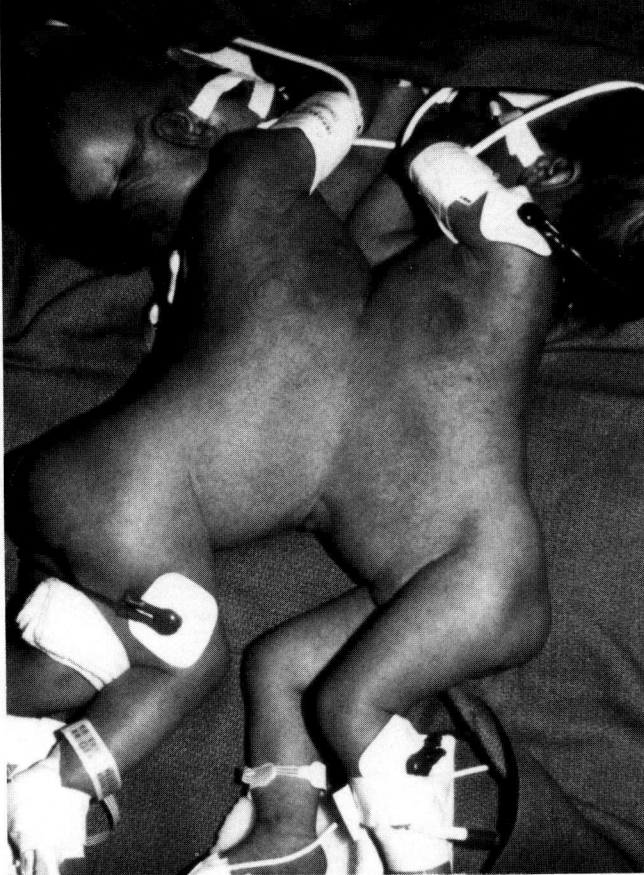

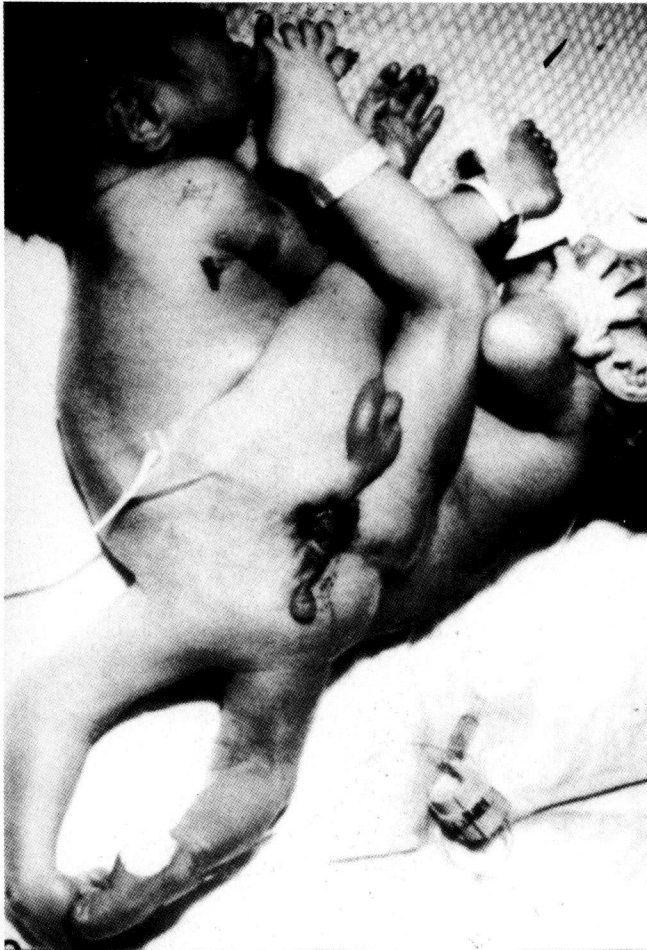

Figure 32.18. Monocephalus tripus dibrachius. Partial duplication of the pelvis, with a third leg. (From Schnaufer L. Conjoined twins. In: Raffensperger JG, ed. Swenson's pediatric surgery, 5th ed. Norwalk, CT: Appleton & Lange, 1990:971.)

Figure 32.20. Ischiopagus twins. (Reproduced with permission from Holder TM, Ashcraft KW. Pediatric surgery. Philadelphia: WB Saunders, 1980:1107.)

Figure 32.19. Thoracopagus twins successfully separated at Egleston Children's Hospital at Emory University in 1985. Both are now living a normal life. (Courtesy of Ricketts R. Egleston Children's Hospital at Emory University, 1985.)

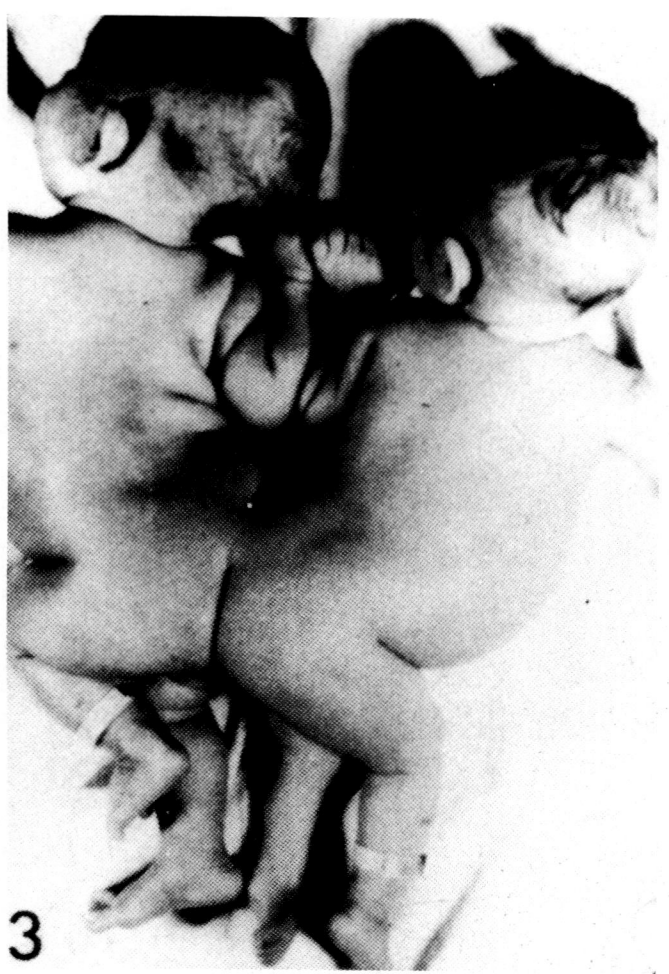

Figure 32.21. Pygopagus twins. (Reproduced with permission from Holder TM, Ashcraft KW. Pediatric surgery. Philadelphia:

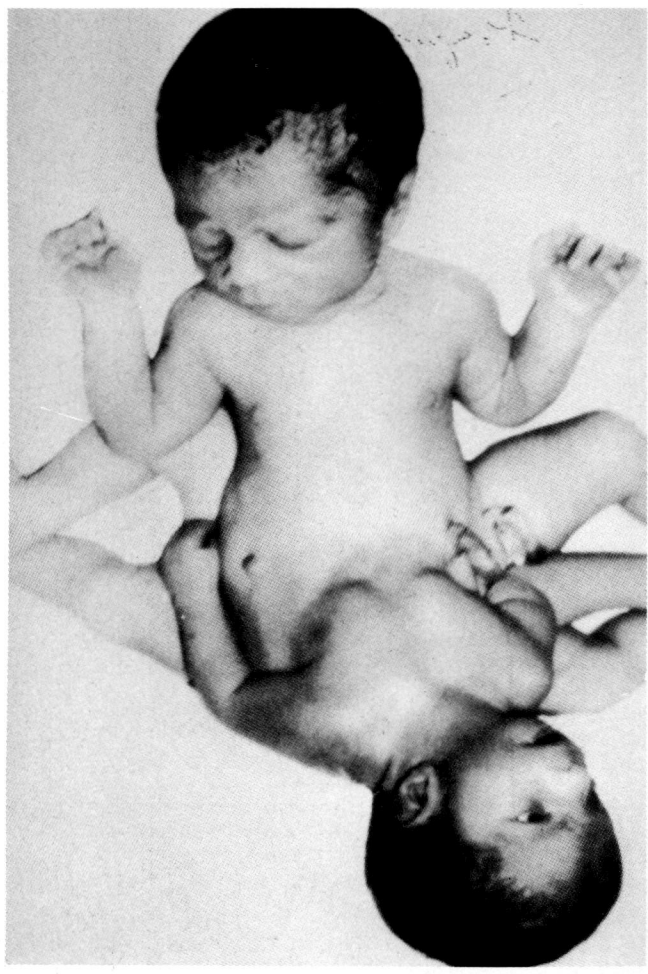

Figure 32.22. Ischiopagus twins. (From Mustard WT et al. Pediatric surgery, 2nd ed. Chicago: Year Book Medical Publishers, 1969:675.)

been improved survivorship of conjoined twins during the past decade.

EDITORIAL COMMENT

Parents of conjoined twins are always anxious to have their babies separated and want both babies to survive. It is no longer acceptable to allow a set of Siamese twins to survive into adulthood as was the case with the original Siamese twins, Chang and Eng Bunker. Nevertheless, in many instances it is simply not possible to separate Siamese twins and have both children survive. In these cir-

cumstances, it is often helpful to explain to the parents that only one child is complete, and in a very real sense, the other part of the twin is like a malignant tumor or teratoma which must be removed to allow one twin to survive. Many anguishing decisions are involved in the treatment of complicated Siamese twins, such as separating twins with three lower extremities in which one twin will obviously have only one leg. In such instances, parents will almost always opt to have the babies separated because they feel a child with one leg can be functional, and indeed, if all that is missing is one leg, such children can have very useful lives (JAH, CAP).

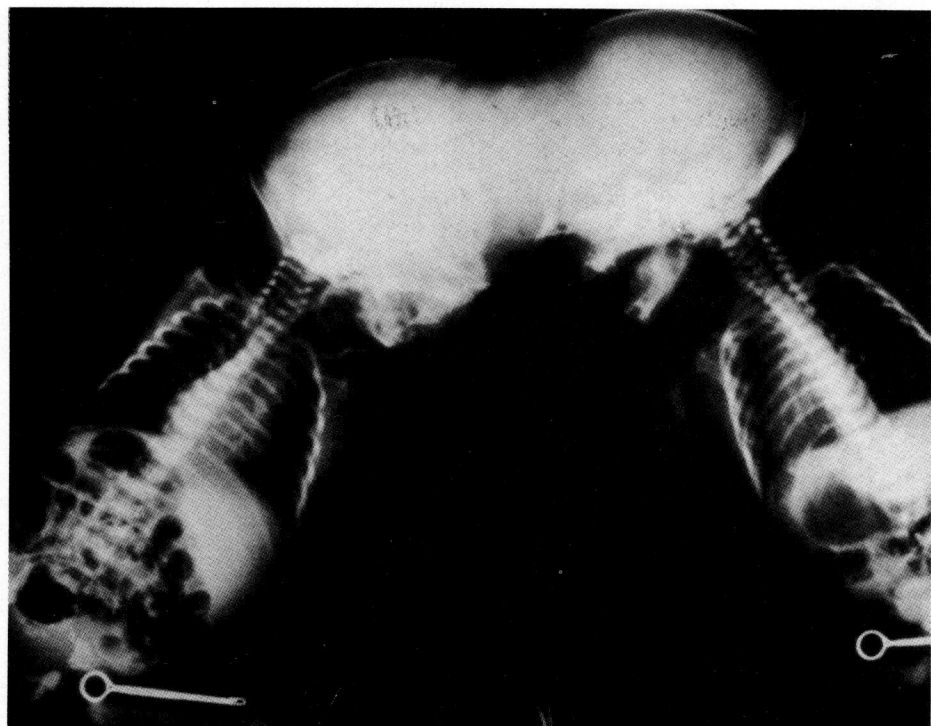

Figure 32.23. Craniopagus twins with connection from brow to vertex. (From Mustard WT et al. Pediatric surgery, 2nd ed. Chicago: Year Book Medical Publishers, 1969:674.)

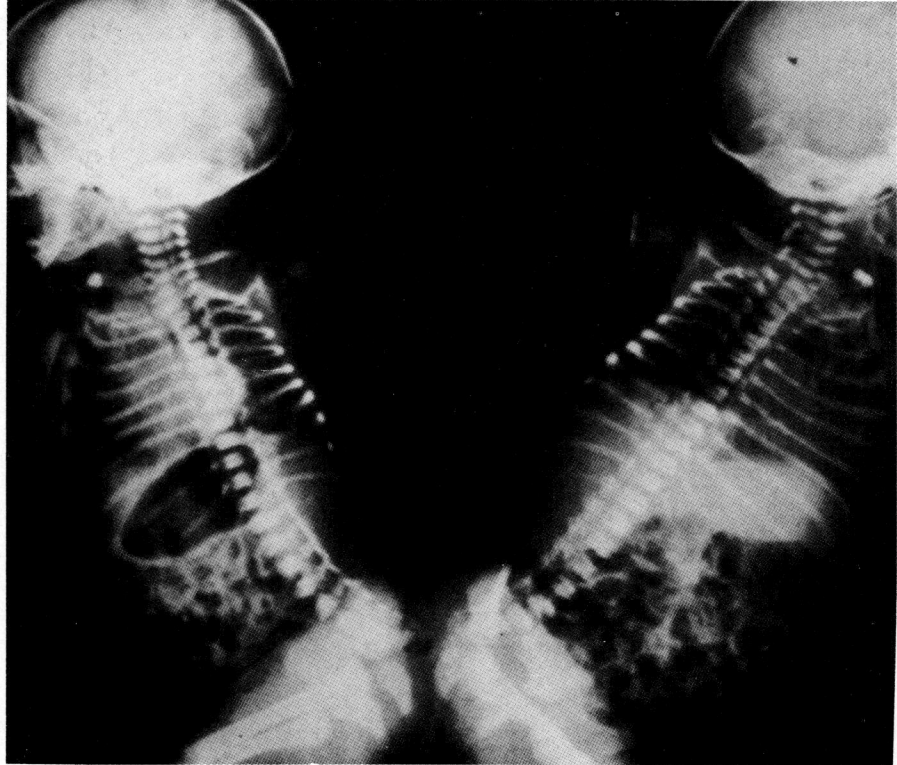

Figure 32.24. Pygopagus twins. (From Mustard WT et al. Pediatric surgery, 2nd ed. Chicago: Year Book Medical Publishers, 1969:673.)

REFERENCES

1. Rock J, Hertig A. The human conceptus during the first two weeks of gestation. Am J Obstet Gynecol 1948;55:6.
2. Hamilton WJ, Mossman HW. Human embryology, 4th ed, Baltimore: Williams & Wilkins, 1960.
3. O'Rahilly R, Miller F. Developmental stages in human embryos. Washington, DC: Carnegie Institution of Washington Publication, 1987:637.
4. Gilbert GS. Pictorial human embryology. Seattle: University of Washington Press, 1989.
5. Schnaufer L. Conjoined twins. In: Raffensperger JG, ed. Swenson's pediatric surgery, 5th ed. Norwalk, CT: Appleton & Lange, 1990:969–978.
6. Spencer R. Conjoined twins: theoretical embryologic basis. Teratology 1992;45:591–602.
7. Zimmerman AA. Embryologic and anatomic considerations of conjoined twins. In: Bergsma D, ed. Birth defects: original article series. Conjoined twins. The National Foundation-March of Dimes, Birth Defects 1967;3(1):18–27.
8. Stockard CR. Developmental rate and structural expressivity. Am J Anat 1921;28:115.
9. Potter EL, Craig JM. Pathology of the fetus in the infant, 3rd ed. Chicago: Year Book Medical Publishers, 1975:1–220.
10. Hirst and Piersol. Human monstrosities. Philadelphia: Lea Brothers, 1891;1:17.
11. Hoyle RM. Surgical separation of conjoined twins. Surg Gynecol Obstet 1990;170:549–562.
12. Guttmacher AF, Nichols BL. Teratology of conjoined twins. In: Bergsma D, ed. Birth defects: original article series. Conjoined twins. The National Foundation-March of Dimes, Birth Defects 1967;3(1):3–9.
13. Rudolph AJ, Michaels JP, Nicholes BL. Obstetric managment of conjoined twins. In: Bergsma D, ed. Birth defects: original article series. Conjoined twins. The National Foundation-March of Dimes, Birth Defects 1967;3(1):28.
14. Shively RE, Vermant MA, Bucholz RD. Separation of craniopagus twins utilizing tissue expanders. Plast Reconstr Surg 1985;76:765–772.
15. Spencer RP, Rockoff ML, Nichols BL, Johnson PC. Radioisotopic flow studies in conjoined twins. In: Bergsma D, ed. Birth defects: original article series. Conjoined twins. The National Foundation-March of Dimes, Birth Defects 1967;3(1):120–122.
16. Ross AJ III, O'Neill JA Jr, Silverman DG, Brousseau DA, Gatti JE, Templeton JM Jr. A new technique for evaluating cutaneous vascularity in complicated conjoined twins. J Pediatr Surg 1985;20:743–746.
17. Ricketts RR, Zubowicz VN. Use of tissue expansion for separation and primary closure of thoracopagus twins. Pediatr Surg Int 1987;2:365–368.
18. Spitz L, Capps SNJ, Kiley EM. Colon xipho-omphaloischiopagus tripus conjoined twins: successful separation following abdominal wall expansion. J Pediatr Surg 1991;26:26–29.
19. Zuker RM, Filler RM, Roopnarine L. Intra-abdominal tissue expansion: an adjunct in the separation of conjoined twins. J Pediatr Surg 1986;21:1198–1200.
20. Walton JM, Gillis DA, Giacomantonio JM, Hayashi AH, Lau HY. Emergency separation of conjoined twins. J Pediatr Surg 1991;26:1337–1340.
21. Pepper CK. Ethical and moral considerations in the separation of conjoined twins: summary of two dialogues between physicians and clergymen. In: Bergsma D, ed. Birth defects: original article series. Conjoined twins. The National Foundation-March of Dimes, Birth Defects 1967;3(1):128–134.
22. Votteler TP. Conjoined twins. In: Welch KJ, Randolph JG, Ravitch MM, O'Neill JA Jr, Rowe MI, eds. Pediatric surgery. Chicago: Year Book Medical Publishers, 1986:771–779.
23. O'Neill JA Jr et al. Surgical experience with thirteen conjoined twins. Ann Surg 1988;208:299–312.

INTRAUTERINE SURGERY FOR THE CREATION AND STUDY OF CONGENITAL ANOMALIES

J. Alexander Haller, Jr. / Charles Paidas

Pour les vaincre, il nous faut de l'audace; encore de l'audace, toujours de l'audace; et la France est sauvé.
—*DANTON*
(*DELIVERED IN THE NATIONAL ASSEMBLY, SEPTEMBER 2, 1792, ON THE DEFENSE OF THE REPUBLIC.*)

General surgeons are, basically, clinical physiologists. Pediatric surgeons have evolved from their general surgery progenitors because they are clinical embryologists as well as physiologists for the newborn. Intrauterine or fetal surgery is a natural research field for those interested in congenital abnormalities because it provides a laboratory approach to the study of the pathophysiology of clinically challenging congenital anomalies, such as diaphragmatic hernia (1, 2) and gastroschisis (3). To serve as a background for this discussion of intrauterine surgery, a brief history of the development of fetal surgery is in order.

BRIEF HISTORY OF INTRAUTERINE SURGERY

The first recorded primitive observation on the living mammalian fetus was by the German anatomist Bichat in 1803. In 1877 two German publications described delivery of guinea pig fetuses with temporary suspension in warm saline. These animals died rapidly and could not be returned to the uterus. In 1918 Mayer (4) first described successful fetal surgery in the form of limb amputation on fetal guinea pigs through a small uterine incision. In that same year it was demonstrated that fetuses undergoing intrauterine surgery could complete normal development and delivery.

The modern era of intrauterine studies began in 1936 with the exquisite studies of Barcroft and his student Dawes (5), who presented a series of papers, describing intrauterine fetal procedures and permitting the accumulation of a large amount of physiologic data which identified them as pioneers in fetal physiology. The lamb was chosen as the animal of choice and introduced the possibility of chronic models of congenital abnormalities. In 1945 Barron (6) introduced the concept of surgical marsupialization of the fetus to the wall of the uterus to decrease amniotic fluid losses and prevent miscarriage. In 1955 Chris Barnard (7), working under his teacher Professor Janney Louw, created a definitive model of congenital anomaly in the form of intestinal atresia by ligating the mesenteric blood vessels of fetal puppies. Although there was a tremendous attrition rate in the 45 experimental animals, with only two live born pups, he established the fact that a so-called congenital anomaly could result from an environmental influence, such as a vascular accident, and introduced a second potential etiology for congenital birth defects in addition to genetic deficiencies. In 1960 Jackson et al. (8) demonstrated a model of continuous monitoring by exteriorized electrodes in fetal puppies which enabled extensive studies of the cardiovascular system of developing animals. In 1964 Silverstein (9, 10) began a series of fundamental studies on developmental immunology and has become a pioneer in the field of fetal immunologic responses.

In the course of these 50 years of modern fetal research, a number of important principles have evolved which make intrauterine surgery a predictably satisfactory research tool. These include the concept that maternal anesthesia does not prohibit fetal viability, although certain anesthetic agents are much safer than others. Experience has demonstrated that the fetus is extremely sensitive to decreased body temperature, to small blood losses, and to excessive amniotic fluid loss during operative manipulation. Any environmental change which creates a need for rapid adjustment on the part of the fetus is likely to result in fetal death. In the course of surgical maneuvers, when fetal respiration occurs in the extrauterine environment, it is impossible to return the fetus to a continuing intrauterine existence. Exposure of the umbilical cord to temperature changes and drying usually results in severe spasm of the umbilical vessels with secondary fetal hypoxia and eventual, if not immediate, death of the animal.

Throughout these studies, it has become apparent that

there is a very wide variation in different species in regard to the hardiness of the fetus to manipulation and exposure. Accumulated data suggests that the sheep fetus is far superior in this regard to other available experimental animals, and the sheep is followed in descending order of hardiness by rabbits, pigs, and dogs.

In 1967 Haller and associates carried out a series of intrauterine operative procedures to elucidate the function of the fetal ductus arteriosus (11). Much experimental work had been done to identify factors responsible for the closure of the ductus arteriosus at birth, but there was the tacit assumption that a closed ductus arteriosus was incompatible with fetal life. A satisfactory technique for the intrauterine ligation of the ductus arteriosus was developed, and the acute and chronic effects of occlusion were studied in fetal dogs.

After ligation of the ductus arteriosus in fetal puppies, electrocardiograph (ECG) leads were attached to their limbs and these were exteriorized through the mother's abdominal incision. In other animals, the fetus was delivered from the uterus and cine-radiographic studies were performed by inserting a catheter into either the external jugular vein or the umbilical vein. Cine-radiographic examinations were made with injections before opening the chest, after thoracotomy, before and after occlusion of the ductus arteriosus, and after inflation of the lungs performed by tracheostomy intubation. Appropriate intralitter controls were simultaneously studied.

The conclusions of the initial studies were that acute and chronic electrocardiographic tracings and measurements of pulmonary artery and left atrial pressures could be carried out successfully. The viability of the fetal puppy after occlusion of the ductus arteriosus could be maintained in utero until normal birth.

Of great interest was the unexpected observation that, while viability was maintained in utero, no fetal animals with the ductus arteriosus occluded were born alive, apparently because of secondary thrombosis of the pulmonary artery. This suggested an hypothesis that the function of the ductus arteriosus in the fetus appears to be the time-honored one of bypassing the lungs and allowing run-off for the right ventricular output, thus ensuring a functionally adequate right ventricle, with the additional suggestion that the ductus also guarantees patency of the main pulmonary artery at the time of birth.

In 1973 another series of intrauterine procedures was carried out to study the effect of coarctation of the aorta on the developing cardiovascular system (12, 13). The model was designed to answer the question, "What is the explanation for the high mortality of preductal coarctation?" Why do some infants with coarctations of the aorta have severe circulatory problems at birth, whereas others are practically asymptomatic?

Using a standard technique for intrauterine surgery in the fetal lamb, preductal and postductal coarctation was created in random animals by tying a ligature over a probe in the preductal position of the aorta to produce a 1-mm lumen, and in the postductal position to produce a 3–5-mm lumen. This distal position would not permit a tighter coarctation because inadequate return of arterial blood to the placenta resulted in a high fetal loss if a severe stenosis was in the postductal position. Spontaneous delivery was allowed in most animals, although a few lambs were delivered by cesarean section. Careful angiographic studies revealed that the ductus arteriosus closed spontaneously in lambs with coarctation in both the preductal and postductal positions. Cardiac catheterization studies in the newborn subjects detected no significant hemodynamic differences between the two positions of the coarctated segment.

The collateral circulation, as measured visually from the aortograms, was not noticeably different in the two groups of animals. This was a surprising finding because it had been the author's hypothesis that the preductal position of the coarctation would not stimulate the development of intrauterine fetal collateral circulation because of the bypass available through the ductus arteriosus. Therefore, at birth, when the patent ductus arteriosus (PDA) closed, there would be inadequate collateral and the baby would die. In contrast, coarctation in the postductal position would put immediate strain on the vascular system necessitating the development of more extensive collateral circulation in the fetus. This, in turn, would permit adequate aortic flow in the newborn baby after closure of the ductus. These events did not take place in this experimental model. Therefore these studies on pre- and postductal coarction of the aorta in fetal lambs did not offer a better explanation for the high mortality associated with preductal coarctation than Abbott's classical one that there are usually intracardiac anomalies associated with preductal coarctation and it is these which cause the high mortality.

In 1974 the perplexing and frustrating problem of the management of infants with gastroschisis was the focus of a model of this anomaly in fetal sheep. This work was carried out at Johns Hopkins University (3). The pathologic anatomy of infants with exposed bowel and gastroschisis has not been carefully studied, nor is there data to explain the dysfunction in peristalsis and the digestive malabsorption which is typical of this condition. Since living human tissue from this anomaly is rarely available for sequential study, an animal model of gastroschisis was designed to help clarify the pathogenesis and pathophysiology of this congenital abnormality.

Gastroschisis was created in fetal lambs by excising a full-thickness disc of abdominal wall, lateral to the umbilical cord. This allowed evisceration of intestine, and the animals were then returned to their intrauterine environment where the exposed bowel remained in contact with the amniotic fluid throughout the remainder of the pregnancy. The results of this study indicated that the experimental model was grossly and microscopically similar to this anomaly in human infants. Histologic studies of the exposed, eviscerated intestine demonstrated interstitial edema without cellular infiltration which appeared to result from contact with amniotic fluid. The specific damage to the myenteric ganglion cells and progressive disappearance of ATP-ase in the muscle of exposed bowel strongly suggested an alteration in neural conduction and a decrease in contractile potential. Preliminary enzyme studies have shown concomitant abnormalities in intracellular enzymes within the mucosa of the exposed bowel, which may well be responsible for malabsorption associated with this condition. Further studies are in progress to define more precisely these enzymatic deficiencies and also to give a better picture of the pathogenesis of bowel damage associated with gastroschisis.

In 1976, studies of pulmonary and ductal hemodynamics in fetal and newborn lambs with simulated diaphragmatic herniae were reported (14). Hypoxemia, acidosis, and persistent pulmonary hypertension were known to be responsible for the high mortality of newborn infants with congenital diaphragmatic hernias. An important factor in this pathophysiology appears to be differential pulmonary blood flow and variable right-to-left shunting through the ductus arteriosus.

A fetal model of posterior (Bochdalek) diaphragmatic hernia was designed to permit studies of pulmonary and ductal hemodynamics in fetal and newborn lambs (14). A silicone polymer balloon was inserted through a small left thoracotomy in fetal lambs of 100 days' gestation. The intrapleural balloon was designed with a 2-cm nipple which protruded through the chest incision and lay subcutaneously. The balloon was inflated through the nipple with 60 cc of saline to simulate herniation of bowel and liver into the left chest.

At term, after the inflated balloon had been in place for 30 to 40 days, the fetus was delivered by cesarean section. Central (preductal) arterial PO_2 was monitored through a carotid arterial catheter and peripheral (postductal) arterial PO_2 via the femoral artery. Pulmonary angiography and technetium microsphere scans were carried out; both studies demonstrated decreased perfusion to the ipsilateral left lung at birth. Following deflation of the balloon, no increase in perfusion occurred immediately; but after 3 weeks, perfusion was markedly improved. Right-to-left shunts via the ductus arteriosus were measured at various times with green dye–dilution techniques.

This model appeared to simulate closely the pathophysiology of diaphragmatic hernia, and preliminary data suggested that a better understanding of this important congenital anomaly would be forthcoming (14–16).

SPECIAL CONSIDERATIONS OF INDIVIDUAL ORGAN SYSTEM ANOMALIES

Congenital Diaphragmatic Hernia

Besides the early studies carried out by Haller (3, 11–14) and associates in Baltimore and deLorimer (1, 2) and associates in San Francisco, little activity was reported until Harrison's group repeated some of the Hopkins' experiments in 1980 using their model of a balloon-filled fetal chest to simulate diaphragmatic hernia and compression of the developing lung (17–21). A similar model was reported by Pringle in 1984 with studies of fetal lung development (22–25). Beginning in 1985 Harrison and his associates, particularly Adzick, reported early prenatal diagnostic findings focused on the diaphragmatic hernia (26). This was rapidly applied to prediction of outcome from these prenatal diagnostic studies and led in 1989 and 1990 to their report of the initial clinical experience of Harrison's group in San Francisco (20, 21). In 1985 Harrison and associates (27) reported their cumulative experience in prenatal diagnosis and related it to the natural history of the fetus with congenital diaphragmatic hernia. Ford (28) reported another human case in 1990.

Urinary Tract Anomalies

Beginning in 1964 Chez and associates (29, 30) reported an observation of fetal renal development and function and developed models of congenital urinary tract obstruction. These were extended in the laboratory of Harrison and associates in the 1980s and led to the initial attempts at clinical correction of obstructed uropathy, which was reported by Crombleholme et al in 1988 (31).

Hydrocephalus and Other Central Nervous System Anomalies

Hydrocephalus was created in the fetal animal by Michejda in 1984 (32). Other studies have followed which have led to a few attempts at clinical correction of continuing hydrocephalus in utero, but most of these clinical reports indicate a very poor outcome with little interruption of the pathophysiologic process. Other studies have been reported on early observations associated with neural tube defects, specifically myelomeningocele. Preliminary studies have been reported by Heffez and associates

(33), who appear to have developed an intrauterine model of meningomyelocele which exposes the fetal sacral neural structures to amniotic fluid, resulting in thickening and fibrosis. This is reminiscent, of course, of the same process in which bowel is exposed to amniotic fluid in the gastroschisis model.

ETHICAL AND PRACTICAL CONSIDERATIONS IN HUMAN INTRAUTERINE SURGERY

Pringle has recently commented in general on some of the ethical issues associated with fetal surgery. Some of the practical considerations are addressed in an unpublished chapter, entitled "Fetal Surgery: Practical Considerations and Current Status," by Pringle from his new base in Wellington, New Zealand. At least one editorial comment has focused on that chapter, which is entitled "Further Considerations Regarding Fetal Surgery" by Haller. The conclusion of Haller's discussion states that "we truly need more experimental primate data before undertaking more extensive human trials." However, if the patients being managed preoperatively, intrauterine, and postoperatively by Harrison's group have truly given uncoerced, informed consent, then the groups' limited and carefully documented *human experiments* may be very helpful to all who are laboring in the vineyard of fetal surgery. These studies could contribute significantly to further understanding of the pathophysiology of congenital diaphragmatic hernia and possibly lead the way toward other clinical applications. Most congenital abnormalities do not result in death of the fetus, and thus studies of intrauterine surgery both prepare the pediatric surgeon technically and increases his understanding of the pathophysiology of anomalies, thus arming him or her for better, more aggressive corrective surgical management immediately after birth of the defective child. This is probably the greatest usefulness of pediatric surgeons' involvement in the fetal laboratory.

And by all means we must paraphrase what Danton stated.

"To conquer we have need to dare, to dare again, always to dare!" And the unborn baby with congenital anomalies perhaps will be saved!

All of us (editors, contributors and consultants) regret that we were born too soon, remembering what a great American, Benjamin Franklin, stated in 1780, "The rapid progress true science now makes, occasions my regretting sometimes that I was born too soon."

John E. Skandalakis, M.D., PhD.

REFERENCES

1. deLorimier AA, Tierney DF, Parker HR: Hypoplastic lungs in fetal lambs with surgically produced congenital diaphragmatic hernia. Surgery 1967;62:12–17.
2. Starrett RW, deLorimier AA. Congenital diaphragmatic hernia in lambs: hemodynamic and ventilatory changes with breathing. J Pediatr Surg 1975;10:575–582.
3. Haller JA Jr, Kehrer BH, Shaker IJ, Shermeta DW, Wyllie RG: Studies of the pathophysiology of gastroschisis in fetal sheep. J Pediatr Surg 1974;9:627–632.
4. Mayer A. Uber die Moglichkeit operativer Eingriffe beim lebenden Saugetierfotus. Zentralbl Gynak 1918;42:773–776.
5. Dawes GS, Mott JC. The vascular tone of the foetal lung. J Physiol 1962;164:465–477.
6. Barron DH. The role of the sensory fibers in the differentiation of the spinal cord in sheep. J Exp Zool 1945;100:431–443.
7. Barnard CN, Louw JH. Congenital intestinal atresia. Lancet 1955;2:1065–1067.
8. Jackson BT, Clarke JP, Egdahl RH. Direct lead fetal electrocardiography with undisturbed fetal maternal relationships. Surg Gynecol Obstet 1960;110:687–692.
9. Silverstein AM, Pendergast RD, Kramer KL. Fetal response to antigenic stimulus. J Exp Med 1964;119–955.
10. Parshall CJ, Silverstein AM. Surgical approaches to the study of fetal immunology in primate animals. Ann NY Acad Sci 1969;162:254–266.
11. Haller JA Jr, Morgan WW Jr, Rodgers BM, Gengos DG, Margulies ST. Chronic hemodynamic effects of occluding the fetal ductus arteriosus. Thorac Cardiovasc Surg 1967;54:770–784.
12. Haller JA Jr, Shaker IJ, Gingell R, Ho CH. Intrauterine production of coarctation of the aorta. J Thorac Cardiovasc Surg 1973;66:343–349.
13. Haller JA Jr, Suzuki H, El Shafie M, Shaker IJ. Intrauterine production of coarctation of the aorta with normal birth and survival. J Pediatr Surg 1973;8:171–174.
14. Haller JA Jr et al. Pulmonary and ductal hemodynamics in studies of simulated diaphragmatic hernia of fetal and newborn lambs. J Pediatr Surg 1976;11:675–680.
15. Kitagawa M, Hislop A, Boyden EA, Reid L. Lung hypoplasia in congenital diaphragmatic hernia: a quantitative study of airway, artery and alveolar development. Br J Surg 1971;58:342–346.
16. Oliver RT, Rupp WM, Telander RL, Kaye MP. Hemodynamics of congenital diaphragmatic hernia in lambs. J Pediatr Surg 1978;13:231–235.
17. Harrison MR, Bressack MA, Churg AM, deLorimier AA. Correction of congenital diaphragmatic hernia in utero. II. Simulated correction permits fetal lung growth with survival at birth. Surgery 1980;88:260–268.
18. Harrison MR, Jester JA, Ross NA. Correction of congenital diaphragmatic hernia in utero. I. The model: intrathoracic balloon produces fatal pulmonary hypoplasia. Surgery 1980;88:174–182.
19. Harrison MR, Ross NA, deLorimier AA. Correction of congenital diaphragmatic hernia in utero. III. Development of a successful surgical technique using abdominoplasty to avoid compromise of umbilical blood flow. J Pediatr Surg 1981;16:934–942.
20. Harrison MR. Fetal diaphragmatic hernia. In: Puri P, ed. Congenital diaphragmatic hernia: Modern Problems in Paediatrics. Basel: Karger, 1989:130–142.
21. Harrison MR et al. Correction of congenital diaphragmatic hernia in utero. V. Initial clinical experience. J Pediatr Surg 1990;25:47–57.
22. Pringle KC, Turner JW, Schofield JC, Soper RT. Creation and repair of diaphragmatic hernia in the fetal lamb: lung development and morphology. J Pediatr Surg 1984;19:131–140.

23. Pringle KC. Fetal lamb and fetal lamb lung growth following creation and repair of a diaphragmatic hernia. Nathanialsz PW, ed. Animal models in fetal medicine. Ithaca, NY: Perinatology Press, 1984:109–148.

24. Pringle KC. Human fetal lung development and related animal models. Clin Obstet Gynecol 1986;29:502–513.

25. Pringle KC. Lung development in congenital diaphragmatic hernia. In: Puri P, ed. Congenital diaphragmatic hernia: Modern Problems in Paediatrics Basel: Karger, 1989;24:28–53.

26. Adzick NS et al. Diaphragmatic hernia in the fetus: prenatal diagnosis and outcome in 94 cases. J Pediatr Surg 1985;20:357–361.

27. Nakayama dK et al. Prenatal diagnosis and natural history of the fetus with a congenital diaphragmatic hernia: initial clinical experience. J Pediatr Surg 1985;20:118–124.

28. Ford WDA. Silastic patch placed via a thoracotomy for fetal repair of diaphragmatic hernia with liver in the chest. Presented at the ninth annual meeting of the International Fetal Medicine and Surgery Society. Rotorua, New Zealand, February 23–28, 1990.

29. Chez RA, Sith FG, Hutchinson DL. Renal function in the intrauterine primate fetus. I. Experimental technique: rate of formation and chemical composition of urine. Am J Obstet Gynecol 1964;90:128–131.

30. Chez RA, Hutchinson DL. The use of experimental surgical techniques in the pregnant *Macaca mulatta*. Ann NY Acad Sci 1969;162:249–253.

31. Crombleholme TM et al. Early experience with open fetal surgery for congenital hydronephrosis. J Pediatr Surg 1988;23:1114–1131.

32. Michejda M, Patronus N, deChiro G, Hodger GD. Fetal hydrocephalus. II. Amelioration of fetal porencephaly by in utero therapy in nonhuman primates. JAMA 1984;251:2548–2552.

INDEX

Page numbers in *italics* denote figures; those followed by "t" denote tables.

Abdominal aorta, 1018, 1024
  coarctation of, 1009
Abdominal defect, 563–577
  classification, 563
  surgical anatomy of umbilical region, 563–564, *564*
  umbilical cord anatomy, 564–565, 565t, *565–568*
  umbilical hernia, 565–568
    anatomy, 565, 567, *569*
    embryogenesis, 567
    incidence, 567
    symptoms, 567
    treatment, 567–568
Abdominal muscle, absence of, with urinary tract defect, 586–588
  anatomy, 586–587
  diagnosis, 588
  incidence, 587
  prognosis, 588
  symptoms, 587
  treatment, 588
Abdominal muscle aplasia, without urinary tract defect, 585–586
Abdominal muscle variation, 577–578
  aponeurotic cleft, of external oblique layer, 577, *577*
  internal oblique muscle, 577–578, *578*
Abdominal wall, anterior, 544–545, *544–545*
Aberrant pancreas, 385–388
  diagnosis, 387–388
  distribution, 385–386, *386*
  embryogenesis, 386–387, *387*
  history, 387
  incidence, 387
  symptoms, 387–388
  treatment, 388
Accessory coronary arteries, 962–963, *963–965*
Accessory diaphragm, 530, *532*, 532–535, *534–535*
  anatomy, 533–534, *534–535*
  diagnosis, 535
  embryogenesis, 534–535
  symptoms, 535
  treatment, 535
Accessory ovary, 756
Accessory spleens, greater omentum, 125
Accessory suprarenal gland, 729–730, 730t, *731*
Achalasia, 100–104, *101*, *103*
Acinus, pancreas, 366–367
Adenomyoma, gallbladder, 323
Adenomyomata, stomach, 174
Adhesions
  gastroduodenal, 176
  greater omentum, congenital, 122
Adrenal hyperplasia, 733
Adrenogenital syndrome, 856, *858–860*, 858–860
Aganglionic bladder, 708
Aganglionic megacolon, congenital. *See* Hirschsprung's disease
Aganglionosis, small intestines, 230–231
Agastria, 154–155, 155t
  diagnosis, 154–155
  embryogenesis, 154
  history, 154

symptoms, 154
treatment, 154–155
Age, gestational
  at malformation occurrence, 7, *8*
  and normal embryonic development, developmental stages, 9–12, 11t
  when developmental errors arise, 7, *8*
Agenesis
  anal, 261
    with fistula, 266
  anorectal, 261, 266
  bladder, *677*
  clitoris, 793
  colon, 245–246
  glans penis, 790–791
  greater omentum, 120
  internal, carotid artery, *1002–1003*, 1003
  kidney, 604–612, *605*
    bilateral, 605–608
      anatomy, 605–606, *606*
      associated anomalies, 606
      diagnosis, 607, 607t
      embryogenesis, 606, *606*
      history, 606–607
      mortality, 607–608
      symptoms, 607
    unilateral, 608–610
      associated anomalies, *605*, 608–609
      diagnosis, 610
      embryogenesis, 609, *610*
      history, 609–610
      incidence, 608
      solitary kidney, 608
      symptoms, 610
      treatment, 610
  lung
    bilateral, 420–421
    unilateral, 429–432
  penis, 789–790, *791*
    embryogenesis, 789
    history, 789–790
    incidence, 789–790
    treatment, 790
  pharynx, median anlage, 50
  spleen, 356–360
  suprarenal glands, 723
  trachea, 421–422
  tracheal, 421–422
Alveolar dysplasia, 444–445
Amastia, *560*, 560–563
Ampulla, pancreas, 373–374, *374*
Ampullary lithiasis, pancreatitis, 374, *374*
Anal
  agenesis, with fistula, 266
  membranous atresia, *265*, 265–266
  stenosis, *265*, *265*
Anastomosis
  arteriovenous, spleen, 356
  esophagus, 79–81
Aneurysm, sinus of Valsalva, 1003–1005, *1004*, 1004t
Angiodysplasia, gastric, 176–178
Annular pancreas, 379–385
  anatomy, 379, *380–381*
  associated anomalies, 379–380
  diagnosis, 382–384, *384*
  embryogenesis, 380–381, *382*
  history, 381

incidence, 381–382
symptoms, 382, *383*
treatment, 384–385
Anomaly, congenital. *See* Congenital anomaly
Anorectal agenesis, 261, 266
Anorectal anomalies
  agenesis, 261
  anal agenesis, 261
    with fistula, 266
  anal defect, 259
  anal stenosis, 259, 261–262
  anatomy, 259–261, *262–264*
  anorectal agenesis, 266
  associated anomalies, 261–262, 264
  atresia, birth prevalence of, 5
  classification, 259–261, *260*, 261t
  cloaca, 266–268
  covered anus, 261
  diagnosis, 269–272, *270–273*
  embryogenesis, 264–266, *265*, *267–268*
  history, 266, 269
  incidence, 261, 264t, 269, 269t, 270, 270t
  membranous atresia, 261
  mortality, 274
  rectal atresia, 261
  symptoms, 269
  treatment, *270–271*, *272–273*
Anterior abdominal wall, 544–545, *544–545*
Anterior body wall, 540–593
  abdominal defect, 563–577
    classification, 563
    surgical anatomy of umbilical region, 563–564, *564*
    umbilical cord anatomy, 564–565, 565t, *565–568*
    umbilical hernia, anatomy, 565, 567, *569*
  abdominal muscle, absence of, with urinary tract defect, 586–588
    anatomy, 586–587
    diagnosis, 588
    history, 587
    prognosis, 588
    symptoms, 587
    treatment, 588
  abdominal muscle aplasia, without urinary tract defect, 585–586
  abdominal muscle variation, 577–578
    aponeurotic cleft, of external oblique layer, 577, *577*
    internal oblique muscle, 577–578, *578*
  amastia, *560*, 560–563
  anomalies of, *545*, 545–588, 546t
  anterior abdominal wall, 544–545, *544–545*
  anterior thoracic wall, 540–544, *541–543*
  defects of
    and ectopia cordis, 551–559
      sternal defect without displacement of heart, 551–552
    embryogenesis, 554–555, *558*
    history, 555–556
    incidence, 556
    prognosis, 557, 559
    sternal defects with ectopia cordis, 552–553, *553*, *556–557*

Anterior body wall—*continued*
  sternal defects without displacement of heart
    absence of sternal elements, 552, *552–553*
    failure of sternal fusion, 552, *554–555*
    symptoms, 556
    treatment, 556–557, *558–559*
  breast
    amastia, *560*, 560–563
    athelia, 560–563
  closure of body wall, critical events in, 545
  congenital anomalies of breast, 559
  development, 540–545, *541–542*
  ectopia cordis, 551–559
  ectopic breast, 560–561, *562*
  exomphalos, 568–574
  gastroschisis, 574–577
    anatomy, 574, *575*
    embryogenesis, 574–576
    history, 576, 576t
    incidence, 576, 576t
    treatment, 576–577
  hydrocele, 578–580
  inguinal hernia, 578–580
  intussusception at umbilicus, 577
  omphalocele, 568–574
    anatomy, 568–569, *570*
    associated anomalies, 569–570, 571t
    diagnosis, 568, 572
    embryogenesis, *547*, 570–571
    etiology, 568
    history, 571, *571–572*
    incidence, 571–572
    massive, 572, *573*
    medium, 572, *573*
    mortality, 573–574
    prognosis, 573–574
    small, 572
    treatment, 572
      conservative, 572–573
  polymastia, 560–563, *561*
  polythelia, 560–563, *561*
  processus vaginalis, incomplete closure, 578–584
    anatomy, 578–580, *579–580*
    definition, 578
    diagnosis, 583
    embryogenesis, *579*, 581
    hernial sac, contents of, 581
    history, 582t, 582–583
    hydrocele, 583
    predisposing conditions, 581–582
    symptoms, 583
    treatment, 583–584
  prune belly syndrome, 585–586
  rib anomalies, 550–551
    associated anomalies, 551
    diagnosis, 551
    Poland's syndrome, 551, *551*
    treatment, 551
    unilateral thoracic wall aplasia, *550*, 550–551
  supernumerary breast, 560–563, *561*
    associated anomalies, 562
    diagnosis, 563
    embryogenesis, 562
    history, 562–563
    number of, 562
    structure of, 561–562
    symptoms, 563
    treatment, 563
  thorax
    anomalies of, 545–559
    dystrophy, 551

transversus abdominis, 578, *578*
varicocele, 584–585
  defined, 584
  scrotal anatomy, 584t, 584–585
    cremaster muscle, 584
    external spermatic fascia, 584
    internal spermatic fascia, 584
    tunica vaginalis, 584
  scrotum
    diagnosis, 585
    embryogenesis, 585
    etiology, 585
    symptoms, 585
    treatment, 585
Anterior thoracic wall, 540–544, *541–543*. *See also* Anterior body wall
  defects of, and ectopia cordis, 551–559
Anus
  agenesis, 261
  covered, 261
  stenosis, 259, 261–262
Aorta
  abdominal, 1018, 1024
    coarctation of, 1009
  arch. *See also* Aortic arch
    atresia, 943–944, *944*
    stenosis, 944–946, *945*
      subvalvular aortic stenosis, 945
      supravalvular aortic stenosis, 944–945, *945*
      valvular aortic stenosis, 945
  thoracic, 976–1025
    anatomy, *986*, 986t–987t, 986–987, 989t
    anomalies of, 988–1025, *990*, 990t, *1018–1019*
      diagnosis, 987–988
      incidence, 1019t
      occupation, birth defect, odds ratio chart, 1022t–1023t
      race, prevalence, 1024t
      sex, prevalence, 1024t
      surgical outcome, 1020t–1021t
    aortic arch, variations in branches of, 988–992, *991*
    aortic trunk, pulmonary trunk, separation, 982–983, *983–985*
    aorticopulmonary septal defect, 1017–1018
    carotid artery, internal, agenesis, *1002–1003*, 1003
    cervical aortic arch, 1001–1003, *1002*
    coarctation of aorta, 1005–1007
    definitive pulmonary trunk, 982
    definitive thoracic aorta, 980–982, *981*
    development, 976–986, *977*
      aortic arches, 976–980, *977–979*, 978t, 980t
      critical events in, 983–984, *986*
    double aortic arch, 993–995, *994*, 994t, *996–997*
    double ductus arteriosus, 1013, *1014*
    ductus arteriosus, absence of, 1013
    interruption of aortic arch, 1007–1009, *1008*
    left aortic arch, with right descending aorta, *997*, 1000
    left ductus arteriosus
      anomalous, 1013, *1014*
      persistent, 1013
    patent ductus arteriosus, 1010–1013, *1011*
    pseudocoarctation of the aorta, 992–993
      anatomy, 992, *992*
      diagnosis, 993

      embryogenesis, 992
      incidence, 992
      symptoms, 993
      treatment, 993
    retroesophageal subclavian artery, *1000*, 1000–1001
    right aortic arch, 994t, 995–1000, *996–998*, 999t
    right ductus arteriosus, 1013
      persistent, 1013
    right-sided aortic elements, persistence of, 993–1001
      classification, 993, *994*
      double aortic arch, 993–995, *994*, *996–997*
      embryogenesis, 993
    sinus of Valsalva, 1003–1005, *1004*, 1004t
      aneurysm of, 1003–1005, *1004*, 1004t
    truncus arteriosus, persistent, 1013–1017, *1015*
    trunk, pulmonary trunk, separation, 982–983, *983–985*
Aortic arch
  cervical, 1001–1003, *1002*
  coarctation of, 1005–1007
  development, 976–980, *977–979*, 978t, 980t
  double, 993–995, *994*, 994t, *996–997*
  interruption of, 1007–1009, *1008*
  left, with right descending aorta, *997*, 1000
  right, 994t, 995–1000, *996–998*, 999t
  variations in branches of, 988–992, *991*
Aorticopulmonary septal defect, 1013–1017, *1015*, 1017–1018
Aplasia
  abdominal muscle, without urinary tract defect, 585–586
  colon, 245–246
  kidney, 604–612, *605*
  lung, unilateral, *428*, 429–432
  pancreas, 369–370, *370*
  rib, unilateral thoracic wall aplasia, *550*, 550–551
  thymus, 47–48
  uterine tube, 827–828, *828*
  uterus, 827–828, *828*
    associated anomalies, 829
    clinical classification, *828*, 830–831, *830–832*
    embryogenesis, 829, *830*
    history, 829
    incidence, 829–830
    prognosis, 833, 833t
    treatment, 831–832
  vagina
    associated anomalies, 829
    clinical classification, *828*, 830–831, *830–832*
    embryogenesis, 829, *830*
    history, 829
    incidence, 829–830
    prognosis, 833, 833t
    treatment, 831–832
Aponeurotic cleft, of external oblique layer, of abdominal, 577, *577*
Appendix, 243t, 244–245, *274–275*, 274–277
  absence of, 275
  diverticula, 276, *276*
  duplication of, 275–276
  epididymis, 775, *778–779*
    torsion of, 777–780, *784*
  heterotopic mucosa, 277

testis, 775, *778–779*
    torsion of, 777–780, *784*
    variations of, 274–275, *275*
    vesiculosa, female reproductive tract, 823
"Apple peel" atresia, small intestines, 203
Arches, branchial, 17–24, *21*, 25t
Arteriohepatic dysplasia, liver, 293
Ask-Upmark kidney, 632–663
Asplenia, 334–336, 337t, 356–357
Asymmetry
    anomalies of, 1054–1057, 1055t
    errors of, 1057
    hemihypertrophy, 1057
    intrauterine growth retardation, 1057
Athelia, 560–563
Atresia
    anal, *265*, 265–266
    aortic, 943–944, *944*
    cervix, 828, *828*
    colon, 246–247, *246–247*
    duodenal, 162, 163t
    esophageal, *158*, 162
        Down's syndrome, 157
    esophagus, 68–72, *71–72*, 79, 80t, 84
        with tracheoesophageal fistula, 71–72, *72*
    extrahepatic biliary, 297–307
    glottic, 407
    infraglottic, 407
    intrahepatic biliary atresia, 292–293
    larynx, 407–408, *409*
        incomplete, 408, *410*
    mitral valve, 940
    panglottic, 407
    peritoneum, "maypole atresia," 127
    pulmonary, 939–940
        tetralogy of Fallot, ventricular septal defect, 941
        ventricular septal defect, 942–943, *942–943*
    pyloric, 162, 163t
    rectal, 261, 266
    small intestines, 200–212
    stomach, 155–159
        Finney pyloroplasty for, 159
        Heinke-Mikulicz pyloroplasty for, 159
    trachea, 421–422
    tricuspid valve, 936–937, *937*
    urethra, 798–800
        anatomy, 798–799
        diagnosis, 800, *800*
        embryogenesis, 799–800
        history, 800
        incidence, 800
        symptoms, 800
        treatment, 800
    uterus
        clinical classification, *828*, 830–831, *830–832*
        embryogenesis, 829, *830*
        history, 829
        incidence, 829–830
        prognosis, 833, 833t
        treatment, 831–832
    vagina, 828, *828*
        associated anomalies, 829
        clinical classification, *828*, 830–831, *830–832*
        embryogenesis, 829, *830*
        history, 829
        incidence, 829–830
        prognosis, 833, 833t
Atrial septal defect, 928, 931, *931*
    clinical aspects, 928, 931
    defined, 928, *931*
    diagnosis, 931

embryology, 928
treatment, 931
Atrioventricular canal division, 918, *921–922*
Atrium
    partition of, 918–920, *922–923*
    pulmonary veins, atrial absorption of, 921–923
    sinus venosus, atrial absorption of, 920–921, *924*
Attachment, abnormal, greater omentum, 120–121, *121*
Auricular pits, congenital, branchial apparatus, 2–33
Autosomal dominant polycystic kidney, *639–640*, 639–644
    diagnosis, 641, *642–643*
    familial tendency, 640
    history, 641
    prognosis, 642, 644, 644t
    symptoms, 641
    treatment, 641–642
Autosomal recessive polycystic kidney, 638–639
Azygous lobe, lung, 432–433

Barrett's esophagus, 98–100, *98–100*, 100
Beckwith-Wiedermann syndrome, 48
Bifid omentum, 122
Bile duct. *See* Common bile duct
Birth weight, gestational age, relationship, 12t
Bladder
    aganglionic, 708
    agenesis, *677*
    anomalies of, 675–712, 676t, *677*
    bilateral duplication, 681–683
        anatomy, 681, *682–683*
        diagnosis, 682
        embryogenesis, 681
        history, 681
        incidence, 681
        symptoms, 682
        treatment, 682–683
    constriction of, 683–685
    development, 671–675
    diverticula, 685–686, *685–686*
    embryogenesis, 675
    exstrophy, 686–688, *687*
        associated anomalies, 686, 688
        diagnosis, 691
        embryogenesis, 688–690, *688–691*
        history, 690
        mortality, 692–693
        prognosis, 692t, 692–693
            for pregnancy, 693
        symptoms, 691
        treatment, 691–692
            palliative therapy, 692
            plastic reconstruction, 692
    formation of, 671–674, *674*, *677*
    frontal duplication, *683*, 683–685
    frontal septa, *682*, 683–685
    hourglass, 684, *684*
    Marion's disease, 708
    multiple septa, 684
    pheochromocytoma, 711
    urachus, 675
Blastocyst, defined, 1066
Bombesin, gastrointestinal peptide ontogeny, 153
Bowel
    mesocolon
        pelvic, 128
        transverse, 128
    small

mesenteries of, 127
mesoappendix, 127
Branchial, term, use of, vs. pharyngeal, 17
Branchial apparatus
    cyst, term, use of, 38
    cystic remnant of, 32–41
    first cleft-pouch defects, 32–35
    first pouch defects, 34–35
    fistula, term, use of, 37
    fistular remnant of, 32–41
    fourth cleft-pouch defects, 37, *37*
    second cleft-pouch defects, 35, *36*
    sinus
        external, term, use of, 37–38
        internal, term, use of, 38
    third cleft-pouch defects, 35, 37, *37*
Branchial arches, of pharynx, 17–24, *21*, 25t
Branchial cleft, of pharynx, 17, *20*, 20–22, 25t
Breast
    amastia, *560*, 560–563
    athelia, 560–563
    congenital anomalies of, 559
    ectopic, 560–561, *562*
    polymastia, 560–563, *561*
    polythelia, 560–563, *561*
    supernumerary, 560–563, *561*
        associated anomalies, 562
        diagnosis, 563
        embryogenesis, 562
        history, 562–563
        number of, 562
        structure of, 561–562
        symptoms, 563
        treatment, 563
Broad ligament
    cysts of, female reproductive tract, 827
    peritoneum, congenital anomalies of, 130–131
Bronchial arteries, variations in, 472–473
Bronchial arteries/veins, development, 454–455
Bronchial tissue, ectopic, 438
Brunner's adenoma, stomach, 173
Bulbourethral gland of Cowper, development, 775, *776*
Bursa, omental, *117*, 118–120

Cake kidney, *622*, 622–623
Calyceal cyst, of kidney, 636
Calyces, extrarenal, 644, *645*
Cardiac lobe, lung, 432
Castleman's disease, 120
Caudal pharyngeal pouch complex, 22
Cecum, 243t, 244–245, *245*
    hyperdescent of, 193, *193*
    inverted, 195, *195*
    mobile, 195
    retroperitoneal, 195, *196*
    undescended, 195, *195*
Cervical aortic arch, 1001–1003, *1002*
Cervix
    atresia, 828, *828*
    teratoma, *1064*
Chagas' disease, esophagus, 100–104
Chest deformity, 545–550, *549*
    complications of, 547–548
    congenital, 545–550
    diagnosis, 549–550
    embryogenesis, 548–549, *549*
    history, 549
    rib, 547
    sternum, 545–547, *546–548*
    symptoms, 549
    treatment, 549–550

Cholecystohepatic triangle, variations in, 327–329
  accessory bile ducts, 329
  cystic artery, 328–329
  right hepatic artery, 327–328
Cholecystokinin, gastrointestinal peptide ontogeny, 153
Choledochocele, common bile duct, 312–314
"Christmas tree" atresia, small intestines, 203
Chromosomal anomalies, birth defect of, as cause of infant death, 4
Chylothorax, 445, 894–895
Classification of congenital anomalies, 6–7
Clitoris
  agenesis, 793
  defect of, 843
  duplication of, 792–795, 794
  hyperplasia, 793
  hypoplasia, 793
Cloaca
  division of, 671, 673–674
  exstrophy, 693–694, 693–695
  formation of, 671, 672
  persistent, anorectal, 266–268
  region, 242–244, 244
Closure of body wall, critical events in, 545
Colon, 242, 243t
  agenesis of, 245–246
  aplasia of, 245–246
  atresia, 246–247, 246–247
    malposition, 246–247
    small left colon syndrome, 247
  bilateral duplications of, 249–251
    anatomy, 249–250, 250
    diagnosis, 251, 251
    embryogenesis, 250
    history, 250
    incidence, 250, 251
    symptoms, 250–251
    treatment, 251
  diverticula, 247–248, 248
  duplications of, 248–251
  Hirschsprung's disease, 252–259
  midline duplications of, 248, 249
Common bile duct, 308–317
  anomalies of, 308–317
    cystic dilation, 312–317, 313
    duplication of, 310–311, 310–312
    ectopia of, 310–312, 312
    variations of, 308–310, 308–310
  pancreas, 372–373
Compression, extrinsic, ureteropelvic junction obstruction, 646
Congenital anomaly
  age at examination, survival rate, epidemiologic data, 5–6, 6
  as cause of infant death, by organ system, 4
  classification of, 6–7
  etiology of, 7
  frequency of, 4
  incidence, epidemiologic data, 2–3, 2–6, 4t–5t, 5–6
  infant mortality from, in United States, 5
  lethality, degree of, epidemiologic data, 5, 5
  multiple, epidemiologic data, 6
  severity, degree of, epidemiologic data, 5
Conjoined twins, 1066–1078
  blastocyst, 1066
  classification, 1066–1067, 1067
  craniopagus classification, 1067

diagnosis, 1068–1068
embryogenesis, 1066
history, 1067, 1067–1077
incidence, 1068
ischiopagus classification, 1066–1067
monovular pregnancy, 1066
monozygotic identical twins, 1066
omphalopagus classification, 1066
polyovular pregnancy, 1066
pygopagus classification, 1066
results of treatment, 1073, 1076
thoracopagus classification, 1066
treatment, 1068–1070, 1073
trophoblast, 1066
Cor triatriatum, 473–474, 473–475
Coronary artery
  accessory, 962–963, 963–965
  aneurysm, 965
  fistula, 969–972, 971, 971t–972t
  pulmonary origin of, 966–968, 969
  "single", 963–964, 965
Coronary vein, anomalies of, 972–973, 973t
Coronary vessels, 958–975. See also Coronary artery, Coronary vein
  abnormal, anatomy of, 968–969, 970
  anomalies of, 959–973, 961, 961t
  development, 958–959, 959–961
    coronary circulation, 958–959
    critical events in, 958–959
  left coronary preponderance, 964, 966–967
  muscle bridge, 965
  origin from contralateral sinus of Valsalva, 964–965
  right coronary preponderance, 964, 966–967
  variations, 959, 961–966, 962t, 963
Corpora cavernosa defect, 792–793, 972
Corpus spongiosum defect, 792–793, 972
Cortical tissue, accessory, 730–732
Covered anus, 261
Cowper's glands, development, 775, 776
Craniopagus classification, conjoined twins, 1067
Cremaster muscle, 584
Cricopharyngeal diverticula, 94
Crossed renal ectopia, 614–617
  anatomy, 614
  diagnosis, 617
  embryogenesis, 610, 615–616, 616
  and fusion, 614–615, 615
  history, 616
  incidence, 616–617
  symptoms, 617
  treatment, 617
  without fusion, 610, 615
Crown-rump length, embryo measurement, 10
Cyst
  branchial apparatus, term, use of, 38
  broad ligament, female reproductive tract, 827
  greater omentum, 122–125
  liver, nonparasitic, 288–291
  lung, congenital, 441–444
  lymphatic, 891–894, 892–893
  mesenteric, 128–129, 128t–131t, 130
  Müllerian duct, 780–784, 785–786
  pancreas, 388t, 388–389
  parathyroid
    anatomy, 44
    embryogenesis, 45–46
    incidence, 45–46
    symptoms, 47
    treatment, 47

parathyroid gland, 44–47
  anatomy of, 44
  diagnosis, 47
  embryogenesis, 45–46
  history/incidence of, 46–47
  symptoms, 47
pharynx, 35
  cervicoaural, 33–34
of prostatic utricle, 780–784, 785–786
spleen, 363
thymic
  anatomy, 48
  diagnosis, 48–49
  embryogenesis, 48
  incidence, 48
  symptoms, 48–49
  treatment, 49, 49t
thymus, 48–49
  anatomy, 48
  embryogenesis, 48
  incidence, 48
  symptoms, 48–49
  treatment, 49, 49t
thyroglossal duct, 59t, 59–60, 60
vitelline, small intestines, 217, 217
Cystic adenoma, kidney, 636
Cystic artery, variation, 326–327, 327, 328–329
Cystic disease, kidney, 626t, 626–644
  autosomal dominant polycystic kidney, 639–640, 639–644
    diagnosis, 641, 642–643
    familial tendency, 640
    history, 641
    prognosis, 642, 644, 644t
    symptoms, 641
    treatment, 641–642
  autosomal recessive polycystic kidney, 638–639
  calyceal cyst, 636
  cystic adenoma, 636
  diverticula, 636
  embryogenesis, 627–628, 628, 630–633
  glomerulocystic disease, 636
  juvenile nephronophthisis complex, 637, 637–638
  multicystic kidney, 629–636, 635
  multiple malformation syndrome, cysts associated with, 644, 644t
  polycystic disease, 638
  simple cyst, 628–629, 634
  sponge kidney, 636–637, 637
Cystic duct
  anomalies of, 324–325, 324–326
  Mirizzi's syndrome, 326, 326
Cystic fibrosis, pancreas, 389–392
Cystic hygroma, 880, 882–888
  anatomy, 882
  associated syndromes, 884–885, 888t
  diagnosis, 887
  history, 883–884
  incidence, 885–886
  location, 882–883, 886–887
  pathogenesis, 883, 888
  prognosis, 888
  symptoms, 886
  treatment, 887–888
Cystic remnants, female reproductive tract, 823, 824

Del Castillo syndrome, 864
Depression deformity, sternum, 545–546, 546–547
Developmental stages, in human embryos, 11t
Diaphragm, 491–539

absence of, 498, *500*, 502
accessory, 530, *532*, 532–535, *534–535*
  anatomy, 533–534, *534–535*
  diagnosis, 535
  embryogenesis, 534–535
  symptoms, 535
  treatment, 535
anomalies, 498t, 498–535, *499*
Bochdalek foramen, hernia through,
    502–510, *503–504*
  anatomy, 502–505, *503–504*
  associated anomalies, 505
  diagnosis, 507–508, *507–509*
  history, 506
  incidence, 506–507
  prognosis, 510
  symptoms, 507–508
  treatment, 508–509
central tendon defect, 515–516, *516*
development, *491–497*, 491–498, 493t
  critical events, 498
esophageal hiatus, enlarged, 499, 501,
    501
esophagus, short, 530
eventration of, 511–515
  anatomy, 511–513, *512–513*, 513t
  diagnosis, 514
  embryogenesis, 513
  history, 513–514
  incidence, 514
  symptoms, 514, *514*
  treatment, 514–515, *515*
fusion defects, 498–516
hernia, 501
  birth prevalence of, 5
  hiatal, 516–530, 517t, *518*
    abdominal esophagus,
      gastroesophageal junction,
      519–521, *520–521*
    complications of, 524–525
    diagnosis, 528–529, *528–529*
    embryogenesis, 525–526, *526–527*
    esophageal hiatus, crura, 521–524,
      522–525
    history, 526–527
    median arcuate ligament, 524, *526*
    symptoms, 527–528
    treatment, 529–531, *531*
  intrauterine surgery, 1081
Morgagni foramen, hernia through, 510–
    511, *510–512*
muscularization, failure of, 498–499
Dieulafoy's disease, 176–177
  stomach, 176
Digestive system, birth defect of, as cause of
    infant death, 4
Diverticulum
  appendix, 276, *276*
  bladder, 685–686, *685–686*
  colon, 247–248, *248*
  concomitant occurrence of, 225
  cystic disease, of kidney, 636
  duodenal, *223*, 223–224
  of esophagus, 93–96, *94*
  giant, 225
  heart, 949–951, *951*
    anatomy, 949, *951*
    associated anomalies, 950–951
    diagnosis, 951
    embryogenesis, 949–950
    heart, 949
    incidence, 950
    treatment, 951
  history, 322
  ileal, 224–225
  jejunal, 224–225

Meckel's
  age, 219
  diagnosis, 219, 219t
  embryogenesis, 218
  familial tendency, 219
  history, 218
  incidence, 218
  inflammatory group, 220
  neoplastic group, 221
  obstruction group, 220, *220*
  peptic ulcer group, 219–220
  sex, 218–219, *219*
  treatment, 221
  umbilical group, 220–221
small intestines, 213–225, *214*, 215
  Meckel's diverticulum, 214–216, *215–
    216*
  non-Meckelian antimesenteric true
    diverticula, 221
  omphaloilial fistula, 213, 215
  primary false diverticula, 221–225
stomach, 164–165
  diagnosis, 165
  embryogenesis, 164
  history, 164
  incidence, 165
  mortality, 165
  symptoms, 165
  treatment, 165
trachea, 427
ureteral, 658–660, *659*
urethra, female, 711
Dorsal enteric remnants, small intestines,
    225–230, *228*, *230–231*
Dorsally facing kidney, *601*, 617
Double aortic arch, 993–995, *994*, 994t,
    996–997
Double crossed renal ectopia, *610*, 615
Double ductus arteriosus, 1013, *1014*
Double-orifice mitral valve, 941
Double superior vena cava, 1038–1040,
    1040–1041
Double ureter, 644t, 649–654, *653*
  accessory ureteric bud, *651*, 652–653
  anatomy, 649–650
  crossing of, *651*, 653
  diagnosis, 654
  ectopic ureteral openings, *651*, 652
  embryogenesis, 652
  incidence, 653t, 653–654
  level of ureter bifurcation, 650, *651–652*
  pathology, 654, 654t
  splitting of ureteric bud, 644t, 652, *653*
  treatment, 654, 655t
  ureteral diverticula, 650, *651*
Down's syndrome, esophageal atresia, 157
Dubois' abscess, thymus, 48
Ducts, aberrant, male reproductive tract,
    775, *778–779*
Ductus arteriosus
  absence of, 1013
  double, 1013, *1014*
  left
    anomalous, 1013, *1014*
    persistent, 1013
  patent, 1010–1013, *1011*
  right, 1013
    persistent, 1013
Ductus deferens, development, 773
Ductus epoophori longitudinalis, female
    reproductive tract, 823–824,
    824
Duodenum
  atresia, 162, 163t
  diverticula, *223*, 223–224
  maldevelopment, 191

papilla
  minor, pancreas, 375
  pancreas, 373, *373*
stenosis, birth prevalence of, 5
Duplication
  greater omentum, 120
  heart, 948–949, *950*
  stomach, 165–169
    anatomy, 165–166, *167*
    diagnosis, 168
    embryogenesis, 166
    history, 166
    incidence, 167–168
    symptoms, 168
    treatment, *168*, 168–169
Dysphagia, esophagus, vascular
    compression, 105–106
Dysplasia
  alveolar, 444–445
  greater omentum, 120
  pancreas, 371

Ebstein's anomaly, of tricuspid valve, 937–
    938, *938*
Ectopia
  accessory thyroid tissue, *60*, 60–61
  breast, 560–561, *562*
  cordis, 554–555, *558*
    associated anomalies, 553–554, *556–
      557*
    history, 555–556
    incidence, 556
    prognosis, 557, 559
    sternal defects with, 552–553, *553*,
      556–557
    symptoms, 556
    treatment, 556–557, *558–559*
  crossed renal
    diagnosis, 617
    embryogenesis, *610*, 615–616, *616*
    history, 616
    incidence, 616–617
    symptoms, 617
    treatment, 617
  endometrium, 840–842
  ovary, and inguinal hernia, 768–769
  renal
    crossed, 614–617
      anatomy, 614
      and fusion, 614–615, *615*
      without fusion, *610*, 615
      double crossed, *610*, 615
      simple, 612–613, *612–613*
      solitary crossed, *610*, 615
      thoracic, 613–614, *614*
  testes, *765*, 766t, 766–768, *767*
  vesicae, birth prevalence of, 5
Egg, postovulatory survival, in humans, 2–3
Embryo
  age of, and developmental stage, 11t
  development, normal, 9–12, *10*, 11t–12t
  measurement of, 9–10, *10*
  size of, 9–11, *10*
Emphysema, lung, congenital, *438*, 438–
    441, 439t, *440*, 441t
Encapsulated small intestine, 193–195, *194*
Endocardial cushion defects, 935–936
  classification, 935
  defined, 935, *935*
  diagnosis, 936
  embryology, 935–936
  incidence, 936
  prognosis, 936
  symptoms, 936
  treatment, 936
Endometrium, ectopic, 840–842

Epididymis, development, 773
Epiploic foramen, peritoneum, 118
Epispadias, male reproductive tract, 800–805
  anatomy, 800–802, *801–802*
  diagnosis, 803, 805
  embryogenesis, 802, *803–804*
  history, 802–803
  incidence, 803
  prognosis, 805
  symptoms, 803
  treatment, 805
Epoophoron, female reproductive tract, 823
Esophagus, *65–68*, 65–106, 69t, *70–74*, 73t, 75t, *76–80*, 81t, 82, 83t, *84–86*, 87t, *88*, 92t, *94*, 96t, *97–101*, *103–104*
  absence of, 69–70, *71*
  achalasia, 100–104, *101*, *103*
    and megaesophagus, 100–104, *101*, *103*
  anomalies, 68–106, 69t, *70–74*, 73t, 75t, *76–80*, 81t–83t, *82*, *84–86*, 86t–87t, *88*, 92t, *94*, 96t, *97–101*, *103–104*
  atresia, 68–83, *71–72*, 79, 80t, 84, *158*, 162
    Down's syndrome, 157
    with tracheoesophageal fistula, 71–72, *72*
  Barrett's, 98–100, *98–100*, 100
  Chagas' disease, 100–104
  congenital short, 530
  cricopharyngeal diverticula, 94
  defects
    diagnosis, 78–79, *78–79*
    embryogenesis, 73–74, *74*
    history, 75–76
    incidence, 76t, 76–77
    mortality, 83
    symptoms, 77, 77t, 77–78
    treatment, 79–83
  development, *65–67*, 65–68
  diverticula of, 93–96, *94*
  dorsal enteric remnants
    in thorax, 89–93, 92t
      diagnosis, 92, 92t
      history, 91
      incidence, 91
      mortality, 93
      symptoms, 91–92
      treatment, 92–93
    thorax, anatomy, 89–91
  dysphagia, vascular compression, 105–106
  embryogenesis, 73–74, *74*
  esophageal web, 84–85, *84–85*
  fistula, 79, 80t
  heterotopic gastric mucosa in, 96–98, *97*
  hiatus, enlarged, diaphragm, 499, *501*, *501*
  laryngotracheoesophageal cleft, 83–84
  lower, functional disturbances of, 95–105, 96t, *97–101*, *103*, *108*
  megaesophagus, 100–104, *101*, *103*
  membranous atresia/stenosis of, 84–85, *84–85*
  reflux, abnormal, idiopathic, congenital, 104–105, *105*
  short, with thoracic stomach, 98–100, *98–100*
  split notochord syndrome, 88–89
  stenosis, 68–73, *72*, 72–73, 84–85
  trachea, anomalies
    diagnosis, 78–79, *78–79*

    incidence, 76t, 76–77
      familial incidence, 76–77
      maternal age, 76
      sex ratio, 76
    symptoms, 77, 77t, 77–78
    treatment, 79–83, 80t, *82*, 82t–83t
    tracheoesophageal fistula, 68–83, *71–74*, 73t, 75t–77t, *76–79*, 81t–83t, *82*
  tubular duplication, 85–88, *86*, 86t–87t
    anatomy, 85–86, *86*
    diagnosis, *86*, 86–87, 87t, *88*
    embryogenesis, 86
    history, 85–86
    incidence, 86
    symptoms, 86, 86t
    treatment, 87–89, *88*
  Zenker's diverticula, 94
Ethical considerations, intrauterine surgery, 1082
Exomphalos, 191, *192*, 568–574
  birth prevalence of, 5
  small intestines, 191, *192*
Exophytic teratoma, *1064*
Exstrophy
  bladder, 686–688, *687*
    associated anomalies, 686, 688
    diagnosis, 691
    embryogenesis, 688–690, *688–691*
    history, 690
    incidence, 690–691
    mortality, 692–693
    prognosis, 692t, 692–693
      for pregnancy, 693
    symptoms, 691
    treatment, 691–692
      palliative therapy, 692
      plastic reconstruction, 692
  cloaca, 693–694, *693–695*
External genitalia
  female, 824–825, *825*
  male, 776–777, *780–782*
Extrahepatic biliary atresia, 297–307
  anatomy, 297–298, *301–302*
  associated anomalies, 302
  diagnosis, 304
  embryogenesis, 298, 301
  etiology, 302, *303*
  history, 302–303
  incidence, 303
  symptoms, 304
  treatment, 304–307, *305*
Extrahepatic biliary tract, vascular relations, variations in, 328t, 329
Extrahepatic duct system
  anomalies of, 297–329, *298*, 298t–301t
  development, 296–297
Extrarenal calyces, 644, *645*

Falciform ligaments, peritoneum, congenital anomalies of, 130
Female reproductive tract, 816–843
  anomalies of, *826*, 826t, 827–843
  cervix, atresia, 828, *828*
  clitoris, defect of, 843
  cystic remnants, 823, *824*
  development, 816–827
    critical events in, 825–827
  ductus epoophori longitudinalis, 823–824, *824*
  ectopic endometrium, 840–842
  external genitalia, 824–825, *825*
  Gartner's canal, 823–824, *824*
  heterotopic cartilage in uterus, 842
  hymen, imperforate, *828*, 828–829
  labia, defect of, 843

  labia minora, fusion, *842*, 842–843
  mesonephric remnants, *823*, 823–824
    appendix vesiculosa, 823
    epoophoron, 823
    paroophoron, 823
    pedunculated hydatid of Morgagni, 823
    Rosenmüller's organ, 823
    tubes of Kobelt, 823
  mesonephric vestiges, disorders associated with, *823–824*, 827
    cysts of broad ligament, 827
    Gartner's canal, dilation of, *824*, 827
    torsion of hydatid of Morgagni, *823*, 827
  Müllerian duct
    duplication of, 833, *833–834*
    incomplete fusion of, 834–840
      complications of pregnancy, *835–836*, 838t, 838–839, *839*
      diagnosis, 839, *842*
      incidence, 837, 838t
      separate hemiuteri with separate vaginae, 834, *834*
      symptoms, 837
      uterus arcuatus, 836, *836*
      uterus didelphys with separate vagina, *834*, 835, 835t
      uterus duplex bicollis, *835*, 836
      uterus duplex unicollis, 836, *836*
      uterus septus, 836, *836*
      uterus unicornis, *835*, 835–836
  Müllerian ducts, development, 816–823, *817–822*
  suprahymenal membrane, 829
  tubal endometrium, 840
  uterus
    aplasia, 827–828, *828*
    duplication, 833–834
    vagina primordia, incomplete fusion, 833–842
  vagina, atresia, 828, *828*
Fertilization age, when developmental errors arise, 7, *8*
Finney pyloroplasty, for stomach atresia, 159
Fissure, lung, absent, 432
Fistula
  branchial apparatus, term, use of, 37
  coronary artery, 969–972, *971*, 971t–972t
  esophagus, 79, 80t
  pharynx, 35
    cervicoaural, 33–34
    remnant, 32–41
  trachea, *427*, 427–429
  tracheoesophageal, 68–83, *71–74*, 73t, 75t–77t, *76–79*, 81t–83t, *82*
    with esophageal atresia, 71–72, *72*
Fold, peritoneal, variations, 147–148, *147–148*
Foramen
  epiploic, peritoneum, 118
  of Winslow, 134–135, *143*
Fossa
  cecal, 133
  intersigmoid, 133–134, *134*
  paraduodenal, 131t, 131–133, *132–134*
Fusion deformity, sternum, 547

Gallbladder
  abnormal position of, 322, *322*
  absence of, *317–318*, 317–319
  adenomyoma, 323
  anomalies of, 297–329, *298*, 298t–301t, 317–324

deformations of, 321–322
development, 296–297, *297*
duplication of, *319,* 319–320
Hartmann's pouch, *321,* 321–322
heterotopic mucosa in, 322–323
hourglass, 321, *321*
hydrops, 319
intrahepatic, 322
mobile, 322
pancreatic, 385
Phrygian cap deformity, 321, *321*
Gartner's canal, 823–824, *824*
dilation of, female reproductive tract, *824,* 827
Gastric angiodysplasia, 176–178, 177t
Gastric mucosa, in esophagus, 96–98, *97*
Gastric mucosal heterotopia, 172–176, *174– 176*
Gastric musculature defects, 169–171
anatomy, 169, *169*
diagnosis, 171, *171*
embryogenesis, 169
history, 169–171, *170*
incidence, 169–171, *170*
symptoms, 171
treatment, 171
Gastric outlet obstruction, 155–159
Gastric teratoma, 176
Gastric volvulus, 172
Gastrin, gastrointestinal peptide ontogeny, 153
Gastrocolic ligament, 118
Gastroduodenal adhesions, 176
Gastroschisis, 574–577
anatomy, 574, *575*
birth prevalence of, 5
embryogenesis, 574–576
history, 576, 576t
incidence, 576, 576t
treatment, 576–577
Gastrosplenic ligament, *348,* 348–349
Genetic sex determination, 849–850, *852– 853*
Genitalia, external
female, 824–825, *825*
male, 776–777, *780–782*
Genitourinary system, birth defect of, as cause of infant death, 4
Gestational age
birth weight, relationship, 12t
at malformation occurrence, 7, *8*
Giant diverticula, 225
Gland
parathyroid, 20–22, 41–47
location of, variations in, 41–43, *42– 43,* 44t
penis, agenesis, 790–791
suprarenal. *See* Suprarenal glands
thyroid, 27–32, *29–31*
developmental stages, 27, 30
partially descended, thyroid, anomaly, 58–59, *59*
Glomerulocystic disease, kidney, 636
Glomerulus formation, 598–599, *602*
Glottic atresia, 407
Glucagon, gastrointestinal peptide ontogeny, 153
Gonad, anomalies of, 748–769, *753,* 753t
absence of ovary, 750–752
anatomy, 750–751, 754t
diagnosis, 752
embryogenesis, 751, 754t
history, 751
symptoms, 752
testes, 752

absence of testis, without feminization, 748–750
anatomy, 748
diagnosis, 749–750
embryogenesis, 748, 754t
history, 748
incidence, 748
symptoms, 748–749
supernumerary testes, 752–755
Greater omentum
accessory spleens, 125
adhesions, congenital, 122
agenesis, 120
cyst, 122–125
duplication, 120
dysplasia, 120
failure to attach, *121,* 121–125, *123–125*
hyperplasia, 120
hypoplasia, 120
infarction, 122–123
omental teratoma, 125
peritoneum, congenital anomalies, 120– 121, *121*
tumors, 122–123, 125
vascular anomalies, 122
Growth retardation, intrauterine, 1057

Hamartoma, of lung, adenomatoid, 444
Hartmann's pouch, gallbladder, *321,* 321– 322
Hashimoto's thyroiditis, 48
Heart, 912–951. *See also* Coronary vessels
anomalies of, 927t, 927–951
aortic atresia, 943–944, *944*
aortic stenosis, 944–946, *945*
subvalvular aortic stenosis, 945
supravalvular aortic stenosis, 944–945, *945*
valvular aortic stenosis, 945
atrial septal defect, 928, 931, *931*
clinical aspects, 928, 931
defined, 928, *931*
diagnosis, 931
embryology, 928
treatment, 931
atrioventricular canal division, 918, *921– 922*
atrium, partition of, 918–920, *922–923*
congenital disease, 927–928, 928t–932t
congenital heart disease, 927–928, 928t– 932t
conotruncal abnormalities, 941–948
development, 912–918, *913–920*
critical events, 926–927
disease, congenital, by age at diagnosis, 6
diverticula, 949–951, *951*
anatomy, 949, *951*
associated anomalies, 950–951
diagnosis, 951
embryogenesis, 949–950
heart, 949
incidence, 950
treatment, 951
duplication of, 948–949, *950*
embryogenesis of conducting system, 926
endocardial cushion defects, 935–936
classification, 935
defined, 935, *935*
diagnosis, 936
embryology, 935–936
incidence, 936
prognosis, 936
symptoms, 936
treatment, 936
mitral valve, 940–941
atresia, 940

double-orifice, 941
embryology, 940
stenosis, 940–941
outflow tract, partition of, 924–926, *926*
parchment, 939
pulmonary atresia, 939–940
ventricular septal defect, 942–943, *942–943*
pulmonary stenosis, 939–940
pulmonary veins, atrial absorption of, 921–923
sinus venosus, atrial absorption of, 920– 921, *924*
tetralogy of Fallot, 942
with absent pulmonary valve, 943
pulmonary atresia, ventricular septal defect, 941
transposition of the great arteries, *946,* 946–947
transposition of the great vessels, congenitally corrected, 947– 948, *948–949*
tricuspid atresia, 936–937, *937*
tricuspid valve
cleft of, 939
duplication of, 939
Ebstein's anomaly, 937–938, *938*
stenosis, 938–939
Uhl's malformation, 939
ventricle, partition of, 923–924, *925*
ventricular septal defect, 931–934
anatomy, 931–933
defined, 931
diagnosis, 934
embryology, 933–934
incidence, 934
prognosis, 934
symptoms, 934
treatment, 934
Heinke-Mikulicz pyloroplasty, for stomach atresia, 159
Hemihypertrophy, 1057
Hemorrhage, suprarenal glands, 723–724
Hepatic artery, variations of, 326–327, *327*
Hepatic ducts, anomalies of, 307–308
absence, common hepatic duct, 307
accessory hepatic ducts, 307, *308*
duplication, common hepatic duct, 307– 308, *308*
hepatocystic duct, 308
subvesicular duct, 308
variations of, 307, *307*
Hepatic segment, of inferior vena cava, absence of, *104,* 1043–1045
Hermaphroditism, 853–873, *862*
classification, 854–866, 856t–857t
diagnosis, 870–871
incidence of, 870, 870t
treatment, 871–872
choice of sex, 871–872
Hernia
diaphragm, 501
intrauterine surgery, 1081
hiatal. *See* Hiatal hernia
incarcerated left paraduodenal, 133, *133*
incarcerated right paraduodenal, 132–133
inguinal
anterior body wall, 578–580
and ectopic ovary, 768–769
hernial sac, contents of, 581
and undescended testes, 761
internal, 134–143, *135–142*
through peritoneal defect
anatomy, 135, 144
classification, 135
diagnosis, 145–146

Hernia—*continued*
    embryogenesis, 144
    incidence, 144
    mortality, 147
    symptoms, 145
    treatment, 147
    through peritoneal defects, 135, 144, 144t, *145–146*
    through, Morgagni foramen, diaphragm, 510–511, *510–512*
    through Bochdalek foramen, diaphragm, 502–510, *503–504*
    umbilical, 565–568
        anatomy, 565, 567, *569*
        embryogenesis, 567
        incidence, 567
        symptoms, 567
        treatment, 567–568
    of Waldeyer, 127
Heterotaxia, 1054–1057, *1055*
Heterotopia, suprarenal, 728–729, *729–730*
Heterotopic cartilage in uterus, 842
Hiatal hernia, 516–530
    abdominal esophagus, gastroesophageal junction, 519–521, *520–521*
    complications of, 524–525
    diagnosis, 528–529, *528–529*
    embryogenesis, 525–526, *526–527*
    esophageal hiatus, crura, 521–524, *522–525*
    history, 526–527
    median arcuate ligament, 524, *526*
    symptoms, 527–528
    treatment, 529–531, *531*
Hirschsprung's disease, 252–259
    age, 255
    anatomy, 252–253, *253*
    associated anomalies, 253
    birth prevalence of, 5
    diagnosis, 255–258, *256–257*
    embryogenesis, 253–254, 254t
    familial tendency, 255
    history, 254–255
    incidence, 255
    mortality, 258–259
    neuropathophysiology, 254
    prognosis, 258–259
    sex, 255
    symptoms, 255–256
    treatment, 258, *258*
His, cervical sinus of, 19, 22
Horseshoe kidney, *618*, 618–622
    anatomy, *618–620*, 619–620
    associated anomalies, 620
    associated conditions, 621
    diagnosis, 622
    embryogenesis, 620–621, *621*
    history, 621
    hydronephrosis, 621
    incidence, 621
    prognosis, 622
    symptoms, 621
    treatment, 622
Hourglass bladder, 684, *684*
Hourglass gallbladder, 321, *321*
Hourglass stomach, 159–160
Hydatid of Morgagni
    pedunculated, female reproductive tract, 823
    torsion of, female reproductive tract, *823*, 827
Hydrocele
    anterior body wall, 583
    processus vaginalis, 578–580
Hydrocephalus, intrauterine surgery, 1081–1082

Hydronephrosis, birth prevalence of, 5
Hydrops, gallbladder, 319
Hygroma
    cystic, 880, 882–888
    renal, 888–889
Hymen, imperforate, *828*, 828–829
Hypernephric syndrome, 856, 858–860
Hyperplasia
    adrenal, 733
    clitoris, 793
    greater omentum, 120
    pancreas, 370–371
    thymus, 48
Hypertrophic stenosis, stomach. *See* Pyloric stenosis
Hypertrophy, pancreas, 370–371
Hypoperistalsis syndrome, megacystis-microcolon-intestinal, small intestines, 231
Hypoplasia
    clitoris, 793
    greater omentum, 120
    kidney, 604–612, *605*, 610–612
        anatomy, 610–611
        diagnosis, 611–612
        embryogenesis, 611, *611*
        incidence, 611
        symptoms, 611
        treatment, 612
    lung
        right, 480–484, *481*
        unilateral, *429*, 429–432, 430t
    pancreas, 369–370, *370*
    suprarenal glands, 728
Hypospadias, 805–811
    anatomy, *805–806*, 805–807
    associated anomalies, 807
    diagnosis, 809, 811
    embryogenesis, 809
    embryology, 807, *808*, 809
    etiology, 807
    incidence, 809
    symptoms, 809
    treatment, 810t, 811

Ileal atresia, birth prevalence of, 5
Ileal diverticula, 224–225
Ima artery, thyroid, anomaly, 53
Imperforate hymen, *828*, 828–829
Incarcerated left paraduodenal hernia, 133, *133*
Incarcerated right paraduodenal hernia, 132–133
Infant mortality
    from birth defects, in United States, 5
    cardiovascular system, birth defect of, as cause of infant death, 4
    central nervous system, birth defect of, as cause of infant death, 4
    chromosomal anomalies, birth defect of, as cause of infant death, 4
    digestive system, birth defect of, as cause of infant death, 4
    genitourinary system, birth defect of, as cause of infant death, 4
    leading causes of, 2–3
    musculoskeletal system, birth defect of, as cause of infant death, 4 56
    respiratory system, birth defect of, as cause of infant death, 4
Inferior vena cava, 1032–1051
    absence of hepatic segment, *104*, 1043–1045
    anomalies of, *1038*, 1038t, 1043–1049

    development, 1032, *1033–1034*, 1034–1037, *1036–1037*
    postrenal, anomalies of, 1045–1049, *1046–1048*
Infraglottic atresia, 407
Inguinal hernia
    anterior body wall, 578–580
    and ectopic ovary, 768–769
    and undescended testes, 761
Insulin, gastrointestinal peptide ontogeny, 153
Internal hernia, 134–143, *135–142*
    through peritoneal defects, 135, 144, 144t, *145–146*
Intersex, atypical idiopathic, female, surgical intervention, 12–13, *12–15*, 15
Intersigmoid fossa, 133–134, *134*
Intestines. *See* Small intestines
Intrahepatic biliary atresia, 292–293
Intrahepatic gallbladder, 322
Intrauterine growth retardation, 1057
Intrauterine surgery, 1079–1083
    diaphragmatic hernia, 1081
    ethical considerations, 1082
    history, 1079–1081
    hydrocephalus, 1081–1082
    urinary tract anomalies, 1081
Intrauterine ulceration, hourglass stomach, 160
Ischiopagus classification, conjoined twins, 1066–1067
Islands of Langerhans, 367–369, *369*

Jackson membrane
    peritoneum, 147–148, *148*
    small intestines, 195, *196*
Jejunal atresia, birth prevalence of, 5
Jejunal diverticula, 224–225
Juvenile nephronophthisis complex, *637*, 637–638

Kartagener's syndrome, *1053*, 1053–1054
Kasai procedure, for biliary atresia, 304–306
Kidney
    adult, 596, 598, 599t, *600–601*
    agenesis, 604–612, *605*
        bilateral, 605–608
            anatomy, 605–606, *606*
            associated anomalies, 606
            diagnosis, 607, 607t
            embryogenesis, 606, *606*
            history, 606–607
            mortality, 607–608
            symptoms, 607
        unilateral, 608–610
            associated anomalies, *605*, 608–609
            diagnosis, 610
            embryogenesis, 609, *610*
            history, 609–610
            incidence, 608
            solitary kidney, 608
            symptoms, 610
            treatment, 610
    anomalies of, 601–663, 604t, *605*
    aplasia, 604–612, *605*
    Ask-Upmark, 632–633
    crossed renal ectopia, 614–617
        anatomy, 614
        diagnosis, 617
        embryogenesis, *610*, 615–616, *616*
        and fusion, 614–615, *615*
        history, 616
        incidence, 616–617
        symptoms, 617

treatment, 617
without fusion, *610*, 615
cystic disease, 626t, 626–644
  autosomal dominant polycystic kidney,
    639–640, 639–644, *642–643*
    diagnosis, 641, *642–643*
    familial tendency, 640
    history, 641
    prognosis, 642, 644, 644t
    symptoms, 641
    treatment, 641–642
  autosomal recessive polycystic kidney,
    638–639
  calyceal cyst, 636
  cystic adenoma, 636
  diverticula, 636
  embryogenesis, 627–628, *628*, *630–633*
  glomerulocystic disease, 636
  juvenile nephronophthisis complex,
    637, 637–638
  multicystic kidney, 629–636, *635*
  multilocular cyst, 629, *635*
  multiple malformation syndrome, cysts
    associated with, 644, 644t
  polycystic disease, 638
  simple cyst, 628–629, *634*
  sponge kidney, 636–637, *637*
development, 594–601, *595*
  critical events in, 601
double, 649–654
double crossed renal ectopia, *610*, 615
embryonic, 594–596, *596–597*
extrarenal calyces, 644, *645*
fused pelvic, 622, 622–623
glomerulus formation, 598–599, *602*
horseshoe, *618*, 618–622
  anatomy, *618–620*, 619–620
  associated anomalies, 620
  associated conditions, 621
  diagnosis, 622
  embryogenesis, 620–621, *621*
  history, 621
  incidence, 621
  prognosis, 622
  symptoms, 621
  treatment, 622
hypoplasia, 604–612, *605*, *610–612*
  anatomy, 610–611
  diagnosis, 611–612
  embryogenesis, 611, *611*
  incidence, 611
  symptoms, 611
  treatment, 612
malrotation of, 617–618
  anatomy, 617
  diagnosis, 618
  dorsally facing, *601*, 617
  embryogenesis, *601*, 617–618
  incidence, 618
  laterally facing, *601*, 617
  symptoms, 618
  treatment, 618
  ventrally facing, *601*, 617
  ventromedially facing, *601*, 617
mesonephric remnant, *598*, 603–604
mesonephros, 594–596, *596–597*
  functional state of, 596, *598*
nephron formation, 600, *603*
pelvic, 614
pronephros, 594–596, *596–597*
renal artery variations, 623–625
  anatomy, 623, *623*
  diagnosis, 625
  embryogenesis, 625
  number of arteries, 265, *620*, 623, 624t
  positions of arteries, 265, *624–625*

symptoms, 625
treatment, 625
simple renal ectopia, 612–613, *612–613*
solitary crossed renal ectopia, *610*, 615
supernumerary, 654–656
  anatomy, 654–655, *656*
  diagnosis, 656
  embryogenesis, 655
  history, 655–656
  incidence, 655–656
  pathology, 656
  symptoms, 656
  treatment, 656
thoracic renal ectopia, 613–614, *614*
ureteropelvic junction obstruction, 644–
    649
  associated anomalies, 646–647
  clinical features, 647–648
  diagnosis, 648
  extrinsic compression, 646
  mucosal fold, 646
  pathogenesis, 645–646
  polyp, 646
  repair, *646*, 649
  secondary etiology, 646
  temporary diversion, 649
Klinefelter's syndrome, 863–864

Labia, defect of, 843
Labia minora, fusion, *842*, 842–843
Laryngomalacia, 410, *411*
Laryngotracheoesophageal cleft, 83–84,
    410–412, *412–413*
Larynx, 405–413
  anomalies, *407*, 407–413, 408t
  atresia, 407–408, *409*
    incomplete, *310*, 408
  development, 405–407, *406–407*
  extrinsic obstruction, 412
  laryngomalacia, 410, *411*
  laryngotracheoesophageal cleft, 410–412,
    412–413
  stenosis, subglottic, 408–410
  web, *310*, 408
Lateral branchial apparatus, anomalies of,
    32–47, 33t, *34–38*, 41t
Laterally facing kidney, *601*, 617
Left aortic arch, with right descending
    aorta, *997*, 1000
Left ductus arteriosus
  anomalous, 1013, *1014*
  persistent, 1013
Left-sided superior vena cava, 1040–1043,
    1042
Lesser omentum
  absence of, 127
  congenital anomalies, 125, 127
Lesser sac, peritoneum, *117*, 118–120
Ligament
  gastrocolic, 118
  peritoneum, congenital anomalies of,
    129–131
  spleen, 346–350
  supracolic, peritoneum, 117
Lingual thyroid, median anlage, thyroid
    anomaly, 57–58
Liver, 282–295
  anomalies of, 285–293, *286*, 286t
  arteriohepatic dysplasia, 293
  development, 282–285, 283t, *283–285*,
    285t
    critical events in, 284
  hemangioendothelioma, congenital,
    hepatic, 293
  hemangioma, congenital, hepatic, 293
  intrahepatic biliary atresia, 292–293

lobulation, anomalies of, 285–288, *287–
    288*
  nonparasitic cyst, 288–291
  polycystic disease, 290–291
  Riedel's lobe, 286, *289*
  solitary cyst, 288–290
  supradiaphragmatic lobes, 286–288,
    289–291
lymphangioma, congenital, hepatic, 293
Lobdell-DiGeorge anomaly, 47–48
Lobulated ovary, 756
Lung
  absent fissure, 432
  agenesis
    bilateral, 420–421
    unilateral, 429–432
  alveolar dysplasia, 444–445
  anomalies, 419–445, 420t, *421*
  aplasia, unilateral, *428*, 429–432
  azygous lobe, 432–433
  cardiac lobe, 432
  chylothorax, 445
  cyst
    congenital, 441–444
    of endothelial origin, 443–444
    of mesothelial origin, 443–444, *444*
    parenchyma, multiple cysts of, 441–442
    solitary, 443, *443*
  development, 414–419, *416–418*, 418t–
    419t
  dorsal lobe, 432
  drainage, anomalous, *474–476*, 475–480,
    476t–477t, *478–479*
  ectopic bronchial tissue, 438
  emphysema, congenital, *438*, 438–441,
    439t, *440*, 441t
  hamartoma, adenomatoid, 444
  hypoplasia, unilateral, *429*, 429–432, 430t
  lobulation, anomalies of, 432–435, *433–
    435*
  pulmonary isomerism, 434–435, *435*
  right, hypoplasia, 480–484, *481*
  scimitar syndrome, 480–484, *481*
  sequestration, 463–470
    anatomy, 463–467, 464t–465t, *465–467*
    diagnosis, 469
    embryogenesis, 467–468
    history, 469
    incidence, 469
    symptoms, 469
    treatment, 470
  tracheal lobe, lobulation anatomy, 433,
    434
  vascular supply to, anomalies, 456t, 456–
    484, *457*
Lymphatic cyst, 891–894, *892–893*
Lymphatic system, 877–895
  anomalies of, 879–895, *880*, 880t
  cancer, 895
  chylothorax, 894–895
  cystic hygroma, 880, 882–888
    anatomy, 882
    associated syndromes, 884–885, 888t
    diagnosis, 887
    history, 883–884
    incidence, 885–886
    location, 882–883, *886–887*
    pathogenesis, 883, *888*
    prognosis, 888
    symptoms, 886
    treatment, 887–888
  development, 877–878, *878–879*
    critical events in, 878
  lymphatic cyst, 891–894, *892–893*
  lymphedema, primary, 889–891, 890t
  renal hygroma, 888–889

Lymphatic system—*continued*
   thoracic duct, variations of, 879–880,
      881–882, 884–886
Lymphedema, primary, 889–891, 890t

Male reproductive tract, 773–811
   anomalies of, 777–811, 783t, *784*
   appendix epididymis, 775, *778–779*
      torsion of, 777–780, *784*
   appendix testis, 775, *778–779*
      torsion of, 777–780, *784*
   bulbourethral gland of Cowper,
      development, 775, *776*
   corpora cavernosa defect, *792–793*, 972
   corpus spongiosum defect, *792–793*, 972
   Cowper's glands, development, 775, *776*
   cyst of prostatic utricle, 780–784, *785–786*
   development, 773–777, *774*
      critical events in, 777
   ducts, aberrant, 775, *778–779*
   ductus deferens development, 773
   duplication of penis, 792–795, *794*
   epididymis development, 773
   epispadias, 800–805
      anatomy, 800–802, *801–802*
      diagnosis, 803, 805
      embryogenesis, 802, *803–804*
      history, 802–803
      incidence, 803
      prognosis, 805
      symptoms, 803
      treatment, 805
   external genitalia, 776–777, *780–782*
   gland penis agenesis, 790–791
   hypospadias, 805–811
      anatomy, *805–806*, 805–807
      associated anomalies, 807
      diagnosis, 809, 811
      embryogenesis, 809
      embryology, 807, *808*, 809
      etiology, 807
      incidence, 809
      symptoms, 809
      treatment, 810t, 811
   mesonephric remnant, 777–784
      wolffian duct, remnants of, 775–777,
         780–782
   Müllerian remnant, 777–784
   paradidymis, 775, *778–779*
   penile urethra, duplication of, 795–798
      anatomy, 795, *798–799*
      diagnosis, 798
      embryogenesis, 796–797
      history, 797
      incidence, 797
      symptoms, 797–798
      treatment, 798
   penis, scrotum, transposition, 795, *796–797*
   penis agenesis, 789–790, *791*
      embryogenesis, 789
      history, 789–790
      incidence, 789–790
      treatment, 790
   phimosis, 791
   prostate gland
      anomalies of, 788–789, *790*
         absence of, 788
         anterior lobe, persistence of, 788, *790*
         heterotopic prostate, 788
         Marion's disease, 788
         prostatic utricle enlargement, 788
         prune belly syndrome, 788–789
      development, 774–775, *776, 778*
   seminal vesicle

      anomalies of, 787–788, *789*
      development, 775, *778*
   urethra
      atresia, 798–800
         anatomy, 798–799
         diagnosis, 800, *800*
         embryogenesis, 799–800
         history, 800
         incidence, 800
         symptoms, 800
         treatment, 800
      development, 774
   vas deferens, anomalies of, 787, *788*
      absence of, 787
      duplication of ductus deferens, 787
   wolffian derivatives, absence of, 784–787,
      787
      anatomy, 784, *787*
      diagnosis, 786
      embryogenesis, 784–785
      history, 785–786
      incidence, 785–786
      symptoms, 786
      treatment, 786
Malrotation of kidney, 617–618
   anatomy, 617
   diagnosis, 618
   dorsally facing, *601*, 617
   embryogenesis, *601*, 617–618
   incidence, 618
   laterally facing, *601*, 617
   symptoms, 618
   treatment, 618
   ventrally facing, *601*, 617
   ventromedially facing, *601*, 617
Marion's disease, 708, 788
"Maypole atresia," peritoneum, 127
Measurement, of embryo, methods, 9–10,
   10
Meckel's diverticulum, 214–216, *215–216*
   age, 219
   diagnosis, 219, 219t
   embryogenesis, 218
   familial tendency, 219
   history, 218
   incidence, 218
   inflammatory group, 220
   neoplastic group, 221
   obstruction group, 220, *220*
   peptic ulcer group, 219–220
   sex, 218–219, *219*
   treatment, 221
   umbilical group, 220–221
Meconium ileus. *See* Pancreas, cystic fibrosis
Megacystis-microcolon-intestinal
      hypoperistalsis syndrome,
      small intestines, 231
Megaesophagus, esophagus, 100–104, *101, 103*
Megaureters, 661–663, *662*
Meige's disease, 890
Mesentery
   congenital anomalies of, *127*, 127–129,
      128t–131t
   cysts, 128t–131t, 128–129, *130*
   dimensions of, 212–213, *213*
   persistent ventral, 195, *196*
   of small bowel, 127
Mesoappendix, 127
Mesocolon
   pelvic, 128
   persistent descending, 195
   transverse, 128
Mesogastrium
   dorsal, peritoneum, greater omentum,
      117–118

   ventral, peritoneum, 117
Mesonephric remnant, *598*, 603–604
   in female reproductive tract, *823*, 823–824
      appendix vesiculosa, 823
   in male reproductive tract, 777–784
Mesonephric remnants, in female
      reproductive tract,
      pedunculated
      hydatid of Morgagni, 823
Mesonephros, 594–596, *596–597*
   functional state of, 596, *598*
   and wolffian duct, remnants of, in male
      reproductive tract, 775–777,
      780–782
Metanephros, 596, 598, 599t, *600–601*
Microgastria, 154–155, 155t
   diagnosis, 154–155
   embryogenesis, 154
   history, 154
   Hunt-Lawrence pouch for, 154
   symptoms, 154
   treatment, 154–155
Mikulicz exteriorization, small intestines,
   210
Milroy's disease, 889–891, 890t
Mirizzi's syndrome, 326, *326*
Mitral valve, 940–941
   atresia, 940
   double-orifice, 941
   embryology, 940
   stenosis, 940–941
Müllerian remnant, in male reproductive
   tract, 777–784
Müllerian duct
   cyst, 780–784, *785–786*
   duplication of, female reproductive tract,
      833, *833–834*
   in female reproductive tract,
      development, 816–823, *817–822*
Mobile gallbladder, 322
Monovular pregnancy, 1066
Monozygotic identical twins, 1066
Mortality, infant
   from birth defects, in United States, 5
   cardiovascular system, birth defect of, as
      cause of infant death, 4
   central nervous system, birth defect of, as
      cause of infant death, 4
   chromosomal anomalies, birth defect of,
      as cause of infant death, 4
   digestive system, birth defect of, as cause
      of infant death, 4
   genitourinary system, birth defect of, as
      cause of infant death, 4
   leading causes of, 2–3
   musculoskeletal system, birth defect of, as
      cause of infant death, 4
   respiratory system, birth defect of, as
      cause of infant death, 4
Motilin, gastrointestinal peptide ontogeny,
   153
Mucosa
   gastric, in esophagus, 96–98, *97*
   heterotopic
      appendix, 277
      gallbladder, 322–323
Mucosal fold, ureteropelvic junction
      obstruction, 646
Mucosal heterotopia, stomach, gastric, 172–
   176, *174–176*
Multicystic kidney disease, 629–636, *635*
Multiple congenital anomaly, epidemiologic
   data, 6
Multiple malformation syndrome, kidney,
   cysts associated with, 644, 644t

Musculature
    absence of, small intestines, 231
    defect, gastric, 169–171

Neck, sinus opening through skin of, 335
Nephron formation, 600, *603*
Neuroblastoma, suprarenal glands, 725–
    727
Neurotensin, gastrointestinal peptide
    ontogeny, 153
Non-Meckelian antimesenteric true
    diverticula, 221
Nontraumatic omental defects, 122
Noonan's syndrome, in male, 866
Normal embryonic development, 9–12, *10,*
    11t–12t
Notochord syndrome, split, 88–89

Oblique muscle, internal, variation, 577–
    578, *578*
Oesophageal atresia, birth prevalence of,
    5
Omentum, 113–127, 114t–115t, *115–118,*
    121, *123–127*
    bifid, 122
    bursa, *117,* 118–120
    greater
        abnormal attachment, 120–121, *121*
        accessory spleens, 125
        adhesions, congenital, 122
        agenesis, 120
        cysts, 122–123, 125
        duplication, 120
        dysplasia, 120
        failure to attach, *121,* 121–125, *123–*
            125
        hyperplasia, 120
        hypoplasia, 120
        infarction, 122–123
        omental teratoma, 125
        peritoneum, congenital anomalies,
            120–121, *121*
        torsion, 122–123, *124*
        tumors, 122–123, 125
        vascular anomalies, 122
    historical overview, 113–114, 114t–
        115t
    lesser, congenital anomalies, 125, 127
        absence of lesser omentum, 127
    nontraumatic defects, 122
    teratoma, greater omentum, 125
Omphalocele, 568–574
    anatomy, 568–569, *570*
    associated anomalies, 569–570, 571t
    diagnosis, 568, 572
    embryogenesis, *547,* 570–571
    etiology, 568
    history, 571, *571–572*
    incidence, 571–572
    internal, small intestines, 193–195, *194*
    massive, 572, *573*
    medium, 572, *573*
    mortality, 573–574
    prognosis, 573–574
    small, 572
    symptoms, 572
    treatment, 572
        conservative, 572–573
Omphaloilial fistula, small intestines, 213,
    215
Omphalopagus classification, conjoined
    twins, 1066
Organ system, birth defect involving, as
    cause of infant death, 4
Osler-Render-Weber syndrome, stomach,
    177

Outlet obstruction, gastric, 155–159
Ovary
    accessory, 756
    descent, 747
    development, 736–748
        critical events in, 748
        indifferent stage, 736–740, *737*
            developing gonad, 737–740, *740–*
                741, 741t
            genital ridge, 737
            primordial germ cell, 736–737, *738–*
                740, 740t
    ectopia
        and inguinal hernia, 768–769
    lobulated, 756
    prenatal differentiation, 745, 747, *749*
    supernumerary, 755–756, *756*
    teratoma, *1062*
    vestigial organs of, 747–748, *750–751*

Pancreas, 366–404
    aberrant, 385–388
    acinus, 366–367
    ampulla, 373–374, *374*
    annular, 379–385
    aplasia, 369–370, *370*
    arterial system, 392–395, *392–395*
    common bile duct, 372–373
    congenital anomalies, 369–399
    cystic fibrosis, 389–392
        associated anomalies, 389–390
        diagnosis, 391, *391*
        embryogenesis, 390
        familial incidence, 390
        history, 390
        mortality, 392
        pathology, 389–390, *390*
        prognosis, 392
        symptoms, 391
        treatment, *391,* 391–392
    cysts, congenital, 388t, 388–389
        multiple, 389
        pseudocysts, 389
        solitary, 388–389
    development, 366–369, *367–368*
    divisum, 378–379, *379*
    ducts, 371–378, *372, 375–378, 376–378*
    duodenal papilla, 373, *373*
        minor, 375
    dysplasia, 371
    gallbladder, 385
    hyperplasia, 370–371
    hypertrophy, 370–371
    hypoplasia, 369–370, *370*
    islands of Langerhans, 367–369, *369*
    lymphatic drainage, 397–399, *399*
    polypeptide, gastrointestinal peptide
        ontogeny, 153
    rotational anomalies, 385
    sphincter of Boyden, 374–375, *375*
    venous drainage, *395,* 395–397, 397t,
        398
Pancreaticocolic ligament, 349
Pancreatitis
    ampullary lithiasis, 374, *374*
    familial, 378
Panglottic atresia, 407
Paradidymis, male reproductive tract, 775,
    778–779
Paraduodenal fossa, peritoneum, 131t,
    131–133, *132–134*
Paraduodenal hernia, 135, 144, 144t, *145–*
    146
Parathyroid cyst, 44–47
    anatomy, 44
    diagnosis, 47

    embryogenesis, 45–46
    history/incidence of, 45–47
    symptoms, 47
    treatment, 47
Parathyroid glands, 20–22, 25–27, 41–47
    color of, 44
    cysts of, 44–47
    history of knowledge of, 41t
    location of, variations in, 41–43, *42–43,*
        44t
    number of, variations in, 43–44
    shapes of, variations in, 44, *45*
    sizes of, variations in, 44
    vascular supply of, 44, 45t, *46–47*
    weight of, 44
Parchment heart, 939
Paroophoron, female reproductive tract,
    823
Patent ductus arteriosus, 1010–1013,
    1011
Patent urachus. *See* Urachus
Pelvic kidney, 614
Pelvic mesocolon, 128
Pelvis
    double, 649–654
    kidney, fused, *622,* 622–623
Penis
    agenesis, 789–790, *791*
        embryogenesis, 789
        history, 789–790
        incidence, 789–790
        treatment, 790
    duplication of, 792–795, *794*
        anatomy, 792–793, *794*
        associated anomalies, 793
        diagnosis, 795
        history, 793, 795
        incidence, 793, 795
        treatment, 795
    scrotum, transposition, 795, *796–797*
    urethra, duplication of
        anatomy, 795, *798–799*
        diagnosis, 798
        embryogenesis, 796–797
        history, 797
        incidence, 797
        symptoms, 797–798
        treatment, 798
Pericardium, 898–911
    anomalies of, 899–909, *901,* 901t
    congenital defects, 899–905
        anatomy, 899, 901, *901–903,* 902t
        associated anomalies, 902
        diagnosis, 904–905
        embryogenesis, 901–902
        history, 902
        incidence, 902–903
        symptoms, 903–904
        treatment, 905
    development, 898–899, *899–900*
        critical events in, 898
    pericardial cysts, diverticula
        anatomy, 905–906
        diagnosis, 907–908
        embryogenesis, 906, *907*
        history, 906–907
        treatment, 908–909
Pericolic hyperfixation, small intestines,
    195, *196*
Peritoneum, 113–149, 114t–115t, *115–118,*
    119t, *121, 123–127,* 128t–
    129t, *130,* 130t–131t, *132–*
    143, 144t, *145–148*
    anatomy, 113–120, 115t, *116–117*
    "apple peel syndrome," 127
    bifid omentum, 122

Peritoneum—*continued*
  broad ligament, congenital anomalies of, 130–131
  Castleman's disease, 120
  "Christmas tree deformity," 127
  compartments, 113–117, *116–117*
  cyst, 122–124
  defects, internal hernia through, 135, 144, 144t, *145–146*
    anatomy, 135, 144
    classification, 135
    diagnosis, 145–146
    embryogenesis, 144
    incidence, 144
    mortality, 147
    symptoms, 145
    treatment, 147
  defined, 113
  embryology, 113–114, *115*
  falciform ligaments, congenital anomalies of, 130
  fold, variations, 147–148, *147–148*
  foramen of Winslow, 134–135, *143*
  fossa
    cecal, 133, *133*
    intersigmoid, 133–134, *134*
  gastrocolic ligament, 118
  greater omentum
    accessory spleens, 125
    congenital adhesions, 122
    congenital anomalies, 120–121, *121*
    cysts, 122–123, 125
    dorsal mesogastrium, *117*, 117–118, 119t
    failure to attach, *121*, 121–125, *123–125*
    omental teratoma, 125
    torsion, 122–123, *124*
    tumors, 122–123, 125
    vascular anomalies, 122
  hernia
    incarcerated left paraduodenal, 133, *133*
    incarcerated right paraduodenal, 132–133
    internal, 134–143, *135–142*
      through peritoneal defects, 135, 144, 144t, *145–146*
      paraduodenal, 135, 144, 144t, *145–146*
    of Waldeyer, 127
  lesser omentum, congenital anomalies, 125, 127
  lesser sac, *117*, 118–120
  ligament, congenital anomalies of, 129–131
  "maypole atresia," 127
  membrane of Jackson, 147–148, *148*
  mesenteric cysts, 128t–131t, 128–129, *130*
  mesenteries
    congenital anomalies of, *127*, 127–129, 128t–131t
    of small bowel, 127
  mesoappendix, 127
  nontraumatic omental defects, 122
  paraduodenal fossa, 131t, 131–133, *132–134*
  paraduodenal hernia, 135, 144, 144t, *145–146*
  pelvic mesocolon, 128
  supracolic compartment, 117, *117*, 119t
  supracolic ligament, 117
  transverse mesocolon, 128
  ventral mesogastrium, 117
Pharyngeal, term, use of, vs. branchial, 17
Pharyngeal pouch complex, 26–27, *28*
Pharynx

agenesis, median anlage, 50
Beckwith-Wiedermann syndrome, 48
branchial arches, 17–24, *21*, 25t
branchial cleft, 17, 20, *20–22*, 25t
caudal pharyngeal pouch complex, 22
cyst, 35
  cervicoaural, 33–34
cystic/fistular remnants of branchial apparatus, 32–41, 33t
development, 17–32, *18–32*, 25t, 42t
  critical events in, 32, 32t
fistula, 35
  cervicoaural, 33–34
  remnant, 32–41
lateral branchial apparatus, anomalies of, 32–47, 33t, *34–38*, 41t
Lobdell-DiGeorge anomaly, 47–48
parathyroid, 20–22, 25–27
  location of, variations in, 41–43, *42–43*, 44t
pouch complex, 26–27, *28*
sinus, cervicoaural, 33–34
sinus opening into, 335
thymus, 22–23, 25–27, *26*, 47–49
thyroid, 27–32, *29–31*, 49–61
Pheochromocytoma, bladder, 711
Phimosis, male reproductive tract, 791
Phrenocolic ligament, 349–350
Phrygian cap deformity, gallbladder, 321, *321*
Poland's syndrome, 551, *551*
Polycystic disease, of kidney, 638
Polymastia, 560–563, *561*
Polyovular pregnancy, 1066
Polyp, ureteropelvic junction obstruction, 646
Polysplenia syndrome, 360–362
Polythelia, 560–563, *561*
Posterior urethral valve, 706–708
  anatomy, 706–707, *707*
  diagnosis, 707–708
  embryogenesis, 707
  history, 707
  incidence, 707
  treatment, 708
Postovulatory survival, of egg, in humans, 2–3
Postrenal inferior vena cava, anomalies of, 1045–1049, *1046–1048*
Pouch complex, pharynx, 26–27, *28*
Practical considerations, intrauterine surgery, 1082
Preduodenal portal vein, small intestines, 231–232, *232*
Pregnancy, splenic, 343
Presplenic fold, 349
Processus vaginalis, incomplete closure, 578–584
  anatomy, 578–580, *579–580*
  definition, 578
  diagnosis, 583
  embryogenesis, *579*, 581
  hernial sac, contents of, 581
  history, 582t, 582–583
  hydrocele, 583
  predisposing conditions, 581–582
  symptoms, 583
  treatment, 583–584
Pronephros, 594–596, *596–597*
Prostate gland
  anomalies of, 788–789, *790*
    absence of, 788
    anterior lobe, persistence of, 788, *790*
    heterotopic prostate, 788
    Marion's disease, 788
    prostatic utricle enlargement, 788

prune belly syndrome, 788–789
development, 774–775, *776*, *778*
Protrusion deformity, sternum, 546–547, *547*
Prune belly syndrome, 585–586
  prostate gland anomaly, 788–789
Pseudocoarctation of the aorta, 992–993
  anatomy, 992, *992*
  diagnosis, 993
  embryogenesis, 992
  incidence, 992
  symptoms, 993
  treatment, 993
Pseudohermaphroditism, 765, 853–873
  classification, 854–866, 856t–857t
  diagnosis, 870–871
  female
    adrenocortical origin, 856, 858–860, *858–860*
    adrenogenital syndrome, 856, 858–860
    extrinsic androgenic influence, 860
    hypernephric syndrome, 856, 858–860
    nonsuprarenal origin, 860
  incidence of, 870, 870t
  male, 860–861, *861*
  treatment, 871–872
    choice of sex, 871–872
Pulmonary atresia, 939–940
  tetralogy of Fallot, ventricular septal defect, 941
  ventricular septal defect, 942–943, *942–943*
Pulmonary circulation
  anomalies, 456t, 456–484, *458–459*
  arterial supply, anomalous, 456–463, *458–459*, *462*
    anatomy, 457–460, *460*
    associated anomalies, 460
    classification, 456–458, *462*
    diagnosis, 461–463
    embryogenesis, 457–460, *461*
    history, 460–461
    incidence, 461
    prognosis, 463
    symptoms, 461–463
    treatment, 463, *463*
  bronchial arteries, variations in, 472–473
  coarctation of pulmonary arteries, 471–472
  crossed pulmonary arteries, 471, *471*
  development, 451–456, *452–453*
    critical events in, 455–456 87
  pulmonary vein
    branches, stenosis, 474–475
    common, stenosis, 473–474, *473–475*
    variations in, 473
  retrotracheal left pulmonary artery, *470*, 470–471
Pulmonary isomerism, 434–435, *435*
Pulmonary origin of coronary arteries, 966–968, *969*
Pulmonary stenosis, 939–940
Pulmonary trunk, 982
  aortic trunk, separation, 982–983, *983–985*
Pulmonary valve, absent, with tetralogy of Fallot, 943
Pulmonary vein
  atrial absorption of, 921–923
  branches of, stenosis, 474–475
  common, stenosis, 473–474
  development, 453–454, *454–455*
Pygopagus classification, conjoined twins, 1066
Pyloric atresia, 162, 163t

Pyloric stenosis
  adult, 163
  infantile
    anatomy, 160
    diagnosis, 161–162, *162*
    history, 161
    incidence, 161
    mortality, 163
    pathogenesis, 160–161, *161*
    Ramstedt's operation for, 162
    symptoms, 161–162
    treatment, 162–163, *163*

Ramstedt's operation, for pyloric stenosis, infantile, 162
Rectum. *See also* Anorectal anomalies
  atresia, 266
  bilateral duplications of, 249–251
    anatomy, 249–250
    diagnosis, 251
    embryogenesis, 250
    history, 250
    incidence, 250
    symptoms, 250–251
    treatment, 251
  Hirschsprung's disease, 252–259
Reflux, esophagus, abnormal, idiopathic, congenital, 104–105, *105*
Renal. *See also* Kidney
  artery variations, 623–625
    anatomy, 623, *623*
    diagnosis, 625
    embryogenesis, 625
    number of arteries, 265, *620*, 623, 624t
    positions of arteries, 265, *624–625*
    symptoms, 625
    treatment, 625
  ectopia
    crossed, 614–617
    simple, 612–613, *612–613*
    thoracic, 613–614, *614*
  hygroma, 888–889
Retrocaval ureter, 656–658
Retroesophageal subclavian artery, *1000*, 1000–1001
Retroiliac ureter, 658, *658*
Retrotracheal left pulmonary artery, *470*, 470–471
Rib
  anomalies, 550–551
    Poland's syndrome, 551, *551*
    unilateral thoracic wall aplasia, *550*, 550–551
  deformity, 547
    and sternum combined, 547
    unilateral thoracic wall aplasia, *550*, 550–551
Riedel's lobe, 286, *289*
Right aortic arch, 994t, 995–1000, *996–998*, 999t
Right ductus arteriosus, 1013
  persistent, 1013
Right hepatic artery, variation in, 327–328
Rosenmüller's organ, female reproductive tract, 823

Sacrococcygeal teratoma, *1062*, 1062–1064
Scimitar syndrome, 480–484, *481*
Scrotum
  anatomy, 584t, 584–585
    cremaster muscle, 584
    external spermatic fascia, 584
    internal spermatic fascia, 584
    tunica vaginalis, 584
  embryogenesis, 585
  penis, transposition, 795, *796–797*

varicocele, 584–585
  defined, 584–585
  diagnosis, 585
  etiology, 585
  symptoms, 585
  treatment, 585
Second epiploic foramen, peritoneum, 117–120
Secretin, gastrointestinal peptide ontogeny, 153
Seminal vesicle
  anomalies of, 787–788, *789*
  development, 775, *778*
Separation, surgical, conjoined twins, 1068–1070, 1073, 1076
Severity, degree of, congenital anomalies, epidemiologic data, 5
Sex chromosomes, role of, 850–851, 853, 853t
Sex determination, 848–876
  anomalies of, 853–873, 854t, *855*
    origin, 866–870, *867–868*, 868t–869t
  Del Castillo syndrome, 864
  hermaphroditism, 853–873, *862*
    classification, 854–866; 856t–857t
    diagnosis, 870–871
    incidence of, 870, 870t
    treatment, 871–872
      choice of sex, 871–872
  Klinefelter's syndrome, 863–864
  Noonan's syndrome, in male, 866
  normal development, 849–853, *850–851*
    critical events in, 853
    genetic sex determination, 849–850, *852–853*
    sex chromosomes, role of, 850–851, 853, 865t
  pseudohermaphroditism, 853–873
    classification, 854–866, 856t–857t
    diagnosis, 870–871
    female
      adrenocortical origin, 856, 858–860, *858–860*
      adrenogenital syndrome, 856, 858–860
      extrinsic androgenic influence, 860
      hypernephric syndrome, 856, 858–860
      nonsuprarenal origin, 860
    incidence of, 870, 870t
    male, 860–861, *861*
    treatment, 871–872
      choice of sex, 871–872
  sexual ambiguity, 853–873
    classification, 853–873, 857t
  single-gene disorder, chart, 849t
  single-gene inheritance, chart, 849t
  Turner's syndrome, 864–866, *865*
Sexual ambiguity, 853–873
  classification, 853–873, 857t
Sinus
  external, branchial apparatus, term, use of, 37–38
  of His, 19, 22
  internal, branchial apparatus, term, use of, 38
  opening into pharynx, 335
  opening through skin of neck, 335
  pharynx, cervicoaural, 33–34
Sinus of Valsalva, aneurysm of, 1003–1005, *1004*, 1004t
Sinus venosus, atrial absorption of, 920–921, *924*
Situs. *See also* Asymmetry
  development, 1052–1054, *1053*
    critical events in, 1053

etiology, 1057
heterotaxia, 1054–1057, *1055*
Kartagener's syndrome, *1053*, 1053–1054
Size of embryo, during normal embryonic development, 9–12, 11t
Small bowel, mesenteries of, 127
Small intestines, 184–241
  anomalies, 190–234, 191t–192t
  atresia, 200–212
    anatomy, 200–201, *201*
    "apple peel," 203
    associated anomalies, 206
    "Christmas tree," 203
    diagnosis, *207–208*, 207–209
    embryogenesis, 203–206, *204–205*
    history, 206
    incidence, 200–203, 206–207
    location, 200–203, 202t–203t
    mortality, 212, 212t
    symptoms, 207
    treatment, *209–210*, 209–212, *211*
  cord, solid, vitelline duct persisting as, 217, *217*
  cystic duplications, 225–230
  development, 184–190, *185–186*
    abdomen return stage, 184–185
    critical events in, 189–190
    fixation stage, 185, *187*, 187–189, *189*, 189t–190t
    herniation stage, 184
  diverticulum, 213–225
    concomitant occurrence of, 225
    duodenal, 223–224
    giant, 225
    ileal, 224–225
    jejunal, 224–225
    Meckel's diverticulum, 214–216, *215–216*
    non-Meckelian antimesenteric true diverticula, 221
    omphaloilial fistula, 213, 215
    primary false diverticula, 221–225
  dorsal enteric remnants, 225–230, *228*, *230–231*
  duodenal aganglionosis, 230–231
  duodenal maldevelopment, 190
  encapsulated small intestine, 193–195, *194*
  exomphalos, 191–192, *192*
  fixation anomalies, 190–200, 191t–192t
    anatomy, 191–196
  hyperdescent of cecum, 193, *193*
  hyperrotation, 193, *193*
  ilial aganglionosis, 230–231
  inverted cecum, 195, *195*
  Jackson's membrane, 195, *196*
  jejunal aganglionosis, 230–231
  length, 212
  megacystis-microcolon-intestinal hypoperistalsis syndrome, 231
  mesentery, dimensions of, 212–213, *213*
  Mikulicz exteriorization, 210
  mixed rotation, 192, *193*
  mobile cecum, 195
  musculature, absence of, 231
  nonrotation, 192, *192*
  pericolic hyperfixation, 195, *196*
  persistent descending mesocolon, 195
  persistent ventral mesentery, 195–196, *196*
  preduodenal portal vein, 231–232, *232*
  retroperitoneal cecum, 195, *196*
  reversed rotation, 192–193, *193*
  rotation anomalies, 190–200, 191t–192t
    treatment, 200
  stenosis

Small intestines—*continued*
  anatomy, 200–201
  associated anomalies, 206
  diagnosis, 207–209
  embryogenesis, 203–206
  history, 206
  incidence, 200–203, 206–207
  location, 200–203, 202t
  mortality, 212
  symptoms, 207
  treatment, *209–210,* 209–212, *211*
  superior mesenteric artery syndrome,
    232–234, *233*
  topographic anatomy of, 212
  tubular duplications, 225–230
  umbilical mucosal remnants, *216,* 216–217
  undescended cecum, 195, *195*
  vitelline cysts, 217, *217*
Solitary crossed renal ectopia, *610,* 615
Somatostatin, gastrointestinal peptide
    ontogeny, 153, 153t
Spermatic fascia
  external, 584
  internal, 584
Sphincter of Boyden, 374–375, *375*
Spinal length, embryo measurement, *10*
Spleen, 334–365
  accessory, 336–338
    greater omentum, 125
  agenesis
    diagnosis, *358,* 358–360, *359*
    embryogenesis, 357–358
    history, 358
    incidence, 358
    mortality, 360
    symptoms, 358
    treatment, 360
  anomalies, 334–336, *336–337,* 337, 337t
  arteriovenous, anastomoses, 356
  artery, 353–355, *353–355*
  asplenia, 334–336, 337t
  borders, 344–345
  cysts, congenital, 363
  development, 334, *335*
  embryology, 346–348
  gastrosplenic ligament, *348,* 348–349
  hypoplasia, 334–336
  ligaments, 346–350
  pancreaticocolic ligament, 349
  peritoneum, 345–346, *346–347*
  phrenocolic ligament, 349–350
  polysplenia syndrome, 360–362
    anatomy, 360, *360*
    associated anomalies, 360–361, *361*
    diagnosis, 362
    embryogenesis, 360, 362, *362*
    history, 362
    incidence, 362
    mortality, 362
    symptoms, 362
    treatment, 362
  presplenic fold, 349
  segmental anatomy, 345, *346*
  shape, 344, *344*
  size, 343–344
  splenocolic ligament, 349
  splenogonadal fusion, 338–343
  splenopancreatic ligament, 349
  splenophrenic ligament, 349
  splenorenal ligament, 349
  surfaces, 344, *344*
  topography, 343–346
  variations, 348
  veins, 353–356, *356*
  wandering, *350,* 350–353, 351t, *352,* 352t
Splenic pregnancy, 343

Splenocolic ligament, 349
Splenogonadal fusion
  anatomy, 338, *339–340*
  associated anomalies, 338–339, 341t–342t
  diagnosis, 340, *343*
  embryogenesis, 339
  symptoms, 339–340, *343*
  treatment, 340–343
Splenopancreatic ligament, 349
Splenophrenic ligament, 349
Splenorenal ligament, 349
Split notochord syndrome, 88–89
Sponge kidney, 636–637, *637*
Standing height, embryo measurement, *10*
Stenosis
  anal, 259, 261–262, 265, *265*
  aortic, 944–946, *945*
  esophagus, 72, 72–73, 84–85
  larynx, subglottic, 408–410
  mitral valve, 940–941
  pulmonary, 939–940
  pulmonary vein
    branches, 474–475
    branches of, 474–475
    common, 473–474, *473–475*
  small intestines, 200–212
  stomach, 155–159
  trachea, 422–425
  tricuspid valve, 938–939
Sternum deformity, 545–547, *546–548*
  depression deformity, 545–546, *546–547*
  fusion deformity, 547
  mixed deformities, 547, *547–548*
  protrusion deformity, 546–547, *547*
Stomach, 150–178, *151–154,* 153t, 155t,
    156–159, 161–164, 163t, *167–
    175,* 177t
  adenomyomata, 174
  agastria, 154–155
    diagnosis, 154–155
    embryogenesis, 154
    history, 154
    symptoms, 154
    treatment, 154–155
  anomalies of, 154–178, 155t
  atresia, 155–159
    anatomy, 155–156, *156*
    diagnosis, 158–159, *158–159*
    Finney pyloroplasty for, 159
    Heinke-Mikulicz pyloroplasty for, 159
    history, 157
    incidence, 157
    mortality, 159
    symptoms, 157–158, *158*
    treatment, 159
  bombesin, gastrointestinal peptide
    ontogeny, 153
  Brunner's adenoma, 173
  cholecystokinin, gastrointestinal peptide
    ontogeny, 153
  development, 150–154, *151–154,* 153t
    critical events in, 154, *154*
  Dieulafoy's disease, 176–177
  diverticula, 164–165
    diagnosis, 165
    embryogenesis, 164
    history, 164
    incidence, 165
    mortality, 165
    symptoms, 165
    treatment, 165
  duplication, 165–169
    anatomy, 165–166, *167*
    diagnosis, 168
    embryogenesis, 166
    history, 166

  incidence, 167–168
    symptoms, 168
    treatment, *168,* 168–169
  gastric angiodysplasia, 176–178, 177t
  gastric mucosal heterotopia, *174–176*
  gastric musculature defects, 169–171
    anatomy, 169, *169*
    diagnosis, 171, *171*
    embryogenesis, 169
    history, 169–171, *170*
    incidence, 169–171, *170*
    symptoms, 171
    treatment, 171
  gastric outlet obstruction, 155–159
  gastric telangiectasia, 176
  gastric teratoma, 176
  gastrin, gastrointestinal peptide ontogeny,
    153
  gastroduodenal adhesions, 176
  gastrointestinal peptides, ontogeny, 153
  glucagon, gastrointestinal peptide
    ontogeny, 153
  hourglass, 159–160
  Hunt-Lawrence pouch, for microgastria,
    154
  insulin, gastrointestinal peptide ontogeny,
    153
  malposition, 171–173, *172–173*
  microgastria, 154–155
    diagnosis, 154–155
    embryogenesis, 154
    history, 154
    symptoms, 154
    treatment, 154–155
  motilin, gastrointestinal peptide
    ontogeny, 153
  neurotensin, gastrointestinal peptide
    ontogeny, 153
  Osler-Render-Weber syndrome, 177
  pancreatic polypeptide, gastrointestinal
    peptide ontogeny, 153
  pyloric stenosis
    adult, 163
    infantile
      anatomy, 160
      diagnosis, 161–162, *162*
      history, 161
      incidence, 161
      mortality, 163
      pathogenesis, 160–161, *161*
      symptoms, 161–162
      treatment, 162–163, *163*
  Ramstedt's operation, for pyloric stenosis,
    infantile, 162
  secretin, gastrointestinal peptide
    ontogeny, 153
  somatostatin, gastrointestinal peptide
    ontogeny, 153
  stenosis, 155–159. *See also* Pyloric stenosis
    anatomy, 155–156
    diagnosis, 158–159, *158–159*
    history, 157
    incidence, 157
    mortality, 159
    symptoms, 157–158, *158*
    treatment, 159
  substance P, gastrointestinal peptide
    ontogeny, 153
  thoracic, short esophagus with,
    congenital, 98–100, *98–100*
Substance P, gastrointestinal peptide
    ontogeny, 153
Subvalvular aortic stenosis, 945
Superior mesenteric artery syndrome, small
    intestines, 232–234, *233*
Superior vena cava, 1032–1051

anomalies of, 1037–1043, *1038*, 1038t
development, 1032–1034, *1033–1035*
double superior vena cava, 1038–1040, *1040–1041*
left-sided, 1040–1043, *1042*
Supernumerary breast
associated anomalies, 562
diagnosis, 563
embryogenesis, 562
history, 562–563
number of, 562
structure of, 561–562
symptoms, 563
treatment, 563
Supernumerary breasts, 560–563, *561*
Supernumerary kidney, 654–656
anatomy, 654–655, *656*
diagnosis, 656
embryogenesis, 655
history, 655–656
incidence, 655–656
pathology, 656
symptoms, 656
treatment, 656
Supernumerary ovarian tissue, 755–756
true ovarian duplication, 755, *756*
Supernumerary ovary, 755–756, *756*
Supernumerary testes, 752–755
anatomy, 752, *755*
diagnosis, 754–755
embryogenesis, 752, 754, *755*
history, 754
symptoms, 754–755
treatment, 755
Supracolic compartment, peritoneum, *117*, 117–118, 119t
Supracolic ligament, peritoneum, 117
Supradiaphragmatic lobes, liver, 286–288, *289–291*
Suprahymenal membrane, female reproductive tract, 829
Suprarenal glands, 718–735
accessory, 729–730, 730t, *731*
adrenal hyperplasia, 733
agenesis, 723
anomalies of, 723–733, *726*, 726t
development, 718–723, *719–725*
critical events in, 723
fusion, 727, *728*
hemorrhage, 723–724
heterotopia, 728–729, *729–730*
hypoplasia, 728
neuroblastoma, 725–727
suprarenal tissue, anomalous location of, 728–733
anatomy, 728–732
accessory cortical tissue, 730–732
accessory suprarenal gland, 729–730, 730t, *731*
suprarenal heterotopia, 728–729, *729–730*
diagnosis, 732–733
embryogenesis, *731*, 732
surgical implications, 732–733
symptoms, 732–733
Suprarenal heterotopia, 728–729, *729–730*
Supravalvular aortic stenosis, 944–945, *945*
Surgical malformation, birth prevalence of, 4–5
Symptoms, musculature, absence of, 231

Tailgut, cystic remnants of, 251–252, 252t
Telangiectasia, gastric, 176
Teratoma, 1054–1065
cervical, *1064*
classification, 1060–1061, 1061t, 1063t

development, 1060
embryogenesis, 1061–1062
exophytic, *1064*
gastric, 176
history, 1062, 1064t
ovarian, *1062*
sacrococcygeal, *1062*, 1062–1064
Testes
associated structures, 741–742, *744*
descent, 742–745, *745–747*, 747t
anomalies of, 759–768
maldescended, 766–768
crossed/transversal ectopia, 766–767, *767*
ectopic sites, *765*, 766–768
perineal ectopia, 766
pubopenile ectopia, *765*, 766, 766t
undescended, 759–766
anatomy, 759, *759*
associated pathology, 760–763
diagnosis, 765
absence, 765
pseudohermaphroditism, 765
testicular ectopia, 765, *765*
embryogenesis, 759–760
fertility, *261–264*, 761–763
history, 763–764
incidence, *764*, 764–765
inguinal hernia, 761
malignancy, 760–761
symptoms, 765
treatment, 765–766, *766*
development, 736–748
critical events in, 748
indifferent stage, 736–740, *737*
developing gonad, 737–740, *740–741*, 741t
genital ridge, 737
primordial germ cell, 736–737, *738–740*, 740t
ectopia, *765*, 766t, 766–768, *767*
epididymis, failure of union, 756–759
anatomy, 756–757, *757–759*
diagnosis, 758–759
embryogenesis, 758
history, 758
incidence, 758
symptoms, 758
testes, 759
fusion, 756
prenatal differentiation, 740–741, *742–743*
supernumerary, 752–755
torsion, 768, *768*
vestigial organs of, 747–748, *750–751*
Tetralogy of Fallot, 942
with absent pulmonary valve, 943
pulmonary atresia, ventricular septal defect, 941
Thoracic aorta, *See* Aorta, thoracic
Thoracic duct, variations of, 879–880, *881–882*, *884–886*
Thoracic dystrophy, 551
Thoracic stomach, short esophagus with, congenital, 98–100, *98–100*
Thoracic wall, anterior, 540–544, *541–543*
Thoracopagus classification, conjoined twins, 1066
Thorax
anomalies of, 545–559
congenital chest deformity, 545–550
complications of, 547–548
diagnosis, 549–550
embryogenesis, 547–548
history, 549
incidence, 549

rib and sternum combined, 547
rib deformity, 547
sternum deformity, 545–547
depression deformity, 545–546, *546–547*
fusion deformity, 547
mixed deformities, 547, *547–548*
protrusion deformity, 546–547, *547*
symptoms, 549
treatment, 550
rib, 550–551. *See also* Rib
unilateral thoracic wall aplasia, *550*, 550–551
dorsal enteric remnants in, 89–93, 92t
anatomy, 89–91
diagnosis, 92, 92t
history, 91
incidence, 91
mortality, 93
symptoms, 91–92
treatment, 92–93
Thymic cyst
anatomy, 48
diagnosis, 48–49
embryogenesis, 48
incidence, 48
symptoms, 48–49
treatment, 49, 49t
Thymus, 22–23, *25–27*, 26, 47–49
aplasia, 47–48
cyst, 48–49
anatomy, 48
embryogenesis, 48
incidence, 48
symptoms, 48–49
treatment, 49, 49t
Dubois' abscess, 48
history of knowledge of, 48–49
hyperplasia, 48
location of, variations in, 49
Thyroglossal duct cyst, 59t, 59–60, *60*
Thyroid, 27–32, *29–31*, 49–61, 50t, *51–60*, 55t–56t, 59t
accessory ectopic tissue, *60*, 60–61
anomalies
artery, 53, *53*
classification of, 50t
ima artery, 53, *53*
lateral, 52
median anlage, 50, 52, *52*, 57–60
agenesis, 50
lingual thyroid, 57–58
thyroid line, 50, 52, *52*
median/lateral anlage involvement, 49–50
partially descended thyroid gland, 58–59, *59*
veins, *53*, 53–54
developmental stages, 27, 30
Hashimoto's thyroiditis, 48
lymphatics, anomaly, 54
nerves, anomalies, 54–57, 55t, *55–57*, 56t
primordium, origin of, 27, *29*
ultimobranchial bodies, relationship, 27–28
Torsion, greater omentum, 122–123, *124*
Trachea
agenesis, 421–422
anomalies, 419–445, 420t
atresia, 421–422
cystic duplication, 435–438, *436*, 437t
development, 414–419, *415–417*
diverticulum, 427
esophagus, anomalies
diagnosis, 78–79, *78–79*

Trachea—*continued*
  incidence, 76t, 76–77
    familial incidence, 76–77
    maternal age, 76
    sex ratio, 76
  symptoms, 77, 77t, 77–78
  treatment, 79–83, 80t–83t, *82*
  fistula, *427*, 427–429
  stenosis, 422–425, *423*, 424t, *425*, 425t
    anatomy, 422–423, *423*
    associated anomalies, 424, 424t
    diagnosis, 424
    embryogenesis, 423, *423*
    history, 424
    incidence, 424
    prognosis, 425
    symptoms, 424
    treatment, 424–425, *425*, 425t
Tracheal lobe, lung, lobulation anatomy,
    433, *434*
Tracheobronchomegaly, 425–427, *426*
Tracheoesophageal fistula, 68–83, *71–74*,
    73t, 75t–77t, *76–79*, 81t–83t,
    82
  with esophageal atresia, 71–72, *72*
Tracheomalacia, 422, 422t–423t
Transposition of the great arteries, *946*,
    946–947
Transposition of the great vessels,
    congenitally corrected, 947–
    948, *948–949*
Transverse mesocolon, 128
Transversus abdominis, body wall layer,
    578, *578*
Tricuspid atresia, 936–937, *937*
Tricuspid valve
  anomalies, 936–939
  cleft of, 939
  duplication of, 939
  Ebstein's anomaly, 937–938, *938*
Triplication of ureter, 652
Trophoblast, 1066
Truncus arteriosus, persistent, 1013–1017,
    1015
Tubes of Kobelt, female reproductive tract,
    823
Tubular duplication, esophagus, 85–88, *86*,
    86t–87t
  anatomy, 85–86, *86*
  diagnosis, *76*, 86–87, 87t, *88*
  embryogenesis, 86
  history, 85–86
  incidence, 86
  symptoms, 86, 86t
  treatment, 87–89, *88*
Tumors, greater omentum, 122–123, 125
Tunica vaginalis, 584
Turner's syndrome, 864–866, *865*
Twins, conjoined. *See* Conjoined twins

Uhl's malformation, 939
Ultimobranchial bodies, thyroid gland,
    relationship, 27–28
Umbilical cord, anatomy, 564–565, 565t,
    565–568
Umbilical fistula, acquired, 679–680
Umbilical hernia, 565–568
  anatomy, 565, 567, *569*
  embryogenesis, 567
  incidence, 567
  symptoms, 567
  treatment, 567–568
Umbilical mucosal remnants, small
    intestines, *216*, 216–217
Umbilical region, anatomy, 563–564, *564*
Umbilicus, intussusception, 577

Unilateral thoracic wall aplasia, rib, *550*,
    550–551
Urachus, 675
  anatomy, 675–678, *677–678*
  anomalies of, 678, *679*
  embryogenesis, 678–680, *679*
    acquired umbilical fistula, 679–680
  history, 680
  patent
    diagnosis, 680–681
    incidence, 680
    symptoms, 680
    treatment, 681
Ureter
  double, 649–654
    accessory ureteric bud, *651*, 652–653
    anatomy, 649–650
    crossing of, *651*, 653
    diagnosis, 654
    ectopic ureteral openings, *651*, 652
    embryogenesis, 652
    incidence, 653t, 653–654
    level of ureter bifurcation, 650, *651–652*
    pathology, 654, 654t
    splitting of ureteric bud, 644t, 652, *653*
    treatment, 654, 655t
    ureteral diverticula, 650, *651*
  ectopic
    anatomy, 695, *696–697*
    diagnosis, *699*, 699–700
    embryogenesis, 696–698, *697–699*
    history, 698
    incidence, 698
    symptoms, 698–699, *699*
    treatment, 700
  retrocaval, 656–658
  retroiliac, 658, *658*
  triplication of, 652
  valve/stricture, *659*, 660–661
  wide, 661–663, *662*
Ureteral diverticula, 658–660, *659*
Ureterocele, 700–704
  anatomy, 700, *701*
  classification, 701–703, *702*
  diagnosis, 703–704
  embryogenesis, 700, *701*
  history, 700–701
  incidence, 701
  symptoms, *701*, 703, *703*
  treatment, 704
Ureteropelvic junction obstruction, 644–
    649
  associated anomalies, 646–647
  clinical features, 647–648
  diagnosis, 648
  extrinsic compression, 646
  mucosal fold, 646
  pathogenesis, 645–646
  polyp, 646
  repair, *646*, 649
  secondary etiology, 646
  temporary diversion, 649
Urethra
  anomalies of, 675–712, 676t, *677*
  atresia, 798–800
    anatomy, 798–799
    diagnosis, 800, *800*
    embryogenesis, 799–800
    history, 800
    incidence, 800
    symptoms, 800
    treatment, 800
  bilateral duplication, 681–683
    anatomy, 681, *682–683*
    diagnosis, 682

embryogenesis, 681
    history, 681
    incidence, 681
    symptoms, 682
    treatment, 682–683
  development, 671–675, 774
    critical events in, 675
  diverticula, female, 711
  duplication of, 708–711, *709–710*
    embryogenesis, 675
    Marion's disease, 708
    penile, duplication of
      anatomy, 795, *798–799*
      diagnosis, 798
      embryogenesis, 796–797
      history, 797
      incidence, 797
      symptoms, 797–798
      treatment, 798
    posterior urethral valve, 706–708
      anatomy, 706–707, *707*
      diagnosis, 707–708
      embryogenesis, 707
      history, 707
      incidence, 707
      treatment, 708
  urachus, 675
  valves, birth prevalence of, 5
  vesicoureteral reflux, *704*, 704–706
    classification, 704–705, *705*
    diagnosis, *705*, 705–706
    treatment, 706, *706*
Urinary tract
  absence of, 603
  anomalies of, 601–663, 604t, *605*
    intrauterine surgery, considerations,
      1081
  upper, duplications of, 649–656, 650t
Uterine tube, aplasia, 827–828, *828*
Uterus
  aplasia, 827–828, *828*
    associated anomalies, 829
    clinical classification, *828*, 830–831,
      830–832
    embryogenesis, 829, *830*
    history, 829
    incidence, 829–830
    prognosis, 833, 833t
    treatment, 831–832
  arcuatus, 836, *836*
  atresia
    clinical classification, *828*, 830–831,
      830–832
    embryogenesis, 829, *830*
    history, 829
    incidence, 829–830
    prognosis, 833, 833t
    treatment, 831–832
  didelphys with separate vagina, *834*, 835,
      835t
  duplex bicollis, *835*, 836
  duplex unicollis, 836, *836*
  duplication, 833–834
  heterotopic cartilage in, 842
  septus, 836, *836*
  unicornis, *835*, 835–836
  vagina primordia, incomplete fusion,
      833–842

Vagina
  aplasia
    associated anomalies, 829
    clinical classification, *828*, 830–831,
      830–832
    embryogenesis, 829, *830*
    history, 829

incidence, 829–830
prognosis, 833, 833t
treatment, 831–832
atresia, 828, *828*
associated anomalies, 829
clinical classification, *828*, 830–831, *830–832*
embryogenesis, 829, *830*
history, 829
incidence, 829–830
prognosis, 833, 833t
treatment, 831–832
primordia, uterus, incomplete fusion, 833–842
Valvular aortic stenosis, 945
Varicocele, 584–585
defined, 584
scrotal anatomy, 584t, 584–585
Vas deferens, anomalies of, 787, *788*
absence of, 787
duplication of ductus deferens, 787
Vascular anomalies, greater omentum, 122
Vascular compression, on esophagus, dysphagia, 105–106

Ventrally facing kidney, *601*, 617
Ventricles, partition of, 923–924, *925*
Ventricular septal defect, 931–934
anatomy, 931–933
defined, 931
diagnosis, 934
embryology, 933–934
incidence, 934
prognosis, 934
pulmonary atresia, 942–943, *942–943*
tetralogy of Fallot, 941
symptoms, 934
treatment, 934
Ventromedially facing kidney, *601*, 617
Vesicoureteral reflux, *704*, 704–706
classification, 704–705, *705*
diagnosis, *705*, 705–706
treatment, 706, *706*
Vitelline cysts, small intestines, 217, *217*

Waldeyer hernia, 127
Wall, body, anterior. *See* Anterior body wall
Wandering spleen, *350*, 350–353, 351t, *352*, 352t

Web, larynx, *310*, 408
Winslow foramen, 134–135, *143*
Wolffian derivatives
absence of, male reproductive tract, 784–787, *787*
male reproductive tract, absence of
anatomy, 784, *787*
diagnosis, 786
embryogenesis, 784–785
history, 785–786
incidence, 785–786
symptoms, 786
treatment, 786
Wolffian duct, and mesonephros, remnants of, in male reproductive tract, 775–777, *780–782*

Xiphopagus classification, conjoined twins, 1066

Zenker's diverticula, 94